Foundations of Maternal-Newborn Nursing

Third Edition

Foundations of Maternal-Newborn Nursing

Third Edition

SHARON SMITH MURRAY, MSN, RN, C
Professor, Health Professions
Golden West College
Huntington Beach, California

EMILY SLONE MCKINNEY, MSN, RN, C
Lecturer, Louise Herrington School of Nursing
Baylor University
Dallas, Texas

TRULA MYERS GORRIE, MN, RN, C
Professor Emeritus
Golden West College
Huntington Beach, California

With 438 Illustrations

W.B. SAUNDERS COMPANY
An Imprint of Elsevier Science
Philadelphia London New York St. Louis Sydney Toronto

W.B. SAUNDERS COMPANY
An Imprint of Elsevier Science

The Curtis Center
Independence Square West
Philadelphia, Pennsylvania 19106

Vice-President Publishing Director: Sally Schrefer
Senior Editor: Michael S. Ledbetter
Senior Developmental Editor: Lisa P. Newton
Project Manager: Linda McKinley
Production Editor: Ellen Forest
Design and Layout: Kathi Gosche

NOTICE
Nursing is an ever-changing field. Standard safety precautions must be followed, but as new research and clinical experience broaden our knowledge, changes in treatment and drug therapy become necessary or appropriate. Readers are advised to check the product information currently provided by the manufacturer of each drug to be administered to verify the recommended dose, the method and duration of administration, and contraindications. It is the responsibility of the treating physician relying on experience and knowledge of the patient to determine dosages and the best treatment for the patient. Neither the Publisher nor the editor assumes any responsibility for any injury and/or damage to persons or property.

The Publisher

Library of Congress Cataloging-in-Publication Data

Murray, Sharon Smith
Foundations of maternal-newborn nursing / Sharon Smith Murray, Emily Slone McKinncy, Truia Myers Gorrie.—3rd ed.
p. cm.
Corrie's name appears first on earlier edition.
Includes bibliographical references and index.
ISBN 0-7216-9435-7
1. Maternity nursing. 1. McKinney, Emily Slone. II. Gorrie, Trula. III. Title.
[DNLM: 1. Maternal-Child Nursing. 2. Family Health. WY 157.3 M984f2002]
RG951 M87 2002
610.73'678—dc21

2001020845

Printed in China

03 04 05 / 9 8 7 6 5 4 3

For Skip, whose love and support makes it all possible
For my daughters, Vicki, Holly, and Shannon, who make me proud
For Marina, Nicholas, and Giovanni, who provide such joy
And to my mother, Clare, who has always shown the way.

S.S.M.

For Michael, the love of my life
For the blessings of our daughters, Cathy and Amy
And to the solid foundation from my mother and late father,
Juanita and Charles Slone

E.S.M.

For the nursing students who have challenged us to
learn something new each day.

S.S.M and E.S.M.

Acknowledgments

The third edition of *Foundations of Maternal-Newborn Nursing* would not have been possible without the contributions of many people. We were very fortunate to work with a group of reviewers who read the manuscript, shared their insights, and encouraged us with their comments:

Brenda Gleason, MSN
Director of Nursing
Iowa Central Community College
330 Avenue M
Fort Dodge, Iowa

Susan Johnson, BSN, MS, RNC
Assistant Professor
The College of St. Catherine
601 25th Avenue South
Minneapolis, Minnesota

Linda Kapinos, MSN, MEd, IBCLC, RNC
Associate Professor of Nursing
Capital Community College
61 Woodland Street
Hartford, Connecticut

Deborah Mary Link, BA, MS, RNC
Assistant Professor of Nursing
The College of St. Catherine
601 25th Avenue South
Minneapolis, Minnesota

Patricia L. Nash, RNC, MSN, NNP
Neonatal Nurse Practitioner
Cardinal Glennon Children's Hospital
1465 South Grand Boulevard
St. Louis, Missouri

Cheryl A. Smith, RNC, MSN
District Clinical Coordinator
DeKalb County Board of Health
445 Winn Way
Decatur, Georgia

Sue G. Thacker, RN, C, BSN, PhD
Wytheville Community College
1000 East Main Street
Wytheville, Virginia

Diane Warner, BA, BSN, MSN
Associate Professor
Community College of Baltimore County at Catonsville
800 South Rolling Road
Baltimore, Maryland

Barbra Welch Manning, RN, MSN, PNP
Northeast Mississippi Community College
Highway 51 N
Senatobia, Mississippi

We give special thanks to Lisa Newton in Editorial who helped organize the project and guide it to completion. Ellen Forest in Book Production helped us refine and clarify our writing with her suggestions and critiques. Jeanne Robertson added to the third edition by designing a new illustration. We also thank Kathi Gosche, Designer, for the beautiful cover and the clear and attractive page layouts.

We thank Michael Ledbetter, Senior Editor, Nursing Division for helping us plan the third edition of our text. Although our book had a successful framework in place, Michael helped us consider changes and additions that improve it for students and teachers.

Finally, we want to thank Trula Myers Gorrie, our co-author on the first two editions of this textbook. Tru has continued to be our colleague, mentor, and coach as we have continued with the third edition. Most of all, Tru is a great friend to us. Although we miss her company as our co-author, we wish Tru only the best as she enjoys a well-earned retirement.

Sharon Smith Murray
Emily Slone McKinney

Our challenge as nursing educators is to keep up with the rapid changes in health care while preparing a student to stay focused on the *care* of nursing. In clinical rotations that seem to grow shorter each year, the nursing faculty must teach the student ways to use the nursing process, drugs, and technology that are beneficial while imparting the values of client-centered care. Our text tries to help the student learn to balance high-touch care with high-tech, often life-saving, care.

Although health care delivery has changed dramatically with more emphasis on outcome management and use of clinical pathways to decrease the length of stay in the birth facility, the family's need for education and support during the childbearing period does not lessen. Nurses have responded to families' needs by developing alternative means of education that use every possible moment before admission and during their stay in the birth facility. A student's clinical experience often includes the home and a variety of community clinics.

An effective textbook must present comprehensive content that can be read with ease because nursing students differ in learning abilities, experience, and primary language. Our objective for the third edition of *Foundations of Maternal-Newborn Nursing* continues to be the presentation of complex material as simply and clearly as possible. We again provide step-by-step instruction in assessments and interventions so that students can function quickly in the clinical area at a beginning level. To this end, proven learning aids, such as summaries, illustrations, tables, and highlights are used generously throughout the book.

CONTENT

Maternity nurses must be flexible to accommodate families from different cultures and who communicate in different languages and hold different health beliefs. Nurses must use critical thinking skills to devise culture-specific care that includes providing necessary education and support. The six elements we consider most important are a scientific base of information, nursing process, communication, client teaching, critical thinking, and cultural diversity.

Scientific Base

Effective nursing care depends on having a sound understanding of the physiologic bases for medical treatments and nursing actions. Although anatomy and physiology courses are part of every curriculum, students often need a review, particularly of the specific content related to childbearing. Because of this, we have incorporated principles of physiology and pathophysiology throughout the book. We have presented these scientific concepts in a clear and understandable manner so that the reader can comprehend the forces underlying both health and dysfunction.

Chapters 4, 5, and 6 provide general information about reproductive physiology, genetics, and the process of conception and fetal development. Chapters 7, 12, 17, and 19 explain physiologic adaptation during pregnancy, birth, and the postpartum period and in the newborn. Part V, Families at Risk during the Childbearing Period, describes the pathophysiological, psychological, and social bases of complications in the mother and in the newborn.

The Nursing Process

The nursing process is the accepted framework for client assessment and analysis of client needs. It is used to plan and provide nursing care and evaluate the client's response to care. Client needs often are a mixture of those for which nurses have the primary accountability and those for which another discipline provides definitive therapy yet for which nurses have some responsibility. Thus when analyzing client needs, we have chosen either a *nursing diagnosis* or a *collaborative problem* depending on whether nurses are primarily responsible for helping the client meet those needs. All nursing diagnoses are drawn from the most recent list of those approved by the North American Nursing Diagnosis Association (NANDA).

The nursing process is treated two ways in our text, in a narrative format and in nursing care plans. In each method we lead the reader through the five steps of the nursing process. In the narrative format, basic information about the condition is presented and general nursing care follows, organized by the steps of the nursing process. Interventions are general rather than client specific and explained by rationales. Because nursing students often have difficulty transferring general information to the care of a specific client, we have created nursing care plans based on scenarios of client situations most often encountered in maternity nursing.

Communication

Although they seldom are included as core content in maternal-newborn nursing texts, communication skills are essential to provide adequate care for a childbearing family. We reinforce the student's previous learning and give practical examples of ways to use communication skills in the maternity setting.

Guidelines and examples of effective communication and potential blocks are reviewed in Chapter 2. Color-highlighted *communication cues* in the text give tips on how to interact with families. Tips include ways to avoid potentially embarrassing situations, role modeling of effective communication styles, and reading nonverbal signals. Communication cues are listed in the index for easy access.

In addition, dialogues throughout the text present realistic possible nurse-client interactions. As the interaction develops, we identify communication techniques and explain the rationale. Because no one is perfect, we occasionally insert communication blocks, identify them, and suggest alternate responses.

Client Teaching

Childbearing families are entitled to comprehensive information about how to achieve the best pregnancy outcome. Nurses are their primary instructors in most areas of maternal-newborn nursing, and they must be well prepared and well organized to be effective. We present client teaching in three ways:

- Teaching-learning principles are discussed in Chapter 2.
- Chapters are organized to highlight key content so that the student can gather information and translate it into client teaching. For example, Chapter 22, Infant Feeding, lays a foundation of basic information, discusses some common problems, identifies relevant assessments, and presents nursing interventions devoted to teaching parents ways to feed their infant successfully.
- Client teaching guidelines are highlighted in *Want to Know* features, which give ideas on ways to answer the most common client questions on a topic. These features are constructed to show students ways to present information in everyday language rather than professional language so that the family will better understand the teaching. For instance, the feature "When to Go to the Hospital or Birth Center" addresses the concern of many expectant parents that they will not recognize onset of labor.

Critical Thinking

Nurses must learn critical thinking skills to overcome habits or impulses that can lead to poor clinical decisions. Chapter 3 discusses steps in critical thinking and describes how critical thinking is used in each step of the nursing process. In addition, critical thinking exercises are presented in two ways. First, exercises based on clinical scenarios of common situations with questions to stimulate critical thinking are placed throughout the text. Answers to the questions follow each exercise to provide reinforcement for student learning. Second, client-specific nursing care plans (described earlier) contain critical thinking exercises that require participation by the student. This makes the care plans interactive and reinforces the concept of critical thinking in clinical practice.

Cultural Diversity

Cultural values are among the most significant factors that influence a woman's perception of childbirth, and effective nursing care must be culture specific. This requires nurses to consider their own cultural values and examine how these values may create conflict with those whose values are different.

Chapter 1 offers an overview of Western cultural values and identifies some areas such as communication and health beliefs that may be sources of conflict. Because many different cultural groups exist in the United States and Canada, emphasis is placed on ways to do a cultural assessment. Plans for care then can show respect for cultural differences and traditional healing practices.

New information is integrated throughout the book in all areas, such as antepartum, nutrition, birth, the postpartum period, and care of the newborn. Chapter 33, Women's Health Care, has a new section on cardiovascular disease in women and its prevention.

The Internet is used by lay people and professionals as a source of health information much more than it was just a few years ago. We provide the addresses for many web sites throughout our text that contain reliable, current information relevant to maternal, newborn, and women's health nursing. Examples of these sites are the March of Dimes, National Institutes of Health, and American Cancer Society.

ORGANIZATION

The third edition of *Foundations of Maternal-Newborn Nursing* is divided into six parts. **Part I, Foundations for Nursing Care of Childbearing Families,** presents an overview of contemporary maternity care including ethical, social, and legal aspects. A review of reproductive anatomy and physiology and the hereditary and environmental factors that affect care are also presented. This material is especially important for students who have not recently completed a full anatomy and physiology course.

Part II, The Family before Birth, begins with conception and fetal development. These chapters also cover the physiologic and psychosocial adaptations to pregnancy and include a thorough explanation of recommended nutrition during pregnancy and after childbirth.

Part III, The Family during Birth, addresses the physiologic processes of birth and nursing care during labor and birth. These chapters include intrapartum fetal monitoring, pain management, and obstetric procedures such as cesarean birth.

Part IV, The Family after Birth, describes care of the new mother and infant. Alternative methods for continuing care, such as home visits and telephone follow-up, also are covered. Separate chapters address infant nutrition and home care of the infant.

Part V, Families at Risk during the Childbearing Period, includes a chapter on the family with special needs such as age-related concerns, childbearing in a substance-abusing or violent environment, birth of an infant with congenital anomalies, and responses to fetal and neonatal death. Additional chapters describe the most common complications of pregnancy, childbirth, and the postpartum and neonatal periods.

Part VI, Other Reproductive Issues, focuses on family planning, care of the infertile couple, and women's health care.

FEATURES

- *Visual Appeal.* The book is visually appealing with numerous up-to-date full color illustrations and photographs that clarify concepts and reinforce learning. Beautiful color pictures also illustrate a childbirth story and cesarean birth.
- *Objectives and Definitions.* Each chapter begins with a list of objectives that spells out the purposes of the chapter. A list of key terms with their definitions follows the objectives. A glossary at the back of the book contains key terms from all chapters and other terms related to this course.
- *Check Your Reading Questions.* Questions to help students monitor their understanding of the material presented are placed at intervals throughout each chapter. Answers to questions are placed in Appendix E so that students can have immediate feedback.
- *Critical Thinking Exercises.* Clinical situations are boxed and set apart to stimulate critical thinking. We believe strongly that immediate feedback is a powerful learning tool, so answers to critical thinking exercises in the text appear at the end of every chapter.
- *Critical to Remember.* Condensed summaries of the essential facts to remember are boxed and set apart to reinforce critical information.
- *Want to Know.* This feature can be used by students who must begin teaching very early in their clinical rotations. These include answers to the most common questions asked by women and parents, often phrased in laymen's terms or as the nurse would actually answer a patient.
- *Procedures.* Illustrated procedures that are specific to maternity and women's health nursing, such as assessment of the uterine fundus, are presented in a step-by-step format with rationales for each step.
- *Drug Guides.* Drug guides for drugs commonly administered in maternity nursing and women's health care are available in appropriate chapters. Information about additional drugs may be given in tables or in the narrative.
- *Complementary and Alternative Therapies.* We have increased the content about these therapies when appropriate throughout the text and it is highlighted with a special heading. Several herbal and botanical preparations have been added to Appendix C, Use of Drugs and Botanical Preparations during Pregnancy and Breastfeeding.
- *Summary of Concepts.* A concise review of content is provided at the end of each chapter. In addition, tables and flow charts are frequently used to summarize complex material.
- *Keys to Clinical Practice.* A description of how to prepare for clinical experience is presented in Appendix D. This feature provides care guides for assessments and interventions for the woman in labor, the woman after childbirth, and the infant. It also provides teaching on key topics such as assisting the inexperienced mother to breastfeed. This feature is designed to help students through their earliest clinical experiences before they have had much theory.
- A CD Companion, prepared by Sue G. Thacker of Wytheville Community College, located in the front of the book, includes interactive case studies, review questions, and fill-in-the-blank and matching exercises designed to test content knowledge and critical thinking skills. A glossary with definitions and sound pronunciations are also included on the valuable CD-ROM.
- A dedicated website, EVOLVE (http://www.evolve.elsevier.com/Murray/foundations/), features WebLinks to current topics related to each chapter of the text and is continually updated with the best topical websites available. The site also includes answers to frequently asked questions, author contact information, and opportunities for feedback.

TEACHING AND LEARNING SUPPORT

- The *Instructor's Electronic Resource CD-ROM,* also prepared by Sue G. Thacker, contains suggested outlines for lectures, extra credit activities, critical thinking exercises, suggestions for teaching-learning activities, a *Test Bank*, and an *Image Collection*. The *Test Bank* provides more than 700 questions that address the content of each chapter and relate to the chapter's objectives. Each item is assigned a cognitive level of knowledge, comprehension, or application. The *Image Collection* provides easy access to over 150 full-color electronic illustrations from the main textbook. Each image in the *Image Collection* can be imported to a slide presentation (such as PowerPoint) to enhance lecture materials.
- The *Study Guide* presents a variety of additional activities designed to help students master content and become more proficient in the clinical area. Review questions at various levels of difficulty are included.

Detailed Table of Contents

1 Maternity Care Today

OBJECTIVES

1. Describe changes in maternity care, from home birth with lay midwives to the emergence of medical management.
2. Compare current settings for childbirth both within and outside the hospital setting.
3. Identify trends that led to the development of family-centered maternity care.
4. Describe current trends that affect perinatal nursing, such as cost containment, outcomes management, evidence-based practice, community-based perinatal care, advances in technology, and increased use of complementary and alternative medicine.
5. Explain changes in family structure and their impact on family functioning.
6. Compare Western cultural values with those of differing cultural groups.
7. Describe the effect of cultural diversity on nursing practice.
8. Discuss the downward trends in infant and maternal mortality rates, and compare current infant mortality rates among specific racial groups and nations.

DEFINITIONS

Antepartum The time during pregnancy before the onset of labor.

Complementary and Alternative Medicine Nonmainstream or unconventional health care treatments and practices that are generally not used in hospitals and often not reimbursed by insurance companies.

Culture Sum of values, beliefs, and practices of a group of people that is transmitted from one generation to the next.

Ethnic Pertaining to religious, racial, national, or cultural group characteristics, especially speech patterns, social customs, and physical characteristics.

Ethnicity Condition of belonging to a particular ethnic group; also refers to ethnic pride.

Ethnocentrism Opinion that the beliefs and customs of one's own ethnic group are superior.

Infant Mortality Rate Number of deaths per 1000 live births that occurs within the first 12 months of life.

Intrapartum The time of labor and childbirth.

Lactation Secretion of milk from the breasts; also describes the time when a child is breastfed.

Maternal Mortality Rate Number of maternal deaths from births and complications of pregnancy, childbirth, and puerperium (the first 42 days after termination of the pregnancy) per 100,000 live births.

Neonatal Mortality Rate Number of deaths per 1000 live births occurring at birth or within the first 28 days of life.

Postpartum The first 6 weeks after childbirth.

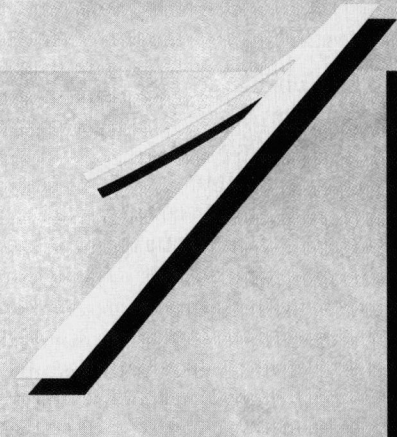

Major changes in maternity care occurred in the first half of the twentieth century as childbirth moved from the home to a hospital setting. Change continues and confusion abounds as health care providers and payers attempt to control the increasing cost of care and the rapid growth of expensive technology. Despite these challenges, health care professionals try to maintain the quality of care.

Alterations in family structure and function and differing cultural beliefs and customs also affect nursing care. Although improvements in health care have resulted in a significant decline in maternal and infant mortality rates in the United States, statistics show a wide disparity between outcomes for whites and nonwhites.

HISTORICAL PERSPECTIVES ON CHILDBEARING

Granny Midwives

Before the twentieth century, childbirth occurred most often in the home with the assistance of a "granny" midwife whose training was obtained through an apprenticeship with a more experienced granny midwife. Physicians were involved in childbirth only if serious problems occurred.

Although many women and infants fared well when a lay midwife assisted with birth in the home, maternal and infant death rates from childbearing were high. The primary causes of maternal death were postpartum hemorrhage, postpartum infection (also known as *puerperal sepsis,* or "childbed fever"), and toxemia, now known as *pregnancy-induced hypertension.* The primary causes of infant death were prematurity, dehydration from diarrhea, and contagious diseases.

Emergence of Medical Management

In the late nineteenth century, technologic developments available to physicians but not midwives led to a decline in home births and an increase in physician-assisted hospital births. Significant discoveries that set the stage for a change in maternity care included the following:

- The discovery by Semmelweis that puerperal infection could be prevented by hygienic practices
- The development of forceps to facilitate birth
- The discovery of chloroform, which was used to control pain during childbirth
- The use of drugs to start or induce labor and increase uterine contractions (augmentation of labor)
- Advances in operative procedures such as cesarean birth

With good intentions to prevent infections, hospitals hurried to develop policies and procedures to meet the needs of physicians and take advantage of technology (Wertz & Wertz, 1992). By 1960, 90% of all births in the United States occurred in hospitals.

Maternity care became highly regimented. Physicians managed all antepartum, intrapartum, and postpartum care. Lay midwifery became illegal in many areas, and nurse-midwifery was not well established. The woman's role in childbirth was seen as passive: the physician "delivered" her infant. The primary functions of nurses were to assist the physician and follow prescribed medical orders after childbirth. Teaching and counseling were not valued nursing functions at that time.

Unlike home births, hospital births hindered bonding between parents and infants. During labor the woman received medication such as "twilight sleep," a combination of a narcotic and scopolamine that provided pain relief but left her disoriented, confused, and heavily sedated. Because of this practice and the lack of knowledge regarding the importance of early contact between parent and child, the mother often did not see her infant for several hours after the delivery. The father was relegated to a waiting area and was not allowed to see the mother until some time after the birth of the infant.

Despite technologic advances and the move from home to hospital, maternal and infant mortality rates declined slowly. The slow decline primarily resulted from problems that could have been prevented, such as poor maternal nutrition, infectious diseases, and inadequate prenatal care. These stubborn problems remained because of inequalities in health care delivery. Affluent families could afford comprehensive medical care early in the pregnancy, but poor families had very limited access to prenatal care or information about childbearing. Two concurrent trends, federal involvement and consumer demands, led to additional changes in maternity care.

Government Involvement in Maternal-Infant Care

The high rates of maternal and infant mortality among indigent women provided the impetus for federal involvement in maternity care. The Sheppard-Towner Act of 1921, the first federally sponsored program, provided funds for state-managed programs for mothers and children. Although the Sheppard-Towner Act was later repealed, it set the scene for future allocation of federal funds. Today the federal government supports several programs to improve the health of mothers, infants, and young children (Table 1-1). Although government funds partially solved the problem of maternal and infant mortality, the distribution of health care remains inequitable. Most physicians practice in urban or suburban areas where the affluent can afford to pay for medical services, but women in rural or inner city areas have difficulty obtaining care. Distribution remains a health care problem today.

The ongoing problem of providing health care for poor women and children left the door open for nurses to expand their roles, and advanced educational programs prepared nurses as certified nurse-midwives

Table 1-1
FEDERAL PROJECTS FOR MATERNAL-CHILD CARE

Program	Purpose
Title V of Social Security Act	Provides funds for maternal-child health programs
National Institute of Health and Human Development	Supports research and education of employees needed for maternal and child health programs
Title V Amendment of Public Health Service Act	Provides comprehensive prenatal and infant care in public clinics by the establishment of the Maternal and Infant Care projects
Title XIX of Medicaid Program	Provides funds to facilitate access to care by pregnant women and young children
Head Start	Provides educational opportunities for low-income children of preschool age
National Center for Family Planning	Acts as a clearinghouse for contraceptive information
Women, Infants, and Children (WIC)	Provides supplemental food and nutrition information
Temporary Assistance to Needy Families (TANF)	Provides temporary money for basic living costs of poor children and their families, with eligibility requirements and time limits varying among states; replaced the Aid to Families with Dependent Children program

(CNM), nurse practitioners, and clinical specialists. (Chapter 2 provides a more complete description of these advanced practice nursing roles.)

Effects of Consumer Demands on Health Care

In the early 1950s, consumers began to insist on their right to be involved in their own health care. Pregnant women were no longer willing to accept only what was offered. They wanted information about planning and spacing their children, and they wanted to know events to expect during pregnancy. Moreover, fathers, siblings, and grandparents wanted to be part of the extraordinary time of pregnancy and childbirth. Parents also wanted more say in the way the birth was accomplished.

Early in the 1950s, Dr. Grantly Dick-Read proposed a method of childbirth that allowed the mother to control her fear and thus to control her pain during labor, allowing for birth without pharmacologic intervention. Additional methods such as Lamaze and Bradley quickly gained favor (see Chapter 11). Moreover, a growing consensus among child psychologists and nurse researchers indicated that the benefits of early, extended parent-newborn contact far outweighed any risks of infection from this contact. As a result, knowledgeable parents insisted that their infants remain with them at all times. The practice of separating the infant from the family was abandoned when infections did not run rampant in nurseries, and family-centered maternity care became the standard.

Development of Family-Centered Maternity Care

Family-centered maternity care describes safe, quality care that recognizes and adapts to both the physical and the psychosocial needs of the family, including the newborn. The goal is to foster family unity while maintaining physical safety.

The basic principles of family-centered care are as follows:

- Childbirth is usually a normal, healthy event in the life of a family.
- Childbirth affects the entire family, and family relationships will need to be restructured.
- Families are capable of making decisions about care, provided that they are given adequate information and professional support.

Family-centered care greatly increased the responsibilities of nurses. Nurses do not only provide physical care and assist physicians, they also now assume a major role in teaching, counseling, and supporting families in their decisions. (See Chapter 2 for additional information about the nurse's role in maternity care.)

CURRENT SETTINGS FOR CHILDBIRTH

Traditional Hospital Setting

In traditional hospital childbirth settings of the past, labor took place in a functional labor room, similar to a small hospital or an emergency department room. When birth was imminent, the mother was moved to a delivery area similar to an operating room. After childbirth, the mother was transferred to a recovery area for 1 to 2 hours of observation and then taken to the postpartum unit, which resembled a standard hospital room. The infant was usually moved to the newborn nursery when the mother was transferred to the recovery area. Mother and infant were reunited when the mother was settled in the postpartum unit. The nurse who cared for the mother in the postpartum unit was rarely the same nurse who cared for her baby. Beginning in the 1970s the father or another significant support person could usually remain with the mother throughout labor, birth, and recovery in this setting.

Although birth in a traditional hospital setting was safe, the setting was impersonal and the multiple moves

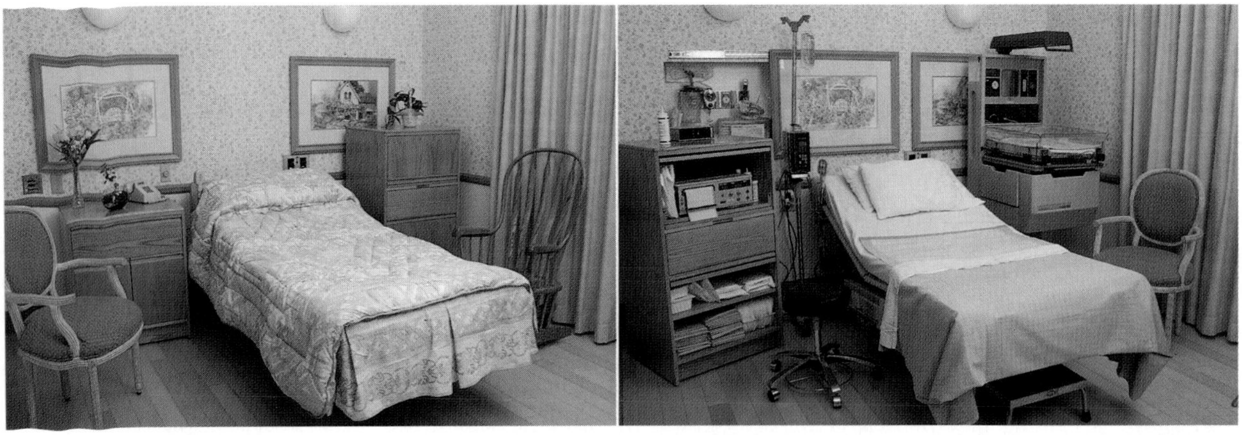

FIGURE 1-1 A typical labor, delivery, and recovery room. Homelike furnishings **(A)** can be adapted quickly to reveal the necessary technical equipment **(B).**

were uncomfortable for the mother. The move from the labor room to the delivery room just before the birth of the baby was particularly difficult for the mother. Furthermore, each move disrupted the family's time together and often separated the parents and infant. Because of these disadvantages, hospitals began to devise settings that were more comfortable and facilitated family participation.

Labor, Delivery, and Recovery Rooms

Today the most common location for hospital birth is the labor, delivery, and recovery (LDR) room. In an LDR room, normal labor, childbirth, and recovery from childbirth take place in one setting (Figure 1-1). Some LDR rooms are quite luxurious, with hardwood floors, paintings, refrigerators, televisions, and video players. Whirlpool baths are available in some facilities. However, the furniture can quickly be transformed into a well-equipped delivery room. Paintings move sideways to expose suction and oxygen apparatus, ceiling spotlights are activated, and wood chests open to reveal fetal monitors and all equipment desired for the birth.

During labor, the woman's significant others are allowed to remain with her. These people may include relatives, friends, and her other children, depending on the policies of the agency and the mother's desires. After she has given birth, the mother typically remains in the LDR room for 1 to 2 hours, after which she is transferred to her postpartum room for the remainder of her hospital stay. The infant may remain with the mother throughout her stay in the LDR room. When the mother is transferred to her postpartum room, the infant may be transferred to the nursery for assessments or may remain with the mother in a mother-baby unit.

The major advantages of LDR rooms are that the setting is more comfortable and homelike and the family can remain with the mother throughout her stay. However, if the family prefers a low-intervention birth, they may regard the technology of the LDR room (fetal monitors, IV fluids) as disadvantages.

Labor, Delivery, Recovery, and Postpartum Rooms

Some hospitals offer rooms similar to LDR rooms in layout and function, with the exception that the mother is not transferred to a postpartum unit after recovery. She and the infant remain in the labor, delivery, recovery, and postpartum (LDRP) room until discharge. The father is encouraged to stay with the mother and infant, and many facilities provide extra beds for overnight stays.

Birth Centers

Freestanding birth centers are designed to provide maternity care to low-risk women outside a hospital setting. In addition to care during childbirth, birth centers also provide antepartum and postpartum care. The mother usually attends classes at the birth center or elsewhere to prepare for childbirth, breastfeeding, and infant care. Both the mother and the infant continue to receive follow-up care during the first 6 weeks after birth. This may include help with breastfeeding problems, a postpartum examination at 4 to 6 weeks, family planning information, and examination of the newborn. Birth is often assisted by CNMs who have provided care for the woman throughout her pregnancy and will continue to provide primary care for the mother and infant.

Birth centers generally charge less than traditional hospitals, which must provide advanced technology that may be unnecessary for low-risk clients. Moreover, women who want a safe, homelike birth in a familiar setting with personnel they have known throughout their pregnancies express a very high rate of satisfaction.

The major disadvantage is that most independent birth centers are not equipped for obstetric emergencies. If unforeseen difficulties develop during labor, the woman must be transferred by ambulance to a nearby hospital to the care of a backup physician who has agreed to perform this role. Although procedures have been designed for these situations, a sudden transfer is frightening for the family.

Home Births

In the United States, only a small number of women give birth at home. Because malpractice insurance for midwives that attend home births is expensive and difficult to obtain, only a small number of CNMs offer this service. Many CNMs have moved their practices to hospitals or birth centers. Mothers who once sought home births have found that they can have many of the advantages of family-centered care in the safe environment of a hospital LDR room or birth center while avoiding the disadvantages and potential dangers of home birth.

Home birth provides the advantage of keeping the family together in its own familiar environment throughout the childbirth experience. When all goes well, birth at home can be a growth-enhancing experience for every family member. Young siblings are not separated from their mothers and are able to establish positive relationships with the new baby immediately after birth. Bonding with the infant is unimpeded by hospital routines, and breastfeeding is highly encouraged and supported. Women who have their babies at home maintain a feeling of control because they actively plan and prepare for each detail of the birth.

However, women who plan a home birth must be screened carefully to ensure their low risk for complications. Opponents of home birth cite the need for immediate, highly technologic care of the woman or infant in case of complications. Even if a hospital is nearby, the transfer time may be too long. Other problems of home birth include the need for the parents to provide a setting and adequate supplies for the birth. In addition, the mother must take care of herself and the infant without the professional help she would have in a hospital setting.

Check Your Reading

1. What two trends created change in maternity care in the last 40 years?
2. How does family-centered maternity care differ from maternity care during the first half of the nineteenth century?
3. How do LDR and LDRP rooms differ from birth centers and home births in their advantages and disadvantages?

CURRENT TRENDS IN MATERNITY CARE

Recently the government, insurance companies, hospitals, and health care providers made a concerted effort to control the increasing cost of health care in the United States. Reform has involved a change in the ways and in which settings money is spent. In the past, most of the health care budget was spent in acute-care settings, in which the facility charged for services after they were provided. Because the facility was paid for any services billed, hospitals had no incentive to be efficient or cost conscious.

Cost Containment

One way in which health care payers have attempted to control costs is with a prospective form of payment; that is, they will no longer pay whatever a hospital charges for a service. Instead, the facility and payers agree in advance on a fixed amount of money for necessary services for specifically diagnosed conditions. An example of this approach is diagnosis-related groups (DRGs).

Diagnosis-Related Groups

DRGs classify related medical diagnoses based on the type or complexity of services generally required by a client with that condition. This method became a standard in 1987 when the federal government set the amount of money that Medicare would pay for each DRG. If a client requires more services than that DRG will pay or if the services are more costly, the hospital must absorb the costs. Conversely, if the hospital delivers the care at less cost than the payment for that DRG, the hospital keeps the remaining money. Hospitals benefit financially if they can reduce the client's length of stay (LOS) in the facility and thereby reduce the costs for service. Although the DRG system originally applied only to Medicare clients, most states have adopted the system for Medicaid payments, and many insurance companies use a similar system.

Managed Care

Health insurance companies also examined the cost of health care and instituted an alternative health care delivery system referred to as *managed* care. Managed care organizations include health maintenance organizations (HMOs) and preferred provider organizations (PPOs). In return for a set fee or premium, HMOs provide relatively comprehensive health services for a group of people enrolled in the organization. Similarly, PPOs are groups of health care providers who agree to provide health services to a specific group of clients on a discounted basis. When the client requires medical treatment, managed care uses strategies such as preadmission authorization to control costs. Prescription medications, although significantly discounted to the consumer, are often limited to a highly restricted formulary without specific additional authorization.

Capitated Care

Capitation may be incorporated into any type of managed care plan. In a pure capitated care plan, the payer of the health insurance (usually the employer or the government) pays a set amount of money each year to a network of primary care providers (PCPs). The contracted amount paid to the PCP may be adjusted for the age and gender of the client group. The PCPs include physicians and often include advanced practice nurses in community clinics or private practices with physicians. In exchange for access to a guaranteed client base, the PCP agrees to provide general health care to each client under contract and pay for all other covered services such as laboratory work, specialist visits, and hospital care.

Capitated plans are of interest to employers and the government because the plans allow payers of health care to predictably budget for health care for a plan year. Health care consumers do not have unexpected financial burdens from illness. The disadvantage for consumers is that they lose most of their freedom of choice regarding their health care providers. PCPs can lose money if they refer too many clients to specialists, who may have no restrictions on their fees, or if they order too many diagnostic tests. Many providers and consumers fear that this method of cost containment will inevitably affect treatment decisions.

Effects of Cost Containment on Maternity Care

As cost containment in health care became essential, insurance plans often mandated that mothers leave the facility within 24 hours after a normal vaginal birth and within 48 hours after a cesarean birth. This policy, in which the decision to discharge the mother was made by the insurance company rather than the woman and her physician or nurse-midwife, was intensely criticized by the press and governmental agencies because problems sometimes developed with mothers or infants after discharge. As a result, legislation was passed that mandates a 48-hour LOS for vaginal deliveries and a 96-hour LOS for cesarean births. A woman may be discharged earlier if she and her physician or nurse-midwife make the joint decision that to do so is in the best interest of herself and her infant. By this legislation an insurance company cannot require a shorter stay.

Unfortunately, 48 hours is still a short time to accomplish the teaching needed before discharge, particularly when the new mother is tired and uncomfortable from the birth. She may or may not have had prenatal classes to prepare her for the care she and her infant will need, and she may not have had prenatal care at all.

However, nurses must examine both sides of the LOS argument. The payer of health care logically questions the reason birthing centers can routinely and safely discharge new mothers in 12 or 24 hours. Payers have good reason to ask for data that support a longer LOS for a normal, anticipated event (Lund, 1997). Nurses and managed care payers alike should examine the reason birthing centers safely accomplish a short LOS for their clients. What additional services and education do they provide that make this possible? What lessons can acute-care facilities learn from low-risk birthing centers? All these areas are ripe for nursing research activities.

Outcomes Management

The determination of providers to lower health care costs while maintaining the quality of care has led to a clinical practice model called *outcomes management.* This systematic method identifies client outcomes and focuses care on interventions that will accomplish the stated outcomes for specific case types, such as the woman who has just given birth or the normal newborn. Clinical pathways are the planning tools used by the health care team to identify and meet stated outcomes.

Clinical Pathways

Clinical pathways, also called *critical paths, care paths,* or *care MAPS (multidisciplinary action plans),* are guidelines developed by each facility in a collaborative process that includes physicians, nurses, and other key professionals. In general, clinical pathways define expected client outcomes, appropriate LOS, and specific interventions by the health care team that help accomplish the stated outcomes. Most clinical pathways also set the time and sequence of interventions of nurses, physicians, and other health care providers for a particular case type.

Variances. Clinical pathways are guidelines meant for clients who are expected to progress along the timeline to meet the expected outcomes. Deviations, or variances, may occur in either the timeline or the expected outcomes. A variance is the difference between the expected event and the reality that occurred. A positive variance occurs when a client progresses more rapidly than expected and is discharged earlier than planned. A negative variance occurs when progress is slower than expected, outcomes are not met within the designated time frame, and the LOS is prolonged. Any variance must be analyzed and the treatment plan adjusted to meet individual or family needs.

Use of Clinical Pathways. In a clinical pathway, assessments, tests, treatments, consultations, and client education are listed in a specific time sequence to accomplish identified outcomes. Figure 1-2 is a clinical pathway that can be used when vaginal births occur in an LDRP room. Outcomes statements have been developed for the prenatal period, labor, childbirth, and postpartum period.

Although this pathway provides insight into the scheduling of assessments and care, it is not meant to teach nursing skills and procedures. For example, outcomes in the first stage of labor state that the woman demonstrates use of breathing and relaxation techniques and the fetus demonstrates normal physiologic parameters. Before students can assess these outcome statements, they must learn breathing and relaxation techniques used during labor and be aware of the normal fetal heart rate and its reaction to uterine contractions.

One purpose of this book is to provide ample information so that students can use clinical pathways in a clinical setting. This involves teaching the reason for performing and the way to perform assessments and interpret the significance of data obtained. The text also provides detailed information about normal values and expected behaviors of clients who are or are not progressing toward the stated outcome. Moreover, the book emphasizes ways to provide information, care, and comfort for childbearing families as they progress along a clinical pathway.

Evidence-Based Practice

Closely related to outcomes management is a change in focus that is often referred to as *evidence-based,* or *research-based,* practice. Nurses and other professionals cannot perform assessments and care solely because "we've always done it that way." They must now rely on research data rather than tradition or habit to determine the optimal techniques and frequencies of assessments and interventions to achieve desired client outcomes in the most cost-effective way. Failure of all nurses to incorporate hard evidence into nursing practice as it becomes available may have numerous undesirable effects, such as the following (Sams & DeGeorges, 1998):

- Significant variations in practice among nurses
- More expensive and less effective care
- Inability of researchers to compare treatments
- Frustration of caregivers and recipients of care

The Association of Women's Health, Obstetric, and Neonatal Nurses (AWHONN) takes an active research role to identify the best practices in a number of areas of this specialty. In appropriate places throughout this text, research evidence to support practice recommendations will be cited.

Another resource for evidence-based practice in perinatal nursing is the Cochrane database, which provides ongoing coordination of research results by an international network of individuals and institutions. The results in the database do not prescribe the policies, procedures, or protocols that a facility should take. However, the critiques of research help identify and distill results from available research so that the best practices may be incorporated into the facility practices.

Community-Based Perinatal Nursing

Because the acute care setting is the most expensive for delivery of health care services, community-based care has increased in all practice areas, including perinatal nursing. Advances in portable technology, such as electronic fetal monitors and infusion pumps for the administration of IV nutrition or subcutaneous medications, allow nurses to perform procedures in the home that were once limited to the hospital. Additionally, women and their families are taught to manage less-severe pregnancy complications at home under the supervision of a nurse, entering the hospital only for periodic checkups or worsening of the problem. Consumers usually prefer home care because of decreased stress on the family when a woman or newborn does not need to be separated from the family support system for hospitalization.

Ample evidence shows that the health care system of the future will be community oriented and involve care for greater numbers of clients in the home and through community agencies. Because home care is a growing part of maternity care, community-based or home care nursing is discussed for specific conditions throughout the text. Public health agencies have existed for many years, and many women obtain all antepartum, postpartum, and neonatal care in these clinics. Other community facilities such as neighborhood health centers, shelters for women and children, school-age mothers' programs, and nurse-managed postpartum centers also provide care to a variety of clients.

Nurses need a broad array of skills to function effectively in community-based care, whether that care takes place in individuals' homes or large clinics. They need to understand the communities in which they practice and the diversity within those communities. Nurses need to develop skills to work with a multidisciplinary team. They are often responsible for assisting clients through high-technology choices and thus need to be proficient in communication and teaching skills.

Perinatal nursing services delivered in a community setting encompass antepartum, postpartum, and neonatal care. Because care is given in an environment that is physically separated from an acute-care institution, nurses must be able to function independently and have superior clinical and critical thinking skills. They should be proficient in interviewing, counseling, and teaching. They assume a leadership role in the coordination of the services a family may require in a complex case, and they frequently supervise the work of other care providers.

YORK HEALTH SYSTEM
YORK, PENNSYLVANIA
CLINICAL PATHWAY
VAGINAL DELIVERY

CLINICAL PATH DAY	EXPECTED PATIENT/ FAMILY OUTCOMES	INTERDISCIPLINARY ASSESSMENT	TESTS	CONSULT
Pre-Natal DATE	□ Prenatal test results available [4] □ 8 or more prenatal visits complete [4] □ Attended baby care and post-partum classes [3] □ Risk assessment complete and referral(s) to appropriate agency made as needed.[5] □ Low risk pregnancy or monitored high risk pregnancy [4] □ ________ □ ________	Each visit-maternal weight; BP; urine dipstick-sugar, protein ketones; FHT S/S of pregnancy complication Perinatal risk assessment Social support Knowledge of self and newborn care Knowledge of warning signs of complications Knowledge of signs of labor	Type and Rh Antibody Screen H and H Sickle cell Rubella RPR HBSAG Trutol or 3h GTT GC, Chlamydia Triple Screen Group B Strep	□ Perinatologist □ Diabetic Educator □ Behavioral Health □ Social Service □ ________ □ ________ □ ________
Admission	□ Demonstrates knowledge of pain management options [1, 2, 3] □ Support person present [2] □ Referral made for identified risk factors □ Admission procedures completed [4] □ ________	Admission assessment Patient needs/desires for pain relief in labor Support system ________ ________	WCBC Type and Rh prn Tube to hold US scan prn ________	□ Perinatologist □ Behavioral Health □ Social Service □ Neonatology □ ________
Labor First Stage	□□□ Achieves desired level of pain relief [1, 2, 3] □□□ Support person present [2] □□□ Referral made for identified maternal/fetal risk during labor □□□ Mother demonstrates normal physiologic parameters [4] □□□ Fetus demonstrates normal physiologic parameters [4] □□□ ________	FHR q 30 min UC q 30-60 min P, R, BP q 2h T q 4° (q2 if ROM) Support system Progress of labor Level of comfort ________	________ ________	□ Neonatology □ ________
Labor Second Stage	□ Pushing effectively [4] □ Support person present {2} □ Referral made for identified maternal/fetal risk during labor [4] □ Mother demonstrates normal physiological parameters [4] □ Fetus demonstrates normal physiological parameters [4] □ ________	FHR q 5 min BP q 30 min Vaginal exam prn ________	________ ________	□ Neonatology □ ________

NAME	INITIALS	NAME	INITIALS

FIGURE 1-2 Clinical pathway for vaginal delivery. (Courtesy Women and Children Services of the York Health System, York, Penn.)

Continued

DOCUMENTATION CODES
Initial=Meets Standard
★=Exception on pathway identified
C=Chronic problems
N=Not applicable

PARENT/FAMILY PROBLEMS
1. Pain r/t childbirth
2. Anxiety r/t childbirth and/or parenting
3. Knowledge deficit r/t childbirth and/or parenting
4. Potential alteration maternal/fetal homeostasis
5. Potential for ineffective parenting
6. ______
7. ______

INTERVENTIONS/ACTIVITIES	MEDS	NUTRITION	EDUCATION AND DC PLANNING
______ ______	Prenatal vitamin, Fe as per order ______ ______	Regular diet ______ ______	Childbirth preparation class Baby care class Breastfeeding class when appropriate Prenatal education
Bed rest with fetal monitor x 30 minutes ______	IV/mini cath ______	NPO with ice chips ______	□ Orient pt/SO/family to L and D area □ Reinforce breathing and relaxation techniques □ ______
Insertion of scalp electrode and IUPC as appropriate Warm/cold compress, massage, position change, ambulates and warm showers prn Encourage to void q 1-2° EFM as ordered Vaginal exam prn Catheterize prn ______ ______	IV as ordered Analgesia prn as ordered Epidural as ordered Induction/augmentation of labor as ordered ______ ______	NPO with ice chips ______	□□□ Reinforce breathing and relaxation technique □□□ Review options for pain management □□□ Encourage support person involvement □□□ Provide explanation of labor progress prn
Position for comfort Catheterize prn Warm/cold compress, massage, position change and void prn ______ ______	IV as ordered Continue epidural as ordered Augmentation of labor as ordered ______ ______	NPO with ice chips ______	□ Assist with pushing □ Encourage support person involvement □ ______ □ ______

NAME	INITIALS	NAME	INITIALS

Illustration continued on following page

FIGURE 1-2 continued

CLINICAL PATH DAY		EXPECTED PATIENT/ FAMILY OUTCOMES	INTERDISCIPLINARY ASSESSMENT	TESTS	CONSULT
Delivery	DATE TIME	□ Deliver live newborn vaginally [4] □ Support person present [2] □ Mother demonstrates normal physiologic parameters □ ______	Fundus, bleeding ______ ______	Cord blood Rh studies when indicated Placenta to pathology as ordered ______	______ ______
Early Recovery	DATE	□ Postpartum parameters stable [4] □ Achieves desired level of pain relief [1] □ ______ □ ______	Temp X 1 P, R, BP, fundus, lochia, bladder, episiotomy q 15 min x 4, and q 30 min x 2 Level of comfort ______	______ ______	______ ______
2-24 Hours	DATE	□□□ Achieves desired level of pain relief [1] □□□ Cares for self and infant [3] □□□ Postpartum parameters stable □□□ Voiding qs [4] □□□ Adequate home support system identified [5] □□□ ______ □□□ ______	T, P, R, BP, Breasts, fundus, lochia, bladder, episiotomy q 4h Readiness to learn Knowledge of self and newborn care Level of comfort Home support system ______	______ ______	______ ______
24-48 Hours	DATE	□□□ Achieves desired level of pain relief [1] □□□ Postpartum parameters stable [4] □□□ Referral made for potential or identified risk (physical/psychosocial) □ Cares for self and infant [3] □□□ ______	T, P, R, BP, bid Breasts, fundus, lochia, bladder, episiotomy q shift WA Level of comfort Readiness to learn Knowledge of self and newborn care ______	WCBC ______ ______	______ ______
Day of Discharge	DATE	□□□ Achieves desired level of pain relief [1] □□□ Postpartum physiological parameters within D/C guidelines [4] □ Patient/SO/family verbalization of D/C instructions [3] □ Postpartum Home Visit not needed based on Interqual Criteria □ Discharge within 2 days after delivery □ ______ □ ______	T, P, R, BP, bid Breasts, fundus, lochia, bladder, episiotomy bid Level of comfort Readiness to learn Pt/SO/family knowledge of self and newborn care ______ ______	______ ______	______ ______

NAME	INITIALS	NAME	INITIALS

NOTE: EACH PATIENT REQUIRES AN INDIVIDUAL ASSESSMENT AND TREATMENT PLAN. THIS CLINICAL PATH IS A RECOMMENDATION FOR THE AVERAGE PATIENT WHICH REQUIRES MODIFICATION WHEN NECESSARY BY THE PROFESSIONAL STAFF.

FIGURE 1-2 continued

Continued

INTERVENTIONS/ACTIVITIES	MEDS	NUTRITION	EDUCATION AND DC PLANNING
Catheterize prn Continue IV Continue epidural or local anesthetic __________ __________	Oxytocin after placenta delivered as ordered □ __________ □ __________	NPO __________ __________	□ Support parent/infant bonding □ __________ □ __________
OOB with assist first time Perineal ice pack q 30 min prn Cath prn Shower __________ __________	Analgesia prn Continue epidural if PPTL Continue IV oxytocin as ordered D/C IV or cap IV □ __________ □ __________	Reg diet as tolerated __________ __________	□ Support parent/infant bonding □ Teach pericare □ __________ □ __________
OOB with assist first time, then OOB ad lib Catheterize per protocol Epifoam, Tucks prn Ice pack prn Sitz bath 12° after delivery prn __________ __________	Analgesia prn __________ __________	Adv to reg diet as tolerated __________ __________	□□□ Initiate and continue maternal/newborn education record, D/C instructions □□□ __________ __________ □□□ __________ __________
OOB ad lib Epifoam, Tucks prn Sitz bath prn __________ __________	Analgesia prn __________ __________	Regular diet __________ __________	□□□ Continue maternal newborn education record □□□ __________ __________ □□□ __________ __________
OOB ad lib Epifoam, Tucks prn Sitz bath prn __________ __________	Analgesia prn □ RhoGAM, when indicated □ Rubella, when indicated __________ __________	Regular diet __________ __________	□ Completion of maternal newborn education record □ Physician discharge instructions □ Support services in community: □ Breastfeeding Support Services □ Perinatal Coaching □ City/State Health □ Other □ D/C after Pt./family review instructions

DISCHARGE DATE	DISCHARGE TIME	DISCHARGED TO	ACCOMPANIED BY □ W/C □ AMBULATE

FIGURE 1-2 continued

Common Types of Perinatal Home Care

Antepartum Home Care. Most preconceptional and low-risk antepartum care takes place in private offices or public clinics. Some common high-risk conditions seen in home-based perinatal nursing include preterm labor, hyperemesis gravidarum (intractable vomiting during pregnancy), bleeding problems, premature rupture of membranes ("bag of waters"), hypertension, and diabetes during pregnancy.

Postpartum and Neonatal Home Care. Even with legislation to limit discharge requirements of managed care agencies, providing the necessary education to new mothers in their own self-care, basic care of their infants, and signs of problems they should report after discharge is a challenge for health care professionals. Before the woman is discharged, hospitals may offer classes, closed-circuit television programs, written materials (often in multiple languages), and individual teaching and demonstration.

After the woman is discharged, various services are offered for home care. These services may include telephone calls, home visits, information lines, and lactation consultations. At the time of discharge, some hospitals provide parents with videotapes of infant care to supplement written materials for later reference. In addition, nurse-managed outpatient clinics provide care for mothers and infants in some areas. (See Chapters 18 and 23 for additional information about home care for mothers and infants.)

Home Care for High-Risk Neonates. Neonatal home care nurses may provide care for infants who are discharged from the acute-care facility with serious medical conditions. Parents of preterm or low-birth-weight infants require a great deal of information and support. Infants with congenital anomalies such as cleft palate may require care adapted to their conditions. Moreover, increasing numbers of technology-dependent infants, such as those who require ventilator assistance, total parenteral nutrition, intravenous medications, and apnea monitoring, are now cared for at home.

The coordination of care for the high-risk newborn is a major challenge for home care nurses. The involvement of multiple specialty providers, such as physicians, nurses, respiratory therapists, and equipment vendors, may result in duplication or fragmentation of services. Duplication of services results in unnecessary costs, and fragmentation of services can result in dangerous gaps in care. (See Chapters 29 and 30 for home care for high-risk infants.)

Standards of Practice for Community-Based Perinatal Nursing

As with other health care, community-based perinatal care must meet guidelines for practice established by the agency itself, accrediting agencies, and appropriate specialty practice organizations.

Agency Standards. Each community health agency is required to have policies, procedures, and protocols to define and guide all elements of care. These standards, which must comply with established national standards, must be kept current and accessible to the nursing personnel.

Organizational Standards. In addition to agency standards, nurses who provide community-based health care must also be aware of organizational standards. The Association of Women's Health, Obstetric, and Neonatal Nurses (AWHONN) is recognized as the national professional organization for perinatal services. AWHONN publishes competency statements, position papers, and practice guidelines. *Didactic Content and Clinical Skills Verification for Professional Nurse Providers of Perinatal Home Care* (1994) provides written statements regarding the scope of services, policies, procedures, and protocols for perinatal home care. Standards set by other professional organizations such as the American College of Obstetricians and Gynecologists, the National Association of Home Care, and the American Academy of Pediatrics may also influence standards for perinatal nurses.

Legal Standards. Professionals that practice in any health care delivery system, including community-based perinatal care, must understand the definition of nursing practice and the rules and regulations that govern its practice. For instance, in most states, home health care agencies and registered nurses must be licensed to provide care. Nurses must also be aware of their scope of practice, which is defined by nurse practice acts. (Chapter 3 gives additional information on legal aspects of nursing.)

Other regulatory bodies, such as the Occupational Safety and Health Administration (OSHA), Food and Drug Administration (FDA), and Centers for Disease Control and Prevention (CDC), also provide guidelines for practice in those areas. Accrediting agencies such as the Joint Commission on Accreditation of Health Care Organizations (JCAHO) and Community Health Accreditation Program (CHAP) give their approval after visiting facilities and observing whether standards are being met in practice. Approval from these accrediting agencies affects reimbursement and funding decisions as well.

Advances in Technology

As with other areas of health care, perinatal care must change constantly to keep pace with technologic advances. Nowhere is technology developing faster than in the fields of information and communication. Health care professionals and their clients have online access to information from a variety of databases. Today's nurse must be as much at ease with a keyboard and mouse as yesterday's nurse was with a pen and clipboard. Fetal monitoring data may not be stored on pa-

Table 1-2
COMPLEMENTARY AND ALTERNATIVE MEDICINE CATEGORIES

Category	Examples
Mind-body medicine: Behavioral, psychologic, social, and spiritual approaches to health	Yoga, relaxation response techniques, meditation, tai chi, hypnotherapy, spirituality, support groups, and biofeedback
Alternative systems of medical practice: Systems developed outside the Western biomedical approach	Traditional Chinese medicine, homeopathy, ayurveda, naturopathy, chiropractic, Native American medicine, and acupuncture
Pharmacologic and biologic treatments	Folk medicine, medicinal plants, processed blood products, and autogenous vaccines
Herbal therapies: Plant-derived preparations used for therapeutic or preventive purposes	Use of plants that have pharmacologic activity, such as ginkgo biloba, ginseng, echinacea, saw palmetto, witch hazel, bilberry, aloe vera, feverfew, and green tea
Diet and nutrition: Dietary approaches and special diets applied as alternative therapies for risk factors or chronic disease in general	Use of vitamins, minerals, and nutritional supplements; cancer and cardiovascular disease diets; possible megadosing, elimination, or excessive intake of certain foods; vegetarian and macrobiotic diets; and diets associated with physicians or others (Pritikin, Atkins diet)
Manual healing methods: Systems based on manipulation and/or movement of the body	Massage, chiropractic, osteopathic manipulation, polarity, reflexology, and therapeutic touch
Bioelectromagnetic applications: Unconventional use of electromagnetic fields for medical purposes	Use of magnets for musculoskeletal and neurologic pain, diathermy, pulsed electromagnetic waves, and transcutaneous electrical nerve stimulation

Modified from American College of Obstetricians and Gynecologists: *Complementary and alternative medicine* (ACOG Committee Opinion Number 227, November 1999), Washington, D.C., The Association; and from the website of the National Center for Complementary and Alternative Medicine, National Institutes of Health.

per at all but instead stored on electronic media. Video and digital imaging technology preserve and recall crisp images that allow image overlay and computerized comparison, often at distant locations. Personal computer systems are linked to share information about staffing, scheduling, and communication. Today's nursing student routinely communicates with instructors by electronic mail (e-mail), receives grades, and completes tests and assignments over the Internet.

Complementary and Alternative Medicine

Complementary and alternative medicine (CAM) is becoming more common, and its use is not restricted to recent immigrants to North America, although some techniques originated thousands of years ago in Eastern cultures. In 1997, nearly 50% of women used CAM. *Complementary and alternative medicine* can be defined as those systems, practices, interventions, modalities, professions, therapies, applications, theories, or claims that are currently not an integral part of the dominant or conventional medical system in North America (American College of Obstetricians and Gynecologists, 1999). The therapies may be used alone (alternative therapy), combined with other therapies, or used in addition to conventional medical therapy (complementary therapy). Table 1-2 gives examples of therapies for complementary or alternative care.

Safety is a major concern in the use of CAM. Many people who use these techniques or substances are self-referred. They may delay necessary care from a conventional physician or nurse-midwife, or they may ingest herbal remedies or other substances that are toxic when combined with conventional medications or when taken in excess. Additionally, because herbs and vitamins are classified as foods rather than medications, they are not heavily regulated, if at all. Thus people may take in variable amounts of active ingredients from these substances. Some lay people do not consider these therapies to be medicine and may not report them to their conventional health care provider, which sets the stage for an interaction between conventional medications and CAM therapies that have pharmacologic properties. Also, many people may not consider some therapies to be alternative because they are considered mainstream in their cultures, in which Western medicine is considered alternative. (See "Cultural Perspectives in Childbearing" on page 16 for more information on health practices used by specific cultures.)

Nurses may find that their professional values do not conflict with many of the CAM therapies. As a profession, nursing supports a self-care and preventive approach to health care in which individuals bear much of the responsibility for their health. Nursing practice has traditionally emphasized a holistic, or body-mind-spirit, model of health that fits with CAM. Nurses may already widely practice some CAM therapies such as therapeutic touch. The rising interest in CAM provides opportunities for nurses to participate in research related to the legitimacy of these treatment modalities.

The National Institutes of Health now has a web page (http://nccam.nih.gov/) to answer questions people may have about CAM. This web page is not an endorsement but is a source of information and classification of these techniques.

Table 1-3
FAMILY TYPES

Family Types	Definition
Traditional (nuclear)	Mother, father, and subadult children (either natural or adopted) living in the same household; single or dual income
Nontraditional	
Single parent	Never-married, divorced, or widowed adult and natural or adopted children
Blended	Parent, stepparent, children, and stepchildren living in the same household
Extended	Nuclear family plus relatives of either or both spouses living in the same household
Communal	Several households of adults and their children living in a common geographic area and working together to achieve the group's goals
Foster	Family members other than biologic or adoptive parents
High risk	Households at increased risk for problems (those below poverty level, headed by a single teenage parent, and with unanticipated stress or an uncertain lifestyle)

Check Your Reading

4. How do cost-containment strategies affect maternal-newborn nursing?
5. What are the functions of clinical pathways?
6. How do standards guide home care?
7. What are possible dangers in the use of complementary and alternative medicine?

THE FAMILY

Families are sometimes categorized into three groups: traditional, nontraditional, and high risk (Table 1-3). In theory, traditional families require care that differs from that needed by nontraditional or high-risk families.

Traditional Families

Traditional families, or nuclear families, are headed by a couple that views parenting as the major priority in their lives and whose energies are not depleted by stressful conditions such as poverty, illness, or substance abuse. Generally, traditional families are motivated to learn all they can about pregnancy, childbirth, and parenting. These families are best served by providing information as the need arises. Traditional families can be single or dual income.

Single-Income Families

In the 1950s and 1960s the idealized single-income American family was epitomized in several long-running television series such as "Leave It to Beaver." This family comprised a father who was the sole provider, a mother who was a homemaker and caregiver, and two children. Today, this family structure represents only a small minority of the nation's families.

Dual-Income Families

Most two-parent families now depend on two incomes. This economic reality has created a great deal of stress on parents, subjecting them to many of the same problems faced by single-parent families. For instance, reliable, competent child care has become a major issue and has increased the stress on traditional families.

Nontraditional Families

Nontraditional families are defined by their unique structure and may be single parent, blended, or extended. As with traditional families, nontraditional families require information. They often benefit from referrals to meet specific needs such as single-parenting classes, classes for parents of multiples, and group classes for adoptive families.

Single-Parent Families

Millions of families are now headed by a single parent, most often the mother, who must function as a homemaker and caregiver and also is often the major provider for the family's financial needs. Divorce is the most common cause of single-parent families, although childbirth among unmarried women is also a major factor.

Single-parent families are more likely to live below the poverty level and are vulnerable to a variety of problems. Parents may feel overwhelmed by the prospect of assuming all child-rearing responsibilities and may be less prepared for illness or unemployment than two-parent families.

Nurses can support and encourage single-parent families with a focus on the unique problems of each specific family. Nurses are often the primary source of information about health care for many of these families and are often instrumental in the initiation of the necessary referrals to social and governmental agencies.

Blended Families

Blended families are formed when divorced or widowed parents remarry and bring children from a previous marriage into the new relationship. Many times the couple desires children with each other, which creates a contemporary family structure commonly described as "yours, mine, and ours." These families may have difficulty forming a cohesive family unit unless they can overcome differences in parenting styles and values. Differing expectations of children's behavior and development and differing beliefs about discipline often cause family conflict.

Extended Families

The extended family includes members from at least three generations living under one roof. This family structure is becoming increasingly common in the United States and has given rise to the term *boomerang families.* This expression refers to single or married adults with children of their own who return to their parents' homes because they either are unable to support their family or want the additional support that grandparents provide for grandchildren. Extended families are vulnerable to generational conflicts and may require education and referral to prevent disintegration of the family unit. However, extended families can also provide a great deal of support for all members.

Homosexual Families

Although homosexual families are relatively uncommon, they are recognized increasingly in the United States. Children in homosexual families may be from previous heterosexual unions, adopted, or conceived by artificial insemination of one or both members of a lesbian couple. These families may face a great many challenges from a community that is unaccustomed to alternative lifestyles.

Adoptive Families

Persons who adopt a child may have problems that biologic parents do not face. Biologic parents have the long period of gestation and the gradual changes of pregnancy to help them adjust emotionally and socially to the birth of a child. The needs of adoptive parents may be overlooked after the end of the adoption process. As with biologic parents, adoptive parents need information, support, and guidance to prepare them to care for the infant and to maintain their own relationship. These parents may be older when the adoption is finalized. Friends in their age group may have children who are much older than the newly adopted child, particularly if the parents adopt an infant. This difference may make adoptive parents feel somewhat out of step with their peers, who are attending soccer and drill team practice while the adoptive parents are changing diapers and doing night feedings.

High-Risk Families

High-risk families include those below the poverty level, those headed by a single teenage parent, and those with unanticipated stress, such as an infant who is preterm, ill, or handicapped. In addition, families with lifestyle problems such as alcoholism, use of illicit drugs, and family violence are considered at high risk for problems in providing adequate care for the infant.

Many high-risk families require specialized services. In such cases the major responsibility of nurses is to refer these families to agencies that can provide comprehensive care. The most common referrals are to social service agencies for financial assistance, crisis intervention, home visits, and drug rehabilitation programs (see Chapter 24).

Characteristics of a Healthy Family

In general, healthy families are able to adapt to changes that occur in the family unit. Pregnancy and childbirth create some of the most powerful changes in a family. The relationship between adults must change to include the care of a helpless infant. Children must learn to share the attention of parents with a new sibling. The healthy, viable family is able to adapt to these changes without undue stress, but the family that is unprepared for change may suffer conflict.

Healthy families exhibit some common characteristics that provide a framework the nurse can use to assess the way all families function. These characteristics include the following:

- Members of healthy families communicate openly with each other to express the concerns and needs of each family member.
- Healthy families remain flexible in role assignment so that if one person is unable to complete the assigned tasks, another member offers assistance.
- Adults in healthy families agree on the basic principles of parenting so that discord about such things as discipline and sleep schedules is minimal.
- Healthy families are adaptable and not overwhelmed by changes that occur in the home and relationships as a result of childbirth. For instance, adaptable families can tolerate less-than-perfect housekeeping, an irregular schedule of meals, and interrupted sleep, all of which are common when an infant is added to the family structure.
- Members of healthy families volunteer assistance without waiting to be asked. Some young parents feel guilty if they must ask for help with the tasks of parenting but are relieved when assistance is offered.

Factors Interfering with Family Functioning

Nurses need to recognize factors that interfere with the family's ability to provide for the individual needs of family members. These factors include lack of financial resources, absence of adequate family support, birth of an infant who requires specialized care, unhealthy habits such as smoking or substance abuse, and inability to make mature decisions that are necessary to provide care for an infant.

Check Your Reading

8. How do structures of traditional and nontraditional families differ?
9. What are four reasons families might be identified as high risk?
10. What are the characteristics of a healthy family?
11. What factors interfere with family functioning?

CULTURAL PERSPECTIVES IN CHILDBEARING

Culture is the sum of the beliefs and values that are learned, shared, and transmitted from generation to generation by a particular group. Cultural values guide the thinking, decisions, and actions of the group, particularly in pivotal events such as childbearing. Ethnicity is the condition of belonging to a particular group that shares race, language and dialect, religious faiths, traditions, values, and symbols, as well as food preferences, literature, and folklore. Cultural beliefs and values vary among different groups, and nurses must be aware that individuals often believe their cultural values and patterns of behavior are superior. This belief, termed *ethnocentrism,* forms the basis for many conflicts that occur when persons from different cultural groups have frequent contact.

Nurses must be aware that culture comprises visible and invisible layers that could be said to resemble an iceberg (Figure 1-3). Observable behaviors can be compared with the visible part—the tip of the iceberg. The history, beliefs, values, and religion are not observed, but they are the hidden foundation on which behaviors are based and can be likened to the large submerged part of the iceberg. A full comprehension of cultural behavior includes knowledge of the hidden beliefs expressed by behaviors.

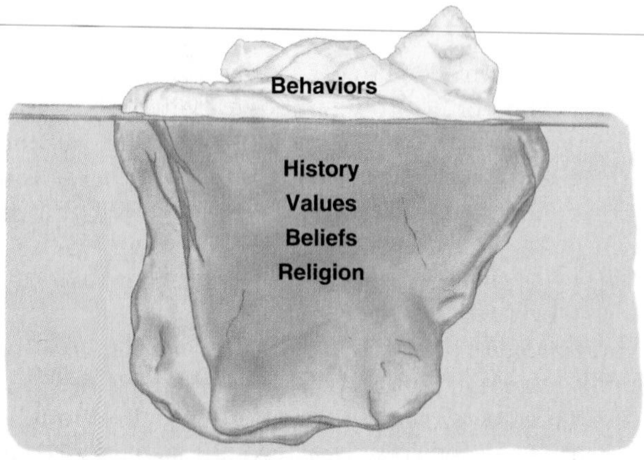

FIGURE 1-3 Visible and hidden layers of culture are like the visible and submerged parts of an iceberg. Many cultural differences are hidden below the surface.

Implications of Cultural Diversity for Perinatal Nurses

Many immigrants and refugees are of childbearing age, which means that perinatal nurses in most localities will provide care for culturally diverse families. To provide effective care, nurses must be aware that culture is among the most significant factors that influence a woman's perception of childbirth.

Western Cultural Beliefs

Nursing practice in the United States is based largely on Western beliefs. Nurses must recognize that these beliefs may differ significantly from those of other societies and that the differences may cause a great deal of conflict.

Leininger (1978) identified seven dominant Western cultural values. These values greatly influence the thinking and action of nurses in the United States but may not be shared by their clients:

1. Democracy is a cultural value not shared by families that believe decisions are made by elders or other higher authorities in the group. Fatalism, or a belief that events and results are predestined, may also affect health care decisions.
2. Individualism conflicts with the values of many cultural groups in which individual goals are subordinated to the greater good of the group.
3. Cleanliness is an American "obsession" that many others view with amazement.
4. Preoccupation with time, which is measured by health care professionals in minutes and hours, is a major source of conflict with those who mark time by different standards such as seasons and body needs.
5. Reliance on machines and equipment may intimidate families who have not reached even minimal comfort with technology.
6. The belief that optimal health is a right is in direct conflict with beliefs in many cultures in the world in which health is not a major emphasis or even an expectation.
7. Admiration of self-sufficiency and financial success may conflict with beliefs of other societies that place less value on wealth and more value on less tangible aspects such as spirituality.

Communication

Communication may also be a source of conflict between "dominant culture" and "other culture" health care professionals. This is particularly true for Southeast Asians, Latinos, African-Americans, and Middle-Eastern immigrants.

Southeast Asians. Language is the greatest barrier to health care for those people from Southeast Asia

(Mattson, 1995). Besides the national languages of Vietnam, Cambodia, and Laos, numerous tribal languages are spoken in each country. People from Southeast Asia also speak softly and avoid prolonged eye contact, which they consider rude, in contrast to the Western belief that eye contact denotes honesty and forthrightness. They invariably show respect to the elderly, priests, and physicians. When medication or therapy is recommended, they seldom say "no." They may accept the prescription or medication sample but not take the medicine, or they may agree to undergo a procedure but not keep the appointment.

Latinos. Latinos include those whose origin is Mexico, Central and South America, and Puerto Rico. Latinos tend to be polite and gracious in conversation. Preliminary social interaction is particularly important, and Latinos may be insulted if a problem is addressed directly without taking time for "small talk." This is counter to the Western value of "getting to the point" and may cause frustration for both the client and the health care worker.

African-Americans. African-Americans sometimes use a communication style that may cause conflict when they seek health care. They may use idioms, colloquial expressions, or speech patterns that are unfamiliar to many health care workers. Nurses must often clarify what is being said so that misunderstandings can be avoided and teaching can be effective.

Middle Easterners. Middle-Eastern immigrants come from a variety of countries, including Lebanon, Syria, Arabia, Egypt, Turkey, Iran, and Palestine. Communication in these countries is an elaborate system, but obtaining information may be difficult because Islam, the primary religion, dictates that family affairs should be kept within the family. Personal information is shared only with personal friends, and health assessment must be done gradually. When interpreters are used, they should be of the same country and religion as the client if possible because of regional differences and hostilities. Because Muslim society tends to be paternalistic, asking the man's permission or opinion when family members require health care is wise.

Cross-Cultural Health Beliefs

More than 100 different ethnocultural groups exist in the United States, and numerous traditional health beliefs are observed among these groups. Culturally based definitions of health are common. Women of Asian origin may view health as the balance of "yin and yang." Those of African or Haitian origin may define health as "harmony with nature." People from Mexico, Central and South America, and Puerto Rico often see health as a balance of "hot and cold."

Traditional Methods to Prevent Illness

The traditional methods of illness prevention rest in the woman's ability to understand the cause of a given illness in her culture. These causes may include the following:

- Agents such as hexes, spells, or the evil eye, which may strike a person (often a child) and cause injury, illness, or misfortune
- Phenomena such as soul loss or accidental provocation of envy, jealousy, or hate of a friend or an acquaintance
- Environmental factors such as bad air and natural events such as solar eclipses

Practices to prevent illness developed from beliefs about the cause of illness. A believer must avoid those persons known to transmit hexes and spells. Elaborate methods are used to prevent inciting envy or jealousy of others and to avoid the evil eye. Protective or religious objects such as amulets with magic powers or consecrated religious objects (such as talismans) are frequently worn or carried to prevent illness. Also, numerous food taboos and traditional combinations are prescribed in traditional belief systems to prevent illness. For instance, people from many ethnic backgrounds eat raw garlic to prevent illness. Those of African origin may consume nonfood substances such as starch to facilitate labor.

Traditional Practices to Maintain Health

Several traditional practices are used to maintain health. Proper clothing such as scarves may prevent drafts and thus maintain the health of a woman who is pregnant and believes she must avoid cool air. Another example is a proper diet. Women of Asian origin eat rice daily. Mental and spiritual health are maintained by activities such as silence, meditation, and prayer. Many people view illness as punishment for breaking a religious code and adhere strictly to religious morals and practices to maintain health.

Traditional Practices to Restore Health

Traditional practices to restore health often conflict with Western medical practice. Some of the most common practices include the use of natural substances such as herbs and plants to treat illness. Religious charms, holy words, and traditional healers may be tried before a medical opinion is sought. Religious medals, prayer cards, and sacrifices may also treat illness.

A variety of substances may be ingested for the treatment of illnesses. The nurse should make an effort to identify the substance and determine whether its active ingredient may alter the effects of prescribed medication.

Dermabrasion, which is the rubbing or irritation of the skin to relieve discomfort, is a common health care practice in some cultures such as the Vietnamese and Cambodian cultures. The most popular form is coining, in which an area is covered with an ointment and the edge of a coin is rubbed over the area. All dermabrasion methods leave marks resembling bruises or burns on the skin and may be mistaken for signs of physical abuse (Mattson, 1995).

Cultural Assessment

All health care professionals must develop skills in performing a cultural assessment so that they can understand the meaning of childbirth in different cultural groups. The following questions might be considered in making such an assessment:

- Is childbearing viewed as a normal process, a time of vulnerability, or a state of illness?
- What are the prescribed practices, customs, and rituals related to diet, activity, and behavior during pregnancy and childbirth?
- What maternal restrictions or precautions are considered necessary during pregnancy and childbirth?
- Who provides support during pregnancy, childbirth, and beyond?
- What are the prescribed practices and restrictions related to care of the newborn?
- Who in the family hierarchy makes health care decisions?
- How is time marked—by minutes and hours or by seasons and body needs?
- What are the views of life and death, including predestination and fatalism?
- How can health care professionals be most helpful?

After such an assessment, plans for care should show respect for cultural differences and traditional healing practices. (Additional information is presented throughout this book relating to culture-specific areas such as nutrition, pregnancy, birth, and the postpartum period.)

Check Your Reading

12. Why is it important for nurses to examine their own cultural values and beliefs?
13. How might communication be a source of conflict?
14. How is culture comparable to an iceberg?

STATISTICS ON MATERNAL AND INFANT HEALTH

Statistics is the science of collecting and interpreting numeric data. In health and medical science, data often focus on mortality rates within a given population. Mortality rates indicate the number of deaths that occur each year by different categories. They are important sources of information about the health of groups of people within a country. They may also be an indication of the value a society places on health care and the kind of health care available to the people.

Maternal and Infant Mortality

Throughout history the number of deaths of women and infants has been high, especially around the time of childbirth. In the United States in 1910, 6 of every 1000 women who gave birth died of causes related to pregnancy and childbirth. In that same year, 130 of every 1000 children died before their first birthday (Simkin, 1989).

Infant and maternal mortality rates began to fall with the improved health of the general population, application of basic principles of sanitation, and increase in medical knowledge. By 1940, major improvements in health care reduced the infant mortality rate to 50% of that of 1910. A further large decrease over the next 10 years resulted from the widespread availability of antibiotics, improvement in public health, and increased prenatal care. Today, mothers seldom die in childbirth and infant mortality rates continue downward. However, this downward trend is greater for whites than for nonwhites.

Maternal Mortality

Because few women today die in childbirth, the maternal mortality rate is now determined by the number of deaths per 100,000 live births instead of per 1000 live births. In 1997 a total of 327 women died in childbirth in the United States for a rate of 8.4 maternal deaths per 100,000 live births. African-American women are more likely to die from birth-related causes than are white women. The 1997 maternal mortality rate for African-American women was 20.8, which is more than three times the rate of 5.8 for white women (National Center for Health Statistics, 1999).

Infant Mortality

Infant mortality rates have been slower to improve than those of maternal mortality. Unlike maternal rates, infant mortality rates are calculated by the number of deaths under 1 year of age per 1000 live births. Between 1950 and 1990, infant mortality dropped from 29.2 to 9.8 deaths per 1000 live births. In 1997 the infant mortality rate was 7.2 per 1000 live births, the lowest ever recorded in the United States. Preliminary data for 1998 show the same rate. The 1997 neonatal mortality rate (death before 28 days of life) was 4.8 deaths per 1000 live births (National Center for Health Statistics, 1999).

Although infant and neonatal mortality rates in the United States have declined overall, the decline for whites has remained significantly greater than that for African-Americans (Figure 1-4). In 1997 the mortality rate for white infants was 6.0. The mortality rate for

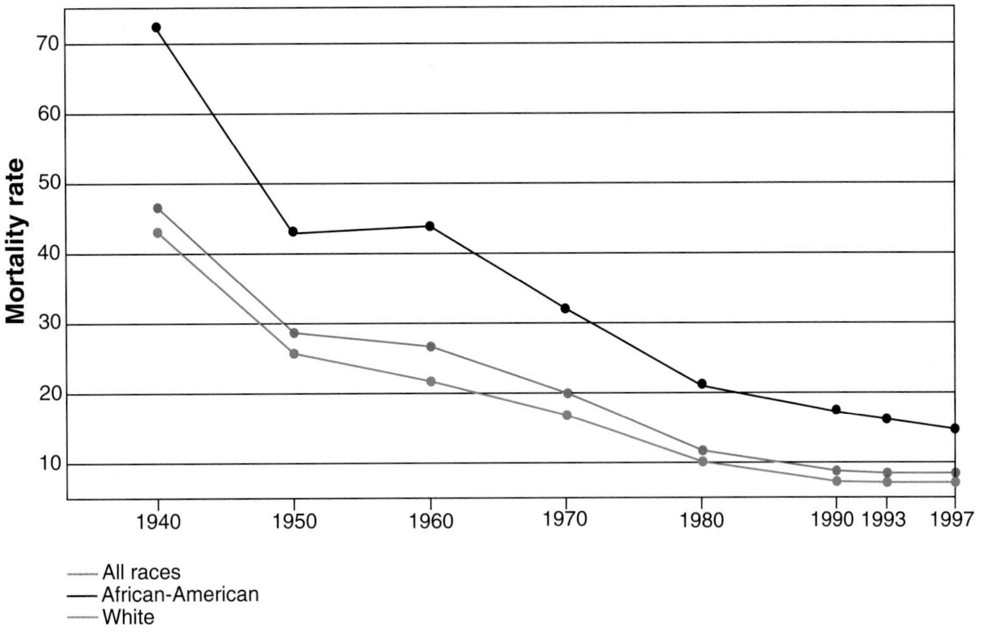

FIGURE 1-4 Infant mortality rates from 1940 to 1997 based on advance report on final mortality statistics. (Courtesy National Center for Health Statistics [1999]. National Vital Statistics Reports 1999; 47:19. Retrieved February 19, 2000, from http://www.cdc.gov/nchs/data/nvs47_19.pdf.)

African-American infants was 14.2 (National Center for Health Statistics, 1999).

Disparity across Racial Groups

The disparity in maternal and infant mortality rates is most obvious between whites and African-Americans, who constitute the largest minority group. The discrepancy is primarily because of greater numbers of low-birth-weight (below 2500 grams) infants among African-Americans. African-American infants have almost twice the risk for low birth weight compared with white infants, and they are twice as likely to die before their first birthday.

Poverty, not race, is the important factor. The rate of poverty is higher for nonwhites than for whites in the United States. People who live below the poverty level are unlikely to be in good health, be well nourished, have adequate housing, or obtain the preventive health care they need. Obtaining care becomes vital during pregnancy and infancy, and lack of care is reflected in the high mortality rates in all categories.

The following *Healthy People 2010* objectives relate to infant mortality in the United States (United States Department of Health and Human Services):

- Reduce infant mortality from the 1998 rate (preliminary data) of 7.2 per 1000 live births to 4.5 per 1000 live births in 2010
- Reduce neonatal mortality from the 1998 rate (preliminary data) of 4.8 per 1000 live births to 2.9 per 1000 live births in 2010
- Reduce the percentage of low-birth-weight infants from 7.6 to 5.0
- Reduce the percentage of very-low-birth-weight infants from 1.4 to 0.9

Infant Mortality across Nations

A country such as the United States, which has one of the highest gross national products in the world, is expected to have one of the lowest infant mortality rates. Yet in 1995, the most recent year for which comparative data among countries are available, the mortality rate in the United States ranked twenty-fifth among developed nations (Table 1-4).

The major reasons for this poor showing are (1) unequal access to health care for women of all socioeconomic levels and (2) the high rate of adolescent pregnancy, which is associated with the low birth weight and complications of prematurity that contribute to infant mortality. Congenital anomalies and sudden infant death syndrome are also leading causes of infant mortality.

Check Your Reading

15. Why is the infant mortality rate so much lower today than at the beginning of the twentieth century?
16. Why are African-American women and infants more likely to die than white women and children?
17. How does the infant mortality rate in the United States compare with the rates in other countries?

Table 1-4
INFANT MORTALITY RATES FOR SELECTED COUNTRIES, 1995

Country	Infant Mortality (per 1000 Live Births)
Finland	3.93
Singapore	4.01
Sweden	4.13
Norway	4.13
Japan	4.26
Hong Kong	4.57
France	4.86
Switzerland	5.05
Denmark	5.07
Germany	5.30
Austria	5.42
Netherlands	5.46
Spain	5.49
Australia	5.66
Belgium	6.05
Italy	6.12
England and Wales	6.14
Canada	6.14
Scotland	6.24
Ireland	6.37
New Zealand	6.68
Israel	6.86
Northern Ireland	7.08
Portugal	7.51
United States	7.59

From US Department of Health and Human Services. (1999). *Health, United States, 1999, with health and aging chartbook,* Hyattsville, MD, Author.

SUMMARY CONCEPTS

- Changes in maternity care in the United States came about as a result of technologic advances, increased knowledge, government involvement, and consumer demands.
- Alternative settings for childbirth are now available in hospitals and freestanding birth centers. Home births are less frequently selected as an alternative.
- Family-centered maternity care, which is based on the principle that families can make decisions about health care if they have adequate information, has greatly increased the role of nurses.
- Outcomes management, which came about as a result of cost-containment strategies, has resulted in new tools to reduce the length of stay for mothers and infants in the birth facility.
- Clinical pathways are interdisciplinary guidelines for assessments and interventions that will accomplish the identified outcomes in the shortest time.
- Students must learn the reason for and the way to perform assessments and interventions so that they can use clinical pathways to determine whether clients are achieving identified outcomes.
- Social trends such as poverty, early unplanned pregnancy, and the increased rate of divorce have altered family structure and function and have increased the need for information and support provided by nurses.
- To provide care for culturally diverse clients, nurses must examine their own beliefs and become familiar with different cultural values and customs.
- Infant and maternal mortality rates have declined dramatically in the last 50 years. However, the United States continues to have a higher infant mortality rate than many other developed nations and variation in mortality rates across ethnic groups is still wide.

REFERENCES & READINGS

American Academy of Pediatrics (AAP) & American College of Obstetricians and Gynecologists (ACOG). (1997). *Guidelines for perinatal care* (4th ed.). Elk Grove Village, IL: Author.

American College of Obstetricians and Gynecologists. (1999). *Complementary and alternative medicine* (ACOG Committee Opinion Number 227, November 1999). Washington, D.C.: Author.

Alexander, G.R., & Kogan, M.D. (1998). Ethnic differences in birth outcomes: The search for answers continues. *Birth,* 25(3), 198-201.

Association of Women's Health, Obstetric, and Neonatal Nurses (AWHONN). (1994a). *Shortened maternity and newborn hospital stays* (position statement). Washington, D.C.: Author.

AWHONN. (1994b). *Didactic content and clinical skills verification for professional nurse providers of perinatal home care.* Washington, D.C.: Author.

Attenborough, R. (1997). The Canadian health care system: Development, reform, and opportunities for nurses. *Journal of Obstetric, Gynecologic, and Neonatal Nursing,* 26(2), 229-234.

Bailey, C. (1994). Education for home care providers. *Journal of Obstetric, Gynecologic, and Neonatal Nursing,* 23(8), 714-719.

Bower, K.A. (1997). Case management and clinical paths: Strategies to support the perinatal experience. *Journal of Obstetric, Gynecologic, and Neonatal Nursing,* 26(3), 329-333.

Buus-Frank, M. (1999). Nurse versus machine: Slaves or masters of technology? *Journal of Obstetric, Gynecologic, and Neonatal Nursing,* 28(4), 433-441.

Callister, L.C. (2000). Cochrane pregnancy and childbirth database: Resource for evidence-based practice. *Journal of Obstetric, Gynecologic, and Neonatal Nursing,* 29(2), 123-128.

Callister, L.C. (1995). Cultural meanings of childbirth. *Journal of Obstetric, Gynecologic, and Neonatal Nursing,* 24(4), 327-334.

Callister, L.C. (1998). Giving birth: Guatemalan women's voices. *Journal of Obstetric, Gynecologic, and Neonatal Nursing,* 27(3), 289-295.

Capitulo, K.L. (1998). The rise, fall, and rise of nurse-midwifery in America. *MCN: Maternal/Child Nursing Journal,* 23(6), 314-321.

Cascio, H. (1998). Medicaid experiments in capitation: What they can teach us about capitation in private managed care. What physicians and patients should know. Retrieved October 2, 1998 from http://home1.gte.net/hcascio/flmchmo/capitate.htm.

Collins, C. (1998). Yoga: Intuition, preventive medicine, and treatment. *Journal of Obstetric, Gynecologic, and Neonatal Nursing,* 27(5), 563-568.

Cox, R.P. (1997). Family health care delivery for the 21st century. *Journal of Obstetric, Gynecologic, and Neonatal Nursing,* 26(1), 109-118.

Dossey, B.M. (1998). Holistic modalities and healing moments. *American Journal of Nursing,* 98(6), 44-47.

Dossey, B.M., & Dossey, L. (1998). Attending to holistic care. *American Journal of Nursing,* 98(8), 35-38.

Elder, K.N., O'Hara, N., Crutcher, T., Wells, N., Graham., & Heflin, W. (1998). Managed care: The value you bring. *American Journal of Nursing,* 98(6), 34-39.

Geissler, E.M. (1998). *Mosby's pocket guide to cultural assessment* (2nd ed.). St. Louis: Mosby.

Gordin, P. (1999). Technology and family-centered perinatal care: Conflict or synergy? *Journal of Obstetric, Gynecologic, and Neonatal Nursing,* 28(4), 401-408.

Henry, J.K. (1997). Community nursing centers: models of nurse-managed care. *Journal of Obstetric, Gynecologic, and Neonatal Nursing,* 26(2), 224-228.

Hoyert, D.L., Danel, I., & Tully, P. (2000). Maternal mortality, United States and Canada: 1982-1997. *Birth,* 27(1), 4-11.

Hutchinson, M.K., & Baqi-Aziz, M. (1994). Nursing care of the childbearing Muslim family. *Journal of Obstetric, Gynecologic, and Neonatal Nursing,* 23(9), 767-772.

Jones, M.L.H., Day, S., Creely, J., Woodland, M.B., & Gerdes, J.B. (1999). Implementation of a clinical pathway system in maternal newborn care: A comprehensive documentation system for outcomes management. *Journal of Perinatal-Neonatal Nursing,* 13(3), 1-20.

Leininger, M. (1978). *Transcultural nursing: Concepts, theories, practices.* New York: John Wiley & Sons.

Lester, N. (1998). Cultural competence: A nursing dialogue (Part One). *American Journal of Nursing,* 98(8), 26-33.

Lester, N. (1998). Cultural competence: A nursing dialogue (Part Two). *American Journal of Nursing,* 98(9), 36-47.

Lowry, L.M., Hays, B.J., Lopez, P., & Hernandez, G. (1998). Care paths: A new approach to high-risk maternal-child home visitation. *MCN: American Journal of Maternal/Child Nursing,* 23(6), 322-328.

Lund, P.Z. (1997). Changing times, shifting paradigms. *AWHONN Lifelines,* 1(6), 38-42.

Martell, L.K. (2000). The hospital and the postpartum experience: A historical analysis. *Journal of Obstetric, Gynecologic, and Neonatal Nursing,* 29(1), 65-72.

Mattson, S. (1995). Culturally sensitive perinatal care for Southeast Asians. *Journal of Obstetric, Gynecologic, and Neonatal Nursing,* 24(4), 335-342.

Mercer, M.M. (1999). Crossing state lines: Are interstate licenses in nursing's future? *AWHONN Lifelines,* 3(1), 21.

Miller, M. (1995). Culture, spirituality, and women's health. *Journal of Obstetric, Gynecologic, and Neonatal Nursing,* 24(3), 257-263.

Nance, T.A. (1995). Intercultural communication: Finding common ground. *Journal of Obstetric, Gynecologic, and Neonatal Nursing,* 24(3), 249-255.

National Center for Health Statistics. (November 1996). *Healthy people 2000 review, 1995-96.* Hyattsville, Md.: Public Health Service.

National Center for Health Statistics. (1999). *National Vital Statistics Reports* (Vol. 47, Number 19). Retrieved February 19, 2000 from http://www.cdc.gov/nchs/data/nvs47_19.pdf.

Nichols, F.H. (2000). History of the women's health movement in the 20th century. *Journal of Obstetric, Gynecologic, and Neonatal Nursing,* 29(1), 56-64.

Ondeck, M. (2000). Historical development. In F.H. Nichols & S.S. Humenick (Eds.), *Childbirth education: Practice, research, and theory* (2nd ed., pp. 18-31). Philadelphia: W.B. Saunders.

Olson, S.L. (1998). Bedside musical care: Applications in pregnancy, childbirth, and neonatal care. *Journal of Obstetric, Gynecologic, and Neonatal Nursing,* 27(5), 569-575.

Pence, M. (1997). Patient-focused models of care. *Journal of Obstetric, Gynecologic, and Neonatal Nursing,* 26(3), 320-326.

Reichert, G.A. (1998). Female circumcision: What you need to know about genital mutilation. *AWHONN Lifelines,* 2(3), 28-34.

Rinker, S.D. (2000). The real challenge: Lessons from obstetric nursing history. *Journal of Obstetric, Gynecologic, and Neonatal Nursing,* 29(1), 100-106.

Sams, L., & DeGeorges, K.M. (1998). Seize the evidence and the opportunity! *AWHONN Lifelines,* 2(3), 15-17.

Schwoebel, A., & Jones, M.L.H. (1999). A clinical pathway system for the neonatal intensive care nursery. *Journal of Perinatal-Neonatal Nursing,* 13(3), 60-69.

Simkin, P. (1989). Childbearing in social context. *Women and Health,* 15(3), 5-21.

Simpson, K.R. (1999). Strategies for developing an evidence-based approach to perinatal care. *MCN: American Journal of Maternal/Child Nursing* 24(3), 122-131.

Starn, J.R. (1998). Energy healing with women and children. *Journal of Obstetric, Gynecologic, and Neonatal Nursing,* 27(5), 576-584.

Tiedje, L.B. (1998). Alternative health care: An overview. *Journal of Obstetric, Gynecologic, and Neonatal Nursing,* 27(5), 557-562.

U.S. Department of Health and Human Services. (January 2000). *Healthy people 2010* (Conference Edition). Washington, D.C. Retrieved February 19, 2000 from http://www.health.gov/healthypeople.

U.S. Department of Health and Human Services. (September 1999). *Health, United States, 1999, with health and aging chartbook.* Hyattsville, MD: The Department.

Ward, S. (1998). Caring and healing in the 21st century. *MCN: American Journal of Maternal/Child Nursing,* 23(4), 210-215.

Wertz, R., & Wertz, D. (1992). *Lying-in: A history of childbirth in America* (2nd ed.). New Haven, CT: Yale University Press.

2 THE NURSE'S ROLE IN MATERNITY CARE

OBJECTIVES

1. Explain the roles of nurses with advanced preparation in maternal-newborn nursing, including the roles of nurse-midwives, nurse practitioners, and clinical specialists.
2. Discuss the roles for nurses in maternity care.
3. Explain the importance of critical thinking in nursing practice, and describe how it may be refined.
4. Relate the five steps of the nursing process to maternal-newborn nursing.
5. Explain how the nursing process relates to critical thinking.
6. Discuss the importance of nursing research in clinical practice.

DEFNITIONS

AMBIGUITY (AMBIGUOUS) Lack of clarity or certainty; having more than one meaning.

ASSUMPTIONS Beliefs taken for granted without examination.

BASELINE DATA Information that describes the status of the client before treatment begins.

BIAS A prejudice that sways the mind.

CESAREAN BIRTH Surgical birth of the fetus through an incision in the abdominal wall and uterus.

DELEGATED NURSING INTERVENTIONS Physician-prescribed nursing actions that require nursing judgment because nurses are accountable for correct implementation; also called *interdependent nursing interventions.* (See also *independent nursing interventions.*)

FETUS The developing baby from 9 weeks after conception until birth; term used in everyday practice to describe a developing baby during pregnancy, regardless of age.

INDEPENDENT NURSING INTERVENTIONS Nurse-prescribed actions used in both nursing diagnoses and collaborative problems. (See also *delegated nursing interventions.*)

INFERENCE The act of drawing a conclusion or making a deduction.

JUDGMENT An opinion.

REFLECTION Meditation, attentive consideration.

SKEPTICISM Doubt in the absence of conclusive evidence.

SUSPEND To delay or bring to a stop temporarily.

VALIDATE To make certain that the information collected during assessment is accurate.

As maternity care changed from regimented care of the mother and newborn to a family-centered approach, maternity nursing evolved to a new level of independence. Nurses who work with childbearing families must be able to communicate and teach effectively. They must be able to think critically and use the nursing process to develop a plan of care that meets the unique needs of each family. They are expected to base their practice on current research and collaborate with other health care providers. Moreover, many nurses complete advanced programs of education that allow them to provide primary care throughout pregnancy and the childbearing experience.

ADVANCED PREPARATION FOR MATERNAL-NEWBORN NURSES

The gradual change to family-centered maternity care and the persistent challenge of providing health care for indigent women and newborns have led to an expanded role for nurses. Many nurses have completed advanced programs of education and are prepared as certified nurse-midwives, nurse practitioners, and clinical specialists.

Certified Nurse-Midwives

Certified nurse-midwives (CNMs) are registered nurses who have completed an extensive program of study and clinical experience. They must pass a certification test administered by the American College of Nurse-Midwives. CNMs are qualified to take complete health histories and perform physical examinations. They can provide complete care during pregnancy, childbirth, and the postpartum period. They attend the mother and infant as long as the mother's progress is normal. CNMs are committed to providing information to prevent problems during pregnancy and preparation for normal pregnancy and childbirth. They spend a great deal of time counseling and supporting the childbearing family. The CNM also provides gynecologic services and family-planning information and counseling. The practice approach of the CNM to childbirth is noninterventionist and supportive and regards pregnancy and birth as a normal process.

The effectiveness of care provided by nurse-midwives has a long history that continues to be validated. In the 1930s the Maternity Center Association, founded to provide care for indigent women, began to educate public health nurses in midwifery. Around the same time, Mary Breckinridge, a nurse-midwife from England, founded the Frontier Nursing Service to provide primary care (including midwifery services) for poor families in the remote mountains of Kentucky.

Despite the proven effectiveness of care, physicians opposed the widespread use of nurse-midwives. For many years, the scope and locations of their practices were restricted. In 1970, however, many restrictions were alleviated when the American College of Obstetricians and Gynecologists and the Nurses' Association of the American College of Obstetricians and Gynecologists (NAACOG)—now known as the Association of Women's Health, Obstetric, and Neonatal Nurses (AWHONN)—issued a joint statement that admitted CNMs as part of the health care team. In 1981, Congress authorized Medicaid payments for the services of CNMs. This measure has greatly increased use of nurse-midwives, particularly in health maintenance organizations (HMOs), birth centers, and some hospitals.

Nurse Practitioners

Nurse practitioners are registered nurses with advanced preparation that allows them to provide primary care for specific groups of clients. They can take a complete health history, perform physical examinations, order and interpret laboratory and other diagnostic studies, and provide primary care for health maintenance and health promotion. Nurse practitioners collaborate with physicians for treatments and medications beyond their scope of practice. Nurse practitioners now specialize in many areas of practice, including maternal-child care. Nurse practitioner programs in all specialties are a popular track for master's degree nursing preparation.

The maternity nurse practitioner, or women's health nurse practitioner, can assess the pregnant woman at prenatal appointments and evaluate the progress of the pregnancy. Although they do not usually attend births, nurse practitioners provide information and care during the postpartum period and provide many women's health services.

Family nurse practitioners (FNPs) are prepared to provide care for all family members, young and old. They care for women during uncomplicated pregnancies and provide follow-up care for the mother and infant after childbirth.

Pediatric nurse practitioners provide health maintenance care for infants and children that do not require the services of physicians. They may see infants at well-baby visits and for common illnesses.

Family planning nurse practitioners usually work in family planning clinics or with physicians in private practice. Major responsibilities include performing pelvic examinations and screening procedures for sexually transmitted diseases and providing family planning services. The family planning nurse practitioner often performs annual examinations and screenings such as Papanicolaou (Pap) tests.

Clinical Nurse Specialists

Maternity, or perinatal, clinical specialists are registered nurses who, through study and supervised practice at the graduate level (master's or doctorate), have become expert in the care of childbearing families. Four major subroles have been identified for clinical nurse specialists: expert practitioner, educator, researcher, and consultant. These professionals often function as clinical leaders, role models, client advocates, and change agents. They also act as consultants to assist other nurses in planning care for difficult problems encountered in the maternity unit. Unlike nurse practitioners, clinical nurse specialists do not provide primary care.

IMPLICATIONS OF CHANGING ROLES FOR NURSES

The roles of perinatal nurses changed once much of perinatal care moved from the acute care settings into community-based settings. Nurses now work in a variety of highly specialized areas such as fetal diagnostic centers, infertility clinics, and facilities offering genetic counseling. Nurses also assume primary responsibility for independent functions such as teaching, counseling, and intervening for a wide variety of nonmedical problems that affect the childbearing family.

Because of the added responsibilities of teaching and counseling, all nurses must develop and maintain additional interpersonal skills. These skills include communication, effective teaching, critical thinking, and the use of the nursing process to identify and intervene for a variety of problems.

Therapeutic Communication

Unlike social communication, therapeutic communication is purposeful, goal directed, and focused. Although it may seem simple, therapeutic communication requires conscious effort and considerable practice. Therapeutic communication is a vital part of all nursing, and techniques are taught early in all curricula. Communication is emphasized throughout this book for three reasons: (1) to review the process, (2) to emphasize the importance of communication in maternal-newborn nursing, and (3) to provide examples for using therapeutic communication with childbearing families.

Guidelines for Therapeutic Communication

Therapeutic communication requires great flexibility and cannot depend on a particular set of learned techniques. However, the following guidelines may prove helpful:

1. A calm setting that provides privacy, reduces distractions, and minimizes interruptions is essential.
2. Interactions should begin with introductions and clarification of the nurse's role: "My name is Claudia Lyall; I am here to complete the discharge teaching that was started yesterday." This introduction acknowledges the nurse's purpose and sets the scene to discuss concerns about the family's discharge from the hospital.
3. Therapeutic communication should be focused and directed toward meeting the needs expressed by the family. One method of focusing the interaction is to begin with an open-ended question: "How do you feel about going home today?" Redirection of the conversation may also be necessary: "Thanks for showing me the beautiful pictures of the baby. I understand you are having a bit of trouble getting him to nurse."
4. Nonverbal behaviors may communicate more powerful messages than the spoken word. For example, facial expressions and eye movements can confirm or contradict what the woman says. Repetitive hand gestures, such as finger tapping and twirling a lock of hair, may indicate frustration, irritation, or boredom. Body posture, stance, and gait can convey energy, depression, or discomfort. Voice tone, pitch, rate, and volume may indicate joy, anger, or fear. Grooming also conveys messages about the way the woman feels about herself. If she is tired or depressed, she may neglect her own grooming, although she may not verbalize a problem.
5. Active listening requires that the nurse "attend" to the words being said and nonverbal clues. Attending behaviors that convey the nurse's interest and a sincere desire to understand include the following:
   - Eye contact, which signals a readiness to interact
   - Relaxed but erect posture with the upper portion of the body inclined toward the client
   - Minimal cues and leads such as nodding, leaning closer, and smiling. Verbal cues include "Uh huh, go on," "Tell me about that," and "Can you give me an example?"
   - Touch, which can be a powerful response when words would break a mood or fail to convey the depth of feeling experienced between the woman and nurse
6. Cultural differences influence communication. In some cultures (such as Chinese, Southeast Asian), prolonged eye contact is confrontational and initiates a great deal of concern. People from some cultures (such as Middle Eastern, Native American) may be uncomfortable with touch and would be disturbed by unsolicited touching.
7. Clarifying communication involves a unique process of the listener receiving the message as the sender intended. The nurse may need to ask questions to clarify a statement. For instance, the nurse may say, "I'm not sure I understand," or "So you are undecided about breastfeeding?"
8. Emotions are part of communication, and nurses must often reflect feelings that are expressed ver-

Table 2-1
COMMUNICATION TECHNIQUES

Definition	Examples
Clarifying: Clearing up or following up to understand both content and feelings expressed, used to check the accuracy of how the nurse perceives the message	"I'm confused about your plans; could you explain...?" "Tell me what you mean when you say you don't feel like yourself." "Are you saying that...?" "Can you tell me more about...?"
Paraphrasing: Restating in words other than those used by the client what the client seems to express; used as a form of clarification	*Example 1* Client: "My boyfriend won't even come into the room for the birth! " Nurse: "It sounds as if you may be angry with him because he won't be here." *Example 2* Client: "I watch my diet, but I am gaining too much weight anyway." Nurse: "You want to control your weight, but your diet isn't working?"
Reflecting: Verbalizing comprehension of what the client said and what she seems to be feeling; linking content and feeling and reflecting the client as a mirror reflects a person without adding the opinion, values, and personality of the nurse	*Example 1* Client: "I don't know what to do. My husband doesn't think a cesarean is needed, but the doctor says the baby is showing some stress." Nurse: "You're confused and frightened because they don't agree?" *Example 2* Woman in early labor: "It was my husband's idea for me to become pregnant. I wasn't too excited about it at first." Nurse *(poor response)*: "I'll bet the dad will be a pushover as a father." (This reflects the nurse's opinion and fails to acknowledge the mother's statement.) Nurse *(better response)*: "Your husband was more excited about the pregnancy than you?"
Silence: Waiting and allowing time for the client to continue; verbal communication need not be constant.	The nurse waits quietly for the client to continue.
Structuring: Creating guidelines or setting priorities	"You said you don't know how to take care of the baby and also that you are afraid of getting pregnant again. What should we talk about first?"
Pinpointing: Calling attention to differences or inconsistencies in statements	"You say you feel wonderful, but I see some tears."
Questioning: Eliciting information directly; using open-ended questions to avoid "yes" or "no" answers and to prevent controlling the answers	"How do you feel about being pregnant?" instead of "Are you happy to be pregnant?"
Directing: Using nonverbal responses or succinct comments to encourage the client to continue	Nod or say "Uh huh." "You were saying..." "Please go on."
Summarizing: Reviewing the main themes or issues that were discussed	"You had two major concerns today. We have talked about breastfeeding and how to bathe the baby today."

bally or nonverbally: "It sounds as if you looked forward to delivery in a birth center and are disappointed that you needed a cesarean birth."

Therapeutic Communication Techniques

Therapeutic communication involves responding and listening, and nurses must learn to use responses that facilitate rather than block communication. These facilitative responses, often called *communication techniques,* focus on both the content of the message and the feeling accompanying the message. Communication techniques include clarifying, reflecting, silence, questioning, and directing (Table 2-1). In addition, nurses must be aware of blocks to communication (Table 2-2).

Check Your Reading

1. How does therapeutic communication differ from social communication?
2. What are the major communication techniques?
3. What are the major blocks to communication?

The Nurse's Role in Teaching and Learning

Nurses can be the most significant teachers on the health care team because of their relationships with clients. Clients often perceive nurses as less threatening than physicians, and they may expect nurses to have

Table 2-2
BEHAVIORS THAT BLOCK COMMUNICATION

Behavior	Example	Alternative
Conveying lack of interest	Looking away or fidgeting	Showing attending behaviors such as eye contact and nodding
Conveying sense of haste	Checking the time or standing near the door	Sitting at the bedside
Displaying closed posture	Crossing the arms over the chest or holding the clipboard in front of body	Having the arms relaxed or leaning forward
Interrupting or finishing sentences	Woman: "I'm not sure how ________." Nurse: "We will have a bath demonstration later."	"Go on ________." "You were saying ________."
Providing false reassurance	"You're going to be okay."	"I sense you are concerned about how to care for the baby. I will help you give the bath today."
Offering inappropriate self-disclosure	To woman in labor: "I was in labor 12 hours, then had a cesarean."	"What concerns you most about labor?"
Giving advice	"You should..." "If I were you, I would..."	"How do you feel about that?" "What do you think is most important?"
Failing to acknowledge comments or feelings	Woman: "I'm sick of being pregnant; I feel like an incubator." Nurse: "You will soon have a beautiful baby."	"You're ready for this to be over?"

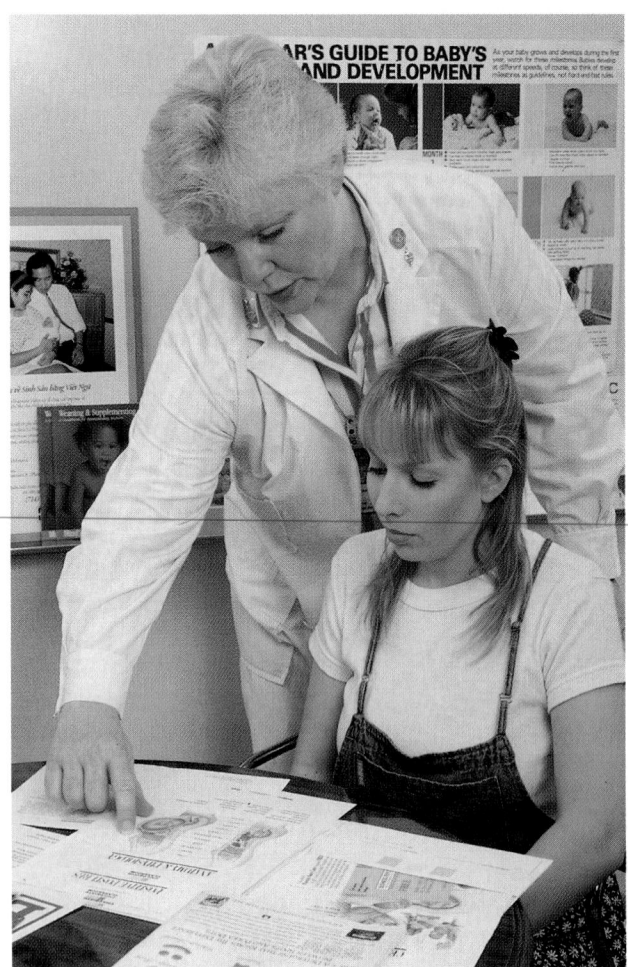

FIGURE 2-1 In the prenatal clinic the nurse teaches a woman in a one-on-one setting.

time to respond to concerns that a physician may find trivial. Nurses teach in several settings, including one-to-one interactions, formal classes, and group discussions (Figure 2-1). To teach effectively, nurses must be familiar with the basic principles of teaching and learning.

Principles of Teaching and Learning

Application of the following principles helps nurses become effective teachers in the childbearing setting:

- Real learning depends on the readiness of the family to learn and the relevance of the content. Fortunately, most childbearing families are highly motivated to learn. The parents want to be effective, and any content relevant to the health of either mother or child is eagerly sought.
- Active participation increases learning. Whenever possible, the learner should be involved in the educational process and not act as a passive listener or viewer. Therefore learning is enhanced when the family and nurse mutually develop goals and time for questions and explanations is ample. A discussion format, in which all can participate, stimulates more learning than a straight lecture.
- Repetition of a skill increases retention and feelings of competence. For example, parents experience real learning when they are allowed to bathe, feed, and diaper the infant more than once. This learning often begins during infant care classes presented during the prenatal period and may continue during home or clinical visits after the mother and infant leave the birth facility.

- Praise and positive feedback are powerful motivators for learning and are particularly important when the family is trying to master a frustrating task such as breastfeeding an unresponsive infant.
- Role modeling is an effective method to demonstrate behavior. Parents benefit greatly from watching a competent nurse respond to their infant. Nurses must be aware that their behaviors are scrutinized carefully at all times and may be copied later.
- Conflicts and frustration impede learning, and they should be recognized and resolved for learning to progress. For instance, couples sometimes do not agree about the way the infant should be fed (breastfeeding versus formula feeding). This issue and the feelings it generates must be acknowledged before teaching about breastfeeding can be effective.
- Learning is enhanced when teaching is structured to present simple tasks before more complex material. For instance, the nurse should teach umbilical cord care, which is simple, before teaching how to bathe and shampoo the infant, which is more difficult.
- A variety of teaching methods are necessary to maintain interest and illustrate concepts. Posters, videos, and printed materials supplement lectures and discussion. Models may be especially useful for teaching family planning or the processes of labor.
- Retention is greater when material is presented in small segments over time. Brief hospital stays do not promote this practice, making follow-up care particularly important.

Factors Influencing Learning

Many factors influence learning, including the developmental level of the family, their primary language, their cultural orientation, and their previous experiences.

Developmental Level. Not surprisingly, teenage parents have different concerns than older parents. Also, younger people usually learn better in different ways than parents in their thirties. For example, very young parents often do not benefit from printed material to the same degree as older parents. However, teenagers often learn well from videos and group discussions with those who share similar problems. To be effective, the nurse must acknowledge this difference and structure teaching-learning sessions to meet the family's primary concerns.

Language. The ability to understand the language in which teaching is presented determines how much the family learns. Although many newly arrived immigrants speak English fairly well, they may not understand the idioms, nuances, medical words, or slang terms that are frequently used. The nurse must create a climate in which families feel free to ask questions when they do not understand.

One helpful method is to ask those who speak a different language to describe what they have learned and how they will use the information. The nurse may also want to determine whether the new information conflicts with the information the parents learned previously.

Culture. Background and culture influence learning. People tend to forget content with which they disagree. For instance, if the family is from a culture that believes the mother should eat certain foods after childbirth, family members may disregard other foods recommended by the nurse. Also, if the recommendations of the family's elders and the teachings of the nurse or physicians conflict, many young parents follow the advice of the elders. Therefore the nurse should determine the cultural beliefs and attempt to reach an understanding about what information will be useful before beginning to teach.

Previous Experiences. Parents who already have children have unique concerns. These families may not need instruction in newborn care, but they may be very concerned about how older children will accept a new infant. They may need advice in checking used toys and equipment to insure the infant's safety.

Physical Environment. The physical environment also influences learning. The hospital room is generally suitable for individual teaching. If group instruction is planned, the instructor should arrange comfortable chairs in a circle so that all persons can hear and participate in face-to-face communication.

Organization and Skill of the Instructor. The instructor must determine the objectives of the class, develop a plan for meeting the objectives, and gather all material before the teaching session begins. If the objective is that participants will observe a bath demonstration, the nurse must decide how to demonstrate the bath, when to present care of the umbilical cord and circumcision, and which major principles should be addressed.

A summary of the major principles discussed is very helpful. For example, after a bath demonstration, the nurse might conclude with "The important points to remember are to prevent the baby from becoming chilled; to be sure the infant doesn't fall; to start at the face, which is the cleanest area; and to bathe the baby's bottom, which is the dirtiest area, last."

Effects of Early Discharge

Although the principles of teaching and learning should be used whenever possible, early discharge of the mother and infant sometimes makes compromise necessary (Figure 2-2). Rarely is there enough time for repetition and return demonstrations of infant care. Many

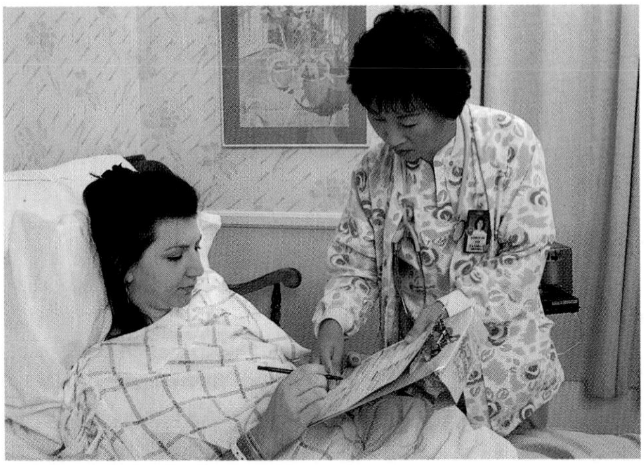

FIGURE 2-2 Often the nurse must condense teaching by using a "check-off" sheet because mothers and infants leave the birth facility within a short time after birth.

families leave the hospital long before they have attained much comfort with infant care.

Innovative methods have been developed to provide a safety net for these families and make them feel more secure. These include follow-up telephone calls, home visits, information lines, videos on infant care, and mother-infant outpatient clinics. Teaching self-care and infant care during the prenatal period is emphasized. This information must be reviewed before the mother and infant leave the birth facility, but review is generally less time consuming than the initial presentation. Printed materials are provided to parents at discharge in addition to the verbal teaching.

The Nurse's Role as Manager

As a result of the short length of stay in the birth facility and cost-containment strategies, the role of nurses has changed from that of primary caregiver to that of manager and teacher. Nurses may provide less direct patient care and delegate tasks, such as giving a bath and taking vital signs, to others. As a result, nurses spend more time teaching families, supervising unlicensed personnel, planning and coordinating care, and collaborating with other professionals and agencies. Nurses are expected to understand the financial squeeze from cost-containment strategies and contribute to their institutions' economic viability. At the same time, they must continue to act as patient advocates and maintain a standard of care (see Chapter 3).

Check Your Reading

4. What are the major principles of teaching and learning?
5. What factors affect learning?

CRITICAL THINKING

Nurses must be concerned with learning and refining the critical thinking skills needed to function in the rapidly changing clinical area. Unlike undirected thinking, during which the mind wanders freely, critical thinking is controlled and directed toward finding solutions or forming opinions. People think critically in their everyday lives as they make decisions about when to pay a bill in relation to its due date and their payday, determining ways to make their grocery dollars go farther, and choosing a car with features that are necessary rather than simply desirable.

For effective critical thinking, nurses must gain insight into their own thought processes and analyze their own thinking by taking it apart for examination and criticism. Critical thinking includes recognizing and acknowledging specific habits and responses that can interfere with productive thinking.

Critical thinking is based on reason rather than preference or prejudice. It also seeks to examine feelings to understand the ways emotions affect thinking. Finally, critical thinking requires the suspension of judgment until evidence is adequate to support inferences or conclusions.

Purpose

The purpose of critical thinking is to identify and overcome habits or impulses that can result in poor decisions or inappropriate actions. In nursing, critical thinking helps nurses make the best clinical judgments. The process begins when nurses realize accumulating a fund of knowledge from texts and lectures is not enough. They must also be able to apply this knowledge to specific clinical situations and thus reach conclusions that provide the most effective care in each situation.

In addition, nurses must also honestly examine their own thought processes for flaws that can lead to inaccurate conclusions or poor judgments. Although this examination requires a great deal of self-analysis, a series of steps makes the process easier. Critical thinking exercises are presented throughout the book to help students develop skills in critical thinking and application of knowledge.

Steps

A series of steps may help clarify the way critical thinking is learned. These steps may be called the *ABCDE's of critical thinking.* They include a recognition of assumptions, an examination of personal biases, an analysis of the amount of pressure for closure, an examination of the way that data are collected and analyzed, and an evaluation of the ways emotions may interfere with critical thinking.

Recognizing Assumptions

Assumptions are ideas, beliefs, or values that are taken for granted without any basis in fact or reason. These unconscious assumptions may lead to unexamined thoughts or unsound actions. For instance, the following assumptions can have negative consequences: "Anyone who wants a job can get one. Teenagers don't listen. Every woman wants a baby."

A list of everything known about a specific situation may be helpful to identify assumptions. Each item on the list should then be analyzed to determine which is true, which could be true, and which is either untrue or lacks enough evidence to determine whether it is true.

Analyzing Biases

Biases are prejudices that sway the mind toward a particular conclusion or course of action on the basis of personal theories or stereotypes. Biases are based on unexamined beliefs, and many are widespread. For instance, "Fat people are lazy. Women are bad drivers. Men are insensitive."

People are often biased against those of different races, religions, or lifestyles. When faced with a predisposition to judge a person or a group of persons, nurses may be wise to ask themselves or their co-workers a series of questions: "Why do you think that? What if this were a different client? What if there were different circumstances? What might someone who disagrees say? What is influencing my thinking?"

Examining the Need for Closure

Many persons look for immediate answers and experience a great deal of anxiety until a solution is found for any problem. In other words, they have very little tolerance for doubt or uncertainty, which is sometimes called *ambiguity.* As a result, they feel pressure to come to a decision or to reach closure as early as possible. This is one of the most important aspects of critical thinking because those who feel pressure to come to an early decision or find a quick solution often do so with insufficient data.

To overcome the pressure to reach an early conclusion, the nurse must make a conscious effort to suspend judgment. This is sometimes called *reflective skepticism.* The first step is to acknowledge the anxiety created by postponed decisions. The next step involves deliberately waiting to make a decision. One method is to follow the example of judges who take information "under advisement" and announce they will "render a decision" at a later date.

Persons who jump to conclusions often stop with one answer. To overcome this tendency, they should always look for a second "right" answer. They could also imagine the problem from the perspective of someone else. They might ask a series of questions: "What alternatives do we have? What else might work? What information supports this? What effect would that have? Is there good evidence to support that decision? Is there reason to doubt that evidence?"

On the other hand, some persons can tolerate a great deal of doubt and uncertainty. They are comfortable with data collection and analysis but feel uncomfortable making decisions. They may procrastinate or postpone the decision for as long as possible. This procrastination may be of little consequence in some situations. For instance, a family might collect information about getting a pet for a considerable time, and the decision may be of slight importance.

On the other hand, failure to make a decision in the clinical area may have serious consequences for clients and their families. Several questions may help overcome the tendency to postpone coming to a decision. "What signs indicate something is wrong? Do I need to do something about it? How much time do I have? What happens if I don't do something about this? What should I do first? What resources can help me?" This step might also be called *priority setting,* and it is one of the most important aspects of critical thinking in nursing.

Becoming Expert in Data Management

Expertise in collecting, organizing, and analyzing data involves developing an attitude of inquiry and learning to live with questions such as "Why? What if? What else? Is this relevant? How does it relate to that? How can I organize the data? Does it form patterns? What can I infer from those patterns?"

Collecting Data. To obtain complete data, nurses must develop skill in verbal communication. Open-ended questions elicit more information than questions that require only a one-word answer. Follow-up questions are often needed to clarify information or pursue a particular thought.

Validating Data. Unclear or incomplete information should be validated. This process may involve rechecking physical signs, collecting additional information, or determining whether a perception is accurate. For instance, the comment "you seem uncomfortable" may result in the client denying or acknowledging discomfort.

Organizing and Analyzing Data. Data are more useful when organized into patterns or clusters. The first step is to separate the relevant data from data that may be interesting but are unrelated to the current situation. For example, the fact that her neighbor is pregnant with twins has little bearing on how a new mother breastfeeds her infant.

The next step is to compare data with expected norms to determine what is within the expected range (normal) and what is not (abnormal). Abnormal results provide cues that can be grouped or clustered so that conclusions can be made. For example, all data that may indicate excessive bleeding, such as pulse rate, blood pressure, amount of vaginal bleeding, and skin color, may seem more meaningful when grouped. Organizing data into clusters often reveals that additional data are needed before a decision can be reached.

Acknowledging Emotions and Environmental Factors

Several emotions and environmental factors can influence critical thinking. For instance, the clinical area is often a noisy, fast-paced, and hectic environment with time limitations and distractions that make calm reflection and reasoning difficult. Fatigue also reduces the ability to concentrate during a 10- to 12-hour shift. Inexperienced nurses and students may lack confidence in their knowledge and often feel anxious, which can reduce their abilities to think critically.

Many nurses, both experienced and inexperienced, have a strong need to protect their self-image. As a result, they become defensive when they have said or done something wrong. This response is a serious barrier to critical thinking, which requires that all health care professionals learn to acknowledge mistakes and become comfortable with constructive criticism.

Extreme emotions such as anger and frustration impede critical thinking by narrowing the focus only to data that support the intense feeling. For example, persons who are extremely frustrated may often repeat the perceived cause of their frustration and may be unable to move on to other information to address the problem.

The first step is to recognize and acknowledge factors or emotions that impede thinking. For example, nurses may find it necessary to say, "I feel flustered by all the activity and need to find a quiet spot for a few minutes of concentration." To develop critical thinking skills, the nurse must learn to admit mistakes and become comfortable saying, "I was wrong." Asking for assistance, verification, or validation is wise when fatigue is a problem or when lack of confidence creates anxiety.

The person who experiences intense frustration or anger must recognize these emotions and their influence on rational thought. A trusted colleague may be asked to point out signs of these emotions such as repetitive vehement comments. Some persons use other methods of control such as visualizations, breathing exercises, and brief, self-imposed "timeouts" from the precipitating situation if possible.

Check Your Reading

6. What is the purpose of critical thinking?
7. What steps may be helpful in refining critical thinking?
8. What is meant by reflective skepticism?

APPLICATION OF THE NURSING PROCESS: MATERNAL-NEWBORN NURSING

The nursing process forms the basis for maternal-newborn nursing, as for all nursing. The nursing process consists of five distinct steps: (1) assessment, (2) analysis, (3) planning, (4) implementation, and (5) evaluation. In maternal-newborn nursing, the nursing process applies to a population that is generally healthy and experiencing a life event that holds the potential for both growth and problems. Much maternal-newborn nursing activity is devoted to the assessment and diagnosis of client strengths and healthy functioning. Interventions often focus on promoting and enhancing these strengths to help families achieve a higher or more satisfying level of wellness. This focus often differs from providing care for clients who are ill, and it presents some difficulty for maternal-newborn nurses when they use the list of predominantly problem-oriented nursing diagnoses provided by the North American Nursing Diagnosis Association (NANDA).

The nursing process is written in the text as a linear, step-by-step process. However, with knowledge and experience, the nurse applies the nursing process in the clinical setting dynamically. For example, the nurse may discover that the woman has a full bladder early in a postpartum assessment. The nurse skips to an intervention and helps the woman to the restroom to urinate before completing the assessment to prevent client discomfort and possible excessive bleeding caused by a full bladder. In another example, the nurse goes to the woman's room to give her an injection of RhoGAM and discovers the woman nursing her baby, who is eagerly suckling for the first time in several hours. Based on critical thinking, the nurse delays the injection (an intervention), which would require that the woman change her position. The nurse realizes that the few minutes required for the infant to complete the feeding are more important than the short delay in giving the injection.

Assessment

Nursing assessment should be accomplished systematically and deliberately and include physiologic data and information related to psychological, social, and cultural considerations. Although the woman or infant may be the primary client, nurses must assess the belief systems, available support, perceptions, and plans of other family members to provide the best nursing care. Two levels of nursing assessment are used to collect comprehensive data: (1) screening assessments and (2) focus assessments.

Screening Assessment

The screening, or database, assessment is usually performed at the initial contact with the client. Its purpose is to gather information about all aspects of the client's health. This information, called *baseline data,* describes the client's health status before interventions begin. It forms the basis for the identification of both strengths and problems.

A variety of methods may be used to organize the assessment. For example, information may be grouped according to body systems. Assessment can also be organized around nursing theory models, such as Roy's adaptation to stress theory or Orem's self-care deficit theory.

Focus Assessment

A focus assessment is used to gather information specifically related to an actual health problem or a problem that the client or family is at risk for acquiring. A focus assessment is often performed at the beginning of a shift and centers on areas relevant to childbearing. For instance, in maternal-newborn nursing the nurse should assess the breasts and nipples because the mother is at risk for problems if she does not have adequate information about breastfeeding or care of the nipples. A focus assessment may also reveal strengths that nursing care will enhance.

Analysis

The data gathered during assessment must be analyzed to identify existing or potential strengths or problems and their causes. Data are validated and grouped in a process of critical thinking to determine cues and inferences. Health needs that nurses can treat independently and for which they are legally accountable are termed *nursing diagnoses.* At present, more than 100 nursing diagnoses have been identified by NANDA.

Nursing Diagnosis

Each nursing diagnosis identified by NANDA consists of the following components:

1. The title offers a concise description of the health problem.
2. Defining characteristics refer to a cluster of signs and symptoms or cues often seen with that particular diagnosis.
3. Etiologic and related factors are factors that can cause or contribute to the problem. The etiology may be pathophysiologic, situational, or maturational. Although the majority of nursing diagnoses address health problems, most wellness diagnoses are in the maternal-infant area. One example of a wellness NANDA nursing diagnosis is "Effective Breastfeeding."

Diagnoses may be actual or risk nursing diagnoses (Table 2-3). Actual nursing diagnoses indicate that the diagnosis exists at the time of assessment and can be validated by the presence of defining characteristics. Risk nursing diagnoses are appropriate when the diagnosis does not exist but the individual or family is at risk to develop it based on contributing factors. Any nursing diagnosis may occur in maternal-newborn nursing, although some diagnostic categories are particularly common (Table 2-4).

Planning

The third step in the nursing process involves planning care for problems that were identified during assessment and reflected in the nursing diagnoses. During this step, nurses set priorities, develop goals or outcomes, and plan interventions to accomplish these goals.

Setting Priorities

Setting priorities includes (1) determining what problems need immediate attention (life-threatening problems) and taking immediate action; (2) determining whether potential problems call for a physician's orders for diagnosis, monitoring, or treatment; and (3) identifying actual nursing diagnoses that take precedence over risk nursing diagnoses.

Establishing Goals and Expected Outcomes

Although the terms *goals* and *expected outcomes* are sometimes used interchangeably, they are different. Generally, broad goals do not state the specific outcome criteria and are less measurable than outcome statements. Broad goals should be linked with more specific and measurable outcome criteria. For example, if the goal is that the parents will demonstrate effective parenting by discharge, expected outcomes that serve as evidence might include prompt, consistent responses to infant signals and competence in bathing, feeding, and comforting the infant.

Certain rules apply to written expected outcomes:

- Outcomes should be stated in client terms. This wording identifies who is expected to achieve the goal. This is usually the woman, infant, or family in the maternal-newborn setting.
- Measurable verbs must be used. For example, *identify, demonstrate, express, walk, relate,* and *list* are observable and measurable verbs. Examples of verbs that are difficult to measure are *understand, appreciate, feel, accept, know,* and *experience.* For instance, "Ms. Brown will experience less anxiety about assuming care of her infant" poses a problem because determining whether she experiences less anxiety is difficult. This outcome can be reworded as "Ms. Brown will state that she feels less anxious about assuming care of her infant and will participate in infant care (umbilical cord, circumcision, bathing) before discharge."
- A time frame is necessary. When is the person expected to perform the action? By the first postpartum day? After teaching? By discharge? Within the second trimester?

Table 2-3

EXAMPLES OF ACTUAL AND RISK NURSING DIAGNOSIS

Actual Nursing Diagnoses Problem	Etiology	Signs and Symptoms
Altered Nutrition: Less Than Body Requirement	Lack of knowledge about nutritional needs during lactation	Weight loss of 5 kg and daily caloric intake <1500 calories
Ineffective Breastfeeding	Nipple trauma	Cracked nipples and reports of discomfort during nursing

Risk Nursing Diagnoses Problem	Risk Factors
Risk for Ineffective Breastfeeding	Lack of knowledge of correct positioning of infant and appropriate breast care
Risk for Altered Nutrition: Less Than Body Requirements	Knowledge deficit of nutritional needs during lactation

Table 2-4

COMMON NANDA-APPROVED NURSING DIAGNOSES USED IN MATERNAL-NEWBORN AND WOMEN'S HEALTH NURSING

Allergy Response, Latex	Infection, Risk for
Anxiety	Knowledge Deficit
Body Image Disturbance	Nausea
Breastfeeding, Effective	Nutrition, Altered: Less Than Body Requirements
Breastfeeding, Ineffective	Nutrition, Altered: More Than Body Requirements
Breastfeeding, Interrupted	Pain
Communication, Impaired Verbal	Parent-Infant Attachment, Risk for Altered
Constipation	Parenting, Altered
Coping, Family: Potential for Growth	Powerlessness
Decisional Conflict	Rape Trauma Syndrome
Family Processes, Altered	Rape Trauma Syndrome: Compound Reaction
Fatigue	Rape Trauma Reaction: Silent Reaction
Fear	Role Performance, Altered
Feeding Pattern, Ineffective Infant	Self-Esteem, Situational Low
Fluid Volume Deficit	Sexuality Patterns, Altered
Health Maintenance, Altered	Skin Integrity, Impaired
Health Seeking Behaviors	Sleep Pattern Disturbance
Home Maintenance Management, Impaired	Temperature, Risk for Altered Body
Hypothermia	Urinary Elimination, Altered
Infant Behavior, Disorganized	Violence, Risk for
Infant Behavior, Potential for Enhanced Organized	

NANDA, North American Nursing Diagnosis Association.

- Goals and expected outcomes must be realistic and attainable. For instance, if a nursing diagnosis of "pain related to inability to cope with uterine contractions and lack of knowledge of the processes of labor" is formulated, a realistic expected outcome might be "The woman will state that her pain during labor remains manageable using techniques learned in childbirth classes." A goal such as "will remain free of pain throughout labor" is not attainable by nursing interventions only and is not realistic.
- Goals and expected outcomes are formed in collaboration with the client and family to ensure their participation in the plan of care.

Developing Nursing Interventions

After the goals and expected outcomes are developed, nurses write nursing interventions that will help the client meet the established outcomes.

Interventions for Actual Nursing Diagnoses. Nursing interventions for actual nursing diagnoses are aimed at reducing or eliminating the causes or related factors. For instance, the nursing diagnosis is "Altered Parenting related to interruption of bonding process secondary to illness of infant as manifested by absences of attachment behaviors (eye contact, holding)." The desired outcome might be that the parents will demonstrate progressive attachment behaviors such as touching, palming, eye contact, and participation in infant care within 1 week. Nursing interventions focus on increasing contact between parents and the infant and facilitating attachment behaviors.

A second example is a nursing diagnosis of "Constipation related to insufficient fluid and fiber intake and inadequate exercise as manifested by painful defecation of small, hard stools." The desired outcome is that the patient will establish a pattern of soft, painless stools occurring at least three times per week. Appropriate nursing interventions seek to increase fluid and fiber intake and initiate a realistic exercise regimen. Interventions for wellness nursing diagnoses promote a greater degree of adaptation in the client.

Interventions for Risk Nursing Diagnoses. Interventions are aimed at (1) monitoring for onset of the problem, (2) reducing or eliminating risk factors, and (3) preventing the problem. For example, the nursing diagnosis for an infant is "Risk for Impaired Skin Integrity related to frequent, loose stools." The planned outcome is that the skin remains intact. Nursing interventions include monitoring the condition of the skin at prescribed intervals for signs of skin impairment and initiating measures to keep the skin clean and dry to reduce the risk of skin impairment.

Implementing Interventions

Implementing nursing interventions may be problematic because written interventions are often not specific. Written nursing interventions should be as specific as physician's orders. When a physician orders "morphine sulfate, 10 mg IM every 3 hours prn for pain," the order specifies the medication to be given, the amount to be given, the method of administration, the time, and the reason. A well-written nursing intervention is equally specific: "Provide 200 ml of fluid (water or juice of choice) q2h while the woman is awake."

Conversely, poorly written interventions, such as "Assist with breastfeeding," provide generalizations rather than specific steps. Specific methods that the nurse should use to assist breastfeeding are more effective. For example, "Demonstrate correct positioning in cradle and football hold at first attempt to breastfeed. Teach mother to elicit rooting reflex by stroking infant's lips with nipple. Demonstrate how to latch infant to nipple, and request a return demonstration before mother is discharged."

Evaluation

The evaluation determines the effectiveness of the plan and its goals or expected outcomes. The nurse must assess the status of the client and compare the current status with the goals or outcome criteria developed during the planning step. The nurse then judges the client's progression toward goal achievement and makes a decision: Should the plan be continued? Modified? Abandoned? Are the problems resolved or the causes diminished? Is another nursing diagnosis more relevant?

The nursing process is dynamic, and evaluation frequently results in expanded assessment and additional or modified nursing diagnoses and interventions. Nurses are cautioned not to view lack of goal achievement as a failure but as a signal to reassess and begin the process anew.

Individualized Nursing Care Plans

Nurses are responsible for documenting nursing diagnoses, expected outcomes, and interventions for each problem. This information is often communicated to colleagues through a written plan of care. Many institutions have standards of care for groups of clients, such as those who have had normal spontaneous vaginal births. However, individual nursing care plans may be necessary on the basis of needs or problems identified during the assessment step of the nursing process. When nurses write individualized plans of care, they implement the plans through interventions that direct the care (Table 2-5).

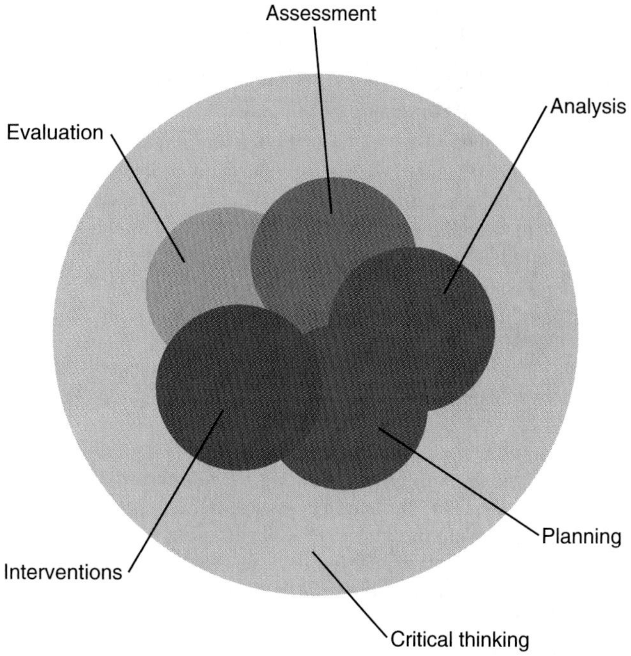

FIGURE 2-3 Relationship between the nursing process and critical thinking.

The Nursing Process Related to Critical Thinking

Although the nursing process and critical thinking are similar and overlap in many respects, major differences exist (Figure 2-3). The five steps of the nursing process provide a logical method for problem solving. Problem solving begins with a specific problem and ends with a solution. Conversely, critical thinking is open ended; it goes before and beyond problem solving. Critical thinking may be triggered by a problem, a positive event, or an opportunity to improve. It focuses on appraisal of the way the individual thinks, and it emphasizes reflective skepticism. Critical thinking is used throughout each step of the nursing process (Table 2-6).

Check Your Reading

9. How does screening assessment differ from focus assessment?
10. How do actual nursing diagnoses differ from risk nursing diagnoses?
11. How should goals and expected outcome criteria be stated?
12. Why are interventions sometimes difficult to implement? How can this difficulty be overcome?

Table 2-5

DEVELOPING INDIVIDUALIZED NURSING CARE THROUGH THE NURSING PROCESS

Although the nursing process is the foundation for maternal-newborn nursing, initially it is a challenging process to apply in the clinical area. It requires proficiency in focus assessments of the new mother and infant and the ability to analyze data and plan nursing care for individual clients and families. Asking questions at each step of the nursing process may be helpful.

Assessment

1. Did some data not fit within normal limits or expected parameters? For example, the client states that she feels "dizzy" when she tries to ambulate.
2. If so, what else should be assessed? (What else should I look for? What might be related to this symptom?) For instance, what are the blood pressure, pulse, skin color, temperature, and amount of lochia if the client feels dizzy?
3. Did the assessment identify the cause of the abnormal data? What are the hemoglobin count, hematocrit value, and estimated blood loss during childbirth?
4. Are other factors present? Did she have medication during labor? When? What medication is the client taking? How long has it been since she has eaten? Is the environment a related factor (crowded, warm, unfamiliar)? Is she reluctant to ask for assistance?

Analysis

1. Are adequate data available to reach a conclusion? What else is needed? (What do you wish you had assessed? What would you look for next time?)
2. What is the major concern? (On the basis of the data, what are you worried about?) The client who is dizzy may fall as she ambulates to the bathroom.
3. What might happen if no action is taken? (What might happen to the client if you do nothing?) She may suffer an injury or a complication.
4. Is there a NANDA-approved diagnostic category that reflects your major concern? How is it defined? Suppose that during analysis, you decide the major concern is that the patient will faint and suffer an injury. What diagnostic category most closely reflects this concern? "Risk for Injury?" Definition: The state in which an individual is at risk for harm because of a perceptual or physiologic deficit, a lack of awareness of hazards, or maturational age)
5. Do this category and definition "fit" this client? Is she at greater risk for a problem than others in a similar situation? Why? What are the additional risk factors?
6. Is this a problem that nurses can manage independently? Are medical interventions also necessary?
7. If the problem can be managed by nurses, is it an actual problem (defining characteristics present) or a risk problem (risk factors present)?

Planning

1. What expected outcomes are desired? That the client will remain free of injury during the hospital stay? That she will demonstrate position changes that reduce the episodes of vertigo?
2. Would the outcomes be clear, specific, and measurable to anyone reading them?
3. What nursing interventions should be initiated and carried out to accomplish these goals or outcomes?
4. Are your written interventions specific and clear? Are action verbs used (*assess, teach, assist*)? After you have written the interventions, look them over. Do they define exactly what is to be done (when, what, how far, how often)? Will they prevent the client from suffering an injury?
5. Are the interventions based on sound rationale? For instance, dehydration possible during labor causes weakness that may result in falls; loss of blood during delivery often exceeds 500 ml, which results in hypotension that is aggravated when the client stands suddenly. A woman who has recently delivered with an epidural block may have lingering effects from this form of labor pain relief.

Implementing Nursing Interventions

1. What are the expected effects of the prescribed intervention? Are adverse effects possible? What are they?
2. Are the interventions acceptable to the client and family?
3. Are the interventions clearly written so that they can be carefully followed?

Evaluation

1. What is the status of the client right now?
2. What were the goals and outcomes? Are they specific? Can they be measured?
3. Compare the current status of the client with the stated goals and outcomes.
4. What should be done now?

NANDA, North American Nursing Diagnosis Association.

Table 2-6
THE USE OF CRITICAL THINKING IN THE NURSING PROCESS

Nursing Process	Critical Thinking Skills
Assessment	Collecting complete data, validating data Clustering data (normal versus abnormal, important versus unimportant, relevant versus irrelevant) Identifying emotions
Analysis	Identifying cues and making inferences Reflecting and suspending judgment Examining thought processes for biases and assumptions Identifying alternatives Determining priorities
Planning	Examining need for closure Searching for alternative solutions Validating plan with client or co-worker Communicating plan Acknowledging defensive behavior
Implementation	Applying knowledge Testing plan Carrying out plan
Evaluation	Examining insights gained Recognizing new ways of thinking or acting Examining options and criteria for action Appraising self and others in the situation

COLLABORATIVE PROBLEMS

In addition to nursing diagnoses, which describe problems that respond to independent nursing actions, nurses must also deal with problems beyond the scope of independent nursing practice. These are sometimes termed *collaborative problems*, which are physiologic complications that usually occur in association with a specific pathologic condition or treatment. Unlike medical diagnoses, collaborative problems represent situations that are the primary responsibilities of nurses.

Nurses monitor clients to detect the onset of complications and collaborate with physicians to manage changes in client status. Both physician-prescribed (delegated) and nursing-prescribed interventions are necessary to minimize complications (Carpenito, 1999). Examples of collaborative problems in maternal-newborn nursing include excessive bleeding after childbirth and labor that begins before term.

Planning

Client goals and expected outcomes are not made for collaborative problems because the nurse's accountability is to detect early changes and manage these problems in conjunction with physicians. Nursing diagnoses have client goals and expected outcomes that reflect the nurse's accountability to achieve or maintain a favorable status after nursing care (Carpenito, 1999).

Collaborative problems should reflect the nurse's responsibility in situations that require delegated nursing interventions. Nursing responsibility in collaborative problems includes the following (Carpenito, 1999):

- Monitoring for signs of complications
- Consulting standing orders, protocols, and physicians if signs of complications are observed
- Performing specific actions to minimize the severity of an event or situation

Interventions

Interventions for collaborative problems include (1) performing assessments to monitor the status of the client and detect signs and symptoms of complications, (2) communicating with the physician when signs and symptoms of complications are noted, (3) performing delegated interventions to prevent or correct the complication, and (4) performing nursing interventions described in the standards of care or policy and procedure manuals.

Evaluation

Although client-centered goals or outcomes are not developed for collaborative problems, the nurse collects and compares data with established norms and judges whether data are within normal limits. If data are not within normal limits, the nurse communicates with the physician for additional direction and implements delegated nursing and independent nursing interventions.

Check Your Reading

13. How do nursing diagnoses differ from collaborative problems?
14. Why are client-centered goals or expected outcomes inappropriate for collaborative problems?

NURSING RESEARCH

As maternal-newborn nursing and the health care system change, nurses are challenged to demonstrate that their work improves client outcomes and is cost effective. To meet this challenge, nurses must generate, participate in, and use research. With the establishment of the National Institute of Nursing Research (NINR) as a full-fledged member of the National Institutes of Health (www.nih.gov/ninr), nurses now have an infrastructure to ensure the support of nursing research and the education of well-prepared nurse researchers. The NINR seeks to establish a scientific basis for care of individuals across the life span. The translation of scientific advances into cost-effective, quality care is inherent to the mission of the NINR.

Clinically based nursing research is increasingly conducted as nurse researchers strive to develop an independent body of knowledge that demonstrates the value of nursing interventions. However, a gap exists between knowledge acquired by the research team and its application to care of the client in the clinical setting.

Students and inexperienced nurses may not participate in research projects, but they must take advantage of the knowledge obtained by researchers. Refereed professional journals such as *Lifelines; Journal of Obstetric, Gynecologic, and Neonatal Nursing; Nursing Research; Journal of Perinatal and Neonatal Nursing;* and *Journal of Neonatal Nursing* (formerly "Neonatal Network"); are good sources of new information in maternal-newborn care that can help nurses provide improved care and demonstrate that their work makes a difference in client outcomes.

SUMMARY CONCEPTS

- Registered nurses with advanced education are prepared to provide primary care for women and children as certified nurse-midwives and nurse practitioners.
- Clinical nurse specialists function as expert practitioners, educators, researchers, and consultants to provide in-depth interventions for many problems encountered in maternity care.
- As maternity care has changed, so have the roles of nurses, who must be adept at communication techniques and communication blocks to meet their responsibilities as educators and counselors.
- A primary responsibility of nurses is to provide information to childbearing families. Nurses must use the principles of teaching and learning to fulfill the role of educator.
- Nurses must refine their critical thinking abilities by examining their own thought processes for flaws that can lead to inaccurate conclusions or poor clinical judgments.
- The nursing process begins with assessment and includes analysis of data that may result in nursing diagnoses. Nurses are legally accountable for identifying and managing independently these problems.
- Collaborative problems are usually physiologic complications that require both delegated, or physician-prescribed, and independent, or nurse-prescribed, interventions.
- Nurses must base their practices on the evidence generated by research. Professional journals are the best sources for the latest research.

REFERENCES & READINGS

Alfaro-LeFevre, R. (1999). *Critical thinking in nursing: A practical approach* (2nd ed.). Philadelphia: W.B. Saunders.

Angelini, D.J. (2000). Obstetric triage and advanced practice nursing. *Journal of Perinatal-Neonatal Nursing,* 13(4), 1-12.

Arnold, E., & Boggs, K. (1999). *Interpersonal relationships: Professional communication skills for nurses* (3rd ed.). Philadelphia: W.B. Saunders.

Beal, J.A. (2000). A nurse practitioner model of practice in the neonatal intensive care unit. *Maternal/Child Nursing Journal,* 25(1), 18-24.

Benner, P., Hooper-Kyriakidis, P., & Stannard, D. (1999). *Clinical wisdom and interventions in critical care.* Philadelphia: W.B. Saunders.

Capitulo, K.L. (1998). The rise, fall, and rise of nurse midwifery in America. *Maternal/Child Nursing Journal,* 23(6), 314-321.

Carpenito, L.J. (1999). *Handbook of nursing diagnosis* (8th ed.). Philadelphia: Lippincott.

Deering, C.G. (1999). To speak or not to speak: Self-disclosure with patients. *American Journal of Nursing,* 99(1), 34-38.

DeGeorges, K.M. (1999). Evidence! Show me the evidence! Untangling the web of evidence-based health care. *AWHONN Lifelines,* 3(3), 47-48.

Fitzgerald, S.M., & Wood, S.H. (1997). Advanced practice nursing: Back to the future. *Journal of Obstetric, Gynecologic, and Neonatal Nursing,* 26(1), 101-107.

Fonteyn, M.E. (1998). *Thinking strategies for nursing practice.* Philadelphia: Lippincott.

Gabay, M., & Wolfe, S.M. (1997). Nurse-midwifery: The beneficial alternative. *Public Health Reports,* 112(5), 386-394.

Gordon, M. (2000). *Manual of nursing diagnosis* (9th ed.). St. Louis: Mosby.

Katz, J.R. (1997). Back to basics: Providing effective patient teaching. *American Journal of Nursing,* 97(5), 33-36.

Kendrick, J.M. (1997). The advanced practice movement in nursing: Impact on perinatal care. *Journal of Perinatal and Neonatal Nursing,* 10(4), 20-27.

Riley, J.B. (2000). *Communication in Nursing* (4th ed.). St. Louis: Mosby.

Roux, G.M, Haas, P., & Sandefur, J.A. (1998). Advanced practice nursing: Two NPs reflect on their roles and responsibilities. *AWHONN Lifelines,* 2(2), 39-42.

Simpson, K.R., & Knox, G.E. (1999). Strategies for developing an evidence-based approach to perinatal care. *Maternal/Child Nursing Journal,* 24(3), 122-131.

Sinclair, B.P. (1997). Advanced practice nurses in integrated health care systems. *Journal of Obstetric, Gynecologic, and Neonatal Nursing,* 26(2), 217-223.

Sperhac, A., & Strodtbeck, F. (1997). Advanced practice nursing: New opportunities for blended roles. *Maternal/Child Nursing Journal,* 22(6), 287-293.

Tucker, D.A., & Flannery, J. (1996). The student process for success: The nursing care plan. *Nurse Educator,* 21(1), 47-50.

3

Ethical, Social, and Legal Issues

OBJECTIVES

1. Apply theories and principles of ethics to ethical dilemmas.
2. Describe how the steps of the nursing process can be applied to ethical decision making.
3. Discuss ethical conflicts related to reproductive issues such as elective abortion, forced contraception, and infertility therapy.
4. Discuss the maintenance of client, institutional, and colleague confidentiality when using electronic communication.
5. Relate how major social issues such as poverty and access to health care affect maternal-newborn nursing.
6. Describe the legal basis for nursing practice.
7. Identify measures to prevent or defend malpractice claims.
8. Describe the nursing implications of current trends in health care.

DEFINITIONS

Bioethics Rules or principles that govern right conduct, specifically those that relate to health care.

Deontologic Theory Ethical theory holding that the right course of action is the one dictated by ethical principles and moral rules.

Emancipated Minor An adolescent younger than the age of majority (usually 18 years) who is considered developmentally competent to make certain medical decisions independent of a parent or guardian.

Ethical Dilemma A situation in which no solution seems completely satisfactory.

Ethics Rules or principles that govern right conduct and distinctions between right and wrong.

Malpractice Negligence by a professional person.

Mutual Recognition Model A model of nurse licensure that would allow nurses to hold licenses in their states of residence and practice in other states that also recognize the home state's license; may be called a *multistate licensure compact.*

Negligence Failure to act in the way a reasonable, prudent person of similar background would act in similar circumstances.

Nurse Practice Acts Laws that determine the scope of nursing practice in each state.

DEFINITIONS—cont'd

STANDARD OF CARE Level of care that can be expected of a professional as determined by laws, professional organizations, and health care agencies.

STANDARDIZED PROCEDURES Procedures determined by nurses, physicians, and administrators that allow nurses to perform duties usually part of the medical practice.

UTILITARIAN THEORY Ethical theory stating that the right course of action is the one that produces the greatest good.

Table 3-1
ETHICAL PRINCIPLES

Beneficence—People are required to do or promote good for others.
Nonmaleficence—People must avoid risking or causing harm to others.
Autonomy—People have the right to self-determination. This includes the right to respect, privacy, and information necessary to make decisions.
Justice—All people should be treated equally and fairly regardless of disease or social or economic status.

Maternal-newborn nurses often grapple with ethical and social dilemmas that affect childbearing families. Nurses must know the way to approach these issues in a knowledgeable and systematic way. Some ethical and social issues result in the passage of laws that regulate reproductive practice. The nurse must understand the legal basis for his or her scope of practice to reduce vulnerability to malpractice claims.

ETHICS AND BIOETHICS

Ethics involves determining the best course of action in a certain situation. Ethical reasoning is the analysis of what is morally right and reasonable. Bioethics is the application of ethics to health care. Ethical behavior for nurses is discussed in codes such as the American Nurses' Association Code for Nurses. Ethical issues have become more complex as technology has created more options in health care. These issues are controversial because agreement over what is right or best does not exist and because moral support is possible for more than one course of action.

Ethical Dilemmas

An ethical dilemma is a situation in which no solution seems completely satisfactory. Opposing courses of action may seem equally desirable, or all possible solutions may seem undesirable. Ethical dilemmas are among the most difficult situations in nursing practice. To find solutions, nurses must apply ethical theories and principles and determine the burdens and benefits of any course of action.

Ethical Theories

Two major theories guide ethical decision making: deontologic and utilitarian. Few people use one theory exclusively. Instead, they make decisions by examining both theories and determining which is most appropriate for the circumstances.

Deontologic Theory. The deontologic approach determines what is right by applying ethical principles and moral rules. It does not vary the solution according to individual situations. One example is the rule "Life must be maintained at all costs and in all circumstances." Strictly used, the deontologic approach would not consider the quality of life or weigh the use of scarce resources against the likelihood that the life maintained would be near normal.

Utilitarian Theory. The utilitarian theory approaches ethical dilemmas by analyzing the benefits and burdens of any course of action to find one that will result in the greatest amount of good. With this theory, appropriate actions may vary according to the situation. This practical approach is concerned more with the consequences of actions than the actions themselves. In its simplest form the utilitarian approach is "The end justifies the means." If the outcome is positive, the method of arriving at that outcome is less important.

Ethical Principles

Ethical principles are also important to solve ethical dilemmas. Four of the most important principles are beneficence, nonmaleficence, respect for autonomy, and justice (Table 3-1). Other important ethical rules, such as accountability and confidentiality, are derived from these four basic principles. Although these principles guide decision making, in some situations the application of one principle conflicts with another principle. In such cases, one principle may outweigh another in importance.

Treatments designed to do good may also cause some harm. For example, a cesarean birth may prevent permanent harm to a fetus in jeopardy. However, the surgery that saves the fetus also harms the mother, causing pain, temporary disability, and possible financial hardship. Both mother and health care providers may decide that the principle of beneficence outweighs the principle of nonmaleficence. If the mother does not want surgery, the principles of autonomy and justice also must be considered. Is the mother's right to determine what happens to her body more or less important than the right of the fetus to fair and equal treatment?

Table 3-2

APPLYING THE NURSING PROCESS TO SOLVE ETHICAL DILEMMAS

Assessment—Gather data to clearly identify the problem and the decisions necessary. Obtain viewpoints of all who will be affected by the decision and applicable legal, agency policy, and common practice standards.
Analysis—Decide whether an ethical dilemma exists. Analyze the situation using ethical theories and principles. Determine whether and how these conflict.
Planning—Identify as many options as possible, their advantages and disadvantages, and which are most realistic. Predict what is likely to happen if each option is followed. Include the option of doing nothing. Choose the solution.
Implementation—Carry out the solution. Determine who will implement the solution and how. Identify all interventions necessary and what support is needed.
Evaluation—Analyze the results. Determine whether further interventions are necessary.

Using Ethical Theories and Principles to Solve Dilemmas

Nurses are often involved in supporting parents when tragedy strikes at birth. They must be knowledgeable of the disease process and the appropriate nursing care in these situations and the support families need when ethical dilemmas arise.

CRITICAL THINKING EXERCISE

The parents of an infant with anencephaly state that they would like to donate the organs from their dying infant to another infant who might live as a result. They believe that in this way their own infant will live on as a part of another baby. Although these transplants have been performed in the past, they are not currently practiced because of ethical concerns.

QUESTIONS:

1. What is the deontologic view of this decision?
2. How would the utilitarian view differ?
3. What ethical principles are involved? If such transplants become routine, what problems might arise?

Many approaches are available to solve ethical dilemmas. Although an approach does not guarantee a right decision, it provides a logical, systematic method for decision making. Because the nursing process is also a method of problem solving, nurses can use a similar approach when faced with ethical dilemmas (Table 3-2).

Decision making in ethical dilemmas may seem straightforward, but it rarely results in answers agreeable to everyone. Many agencies therefore have bioethics committees to formulate policies for ethical situations, provide education, and help make decisions in specific cases. The committees include a variety of professionals such as nurses, physicians, social workers, ethicists, and clergy members. The family members most closely affected by the decision also participate if possible. A satisfactory solution to ethical dilemmas is more likely to occur when a variety of people work together.

Check Your Reading

1. What is the difference between ethics and bioethics?
2. How does the deontologic theory differ from the utilitarian theory?
3. When might two ethical principles conflict?
4. How do the steps of the nursing process relate to ethical decision making?

Ethical Issues in Reproduction

Reproductive issues often involve conflicts in which a woman behaves in a way that may cause harm to her fetus or is disapproved of by some or most members of society. Conflicts between a mother and fetus occur when the mother's needs, behavior, or wishes may injure the fetus. The most obvious instances involve abortion, substance abuse, and a mother's refusal to follow the advice of caregivers. Health care workers and society may respond to such a woman with anger rather than support. However, the rights of both mother and fetus must be examined.

Elective Abortion

Abortion was a volatile legal, social, and political issue even before the *Roe v. Wade* decision by the United States Supreme Court in 1973. Before that time, states could outlaw abortion within their boundaries. In *Roe v. Wade* the Supreme Court stated that abortion was legal in the United States and that existing state laws prohibiting abortion were unconstitutional because they interfered with the mother's constitutional right to privacy. This decision stipulated that (1) a woman could obtain an abortion at any time during the first trimester, (2) the state could regulate abortions during the second trimester only to protect the woman's health, and (3) the state could regulate or prohibit abortion during the third trimester, except when the mother's life might be jeopardized by continuing the pregnancy.

For many people, the woman's constitutional right to privacy conflicts with the fetus' right to life. However, the Supreme Court did not rule on when life begins. This omission provokes debate between those who believe life begins at conception and those who believe life begins when the fetus is viable, or capable of living outside the uterus. Those who believe life begins at conception may be opposed to abortion at any time

Table 3-3

SUPREME COURT DECISIONS ON ABORTION SINCE *ROE v. WADE*

1976—States cannot give a husband veto power over his spouse's decision to have an abortion.

1977—States do not have an obligation to pay for abortions as part of government-funded health care programs. (This is considered by abortion rights advocates to be unfair discrimination against poor women who are unable to pay for an abortion.)

1979—Physicians have broad discretion in determining fetal viability, and states have leeway to restrict abortions of viable fetuses.

1979—States may require parental consent for minors seeking abortions if an alternative (such as judge's approval) is also available.

1989—Upheld a Missouri law barring abortions performed in public hospitals and clinics or performed by public employees. Also required physicians to conduct tests for fetal viability at 20 weeks of gestation.

1990—States may require notification of both parents before a person under the age of 18 years has an abortion. A judge can authorize the abortion without parental consent.

1992—Validated a Pennsylvania law imposing restrictions on abortions. The restrictions upheld include the following:

- A woman must be told about fetal development and alternatives to abortion.
- She must wait at least 24 hours after this explanation before having an abortion.
- Unmarried women under the age of 18 must obtain consent from their parents or a judge.
- Physicians must keep detailed records of each abortion, subject to public disclosure.
- Struck down only one requirement of the Pennsylvania law: that a married woman must inform her husband before having an abortion.

1993—Rescinded the so-called gag rule, which restricted counseling that health care professionals (with the exception of physicians) could provide at federally funded family planning clinics.

1995—Upheld a ruling that states cannot withhold state funds for abortions in case of pregnancies resulting from rape or incest or when the mother's life is in danger.

during pregnancy. Those who believe life begins when the fetus is viable (20 to 26 weeks of gestation) may oppose abortion after that time. Nurses need to understand abortion laws and the conflicting beliefs that divide society on this issue.

Conflicting Beliefs about Abortion. Some people believe abortion should be illegal at any time because it deprives the fetus of life. In contrast, others believe that women have the right to control their reproductive functions and that political discussion of reproductive rights is an invasion of a woman's most private decisions.

Belief That Abortion Is a Private Choice. Central to political action to keep abortion legal is the conviction that women have the right to make decisions about their reproductive functions on the basis of their own ethical and moral beliefs and that the government has no place in these decisions. Many women who support this view state that they would not choose abortion for themselves. Still, they support the right of each woman to make her own decision and view government action as interference in a very private part of women's lives. Many people who support legal abortions prefer to call themselves *pro-choice* rather than *pro-abortion* because they believe that *choice* more accurately expresses their philosophical and political position.

Each year, more than 1.2 million legal abortions are performed in the United States. In 1996 the rate was 22.9 abortions for every 1000 women aged 15 to 44 years. This translates into 1.37 million induced abortions in that year, the latest for which statistics are available (Ventura, et al., 2000). Many abortions are obtained by minors. Advocates of the legal right to abortion point out that abortion, either legal or illegal, has always been a reality of life and will continue regardless of legislation or judicial rulings. Advocates also express concern about the unsafe conditions that accompany illegal abortion, citing the deaths that resulted from illegal abortions performed before the *Roe v. Wade* decision.

Belief That Abortion Is Taking a Life. Many people believe that legalized abortion condones taking a life and feel morally bound to protect the lives of fetuses. This position is called *pro-life.* The term has become emotionally charged, and some believe it polarizes opinion and implies that those who do not agree with the antiabortion position are not concerned about life or are "anti-life."

Persons opposed to abortion have demonstrated their commitment by organizing as a potent political force. They have willingly been arrested for civil disobedience when they attempted to prevent admissions to clinics that perform abortions.

Legal Aspects of Roe v. Wade. Abortion has been a complex legal issue, and the Supreme Court has made major decisions that affect abortion law since 1973. Some decisions have strengthened the original *Roe v. Wade* ruling, and others have weakened it (Table 3-3). Legislation introduced in 1995 that banned late-term abortions received a presidential veto because it did not provide an exception when the mother's health is at risk.

Other versions of this bill will probably be introduced and, if passed, may come before the Supreme Court.

Political Aspects of Abortion. The abortion question is one of the primary issues confronting political candidates, who are often asked to explain their stand on abortion. Abortion-rights advocates emphasize that their message is to keep government out of the daily lives of citizens and that abridging women's right to abortion is unconstitutional. Antiabortion leaders will probably continue a confrontational strategy to bring attention to their point of view. In addition, they will continue to try to pass legislation that would hinder abortion by any means possible.

Implications for Nurses. Nurses have several responsibilities that cannot be ignored in the conflict about abortion. First, they must be informed about the complexity of the abortion issue from a legal and an ethical standpoint and know the regulations and laws in their state. Second, they must realize that for many people, abortion is an ethical dilemma that results in confusion, ambivalence, and personal distress. Next, they must also recognize that for many others, the issue is not a dilemma but a fundamental violation of the personal or religious views that give meaning to their lives. Finally, nurses must acknowledge the sincere convictions and strong emotions of those on all sides of the issue.

Personal Values. Nurses respond to abortion issues in ways that illustrate the complexity of the issue and the ambivalence it often produces. For instance, some nurses have no objection to participation in abortions. Others do not assist with abortions but may care for women after the procedure. Some nurses assist with a first-trimester abortion but may object to later abortions. Many nurses are comfortable assisting in abortion if the fetus has severe anomalies but are uncomfortable in other circumstances. Some nurses feel that they could not provide care before, during, or after an abortion but that they are bound by conscience to try to dissuade a woman from the decision to abort.

Professional Obligations. Nurses have no obligation to support a position with which they disagree. The nursing practice acts of many states allow nurses to refuse to assist with the procedure if it violates their ethical, moral, or religious beliefs. However, nurses are obligated to disclose this information before they are employed in an institution that performs abortions. For a nurse to withhold this information until assigned to care for a woman having an abortion and then refuse to provide care is unethical. As always, nurses must respect the decisions of women who look to nurses for care. If nurses believe they are not able to provide compassionate care because of personal convictions, they must inform a supervisor so that appropriate care can be arranged.

Check Your Reading

5. How did the *Roe v. Wade* ruling affect state laws related to abortion in the United States?
6. What are the major conflicting beliefs about abortion?
7. What are some Supreme Court decisions that have modified the *Roe v. Wade* ruling?
8. What are nurses' responsibilities if they are morally opposed to abortion?

Mandated Contraception

The availability of long-term contraception (e.g., implants) has led to speculation about whether certain women should be forced to use this method of birth control. In fact, the procedure has already been used as a condition of probation, allowing women accused of child abuse to avoid jail terms. Legislative efforts have been made to require women who receive public assistance to use the implants.

Some people believe that mandated contraception is a reasonable way to prevent additional births to women who are considered unsuitable parents and decrease government expenses for dependent children. However, this punitive approach to social problems does not provide long-term solutions. In addition, coercing poor women to use birth control to limit the money spent supporting them is both legally and ethically questionable. Such a practice interferes with a woman's constitutional rights to privacy, reproduction, refusal of medical treatment, and freedom from cruel and unusual punishment. In addition, hormone implants may pose health risks to the woman. Other methods to limit unwanted pregnancies, such as access to free or low-cost information on family planning, would be more appropriate.

Fetal Injury

If a mother's actions cause injury to her fetus, the question of whether she should be restrained or prosecuted has legal and ethical implications. In some instances, courts have issued jail sentences to women who have caused or who may cause injury to the fetus. This response punishes the woman and places her in a situation in which she cannot further harm the fetus. In other cases, women have been forced to undergo cesarean births against their will when physicians have testified that such a procedure was necessary to prevent injury to the fetus.

The state has an interest in protecting children, and the Supreme Court has ruled that a child has the right to begin life with a sound mind and body. Many state laws require reporting evidence of prenatal drug exposure. Women have been charged with negligence, involuntary manslaughter, delivery of drugs to a minor, and child endangerment.

However, forcing a woman to behave in a certain way because she is pregnant violates the principles of autonomy, self-determination of competent adults, bodily integrity, and personal freedom. Because of fear of prosecution, this practice could impede, not advance, health care during pregnancy.

The punitive approach to fetal injury also raises the question of how much control the government should have over a pregnant woman. Laws could be passed to mandate maternal human immunodeficiency virus (HIV) testing, fetal testing, use of tocolytics for preterm labor, intrauterine surgery, or even the foods the woman eats during pregnancy. The decision of just how much control should be allowed in the interests of fetal safety is difficult.

Fetal Therapy

Fetal therapy is becoming more common as techniques improve and knowledge grows. Although intrauterine blood transfusions are relatively standard practice in some areas, fetal surgery is still relatively uncommon.

The risks and benefits of surgery for major fetal anomalies must be considered in every case. Even when surgery is successful, the fetus may not survive, may have other serious problems, or may be born preterm. The mother may require weeks of bedrest and a cesarean birth. Yet despite the risks, successful surgery may result in birth of an infant who could not otherwise have survived.

Parents need help to balance the potential risks to the mother and the best interests of the fetus. They might feel pressured to have surgery or other fetal treatment they do not understand. As with any situation involving informed consent, women need adequate information before making a decision. They should understand whether procedures are still experimental, what are the chances of success, and what alternatives are available.

Issues in Infertility

Infertility Treatment. Perinatal technology has found ways for some infertile couples to bear children (see Chapter 32). The ethical concerns with this technology include the high cost and overall low success of some treatments. Because many of these costs are not covered by insurance, their use is limited to the affluent. Another questionable aspect is the high price of research on techniques that will benefit only a few. Some think that the money should be spent on research that will help a greater number of people. Even with highly technologic infertility treatment, many couples never give birth. Also, when treatment is successful, the risk of multiple births and premature infants is increased, which leads to extensive complications and expensive care. Because of couples' emotional vulnerability and the intense competition for their business, clients can be easily misled by advertised success rates and overlook the risks involved in infertility therapy (Reame, 1999).

Other ethical concerns focus on the fate of unused embryos. Should they be frozen for later use by the woman or someone else or used in genetic research? What if the parents divorce or die? Who should make these decisions? In multiple pregnancies with more fetuses than can be expected to survive intact, reduction surgery may be used to destroy one or more fetuses for the benefit of those remaining. The ethical and long-term psychologic implications of this procedure are also controversial.

Assisted reproductive techniques now allow postmenopausal women to become pregnant. What are the ethical implications of giving birth to children who may very well be orphaned at an early age or, at best, have a mother who is several decades older than their peers' mothers? Should the age and health of the parents be a factor in determining whether this treatment is offered? Should a consideration be the risk these women face for complications that might result in unhealthy infants?

Surrogate Parenting. In surrogate parenting a woman agrees to bear an infant for another woman. Conception may take place outside the body using ova and sperm from the couple who wish to become parents. These so-called test-tube babies are then implanted into the surrogate mother, or the surrogate mother may be inseminated artificially with sperm from the intended father.

Cases in which the surrogate mother has wanted to keep the child have created controversy. No standard regulations govern these cases, which are decided individually. Ethical concerns involve who should be a surrogate mother, what her role should be after birth, and who should make these decisions. Screening of parents and surrogates is necessary to determine whether they are suited for their roles. Who should perform the screening? Should it be left to the private interests of those involved, or should the government become involved? Answers to these questions are not definite at this time.

An issue closely related to surrogate parenting is the use of donor gametes. Will the use of donor gametes violate religious or moral beliefs of the parents? Does the child thus conceived have a right to know the identity of the biologic parents? What are the rights of the biologic parents? What about the ethics involved in the selling of gametes?

Check Your Reading

9. What dangers are involved in punitive approaches to ethical and social problems?
10. What problems are involved in the use of advanced reproductive techniques?

Privacy Issues

Many people are concerned about the possible misuse of their health information. They may fear that health information in the wrong hands, whether that information is accurate or not, may cost them a job, promotion, loan, or something equally valuable.

Government Regulations

The Health Insurance Portability and Accountability Act (HIPAA) of 1996 was designed to reduce fraud in the insurance industry and make it simpler for people to remain insured if they move from one job to another. Also within HIPAA's provisions was the mandate that Congress pass a law to protect the privacy of personal medical information by August 1999. Congress failed to do so, and the U.S. Department of Health and Human Services (HHS) Secretary proposed interim regulations in October 1999 to protect personal medical privacy as required by HIPAA. The HHS regulations provide consumers with significant new power over their records, including the right to see and correct their records, the application of civil and criminal penalties for violations of privacy standards, and protection against deliberate or inadvertent misuse or disclosure (U.S. Department Health and Human Services, 1999). The HHS regulations will cease to exist if Congress passes a law to replace them.

Online Communications. Client health data are rapidly being converted to computerized format. Although this allows nearly instant exchange of data between providers in an emergency situation, it also has the potential of greater violation of privacy than data maintained on paper. Terminals are often placed conveniently in hallways or client rooms to facilitate entry and retrieval of information for staff. The nurse must remember that this information may also be easily accessed by a computer-savvy client or family.

Nurses must take care to avoid violating client confidentiality when using electronic client data formats. For example, nurses must log off terminals when finished so that unauthorized people cannot gain access to the system. Passwords should remain secret and committed to memory and should not be words that another person can easily guess. Any suspected loss of a password should be promptly reported to the system administrator. Some systems require regular changes of passwords or combinations of letters and numbers to overcome some of these "word" problems. Screen savers that require a password to reenter the system further protect confidentiality.

Internet discussion lists allow nurses to exchange information and nursing care tips that can promote good practice. These forums also have the potential to allow lapses of client or institutional confidentiality because their communications cannot be considered private. When participating in discussion lists or using e-mail, nurses must respect the confidentiality of clients, colleagues, and institutions. Institutional documents such as chart forms, policies, and procedures should not be shared without the facility's approval. A personal message should not be forwarded without the original sender's permission.

SOCIAL ISSUES

Nurses are exposed to many social issues that influence health care and often have ethical implications. Some issues that affect maternity care include poverty, homelessness, access to care, and allocation of funds.

Poverty

Although the poverty rate for the United States dropped slightly in 1998, poverty remains an underlying factor in problems such as inadequate access to health care and homelessness. Minority children and families headed by women with children under 18 have higher poverty rates (U.S. Census Bureau, 1999). Families headed by women had the highest poverty rate in 1998 (29.9%) and comprised the majority of all indigent families (53%). Because of adverse living conditions and poor health care, infants born to low-income women are more likely to begin life with problems such as low birth weight. Poverty continues to influence the health of poor women and children because health care is less available to them.

Poverty tends to breed poverty. In poor families, children may leave the educational system early, making them less likely to learn skills necessary to obtain good jobs. Childbearing at an early age is common and further interferes with education and the ability to work. The cycle of poverty may continue from one generation to the next as a result of hopelessness and apathy (Figure 3-1).

Even people with incomes above the poverty level may not be able to pay for health care because of rising costs. The working poor have jobs but receive wages that barely meet their day-to-day needs. These jobs often do not offer health insurance, or high, unaffordable health insurance premiums may be the only option. The working poor have little opportunity to save for emergencies such as serious illness. Nationwide in 1995, 16.5% of the population under age 65 years had no health insurance (National Center for Health Statistics, 1997). Millions of other people have only limited insurance and would not be able to survive financially in the event of serious illness. People without insurance seek care only when absolutely necessary. Health maintenance and illness prevention may seem costly and unnecessary to them. Some receive no health care during pregnancy until they arrive at the hospital for birth.

Various government programs are available to help the poor. One such program is Temporary Assistance to Needy Families (TANF), which provides money for basic living costs of indigent children and their families. Created by the Welfare Reform Law of 1996, this re-

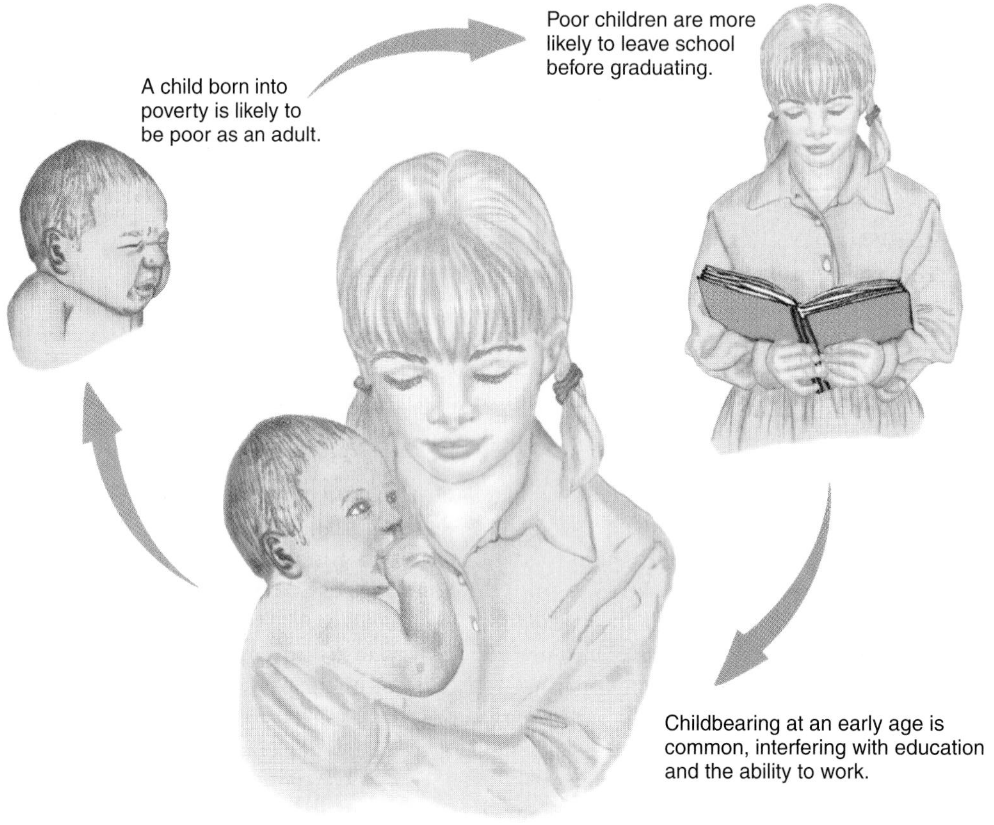
A child born into poverty is likely to be poor as an adult.
Poor children are more likely to leave school before graduating.
Childbearing at an early age is common, interfering with education and the ability to work.

FIGURE 3-1 The cycle of poverty.

placed the Aid to Families with Dependent Children (AFDC) program of the older welfare system. TANF imposes time limits on the aid given to the family, unlike AFDC. Eligibility requirements, income limits, allowances for homelessness, and time limitations vary among states. (Additional state information can be found at the Department of Health and Human Services' website at www.acf.dhhs.gov/programs/ofa/.)

Homelessness

Families, many of which are composed of single women and their children, are the fastest-growing group of homeless people. Their health problems may include substance abuse, malnutrition, tuberculosis, HIV infection, and sexually transmitted diseases (STDs). Other problems include rape, assault, and a high rate of pregnancy among homeless teens. Infants born to homeless women are subject to a lower birth weight and greater likelihood of neonatal mortality (Beal & Redlener, 1995).

Pregnancy and birth, especially involving teenage parents, are important contributing causes for becoming homeless. Pregnancy interferes with a woman's ability to work and may decrease her income to the point at which she loses her housing. Without child care or a home address, she may have less chance of obtaining and keeping employment. In addition, her children are more likely to be ill because of inadequate food and shelter. Without money to pay for insurance or early health care, the chance that children will need hospitalization increases.

Access to Health Care

The United States ranks twenty-fifth in infant mortality compared with other developed countries (see Chapter 1). Data for 1997 showed that for every 1000 live births in the United States, 7.2 infants died before their first birthday. This is approximately 80 infants each day (National Center for Health Statistics, 1999). Many of these deaths are related to low birth weight and other prenatal factors.

Prenatal Care in the United States

Prenatal care is widely accepted as an important element in a good pregnancy outcome. In 1997, 18.1% of mothers with live-born infants did not receive prenatal care during their first trimester of pregnancy (National Center for Health Statistics, 1999). Prenatal care is often poor because health care is not easily available. Lack of access to prenatal care contributes to the high infant mortality rate and the large number of low-birth-weight infants born each year in the United States. Because preterm infants are the largest category of those needing intensive care, millions of dollars could

Table 3-4

FACTORS RELATED TO LACK OF ACCESS TO HEALTH CARE

Poverty
Unemployment
Lack of medical insurance
Adolescence
Minority group membership
Inner city residence
Rural residence
Unmarried mother status
Less than high school education
Inability to speak English

be saved each year by ensuring adequate prenatal care. Even a small improvement in an infant's birth weight decreases complications and hospital time.

Table 3-4 summarizes factors that interfere with access to care. Many factors overlap; for example, poverty is often associated with the other characteristics listed. In the United States, minority women are more likely to be indigent, less likely to obtain adequate prenatal care, and more likely to die in childbirth when compared with white women.

Adolescent pregnancy is also associated with many factors listed in Table 3-4. In the United States, adolescent pregnancy rates have fallen slightly but remain high, with approximately 1352 teens giving birth daily (March of Dimes Birth Defects Foundation, 2000). The 1997 birth rate for teenagers declined to 52.3 births per 1000 women aged 15 to 19 years. Teen mothers are less likely to complete their education and more likely to be poor than adult mothers.

In some situations, women can obtain prenatal care but choose not to do so. These women may not understand the importance of the care or may deny they are pregnant. Some have had such unsatisfactory past experiences with the health care system that they avoid it as long as possible. Others want to hide substance use or other habits from disapproving health care workers. When women have overwhelming problems, prenatal care is not a priority for them. Language and cultural differences also play a part in whether a woman seeks prenatal care. Although these are not access issues as such, they must be addressed to improve health care.

Government Programs for Health Care

Medicaid. More than 46% of all money spent on health care in 1995 was publicly funded (National Center for Health Statistics, 2000). One government program that increases access to health care is Medicaid, which has existed since 1965. Medicaid provides health care for indigent persons, older adults, and persons with disabilities. Pregnant women and young children are especially targeted. Medicaid is funded by both the federal and the state governments. The states administer the program and determine which services are offered. Although the qualifying level of poverty varies among states, all women whose income is below 133% of the current federal poverty level are eligible for perinatal care.

Medicaid has a number of problems. Determination of a client's eligibility often takes weeks. The woman must fill out lengthy, complicated forms; provide documentation of income; and then wait for determination of eligibility. If a woman is not already enrolled at the beginning of her pregnancy, she is unlikely to finish the process in time to receive the early prenatal care so beneficial to a good pregnancy outcome.

Some physicians are unwilling to care for Medicaid clients who may be at higher risk. Many are especially unwilling if the reimbursement rate for physicians and hospitals is slow and less than that paid by other insurers. Physicians may be less inclined to accept high-risk, lower-paying clients because of the continual concern about malpractice suits.

Women who do not have private insurance may receive prenatal care at public clinics. However, such clinics are often understaffed and have large numbers of clients. Clinics may be located in areas not easily accessible to pregnant women who have transportation problems. Long waits for appointments may require time off from work, resulting in loss of pay for an hourly worker. A mother may not be able to find child care for older children while she visits the clinic. These problems decrease the chance that women will take steps to obtain care.

Shelters and Health Care for the Homeless. Federal funding has assisted homeless people with shelter and health care. However, as with other indigent people, the homeless have difficulties in obtaining health care because of lack of transportation, inconvenient hours, and poor continuity of care.

Quality and quantity of care in clinics may be poor because of inadequate funding. Nurses have been instrumental in opening shelters, clinics, and outreach services for the homeless, with nurse practitioners often playing a major role. Nurses also help inform the public and legislatures about the needs of the homeless.

Innovative Programs. Innovative programs to ensure that all women receive good prenatal care are necessary to help improve pregnancy outcomes. Many different programs are available in various areas of the country. Some outreach programs are designed to improve health in women who traditionally do not seek prenatal care. Bilingual health care workers and bilingual educational classes are part of some programs. Many programs employ certified nurse practitioners (CNPs) and are located in schools, shopping centers, churches, workplaces, and neighborhoods that are easily accessible to clients. Mobile vans outfitted with basic equipment bring prenatal care to women who are unable or unwilling to attend care at fixed locations or in more distant neighborhoods. (Such vans often provide neighborhoods with additional programs such as dental care, immunizations, well-child care, women's health care, and screening mammography.) Because the number of programs is insufficient to meet the need, more are necessary to make adequate health care for women and children a reality.

Allocation of Health Care Resources

In 1997 the United States spent $1.09 trillion, or 13.5% of its gross domestic product, on health care (National Center for Health Statistics, 2000). Expenditures for health care continue to rise. Areas that must be addressed include ways to provide care for indigent persons, the uninsured or underinsured, and those with long-term care needs. Distribution of the limited funds available for health care among all these areas is a major concern.

The 1997 Balanced Budget Act has had a major impact on health care facilities, including those that provide maternal-newborn care. The act seeks to limit Medicare fraud, extend the life of Medicare funds, and improve the benefits for staying healthy. The act also included changes in the Medicaid policies and the institution of a State Children's Health Insurance Program. Because the health care for a large percentage of any facility's clients is likely to be publicly funded by Medicare and Medicaid, the impact of the Balanced Budget Act cannot be ignored by nurses. This act has further limited income to hospitals and community agencies from the public sector, requiring that nurses work with even fewer financial resources than they did just a few years ago. However, the act's emphasis on preventive care also provides an opportunity for nurses to become innovators in such programs. (Additional information on the act can be found at the Health Care Financing Administration's website at www.hcfa.gov/init/bba/bbaintro.htm.)

Care versus Cure

One problem to be addressed is whether the focus of health care should be on preventive and caring measures or cures for disease. Medicine has traditionally centered more on treatment and cure than prevention and care. Yet prevention avoids suffering and is also less expensive than treating diseases after diagnosis.

The focus on cure has resulted in great technologic advances that have enabled some people to live longer, healthier lives. However, financial resources are limited, and the costs of expensive technology must be balanced against the benefits obtained. Indeed, the cost of one organ transplant would pay for prenatal care for many low-income mothers.

Although low-birth-weight infants comprise a small percentage of all newborns, they require a large percentage of total hospital expenditures. The expenses of one preterm infant for a single day in an intensive care nursery are more than enough to pay for care of the mother throughout her pregnancy and birth. Yet if the mother had received prenatal care early and regularly, the infant might not have needed intensive care.

In addition, quality of life issues are important in regard to technology. Neonatal nurseries are able to keep alive very-low-birth-weight babies because of advances in knowledge. Some of these infants go on to lead normal or near-normal lives. Others gain time but not quality of life. Families and health care professionals face difficult decisions about when to treat, when to end treatment, and how to recognize that the suffering outweighs the benefits.

Health Care Rationing

Modern technology has greatly influenced health care rationing. Some argue that such rationing does not exist, but it occurs whenever some people have no access to care and money is insufficient for all people to equally share the available technology. Advanced medical care often benefits only a small number of people but at great cost. Health care is also rationed when it is more freely given to those who have money to pay for it than to those who do not.

Many questions will need answers as the costs of health care increase faster than the funds available. Is health care a fundamental right? Should a certain level of care be guaranteed to all citizens? What should that care entail? Should the cost of treatment and its effectiveness be considered when the amount covered by government or third-party payers is decided? Nurses will be instrumental in finding solutions to these vital questions.

Check Your Reading

11. How do poverty and inadequate prenatal care affect infant mortality and morbidity?
12. How has the Balanced Budget Act of 1997 affected nursing practice?
13. How does a decision to spend money on technology sometimes conflict with issues of disease prevention?

LEGAL ISSUES

The legal foundation for the practice of nursing provides safeguards for clients and sets standards by which nurses can be evaluated. Nurses need to understand the way the law applies specifically to them. When nurses do not meet the standards expected, they may be held legally accountable.

Safeguards for Health Care

Three categories of safeguards determine the law's view of nursing practice: (1) nurse practice acts, (2) standards of care set by professional organizations, and (3) rules and policies set by the institution employing the nurse.

Nurse Practice Acts

Every state has a nurse practice act that determines the scope of practice of registered nurses in that state. Nurse practice acts define what the nurse is allowed to do when caring for clients. The acts also specify what the nurse is expected to do when providing care. Some parts of the law may be very specific. Others are stated broadly enough to allow flexible interpretation of the role of nurses. Nurse practice acts vary among states, and nurses must understand these laws wherever they practice. Nurses should have a copy of the nurse practice act for their state and refer to it for questions about their scope of practice. Most state nurse practice acts are also available on the Internet. The website of the National Council of State Boards of Nursing (NCBSN) (www.ncsbn.org) has information on nurse practice acts for all states, territories, and the District of Columbia, as well as other information related to licensing and practice.

Laws relating to nursing practice also delineate methods, called *standardized procedures,* by which nurses may assume certain duties commonly considered part of medical practice. The procedures are written by committees of nurses, physicians, and administrators. They specify the nursing qualifications required for practicing the procedures, define the appropriate situations, and list the education required. Standardized procedures allow the role of the nurse to change to meet the needs of the community and expanding knowledge.

A number of states have adopted a mutual recognition model, or a multistate licensure compact, for nursing licensure proposed by the NCSBN (National Council of State Boards of Nursing, 1997, 1998). States involved in the compact agree to recognize an unrestricted license to practice nursing issued by another state in the compact. This gives the license holder the authority to practice in the state in which the license was issued and those states that recognize the license. The nurse must abide by the rules and regulations in each state. Some advantages include reduced duplication and more cost-effective interstate practice.

Concerns have been raised about the NCSBN interstate compact model by the Association of Women's Health, Obstetric, and Neonatal Nurses (AWHONN), the major organization for maternal-newborn and women's health nurses (AWHONN, 1999a). This organization recognizes that nursing practice must change to facilitate telehealth, transport nursing, and greater mobility of nurses. However, AWHONN opposes the proposed compact model for several reasons, including concerns about constitutionality; licensure changes from the state of practice to the state of residence, possibly making it more difficult for consumers to file complaints; and confidentiality of malpractice or complaint data filed against nurses in a centralized database maintained by NCSBN. Additional concerns include increased costs if a claim must be defended in multiple jurisdictions.

Standards of Care

Court decisions have generally held that nurses must practice according to established standards and health agency policies in addition to nurse practice acts. Standards of care are set by professional associations and describe the level of care that can be expected from practitioners. For example, perinatal nurses are held to the national standards published by AWHONN, which are based on research and the agreement of experts. AWHONN also publishes practice resources, position statements, and other guidelines for nurses. Nurses should be familiar with the latest standards of care that cover their own practices.

Agency Policies

Each health care agency sets specific policies, procedures, and protocols that govern nursing care. All nurses should be familiar with those that apply in the agencies in which they work. Nurses are frequently involved in writing and revising nursing policies and procedures. In the event of a malpractice claim, the applicable policy, procedure, or protocol is likely to be used as evidence. The case of the professionals is strengthened if all agency policies were followed properly. These policies should be revised and updated regularly.

Malpractice

Negligence is the failure to perform the way a reasonable, prudent person of similar background would act in a similar situation. Negligence may consist of doing something that should not be done or failing to do something that should be done.

Malpractice is negligence by professionals, such as nurses and physicians, in the performance of their duties. Nurses may be accused of malpractice if they do not perform according to established standards of care and in the manner of a reasonable, prudent nurse with similar education and experience in a similar situation. Four elements must be present to prove negligence: duty, breach of duty, damage, and proximate cause.

Prevention of Malpractice Claims

Malpractice claims continue to be a major cost in health care. As a result of awards from such claims, the cost of malpractice insurance has risen for all health care workers. In addition, more health care workers practice defensively and accumulate evidence that their actions are in the client's best interest. For example, nurses must be careful to include detailed data on charts. This responsibility is especially important in perinatal nursing because most suits occur in this area.

CRITICAL TO REMEMBER

Elements of Negligence

Duty—The nurse must have a duty to act or give care to the client. It must be part of the nurse's responsibility.

Breach of duty—A violation of that duty must occur. The nurse fails to conform to established standards in performing that duty.

Damage—An actual injury or harm to the client as a result of the nurse's breach of duty must occur.

Proximate cause—The nurse's breach of duty must be proved to be the cause of harm to the client.

Many reasons exist for perinatal malpractice claims. Complications are usually unexpected because parents view pregnancy and birth as normal. The birth of a child with a problem is a tragic surprise, and they may look for someone to blame. Although very small preterm infants now survive, some have long-term disabilities that require expensive care. Statutes of limitations vary in different states, but plaintiffs often have more than 20 years for lawsuits that involve a newborn. Therefore the period during which a malpractice suit may be filed is longer.

Health care agencies and individual nurses must work together to prevent malpractice claims. Nurses are responsible and accountable for their own actions. Therefore they must be aware of the limits of their knowledge and scope of practice, and they must practice within those limits.

Prevention of claims is sometimes referred to as *risk management* or *quality assurance*. Although prevention of all malpractice claims may not be possible, nurses can help prevent malpractice judgments against themselves by following guidelines for informed consent, refusal of care, and documentation; acting as a client advocate; and maintaining their levels of expertise.

Informed Consent

When clients receive adequate information, they are less likely to file malpractice suits. Informed consent is an ethical concept that has been enacted into law. Clients have the right to decide whether to accept or reject treatment options as part of their right to function autonomously. To make wise decisions, they need full information about treatments offered.

CRITICAL TO REMEMBER

Requirements of Informed Consent

Client's competence to consent
Full disclosure of information needed
Client's understanding of information
Client's voluntary consent

Competence. Certain requirements must be met before consent is considered informed. First, the client must be competent, or able to think through a situation and make rational decisions. Infants, children, and clients who are comatose or severely mentally retarded are incapable of making such decisions. A client who has received drugs that impair the ability to think is temporarily incompetent. In these cases, another person is appointed to make decisions for the client.

In most states the age of majority, the age at which the person can give consent to medical treatment, is 18 years. However, in some states, younger adolescents can consent independently to some treatments, such as those for mental illness, abortions, contraceptives, drug abuse, and STDs. Pregnant adolescents may be considered emancipated minors in some states as well. Nurses must be familiar with laws governing age of consent in their jurisdiction.

Another exception to the usual requirement of informed consent is in emergency circumstances because consent is considered to be implied (Cady, 2000b). Treatment may proceed if evidence that the client does not want the treatment is lacking. *Emergency* may be specifically defined by state law and is usually restricted to unforeseen conditions that, if uncorrected, would result in severe disability or death. Emergency consent applies only for the emergency condition and does not extend to any other nonemergent, coexisting condition.

Full Disclosure. The second requirement is full disclosure of information, including details of what the treatment entails, the expected results, and the meaning of those results. The risks, side effects, benefits, and other treatment options must be explained to clients. The client also must be informed about the consequences if no treatment is chosen.

Understanding of Information. The third requirement is that the client must comprehend information about proposed treatment. Health professionals must explain the facts in terms the person can understand. If a client does not speak English, an interpreter is required. A hearing-impaired client must have a sign-language interpreter of the appropriate level to sign all explanations before consent is given. If the information to be provided or obtained is sensitive, foreign language or sign language interpreters should not be family or friends because these people may interpret selectively rather than objectively. Additionally, client confidentiality is compromised when nonprofessional interpreters are used for sensitive information. Nurses must be client advocates when they find a client does not fully understand or has questions about a treatment. If it is a minor point, the nurse may be able to explain it. Otherwise the nurse must inform the physician that the client's misconceptions need to be clarified.

Voluntary Consent. The fourth requirement is that clients must be allowed to make choices voluntarily without undue influence or coercion from others. Although others can give information, the client alone makes the decision. Clients should not feel pressured to choose in a certain way, and they should not believe that their future care depends on their decision.

Refusal of Care

Sometimes clients decline treatment offered by health care workers. Clients refuse treatment when they believe that the benefits of treatment are insufficient to balance the burdens of the treatment or their quality of life after treatment. Clients have the right to refuse care, and they can withdraw agreement to treatment at any time. When a person makes this decision, a number of steps should be taken.

First, the physician or nurse should establish that the client understands the treatment and consequences of refusal. If the physician is unaware of the client's decision, the nurse should notify that physician accordingly. The nurse documents the refusal, explanations given to the client, and notification of the physician on the chart. If the treatment is considered vital to the client's well-being, the physician discusses the need with the client and documents the results. Opinions by other physicians may be offered to the client as well.

Clients may be asked to sign forms indicating that they understand the possible results of rejecting treatment. This measure is to defend any subsequent lawsuit in which a client claims lack of knowledge of the possible results of a decision. If no ethical dilemma exists, the client's decision stands.

In cases of an ethical dilemma, a referral may be made to the hospital ethics committee. In rare situations the physician may seek a court ruling to force treatment. For example, if a woman refuses a cesarean birth, her decision may gravely harm the fetus. This situation is the only legal instance in which a person is forced to undergo surgery for the health of another. Indigent or minority women are more likely to have a court-ordered cesarean birth (Lindgren, 1996). However, court action is avoided if possible because it places the woman and her caregiver in adversarial positions. In addition, it invades the woman's privacy and interferes with her autonomy and right to informed consent. If legally mandated surgery became widespread and caused women to avoid health care during pregnancy, the resulting harm would affect more women and infants than would be protected by the surgery.

Coercion is illegal and unethical in obtaining consent. Even though the nurse may strongly believe that the client should receive the treatment, the client should not feel forced to submit to unwanted procedures. Nurses must be sure that personal feelings do not adversely affect the quality of their care. Clients have the right to good nursing care, regardless of their decisions to accept or reject treatment.

Documentation

Documentation is the best evidence that a standard of care has been maintained. It includes nurses' notes, fetal monitoring strips, electronic data, flow sheets, care paths, and any other data recorded in the chart. In many instances, notations on hospital records are the only proof that care has been given. Unfortunately, accurate and thorough documentation is the most common area lacking in malpractice cases (Simpson & Chez, 1996). When documentation is not present, juries tend to assume that care was not given.

Documentation must be specific and complete in perinatal nursing. This careful step is critical because of the long statute of limitations when a newborn is involved. Nurses are unlikely to remember situations that happened years in the past and, if sued, must rely on their documentation to explain their care. Documentation must show that nurses assessed the client appropriately, continually monitored for problems, identified problems and instituted correct interventions, and reported changes in the client's condition to the primary care provider.

Documenting Fetal Monitoring. Fetal monitor strips, or electronic storage, are important sources of information about the mother and fetus during labor and birth. Nurses record a great deal of information about nursing care on the monitor strip. Sometimes the client requires the nurse's full attention, and completion of other charting must be delayed temporarily. In this situation the nurse's notes on the monitor strip provide the basis for later charting.

Although monitor strips are a legal part of the chart, paper strips may become lost or separated from the chart and electronic media may be erased. These risks increase the importance of nurses recording summaries about the fetal condition in the flowsheets at appropriate intervals. Complete, detailed charting ensures that the nurse's actions will be apparent many years later in a court, even without the monitor strip.

Documenting Discharge Teaching. Discharge teaching is important to ensure that clients know how to take care of themselves and their infants after they leave the facility. To prevent or defend lawsuits, nurses must document the teaching they perform and the client's understanding of that teaching. Various documentation forms verify teaching and the degree of understanding about important topics. The nurse should also note the need for reinforcement and the method of providing that reinforcement.

Documenting Incidents. Another form of documentation used in risk management is the incident report, sometimes called a *quality assurance report* or *variance report.* The nurse completes a report when something occurs that might result in legal action, such as injury to a client, visitor, or staff member. The report warns the agency's legal department that a problem may exist. It also identifies situations that might endanger clients in the future. Incident reports are not a part of the client's chart and should not be referred to on the chart. When an incident occurs, documentation on the chart should include the same type of factual information on the client's condition that would be recorded in any other situation.

Cameras in the Birthing Room

Another issue is that of cameras (primarily videocameras) in the birthing or operating room. Although the videos are a precious memento of the birth for families, health care providers (and especially their insurers) are concerned that the videotapes or photos may be used as evidence in any malpractice action against the provider. Some institutions have prohibited photography altogether in the birth setting, and others limit photography to before and immediately after birth but not during the birth itself. Many facilities require clients to sign forms stating that the photos or videotapes cannot be used in legal action and placing other restrictions on photography. However, videotapes and photographs can help defend the providers in a malpractice case by showing that the standard of care was met.

The nurse must determine the woman's wishes regarding photography so that friends or family do not unintentionally photograph her against her wishes. The woman and her partner should be made aware of any facility policies about photography during pregnancy so that they are aware of restrictions before birth. The labor record should note that a video recording was made, by whom the recording was made, and who will maintain possession of the video. This note makes the video discoverable evidence by the facility in a future legal action (Cesario, 1998). Staff must be careful of their speech and facial expressions when they are being videotaped and avoid any conversations that could sound unprofessional if taken out of context or facial expressions that do not match what the charted notes say.

The Nurse as Client Advocate

The plaintiff may win a malpractice suit if the nurse fails in the role of client advocate. Nurses are ethically and legally bound to act as the client's advocate. When nurses feel that the client's best interests are not being served, they are obligated to seek help from appropriate sources. This usually involves taking the problem through the facility's chain of command. The nurse consults a supervisor and the client's physician. If the results are not satisfactory, the nurse continues through administrative channels to the director of nurses, hospital administrator, and chief of the medical staff if necessary. All nurses should know the chain-of-command process for their workplaces.

Nurses must document their efforts to seek help for clients. For example, when postpartum clients are experiencing excessive bleeding, nurses document the methods used to control the bleeding. They also document each time they call the physician, the information given to the physician, and the response received. When nurses cannot contact the physician or do not receive adequate instructions, they should document their efforts to seek instruction from others such as the supervisor. They should also complete an incident report. Nurses must continue their efforts until the client receives the care needed.

Maintaining Expertise

The nurse can also reduce malpractice liability by maintaining expertise. To ensure that nurses maintain their expertise to provide safe care, most states require proof of continuing education for renewal of nursing licenses. Nursing knowledge grows and changes rapidly, and all nurses must keep current. New information from classes, conferences, and professional publications can help nurses perform as would a reasonably prudent peer. Nurses should analyze research articles to determine whether changes in client care are indicated by the research evidence.

Employers often provide continuing education classes for their nurses through conferences, satellite TV systems, computer networks, and other means. Membership in professional organizations, such as state branches of the American Nurses' Association or specialty organizations like AWHONN, gives nurses access to new information through publications, nursing conferences, and other educational offerings. Continuing nursing education is also widely available on the Internet.

Expertise is a concern when nurses are "floated" or required to work with clients who have needs different from those of their usual clients. A nurse may be floated from one maternal-newborn setting to another or to a nonmaternity setting. In these situations, nurses need cross-training; in other words, orientation and education to perform care safely in new areas. The employer must provide appropriate cross-training for nurses who float. Nurses who work outside their usual expertise must assess their own skills and avoid performing tasks or taking responsibilities in areas until they have been educated to be competent in those areas.

Check Your Reading

14. How do state boards of nursing safeguard clients?
15. How do standards of care and agency policies influence judgments about malpractice?
16. How can standards of care be used to help defend malpractice claims against nurses?

COST CONTAINMENT AND DOWNSIZING

Measures to lower health care costs continue to directly and indirectly affect nurses' work. Two measures of special concern are the use of unlicensed assistive personnel and short lengths of stay (LOS) for clients.

Delegation to Unlicensed Assistive Personnel

In an effort to reduce health care costs, facilities have increased the use of unlicensed assistive personnel to perform direct client care and decreased the number of supervising nurses. An unlicensed person may be trained to do everything from housekeeping tasks to drawing blood and other diagnostic testing to giving medications, all in the same day. This practice raises grave concerns about the quality of care that clients receive when the nurse becomes responsible for the care of more clients but must rely on unlicensed persons to perform much of this care.

Nurses must be aware that they remain legally responsible for client assessments and must make the critical judgments necessary to ensure client safety when delegating tasks to unlicensed personnel. Nurses must know the capabilities of each unlicensed person who is caring for clients and must supervise them sufficiently to ensure their competence. The American Nurses Association, AWHONN, and state boards of nursing have issued statements to help nurses understand their roles in working with unlicensed assistive personnel (American Nurses Association, 1994; AWHONN, 1997).

Short Length of Stay

Regardless of the client's diagnosis the time from admission to discharge is as short as possible to keep costs in check. New mothers and infants have been especially targeted by third-party payers because birth is considered a normal event that does not require a long LOS. When discharge within 24 hours of vaginal birth was mandated by many third-party payers, health care professionals were apprehensive about client safety. Discharge after cesarean birth has been as early as the second morning after surgery.

A backlash has occurred against the mandated short stays for clients who have vaginal and cesarean births. In 1996, federal legislation was passed to require insurance companies to allow the option of a 48-hour hospital LOS after vaginal birth and a 4-day LOS after cesarean birth. Discharge may be earlier if deemed appropriate after discussion between the physician and client. Although not required by federal law, many states mandate prompt follow-up for early discharge in the client's home, an office, or a clinic. Some third-party payers voluntarily cover home visits for mothers who opt for earlier discharge because of the lower total cost for the home visit plus a short hospital LOS.

Concerns about Early Discharge

Health care professionals are concerned about women's ability to care for themselves and their infants so soon after birth. Women may be exhausted from a long labor or illness and unable to absorb all the information nurses attempt to teach before discharge. Once home, many women must also care for other children, often without the assistance of family members or friends.

During the time mothers remain in the birth facility, nurses are able to detect early signs of maternal or infant complications that may not be evident to parents. Mothers at home may not recognize development of serious maternal or neonatal infection or jaundice, and care may be delayed until the illness is severe. The ethical and legal implications of sending a mother home before she is ready to adequately care for herself and her newborn are very real concerns for nurses who must balance cost constraints with client needs.

Methods to Deal with Short Lengths of Stay

Early discharge is both a challenge and an opportunity for nurses. More teaching must occur during pregnancy when the mother's physical needs do not interfere with her ability to comprehend the new knowledge. In the birth facility, careful documentation and notification of the primary care provider is essential so that clients are not discharged inappropriately if abnormal findings develop. Methods of follow-up such as home visits, phone calls, and return visits to the birth facility for nursing assessments after discharge can identify complications early when they can be dealt with most effectively.

Phone call follow-up, sometimes called *telephone triage,* is the least expensive of these alternatives. However, the nurse does not see or physically examine the client or her infant. For this reason, hospitals offering phone follow-up to early discharge must have carefully designed protocols that are precisely followed, reviewed, and updated regularly (Cady, 1999c). Documentation should be kept on a form developed for this purpose. Any instructions given to the client (recommended actions if problems arise, if a minor problem does not improve, or if a problem worsens during phone triage) must be documented.

Check Your Reading

17. What concerns do nurses have about unlicensed personnel?
18. Why is early discharge a concern for nurses?
19. What are important points in phone-call triage?

SUMMARY CONCEPTS

- Ethical dilemmas are a difficult area of practice and are best solved by applying ethical theories and principles and the steps of the nursing process.
- When ethical principles of beneficence, nonmaleficence, autonomy, and justice result in ethical dilemmas, the nursing process may be used to guide ethical decision making.
- Elective abortion is a controversial issue that generates strong feelings in two opposing factions in the United States. Decisions by the Supreme Court have limited or upheld the right of states to impose restrictions on abortion.
- Nurses must examine their beliefs and come to personal decisions about abortion before they are faced with the situation in their own practices.
- When using online communications to transmit data about clients, colleagues, or facilities, nurses must be careful not to violate confidentiality and to maintain ethical conduct.
- Punitive approaches to ethical and social problems may prevent women from seeking adequate prenatal care.
- Issues in fetal therapy include weighing of the risks and benefits for the mother versus those for the fetus and determination of whose rights should prevail.
- Issues in infertility concern the high cost and low success rate of some treatments, the fate of unused embryos and multiple fetuses, and the rights of surrogate parents.
- Poverty is a major social issue that underlies allocation of health care resources, access to prenatal care, government programs to increase health care to indigent women and children, and health care rationing.
- Nurses are expected to perform in accordance with nurse practice acts, standards of care, and agency policies. Doing so provides the best prevention of or defense against malpractice claims.
- Nurses can help defend malpractice claims by following guidelines for informed consent, refusal of care, and documentation and by maintaining their levels of expertise.
- To give informed consent, the client must be competent, receive full information, understand that information, and consent voluntarily.
- Complete documentation is the best evidence that the standard of care received by a client was met. Therefore nurses must ensure their documentation accurately reflects the care given.
- Continuing pressures on optimal nursing practice include use of unlicensed assistive personnel and short lengths of stay.

ANSWERS TO CRITICAL THINKING QUESTIONS

1. The deontologic view is that taking organs necessary for life from one human being to give to another is wrong, even when the donor cannot survive. This view disapproves of aggressive treatment necessary to maintain perfusion to the organs until a recipient is located because treatment does not help the dying infant and may increase suffering. This concern invokes the principle of nonmaleficence.
2. The utilitarian view is that anencephalic infants cannot survive but that their organs could provide great benefit to other infants (beneficence). Because this family feels strongly that helping other infants allows good to come from their own tragedy, the greatest good would be for an organ transplant.
3. Potential problems include the possibility that transplants might someday be required, even against the parents' will, which might deny them autonomy in making decisions for their child's benefit. A woman might be forced to carry a pregnancy to term so that the organs could be harvested, even if the parents would rather terminate the pregnancy. If anencephalic infants are used for organ donation, people with profound mental retardation or persistent vegetative states might be placed in the same situation. Choosing infants to benefit would also be a concern, involving principles of justice. An overriding concern would be determining who would make the decisions necessary.

REFERENCES & READINGS

American College of Physicians & American Society of Internal Medicine. (1999). *No health insurance? It's enough to make you sick. Scientific research linking the lack of health coverage to poor health.* Philadelphia: Author.

American Nurses Association. (1994). *Registered professional nurses and unlicensed assistive personnel.* Washington, D.C.: Author.

Association of Women's Health, Obstetric, and Neonatal Nurses. (AWHONN). (1999a). *Position statement: Issue: Interstate compact for mutual recognition of state licensure.* Washington, D.C.: Author.

AWHONN. (1999b). *Position statement: Issue: Nurses' rights and responsibilities related to abortion and sterilization.* Washington, D.C.: Author.

AWHONN. (1995a). *The role of the nurse in clinical ethical decision making.* Washington, D.C.: Author.

AWHONN. (1997). *Position statement: Issue: The role of unlicensed assistive personnel in the nursing care for women and newborns.* Washington, D.C.: Author.

AWHONN. (1995b). Shortened maternity, newborn stay issue gaining momentum. *AWHONN Voice,* 3(9), 13, 20.

Beal, A.C., & Redlener, I. (1995). Enhancing perinatal outcome in homeless women: The challenge of providing comprehensive health care. *Seminars in Perinatology,* 19(4), 307-313.

Brent, N.J. (1997). Reproductive and family concerns. In N.J. Brent (Ed.), *Nurses and the law: A guide to principles and applications* (pp. 211-236). Philadelphia: W.B. Saunders.

Cady, R. (1999a). Anencephalics as organ donors: Where do we stand? *MCN: The American Journal of Maternal/Child Nursing,* 24(1), 51.

Cady, R. (1999b). Staffing problems and their legal consequences. *MCN: The American Journal of Maternal/Child Nursing,* 24(6), 313.

Cady, R. (1999c). Telephone triage—avoiding the pitfalls. *MCN: The American Journal of Maternal/Child Nursing,* 24(4), 209.

Cady, R. (2000a). Informed consent for adult patients, part 1. A review of basic principles. *MCN: The American Journal of Maternal/Child Nursing,* 25(2), 106.

Cady, R. (2000b). Informed consent for adult patients, part 2. *MCN: The American Journal of Maternal/Child Nursing,* 25(3), 164.

Cesario, S.K. (1998). Should cameras be allowed in the delivery room? *MCN: The American Journal of Maternal/Child Nursing,* 23(2), 87-91.

Chally, P.S., & Loriz, L. (1998). Ethics in the trenches: Decision making in practice. *American Journal of Nursing,* 98(6), 17-20.

Douglas, M.R. (1997). Ethics and nursing practice. In N.J. Brent (Ed.), *Nurses and the law: A guide to principles and application* (pp. 187-210). Philadelphia: W.B. Saunders.

Driscoll, K.M. (1998). Legal aspects of perinatal care. In C. Kenner, J.W. Lott, & A.A. Flandermeyer (Eds.), *Comprehensive neonatal nursing, a physiologic perspective* (pp. 32-45). Philadelphia: W.B. Saunders.

Eitel, D.R., Yankowitz, J., & Ely, J.W. (1999). Legal implications of birth videos. *Obstetrical and Gynecological Survey,* 54(1), 22-24.

Ferguson, S.L., & Engelhard, C.L. (1997). Short stay: The art of legislating quality and economy. *AWHONN Lifelines,* 1(1), 17-23.

Freda, M.C., DeVore, N., Valentine-Adams, N., Bombard, A., & Merkatz, I.R. (1998). Informed consent for maternal serum alpha-fetoprotein screening in an inner city population: How informed is it? *Journal of Obstetric, Gynecologic, and Neonatal Nursing,* 27(1), 99-106.

Gardner, S.L., & Hagedorn, M.E. (1997). Holding nurses accountable. AWHONN *Lifelines,* 1(1), 55-56.

Goldsmith, J. (2000). How will the internet change our health system? *Health Affairs,* 19(1), 148-156.

Guyer, B., Strobino, D.M., Ventura, S.J., MacDorman, M., & Martin, J.A. (1996). Annual summary of vital statistics 1995. *Pediatrics,* 98(6), 1007-1019.

Jadad A.R. (1999). Promoting partnerships: Challenges for the internet age. *British Medical Journal,* 319(7212), 761-764.

Johnson, S.A. (1992). Ethical dilemma: A patient refuses a life-saving cesarean. *MCN: The American Journal of Maternal/Child Nursing,* 17(3), 121-125.

Koniak-Griffin, D. (1999). Strategies for reducing the risk of malpractice litigation in perinatal nursing. *Journal of Obstetric, Gynecologic, and Neonatal Nursing,* 28(3), 291-299.

Ladebauche, P. (1995). Limiting liability to avoid malpractice litigation. *MCN: The American Journal of Maternal/Child Nursing,* 20(6), 339.

Lescale, K.B., Inglis, S.R., Eddleman, K.A., Peeper, E.Q., Chervenak, F.A., & McCullough, L.B. (1996). Conflicts between physicians and patients in non-elective cesarean delivery: Incidence and the adequacy of informed consent. *American Journal of Perinatology,* 13(3), 171-176.

Lindgren, K. (1996). Maternal-fetal conflict: Court-ordered cesarean section. *Journal of Obstetric, Gynecologic, and Neonatal Nursing,* 25(8), 653-656.

Locher, A.W. (1996). Ethics, women with HIV, and procreation: Implications for nursing practice. *Journal of Obstetric, Gynecologic, and Neonatal Nursing,* 25(6), 564-569.

Mahlmeister, L. (1999). Professional accountability and legal liability for the team leader and charge nurse. *Journal of Obstetric, Gynecologic, and Neonatal Nursing,* 28(3), 300-309.

Mahlmeister, L., & Van Mullem, C. (2000). The process of triage in perinatal settings: Clinical and legal issues. *Journal of perinatal and neonatal nursing,* 13(4), 13-30.

March of Dimes Birth Defects Foundation. (1993). *Toward improving the outcome of pregnancy: The 90s and beyond.* White Plains, N.Y.: Author.

March of Dimes Birth Defects Foundation. (2000). On an average day in the United States. Prepared by the March of Dimes Perinatal Data Center, 2000. Retrieved May 10, 2000 from http://www.modimes.org/HealthLibrary2/factsfigures/avgday.htm.

McCartney, P.R. (2000). Nettiquette: Maintaining confidentiality privacy on discussion lists. *AWHONN Lifelines,* 4(1), 28-33.

McGregor, L.A. (1998). Unlicensed assistive personnel: Getting it right from the beginning. *MCN: The American Journal of Maternal/Child Nursing,* 23(2), 65-69.

McRae, M.J. (1999). Fetal surveillance and monitoring: Legal issues revisited. *Journal of Obstetric, Gynecologic, and Neonatal Nursing,* 28(3), 310-319.

Muscari, M.E. (1998). When can an adolescent give consent? *American Journal of Nursing,* 98(5), 18-19.

National Center for Health Statistics. (2000). *Fastats: Health Expenditures.* Retrieved May 12, 2000 from http://www.cdc.gov/nchs/fastats/hexpense.htm.

National Council of State Boards of Nursing. (1998). Mutual recognition model for nursing regulation: Frequently asked questions. *Issues,* 19(1). Chicago, IL: Author.

National Council of State Boards of Nursing (1998). Boards of nursing adopt revolutionary change for nursing regulation. *Issues,* 18(3). Chicago, IL: Author.

Penticuff, J. (1996). Ethical dimensions in genetic screening: A look into the future. *Journal of Obstetric, Gynecologic, and Neonatal Nursing,* 25(9), 785-789.

Peter, E. (2000). Commentary: Ethical conflicts or political problems in intrapartum nursing care? *Birth* 27(1), 46-47.

Raines, D.A. (2000). Making mistakes: Prevention is key to error-free health care. *AWHONN Lifelines,* 4(1), 35-39.

Ray, M.M. (1999). Crossing state lines: Are interstate licenses in nursing's future? *AWHONN Lifelines,* 3(1), 21-22.

Reame, N. (1999). Informed consent issues in assisted reproduction. *Journal of Obstetric, Gynecologic, and Neonatal Nursing,* 28(3), 331-338.

Rhodes, A.M. (1996b). Drug use during pregnancy. *MCN: The American Journal of Maternal/Child Nursing,* 21(3), 127.

Rhodes, A.M. (1996c). Testing the standards of death. *MCN: The American Journal of Maternal/Child Nursing,* 21(2), 109.

Rhodes, A.M. (1997a). Liability for unlicensed assistive personnel, part I. *MCN: The American Journal of Maternal/Child Nursing,* 22(5), 269.

Rhodes, A.M. (1997b). Viable fetus vs. drug-abusing mother. *MCN: The American Journal of Maternal/Child Nursing,* 22(3), 127.

Rostandt, D.M., & Cady, R.F. (2000). HIV and women: Understand your responsibilities; reduce your risk. *AWHONN Lifelines,* 3(6), 35-38.

Simpson, K.R., & Chez, B.F. (1996). Professional and legal issues. In K.R. Simpson & P.A. Creehan (Eds.), *AWHONN's perinatal nursing* (pp. 15-25). Philadelphia: J.B. Lippincott.

Simpson, K.R. (1997). Unlicensed assistive personnel: What nurses need to know. *AWHONN Lifelines,* 1(3), 26-31.

Sleutel, M.R. (2000). Intrapartum nursing care: A case study of supportive interventions and ethical conflicts. *Birth,* 27(1), 38-45.

Southwell, S.M., & ArcherDuste, H. (1998). Ethical aspects of perinatal care. In C. Kenner, J.W. Lott, & A.A. Flandermeyer (Eds.), *Comprehensive neonatal nursing: A physiologic perspective* (pp. 13-31). Philadelphia: W.B. Saunders.

Tabone, S. (2000). Redefining confidentiality in an on-line world. *Texas Nursing,* 74(3), 4-5.

Taylor, D.L., & Woods, N.F. (1996). Changing women's health, changing nursing practice. *Journal of Obstetric, Gynecologic, and Neonatal Nursing,* 25(9), 791-802.

Tiedje, L.B. (1998). Ethical and legal issues in the care of substance-using women. *Journal of Obstetric, Gynecologic, and Neonatal Nursing,* 27(1), 92-98.

United States Census Bureau. (1999). *Poverty in the United States: 1998.* Retrieved May 9, 2000, from http://www.census.gov//prod/99pubs/p60-207.pdf.

Urbanski, P.K. (1997). Getting the "go ahead": Helping patients understand informed consent. *AWHONN Lifelines,* 1(3), 45-48.

United States Department of Health and Human Services. (September 1999). *Health, United States, 1999, with health and aging chartbook.* Hyattsville, MD: Author.

United States Department of Health and Human Services. (October 29, 1999). *HHS Proposes First-Ever National Standards To Protect Patients' Personal Medical Records.* Press Release. Retrieved June 8, 2000 from http://www.hhs.gov/news/press/1999/pres/991019.html.

Ventura, S.J., Mosher, W.D., Curtin, S.C., Abma, J.C., & Henshaw, S. (2000). *Trends in pregnancies and pregnancy rates by outcome: Estimates for the United States, 1976-1996.* National Center for Health Statistics, Vital Health Statistics, 21(56), 1-2.

Wegman, M.E. (1996). Infant mortality: Some international comparisons. *Pediatrics,* 98(6), 1020-1027.

York, R., Grant, C., Gibeau, A., Beecham, J., & Kessler, J. (1996). A review of problems of universal access to prenatal care. *Nursing Clinics of North America,* 31(2), 279-292.

4 Reproductive Anatomy and Physiology

OBJECTIVES

1. Explain female and male sexual development from prenatal life through sexual maturity.
2. Describe the normal anatomy of the female and male reproductive systems.
3. Explain the normal function of the female and male reproductive systems.
4. Explain the normal structure and function of the female breast.

DEFINITIONS

Amenorrhea Absence of menstruation. Primary amenorrhea is a delay of the first menstruation and secondary amenorrhea is cessation of menstruation after its initiation.

Cilia Hairlike processes on the surface of a cell that beat rhythmically to move the cell or to move fluid or other substances over the cell surface.

Climacteric Endocrine, body, and psychic changes occurring at the end of a woman's reproductive period (informally called *menopause*).

Coitus Sexual union between a male and a female.

Fornix (pl. *fornices*) An arch or pouchlike structure at the upper end of the vagina (also called a *cul-de-sac*).

Gamete Reproductive cell; in the female an ovum and in the male a spermatozoon.

Genetic Sex Sex determined at conception by union of two X chromosomes (female) or an X and a Y chromosome (male) (also called *chromosomal sex*).

Gonad Reproductive (sex) gland that produces gametes and sex hormones. The female gonads are ovaries and the male gonads are testes.

Gonadotropic Hormones Secretions of the anterior pituitary gland that stimulate the gonads, specifically follicle-stimulating hormone and luteinizing hormone. Chorionic gonadotropin is secreted by the placenta during pregnancy.

Graafian Follicle A small sac within the ovary that contains the maturing ovum.

Menarche Onset of menstruation; average age is 13 years.

Menopause Permanent cessation of menstruation during the climacteric.

DEFINITIONS — cont'd

PUBERTY Period of sexual maturation accompanied by the development of secondary sex characteristics and the capacity to reproduce.

RUGA (PL. *RUGAE*) Ridge or fold of tissue, as on the male's scrotum and in the female's vagina.

SECONDARY SEX CHARACTERISTICS Physical differences between mature males and females that are not directly related to reproduction.

SOMATIC SEX Gender assignment as male or female on the basis of form and structure of the external genitalia.

SPERMATOGENESIS Formation of male gametes (sperm) in the testes.

SPINNBARKEIT Clear, slippery, stretchy quality of cervical mucus during ovulation.

An understanding of the structure and function of the reproductive organs is necessary for effective nursing care of women during and after their reproductive years and for couples that require family planning or infertility care. This chapter reviews basic prenatal development, sexual maturation, and the structure and function of female and male reproductive systems. Because of its emphasis in this book, the female reproductive system is discussed most extensively.

SEXUAL DEVELOPMENT

Sexual development begins at conception when the genetic sex is determined by the union of an ovum and a sperm. During childhood the sex organs are inactive. They become active during puberty as the person begins sexual maturation.

Prenatal Development

The mother's ovum carries a single X chromosome. Each of the father's spermatozoa carries either an X chromosome or a Y chromosome. If an X-bearing spermatozoon fertilizes the ovum, the offspring's genetic sex is female. If a Y-bearing spermatozoon fertilizes the ovum, a male offspring results.

Although genetic sex is determined at conception, the reproductive system of both males and females is similar, or sexually undifferentiated, for the first 6 weeks of prenatal life. During the seventh week, differences between males and females appear in the internal structures. The external genitalia continue to look similar until the ninth week, when these outer structures begin to change. Differentiation of the external sexual organs is complete at about 12 weeks' gestational age.

The basic trend for prenatal sexual development is to have female structures. Presence of only a small part of the Y chromosome (the short arm) changes this trend and directs the early (primitive) sex cells to become testes. Absence of the critical part of the Y chromosome allows the primitive sex cells to continue on their course of becoming ovaries (see Chapter 6).

During fetal life, both ovaries and testes secrete their primary hormones, which are estrogen and testosterone, respectively. Testosterone causes development of male sex organs and external genitalia, and its absence results in development of female sex characteristics. Although estrogen is secreted by the fetal ovary, the hormone is not required to initiate development of female sex structures.

Childhood

The sex glands of girls and boys are inactive during infancy and childhood. At sexual maturity the hypothalamus stimulates the anterior pituitary gland to produce hormones, which in turn stimulate sex hormone production by the gonads.

Sexual Maturation

Puberty refers to the time during which the reproductive organs become fully functional. It is not a single event but a series of changes that occurs over several years during late childhood and early adolescence. Primary sex characteristics relate to the maturation of those organs directly responsible for reproduction. Examples of primary sex characteristics are maturation of ova in the ovaries and production of sperm in the testes. Secondary sex characteristics are changes in other systems that differentiate females and males but do not directly relate to reproduction (Table 4-1).

Initiation of Sexual Maturation

Not all factors that initiate sexual maturation are known. Secretions of the hypothalamus, anterior pituitary, and gonads all play a part. The hypothalamus can secrete gonadotropin-releasing hormone (GnRH) to initiate puberty during infancy and early childhood, but it does not do so in significant amounts until late childhood. Production of even tiny quantities of sex hormones by the young child's ovaries or testes inhibits secretions of the hypothalamus, preventing premature onset of puberty. Maturation of another brain area, as yet unknown, probably triggers the hypothalamus to initiate puberty (Guyton & Hall, 2000).

The maturing child's hypothalamus gradually increases production of GnRH beginning around age 8. The level of GnRH increases slowly until it reaches a level adequate to stimulate the anterior pituitary to increase its production of follicle-stimulating hormone (FSH) and luteinizing hormone (LH). The ovaries and testes increase production of sex hormones and begin maturing gametes in response to higher levels of FSH and LH. The sex hormones also induce development of secondary sex characteristics. (Table 4-2 presents the major hormones that play a role in reproduction.)

Table 4-1
COMPARISON OF SECONDARY SEX CHARACTERISTICS IN FEMALES AND MALES

Females	Males
Development of glandular and ductal systems in the breast; deposition of fat selectively in the breast, buttocks, and thighs, resulting in a rounded figure	50% greater muscle mass
Wide, round pelvis	Narrow, upright, and heavier pelvis
Pubic and axillary hair	Pubic and axillary hair; facial and chest hair; increased amount of hair on the upper back in some males; male pattern baldness, beginning on the top of the head
Soft, smooth skin texture	Coarser skin
Higher-pitched voice	Deeper voice

The age at which changes of puberty begin and the time required to complete these changes vary among individuals. The hormonal changes of puberty begin about 6 months to 1 year earlier in girls than in boys. The growth spurt that occurs with puberty also begins earlier for girls than for boys. The obvious changes of puberty in girls, such as breast development, begin an average of 2 years before changes in boys. Changes of puberty occur in an orderly sequence in both genders. Increases in height and weight are dramatic during puberty but slow after puberty until mature heights and weights are attained. The nutritional state can also influence the start of puberty, with earlier onset in well-nourished children.

Female Puberty Changes

As girls mature, the anterior pituitary gland secretes increasing amounts of FSH and LH in response to the hypothalamic secretion of GnRH. These two pituitary secretions stimulate secretion of estrogens and progesterone by the ovary, resulting in maturation of the reproductive organs and breasts and development of secondary sex characteristics. The first noticeable change of puberty in girls, development of the breasts, begins at an average age of 10.9 years, with a low of 8.9 years and a high of 12.9 years (Behrman, et al., 2000).

Breast Changes. Initially, the nipple enlarges and protrudes. The areola surrounding the nipple enlarges and becomes somewhat protuberant, although less so than the nipple. These changes are followed by growth of the glandular and ductal tissue. Fat is deposited in the breasts to give them the characteristic rounded female appearance. During puberty a girl's breasts often develop at different rates, resulting in a lopsided appearance until one breast catches up with the other.

Body Contours. The pelvis widens and assumes a rounded, basinlike shape that favors passage of the fetus during childbirth. Fat is deposited selectively in the hips, giving them a rounder appearance than that of the male.

Body Hair. Pubic hair first appears downy and becomes thicker as puberty progresses. Axillary hair appears near the time of menarche. The texture and quantity of pubic and axillary hair vary among women and ethnic groups. Women of African descent usually have body hair that is coarser and curlier than that of white women. Asian women often have sparser body hair than women of other racial groups.

Skeletal Growth. The girl grows taller for several years during early puberty in response to estrogen stimulation. The growth spurt begins about 1 year after initial breast development. Estrogen's other powerful effect on the skeleton is to cause the epiphyses (growth areas of the bone) to unite with the shaft of the bones, which eventually stops growth in height.

Reproductive Organs. The girl's external genitalia enlarge as fat is deposited in the mons pubis, labia majora, and labia minora. The vagina, uterus, fallopian tubes, and ovaries grow larger. In addition, the vaginal mucosa changes, becoming more resistant to trauma and infection in preparation for sexual activity. Cyclic changes in the reproductive organs occur during each female reproductive cycle.

Menarche. About 2 to 2.5 years after the beginning of breast development, girls experience their menarche, or first menstrual period. Early menstrual periods are often irregular and scant. These early menstrual cycles are not usually fertile because ovulation occurs inconsistently. Fertile reproductive cycles require preparation of the uterine lining precisely timed with ovulation. However, ovulation may occur during any female reproductive cycle, including the first. The sexually active girl can conceive even before her first menstrual period.

Delayed onset of menstruation is called *primary amenorrhea* if the girl's periods have not begun within 2 years after the onset of breast development or by age 16 or if the girl is more than 1 year older than her mother or sisters were when their menarche occurred.

Table 4-2

MAJOR HORMONES IN REPRODUCTION

Produced by	Target Organs	Action in Females	Action in Males
GONADOTROPIN-RELEASING HORMONE (GnRH)			
Hypothalamus	Anterior pituitary	Stimulates release of FSH and LH, initiating puberty and sustaining female reproductive cycle. Release of GnRH is pulsatile (rhythmic, pulsating).	Stimulates release of FSH and LH, initiating puberty. Release of GnRH is pulsatile.
FOLLICLE-STIMULATING HORMONE (FSH)			
Anterior pituitary	Female: ovaries Male: testes	1. Stimulates production of estrogens and progesterone 2. Stimulates growth and maturation of graafian follicles before ovulation	Stimulates sperm formation
LUTEINIZING HORMONE (LH)			
Anterior pituitary	Female: ovaries Male: testes	1. Stimulates final maturation of follicle 2. Causes ovulation with surge of LH about 14 days before next expected menstrual period 3. Stimulates transformation of graafian follicle into corpus luteum, which continues secretion of estrogens and progesterone for about 12 days if ovum is not fertilized (with fertilization, placenta gradually assumes secretion of estrogen and progesterone)	Stimulates testes to secrete testosterone, most of which is secreted in the Leydig cells
ESTROGENS			
1. Ovaries and corpus luteum (female) 2. Placenta (pregnancy) 3. Small quantities from testosterone in testes and from other tissues, especially the liver (males)	Female: internal and external reproductive organs and breasts Male: testes	1. Reproductive organs: Stimulate maturation at puberty, endometrium before ovulation 2. Breasts: Induce growth of glandular (milk-secreting) and ductal (milk-carrying) tissue, initiate deposition of fat at puberty 3. Stimulate growth of long bones but cause closure of epiphyses (growth plates), limiting mature height 4. Pregnancy: Stimulate growth of uterus and breast tissue, inhibit active milk secretion until after the placenta is expelled, relax pelvic ligaments	Facilitates normal sperm formation

PROGESTERONE			
1. Ovary, corpus luteum 2. Placenta	Female: uterus and breasts	1. Stimulates secretion of endometrial glands, causes endometrial vessels to become highly dilated and tortuous (twisting around) in preparation for possible embryo implantation 2. Pregnancy: Induces growth of cells of fallopian tubes and uterine lining to nourish embryo, decreases contractions of uterus, prepares breasts for lactation but inhibits active prolactin secretion until after birth	N/A
PROLACTIN			
Anterior pituitary	Female breasts	Stimulates secretion of milk (lactogenesis); estrogen and progesterone inhibit active milk secretion until the placenta is expelled; newborn suckling maintains prolactin secretion to maintain milk production	N/A
OXYTOCIN			
Posterior pituitary	Female: uterus and breasts Sexual organs (males)	1. Stimulates uterine contractions during birth to expel the fetus and stimulates contractions after birth to compress uterine blood vessels and control bleeding 2. Stimulates let-down, or milk-ejection, reflex during breastfeeding	N/A
TESTOSTERONE			
Testes (male) Adrenal glands (female) Ovaries (female)	Male: sexual organs	1. Causes growth of pubic and axillary hair at puberty from small quantities of androgenic (masculinizing) hormones released from the adrenal glands 2. Is converted to estrogen, like most androgens	1. Induces development of male sex organs in fetus (regardless of chromosome composition, female fetus results without testosterone stimulation), stimulates descent of testes 2. Induces growth and division of the cells that mature sperm 3. Induces development of male secondary sex characteristics (deeper voice, pelvic type, body and facial hair, male-pattern baldness)

N/A, Not applicable.

Secondary amenorrhea describes absence of menstruation for at least three cycles after regular cycles have been established or for 6 months (Kim, 2000). Both primary and secondary amenorrhea are more common in females who are thin. Women who are competitive athletes or ballet dancers or suffer from eating disorders (such as anorexia nervosa, bulimia) may have too little fat to produce enough sex hormones to stimulate ovulation and menstruation. Pregnancy is also a common cause of secondary amenorrhea. Both primary and secondary amenorrhea may result from inadequate pituitary stimulation of the ovary or failure of the ovary to respond to pituitary stimulation. Amenorrhea also may be caused by excessive androgenic hormones from the adrenal glands, which have a masculinizing effect.

Male Puberty Changes

Secretion of GnRH by the hypothalamus stimulates secretion of LH and FSH from the anterior pituitary. LH and FSH then stimulate secretion of testosterone and eventually cause spermatogenesis in the maturing adolescent. Testosterone stimulates development of a boy's reproductive organs and secondary sex characteristics. The first outward sign of puberty is growth of the testes, which may begin as early as 9.5 years. Penile development occurs at an average age of 10.5 years, with a low of 9.2 years and a high of 13.7 years (Behrman, et al., 2000). The skin of the scrotum thins and darkens.

Nocturnal Emissions. Often called *wet dreams,* nocturnal emissions commonly occur during the teenage years. The boy experiences a spontaneous ejaculation of seminal fluid during sleep, often accompanied by dreams with sexual content. Boys should be prepared for this normal occurrence so that they do not feel abnormal or ashamed or fear that they have an infection or other problem.

Body Hair. Pubic hair growth begins at the base of the penis. Gradually, the hair coarsens and grows upward and in the midline of the abdomen. About 2 years later, axillary hair appears. Facial hair begins as a fine, downy mustache and progresses to the characteristic beard of the adult male. In most boys, chest hair develops, and some boys have hair on their upper backs. The amount and character of body hair vary among men of different racial groups, with Asian and Native American men often having less than white or African men. The quantity and character of body hair among men of the same racial group also vary.

Body Composition. Because of the influence of testosterone, men develop a greater average muscle mass than women. At maturity, a man's muscle mass exceeds the woman's by an average of 50%, explaining the biologic advantage of men in tasks requiring muscle strength.

Skeletal Growth. Testosterone causes boys to undergo a rapid growth spurt, especially in height. A boy's linear growth begins about 1 year later than a girl's and lasts longer. Testosterone eventually causes union of the epiphysis with the shaft of long bones, as estrogen does in girls. However, the height-limiting effect of testosterone is not as strong as that of estrogen in females, with the result that boys grow in stature for several years longer than girls. The male's greater average height at maturity is the combined result of beginning the growth spurt at a slightly later age and continuing it for a longer time.

A boy's shoulders broaden as his height increases. His pelvis assumes a more upright shape, with narrower diameters and heavier composition than the female's. A man's pelvis is structurally suited for tasks requiring load bearing.

Voice Changes. Hypertrophy of the laryngeal mucosa and enlargement of the larynx cause the male's voice to deepen. Before reaching their lower tones at maturity, many boys experience embarrassing "cracking" or "squeaking" of their voices when they speak.

Decline in Fertility

A woman's ability to reproduce decreases over a period called the *climacteric.* In most women the climacteric occurs between ages 45 and 50. At this time, maturation of ova and production of ovarian hormones gradually decline. The external and internal reproductive organs atrophy somewhat as well. *Menopause* is the term used to describe the final menstrual period. However, *menopause* and *climacteric* are often used interchangeably to describe the entire gradual process of change. Perimenopause is the time from onset of symptoms associated with the climacteric until at least 1 year after the last menstrual period. (See Chapter 33 for more information about the woman's needs during this phase of her life.)

Men do not experience a distinct marker event like menopause. Their production of testosterone and sperm gradually declines, but men in their 50s, 60s, and beyond may still be able to father children.

Check Your Reading

1. What are the first noticeable changes of puberty in girls and boys?
2. What are common differences in body hair characteristics among adult females and males of different races?
3. What are basic differences between the mature male and female pelves?
4. Why do males generally attain greater mature height than females?
5. What are common male and female secondary sex characteristics?

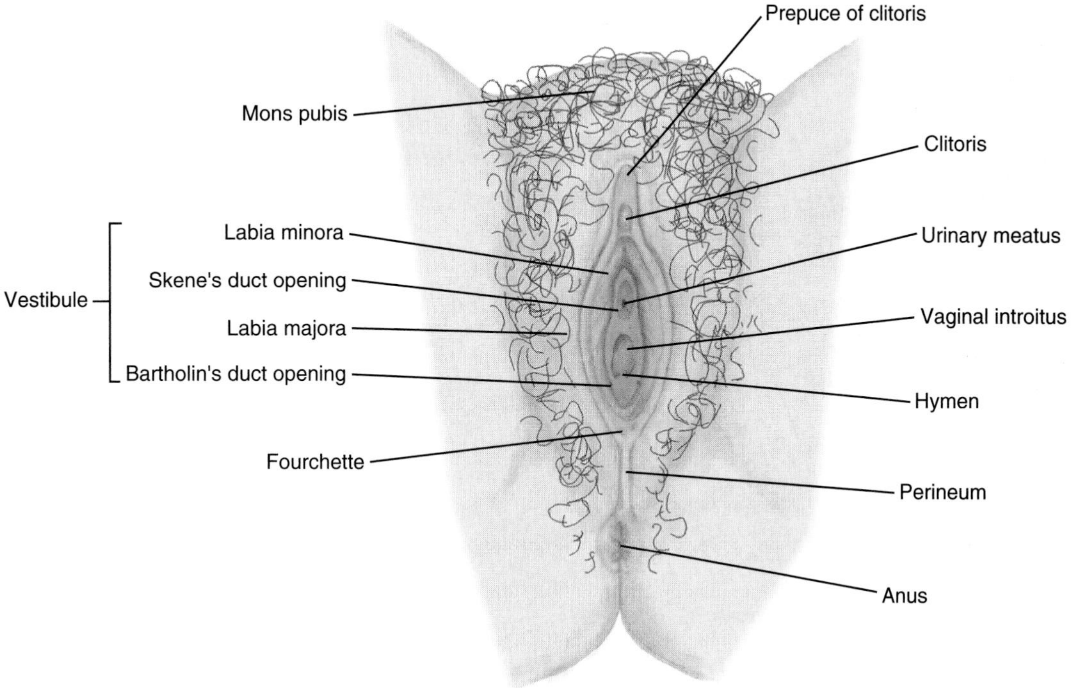

FIGURE 4-1 External female reproductive structures.

Table 4-3
FUNCTIONS OF FEMALE REPRODUCTIVE AND ACCESSORY ORGANS

Organ	Function
Vagina	1. Provides the passageway for the menstrual flow 2. Is the female organ for coitus; receives the male penis during coitus 3. Provides the passageway for the fetus during birth
Uterus	Houses and nourishes the fetus to sufficient maturity to function outside the mother's body, propels fetus to outside
Fallopian tube	1. Provides passageway for ovum as it travels from ovary to uterus 2. Is the site of fertilization
Ovaries	1. Secrete estrogens and progesterone 2. Contain ova within follicles for maturation during the woman's reproductive life
Breasts	
Alveoli	Secrete milk after childbirth (acinar cells within alveoli)
Lactiferous ducts and sinuses	Collect milk from alveoli and conduct it to the outside

FEMALE REPRODUCTIVE ANATOMY

The nurse needs a basic knowledge of the structure and function of the external and internal reproductive organs to understand their roles in pregnancy and childbirth (Table 4-3).

External Female Reproductive Organs

Collectively, the external female reproductive organs are called the *vulva*. These structures include the mons pubis, labia majora and minora, clitoris, structures of the vestibule, and perineum (Figure 4-1).

Mons Pubis

The mons pubis is the rounded, fleshy prominence over the symphysis pubis that forms the anterior border of the external reproductive organs. It is covered with varying amounts of pubic hair.

Labia Major and Minora

The labia majora are two rounded, fleshy folds of tissue that extend from the mons pubis to the perineum. They have a slightly deeper pigmentation than surrounding skin and are covered with pubic hair. The labia majora protect the more fragile tissues of the external genitalia.

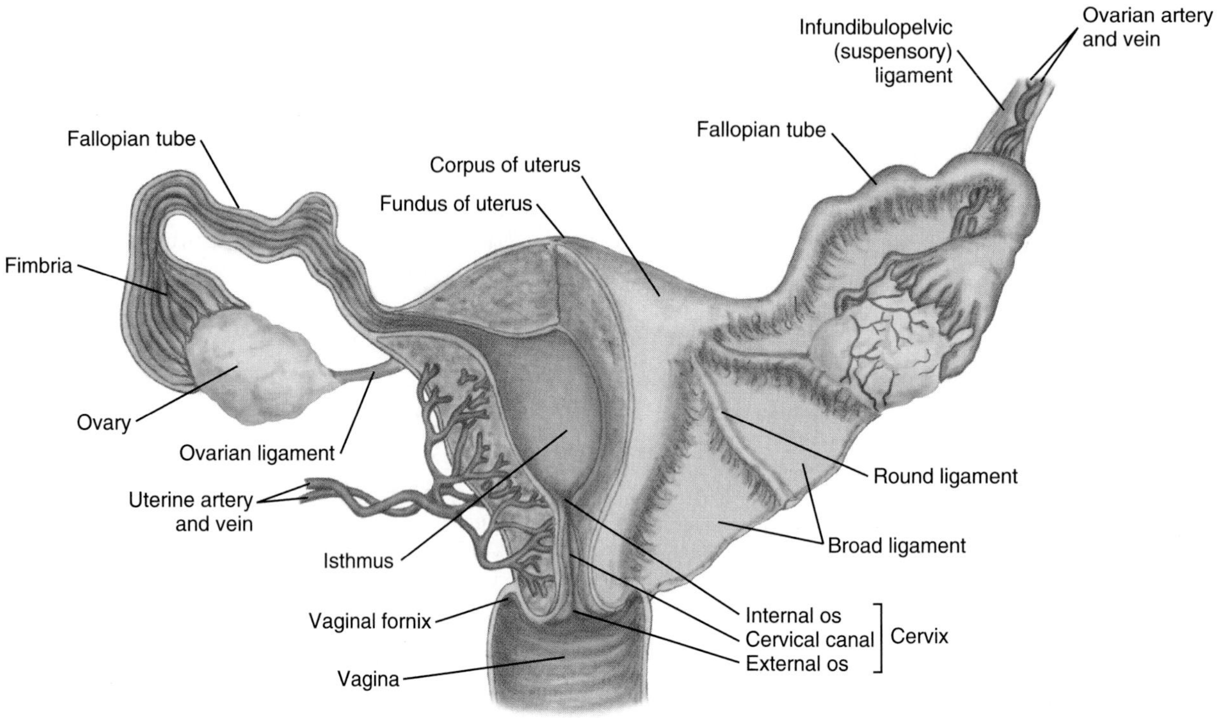

FIGURE 4-2 Internal female reproductive structures, anterior view.

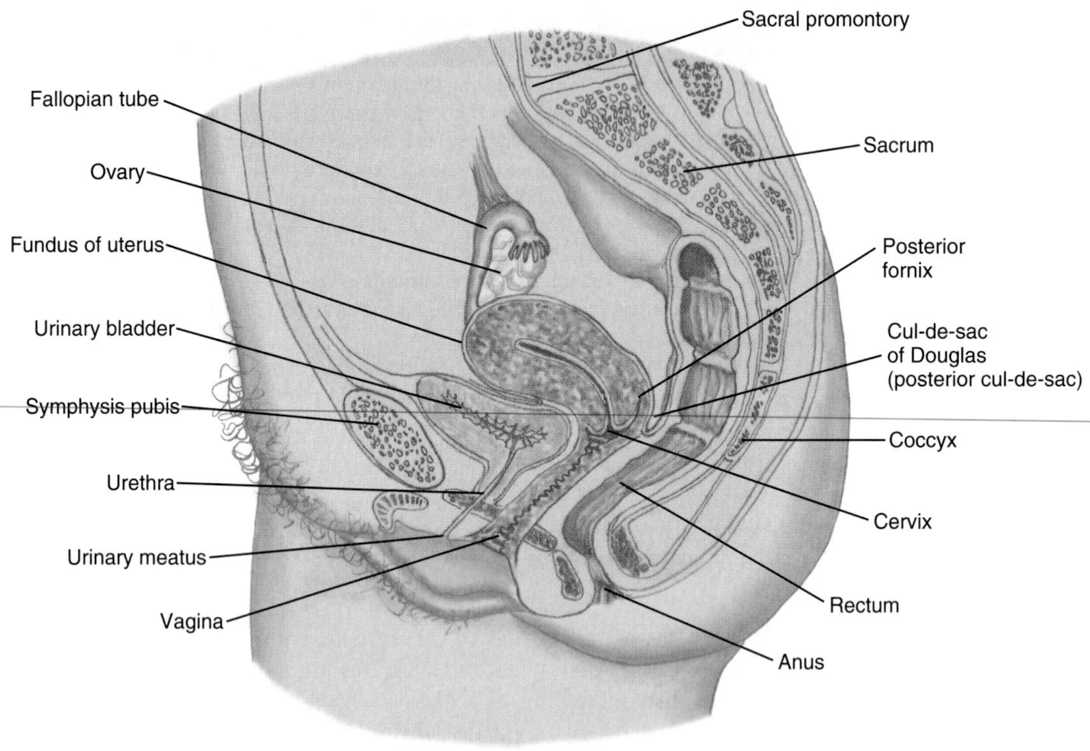

FIGURE 4-3 Internal female reproductive structures, midsagittal view.

The labia minora run parallel to and within the labia majora. The labia minora extend from the clitoris anteriorly and merge posteriorly to form the fourchette, which is the posterior rim of the vaginal introitus, or vaginal opening. The labia minora do not have pubic hair. They are highly vascular and respond to stimulation by becoming engorged with blood.

Clitoris

The clitoris is a small projection at the anterior junction of the two labia minora. This structure is composed of highly sensitive erectile tissue similar to that of the penis. The labia majora merge to form a prepuce over the clitoris.

Vestibule

The *vestibule* refers to structures enclosed by the labia minora. The urinary meatus, vaginal introitus, and ducts of Skene's and Bartholin's glands lie within the vestibule. Skene's, or periurethral, glands provide lubrication for the urethra. Bartholin's glands provide lubrication for the vaginal introitus, particularly during sexual arousal.

The vaginal introitus is surrounded by erectile tissue. During sexual stimulation, blood flows into the erectile tissue, allowing the introitus to tighten around the penis. This adds a massaging feeling that heightens the male's sexual sensations and encourages ejaculation.

The hymen is a thin fold of mucosa that partially separates the vagina and vestibule. The intactness or lack thereof of the hymen is not a criterion of virginity. The hymen may be broken by injury, tampon use, intercourse, or childbirth.

Perineum

The perineum is the most posterior part of the external female reproductive organs. The perineum extends from the fourchette anteriorly to the anus posteriorly. It is composed of fibrous and muscular tissues that provide support for pelvic structures. The perineum may be lacerated during childbirth, or it may be incised to enlarge the vaginal opening in a procedure called an *episiotomy.*

Internal Female Reproductive Organs

The internal reproductive structures are the vagina, uterus, fallopian tubes, and ovaries (Figures 4-2 and 4-3). These organs are supported and contained within the bony pelvis.

Vagina

The vagina is a tube of muscular and membranous tissue about 8 to 10 cm long that lies between the bladder anteriorly and the rectum posteriorly. The vagina connects the uterus above with the vestibule below. The vaginal lining has multiple folds, or rugae, and a muscular layer capable of marked distention during childbirth. The vagina is lubricated by secretions of the cervix (the lowermost part of the uterus) and Bartholin's glands.

The vagina does not end abruptly at the uterine opening but arches to form a pouchlike structure called the *vaginal fornix.* Each fornix is described by its location: anterior, posterior, and lateral.

The vagina has three major functions: (1) it allows discharge of the menstrual flow; (2) it is the female organ of coitus; and (3) it allows passage of the fetus from the uterus to outside the mother's body during childbirth.

Uterus

The uterus is a hollow, thick-walled, muscular organ shaped like a flat, upside-down pear. The uterus houses and nourishes the fetus until birth and then contracts rhythmically during labor to expel the fetus. Each month, the uterus is prepared for a pregnancy, regardless of whether conception occurs.

The uterus measures about 7.5 × 5 × 2.5 cm and is larger in women who have borne children. It is suspended above the bladder and is anterior to the rectum. Its normal position is anteverted (rotated forward) and slightly anteflexed (flexed forward).

Divisions of the Uterus. The uterus has three divisions: the corpus, isthmus, and cervix.

Corpus. The corpus, or body, is the upper division of the uterus. The uppermost part of the uterine corpus, above the area where the fallopian tubes enter the uterus, is the fundus of the uterus.

Isthmus. A narrower transition zone, the isthmus, is located between the corpus of the uterus and cervix. During late pregnancy the isthmus elongates and is known as the *lower uterine segment.*

Cervix. The cervix is the tubular "neck" of the lower uterus and is about 2 to 3 cm in length. During labor the cervix effaces (thins) and dilates (opens) to allow passage of the fetus. The os is the opening in the cervix between the uterus and vagina. The upper and lower cervix are marked by the internal and external os, respectively. The external os of a childless woman is round and smooth. After vaginal birth, the external os has an irregular, slitlike shape and may have tags of scar tissue.

Layers of the Uterus. The uterus has three layers: the perimetrium, myometrium, and endometrium.

Perimetrium. The perimetrium is the outer peritoneal layer of serous membrane that covers most of the uterus. Laterally, the perimetrium is continuous with the broad ligaments on either side of the uterus.

Myometrium. The myometrium is the middle layer of thick muscle. Most muscle fibers are concentrated in the upper uterus, and their number diminishes progressively toward the cervix. The myometrium con-

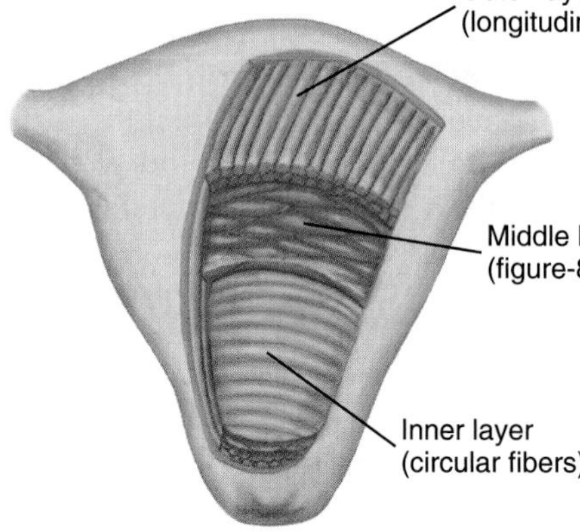

FIGURE 4-4 Layers of the myometrium showing the three types of smooth muscle fiber.

tains three types of smooth muscle fiber, each suited to specific functions in childbearing (Figure 4-4):

1. Longitudinal fibers are found mostly in the fundus and are designed to expel the fetus efficiently toward the pelvic outlet during birth.
2. Interlacing figure-8 fibers comprise the middle layer. These fibers contract after birth to compress blood vessels that pass between them to limit blood loss.
3. Circular fibers form constrictions where the fallopian tubes enter the uterus and surround the internal cervical os. Circular fibers prevent reflux of menstrual blood and tissue into the fallopian tubes, promote normal implantation of the fertilized ovum by controlling its entry into the uterus, and retain the fetus until the appropriate time of birth.

Endometrium. The endometrium is the inner layer of the uterus. It responds to the cyclic variations of estrogen and progesterone during the female reproductive cycle (see p. 66). The endometrium has two layers:

1. The basal layer is the area nearest the myometrium that regenerates the functional layer of the endometrium after each menstrual period and after childbirth.
2. The functional layer lies above the basal layer and contains the endometrial arteries, veins, and glands; this layer is shed during each menstrual period and after childbirth in the lochia.

Fallopian Tubes

The fallopian tubes, also called *oviducts,* are 8 to 14 cm long and quite narrow (2 to 3 mm at their narrowest and 5 to 8 mm at their widest). They are a pathway for the ovum between the ovary and uterus. Fertilization occurs in the fallopian tubes. Each fallopian tube enters the upper uterus at the cornu, or horn, of the uterus.

The fallopian tubes are lined with folded epithelium containing cilia that beat rhythmically toward the uterine cavity to propel the ovum through the tube. The rough, folded surface of its lining and small diameter make the fallopian tube vulnerable to blockage from infection or scar tissue. Tubal blockage may result in sterility or a tubal pregnancy because the fertilized ovum cannot enter the uterus for proper implantation.

The fallopian tubes have the following four divisions:

1. The interstitial portion runs into the uterine cavity and lies within the uterine wall.
2. The isthmus is the narrow part adjacent to the uterus.
3. The ampulla is the wider area of the tube lateral to the isthmus, where fertilization occurs.
4. The infundibulum is the wide, funnel-shaped terminal end of the tube. Fimbria are fingerlike processes that surround the infundibulum.

The fallopian tubes are not directly connected to the ovary. At ovulation the ovum is expelled into the abdominal cavity. Wavelike motions of the fimbria draw the ovum into the tube. However, the tubal isthmus remains contracted until 3 days after conception to allow the fertilized ovum to develop within the tube. Initial growth of the fertilized ovum within the fallopian tube promotes its normal implantation in the upper uterus.

Ovaries

The ovaries are the female gonads, or sex glands. They have two functions: (1) sex hormone production and (2) maturation of an ovum during each reproductive cycle.

The ovaries secrete estrogen and progesterone in varying amounts during a woman's reproductive cycle to prepare the uterine lining for pregnancy. Ovarian hormone secretion gradually declines to very low levels during the climacteric.

At birth the ovary contains all the ova it will ever have. About 1 million immature ova are present at birth. Many of these degenerate during childhood, and at puberty, 200,000 to 400,000 viable ova remain. Many ova begin the maturation process during each reproductive cycle, but most never reach maturity. During a woman's reproductive life, only about 400 of the ova ever mature enough to be released and fertilized. By the time a woman reaches the climacteric, almost all her ova have been released during ovulation or have regressed. The few remaining ova are unresponsive to stimulating hormones and do not mature.

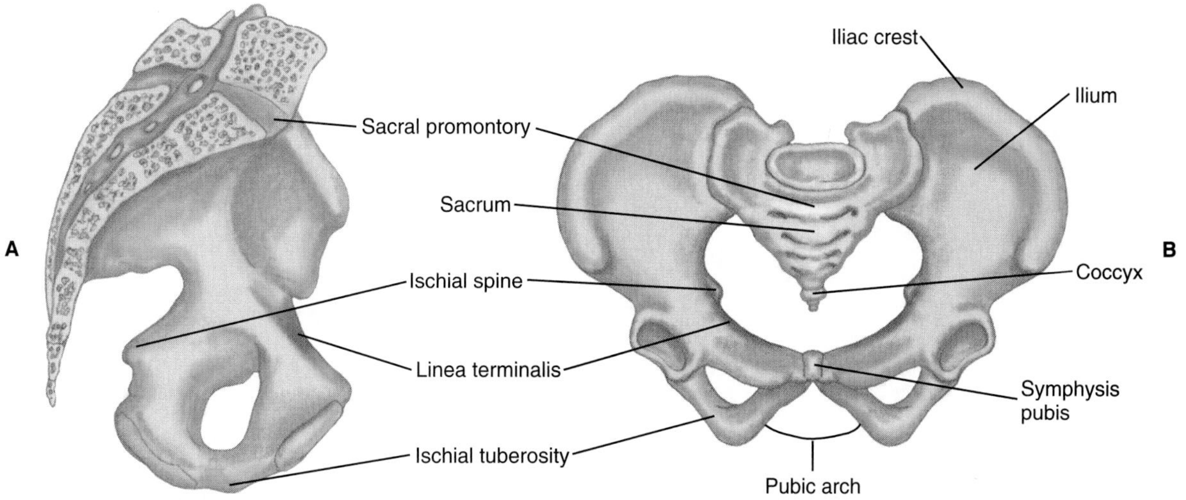

FIGURE 4-5 Structures of the bony pelvis, shown in lateral **(A)** and anterior **(B)** views.

Check Your Reading

6. What is the vulva? Describe the location of each of these external female organs: labia majora and minora, clitoris, urinary meatus, vaginal introitus, hymen, and perineum.
7. What are the three divisions of the uterus? Where is the fundus located?
8. Describe the three myometrial layers of the uterus. What is the function of each layer?
9. How do the fallopian tubes conduct the ovum from the ovary to the uterus? Why does the fertilized ovum first grow within the fallopian tube?
10. What are the two functions of the ovaries?

Support Structures

The bony pelvis supports and protects the lower abdominal and internal reproductive organs. Muscles and ligaments provide added support for the internal organs of the pelvis against the downward force of gravity and increases in intraabdominal pressure.

Pelvis

The bony pelvis is a basin-shaped structure at the lower end of the spine (Figure 4-5). Its posterior wall is formed by the sacrum. The side and anterior pelvic walls are composed of three fused bones: the ilium, ischium, and pubis.

The linea terminalis, also called the *pelvic brim* or *ileopectineal line,* is an imaginary line that divides the upper, or false, pelvis from the lower, or true, pelvis. The false pelvis provides support for the internal organs and the upper part of the body. The true pelvis is most important during childbirth (see Chapter 12).

Muscles

Paired muscles enclose the lower pelvis and provide support for internal reproductive, urinary, and bowel structures (Figure 4-6). In addition, a fibromuscular sheet, the pelvic fascia, provides support for the pelvic organs. Vaginal and urethral openings are located in the pelvic fascia.

The levator ani is a collection of three pairs of muscles: the pubococcygeus, which is also called the *pubovaginal muscle* in the female; the puborectal; and the iliococcygeus. These muscles support internal pelvic structures and resist increases in the intraabdominal pressure.

The ischiocavernosus muscle extends from the clitoris to the ischial tuberosities on each side of the lower bony pelvis. The two transverse perineal muscles extend from fibrous tissue of the perineum to the two ischial tuberosities, stabilizing the center of the perineum.

Ligaments

Seven pairs of ligaments maintain the internal reproductive organs and their nerve and blood supplies in their proper positions within the pelvis (see Figure 4-2).

Lateral Support. Paired ligaments stabilize the uterus and ovaries laterally and keep them in the midline of the pelvis. The broad ligament is a sheet of tissue extending from each side of the uterus to the lateral pelvic wall. The round ligament and fallopian tube mark the upper border of the broad ligament, and the lower edge is bounded by the uterine blood vessels. Within the two broad ligaments are the ovarian ligaments, blood vessels, and lymphatics.

The right and left cardinal ligaments provide support to the lower uterus and vagina. They extend from the lateral walls of the cervix and vagina to the side walls of the pelvis.

The two ovarian ligaments connect the ovaries to the lateral uterine walls. The infundibulopelvic (suspensory) ligaments connect the lateral ovary and distal

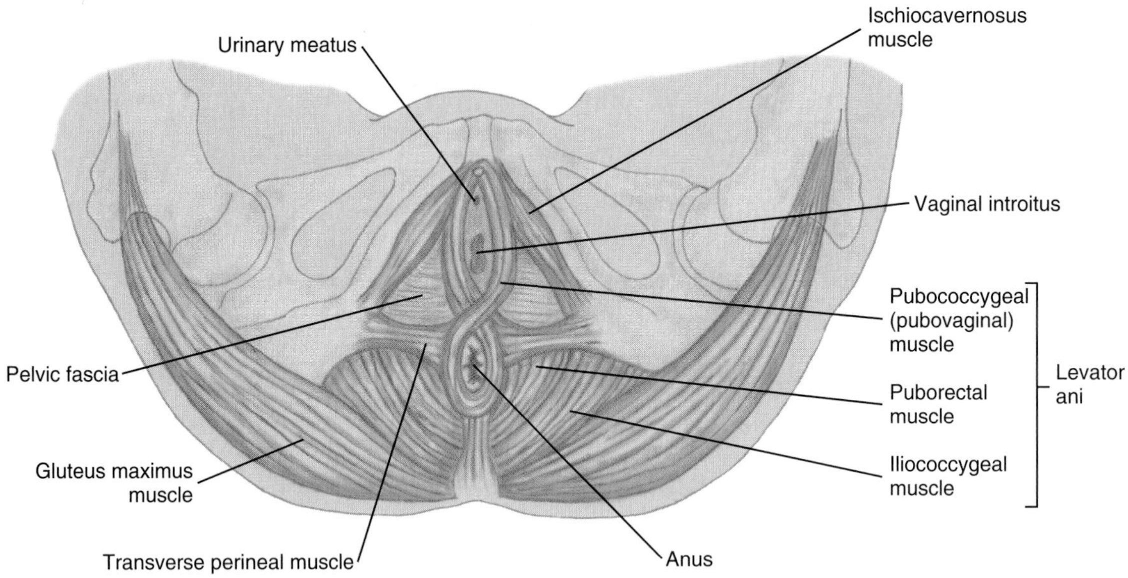

FIGURE 4-6 Muscles of the female pelvic floor.

fallopian tubes to the pelvic side walls. The infundibulopelvic ligament also carries the blood vessel and nerve supply for the ovary.

Anterior Support. Two pairs of ligaments provide anterior support for the internal reproductive organs. The round ligaments connect the upper uterus to the connective tissue of the labia majora. These ligaments maintain the uterus in its normal anteflexed position and help direct the fetal presenting part against the cervix during labor.

The pubocervical ligaments support the cervix anteriorly. They connect the cervix and interior surface of the symphysis pubis.

Posterior Support. The uterosacral ligaments provide posterior support, extending from the lower posterior uterus to the sacrum. These ligaments also contain sympathetic and parasympathetic nerves of the autonomic nervous system.

Blood Supply

The uterine blood supply is carried by the uterine arteries, which are branches of the internal iliac artery. These vessels enter the uterus at the lower border of the broad ligament near the isthmus of the uterus. The vessels branch downward to supply the cervix and vagina and upward to supply the uterus. The upper branch also supplies the ovaries and fallopian tubes. The vessels are coiled to allow for elongation as the uterus enlarges and rises from the pelvis during pregnancy. Blood drains into the uterine veins and from there into the internal iliac veins.

Additional ovarian and tubal blood supply is carried by the ovarian artery, which arises from the abdominal aorta. The ovarian blood supply drains into the two ovarian veins. The left ovarian vein drains into the left renal vein, and the right ovarian vein drains directly into the inferior vena cava.

Nerve Supply

Most functions of the reproductive system are under involuntary, or unconscious, control. Nerves of the autonomic nervous system from the uterovaginal plexus and inferior hypogastric plexus control automatic functions of the reproductive system.

Sensory and motor nerves that innervate the reproductive organs enter the spinal cord at the T12 through L2 levels. These nerves are important for pain management during childbearing (see Chapter 15).

Check Your Reading

11. Where is the true pelvis located?
12. What are the purposes of the muscles of the pelvis? What are the purposes of the ligaments?

FEMALE REPRODUCTIVE CYCLE

The *female reproductive cycle* describes the regular and recurrent changes in the anterior pituitary secretions, ovaries, and uterine endometrium that are designed to prepare the body for pregnancy (Figure 4-7). Associated changes in the cervical mucus promote fertilization during each cycle. The female reproductive cycle is often called the *menstrual cycle* because men-

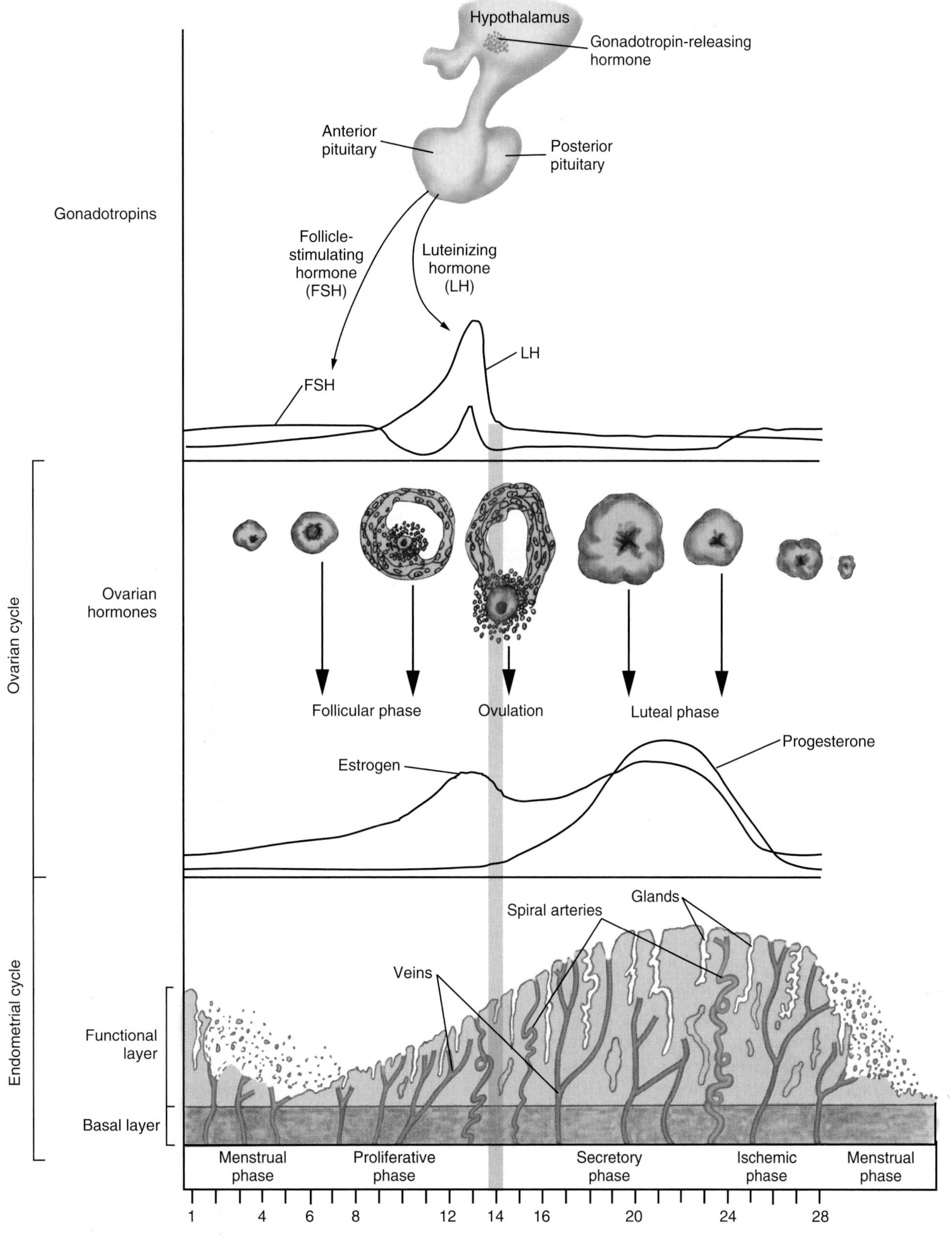

FIGURE 4-7 The female reproductive cycle showing the changes in hormone secretion from the anterior pituitary and interrelated changes in the ovary and uterine endometrium.

struation provides a marker for each cycle's beginning and end if pregnancy does not occur.

The female reproductive cycle is driven by a feedback loop between the anterior pituitary and ovaries. A feedback loop is a change in the level of one secretion in response to a change in the level of another secretion. The feedback loop may be positive, in which rising levels of one secretion cause another to rise, or negative, in which rising levels of one secretion cause another to fall.

The duration of the cycle is about 28 days, although it may range from 20 to 45 days (Guyton & Hall, 2000). Significant deviations from the 28-day cycle are associated with reduced fertility. The first day of the menstrual period is counted as day 1 of the woman's cycle. The female reproductive cycle is further divided into two cycles that reflect changes in the ovaries and uterine endometrium.

Ovarian Cycle

In response to GnRH from the woman's hypothalamus, the anterior pituitary secretes FSH and LH. These secretions stimulate the ovaries to mature and release an ovum and secrete additional hormones that will prepare the endometrium for implantation of a fertilized ovum. The ovarian cycle consists of three phases: the follicular, ovulatory, and luteal.

Follicular Phase

The follicular phase is the period during which an ovum matures. It begins with the first day of menstruation and ends about 14 days later in a 28-day cycle. The length of this phase varies more among different women than do the lengths of the other two phases. The fall in estrogen and progesterone secretion by the ovary just before menstruation stimulates secretion of FSH and LH by the anterior pituitary. As the FSH and LH levels rise slightly, 6 to 12 graafian follicles, each containing an immature ovum, begin to grow. Each follicle secretes fluid containing high levels of estrogen, which accelerates maturation by making the follicle more sensitive to the effects of FSH. Eventually, one follicle outgrows the others to reach maturity. The mature follicle secretes large amounts of estrogen, which depresses FSH secretion. The dip in FSH secretion just before ovulation blocks further maturation of the less-developed follicles. Occasionally, more than one follicle matures and releases its ovum, which can lead to a multifetal pregnancy. Women who take fertility drugs usually intentionally mature and release multiple ova for assisted reproductive techniques (see Chapter 32).

Ovulatory Phase

Near the middle of a 28-day reproductive cycle and about 2 days before ovulation, LH secretion rises markedly. Secretion of FSH also rises but to a lesser extent than that of LH. These surges in LH and FSH cause a slight fall in follicular estrogen production and a rise in progesterone secretion, which stimulates final maturation of a single follicle and release of its ovum. Ovulation marks the beginning of the luteal phase of the female reproductive cycle and occurs about 14 days before the next menstrual period.

The mature follicle is a mass of cells with a fluid-filled chamber. A smaller mass of cells houses the ovum within this chamber. At ovulation a blisterlike projection called a *stigma* forms on the wall of the follicle, the follicle ruptures, and the ovum with its surrounding cells is released from the surface of the ovary, where it is picked up by the fimbriated end of the fallopian tube for transport to the uterus.

Luteal Phase

After ovulation and under the influence of LH, the remaining cells of the old follicle persist for about 12 days as a corpus luteum. The corpus luteum secretes estrogen and large amounts of progesterone to prepare the endometrium for a fertilized ovum. During this phase, levels of FSH and LH decrease in response to higher levels of estrogen and progesterone. If the ovum is fertilized, it secretes a hormone (chorionic gonadotropin) that causes persistence of the corpus luteum to maintain an early pregnancy. If the ovum is not fertilized, FSH and LH fall to low levels and the corpus luteum regresses. Decline of estrogen and progesterone with corpus luteum regression results in menstruation as the uterine lining breaks down.

The loss of estrogen and progesterone from the corpus luteum at the end of one cycle stimulates the anterior pituitary to again secrete more FSH and LH, initiating a new female reproductive cycle. The old corpus luteum is replaced by fibrous tissue called the *corpus albicans.*

Endometrial Cycle

The uterine endometrium responds to ovarian hormone stimulation with cyclic changes. Three phases mark the changes in the endometrium: the proliferative, secretory, and menstrual.

Proliferative Phase

The proliferative phase occurs as the ovum matures and is released during the first half of the ovarian cycle. After completion of a menstrual period the endometrium is very thin. The basal layer of endometrial cells remains after menstruation. These cells multiply to form new endometrial epithelium and endometrial glands under the stimulation of estrogen secreted by the maturing ovarian follicles. Endometrial spiral arteries and endometrial veins elongate to accompany thickening of the functional endometrial layer and nourish the proliferating cells. As ovulation approaches, the endometrial glands secrete a thin, stringy mucus that aids entry of sperm into the uterus.

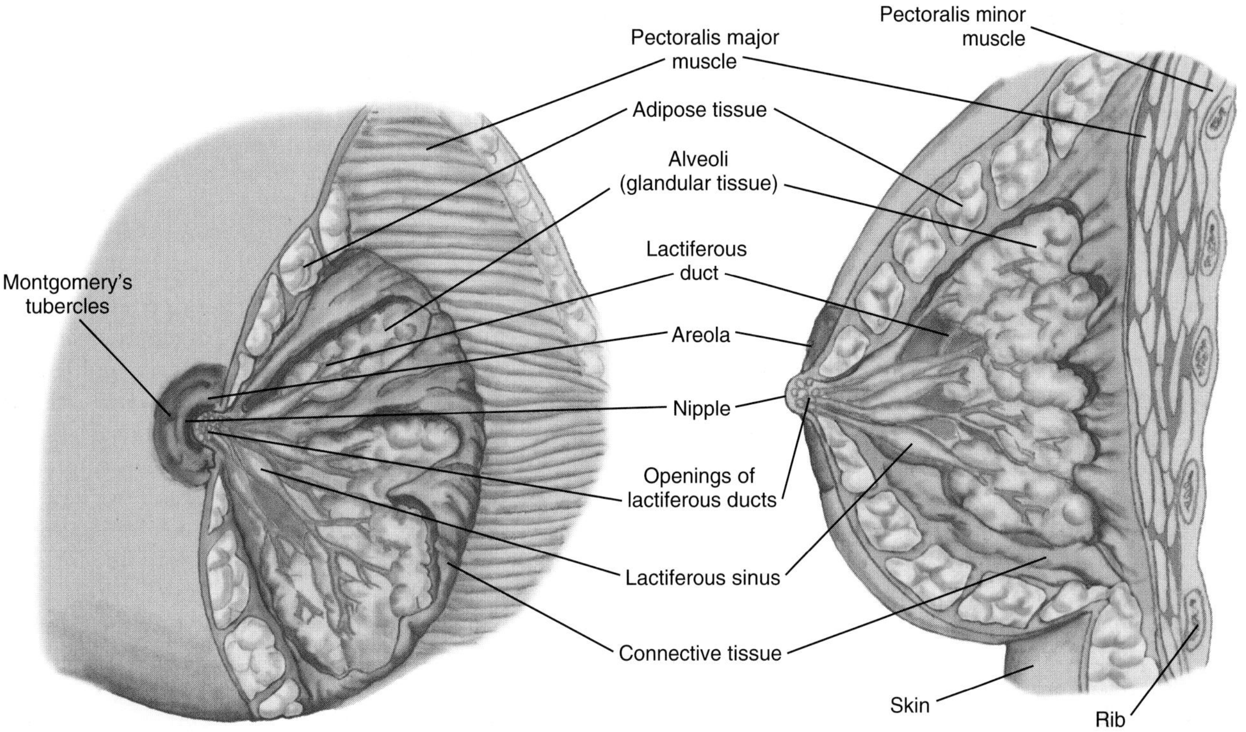

FIGURE 4-8 Structures of the female breast.

Secretory Phase

The secretory phase occurs during the last half of the ovarian cycle as the uterus is prepared to receive a fertilized ovum. The endometrium continues to thicken under the influence of estrogen and progesterone from the corpus luteum, reaching its maximum thickness of 5 to 6 mm. The blood vessels and endometrial glands become twisted and dilated.

Progesterone from the corpus luteum causes the thick endometrium to secrete substances to nourish a fertilized ovum. Large quantities of glycogen, proteins, lipids, and minerals are stored within the endometrium, awaiting arrival of the ovum.

Menstrual Phase

If fertilization does not occur, the corpus luteum regresses and its production of estrogen and progesterone falls. About 2 days before the onset of mensturation, vasospasm of the endometrial blood vessels causes the endometrium to become ischemic and necrotic. The necrotic areas of endometrium separate from the basal layers, resulting in the menstrual flow. The duration of the menstrual phase is about 5 days.

During a menstrual period, women lose about 40 ml of blood. Because of the recurrent loss of blood, many women are mildly anemic during their reproductive years, especially if their diets are low in iron.

Changes in Cervical Mucus

During most of the female reproductive cycle, the mucus of the cervix is scant, thick, and sticky. Just before ovulation, cervical mucus becomes thin, clear, and elastic to promote passage of sperm into the uterus and fallopian tube, where they can fertilize the ovum. *Spinnbarkeit* refers to the elasticity of cervical mucus. A woman may assess the elasticity of her cervical mucus to either avoid or promote conception (see Procedure 33-1).

Check Your Reading

13. Which ovarian structures secrete estrogen and progesterone during the female reproductive cycle?
14. What three ovarian phases occur during each female reproductive cycle?
15. How does the uterine endometrium change during a woman's reproductive cycle?
16. Why is it important for the cervical mucus to become thin, clear, and elastic around the time of ovulation?

THE FEMALE BREAST

Structure

The breasts, or mammary glands, are not directly functional in reproduction, but they secrete milk after childbirth to nourish the infant. The small, raised nipple is located at the center of each breast (Figure 4-8). The nipple is composed of sensitive erectile tissue and may respond to sexual stimulation. A larger circular areola surrounds the nipple. Both the nipple and areola are darker than surrounding skin. Montgomery's tubercles are sebaceous glands in the areola. They are inactive and not obvious except during pregnancy and lactation, when they enlarge and secrete a substance that keeps the nipple soft.

Within each breast are lobes of glandular tissue that secrete milk. These lobes are arranged in a pattern similar to spokes of a wheel around the hub. Between 15 and 20 of these lobes are arranged around and behind the nipple and areola. Fibrous tissue and fat in the breast support the glandular tissue, blood vessels, lymphatics, and nerves.

Alveoli are small sacs that contain acinar cells to secrete milk. The acinar cells extract the necessary substances from the mammary blood supply to manufacture milk when the breasts are properly stimulated by the anterior pituitary gland. Myoepithelial cells surround the alveoli to contract and eject the milk into the ductal system when signaled by secretion of the hormone oxytocin from the posterior pituitary gland.

The alveoli drain into lactiferous ducts, which connect to drain milk from all areas of the breast. The lactiferous ducts become wider under the areola and are called *lactiferous sinuses* in this area. The lactiferous sinuses narrow again as they open to the outside in the nipple.

Function

The breasts are inactive until puberty, when rising estrogen levels stimulate growth of the glandular tissue. In addition, fat is deposited in the breasts, resulting in the mature female contour. The amount of fat is the major determinant of breast size; the amount of glandular tissue is similar for all mature women. Thus breast size is unrelated to the amount of milk a woman can produce during lactation.

During pregnancy, high levels of estrogen and progesterone produced by the placenta stimulate growth of the alveoli and ductal system to prepare them for lactation. Prolactin secretion by the anterior pituitary gland stimulates milk production during pregnancy, but this effect is inhibited by estrogen and progesterone produced by the placenta. Inhibiting effects of estrogen and progesterone stop when the placenta is expelled after birth, and active milk production occurs in response to the infant's nursing.

Check Your Reading

17. What is the function of Montgomery's tubercles?
18. How is a woman's breast size related to the amount of milk she can produce?
19. Why is milk not actively secreted during pregnancy?

MALE REPRODUCTIVE ANATOMY AND PHYSIOLOGY

External Male Reproductive Organs

The male has two external organs of reproduction, the penis and scrotum (Figure 4-9).

Penis

The penis has two functions. As part of the urinary tract, it carries urine from the bladder to the exterior during urination. As a reproductive organ, the penis deposits semen into the female vagina during coitus.

The penis is composed mostly of erectile tissue, which is spongy tissue with many small spaces inside. The three areas of erectile tissue are the corpus spongiosum, which surrounds the urethra, and two columns of the corpus cavernosum on each side of the penis.

The penis is flaccid most of the time because the small spaces within the erectile tissue are collapsed. During sexual stimulation, arteries within the penis dilate and veins are partly occluded, trapping blood in the spongy tissue. Entrapment of blood within the penis causes erection and enables the man to penetrate the vagina during sexual intercourse.

The glans is the distal end of the penis. The urinary meatus is centered in the end of the glans. The loose skin of the prepuce, or foreskin, covers the glans. The prepuce may be removed during circumcision, a surgical procedure usually performed during the newborn period, although it may be performed later. The glans is very sensitive to tactile stimulation, which adds to a man's sensation during coitus.

Scrotum

The scrotum is a pouch of thin skin and muscle suspended behind the penis. The skin of the scrotum is somewhat darker than the surrounding skin and is covered with small ridges called *rugae.* The scrotum is divided internally by a septum. One of the male gonads (testicle) is contained within each pocket of the scrotum.

The scrotum's main purpose is to keep the testes cooler than the core body temperature. Formation of normal male sperm requires that the testes not be too warm. A cremaster muscle is attached to each testicle to either draw them closer to the body for warming or relax them and allow them to fall from the body for cooling.

Internal Male Reproductive Organs

The functions of the male external and internal organs are summarized in Table 4-4.

Testes

The male gonads, or testes, have two functions: (1) they serve as endocrine glands and (2) they produce male gametes, or sperm, also called *spermatozoa.*

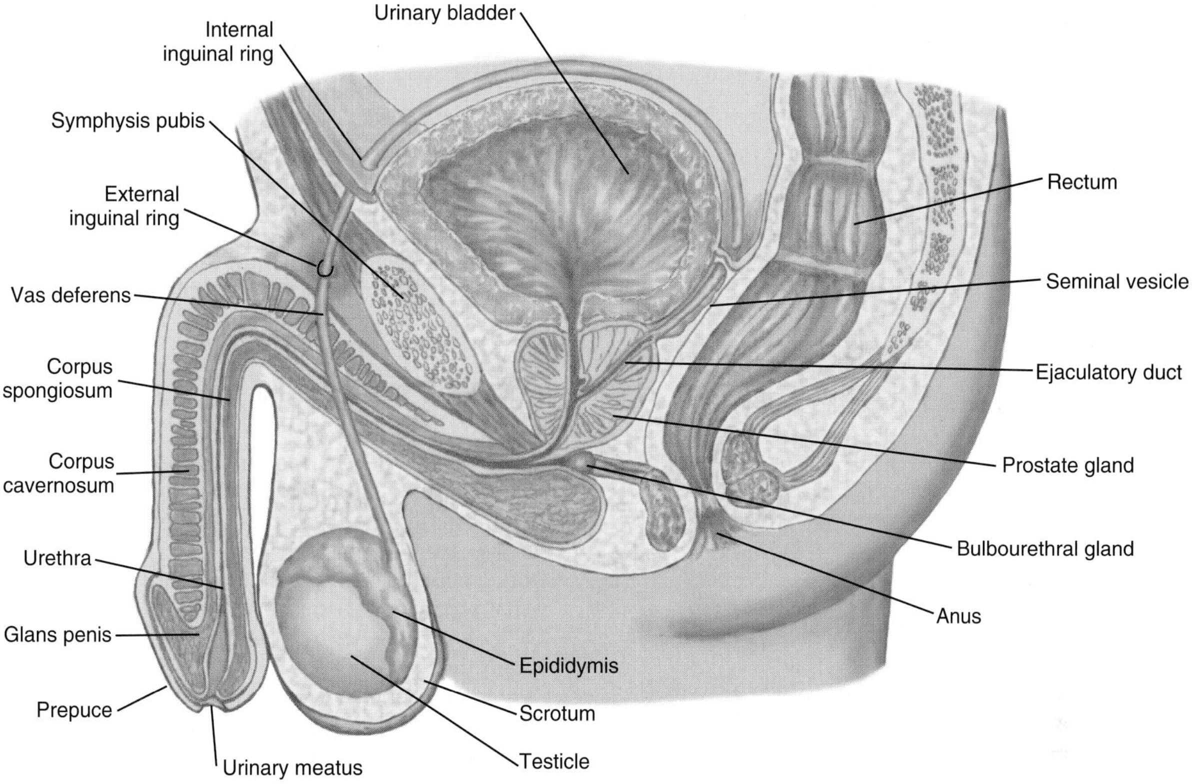

FIGURE 4-9 Structures of the male reproductive system, midsagittal view.

Table 4-4

FUNCTIONS OF MALE REPRODUCTIVE AND ACCESSORY ORGANS

Organ	Function
Penis	1. Conduit for urine from bladder 2. Male organ of sexual intercourse
Scrotum	Housing of testes and maintenance of their temperature at a level cooler than the trunk of the body, thus promoting normal sperm formation
Testes	1. Endocrine glands that secrete the primary male hormone (testosterone) 2. Sperm formation
Seminiferous tubules	Location of spermatogenesis within the testes
Epididymis	1. Storage of some sperm 2. Final sperm maturation 3. The location where sperm develop the ability to be motile
Vas deferens	1. Storage of sperm 2. Conduction of sperm from the epididymis to the urethra
Seminal vesicles, prostate, and bulbourethral glands	Secretion of seminal fluids that carry sperm and provide for the following: 1. Nourishment of sperm 2. Protection of sperm from the hostile acidic environment of the vagina 3. Enhancement of the motility of sperm 4. Washing of all sperm from the urethra

Androgens (male sex hormones) are the primary endocrine secretions of the testes. Androgens are produced by Leydig cells of the testes. The primary androgen produced by the testes is testosterone.

Unlike the female, who experiences a cyclic pattern of hormone secretion, the male secretes testosterone in a relatively even pattern. A feedback loop with the hypothalamus and anterior pituitary stabilizes testosterone levels. A small amount of testosterone is converted to estrogen in the male and is necessary for sperm formation.

Spermatogenesis occurs within tiny coiled tubes, the seminiferous tubules of the testes (Figure 4-10). Leydig cells are interstitial cells that support the seminiferous tubules and secrete testosterone, which is necessary to form new cells that will mature into sperm. Sertoli cells

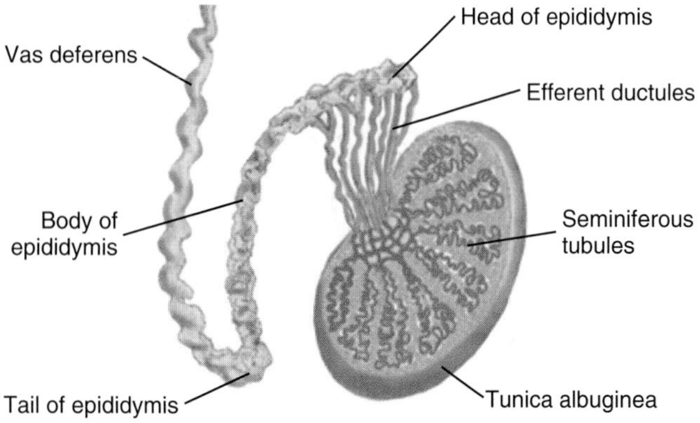

FIGURE 4-10 Internal structures of the testis. Initial production of sperm begins within the tiny, coiled seminiferous tubules. Immature sperm pass from the seminiferous tubules to the epididymis and then to the vas deferens. During their passage through these structures, the sperm mature and acquire the ability to propel themselves.

within the seminiferous tubules respond to FSH secretion by nourishing and supporting sperm as they mature. Unlike the female, who has a lifetime supply of ova in her gonads at birth, the male does not begin producing sperm until puberty. The normal male produces new sperm throughout life, although production declines with age.

At ejaculation, about 40 to 300 million sperm are deposited in the vagina (Surrey, 1998). This large number is needed for normal fertility, although a single sperm fertilizes the ovum. Only a few sperm ever reach the fallopian tube, where an ovum may be available for fertilization. When the first sperm penetrates the ovum, changes within the ovum prevent other sperm from also fertilizing it (see Chapter 6.)

Accessory Ducts and Glands

From the seminiferous tubules, sperm pass into the epididymis within the scrotum for storage and final maturation. In the epididymis, sperm develop the ability to be motile, although secretions within the epididymis inhibit actual motility until ejaculation occurs.

The epididymis empties into the vas deferens, where larger numbers of sperm are stored. The vas deferens then leads upward into the pelvis, then downward toward the penis through the internal and external inguinal rings. Within the pelvis the vas deferens joins the ejaculatory duct before connecting to the urethra.

Three glands—the seminal vesicles, prostate, and bulbourethral gland—secrete seminal fluids that carry sperm into the vagina during intercourse. The seminal fluid has four functions: (1) nourish the sperm, (2) protect the sperm from the hostile pH (acidic) environment of the vagina, (3) enhance the motility of the sperm, and (4) wash the sperm from the urethra so that the maximum number are deposited in the vagina.

Check Your Reading

20. What are the two functions of the penis?
21. What two types of erectile tissue are in the penis? What is their function?
22. Why is it important for the testes to be contained within the scrotum?
23. What are the two functions of the testes?

SUMMARY CONCEPTS

- Initial prenatal development of the reproductive organs is similar for both males and females. If a critical part of the Y chromosome is not present at conception, female reproductive structures will develop.
- During puberty, the reproductive organs become fully functional and secondary sex characteristics develop.
- The external changes of puberty begin about 2 years earlier in girls than in boys.
- Females are generally shorter than males because they begin their growth spurt at an earlier age and complete it more quickly than boys.
- The onset of menstruation (menarche) is an obvious marker of puberty in girls.
- Girls often do not ovulate in early menstrual cycles, although they can ovulate even before the first cycle. Therefore a girl can become pregnant before her first menstrual period if she is sexually active.
- The onset of puberty is more subtle in boys than in girls, beginning with growth of the testes and penis.
- Boys may have nocturnal emissions of seminal fluid, which may be distressing unless they are educated that these events are normal and expected.
- At birth, a girl has all the ova she will ever have. New ova are not formed after birth; almost all are depleted when the woman reaches the climacteric.
- The female reproductive cycle is often called the *menstrual cycle.* It includes changes in the anterior pituitary gland, ovaries, and uterine endometrium to prepare for a fertilized ovum. The character of cervical mucus also changes to encourage fertilization.
- Breast size is unrelated to glandular tissue or the quantity or quality of milk a woman can produce for her infant after childbirth. Breast size is primarily related to the amount of fat present.
- For normal sperm formation, a man's testes must be cooler than his core body temperature.
- Seminal fluids secreted by the seminal vesicles, prostate, and bulbourethral glands nourish and protect the sperm, enhance their motility, and ensure that most sperm are deposited in the vagina during sexual intercourse.

REFERENCES & READINGS

Blackburn, S.T., & Loper, D.L. (1992). *Maternal, fetal, and neonatal physiology.* Philadelphia: W.B. Saunders.

Cunningham, F.G., MacDonald, P.C., Gant, N.F., Leveno, K.J., Gilstrap, L.C., Hankins, G.D.V., et al. (1997). *Williams obstetrics* (20th ed.). Norwalk, CT: Appleton & Lange.
Georges, J.M. (2000). Female genital and reproductive function. In L.C. Copstead & J. Banasik (Eds.), *Pathophysiology: Biological and behavioral perspectives* (2nd ed., pp. 648-666). Philadelphia: W.B. Saunders.
Guyton, A.C., & Hall, J.E. (2000). *Textbook of medical physiology* (10th ed.). Philadelphia: W.B. Saunders.
Kim, M.H. (2000). Secondary amenorrhea. In F.P. Zuspan & E.J. Quilligan (Eds.), *Current therapy in obstetrics and gynecology* (5th ed., pp. 146-150). Philadelphia: W.B. Saunders.
Mikkelsen, D., & Cagle, C.S. (2000). Male genital and reproductive function. In L.C. Copstead & J. Banasik (Eds.), *Pathophysiology: Biological and behavioral perspectives* (2nd ed., pp. 708-725). Philadelphia: W.B. Saunders.
Moore, K.L., & Persaud, T.V.N. (1998). *The developing human* (6th ed.). Philadelphia: W.B. Saunders.
Needlman, R.D. (2000). Adolescence. In R.E. Behrman, R. M. Kliegman, & H. B. Jenson (Eds.), *Nelson Textbook of Pediatrics* (16th ed., pp. 52-57). Philadelphia: W.B. Saunders.
Riddick, D.H. (2000). Primary amenorrhea. In F.P. Zuspan & E.J. Quilligan (Eds.), *Current therapy in obstetrics and gynecology* (5th ed., pp. 143-146). Philadelphia: W.B. Saunders.
Surrey, E.S., Lu, J.K.H., & Joot, P.J. (1998). The menstrual cycle, ovulation, fertilization, implantation, and the placenta. In N.F. Stacker & J.G. Moore (Eds.), *Essentials of obstetrics and gynecology* (3rd ed., pp. 59-76). Philadelphia: W.B. Saunders.

5

Hereditary and Environmental Influences on Childbearing

OBJECTIVES

1. Describe the structure and function of normal human genes and chromosomes.
2. Give examples of ways to study genes and chromosomes.
3. Explain some of the benefits and ethical implications of the Human Genome Project.
4. Describe the characteristics of single gene traits and their transmission from parent to child.
5. Relate chromosomal abnormalities to spontaneous abortion and birth defects in the infant.
6. Explain characteristics of multifactorial birth defects.
7. Identify environmental factors that can interfere with prenatal development and ways to prevent or reduce their effects.
8. Describe the process of genetic counseling.
9. Explain the role of the nurse in caring for individuals or families with concerns about birth defects.

DEFINITIONS

Allele An alternate form of a gene.

Autosome Any of the 22 pairs of chromosomes other than the sex chromosomes.

Birth Defect An abnormality of structure, function, or body metabolism present at birth that results in physical or mental disability or is fatal (March of Dimes Birth Defects Foundation, 1999a).

Congenital Present at birth.

Diploid Having a pair of chromosomes (46 in humans) that represents one copy of every chromosome from each parent; the number of chromosomes normally present in body cells other than gametes.

DEFINITIONS—cont'd

Familial Presence of a trait or condition in a family more often than would be expected by chance alone.

Gamete Reproductive cell or germ cell; in the female an ovum and in the male a spermatozoon.

Gene Segment of DNA that directs the production of a specific product needed for body structure or function.

Genetic Pertaining to the genes or chromosomes.

Genotype Genetic makeup of an individual.

Haploid Having one copy of a chromosome from each pair (23 in humans, or half the diploid number); normal for gametes.

Heterozygous Having two different alleles for a genetic trait.

Homologous Chromosomes that pair during meiosis, one received from the person's mother and one from the father.

Homozygous Having two identical alleles for a genetic trait.

Karyotype A display of a cell's chromosomes, arranged from largest to smallest pairs.

Monosomy Presence of only one of a chromosome pair in every body cell.

Mutation Alteration in DNA sequence in a gene, usually one that adversely affects its function.

Pedigree A graphic representation of a family's medical and hereditary history and the relationships among the family members (also called a *genogram*).

Phenotype The outward expression of a person's genetic makeup; observed characteristics produced by the interaction of genes and environment.

Polymorphism Alternate form of a gene found in the population at a frequency greater than 1%.

Polyploidy Having additional full sets of chromosomes, such as 69 or 92.

Sex Chromosome The X or Y chromosome; females have two X chromosomes and males have one X and one Y chromosome.

Somatic Cells Body cells other than the gametes, or germ cells.

Teratogen An environmental agent that can cause defects in a developing fetus during pregnancy.

Translocation Exchange of genetic material between nonhomologous chromosomes.

Trisomy Presence of three copies of a chromosome in each body cell.

Hereditary and environmental forces shape a person's development from before conception until death. As people learn more about genes and their influences on the body's function, they are discovering that genes have more influence on health and disease than was previously thought. The nurse needs a basic knowledge of these forces to better understand disorders evident at birth and those that develop later in life. This chapter reviews the basics of hereditary influences on development and the impact of environmental factors in causing birth defects. The nursing role in relation to genetic knowledge is also discussed.

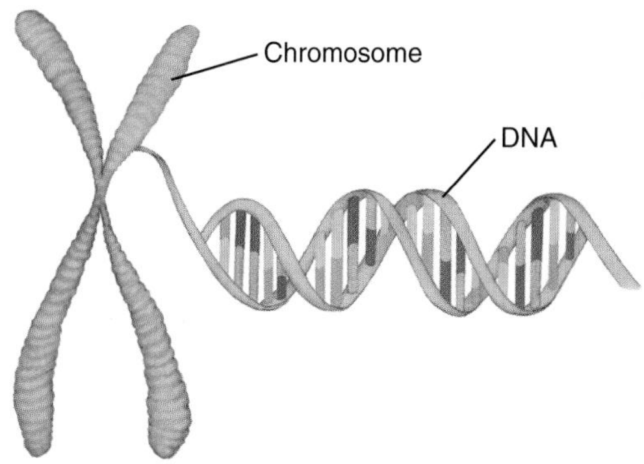

FIGURE 5-1 The DNA helix is the building block of genes and chromosomes.

HEREDITARY INFLUENCES

Hereditary influences on development result from the directions for cellular functions provided by genes that comprise the 46 chromosomes in every somatic cell. Disorders can result if too much or too little genetic material is present in the cells and if one or more genes are abnormal and provide incorrect directions.

Structure of Genes and Chromosomes

A review of the structure of genes and chromosomes aids in understanding the reasons for the occurrence of disorders. Chromosomes are composed of genes that in turn are composed of deoxyribonucleic acid, or DNA (Figure 5-1).

DNA

DNA is the building block of genes and chromosomes. Its three units are (1) a sugar (deoxyribose), (2) a phosphate group, and (3) one of four nitrogen bases (adenine, thymine, guanine, and cytosine).

DNA resembles a spiral ladder, with a sugar and a phosphate group forming each side of the ladder and a pair of nitrogen bases forming each rung. The four bases of the DNA molecule pair in a fixed way, allowing the DNA to be accurately duplicated during each cell division.

- Adenine pairs with thymine.
- Guanine pairs with cytosine.

The DNA also directs manufacture of proteins needed for cell function. The sequence of bases within the DNA determines which amino acids will be assembled to form a protein and the order in which they will be assembled for cell processes. Some proteins form the structure of body cells, whereas others are enzymes that control metabolic processes within the cell. If the sequence of nitrogen bases in the DNA is incorrect or some bases are missing or added in critical places, a defect in body structure or function may result.

Bases are arranged in groups of three called *codons* for translation into a specific amino acid in the cell. For example, a triplet base codon may consist of the bases GCC (guanine, cytosine, cytosine), which tells the cell to produce the amino acid alanine. Other codons, known as *stop codons,* signal the end of a gene sequence.

Genes

A gene is a segment of DNA that directs the production of a specific product needed for body structure or function. Humans may have as many as 100,000 genes, but not all genes function at the same time. Some are active only during prenatal life; others become functional at various times after birth.

Genes that code for the same trait often have two or more alternate forms, or alleles. Familiar examples of alleles are the ABO blood types. Normal alleles provide genetic variation and sometimes a biologic advantage. If an allele occurs at least 1% of the time in the population, it is deemed a *polymorphism.*

Some changed gene forms, or mutations, may be harmless, but many are harmful, such as those that cause the production of abnormal hemoglobin in sickle cell disease. Mutations may cause harm by the following actions:

- Substituting incorrect bases for the normal bases
- Interrupting the normal gene sequence or stopping it prematurely
- Duplicating some bases or entire gene sequences
- Adding or subtracting some bases within those making up a gene's sequence of bases, which will alter the amino acids it causes to be assembled

A mutation may occur in gametes or somatic cells. If the mutation occurs in a gamete, the mutation can be transmitted from one generation to the next. Mutations occurring in somatic cells are often associated with malignant change, but they are not transmitted from generation to generation.

Genes are too small to be seen under a microscope, but they can be studied in several ways:

- By measuring the products that they direct cells to produce, such as an enzyme or other substance
- By directly studying the gene's DNA
- By analyzing the gene's close association (linkage) with another gene that can be studied in one of the previous two ways

The tissue used for study of a gene depends on where the gene product is present in the body and the available technology. These tissues may include blood, skin cells, hair follicles, and fetal cells from the amniotic fluid or chorionic villi.

Genes that can be identified by direct analysis of DNA can be studied in any cells containing a nucleus, even if the gene product is not present in that tissue. Although not always used, DNA analysis of the blastomere (eight-cell stage of prenatal development) can be used to select embryos to be implanted in the uterus after in vitro fertilization. This prevents implantation of embryos with a specific gene defect or common chromosome defects.

Human Genome Project. The Human Genome Project is a massive international effort begun in 1990 to identify all genes contained in the 46 human chromosomes. A working draft of the human genetic code was completed in 2000, with full sequencing expected to be completed by the end of 2003 (U.S. Department of Energy, 2000). The goals of the project are the following:

- To identify all the genes in the human DNA
- To determine the sequences of the 3 billion base pairs that comprise the human DNA
- To store the information in databases
- To develop tools for data analysis
- To address the ethical, legal, and social issues that may arise from the project

(For an update on the project and other information, visit its website at http://www.ornl.gov/TechResources/Human_Genome/home.html.)

The potential human implications of the Human Genome Project are enormous. They include the following:

- Identifying the DNA alteration in the gene that causes a disorder may lead to a direct test to determine the presence of the disorder in or the carrier status of an individual. This type of testing is more accurate than biochemical or similar tests to identify people who are carriers or affected.
- Molecular testing for some genes can be done for anyone, not just for those with a family history of a genetic problem. Many current DNA studies require multiple family members for linkage analysis, limiting usefulness if family members are deceased or refuse to participate, if family members are few, and if the person is adopted.
- Information obtained in preconception or prenatal testing has greater accuracy for making reproductive decisions. Rather than assessment of tissue for the product of a gene (for example, an enzyme, which is subject to a greater degree of error), the actual gene can be directly identified.
- Predisposition testing can identify genetic susceptibility for a disorder, allowing lifestyle changes or interventions such as more frequent diagnostic tests for earlier identification of a disease when it is most treatable.
- Gene therapy, which entails modifying the defective gene itself rather than merely compensating for an

Table 5-1

ETHICAL ISSUES CREATED BY GREATER GENETIC KNOWLEDGE

- *Should testing be offered for a genetic disease for which no treatment is available? What if the disease is fatal? Should testing be required if a person may carry a diagnosable disorder that they might pass on to their children, even if they do not want the test?*
  Huntington's disease is an example of a genetic disease that can be diagnosed. It has serious effects, with a fatal outcome. Should testing be offered? Should it be required before the person is allowed to reproduce?
- *The ability to substitute one human gene for another may be in the future. Although this has the potential for preventing or curing a genetic disorder, it could also be used to substitute or enhance traits such as eye color, height, or even intelligence. Should the technology be restricted to only those genes that have serious negative effects on body function, or should this technology be used to substitute for any available gene the parents desire? Who should have access to this expensive technology?*
  Artificial chromosomes carrying desired genes are now being developed for animal research (Vastag, 2000). The process may ultimately be refined so that altered genes are available for humans. If these were altered in gametes, the altered gene would be passed to future generations. What are the added implications of this technology?
- *Who should own and control genetic information? Does an insurer have the right to a person's genetic information to assess risk and thus set more accurate rates? Or is this information private? Should this information be disregarded for everyone when insurance rates are set?*
  Geneticists may have the ability to identify conditions that a person will develop in the future even if the problem is not present. Examples include hypertension, diabetes, and heart disease. If an insurance company knows that the person will develop this disorder, rates would be higher or coverage would be denied. If an employer has this information, the person might not be hired to avoid raising insurance costs for the company. Yet the reverse could be true. Genetic testing might prove that a person *would not* develop a disorder, thus gaining them lower rates. If genetic testing before being insured is not permitted, is it right that all persons insured by a company subsidize those who develop disorders that could have been determined before being insured by paying higher rates?
- *How should issues of racial or ethnic identification be handled? What if their parentage is not what they have always thought?*
  Discoveries in the process of genetic analysis may determine that a person is not of the racial identity previously thought, or a person might discover that a parent is not the biologic parent. What should be done if information of this nature is uncovered? What are possible implications for self-image and identity? How might other members of the family be involved in the unexpected discovery?

abnormal gene product, might be possible for some disorders.
- In the future, medication may be tailored to a person's genetic makeup.

Today's nurse must expect development of genetic prediction, diagnosis, and therapy for disorders never known to have a genetic basis. At the same time, the explosion of knowledge about the genetic basis for disease raises many legal and ethical issues for which answers are not available. As the knowledge base grows, the following new issues are likely to emerge:

- Genetic information has implications for others in the affected person's family, raising privacy issues.
- Identification of genetic problems could lead to poor self-esteem, guilt, excessive caution, or conversely, a reckless lifestyle.
- Presymptomatic identification of genetically influenced illness would be a source of long-term anxiety.
- Genetic knowledge could affect a person's choice of a partner.
- Discrimination is a real possibility, such as the imposition of high insurance rates, denial of insurance coverage, or decision not to hire a qualified, but genetically compromised, person. A person might be discriminated against for conditions that might occur, not for conditions that already have occurred.

Table 5-1 raises some questions to consider related to the rapid expansion of knowledge in genetics.

Chromosomes

Genes are organized in 46 paired chromosomes in the nucleus of somatic cells. A gene can be likened to a single bead; a chromosome is like a string of beads. Each chromosome is composed of varying numbers of genes. A total of 22 chromosome pairs are autosomes, and the twenty-third pair comprises the sex chromosomes. Added, missing, and structurally abnormal chromosomes are usually harmful.

Mature gametes have half the chromosomes (23) of other body cells. One chromosome from each pair is distributed randomly in the gametes, allowing variation of genetic traits among people. When the ovum and sperm unite at conception, the total is restored to 46 paired chromosomes.

Cells for chromosomal analysis must have a nucleus and be living. Chromosomes can be studied using any of several types of cells: white blood cells, skin fibroblasts, bone marrow cells, and fetal cells from the chorionic villi of the placenta or suspended in amniotic fluid.

Unlike genes, chromosomes can be seen under the microscope but only during cell division. Specimens must be obtained and preserved carefully to provide enough living cells for chromosomal analysis. Temperature extremes, blood clotting, and the addition of

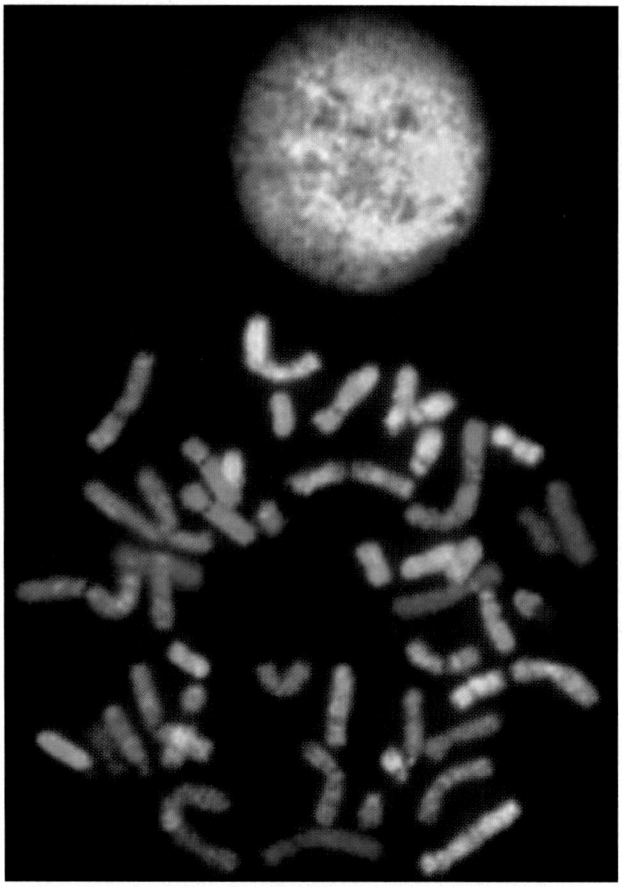

FIGURE 5-2 Before arrangement in a karyotype, chromosomes appear jumbled. (From Jorde, L.B., Carey, J.C., Bamshad, M.J., & White, R.L. [1999]. *Medical genetics* [2nd ed., color plate 5, following p. 116]. St. Louis: Mosby.)

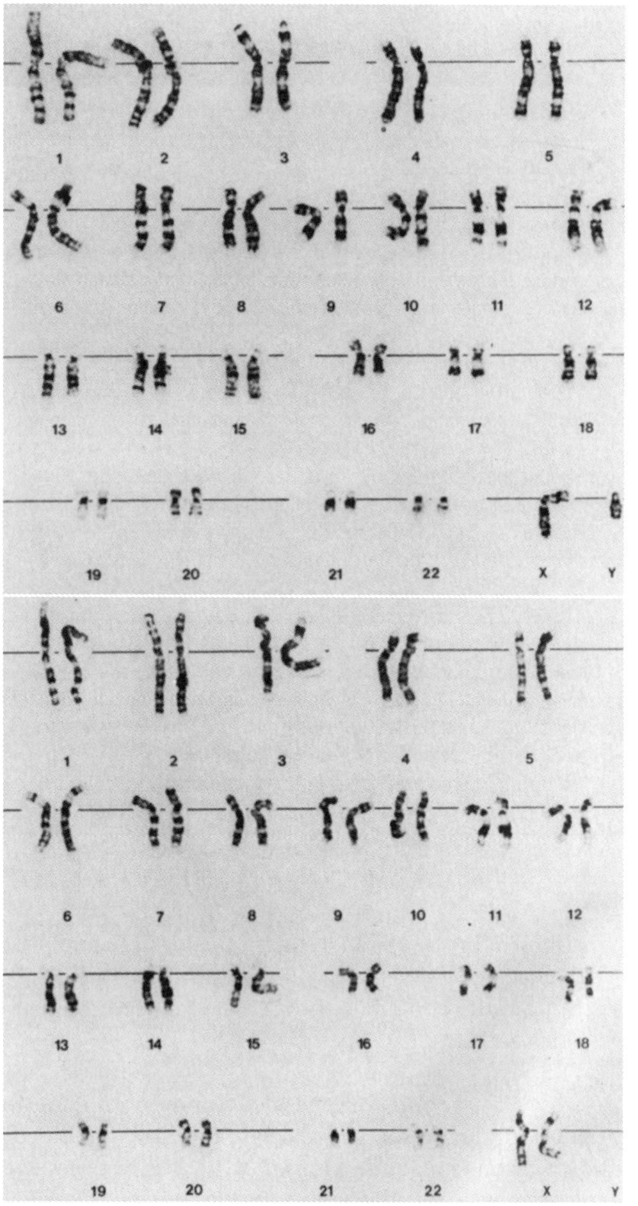

FIGURE 5-3 Chromosomes arranged in karyotypes. **A,** Normal male karyotype: 46,XY. **B,** Normal female karyotype: 46,XX. (From Knuppel, R.A., & Drukker, J.E. [1993]. *High-risk pregnancy: A team approach* [p. 666]. Philadelphia: W.B. Saunders.)

improper preservatives can kill the cells and render them useless for analysis.

Chromosomes look jumbled before they are arranged into a karyotype (Figure 5-2). Systematic study is possible using photography or computer imaging of prepared chromosomes and then arranging them into a karyotype (Figure 5-3). In a karyotype, autosomal pairs are arranged from largest to smallest. Letters describe groups of similar size and appearance. Sex chromosomes usually are arranged in a separate group.

A person's karyotype is abbreviated by a combination of numbers and letters. A number describes the total number of chromosomes, followed by either an XX to indicate the sex chromosomes are female or XY to indicate they are male. Thus the chromosome complement is abbreviated 46,XX for a normal female and 46,XY for a normal male. If the chromosome number is abnormal, such as that in Down syndrome, which has an extra 21 chromosome, an added abbreviation indicates the abnormality: 47 (total number of chromosomes), XY (male), +21 (the number that describes the added chromosome). Other abbreviations describe karyotypes with missing or structurally altered chromosomes.

A way to more finely analyze chromosomes makes use of fluorescent-labeled DNA probes that attach to specific chromosomes. This technique is called *fluorescent in-situ hybridization* and permits testing for added, missing, or rearranged chromosome material that otherwise may not be visible microscopically. Another more specific chromosome analysis is the comparative genomic hybridization used to identify losses or duplications of specific chromosome regions, which often occurs in tumor cells (Jorde, et al., 1999). A spectral karyotype is a method in which each chromosome is colored differently. The value of this technique is that small rearrangements, losses, or gains of chromosome material can more readily be seen.

Check Your Reading

1. What is the relationship among DNA, genes, and chromosomes?
2. Can genes be studied by examining them under a microscope? Why or why not? What methods are used to study them?
3. Why do cell specimens for chromosomal analysis have to be alive, regardless of the tissue used?
4. What do each of these abbreviations mean: 46,XY and 46,XX? How are chromosome abnormalities described?

Transmission of Traits by Single Genes

Inherited characteristics are passed from parent to child by the genes in each chromosome. These traits are classified according to whether they are dominant (strong) or recessive (weak) and whether the gene is located on one of the autosome pairs or on the sex chromosomes. Both normal and abnormal hereditary characteristics are transmitted by these mechanisms.

Because humans have pairs of matched chromosomes, excepting the sex chromosomes in the male, they have one allele for a gene at the same location on each member of the chromosome pair. The paired alleles may be identical (homozygous) or different (heterozygous).

Some genes, both normal and abnormal, occur more frequently in certain groups than in the population as a whole. For example, the gene that causes Tay-Sachs disease is carried by about 1 of every 30 (3.3%) American Jews, a rate approximately 100 times its occurrence in the general population. Persons of French-Canadian ancestry and members of the Cajun population in Louisiana are similarly at risk (March of Dimes, 2000). Because the abnormal gene occurs more frequently in these groups, their incidence of Tay-Sachs disease is also higher. Other disorders that are more common in certain ethnic groups are cystic fibrosis, which occurs primarily in whites of northern European descent, and sickle cell disease, which occurs more frequently in people of African descent.

Dominance

Dominance describes the way a person's genetic composition is translated into the phenotype, or observable characteristics. In the case of a dominant gene, one copy is enough to cause the trait to be expressed. For example, in the ABO blood system, genes for types A and B are dominant. Therefore a single copy of either of these genes is enough for it to be expressed in the person's blood type.

Two identical copies of a recessive gene are required for the trait to be expressed. The gene for blood group O is recessive. Laboratory testing identifies a person's blood group as O only if that person receives a gene for blood group O from both parents. If the person receives a gene for group O from one parent and group A from the other parent, group A is expressed in laboratory blood typing.

On the basis of dominant and recessive forms of a gene, a person with group A blood can have one of two possible combinations of gene alleles:

- Two group A alleles
- One group A allele and one group O allele

Other alleles are equally dominant. The person who receives a gene for blood group A from one parent and group B from the other will have type AB blood because both alleles are equally dominant and expressed in blood typing.

Dominance and recessiveness are relative qualities for many genes. Some people with a single copy of an abnormal recessive gene (carriers) may have a lower than normal level of the gene product (for example, an enzyme) that can be detected by biochemical methods. These people usually do not have overt disease because the normal copy of the gene produces enough of the required product to allow normal or near-normal function.

Chromosome Location

Genes located on autosomes are either autosomal dominant or autosomal recessive, depending on the number of identical copies of the gene needed to produce the trait. However, genes located on the X chromosome are paired only in females because males have one X and one Y chromosome.

A female with an abnormal recessive gene on one of her X chromosomes usually has a normal gene on the other X chromosome that compensates and maintains relatively normal function. However, the male is at a disadvantage if his only X chromosome has an abnormal gene. The male has no compensating normal gene because his other sex chromosome is a Y. The abnormal gene is expressed in the male because it is unopposed by a normal gene.

Patterns of Single Gene Inheritance

Three major patterns of single gene inheritance are (1) autosomal dominant, (2) autosomal recessive, and (3) X-linked (Table 5-2). Few genes are found on the Y chromosome, primarily the one that causes the embryo to differentiate into a male. Because very few Y-linked traits have been identified, these will not be discussed.

> Be cautious when referring to the illustration of a family's genetic history as a *pedigree.* Some people may be offended because they associate that word with animals. Although the word *pedigree* is widely used among genetic professionals, the nurse may need to interpret it for the client. For example, when taking a genetic family history, the nurse might say, "I'm going to use several symbols to depict your family tree and its members' health histories. This diagram is often called a *pedigree.*"

Table 5-2

SINGLE GENE TRAITS

Pedigree Symbols

A pedigree is a way to symbolically represent a family's medical history and the relationships of its members to one another. It can help identify patterns of inheritance that may help distinguish one type of disorder from another.

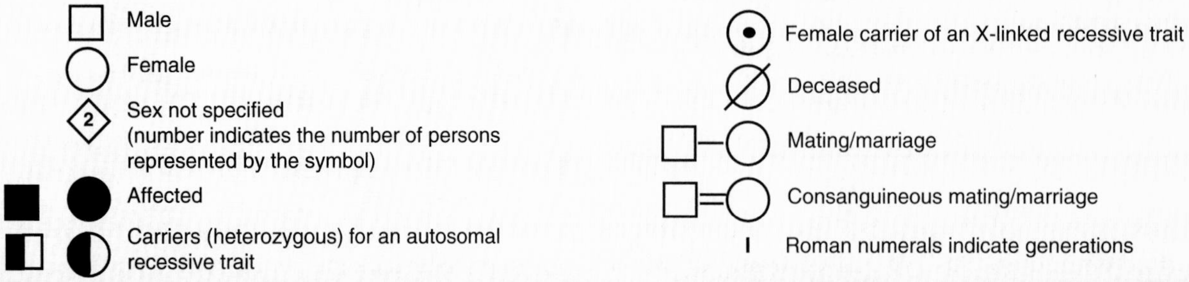

Characteristics	Transmission of Trait from Parent to Child	Examples
AUTOSOMAL DOMINANT		
A single copy of the gene is enough to produce the trait. Males and females are equally likely to have the trait. The trait often appears in every generation of a family, although family members having the trait may have widely varying manifestations of it. It may have multiple and seemingly unrelated effects on body structure and function.	A parent with the trait has a 50% (1 in 2) chance of passing the trait to the child. The trait may arise as a new mutation from an unaffected parent. Children who receive the mutated gene in their germline (gametes) can transmit it to future generations.	Examples of normal traits include blood groups A and B and Rh-positive blood factor. Examples of abnormal traits include Huntington's disease and neurofibromatosis.

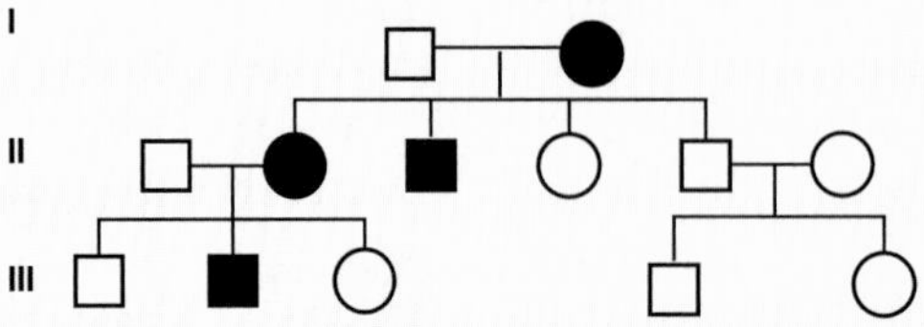

Characteristics	Transmission of Trait from Parent to Child	Examples
AUTOSOMAL RECESSIVE		
Two autosomal recessive genes are required to produce the trait. Males and females are equally likely to have the trait. There is often no prior family history of the disorder before the first affected child. If more than one family member is affected, they are usually full siblings. Consanguinity (blood relationship) of the parents increases the risk for the disorder.	Unaffected parents are carriers of the abnormal autosomal recessive trait. Children of carriers have a 25% (1 in 4) chance for receiving both copies of the defective gene and thus having the disorder. Children of carriers have a 50% (1 in 2) chance of receiving one copy of the gene and being carriers like the parents.	Examples of normal traits include blood group O and Rh-negative blood factor. Examples of abnormal traits include Tay-Sachs disease, sickle cell disease, and cystic fibrosis.

Table 5-2

SINGLE GENE TRAITS—cont'd

Characteristics	Transmission of Trait from Parent to Child	Examples
AUTOSOMAL RECESSIVE—CONTINUED		
Disorders are more likely to occur in groups isolated by geography, culture, religion, or other factors. Some autosomal recessive disorders are more common in specific ethnic groups.	Children of carriers have a 25% (1 in 4) chance of receiving both copies of the normal gene. They are neither carriers nor affected.	

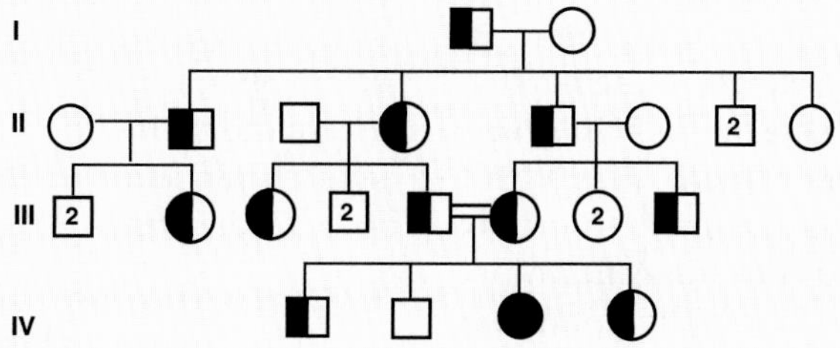

Characteristics	Transmission of Trait from Parent to Child	Examples
X-LINKED RECESSIVE		
Although recessive, only one copy of the gene is needed to cause the disorder in the male, who does not have a compensating X without the trait. Males are affected with rare exceptions. Females are carriers of the trait but not usually adversely affected. Affected males are related to one another through carrier females. Affected males do not transmit the trait to their sons.	Males who have the disorder transmit the gene to the following: • 100% of their daughters • None of their sons Sons of carrier females have a 50% (1 in 2) chance of being affected. They also have a 50% chance of being unaffected. Daughters of carrier females have a 50% (1 in 2) chance of being carriers like their mothers. They also have a 50% chance of being neither affected nor carriers. An abnormal X-linked recessive gene also may arise by mutation.	Examples include color-blindness, Duchenne's muscular dystrophy, and hemophilia A.

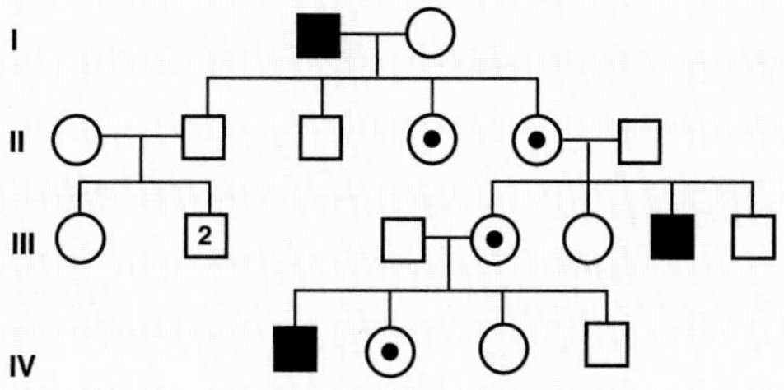

Single gene traits have mathematically predictable and fixed rates of occurrence. For example, if a couple has a child with an autosomal recessive disorder, the risk that future children will have the same disorder is one in four (25%) at every conception. The risk is the same at every conception, regardless of how many of a couple's children have been affected.

Autosomal Dominant Traits

An autosomal dominant trait is produced by a dominant gene on a nonsex chromosome. The expression of abnormal autosomal dominant genes may result in multiple and seemingly unrelated effects in the person. The gene's effects also may vary substantially in severity, leading a family to believe incorrectly that a trait skips a generation. A careful physical examination may reveal subtle evidence of the trait in each generation. In other cases, some people may carry the dominant gene but have no apparent expression of it in their physical makeup.

In some autosomal dominant disorders, such as Huntington's disease, those with the gene will always have the disease if they live to the age when the disorder becomes apparent. In other disorders, only a portion of those carrying the gene ever exhibit the disease.

New mutations account for the introduction of abnormal autosomal dominant traits into a family that has no prior history. In this case, parents of the child are normal because their body cells do not have the altered gene. Men over age 40 who father children are more likely to have offspring with a new autosomal dominant mutation (Jorde, et al., 1999).

CRITICAL TO REMEMBER

Single Gene Abnormalities

- A person affected with an autosomal dominant disorder has a 50% chance of transmitting the disorder to each biologic child.
- Two healthy parents who carry the same abnormal autosomal recessive gene have a 25% chance of having a child affected with the disorder caused by this gene.
- Parental consanguinity increases the risk for having a child with an autosomal recessive disorder.
- One copy of an abnormal X-linked recessive gene is enough to produce the disorder in a male.
- Abnormal genes can arise as new mutations. If these mutations are in the gametes, they are transmitted to future generations.

The person who is affected with an autosomal dominant disorder is usually heterozygous for the gene; that is, the person has a normal gene on one chromosome and an abnormal gene on the other chromosome of the pair. Occasionally a person receives two copies of the same abnormal autosomal dominant gene. Such an individual is usually much more severely affected than someone with only one copy.

Autosomal Recessive Traits

An autosomal recessive trait occurs if a person receives two copies of a recessive gene carried on an autosome. Everyone is estimated to carry up to five lethal autosomal recessive genes without manifesting the disorder because they have a compensating normal gene (Jorde, et al., 1999). Because the probability that two unrelated people share even one of the same abnormal genes is low, the incidence of autosomal recessive diseases is relatively low in the general population.

Situations that increase the likelihood of two parents sharing the same abnormal autosomal recessive gene are the following:

- Consanguinity (blood relationship of the parents)—Blood relatives have more genes in common, including abnormal ones.
- Groups that are isolated by culture, geography, religion, or other factors—The isolation allows abnormal genes to become concentrated over the years and occur at a greater frequency than in more diverse groups.

Many autosomal recessive disorders are severe, and affected persons may not live long enough to reproduce. Two notable exceptions are phenylketonuria and cystic fibrosis. Improved care of people with these disorders has allowed them to live into the reproductive years. If one member of the couple has the autosomal recessive disorder, all their children will be carriers. Their risk for having similarly affected children is also higher depending on the prevalence of the abnormal gene in the general population and the likelihood that their mate is a carrier.

X-Linked Traits

X-linked recessive traits are more common than X-linked dominant traits and are the only X-linked pattern discussed in this chapter. Gender differences in the occurrence of X-linked recessive traits and the relationship of affected males to one another are important factors that distinguish these disorders from autosomal dominant and recessive disorders. In general, males are the only ones to show full effects of an X-linked recessive disorder because their only X chromosome has the abnormal gene on it. Females can show the full disorder in two uncommon circumstances:

- If a female has a single X chromosome (Turner's syndrome)
- If a female child is born to an affected father and a carrier mother

X-linked recessive disorders can be relatively mild, such as colorblindness, or they may be severe, such as hemophilia. In addition, those having the disorder may be affected with varying degrees of severity.

Check Your Reading

5. If a parent has an autosomal dominant disorder, what is the chance that the child will have the same disorder?
6. Why would parents who are first cousins be more likely to have a child with an autosomal recessive disorder?
7. If each member of a couple carries a gene for an autosomal recessive disorder, what is the chance that the children will have the disorder? What is the chance that the children will be carriers? What is the chance that the children will not receive the abnormal gene from either parent?
8. Why are males more often affected with X-linked recessive disorders? If a female carries an X-linked recessive disorder such as hemophilia, what are the chances that her sons will have the disorder? What is the chance that her daughters will be carriers?

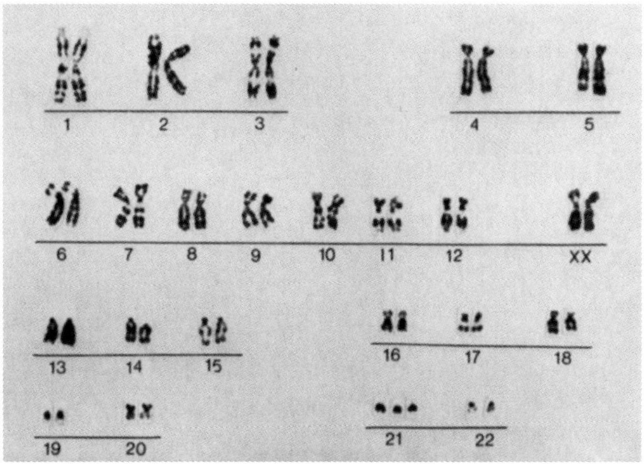

FIGURE 5-4 Karyotype of a female with trisomy 21 (Down syndrome: 47,XX, +21). (From Hacker, N., & Moore, J.G. [1998]. *Essentials of obstetrics and gynecology* [3rd ed., p. 124]. Philadelphia: W.B. Saunders.)

Chromosomal Abnormalities

Chromosomal abnormalities can be numerical or structural. They are quite common (50% or more) in the embryo or fetus that is spontaneously aborted. Chromosomal abnormalities often cause major defects because they involve deletion or duplication of many genes.

Numerical Abnormalities

Numerical chromosomal abnormalities involve added or missing single chromosomes or multiple sets of chromosomes. Trisomy and monosomy are numerical abnormalities of single chromosomes. *Polyploidy* describes abnormalities involving full sets of chromosomes.

CRITICAL TO REMEMBER

Chromosome Abnormalities

Chromosome abnormalities are either numerical or structural.

Numerical	Structural
Entire single chromosome added (trisomy)	Part of a chromosome missing or added
Entire single chromosome missing (monosomy)	Rearrangements of material within chromosome(s)
One or more added sets of chromosomes, resulting in cells containing 69 or 92 chromosomes	Two chromosomes that adhere to each other
	Fragility of a specific site on the X chromosome

Trisomy. A trisomy exists when each body cell contains an extra copy of one chromosome, bringing the total number to 47 (Figure 5-4). Each chromosome is normal, but there are too many in each cell. The most common trisomy is Down syndrome, or trisomy 21. In Down syndrome, each cell has three copies of chromosome 21. Trisomies of chromosomes 13 and 18 are less common and have more severe effects. The incidence of bearing children with trisomies increases with maternal age, so most women who are 35 years old or older and become pregnant are offered prenatal diagnosis to determine whether the fetus has Down syndrome or another trisomy.

Infants with Down syndrome have characteristic features that are usually noticed at birth (Figure 5-5). Chromosomal analysis is performed during the neonatal period to confirm the diagnosis and determine whether Down syndrome is caused by trisomy 21 or a rarer chromosomal anomaly that involves a structural rather than numerical abnormality of chromosome 21.

Children with Down syndrome reach developmental milestones more slowly than normal children. They are mentally retarded, although the severity varies, just as intelligence varies in the general population. Early intervention programs and regular medical care help these children reach their full ability and manage the physical problems associated with Down syndrome.

Monosomy. A monosomy exists when each body cell has a missing chromosome, with a total number of 45. The only monosomy compatible with postnatal life is Turner's syndrome, or monosomy X (Figure 5-6). Over 99% of conceptions with the 45, XO karyotype are lost in spontaneous abortion (Jorde, et al., 1999). The person with Turner's syndrome has a single X chromosome and is always female.

Large cystic masses on either side of the neck (cystic hygromas) may be found on routine ultrasound exam and lead to the diagnosis. Liveborn infants have excess

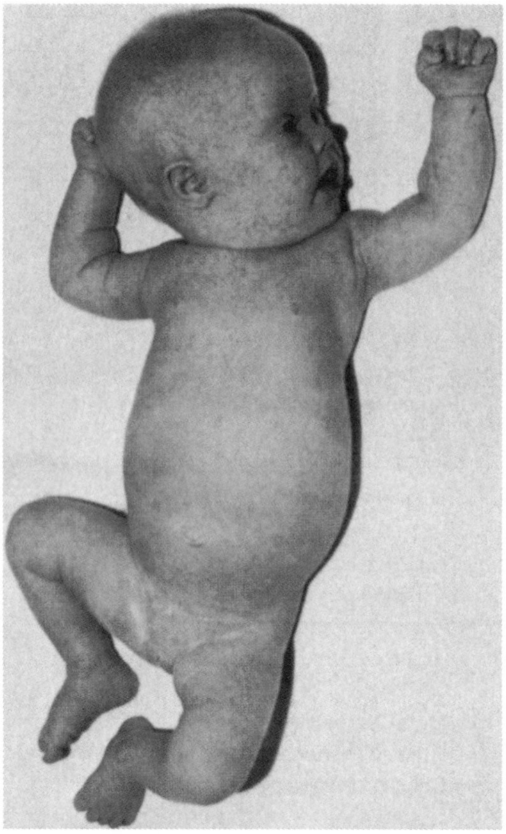

FIGURE 5-5 Newborn with several characteristic features of Down syndrome. Note that the infant has less flexion of her extremities and a flat face and occiput. (From Jones, K.L. [1997]. *Smith's recognizable patterns of human malformation* [5th ed., p. 11]. Philadelphia: W.B. Saunders.)

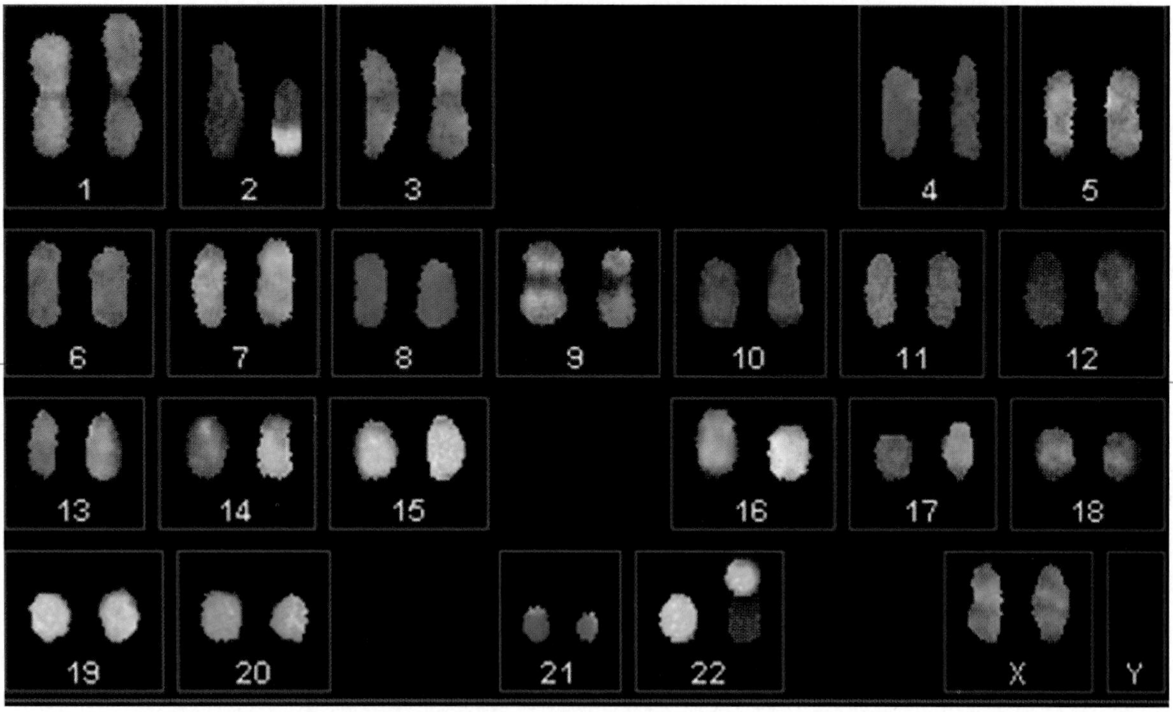

FIGURE 5-6 Spectral karyotype of a chromosome rearrangement. Because each chromosome is a different color and size, the exchange of a portion of chromosome 2 (brown) with a portion of chromosome 22 (yellow) is apparent. Genetic information may have been lost or duplicated in the process, or gene sequences may have been interrupted. (From Jorde, L.B., Carey, J.C., Bamshad, M.J., & White, R.L. [1998]. *Medical genetics* [2nd ed., color plate 6, following p. 116]. St. Louis: Mosby.)

skin around the neck left from the hygromas and edema that is most noticeable in the hands and feet during infancy. If Turner's syndrome is not identified and treated during infancy or childhood, an affected girl will remain very short and not have menstrual periods or develop secondary sex characteristics. Children with Turner's syndrome usually have normal intelligence, although they may have difficulty with spatial relationships or the solving of visual problems such as reading a map. The girl may have a broad, shieldlike chest with widely spaced nipples. Her kidneys may be joined at their upper poles (horseshoe kidney), and coarctation of the aorta may require corrective surgery.

Polyploidy. Polyploidy may occur when gametes do not halve their chromosome number during meiosis and retain both members of the pair or when two sperm fertilize an ovum simultaneously. The result is an embryo with one or more extra sets of chromosomes. The total number of chromosomes is a multiple of the haploid number of 23 (69 or 92 total chromosomes). Polyploidy usually results in an early spontaneous abortion but may occasionally be seen in a liveborn infant. This abnormality may be found in chorionic villus sampling (see Chapter 10) and may reflect an abnormality of the chorionic villi rather than the fetus.

Structural Abnormalities

Chromosomal abnormalities may involve the structure of one or more chromosomes. Part of a chromosome may be missing or added, or DNA within the chromosome may be rearranged. Some of these rearrangements are common harmless variations. Others are harmful because important genetic material is lost or duplicated in the structural abnormality or the position of the genes in relation to other genes is altered so that normal function is not possible.

Another structural abnormality occurs when all or part of a chromosome is attached to another (translocation). Many people with a translocation chromosomal abnormality are clinically normal because the total of their genetic material is normal or balanced. If a parent has a balanced translocation, the offspring may have completely normal chromosomes or a balanced translocation like the parent. However, the offspring may receive too much or too little chromosomal material and be spontaneously aborted or have birth defects.

Balanced translocations are usually discovered when amniocentesis reveals a translocation in the fetus or during infertility evaluations if a history of recurrent spontaneous abortions is reported. Either balanced or unbalanced chromosomal translocations may occur spontaneously in the offspring of parents who have no translocation.

Fragile X syndrome is an X-linked chromosomal abnormality. The syndrome was so named because a site on the X chromosome demonstrates breaks and gaps when the cells are grown in a medium deficient in folic acid. The syndrome is now usually diagnosed by molecular DNA studies. As in other X-linked traits, males are more severely affected than females, who have a compensating X chromosome that is usually normal. Fragile X syndrome is the most common form of male mental retardation (Hall, 2000a).

Check Your Reading

9. What is a chromosomal trisomy? Name a common trisomy.
10. What is a chromosomal monosomy? Which monosomy is compatible with life?
11. Why are structural chromosomal abnormalities often harmful?
12. What are the possible outcomes of the offspring of a parent who has a balanced chromosomal translocation?

MULTIFACTORIAL DISORDERS

Multifactorial disorders result from an interaction of genetic and environmental factors. The genetic tendency toward the disorder is modified by the environment. These interactions may either positively or negatively influence prenatal and postnatal development. For example, two embryos may have an equal genetic susceptibility for the development of a disorder such as spina bifida (open spine). However, the disorder will not occur unless an environment that favors its development, such as deficient maternal intake of folic acid, also exists.

Characteristics

Multifactorial birth defects are typically (1) present and detectable at birth and (2) isolated defects rather than defects that occur with unrelated abnormalities. However, a multifactorial defect may cause a secondary defect. For example, infants with spina bifida often have hydrocephalus (abnormal collection of spinal fluid within the brain) as well. The hydrocephalus is not a separate defect but one that occurs because the primary defect—abnormal development of the spine and spinal cord—disrupts spinal fluid circulation, allowing the fluid to build up within the brain's ventricular system.

The infant who has defects other than those associated with disrupted central nervous system development probably does not have a multifactorial disorder. In this case the spina bifida is more likely to be part of

CRITICAL TO REMEMBER

Multifactorial Birth Defects

- Multifactorial defects are some of the most common birth defects encountered in maternity and pediatric nursing practice.
- They are a result of interaction between a person's genetic susceptibility and environmental factors during prenatal development.
- These are usually single, isolated defects, although the primary defect may cause secondary defects.
- Some occur more often in certain geographic areas.
- A greater risk of occurrence exists with the following:
  - Several close relatives have the defect, whether mild or severe.
  - One close relative has a severe form of the defect.
  - The defect occurs in a child of the less frequently affected gender.
- Infants who have several major or minor defects that are not directly related probably do not have a multifactorial defect but have another syndrome, such as a chromosomal abnormality.

a syndrome that may pose a much different risk for recurrence in a future child.

Multifactorial disorders are some of the most common birth defects that a maternal-child nurse encounters. Examples include the following:

- Many heart defects
- Neural tube defects such as anencephaly (absence of most of the brain and skull) and spina bifida
- Cleft lip and cleft palate
- Pyloric stenosis

Risk for Occurrence

Unlike single gene traits, multifactorial disorders are not associated with a fixed risk of occurrence or recurrence in a family. The risks are an average rather than a constant percentage. Factors that may affect the risk are as follows:

1. Number of affected close relatives—Risk increases as the number of affected close relatives (parent, full sibling, or child) increases.
2. Severity of the disorder in affected family members—For example, bilateral cleft lip is associated with a higher risk for recurrence in a close relative than is a unilateral cleft lip.
3. Gender of the affected person(s)—For example, pyloric stenosis occurs five times as often in males as in females. The couple who has a daughter with pyloric stenosis faces a higher risk for recurrence with subsequent children because the genetic influence for development of the defect is greater if a female develops it.
4. Geographic location—The risk for some disorders, such as neural tube defects, is higher in some locations than others. Neural tube disorders have shown greater prevalence in some areas such as the Rio Grande Valley area in Texas.
5. Seasonal variations—Seasonal variations are noted with some multifactorial disorders.

If multifactorial disorders had no environmental component, the risk for occurrence and recurrence would be a precise percentage rather than a range. However, if no genetic component exists (if the disorder were totally related to environment), the ability to predict the risk for occurrence or recurrence would be minimal.

ENVIRONMENTAL INFLUENCES

Environment may positively influence prenatal development, such as good nutrition that supplies all necessary raw materials for fetal growth. However, some environmental influences are harmful, such as teratogens and mechanical forces that disrupt development.

Environmental influences on childbearing are those that are not now known to have a genetic component. At one time the placenta was thought to be a shield against harmful agents within a pregnant woman's body. Now the fact that most agents can cross the placenta and affect the developing fetus is recognized.

Teratogens

Teratogens are agents in the fetal environment that either cause or increase the likelihood that a birth defect will occur. Some drugs have been definitely established as safe or harmful. For most agents, however, their potential for harming the fetus is not clear. Several factors make it difficult to establish the teratogenic potential of an agent:

1. Retrospective study—Investigators must rely on the mother's memory about substances she ingested or was exposed to during pregnancy. The conclusion that a specific agent is harmful and the ways in which it harms the fetus is only possible when many cases are collected in which the exposure history is similar and the birth defects are also similar.
2. Timing of exposure—Agents may be harmful at one stage of prenatal development but not at another.
3. Different susceptibility of organ systems—Some agents affect only one fetal organ system, or they affect one system at one stage of development and another at a different stage of development.
4. Noncontrolled fetal exposure—Exposures cannot be controlled to eliminate extraneous agents or ensure a consistent dose. Interactions with other

Table 5-3
ENVIRONMENTAL SUBSTANCES KNOWN OR THOUGHT TO HARM THE FETUS

Alcohol	Syphilis
Aminoglycosides	Toxoplasmosis
Antineoplastic agents	Varicella
Antithyroid drugs	Lithium
Cocaine	Mercury
Diethylstilbestrol	Phenytoin
Folic acid antagonists	Retinoic acid
Infections	Tetracycline
Cytomegalovirus	Tobacco
Herpes simplex virus	Trimethadione
Human immunodeficiency virus	Valproic acid
Rubella	Warfarin

agents may reduce or compound the fetal effects. An agent that is toxic at one dose may have no apparent effect at another.

5. Placental transfer—Agents vary in their ability to cross the placenta.
6. Individual variations—Fetuses show varying susceptibility to harmful agents.
7. Nontransferability of animal studies—Results of animal studies cannot always be applied to humans. Agents that do not harm animal fetuses may damage the human embryo or fetus.

Teratogens typically cause more than one defect, which distinguishes teratogenic defects from multifactorial disorders. However, children affected by single gene and chromosome defects are also likely to have multiple defects. Therefore clinicians consider single gene disorders, chromosomal abnormalities, and effects of teratogenic agents when trying to diagnose an infant born with multiple anomalies.

Hundreds of individual agents are either known or suspected teratogens (Table 5-3). Types of teratogens include the following:

- Maternal infectious agents (for example, viruses, bacteria)
- Drugs and other substances used by the woman (for example, therapeutic agents, illicit drugs, tobacco, alcohol)
- Pollutants, chemicals, and other substances to which the mother is exposed in her daily life
- Ionizing radiation
- Maternal hyperthermia
- Effects of maternal disorders such as diabetes mellitus and phenylketonuria

Theoretically, all or some of the risk to the developing fetus can be eliminated by avoiding exposure to the agent or changing the fetal environment in some way.

Preventing Fetal Exposure

Ideally, prevention of exposure to harmful influences begins before conception because all major organ systems develop early in pregnancy, often before a woman realizes that she is pregnant. To avoid some agents such as alcohol and illicit drugs, pregnant women must be committed to make substantial lifestyle changes.

Infections. Rubella immunization at least 3 months before pregnancy virtually eliminates the risk that the mother will contract this infection, which can damage the fetus severely. For infections that cannot be prevented by immunization, the nurse can counsel the woman to avoid situations in which acquiring the disease is more likely (see Chapters 26 and 30).

Drugs and Other Substances. The United States Food and Drug Administration has established pregnancy categories for therapeutic drugs based on their potential to harm the fetus. The categories range from A through D and X. Class A drugs have no demonstrated fetal risk in well-controlled studies. At the opposite end, pregnancy category X drugs are well established as being harmful. The physician must balance the woman's need for the drug's therapeutic effects against the fetal need to avoid exposure to it (see Appendix C).

Establishing whether an illicit drug can cause prenatal damage is especially difficult because women who use illegal drugs often have other problems that complicate analysis of fetal effects. For example, these women may use multiple drugs and often have poor nutrition, untreated sexually transmitted diseases, inadequate prenatal care, and stressful lives. In addition, the purity of illicit drugs is unlikely and substances used to dilute them may themselves be harmful.

The best action is for the woman to eliminate use of nontherapeutic drugs and substances such as alcohol. If she takes therapeutic drugs, the physician may be able to prescribe an alternative drug with a lower risk to the fetus or may eliminate nonessential therapeutic drugs such as acne medications.

The pregnant woman who abuses drugs presents a complicated picture because maintenance of her drug habit usually takes priority over her health needs. She often has late or no prenatal care, increasing the likelihood that fetal damage occurred long before she encountered health care professionals.

Ionizing Radiation. Nonurgent radiologic procedures may be done during the first 2 weeks after the menstrual period begins, before ovulation occurs. For urgent procedures during pregnancy, the lower abdomen should be shielded with a lead apron if possible. The radiation dose is kept as low as possible to reduce fetal exposure.

Maternal Hyperthermia. An important teratogen is maternal hyperthermia. The mother's temperature may rise unavoidably during illness. Nurses should caution pregnant women to avoid deliberate exposure to heat sources such as saunas and hot tubs. Temperatures vary widely among public hot tubs, and a specific guideline for duration of exposure is difficult. The important factor is how high the woman's body temperature rises and for how long, not just the sauna or hot tub temperature.

Manipulating the Fetal Environment

Appropriate medical therapy can help a woman prevent fetal damage that could result from her illness. For example, a woman who has diabetes should try to keep her blood glucose levels normal and stable before and during pregnancy for the best possible fetal outcomes. A woman with phenylketonuria (PKU) should return to her special phenylalanine-free diet before conception to prevent high levels of phenylalanine in her body that will damage the fetus.

All women of childbearing age should take at least 400 mcg (0.4 mg) of folic acid daily before conception because this has been found to reduce the incidence of neural tube defects by 50% to 70%. Women who have had a child with a neural tube defect should take a higher amount of folic acid after consulting with their health care provider. In January 1999 the Centers for Disease Control and Prevention, March of Dimes Birth Defects Foundation, and National Council on Folic Acid began a national campaign to educate women about the importance of consuming adequate folic acid every day. Recent Gallup polls sponsored by the March of Dimes show that in 1998, only 13% of women knew that adequate folic acid intake could reduce the risk for neural tube defects (Mersereau, 2000). The neural tube closes during the fourth week after conception, often before the woman knows she is pregnant. Nurses can help make women aware of their need for a supplement of folic acid before conception to help reduce this serious birth defect.

Mechanical Disruptions to Fetal Development

Mechanical forces that interfere with normal prenatal development include oligohydramnios and fibrous amniotic bands.

Oligohydramnios, an abnormally small volume of amniotic fluid, reduces the cushion surrounding the fetus and may result in deformations such as clubfoot. Prolonged oligohydramnios can interfere with fetal lung development because it does not allow normal branching and development of the alveoli. Oligohydramnios may not be the primary fetal problem; rather, it may be related to other fetal anomalies.

Fibrous amniotic bands may result from tears in the inner sac (amnion) of the fetal membranes and can result in fetal deformations or intrauterine limb amputation. Fibrous bands are usually sporadic and unlikely to recur. Because these bands can cause multiple defects, they may be confused with birth defects from other causes such as chromosome and single gene abnormalities.

Check Your Reading

13. What are the usual characteristics of multifactorial disorders?
14. What factors can vary the likelihood that a multifactorial disorder will occur or recur?
15. How can a woman avoid exposing her fetus to teratogens?
16. Why should a woman with phenylketonuria adhere to a low-phenylalanine diet before and during pregnancy?
17. Why is adequate folic acid intake before conception important?

GENETIC COUNSELING

Genetic counseling provides services to help people understand the genetic disorder about which they are concerned and the risk of its occurrence in their family. Those concerned about multifactorial or environmental hazards can receive up-to-date information at most centers as well.

Availability

Genetic counseling is often available through university medical centers. State departments of mental health and mental retardation and rehabilitation services also may provide counseling services. Local chapters of the March of Dimes are an important source of information about birth defects and counseling sites. Also, organizations that focus on specific birth defects provide valuable support and assistance in obtaining needed services for individuals and families affected by the disorder.

Focus on the Family

Genetic counseling focuses on the family rather than the individual. One family member may have a birth defect, but study of the entire family is often needed for accurate counseling. This may involve obtaining medical records and performing physical examinations and laboratory studies on numerous family members. Counseling is impaired if family members are unwilling to provide their medical records and agree to examinations and laboratory studies. In addition, those who seek counseling may be unwilling to request cooperation from other family members or share newly acquired genetic information.

Table 5-4

DIAGNOSTIC METHODS THAT MAY BE USED IN GENETIC COUNSELING

- Preconception screening
  - Family history to identify hereditary patterns of disease or birth defects
  - Examination of family photographs
  - Physical examination for obvious or subtle signs of birth defects
  - Carrier testing
    - Persons from ethnic groups with a higher incidence of some disorders
    - Persons with a family history suggesting that they may carry a gene for a specific disorder
  - Chromosomal analysis
  - DNA analysis
- Prenatal diagnosis for fetal abnormalities
  - Chorionic villus sampling
  - Amniocentesis
  - Ultrasonography
  - Percutaneous umbilical blood sampling
- Postnatal diagnosis for an infant with a birth defect
  - Physical examination and measurements
  - Imaging procedures (for example, ultrasonography, radiography, echocardiography)
  - Chromosomal analysis
  - DNA analysis
  - Biochemical tests for metabolic disorders (for example, phenylketonuria, cystic fibrosis)
  - Hemoglobin analysis for disorders such as sickle cell disease
  - Immunologic testing for infections
  - Autopsy

Process of Genetic Counseling

Genetic counseling is often a slow process that is not always straightforward. Several visits spread over months may be needed. Tests for rare disorders may be performed at only one or a few laboratories in the world, and several weeks may be needed to complete them. Despite a comprehensive evaluation, a diagnosis may never be established. An accurate diagnosis is crucial to provide families with the best information about the risks for a specific birth defect, prognosis for one affected, and options available to prevent or manage the disorder (Table 5-4). Even if the counseling does not provide clear information, expanding knowledge may allow a definite diagnosis later, and families are encouraged to contact the center for updates.

Individuals or families may request genetic counseling before or during pregnancy or after a child has been born with a defect. A genetic evaluation may include many factors:

- A complete medical history of the affected person, including prenatal and perinatal history
- The medical history of other family members
- Laboratory, imaging, and other studies
- Physical assessment of a child with the birth defect and other family members as needed
- Examination of photographs, particularly for family members who are deceased or unavailable
- Construction of a pedigree to identify relationships among family members and their relevant medical history

If a diagnosis is established, genetic counseling educates the family about the following:

- What is known about the cause of the disorder
- The natural course of the disorder
- The likelihood that the disorder will occur or recur in other family members
- Availability of prenatal diagnosis for the disorder
- The ways a couple may be able to avoid having an affected child
- Availability of treatment and services for the person with the disorder

Genetic counseling is nondirective; that is, the counselor does not tell the individual or parents what decision to make but educates them about options for dealing with the disorder. However, families often subjectively interpret the counseling. Some parents may regard a 50% risk of occurrence or recurrence as low, whereas others may think that a 1% risk is unacceptably high. Also, the family's values and beliefs influence whether they seek counseling and what they do with the information provided.

When risks and probabilities are discussed, these numbers must be stated in terms the individual or parents can understand and their understanding must be verified. A 1 in 100 risk may sound higher to many people than a 1 in 5 risk. However, when the same numbers are framed in terms of percentages, the 1% risk is obviously much lower than the 20% risk.

Supplemental Services

Comprehensive genetic counseling includes services of professionals from many disciplines, such as biology, medicine, nursing, social work, and education. These professionals provide family support and referrals to parent support groups, grief counseling, and intervention for problems that accompany the birth of a child with a birth defect, such as socioeconomic and family dysfunction.

NURSING CARE OF FAMILIES CONCERNED ABOUT BIRTH DEFECTS

Nurses have an important role in helping families that are concerned about birth defects. Some nurses work directly with family members who are undergoing genetic counseling. Many more nurses are generalists who bring their knowledge about birth defects and

PARENTS WANT TO KNOW About Birth Defects

How can this birth defect be genetic? No one else in our family has ever had anything like it.

Autosomal recessive disorders are carried by parents who themselves are unaffected. The abnormal gene may have been passed down through many generations, but the risk for an affected child is nonexistent until two carrier parents mate.

Isn't the chance that this birth defect will happen to another of our children only one in a million?

Autosomal recessive disorders have a 25% (1 in 4) chance of recurring in children of the same parents. Autosomal dominant disorders may pose a 50% risk for recurrence unless they resulted from a new mutation in the parental germ cells.

Isn't this birth defect very likely to recur? We'd better not have any more children.

Some birth defects are associated with a relatively high risk of recurrence; others have a relatively low risk. Prenatal diagnosis may offer parents a way to avoid having an affected child, or some disorders may be treated before birth. New genetic knowledge may provide therapies not available just a short time ago.

Because we've already had a child with this birth defect (an autosomal recessive defect), will the next three be normal?

If both parents are carriers for an autosomal recessive disorder, there is a 25% (1 in 4) risk that is constant with each conception. The chance that their children will be neither affected nor carriers is equal.

If I have an amniocentesis or other prenatal diagnostic test, can the test detect all birth defects?

Although many disorders can be prenatally diagnosed, not all can be diagnosed in the same fetus. Testing is offered for one or more specific disorders after a careful family history is taken to determine appropriate tests.

If the prenatal test is normal, will my baby be normal?

Normal results from prenatal testing exclude those specifically tested disorders. Every healthy couple has about a 5% risk of having a child with a birth defect, some of which are not obvious at birth. This baseline risk remains, even if all prenatal test results are normal.

Will I have to have an abortion if my prenatal tests show that my baby is abnormal?

Abortion may be an option for parents whose fetus is affected with a birth defect, but most parents are reassured by normal test results. If results are abnormal, some parents appreciate the time to prepare for a child with special needs. Better medical management can be planned for a newborn who is expected to have problems. Prenatal diagnosis gives many parents the confidence to have children despite their increased risk for having a child with a birth defect.

their prevention to those they encounter in everyday practice.

Nurses as Part of a Genetic Counseling Team

Many genetic counseling teams include nurses. Genetic nursing may include the following:

- Providing counseling after additional education in this area
- Guiding a woman or couple through prenatal diagnosis
- Supporting parents as they make decisions after receiving abnormal prenatal diagnostic results
- Helping the family deal with the emotional impact of a birth defect
- Assisting parents who have had a child with a birth defect to locate needed services and support
- Coordinating services of other professionals, such as social workers, physical and occupational therapists, psychologists, and dietitians
- Helping families find appropriate support groups to help them cope with the daily stresses associated with a child who has a birth defect

Nurses in General Practice

Nurses who work in women's health care, antepartum, intrapartum, newborn, and pediatric settings often encounter families who are concerned about birth defects. These families may include a member with a birth defect. Other families may believe that they have an increased risk for having a child with a birth defect. Generalist nurses provide care and support that complements those of nurses who work on a genetic counseling team.

Women's Health Nurses

The nurse who provides care in women's health may encounter families who should be referred for genetic counseling. The ideal time to provide counseling is before conception so that the childbearing couple has more options if risks are identified.

The primary nursing role is to identify families who might benefit from counseling before conception. For example, the nurse may identify a woman who belongs to a group in which the sickle cell gene is more frequent and arrange for testing to determine her carrier status. If testing reveals that she is a carrier for the gene, the woman can be advised that she could conceive a child with sickle cell disease if her partner is also a carrier. If her partner has not been tested, the nurse can arrange for his testing.

Antepartum Nurses

During the initial antepartum interview, the nurse may identify the pregnant woman or family who may bene-

Table 5-5

REASONS FOR REFERRAL TO A GENETIC COUNSELOR

Pregnant women who will be 35 years of age or older when the infant is born
Men who father children after age 40
Members of a group with an increased incidence of a specific disorder
Carriers of autosomal recessive disorders
Women who are carriers of X-linked disorders
Couples related by blood (consanguineous relationship)
Family history of birth defect or mental retardation
Family history of unexplained stillbirth
Women who experience multiple spontaneous abortions
Pregnant women exposed to known or suspected teratogens or other harmful agents either before or during pregnancy
Pregnant women with abnormal prenatal screening results, such as alpha-fetoprotein, triple screen, and suspicious ultrasound findings

fit from genetic counseling. The antepartum nurse also assists families with decision making, teaching, and emotional support.

Identifying Families for Referral. Nurses in antepartum settings often identify a woman or family for whom referral for genetic counseling is appropriate (Table 5-5). The personal and family history of the woman and her partner may reveal factors that increase their risks for having a child with a birth defect. In addition to the usual medical history about disorders such as hypertension and diabetes, the woman should be questioned about a family history of birth defects, diseases that seem to "run in the family," mental retardation, and developmental delay.

> Some people are reluctant to disclose that they have a family member with mental retardation or a birth defect. The nurse can gently probe for sensitive information by asking questions about whether any family members have learning problems or are "slow." The use of words that are lay oriented often elicits more information than clinical terms that may seem harsh.

Helping the Family Decide about Genetic Counseling. If genetic counseling is appropriate, the physician or nurse-midwife discusses it with the woman and refers the family to an appropriate center. However, the final decision rests with the family. The nurse can help the family weigh issues that are important to them as they decide.

Genetic counseling can raise issues that are uncomfortable, such as whether to undergo prenatal diagnosis, what to do if a condition cannot be prenatally diagnosed, and what options are acceptable if prenatal diagnosis shows abnormal results. Counseling may open family conflicts if information from other family members is needed or if family values differ on issues such as abortion of an abnormal fetus. In addition, the tests can show unexpected results (Table 5-6).

Table 5-6

PROBLEMS ENCOUNTERED IN GENETIC COUNSELING AND PRENATAL DIAGNOSIS

Inadequate medical records
Family members' refusal to share information
Records that are incomplete, vague, or uninformative
Inconclusive testing
Too few family members available when family studies are needed
Inadequate number of live fetal cells obtained during amniocentesis
Failure of fetal cells to grow in culture
Ambiguous prenatal test results that are neither clearly normal nor clearly abnormal
Unexpected results from prenatal diagnosis
Discovery of an abnormality other than the one for which the person was tested
Nonpaternity revealed
Inability to determine the severity of a prenatally diagnosed disorder
Inability to rule out all birth defects
Misunderstanding of the mathematical risk as it is presented

Teaching about Lifestyle. Nurses can teach a pregnant woman about harmful factors in her lifestyle that can be modified to reduce the risk of defects to offspring. The nurse can support the woman in making lifestyle changes that may be difficult, such as stopping alcohol consumption, reducing or eliminating smoking, and improving her diet. Using liberal praise can motivate a woman to continue her efforts to promote an optimal outcome. However, a negative attitude from nurses or other professionals may make her feel like a failure, and she may abandon her efforts to create a healthier lifestyle.

Providing Emotional Support. Until they know that prenatal test results are normal, many women delay telling friends or family about their pregnancy or investing emotionally in their pregnancy. When results are abnormal, women face more difficult decisions about whether to terminate or continue the pregnancy.

Helping the Family Deal with Abnormal Results. Because prenatal diagnostic tests are performed to detect disorders involving serious physical and often

Therapeutic Communication

Assisting a Woman Who May Benefit from Genetic Counseling

Paula Crandall is a 41-year-old white woman who is 8 weeks pregnant with her first child after more than 10 years of infertility. Barbara Glenn is a nurse who works with Paula's obstetrician.

Paula: I know all about the risks at my age. I'm not so much worried about my own health but the baby's.

Barbara: You seem to be concerned that the baby might not be all right. *(Clarifying)*

Paula: Sure, what woman wouldn't be? I know I'm more likely to have a baby with Down syndrome at my age.

Barbara: Yes, the risks of having an infant with a chromosomal abnormality increase after the mother is 35 years old. Do you want prenatal diagnosis to see if the fetus has this kind of problem? *(Paraphrasing and giving information. Barbara also uses a closed-end question that tends to block communication because it is usually answered with a simple "yes" or "no.")*

Paula: Oh, yes. I know what's available from surfing the Internet. When we waited so long to have children, I just assumed that I'd have whatever tests were recommended. I just don't know . . .

Barbara: You're reconsidering prenatal testing now? *(Reflecting)*

Paula: Well, not exactly reconsidering . . . It's just that I've waited so long for a baby, and this may be our only one.

Barbara: [Waiting quietly but attentively because Paula seems to be thinking.] *(Using silence)*

Paula: I'm just worried about testing. I know prenatal tests have a low risk, but what if I lose a normal baby? It took me so long to finally get pregnant, and I'm running out of time. I might not get another chance.

Barbara: It must be a very difficult decision. *(Reflecting)*

Paula: It is. Even if I have testing and the baby has Down syndrome, I'm not so sure I'd have an abortion. The outlook for people with Down syndrome is much better than it used to be. Why have testing if I wouldn't do anything about an abnormal baby?

Barbara: You certainly have some valid concerns. How does your husband feel about testing? *(Questioning using an open-ended question)*

Paula: Oh, Bill is all for it. He keeps reminding me that the baby is probably normal and that I probably won't have a miscarriage if I have testing. His cousin had a child with Down syndrome, and Bill doesn't think we should knowingly bring a child with a serious birth defect into the world. What would you do if you were in my place?

Barbara: I can't answer that question because I'm not in your place. Let's review some of the issues so you can make the best decision for yourself and your family. First, you know you have an increased risk for having a baby with a chromosomal defect such as Down syndrome because of your age. Second, the odds that the baby will be normal are much higher than the risk that the baby will be abnormal. Third, amniocentesis poses a small but real risk of causing a miscarriage. Fourth, you are undecided about whether you would terminate a pregnancy if the fetus were abnormal. Another issue that you haven't specifically mentioned is time. Depending on whether you choose chorionic villus sampling, which needs to be done in about 2 weeks, or amniocentesis, which should be done about 8 weeks from now, you don't have a long time to decide. *(Summarizing)*

Paula: I know. I'm running out of time in more ways than one.

Barbara: If you like, I can set up an appointment with a genetic counselor. The counselor can provide you with the most accurate assessment of your risk for having a child with a birth defect and also the risks of any indicated prenatal diagnosis procedure. Then you can decide whether or not to have testing.

Paula: I think I'd like that, as long as I don't have to be committed to a particular decision before I go.

mental effects, the woman whose test results are abnormal must confront painful decisions. For many of these disorders, no effective prenatal or postnatal treatment exists. In many cases, only two choices are available: to continue or terminate the pregnancy. In addition, the decision to terminate a pregnancy must be made in a short time. Failure to make a decision is effectively a decision to continue the pregnancy. Although the physician or genetic counselor discusses abnormal results and available options, the nurse reinforces the information given to these anxious families and supports them.

When test results are abnormal, nurses can expect the couple to grieve. Even if a pregnancy was unplanned, the woman who reaches the time of prenatal diagnosis has already made the initial decision to continue the pregnancy. If results are abnormal, she must decide again if she will continue or end the pregnancy. Women who continue their pregnancies grieve over losing the expected normal infant.

Intrapartum and Neonatal Nurses

Nurses working in intrapartum and neonatal settings encounter families who have given birth to an infant with a birth defect that was often unexpected. Stillborn infants sometimes have birth defects that contributed to their intrauterine death. Besides the loss of their baby, these parents face additional pain because of the associated abnormality. An autopsy may be performed to document all anomalies and to establish the most accurate diagnosis of the birth defect for future counseling (see Chapter 24).

Nurses who care for these families in the intrapartum and neonatal settings will find the parents anxious, depressed, and sometimes hostile because of the unexpected event. The family's usual coping mechanisms may be inadequate for the situation, or new coping mechanisms have not been developed. Various diagnostic studies are often recommended soon after the birth of an abnormal infant to establish a diagnosis and give parents accurate information about the disorder and their options. However, a high anxiety level reduces their ability to understand the often massive amount of information received. The nurse is in the best position to evaluate the family's perception of the problem, help them understand the diagnostic tests, reinforce correct information, and correct misunderstandings. In addition, the nurse is often most therapeutic by simply being an available, active listener, helping to ease the family's pain over the event.

Nurses should encourage families to contact lay support groups, which are significant sources of support because members fully understand the daily problems encountered in the care of a child with a birth defect. They can help the parents deal with the stress and chronic grief associated with prolonged care of these children. Support groups also can help the parents see the positive aspects and victories when caring for their special-needs child. Many support groups have Internet sites that offer help to parents in any location.

Pediatric Nurses

Children with birth defects typically have numerous recurrent medical problems. They usually are hospitalized more often and for longer periods than children without birth defects. They may have to travel to specialized hospitals for care, adding to the family's stress. Their families often have large expenses for medical care and equipment that are not covered by insurance or public assistance programs. Income may be lost because one parent, usually the mother, stops working to care for the child.

Family dysfunction is common, and the strain of having a child with a serious birth defect may lead to divorce. Siblings often feel left out of their parents' attention because the needs of this child demand so much of their time.

The pediatric nurse can reduce the family's stress by helping them locate appropriate support services. The nurse can contact social services departments to help the family find financial and other resources needed to care for the child. If parents have not connected with a lay support group, the pediatric nurse can encourage them to do so.

SUMMARY CONCEPTS

- The 46 human chromosomes are long strands of DNA, each containing up to several thousand individual genes.
- With the exception of those genes located on the X and Y chromosomes in males, genes are inherited in pairs that may be identical or different. Some genes are dominant, and some are recessive.
- Many genes can be analyzed by the products they produce, their DNA, or their close association with another gene that is more easily analyzed.
- The Human Genome Project seeks to map the base-pair sequences of all 46 of the human chromosomes by 2003. There are many potential benefits to this undertaking, as well as many legal, social, and ethical issues that may be raised.
- Cells for chromosome analysis must be living. Specimens must be handled carefully to preserve their viability.
- Chromosome abnormalities are either numerical, with the addition or deletion of an entire chromosome or chromosomes, or structural, with deletion, addition, rearrangement, or fragility of the chromosome material.
- Single gene disorders are associated with a fixed risk of occurrence or recurrence. The type of single gene abnormality (autosomal dominant, autosomal recessive, or X-linked) determines the risk.
- Multifactorial disorders occur because of a genetic predisposition combined with environmental factors.
- The risk for occurrence or recurrence of multifactorial disorders is not fixed but varies according to the number of close relatives that are affected, severity of the defect in affected persons, gender of the affected person, and geographic locale. Seasonal variations may affect the risk for some disorders.
- Relatively few agents that can enter the fetal environment are known to be definitely teratogenic or definitely safe.
- The risk for fetal damage from environmental agents can be decreased by reducing exposure to the agent or manipulating the fetal environment.
- The purpose of genetic counseling is to educate individuals or families with accurate information so that they can make informed decisions about reproduction and appropriate care for affected members.
- The nurse cares for people with concerns about birth defects by identifying those needing referral, teaching, coordinating services, and offering emotional support.

REFERENCES & READINGS

Alteneder, R.R., Kenner, C., Greene, D., & Pohorecki, S. (1998). The lived experience of women who undergo prenatal diagnostic testing due to elevated maternal serum alpha-fetoprotein screening. *MCN: American Journal of Maternal/Child Nursing,* 23(4), 180-186.

American Academy of Pediatrics & American College of Obstetricians and Gynecologists. (1997). *Guidelines for perinatal care* (4th ed.). Washington, D.C.: Author.

American College of Obstetricians and Gynecologists. (1995). Genetic technologies. *ACOG Technical Bulletin number 208.* Author.

American College of Obstetricians and Gynecologists. (2000). Maternal phenylketonuria. *ACOG Committee Opinion number 230.* Author.

Banasik, J.L. (2000a). Genetics and developmental disorders. In L.C. Copstead & J.L. Banasik (Eds.), *Pathophysiology: Biological and behavioral perspectives* (2nd ed., pp. 110-133). Philadelphia: W.B. Saunders.

Banasik, J.L. (2000b). Molecular genetics and tissue differentiation. In L.C. Copstead & J.L. Banasik (Eds.), *Pathophysiology: Biological and behavioral perspectives* (2nd ed., pp. 62-109). Philadelphia: W.B. Saunders.

Dorinzi, D. (1999). Learning about genetic risk. *AWHONN Lifelines,* 3(5), 49-52.

Farndon, P.A., & Kilby, M.D. (1999). Genetics, risks and genetic counseling. In D.K. James, P.J. Steer, C.P. Weiner, & B. Gonik (Eds.), *High-risk pregnancy: Management options* (2nd ed., pp. 23-38). London: W.B. Saunders.

Fletcher, J.C. (1998). Ethical issues in reproductive genetics. *Seminars in Perinatology,* 22(3), 189-197.

Fox, M., & Garber, A. (1998). Genetic evaluation and teratology. In N.H. Hacker & J.G. Moore (Eds.), *Essentials of obstetrics and gynecology* (3rd ed., pp. 123-139). Philadelphia: W.B. Saunders.

Evans, M., & Johnson, M.P. (2000). Genetic counseling, screening, and diagnosis. In S.B. Ransom, M.P. Dombrowski, S.G. McNeeley, K.S. Moghissi, & A.R. Munkarah (Eds.), *Practical strategies in obstetrics and gynecology* (pp. 213-223). Philadelphia: W.B. Saunders.

Grabowski, G.A., & Whitsett, J.A. (2000). Gene therapy. In R.E. Behrman, R.M. Kliegman, & H.B. Jenson (Eds.), *Nelson textbook of pediatrics* (16th ed., pp. 333-341). Philadelphia: W.B. Saunders.

Grimes, D.A., & Snively, G.R. (1999). Patients' understanding of medical risks: Implications for genetic counseling. *Obstetrics and Gynecology,* 93(6), 910-914.

Guyton, A.C., & Hall, J.E. (1996). *Textbook of medical physiology* (9th ed.). Philadelphia: W.B. Saunders.

Hall, J.G. (2000a). Chromosomal clinical abnormalities. In R.E. Behrman, R.M. Kliegman, & H.B. Jenson (Eds.), *Nelson textbook of pediatrics* (16th ed., pp. 325-333). Philadelphia: W.B. Saunders.

Hall, J.G. (2000b). Genetic counseling. In R.E. Behrman, R.M. Kliegman, & H.B. Jenson (Eds.), *Nelson textbook of pediatrics* (15th ed., p. 327). Philadelphia: W.B. Saunders.

Howse, J. (1999). Stopping neural tube defects: Nurses and folic acid partner for patient awareness. *AWHONN Lifelines* 3(3), 10-11.

Hueppchen, N.A., & Pressman, E.K. (1999). Preconception care: Planning for a healthy pregnancy: Strategies to minimize risk to mother and child. *Women's Health in Primary Care,* 2(4), 259-274.

Jones, K.L. (1999). Effects of therapeutic, diagnostic, and environmental agents. In R.K. Creasy & R. Resnik (Eds.), *Maternal-fetal medicine: Principles and practice* (4th ed., pp. 132-144). Philadelphia: W.B. Saunders.

Jones, O.W., & Cahill, T.C. (1999). Basic genetics and patterns of inheritance. In R.K. Creasy & R. Resnik (Eds.), *Maternal-fetal medicine: Principles and practice* (4th ed., pp. 1-39). Philadelphia: W.B. Saunders.

Jorde, L.B., Carey, J.C., Bamshad, M.J., & White, R.L. (1999). *Medical genetics.* St. Louis: Mosby.

Kopala, B. (1997). The Human Genome Project: Issues and ethics. *MCN: American Journal of Maternal/Child Nursing* 22(1), 9-15.

March of Dimes Birth Defects Foundation. (1999a). *Fact sheet: Birth defects.* Retrieved May 19, 2000 from http://www.modimes.org/HealthLibrary2/FactSheets/Birth_Defects.htm.

March of Dimes Birth Defects Foundation. (1999b). *Fact sheet: Sickle cell disease.* Retrieved May 22, 2000 from http://www.modimes.org/HealthLibrary2/FactSheets/Sickle_Cell_Disease.htm.

March of Dimes Birth Defects Foundation. (2000). *Fact sheet: Tay Sachs disease.* Retrieved May 22, 2000 from http://www.modimes.org/HealthLibrary2/FactSheets/Tay_Sachs_Disease.htm.

March of Dimes Resource Center. (1999). *Folic acid.* Wilkes-Barre, PA: Author.

Mereseau, P.W. (2000). Preventing birth defects: A national campaign. *Small Talk* 12(2), 1-2, 4-5. Retrieved May 24, 2000 from cdc.gov/nceh/cddh/folic/smalltalk.htm.

Moore, K.L. & Persaud, T.V.N. (1998). *Before we are born: Essentials of embryology and birth defects* (5th ed.). Philadelphia: W.B. Saunders.

National Human Genome Research Institute & National Institutes of Health. (1998). Ethical, legal and social implications research: Goals and related research questions and education activities for the next five years of the U.S. Human Genome Project. Retrieved May 26, 2000 from http://www.nygri.nih.gov/98plan.

Penticuff, J.H. (1996). Ethical dimensions in genetic screening: A look into the future. *Journal of Obstetric, Gynecologic, and Neonatal Nursing,* 25(9), 785-789.

Rhodes, A.M. (1995). Liability for failure to offer prenatal AFP testing. *MCN: American Journal of Maternal/Child Nursing,* 20(3), 169.

Rogee, S.A. (1999). Genetics and discrimination: How nurses can help women make smart choices. *AWHONN Lifelines,* 3(3), 17-18.

Rogers, J., & Davis, B.A. (1995). How risky are hot tubs and saunas for pregnant women? *MCN: American Journal of Maternal/Child Nursing,* 20(3), 137.

Schröck, S., Du Manoir, S., Veldman, T., Schoell, B., Wienberg, J, Ferguson-Smith, M.A., Ning, Y., Ledbetter, D.H., Bar-Am, I., Soenksen, D., Garini, Y., & Ried, T. *New methods for karyotyping.* Retrieved May 23, 2000 from www.biology.arizona.edu/human_bio/current/new_karyotyping.html.

Scioscia, A.L. (1999). Prenatal diagnosis of genetic disorders. In R.K. Creasy & R. Resnik (Eds.), *Maternal-fetal medicine: Principles and practice* (4th ed., pp. 40-62). Philadelphia: W.B. Saunders.

Shapiro, L.J. (2000a). Patterns of inheritance. In R.E. Behrman, R.M. Kliegman, & H.B. Jenson (Eds.), *Nelson textbook of pediatrics* (16th ed., pp. 321-325). Philadelphia: W.B. Saunders.

Shapiro, L.J. (2000b). The molecular basis of genetic disorders. In R.E. Behrman, R.M. Kliegman, & H.B. Jenson (Eds.), *Nelson textbook of pediatrics* (16th ed., pp. 313-317). Philadelphia: W.B. Saunders.

Shapiro, L.J. (2000c). Molecular diagnosis of genetic diseases. In R.E. Behrman, R.M. Kliegman, & H.B. Jenson (Eds.), *Nelson textbook of pediatrics* (16th ed., pp. 317-321). Philadelphia: W.B. Saunders.

Slaughter, L. (1997). Ensuring protection from genetic discrimination in health insurance. *Lifelines,* 1(3), 23.

Verstag, B. (2000). Tinker with our genetic future? Not yet, say experts. *Journal of the National Cancer Institute,* 92: 518-520.

Verma, L., Macdonald, F., Leedham, P., McConachie, M., Dhanjal, S., & Hulten, M. (1998). Rapid and simple DNA diagnosis of Down's syndrome. *Lancet,* 352(9121), 9-12.

Ward, K. (1999). Prenatal diagnosis and genetics. In J.R. Scott, P.J. DiSaia, C.B. Hammond, & W.N. Spellacy (Eds.), *Danforth's obstetrics and gynecology* (8th ed., pp. 173-195). Philadelphia: Lippincott, Williams and Wilkins.

Williams, J.K., & Lea, D.H. (1995). Applying new genetic technologies: Assessment and ethical considerations. *Nurse Practitioner,* 20(7), 16-26.

6 Conception and Prenatal Development

OBJECTIVES

1. Describe formation of the female and male gametes.
2. Relate ovulation and ejaculation to the process of human conception.
3. Explain implantation and nourishment of the embryo before development of the placenta.
4. Describe normal prenatal development from conception through birth.
5. Explain structure and function of the placenta, umbilical cord, and fetal membranes.
6. Describe the occurrence of common deviations from normal conception and prenatal development.
7. Describe prenatal circulation and the circulatory changes after birth.
8. Explain the mechanisms and trends in multifetal pregnancies.

DEFINITIONS

Autosome Any of the 22 pairs of chromosomes other than the sex chromosomes.

Conceptus Cells and membranes resulting from fertilization of the ovum at any stage of prenatal development.

Corpus Luteum Graafian follicle cells remaining after ovulation that produce estrogen and progesterone.

Diploid The number of chromosomes (46 in humans) normally present in body cells other than gametes that represents one copy of every chromosome from each parent.

Ejaculation Expulsion of semen from the penis.

Embryo The developing baby from the beginning of the third week through the eighth week after conception.

Endometrium Lining of the uterus.

Fertilization Prenatal age of the developing baby, calculated from the date of conception. (Also called *postconceptional age.*)

Fetus The developing baby from 9 weeks after conception until birth; used in everyday practice to describe a developing baby during pregnancy, regardless of age.

Gamete Reproductive cell; in the female an ovum and in the male a spermatozoon.

DEFINITIONS—cont'd

Gestational Age Prenatal age of the developing baby (measured in weeks) calculated from the first day of the woman's last menstrual period; about 2 weeks longer than the fertilization age. (Also called *menstrual age.*)

Graafian Follicle A small sac within the ovary that contains the maturing ovum.

Haploid Usually occurs in gametes; refers to one copy of a chromosome from each pair (23 in humans, or half the diploid number).

Meiosis Reduction cell division in gametes that halves the number of chromosomes in each cell.

Mitosis Cell division in body cells other than the gametes.

Nidation Implantation of the fertilized ovum (zygote) in the uterine endometrium.

Oogenesis Formation of gametes (ova) in the female.

Ovulation Release of the mature ovum from the ovary.

Placenta Fetal structure that provides nourishment and removes wastes from the developing baby and secretes hormones necessary for the continuation of pregnancy.

Sex Chromosome The X or Y chromosome. Females have two X chromosomes; males have one X and one Y chromosome.

Somatic Cells Body cells other than the gametes, or germ cells.

Spermatogenesis Formation of male gametes (sperm) in the testes.

Teratogen An agent that can cause defects in a developing baby during pregnancy.

Zygote The developing baby from conception through the first week of prenatal life.

A basic understanding of conception and prenatal development helps the nurse provide care to parents during normal childbearing and better understand problems such as infertility and birth defects. This chapter addresses formation of the gametes, the process of conception, prenatal development, and important auxiliary structures that support normal prenatal development. The reason for the occurrence of multifetal pregnancy (for example, twinning) is also discussed.

GAMETOGENESIS

Gametogenesis is the development of ova in the woman and sperm in the man (Table 6-1). Production of gametes requires a different process than formation of somatic cells. Somatic cells reproduce by a process called *mitosis.* Each somatic cell has 46 paired chromosomes: 22 pairs of autosomes and 1 pair of sex chromosomes. During mitosis the cell divides into two new cells, each having 46 chromosomes like the parent cell.

Gametogenesis requires a special reduction division called *meiosis.* Unlike mitosis, in which the diploid number of chromosomes is retained in the new cells, meiosis halves the number of chromosomes to arrive at the haploid number. Only one of each chromosome pair (22 autosomes and 1 sex chromosome) is directed to the gamete. Also, with the exception of the X and Y chromosomes in the male, each chromosome exchanges some material with its mate so that the new chromosome in the gamete contains some material from the mother and some from the father. This process, which is called *crossing over,* allows variation in genetic material while keeping constant the total amount of chromosome material from generation to generation. When the sperm and ovum unite at conception, the "halves" form a new cell and restore the chromosome number to 46.

Oogenesis

Oogenesis is the formation of female gametes (Figure 6-1, *A*) within the ovary. Oogenesis begins during prenatal life when primitive ova (oogonia), like all other cells, multiply by mitosis. Each oogonium contains 46 chromosomes, as do other body cells. Before birth these oogonia enlarge to form primary oocytes, each surrounded by a layer of follicular cells. These are called *primary follicles.* The primary oogonium begins its first meiotic division during fetal life but does not complete the process until puberty. The primary follicle and its oogonium, which still contains 46 chromosomes, remain dormant throughout childhood.

The female fetus has all the ova she will ever have by the thirtieth week of gestation. Many of these ova regress during childhood. When a girl's reproductive cycles begin at puberty, some of the primary follicles present at birth begin maturing. The process of gamete maturation continues throughout her reproductive years until the climacteric, which is sometimes called the *change of life.*

When the oocyte matures, two meiotic divisions reduce the chromosome number from 46 paired to 23 unpaired chromosomes: 22 autosomes and 1 X chromosome. Shortly before ovulation, the primary oocyte completes its first meiotic division, which began during fetal life. The result is a secondary oocyte that now contains 23 chromosomes. The primary cell's cytoplasm is divided unequally with this division, and most of it is retained by the secondary oocyte. The remainder of cytoplasm plus the other half of the chromosomes go into a tiny, nonfunctional polar body that soon degenerates.

At ovulation, the secondary oocyte begins dividing again (second meiotic division) to form a mature ovum. The second meiotic division is prolonged, and the mature ovum remains suspended in metaphase, the

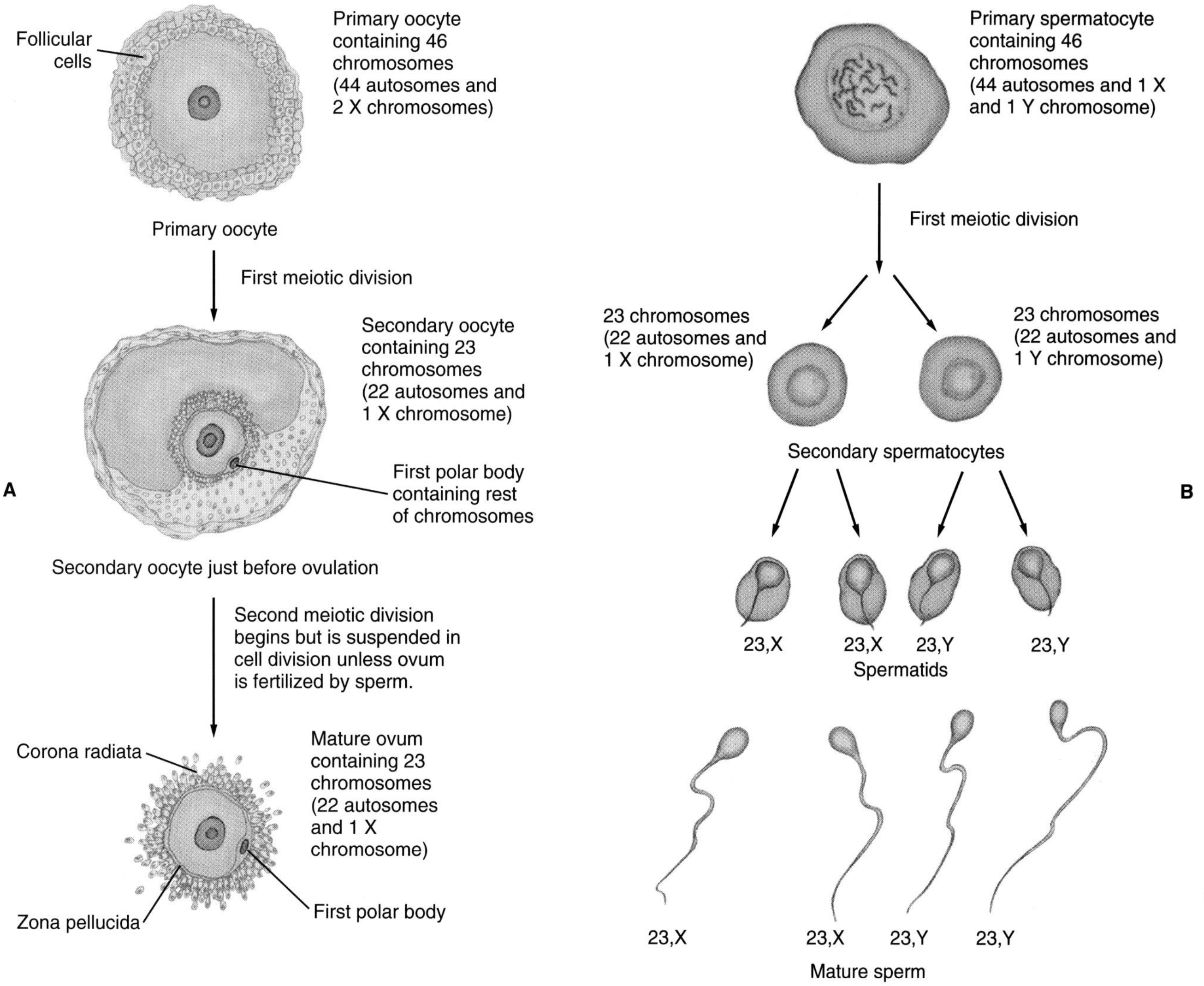

FIGURE 6-1 Gametogenesis. **A,** Formation of the mature ovum. **B,** Formation of mature sperm.

Table 6-1

COMPARISON OF FEMALE AND MALE GAMETOGENESIS

Factor	Oogenesis	Spermatogenesis
Time during which primary germ cells are produced	Fetal life with no other ova developing after about 30 weeks of gestation	Continuously after puberty
Hormones controlling process	GnRH FSH LH Estrogen	GnRH FSH LH Testosterone Estrogen (small amounts converted from testosterone) Growth hormone
Number of mature germ cells that develop from each primary cell	One	Four
Quantity	One during each reproductive cycle of about 28 days	40 to 300 million released with each ejaculation
Size	Large, visible to naked eye, abundant cytoplasm to nourish embryo until implantation	Tiny compared with ovum, little cytoplasm, head consisting of almost all nuclear material (chromosomes)
Motility	Relatively nonmotile, carried along by action of cilia and currents within fallopian tubes	Independently motile by means of whiplike tail, mitochondria in middle piece providing energy for motility
Chromosome complement	23 total: 22 autosomes plus 1 X sex chromosome	23 total: 22 autosomes plus either an X or a Y sex chromosome

GnRH, Gonadotropin-releasing hormone; *FSH,* follicle-stimulating hormone; *LH,* luteinizing hormone.

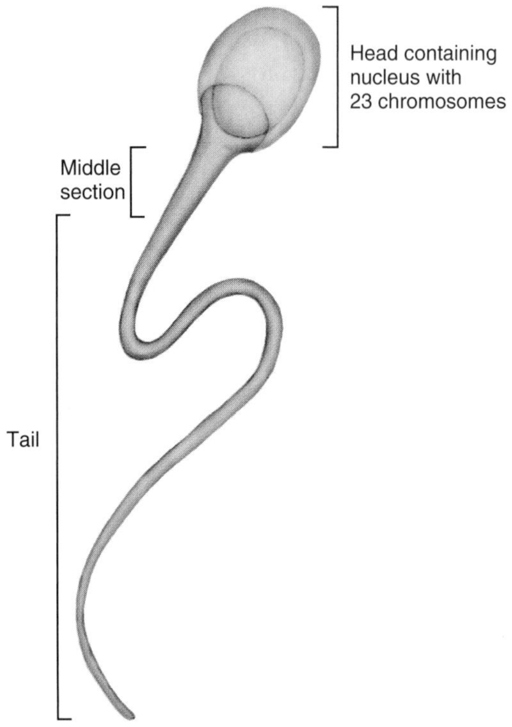

FIGURE 6-2 Mature sperm.

middle part of cell division. If fertilization occurs, the second meiotic division is completed, resulting in a mature ovum that also contains 23 chromosomes and a second tiny polar body that degenerates. If the ovum is not fertilized, it does not complete the second meiotic division and degenerates. In oogenesis, one primary oocyte results in a single mature ovum.

When the mature ovum is released from the ovary, it is surrounded by two layers: the zona pellucida and the cells of the corona radiata. These layers protect the ovum and prevent fertilization by more than one sperm. For fertilization to occur, the sperm must penetrate these two layers to reach the ovum's cell nucleus.

Spermatogenesis

Spermatogenesis (Figure 6-1, *B*) begins during puberty in the male and requires about 70 days to complete. Primitive sperm cells, or spermatogonia, develop during the prenatal period and begin multiplying by mitosis during puberty. Unlike the female, the male continues to produce new spermatogonia that can mature into sperm throughout his lifetime. Although male fertility gradually declines with age, men can father children in their 50s, 60s, and beyond.

Each spermatogonium contains 46 paired chromosomes, like other body cells. In the mature male a spermatogonium enlarges to become a primary spermatocyte that still contains all 46 chromosomes. The first meiotic division forms two secondary spermatocytes and reduces the number to 23 unpaired chromosomes: 22 autosomes and 1 X or Y sex chromosome. Each secondary spermatocyte divides again in the second meiotic division to form two spermatids. Therefore 50% of the four spermatids that result from the two meiotic divisions of the spermatogonium carry an X chromosome and 50% carry a Y chromosome. The spermatids gradually evolve into mature sperm.

The gamete from a male determines the gender of the new baby because the ovum carries only an X chromosome. Each mature sperm contains 23 chromosomes: 22 autosomes and either an X or a Y chromosome. If an X-bearing spermatozoon fertilizes the ovum, the baby is a girl. If a Y-bearing spermatozoon fertilizes the ovum, the baby is a boy.

The mature sperm has three major sections: a head, middle portion, and tail (Figure 6-2). The head is almost entirely a cell nucleus and contains the male chromosomes that join the chromosomes of the ovum. The middle portion supplies energy for the tail's whiplike action. The movement of the tail propels the sperm toward the ovum.

Check Your Reading

1. What is the purpose of meiosis in the gametes?
2. How many mature ova can be produced by each oogonium? When does meiosis occur in the female?
3. How many mature spermatozoa can be produced by each spermatogonium? When does meiosis occur in the male?

CONCEPTION

Conception requires interaction of many factors, including correct timing between release of a mature ovum at ovulation and ejaculation of enough healthy, mature, motile sperm into the vagina. Although exact viability is unknown, the ovum may survive no longer than 24 hours after its release at ovulation. Most sperm survive no more than 24 hours in the female reproductive tract, although some remain fertile up to 72 hours.

Preparation for Conception in the Female

Before ovulation, several oocytes begin to mature under the influence of follicle-stimulating hormone (FSH) and luteinizing hormone (LH) from the woman's anterior pituitary gland. Each maturing oocyte is contained within a sac called the *graafian follicle,* which produces estrogen and progesterone to prepare the endometrium for a possible pregnancy. Eventually, one follicle outgrows the others. The less mature oocytes permanently regress.

Release of the Ovum

Ovulation occurs about 14 days before a woman's next menstrual period would begin. The follicle develops a weak spot on the surface of the ovary and ruptures, releasing the mature ovum with its surrounding cells onto the surface of the ovary. The collapsed follicle is transformed into the corpus luteum, which maintains high estrogen and progesterone secretion necessary to make final preparation of the uterine lining for a fertilized ovum.

Ovum Transport

The mature ovum is released on the surface of the ovary, where it is picked up by the fimbriated (fringed) ends of the fallopian tube. The ovum is transported through the tube by the muscular action of the tube and movement of cilia within the tube. Fertilization normally occurs in the distal third of the fallopian tube (ampulla) near the ovary. The ovum, fertilized or not, enters the uterus about 3 days after its release from the ovary.

Preparation for Conception in the Male

The male preparation for fertilizing the ovum consists of ejaculation, movement of the sperm in the female reproductive tract, and preparation of the sperm for actual fertilization.

Ejaculation

When a male ejaculates during sexual intercourse, 40 to 300 million sperm are deposited in the upper vagina and over the cervix, 50% to 90% of which are morphologically normal. The sperm are suspended in 2 to 5 ml of seminal fluid, which nourishes and protects the sperm from the acidic environment of the vagina (Surrey, et al., 1998). Many sperm are lost as the ejaculate drips from the vaginal introitus. Other sperm are inactivated by acidic vaginal secretions or digested by vaginal enzymes and phagocytes. The seminal fluid coagulates slightly after ejaculation to hold the semen deeply in the vagina. Many sperm are relatively immobile for about 15 to 30 minutes until other seminal enzymes dissolve the coagulated fluid and allow the sperm to begin moving upward through the cervix.

Transport of Sperm in the Female Reproductive Tract

The whiplike movement of the tails of spermatozoa propels them through the cervix, uterus, and fallopian tubes. Uterine contractions induced by prostaglandins in the seminal fluid enhance movement of the sperm toward the ovum. Only sperm cells enter the cervix. The seminal fluid remains in the vagina.

Many sperm are lost along the way. Some are digested by enzymes and phagocytes in the female reproductive tract, whereas others simply lose their direction, moving into the wrong tube or past the ovum and out into the peritoneal cavity. Fewer than 200 reach the fallopian tube where the ovum waits (Surrey, et al., 1998).

Preparation of Sperm for Fertilization

Sperm are not immediately ready to fertilize the ovum when they are ejaculated. During the trip to the ovum, the sperm undergo changes that enable one of them to penetrate the protective layers surrounding the ovum, a process called *capacitation.* During capacitation a glycoprotein coat and seminal proteins are removed from the acrosome, which is the tip of the sperm head. After capacitation the sperm look the same but are more active and can better penetrate the corona radiata and zona pellucida surrounding the ovum.

Sperm must also undergo an acrosome reaction to further prepare them to fertilize the ovum. The sperm that reach the ovum release hyaluronidase and acrosin to digest a pathway through the corona radiata and zona pellucida. Their tails beat harder to propel them toward the center of the ovum. Eventually, one spermatozoon penetrates the ovum.

Fertilization

Fertilization occurs when one spermatozoon enters the ovum and the two nuclei containing the parents' chromosomes merge (Figure 6-3).

Entry of One Spermatozoon into the Ovum

Entry of a spermatozoon into the ovum has three results. First is the zona reaction, in which changes in the zona pellucida surrounding the ovum prevent other sperm from entering. Second, the cell membranes of the ovum and sperm fuse and break down, allowing the contents of the sperm head to enter the cytoplasm of the ovum. Third, the ovum, which has been suspended in the middle of its second meiotic division since just before ovulation, completes meiosis. This results in a nucleus with 23 chromosomes and the expulsion of a second nonfunctional polar body. The mature ovum now contains 23 unpaired chromosomes (22 autosomes and 1 X chromosome) in its nucleus.

Fusion of the Nuclei of Sperm and Ovum

Once a spermatozoon has penetrated the ovum, fusion of their nuclei begins. The sperm head enlarges and the tail degenerates. The nuclei of the gametes move toward the center of the ovum, where the membranes surrounding their nuclei touch and dissolve. The 23 chromosomes from the sperm mingle with the 23 from the ovum, restoring the diploid number to 46. Fertilization is complete, and cell division can begin when the nuclei of the sperm and ovum unite.

Check Your Reading

4. Where does fertilization usually occur?
5. What are the purposes of the seminal fluid?
6. What occurs when a spermatozoon penetrates the ovum?
7. When is fertilization complete and a new human conceived?

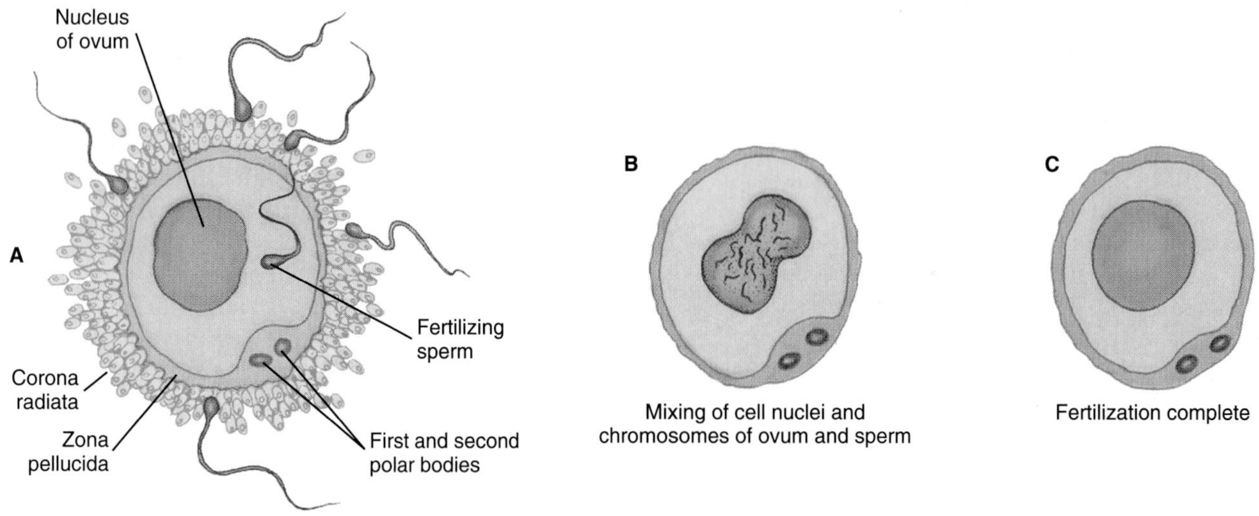

FIGURE 6-3 Process of fertilization. **A,** A sperm enters the ovum. **B,** The 23 chromosomes from the sperm mingle with the 23 chromosomes from the ovum, restoring the diploid number to 46. **C,** The fertilized ovum is now called a *zygote* and is ready for the first mitotic cell division.

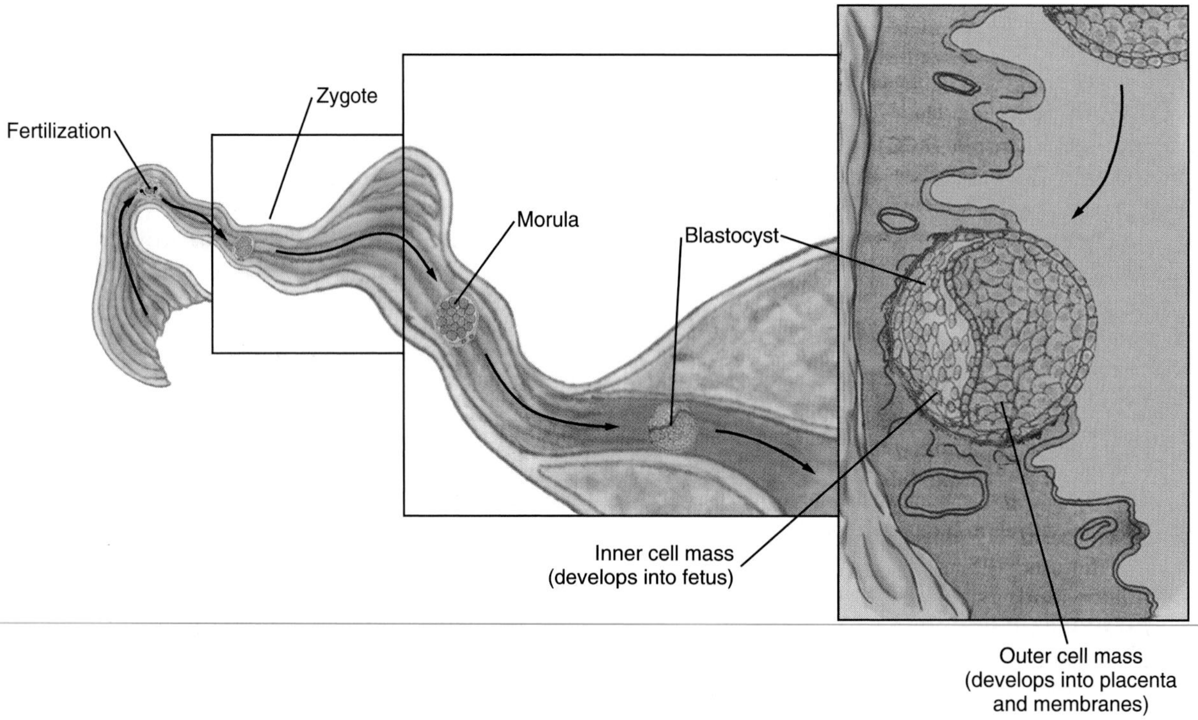

FIGURE 6-4 Prenatal development from fertilization through implantation of the blastocyst. Implantation gradually occurs from the sixth through the tenth day. Implantation is complete on the tenth day.

PREEMBRYONIC PERIOD

The preembryonic period is the first 2 weeks after conception (Figure 6-4). Around the fourth day after conception, the fertilized ovum, now called a *zygote,* enters the uterus.

Initiation of Cell Division

The zygote divides into 2, then 4, then 8 cells, and so on. Until the 16-cell stage, the cells become tightly compacted with each division so that they occupy about the same amount of space as the original zygote. When the conceptus is a solid ball of 12 to 16 cells, it is called a *morula* because it resembles a mulberry.

The outer cells of the morula secrete fluid, forming a blastocyst, a sac of cells with an inner cell mass placed off center within the sac. The inner cell mass develops into the fetus. Part of the outer layer of cells develops as the placenta and fetal membranes.

Entry of the Zygote into the Uterus

The blastocyst enters the uterus when it contains about 100 cells. It lingers in the uterus another 2 to 4 days before beginning implantation. The endometrium, now called the *decidua,* is in the secretory phase of the reproductive cycle, 1½ weeks before the woman would otherwise begin her menstrual period. The endometrial glands are secreting at their maximum, providing rich fluids to nourish the conceptus before placental circulation is established. The endometrial spiral arteries are well developed in the secretory phase, providing easy access for development of the placental blood supply.

Implantation in the Decidua

The conceptus carries a small supply of nutrients for early cell division. However, implantation at the proper time and location in the uterus is critical for continued development. Implantation, or nidation, is a gradual process that occurs between the sixth and tenth days after conception. During the relatively long process of implantation, embryonic structures continue to develop.

Maintaining the Decidua

Implantation and survival of the conceptus require a continuing supply of estrogen and progesterone to maintain the decidua in the secretory phase. The zygote secretes human chorionic gonadotropin (hCG) to signal the woman's body that a pregnancy has begun. Production of hCG by the conceptus causes the corpus luteum to persist and continue secretion of estrogen and progesterone until the placenta takes over this function.

Location of Implantation

The conceptus must be in the right place at the right time for normal implantation to occur. The site of implantation is important because that is where the placenta develops. Normal implantation occurs in the upper uterus, slightly more often on the posterior wall than the anterior wall (Moore and Persaud, 1998a). The upper uterus is the best area for implantation and placental development for three reasons:

- The upper uterus is richly supplied with blood for optimal fetal gas exchange and nutrition.
- The uterine lining is thick in the upper uterus, preventing the placenta from attaching too deeply into the uterine muscle and facilitating easy expulsion of the placenta after birth.
- Implantation in the upper uterus limits blood loss after birth because strong interlacing muscle fibers in this area compress open endometrial vessels after the placenta detaches.

Mechanism of Implantation

Enzymes produced by the conceptus erode the decidua, tapping maternal sources of nutrition. Primary chorionic villi are tiny projections on the surface of the conceptus extending into the decidua basalis that lies between the conceptus and the wall of the uterus. The chorionic villi eventually form the fetal side of the placenta. The decidua basalis forms the maternal side of the placenta (see p. 110, Figure 6-7, *A*).

At this early stage, nutritive fluid passes to the embryo by diffusion (the passive movement across a cell membrane from an area of higher concentration to one of lower concentration) because the circulatory system is not yet established. The conceptus is fully embedded within the mother's uterine decidua by 10 days, and the site of implantation is almost invisible.

As the conceptus implants, usually near the time of the next expected menstrual period, a small amount of bleeding ("spotting") may occur at the site. Implantation bleeding may be confused with a normal menstrual period, particularly if the woman's menstrual periods are usually light.

Check Your Reading

8. When does implantation occur?
9. What are the advantages of implantation in the upper uterine?
10. How is the embryo nourished before the placenta develops?

EMBRYONIC PERIOD

The embryonic period of development extends from the beginning of the third week through the eighth week after conception (Figure 6-5). Basic structures of all major body organs are completed during the embryonic period (Table 6-2).

Differentiation of Cells

The embryo progresses from undifferentiated cells with essentially identical functions to differentiated, or specialized, body cells. By the end of the eighth week, all major organ systems are in place and many are functioning, although in a simple way.

Development of the specialized structures is controlled by three factors: (1) genetic information in the chromosomes received from the parents, (2) interaction between adjacent tissues, and (3) timing. Although basic instructions are carried within the chromosomes, one tissue may induce change toward greater specialization in another but only if a signal between the two tissues occurs at a specific time during development. In this way, structures develop with appropriate sizes and relationships to each other.

During the embryonic period, structures are vulnerable to damage from teratogens because they are devel-

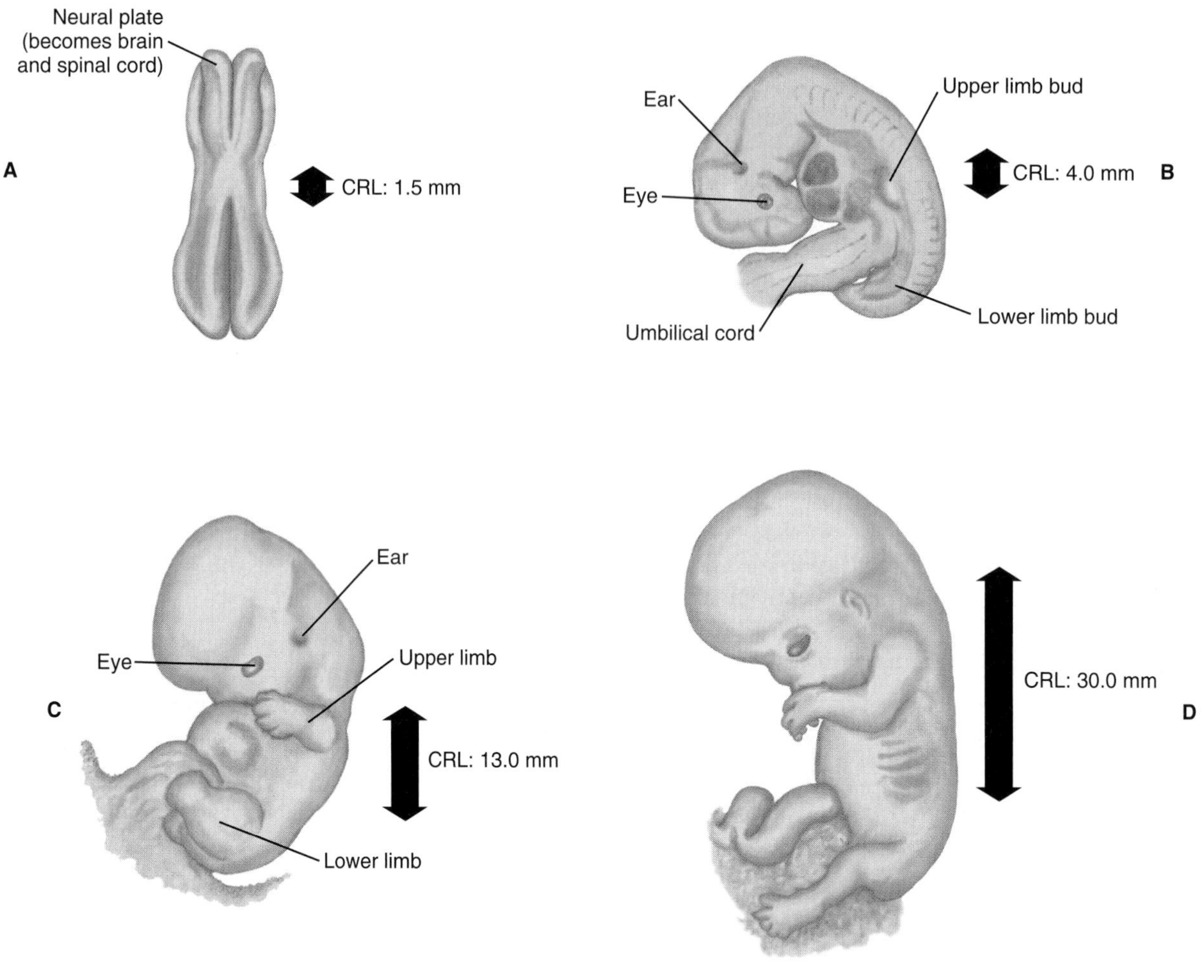

FIGURE 6-5 Embryonic development from the third through eighth weeks after fertilization. **A,** Week 3. **B,** Week 4. **C,** Week 6. **D,** Week 8. (*CRL,* Crown-to-rump length.)

oping rapidly. Normal development of one structure often requires normal and properly timed development of another structure. Unfortunately, a woman may not realize she is pregnant during this sensitive time. For this reason the possibility of pregnancy should be explored with her before the prescription of drugs or administration of diagnostic procedures such as radiography. Some agents may be damaging at one time during pregnancy but not at another. Others may be damaging at any time during pregnancy (see Appendix C).

Weekly Developments

Development occurs simultaneously in all embryonic organ systems. Development of the embryo and fetus proceeds in a cephalocaudal (head-to-toe) and central-to-peripheral direction. Generalized to specific development continues as refinement of organs occurs. This developmental pattern continues after birth.

Full term ranges from 36 to 40 weeks of fertilization age, or 38 to 42 weeks of gestational age (after last menstrual period). Because conception occurs about 2 weeks after the first day of the last menstrual period in most women who have 4-week cycles, the fertilization age, used in this chapter, is about 2 weeks shorter than the gestational age. However, gestational age is most commonly used in practice because the last menstrual period provides a known marker, whereas most women do not know exactly when they conceived.

Week 2

Implantation is complete by the end of the second week after fertilization. The most growth occurs in the outer cells, or trophoblast, which eventually becomes the fetal part of the placenta. The inner cell mass that will develop into the baby becomes flattened into the embryonic disk. Cells that eventually form part of the fetal membranes develop.

Week 3

Many women miss their first menstrual period during the third week after conception. The embryonic disk develops three layers called *germ layers* that in turn

Table 6-2

PRENATAL DEVELOPMENT BASED ON FERTILIZATION AGE*

Nervous/Sensory System	Cardiorespiratory System	Digestive System	Genitourinary System	Musculoskeletal System	Integumentary System
3 weeks: 1.5 mm CRL					
Flat neural plate begins closing to form neural tube. Neural tube still open at each end.	Heart consists of two parallel tubes that fuse into a single tube. Contractions of heart tube begin in a wavelike manner. Chorionic villi of early placenta connect with heart.	Endoderm (inner germ layer) will become digestive tract.		Paired, cube-shaped swellings (somites) appear and will form most of the head and trunk skeleton. Muscle, bone, and cartilage develop from mesoderm.	Epidermis (outer skin layer) will develop from ectoderm (outer germ layer). Dermis (deep skin layer) and connective tissue will develop from mesoderm (middle germ layer).
4 weeks: 4.0 mm CRL					
Neural tube is closed at each end. Cranial end of neural tube will form brain and caudal end will form spinal cord. Eye development begins as an outgrowth of forebrain. Nose development begins as two pits. Inner ear begins developing from hind brain.	Heart begins partitioning into four chambers and begins beating in a coordinated way. Blood circulating through embryonic vessels and chorionic villi. Tracheal development begins as a bud on the upper gut and branches into two bronchial buds.	Primitive gut develops as embryo folds laterally. Stomach begins as a widening of the tube-shaped primitive gut. Liver, gallbladder, and biliary ducts begin as a bud from primitive gut.	Primordial germ cells (reproductive cells) are present on embryonic yolk sac.	Upper limb buds are present and look like flippers. Lower limb buds appear. Upper limbs develop and become refined earlier than lower limbs.	Mammary ridges that will develop into mammary glands appear.
6 weeks: 13 mm CRL					
Pituitary gland and cranial nerves develop. Head is sharply flexed because of rapid brain growth. Eyelid development begins. External ear development begins in neck region as six swellings.	Blood formation is primarily in liver. Three right and two left lung lobes develop as outgrowths of the right and left bronchi.	Most intestines are contained within the umbilical cord because the liver and kidneys occupy most of the abdominal cavity. Stomach nears its final form. Development of upper and lower jaws begins.	Kidneys are near bladder in the pelvis. Kidneys occupy much of the abdominal cavity. Primordial germ cells are incorporated into developing gonads. Male and female gonads appear identical.	Arms are paddle shaped and fingers are webbed. Feet and toes develop similarly but a few days later than arms and hands. Bones are cartilaginous, but ossification of skull begins.	Mammary glands begin development. Tooth buds for primary (deciduous) teeth begin developing.
8 weeks: 30 mm CRL					
Spinal cord stops at end of vertebral column. Taste buds begin developing. Eyelids fuse. Ears have final form but appear low set because of the small mandible.	Heart has partitioned into four chambers. Heartbeat detectable with ultrasound. Additional branching of bronchi occurs.	Stomach has reached final form. Lips are fused. Some intestines remain in umbilical cord.	Testes begin developing under influence of Y chromosome. Ovaries will develop if a Y chromosome is not present. External genitalia begin to differentiate but still appear quite similar.	Fingers and toes are still webbed but are distinct by end of eighth week. Bones begin to ossify. Joints resemble those of adults.	

CRL, Crown-rump length.
*Fertilization age is about 2 weeks less than gestational age.

Continued

Table 6-2

PRENATAL DEVELOPMENT BASED ON FERTILIZATION AGE—cont'd

Nervous/Sensory System	Cardiorespiratory System	Digestive System	Genitourinary System	Musculoskeletal System	Integumentary System
10 WEEKS: 61 MM CRL WEIGHT: 14 G					
Head flexion is still present but less pronounced. Eyelids are closed and fused. Top of external ear is slightly below eye level.	A heartbeat may be detected with Doppler transducer. Blood is produced in spleen and lymphatic tissue.	Intestines are contained within abdominal cavity as growth of this cavity catches up with digestive system development. Digestive tract is patent from mouth to anus.	Kidneys are in their adult position. Male and female external genitalia have different appearance but are still easily confused.	Toes are distinct. Soles of feet face each other.	Fingernails begin developing. Tooth buds for permanent teeth begin developing below those for primary teeth.
12 WEEKS: 87 MM CRL WEIGHT: 45 G					
Surface of brain is smooth and without sulci (grooves) or gyri (convolutions). Nasal septum and palate complete development.	Heartbeat should be detected with Doppler transducer.	Sucking reflex is present. Bile is formed by liver.	Kidneys begin producing urine. Male and female external genitalia can be distinguished by appearance.	Limbs are long and thin. Involuntary muscles of viscera develop.	Downy lanugo begins developing at end of this week.
16 WEEKS: 140 MM CRL WEIGHT: 200 G					
	Pulmonary vascular system is developing rapidly.	Fetus swallows amniotic fluid and produces meconium (bowel contents).	Urine is excreted into amniotic fluid.	Lower limbs reach final relative length and are longer than upper limbs. A woman who has been pregnant before may begin to feel fetal movements.	External ears have enough cartilage to stand away from head somewhat. Blood vessels are easily visible through the delicate skin. Fingerprints are developing.
20 WEEKS: 160 MM CRL WEIGHT: 460 G					
Myelination of nerves begins and continues through first year of postnatal life.	Heartbeat can be detected with regular (nonelectronic) fetoscope. Surfactant (to reduce surface tension in alveoli) production begins.	Peristalsis is well developed.	More than 40% of nephrons are mature and functioning. Testes are contained in abdomen but begin descent toward scrotum. Primordial follicles of ovary develop.	Fetal movements are felt by mother and may be palpable by an experienced examiner.	Skin is thin and covered with vernix caseosa. Brown fat production is complete. Nipples begin development.

CRL, Crown-rump length.

Table 6-2

PRENATAL DEVELOPMENT BASED ON FERTILIZATION AGE—cont'd

Nervous/Sensory System	Cardiorespiratory System	Digestive System	Genitourinary System	Musculoskeletal System	Integumentary System
24 WEEKS: 230 MM CRL WEIGHT: 820 G					
Spinal cord ends at level of first sacral vertebra because of more rapid growth of vertebral canal.	Primitive thin-walled alveoli (air sacs) have developed and are surrounded by capillary network. Surfactant production continues. Respiration is possible, but most fetuses die if born at this time. Some born at the end of this period may survive with aid of artificial surfactant.			Fetus is active. Fetal movements become progressively more noticeable to both mother and examiner.	Body appearance is lean. Skin is wrinkled and red. Fingerprints and footprints have developed. Fingernails are present. Eyebrows and lashes are present.
28 WEEKS: 230 MM CRL WEIGHT: 1300 G					
Major sulci and gyri are present. Eyelids are no longer fused after 26 weeks. Fetus responds to bitter substances on tongue.	Erythrocyte formation shifts completely to bone marrow. Alveoli, surfactant, and capillary networks are sufficient to allow respiratory function, although respiratory problems may occur. Many infants born at this time survive with intensive care.		Testes begin descent into scrotum.		Skin is slightly wrinkled but is smoothing out as subcutaneous fat is deposited under it.
32 WEEKS: 230 MM CRL WEIGHT: 2100 G					
			Testes enter scrotum.		Skin is smooth and pigmented. Large vessels are visible beneath skin. Fingernails reach fingertips. Lanugo is disappearing.
38 WEEKS: 230 MM CRL WEIGHT: 3400 G					
Sulci and gyri are developed. Visual acuity is about 20/600 at birth.	Newborn has about one-eighth to one-sixth the number of alveoli of an adult. Ability to exchange gas is well developed.		Both testes are usually palpable in scrotum at birth. The newborn girl's ovaries contain about 1 million follicles. No new ones are formed after birth.		Fetus is plump and skin is smooth. Vernix caseosa is present in major body creases. Lanugo is present on shoulders and upper back only. Fingernails extend beyond the fingertips. Ear cartilage is firm.

Table 6-3
DERIVATIVES OF THE THREE GERM LAYERS

Ectoderm	Mesoderm	Endoderm
Brain and spinal cord	Cartilage	Lining of gastrointestinal and respiratory tracts
Peripheral nervous system	Bone	Tonsils
Pituitary gland	Connective tissue	Thyroid
Sensory epithelium of the eye, ear, and nose	Muscle tissue	Parathyroid
	Heart	Thymus
Epidermis	Blood vessels	Liver
Hair	Blood cells	Pancreas
Nails	Lymphatic system	Lining of urinary bladder and urethra
Subcutaneous glands	Spleen	Lining of ear canal
Mammary glands	Kidneys	
Tooth enamel	Adrenal cortex	
	Ovaries	
	Testes	
	Reproductive system	
	Lining membranes (pericardial, pleural, and peritoneal)	

give rise to major organ systems of the body (Table 6-3). The three germ layers are the ectoderm, mesoderm, and endoderm.

The central nervous system begins developing during the third week. A thickened flat neural plate appears, extending toward the end of the embryonic disk that will become the head. The neural plate develops a longitudinal groove that folds to form the neural tube. At the end of the third week the neural tube is fused in the middle but still open at each end.

Early heart development consists of a pair of parallel heart tubes that run longitudinally and join. The primitive heart begins beating at 21 to 22 days in a way that results in a wavelike flow of blood. By the end of the fourth week, coordinated contractions result in the unidirectional flow of blood that characterizes the mature heart. Vessels developing in the chorionic villi and membranes join the heart tube. Primitive blood cells arise from the endoderm lining the distal blood vessels.

Week 4

The shape of the embryo changes during the fourth week after conception. It folds at the head and tail end and laterally, resembling a C-shaped cylinder. A "tail" is apparent during the embryonic period because the brain and spinal cord develop more rapidly than other systems. The tail disappears as the rest of the body catches up with growth of the central nervous system. The neural tube closes during the fourth week. If the neural tube does not close, defects such as anencephaly and spina bifida result.

Formation of the face and upper respiratory tract begins. Beginnings of the internal ear and the eye are apparent. The upper extremities appear as buds on the lateral body walls. Because the embryo is sharply flexed anteriorly, the heart is near the embryo's mouth. Partitioning of the heart into four chambers begins during the fourth week and is completed by the end of the sixth week.

The lower respiratory tract begins growth as a branch of the upper digestive tract, which is a simple tube at this time. Gradually, the esophagus and trachea complete separation. The trachea branches to form the right and left bronchi. These bronchi in turn branch to form the three lobes of the right lung and two lobes of the left lung. Continued branching of the bronchi eventually forms the terminal air sacs, or alveoli. The alveoli proliferate and become surrounded by a rich capillary network that enables oxygen and carbon dioxide exchange at birth.

Week 5

The head is very large because the brain grows rapidly during the fifth week after fertilization. The heart is beating and developing four chambers. Upper limb buds are paddle shaped with obvious notches between the fingers. Lower limbs form slightly later than upper ones. Lower limbs are also paddle shaped, but the area between the toes is not as well defined as the division between the fingers.

Week 6

The rapidly developing head is bent over the chest. The heart reaches its final four-chambered form. Upper and lower extremities continue to become more defined.

The eyes continue to develop, and the beginnings of the external ears appear as six small bumps on each side of the neck. Facial development begins with eyes, ears, and nasal pits that are widely separated and aligned with the body walls. Gradually the embryo grows so that the face comes together in the midline and the external ears assume their proper position on the sides of the head.

Week 7

General growth and refinement of all systems occur seven weeks after conception. The face becomes more human looking. The eyelids begin to grow, and the extremities become longer and better defined. The trunk elongates and straightens, although a C-shaped spinal curve is still present in the newborn at birth.

The intestines have been growing faster than the abdominal cavity during the embryonic period. The relatively large liver and kidneys also occupy much of the abdominal cavity. Therefore most of the intestines are contained within the umbilical cord while the abdominal cavity grows to accommodate them. The abdomen is large enough to contain all its normal contents by 10 weeks.

Week 8

The embryo has a definite human form, and refinements to all systems continue. The ears are low set but approaching their final location. The eyes are pigmented but not yet fully covered by eyelids. Fingers and toes are stubby but well defined. The external genitalia begin to differentiate, but male and female characteristics are not distinct until 10 weeks after conception, or 12 weeks after the woman's last menstrual period.

Check Your Reading

11. Why is the embryo particularly susceptible to damage from teratogens?
12. How does the lower respiratory tract develop?
13. Why are the intestines mostly contained within the umbilical cord until the tenth week?

FETAL PERIOD

The fetal period is the longest part of prenatal development. It begins 9 weeks after conception and ends with birth. All major systems are present in their basic form. Dramatic growth and refinement in the structure and function of all organ systems occur during the fetal period (Figure 6-6). Teratogens may damage already formed structures but are less likely to cause major structural alterations. The central nervous system is vulnerable to damaging agents through the entire pregnancy. (In this discussion, *weeks of gestation* refer to weeks after conception. Add 2 weeks to obtain the approximate weeks from the woman's last menstrual period.)

Weeks 9 through 12

The head is about half the total length of the fetus at the beginning of this period. The body begins growing faster than the head, changing the proportions. The extremities approach their final relative lengths, although the legs remain proportionately shorter than the arms. The first fetal movements begin but are too slight for the mother to detect.

The face is broad with a wide nose and widely spaced eyes. The eyes close at 10 weeks and reopen at about 26 to 28 weeks. The ears appear low set because the mandible is still small.

The intestinal contents that were partly contained within the umbilical cord enter the abdomen as the capacity of the abdominal cavity catches up with them in size. Blood formation occurs primarily in the liver during the ninth week but shifts to the spleen by the end of the twelfth week. The fetus begins producing urine during this period and excretes it into the amniotic fluid.

Internal differences in males and females begin to be apparent in the seventh week. External genitalia look similar until the end of the ninth week. By the end of the twelfth week, the fetal gender can be determined by the appearance of the external genitalia.

Weeks 13 through 16

The fetus grows rapidly in length, so the head becomes smaller in proportion to the total length. Movements strengthen, and some women, particularly those who have been pregnant before, are able to detect them. This phenomenon is referred to as *quickening*. The face looks human because the eyes face fully forward. The ears near their final position at the sides of the head and in line with the eyes.

Weeks 17 through 20

Fetal movements feel like fluttering or "butterflies." Some women may not recognize these subtle sensations.

Changes in the skin and hair are evident. Vernix caseosa, a fatty, cheeselike secretion of the fetal sebaceous glands, covers the skin to protect it from constant exposure to amniotic fluid. Lanugo is fine, downy hair that covers the fetal body and helps the vernix adhere to the skin. Both vernix and lanugo diminish as the fetus reaches term. Eyebrows and head hair appear.

Brown fat is a special heat-producing fat deposited during this period that helps the newborn maintain temperature stability after birth. It is located on the back of the neck, behind the sternum, and around the kidneys.

Weeks 21 through 24

While continuing to grow and gain weight, the fetus still appears thin because of minimal subcutaneous fat. The skin is translucent and red because the capillaries are close to its fragile surface.

The lungs begin to produce surfactant, a surface-active lipid substance that facilitates lung expansion and makes it easier for the baby to breathe after birth.

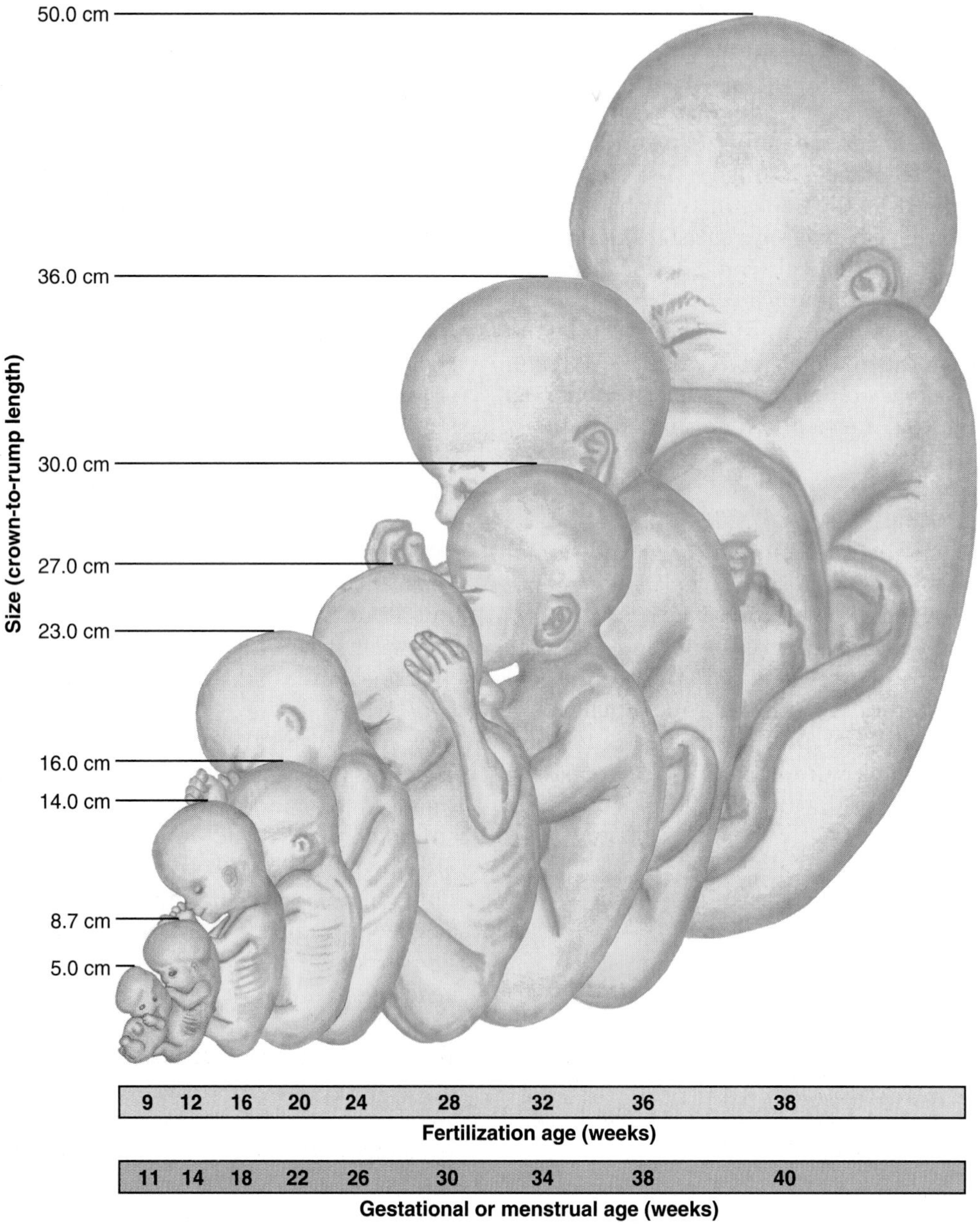

FIGURE 6-6 Fetal development from 9 weeks through 38 weeks of fertilization age. The gestational age, measured from the first day of the last menstrual period, is about 2 weeks longer than the fertilization age.

Surfactant reduces surface tension in the lung alveoli and prevents them from collapsing with each breath. Production of surfactant begins at about 20 weeks but does not reach levels to permit easy survival outside the uterus until 26 to 28 weeks after conception. Surfactant production increases during late pregnancy, particularly during the last 2 weeks (Moore & Persaud, 1998a). Use of artificial surfactant has allowed some newborns born at early gestations to survive, however.

The capillary network surrounding the alveoli is increasing but still very immature, although some gas exchange is possible. A fetus born at this time is unlikely to survive because adequate gas exchange is not possible. Other systems are extremely immature as well.

Weeks 25 through 28

The fetus may survive if born during this period because of maturation of the lungs, pulmonary capillaries, and central nervous system. The fetus becomes plumper with smoother skin as subcutaneous fat is deposited under the skin. The skin gradually becomes less red. The eyes, which were closed during the ninth week, reopen. Head hair is abundant. Blood formation shifts from the spleen to the bone marrow.

During early pregnancy the fetus floats freely within the amniotic sac. However, the fetus usually assumes a head-down position during this time for two reasons:

- The uterus is shaped like an inverted egg. The overall shape of the fetus in flexion is similar, with the head being the small pole of the egg shape and the buttocks, flexed legs, and feet being the larger pole.
- The fetal head is heavier than the feet, and gravity causes the head to drift downward in the pool of amniotic fluid.

The head-down position is also most favorable for normal birth.

Weeks 29 through 32

The skin is pigmented according to race and is smooth. Larger vessels are visible over the abdomen, but small capillaries cannot be seen. Toenails are present, and fingernails extend to the fingertips. The fetus has more subcutaneous fat, which rounds the body contours. If the fetus is born during this period, chances of survival are good.

Weeks 33 through 38

Growth of all body systems continues until birth, but the rate of growth slows as full term approaches. The fetus is mainly gaining weight. The pulmonary system matures to enable efficient and unlabored breathing after birth.

The well-nourished term fetus is rotund with abundant subcutaneous fat. At birth, boys are slightly heavier than girls. The skin is pink to brownish pink, depending on race. Lanugo may be present over the forehead, upper back, and upper arms. Vernix often remains in major creases such as the groin and axillae.

The testes are in the scrotum. Breasts of both male and female infants are enlarged, and breast tissue is palpable beneath the areola and nipple.

Check Your Reading

14. What is the difference between fertilization age and gestational age? Which term is more commonly used and why?
15. Why does the fetus usually assume a head-down position in the uterus?
16. What is the purpose of each of these fetal structures or substances: Vernix caseosa? Lanugo? Brown fat? Surfactant?

AUXILIARY STRUCTURES

Three auxiliary structures sustain the pregnancy and permit normal prenatal development: the placenta, the umbilical cord, and fetal membranes. These structures develop simultaneously with the baby's development.

Placenta

The placenta is a thick, disk-shaped organ. The placenta has two components, maternal and fetal (Figure 6-7). It is involved in (1) metabolic functions, (2) transfer functions, and (3) endocrine functions. The fetal side is smooth, with branching vessels covering the membrane-covered surface. The maternal side is rough where it attaches to the uterus (see Figure 12-14, *A*).

The umbilical cord is normally inserted on the fetal side of the placenta, near the center. However, it may insert off center or even out on the fetal membranes (Figure 6-8).

During early pregnancy, the placenta is larger than the embryo or fetus. However, the fetus grows faster than the placenta, so the placenta is about one sixth the weight of the fetus at the end of a term pregnancy.

Maternal Component

Development. When conception occurs, cells of the endometrium undergo changes that promote early nutrition of the embryo and enable most of the uterine lining to be shed after birth. These changes convert endometrial cells into the decidua. In addition to providing nourishment for the embryo, the decidua may protect the mother from uncontrolled invasion of fetal placental tissue into the uterine wall.

The three decidual layers are (1) the decidua basalis, which underlies the developing embryo and forms the maternal side of the placenta; (2) the decidua capsularis, which overlies the embryo and bulges into the uterine cavity as the embryo and fetus grow; and (3) the decidua parietalis, which lines the rest of the uterine cavity. By about 22 weeks of gestation, the decidua capsularis fuses with the decidua parietalis, filling the uterine cavity.

Circulation in the Maternal Side. Maternal and fetal blood normally do not mix in the placenta, although they flow very close to each other. Exchange of substances between mother and fetus occurs within the intervillous spaces of the placenta. While in the intervillous space, the mother's blood is briefly outside her circulatory system. About 150 ml of maternal blood is contained within the intervillous space. Blood in the intervillous space is changed about three to four times per minute, requiring circulation of 450 to 750 ml per minute for placental perfusion.

Maternal blood spurts into the intervillous spaces through 80 to 100 spiral arteries in the decidua. After the oxygenated and nutrient-bearing maternal blood washes over the chorionic villi containing the fetal vessels, it returns to the maternal circulation through the endometrial veins for elimination of fetal waste products.

Fetal Component

Development. The fetal side of the placenta develops from the outer cell layer (trophoblast) of the blastocyst at the same time the inner cell mass develops into the

A

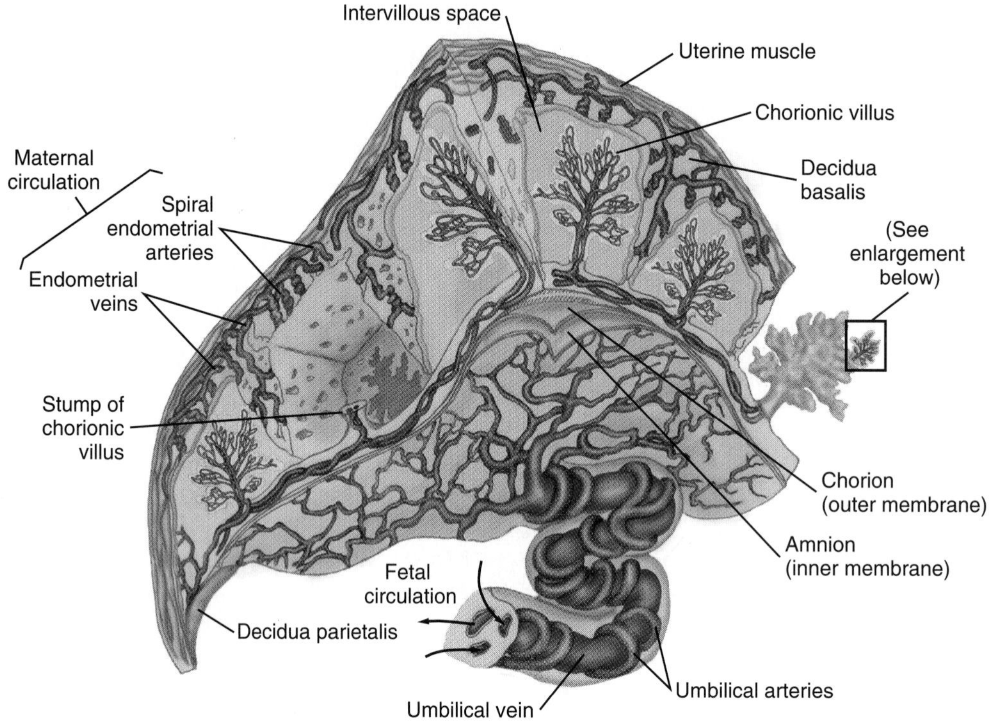

B

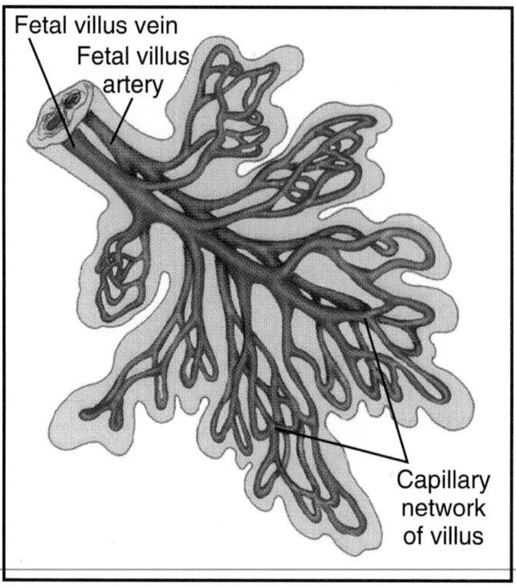

FIGURE 6-7 **A,** Placental structure showing relationship of placenta, fetal membranes, and uterus. Arrows indicate the direction of blood flow between the fetus and placenta through the umbilical arteries and vein. Blood from the woman bathes the fetal chorionic villi within the intervillous spaces to allow exchange of oxygen, nutrients, and waste products without gross mixing of maternal and fetal blood. **B,** Structure of a chorionic villus showing its fetal capillary network.

embryo and fetus. The primary chorionic villi are the initial structures that eventually form the fetal side of the placenta.

Circulation in the Fetal Side. The umbilical cord contains the umbilical arteries and vein to transport blood between the fetus and placenta. Chorionic villi are bathed by oxygen- and nutrient-rich maternal blood in the maternal intervillous spaces. Each chorionic villus is supplied by a tiny fetal artery carrying deoxygenated blood and waste products from the fetus. The vein of the chorionic villus returns oxygenated blood and nutrients to the embryo and fetus.

Capillaries in the chorionic villi are separated from actual contact with the mother's blood by the membranes of each villus. This arrangement allows contact close enough for exchange and prevents mixing of maternal and fetal blood. The closed fetal circulation is im-

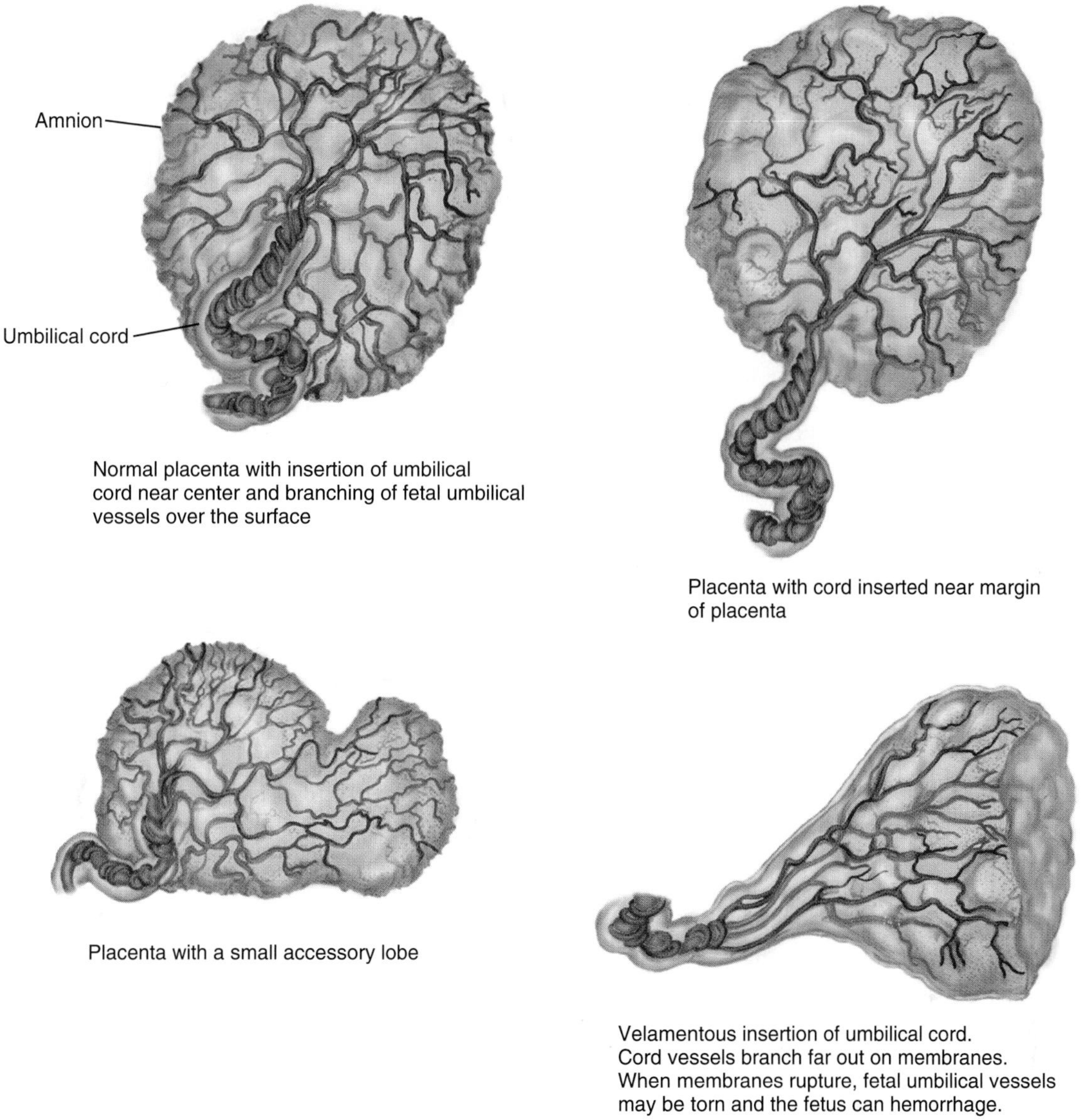

Amnion
Umbilical cord
Normal placenta with insertion of umbilical cord near center and branching of fetal umbilical vessels over the surface
Placenta with cord inserted near margin of placenta
Placenta with a small accessory lobe
Velamentous insertion of umbilical cord. Cord vessels branch far out on membranes. When membranes rupture, fetal umbilical vessels may be torn and the fetus can hemorrhage.

FIGURE 6-8 Placental variations.

portant because the blood types of mother and fetus may not be compatible.

The placental arteries and veins converge in the blood vessels of the umbilical cord. Two umbilical arteries and one umbilical vein transport blood between the fetus and the fetal side of the placenta. Blood is circulated to and from the fetal side of the placenta by the fetal heart.

Metabolic Functions

The placenta produces some nutrients needed by the embryo and for its own functions. Substances synthesized include glycogen, cholesterol, and fatty acids (Moore & Persaud, 1998).

Transfer Functions

Exchange of oxygen, nutrients, and waste products across the chorionic villi occurs through several methods (Table 6-4). Placental transfer of harmful substances also may occur. Most substances that enter the mother's bloodstream can enter the fetal circulation, and many agents enter it almost immediately.

Gas Exchange. Respiration is a key function of the placenta. Oxygen and carbon dioxide pass through the placental membrane by simple diffusion. The average oxygen-partial pressure (Po_2) of maternal blood in the intervillous space is 50 mm Hg. The average blood Po_2 in the umbilical vein (after oxygenation) is about 30 mm Hg (Guyton, 2000).

The fetus can thrive in this low-oxygen environment for three reasons:

- Fetal hemoglobin can carry 20% to 50% more oxygen than adult hemoglobin.

Table 6-4
MECHANISMS OF PLACENTAL TRANSFER

Mechanism	Description	Examples of Substances
Simple diffusion	Passive movement of substances across a cell membrane from an area of higher concentration to one of lower concentration	Oxygen and carbon dioxide Carbon monoxide Water Urea and uric acid Most drugs and their metabolites
Facilitated diffusion	Passage of substances across a cell membrane by binding with carrier proteins that assist transfer	Glucose
Active transport	Transfer of substances across a cell membrane against a pressure or electrical gradient or from an area of lower concentration to one of higher concentration	Amino acids Water-soluble vitamins Minerals: Calcium, iron, iodine
Pinocytosis	Movement of large molecules by ingestion within cells	Maternal IgG class antibodies Some passage of maternal IgA antibodies

IgA, Immunoglobin A; *IgG*, immunoglobin G.

- The fetus has a higher oxygen-carrying capacity because of a higher average hemoglobin (14.5 to 22.5 g/dl) and hematocrit value (about 48% to 69%).
- Hemoglobin can carry more oxygen at low carbon dioxide–partial pressure (PCO_2) levels than it can at high ones (Bohr effect). Blood entering the placenta from the fetus has a high PCO_2, but carbon dioxide diffuses quickly to the mother's blood, where the PCO_2 is lower, reversing the levels of carbon dioxide in maternal and fetal bloods. Therefore the fetal blood becomes more alkaline and the maternal blood becomes more acidic. This allows the mother's blood to give up oxygen and the fetal blood to combine with oxygen readily.

Fetal PCO_2 is only about 2 to 3 mm Hg higher than that of maternal blood. However, carbon dioxide is very soluble, allowing it to pass across the placental membrane into maternal blood at this low pressure gradient.

Nutrient Transfer. The growing fetus requires a constant supply of nutrients from the pregnant woman. Glucose, fatty acids, vitamins, and electrolytes pass readily across the placenta. Glucose is the major energy source for fetal growth and metabolic activities.

Waste Removal. In addition to carbon dioxide, urea, uric acid, and bilirubin are readily transferred from fetus to mother for disposal. Because the normal placenta removes wastes for the fetus, metabolic defects such as phenylketonuria are usually not evident until after birth.

Antibody Transfer. Many of the immunoglobulin G (IgG) class of antibodies are passed from mother to fetus through the placenta. This confers passive (temporary) immunity to the fetus against diseases such as measles if the mother is immune to them. Passage of antibodies against disease is beneficial because the newborn does not produce antibodies for several months after birth. The preterm infant has little protection from maternal antibodies because they are transferred during late pregnancy.

Passage of antibodies from expectant mother to fetus is not always beneficial. If maternal and fetal blood types are not compatible, the mother may already have or may produce antibodies against fetal erythrocytes. The mother's antibodies may then destroy the fetal erythrocytes, causing fetal anemia or even death. This situation may occur if the mother is Rh-negative and the fetus is Rh-positive.

Transfer of Maternal Hormones. Most maternal protein hormones do not reach the fetus in significant amounts. The female fetus exposed to androgenic hormones may have masculinization of her genitalia, and her true gender may be difficult to determine at birth.

Diethylstilbestrol was given to prevent spontaneous abortion in the late 1940s through the early 1960s but was ineffective for this purpose. However, females prenatally exposed to the drug have a higher incidence of vaginal carcinoma, infertility, spontaneous abortion, preterm labor, and other reproductive problems.

Endocrine Functions

The placenta produces several hormones necessary for normal pregnancy. hCG causes the corpus luteum to persist for the first 6 to 8 weeks of pregnancy and secrete estrogens and progesterone. As the placenta develops further, it takes over estrogen and progesterone production and the corpus luteum regresses. When a Y chromosome is present in the male fetus, hCG also causes the fetal testes to secrete testosterone necessary for normal development of male reproductive structures.

Human placental lactogen, also called *human chorionic somatomammotropin,* is a placental hormone that promotes normal nutrition and growth of the fetus and maternal breast development for lactation. The hormone decreases maternal insulin sensitivity and glucose use, making more glucose available for fetal nutrition.

Steroid hormones secreted by the placenta include estrogens and progesterone. Estrogens cause enlargement of the woman's uterus, enlargement of the breasts, growth of the ductal system of the breasts, and enlargement of the external genitalia. Estriol is the most plentiful estrogen produced during pregnancy.

Progesterone is essential for normal continuation of the pregnancy. Functions of progesterone include the following:

- Causes secretory changes in the endometrium, providing nourishment as the conceptus enters the uterus
- Causes the changes in endometrial cells that convert them into the larger and thicker cells of the decidua, which characterize pregnancy
- Reduces muscle contractions of the uterus to prevent spontaneous abortion
- May induce some immune tolerance in the mother's body for the conceptus
- Acts with estrogens and other hormones to cause growth of the breasts, budding of the alveoli that will secrete milk, and development of secretory characteristics in the alveolar cells

Other hormones produced by the placenta include human chorionic thyrotropin and human chorionic adrenocorticotropin.

Check Your Reading

17. Which structure takes over the functions of the corpus luteum?
18. What is the purpose of the intervillous spaces of the placenta?
19. Why must fetal and maternal blood not actually mix?
20. What factors enable the fetus to thrive in a low-oxygen environment?
21. What are the purposes of these placental hormones: hCG? Human placental lactogen? Estrogen? Progesterone?

Fetal Membranes and Amniotic Fluid

The two fetal membranes are the amnion (inner membrane) and the chorion (outer membrane). The two membranes are so close as to be one (the "bag of waters"), but they can be separated. If the membranes rupture in labor, amnion and chorion usually rupture together, releasing the amniotic fluid within the sac.

The amnion is continuous with the surface of the umbilical cord, joining the epithelium of the fetus' abdominal skin. Chorionic villi proliferate over the entire surface of the gestational sac for the first 8 weeks after conception. A conceptus observed at this time looks like a shaggy sphere with the embryo suspended inside. As the embryo grows, it bulges into the uterine cavity. The villi on the outer surface gradually atrophy and form the smooth-surfaced chorion. The remaining villi continue to branch and enlarge to form the fetal side of the placenta.

Amniotic fluid protects the growing fetus and promotes normal prenatal development. Amniotic fluid protects the fetus by the following actions:

- Cushioning against impacts to the maternal abdomen
- Providing a stable temperature

Amniotic fluid promotes normal prenatal development by the following actions:

- Allowing symmetric development as the major body surfaces fold toward the midline
- Preventing the membranes from adhering to developing fetal parts
- Allowing room and buoyancy for fetal movement

Amniotic fluid is derived from two sources: (1) fetal urine and (2) fluid transported from the maternal blood across the amnion. Castoff fetal epithelial cells and vernix are suspended in the amniotic fluid. The water of the amniotic fluid changes by absorption across the amnion, returning to the mother. The fetus also swallows amniotic fluid and absorbs it in the digestive tract. Waste products are returned to the placenta through the umbilical arteries.

The volume of amniotic fluid increases during pregnancy and is about 500 to 1500 ml at term (Guyton, 2000; Blackburn & Loper, 1992). An abnormally small quantity of fluid (less than 50% of the amount expected for gestation, or under 500 ml at term) is called *oligohydramnios* and may be associated with poor fetal lung development and malformations that result from compression of fetal parts. Oligohydramnios may occur because the kidneys fail to develop, urine excretion is blocked, or placental blood flow is inadequate. Hydramnios (also called *polyhydramnios*) is the opposite situation, in which the quantity may exceed 2000 ml. Hydramnios may occur when the fetus has a severe malformation of the central nervous system or gastrointestinal tract that prevents the normal fetal cycle involving ingestion of amniotic fluid.

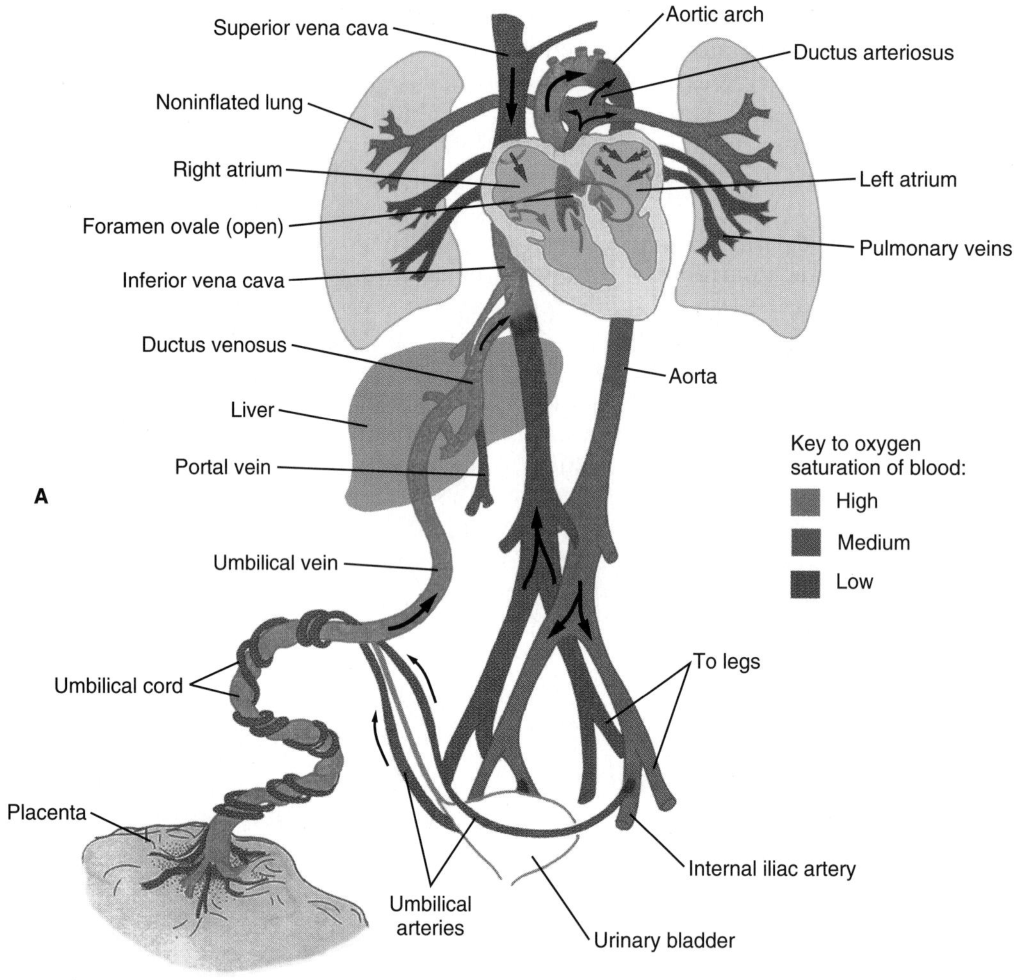

FIGURE 6-9 **A,** Fetal circulation. Three shunts allow most blood from the placenta to bypass the fetal lungs and liver, ductus venosus, ductus arteriosus, and foramen ovale.

FETAL CIRCULATION

The course of fetal blood circulation is from the fetal heart, to the placenta for exchange of oxygen, nutrients, and waste products, and back to the fetus for delivery to fetal tissues (Figure 6-9, *A*).

Umbilical Cord

The fetal umbilical cord is the lifeline between the fetus and placenta. It has two arteries that carry deoxygenated blood and waste products away from the fetus to the placenta, where these substances are transferred to the mother's circulation. The umbilical vein carries freshly oxygenated and nutrient-laden blood from the placenta back to the fetus. The umbilical arteries and vein are coiled within the cord to allow them to stretch and prevent obstruction of blood flow through them. The entire cord is cushioned by a soft substance called *Wharton's jelly* to prevent obstruction resulting from pressure.

Fetal Circulatory Circuit

Because the fetus does not breathe air, several alterations of the postnatal circulatory route are needed (see Figure 6-9, *A*). Also, the fetal liver does not have the metabolic functions that it will have after birth because the mother's body performs these functions. Three shunts in the fetal circulatory system allow blood with the highest oxygen content to be sent to the fetal heart and brain: the ductus venosus, foramen ovale, and ductus arteriosus. At birth the infant's lungs oxygenate the blood, the placenta is removed from the circulatory path, and the liver must perform its metabolic functions, so all three shunts are converted to functions unrelated to circulating the blood.

Oxygenated blood from the placenta enters the fetal body through the umbilical vein. About half the blood

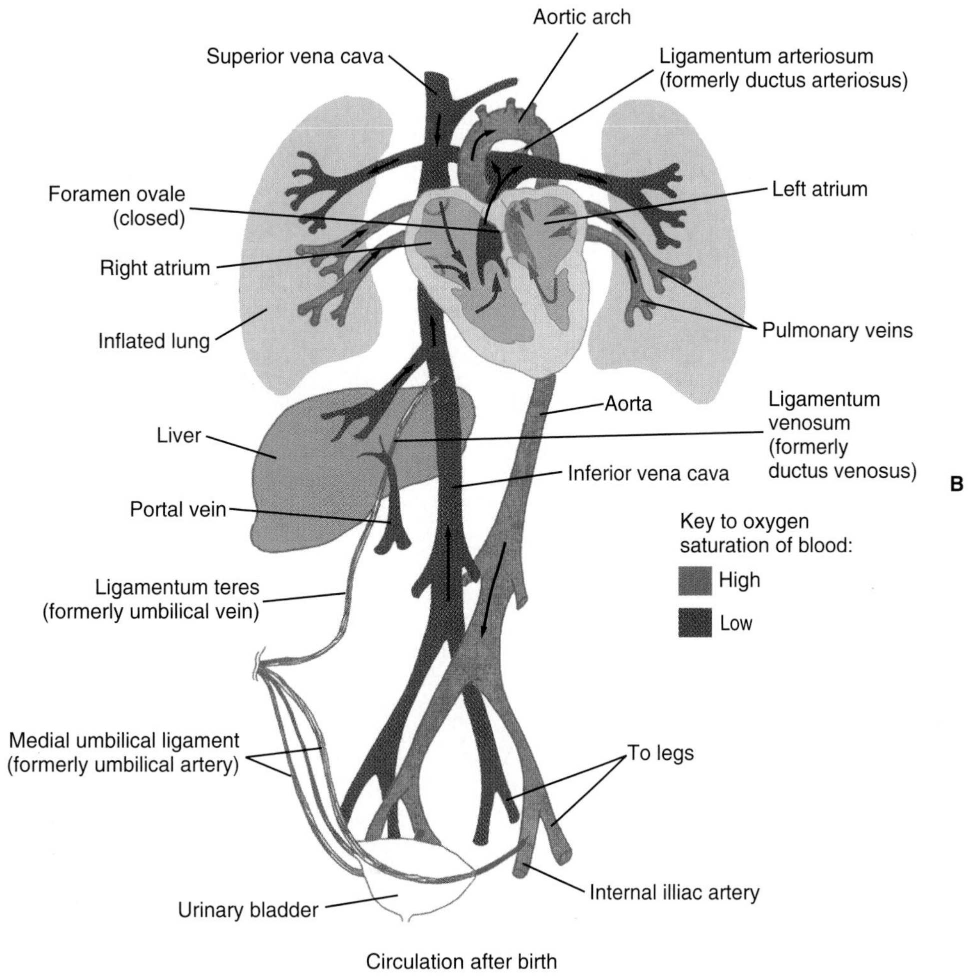

FIGURE 6-9, cont'd **B,** Circulation after birth. Note that the fetal shunts have closed. The umbilical vessels (ductus venosus and ductus arteriosus) will be converted to ligaments.

goes through the liver, and the rest bypasses the liver and enters the inferior vena cava through the first shunt, the ductus venosus. The blood then enters the right atrium and joins with deoxygenated blood from the lower body and head. Most of the blood passes directly into the left atrium through the second shunt, the foramen ovale, where it mixes with the small amount of blood returning from the lungs. Blood is pumped from the left ventricle into the aorta to nourish the body. A small amount of blood from the right ventricle is circulated to the lungs to nourish the lung tissue. The rest of the blood from the right ventricle joins oxygenated blood in the aorta through the third shunt, the ductus arteriosus. The head and upper body receive the greatest amount of oxygenated blood.

The muscle wall of the right side of the fetal heart is thicker than that of the left because resistance to blood flow through the uninflated lungs is high, similar to the resistance in other parts of the fetal body. When the infant begins breathing after birth, resistance to pulmonary blood flow falls dramatically and the right side of the heart does not need to be as thick. During infancy the thickness of the right heart gradually decreases (Moore & Persaud, 1998).

Changes in Blood Circulation after Birth

Fetal circulatory shunts are not needed after birth because the infant oxygenates blood in the lungs and is not circulating blood to the placenta (Figure 6-9, *B*). As the infant breathes, blood flow to the lungs increases, pressure in the right heart falls, and the foramen ovale closes. The ductus arteriosus constricts as the arterial oxygen level rises. The ductus venosus constricts when flow of blood from the umbilical cord stops.

Transition to the postnatal circulatory pattern is gradual. Functional closure begins when the infant

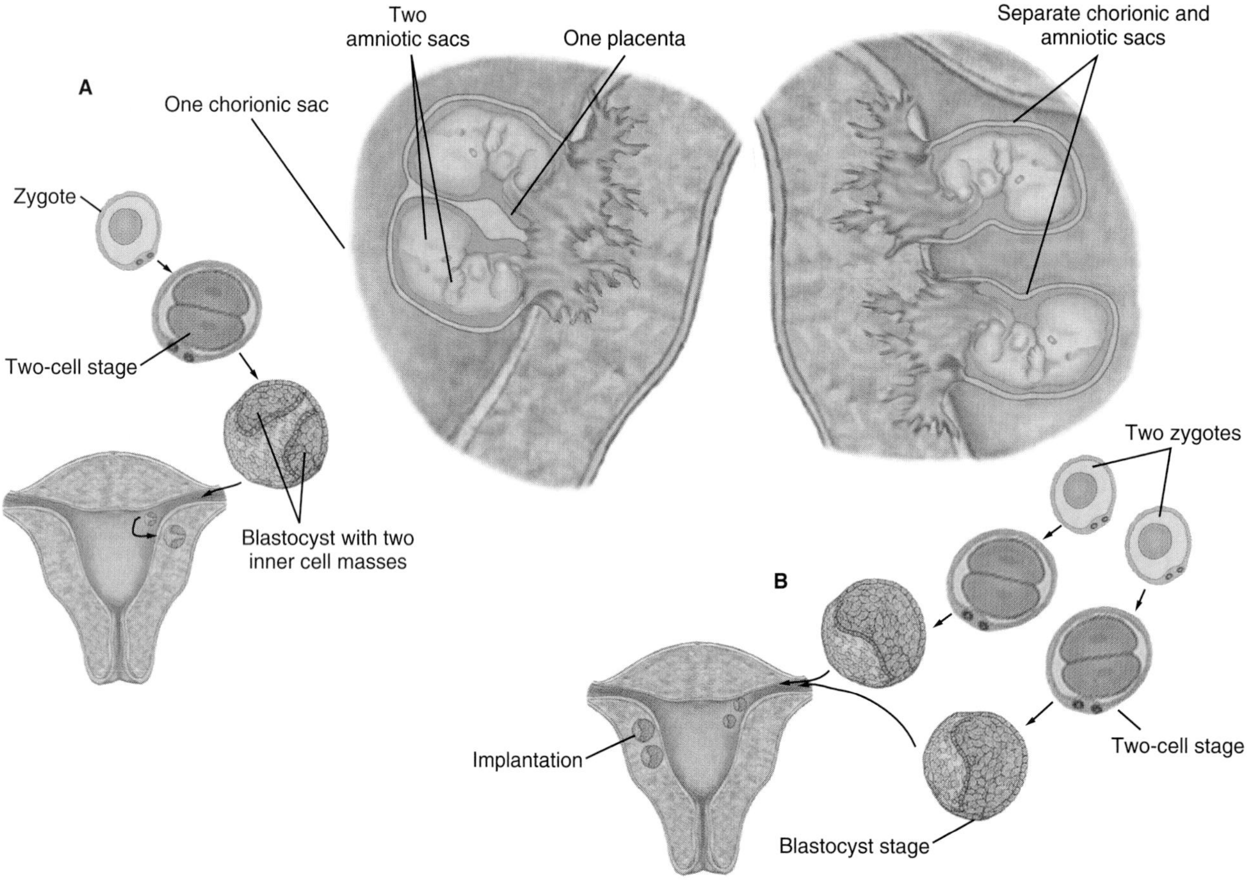

FIGURE 6-10 **A,** Monozygotic twinning. The single inner cell mass divides into two inner cell masses during the blastocyst stage. These twins have a single placenta and chorion, but each twin develops in its own amnion. **B,** Dizygotic twinning. Two ova are released during ovulation, and each is fertilized by a separate spermatozoon. The ova may implant near each other in the uterus, or they may be far apart.

breathes and the cord is cut, removing the placenta from the circulation. The foramen ovale and ductus venosus are permanently closed as tissue proliferates in these structures. The ductus venosus becomes a ligament, as do the umbilical vein and arteries (see Table 19-1).

Check Your Reading

22. What are the purposes of the fetal membranes and amniotic fluid?
23. Trace the path of fetal circulation from the placenta through the fetal body and back to the placenta.

MULTIFETAL PREGNANCY

The incidence of multifetal pregnancy (multiple gestation) is increasing in the United States. Much of the increase is due to a rise in maternal age, when women naturally are more likely to have twins, and infertility treatments that induce multiple ovulation. The 1998 twin birth rates were 6% higher than in 1997, at 38.1 per 1000 live births (2.8% of all births). The greatest rise in twin births has been among women aged 30 years and older. Triplet and higher-order multiple births rose 423% between 1980 and 1998 to 193.5 per 100,000 live births in 1998 (National Center for Health Statistics, 2000).

Twinning is the most common form of multifetal pregnancy. The same processes that occur in twin pregnancies also may occur in higher-order multiple gestations. Twins are often called *identical* or *fraternal* by lay people but are more accurately described by their zygosity, or the number of ova and sperm involved. The two types of twins are monozygotic and dizygotic (Figure 6-10).

Monozygotic Twinning

Monozygotic twins are conceived by the union of a single ovum and spermatozoon, with later division of the conceptus into two. Monozygotic twins have identical genetic complements and are the same gender. However, they may not always look identical at birth because one twin may have grown much larger than the other or one may have a birth defect such as a cleft lip. Monozygotic twinning occurs essentially at random (about 3 to 5 per 1000 pregnancies), and a hereditary or racial component is not well established (Stoll & Kliegman, 2000).

Monozygotic twinning occurs when a single conceptus divides early in gestation. In most cases (about 70%) of monozygotic twins the blastocyst is formed with two inner cell masses instead of one. If this occurs, the fetuses have two amnions (inner membranes) but a single chorion (outer membrane).

If the conceptus divides earlier, two separate but identical morulas (and then blastocysts) develop and implant separately. These monozygotic twins have two amnions and two chorions. Although the placentas develop separately, they may fuse and appear as one at birth. The chorions also may fuse during prenatal development. Therefore an examination of the placenta and membranes after birth cannot always establish whether twins are monozygotic or dizygotic, and specialized tests may be required.

Late separation of the inner cell mass may result in twins having a single amnion and a single chorion. These twins often die because their umbilical cords become entangled. Incomplete separation of the inner cell mass may result in conjoined (formerly called "Siamese") twins.

Dizygotic Twinning

Dizygotic twins arise from two ova that are fertilized by different sperm. Dizygotic twins may be the same or different gender, and they may not have similar physical traits.

Dizygotic twinning may be hereditary in some families, presumably because of an inherited tendency of the females to release more than one ovum per cycle. Women of some races are more likely to have dizygotic twins as well. United States data for 1998 show that the rate of twinning is highest for non-Hispanic black women at 31.3 per 1000 (1 in 32) live births compared with 30.2 per 1000 (1 in 34) live births for non-Hispanic white women. The Hispanic twin birth rate is lower at 20.4 per 1000 (1 in 49) live births (National Center for Health Statistics, 2000). Asian women have a considerably lower rate for spontaneous twinning—about 1 in 150 for Japanese women and 1 in 300 for Chinese women (Stoll & Kliegman, 2000).

Women who conceive after age 40 have an increased incidence of dizygotic twin births because multiple ova are more likely to be released as the climacteric approaches. Fertility treatments that induce ovulation also lead to an increased incidence of dizygotic multifetal gestations.

Because dizygotic twins arise from two separate zygotes, their membranes and placentas are separate. The membranes, the placentas, or both may fuse during development if they implant closely. Dizygotic twins are not conjoined because they do not involve division of a single cell mass into two but arise from two separate conceptions.

Other Multifetal Gestations

Pregnancies resulting in more offspring than twins may arise from a single zygote or a combination of a single and multiple zygotes, or each may arise from a separate zygote. Multifetal pregnancies pose much greater hazards to both expectant mother and fetuses. The incidence of long-term handicaps is higher as the number of fetuses increases.

Check Your Reading

24. How do monozygotic twins occur?
25. Why can examination of the placenta and membranes in a multifetal pregnancy not always establish whether they are monozygotic or dizygotic?
26. Why are dizygotic twins often of different genders?

SUMMARY CONCEPTS

- The purpose of gametogenesis is to produce ova and sperm that have half the full number of chromosomes, or 23 unpaired chromosomes. When an ovum and sperm unite at conception, the number is restored to 46 paired chromosomes.
- The female has all the ova she will ever have at 30 weeks of prenatal gestation. No other ova are formed after this time.
- One primary oocyte can mature into one mature ovum that contains 23 unpaired chromosomes (22 autosomes and 1 X chromosome).
- A male can continuously produce new sperm from puberty through the rest of his life, although fertility gradually declines after age 40.
- One primary spermatocyte can result in production of four mature sperm. Two of the mature sperm have 22 autosomes and 1 X sex chromosome. Two have 22 autosomes and 1 Y sex chromosome.
- The male determines the baby's gender because only sperm carry either an X or Y sex chromosome. The female can contribute only an X chromosome to the baby.
- The basic structure of all organ systems is established during the first 8 weeks of pregnancy. Teratogens during this period may cause major structural and functional damage to the developing organs.
- The fetal period is one of growth and refinement of already established organ systems. Teratogens can still damage the fetus but are less likely to cause major structural damage. They may still cause major functional damage.

- The placenta is an embryonic or a fetal organ with metabolic, respiratory, and endocrine functions.
- Transfer of substances between mother and embryo or fetus occurs by four mechanisms: simple diffusion, facilitated diffusion, active transport, and pinocytosis.
- Most substances in the maternal blood can be transferred to the fetus.
- The fetal membranes contain the amniotic fluid, which cushions the fetus, allows normal prenatal development, and maintains a stable temperature.
- The umbilical cord is the lifeline between the fetus and the placenta. Two umbilical arteries carry deoxygenated blood and waste products to the placenta for transfer to the mother's blood. One umbilical vein carries oxygenated and nutrient-rich blood to the fetus. Coiling of the vessels and enclosure in Wharton's jelly reduce the risk of obstruction of the umbilical vessels.
- Three fetal circulatory shunts are needed to partially bypass the fetal liver and lungs: the ductus venosus, foramen ovale, and ductus arteriosus. These structures close functionally after birth but are not closed permanently until several weeks or months later.
- Multifetal pregnancy may be monozygotic or dizygotic. Twins are the most common form of multifetal pregnancy.
- Examination of the placenta and membranes alone cannot conclusively establish whether multiple fetuses are monozygotic or dizygotic.
- Dizygotic twins are more likely to occur in certain families and racial groups and especially in mothers older than 40 years and women who take fertility treatments to induce ovulation.

REFERENCES & READINGS

Benirschke, K. (1999). Multiple gestation: Incidence, etiology and inheritance. In R.K. Creasy & R. Resnik (Eds.), *Maternal-fetal medicine: Principles and practice* (4th ed., pp. 598-615). Philadelphia: W.B. Saunders.

Benirschke, K. (1999). Normal development. In R.K. Creasy & R. Resnik (Eds.), *Maternal-fetal medicine: Principles and practice* (4th ed., pp. 63-71). Philadelphia: W.B. Saunders.

Bernstein, D. (2000). Developmental biology of the cardiovascular system. In R.E. Behrman, R.M. Kliegman, & H.B. Jenson (Eds.), *Nelson textbook of pediatrics* (16th ed., pp. 1337-1343). Philadelphia: W.B. Saunders.

Blackburn, S.T., & Loper, D.L. (1992). *Maternal, fetal, and neonatal physiology: A clinical perspective.* Philadelphia: W.B. Saunders.

Borgida, A.F., & Rodis, J.F. (2000). Twin pregnancy. In E.J. Quilligan & F.P. Zuspan (Eds.), *Current therapy in obstetrics and gynecology* (5th ed., pp. 364-368). Philadelphia: W.B. Saunders.

Carsten, M.E. (1998). Endocrinology of pregnancy and parturition. In N.F. Hacker & J.G. Moore (Eds.), *Essentials of obstetrics and gynecology* (3rd ed., pp. 76-83). Philadelphia: W.B. Saunders.

Guyton, A.C., & Hall, J.E. (2000). *Textbook of medical physiology* (10th ed.). Philadelphia: W.B. Saunders.

Kellogg, B. (2000a). Fetal development. In S. Mattson & J.E. Smith (Eds.), *Core curriculum for maternal-newborn nursing* (2nd ed., pp. 36-54). Philadelphia: W. B. Saunders.

Kellogg, B. (2000b). Placental development and functioning. In S. Mattson & J.E. Smith (Eds.), *Core curriculum for maternal-newborn nursing* (2nd ed., pp. 55-67). Philadelphia: W. B. Saunders.

Moore, K.L., & Persaud, T.V.N. (1998a). *Before we are born: Essentials of embryology and birth defects* (5th ed.). Philadelphia: W.B. Saunders.

Moore, K.L., & Persaud, T.V.N. (1998a). *The developing human: Clinically-oriented embryology.* Philadelphia: W.B. Saunders.

Moore, K.L., Persaud, T.V.N., & Shiota, K. (1994). *Color atlas of clinical embryology.* Philadelphia: W.B. Saunders.

National Center for Health Statistics. (2000). Births: Final data for 1998. *National Vital Statistics Reports,* 48(3), 2.

Stables, D. (1999). *Physiology in childbearing with anatomy and related biosciences.* Edinburgh: Balliere-Tindall.

Stoll, B.J., & Kliegman, R.M. (2000). The high-risk infant: multiple pregnancies. In R.E. Behrman, R.M. Kliegman, & H.B. Jenson (Eds.), *Nelson textbook of pediatrics* (16th ed., pp. 475-477). Philadelphia: W.B. Saunders.

Surrey, E.S., Lu, J.K.H., & Toot, P.J. (1998). The menstrual cycle, ovulation, fertilization, implantation, and the placenta. In N.F. Hacker & J.G. Moore (Eds.) *Essentials of obstetrics and gynecology* (3rd ed., pp. 59-76). Philadelphia: W.B. Saunders.

7

Physiologic Adaptations to Pregnancy

OBJECTIVES

1. Describe the physiologic changes that occur during pregnancy.
2. Differentiate presumptive, probable, and positive signs of pregnancy.
3. Compute gravida, para, and estimated date of delivery.
4. Describe initial antepartum assessments in terms of history, physical examination, and risk assessment.
5. Identify subsequent antepartum assessments.
6. Discuss maternal adaptation to multifetal pregnancy.
7. Describe the common discomforts of pregnancy in terms of causes and preventive and relief measures.
8. Explain cultural assessment and negotiation.
9. Discuss the nursing process and critical thinking skills needed to develop nursing care plans for the most common problems and discomforts of pregnancy.

DEFINITIONS

Abortion Spontaneous or elective termination of pregnancy before the twentieth week of gestation based on the date of the last menstrual period. Spontaneous abortion is frequently termed *miscarriage* by the lay public.

Amenorrhea Absence of menstruation; primary amenorrhea being a delay of the first menstruation and secondary amenorrhea being cessation of menstruation after its initiation.

Braxton Hicks Contractions Irregular, mild uterine contractions that occur throughout pregnancy and become stronger in the last trimester.

Chadwick's Sign Bluish discoloration of the cervix, vagina, and labia during pregnancy as a result of increased vascular congestion.

Chloasma Brownish pigmentation of the face during pregnancy; also called *melasma* and "mask of pregnancy."

Colostrum Breast fluid secreted during pregnancy and the first week after childbirth.

Diastasis Recti Separation of the longitudinal muscles of the abdomen (rectus abdominis) during pregnancy.

DEFINITIONS—cont'd

Goodell's Sign Softening of the cervix, uterus, and vagina during pregnancy.

Gravida A woman who is or has been pregnant, regardless of the duration of the pregnancy.

Hegar's Sign Softening of the lower uterine segment that allows it to be easily compressed by the sixth week of pregnancy.

Hyperemia Excess of blood in a part of the body.

Multigravida A woman who has been pregnant more than once.

Multipara A woman who has given birth two or more times at more than 20 weeks of gestation.

Nullipara A woman who has never completed a pregnancy beyond 20 weeks of gestation.

Para Number of pregnancies that have progressed past 20 weeks at delivery, whether the fetus was born alive or stillborn; refers to number of pregnancies, not number of fetuses.

Physiologic Anemia of Pregnancy Decrease in hematocrit values caused by dilution of erythrocytes by expanded plasma volume rather than by an actual decrease in erythrocytes or hemoglobin.

Postterm Birth One that occurs after the forty-second week of gestation.

Preterm Birth One that occurs after the twentieth week and before the start of the thirty-eighth week of gestation.

Primigravida A woman who is pregnant for the first time.

Primipara A woman who has given birth once after a pregnancy of at least 20 weeks.

Striae Gravidarum Irregular reddish streaks resulting from tears in connective tissue; generally appear on the woman's abdomen, breasts, and thighs during pregnancy.

Term Birth One that occurs between the thirty-eighth and forty-second weeks of gestation.

Trimester A division of pregnancy into three equal parts of 13 weeks each.

From the moment of conception, important changes occur in the pregnant woman's body that are necessary to support and nourish the fetus, prepare the woman for childbirth and lactation, and maintain her health. Pregnant women are often puzzled by the physical changes and unprepared for any associated discomforts. Many pregnant women rely on nurses to provide accurate information and compassionate guidance throughout their pregnancies. To respond effectively, nurses must understand not only the physiologic changes but also the ways these changes affect the daily lives of expectant mothers.

CHANGES IN BODY SYSTEMS

Although pregnancy challenges each body system to adapt to increasing demands of the fetus, the most obvious changes are in the reproductive system.

Reproductive System

Uterus

Growth. Perhaps the most dramatic change during pregnancy occurs in the uterus, which before conception is a small, pear-shaped organ entirely contained in the pelvic cavity. Before pregnancy the uterus weighs approximately 50 to 70 g (1.8 to 2.5 oz) and has a capacity of about 10 ml (one third of an ounce). By the end of pregnancy the uterus extends to the level of the xiphoid process, weighs approximately 1000 g (2.2 lb), and has sufficient capacity (about 5000 ml) for the fetus, placenta, and amniotic fluid.

Uterine growth occurs as the result of hyperplasia and hypertrophy. During the first trimester, growth is mainly caused by hyperplasia and the formation of new cells resulting from stimulation of the myometrium by estrogen (Resnik, 1999). During the second and third trimesters, uterine growth results from hypertrophy as the muscle fibers stretch in all directions to accommodate the growing fetus. In addition to muscle growth, fibrous tissue accumulates in the outer muscle layer of the uterus and the amount of elastic tissue increases. These changes greatly increase the strength of the muscle wall.

Muscle fibers in the myometrium increase in both length and width. As a result, by the third trimester the uterine muscles are thin and the fetus can be easily palpated through the abdominal wall. As the uterus expands into the abdominal cavity, it gradually rotates to the right, displacing the intestine upward and laterally. The rotation is probably the result of pressure of the rectosigmoid colon on the left side of the pelvis.

Pattern of Uterine Growth. The uterus grows in a predictable pattern that provides information about fetal growth and helps to confirm the expected date of delivery (EDD), sometimes called the *expected date of birth (EDB)* (Figure 7-1). For instance, by 12 weeks of gestation the uterus extends out of the maternal pelvis and can be palpated above the symphysis pubis. At 16 weeks the fundus reaches midway between the symphysis pubis and the umbilicus. At 20 weeks the fundus is located at the umbilicus.

By 36 weeks the fundus reaches its highest level at the xiphoid process. It pushes against the diaphragm, and the expectant mother may experience shortness of breath, even during rest. By 40 weeks the fetal head descends into the pelvic cavity, and the uterus sinks to a lower level. This descent of the fetal head is called *lightening* because it reduces pressure on the diaphragm and makes breathing easier.

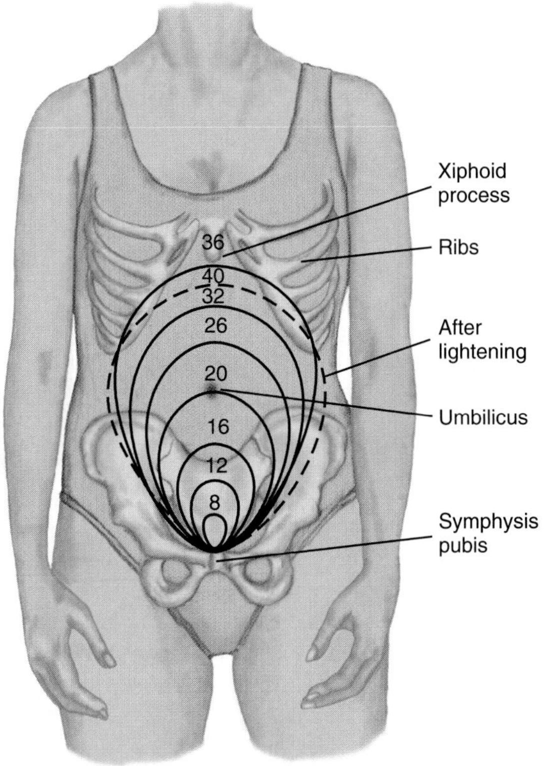

FIGURE 7-1 Uterine growth pattern during pregnancy.

Contractility. Throughout pregnancy the uterus undergoes irregular, painless contractions called *Braxton Hicks contractions.* During the contraction the uterus temporarily tightens and becomes firm. It then returns to its original relaxed state. During the first two trimesters the contractions are infrequent. During the third trimester the contractions occur more frequently and may cause some discomfort. These are termed *false labor* when they are mistaken for the onset of early labor.

Uterine Blood Flow. As the uterus increases in size, blood flow increases dramatically. In early pregnancy when the uterus and placenta are relatively small, most blood flow is to the myometrium and endometrium. As pregnancy continues, the delivery of most substances needed for fetal growth and removal of metabolic wastes depends on adequate perfusion of the placental intervillous spaces. Maternal blood carried by the myometrial arteries enters the intervillous spaces, where oxygen and nutrients are transferred to the chorionic villi and hence to the fetus. Metabolic wastes from the fetus diffuse into venous structures of the mother (see Chapter 6).

Cervix

The cervix also undergoes significant changes after conception. The most obvious changes occur in color and consistency. In response to the increasing levels of estrogen the cervix becomes congested with blood (hyperemic), resulting in the characteristic bluish color that extends to include the vagina and labia. This discoloration, referred to as *Chadwick's sign,* is one of the earliest signs of pregnancy.

The cervix is largely composed of connective tissue that softens when the collagen fibers decrease in concentration. Before pregnancy the cervix has a consistency similar to that of the tip of the nose. After conception the cervix feels more like the lobe of the ear. The cervical softening is referred to as *Goodell's sign.*

A less obvious change occurs as the cervical glands proliferate during pregnancy and the glandular walls become thin and widely separated. As a result, the endocervical tissue resembles a honeycomb that fills with mucus secreted by the cervical glands. The mucus forms a plug in the cervical canal. This plug blocks the ascent of bacteria from the vagina into the uterus during pregnancy and protects the membranes and fetus from infection (Figure 7-2). The mucous plug remains in place until the onset of labor when the cervix begins to thin and dilate, allowing the mucous plug to be expelled. One of the earliest signs of labor may be "bloody show," which consists of the mucous plug and a small amount of blood produced by disruption of the cervical capillaries as the mucous plug is dislodged.

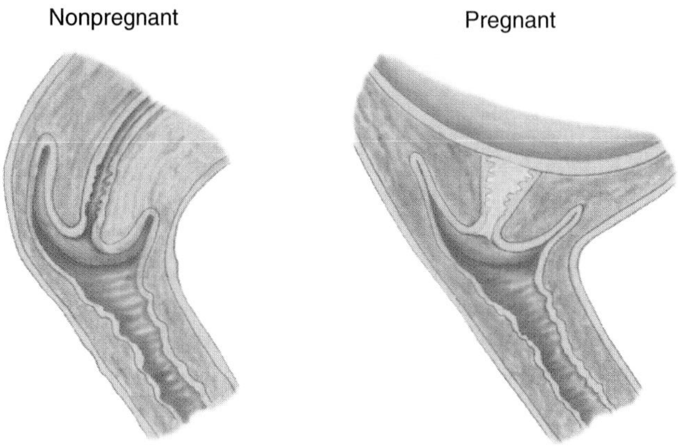

FIGURE 7-2 Cervical changes that occur during pregnancy. Note enlargement of spaces in cervical mucosa, which are filled with a thick mucous plug.

Vagina and Vulva

Changes of the vagina result from increased vascularity and are somewhat similar to those of the cervix. Softening of the abundant connective tissue allows the vagina to distend during childbirth. Because of hyperemia, the vaginal walls, like the cervix, appear blue or purple. The vaginal mucosa thickens, and vaginal rugae (folds) become very prominent.

Vaginal cells contain increasing amounts of glycogen, which causes rapid sloughing and increased vaginal dis-

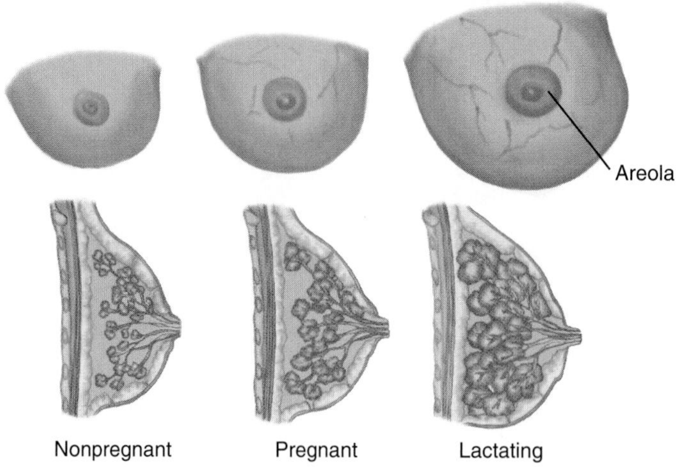

FIGURE 7-3 Breast changes that occur during pregnancy. The breasts increase in size and become more vascular, the areolae become darker, and the nipples become more erect.

charge. The pH of the vaginal discharge is acidic (3.5 to 6.0) because of the increased production of lactic acid that results from the action of *Lactobacillus acidophilus* on glycogen in the vaginal epithelium (Cunningham, et al., 1997). The acidic condition works to prevent growth of harmful bacteria found in the vagina. However, the glycogen-rich environment favors the growth of *Candida albicans* and persistent yeast infections (candidiasis) are common during pregnancy.

Increased vascularity, edema, and connective tissue changes make the tissues of the vulva and perineum more pliable. Pelvic congestion during pregnancy can lead to heightened sexual interest and increased orgasmic experiences.

Ovaries

Once conception occurs, the major function of the ovaries is to secrete progesterone for the first 6 to 7 weeks of pregnancy. Progesterone is called the "hormone of pregnancy," and adequate amounts must be available from the earliest stages to maintain pregnancy. The corpus luteum secretes progesterone until the placenta is developed and then regresses because it is no longer needed. The placenta secretes progesterone throughout the rest of pregnancy.

Ovulation ceases during pregnancy because the high circulating levels of estrogen and progesterone inhibit the release of follicle-stimulating hormone (FSH) and luteinizing hormone (LH), which are necessary for ovulation.

Breasts

During pregnancy the breasts change in both size and appearance (Figure 7-3). Estrogen and progesterone cause this increase in size. Estrogen stimulates the growth of mammary ductal tissue, and progesterone promotes the growth of lobes, lobules, and alveoli. The breasts become highly vascular, with a delicate network of veins often visible just beneath the surface of the skin. If the increase in breast size is extensive, striations ("stretch marks") similar to those that occur on the abdomen may develop.

Characteristic changes in the nipples and areolae occur during pregnancy. The nipples increase in size and become more erect, and the areolae become larger and more pigmented. The degree of pigmentation varies with the complexion of the expectant mother. Women with very light complexions exhibit less change in pigmentation than those with darker skin. Sebaceous glands called *tubercles of Montgomery* become more prominent during pregnancy and secrete a substance that lubricates the nipples. In addition, a thin, yellowish breast fluid, or colostrum, is present beginning in the second trimester and can readily be expressed by the third trimester.

Check Your Reading

1. What is the expected uterine growth at 20 weeks of gestation compared with that at 36 weeks of gestation?
2. How does uterine blood flow change during pregnancy?
3. What is the major purpose of progesterone?
4. What is the purpose of the cervical mucous plug?
5. How do the breasts change in size and appearance during pregnancy?

Cardiovascular System

During pregnancy, alterations occur in heart size and position, blood volume, blood flow, and blood components.

Heart

Heart Size and Position. Cardiac changes are minor and reverse soon after childbirth. The muscles of the heart (myocardium) enlarge slightly because of the increased workload during pregnancy. The heart is pushed upward and toward the left as the uterus elevates the diaphragm during the third trimester. As a result of the change in position, the locations for auscultation of heart sounds may be shifted upward and laterally in late pregnancy.

Heart Sounds. During pregnancy, some heart sounds may be so altered that they would be considered abnormal in a nonpregnant state. The changes are first heard between 12 and 20 weeks of gestation and continue for 2 to 4 weeks after childbirth. The most common variations in heart sounds include splitting of the first heart sound and a systolic murmur that is found in 90% of pregnant women (Cunningham, et al., 1997). The murmur is best heard at the left sternal border. A third heart sound also is often present.

Blood Volume

Total blood volume is a combination of plasma and solutes such as red blood cells, white blood cells, and platelets. Total blood volume increases about 45% during pregnancy.

Plasma Volume. Plasma volume increases progressively from 6 to 8 weeks of gestation to 4700 to 5200 ml at 32 weeks. This increase is 45% (1200 to 1600 ml) above nonpregnant values (Monga, 1999). The exact reason for plasma volume increase is unclear but may be related to estrogen stimulation of the renin-angiotensin-aldosterone system, which stimulates sodium and water retention.

Although the cause of plasma volume expansion is poorly understood, the increased volume is clearly needed for two reasons: (1) to transport nutrients and oxygen to the placenta, where they become available for the growing fetus, and (2) to meet the demands of the expanded maternal tissue in the uterus and breasts. An additional benefit of hypervolemia is that it provides a reserve to protect the pregnant woman from the adverse effects of blood loss that occurs during childbirth.

Dilution of red blood cells by plasma also may have a protective function. By decreasing blood viscosity, dilution may counter the tendency to form clots (thrombi) that can obstruct blood vessels and cause serious complications (see Chapter 28).

Red Blood Cell Volume. Red blood cell mass increases by 250 to 450 ml, which is about 20% to 30% above prepregnancy values (Monga, 1999). Although both red blood cell volume and plasma volume expand, the increase in plasma volume is more pronounced and occurs earlier. The resulting dilution of red blood cell mass causes a decline in maternal hematocrit. This condition is frequently called *physiologic anemia,* or *pseudoanemia of pregnancy,* because it reflects dilution of red blood cells in greatly expanded plasma volume and does not indicate true anemia. However, physiologic anemia should not be dismissed as unimportant. Frequent laboratory examinations may be needed to distinguish between physiologic and true anemia. Generally, iron deficiency anemia does not exist unless the hemoglobin is 10.5 g/dl or lower (Duffy, 1999) or the hematocrit is less than 33%.

Iron supplementation is necessary if hemoglobin or hematocrit falls below these levels. Iron supplementation is often associated with constipation.

Cardiac Output

A major consequence of expanded vascular volume during pregnancy is an increase in cardiac output. Cardiac output is the amount of blood discharged from the heart each minute, based on stroke volume (the amount of blood pumped from the heart with each contraction) and heart rate (the number of times the heart beats each minute). Cardiac output rises rapidly during the first trimester and increases about 40% by 20 to 24 weeks of pregnancy, with little change afterward (Nuwayhid, Nguyen, & Khraibi, 1999). The increase in cardiac output is primarily the result of a gain in stroke volume, but the heart rate also rises about 15 to 20 beats per minute (Monga, 1999).

Peripheral Vascular Resistance

Peripheral vascular resistance falls during pregnancy. This change is likely because of (1) smooth muscle relaxation in vessel walls resulting from the effects of progesterone; (2) the addition of the uteroplacental unit, which provides a greater area for circulation; (3) fetal heat production, which may produce vasodilation; and (4) increased synthesis of prostaglandins that cause resistance to circulating vasoconstrictors such as angiotensin II and norepinephrine.

Blood Pressure

The effect of decreased peripheral vascular resistance is that blood pressure remains stable during pregnancy despite the increase in blood volume. Systolic pressure remains largely unchanged if it is measured with the woman in a sitting or standing position. Diastolic pressure may decrease (about 10 mm Hg) by 28 weeks of gestation and return to usual levels by term.

If the blood pressure is measured with the woman lying on her left side, both systolic and diastolic decrease slightly, especially from 24 to 32 weeks of gestation, but then rise to nonpregnant levels by the end of pregnancy (Monga, 1999).

Effect of Position. Because the blood pressure is affected by position during pregnancy, agencies need to standardize the way blood pressure is taken. The woman's position and pressure should be recorded so that the site of evaluation remains consistent. In addition, controversy continues about whether Korotkoff's

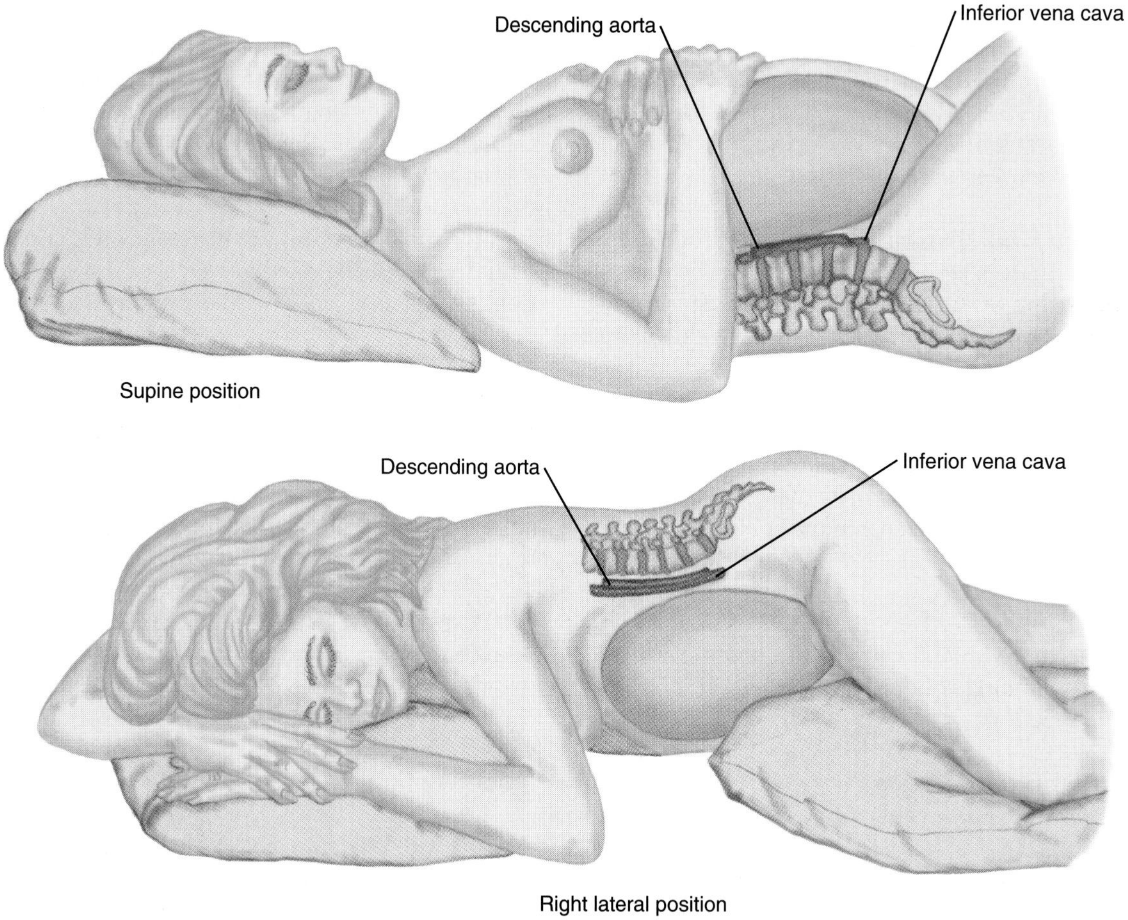

FIGURE 7-4 Supine hypotensive syndrome. When the woman is in the supine position, the weight of the gravid uterus partially occludes the vena cava and the descending aorta. A lateral recumbent position corrects supine hypotension.

fifth phase (disappearance of sound) correlates better with the true diastolic pressure than does the fourth (muffling) phase. Facilities should select the phase to be used and remain consistent throughout the prenatal, intrapartum, and postpartum periods. Blood pressures of 140/90 require additional evaluations.

Supine Hypotension. When the pregnant woman is in the supine position, particularly in the second and third trimesters, the weight of the gravid (pregnant) uterus partially occludes the vena cava and the descending aorta (Figure 7-4). The occlusion impedes return of blood from the lower extremities and consequently reduces cardiac return, cardiac output, and blood pressure. This supine hypotensive syndrome is also called *vena cava syndrome.* However, occlusion of the aorta also causes decreased blood pressure in the lower extremities, and thus a more precise term is *supine hypotensive syndrome.* Symptoms include faintness, lightheadedness, dizziness, and agitation. Some may experience syncope, a brief lapse in consciousness. Blood flow through the placenta is also decreased if the woman remains in the supine position for a prolonged time, which could result in fetal hypoxia.

A lateral recumbent position alleviates the pressure on the blood vessels and quickly corrects supine hypotension. Women should be advised to rest in a side-lying position to prevent or correct the occurrence of supine hypotension. If they must assume a supine position for fetal surveillance testing, a wedge or pillow under the right hip may be effective in decreasing supine hypotension.

Blood Flow

Four major changes in blood flow occur during pregnancy:

1. Blood flow is altered to include the uteroplacental unit. Approximately 500 ml/min is required to perfuse the placenta adequately.
2. Approximately 30% more blood must circulate through the maternal kidneys to remove the increased metabolic wastes generated by the mother and the fetus.

3. The woman's skin requires increased circulation to dissipate heat generated by increased metabolism during pregnancy.
4. The weight of the expanding uterus on the inferior vena cava and iliac veins partially obstructs blood return from veins in the legs, and blood pools in the deep and superficial veins of the legs. The resulting stasis of blood exerts pressure on the veins and cause the veins to become distended. Prolonged engorgement of the veins of the lower legs may result in varicose veins of the legs, vulva, or rectum (hemorrhoids).

Blood Components

Erythrocytes, leukocytes, and clotting factors increase during pregnancy. Erythrocytes increase by 20% to 30%, reflecting accelerated production of erythrocytes rather than prolonged red cell life. The gain in erythrocytes greatly increases the maternal demand for iron, which is necessary for hemoglobin formation.

Although iron absorption and iron-binding power are increased during pregnancy, sufficient iron is not always supplied by the woman's diet. Iron supplementation is necessary to promote hemoglobin synthesis and thus ensure sufficient erythrocyte production to prevent the development of iron-deficiency anemia (see Chapter 25).

Beginning in the first trimester, leukocytes increase from an average prepregnancy level of 5000 cells/mm^3 to an average of 9000 to 15,000 cells/mm^3, primarily because of an increase in neutrophils. Leukocytes increase further during labor but fall to the normal nonpregnant level by the sixth postpartum day (Kilpatrick & Laros, 1999).

Several clotting factors are elevated during pregnancy, particularly plasma fibrinogen (factor I), which rises about 50%. Elevated fibrinogen levels increase the ability to form clots, which offers some protection from hemorrhage during childbirth but also increases the risk of clot formation (thrombus) in the legs and the development of thrombophlebitis. The risk is a particular concern if the woman must stand or sit for prolonged periods with stasis of blood in the veins of the legs (see Appendix B).

Check Your Reading

6. How does the cause of physiologic anemia or pseudoanemia differ from iron deficiency anemia?
7. Why is circulation to the kidneys and skin increased during pregnancy?
8. Why do some pregnant women feel faint when they are in a supine position?
9. Why is standardizing techniques for taking blood pressure important?

Respiratory System

The major respiratory changes in pregnancy are the result of three factors: increased oxygen consumption, hormonal factors, and physical effects of the enlarging uterus.

Oxygen Consumption

Oxygen consumption increases by about 15% to 20% in pregnancy. Half the oxygen is used by the fetus, and the rest is consumed by the uterus, breast tissue, and increased maternal respiratory and cardiac demands. The woman breathes more deeply to compensate for the increased need for oxygen, although her respiratory rate remains unchanged. As a result, the tidal volume (the volume of gas moved into or out of the respiratory tract with each breath) and respiratory minute volume (the volume of air inspired or expired in 1 minute) increase by about 40%.

As a consequence of the elevated minute volume, the partial pressure of carbon dioxide (PCO_2) is lowered. The resulting respiratory alkalosis is partially compensated by renal excretion of bicarbonate. Decreased partial pressure of PCO_2 also promotes the transfer of carbon dioxide from fetal to maternal circulation.

Hormonal Factors

Progesterone. Progesterone is considered a major factor in the respiratory changes of pregnancy. It helps decrease airway resistance by relaxing the smooth muscle in the respiratory tract. Progesterone is also believed to raise the sensitivity of the respiratory center (medulla oblongata) to carbon dioxide, thus stimulating the increase in minute ventilation and lowering the PCO_2. These two factors are responsible for the heightened awareness of the need to breathe, or dyspnea, experienced by many women during pregnancy.

Estrogen. Estrogen causes increased vascularity of the mucous membranes of the upper respiratory tract. As the capillaries become engorged, edema and hyperemia develop within the nose, pharynx, larynx, and trachea. This congestion gives rise to several conditions commonly seen during pregnancy, such as nasal and sinus stuffiness, epistaxis (nosebleeds), and changes in the voice. Increased vascularity also causes edema of the eardrum and eustachian tubes and may result in a sense of fullness in the ears or earaches.

Physical Changes

By the third trimester the enlarging uterus lifts the diaphragm by about 4 cm (1.6 in), which prevents the lungs from expanding as fully as they normally do. The ribs flare, the substernal angle widens, and the circumference of the chest expands by about 6 cm (2.5 in) to compensate for the reduced space. Breathing becomes thoracic rather than abdominal, adding to the dyspnea experienced by many women.

Gastrointestinal System

The gastrointestinal system undergoes changes that are clinically significant because they may cause discomfort for the expectant mother.

Mouth

Elevated levels of estrogen cause hyperemia of the tissues of the mouth and gums and may lead to gingivitis and bleeding gums. Some women develop severe vascular hypertrophy of the gums, which appear reddened and swollen and bleed easily. The condition regresses spontaneously after childbirth.

Some women experience ptyalism, or excessive salivation, that is unpleasant and embarrassing. The cause of ptyalism appears to be stimulation of the salivary glands by the ingestion of starch (Cunningham, et al., 1997). Small, frequent meals and use of chewing gum and oral lozenges offer limited relief for some women.

Many women think that pregnancy adversely affects the teeth. However, the teeth do not lose minerals to the fetus and remain unaffected by pregnancy.

Esophagus

The lower esophageal sphincter tone decreases during pregnancy primarily because of the relaxant activity of progesterone on the smooth muscles. The reduced tone allows reflux of acidic stomach contents into the esophagus and produces heartburn, or pyrosis.

Stomach and Small Intestine

Elevated levels of progesterone relax all smooth muscle, leading to decreased tone and motility of the gastrointestinal tract. The stomach and small intestine take longer to empty, allowing additional time for nutrient absorption. This slowed process benefits the growing fetus but may contribute to the nausea experienced by many expectant mothers.

Large Intestine

Decreased motility in the large intestine allows time for more water to be absorbed, which tends to make the stools hard and may lead to constipation. Constipation may cause or exacerbate hemorrhoids if the expectant mother must strain to have bowel movements.

Liver and Gallbladder

Although the size of the liver and gallbladder remains unchanged during pregnancy, functional changes occur largely because of the effects of progesterone. The gallbladder becomes hypotonic and emptying time is prolonged, resulting in thicker bile that can predispose to the development of gallstones. Reduced gallbladder tone also leads to a tendency to retain bile salts, which can lead to itching (pruritus).

The enlarging uterus pushes the liver upward and backward during the last trimester and also alters liver function. Levels of serum alkaline phosphatase and serum cholesterol almost double by the end of pregnancy, whereas levels of serum albumin fall gradually. These changes are primarily because of the effect of estrogen and hemodilution.

Urinary System

Bladder

During the first trimester the uterus begins to expand within the pelvic cavity. Expansion applies pressure to the bladder, causing the woman to experience frequency and urgency of urination. During the second trimester the uterus extends into the abdominal cavity, relieving pressure on the bladder and decreasing the urge to void. In addition, bladder capacity almost doubles as the bladder, like all smooth muscle, relaxes in response to increasing levels of progesterone.

Bladder mucosa also becomes congested with blood, and the bladder walls become hypertrophied as a result of stimulation from estrogen. Decreased drainage of blood from the base of the bladder results in edema of its tissues and renders the area susceptible to trauma and infection during childbirth.

Late in the third trimester, lightening causes the fetus to settle into the pelvis and press against the bladder. Once again the woman experiences frequency, urgency, and nocturia. Although frequency and urgency are normal during early and late pregnancy, they are also signs of infection and, if accompanied by burning sensations or pain, are cause for assessment for urinary tract infection.

Kidneys and Ureters

Changes in Size and Shape of the Kidneys. During pregnancy the kidneys change in both size and shape because dilation of the renal pelves, calyces, and ureters occurs above the pelvic brim. The dilation is caused by (1) the effect of progesterone, which relaxes the walls of the ureters and makes them more distensible, and (2) compression of the ureters between the enlarging uterus and the bony pelvic brim. As the flow of urine through the ureters is obstructed, particularly on the right side (the left ureter being cushioned by the sigmoid colon), the ureters dilate and apply hydrostatic pressure against the renal pelvis, which also dilates. The resulting stasis of urine is clinically significant because it allows time for bacteria to multiply and increases the risk of urinary tract infection during pregnancy.

Functional Changes of the Kidneys. Renal plasma flow, or the total amount of plasma to flow through the kidneys, increases significantly. This change results from increases in plasma volume and cardiac output. The glomerular filtration rate, the rate at which water and dissolved substances are filtered in the glomerulus, increases by as much as 50% by the end of the first trimester. This elevation results from the rise in renal plasma flow and decreased colloid osmotic pressure caused by a reduction in the concentration of plasma proteins.

The increases in renal plasma flow and glomerular filtration rate are necessary to excrete additional metabolic waste from the mother and fetus, but they also affect the excretion of glucose. As the glomerular filtration rate increases, the filtered load of glucose exceeds the ability of the renal tubules to reabsorb it, and glucose spills into the urine. Therefore glycosuria is common during pregnancy, particularly after consumption of foods such as candy and cookies that are high in simple sugars. Furthermore, small quantities of amino acids and water-soluble vitamins are excreted. Bacteria thrive in urine that is rich in nutrients, and thus glycosuria is another reason for the increased incidence of urinary tract infections during pregnancy.

Tests of renal function may be misleading during pregnancy. As a result of increased glomerular filtration rate, plasma concentrations of both creatinine and urea normally decline.

Check Your Reading

10. How does the respiratory system compensate for the pressure exerted on the diaphragm by the enlarging uterus?
11. Why do some women experience dyspnea during pregnancy?
12. How does pregnancy affect the gastrointestinal system?
13. Why are pregnant women at increased risk for urinary tract infection?

Integumentary System

Skin

Circulation to the skin increases during pregnancy and encourages activity of the sweat and sebaceous glands. Pregnant women feel warmer and perspire more, particularly during the last trimester. Accelerated activity by the sebaceous glands fosters the development of facial blemishes, which are usually reduced by careful cleansing of the face several times each day. Additional changes include hyperpigmentation and vascular changes in the skin.

Hyperpigmentation. Increased pigmentation may begin as early as the second month when estrogen and progesterone cause elevated levels of melanocyte-stimulating hormone. Women with dark hair or skin exhibit more hyperpigmentation than women with very light skin.

Areas of pigmentation include brownish patches called *chloasma* that usually involve the forehead, cheeks, and bridge of the nose. This sign is commonly called the "mask of pregnancy." It may also occur in nonpregnant women taking oral contraceptives. A dark line of pigmentation (linea nigra) may also extend from the symphysis pubis to the umbilicus or above. Preexisting moles become darker, and the areolae become darker as pregnancy progresses. Hyperpigmentation usually disappears after childbirth when the levels of estrogen and progesterone decline.

Cutaneous Vascular Changes. Blood vessels dilate and proliferate during pregnancy. This change is thought to be largely because of the effect of estrogen. Changes in surface blood vessels are obvious during pregnancy, especially in white women. These include angiomas (vascular spiders, telangiectasis) that appear as tiny red elevations branching in all directions and appear most often on the face, neck, upper chest, and arms. Redness of the palms or soles of the feet, known as *palmar erythema,* also occurs in many white women and some African-American women. Vascular changes often occur simultaneously, and although they may be emotionally distressing for the expectant mother, they are clinically insignificant and usually disappear shortly after childbirth.

Connective Tissue

Linear tears may occur in the connective tissue, most often on the abdomen, breasts, and buttocks, appearing as slightly depressed, pink to purple streaks called *striae gravidarum* or "stretch marks" (Figure 7-5). Women are concerned about striae because they do not disappear after childbirth, although the marks fade to silvery lines. Laser therapy is sometimes used after childbirth to reduce or eliminate severe striae. Many women claim that striae can be prevented by massage with oil or vitamin E, but the effectiveness of this treatment has not been documented. Antipruritic ointments may be effective in controlling the itching that accompanies severe striae.

Hair and Nails

Because fewer follicles are in the resting phase, hair grows more rapidly and less hair falls out during pregnancy. After childbirth, hair follicles return to normal activity, and many women become concerned at the rate of hair loss that may peak about 3 to 4 months after childbirth (Rapini & Jordan, 1999). They should be reassured that more follicles have returned to the normal resting phase and excessive hair loss will not continue.

Nail growth increases during pregnancy. Many women notice thinning and softening of the nails as pregnancy progresses, although reasons for these changes are unclear.

Musculoskeletal System

Postural Changes

Musculoskeletal changes are progressive. They begin in the second trimester when maternal hormones (such as relaxin, progesterone) initiate gradual softening of the

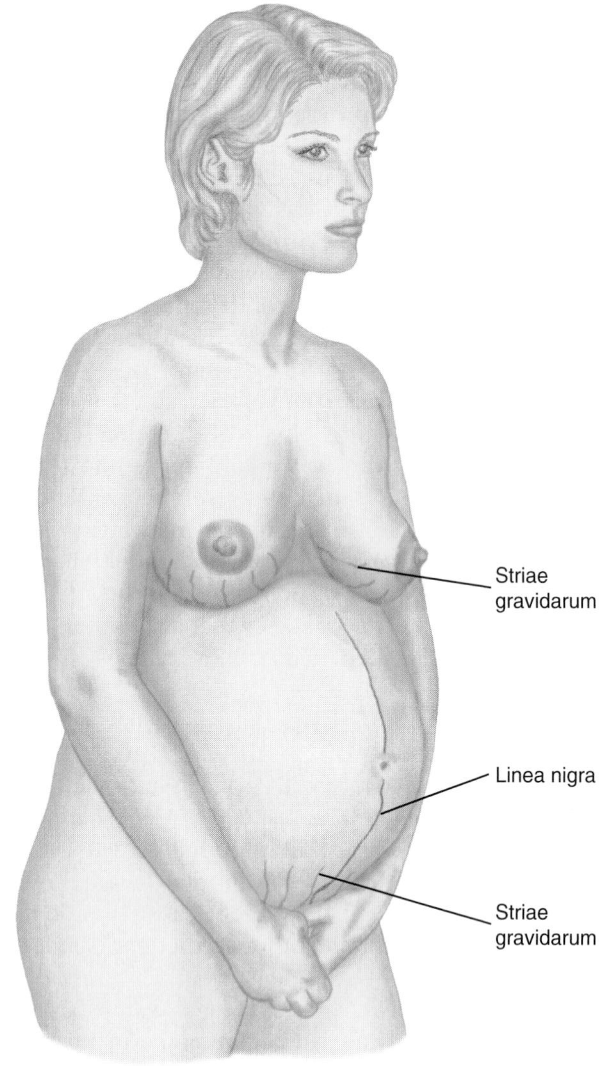

FIGURE 7-5 Striae gravidarum are linear tears that may occur in the connective tissue. Linea nigra, a pigmented line from above the umbilicus to the symphysis pubis, may also appear.

pelvic ligaments and joints to facilitate passage of the fetus through the pelvis during birth. Relaxation of the pelvic joints creates pelvic instability, and the pregnant woman assumes a wide stance. The "waddling" gait of pregnancy occurs because of muscle fatigue and an effort to compensate for a changing center of gravity.

During the third trimester, as the uterus increases in size, the expectant mother must lean backward to maintain her balance. This creates a progressive lordosis, or curvature of the lower spine (Figure 7-6). The strain on the muscles and ligaments of the back often causes backache.

Abdominal Wall

Pregnancy also affects the abdominal muscles, which may be stretched beyond their capacity during the third trimester, causing the rectus abdominis muscles to separate (diastasis recti). The extent of the separation varies from slight and not clinically significant to severe, when a large portion of the uterine wall is covered only by skin and fascia (see Chapter 17).

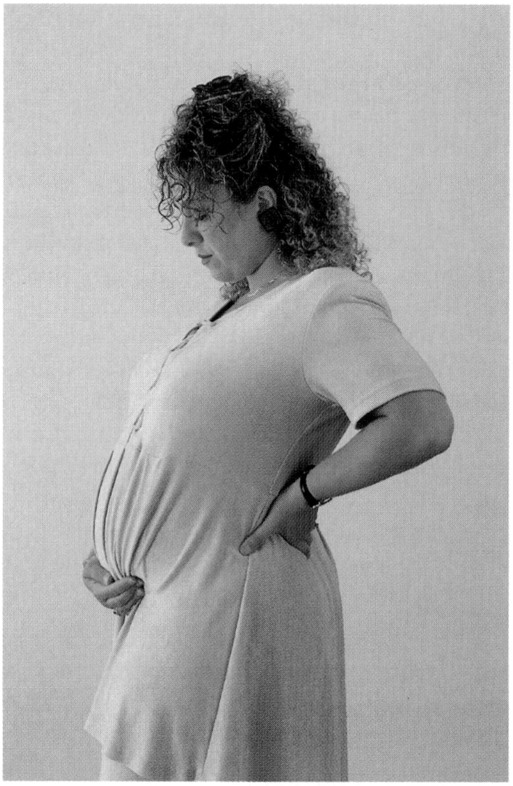

FIGURE 7-6 Lordosis increases by the third trimester as the uterus grows larger, and the woman must lean backward to maintain her balance.

Endocrine System

Numerous changes in hormones occur in pregnancy (Table 7-1).

Pituitary Gland

Most hormones from the pituitary gland are suppressed during pregnancy. The hormones FSH and LH, which are normally produced to stimulate ovulation in the nonpregnant woman, are unnecessary during pregnancy, and the growth hormone from the anterior pituitary also appears to decrease during pregnancy. However, prolactin increases to prepare the breasts to produce milk.

The posterior pituitary secretes oxytocin, the second hormone involved in lactation. Oxytocin stimulates the milk-ejection reflex after childbirth. Oxytocin also stimulates contractions of the uterus, but this action is inhibited during pregnancy by progesterone, which relaxes the smooth muscle fibers of the uterus. After childbirth, progesterone levels decline, and oxytocin plays an important role in keeping the uterus contracted and thus preventing excessive bleeding.

Table 7-1
HORMONES RELATED TO PREGNANCY

Hormone	Source	Major Effects
ESTROGEN	Ovary, placenta	Stimulates uterine development to provide an environment for the fetus, stimulates the breasts in preparation for lactation
PROGESTERONE	Ovary, placenta	Maintains the uterine lining for implantation, relaxes all smooth muscle including the uterus, develops acini cells and lobes to prepare the breasts for lactation
HUMAN PLACENTAL LACTOGEN	Placenta	Stimulates metabolism of glucose and converts glucose to fat; acts as an antagonist to insulin
HUMAN CHORIONIC GONADOTROPIN	Trophoblasts (placenta)	Prevents involution of the corpus luteum, which maintains production of progesterone until the placenta is formed
RELAXIN	Ovary, placenta	Softens muscles and joints of pelvis
FOLLICLE-STIMULATING HORMONE	Anterior pituitary	Initiates maturation of ovum, necessary for conception, is suppressed during pregnancy
LUTEINIZING HORMONE	Anterior pituitary	Stimulates ovulation of the mature ovum in the nonpregnant state
MELANOCYTE-STIMULATING HORMONE	Anterior pituitary	Increases during pregnancy, produces hyperpigmentation
OXYTOCIN	Posterior pituitary	Stimulates uterine contractions to initiate labor, stimulates the milk-ejection reflex
PROLACTIN	Anterior pituitary	Serves as the primary hormone of milk production
ALDOSTERONE	Adrenals	Increases during pregnancy to conserve sodium and maintain fluid balance
CORTISOL	Adrenals	Increases during pregnancy, is active in metabolism of glucose and fats, may be helpful in preventing rejection of pregnancy because of its antiinflammatory effect
THYROXINE	Thyroid	Increases during pregnancy to stimulate basal metabolic rate

Thyroid Gland

Early in the first trimester, a rise in total thyroxine (T_4) occurs along with a corresponding gain in thyroxine-binding protein. The increased amounts of T_4 bind readily with the thyroxine-binding proteins, and the serum level of unbound T_4 remains stable. These changes produce slight enlargement in the size of the thyroid gland and an increase in basal metabolic rate (BMR). The BMR increases by 20% to 25% during pregnancy, causing greater cardiac output, pulse rate, and heat intolerance. The BMR returns to normal within a few weeks after childbirth.

Parathyroid Glands

The metabolism of calcium and phosphorus depends on the secretion of parathyroid hormone. During pregnancy, fetal demands for calcium and phosphorus increase, and the maternal parathyroid glands respond by producing additional parathyroid hormone. Parathyroid hormone generally acts to improve absorption of calcium from the intestine, decrease renal losses, and mobilize calcium from bone. During pregnancy, however, no loss of bone density occurs despite the increase in parathyroid activity. The skeleton appears to be protected by increased levels of calcitonin and estrogen, which interfere with the action of parathyroid hormone on bone.

Pancreas

Significant changes in the pancreas during pregnancy are the result of alterations in maternal blood glucose levels and consequent fluctuations in insulin production. The fetus draws glucose from the maternal supply. In addition, the fetus draws amino acids from maternal circulation and thereby inhibits the mother's ability to synthesize glucose. During the first trimester the combination of increasing glucose demand by the fetus and a declining supply of glucose results in a fall in maternal blood glucose levels. Consequently, during this time the islets of Langerhans produce less insulin.

During the second trimester, maternal tissue sensitivity to insulin begins to decline, mainly because of the effects of hormones such as human placental lactogen, prolactin, progesterone, and cortisol. As a consequence of the tissue resistance to insulin, postprandial (after a meal) blood glucose levels rise. A higher blood glucose level has two major effects: (1) it makes more glucose available for fetal energy needs, and (2) it stimulates the pancreas of a healthy woman to produce additional insulin. Insulin production more than doubles during meals and is 30% higher than usual by the third trimester to meet the insulin needs (Moore, 1999). Inadequate insulin production results in gestational diabetes (see Chapter 26).

Adrenal Glands

The adrenal glands enlarge only slightly during pregnancy. Significant changes occur in two adrenal hormones: cortisol and aldosterone. Although production of cortisol does not increase during pregnancy, the unbound level of cortisol is elevated. The specific plasma protein (transcortin) that binds to cortisol also is elevated. Cortisol regulates carbohydrate and protein metabolism. It stimulates gluconeogenesis (formation of glycogen from noncarbohydrate sources such as amino and fatty acids) whenever the supply of glucose is inadequate to meet the body's needs for energy.

Aldosterone regulates the absorption of sodium from the distal tubules of the kidneys and has been called the "great sodium saver." Aldosterone production is increased during pregnancy to overcome the salt-wasting effects of progesterone. Aldosterone thereby maintains the necessary level of sodium in the greatly expanded blood volume. Aldosterone is closely related to water metabolism (see p. 131).

Changes Caused by Placental Hormones

Human Chorionic Gonadotropin. In early pregnancy, human chorionic gonadotropin (hCG) is produced by the trophoblastic cells surrounding the developing embryo. The primary function of hCG in early pregnancy is to stimulate the corpus luteum to produce progesterone and estrogen until the placenta is sufficiently developed to assume this function. The presence of this hormone produces positive pregnancy tests.

Estrogen. Although estrogen is produced by the ovaries during the menstrual cycle and by the corpus luteum for the first few weeks of pregnancy, it is produced primarily by the placenta after the sixth or seventh week of pregnancy. Estrogen has numerous functions during pregnancy: (1) it stimulates uterine growth and increases blood supply to uterine vessels, (2) it aids in developing the ductal system in the breasts in preparation for lactation, and (3) it is associated with hyperpigmentation, vascular changes in the skin, increased activity of the salivary glands, and hyperemia of the gums and nasal mucous membranes.

Progesterone. Progesterone is produced first by the corpus luteum and then by the fully developed placenta. Progesterone is the most important hormone of pregnancy. Its major functions include the following:

- Maintaining the endometrial layer for implantation of the fertilized ovum
- Preventing spontaneous abortion by relaxing smooth muscles of the uterus
- Stimulating the development of the lobes and lobules in the breast in preparation for lactation
- Facilitating the deposit of maternal fat stores, which provide a reserve of energy for pregnancy and lactation

Progesterone relaxes not only the smooth muscle of the uterus but also all other smooth muscle. Consequently, progesterone is associated with decreased motility of the bowel, dilation of the ureters, and increased bladder capacity. Progesterone raises the respiratory sensitivity to carbon dioxide and thus stimulates increased ventilation.

Human Placental Lactogen. Human placental lactogen (hPL), also called *human chorionic somatomammotropin (hCS),* is present during early pregnancy and increases steadily throughout pregnancy. Its primary function is to increase the availability of glucose for the fetus, who needs a constant supply for growth and development. hPL does this by decreasing the sensitivity of maternal cells to insulin, which decreases maternal metabolism of glucose, thereby freeing glucose for transport to the fetus. In addition, hPL encourages the quick metabolism of free fatty acids to provide energy for the pregnant woman.

Relaxin. Relaxin is produced by the corpus luteum and placenta and is present by the first missed menstrual period. Relaxin inhibits uterine activity, softens connective tissue in the cervix, relaxes pelvic joints, and stimulates growth of the breasts.

Changes in Metabolism

Weight Gain. Because a correlation between infant mortality and low birth weight has been documented, women are encouraged to gain an average of 25 to 35 pounds during pregnancy (see Table 9-1). The fetus, placenta, and amniotic fluid make up less than half the recommended weight gain. The remainder is found in the increased size of the uterus and breasts, increased blood volume, increased interstitial fluid, and maternal stores of subcutaneous fat (see Figure 9-1).

Water Metabolism. The required amount of water increases during pregnancy to meet the needs of the fetus, placenta, amniotic fluid and increased blood volume. Fluid balance depends on adequate concentrations of sodium, and the kidneys must compensate for the many factors favoring excretion of sodium during pregnancy. For example, increased glomerular filtration rate, decreased concentration of plasma proteins, and increased progesterone levels all result in an increase in sodium excretion. On the other hand, increased concentrations of estrogen, cortisol, prolactin, and aldosterone all tend to promote the reabsorption of sodium. The net effect of the combined hormonal action is the maintenance of the sodium balance.

Dependent Edema. Because of hemodilution, colloid osmotic pressure slightly decreases, favoring the development of edema during pregnancy. Edema further increases toward term when the weight of the uterus compresses the veins of the pelvis. This process delays venous return, causing the veins of the legs to become distended, and increases venous pressure, resulting in additional fluid shifts from the vascular compartment to interstitial spaces.

Edema of the feet and ankles is obvious at the end of the day (particularly if a pregnant woman stands for prolonged periods), and the force of gravity contributes to the pooling of blood in the veins of the legs. Dependent edema is clinically insignificant. However, if edema of the face or hands is noted, the nurse should assess for hypertension and proteinuria to identify signs of pregnancy-induced hypertension.

Carpal Tunnel Syndrome. Fluid retention is also associated with carpal tunnel syndrome, believed to result when edema compresses the median nerve at the point where it passes through the carpal tunnel of the wrist. Symptoms include soreness, weakness, and tenderness of the muscles of the thumb. The condition usually resolves when the pregnancy ends.

Carbohydrate Metabolism. Carbohydrate metabolism changes markedly during pregnancy because more insulin is required as pregnancy progresses. As hormones such as progesterone and hPL cause maternal tissue resistance to insulin, an enzyme called *insulinase,* which is produced by the placenta, speeds up the breakdown of insulin.

Insulin is essential for the metabolism of glucose and maintenance of proper blood glucose levels. A protective mechanism that allows an ample supply of glucose for transfer to the fetus decreases the mother's ability to use insulin. However, the mother's pancreas must produce more insulin so that she can continue to metabolize enough glucose to meet her own energy needs and prevent hyperglycemia. Hyperglycemia occurs when blood glucose levels exceed available insulin, which is needed to transport glucose into cells.

For most women, hyperglycemia is not a problem and insulin production is increased, particularly during the second and third trimesters. In some women, however, insulin production cannot be increased, and these women experience periodic hyperglycemia. This condition is called *gestational diabetes mellitus* (see Chapter 26).

Check Your Reading

14. What causes the progressive changes in posture and gait during pregnancy?
15. Why is progesterone called the "hormone of pregnancy"?
16. Why do maternal needs for insulin change during pregnancy?

CONFIRMATION OF PREGNANCY

Confirmation of pregnancy has become much simpler since the development of ultrasonography, which makes it possible to view the fetal outline and observe the fetal heartbeat very early in pregnancy. Traditionally, the diagnosis of pregnancy has been based on symptoms experienced by the woman and signs observed by a physician, nurse-midwife, or nurse practitioner.

Figure 7-7 summarizes fetal and maternal changes that occur throughout pregnancy. These signs and symptoms are grouped into three classifications: presumptive, probable, and positive indications of pregnancy. A diagnosis of pregnancy cannot be made solely on the presumptive or probable signs because other causes may exist (Table 7-2).

Presumptive Indications of Pregnancy

Presumptive indications can also be termed *subjective changes* because they are experienced and reported by the woman. Presumptive changes are the least reliable

Text continued on p. 136

Table 7-2

INDICATIONS OF PREGNANCY AND OTHER POSSIBLE CAUSES

Sign or Symptom	Other Possible Causes
PRESUMPTIVE INDICATORS	
Amenorrhea	Emotional stress, strenuous physical exercise, endocrine problems, chronic disease, early menopause
Nausea and vomiting	Gastrointestinal virus, food poisoning, emotional stress
Fatigue	Illness, stress, sudden changes in lifestyle
Urinary frequency	Urinary tract infections
Breast and skin changes	Premenstrual changes, use of oral contraceptives
Cervical color changes	Infection or hormonal imbalance
Quickening	Abdominal gas, peristalsis, pseudocyesis (false pregnancy)
PROBABLE INDICATIONS	
Abdominal enlargement	Abdominal or uterine tumors
Cervical softening	Hormonal imbalance
Ballottement	Uterine or cervical polyps
Braxton Hicks contractions	Soft uterine fibroids (myomas)
Palpation of fetal outline	Large leiomyoma (possibly feeling like the fetal head), small, soft leiomyoma (possibly simulating fetal body parts)
Positive pregnancy tests	Use of certain medications (e.g., antianxiety, anticonvulsant drugs), premature menopause, blood in urine, malignant tumors that produce human chorionic gonadotropin
POSITIVE INDICATIONS	
Auscultation of fetal heart sounds	
Fetal movements felt by examiner	
Visualization of embryo or fetus	

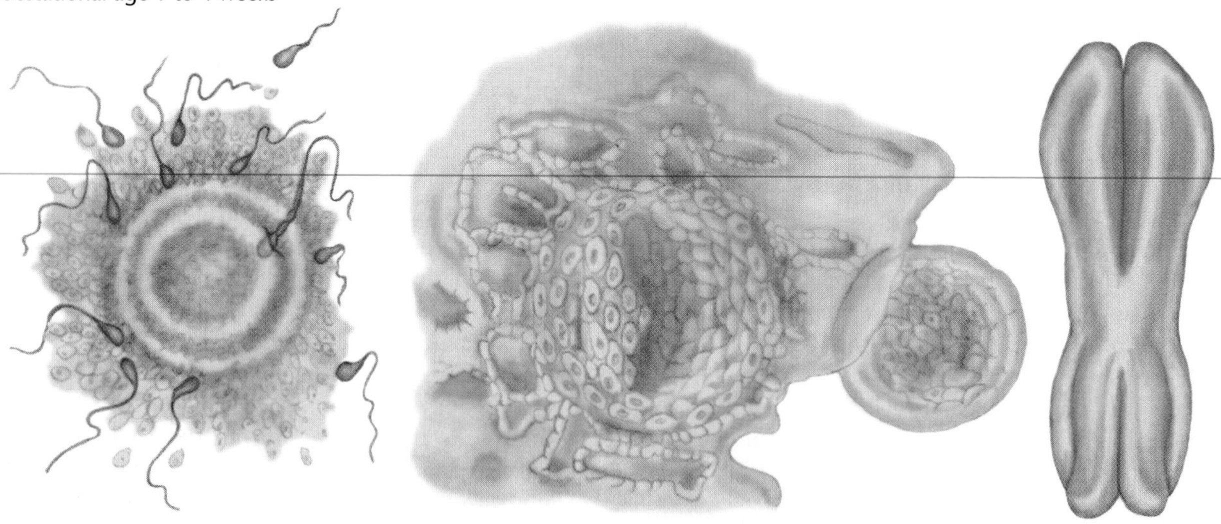

Gestational age 1 to 4 weeks
Woman's basal body temperature elevated; hCG elevated; pregnancy tests positive.
Crown-to-rump length 4 mm. Fertilization, implantation. Preembryonic stage.

FIGURE 7-7 Fetal growth and development and maternal responses based on the date of the last menstrual period.

Gestational age 5 to 8 weeks

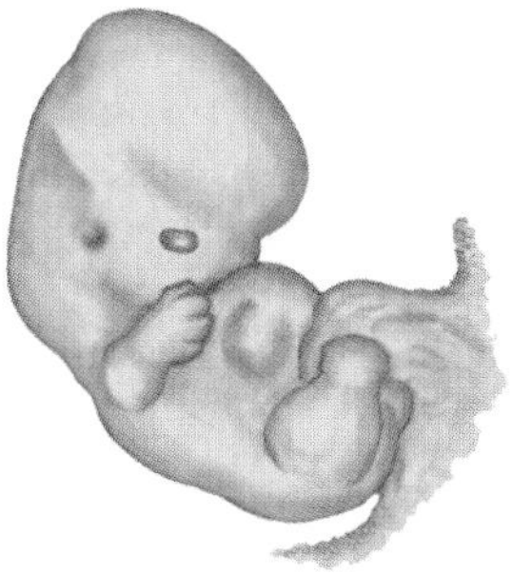

Crown-to-rump length 13 mm. Embryonic stage. Heart developed, beginning to pump. Arm and leg buds present. Head large, with facial features beginning to form.

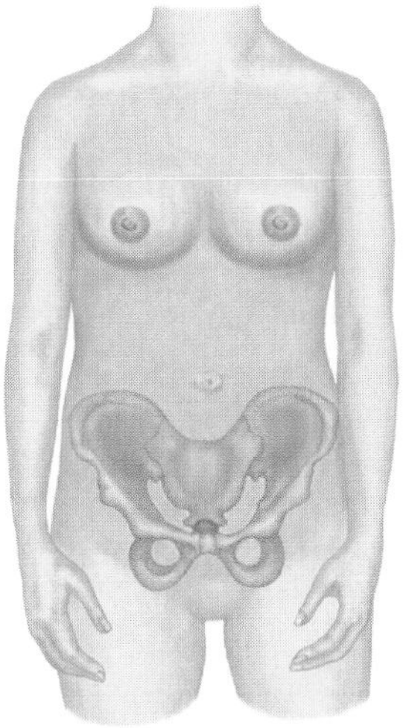

Woman misses menstrual period. Nausea; fatigue. Tingling of breasts. Uterus is size of a lemon; positive Chadwick's, Goodell's and Hegar's signs. Urinary frequency as enlarging uterus presses on the bladder; increased vaginal discharge.

Gestational age 9 to 12 weeks

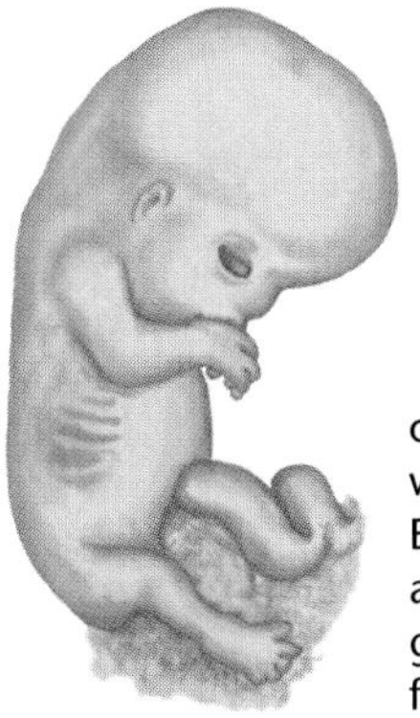

Crown-to-rump length 6 to 7 cm. Fetal stage begins at 10 weeks after last menstrual period. Extremities developed; fingers and toes differentiated; external genitalia show signs of male or female sex. Weight 14 g (0.5 oz).

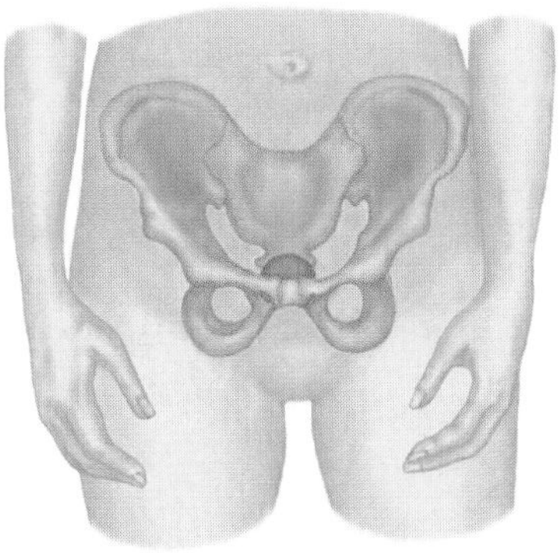

Nausea decreases after 12 weeks. Uterus is size of an orange; palpable above symphysis pubis. Vulvar varicosities may appear.

Gestational age 13 to 16 weeks

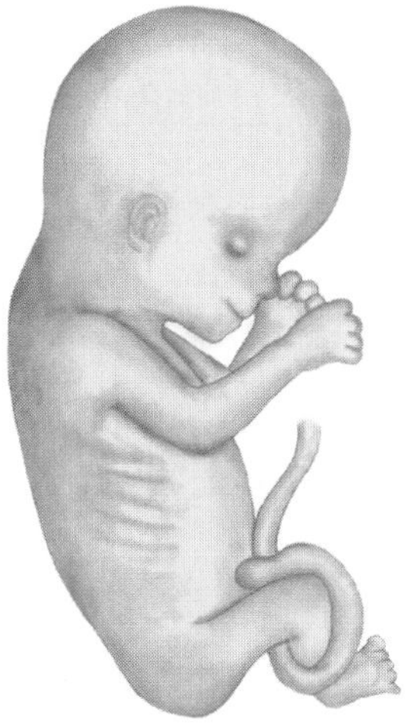

Crown-to-rump length 12 cm. Weight 110 g. Fetus begins to move. Head and thorax can be identified by ultrasound; sexual organs formed. Urine formation begins.

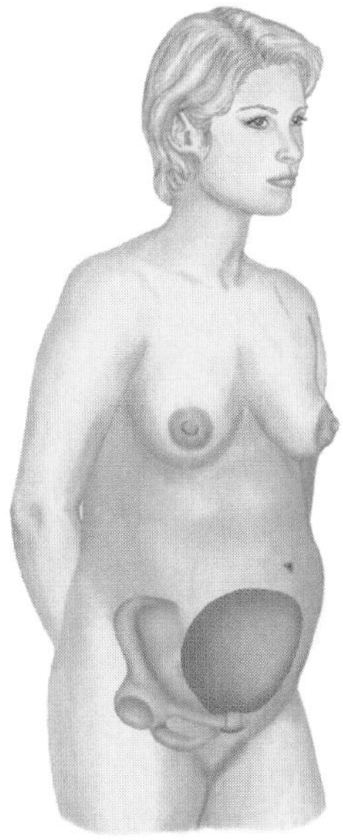

Fetal movements may be felt. Uterus has risen into the abdomen; fundus midway between symphysis pubis and umbilicus. Urinary frequency decreases; blood volume increases; uterine souffle heard.

FIGURE 7-7, cont'd For legend see opposite page.

Continued

Gestational age 17 to 20 weeks

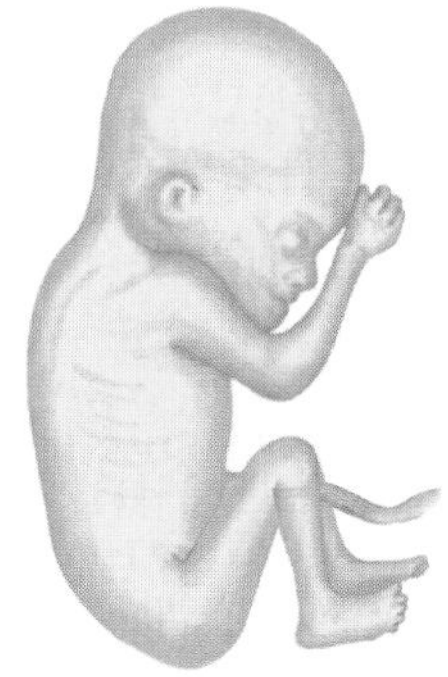

Crown-to-rump length 16 cm. Weight 320 g. Heart beat can be heard with fetoscope or electronic device. Meconium begins collecting in bowel. Period of very rapid growth.

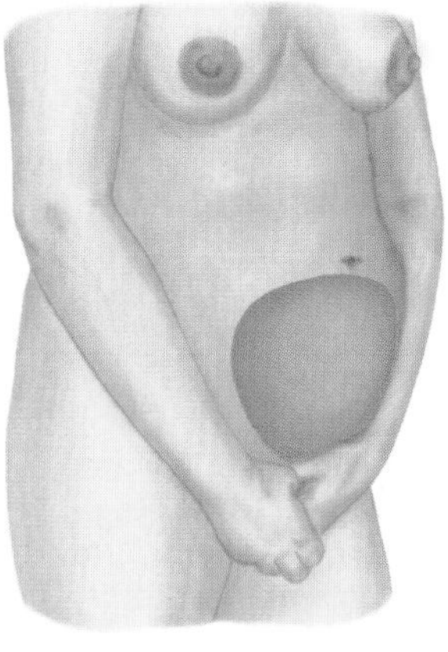

Skin pigmentation increases: areolae darken; chloasma and linea nigra may be obvious. Colostrum may be expressed. Braxton Hicks contractions palpable. Fundus at level of umbilicus.

Gestational age 21 to 24 weeks

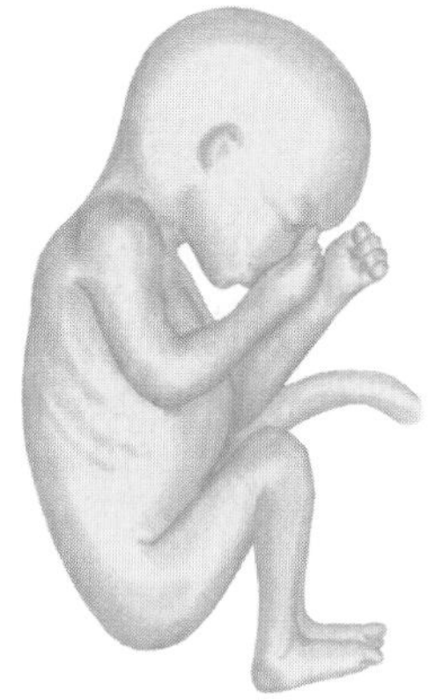

Crown-to-rump length 21 cm. Weight 630 g. Skin wrinkled and red; vernix present; head and body covered with lanugo.

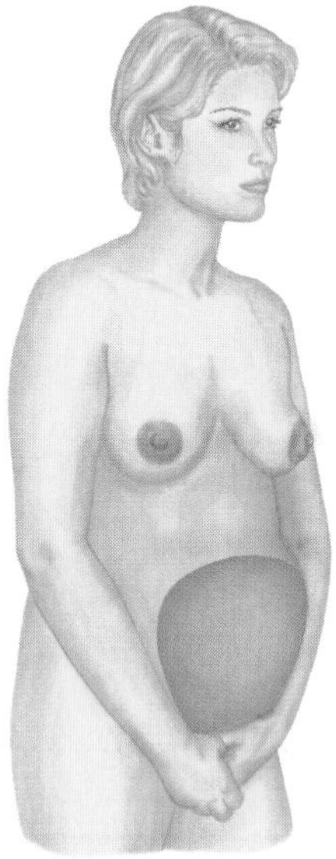

Relaxation of smooth muscles of veins and bladder increases the chance of varicose veins and urinary tract infections. Woman is more aware of fetal movements.

Gestational age 25 to 28 weeks

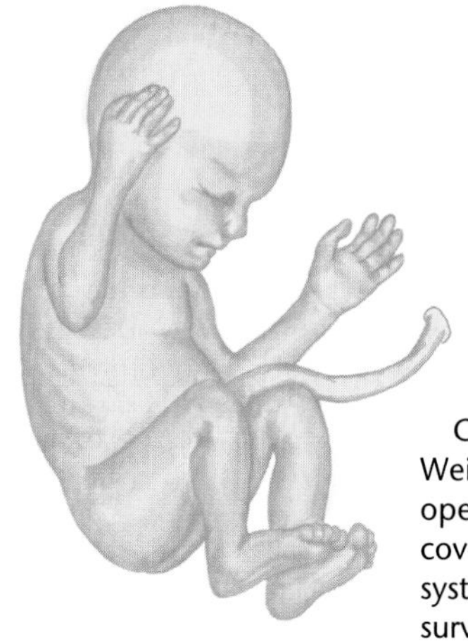

Crown-to-rump length 25 cm. Weight 1000 g. Eyes partially open; eyelashes present. Skin covered with vernix. Respiratory system immature, but fetus may survive if born.

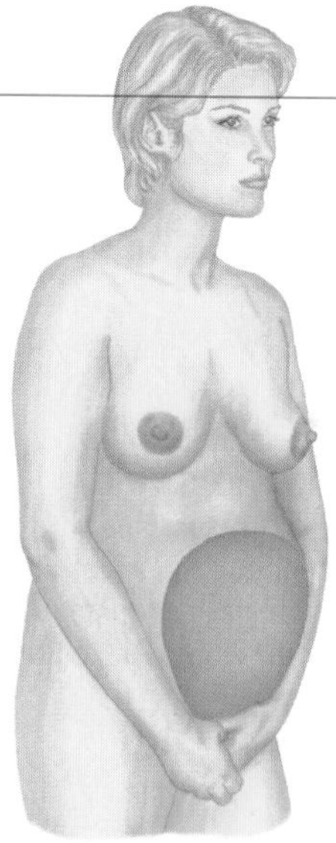

Period of greatest weight gain and lowest hemoglobin level begins. Fundal height is 3 to 4 fingerbreadths above umbilicus. Lordosis may cause backache.

FIGURE 7-7, cont'd For legend see page 132.

Gestational age 29 to 32 weeks

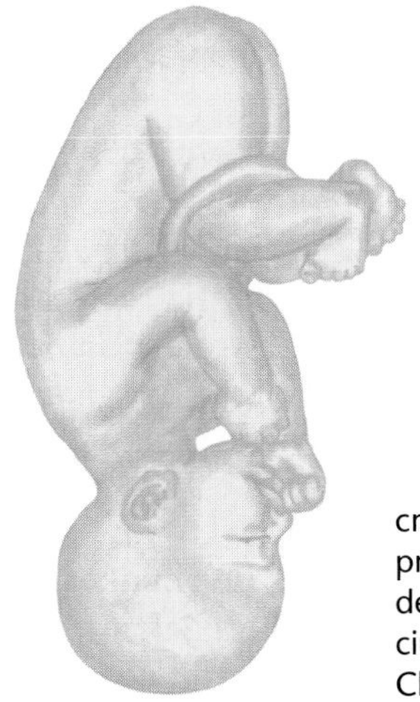

Crown-to-rump length 28 cm. Weight 1700 g. Toenails present. Body filling out, testes descending. Iron, nitrogen, calcium stored. Vernix covers body. Chances of survival improving.

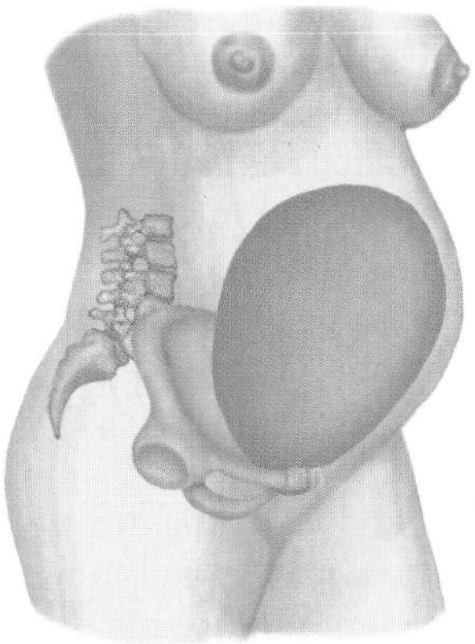

Heartburn common as uterus presses on diaphragm and displaces stomach. Braxton Hicks contractions more noticeable. Lordosis increases; waddling gait develops as relaxin softens pelvic joints.

Gestational age 33 to 36 weeks

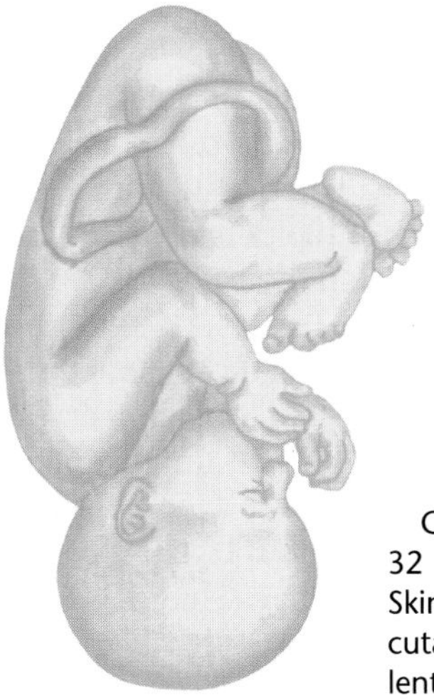

Crown-to-rump length 30 to 32 cm. Weight 2000 to 2500 g. Skin thicker, less wrinkled as subcutaneous fat accumulates. Excellent chance for survival.

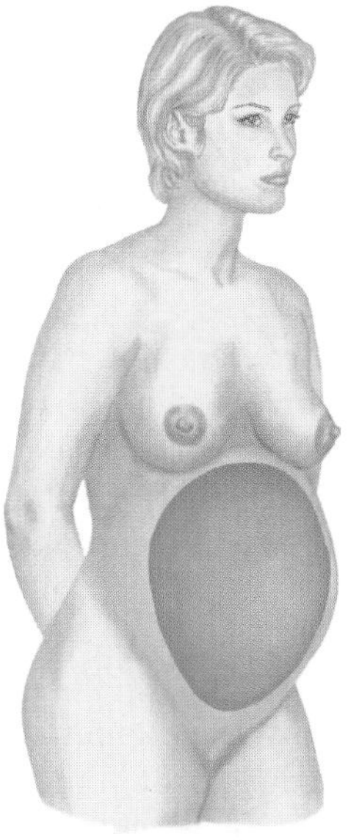

Shortness of breath caused by upward pressure on diaphragm; woman may have difficulty finding a comfortable position for sleep. Umbilicus protrudes. Varicosities more pronounced; pedal or ankle edema may be present. Urinary frequency noted following lightening when presenting part settles into pelvic cavity.

Gestational age 37 to 40 weeks

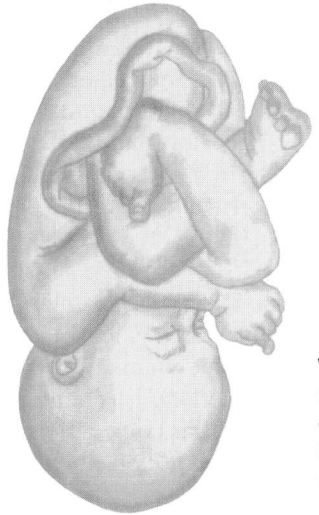

Crown-to-rump length 36 cm. Weight 3400 g. Body plump; lanugo remains only over shoulders; nails extend beyond nail beds; testes within scrotum; female labia well developed; labia majora cover labia minora.

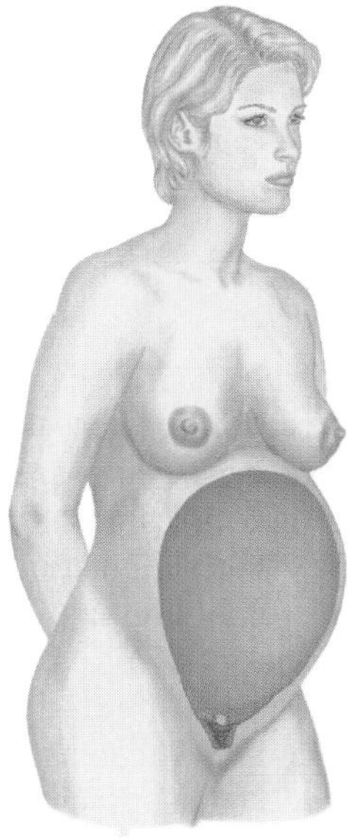

Woman is uncomfortable; looking forward to birth of baby. Cervix softens, begins to efface; mucus plug is often lost.

FIGURE 7-7, cont'd For legend see page 132.

indicators of pregnancy because any can be caused by conditions other than pregnancy.

Amenorrhea

Absence of menstruation in a woman who regularly menstruates is one of the first changes noted and strongly suggests that conception has occurred in a sexually active woman. Menses cease after conception because progesterone and estrogen, which are secreted from the corpus luteum, maintain the endometrial lining in preparation for implantation of the fertilized ovum.

Nausea and Vomiting

Many women experience nausea and vomiting during early pregnancy, generally beginning about 6 weeks after the last menstrual period. These symptoms usually disappear spontaneously by about 16 weeks (Cunningham, et al., 1997). Nausea and vomiting are believed to be caused by the increased levels of hormones (such as hCG, estrogen), decreased gastric motility (an effect of progesterone), and relative hypoglycemia resulting from night-long fasting.

Fatigue

Many pregnant women experience extraordinary fatigue and drowsiness during the first trimester. The direct cause is unknown. However, fatigue may be related to periodic hypoglycemia that occurs because glucose is transferred from the mother to the fetus to provide energy for rapid development.

Urinary Frequency

Urinary frequency is first noticed by the expectant mother in the first few weeks of pregnancy when pressure is exerted on the bladder by the expanding uterus, causing the urge to void. This symptom abates during the second trimester when the uterus expands into the abdominal cavity. Late in the third trimester the fetus settles into the pelvic cavity, and the woman once again experiences frequency and urgency of urination as the uterus presses against the bladder.

Breast and Skin Changes

Breast changes occur early, around the sixth week of pregnancy. The expectant mother experiences breast tenderness, feelings of fullness, and increased size and pigmentation of the areolae. Breast changes result from the influence of estrogen and progesterone, which stimulates the lobes and ducts to prepare for lactation.

Many women observe increased pigmentation of the skin (such as chloasma, linea nigra, darkening of the areolae of the breasts) during pregnancy. These skin changes are the result of increased levels of melanocyte-stimulating hormone, which is an effect of estrogen.

Fetal Movement

Unlike other presumptive indications of pregnancy, fetal movement (quickening) is not perceived until the second trimester. Between 16 and 20 weeks of gestation the expectant mother first notices subtle fetal movements, which gradually increase in intensity.

Probable Indications of Pregnancy

Probable indications of pregnancy are objective findings that can be documented by an examiner. They are primarily related to physical changes in the reproductive organs. Although these signs are stronger indicators of pregnancy, a positive diagnosis of pregnancy cannot be made on the basis of objective findings.

Abdominal Enlargement

Enlargement of the abdomen during the childbearing years is a fairly reliable indication of pregnancy, particularly if it corresponds with a slow, gradual increase in uterine growth (see Figure 7-1). Evidence of pregnancy is even more reliable when uterine growth is accompanied by amenorrhea.

Changes in the Cervix

Color. The cervix changes from pink to a dark bluish violet. This color change, called *Chadwick's sign,* also extends to the vagina and labia. The bluish color is because of increased vascularity of the pelvic organs and is one of the earliest signs of pregnancy.

Consistency. In the early weeks of pregnancy the cervix softens as a result of pelvic vasocongestion (Goodell's sign). Cervical softening is noted during pelvic examination. Around the sixth week of pregnancy the lower uterine segment is so soft that it can be compressed to the thinness of paper. This degree of softness is called *Hegar's sign* (Figure 7-8). Therefore the uterus can be easily flexed against the cervix (McDonald's sign).

Changes in the Uterus

Ballottement. Near midpregnancy a sudden tap on the cervix during vaginal examination may cause the fetus to rise in the amniotic fluid and then rebound to its original position (Figure 7-9). This movement, called *ballottement,* is a strong indication of pregnancy, but it may also be caused by other factors such as uterine or cervical polyps.

Braxton Hicks Contractions. Irregular, painless contractions occur throughout pregnancy, although many expectant mothers do not notice them until the third trimester. Braxton Hicks contractions are not positive signs of pregnancy because similar contractions may occur with other conditions such as soft uterine leiomyomas (fibroids).

Palpation of the Fetal Outline. An experienced practitioner is able to palpate (feel) the outlines of the fetal body by midpregnancy. Outlining the fetus becomes easier as the pregnancy progresses and the uter-

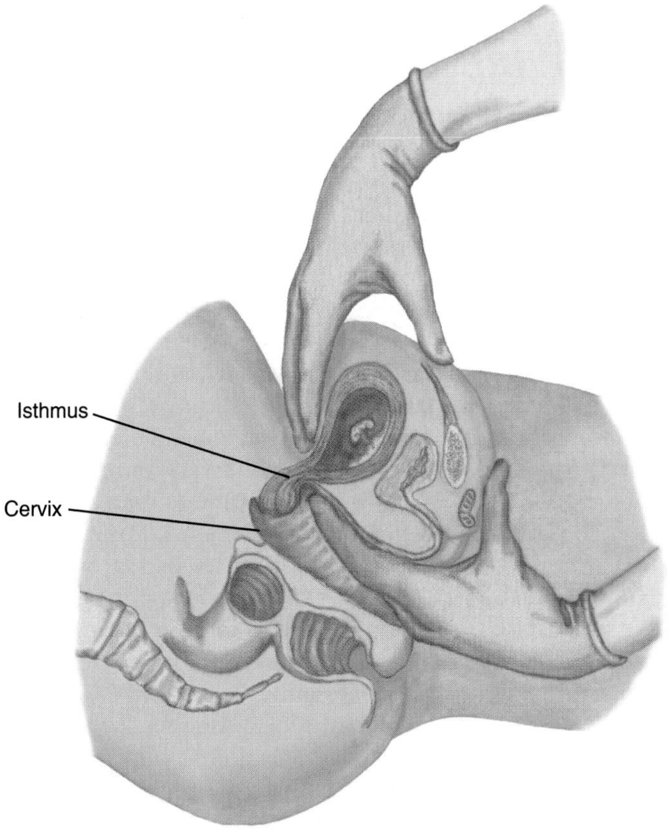

FIGURE 7-8 Hegar's sign demonstrates softening of the isthmus of the cervix.

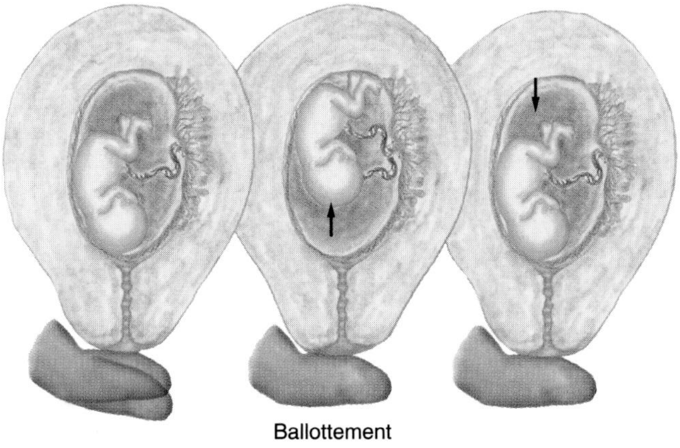

FIGURE 7-9 When the cervix is tapped, the fetus floats upward in the amniotic fluid. A rebound is felt by the examiner when the fetus falls back.

ine walls thin to accommodate the growing fetus. Occasionally, large leiomyomas may feel like the fetal head, or small, soft leiomyomas may simulate small parts of the fetus and may result in a false diagnosis of pregnancy.

Uterine Souffle. A soft, blowing sound that corresponds to the maternal pulse may be auscultated over the uterus (uterine souffle). This sound is because of blood circulation through the placenta and corresponds to the maternal pulse. Therefore the rate of the maternal pulse must be checked simultaneously to identify uterine souffle. Uterine souffle differs from funic souffle, the soft purring sound heard over the umbilical cord that corresponds to the fetal heart rate.

Pregnancy Tests

Pregnancy tests detect hCG or the beta subunit of hCG, which is secreted by the placenta and present in the blood and urine of the pregnant woman shortly after conception. Some tests can be accurate as early as 1 week after fertilization.

Home Pregnancy Tests. Pregnancy tests used in the home identify hCG in maternal urine. They are available for purchase over the counter and are uncomplicated and convenient. Home-test kits are capable of greater than 97% accuracy, but their instructions must be followed precisely to obtain accurate results (Cunningham, et al., 1997).

When pregnancy test results are reported as negative and the woman is in fact pregnant, the results are called *false-negative.* Tests with negative results should be repeated in 2 weeks if the woman believes she may be pregnant. The primary causes of false-negative results are the following:

- A test performed too soon
- Urine that is too dilute
- Impending spontaneous abortion
- Ectopic pregnancy
- Improper use of the test

Results are called *false-positive* when test results are positive and pregnancy has not occurred. The major causes of false-positive test results are the following:

- Error in reading
- Presence of protein or blood in the urine
- Recent pregnancy
- Recent first trimester abortion
- Drug interference (such as marijuana, methadone, phenothiazine, aspirin in large quantities)

Immunometric Tests. Immunometric tests specifically test for the presence of the beta subunit of hCG. The tests are inexpensive and are positive within 1 week of implantation (Stewart, 1998). Some are available for home use without prescription.

Radioimmunoassay Tests. Because radioimmunoassay tests use radioactively labeled markers to detect antibodies against beta subunit hCG in blood or urine, they must be performed in a laboratory. This causes them to be more expensive than immunometric tests. They are accurate as early as 1 week after conception.

Positive Indications of Pregnancy

Only three signs are accepted as positive confirmation of pregnancy: auscultation of fetal heart sounds, fetal movement felt by an examiner, and visualization of the fetus with sonography.

Auscultation of Fetal Heart Sounds

Fetal heart sounds can be heard with a fetoscope by 18 to 20 weeks of gestation. The electronic Doppler scan amplifies fetal heart sounds so that they may be audible by 10 to 12 weeks of gestation. (The fetoscope and Doppler transducer are illustrated in Chapter 14.)

The fetal heartbeat must be heard and distinguished from the maternal pulse to make a positive diagnosis of pregnancy. The fetal heart rate depends on gestational age. The fetal heart rate is in the range of 160 to 170 beats per minute in the first trimester but slows with fetal growth (DuBose, 1996). It should be auscultated during palpation of the radial pulse of the expectant mother. The fetal heart rate is muffled by amniotic fluid, so the sound has been likened to a clock ticking behind a pillow. The location changes because the fetus moves freely in the amniotic fluid.

Fetal Movements Felt by Examiner

Fetal movements vary from faint flutterings in early pregnancy to the characteristic kick or thrust of later pregnancy. These movements are considered a positive sign of pregnancy when felt by an experienced examiner who is not likely to be deceived by similar sensations produced by peristalsis in the large intestine.

Visualization of the Fetus

Transabdominal ultrasound examination is frequently used to confirm pregnancy as early as 5 to 6 weeks of gestation. This procedure involves placing an ultrasound transducer (probe) on the lower abdomen to detect the gestational sac, which is readily identifiable in the maternal pelvis. Movements of the fetal heart are also discernible. By the fourteenth week the fetal head and thorax can be identified (see Chapter 10).

Positive confirmation of pregnancy is possible even earlier with transvaginal ultrasonography. The gestational sac is obvious by 10 days after implantation (16 days after ovulation) when an ultrasound probe is placed in the vagina (Cunningham, et al., 1997).

Check Your Reading

17. How do presumptive and probable indications of pregnancy differ?
18. Why is "fetal" movement felt by the pregnant woman not a positive sign of pregnancy?
19. What are the most common causes of false-negative pregnancy tests?

ANTEPARTUM ASSESSMENT AND CARE

The objective of antepartum care is to ensure that every wanted pregnancy culminates in the birth of a healthy infant without impairing the health of the mother. Three basic components of antepartum care are early and continuing risk assessments, health promotion, and medical and psychosocial interventions. Inadequate antepartum care is associated with low birth weight and an increased incidence of prematurity in neonates. A strong correlation has been found between these two complications and increased infant mortality.

Antepartum care is considered adequate when it begins in the first trimester of pregnancy and continues on a regular basis thereafter. In addition to the collection and evaluation of laboratory values and physical measurements, prenatal care should also provide health education, counseling, and social support.

Approximately 75% of American women begin antepartum care in the first trimester. The United States Department of Health and Human Services (2000) goal for the year 2010 is for at least 90% of American women to commence antepartum care in the first trimester.

A clinical pathway for prenatal care provides guidelines and a time sequence for specific assessments and interventions (Figure 7-10). A pathway does not detail the way to perform assessments or interventions or interpret laboratory or test values, nor does it discuss the significance of specific data. Instead, it allows a multidisciplinary team comprised of nurses, nurse-midwives, physicians, social workers, nutritionists, and counselors to coordinate care for each woman. The most common family problems and risk factors are listed at the top of the pathway and alert the team that additional assessments or care may be required.

Preconception Visit

Ideally, the first visit takes place before conception with a complete history and physical exam. The woman is assessed for any health problems (such as diabetes, sexually transmissible infections), habits (such as use of alcohol or drugs), or social problems (such as domestic violence) that might unfavorably affect pregnancy. She is asked about her use of prescription and over-the-counter drugs. Medications for chronic health problems can be changed if they may be problematic during pregnancy. Screening for rubella is performed and the vaccine is given with instructions to wait at least 3 months before conception. The woman is advised to consume 400 micrograms of folic acid daily before conception to decrease the risk of neural tube defects.

Initial Prenatal Visit

If a preconception visit has occurred recently, many initial prenatal assessments will have been completed

Table 7-3
CALCULATION OF GRAVIDA AND PARA

A useful method for calculating gravida and para is to divide pregnancy outcome into the number of term births, preterm births, abortions, and living children. The acronym GTPAL is helpful: G = gravida, T = term, P = preterm, A = abortions, L = living children.

The following examples illustrate the use of this method to obtain complete information.

- Sally Lam is pregnant for the fifth time. She had two elective abortions in the first trimester. She has a son who was born at 40 weeks' gestation and a daughter who was born at 36 weeks'. She is gravida 5, para 2 and T = 1 (the son born at 40 weeks'); P = 1 (the daughter born at 36 weeks'), A = 2, L = 2. The two abortions are counted in the gravida but not included in the para because they occurred before 20 weeks'.
- Kathleen Eber gave birth to twins at 36 weeks' and to a stillborn infant at 24 weeks'. Approximately 2 years later, she experienced a spontaneous abortion at 12 weeks'. If pregnant now, she is gravida 4, para 2 (the twins counting as 1 parous experience and the stillborn counting as 1), and T = 0 (pregnancies not to term), P = 2 (the twins, born at 36 weeks', counting as 1 preterm birth and the stillborn infant born at 24 weeks' also counting as 1), A = 1, L = 2.

at that time. If not, a thorough history and physical examination must be completed. The primary objectives of the first antepartum examination are as follows:

- To verify or rule out pregnancy
- To evaluate the pregnant woman's physical health relevant to childbearing
- To assess the growth and health of the fetus
- To establish baseline data for comparison with future observations
- To establish trust and rapport with the childbearing family
- To evaluate the psychosocial needs of the woman and her family
- To assess the need for counseling or teaching
- To negotiate a plan of care to ensure both a healthy mother and a healthy baby

History

Obstetric History. The obstetric history provides essential information about previous pregnancies that may alert the physician or nurse-midwife to possible problems in the present pregnancy. The usual components of this history are the following:

- Gravida, para, abortions, and living children
- Weight of infants at birth and length of gestation
- Labor experience, type of delivery, location of birth, and name of attending physician or midwife
- Type of anesthesia and any difficulties
- Maternal complications such as hypertension, diabetes, infection, and bleeding
- Complications with the infant
- Method of infant feeding planned (breastfeeding or formula)
- Special concerns

Gravida refers to the number of pregnancies the woman has had of any length. *Para* refers to the number of pregnancies that have progressed past 20 weeks at delivery. This term does not indicate whether the fetus was born alive or was stillborn. *Parity* refers to the number of pregnancies rather than the number of fetuses or infants. Thus a woman who gives birth to twins after her first pregnancy will be a gravida 1, para 1 if the birth occurred after 20 weeks of gestation.

Information is incomplete if only gravida and para are considered. Pregnancy outcomes can be described with the GTPAL acronym: gravida (G), term births (T), preterm births (P), abortions (A), and live births (L) (Table 7-3).

Nurses must exercise caution when discussing gravida and para with the expectant mother in the presence of her family or significant other. Although the antepartum record indicates a previous pregnancy or childbirth, she may not have shared this information with her family and her right to privacy could be jeopardized by probing questions. The pregnancy may have terminated in elective or spontaneous abortion or in the birth of an infant who was placed for adoption. The confidentiality of the pregnant woman must be protected in both instances.

Menstrual History. A complete menstrual history is necessary to establish the estimated date of delivery (EDD). Common practice is to estimate the EDD on the basis of the first day of the last menstrual cycle, although ovulation and conception occur approximately 2 weeks after the beginning of menstruation in a regular 28-day cycle. The average duration of pregnancy from the first day of the last normal menstrual period is 40 weeks, or 280 days.

Nagele's rule is often used to establish the EDD. This method involves subtracting 3 months, adding 7 days to the first day of the last normal menstrual period (LNMP), and correcting the year.

For example: LNMP August 30, 2001
Subtract 3 months = May 30, 2001
Add 7 days and change the year = June 6, 2002

Many health care providers also use a gestational calculator or wheel to quickly calculate EDD, although some wheels are prone to error (Cunningham, et al.,

DEMOGRAPHIC LABEL

EDC ________

YORK HEALTH SYSTEM
YORK, PENNSYLVANIA
PRENATAL CARE
CLINICAL PATHWAY

PRETERM LABOR RISK
1. ☐ Substance abuse
2. ☐ Prior preterm delivery
3. ☐ >2 abortions
4. ☐ <90 lb prepregnancy weight
5. ☐ Placental anomaly
6. ☐ STD current pregnancy
7. ☐ Multiple gestation
8. ☐ Persistent bleeding
9. ☐ Incompetent cervix

DOCUMENTATION CODES
Initialed box=Meets standard ★=Exception on pathway identified N=Not applicable

CONSULTS/PROBLEM MANAGEMENT FOR PATIENTS INCLUDE:
- Social Service prn
- Perinatologist prn
- Genetic Counseling prn
- Nutritionist prn
- WIC prn
- Pastoral Care prn
- Lactation Consultant prn (3rd trimester)

STANDARD OF CARE FOR PRENATAL PATIENTS INCLUDES:
- Activity ad lib
- Diet to meet needs of pregnancy
- Prenatal vitamins
- $FeSO_4$, if needed

	Clinical Path Visits	Expected Patient/ Family Outcomes	Multidisciplinary Assessment (Refer to STD-0011)	Tests	Education & DC Planning (Refer to STD-0011)
Nurse Interview	Date ________ ________ ________ ________ ________ ________	☐ Referrals made as indicated following prenatal standard of care ☐ Verbalizes understanding of normal vs. abnormal signs and symptoms of pregnancy ☐ Verbalizes agreement to complete labs, obtain prenatal vitamins and keep scheduled appointments ☐ Verbalizes signs and symptoms of preterm labor ☐ No risk factors PTL identified ☐ ________	• Refer to Standard 0011-Nurse interview • Weight, height • Physical, psych/social, behavioral, nutritional risk factors • Knowledge of normal vs. abnormal signs and symptoms of pregnancy • Premature labor risk assessment ________	• CCMS-UA, for nitr/leuk/ glucose, C and S if applicable • Prenatal group ________ • HIV • Sickle cell if applicable • Dating ultrasound scheduled ________	☐ Childbirth ed., baby care and postpartum classes. Exercise during pregnancy. Effects of risk factors on pregnancy. Sexuality during pregnancy. Nutrition education. Normal effects of pregnancy on the body. Fetal growth/development. S and S of complications/preterm labor. Preadmission form. Contraceptives/STD Prevention/HIV counseling. Schedule return-to-clinic appointment. Orient to clinic hours/physical setup, emergency protocol. ________
	RN Name				
1st OB Exam	________ ________ ________ ________	☐ Prenatal group tests within normal limits ☐ Demonstrates measures to relieve normal complaints of pregnancy ☐ No change in preterm labor risk factors ☐ ________	• Signs and symptoms of normal physical changes, complications • Behavioral risks • BP, weight • Urine dipstick for sugar/ ketone/protein • Fetal heart sounds • Fundal height • Pelvimetry ________	• Pap • GC • Chlamydia (if indicated) • Wet smear bacterial/ trich./vaginosis, vaginal ph and Whiff Test ________	
	RN Name				

	Date				
(1-14 Weeks)		☐ Demonstrates measures to relieve the normal complaints of pregnancy during 1st trimester ☐ Established exercise routine ☐ Exhibits minimum weight loss/gain ☐ 1st trimester test results within normal limits ☐ Avoids or demonstrates decrease in risk associated behavior (ie. smoking) ☐ No change in preterm labor risk factors ☐ Takes prenatal vitamins ☐ ____	• Signs and symptoms of normal physical changes, complications • Behavioral risks • BP, weight • Urine dipstick for sugar, ketone, protein • Fetal heart sounds • Fundal height ____		☐ Reinforce (STD-0011) (Prenatal Standard of Care) Importance of compliance ____
	RN Name				
(15-28 Weeks)		☐ Demonstrates measures to relieve the normal complaints of pregnancy during 2nd trimester. ☐ Exhibits normal weight gain. ☐ 2nd trimester test results within normal limits. ☐ Continues exercise routine. ☐ Avoids risk-associated behavior. ☐ Demonstrates self-palpation technique and verbalizes signs and symptoms of preterm labor. ☐ No change in preterm labor risk factors. ☐ ____	• Signs and symptoms of normal physical changes, complications including: • Behavioral risks • BP, weight • Urine dipstick for sugar/ketone/protein • Fetal heart sounds, fundal height • Fundal movement at 16-20 weeks • Premature labor ____	• Triple Screen (16 to 19 weeks) • Ultrasound, as needed • Fibronectin (24 to 26 weeks) ORDER AT 26 WEEKS: • Trutol • Antibody screen (Rh Neg) • Repeat WCBC • RhoGAM at 28 weeks, if indicated ____	☐ Fetal growth/development for 2nd tri. Encourage childbirth, baby care and postpartum classes Reinforce (STD-0011) (Prenatal Standard of Care) Review S and S of preterm labor at 24 week appointment Importance of compliance Home visit ____
	RN Name				
(29-42 Weeks)		☐ Demonstrates measures to relieve the normal complaints of pregnancy during 3rd trimester. ☐ Exhibits normal weight gain. ☐ Continues exercise routine. ☐ Normal physical changes of pregnancy w/o complications. ☐ Avoids risk-associated behaviors. ☐ Attends childbirth, baby care and postpartum classes ☐ Responds appropriately to signs and symptoms of preterm labor or other complications when indicated. ☐ Performing nipple preparation, if needed. ☐ No change in preterm labor risk factors. ☐ ____	• Signs and symptoms of normal physical changes, complications including: • Behavioral risks • BP, weight • Urine dipstick for sugar/ketone/protein • Fetal heart sounds, fundal height • Fetal movement • Planned method of infant feeding • Nipple exam, if planning to breast feed • Premature labor ____	• Ultrasound as needed ORDER AT 36 WEEKS: • Recto vaginal cultures for GBS Order at 41 Weeks: • NST and AFI Biweekly (amniotic fluid index) ____	☐ Fetal growth/development for 3rd trimester Review signs and symptoms and admission procedures for normal labor at 36 weeks. Reinforce (STD-0011) (Prenatal Standard of Care) Review S and S of preterm labor Importance of compliance Update perinatal risk assessment Childbirth education, babycare and postpartum classes Tubal forms, if indicated by 34 weeks Treatment for inverted nipples if indicated Home visit ____
	RN Name				

FIGURE 7-10 The prenatal clinical pathway identifies outcomes, assessments, interventions, and consultations performed during pregnancy. (Courtesy Women and Children Services of the York Health System, York, Pennsylvania. Modified with permission.)

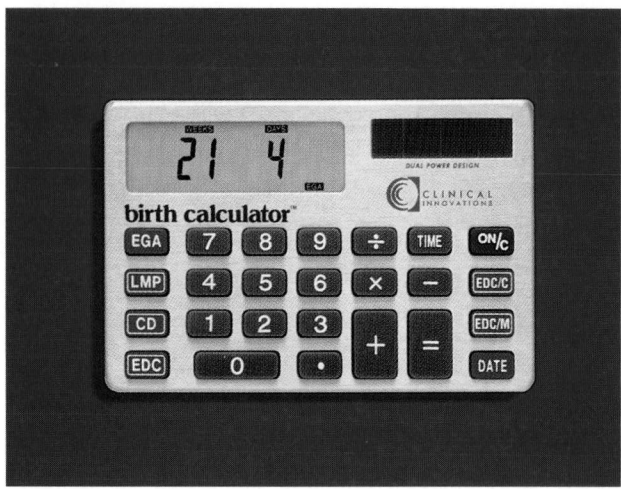

FIGURE 7-11 Electronic birth calculator used to compute the estimated due date, appointments, and specific tests. (Courtesy Clinical Innovations, Murray, Utah.)

1997). Newer methods include electronic calculators (Figure 7-11) that compute the EDD, gestational age, and future dates for procedures such as ultrasound examinations and Rh immunizations. These methods may be inaccurate in some situations. For example, Nagele's rule is less accurate when the woman's menstrual cycle is very irregular. Many woman have one or more ultrasounds during pregnancy. Ultrasound measurements taken early in pregnancy can more accurately determine the gestational age.

CRITICAL THINKING EXERCISE

Wilma Turner gave birth to twin girls at 38 weeks of gestation 3 years ago. She had a spontaneous abortion last year at 12 weeks of gestation and thinks she may be pregnant now because she has missed a menstrual period and is experiencing morning sickness. Wilma's last normal menstrual period began June 22.

QUESTIONS:

1. If Wilma is pregnant now, what would be the gravida and para?
2. Explain to Wilma the reasons that amenorrhea and morning sickness are not positive indications of pregnancy.
3. Use Nagele's rule to compute the EDD.

Contraceptive History. Some forms of contraception may impose a risk on the fetus, mother, or both. Therefore a detailed history of contraceptive methods is needed. Very recent use of oral contraceptives before pregnancy or continued use during early unrecognized pregnancy remains a source of concern because of the effect of estrogens and some synthetic progestins on the sexual organs of the fetus (Briggs, et al., 1998). Some physicians advise women in preconception counseling to stop oral contraception and use alternative contraceptive methods (such as condoms, diaphragm) for 3 months before conceiving.

Intrauterine devices, which are not widely used in the United States, can cause complications. If pregnancy occurs with an intrauterine device in place, abortion, premature delivery, and puncture of the uterus are serious risks.

Medical and Surgical History. Chronic conditions such as diabetes mellitus, hypertension, and renal disease can affect the outcome of the pregnancy and must be investigated. Infections, surgical procedures, and trauma that may complicate the pregnancy or childbirth should be documented. The history should include the following:

- Age, race, and ethnic background (relevant for groups at high risk for specific genetic problems such as sickle cell anemia, thalassemia, and Tay-Sachs disease)
- Childhood diseases and immunizations
- Chronic illnesses such as asthma and heart disease (onset and treatment)
- Previous illnesses, surgical procedures, and injuries (particularly of the pelvis and back)
- Previous infections such as hepatitis, sexually transmissible diseases, tuberculosis, and presence of group B streptococcus
- History of and treatment for anemia
- Medications such as prescription or over-the-counter drugs and reasons for use
- Bladder and bowel function (problems or changes)
- Amount of caffeine consumed each day (such as coffee, tea, chocolate, soft drinks)
- Tobacco use (number of years and number of packs per day)
- Use of drugs (name, amount, date, and time of last use)
- Overall health and energy
- Appetite, general nutrition, and history of eating disorders
- Contact with domestic pets, particularly cats, which increases the risk of infections such as toxoplasmosis
- Allergies and drug sensitivities
- Occupation and related risk factors

Family History. A family history provides valuable information about the general health of the family, including chronic diseases such as diabetes and heart disease and infections such as tuberculosis and hepatitis. In addition, it may reveal information about patterns of genetic or congenital anomalies.

Partner's Health History. The partner's history helps determine whether the father of the expected child or his family has a history of significant health problems such as genetic abnormalities, chronic diseases, and infections. Use of drugs such as cocaine and alcohol may affect the ability of the family to cope with pregnancy and childbirth. Tobacco use by the father is of concern because both the mother and the infant are at risk for upper respiratory complications as a result of passive smoking.

In addition, the blood type and Rh factor of the father are important if the mother is Rh negative and if blood incompatibility between the mother and fetus is possible.

Psychosocial History. The psychosocial history should be completed during the initial visit (see Chapter 8).

Physical Examination

Because many women have never had a complete physical examination, a thorough evaluation of all body systems is necessary to detect previously undiagnosed physical problems that may affect the pregnancy outcome. A complete examination also allows the examiner to establish baseline levels that will guide the treatment of the expectant mother and fetus throughout pregnancy.

Vital Signs

Blood Pressure. The method for obtaining blood pressure should be as standardized as possible because position affects blood pressure in the pregnant woman. Blood pressure should be obtained in the sitting position with the arm supported in a horizontal position at heart level. Documentation should include the position, arm used, and pressures obtained. Ideally, documentation also should indicate whether Korotkoff's fourth phase (muffling) or fifth phase (disappearance of sound) is used because pressures are 5 to 10 mm Hg higher if the fourth phase is used.

Pulse. The normal pulse rate is 60 to 90 BPM. Tachycardia is associated with anxiety, hyperthyroidism, and infection and should be investigated. Apical pulse should be assessed for at least 1 minute to determine the amplitude and regularity of the heartbeat. Pedal pulses are assessed to determine the presence of circulatory problems in the legs. Pedal pulses should be strong, equal, and regular.

Respiratory Effort. Respiratory rate during pregnancy is in the range of 16 to 24 BPM. Tachypnea may indicate respiratory infection or cardiac disease. Breath sounds should be equal bilaterally, chest expansion should be symmetric, and lung fields should be free of all abnormal breath sounds.

Temperature. Normal temperature during pregnancy is 36.2° C to 37.6° C (98° F to 99.6° F). Increased temperature suggests infection and may require medical management.

Cardiovascular System

Venous Congestion. Additional assessment of the cardiovascular system includes observation for venous congestion, which can develop into varicosities. Venous congestion is most commonly noted in the legs, vulva, and rectum.

Edema. Edema of the legs may be a benign condition that reflects pooling of blood in the extremities, which results in a shift of intravascular fluid into interstitial spaces. When pressure exerted by a finger or thumb leaves a persistent depression, it is termed *pitting edema* (see Figure 17-9). Edema of the hands or face necessitates further assessment for signs of pregnancy-induced hypertension.

Musculoskeletal System

Posture and Gait. Body mechanics and changes in posture and gait should be addressed. Body mechanics during pregnancy may produce strain on the muscles of the lower back and legs.

Height and Weight. An initial weight is needed to establish a baseline for weight gain throughout pregnancy. Weight should be compared with the ideal weight-for-height chart to determine whether the expectant mother is at her target weight. Preconception weight lower than 45 kg (100 lb) or height under 150 cm (60 in) is associated with preterm labor and low-birth-weight infants. Preconception weight higher than 90 kg (200 lb) is associated with increased incidence of gestational diabetes, pregnancy-induced hypertension, neural tube defects, cesarean birth, and postpartum infection (Morin, 1998). Recommendations for weight gain during pregnancy are often made based on the woman's body mass index (see Chapter 9).

Pelvic Measurements. The bony pelvis is evaluated early in the pregnancy to determine whether the diameters are adequate to permit vaginal delivery (see Chapter 12).

Abdomen. The contour, size, and muscle tone of the abdomen should be assessed. Fundal height should be measured if the fundus is palpable above the symphysis pubis. The bladder must be empty before the measurement is taken to ensure accuracy. The MacDonald method of measurement involves the woman lying on her back with her knees slightly flexed. The top of the fundus is palpated, and a tape is stretched from the top of the symphysis pubis over the abdominal curve to the top of the fundus (Figure 7-12).

From 22 weeks to term, the fundal height, which is measured in centimeters, is roughly equal (± 2 cm) to the gestational age of the fetus in weeks (Hobel, 1998). If fundal height exceeds weeks of gestation, additional assessment is necessary to investigate the cause for the unexpected uterine size. For example, more than one fetus may be present, or the EDD may be incorrect and the pregnancy is further advanced than previously thought.

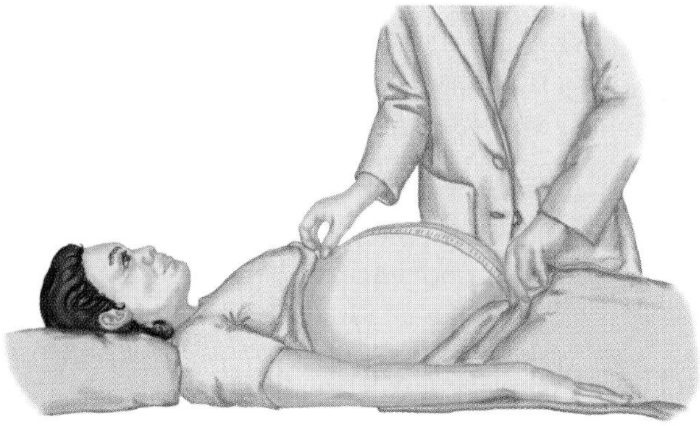

FIGURE 7-12 Uterine measurements include the distance between the upper border of the symphysis pubis and the top of the fundus.

If fundal height is less than expected on the basis of gestational age, the EDD must be confirmed. If dates are accurate, further assessment may be necessary to determine whether the fetus is experiencing inadequate growth.

Fetal heart rate should be counted and documented if the pregnancy is advanced enough to hear fetal heart tones.

Neurologic System

A complete neurologic assessment is not necessary for young women who are free of signs or symptoms indicating a problem. However, deep tendon reflexes should be evaluated because hyperreflexia is associated with complications of pregnancy. (See Procedure 25-1 for assessment of deep tendon reflexes.)

Integumentary System

Skin color should be consistent with racial background. Pallor may indicate anemia. Jaundice may indicate hepatic disease. Lesions, bruising, rashes, areas of hyperpigmentation (such as chloasma, linea nigra) related to pregnancy, and stretch marks (striae) should be noted. Nail beds should be pink with instant capillary return.

Endocrine System

The thyroid enlarges slightly during the second trimester. However, gross enlargement or tenderness may indicate hyperthyroidism and requires further medical evaluation.

Gastrointestinal System

Mouth. Mucous membranes should be pink, smooth, glistening, and uniform. The lips should be free of ulcerations. The gums may be red, tender, and edematous as a result of the effects of increased estrogen, which produces hyperplasia. The teeth should be in good repair. The woman should be referred for regular dental care because periodontal disease may result in infections that precipitate preterm labor. The second trimester may be the most comfortable time for dental care.

Intestine. A warm stethoscope for assessing bowel sounds is most comfortable for the pregnant woman. Bowel sounds may be diminished because of the effects of progesterone on smooth muscle. The examination is an excellent time for the examiner to ask about problems with constipation. Bowel sounds are often increased if a meal is overdue or diarrhea is present.

Urinary System

Urine collected for testing should always be a clean-catch midstream sample. Urine is tested to detect signs of urinary tract infection and substances in the urine that may indicate a problem.

Protein. Protein should not be present in urine. Its presence may indicate contamination by vaginal secretions, kidney disease, or pregnancy-induced hypertension.

Glucose. Small amounts of glucose may indicate physiologic "spilling" that occurs during normal pregnancy. Larger amounts require glucose screening of the blood.

Ketones. Ketones may be found in the urine after heavy exercise or as a result of inadequate intake of food and fluid.

Bacteria. Increased bacteria in the urine is associated with urinary tract infection, which is common during pregnancy.

Reproductive System

Breasts. Breast size, symmetry, condition of nipples, and presence of colostrum should be noted. Any lumps, dimpling of the skin, or asymmetry of the nipples requires further evaluation.

External Reproductive Organs. The skin and mucous membranes of the perineum, vulva, and anus are inspected for excoriations, growths, ulcerations, lesions, varicosities, warts, chancres, and perineal scars. Enlargement, tenderness, redness, or discharge of Bartholin's glands or Skene's glands may indicate gonorrheal or chlamydial infection. The examiner should obtain a specimen for culture of any discharge from lesions or inflamed glands to determine the causative organisms and provide effective care.

Internal Reproductive Organs. A speculum inserted into the vagina permits the examiner to view the walls of the vagina and the cervix. The cervix should be pink in a nonpregnant woman and bluish in a pregnant woman (Chadwick's sign). The external cervical os is closed in primigravidas, but one fingertip may be admitted in multiparas. The cervix feels relatively firm except during pregnancy, when marked softening is

Table 7-4
COMMON LABORATORY TESTS

Test	Purpose	Significance
Blood grouping	To determine blood type	Mother may need blood replacement
Hemoglobin (Hgb) or hematocrit (Hct)	To detect anemia	Requires iron supplementation if Hgb <10.5 g/dl or Hct <32%
Complete blood count (CBC)	To detect infection or cell abnormalities	Requires follow-up if 15,000/mm³ or more white blood cells or decreased platelets
Rh factor and antibody screen	To test for possible maternal-fetal blood incompatibility	Requires additional testing and treatment if the mother is Rh-negative and the father is Rh-positive or if antibodies are present
Venereal Disease Research Laboratory (VDRL) test or rapid plasma reagin (RPR)	To screen for syphilis	Requires treatment if positive, requires retest at 36 weeks' gestation
Rubella titer	To determine immunity	Is not immune if titer of 1:8 or less, requires retest during pregnancy, requires immunization postpartum if mother not immune
Skin test	To screen for tuberculosis	Requires referral for additional testing or therapy if mother tests positive
Hemoglobin electrophoresis	To screen for sickle cell trait in African-American clients	Requires checking the positive-testing mother's partner; the infant is at risk only if both parents are positive
Hepatitis B screen	To detect presence of antigens in maternal blood	If present, requires administration of hepatitis immune globulin and vaccine to infant soon after birth
Human immunodeficiency virus (HIV) screen	To detect HIV antibodies (a voluntary test encouraged at the first visit)	If positive, requires retesting, counseling, and treatment during pregnancy to greatly lower infant infection
Urinalysis	To detect infection, renal disease, and diabetes	Requires further assessment if test shows protein (renal damage, pregnancy-induced hypertension), ketones (fasting), or bacteria (infection)
Papanicolaou (Pap) test	To screen for cervical neoplasia	Requires treatment and referral if abnormal cells are present
Cervical culture	To detect group B streptococci and sexually transmissible diseases	Requires treatment and retesting as necessary, requires administration of antibiotics during labor
Maternal serum alpha-fetoprotein Triple screen	To screen for fetal anomalies	Requires investigation of high (neural tube defects) or low (Down syndrome) levels
Maternal blood glucose	To screen for gestational diabetes	Requires recommendation of a 3-hour glucose tolerance test if levels are elevated

noted (Goodell's sign). Routine cervical cultures for gonorrhea and chlamydial infection are standard practice during initial pregnancy examination at most agencies. The examiner also collects a specimen for a Papanicolaou (Pap) smear, a screening test for cervical cancer.

A bimanual examination involves the use of both hands to palpate the internal genitalia. The examiner palpates the uterus for size, contour, tenderness, and position. The uterus should be movable between the two examining hands and should feel smooth. The ovaries, if palpable, should be about the shape and size of almonds and not tender.

Laboratory Data

Table 7-4 lists laboratory examinations commonly performed during pregnancy and the purpose and significance of each test.

Check Your Reading

20. Why is a medical-surgical history and an obstetric history necessary?
21. How should blood pressure be obtained and documented? Why is documentation of the position of the woman during blood pressure readings important during pregnancy?
22. How does fundal height relate to gestational age?

Risk Assessment

Risk assessment begins at the initial visit when the health care team identifies factors that put the expectant mother or fetus at risk for complications and thus require specialized care (Table 7-5). Because not all factors present equal threats, many agencies use a risk-

Table 7-5
HIGH-RISK FACTORS IN PREGNANCY

Factors	Implications
DEMOGRAPHIC FACTORS	
<16 years or >35 years	Increased risk for preterm labor, pregnancy-induced hypertension, and congenital anomalies
Low socioeconomic status or dependence on public assistance	Increased risk for preterm labor and low-birth-weight infants
Nonwhite race	Doubled incidence of infant and maternal death compared with whites
Multiparity (>4 pregnancies)	Increased risk of pregnancy loss, antepartum or postpartum hemorrhage, and cesarean birth
SOCIAL-PERSONAL FACTORS	
Weight <45 kg (100 lb)	Association with low-birth-weight infant
Weight >90 kg (200 lb)	Increased risk for pregnancy-induced hypertension, difficult labor, large-for-gestational-age infant, and cesarean birth
Height <154 cm (5 feet)	Increased incidence of cesarean birth resulting from cephalopelvic disproportion
Smoking	Increased risk for preterm birth and low birth weight
Use of alcohol or addicting drugs	Increased risk of congenital anomalies, neonatal withdrawal syndrome, and fetal alcohol syndrome
OBSTETRIC FACTORS	
Birth of previous infant >4000 g (8.5 lb)	Increased need for cesarean birth; increased risk for infant birth injury, neonatal hypoglycemia, and maternal gestational diabetes
Previous stillborn infant	Maternal psychological distress
Rh sensitization	Fetal anemia, erythroblastosis fetalis, and kernicterus
EXISTING MEDICAL CONDITIONS	
Diabetes mellitus	Increased risk of pregnancy-induced hypertension, cesarean birth, small or large infant for gestational age, neonatal hypoglycemia, fetal or neonatal death; increased incidence of congenital anomalies
Thyroid disorder	
Hypothyroidism	Increased incidence of spontaneous abortion, congenital anomalies, and congenital hypothyroidism
Hyperthyroidism	Maternal risk of pregnancy-induced hypertension, thyroid storm, or postpartum hemorrhage; neonatal risk of thyrotoxicosis
Cardiac disease	Maternal risk for cardiac decompensation and increased death rate; increased risk for fetal and neonatal death
Renal disease	Maternal risk for renal failure and preterm delivery; fetal risk for intrauterine growth retardation
Concurrent infections	Severe fetal implications (e.g., heart disease, blindness, deafness, bone lesions) if maternal disease in the first trimester; increased incidence of spontaneous abortion or congenital anomalies associated with some infections

scoring tool to determine degree of risk. Although risk scoring is a valuable method for identifying the high-risk pregnancy, it cannot be relied on to predict problems or the absence of complications every time.

Many women identified as high risk give birth to healthy term infants. Furthermore, risk factors change as pregnancy progresses, and risk assessment must be updated throughout pregnancy. Gestations categorized as low risk at the initial assessment may later become high risk.

Subsequent Assessments

Ongoing antepartum care is important to the successful outcome of pregnancy. The recommended schedule for prenatal assessment in an uncomplicated pregnancy is as follows:

Conception to 28 weeks—every 4 weeks
29 to 36 weeks—every 2 to 3 weeks
37 weeks to birth—weekly

Vital Signs. Deviations from the baseline value in blood pressure, pulse, or respiratory rate indicate the need for further assessment. Temperature should remain within normal limits.

Weight. Weight should be plotted to document the occurrence of the expected pattern of weight gain.

Inadequate weight gain may signify that the pregnancy is not as advanced as was initially thought or the fetus is not growing as expected. Sudden, rapid weight gain may indicate fluid retention and the need for further assessment for pregnancy-induced hypertension (see Chapter 9).

Urinalysis. Urine is tested at each visit for the presence of protein, glucose, and ketones. A screen for bacteria may be repeated at 26 to 30 weeks' if the woman has a history or symptoms of urinary tract infection. The urine may be checked for nitrites with a dipstick. If the urine is positive for nitrites, infection may be present and a urine culture performed.

Glucose Screen. The blood glucose level is screened between 24 and 28 weeks of gestation using a 50-g glucose load followed by a 1-hour plasma glucose determination. If the result is 140 mg/dl or higher, additional testing with a glucose tolerance test is needed. The woman receives a 3-hour, 100-g glucose tolerance test to determine whether she has gestational diabetes (Dickerson & Chez, 1999).

Fundal Height. Measuring fundal height is an inexpensive and noninvasive method of evaluating fetal growth and confirming gestational age.

Leopold's Maneuvers. Leopold's maneuvers provide a systematic method for palpating the fetus through the abdominal wall during the later part of pregnancy. These maneuvers provide valuable information about location and presentation of the fetus (see Chapter 13).

Fetal Heart Rate. The fetal heart rate may be heard with a Doppler transducer in early pregnancy or with a fetoscope in later pregnancy (see Figure 14-1). The location of the fetal heart sounds provides information that may help determine the position in which the fetus is entering the pelvis. For instance, fetal heart tones heard in an upper quadrant of the abdomen suggest that the fetus is in a breech presentation.

Fetal Activity. Fetal movements (quickening) are first noticed by the expectant mother at 16 to 20 weeks of gestation and gradually increase in frequency and strength. In the last trimester the woman may be asked to count fetal body movements, commonly called *kick counts,* using various methods. In general, fetal activity indicates a physically healthy fetus. Therefore fetal activity is a reassuring sign.

Pelvic Examination. During the last month of pregnancy the physician or midwife may perform a pelvic examination to determine cervical changes. The descent of the fetus and the presenting part can also be assessed at this time.

Multifetal Pregnancy

A *multifetal pregnancy* may be defined as any pregnancy in which two or more embryos or fetuses exist simultaneously (see Chapter 6).

Diagnosis

Maternal symptoms of multifetal pregnancy include the woman's sensations of feeling larger than with previous pregnancies and excessive fetal movements. Excessive weight gain and rapid uterine growth also increase the suspicion that more than one fetus is present. Fundal height is often 4 cm larger than expected on the basis of gestational age computed from the last menstrual period (see Figure 7-12).

Maternal history may be helpful in making the diagnosis. A maternal family history that includes nonidentical twins slightly increases the chance of twins. The older mother is also more likely to have nonidentical twins. Recent administration of fertility drugs such as clomiphene greatly increases the chance of multifetal pregnancy.

When more than one fetus is suspected, diagnosis should be confirmed by sonography. Separate gestational sacs may be seen as early as 6 weeks of gestation. Multiple fetal parts may be visible by the tenth week.

Maternal Adaptation to Multifetal Pregnancy

The degree of maternal physiologic change is greater with multiple fetuses than with a single fetus. For instance, blood volume increases 500 ml more than the amount needed for a single fetus. This increase heightens the workload of the heart and may contribute to fatigue and activity intolerance. The additional size of the uterus intensifies the mechanical effects of pregnancy. The uterus may achieve a volume of 10 L or more and weigh more than 20 lb (Cunningham, et al., 1997). The weight increases respiratory difficulty because the overdistended uterus causes greater elevation of the diaphragm.

The uterus may also cause more compression of the large vessels, resulting in more pronounced and earlier supine hypotension. Greater compression of the ureters can occur, and maternal edema and proteinuria are common. Compression of the bowel makes constipation a persistent problem.

Antepartum Care in Multifetal Pregnancy

Early diagnosis of multifetal pregnancy allows time for the family to be educated about the many ways in which the pregnancy will differ from those involving a single fetus. Special antepartum classes can explain the need for increased nutrition, rest, and fetal monitoring. Instruction about signs of preterm labor, a common complication, should begin early. Discussions of the possible need to reduce activity and the potential family stress caused by a high-risk pregnancy should also be included.

Women with multifetal pregnancies have more frequent antepartum visits to allow early detection of common complications such as anemia, hypertension, premature labor, and congenital anomalies. Visits may be scheduled biweekly at 20 weeks of gestation and weekly at 24 weeks.

Diet also must be considered. The need for calories, iron, vitamins, and folic acid is higher than for single-fetus pregnancies. The Institute of Medicine has recommended that the target weight gain at term for women carrying twins should be 16 to 20.5 kg (35 to 45 lb).

Check Your Reading

23. What are major risk factors during pregnancy?
24. What is the recommended schedule for subsequent antepartum visits?
25. How does maternal adaptation differ in multifetal pregnancies?

Common Discomforts of Pregnancy

Many women experience discomforts of pregnancy that are not serious but detract from the woman's feeling of comfort and well-being. (Measures to help relieve these discomforts are discussed in "Women Want to Know: How to Overcome the Common Discomforts of Pregnancy.")

Nausea and Vomiting

The nausea and vomiting of pregnancy is frequently called *morning sickness* because these symptoms are more acute on arising. However, they may occur at any time and continue throughout the day. Morning sickness occurs in more than 50% of pregnant women in Western societies (Kronenberg, Murphy, & Wade, 1999). Women need reassurance that nausea and vomiting is common and that the condition is temporary. Morning sickness must be distinguished from hyperemesis gravidarum, a severe state of vomiting accompanied by weight loss, dehydration, electrolyte imbalance, and ketosis (see Chapter 25).

Although the cause of nausea and vomiting is unknown, these symptoms are believed to be related to increased levels of hCG and estrogen, as well as periodic hypoglycemia. Symptoms may be aggravated by odors (such as from cooking) and fatigue. Emotional factors may also be implicated. Women under emotional stress are more likely to experience nausea.

Nausea usually ends by the second trimester, but some women experience it longer. Severity of vomiting may be related to its duration throughout the pregnancy (Zhou, O'Brien, & Relyea, 1999). Nausea and vomiting that interferes with the woman's intake of nutrients may decrease nutrients available to the fetus. Various alternative therapies are available for the relief of nausea.

WOMEN WANT TO KNOW *How to Overcome the Common Discomforts of Pregnancy*

Nausea and Vomiting

- Eat dry crackers or toast before arising in the morning and then get out of bed slowly.
- Eat dry crackers every 2 hours to prevent an empty stomach, or eat five or six small meals per day rather than three full meals.
- Take fluids separately from meals.
- Avoid fried, greasy, or spicy foods and foods with strong odors such as onion and cabbage.
- Experiment with different foods that may be helpful, such as ginger, peppermint, or tart and salty combinations.

Heartburn

- Eat several small meals daily and avoid fatty foods.
- Curtail smoking and coffee drinking, which stimulate acid formation in the stomach.
- Sit upright to reduce reflux and relieve symptoms. Do not lie down for at least 1 hour after eating.
- Avoid eating or drinking at bedtime and sleep with an extra pillow under the head and shoulders.
- Try deep breathing and sipping water to help relieve the burning sensation.
- Use antacids but avoid those that are high in sodium (such as AlkaSeltzer, baking soda) because excessive sodium may result in fluid retention and electrolyte imbalance. Antacids high in calcium (such as Tums, Alkamints) provide relief but may cause rebound hyperacidity.

Backache

- Maintain correct posture with the head up and the shoulders back.
- When picking up objects, squat rather than bend from the waist.
- When sitting, use foot supports, arm rests, and pillows behind the back.
- Exercise: Tailor sitting, shoulder circling, and pelvic rocking strengthen the back and help prepare for labor.

Round Ligament Pain

- Use good body mechanics and avoid very strenuous exercise.
- Avoid stretching and twisting at the same time. When getting out of bed, first turn on the side and then arise.
- Bend toward the pain, squat, or bring the knees up to the chest to relieve pain by relaxing the ligament.

Urinary Frequency

Performing Kegel's exercises helps maintain bladder control:

- Identify the muscles to be exercised when stopping the flow of urine midstream. However, do not perform the exercise while urinating because urinary retention increases the risk of urinary tract infection.
- Contract the muscles around the vagina and hold for 10 seconds. Relax for at least 10 seconds.
- Repeat the contraction-relaxation cycle 30 times each day.

Varicosities

The key to treatment is to prevent pooling of blood in the large veins of the legs:

- Avoid constricting clothing. Refrain from crossing the legs at the knees because this position impedes blood return from the legs.
- Take frequent rest periods with the legs elevated above the level of the hips.
- Wear support hose or elastic stockings that reach above the varicosities, and apply them before getting out of bed each morning. Putting them on later makes them less effective because pooling begins on rising.
- If working in one position for prolonged periods is necessary, walk around for a few minutes at least every 2 hours. This stimulates blood flow and relieves discomfort.

Hemorrhoids

- To prevent hemorrhoids, try to establish a regular pattern of bowel elimination that does not require straining. Drink plenty of water, eat foods rich in fiber, and exercise regularly.
- To relieve existing hemorrhoids, take frequent, tepid baths. Apply cool witch hazel compresses or anesthetic ointments. Use a side-lying position with the hips elevated on a pillow.
- Gently push the hemorrhoids back into the rectum. To do so, put on a latex glove and lubricate the index finger. Maintain pressure for 1 to 2 minutes.
- If pain or bleeding persists, call the physician or midwife.

Constipation

Self-care measures generally are as effective as laxatives, but they are most beneficial because they do not interfere with absorption of nutrients or lead to laxative dependency:

- Drink at least eight glasses of water each day. These should not include coffee, tea, or carbonated drinks because of their diuretic effect. After drinking one of these beverages, drink a glass of water to counteract its diuretic effect.
- Additional fiber in the diet helps maintain bowel elimination. Foods high in fiber include unpeeled fresh fruits and vegetables, whole-grain cereals, bran muffins, oatmeal, baked potatoes with skins, and fruit juices. Four pieces of fruit and a large salad provide enough fiber requirements for 1 day.
- Restrict cheese consumption, which causes constipation.
- Curtail the intake of sweets, which increases bacterial growth in the intestine and can lead to flatulence.
- Do not discontinue taking iron supplements if they have been prescribed. If constipation persists, consult the health care provider for advice about bulk-forming laxatives or fecal wetting agents.
- A brisk walk of at least 1 mile per day is one of the best exercises to stimulate peristalsis and improve muscle tone. Swimming and riding a stationary bicycle also are helpful.
- Establish a regular pattern by allowing a consistent time each day for elimination. One hour after meals is ideal to take advantage of the gastrocolic reflex (the peristaltic wave in the colon that is induced by taking food into the fasting stomach). Using a footrest during elimination provides comfort and decreases straining.

Leg Cramps

- To prevent cramps, elevate the legs frequently during the day to improve circulation.
- To relieve cramps, extend the affected leg, keeping the knee straight. Bend the foot toward the body, or ask someone to assist. Stand and apply pressure on the affected leg. Either measure lengthens the affected muscles and relieves cramping.
- Avoid unnecessary foods high in phosphorus, such as soft drinks. Restricting milk intake and taking supplemental calcium or taking magnesium may provide relief, but these measures should be initiated only with advice of the physician or nurse-midwife.

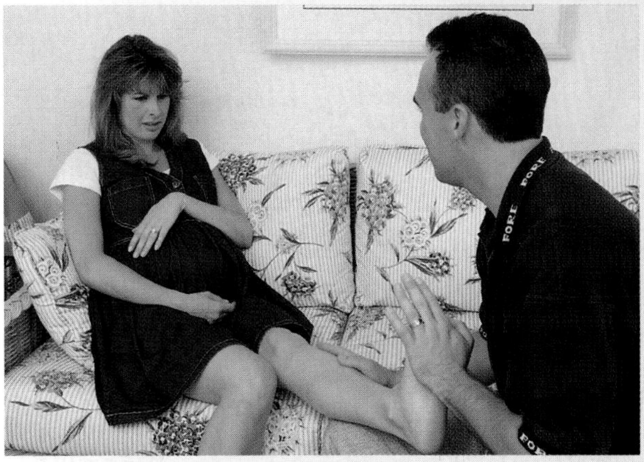

A 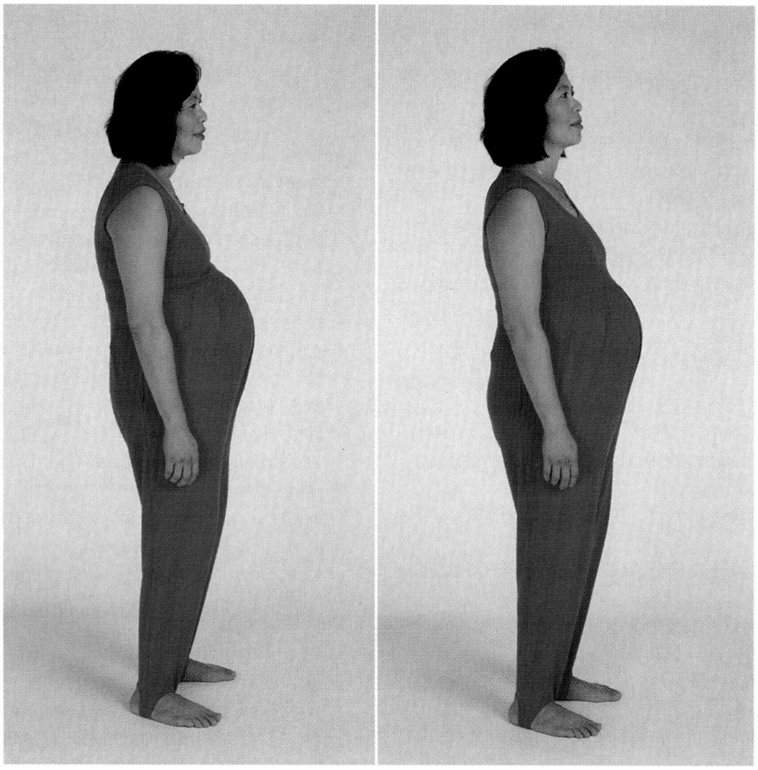 B

FIGURE 7-13 Posture during pregnancy may cause or alleviate backache. **A,** Incorrect posture. The neck is jutting forward, the shoulders are slumping, and the back is sharply curved, creating back pain and discomfort. **B,** Correct posture. The neck and shoulders are straight, the back is flattened, and the pelvis is tucked under and slightly upward.

A 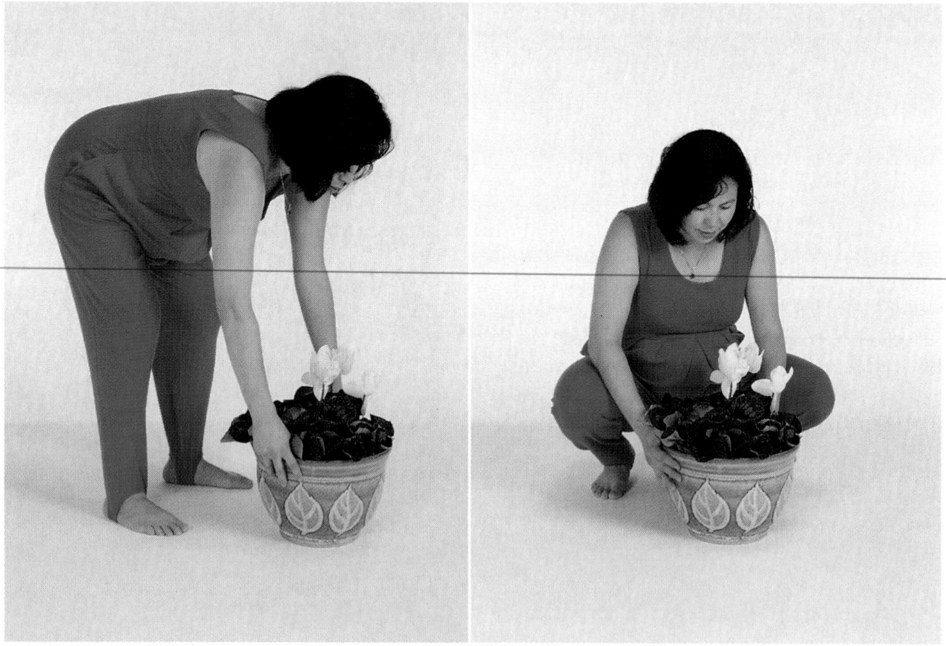 B

FIGURE 7-14 Techniques for lifting. Squatting places less strain on the back. **A,** Incorrect technique. Stooping or bending places a great deal of strain on muscles of the lower body. **B,** Correct technique. Squatting and moving the object close permits the stronger muscles of the legs to do the lifting.

Complementary/Alternative Therapy

Nausea in Pregnancy

Acupressure over the Neiguan acupuncture point (approximately three fingerwidths above the wrist crease on the inner arm)—Devices that apply an electrical impulse over this point available by prescription; devices that apply pressure alone available over the counter.
Combinations of salty and tart foods such as potato chips and lemonade or green apples
Peppermint (tea or candy)
Ginger (tea, cookies, soda, capsules)
Vitamin B_6 (pyridoxine)—Dosage to be checked with the primary caregiver

Heartburn

Heartburn is an acute burning sensation in the epigastric and sternal regions. It may be associated with other gastrointestinal symptoms such as frequent belching, nausea, and epigastric pressure.

Heartburn occurs when reverse peristaltic waves cause regurgitation of acidic stomach contents into the esophagus. The underlying causes are diminished gastric motility and displacement of the stomach by the enlarging uterus. Improper diet and nervous tension may be precipitating factors.

Backache

Backache is a common complaint during the third trimester. Prevention of backache with correct posture and body mechanics is a primary focus (Figure 7-13). Stooping or bending puts a great deal of strain on the muscles of the lower back. Instruction should include correct and incorrect methods for lifting (Figure 7-14) and exercises to relax the shoulders and thighs and help prevent backache (Figure 7-15).

Round Ligament Pain

Round ligament pain is a sharp pain in the side or inguinal area, usually on the right side, that occurs because of softening and stretching of the ligament from hormones and uterine growth. The right round ligament is stretched more than the left because the uterus turns slightly to the right during pregnancy. The woman should be instructed to apply heat and lie on her right side to help relieve the pain.

Urinary Frequency

Although urinary frequency is a common complaint of women during the first trimester and near term, the condition is temporary and is managed by most women without undue distress. Kegel exercises are sometimes recommended to help maintain bladder control.

Varicosities

Varicosities are usually confined to the legs but may involve the veins of the vulva or rectum (hemorrhoids). Varicosities most often occur in women with a family history of varicose veins and are more likely to be a problem for obese women and multiparas. Symptoms depend on the degree of engorgement and range from barely noticeable blemishes with minimal discomfort at the end of the day to large, tortuous veins that produce severe discomfort with any activity.

Varicosities are common in pregnancy because the weight of the uterus partially compresses the veins returning blood from the legs. As blood pools, the vessels dilate and the valves in the veins become stretched and incompetent. This process results in even more pooling, and in time the veins may become engorged, inflamed, and painful. Varicose veins are exacerbated by prolonged standing, during which the force of gravity makes blood return more difficult.

Hemorrhoids. Hemorrhoids are varicosities of the rectum and may be external (outside the anal sphincter) or internal (above the sphincter). Some common causes of hemorrhoids are vascular engorgement of the pelvis, constipation, straining at stool, and a prolonged sitting or standing position. The pushing that occurs during the second stage of labor exacerbates the problem, which may continue into the postpartum period.

Constipation

Occasional constipation is not harmful, although it can cause feelings of abdominal fullness and flatulence and aggravate painful hemorrhoids. Intestinal motility is reduced during pregnancy as a result of progesterone, which benefits the expectant mother and the fetus by allowing additional time for nutrient absorption. It also allows more time for water absorption from the large intestine, which can result in hard, dry stools and decreased frequency of bowel movements. Iron supplementation often increases constipation.

Leg Cramps

Painful contractions of the muscles of the lower legs occur most often during sleep when the muscles are relaxed. Cramps are also likely to occur when the woman stretches and extends her feet. Leg cramps may be caused by an imbalance of serum calcium and phosphorus, but this has not been proved. Low magnesium levels may also be a cause (Fagen, 2000). A 1:1 ratio of calcium to phosphorus is desirable but difficult to achieve during pregnancy when many women consume large amounts of dairy products that are high in calcium. Venous congestion in the legs during the third trimester also contributes to leg cramps.

Shoulder circling

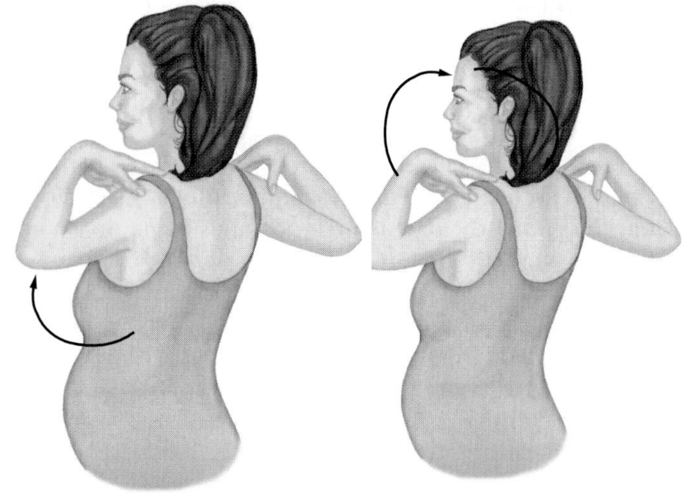

The fingertips are placed on the shoulders, then the elbows are brought forward and up during inhalation, back and down during exhalation. Repeat five times.

Tailor sitting

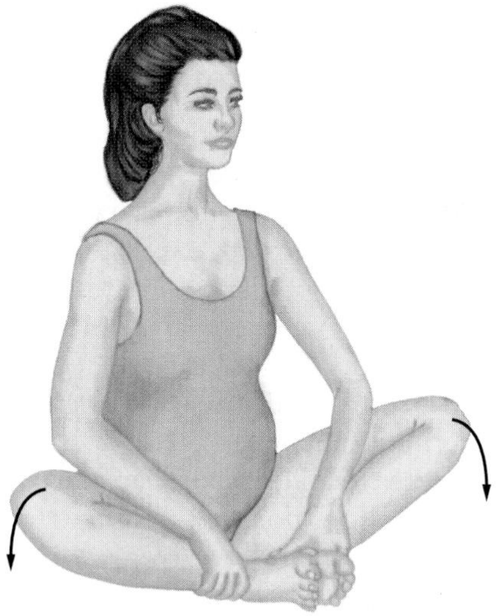

The woman uses her thigh muscles to press her knees to the floor. Keeping her back straight, she should remain in the position for 5 to 15 minutes.

Pelvic tilt or pelvic rocking

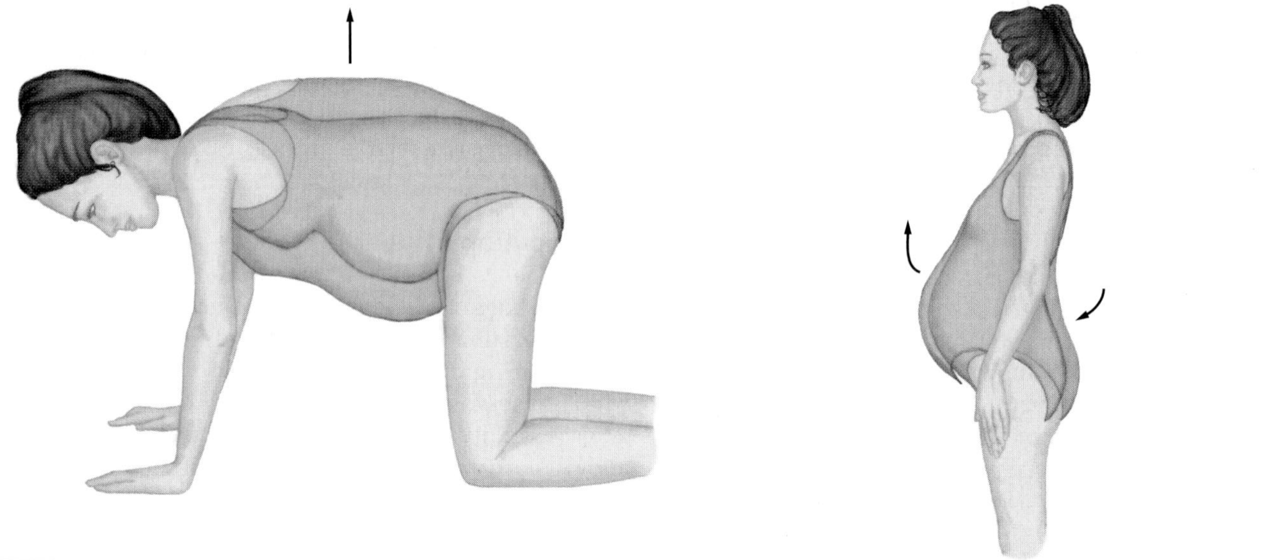

This exercise can be performed on hands and knees, with the hands directly under the shoulders and the knees under the hips. The back should be in a neutral position, not hollowed. The head and neck should be aligned with the straight back. The woman then presses up with the lower back and holds this position for a few seconds, then relaxes to a neutral position. Repeat 5 times. The exercise may also be performed in a standing position when the pelvis is rotated forward to flatten the lower back.

FIGURE 7-15 Exercises to prevent backache.

Cultural Considerations

Although the physical changes of pregnancy are fairly universal, culture often determines the health beliefs, values, and expectations of the family when a woman becomes pregnant (see Chapter 8).

Check Your Reading

26. What causes morning sickness?
27. How can backache be alleviated during pregnancy?

APPLICATION OF THE NURSING PROCESS: FAMILY RESPONSES TO PHYSICAL CHANGES OF PREGNANCY

The nursing process focuses on identifying each family's unique responses to the physiologic changes of pregnancy, determining factors that might interfere with the ability to adapt to changes that occur, and finding solutions to problems that are identified.

Assessment

Assess the family's responses to the physiologic processes of pregnancy and explore the family's preparation for the birth. Use structured interviews and planned teaching sessions, as well as more informal discussions that occur spontaneously during the initial or subsequent assessments. Review the history and physical examination to obtain important data. Information may come from not only the expectant mother but also the spouse and other significant family members.

Analysis

When analyzing data, nurses must use all their critical thinking skills before coming to a conclusion about the most significant nursing diagnoses (Table 7-6). One of the most common errors is an unexamined assumption. Nurses may assume that all families experience the same concerns during pregnancy. Such an assumption may lead to diagnoses that are irrelevant to the actual problems of a specific family.

In maternal-newborn nursing the nursing process must be adapted to a generally healthy population experiencing a life event that holds the possibility for growth and problems. Unlike medical-surgical nursing, much maternal-newborn nursing activity is devoted to assessing, diagnosing, and promoting family strengths and healthy functioning (see Nursing Care Plans 7-1 and 7-2).

Many problem-oriented nursing diagnoses do not address the healthy family preparing for the birth of a child. Most families express an intense desire to protect the health of the unborn child and well-being of the mother. Perhaps the most encompassing nursing diagnosis for the prenatal period is "Health-Seeking Behaviors: prenatal care and health practices that provide optimal benefit to the fetus and mother."

Table 7-6

COMMON NURSING DIAGNOSES
Activity Intolerance
Altered Family Processes
Altered Health Maintenance
Altered Sexuality Patterns
Constipation
Diversional Activity Deficit
* Fatigue
Fluid Volume Deficit
* Health-Seeking Behavior
Pain (backache)
* Risk for Altered Nutrition: Less than Body Requirements
Risk for Altered Nutrition: More than Body Requirements
Risk for Injury
Sleep Pattern Disturbance

* Nursing diagnoses that are explored in this chapter

Planning

Goals for this nursing diagnosis are that the expectant mother, the family, or both will do the following:

- Demonstrate knowledge of practices that promote the safety and well-being of the mother and fetus throughout pregnancy
- Describe measures that provide relief from the common discomforts of pregnancy
- Describe a realistic plan during the first trimester to modify behaviors or habits that could adversely affect the health of the mother and fetus

Interventions

After the initial assessment the woman is usually not seen by the health care provider for 4 weeks. She and her family must be instructed about signs and symptoms that indicate a serious danger. Any such signs or symptoms should be reported immediately ("Critical to Remember: Danger Signs of Pregnancy").

CRITICAL TO REMEMBER

Danger Signs of Pregnancy

- Vaginal bleeding with or without discomfort
- Rupture of membranes (escape of fluid from the vagina)
- Swelling of the fingers (such as rings becoming tight) or puffiness of the face or around the eyes
- Continuous pounding headache
- Visual disturbances (such as blurred vision, dimness, spots before the eyes)
- Persistent or severe abdominal pain
- Chills or fever
- Painful urination
- Persistent vomiting
- Change in frequency or strength of fetal movements

NURSING CARE PLAN 7-1

Discomfort During Early Pregnancy

Assessment: Maria Gomez, a thin, 18-year-old primigravida of 8 weeks' gestation, has dry, cracked lips and a pulse rate of 90 when she arrives at the prenatal clinic. She states that she is experiencing nausea with occasional vomiting throughout the day. She reports that the nausea is intensified by the odor of cooking food and she has little appetite. Although she is always thirsty, she restricts fluids because "they make me sicker." Her urine sample is concentrated, with a specific gravity of 1.030.

Nursing Diagnosis: Risk for Altered Nutrition: Less than Body Requirements related to nausea, vomiting, and anorexia.

Critical Thinking: Were all data considered? Organize data and develop a second diagnosis. State outcomes for that diagnosis, and identify at least two interventions.

Answer: No. All data should be grouped and analyzed. For example, nausea throughout the day, occasional vomiting, and anorexia support the stated nursing diagnosis. Dry lips, tachycardia, thirst, and concentrated urine, however, are not analyzed. These data suggest a second nursing diagnosis: Risk for Fluid Volume Deficit related to inadequate intake of fluids and fluid loss through vomiting.

Goals/Outcome Criteria Include:
1. Increase intake of fluids to 2000 ml/day
2. Maintain urine specific gravity within normal range
3. Demonstrate no signs or symptoms of dehydration

Interventions Include:
1. Suggest alternative fluids, such as Jello, frozen juice bars, ice cream, pudding, and watermelon.
2. Recommend frequent small amounts of ice chips or clear liquids.
3. Emphasize the importance of taking frequent small amounts of water instead of coffee or tea, which act as diuretics.
4. Ask Maria to return within 2 days if she is unable to retain recommended amounts of fluid. Waiting until the next scheduled prenatal visit is not prudent if she is dehydrated.

Goals/Outcome Critieria:
Maria will do the following:
1. Maintain adequate intake of calories and nutrients to meet her needs, as evidenced by sufficient energy to carry on the activities of daily living, and a continuous pattern of weight gain during pregnancy (see Chapter 9)
2. Report less nausea and a decrease in the episodes of vomiting

Intervention	Rationale
1. Recommend that she eat two dry crackers half an hour before arising in the morning and that she get out of bed slowly.	1. Food counteracts hypoglycemia resulting from night-long fasting and prevents an initial episode of nausea that may become difficult to control.
2. Suggest that she eat a high-protein bedtime snack, such as cottage cheese or half a turkey sandwich on whole wheat bread.	2. Proteins are metabolized at a slower rate, helping prevent morning hypoglycemia.
3. Instruct Maria to eat small, dry meals five to six times a day rather than three large ones.	3. Frequent dry meals prevent the stomach from becoming empty and decrease the feeling of nausea.
4. Suggest that fluids be taken separately and that she brush her teeth often.	4. Fluids overstretch the stomach and may precipitate vomiting. Brushing her teeth often removes bad tastes in the mouth.
5. Recommend that she eat a dry cracker, unbuttered popcorn, or dry toast every 2 hours.	5. Nausea is more intense when the stomach is empty.
6. Suggest that she avoid fried or greasy foods, highly-seasoned foods, or foods with strong odors. Suggest that she try ginger teas or combinations of salty and tart flavors.	6. Odors and greasy textures are associated with nausea and increased episodes of vomiting. Some women find various foods or combinations helpful.
7. Teach Maria to keep a record of daily intake of food and fluids, episodes of vomiting, and measures that reduce nausea.	7. Determining whether adequate nutrients and fluids are being retained and identifying the most helpful measures to control nausea is essential.
8. Suggest that she experiment with soups, eggnogs, and vegetable drinks.	8. These foods are high in nutrients and are often tolerated well when taken separately.
9. Reassure her that nausea and vomiting usually disappear by the second trimester and do not indicate a problem with the pregnancy.	9. Knowing that the condition is self-limiting and does not threaten the fetus reduces anxiety.
10. Assess Maria's weight at each prenatal visit and compare weight gain with that expected for the weeks of gestation.	10. If weight gain is normal, the focus remains on relieving the discomfort of nausea and vomiting. If weight gain is too low or signs of dehydration are present, refer her for medical management.

Evaluation: Periodic nausea and vomiting continued throughout the first trimester but ceased during the second trimester. At 20 weeks, Maria appears well hydrated and has gained 4.5 kg (approximately 10 lb).

Assessment: Maria also says that she is often very tired during the day even though she is sleeping 8 to 10 hours at night. Fatigue concerns her because she is employed and must keep her mind on her work.

Nursing Diagnosis: Fatigue related to inadequate rest periods to accommodate the physiologic demands of pregnancy.

Critical Thinking: What assumption has the nurse made? What other factors should be considered before this diagnosis is made?

Answer: Although extraordinary fatigue is common in early pregnancy, nurses must not assume that pregnancy is the only cause. Additional data, such as hemoglobin and hematocrit levels, should be obtained before this diagnosis is made. Information about increasing iron-rich foods or iron supplementation may be necessary.

Goals/Outcome Criteria:
Maria will do the following:
1. Identify methods to cope with fatigue, such as negotiating a flexible work schedule or time for short rest periods while continuing employment during pregnancy.
2. Report increased energy by the end of the first trimester.

Intervention	Rationale
1. Acknowledge the fatigue and reassure Maria that this is self-limiting and a common experience during the first months because of the change in hormone levels.	1. Reassurance helps alleviate the concern that fatigue indicates a problem with her pregnancy.
2. Recommend that she lie down or sit comfortably with feet elevated for a few minutes every 2 hours and consciously relax the muscles of the legs, abdomen, and shoulders.	2. This position renews energy even though sleep is not possible.
3. Suggest that she try deep breathing and visualizing a favorite location or pastime whenever possible. Progressive relaxation—conscious tensing and relaxing of groups of muscles beginning with those in the feet and working upward toward the head—may be helpful.	3. These exercises relieve physical tension that adds to fatigue and also provide mental distraction.
4. Recommend that she get as much sleep as she feels she needs when possible. Adequate rest may involve curtailing social activities and tasks that can be postponed.	4. Although recreation is important, the need for sleep is overwhelming for some women during the first weeks of pregnancy.
5. Encourage her to explore a flexible schedule or routine with her employer.	5. Often a very short nap in the morning or afternoon is all that is needed to continue to function effectively.
6. Recommend that she enlist the assistance of family, significant other, and friends with home responsibilities.	6. Assistance can free her of all but the most essential tasks during this time.

Critical Thinking: What additional interventions are necessary if the hemoglobin level and hematocrit are low?

Answer: If low levels of hemoglobin and hematocrit indicate that the client is anemic, the physician or nurse-midwife should be notified so that iron supplementation can be started.

Evaluation: Maria was able to negotiate two short rest periods each day and, at 12 weeks of gestation, continues to use learned techniques to renew energy. Maria relates increased energy at the third prenatal visit (16 weeks).

Although making the expectant mother aware of the danger signs of pregnancy is crucial, the nurse must take care not to frighten her. Avoid the term *danger signs* when talking to the woman and her family because it may be frightening. It is less frightening to say "The signs I am about to explain to you are rare, but if you see them, notify the physician (or nurse-midwife) at once because they require immediate attention."

Teaching Health Behaviors

Bathing. Daily bathing protects pregnant women from infections that may develop if bacteria normally present on the skin are allowed to remain and multiply. Bathing also promotes comfort by dissipating heat produced by increased metabolism. The woman should be cautioned to use nonskid pads in the tub or shower during the last trimester, during which balance is altered by a changing center of gravity.

NURSING CARE PLAN 7-2
Self-Care during Pregnancy

Assessment: Paula Orne, a primigravida of 28 weeks of gestation, has numerous questions about self-care. She is a courier and drives many hours each day. She is concerned about safety while driving. She also asks what sexual activity is allowed, and she is concerned because her partner continues to smoke.

Nursing Diagnosis: Health-Seeking Behaviors: Prenatal care related to travel, sexual activity, and effects of passive smoking

Outcome Critieria:
Paula will do the following:
1. Describe measures to decrease discomfort and promote safety while traveling by next visit
2. Continue mutually satisfactory sexual activity during pregnancy
3. Modify the environment to eliminate exposure to passive smoking by (specific date)

Intervention	Rationale
1. Recommend that Paula use car lap and shoulder restraints throughout pregnancy. Suggest that she keep the lap restraint under the abdomen.	1. Use of restraints prevents ejection from the car in case of an accident. The most serious injuries are sustained when a person is ejected at impact.
2. Suggest that she stop the car at least every 2 hours to walk for a few minutes and perform some gentle shoulder and upper body stretches. She should also empty her bladder at each stop.	2. Frequent stops improve circulation and relieve the muscles involved in prolonged sitting and driving. Frequent voiding promotes comfort and prevents bladder infection resulting from stasis of urine.
3. Suggest that she drink a glass of water at each stop but avoid sweet drinks and caffeinated beverages.	3. Sweet drinks increase thirst, and caffeine drinks act as diuretics and increase thirst. Water refreshes and prevents dehydration.
4. Determine the client's specific concerns about sexuality and respond to those in particular.	4. Concerns vary among couples. Some couples worry about harming the fetus or causing discomfort for the mother.
5. Reassure her that sexual activity poses no harm to either the mother or the fetus in a normal pregnancy. Explain the anatomy of the vagina, cervix, and uterus. Suggest she bring her partner to the next visit if he has concerns.	5. Knowledge of the separation between the vagina and fetus may relieve concern about the safety of vaginal intercourse during pregnancy.
6. Suggest that alternative positions, such as side-lying, women-superior, and rear-entry, be used during the third trimester.	6. The male-superior position becomes uncomfortable for the woman when the uterus is large and heavy, and it increases the risk of supine hypotension.
7. Discuss the danger of passive smoking, and recommend that the partner curtail smoking in the house, car, and other enclosed areas. This limitation is important during pregnancy and also after the infant is born.	7. Toxins in cigarette smoke affect those in the vicinity as well as the one who is smoking.

Evaluation: Paula uses both shoulder and lap restraints and says she feels more comfortable while driving. She relates mutually satisfying sexual experiences. Her partner agrees to curtail smoking in Paula's presence.

Hot Tubs and Saunas. Although warm baths and showers help relax tense and tired muscles, pregnant women should avoid saunas and hot tubs, which may produce maternal hyperthermia. Maternal hyperthermia, particularly during the first trimester, has been associated with fetal anomalies such as central nervous system defects (Rogers & Davis, 1995).

Douching. Despite increased vaginal discharge, no hygienic need exists for douching before, during, or after pregnancy. The only exception is an order by a physician or nurse-midwife to treat a specific problem. In that case, guidelines must be carefully followed to prevent the possibility of injury (Cunningham, et al., 1997).

- Bulb-type syringes have been associated with deaths of women caused by air embolism and therefore should never be used.
- Douche bags should not be elevated more than 2 feet above the hips to prevent excessive force of the fluid.
- The nozzle should not be inserted more than 3 inches into the vagina.

Breast Care. Instruct the expectant mother to wash her breasts and nipples with clear water and avoid soap, which removes the natural lubricant that forms on the nipples. Advise all clients to wear bras that fit well and support the breasts, preventing loss of muscle tone that can occur as the breasts become heavier during pregnancy. Wide bra straps distribute the weight evenly across the shoulders and provide greater comfort.

Inform the couple that breast stimulation, which increases oxytocin secretion and thus initiates uterine contractions, is unsafe if the woman has a history of preterm labor or existing signs of preterm labor. These signs include uterine contractions that increase in frequency or intensity, rhythmic pelvic pressure, and uterine contractions that assume a regular pattern.

Clothing. Recommend practical, comfortable, and nonconstricting clothing. Tight jeans or panty hose that may constrict venous circulation should be worn only for short periods. Low heels are preferred because they do not interfere with balance. High heels increase the curvature of the lower spine (lordosis) that is prevalent during the last trimester.

Exercise. Exercise during pregnancy is generally beneficial. Regular exercise can strengthen muscles, reduce backache, and provide a feeling of well-being. Exercise, especially in the first two trimesters, may help prevent cesarean delivery (Bungum, et al., 2000). However, the amount and type of exercise recommended depend on the physical condition of the woman and the stage of pregnancy.

Walking is perhaps the ideal exercise because it stimulates muscular activity of the entire body, gently increases respiratory and cardiovascular effort, and does not result in fatigue or strain. Swimming and water exercises are excellent forms of exercise during pregnancy because the buoyancy of the water helps prevent injuries.

Women should not begin strenuous exercise programs or intensify training during pregnancy. A major concern with vigorous exercise is the possibility that it will divert blood supply from the placenta to maternal muscles and thus deprive the fetus of needed oxygen. Vigorous exercise also increases circulating catecholamines, which cause visceral vasoconstriction and decreased placental circulation.

Women who have followed an exercise routine before pregnancy can be advised to continue low-impact exercise during pregnancy. Expectant mothers should curtail any activity that causes undue fatigue or poses the threat of injury. This caution may mean that an activity that is safe in the first trimester may not be safe in the third trimester. Suggest that the expectant mother avoid sports requiring balance and postpone undertaking a new sport until after childbirth.

As pregnancy progresses, the woman may need to reduce the level of exercise to prevent physiologic stress. The pregnant woman should avoid exercise in the supine position after the first trimester because this position is associated with decreased cardiac output. Exercise should be stopped if the woman feels extreme fatigue or dizziness or becomes very short of breath. Instruct her to take her pulse every 10 to 15 minutes and not exceed a target heart rate that has been determined in consultation with her health care provider.

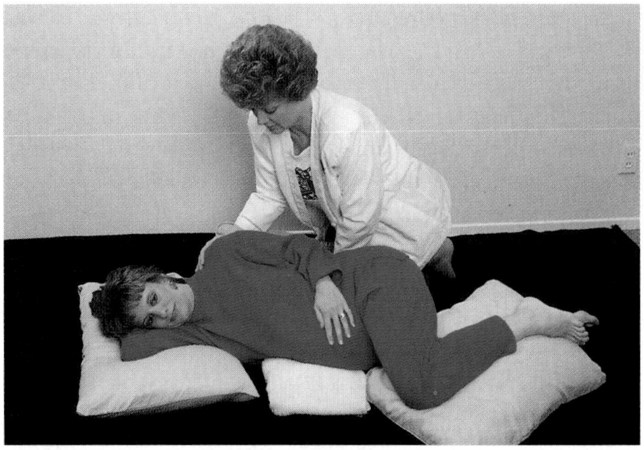

FIGURE 7-16 During the third trimester, pillows supporting the abdomen and back provide a comfortable position for rest.

Pregnant women should include a period of warm-up and stretching exercises in each exercise session. They must avoid becoming overheated because heat is transmitted to the fetus. A cool-down period of mild activity should conclude each exercise session. Emphasize the importance of taking liquids before, during, and after exercise to prevent dehydration.

Sleep and Rest. Finding a comfortable position for rest becomes a problem in the third trimester. Pillows can be used to support the abdomen and back and provide the best opportunity for sleep (Figure 7-16). Emphasize that frequent rest periods are beneficial, even if the woman does not fall asleep.

Employment. Most women of childbearing age in the United States are employed outside the home, and most continue to work during pregnancy. Whether the expectant mother can or should work depends on the presence of environmental toxins and industrial hazards and the level of physical activity involved.

Maternal Safety. Work should not lead to undue fatigue. Frequent rest periods with the feet elevated are essential. Jobs that require constant standing or sitting are very tiring, and the pregnant woman should change positions often or walk briefly to stimulate circulation and reduce fatigue. Tasks that require balance may be hazardous because the uterus enlarges and the center of gravity shifts. Suggest curtailing these jobs during the last trimester.

Working women often have many home responsibilities that, for some, do not decrease during pregnancy. The fatigue and stress of the home and employment workload may increase the incidence of problems during pregnancy (Luke, et al., 1999). Recommend that the expectant mother adapt her home and employment workloads as needed during pregnancy to reduce fatigue and stress.

Exposure to Teratogens. The problem of intrauterine exposure to toxic substances is a major concern in many industries. Exposure is a particular concern during the first trimester, which is the period of organogenesis. Advise clients to investigate their own occupational hazards. For example, hairdressers are exposed to toxic substances in hair dyes and aerosol sprays; painters and printers may be exposed to benzene, lead, and toluene; nurses and hospital personnel may be exposed to radiation; and anesthetic gases; and laundry and dry cleaning workers may be exposed to fetotoxic compounds. In addition, some women are exposed to smoke from other people's cigarettes (passive smoking) in the workplace. Passive smoking is known to be harmful to both mother and fetus.

Sexual Activity. Sexual intercourse is generally agreed to be safe for the healthy pregnant woman (see Chapter 8).

Travel. Although travel by car is generally safe, it may cause discomfort or fatigue. Frequent stops are necessary to allow the expectant mother to empty her bladder and walk. She must fasten the seat belt snugly with the lap belt below her abdomen. This position is uncomfortable for some women, and it causes concern about internal injuries in the event of collision. However, wearing the belt is much safer than leaving it off and risking ejection from the vehicle during an accident.

Travel by plane and train is generally safe, although some physicians discourage air travel after 26 weeks of gestation. If travel is necessary, the woman should be advised to walk frequently to maintain adequate peripheral circulation. The woman should not travel to remote locations where adequate medical care is unavailable.

Immunizations. In general, immunizations using live virus vaccines (such as measles, mumps, rubella, oral polio) are contraindicated during pregnancy because they may have teratogenic effects on the fetus. The pregnant woman should consult her physician or nurse-midwife about which immunizations are safe during pregnancy. The woman should also be advised to divulge that she is pregnant before a vaccine is administered.

Teaching about the Common Discomforts of Pregnancy

Although pregnancy is a state of health, the numerous physiologic changes that occur during pregnancy often cause physical discomforts for which medical care does not exist. Relief depends on self-help measures that informed nurses are expected to teach. (See Figures 7-14 to 7-16 and "Women Want to Know: How to Overcome the Common Discomforts of Pregnancy.")

Teaching Necessary Lifestyle Changes

Many expectant parents are willing to make changes in lifestyle to avoid adversely affecting the fetus. For example, use of tobacco, alcohol, and illegal drugs should be curtailed during pregnancy. In addition the use of over-the-counter medications and prescription drugs should be discussed.

Prescription and Over-the-Counter Drugs. Advise pregnant women to consult with their health care providers before taking any drugs. This precaution is important for over-the-counter and prescription drugs. Explain that information is inadequate in regard to safe use of some medications during pregnancy. When prescription drugs are necessary, their risks and benefits must be considered. In general, the health care provider must weigh the risks against the benefits and decide whether a drug can safely be used or changes are necessary.

Tobacco. In 1997, 13.2% of women reported smoking during their pregnancies (Guyer, 1999). Although this statistic shows improvement over past numbers, the nurse must make every effort to motivate the expectant mother to stop smoking and avoid contact with other smokers. Pregnant women who smoke have smaller infants and an increased incidence of preterm births. In addition, developmental problems such as short attention span and lower cognitive skills are also more common in children whose mothers smoked during pregnancy.

Smoking tobacco affects fetal development for several reasons:

- Nicotine causes vasoconstriction of vessels in the placenta.
- Carbon monoxide, which is released in tobacco smoke, inactivates maternal and fetal hemoglobin, which is essential to transport oxygen to the fetus.
- Maternal appetite is decreased, causing inadequate intake of calories.
- Plasma volume, needed to transport nutrients and oxygen to the fetus, is decreased.

Alcohol. Alcohol is a known teratogen, and maternal alcohol use is a leading cause of mental retardation in the United States. Alcohol produces a characteristic cluster of developmental anomalies known as *fetal alcohol syndrome.* Children with fetal alcohol syndrome exhibit a typical pattern of prenatal and postnatal growth retardation with characteristic facial, cardiovascular, and limb defects (see Figure 24-3). These children also exhibit cognitive and fine-motor dysfunctions that are tragic and irreversible.

Conclusive data about fetal effects of social or moderate drinking are not available. Therefore the best advice for women who are pregnant or who plan to become pregnant is to abstain from all alcohol (see Chapter 24).

Illegal Drugs. Use of so-called street drugs such as cocaine, heroin, and methamphetamine is harmful to the fetus. The pregnant woman should be advised to discontinue all illicit drug use (see Chapters 24 and 30).

Evaluation

Interventions can be considered to effectively meet the established outcomes if the mother and her family (1) discuss and practice self-care measures taught them to promote safety and health of the mother and fetus, (2) verbalize knowledge of methods that help relieve common discomforts of pregnancy, and (3) identify a plan early in pregnancy to modify habits that could adversely affect health, such as curtailing the use of alcohol or tobacco. If interventions are ineffective, the nurse collaborates with the family to define new plans and work out additional interventions.

Antepartum Home Care Nursing

Economic constraints in health care often limit or prevent antepartum nursing care for clients in the home setting. Home visits for women who have no complications are not common in the United States. Women with specific high-risk conditions that can be cared for in the home setting may receive home visits to help them manage intravenous fluids or other aspects of care.

SUMMARY CONCEPTS

- Pregnancy causes a predictable pattern of uterine growth that provides information about fetal development and helps to confirm the expected date of birth. In general, the uterus can be palpated at the level of the umbilicus at 20 weeks of gestation and at the xiphoid process by 36 weeks.
- Thick mucus fills the softened connective tissue in the cervical canal and protects the fetus from infection caused by bacteria ascending from the vagina.
- Plasma volume expands faster and to a greater extent than red blood cells, resulting in a dilution of hemoglobin concentration. This condition is referred to as *physiologic (pseudo) anemia* because the low levels of hemoglobin and hematocrit are the result of dilution and do not reflect an inadequate number of red blood cells.
- Blood flow alters during pregnancy to include the uteroplacental unit. Increased renal plasma flow results in increased glomerular filtration rate, which effectively removes additional metabolic wastes produced by the mother and the fetus but often results in "spilling" of glucose and other nutrients in the urine. Increased blood flow to the skin attempts to reduce the additional heat generated by the fetus and the increased maternal metabolic rate.
- The gravid uterus partially occludes the vena cava and descending aorta when the mother rests in a supine position. The occlusion causes supine hypotensive syndrome, which can be prevented or corrected when she assumes a lateral position.
- During the last trimester the uterus pushes the diaphragm upward, decreasing lung capacity. To compensate, the ribs flare, the substernal angle widens, and the circumference of the chest increases.
- Alterations in hormones during pregnancy may result in discomfort for the mother. Increased hCG and estrogen are associated with nausea in early pregnancy. Increased progesterone is associated with relaxation of smooth muscles, including those of the ureters, bladder, and bowel. Resulting stasis of urine, rich in nutrients, increases the risk of urinary tract infections. Decreased bowel motility is a major cause of constipation during pregnancy.
- Alterations in hormones are also responsible for cutaneous changes such as hyperpigmentation.
- The expanding uterus and the hormone relaxin result in progressive changes that can lead to muscle strain and backache during the last trimester.
- Progesterone is called the "hormone of pregnancy" because it maintains the uterine lining for implantation of the blastocyst, prevents uterine contractions during pregnancy, which could result in spontaneous abortion, and helps prepare the breasts for lactation.
- Presumptive and probable signs of pregnancy may be caused by conditions other than pregnancy and thus cannot be considered positive or diagnostic signs. Positive signs can have no other cause.
- A complete history and physical examination are necessary at the initial antepartum visit to determine the potential risks to the mother and fetus and obtain baseline data for a plan of care.
- Risk assessment begins at the initial visit and continues throughout pregnancy because gestations that are categorized as low risk in early pregnancy may later become high risk.
- Multifetal pregnancies impose greater physiologic changes than a single-fetus pregnancy and require extra vigilance to detect possible complications.
- Families need information related to self-care and health promotion and information to deal with the common discomforts of pregnancy, which do not require or respond to medical management.
- Nurses must use the nursing process and critical thinking skills to assist the parents to make necessary changes in their lifestyles.

ANSWERS TO CRITICAL THINKING QUESTIONS

1. If pregnant now, Wilma is gravida 3, para 1 (the twin birth counts as one parous experience). If the acronym GTPAL is used, more complete information can be recorded: G = 3, T = 1, P = 0 (no preterm infants), A = 1 (one pregnancy ending before 20 weeks of gestation), L = 2 (living twins).
2. Amenorrhea and nausea and vomiting are only presumptive (subjective) indications of pregnancy because they can be caused by conditions other than pregnancy.
3. Count back 3 months to March 22, and add 7 days. This brings the date to March 29. Correct the year to 2002. Wilma's EDD is March 29, 2002.

REFERENCES & READINGS

American Academy of Pediatrics & American College of Obstetricians and Gynecologists. (1997). *Guidelines for perinatal care* (4th ed.). Elk Grove Village, IL: Author.

American College of Obstetricians and Gynecologists (ACOG). (1994). *Exercise during pregnancy and the postnatal period.* Washington, D.C.: Technical Bulletin number 189.

American College of Obstetricians and Gynecologists (ACOG). (1996). *Guidelines for women's health care.* Washington, D.C.: Author.

Andres, R.L., & Jones, K.L. (1999). Social and illicit drug use in pregnancy. In R.K. Creasy & R. Resnik, *Maternal-fetal medicine: Principles and practice* (4th ed., pp. 145-164). Philadelphia: W.B. Saunders.

Association of Women's Health, Obstetric, and Neonatal Nurses (AWHONN). (1999). *Standards and guidelines for professional nursing practice in the care of women and newborns* (5th ed.). Washington, D.C.: Author.

Barron, M.L. (1998). *Nursing assessment of the pregnant woman: Antepartal screening and laboratory evaluation.* White Plains, NY: March of Dimes Birth Defects Foundation.

Beal, M.W. (1999). Acupuncture and acupressure: Applications to women's reproductive health care. *Journal of Nurse-Midwifery,* 44(3), 217-229.

Blackburn, S.T., & Loper, D.L. (1992). *Maternal, fetal, and neonatal physiology.* Philadelphia: W.B. Saunders.

Bond, L. (2000). Physiology of pregnancy. In Mattson, S. & Smith, J.E. (Eds.), *Core curriculum for maternal-newborn nursing* (2nd ed., pp. 85-100). Philadelphia: W.B. Saunders.

Briggs, G.G., Freeman, R.K., & Sumner, J.Y. (1998). *Drugs in pregnancy and lactation* (5th ed.). Baltimore: Williams & Wilkins.

Bungum, T.J., Peaslee, D.L., Jackson, A.W., & Perez, M. (2000). Exercise during pregnancy and type of delivery in nulliparae. *Journal of Obstetric, Gynecologic, and Neonatal Nursing,* 29(3), 258-264.

Carl, D.L., Roux, G. & Matacale, R. (2000). Exploring dental hygiene and perinatal outcomes—oral health implications for pregnancy and early childhood. *AWHONN Lifelines,* 4(1), 23-27.

Corrarino, J.E., Walsh, P.J., & Anselmo, D. (1999). A program to educate women who test positive for the hepatitis B virus during the perinatal period. *MCN: The American Journal of Maternal/Child Nursing,* 24(3), 151-155.

Cunningham, F.G., MacDonald, P.C., Gant, N.F., Leveno, K.J., Gilstrap, L.C., Hankins, G.D.V., & Clark, S.L. (1997), *Williams obstetrics* (20th ed.). Norwalk, CT: Appleton & Lange.

Dickerson, V.M., & Chez, R.A. (1999). Normal pregnancy and prenatal care. In J.R. Scott, P.J. DiSaia, C.B. Hammond, & W.N. Spellacy, *Danforth's obstetrics and gynecology* (8th ed., pp. 65-82.) Philadelphia: Lippincott.

DuBose, T.J. (1996). First trimester. In T.J. DuBose, *Fetal sonography* (pp. 389-425). Philadelphia: W.B. Saunders.

Duerbeck, N.B. & Reed, K.L. (1998). Pregnancy and lactation. In L.A. Wallis (Ed.), *Textbook of women's health* (pp. 663-674). Philadelphia: Lippincott-Raven.

Duffy, T.P. (1999). Hematologic aspects of pregnancy. In G.N. Burrow & T.F. Ferris (Eds.), *Medical complications during pregnancy* (5th ed., pp. 79-95). Philadelphia: W.B. Saunders.

Ellings, J.M., & Bowers, N.A. (1999). Prenatal care and multiple pregnancy. *Journal of Obstetric, Gynecologic, and Neonatal Nursing,* 27(4), 457-465.

Fagen, C. (2000). Nutrition during pregnancy and lactation. In L.K. Mahan, & S. Escott-Stump, *Krause's food, nutrition, and diet therapy* (10th ed., pp. 167-195). Philadelphia: Saunders.

Flake, D.J. (2000). HIV testing during pregnancy—building the case for voluntary testing. *AWHONN Lifelines,* 4(1), 13-16.

Freels, D.L., & Coggins, M. (2000). Acupressure at the Neiguan P6 point for treating nausea and vomiting in early pregnancy: An evaluation of the literature. *Mother Baby Journal,* 5(3), 17-22.

Fuhrman, L. (2000). Common dermatoses of pregnancy. *Journal of Perinatal & Neonatal Nursing,* 4(1), 1-16.

Georges, J.M. (2000). Female genital and reproductive function. In L.C. Copstead & J.L. Banasik, *Pathophysiology: Biological and behavioral perspectives* (2nd ed., pp. 742-760). Philadelphia: W.B. Saunders.

Guyer, B., Hoyert, D.L., Martin, J.A., Ventura, S.J., MacDorman, M.F., & Strobino, D.M. (1999). Annual summary of vital statistics, 1998. *Pediatrics,* 104(6), 1229-1245.

Gookheart, H. (1999). The skin and hair during pregnancy. *Women's Health in Primary Care,* 2(7), 569-570.

Hartmann, S., & Bung, P. (1999). Physical exercise during pregnancy—physiological considerations and recommendations. *Journal of Perinatal Medicine,* 27, 204-215.

Hobel, C.J. (1998). Prenatal care. In N.F. Hacker & J.G. Moore, *Essentials of obstetrics and gynecology* (3rd ed., pp. 111-122). Philadelphia: W.B. Saunders.

Hutchinson, M.K., & Baqi-Aziz, M. (1994). Nursing care of the childbearing Muslim family. *Journal of Obstetric, Gynecologic, and Neonatal Nursing,* 23(9), 767-771.

Kilpatrick, S.J., & Laros, R.K. (1999). Maternal hematologic disorders. In R.K. Creasy & R. Resnik, *Maternal-fetal medicine: Principles and practice* (4th ed., pp. 935-963). Philadelphia: W.B. Saunders.

Kronenberg, F., Murphy, P.A., & Wade, C. (1999). Complementary/alternative therapies in select populations: Women. In J.W. Spencer & J.J. Jacobs, *Complementary/alternative medicine: An evidence-based approach,* (pp. 340-362). St. Louis: Mosby.

Larson, L., & Star, J. (1999). Answering your pregnant patient's most common questions. *Women's Health in Primary Care,* 2(7), 519-530.

Lee, K.A., & Zafke, M.E. (1999). Longitudinal changes in fatigue and energy during pregnancy and the postpartum period. *Journal of Obstetric, Gynecologic, and Neonatal Nursing,* 28(2), 183-191.

Luke, B., Avni, M., Min, L., & Misiunas, R. (1999). Work and pregnancy: The role of fatigue and the "second shift" on antenatal morbidity. *American Journal of Obstetrics & Gynecology,* 185(5), Part 1, 1172-1179.

Malone, S.F., & D'Alton, M.E. (1999). Multiple gestation: Clinical characteristics and management. In R.K. Creasy & R. Resnik, *Maternal-fetal medicine: Principles and practice* (4th ed., pp. 598-615). Philadelphia: W.B. Saunders.

Meikle, S.F., Orleans, M., Leff, M., Shain, R., & Gibbs, R.S. (1995). Women's reasons for not seeking prenatal care: Racial and ethnic factors. *Birth,* 22(2), 81-86.

Monga, M. (1999). Cardiovascular and renal adaptation to pregnancy. In R.K. Creasy & R. Resnik, *Maternal-fetal medicine: Principles and practice* (4th ed., pp. 783-792). Philadelphia: W.B. Saunders.

Moore, T.R. (1999). Diabetes in pregnancy. In R.K. Creasy & R. Resnik, *Maternal-fetal medicine: Principles and practice* (4th ed., pp. 964-995). Philadelphia: W.B. Saunders.

Morin, K.H. (1998). Perinatal outcomes of obese women: a review of the literature. *Journal of Obstetric, Gynecologic, and Neonatal Nursing, 27*(4), 431-440.

Murphy, P.A. (1998). Alternative therapies for nausea and vomiting of pregnancy. *Obstetrics & Gynecology, 91*(1), 149-154.

Nuwayhid, B., Nguyen, T., & Khraibi, A. (1999). Maternal physiology. In N.F. Hacker & J.G. Moore (Eds.), *Essentials of obstetrics and gynecology* (3rd ed., pp. 85-99). Philadelphia: W.B. Saunders.

Priddy, K.D. (1997). Immunologic adaptations during pregnancy. *Journal of Obstetric, Gynecologic, and Neonatal Nursing, 26*(4), 388-394.

Rapini, R.P., & Jordon, R.E. (1999). The skin and pregnancy. In R.K. Creasy & R. Resnik, *Maternal-fetal medicine: Principles and practice* (4th ed., pp. 1120-1127). Philadelphia: W.B. Saunders.

Resnik, R. (1999). Anatomic alterations in the reproductive tract. In R.K. Creasy & R. Resnik, *Maternal-fetal medicine: Principles and practice* (4th ed., pp. 90-94). Philadelphia: W.B. Saunders.

Rogers, J., & Davis, B.A. (1995). How risky are hot tubs and saunas for pregnant women? *MCN: The American Journal of Maternal/Child Nursing, 20*(3), 137-140.

Simpson, K.R., & Creehan, P.A. (1996). *AWHONN perinatal nursing.* Philadelphia: Lippincott-Raven.

Smith, S. (2000). Exercise. In F.H. Nichols & S.S. Humenick, *Childbirth education: Practice, research, and theory* (2nd ed., pp. 463-475). Philadelphia: W.B. Saunders.

Spector, R.E. (2000). *Cultural diversity in health and illness* (4th ed.). Norwalk, CT: Appleton & Lange.

Stables, D. (2000). *Physiology in childbearing.* Edinburgh: Bailliere Tindall.

Stewart, F. (1998). Pregnancy testing and management of early pregnancy. In R. Hatcher, J. Trussell, F. Stewart, W. Cates, G.K. Stewart, F. Guest, & D. Kowal, *Contraceptive technology* (17th ed., pp. 635-652). New York: Ardent Media.

Thorpe, J.M., Norton, P.A., Wall, L.L., Kuller, J.A., Eucker, B., & Wells, E. (1999). Urinary incontinence in pregnancy and the puerperium: A prospective study. *American Journal of Obstetrics & Gynecology, 181*(2), 266-273.

Tomlinson, M.W. (2000). Overview of routine prenatal care. In S.B. Ransom et al. (Eds.), *Practical strategies in obstetrics and gynecology* (pp. 199-211). Philadelphia: W.B. Saunders.

Turner, M.L.C. (1999). The skin in pregnancy. In G.N. Burrow & T.F. Ferris (Eds.), *Medical complications during pregnancy* (5th ed., pp. 453-468). Philadelphia: W.B. Saunders.

U.S. Department of Health and Human Services. (2000). *Healthy people 2010* (Conference ed. in 2 volumes). Washington, D.C.: Author.

Zhou, Q., O'Brien, B., & Relyea, J. (1999). Severity of nausea and vomiting during pregnancy: What does it predict? *Birth, 26*(2), 108-114.

8 PSYCHOSOCIAL ADAPTATIONS TO PREGNANCY

OBJECTIVES

1. Describe the psychological responses of the expectant mother to pregnancy.
2. Identify the process of role transition.
3. Explain the maternal tasks of pregnancy.
4. Describe the developmental processes that a man completes to make the transition to the role of father.
5. Describe the responses of prospective grandparents and siblings to pregnancy.
6. Discuss factors influencing psychosocial adaptation to pregnancy, such as age, parity, and socioeconomic status.
7. Describe the ways in which these factors affect nursing practice.
8. Explain cultural influences on pregnancy and cultural assessment and negotiation.

DEFINITIONS

AMBIVALENCE Simultaneous conflicting emotions, attitudes, ideas, or wishes.

ATTACHMENT Development of strong affectional ties as a result of interaction between an infant and a significant other (such as mother, father, sibling, caretaker).

BODY IMAGE Subjective image of a person's own physical appearance and capabilities; derived from that person's own observations and the evaluation of significant others.

BONDING Development of a strong emotional tie of a parent to a newborn; also called *claiming,* or *binding in.*

COUVADE Pregnancy-related rituals or a cluster of symptoms experienced by some prospective fathers during pregnancy and childbirth.

DEVELOPMENTAL TASK A necessary step in growth and maturation that must be completed before additional growth and maturation are possible.

DISTURBANCE IN BODY IMAGE A person's negative feelings about the characteristics, functions, and self-limits of his or her body.

FANTASY Mental images formed to prepare for the birth of a child.

INTROVERSION Inward concentration on the self and body.

DEFINITIONS—cont'd

MIMICRY Copying the behaviors of other pregnant women or mothers as a method of "trying on" the role of advanced pregnancy or motherhood.

NARCISSIM Undue preoccupation with the self.

ROLE TRANSITION Changing from one pattern of behavior and one image of self to another.

Becoming a parent who is capable of loving and caring for a totally dependent infant is more than a biologic event. This process begins before conception and involves major changes in the expectant mother, her partner, and the entire family. Although each couple adapts to pregnancy in a unique way, the psychological responses of prospective parents change as the pregnancy progresses. Thus although the initial reaction may be uncertain, by the time the infant is born, the woman and her partner have completed developmental tasks allowing them to become parents in the true sense of the word. Both social and cultural factors influence their adjustment to pregnancy.

MATERNAL PSYCHOLOGICAL RESPONSES

A woman's psychological response to pregnancy changes with time. Initially, she may be uncertain or ambivalent about the pregnancy, and her primary focus is on herself. Gradually her focus shifts, and she becomes increasingly concerned about protecting and providing for the fetus.

First Trimester

Uncertainty

During the early weeks the woman is unsure whether she is pregnant and tries to confirm it. She observes her body carefully for changes that indicate she is pregnant. She may confer with family and friends about the probability and may use an over-the-counter pregnancy test kit for validation.

Reaction to the uncertainty of pregnancy depends on the individual. A woman may be eager to find confirming signs, or she may dread the possibility and hope for signs indicating she is not pregnant. Usually she seeks confirmation from a physician, certified nurse-midwife, or nurse practitioner within 12 weeks of the first missed menstrual period.

Ambivalence

Once the pregnancy is confirmed, most women have conflicting feelings, or ambivalence, about being pregnant. Many feel that this is not the right time, even if the pregnancy is wanted and planned. Women who had planned to become pregnant often say they thought it would take longer for the pregnancy to become a reality. Many pregnancies are desired but unplanned, and these women may wish they had completed some specific plan or goal before becoming pregnant.

Many women examine the meaning of the pregnancy in terms of changes that must be made in their lives and what they must give up as a result of the pregnancy. If it is her first pregnancy, the woman may worry about the added responsibility and feel unsure of her ability to be a good parent. Some women worry about the ways in which this pregnancy will affect their relationship with other children or the father.

The Self as Primary Focus

Throughout the first trimester the woman's primary focus is on herself, not the fetus. Early physical responses to pregnancy, such as nausea and fatigue, confirm that something is happening to her, but the fetus seems vague and unreal. Because she has not gained weight to confirm a growing, developing fetus, she probably says "I am pregnant" rather than "I am going to have a baby."

Physical changes and increased hormone levels may cause emotional lability (unstable moods). Her mood can change quickly from contentment to irritation or from optimistic planning to an overwhelming need for sleep. This may be confusing to her partner, who is accustomed to a more stable relationship. The nurse should tell the couple that mood changes are normal and do not necessarily indicate problems.

Second Trimester

Physical Evidence of Pregnancy

During the second trimester, physical changes occur in the expectant mother that make the fetus "real." The uterus grows rapidly and can be palpated in the abdomen, weight increases, and breast changes are obvious. Most important, the woman feels the fetus move (quickening), which confirms that a life is developing within the uterus. As a result, she no longer thinks of the fetus as simply a part of her body but now perceives it as separate although entirely dependent on her. Now she might say "I am going to have a baby" (Figure 8-1).

The Fetus as Primary Focus

During the second trimester the fetus becomes the woman's major focus. The discomforts of the first trimester have usually abated and her size does not alter her activity. She is now concerned about producing a healthy infant. She generally seeks information about nutrition and fetal development. She experiences a feeling of creative energy and satisfaction.

Narcissism and Introversion

During this time, many women become increasingly concerned about their ability to protect and provide for the fetus. This concern is often manifested as narcis-

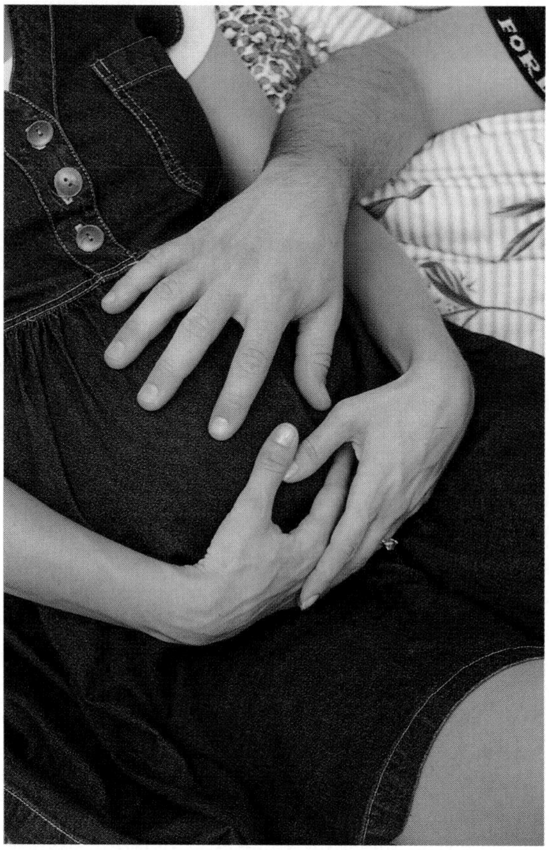

FIGURE 8-1 Fetal movement, or quickening, confirms that a separate life is developing.

sism and introversion. Selecting exactly the right foods to eat or the right clothes to wear may assume much importance. Some women lose interest in their jobs, which may seem alien to the events taking place in their bodies. They may be less interested in current events as they concentrate on the pregnancy, or they may become fearful that world events threaten them and therefore present a danger to the fetus.

The primigravida wonders about the infant. She looks at baby pictures of herself and her partner and wants to hear stories about themselves as infants. Although multiparas know more about infants in general, they are interested in this infant and concerned with this child's acceptance by siblings and grandparents.

Body Image

Rapid and profound changes take place in the body during the second trimester. Changes in body size and contour are obvious and include bulging of the abdomen, thickening of the waist, and enlargement of the breasts. The changes may be welcomed because they signify growth of the fetus, creating pride in the woman and her partner. For some women, however, the change in body size and shape, coupled with hyperpigmentation of the skin and striae gravidarum, may contribute to a negative body image. In addition, changes in body function such as altered balance, less physical endurance, and discomfort in the pelvis and lower back areas may also contribute to a negative body image (Nursing Care Plan 8-1).

Changes in Sexuality

Despite the need for information, most women are reluctant to initiate a discussion about sexual activity. Furthermore, most health professionals do not introduce the topic. They may fear offending the client or may be uncomfortable with their own sexuality and are embarrassed to begin a discussion. They may lack time for any but the most pressing assessments. The result may be that an important aspect of care is ignored.

> A broad opening statement may help initiate discussion about sexual activity, such as "Sometimes couples are concerned about having sex during pregnancy." Such statements provide a method of introducing the subject in a way that the woman feels comfortable to pursue it or to let it drop.

The expectant couple should be made aware of the normal changes in sexual desire that occur during pregnancy and the importance of communicating their feelings openly with each other to find solutions to problems. The nurse can reassure the couple that their feelings are normal.

The sexual interest and activity of pregnant women and their partners are unpredictable and may increase, decline, or remain unchanged. The fact that she does not have to worry about pregnancy or contraception may give the woman a sense of freedom and increase sexual activity. The woman's physical comfort and sense of well being are closely linked to her interest in sexual activity.

During the first trimester, freedom from the worry of becoming pregnant may enhance sexual interest. However, physical complaints such as nausea, fatigue, and breast tenderness may interfere with erotic feelings. Fear of miscarriage may cause couples to avoid intercourse, particularly if the woman has previously lost a pregnancy. Guilt and anxiety may develop if sexual activity is curtailed. Nurses can help reassure the couple that no evidence links intercourse to early pregnancy loss when no other complications are present.

As a result of pelvic vasocongestion, women experience increased sensitivity of the labia and clitoris and increased vaginal lubrication during the second trimester. These changes, coupled with a general feeling of well-being and energy, may increase the sexual responsiveness of many women. Orgasm may occur more frequently and with greater intensity during pregnancy because of these changes.

During the third trimester the "missionary position" (male on top) may cause discomfort from abdominal pressure. Heartburn, indigestion, and supine hypoten-

NURSING CARE PLAN 8-1

Body Image during Pregnancy

Assessment: Dolores White is a 34-year-old primigravida in the 26th week of pregnancy. Both she and her husband have been runners for several years. Dolores stopped running 6 months ago and reports that she now walks "like other old ladies." She verbalizes concern about her size and says she feels "awkward and ugly." She states, "I hate the way I look! I can't wait to get back into shape."

Nursing Diagnosis: Body Image Disturbance related to changes in body size, contour, and function.

Expected Outcomes:
Dolores will do the following:

1. Make statements that indicate acceptance of expected body changes throughout the rest of her pregnancy.
2. Express her feelings about body changes to her husband and the health care team by (date).
3. Set realistic goals for weight loss and the resumption of a running program after childbirth.

Intervention	Rationale
1. Acknowledge Dolores' feelings. "I can see you are disappointed at not being able to run and concerned about how your body has changed as a result of pregnancy."	1. Feelings must be acknowledged, reflected, and dealt with before the underlying cause can be addressed.
2. Clarify her concerns. "You've always been an athlete. Women often wonder if changes in pregnancy will affect them permanently."	2. An unvoiced concern may be that pregnancy will change the woman from athlete to mother. This altered perception of herself causes fear, grief, or both.
3. Suggest that she share her feelings with her husband and seek his support. Model this interaction if necessary: "I feel awkward and left out of a big part of our lives. I need some reassurance from you now."	3. Although the woman may assume the partner observes and understands when negative feelings exist, this may not be true.
4. Explain the expected pattern of weight gain from 26 weeks to term gestation and correlate this with the growth and development of the fetus.	4. Understanding that weight gain indicates the fetus is growing and knowledge of the expected weight gain may allay unexpressed fears of excessive weight gain.
5. Help Dolores make realistic plans to lose weight and recover her strength and endurance after childbirth. a. Discuss the expected pattern of weight loss after childbirth: an initial weight loss of 10 to 12 pounds. An additional 5 to 8 pounds may be lost in the first few postpartum days. Many women return to their prepregnancy weight within 6 months. b. Demonstrate graduated exercises that increase muscle tone and strength. c. Explain the purpose of adipose tissue gained during pregnancy and discuss a diet that meets her needs for breastfeeding.	5. Adipose tissue provides a needed source of energy after childbirth and during lactation. Many women are relieved to know that there is a purpose and the added weight will be lost gradually. Breastfeeding requires at least 500 additional calories per day.

Evaluation: Dolores begins to speak with pride about how big the baby is growing. She reports her husband shows increased concern about her feelings since she shared her feelings with him. She begins to plan a realistic schedule of diet and exercise for after the birth.

sive syndrome also increase in this position. The pressure of the fetus low in the pelvis may add to discomfort. In addition, fatigue, ligament pain, urinary frequency, and shortness of breath may be problems. As they become larger, some women believe their bodies are ugly and may worry about their partners' reactions to their increased size.

The nurse can suggest alternative positions such as female superior, side-lying, or rear-entry for intercourse. The side-lying position may be the most comfortable and require the least amount of energy during the third trimester. Hugging, cuddling, kissing, and mutual massage or masturbation are other ways to express affection without vaginal intercourse. Sexual response varies widely among males. Some men report heightened feelings of sexual interest, but others perceive the woman's body in late pregnancy as unattractive and erotic feelings decrease. In addition, fear of harming the fetus or causing discomfort during pregnancy may interfere with sexual activity.

The couple should be instructed to avoid all sexual activity if the risk for preterm labor is high. They may be able to cope with this change if they understand that uterine contractions can be initiated by nipple stimulation, orgasm, and semen. Bleeding, an incompetent cervix, and the rupture of membranes are other con-

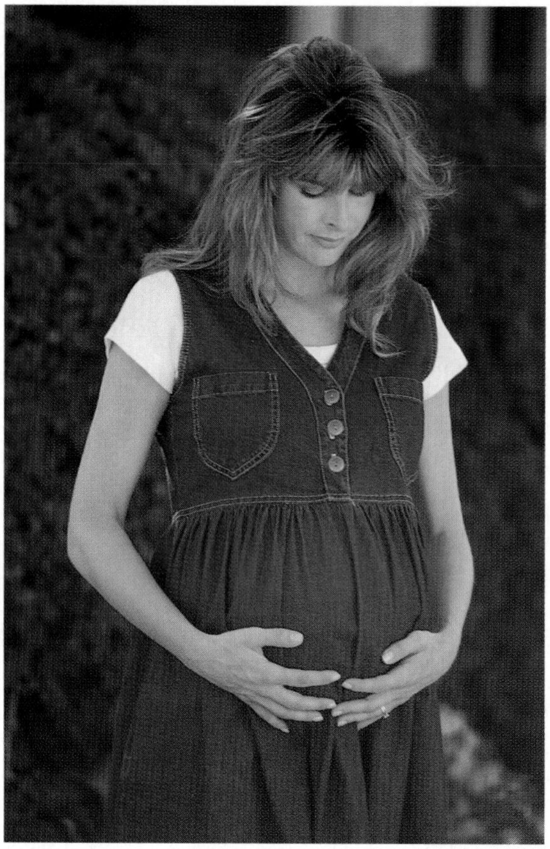

FIGURE 8-2 During the third trimester the mother feels increasingly vulnerable. She cradles her fetus to signify her protectiveness.

traindications for intercourse. In addition, blowing into the vagina must be avoided as it may cause an air embolus (Mullaly, 2000).

Third Trimester

Vulnerability

The sense of well-being and contentment that dominates the second trimester gives way to increasing feelings of vulnerability during the third trimester, particularly during the seventh month of pregnancy. Pregnant women often feel that the precious baby may be lost or harmed if not protected at all times (Figure 8-2). Many mothers have fantasies or nightmares about harm coming to the infant and become very cautious as a result. They may avoid crowds because they feel unable to protect the infant from infectious diseases or potential physical dangers.

Increasing Dependence

The expectant mother often becomes increasingly dependent on her partner in the last weeks of pregnancy. She may insist that he carry a beeper, or she may call his place of work several times during the day just to be sure that he is available. Her need for love and attention from her partner is even more pronounced in late pregnancy. She needs to be certain of his support and availability. When she is assured of his concern and willingness to provide assistance, she feels more secure and able to cope.

Although the woman may not be able to explain the increasing dependence, she expects her partner to understand the feeling and may become angry if he is not sympathetic. The nurse can encourage couples to discuss their fears and feelings openly so that misunderstandings can be avoided.

Preparation for Birth

Gradually, the feelings of vulnerability decrease as the woman comes to terms with her situation. The fetus continues to grow, and fetal movements are no longer gentle. Pokes, jabs, and kicks are intrusive expressions of the baby's crowded condition and increasing activity. The woman's relationship with the fetus changes as she acknowledges that although she and the fetus are interrelated, the baby is a pervasive presence and not a part of herself. Although she may not consciously acknowledge the increasing feelings of separateness, she longs to see the baby and become acquainted with her child.

Most pregnant women are concerned with their ability to determine when they are in labor. They review the signs of labor and question friends and family members who have given birth. Many couples worry that they will not get to the hospital or clinic in time for the birth, and they may be concerned about coping with labor.

During the last several weeks the woman becomes increasingly concerned with her due date and the experience of labor and delivery. Some women fear labor and dread the due date, whereas others are so uncomfortable that they look forward to that day as the exact day the birth will occur.

During the third trimester an expectant mother may say "I am going to be a mother" as she prepares for the infant (Table 8-1). Providing clothing and a place for the infant to sleep and negotiating the sharing of household tasks with her partner are among the plans made at this time. In addition, many couples complete childbirth education classes at this time (see Chapter 11).

Check Your Reading

1. Why might an expectant mother say "I am pregnant" during the first trimester and "I am going to be a mother" late in pregnancy?
2. How might pregnancy affect sexual responses of the mother and father?

Table 8-1
PROGRESSIVE CHANGES IN MATERNAL RESPONSES TO PREGNANCY

First Trimester	Second Trimester	Third Trimester
Emotional Response		
Uncertainty, ambivalence, focus on self	Wonder, increased narcissim, introversion, concern about body and changes in sexuality	Vulnerability, increased dependence, acceptance that fetus is separate but totally dependent
Physical Validation		
No obvious signs of fetal growth	Quickening	Obvious fetal growth, discomfort, decreased maternal activity
Role		
May begin to seek safe passage for self and fetus	Seeks acceptance of fetus and her role as mother	Prepares for birth
"Self" Statement		
"I am pregnant."	"I am going to have a baby."	"I am going to be a mother."

Maternal Role Transition

Becoming a mother involves more than giving birth and providing physical care for the newborn. Mothering also involves intense feelings of love, tenderness, and devotion that endure over a lifetime. How does a woman learn to be a mother?

The transition into mothering begins during pregnancy and increases with gestational age. An early task of pregnancy is to accept the intrusion of the fetus, then move to developing love for the child as an independent being (Mercer & Ferketich, 1994a). The greatest increase in maternal-fetal attachment seems to occur after quickening, which is when the mother begins to differentiate herself from the fetus (Bloom, 1995). A pregnant woman prepares for becoming a mother by contemplating her life as a woman with a child. She thinks about the characteristics she wishes to have as a mother and anticipates life changes that will be necessary.

Steps in Maternal Role Taking

Rubin (1984) observed specific steps that provide a framework for understanding the process of maternal role taking: mimicry, role play, fantasy, the search for a role fit, and grief work.

Mimicry

Mimicry involves women observing and copying the behavior of other women who are pregnant or mothers in an earnest attempt to discover the characteristics of the role. Mimicry often begins in the first trimester when the woman may prematurely wear maternity clothes to understand the feelings of women in more advanced pregnancy and see others' reactions to her. She may also mimic the waddling gait or posture of a woman who is close to delivery long before these changes are necessary for her.

Role Play

Role play consists of acting out some aspect of actual maternal actions. The pregnant woman searches for opportunities to hold or care for infants in the presence of another person. She does this to evaluate not only her comfort in the situation but also the response of the observer. Role playing gives her an opportunity to "practice" the expected role and receive validation from the observer. She is particularly sensitive to the responses of her partner and her own mother.

Fantasy

Fantasies allow the woman to try a variety of possibilities and daydream or "try on" a variety of behaviors. Fantasies often concern the infant's gender, physical and psychological traits, behavior, and the effect on all family members (Sorenson & Schuelke, 1999). The woman may daydream about taking her child to the park or holding, reading to, or playing music to the child. She may also have vivid dreams at night.

At times, fantasies are fearful. What happens if something is wrong with the infant? What if the baby cries and will not stop? Fearful fantasies often provoke a pregnant woman to respond to the fears by seeking information or reassurance. For instance, she may ask her partner if he will love the baby even if it is not perfect, or she may strive to learn all she can about caring for a baby that is difficult to console.

Fantasies may change during each trimester and may be different for primigravidas and multigravidas. Women have the most frequent fantasies during the third trimester. Listening to women's fantasies helps the nurse show the woman acceptance and understanding. In addition, it provides a means of identifying potential concerns that may need further discussion.

The Search for a Role Fit

The search for a role fit is a process that occurs once the woman has built up a set of role expectations for herself and internalized a view of the behavior of a "good" mother. She then observes the behaviors of mothers and compares them with her own expectations of herself. She imagines herself acting in the same way and either rejects or accepts the behaviors, depending on how well they fit her idea of what is right. This process implies that the woman has explored the role of mother long enough to have developed a sense of herself in the role and to be able to select behaviors that reaffirm her idea of fulfilling the role.

Grief Work

Although grief work seems incongruous with maternal role taking, women often experience a sense of sadness when they realize that they must give up certain aspects of their previous selves and can never go back. A mother will never again be a carefree woman without a child. She must relinquish some of her old patterns of behavior so that she can move into the new identity as mother of an infant. Even simple things such as going shopping or to the movies will require planning to include the infant or finding alternative care. Changes may be particularly difficult for the adolescent mother, who is unused to planning and may have to give up or change school plans as well.

Maternal Tasks of Pregnancy

To become mothers, pregnant women spend a great deal of time and energy learning new behaviors. In addition, as a woman works to establish a relationship with the infant, she must also reorder her relationship with her partner and family. This psychological work of pregnancy has been grouped into four maternal tasks of pregnancy: (1) seeking safe passage for herself and baby through pregnancy, labor, and childbirth; (2) securing acceptance of the baby and herself by her partner and family; (3) learning to give of herself; and (4) developing attachment and interconnection with the unknown child (Rubin, 1984).

Seeking Safe Passage

Seeking safe passage for herself and her baby is the woman's primary task. If she cannot be assured of that safety, she cannot move on to the other tasks. Behaviors that ensure safe passage include seeking the care of a physician or certified nurse-midwife and following recommendations about diet, vitamins, rest, and subsequent visits to the office or clinic.

In addition, the pregnant woman must adhere to cultural practices that ensure the safety of herself and the infant. For instance, some Southeast Asian women avoid contact with scissors and knives because they fear sharp instruments may cause cleft lip or spontaneous abortion (Mattson & Lew, 1995).

Securing Acceptance

Securing acceptance is a process that begins in the first trimester and continues throughout pregnancy. The process involves reworking relationships so that the important persons in the family accept the woman in the role of mother and welcome the baby into the family constellation. For example, she and the father of the baby must give up an exclusive relationship and make a place in their lives for a child. The woman feels valued and comforted when her partner expresses pride and joy in the pregnancy. This feeling is so important that many women retain a memory of the partner's reaction to the announcement of pregnancy for many years. Women with supportive partners are more likely to report the pregnancy as wanted (Kroelinger & Oths, 2000).

Obtaining acceptance from others also helps the woman focus on the physical needs of pregnancy. Support by the father has been correlated with adequacy of prenatal care. Other sources of social support, such as relatives and friends, are associated with improved prenatal health behaviors (Schaffer & Lia-Hoagberg, 1997).

Women's childhood relationships with their own mothers have been shown to be particularly important in the development of maternal attachment (Mercer & Ferketich, 1994a). The pregnant woman gains energy and contentment when acceptance and support are freely offered by her mother (Figure 8-3).

Problems may occur if the family strongly desires a child with particular characteristics and the woman feels that the family may reject an infant who does not meet the criteria. For example, if family members wish for a boy, will they accept a girl? Women who receive unconditional acceptance experience the least anxiety (Mercer, 1990).

Learning to Give of Herself

Giving is one of the most idealized components of motherhood, but it also must be learned. Learning to give begins in pregnancy when the woman allows her body to give space and nurturing to the fetus. She also observes giving in others and then tests her own ability to derive pleasure from giving. This test most often takes the form of providing food or care for her family. Their acceptance and enjoyment of the "gift" enhance her pleasure and strengthen the role. She may explore further by making and giving small gifts to friends, especially those who are pregnant, and she feels pride and delight when the gift is appreciated.

Pregnant women also learn to give by receiving. Gifts received at "baby showers" are more than needed items. They also confirm continued interest and com-

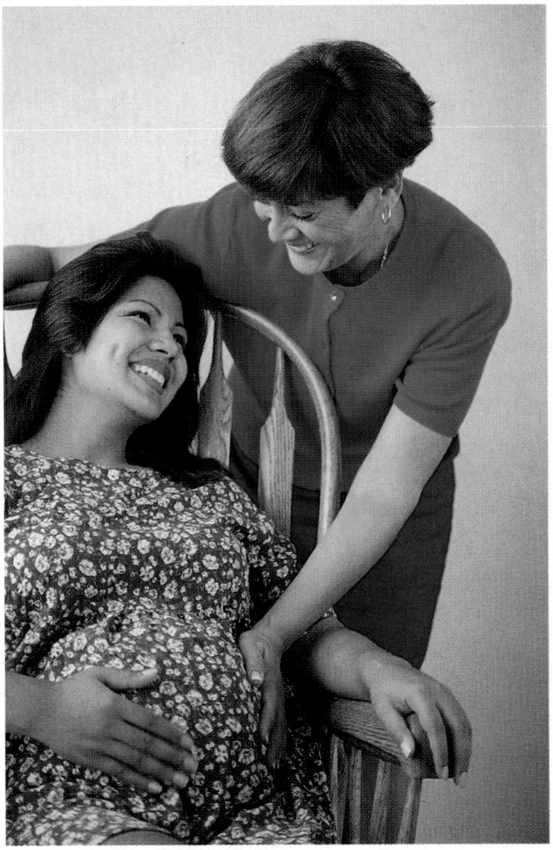

FIGURE 8-3 The bond between a pregnant woman and her own mother is particularly important to the young mother.

mitment from friends and family and enhance the ability of the woman to give. Intangible gifts from others, such as companionship, attention, and support, help increase her energy and affirm the importance of giving.

Committing Herself to the Unknown Child

The process of attachment begins in early pregnancy when the woman accepts or "binds in" to the idea that she is pregnant, although the baby is not yet real to her. During the second trimester the baby becomes real when quickening occurs, and feelings of love and attachment surge. A special, exclusive relationship develops between the woman and fetus that simulates a secret, romantic love.

Mothers report feedback from their unborn infants during the third trimester and describe unique characteristics of the fetus with regard to sleep-wake cycles, temperament, and communication. Love of the infant becomes possessive and leads to feelings of vulnerability. The woman integrates the role of mother into her image of herself. She becomes comfortable with the idea of herself as mother and finds pleasure in contemplating the new role (Mercer & Ferketich, 1994b). Her unconditional acceptance of the infant is an important accomplishment by the third trimester (Mullaly, 2000).

Check Your Reading

3. What does "looking for a fit" mean in role transition?
4. Why is grief work part of maternal role transition?
5. How does the pregnant woman seek safe passage for herself and the baby?

PATERNAL ADAPTATION

Expectant fathers do not experience the biologic processes of pregnancy, but they also must make major psychosocial changes to adapt to a new role. These changes may be more difficult because the male partner is often neglected by both the health care team and his peer group when attention is focused on the woman.

Variations in Paternal Adaptation

Wide variations exist in paternal responses to pregnancy. Some men are emotionally invested and comfortable as full partners and wish to explore every aspect of pregnancy, childbirth, and parenting. Others are more task oriented and view themselves as managers. They may direct the woman's diet and rest periods and act as coaches during childbirth but remain detached from the emotional components. Other men are more comfortable as observers and prefer not to participate. Some men are culturally conditioned to see pregnancy and childbirth as "women's work" and may not be able to express their true feelings about pregnancy and fatherhood.

Research indicates that a stable relationship with their partners, financial security, and a sense of closure to the childless part of the couple's relationship contribute to readiness for fatherhood (Tiller, 1995). Additional factors influencing a man's adaptation to pregnancy and childbirth include his relationship with his own father, previous experience with children, and confidence in his ability to care for the infant.

Developmental Processes

The responses of the expectant father are dynamic, progressing through phases that are subject to individual variation. Jordan (1990) describes three developmental processes that an expectant father must address:

- Grappling with the reality of pregnancy and the new child
- Struggling for recognition as a parent from his family and social network
- Making an effort to be seen as relevant to childbearing

The Reality of Pregnancy and the Child

The pregnancy and the child must become real before a man can take on the identity of father. The process

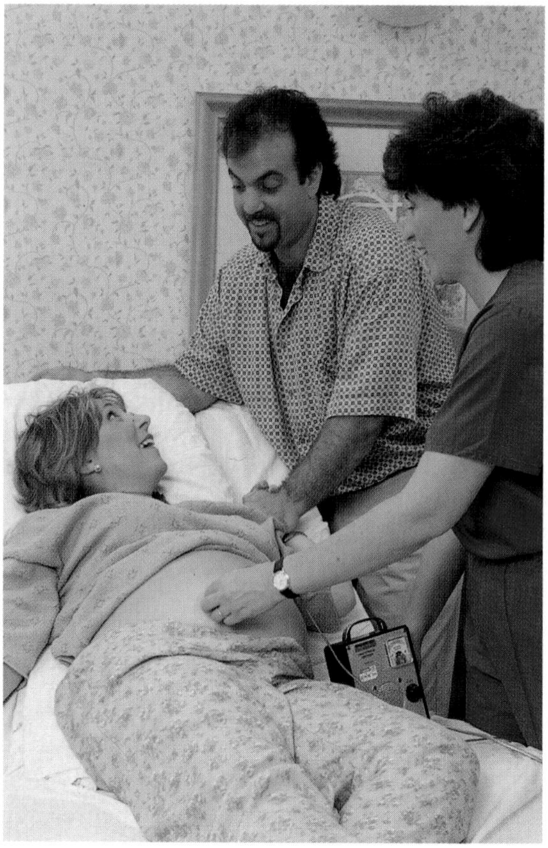

FIGURE 8-4 The existence of the fetus becomes real (a reality booster) for the father when he hears the fetal heartbeat through the transducer.

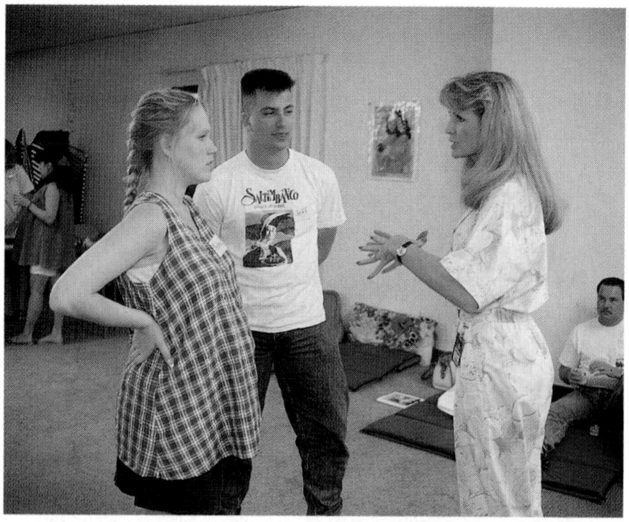

FIGURE 8-5 The nurse who views the mother-father-child as one client provides parents with the greatest opportunity to learn infant care and parenting skills.

requires time and is often incomplete until the birth. Initially, the pregnancy is a diagnosis only, and changes in the expectant woman's behavior, such as nausea and fatigue, are perceived as symptoms of illness that have little to do with having a baby.

A man's initial reaction to the announcement of pregnancy may be pride and joy, but he often experiences the same ambivalence that his partner experiences, particularly if he is unprepared for the added responsibility or commitment. Various experiences act as catalysts or "reality boosters" that make the child more real (Figure 8-4). The most frequently mentioned experiences are hearing the baby's heartbeat, feeling the infant move, and seeing the fetus on a sonogram. Once they can feel the fetus move, many expectant fathers invent a nickname and talk to the fetus. Almost all describe specific behaviors of their unborn child (Ferketich & Mercer, 1995).

Preparing the nursery or a space in the home and accumulating supplies for the new addition also reinforce the reality of the forthcoming child. These tasks often represent the first time that the expectant father has the opportunity to do something for the child directly. The birth itself is the most powerful "reality booster," and the infant becomes real to the father when he has an opportunity to see and hold the infant.

The Struggle for Recognition as a Parent

Men are often viewed by others as helpmates but not parents in their own right. During pregnancy and childbirth, their primary responsibility is to support their partners. Many men are upset that their feelings are seldom validated and that they may not be recognized as parents as well as helpers. Some men accept that the focus should be on their partners, but others are frustrated by the lack of understanding of their own experiences.

Expectant mothers play an important role in helping their partners gain recognition as parents. Women who openly share their physical sensations and emotions help their partners to feel that they are part of the process. These women often refer to it as "our" pregnancy and "our" child rather than as "my" pregnancy or "my" child. They also insist on including their partners in all discussions and decisions.

Nurses must learn to view the mother-father-child as the client and not focus exclusively on the mother and fetus. Men may be concerned about the physical symptoms experienced by expectant mothers. The nurse should encourage men to ask questions about their partners' pregnancies. These men are entitled to as much advice and reassurance as expectant women (Figure 8-5).

The Role of the Involved Father

Men use various means to create parenting roles that are comfortable for them. They may seek closer ties with their own fathers to reminisce about their own childhoods. They may fantasize about their relationships with their children as they grow up. Some men change their self-images and even their appearances to fit their new images (Mullaly, 2000).

Expectant fathers also observe men who are already fathers and "try on" fathering behaviors to determine whether they are comfortable and fit their own concepts of the father role. In addition, many men assertively seek information about infant care and growth and development so that they will be prepared for their new responsibilities.

Parenting Information

Studies indicate that fathers believe they receive inadequate parenting information in prenatal classes (Tiller, 1995). Although adequate information is usually presented, fathers may not be ready for the information at the time it is provided. As a result, they may be unprepared to care for their infants and have unrealistic expectations of newborns. Nurses must review information about infant care and growth and development after birth when the information is immediately relevant.

Couvade

The term *couvade* refers to pregnancy-related symptoms and behavior in expectant fathers. In primitive cultures, couvade took the form of rituals involving special dress, confinement, limitations of physical work, avoidance of certain foods, sexual restraint, and in some instances, performance of "mock labor."

In modern practice, expectant fathers sometimes experience physical symptoms similar to those experienced by pregnant women, such as loss of appetite, nausea and vomiting, headache, fatigue, and weight gain. Symptoms may be caused by stress, anxiety, or empathy for the pregnant partner. Although the symptoms are almost always unobserved by the health care team, anticipatory guidance is beneficial for both partners.

Check Your Reading

6. What are "reality boosters"? Why are they important for the expectant father's adjustment?
7. How can nurses help men in their struggle for recognition as parents?
8. Why should information relating to newborn care presented in prenatal classes be repeated after the infant is born?

ADAPTATION OF GRANDPARENTS

The initial reaction of grandparents depends on several factors such as their ages, the number and spacing of other grandchildren, and their perceptions of the role of grandparents.

Age

Age is a major determining factor in the emotional responses of prospective grandparents. By the time they become grandparents, many people have already dealt with their feelings about aging and react with joy when they find they are to become grandparents. They look forward to being able to love grandchildren, who signify the continuity of life and family.

Younger grandparents may not be happy with the stereotype of grandparents as older persons. They may experience conflict when they must resolve their self-image with the stereotype. They often have career responsibilities and may not be accessible because of the continuing demands of their own lives.

Number and Spacing of Other Grandchildren

The number and spacing of other grandchildren determine grandparents' reactions. A first grandchild may be an exciting event that creates great joy. If the grandparents already have other grandchildren, another may be welcomed, but the excitement is often less than for the first grandchild. The subdued reaction may be disappointing to the couple, who may desire the same excited reaction as that expressed for the first grandchild.

Perceptions of the Role of Grandparents

Grandparents' beliefs about their importance to grandchildren vary widely. Many grandparents see their relationships with grandchildren as second in importance only to the parent-child relationship. They want to be involved in the pregnancy, and grandmothers often engage in rituals such as shopping and gift-giving showers that confirm their role as important participants. Many grandparents are intimately involved in child care and offer unconditional love to the child. They offer to care for older children while the mother gives birth, and they assist during the first weeks after childbirth.

In the past, grandparents were often looked to for advice about childbearing and child rearing. Health care workers have become the "experts," and many grandparents have difficulty adjusting to this change. If the issue is not recognized, distance may develop as the grandparents withdraw, sensing that their participation is no longer valued. Other grandparents worry about their lack of familiarity with modern ways of childbearing and parenting.

> Nurses can assist families to verbalize their feelings with statements such as "It may seem that the grandparents aren't interested in the baby, but that may not be their real feeling. Perhaps they are uneasy about what their role should be and being responsible for care of the child. If you let them know that you will care for the baby but want them to share in the joy the child brings, they may be less concerned."

On the other hand, some contemporary grandparents plan little participation in pregnancy or child care. A frequently heard comment is "I have raised my children, and I don't plan to do it again." This attitude often results in conflict with the parents, who are hurt and wish for the grandparents' help during the third trimester and after the birth.

Parents and grandparents may need to negotiate ways in which the grandparents can be involved without feeling that they must assume care of the child. For instance, the couple may need suggestions to help the grandparents participate in family gatherings that do not involve baby-sitting or child care (see Chapter 11).

ADAPTATION OF SIBLINGS

Toddlers

Sibling adaption to the birth of an infant depends largely on age and developmental level. Very young children (2 years or younger) are unaware of the maternal changes occurring during pregnancy and are unable to understand that a new brother or sister is going to be born. Because toddlers have little perception of time, many parents delay telling them that a baby is expected until shortly before the birth.

Although preparing very young children for the birth of a baby is difficult, the nurse can make suggestions that may prove helpful. Any changes in sleeping arrangements should be made several weeks before the birth so that the child does not feel displaced by the new baby. Parents can prepare family and friends for the toddler's feelings of jealousy and resentment when the young child must share time and attention with a baby.

Until children feel secure in the affection of their parents, expecting 2-year-olds to welcome a new "stranger" is not realistic. Frequent reassurances of parental love and affection are of primary importance. The parents can be taught to accept strong feelings that the toddler expresses, such as anger, jealousy, and frustration, without judgment and to continue to reinforce the child's feelings of being loved (see Chapter 18).

Older Children

Older children are more aware of changes in the mother's body that show a baby is to be born. They may be interested in observing the mother's abdomen, feeling the fetus move, and listening to the heartbeat. They may have questions about the way the fetus develops, the way it started, and the way it will get out of the abdomen. Although they look forward to the baby's arrival, they may expect the infant to be a full-fledged playmate and may be shocked when the infant is small and helpless.

School-age children benefit from being included in preparations for the new baby. They enjoy following the development of the fetus, preparing space for the infant to sleep, and accumulating supplies the infant will need. The children should be encouraged to feel the fetus move, and many come close to the mother's abdomen and talk to the fetus. Older children also gain a sense of security and enjoy time alone with parents (Figure 8-6).

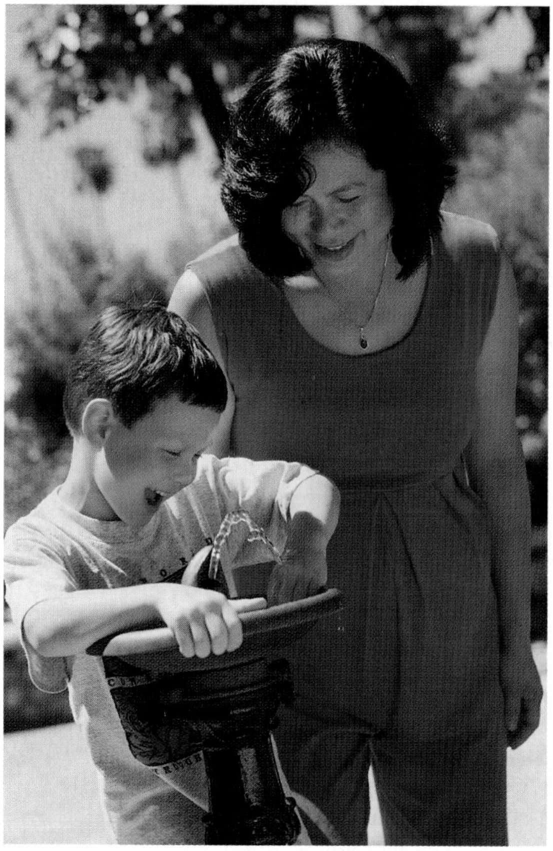

FIGURE 8-6 A pregnant woman who spends time with an older child can provide affection and a sense of security.

Young children (3 years and older) can benefit from sibling classes. They are encouraged to bring a doll to simulate caring for the infant. The classes also provide an opportunity for them to discuss what changes the new baby will mean for the family (see Chapter 11).

In some settings, children as young as 3 years old are permitted to be with the mother during childbirth. If young children are to be present, they should attend a class that prepares them for the event. During the birth a familiar person should be available to explain what is taking place and to comfort or remove them if events become overwhelming.

Adolescents

The response of adolescents also depends on their developmental level. Some adolescents are embarrassed because the pregnancy confirms the continued sexuality of their parents. They may be repelled by the obvious physical changes. Many adolescents are immersed in their own developmental tasks that involve loosening ties to their parents and coming to terms with their own sexuality. They may be indifferent to the pregnancy unless it directly affects them or their activities. Other adolescents become very involved and want to help with preparations for the baby.

Check Your Reading

9. What determines the response of grandparents to the pregnancy?
10. How does the response to pregnancy differ for a toddler, a preschool child, and an adolescent?
11. How can parents prepare siblings for the addition of a newborn to the family?

FACTORS INFLUENCING PSYCHOSOCIAL ADAPTATIONS

Age

Pregnancy presents a challenge for teenagers who, as expectant parents, must cope with the conflicting developmental tasks of pregnancy and adolescence at the same time. The major developmental task of adolescence is to form and become comfortable with a sense of self. On the other hand, one of the major tasks of pregnancy involves learning to "give of self," a process that includes sacrificing personal desires for the benefit of the fetus. Giving is particularly difficult for young adolescents, who may not be able to perceive the fetus as real (Bloom, 1995).

Nurses who work with pregnant teenagers should help them adjust to their changing bodies and the increasing presence of the developing fetus. Adolescents also need prompting to follow a lifestyle that promotes the best outcomes for them and their infants (see Chapter 24).

Absence of a Partner

The proportion of single women who become pregnant is increasing. Although some unmarried women have the financial and emotional support of a partner, many do not. These women have unique concerns, especially in the first and second trimesters. For instance, they experience more stress about telling their family and friends about the pregnancy. They may have to enlist more social support to substitute for that of a partner. They may have legal concerns such as whom to list as the father on birth records and what arrangements must be made to allow paternal contact with the infant.

Single women without partners often live below the poverty level. They are more likely to delay prenatal care until the second or third trimester and are at increased risk for pregnancy complications and delivery of a low-birth-weight infant.

Nurses must recognize the single mother's needs for accessible and affordable prenatal care. In addition, nurses must be prepared to offer specialized supportive care for single mothers. Necessary social services may include Medicaid, food stamps, and transportation to the prenatal clinic.

Some women are single by choice and may have been inseminated to achieve pregnancy. These women usually have fewer financial concerns because the pregnancy is planned. Like other single mothers, the presence of support persons in their lives will be an important determinant in their adaptations to pregnancy (Mullaly, 2000).

Multiparity

The assumption that a multipara needs less help than a first-time mother is inaccurate. Pregnancy tasks are actually much more complex for the multipara than for the primigravida. When dealing with the task of negotiating safe passage for herself and the infant, the multipara does not have time to take special care of herself as she did during the first pregnancy. She is more likely to experience fatigue and may have serious worries about the children accepting the infant and finding time and energy for additional responsibilities. When seeking acceptance of the new baby, the multipara may find the family less excited than they were for the first child. The couple's celebration is also more subdued.

The woman spends a great deal of time working out a new relationship with the first child, who often becomes demanding. This behavior may foster feelings of guilt as she tries to expand her love to include the second child. Developing attachment for the coming baby is hampered by feelings of loss between herself and the first child. She senses that the child is growing up and away from her, and she may grieve for the loss of their special relationship.

CRITICAL THINKING EXERCISE

Emma H., a 24-year-old gravida 2 of 32 weeks' gestation, appears apathetic and tired when she arrives at the prenatal clinic. She states that she is concerned about whether her 2-year-old son will accept the new baby and sometimes feels guilty that she is having this baby so soon.

Sara N., age 28, also has a prenatal visit. She is in her twenty-eighth week of pregnancy and has children who are 2, 4, and 6 years old.

QUESTIONS:

1. How will the concerns of these multiparas differ from those of a primipara?
2. How might the tasks of pregnancy differ between the two women?
3. What measures can each mother take to prepare other children before the new baby arrives?

Table 8-2
IMPACT OF SOCIOECONOMIC FACTORS ON FAMILY'S RESPONSE TO PREGNANCY

Affluent	Middle Class	Working Poor and Unemployed	New Poor
RESOURCES			
Is confident of ability, has financial protection from economic fluctuations, owns or rents home in a safe neighborhood, has health insurance or can pay for health care, able to provide enriched environment	Has relative security but fewer reserves and more debt, owns or rents home in relatively safe neighborhood, depends on employment for health insurance	Lacks skills and bargaining power, is most vulnerable to economic fluctuations, struggles for basic needs	Was previously self-sufficient but has lost prior resources, may have recently lost job and insurance, is unused to public assistance
VALUE PLACED ON HEALTH CARE			
Values preventive care	Values health care but must rely on health insurance related to employment	May value health care but often does not see a way to improve situation	Values health care but may no longer have finances to access it
TIME ORIENTATION			
Seeks prenatal care early	Is future oriented and seeks early prenatal care, makes plans to provide best possible care and education for children	Meets present needs first, but often seeks prenatal care late, has an uncertain future	Has a middle-class time orientation but must meet present needs, may begin prenatal care late

Nurses must remember that multiparas may need more help and understanding than primigravidas. The nurse cannot assume that the process is "old hat" and that information about labor, breastfeeding, and infant care is not needed. Special assistance may be necessary to help a multipara integrate an additional infant into the family structure.

Socioeconomic Status

One of the greatest influences on childbearing practices is the socioeconomic status of the family (Table 8-2). *Socioeconomic status* refers to the resources of the family to meet the needs for food, shelter, and health care. Socioeconomic status can be divided into the affluent, middle class, working poor, and new poor.

The Affluent

Affluent families have resources to provide for their needs and purchase health care. They have a good income, secure shelter in a safe neighborhood, and the education and reserves to protect themselves from economic fluctuations. They are able to provide an enriched environment for children, and they can pay for health care through either private means or insurance.

The affluent family's attitudes toward health care reflect their ability to pay. They believe they deserve the best in health care and respect from health care providers, and they expect to be active participants in their care. They are future oriented and thus value preventive care. In general, they seek early, regular antepartum care and comply with recommendations of the health care providers.

The Middle Class

The middle class comprises the largest group of families in the United States. In fact, most health care workers fit into this class. Although these families do not have the reserves of the affluent, they generally are able to rent or own their homes in relatively safe neighborhoods. They have adequate food and either education or skills that assist them to obtain and keep jobs for long periods. They often share child care with family and neighbors and develop a network of people who rely on each other for support and assistance.

Middle-class families rely on group insurance, obtained as part of their salaries, to shield themselves from exorbitant health care costs. A major concern is loss of a job that results in loss of health insurance.

These families are future oriented and seek health care early in pregnancy. They prepare for the birth and make plans to provide for their children's security and education.

The Working Poor and Unemployed

The working poor and unemployed include unskilled or unemployed workers who live with a great deal of uncertainty. They work for low wages and are often the last hired and the first fired. They often live below the

NURSING CARE PLAN 8-2

Socioeconomic Problems during Pregnancy

Assessment: Theresa Matheny, a 19-year-old primigravida, is seen for initial prenatal care at 24 weeks of gestation. She took the day off from work in a factory and rode the bus to the clinic. She is currently living with an unmarried sister who receives Temporary Assistance for Needy Families. During the interview, Theresa states that she will not be able to keep clinic appointments because she cannot afford to take more time off until the baby comes. She is unmarried and states that the father of the baby is "gone." She says that she is healthy and only needs to find someone to deliver the baby.

Nursing Diagnosis: Risk for Altered Health Maintenance related to lack of a plan to obtain regular prenatal care and knowledge deficit of the importance of care.

Expected Outcomes:
During the first prenatal visit, Theresa will do the following:
1. Verbalize a plan for regular prenatal care.
2. Describe the benefits of regular prenatal care.

Intervention	Rationale
1. Emphasize the reasons regular prenatal care is essential: a. To monitor the growth and development of the baby b. To evaluate Theresa's health, which directly affects the health of the fetus c. To detect problems and intervene before they become severe.	1. Preventive care is often not a priority when the client has conflicting needs for food and shelter. Many women are unaware that some complications such as pregnancy-induced hypertension and gestational diabetes, which may be detected and treated in early pregnancy, are serious hazards if they remain undetected.
2. Assist Theresa in devising a plan to obtain regular prenatal care: a. Provide her with a list of prenatal clinics near her home or place of work and the hours they are open b. Discuss transportation services and determine whether family or friends can help her keep prenatal appointments. c. Explore dates, times, and alternatives until she finds a schedule that works for her d. Obtain a list of phone numbers (e.g., friends, family, employer) where she can be reached for follow-up.	2. Some clinics are open on weekends and evenings to accommodate working women. Unreliable transporation is a major reason for failure to keep scheduled appointments, and clinic schedules that allow some flexibility are helpful. Interest in a client's individual situation is highly motivating for her to find a way to continue prenatal care.

Evaluation: Theresa shows interest in finding a way to have regular prenatal care. She makes an appointment for the next visit. If she misses scheduled appointments, follow-up phone calls to arrange alternative appointments may be necessary.

Critical Thinking: Although this diagnosis addresses Theresa's problem with managing prenatal care, what additional assessments should be made to determine the way she is managing the psychosocial concerns of pregnancy? What additional nursing diagnosis might be relevant?

Answer: The nurse should assess Theresa's progress with the tasks of pregnancy. She has made the first step in seeking safe passage, but other tasks need attention, such as securing the acceptance of her family and learning to give of herself. In addition, signs that she is developing attachment for the fetus are particularly important. An additional nursing diagnosis might be Risk for Altered Parenting related to lack of support from significant others or the presence of financial stress.

poverty level and barely have enough to survive. Many have difficulty meeting the basic needs for food and shelter, and some become homeless families. They have few financial resources, and their limited skills give them little bargaining power.

Attitudes related to health care differ from those of the more affluent (Nursing Care Plan 8-2). Because of economic uncertainty, they place more emphasis on meeting present needs rather than future goals. As a result, they place less value on preventive (future-oriented) care. This often causes them to postpone prenatal care until the second or even the third trimester.

The New Poor

The new poor comprise an expanding group of individuals and families who were previously self-sufficient but are now without resources because of such circumstances as loss of a job or health care insurance. These people must find their way into a health care system that is unfamiliar and frightening.

The values of the new poor are those of the middle class: self-sufficiency, hard work, and pride in their ability to succeed. Seeking public assistance is very difficult for this group. These families are devastated when they encounter the lack of respect and rudeness that may occur when some health care workers interact with families unable to pay for health care.

Barriers to Prenatal Care

The value of prenatal care has been extensively documented. Women who receive inadequate prenatal care are more likely to have poor pregnancy outcomes such as higher rates of low-birth-weight babies and increased infant mortality rates. However, women's access to prenatal care is limited by financial, systemic, and attitudinal barriers.

Financial barriers are one of the most important factors limiting prenatal care. Many women have either no insurance or insufficient insurance to cover maternity care. Although Medicaid finances prenatal care for indigent women, the enrollment process is so burdensome that some women do not register (Maloni, et al., 1996). Others may not know ways to access this resource.

Systemic barriers include negative institutional practices that interfere with consistent care. For instance, women must often wait 6 to 8 weeks for their first visit. Prenatal visits are usually scheduled during daytime hours that conflict with working women's schedules. In addition, child care is rarely available, and women who must find child care are torn between being a mother and keeping clinic appointments.

An important barrier to health care results from the unsympathetic attitude of some health care workers toward those who are unable to pay for prenatal care. Poor families may experience long delays, hurried examinations, rudeness, and arrogance from members of the health care team in public clinics. Many pregnant women report waiting 3 to 4 hours for an examination that lasts only a few minutes. Many never see the same health care provider more than once. These women may not keep clinic appointments because they do not see the importance of the hurried examinations.

Nurses must understand the importance of treating each family with respect and consideration. They must insist that poor families who are unable to pay receive the same standard of care as families who can pay. To do this, nurses can work to determine which barriers apply to the clients with whom they work and find ways to meet the needs of the specific population being served. Scheduling prenatal visits in the evening or on weekends, setting aside times for walk-in prenatal visits, and offering other services such as applications for Medicaid and the Women, Infants, and Children Supplemental Food Program (WIC) might increase use of prenatal services (Beckmann, Buford, & Witt, 2000).

Some women may not obtain early prenatal care because they do not want the pregnancy confirmed, do not want anyone to know about the pregnancy, or are considering an abortion. One study found that only 17.5% of women who did not want to be pregnant began prenatal care during the first trimester. Poor housing and use of substances also decreased early prenatal care (Pagnini & Reichman, 2000). Women who are depressed and those who do not believe their actions influence the health of the fetus are also less likely to be concerned about health behaviors such as eating well and avoiding smoking and alcohol use (Walker, Cooney, & Riggs, 1999).

Many women rely on advice from family and friends during pregnancy, and some do not believe that prenatal care is important, especially when they have no obvious problems with the pregnancy. Other reasons may include the lack of child care, inability to take time off from work for financial reasons and lack of job security, and lack of transportation.

Cultural Influences on Childbearing

More different cultural groups live in the United States than anywhere else in the world. Each culture has its own health and healing belief system for major life events such as pregnancy and childbirth. The success of health care depends on its ability to fit in with the beliefs of those being served. Therefore ignorance of culturally divergent beliefs may lead to failure in health care delivery. Some groups with beliefs that differ significantly from those of the dominant culture include Native Americans, Hindus (largely from India), Muslims, and Filipinos.

Culturally Divergent Groups

Southeast Asians are a large group of immigrants from Cambodia, Vietnam, and Laos. Another large group, Latinos, comes directly or has ancestry from Mexico, Puerto Rico, Cuba, El Salvador, the Dominican Republic, and other Latin American countries. The term *Latino* indicates common background in Spanish language and customs but is not accepted by all groups. Some prefer Hispanic, Mexican-American, Chicano, or La Raza (the race).

The term *African-American* includes those with a common background in African languages and customs. Generalizations about the cultural aspects of pregnancy for African-Americans are particularly difficult. Many have been in the United States for generations, and their health beliefs do not differ significantly from those held by whites. New immigrants from Africa, however, often retain some of the cultural beliefs of their countries of origin.

Differences within Cultures

Wide variations of beliefs and practices exist within each culture, and nurses must recognize that not all people sharing a culture have identical beliefs. Those who have lived in Western societies for years or generations often do not exhibit behaviors prescribed by their cultures. Nurses must be careful not to stereotype families or expect a certain set of behaviors from every family in a particular cultural group. Individual differences are as important as cultural variations.

Cultural Differences Causing Conflict

Cultural differences that cause conflict between health care workers and families during pregnancy are observed most often in the areas of health care beliefs, communication, and time orientation.

Health Beliefs

For many cultures, health is the balance of mind, body, and spirit. Health-promoting behaviors are the actions used in each of these dimensions to maintain health, prevent illness, and restore health (Spector, 2000).

Health Maintenance. Practices to maintain health include wearing proper clothing, which is believed by some Latina women to ensure a safe birth. Although Korean women often follow a combination of western and traditional practices, they may follow taekyo, or prenatal care of the fetus through rituals and taboos. This includes avoidance of unclean things because they might result in a difficult childbirth (Howard & Berbiglia, 1997). Women must avoid contact with illness and death in many cultures and may not attend funerals during pregnancy. They also must surround themselves with beautiful things and positive people (Shilling, 2000). Guatemalan women believe that strong emotions such as anger will affect the fetus (Callister & Vega, 1998). Other examples include a specific diet for pregnancy (see Chapter 9). For instance, women from Southeast Asia may eat rice daily. Many groups also believe that concentration, silence, prayer, and meditation maintain mental and spiritual health.

Belief in Fate. Some cultures (such as Southeast Asian, Middle Eastern) promote a strong belief in fate. Women often believe that the only way in which they can affect the outcome of pregnancy is by eating correctly and observing the taboos of their culture. Because of this belief, getting women to seek early and regular prenatal care is sometimes difficult. In addition, women in many cultures do not seek early prenatal care because they view childbearing as normal rather than something requiring care by a physician.

Preventing Illness. Practices that prevent illness include the use of protective religious objects and charms, such as amulets and talismans. Some women also believe that certain foods can prevent illness. For instance, people in many cultures eat raw garlic or onion or adhere to numerous food taboos and prescribed combinations of foods. Strict adherence to religious codes, morals, and practices is also believed to prevent illness.

Modesty. Fear, modesty, and a desire to avoid examination by men may keep some women from seeking health care during pregnancy. In many cultures (such as Muslim, Hindu, Latino), exposure of the genitals to men is considered demeaning. Nurses must remember that the reputations of women from these cultures depend on their demonstrated modesty. If necessary, female physicians or nurse practitioners can perform examinations. If this is not possible, the woman should be carefully draped with her legs completely covered. A female nurse needs to remain with the woman at all times. Obtaining permission from the husband may be necessary before any examination or treatment can be performed.

Female Genital Mutilation. Female genital mutilation is also called *female circumcision.* It involves clitoridectomy (removal of the clitoris and part of the labia minora) or infibulation (removal of the clitoris, labia minora, and all or part of the labia majora) and is usually performed at some time during childhood. The procedure is widely practiced in parts of Africa and some areas of the Middle East (AAP, 1998). The practice has been associated with premarital chastity and is a prerequisite for marriage in some African cultures. Female genital mutilation is illegal in some countries, including the United States.

Some women who have had the procedure now live in North America. Nurses and physicians must be knowledgeable about the custom and prepared for the woman to have abnormal-looking genitals. Pelvic examination is very painful because the introitus is so small and inelastic scar tissue makes the area especially sensitive.

Nurses must make sure that pelvic examinations are as comfortable as possible, maintaining utmost privacy, draping the woman to provide maximal coverage, and assisting her in locating a health care provider with whom she is comfortable. The woman may not give any verbal or nonverbal sign of pain, but this lack of response does not indicate an absence of pain.

Restoring Health. Traditional ways to restore health include natural folk medicine such as herbs and plants. Women may often use charms, holy words and actions, and traditional healers before seeking other medical advice. Latinas may consult with *curanderas* (faith healers), who work with women to keep a balance between hot and cold and to relieve them of their sins, which may be the basis for illness. Africans and Haitians may rely on folk medicine that includes witchcraft, voodoo, and magic.

To be certain that all essential information about folk medicine is obtained, nurses should inquire whether the client is taking folk remedies with questions such as "What do pregnant women take to protect themselves and the baby? How often and how much of this do you take? What special foods and drinks are important?"

Communication

Language. Language is a major barrier to health care. Numerous dialects within many languages can make it difficult to find competent interpreters. The ideal is to have trained interpreters that are preferably women. Other persons may be used if necessary, but considerations of confidentiality, the use of medical jargon, and the possible need to discuss sensitive issues indicate the need for professional interpreters.

Adults who came to the United States as children may speak English well and can interpret for their parents and grandparents. Other family members or friends, as well as co-workers in the clinic or hospital, may be helpful but not fluent. They may misunderstand instructions, particularly if medical jargon is used (Nursing Care Plan 8-3).

Most African-Americans speak English, but variations in pronunciation, grammar, and sentence structure may make communication difficult. The dialect spoken by African-Americans is sometimes labeled "Black English." Nurses who work with African-Americans must realize that English as spoken by African-Americans is a different dialect rather than an unacceptable form of English and avoid labeling and stereotyping those who speak it.

Nurses must also clarify the meaning of slang terms. For example, the words *chilly* and *chillin* imply sophistication, much like the Standard English slang use of the word *cool* (Cherry & Giger, 1999).

Communication Style. Styles in communication differ among cultures. For example, among Asians, nodding and smiling do not necessarily denote agreement or even understanding but simply mean "Yes, I hear you." When presenting information, the nurse should validate the person's understanding by requesting the listener to repeat the information: "Tell me what you understood" or "Show me what you learned."

Latinas are traditionally diplomatic and tactful. They frequently engage in "small talk" before bringing up questions they may have about their care. Nurses must remember that small talk is a valuable use of time. It establishes rapport and often helps to accomplish the goals of care.

Native Americans often converse in a low tone that may be difficult to hear in a noisy setting. They may consider note-taking taboo and expect the caregiver to remember what is said (Spector, 2000).

Eye Contact. Southeast Asians believe that eye contact shows disrespect (Mattson & Lew, 1995). Eye avoidance sometimes frustrates health care personnel who believe that eye contact denotes honesty. Eye behavior is also important when nurses deal with Latino infants and children. *Mal ojo* (evil eye) is a sudden unexplained illness that may occur when an individual with special powers admires a child too openly. Eye contact between a woman and man may be considered seductive by those from Middle Eastern cultures.

Touch. Touch is also an important component of communication. Some Native Americans avoid shaking hands but lightly touch the hand of the person they are greeting. In some cultures (such as Hindu, Muslim), touch by a woman other than the wife is offensive. In contrast, women from Haiti find touch supportive and reassuring, and gentle touch is particularly important during labor and birth. Nurses must remain sensitive to the response of the person being touched and should refrain from touching if the person indicates it is not welcomed.

Time Orientation

Time orientation can create conflict between health care professionals, who parcel out care in discrete units of time measured in minutes, and groups who keep time by the progress of the sun or seasons. Middle Eastern women, Latinas, and African-American women tend to emphasize the moment rather than the future. This attitude causes conflicts in a health care setting where tests or appointments are scheduled at particular times. If a woman does not place the same importance on keeping appointments, she may encounter anger and frustration in the health care setting that leaves her bewildered and ashamed.

Culturally Competent Nursing Care

Culturally competent nursing care requires an awareness of, sensitivity to, and respect for the diversity of the clients served. It involves assessment of the family's culture and cultural negotiation when necessary.

Cultural Assessment

Although nurses cannot know all the specific aspects of every culture, they must be aware of the predominant cultures seen in their practice area and become adept at performing cultural assessment. Some specific questions may elicit information that helps the nurse understand the family's beliefs about appropriate care during pregnancy:

- How will you and your family prepare for the baby?
- What concerns do you have about the pregnancy?
- What would provide the greatest assistance?

NURSING CARE PLAN 8-3

Language Barrier during Pregnancy

Assessment: Thuy Pham, a young Vietnamese primigravida of 26 weeks' gestation, speaks very little English. She listens quietly to the nurse's health care instructions, and although she appears confused, she asks no questions. Her husband, Bao Nguyen, nods and smiles frequently but has difficulty responding to questions about his wife's health.

Critical Thinking: Why must additional assessments be made before a nursing diagnosis can be formulated?

Answer: Nodding and smiling do not always mean that persons from Southeast Asia understand health teaching. Instead, these actions may simply indicate that the information has been heard or Mr. Nguyen is polite and does not want the nurse to feel inadequate as an instructor. Before assuming that Mr. Nguyen can translate health care teaching for his wife, the nurse must validate his learning by asking him to explain it himself.

Nursing Diagnosis: Impaired Verbal Communication related to foreign language barriers.

Expected Outcomes:
Throughout the pregnancy, the family will do the following:
1. Keep scheduled appointments.
2. Demonstrate ability to follow health care instructions.
3. Verbalize basic needs and concerns.

Intervention	Rationale
1. Assess the couple's ability to speak, read, and write in English and determine whether they are fluent in other languages.	1. People can often read a language better than they can speak it. Knowing that many Vienamese also speak Chinese or French helps locate an interpreter.
2. Obtain the assistance of a fluent interpreter. a. Establish a list of bilingual staff members in all areas of the facility who are willing to interpret and be educated about the importance of confidentiality and exactness. b. Enlist the aid of family members or friends who can interpret for the couple if a professional interpreter is not available. c. Use interpreters to develop written material in the most commonly spoken languages by making printed instructions for common teaching topics and using cards with common questions and answers.	2. A fluent interpreter is essential because Vietnamese persons do not always reveal when they do not understand instructions, which may hinder follow-up questions. Printed instructions reinforce information that was given verbally and may answer unasked questions. Communication cards convey interest in communicating and provide a means of eliciting basic information.
3. Speak quietly, and use the same interpreter whenever possible.	3. Soft speech protects the privacy and modesty of the patient. A natural response when people do not understand is to raise the voice, but this may convey impatience or anger.
4. Consider nonverbal factors when communicating. a. Speak slowly and smile. b. Keep an open posture. Avoid crossing the arms over the chest or turning away from the family. c. Determine Thuy's response to light touch on the arm, and either use or avoid touch depending on her response. d. Attend carefully to what the family says by nodding, leaning forward, or encouraging continued talk with frequent "uh huhs". e. Do not expect prolonged eye contact.	4. Even subtle body language can indicate interest and empathy or impatience, annoyance, or a desire to escape. Touch and eye contact are sensitive cultural variables, and nurses must be aware that they are not always welcomed.
5. Locate prenatal classes that are taught in Vietnamese. Explain what is included and encourage the couple to attend.	5. Information is more easily learned in a person's own language. Appropriate cultural concerns are likely to be discussed in classes taught in Vietnamese.

Evaluation: Thuy kept each prenatal appointment. She brought her husband or a friend with her to translate. She followed all recommendations and asked many questions.

- Where do you obtain most health care information?
- What foods are encouraged or discouraged?
- Where will the baby be born? Who will assist in the birth of the baby?
- Who will help you at home during the pregnancy and after birth?

Cultural Negotiation

Cultural negotiation involves providing information while acknowledging that the family may hold different views than the nurse. If the family indicates that the information would be helpful, it can be incorporated into the teaching plan.

> If the family indicates that the information is not helpful or is harmful in their opinion, the conflict must be acknowledged openly and clarified. "I sense that you are unsure of this. Help me understand your reluctance to try it." After allowing the family to express their beliefs, the nurse explains the reason the recommendation is valid and works with the family to find a compromise.

Cultural negotiation also involves sensitivity to specific concerns. For example, nurses must be aware of Islamic laws governing modesty when caring for Muslim women. Muslim women must cover their hair, body, arms to the wrist, and legs to the ankles at all times when in the presence of a man. She is not to be alone in the presence of a man other than her husband or a male relative.

Muslim women prefer a female health care provider and should be informed of the availability of female caregivers. Adequate drapes and covers should be available to allow covering all areas of the body except those that must be exposed for examination. In addition, the woman's husband, a female friend, or a male relative should be allowed to be present during examinations.

When talking to the woman's significant others, the nurse must be sure to call them by the correct name. For example, Vietnamese women do not usually change their names when they marry. Therefore the husband and wife will have different last names.

Check Your Reading

12. Why do many poor women delay seeking health care until the second or third trimester?
13. How do the attitudes of health care workers affect the care of poor families?
14. What are some cultural differences that may cause conflict between health care workers and clients?
15. What is meant by the term *cultural negotiation?*

APPLICATION OF THE NURSING PROCESS: PSYCHOSOCIAL CONCERNS

Assessment

The purpose of a psychosocial assessment is to monitor the adaptation of the family to pregnancy, which some consider a maturational "crisis" that requires a major transition in role function and relationships. Although not all agree that pregnancy is a crisis, it does initiate change and stress. The family's ability to cope is a primary concern. For some families, pregnancy offers the potential for growth. For others, an alteration in family processes requires guidance and information. More specific needs are discovered during a thorough psychosocial assessment (Table 8-3). Some data, such as age, gravida, para, and general health status, are obtained during the physical assessment.

Analysis

Critical thinking is extremely important when analyzing psychosocial data that may be open to several interpretations. Nurses must be careful to examine their own assumptions and biases about proper responses to pregnancy. They must resist the urge to form an opinion before obtaining adequate information. In addition, they must validate data, particularly when assessing clients of different cultural backgrounds.

Nursing diagnoses are based on data obtained during individual assessments and can vary among families (Table 8-4). Most families strive to maintain the health of the expectant mother and fetus and complete developmental tasks that allow the couple to become parents. Perhaps the most encompassing nursing diagnosis is "Family Coping: Potential for Growth," which relates to the readiness and desire to meet added family needs and assume parenting roles.

Planning

Goals related to family coping include the following:

- The family will verbalize emotional responses that are appropriate to each trimester.
- The family will verbalize methods that assist the expectant parents to complete the developmental processes of pregnancy.
- The family will identify cultural factors that may produce conflicts and collaborate to reduce those conflicts.

Interventions

Providing Information

Information and guidance is necessary to prepare prospective parents for the progressive changes that occur during pregnancy and reassure them that their feel-

Table 8-3

PSYCHOSOCIAL ASSESSMENT

Findings (Normal and Unusual)*	Sample Questions	Nursing Implications
PSYCHOLOGICAL RESPONSE		
First trimester: uncertainty, ambivalence, mood changes, self as primary focus Second trimester: wonder, joy, focus on fetus Third trimester: vulnerability, preparation for birth (fear, anger, apathy, lack of preparation)	"How do you and your partner feel about being pregnant?" "How will your lives change as a result of being pregnant?" "How do you feel about the changes in your body?" "What preparations have you made for the baby?"	Use active listening and reflection to establish a sense of trust. Reevaluate negative responses (fear, apathy, anger) in subsequent assessments.
AVAILABILITY OF RESOURCES		
Financial concerns (lack of funds or insurance), availability (family is geographically or emotionally unavailable) and response of grandparents, friends, and family	"What are your plans for prenatal care and birth?" "How do your parents feel about being grandparents?" "Who else can you depend on besides the family?" "Who provides strength when there is a problem?"	Determine adequate funds and refer to resources such as a public clinic for care and WIC for food. Help the couple discover alternative resources if the family is unavailable. Identify family conflicts early to allow time for resolution.
CHANGES IN SEXUAL PRACTICES		
Mutual satisfaction with changes (excessive concern with comfort or safety)	"How have sexual patterns or satisfaction changed?" "How do you cope with the changes?" "What concerns you most?"	Offer reassurance that intercourse is usually safe. Suggest alternative positions and open communication
EDUCATIONAL NEEDS		
Many questions about pregnancy, childbirth, and infant care (no questions, absence of interest in educational programs)	"How do you feel about caring for an infant?" "What are your major concerns?" "Whom do you count on for information?"	Respond to priority needs that are expressed. Refer couple to appropriate child and parenting classes.
CULTURAL INFLUENCES		
Ability of either the woman or her family to speak English or availability of fluent interpreters, culture influences support a healthy pregnancy and infant (harmful cultural beliefs or health practices)	"What foods are recommended during pregnancy?" "What practices are recommended?" "What is forbidden?" "What is most important to you in your care?" "How do your religious beliefs affect pregnancy?"	Locate fluent interpreters if needed. Avoid labeling beliefs as superstitions. Reinforce beliefs that promote a good pregnancy outcome. Elicit help from accepted source of information to overcome harmful practices.

* Findings that require additional assessment or intervention are shown in parentheses.

Table 8-4

COMMON NURSING DIAGNOSES USED IN PREGNANCY

*Risk for Altered Health Maintenance	* Impaired Verbal Communication
Altered Family Processes	Knowledge Deficit
Altered Role Performance	Personal Identity Disturbance
Altered Sexuality Patterns	Risk for Altered Parenting
* Body Image Disturbance	Risk for Injury
* Family Coping: Potential for Growth	Situational Low Self-Esteem
Impaired Home Maintenance Management	

* Nursing diagnoses explored in this chapter.

ings and behaviors are normal. Guidance also gives them an opportunity to ask questions and explore their feelings. Common subjects include:

- The emotional changes that occur during pregnancy (such as ambivalence, introversion, increased feelings of vulnerability)
- The developmental tasks of the mother (such as seeking safe passage, securing acceptance, forming an attachment with the unknown baby)
- Role transition (such as mimicry, role playing, fantasy, grief work)
- The developmental processes of the prospective father (such as grappling with the reality, struggling for recognition as a parent, creating the role of involved father)

Discussion of Resources

Initiate a discussion of the adequacy of the financial situation and support systems and help couples without financial resources or insurance coverage to obtain convenient prenatal care. This concern is particularly important for the new poor, who have little knowledge of gaining access to government-sponsored care. Emotional resources include those that assist the new family to adjust to the demands of pregnancy and parenting.

Discuss the responses and participation of the grandparents. Although emotional responses vary, the family unit is strengthened and the attachment of the grandparents to the child is enhanced when grandparents actively participate in the pregnancy.

If family members who traditionally offer support in times of stress are unavailable, refer the prospective parents to community resources such as support groups and childbirth education, sibling, breastfeeding, and new parenting classes.

Family Preparation for Birth

During the last trimester, discuss lifestyle changes that will occur when the infant is born. Unanticipated changes that accompany this dramatic life event may add stress and lead to disruption in family processes. Help the prospective parents make practical plans for the infant, such as obtaining clothing, finding a place to sleep, and choosing the method of feeding.

Siblings should also be prepared several weeks or even months before the birth. The response of children depends on their ages and developmental levels. Older children (older than 4 years) often benefit from participating in prenatal care and planning for the baby. Younger children have a poor concept of time and can be prepared for the arrival of a new baby shortly before the birth.

Suggest that the expectant parents determine the way they will work out the division of household and parenting tasks and help them decide what they will do about child care if the mother must return to work after childbirth. If these issues are not resolved, the couple can experience frustration and anger when one parent, usually the mother, assumes total care of the infant and attempts to complete all household tasks. In addition, exhaustion and frustration can overwhelm the joys of parenting when one parent must provide all care.

Communication Technique Models

When disagreements are evident, discussing and modeling therapeutic communication techniques that include all significant family members can be helpful as the family prepares for the birth. Techniques to clarify, summarize, and reflect feelings can defuse negative feelings that might result in family disruption (see Chapter 2).

Identification of Conflicting Cultural Factors

Explore possible areas of conflict related to cultural beliefs and health practices that affect pregnancy.

> Expectant mothers are reassured when nurses support beneficial health beliefs before confronting them with concerns. For example, "Eating many vegetables is so good for you and the baby. I am worried, though, because you missed your last appointment."

If conflict results from differences in time orientation, acknowledge the problem, convey understanding of the differences, and emphasize the importance of calling when appointments cannot be kept. Many families do not realize that when they miss appointments, another family misses the opportunity for health care.

Evaluation

When the family verbalizes concerns and emotions throughout pregnancy, the initial goal is met. Continued interest and involvement of the partner and significant family members are evidence that the family has completed the developmental tasks of pregnancy. Participation of the family with health care workers to find a compromise when differing cultural beliefs cause conflict confirms that the family will identify and initiate measures to reduce conflicts.

SUMMARY CONCEPTS

- Maternal psychological responses progress during pregnancy from uncertainty and ambivalence to feelings of vulnerability and preparation for the birth of the infant.
- As the fetus becomes real, usually in the second trimester, maternal focus shifts from the self to the fetus and the woman turns inward to concentrate on the processes taking place in her body.

- Changes in the maternal body during pregnancy may result in a negative body image that affects sexual responses. This change may be especially troubling if the couple does not discuss emotions and concerns related to the changes in sexuality.
- Making the transition to the role of mother involves mimicking the behavior of other mothers, fantasizing about the baby, grieving for the loss of previous roles, and developing a sense of self as mother.
- To complete the maternal tasks of pregnancy the woman must take steps to seek safe passage for herself and the infant, gain acceptance of significant persons, and form an interconnection and attachment to the unknown child.
- Paternal responses change throughout pregnancy and depend on the ability to perceive the fetus as real, gain recognition for the role of parent, and create a role as involved father.
- The most powerful reality boosters for the expectant father during pregnancy are hearing the fetal heartbeat, feeling the fetus move, and viewing the infant on a sonogram.
- In primitive cultures, *couvade* refers to pregnancy-related rituals performed by the man. In modern society, it often refers to a cluster of pregnancy-related signs and symptoms experienced by the man.
- The response of grandparents to pregnancy depends on their ages, the number and ages of other grandchildren, and their beliefs about the role of grandparents.
- The response of siblings to pregnancy depends on their ages and developmental levels.
- Completing the developmental tasks of pregnancy is more difficult for multiparas because they have less time, experience more fatigue, and must negotiate a new relationship with the older child or children.
- Socioeconomic status is a major factor in determining health practices during pregnancy. Poor families have competing priorities for food and shelter and seek prenatal care late in pregnancy.
- Cultural differences can create major conflicts between expectant families and health care workers. Language, time orientation, and health beliefs are the areas in which conflicts are most likely to occur.

ANSWERS TO CRITICAL THINKING QUESTIONS

1. These women will have more concerns about lack of time and increased fatigue. In addition, they will have concerns about the effect of another baby on their other children and their time and energy to meet the needs of all children.
2. Although both have 2-year-olds, Ms. H. will be concerned about her son's response to sharing her time and attention. Ms. N. has experienced this before and may be more worried about the effect of another baby on her economic situation.
3. Suggest that any changes in sleeping arrangements be made early so that other children will not feel displaced by the infant. Recommend that they plan ways to have time alone with the older child(ren) when the baby arrives, and review measures to reduce sibling rivalry. Ask Ms. N. about measures that were helpful when her last two children were born and suggest that she involve the older children in preparing for the new baby.

REFERENCES & READINGS

Alteneder, R.R., & Hartzell, D. (1997). Addressing couples' sexuality concerns during the childbearing period: Use of the PLISSIT model. *Journal of Obstetric, Gynecologic, and Neonatal Nursing* 26(6), 651-658.

American College of Obstetricians. (1999). *ACOG educational bulletin no. 255: Psychosocial risk factors: Perinatal screening and intervention.* Washington, D.C.: Author.

American College of Obstetricians and Gynecologists (ACOG). (1998). Cultural competency in health care. (ACOG Committee Opinion 201). Author.

American Academy of Pediatrics (AAP), Committee on Bioethics. (1998). Female genital mutilation. *Pediatrics,* 102(1), 153-156.

Association of Women's Health, Obstetric, & Neonatal Nurses (AWHONN). (2000). Nurse providers of perinatal education: Competencies and program guide. Washington, D.C.: Author.

Beckmann, C.A., Buford, T.A., & Witt, J.B. (2000). Perceived barriers to prenatal care services. *American Journal of Maternal/Child Nursing,* 25(1), 43-46.

Bloom, K.C. (1995). The development of attachment behaviors in pregnant adolescents. *Nursing Research,* 44(5), 284-289.

Callister, L.C., & Vega, R. (1998). Giving birth: Guatemalan women's voices. *Journal of Obstetric, Gynecologic, and Neonatal Nursing,* 27(3), 289-295.

Cherry, B., & Giger, J.N. (1999). African Americans. In J.N. Giger & R.E. Davidhizar (Eds.), *Transcultural nursing* (3rd ed., pp. 107-201). St. Louis: Mosby.

Choudhry, U.K. (1997). Traditional practices of women from India: Pregnancy, childbirth, and newborn care. *Journal of Obstetric, Gynecologic, and Neonatal Nursing* 26(5), 533-539.

Clement, S. (Ed.) (1998). *Psychological perspectives on pregnancy & childbirth.* Edinburgh: Churchill Livingstone.

Ferketich, S.L., & Mercer, R.T. (1995). Paternal-infant attachment of experienced and inexperienced fathers during infancy. *Nursing Research,* 44(1), 31-37.

Galanti, G. (1997). Caring for patients from different cultures (2nd ed.). Philadelphia: University of Pennsylvania Press.

Geissler, E.M. (1998). *Cultural assessment* (2nd ed.) St. Louis: Mosby.

Gennaro, S., Kamwendo, L.A., Mbweza, E., & Kershbaumer, R. (1998). Childbearing in Malawi, Africa. *Journal of Obstetric, Gynecologic, and Neonatal Nursing,* 27(2), 191-196.

Gibeau, A.M. (1998). Female genital mutilation: When a cultural practice generates clinical and ethical dilemmas. *Journal of Obstetric, Gynecologic, and Neonatal Nursing,* 27(1), 85-91.

Gichia, J.E.U. (2000). African-American women's preparation for motherhood. *MCN: American Journal of Maternal Child Nursing,* 25(2), 86-91.

Howard, J.Y., & Berbiglia, V.A. (1997). Caring for childbearing Korean women. *Journal of Obstetric, Gynecologic, and Neonatal Nursing,* 26(6), 665-671.

Hutchinson, M.K., & Baqi-Aziz, M. (1994). Nursing care of the childbearing Muslim family. *Journal of Obstetric, Gynecologic, and Neonatal Nursing,* 23(9), 767-771.

Jordan, P.L. (1990). Laboring for relevance: Expectant and new fatherhood. *Nursing Research,* 39(1), 11-16.

Kroelinger, C.D., & Oths, K.S. (2000). Partner support and pregnancy wantedness. *Birth, 27*(2), 112-119.
Lodgson, M.C. (2000). *Social support for pregnant and postpartum women.* Washington, D.C.: AWHONN.
Maloni, J.A., Cheng, C.Y., Liebl, C.P., & Maier, J.S. (1996). Transforming prenatal care: Reflections on the past and present with implications for the future. *Journal of Obstetric, Gynecologic, and Neonatal Nursing, 25*(1), 17-23.
Mattson, S. (2000). Ethnocultural considerations in the childbearing period. In S. Mattson & J. E. Smith (Eds.), *Core curriculum for maternal-newborn nursing* (2nd ed., pp. 70-84). Philadelphia: W.B. Saunders.
Mattson, S. (2000). Providing culturally competent care: Strategies and approaches for perinatal clients. *AWHONN Lifelines,* 4(5), 39-41.
Mattson, S. (2000). Striving for cultural competence: Providing care for the changing face of the U.S. *AWHONN Lifelines,* 4(3), 48-52.
Mattson, S. (2000). Working toward cultural competence: Making the first steps through cultural assessment. *AWHONN Lifelines,* 4(4), 41-43.
Mattson, S., & Lew, L. (1995). Culturally sensitive perinatal care for Southeast Asians. *Journal of Obstetric, Gynecologic, and Neonatal Nursing,* 24(4), 335-341.
Mayberry, L.J., Affonso, D.D. Shibuya, J., & Clemmens, D. (1998). Integrating cultural values, beliefs, and customs into pregnancy and postpartum care: Lessons learned from a Hawaiian public health nursing project. *Journal of Perinatal Neonatal Nursing,* 13(1), 15-26.
Meikle, S.F., Orleans, M., Leff, M., Shain, R., & Gibbs, R.S. (1995). Women's reasons for not seeking prenatal care: Racial and ethnic factors. *Birth,* 22(2), 81-86.
Mercer, R.T. (1990). *Parents at risk.* New York: Springer.
Mercer, R.T. (1995). *Becoming a mother: Research on maternal identity from Rubin to the present.* New York: Springer.
Mercer, R.T., & Ferketich, S.L. (1994a). Maternal-infant attachment of experienced and inexperienced mothers during infancy. *Nursing Research,* 43(6) 344-351.
Mercer, R.T., & Ferketich, S.L. (1994b). Predictors of maternal role competence by risk status. *Nursing Research,* 43(1), 38-43.
Midmer, D. (2000). Psychosocial support for childbearing families. In H. Nichols & S.S. Humenick. *Childbirth education: Practice, research, and theory* (2nd ed., pp. 476-500). Philadelphia: W.B. Saunders.
Mikhail, B.I. (1999). Perceived impediments to prenatal care among low-income women. *Western Journal of Nursing Research,* 21(3), 335-355.
Mullaly, L.M. (2000). Psychology of pregnancy. In Mattson, S., & Smith, J.E. (Eds.) *Core curriculum for maternal-newborn nursing* (2nd ed. , pp. 101-114). Philadelphia: W.B. Saunders.
Pagnini, D.L., & Reichman, N.E. (2000). Psychosocial factors and the timing of prenatal care among women in New Jersey's HealthStart program. *Family Planning Perspectives,* 32(2), 56-64.
Reichert, G.A. (1998). Female circumcision: What you need to know about genital mutilation. *AWHONN Lifelines,* 2(3), 29 34.
Rubin, R. (1975). Maternal tasks in pregnancy. *MCN: Maternal Child Nursing Journal,* 4(3), 143-153.
Rubin, R. (1984). *Maternal identity and the maternal experience.* New York: Springer.
Schaffer, M.A., & Lia-Hoagberg, B. (1997). Effects of social support on prenatal care and health behaviors of low-income women. *Journal of Obstetric, Gynecologic, and Neonatal Nursing* 26(4), 433-440.
Shilling, T. (2000). Cultural perspectives on childbearing. In F.H. Nichols & S.S. Humenick. *Childbirth education: Practice, research, and theory* (2nd ed., pp. 138-154). Philadelphia: W.B. Saunders.
Sorenson, D.S., & Schuelke, P. (1999) Fantasies of the unborn among pregnant women. *MCN: American Journal of Maternal Child Nursing,* 24(2), 92-97.
Spector, R.E. (2000). Cultural diversity in health and illness (5th ed.). Norwalk, CT: Appleton & Lange.
Stark, M.A. (2000). Is it difficult to concentrate during the 3rd trimester and postpartum? *Journal of Obstetric, Gynecologic, and Neonatal Nursing,* 29(4), 378-389.
Sullivan-Lyons, L. (1998). Men becoming fathers: "Sometimes I wonder how I'll cope." In S. Clement. *Psychological perspectives on pregnancy and childbirth.* (pp. 227-243.) Edinburgh: Churchill Livingstone.
Tiller, C.M. (1995). Father's parenting attitudes during a child's first year. *Journal of Obstetric, Gynecologic, and Neonatal Nursing,* 24(6), 508-514.
Walker, L.O., Cooney, A.T., & Riggs, M.W. (1999). Psychosocial and demographic factors related to health behaviors in the first trimester. *Journal of Obstetric, Gynecologic, and Neonatal Nursing,* 28(6), 606-614.
Wheatley, S. (1998). Psychosocial support in pregnancy. In S. Clement (Ed.). *Psychological perspectives on pregnancy and childbirth* (pp. 45-59). Edinburgh: Churchill Livingstone.
White, M.B. (1998). Men's concerns during pregnancy, part 1: Reevaluating the role of the expectant father. *International Journal of Childbirth Education,* 13(2), 14-17.
Wilkerson, N.N., & Shrock, P. (2000). Sexuality in the perinatal period. In F.H. Nichols & S.S. Humenick. *Childbirth education: Practice, research, and theory* (2nd ed. , pp. 48-65.) Philadelphia: W.B. Saunders.
Willis, W.O. (1999). Culturally competent nursing care during the perinatal period. *Journal of Perinatal Neonatal Nursing,* 13(1), 45-58.
Zwelling, E. (2000). The pregnancy experience. In F.H. Nichols & S.S. Humenick. *Childbirth education: Practice, research, and theory* (2nd ed. , pp. 35-47.) Philadelphia: W.B. Saunders.

9 NUTRITION FOR CHILDBEARING

OBJECTIVES

1. Explain the importance of adequate nutrition and weight gain during pregnancy.
2. Compare the nutrient needs of pregnant and nonpregnant women.
3. Describe common factors that influence a woman's nutritional status and choices.
4. Describe the effects of common nutritional risk factors on nutritional requirements during pregnancy.
5. Compare the nutritional needs of the postpartum woman who is breastfeeding with those of the woman who is not breastfeeding.
6. Apply the nursing process to nutrition during pregnancy, the postpartum period, and lactation.

DEFINITIONS

ANOREXIA NERVOSA Refusal to eat because of a distorted body image and feeling of obesity.

BULIMIA Eating disorder characterized by ingestion of large amounts of food followed by purging behavior such as induced vomiting or laxative abuse.

DIETARY REFERENCE INTAKES A label for several terms that estimate nutrient needs, including recommended dietary allowance, adequate intake, tolerable upper intake level, and estimated average requirement.

ESSENTIAL AMINO ACIDS Amino acids that cannot be synthesized by the body and must be obtained from foods.

GYNECOLOGIC AGE The number of years since menarche (first menstrual period).

HEME IRON Iron obtained from meat, poultry, or fish sources; the form most usable by the body.

INCOMPLETE PROTEIN FOOD Food that does not contain all the essential amino acids.

KILOCALORIE A unit of heat; used to show the energy value in foods (commonly called *calorie*).

LACTO-OVOVEGETARIAN A vegetarian whose diet includes milk products and eggs.

LACTOSE INTOLERANCE Inability to digest most dairy products because of a deficiency of the enzyme lactase.

LACTOVEGETARIAN A vegetarian whose diet includes milk products.

NONHEME IRON Iron obtained from plant sources.

NUTRIENT DENSITY The quality of protein, vitamins, and minerals per 100 calories in foods.

OVOVEGETARIAN A vegetarian whose diet includes eggs.

PICA Ingestion of a nonfood substance such as laundry starch, dirt, and ice.

DEFINITIONS—cont'd

Recommended Dietary Allowances Levels of nutrient intake considered to meet the needs of healthy individuals.

Vegan A complete vegetarian who does not eat any animal products.

Vegetarian An individual whose diet consists wholly or mostly of plant foods and who avoids animal food sources.

At no other point in a woman's life is nutrition as important as during pregnancy and lactation. At this time she must nourish not only her own body but also that of her baby. Nutrition may affect the size of the fetus and determine whether it has adequate stores of some nutrients after birth. If the woman fails to consume sufficient nutrients during pregnancy, her own stores of some nutrients may be depleted to meet the needs of the fetus, who also may be deprived of essential nutrients.

The nurse can provide women with education about nutritional needs on a continuing basis during office and clinic visits throughout the childbearing period. Nurses are often able to offer nutrition counseling before conception for women who are considering becoming pregnant. This counseling increases the chances that a woman is nutritionally healthy at the time of conception and will continue to practice good nutrition throughout pregnancy. It may also increase the level of nutrition the woman provides her entire family. Therefore nutritional education is an essential part of nursing care.

WEIGHT GAIN DURING PREGNANCY

Weight gain during pregnancy, especially after the first trimester, is an important determinant of fetal growth. Low birth weight (less than 2500 g), preterm labor, and increased risk of fetal and newborn mortality and morbidity have been associated with insufficient weight gain during pregnancy. Poor maternal weight gain indicates lower caloric intake and low intake of other important nutrients.

Excessive weight gain is associated with higher risk for macrosomia (large babies), prolonged second stage labor, and cesarean birth (Abrams & Pickett, 1999; Strychar, et al., 2000). Gaining more than the recommended weight during pregnancy influences the woman's functional ability in tasks such as child care and household activities during the third trimester (Tulman, Morin, & Fawcett, 1998).

The nutrient intake that comprises the weight gain is even more important than the weight gain itself. Weight gain from a diet lacking in essential nutrients is not as beneficial as weight gain from a balanced diet.

Recommendations for Total Weight Gain

Recommendations for weight gain during pregnancy have changed considerably over the years. In the late nineteenth century, rickets, a disease of the bones from calcium and vitamin D deficiency, caused some women to have small, distorted pelves. Restricted weight gain kept the fetus small and facilitated delivery. Later, weight gain was limited because of the belief that large gains caused pregnancy-induced hypertension, which is now known to be inaccurate.

Recommendations for weight gain in pregnancy are based on the woman's prepregnancy weight for her height or body mass index (BMI). BMI is calculated by dividing the weight in kilograms by the height in meters squared. Another method is to divide the weight in pounds by the height in inches squared and multiplying the result by 704.5. For example, if a woman weighs 56 kg (124 lb) before pregnancy and is 1.63 meters (64 inches) tall, her BMI is 21, which shows normal weight for height.

The recommended weight gain during pregnancy is 11.5 to 16 kg (25 to 35 lb) for women who begin pregnancy at normal weight (a BMI between 19.8 and 26). This amount is believed to reduce intrauterine growth restriction caused by inadequate maternal intake. The range allows for individual differences because no precise weight gain is appropriate for every woman. It provides a target while allowing for variations in individual needs.

Suggested gains vary according to the woman's BMI before pregnancy (Table 9-1). Prepregnancy weight below 45 kg (100 lb) is associated with preterm labor and low-birth-weight infants. Women who have low BMIs (less than 19.8) should gain more during pregnancy to meet the needs of pregnancy and normalize their weight.

In the past, obese women (BMI above 29) were told to gain little or even lose weight during pregnancy. Prepregnancy weight above 90 kg (200 lb) is associated with increased incidence of gestational diabetes, pregnancy-induced hypertension, neural tube defects, cesarean birth, and postpartum infection (Morin, 1998). The current recommended gain for overweight women (BMI above 26 to 29) is at least 15 lb, which is equivalent to the weight of the products of conception (such as fetus, placenta). This provides sufficient nutrients for the fetus. The weight gain for obese women (BMI above 29) should be individually determined. Women who are shorter than 62 inches (157 cm) may not need to gain as much as taller women and should gain only to the lower limits of the recommended range. Young adolescents need to gain to the upper end of the range to provide for their own growth during pregnancy and that of the fetus.

Table 9-1

RECOMMENDED WEIGHT GAIN DURING PREGNANCY

Weight before Pregnancy	Total Gain	Total Gain (First Trimester)	Weekly Gain (Second and Third Trimesters)
Normal weight (BMI 19.8 to 26.0)	11.5 to 16 kg (25 to 35 lb)	1.6 kg (3.5 lb)	0.44 kg (0.97 lb)
Underweight (BMI < 19.8)	12.5 to 18 kg (28 to 40 lb)	2.3 kg (5 lb)	0.49 kg (1.07 lb)
Overweight (BMI > 26 to 29)	7 to 11.5 kg (15 to 25 lb)	0.9 kg (2 lb)	0.3 kg (0.67 lb)
Obese (BMI > 29.0)	At least 6.8 kg (15 lb)	Individually determined	Individually determined
Twin pregnancies	16 to 20.5 kg (35 to 45 lb)	1.6 kg (3.5 lb)	0.75 kg (1.5 lb)

Modified from National Academy of Sciences. (1990). *Nutrition during pregnancy, Part I: Weight gain.* Washington, D.C.: National Academy Press.

Another variation is the woman who is pregnant with more than one fetus. Infants of a multifetal pregnancy are often born before term and tend to weigh less than those born of single pregnancies. A greater weight gain in the mother may help prevent low birth weight.

Pattern of Weight Gain

The pattern of weight gain is as important as the total increase in weight. Inadequate early weight gain may be associated with infants who are small for their gestational ages whereas poor gain late in pregnancy is associated with preterm labor even when total weight gain is within normal range (Scholl & Hediger, 1995). Early and adequate prenatal care allows assessment of weight gain on a weekly basis throughout pregnancy. The general recommendation is an increment of about 1.6 kg (3.5 lb) during the first trimester when the mother may be nauseated and the fetus needs fewer nutrients for growth. During the rest of the pregnancy the expected weight gain is 0.44 kg (nearly 1 lb) per week.

Maternal and Fetal Distribution

Women often wonder why they should gain so much weight when the fetus weighs only 3 to 3.6 kg (7 to 8 lb). The nurse should explain the distribution of weight and the dangers of poor weight gain to help them understand (Figure 9-1).

Factors Influencing Weight Gain

The nurse can positively influence the expectant mother's weight gain by teaching her the importance of her diet for fetal growth. A discussion of the effects of maternal intake on fetal growth and storage of nutrients often motivates women to improve their nutrition. Knowing about factors that may negatively influence nutrient intake and weight gain helps the nurse devise plans for improving nutrition.

Women at risk for inadequate weight gain include those who are young, unmarried, in a low-income

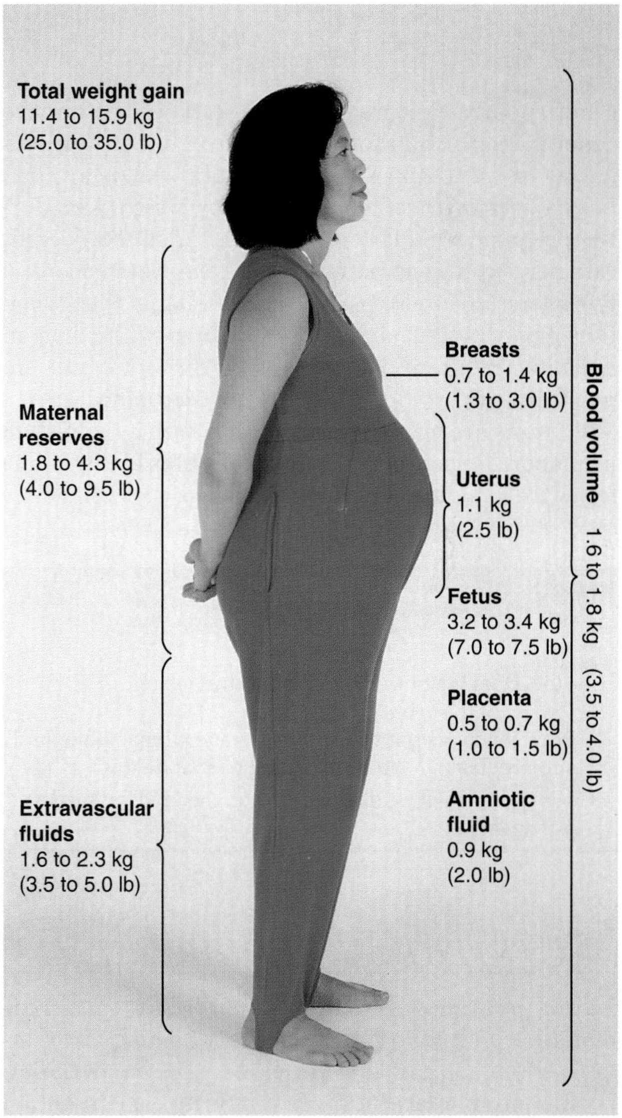

FIGURE 9-1 Distribution of weight gain in pregnancy. The numbers represent a general distribution because variation among women is great. The component with the greatest fluctuation is the amount of weight increase attributed to extravascular fluids (edema) and maternal reserves of fat.

Table 9-2
EXTRA FOODS NEEDED TO MEET PREGNANCY NEEDS

Energy (kcal)	1 banana, 1 carrot, 1 slice bread, *and* 1 glass low-fat milk
Protein	2 oz meat, fish, or poultry; or 2 cups milk; or 2 oz cheddar cheese; or ½ cup cottage cheese; or 1 cup brown rice *and* 1 block (4 oz) tofu; or 1 cup beans
Iron	3 oz red meat, *and* 1 cup lima beans, *and* ½ cup bran flakes with raisins, *and* 2 slices bread, *and* ½ cup cooked spinach, *and* 1 cup broccoli
Thiamine	½ cup bran flakes, or 1 cup peanuts, or ¾ ounce sunflower seeds, or 3 oz pork, or 1 cup rice or macaroni
Riboflavin	1 cup milk, yogurt, or cottage cheese; or ½ cup enriched cereal; or 2 eggs; or 5 oz poultry or meat; or 1 cup broccoli; or 1 cup spinach
Niacin*	1 T peanut butter, or 4 slices bread, or 3 to 4 oz meat
Vitamin C	⅓ cup cabbage, or ½ cup lima beans, or 1 cup loose-leaf lettuce, or ¼ cup tomato juice, or 1 apple

AI, Adequate intake; other values are for RDA. *T*, tablespoon.
*Niacin is also made by the body by tryptophan. From Mahan, L.K., & Escott-Stump, S. (2000). *Krause's food, nutrition, and diet therapy* (10th ed.). Philadelphia: W.B. Saunders; and from Grodner, M., Anderson, S.L., & DeYoung, S. (2000). *Nutrition, a nursing approach* (2nd ed.). St. Louis: Mosby.
Examples of foods that would meet the additional requirements for pregnancy for women between ages 19-30.

group, poorly educated, of short stature, and in poor general health and those who receive insufficient prenatal care. African-American, Southeast Asian, and Latina women are at more risk for low weight gain during pregnancy than white women. Adequate weight gain may be more important for African-Americans and teenagers, who tend to have smaller infants even when they gain the same amount of weight as white women and older mothers. The reasons for this difference are not fully understood (Institute of Medicine, 1990). Multiparas are at higher risk for low weight gain than primaparas. Smoking and substance abuse may interfere with food intake and weight gain.

Check Your Reading

1. How does weight gain in the mother relate to the birth weight of the infant?
2. How much weight should the average woman gain during pregnancy? What factors might change this?
3. What pattern of weight gain is recommended for the average woman?

NUTRITIONAL REQUIREMENTS

During pregnancy, nutrient needs increase to meet the demands of the mother and fetus. The amount of increase for each nutrient varies. In most cases the increases are not large and are relatively easy to obtain through the diet (Table 9-2).

Dietary Reference Intakes

In the past, most recommendations for nutrient intakes in the United States were given as recommended dietary allowances (RDAs) set by the Food and Nutrition Board of the National Research Council. Ongoing studies of nutrient needs have led the board to combine the RDA with several other terms under the label *dietary reference intakes (DRIs)* to estimate nutrient needs. These studies will continue until DRIs are set for all nutrients. DRIs include four categories:

- Recommended dietary allowance (RDA)—The amount of a nutrient that is sufficient to meet the needs of almost all (97% to 98%) healthy people of each gender in an age group
- Adequate intake (AI)—The nutrient intake assumed to be adequate when an RDA cannot be determined; based on an observed average or experimentally set intake that appears to sustain nutritional status
- Tolerable upper intake level (UL)—The highest amount of a nutrient that can be taken without probable adverse health effects by most people
- Estimated average requirement (EAR)—The amount of a nutrient estimated to meet the needs of 50% of the healthy people in an age group

Tables of recommendations are based on a reference individual, a hypothetical person of medium size. These tables are used to calculate nutrient needs based on age, gender, and size. For example, the reference woman for ages 19 to 30 years is 163 cm (64 inches) tall and weighs 61 kg (133 lb). Actual needs of individuals, particularly for calories and protein, may vary according to body size, previous nutritional status, and usual activity level.

Energy

The energy provided by foods for body processes is calculated in kilocalories. Kilocalories (commonly called *calories*) are obtained from carbohydrates and proteins, which provide 4 calories in each gram, and fats, which provide 9 calories in each gram.

Carbohydrates

Carbohydrates may be simple or complex. The most common simple carbohydrate is sucrose (table sugar), which is a source of energy but does not provide other nutrients. Fruits and vegetables also contain simple sugars and other nutrients. Complex carbohydrates are present in starches such as cereals, which supply vitamins, minerals, energy, and fiber. They should be the major source of carbohydrates in the diet because of their value in providing other nutrients.

Another type of carbohydrate is fiber, which is the nondigestible product of plant foods and an important source of bulk in the diet. Fiber absorbs water and stimulates peristalsis, causing food to pass more quickly through the intestines. Fiber helps prevent constipation and also slows gastric emptying, causing a sensation of fullness.

Fats

Fats provide energy and fat-soluble vitamins. When reducing calories is necessary, reduction but not elimination of carbohydrates and fats is important. If carbohydrate and fat intake provide insufficient calories, the body uses protein to meet energy needs. This use decreases the amount of protein available for building and repairing tissue.

Women often restrict fat to prevent weight gain. However, essential fatty acids such as DHA, an omega-3 fatty acid, help in formation of the placenta, fetal brain development, and fetal visual function. DHA is transferred to the infant after birth during breastfeeding. Women should be encouraged to include fish and red meat containing these fatty acids in their diets several times per week (Brooks, Mitchell, & Steffenson, 2000).

Calories

Approximately 85,000 additional calories are needed during pregnancy (Worthington-Roberts, 1997a). These extra calories furnish energy for production and maintenance of the fetus, placenta, added maternal tissues, and increased basal metabolic rate. The RDA for women of childbearing age is approximately 2200 calories per day. Although additional calories are not particularly needed during the early weeks of pregnancy, another 300 calories are necessary each day after that time. A 300-calorie increase can be achieved relatively easily with a variety of foods and only a small increase in food.

Nutrient density, the quality of the various nutrients in each 100 calories of food, must be considered when adding calories. Foods of high nutrient density have large amounts of quality nutrients per serving. During pregnancy the increased need for most nutrients may not be met unless calories are selected carefully. The term *empty calories* refers to foods that are high in calories but low in other nutrients. Many snack foods contain excessive calories and low nutrient density and are high in fat and sodium (Table 9-3). Increased calories should be "spent" on foods that provide the nutrients needed in increased amounts during pregnancy.

Table 9-3
HIGH-SODIUM FOODS*

Products that contain the words *salt* and *sodium,* such as table salt, onion salt, monosodium glutamate, and bicarbonate of soda (baking soda)
Foods that taste salty, including snack foods like popcorn, potato chips, pretzels, and crackers
Condiments and relishes such as catsup, horseradish, mustard, soy sauce, bouillon cubes, pickles, and green and black olives
Smoked, dried, and processed foods such as ham, bacon, lunch meats, and corned beef
Canned soups, meats, and vegetables unless the label states that the contents are low in sodium
Packaged mixes for sauces, gravies, cakes, and other baked foods

*During pregnancy, foods high in sodium should be consumed in moderation. Expectant mothers should be taught to read labels and avoid products in which sodium is listed among the first ingredients.

Protein

Protein is necessary for metabolism, tissue synthesis, and tissue repair. The RDA for adults is 0.75 g of protein per kilogram of body weight. This requirement averages to a daily need of 44 to 50 g for females depending on age and size. During pregnancy a daily protein intake of 60 g (10 to 16 g more than nonpregnancy RDAs) is recommended because of expansion of blood volume and growth of maternal and fetal tissues.

Protein is generally abundant in diets in most industrialized nations, and many women obtain more than the required amount of this nutrient. Diets low in caloric intake may also be low in protein, however. If calories are low and protein is used to provide energy, fetal growth may be impaired.

The nurse should counsel women at risk for protein deficiency about ways to determine protein intake and increase food sources of protein. When a woman needs to increase her protein intake, she should eat more high-protein foods rather than use high-protein powders and drinks. Protein substitutes increase protein but do not have the other nutrients provided by foods (see Table 9-2).

Vitamins

Although most people do not eat as much of every vitamin each day as they should, true deficiency states are uncommon in North America. During pregnancy, women usually get enough of most vitamins in their diets. However, they may not eat enough foods high in vitamins B_6, D, and E and folic acid to obtain the recommended levels (Table 9-4).

Table 9-4
VITAMINS AND MINERALS

Adult Females: Nonpregnant	Pregnancy/ Lactation	Sources	Purpose	Importance in Pregnancy
Fat Soluble Vitamins				
Vitamin A				
800 RE (RDA)	800/1300 RE (RDA)	Include green leafy and dark yellow vegetables, liver, whole and fortified low-fat and skim milk, egg yolk, butter and fortified margarine	Is important for vision and cell reproduction, growth, and functioning in skin and mucous membranes	Is important for fetal growth and cell differentiation; may result in spontaneous abortions or serious fetal defects if intake is excessive. It is important to avoid isotretinoin (Accutane) for acne treatment during pregnancy to prevent fetal defects
Vitamin D				
Age 14 to 50: 5 mcg (AI)	5/5 mcg (AI)	Include fortified milk, margarine, and soy products; butter; egg yolks; is synthesized in skin with exposure to sunlight; recommend supplement use for vegans who are not exposed to sun and do not eat fortified foods	Is necessary for metabolism of calcium and prevention of rickets	May cause neonatal hypocalcemia, hypoplasia of tooth enamel, and maternal osteomalacia (softening of the bones) if intake is inadequate, hypercalcemia and possible fetal deformities if intake is excessive; is important to recommend cautious use of supplements
Vitamin E				
Age 14 to 50: 15 mg (RDA)	5/19 mg (RDA)	Include vegetable oils, whole grains, nuts, and green leafy vegetables	Acts as an antioxidant; is important for tissue growth and integrity of cells (particularly red blood cell membranes)	Is rarely deficient in pregnant women; can cause anemia in the mother and fetus
Vitamin K				
Age 15 to 18: 55 mcg, age 19 to 24: 60 mcg, age 25 to 50: 65 mcg (RDA)	65/65 mcg (RDA)	Include green leafy vegetables; is also produced by normal bacterial flora in the small intestine	Is necessary for clotting	Temporary deficiency in newborns alleviated by receiving one dose by injection at birth to prevent hemorrhage
Water-Soluble Vitamins				
Vitamin B_6 (pyridoxine)				
Age 14 to 18: 1.2 mg; age 19 to 50: 1.3 mg (RDA)	1.9/2.0 mg (RDA)	Include chicken, fish, liver, pork, eggs, peanuts, and whole grains; recommend supplements to vegans with low intake	Is important in amino acid metabolism and blood, hormone, and immune function	Is important for increased metabolism of amino acids during pregnancy
Vitamin B_{12}				
2.4 mcg (RDA)	2.6/2.8 mcg (RDA)	Include meat, fish, eggs, milk, and forti-	Is important for cell division and protein	Is important for increased formation

Folic Acid				
400 mcg (RDA)	600/500 mcg (RDA)	May be lost in cooking (see Table 9-5)	Is important for cell replication and metabolism and prevention of megaloblastic anemia	Is important for expanded blood volume and tissue growth; may cause spontaneous abortion and neural tube defects if deficiency during the first 6 weeks of pregnancy
Thiamine				
Age 14 to 18: 1.0 mg, age 19 to 50: 1.1 mg (RDA)	1.4 mg (RDA)	Include pork, whole and enriched grain products, milk, legumes, organ meats, corn, seeds, and nuts	Forms coenzymes necessary to release energy	Is increased as a result of greater intake of calories
Riboflavin				
Age 14 to 18: 1.0 mg, age 19 to 50: 1.1 mg (RDA)	1.4/1.6 mg (RDA)	Include milk, pork, beef, enriched grain products, and deep green vegetables	Forms coenzymes necessary to release energy	Is increased as a result of greater intake of calories
Niacin				
14 mg (RDA)	18/17 mg (RDA)	Include meats, legumes, fish, poultry, and enriched grains	Forms coenzymes necessary to release energy	Is increased as a result of greater intake of calories
Vitamin C				
Age 14 to 18: 65 mg, age 19 to 50: 75 mg (RDA)	Age 18 and under: 80/115 mg; age older than 18: 85/120 mg (RDA)	Include citrus fruit, peppers, strawberries, cantaloupe, green leafy vegetables, tomatoes, and potatoes; is destroyed by heat and oxidation	Is important in collagen formation, tissue integrity, healing, immune response, and metabolism; may result in scurvy if severe deficiency	Is necessary for formation of fetal tissue; increased amounts are necessary for smoking, drug or alcohol abuse, and aspirin use
Minerals				
Iron				
15 mg (RDA)	30/15 mg (RDA)	Include meats, green leafy vegetables, eggs, grain products, tofu, legumes, nuts, and blackstrap molasses	Is important for the formation of hemoglobin and enzymes for metabolism	Is important for expanded maternal blood volume, formation of fetal red blood cells, and storage in the fetal liver for use after birth
Calcium				
Age 14 to 18: 1300 mg; age 19 to 50: 1000 mg (AI)	Age 18 and younger: 1300/1300 mg, older than 18: 1000/1000 mg (AI)	Include dairy products, salmon and sardines with bones, legumes, nuts, dried fruits, dark green leafy vegetables, tofu, and broccoli	Is needed in bone formation, cell membrane permeability, coagulation, and neuromuscular function	It is important for mineralization of fetal bones and teeth

AI, Adequate intake; *RE,* retinol equivalents (1 RE = 3.33 IU); *RDA,* recommended daily allowances.

Data from Food & Nutrition Board (FNB), National Academy of Sciences (1989). *Recommended dietary allowances* (10th ed.), Washington, D.C.: National Academy Press; Institute of Medicine (IOM), FNB (1998). *Dietary reference intakes for thiamin, riboflavin, niacin, vitamin B_6, folate, vitamin B_{12}, pantothenic acid, biotin, and choline.* Washington, D.C.: National Academy Press; IOM, FNB (1997). *Dietary reference intakes for calcium, phosphorus, magnesium, vitamin D, and fluoride,* Washington, D.C.: National Academy Press; and IOM, FNB (2000). *Dietary reference intakes for vitamin C, vitamin E, selenium, and carotenoids.* Washington, D.C.: National Academy Press.

Continued

Table 9-4

VITAMINS AND MINERALS—cont'd

Adult Females: Nonpregnant	Pregnancy/ Lactation	Sources	Purpose	Importance in Pregnancy
		Minerals—cont'd		
PHOSPHORUS				
Age 14 to 18: 1250 mg, age 19 to 50: 700 mg (RDA)	Age 18 and younger: 1250/1250 mg, older than 18: 700/700 mg (RDA)	Include dairy products and lean meat; is found in high amounts in processed foods, snacks, and carbonated drinks	Is needed with calcium for bone formation and cell metabolism	Is important for mineralization of fetal bones and teeth; results in binding of calcium in intestines and prevention of calcium absorption if intake is excessive
ZINC				
12 mg (RDA)	15/19 mg (RDA)	Include meat, poultry, seafood, eggs, nuts, seeds, legumes, wheat germ, whole grains, and yogurt	Is used in cell differentiation and reproduction, DNA and RNA synthesis, metabolism, and acid-base balance	Is important for fetal and maternal tissue growth
MAGNESIUM				
Age 14 to 18: 360 mg, age 19 to 30: 310 mg, age 31 to 50: 320 mg (RDA)	Age 18 and younger: 400/360 mg, older than 18: 350/ 310 mg (RDA)	Include whole grains, nuts, legumes, dark green vegetables, scallops, and oysters; is found in small amounts in many foods	Is important in cell growth and neuromuscular function; activates enzymes for metabolism of protein and energy	Is the same as for nonpregnancy state; may interfere with absorption of iron if intake is excessive
IODINE				
150 mcg (RDA)	175/200 mcg (RDA)	Include seafood and iodized salt	Is important in thyroid function	May cause abortion, stillbirth, congenital hypothyroidism,and neurologic conditions if deficient

Table 9-5
FOODS HIGH IN FOLIC ACID

Food	Micrograms per 1-Cup Serving
Black beans	256
Kidney beans	229
Pinto beans	294
Refried beans	150
Peanuts	181
Orange (whole)	44
Orange juice	109
Asparagus	176
Peas (cooked from frozen)	94
Broccoli	78
Lettuce (such as Romaine)	60
Spinach (raw)	109
(cooked from frozen)	204

Data from Mahan, L.K., & Escott-Stump, S. (2000). *Krause's food, nutrition, and diet therapy.* (10th ed.). Philadelphia: W.B. Saunders.

Fat-Soluble Vitamins

Fat-soluble vitamins include vitamins A, D, E, and K. Because these vitamins can be stored in the liver, deficiency states are not as likely to occur as with the water-soluble vitamins. However, excessive intakes of fat-soluble vitamins can be toxic. For example, excessive vitamin A can cause fetal defects. The nurse should inquire about vitamins and medications taken by pregnant women and counsel them about the dangers of excess vitamins.

Water-Soluble Vitamins

Water-soluble vitamins (such as B_6, B_{12}, C, folic acid, thiamine, riboflavin, niacin) are easily transferred from food to water during cooking. Foods should be steamed, microwaved, or prepared in only small amounts of water. The remaining water can be used in other dishes such as soups. Water-soluble vitamins are not stored in the body as easily as fat-soluble vitamins and therefore should be included in the daily diet. Because excess amounts are excreted in the urine, the chance of toxicity from ingestion of excessive amounts is less. Vitamin C is supplemented in many juices, and riboflavin, vitamin B_{12}, and niacin are supplemented in many breads and cereals. Diets are less likely to be low in these nutrients.

Folic Acid

Folic acid (also called *folate*) can decrease the occurrence of neural tube defects in newborns. Adequate intake of folic acid is especially important just before conception and during the first 4 weeks after conception, at which time the neural tube is closing. Because many pregnancies are unplanned, all women of childbearing age should consume at least 400 mcg of folic acid every day. If all women consumed this amount daily beginning at least 1 month before pregnancy, the incidence of neural tube defects would decrease as much as 70% (Howse, 1999). Women who have given birth to an infant with a neural tube defect should take higher doses of folic acid (Table 9-5).

A national goal for the year 2010 is to reduce the incidence of neural tube defects to 3 per 10,000 live births from a baseline of 6 per 10,000 in 1996. Another goal is to increase the proportion of pregnancies that begin at an optimum folic acid level. Data from 1991 to 1994 showed that only 21% of nonpregnant women between the ages of 15 and 44 years consumed at least 400 mcg of folic acid daily. The goal is to elevate this to 80% by 2010 (U.S. Department of Health and Human Services, 2000).

Check Your Reading

4. How many more calories should a woman consume each day during pregnancy?
5. How much protein is recommended during pregnancy?
6. Which vitamins are most likely to be low in the diets of pregnant women?
7. Which vitamins are in the fat-soluble and water-soluble groups? What is the difference in the way the body stores them?
8. Why should all childbearing-age women consume 400 mcg of folic acid daily?

Minerals

Although most minerals (see Table 9-4) are supplied in adequate amounts in normal diets, the intake of iron, calcium, zinc, and magnesium may drop below recommended levels for pregnancy (Institute of Medicine, 1990).

Iron

Iron is important in the formation of hemoglobin to carry oxygen throughout the body, and it helps form some enzymes necessary for metabolism. During pregnancy, additional iron is needed for the 20% to 30% increase in maternal red blood cells and transfer to the fetus for storage and production of red blood cells. The woman needs 500 mg of iron during pregnancy in addition to the 300 mg that are transferred to the fetus and the 200 mg used for normal daily losses (Monga, 1999).

Full-term infants are seldom anemic at birth. However, they may later develop anemia if storage of iron during fetal life is not enough to last 4 to 6 months after birth.

Iron is probably the only nutrient that cannot be supplied completely and easily by the diet during pregnancy. Iron is present in many foods, but large amounts of these foods are required to provide enough iron for pregnancy needs (see Tables 9-4 and 9-6).

Table 9-6
FOODS HIGH IN IRON*

Food and Amount	Average Amounts of Iron Supplied (mg)
MEATS (3 OZ)	
Liver	5.3
Red meats (avg)	2.5
POULTRY	
Chicken	0.9
Turkey	1.4
LEGUMES (½ CUP)	
Kidney beans	2.3
Lentils	2.1
Peanuts	1.4
Sunflower seeds	7.6
Chickpeas (garbanzo beans)	2.4
Black-eyed peas	1.8
Lima beans, baby	1.7
Peas	1.1
EGGS	
Eggs (each)	1.0
GRAINS (1 CUP)	
Rice	1.8
Bran flakes	6.8
(with raisins)	9.0
Oatmeal	1.6
Bread (slice)	0.9
FRUITS	
⅓ cup raisins	1.0
4 prunes	1.2
½ cup dried apricots	3.0
VEGETABLES (1 CUP)	
Asparagus (frozen)	1.2
Broccoli	1.8
Collards	1.9
Spinach (raw)	1.5
(cooked from frozen)	2.9
OTHER	
Tofu (2.5 × 2.75 × 1 inch)	2.3

Data from Mahan, L.K., & Escott-Stump, S. (2000). *Krause's food, nutrition, and diet therapy.* (10th ed.). Philadelphia: W.B. Saunders.
*The recommended daily allowance for iron during pregnancy is 30 mg. Although many women do not eat enough iron-containing foods in their daily diets to meet this need and instead take supplements, iron in foods is often better absorbed. Therefore the nurse should suggest ways a woman can increase her dietary iron.

The average American diet contains only about 6 mg of iron for each 1000 calories of food. The nonpregnant woman would have to eat approximately 2500 calories daily and the pregnant woman would need as much as 5000 calories to meet her iron needs (Worthington-Roberts, 1997b). In addition, some women restrict their intake of meats and grains in an effort to cut down on fat and calories. Thus many adult women do not meet their daily nonpregnancy requirements for iron and are already anemic or have low iron stores when they begin pregnancy.

Absorption of iron is affected by many other substances. Calcium and phosphorus in milk and tannin in tea decrease iron absorption from plant sources (called *nonheme iron*) if they are consumed during the same meal. Coffee binds iron, preventing it from being fully absorbed. Foods cooked in cast-iron pans contain more iron. Foods containing ascorbic acid and meats eaten with other iron-containing foods may increase absorption. Iron from meat (called *heme iron*) is more readily absorbed than iron from plants and less affected by other foods.

Physicians and nurse practitioners often prescribe iron supplements of 30 mg daily during pregnancy because obtaining enough iron in the diet is difficult. Supplementation should begin during the second trimester when the need increases. The expectant mother can also tolerate the iron better because morning sickness usually ends by this time.

Iron taken between meals is absorbed more completely, but many women find iron difficult to tolerate without some food. Iron taken at bedtime may be easier to tolerate. Milk, tea, coffee, eggs, and antacids taken with iron decrease absorption, but iron taken with a vitamin C source such as orange juice may increase absorption. Side effects occur more often with higher doses and include nausea, vomiting, heartburn, epigastric pain, constipation, and diarrhea. (Anemia during pregnancy is discussed in Chapter 26.)

Women should be reminded to keep iron and all other medicines out of the reach of children. Accidental iron overdose is a leading cause of childhood poisoning.

Calcium

Calcium is necessary for bone formation, maintenance of cell membrane permeability, coagulation, and neuromuscular function. Calcium is transferred to the fetus (especially in the last trimester) and is important for mineralization of fetal bones and teeth. Calcium absorption increases during the second trimester.

The pregnant woman's diet must provide enough calcium for her own and the fetus' needs to prevent loss from her bones. The pregnancy daily calcium requirement (1300 mg for women under age 18 and 1000 mg for those 18 and older) is the same as that recommended for nonpregnant women.

Because calcium is absorbed more efficiently during pregnancy and the total amount of calcium required is only a small part of that stored in the bones, mineralization of the woman's bones is not usually reduced significantly. However, in women with poor diets, more than one fetus, or closely spaced pregnancies, stores may be depleted. A common myth is that calcium is removed from the teeth during pregnancy, leading to excessive decay. In reality, calcium in the teeth is stable and not affected by pregnancy.

PREGNANT WOMEN WANT TO KNOW ***About Vitamins and Minerals***

- Take only vitamin and mineral supplements prescribed by a physician, nurse practitioner, or certified nurse-midwife. Over-the-counter supplements may not be formulated to meet your individual needs and could be harmful to you and your baby.
- Take iron on an empty stomach if possible. If you have nausea, heartburn, constipation, or diarrhea, try taking your iron at different times of the day such as at bedtime or 1 to 2 hours after meals. To increase absorption, take iron with orange juice or another source of vitamin C. Do not take iron with calcium supplements, milk, eggs, tea, and coffee because these substances decrease absorption.
- Keep all vitamin and mineral supplements away from children because they may cause accidental poisoning.

Table 9-7

CALCIUM SOURCES APPROXIMATELY EQUIVALENT TO 1 CUP OF MILK*

1 cup yogurt
1½ oz hard cheese
2 cups low-fat cottage cheese
1¾ cup ice cream or ice milk
3 cup sherbet
2¼ cup peanuts
1 cup almonds
9 oz sunflower seeds
2 cup refried beans
3 pieces (2.5 × 2.75 × 1 inch) tofu (soybean curd)
1¾ cup broccoli
1½ cup cooked kale
1 cup cooked collard greens
1⅓ cup oysters
4 oz salmon with bones
2½ oz sardines with bones
7 corn tortillas
5 tsp blackstrap molasses

*This list can be used to counsel women who are vegans or lactose intolerant. Lactose-intolerant women can often tolerate yogurt and cheese without distress. Although the amounts of some foods listed are more than would be likely to be eaten within 1 day, they serve for comparison.

Data from Mahan, L.K., & Escott-Stump, S. (2000). *Krause's food, nutrition, and diet therapy.* (10th ed.). Philadelphia: W.B. Saunders.

Dairy products are the best source of calcium. Whole, low-fat, and skim milk all contain the same amount of calcium and may be used interchangeably to increase or reduce calorie intake. However, women with lactose intolerance (lactase deficiency resulting in gastrointestinal problems when dairy products are consumed) need other sources of calcium.

Calcium is also present in legumes, nuts, dried fruits, dark green leafy vegetables, and broccoli (Table 9-7). Although spinach contains calcium, it also contains oxalates that decrease calcium availability and thus is not a good source. Canned salmon and sardines with bones also provide calcium. Blackstrap molasses and tofu processed with calcium sulfate are sources for vegans. Caffeine increases the excretion of calcium and decreases intestinal absorption.

Women who do not eat dairy products for cultural reasons, because of lactose intolerance, because they avoid animal products, or for other reasons should take supplements. Women younger than 25 years whose diets are low in calcium may need supplements during pregnancy because bone density is not complete and lack of available calcium may interfere with adequate bone formation in the mother. To ensure absorption of calcium, women should take supplements with meals and separately from iron supplements.

Nutritional Supplementation

Purpose

Food is the best source of nutrients. Women generally do not need routine vitamin and mineral supplements during pregnancy unless their diets are inadequate (Institute of Medicine, 1990). The exception is iron, which is unlikely to be obtained in adequate amounts through normal food intake. Expectant mothers who are vegetarians or lactose intolerant or have special problems in obtaining nutrients through diet alone may need vitamin and mineral supplements. Assessment of each woman's individualized needs determines whether supplementation is appropriate.

Disadvantages and Dangers

Routine supplementation with vitamin-mineral capsules or tablets is very common during pregnancy, but the practice may cause problems. Commonly used supplements provide from 50% to 150% of the RDA for the vitamins and minerals they contain. In some cases the interaction among certain nutrients may interfere with their absorption and use. For example, a high calcium intake decreases absorption of iron and zinc. Excessive intake of vitamin C inhibits absorption and metabolism of vitamin B_{12}.

Because they believe supplements are a harmless way to improve their diets, some women take large amounts without consulting a physician or in addition to prescribed supplements. Women should be advised that extra vitamins and minerals may cause deficiencies. The physician, nurse midwife, or nurse practitioner can suggest ways to increase intake if necessary and still maintain a balance.

The use of supplements in addition to food may increase the intake of some nutrients to doses much

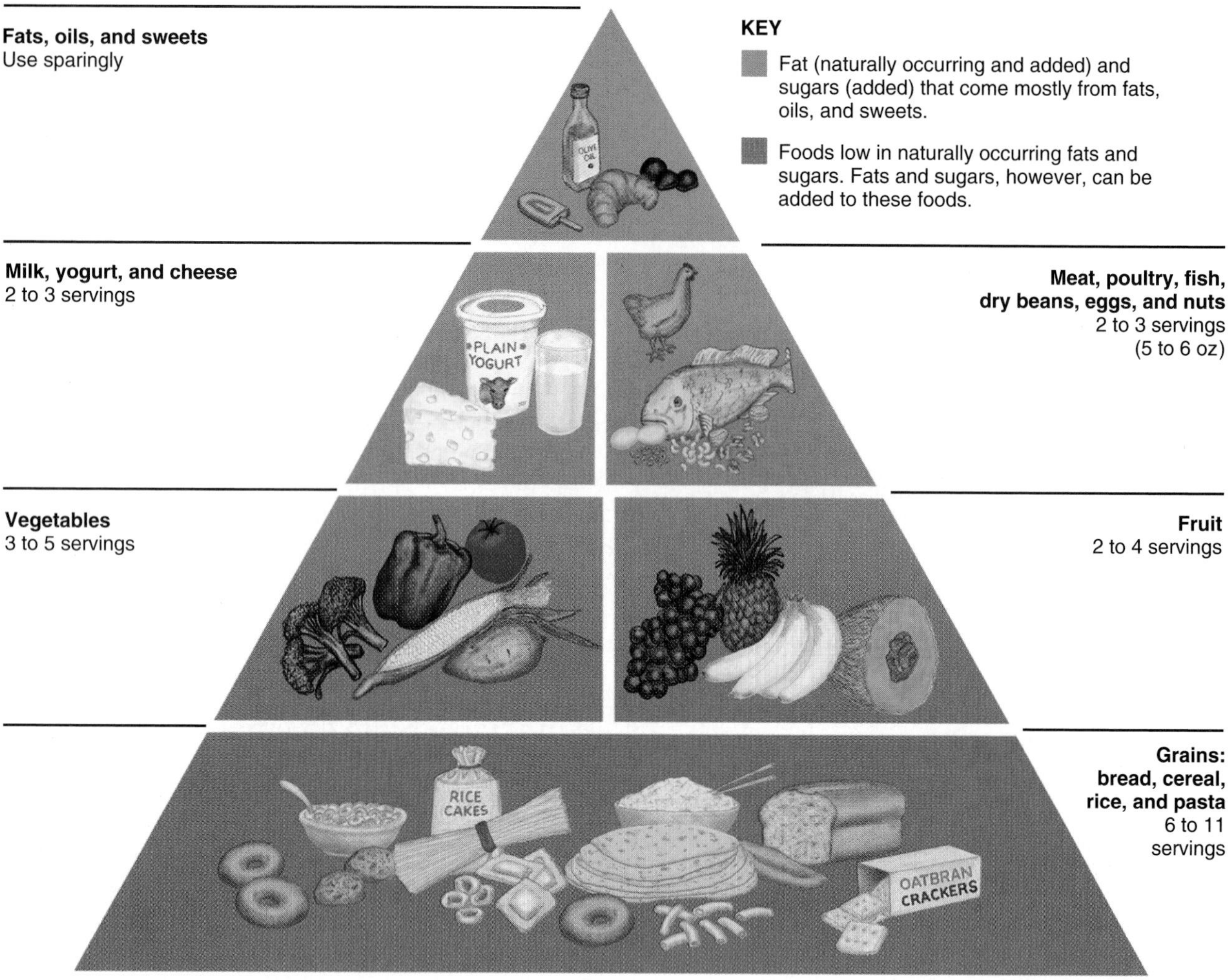

FIGURE 9-2 The food guide pyramid. (Adapted from U.S. Department of Agriculture, 1992.)

higher than the recommended amounts. Excessive amounts of some vitamins and minerals may be toxic to the fetus. Vitamin A can cause craniofacial, central nervous system, and cardiac defects in the fetus when taken in large amounts (Worthington-Roberts, 1997a). High levels of vitamin A are taken by women using the drug isotretinoin (Accutane) for acne.

The pregnancy risk category changes from A (no evidence of fetal risk) to C (animal studies showing adverse effects but good studies on humans not available) for vitamins such as E, thiamine, riboflavin, niacin, B_6, folic acid, and B_{12} when recommended doses for pregnancy are exceeded (LeMone, 1999). Other nutrients that may cause harm in excessive amounts include vitamins C and D and the minerals iron and zinc.

Some women believe their nutrient needs can be met in supplement form and are less concerned about their food intake. Supplements do not contain protein and calories and may lack many necessary nutrients. Nurses must emphasize that supplements are not food substitutes and do not contain all the nutrients needed during pregnancy. In fact, not all nutrients that are important to pregnancy and provided by foods are known.

Water

Water is important during pregnancy for the expanded blood volume and as part of the increased maternal and fetal tissues. Women should drink at least eight 8-ounce glasses of fluids each day, with water constituting most fluid intake. Fluids low in nutrients (such as carbonated beverages, coffee, tea, juice drinks that contain high amounts of sugar and little real juice) should be limited because they are filling and replace other more nutritional foods and drinks.

Food Guide Pyramid

The U.S. Department of Agriculture (USDA) food pyramid (Figure 9-2) provides a guide for healthy eating for adults and children. It can also be adapted to serve as a guide during pregnancy (Figure 9-3). (Table 9-8 lists portion sizes per serving.)

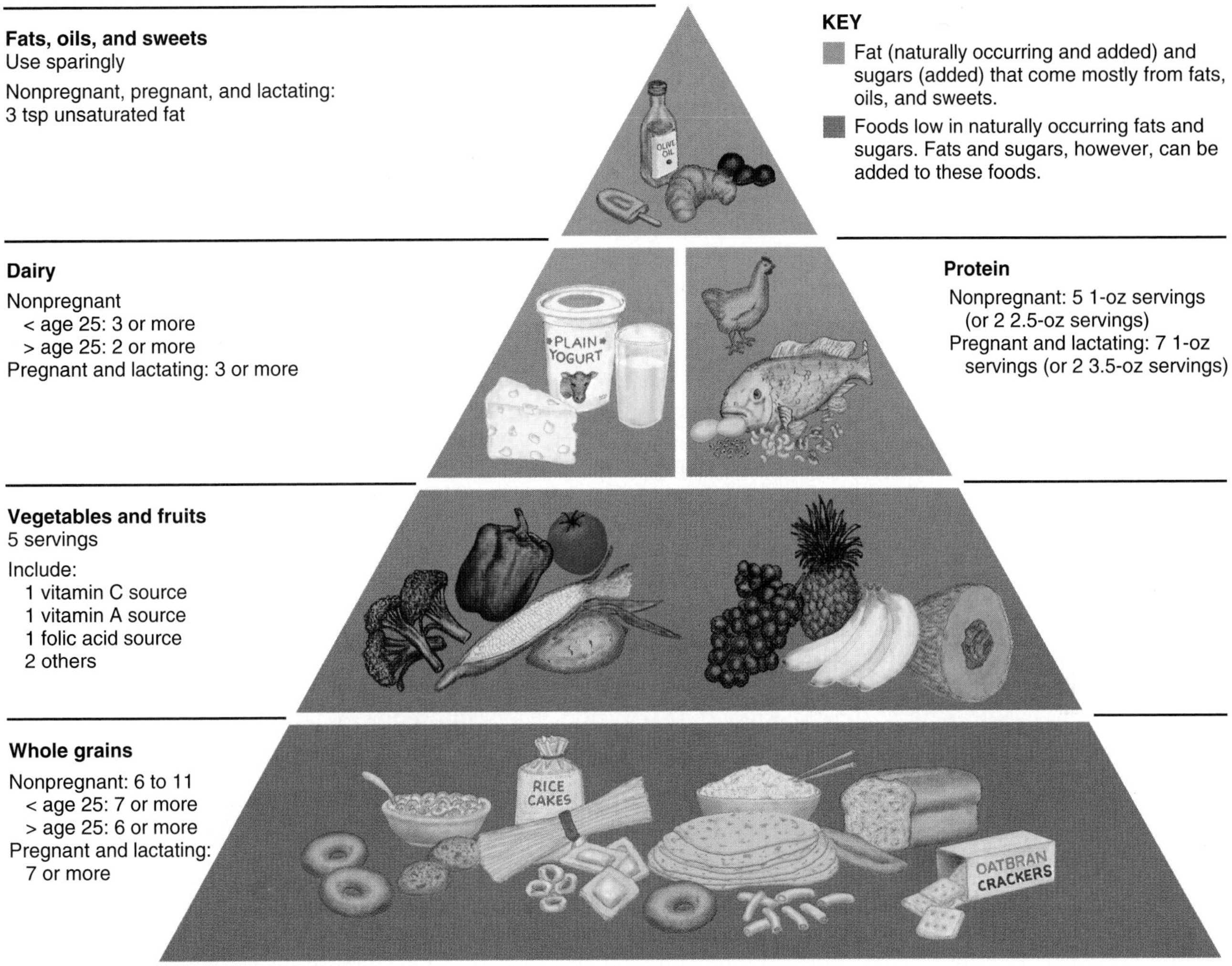

FIGURE 9-3 Nutrient needs during pregnancy and lactation. Eating *at least* the number of servings listed meets the minimal nutrient need for pregnancy. Additional calories may be necessary to meet individual requirements. (Modified from California Department of Health Services, Maternal and Child Health. [1990]. *Nutrition during pregnancy and the postpartum period: A manual for health care professionals, summary.* Sacramento, CA: Author, and from U.S. Department of Agriculture, 1992.)

Table 9-8

FOOD GROUP EXAMPLES AND PORTION SIZES

Dairy Products

1 cup milk or yogurt, 1½ oz or ⅓ cup grated hard cheese, 2 cups cottage cheese

Protein Sources to Make 1-oz Serving

1 oz or ¼ cup chopped meat, poultry, fish, ½ cup cooked legumes, 1 egg, 3 oz tofu, 2 T peanut butter

Vegetables and Fruits

Serving size for all fruits and vegetables: 1 medium piece or ½ cup cooked or chopped raw, ¾ cup juice, 1 lettuce leaf
Vitamin C source: orange juice, strawberries, cabbage, kiwi, orange, mango
Vitamin A source: deep yellow or dark green leafy: carrot, sweet potato, apricots (3), spinach, broccoli
Folic acid source: beans, oranges, dark green leafy
Other fruits and vegetables: green beans, corn, apple, banana, pear

Whole Grains

Breads (1 slice), cereals (½ to ¾ cup), rice and pastas (½ cup)

Unsaturated Fats

1 tsp

Whole Grains

At the base of the pyramid are breads, cereals, rice, and pastas. They provide complex carbohydrates, fiber, vitamins, and minerals. Whole grains provide more nutrients than processed grain products. Although foods can be enriched to replace some nutrients lost during processing, zinc, vitamin B_6, magnesium, and vitamin E may not be replaced by enrichment. The USDA recommends 6 to 11 servings of this group for healthy adults over age 25. Pregnant women should have at least 7 servings.

Vegetables and Fruits

Vegetables and fruits form the next two groups of the pyramid and are important sources of vitamins, minerals, and fiber. At least one food that provides vitamin C, one that provides vitamin A, and one that provides folic acid are important selections from the fruit and vegetable group each day. Healthy adults should have at least five servings of fruits and vegetables, with a range of three to five servings of vegetables and two to four servings of fruits. The pregnant or lactating woman also needs at least five servings of fruits and vegetables and should include sources of vitamin C, vitamin A, and folic acid daily.

Dairy Foods

Dairy foods include foods such as milk, yogurt, and cheese. They contain approximately the same nutrient values whether they are whole (4% fat), low fat (2% fat), or nonfat (skim), but the latter two have fewer calories and less fat. Dairy products are especially good sources of calcium. Adults older than age 25 need two to three servings from this group. Younger women and those who are pregnant or lactating need at least three servings.

In the past, calcium supplements and decreased milk intake were recommended to prevent leg cramps from an imbalance of calcium and phosphorous in the diet. However, the effectiveness of this treatment has not been proved (Worthington-Roberts, 1997b; Fagen, 2000). Because milk provides a large number of nutrients, women generally should not limit intake during pregnancy.

Protein

Many adults think of meat, poultry, fish, and eggs as the only sources of protein. However, legumes (dried beans and peas), nuts, and soybean products such as tofu are also good sources. Adults should consume 5 to 6 oz. Pregnant and lactating women need at least 7 oz of protein foods. A typical portion of meat, fish, and poultry varies in size and may contain several ounces. A 3-oz portion is about the size of a deck of playing cards.

Other Elements

The tip of the pyramid represents fats, oils, and concentrated sugars, which should be used sparingly. They provide calories for energy but few other nutrients. An adequate allowance for this group is 3 teaspoons of unsaturated fats.

Check Your Reading

9. Which minerals are often below the recommended amounts in the diets of pregnant women?
10. Why is routine use of vitamin-mineral supplements unnecessary and possibly dangerous?
11. How much fluid should a woman drink each day during pregnancy?
12. How many servings of each food pyramid group are recommended during pregnancy?

FACTORS INFLUENCING NUTRITION

Cultural background, age, and knowledge about nutrition influence the food choices women make and their nutritional status. The nurse must consider these factors when counseling women about their diets.

Culture

Food is important in all cultures and often has special meaning during pregnancy and childbirth when certain foods may be favored or discouraged. Nurses need to be aware of the habits of a variety of cultures to provide culturally appropriate nutritional counseling. Before making assumptions about the influence of a woman's culture on her diet, the nurse must assess each woman individually. Not all women follow food practices considered typical for their culture. Variations among members of a culture may be attributable to diverse practices found in different areas of their countries of origin.

The nurse should assess the woman's age, her length of time in America, and whether she has adopted any prevalent American eating habits. Greater exposure to an American diet may cause younger members of a group to make more dietary changes than older relatives. Some women who follow an American diet may return to some aspects of their cultures' traditional diets during pregnancy because they believe it helps prevent harm to the fetus.

Nurses often use pamphlets as part of nutritional teaching and may be able to obtain them in various languages.

> The nurse should be certain that the woman can read her own language before giving her written materials. People may not readily admit that they cannot read. In addition, the translation may be too complicated for the woman with little education to understand. Having an interpreter discuss the material with the woman helps discover whether she can read and aids in other teaching.

Table 9-9

COMMON "HOT" AND "COLD" FOODS: SOUTHEAST ASIAN AND LATINO DIETS*

Southeast Asian	
Hot (Yang) Foods	**Cold (Yin) Foods**
Peppers and onions	Most fruits and juices
Meat and poultry	Flour
Fish and fish sauce	Cold fluids
Broth	Sour foods
Eggs	
Spices and sweets	
Latino	
Hot Foods	**Cold Foods**
Potatoes, peas, onions, and chili peppers	Most fruits and vegetables
Cheese and evaporated milk	Milk
Chicken and lamb	Fish
Flour tortillas	Corn tortillas
Chickpeas and kidney beans	Green and red beans

*Although variations exist within cultural groups, foods considered "hot" are used for conditions thought to be "cold" and vice versa. These customs influence what women are willing to eat during pregnancy and illness and must be respected as part of nursing care.

Many cultures believe that certain foods, conditions, and medicines are "hot" or "cold" and must be balanced to preserve health (Table 9-9). In Asian cultures, this belief is referred to as *yin* (cold) and *yang* (hot) and may influence what the mother eats during pregnancy and the postpartum period.

Food taboos may influence what some women eat during the childbearing period. For example, Korean women may avoid chicken, pork, and blemished fruits during pregnancy. These foods are thought to have a harmful effect on the infant's physical appearance.

Cultural preferences for foods are extremely varied. For instance, some African-Americans follow a diet similar to that of people living in the southeastern United States. This diet includes foods such as okra, collards, mustard greens, ham hocks, black-eyed peas, and hominy or grits. However, the diet of other African-Americans varies according to the geographic area in which they live.

Iron-deficiency anemia occurs in 15% of African-American women of childbearing age compared with 10% of white women (U.S. Department of Health and Human Services, 2000). Lactose intolerance is common, resulting in lack of calcium if other sources are not present in the diet. Intake of high-sodium and fried foods may present health problems.

Some Jewish women follow a strictly kosher diet. This diet includes meat processed to remove all blood, meat only from animals with cloven hooves, and avoidance of milk and meat in the same meal. Muslim women do not eat pork and may wish to fast on certain days. However, the religion exempts pregnant and nursing women from obligatory fasting.

The diet of Native American women may contain corn, beans, and squash but lack fresh fruits and vegetables. Lactose intolerance is common, and meat intake is low. Fat, carbohydrate, sodium, and sugar intake are often high. Low-income Native Americans living on reservations may receive foods such as white flour, cornmeal, white rice, and processed meats from federal programs. However, some Native Americans take in less than two thirds of the RDA for calories, calcium, iron, iodine, riboflavin, and vitamins A and C (Davis & Sherer, 1994).

Food preferences for Southeast Asians and Latinos are examples of the influence of culture on diet. Immigrants and refugees from Southeast Asia are the newest large group of people to come into the United States. They are likely to continue diets similar to those from their homelands. Latinos are a large minority group in the United States and nurses throughout the United States need information about Latino food preferences.

Southeast Asian Dietary Practices

The term *Southeast Asian* refers to people from Cambodia, Laos, and Vietnam who came to the United States beginning in the mid-1970s. The majority settled in western states, but smaller numbers found homes elsewhere in the country.

Southeast Asian cooking methods include searing fresh vegetables quickly with small portions of meat, poultry, or fish in a little oil over high heat. Meals cooked in this manner are low in fat and retain vitamins. Most meals are accompanied by rice, which increases the intake of complex carbohydrates. A salty fish sauce called *nuoc mam* and fresh vegetables are part of most meals.

Many Southeast Asians have adapted their dietary habits to more American ways. Increased intake of eggs, beef, pork, and bread has added nutrients but also fat to the diet. Candy, soft drinks, sweet snacks, butter or margarine, and fast foods have been less favorable influences because they are low in nutrients but high in sugar or fat (Williams, 1999).

Effect of Culture on Diet during Childbearing

In Southeast Asian cultures, pregnancy (especially the third trimester) is considered "hot" and the woman is encouraged to eat "cold" foods to maintain a balance of hot and cold. During pregnancy, she eats more sour foods, fruits, noodles, and sweets and avoids fish, excessively salty or spicy foods, alcohol, and rice. She does not eat unfamiliar foods for fear that they may harm her or her fetus.

The postpartum period is considered "cold," partly because of the loss of blood, which is "hot." Mothers avoid losing more heat, which they believe would negatively affect their health. They stay warm physically and may refuse to shower for fear of exposure to cold. They choose "hot" foods to eat, including rice with fish sauce, broth, salty meats, fish, chicken, and eggs. They may refuse cold drinks but welcome hot fluids, requesting tea or even plain hot water. Families frequently bring food to the mother while she is in the hospital because hospital food may not meet her preferences.

The diet of Southeast Asians, especially those with low incomes, may be high in sodium but below recommended levels for energy, calcium, iron, zinc, magnesium, and vitamins B_6 and D. These deficiencies may be of special concern during pregnancy. The woman can often increase her intake of needed nutrients without deviating greatly from her usual diet.

Increasing Nutrients with Traditional Foods

Milk products are not part of the traditional Southeast Asian diet, and lactose intolerance is common. However, intake of commonly used dark green leafy vegetables such as mustard greens, bok choy, and broccoli increases levels of calcium, iron, magnesium, and folic acid. Tofu contains good amounts of calcium and iron. A broth made from pork or chicken bones soaked in vinegar, which removes calcium from the bones, is frequently taken. If the mother avoids fortified milk, she may need vitamin D supplementation. An increased intake of meats and poultry elevates levels of vitamin B_6 and zinc.

Latino Dietary Practices

Spanish-speaking people such as Mexican-Americans, Puerto Ricans, and Cuban-Americans are often referred to as *Latinos* or *Hispanics*. This major minority group in the United States continues to grow. Mexican-Americans comprise the largest share of the group. Although many live in the southwestern United States and Florida, they are located throughout the country. Like Asians, Latinos follow the theories of "hot" and "cold" foods and conditions. They also consider pregnancy to be "hot" and the postpartum period to be "cold" and adjust the diet accordingly.

Dried beans (especially pinto beans) are a staple of the Mexican-American diet and are part of most meals as refried beans, served alone, or mixed with other foods such as rice. The most common meats are beef, pork, and chicken. The major grain is corn, which is ground and made into a dough called *masa* to make corn tortillas. The corn is treated with lime and is a good source of calcium. Corn and flour tortillas are eaten with most meals. Rice is also an important grain. Although milk is not commonly used except for infants, cheese is part of many dishes.

Chili peppers and tomatoes are the most common vegetables in Latino diets. Others include beets, cabbage, chayotes, bell peppers, and string beans. Green leafy and yellow vegetables are seldom used. Oranges, bananas, canned peaches, pumpkin, and avocado are common fruits.

Foods are often hot, spicy, and fried. The diet is high in fiber and complex carbohydrates. However, it tends to be high in calories and fat, leading many Mexican-Americans to become overweight. The diet may be low in iron, calcium, and vitamins A and D, which should be increased through foods or supplements during pregnancy.

Puerto Rican and Cuban diets are similar to that of Mexican-Americans with the addition of tropical fruits and vegetables from the homeland when available. Viandas, which are starchy fruits and vegetables like plantain, green bananas, sweet potatoes, yams, and breadfruit are common. They may be cooked with codfish and onion. Guava, papaya, mango, and eggplant also are used when available.

Check Your Reading

13. When the nurse assesses cultural influences on nutrition during pregnancy, what factors must be considered?
14. Compare the diet of Southeast Asian women with that of Latina women.

Age

Extremes of age may influence the nutritional needs of pregnancy. The adolescent who is not fully mature needs nutritional support for her own growth. Older women who are in good health have the same nutritional requirements as younger pregnant women. They may have more knowledge about nutrition through life experiences or need as much teaching as younger women. They are more likely to be financially secure than very young women.

Nutritional Knowledge

Information about nutrition is readily available to those who read popular books and magazine articles about the subject. Even women who have not been attentive to their diets before pregnancy often try to learn about the relationship between what they eat and the effect on the fetus once pregnancy is confirmed. Although women know they should "eat well" during pregnancy, they may have little idea of the meaning. Some women lack basic understanding of nutrition and have misconceptions based on common food myths that interfere with good nutritional choices. These expectant mothers need help from nurses when learning about nutrition.

NUTRITIONAL RISK FACTORS

Factors that may interfere with a woman's ability to meet the nutritional needs of pregnancy include poverty, adolescence, vegetarianism, lactose intolerance, nausea and vomiting ("morning sickness"), anemia, abnormal prepregnancy weight, eating disorders, pica, multiparity, and substance abuse.

Socioeconomic Status

Poverty

Low-income women may have deficient diets because of lack of financial resources and nutritional education. Carbohydrate foods are often less expensive than meats, dairy products, fruits, and vegetables. Therefore the diet may be high in calories but low in vitamins and minerals. A referral to Temporary Assistance to Needy Families (TANF) or the Special Supplemental Food Program for Women, Infants, and Children (WIC) may be helpful if a woman's food intake is inadequate because of lack of money. Vitamin and mineral supplementation may be important for her, especially if her diet is likely to be inconsistent.

Food Supplement Programs

The WIC program is administered by the USDA to provide nutritional assessment, counseling, and education to low-income women and children under the age of 5 years who are at nutritional risk. The program also provides food vouchers for foods such as milk, cheese, eggs, iron-fortified cereal, fruit juice, dried beans, peanut butter, and formula to qualified women and their children. Eligibility is based on an income below 185% of the federal poverty level. Women are eligible throughout pregnancy and for 6 months after birth if formula feeding or 1 year if breastfeeding.

Women from other cultures who receive WIC might not use their food vouchers for unfamiliar foods. For example, Chinese women might not use the vouchers for cheese but might increase their intake of foods that are not usually part of the Asian diet, such as milk, beans, and cereal (Horswill & Yap, 1999).

Adolescence

Adolescent pregnancies are associated with higher risk for complications for both the expectant mother and the fetus. Adolescents at greatest risk for problem pregnancies are those who are the youngest in terms of gynecologic age (number of years since menarche) and those who are still growing. Girls who become pregnant less than 2 years after menarche are not anatomically and physiologically mature, and they require more nutrients to meet their needs than older adolescents. Those with a gynecologic age of 4 years are usually physically mature and have nutritional demands similar to those of older women (Worthington-Roberts & Rees, 1997).

Maternal growth may interfere with placental blood flow and transfer of nutrients to the fetus. As a result, the adolescent mother may add weight and fat to her own body rather than use it for support of the fetus. This leads to a tendency to have smaller infants even with good weight gains in the mother (Spear, 2000). Weight gain for the pregnant adolescent should be in the upper part of the range suggested for her BMI.

Nutrient Needs

Nutrient needs for adolescents older than age 18 are the same as those for older women during pregnancy. Adolescents age 18 and younger need more calcium and magnesium to meet their own growth needs. Individualized assessment of gynecologic age, nutritional status, and daily diet may indicate the need for increases in other areas. Increased amounts of energy, protein, and iron may be necessary for some younger adolescents.

Common Problems

The diets of teenagers before and during pregnancy are often low in needed vitamins and minerals. Supplements may be prescribed, but the adolescent may not take them regularly. This combination of poor intake and unreliable supplementation may further deplete nutrient stores and general nutrition.

Peer pressure is an important influence on nutritional status. Adolescents are often concerned about body image. If weight is a major focus for a teenager and her peers, she is more likely to restrict calories to prevent weight gain during pregnancy. Teenagers tend to skip meals, especially breakfast. The fetus requires a steady supply of nutrients, and the expectant mother's stores may be used if intake is not sufficient to meet energy needs.

Because snacks provide as much as one fourth of the caloric intake of the adolescent girl, they should be rich in nutrients (Worthington-Roberts & Rees, 1997). Fast foods from restaurants or snack machines are a significant part of many teenagers' diets. Although occasional consumption of these foods is not harmful, fast foods are often high in calories, fat, and sodium but low in vitamins, minerals, and fiber. Fast foods that do not make her appear different from her peers but are still able to meet her added nutrient needs are important for the pregnant adolescent. (See Nursing Care Plan for strategies to educate and encourage the pregnant adolescent about nutrition.)

Teaching the Adolescent

Teaching the adolescent about nutrition can be a challenge for nurses. Establishing an accepting, relaxed atmosphere and showing willingness to listen to the teenager's concerns are essential. The teenager's lifestyle, pattern of eating, and food likes and dislikes should be explored first. The nurse must consider these factors in determining whether changes are necessary in the diet.

The adolescent's home life may affect her nutritional status. She may live at home with a mother who does the cooking, and the whole family may eat together. Or she may eat with the family only occasionally because she is often away at mealtimes. Some pregnant adolescents are homeless or in unstable situations. The number of other people in the home and the sufficiency of the food available affect the dietary intake.

NURSING CARE PLAN 9-1

Nutrition for the Pregnant Adolescent

Assessment: Vicki, age 15, is 20 weeks pregnant and has gained 4.5 kg (10 lb). She attends school and lives at home but usually cooks for herself because "I don't like the stuff Mom cooks." She skips breakfast and eats from snack machines during breaks at school. She goes to fast food restaurants for lunch and after-school snacks. Vicki says she is disgusted with how heavy she is and wants to go on a diet to lose some weight or "I'm going to look like a blimp!" Her hemoglobin level is 10.4 g/dl. She listens with interest when the nurse discusses nutrition, especially when weight is mentioned. Her statements show concern about her baby's needs. Vicki was at a normal weight before her pregnancy, and a weight gain of approximately 16 kg (35 lb) is appropriate for her. Her gynecologic age is 2.5 years.

Nursing Diagnosis: Altered Nutrition: Less Than Body Requirements related to concern about weight gain and diet choices inadequate to meet nutrient requirements of adolescent pregnancy.

Critical Thinking: What other information does the nurse need to complete the assessment?

Answer: A 24-hour diet history is necessary for a better understanding of Vicki's diet. The nurse should also ask about her likes and dislikes to make a meaningful diet plan for Vicki.
The diet history reveals Vicki eats few dairy foods, although she says she does not dislike them. She has no real food dislikes.

Goals/Expected Outcomes:
Vicki will do the following:
1. Explain the weight gain pattern and intake from each food group optimal for adolescent pregnancy.
2. List foods she can choose at fast food restaurants that meet her nutrient needs and allow her to feel part of her peer group.
3. Gain approximately 0.44 to 0.57 kg (1 to 1.25 lb) per week for the rest of her pregnancy.
4. Maintain a hemoglobin level above 10.5 g/dl throughout her pregnancy.

Intervention	Rationale
1. Praise Vicki for her interest in nutrition and her concern about gaining too much weight.	1. Praise helps foster rapport and may focus attention on learning.
2. Discuss the reasons for appropriate weight gain during pregnancy and its effect on the fetus. Explain the needs of the adolescent who is not finished growing and the importance of preventing the problems associated with low birth weight in the infant	2. The adolescent may not understand the way diet affects the fetus and herself during pregnancy. An explanation of the potential effects of her actions will increase the expectant mother's interest in nutrition.
3. Assist Vicki in comparing her food intake with the recommended servings from each food group. Point out areas of strength and praise her for these.	3. Active involvement of the learner and positive reinforcement help increase motivation.
4. Ask Vicki what problems she sees in her diet. Point out areas she may have missed. Explain the effect that lack of specific nutrients may have on the fetus.	4. Adolescents learn best when they see that the material applies to them.
5. Discuss the high caloric intake of fast foods in relation to her present diet and explain the concept of nutrient density in terms of "spending calories" to "buy" nutrients needed during pregnancy.	5. Relating information to concepts already understood increases understanding.
6. Using Vicki's food likes and dislikes, identify low-calorie foods she would like that meet her nutrient needs. Point out fruits and vegetables high in vitamins A and C yet low in calories.	6. Individualizing the recommended diet to meet the woman's likes and dislikes increases compliance.
7. Suggest nutritional foods that Vicki could choose at fast food restaurants and ask which ones are acceptable to her.	7. The adolescent needs to feel that she is part of her peer group. Including her input on what she likes to eat may increase her compliance.
8. Discuss the importance of breakfast during pregnancy. Explain that the fetus needs a steady supply of nutrients, especially in the morning after the long fast during the night.	8. Prolonged periods without maternal food intake can lead to a state of ketosis that is hostile to the fetus.
9. Discuss breakfast foods that Vicki likes. Point out the nutrients found in whole grain breads and cereals (such as protein, iron, B vitamins) and their importance.	9. Whole grains are often part of a well-balanced breakfast.
10. Suggest that Vicki eat foods not usually considered breakfast foods. For example, cold pizza provides calcium and protein.	10. Nontraditional methods of meeting the adolescent's nutritional needs may be very effective.

Intervention—cont'd	Rationale
11. Suggest foods high in nutrient density that are available from snack dispensers. Ask which of these are acceptable to Vicki.	11. Adolescents are unlikely to give up foods that help them feel part of their peer group.
12. After explaining their importance to her and her baby, ask Vicki whether she is willing to eat more dairy products. Help her choose those she will eat to meet her needs.	12. Compliance is increased when clients maintain a feeling of control.
13. Ask Vicki whether she is taking and tolerating her vitamin-mineral supplements. Offer suggestions on ways to deal with any problems she is having in this area. Reinforce the importance of consistent intake.	13. Adolescents generally need supplements but may be inconsistent in taking them, especially if they experience side effects.
14. Ask Vicki to bring in another 24-hour diet history on her next visit.	14. Reassessment of dietary intake identifies new or continuing problems.
15. Ask Vicki to share ways she has found to meet her diet needs that you could tell other teenagers. Ask for feedback on the methods discussed.	15. Feeling that her thoughts and ideas are valued by the nurse is important for the adolescent.

Evaluation: Vicki gains 1.8 to 2.7 kg (4 to 6 lb) per month throughout the rest of her pregnancy for a total weight gain of 15 kg (33 lb). Her reported dietary intake shows that she is meeting the recommendations for each food group. She brings back ideas about ways to eat fast foods healthfully and seems to like educating the nurse about teenage diet preferences. Her hemoglobin level rises to 11 g/dl. A healthy 3.4 kg (7.5 lb) baby girl is born at term.

When making suggestions, the nurse should focus on necessary changes only. If an adolescent believes she must eliminate all her favorite foods, she is likely to rebel. Suggestions should be kept to a minimum, and snacks should be included in the meal plan. Asking for the adolescent's input increases the likelihood that she will follow suggestions. When changes are necessary the nurse should explain the reasons they are important for both the fetus and the expectant mother. Teenagers, like other pregnant women, often make changes for the sakes of their unborn children that they would not consider for themselves alone.

The need to be like her peers is of major importance to the adolescent, especially when she is going through the changes of pregnancy. With education about appropriate choices, she can eat fast foods with her friends and still maintain a nourishing diet. Various examples of alternatives from which she can choose should be very helpful (Table 9-10 and "Pregnant Adolescents Want to Know").

Table 9-10
NUTRITIOUS CHOICES FROM SNACK MACHINES*

Food	Nutrients Provided
Yogurt and white or chocolate milk	Protein and calcium
Fruit juices and fresh fruits (such as apples, oranges)	Vitamins and fiber
Popcorn (best without butter and salt)	Fiber
Peanuts	Protein
Granola and granola bars	Fiber and protein
Crackers and cheese	Protein and calcium
Crackers and peanut butter	Protein

*Snack machines generally dispense foods high in calories, fats, and sodium and low in nutrients. Although the foods listed here are somewhat high in calories, they also provide other worthwhile nutrients.

Vegetarianism

Although the knowledgeable vegetarian may eat a highly nutritional diet, she is at higher risk during pregnancy when her nutrient intake must nourish the fetus and herself. If she is new to vegetarian food practices, uninformed about pregnancy needs, or careless with her diet, she could fail to meet her nutrient needs. Guidelines for vegetarians during pregnancy are similar to the food pyramid groups for nonvegetarians and easy to remember when planning the daily diet (Table 9-11).

Table 9-11
FOOD PLAN FOR PREGNANT VEGETARIANS

Food	Number of Servings/Day
Whole and enriched grains	7
Green and yellow vegetables	3 to 5
Fruits, including vitamin C	3
Dairy products	3
Legumes, soy products, and meat substitutes	2 to 3

Vitamin and mineral supplements may be necessary according to individual needs. Those who do not use dairy products need to increase sources of calcium and may need supplementation.

Vegetarianism occurs in a variety of forms. Vegans avoid all animal products and may have the most dif-

PREGNANT ADOLESCENTS WANT TO KNOW: How Can I Eat Fast Foods and Still Maintain a Good Diet?

- Add cheese to hamburgers to increase calcium and protein. Include lettuce and tomato for vitamins A and C.
- Avoid dressings on hamburgers because they tend to be high in calories and fat.
- To reduce fat and calories, choose broiled, roasted, and barbecued foods (such as chicken breast, roast beef). Avoid fried foods (such as French fries, fried zucchini, onion rings) because they are high in fat and the high heat may destroy some vitamins. Breaded foods like chicken nuggets and breaded clams are high in calories and absorb more oil if they are fried.
- Baked potatoes with broccoli, cheese, and meat fillings provide better nutrition than French fries or even baked potatoes with sour cream and butter.
- Pizza is high in calories, but the cheese provides protein and calcium. Ask for vegetable toppings or add a salad to increase vitamins.
- Salad bars are often available at fast food restaurants and provide vitamins and minerals without adding too many calories. Use only a small amount of salad dressing, which is high in fat.
- Milk, milkshakes, and orange juice provide more nutrients than carbonated beverages, which are high in sodium, phosphorus, and calories. Too much sodium may increase swelling of the ankles. Too much phosphorus may lead to leg cramps.
- Avoid pickles, olives, and other salty foods. Add only small amounts of salt to foods to prevent or decrease swelling.

ficulty meeting their nutrient needs. Their diet may be lacking in adequate iodine, calcium, iron, zinc, riboflavin, and vitamins D and B_{12} (Peckenpaugh & Poleman, 1999). Vegans must pay particular attention to obtaining these nutrients in food or supplement form. Meeting their nutrient needs is easier for lactovegetarians, ovovegetarians, and lacto-ovovegetarians.

Although not true vegetarianism, the elimination of red meats from the diet to decrease intake of saturated fats and cholesterol is a growing trend. Women who follow this type of diet usually eat small amounts of chicken, fish, and dairy products. The needs of women who follow any form of vegetarianism are different during pregnancy.

Meeting the Nutritional Requirements of Pregnancy

Energy. Vegetarian diets are low in calories and fat and may not meet energy needs of pregnancy. The diets are high in fiber and may cause a feeling of fullness before enough calories are eaten. A pregnant woman can increase caloric intake by eating snacks between meals and foods with higher caloric content. If carbohydrate and fat intake are too low, her body may use protein for energy, making it unavailable for other purposes.

Protein. Protein intake is a concern in all vegetarian diets. "Complete" proteins, which contain all the essential amino acids the body cannot synthesize from other sources, are an indispensable part of the diet. Animal proteins are complete, but vegetable proteins lack one or more of the essential amino acids. Combining incomplete plant proteins with other plant foods that have complementary amino acids allows intake of all essential amino acids. Dishes that combine grains (such as wheat, rice, corn) with legumes (such as garbonzo, navy, kidney, pinto, or soy beans and peas, peanuts) provide complete proteins. Tofu, made from soybeans, is often used by vegetarians to provide protein.

Incomplete proteins can also be combined with small amounts of complete protein foods such as cheese to provide all amino acids. Therefore women who include even small amounts of animal products have less difficulty meeting their protein needs.

Calcium. Vegetarians who include milk products in their diet may meet their pregnancy needs for calcium. Vegans obtain calcium from vegetables, but their high-fiber diet may interfere with calcium absorption. Calcium-fortified soy products such as soy milk and tofu may meet the requirements, or calcium supplements may be necessary. Vitamin D supplementation is especially important if the woman drinks no milk and has little exposure to sunlight. Soy milks may be enriched with vitamin D.

Iron. Iron in the vegetarian diet is poorly absorbed because of the lack of heme iron from meats, which improves absorption. Iron supplementation is particularly important for vegetarian women during pregnancy.

Zinc. Because the best sources of zinc are meat and fish, vegans may be deficient in this mineral. They usually need zinc supplements to meet their needs.

Vitamin B_{12}. Vitamin B_{12} is obtained only from animal products. Because vegetarian diets contain large amounts of folic acid, the development of anemia from inadequate intake of vitamin B_{12} may not be apparent at first. Vegans may eat fortified foods such as soy products or take supplements.

Vitamin A. Vitamin A is generally abundant in vegetarian diets. If a pregnant woman receives a multiple vitamin–mineral supplement, she may take in excessive amounts of vitamin A, causing toxicity with anorexia, irritability, hair loss, and dry skin and damage to the fetus. Supplementation should be individualized for each woman based on her diet and needs.

Lactose Intolerance

Intolerance to lactose is caused by a deficiency of lactase, a small intestine enzyme necessary for absorption of lactose, a milk sugar. Some degree of lactose intolerance is normal for most of the world's population after early childhood. This includes many African-American, Latina, Asian, Native American, and Middle Eastern women. Although women with lactose intolerance may tolerate cultured and fermented milk products such as aged cheese, buttermilk, and yogurt, symptoms may occur after drinking as little as 1 cup of milk. Symptoms include nausea, bloating, flatulence, diarrhea, and intestinal cramping.

Although the ability to tolerate lactose may increase during pregnancy, women who avoid dairy foods are at risk for not meeting the recommended amounts of calcium unless they get enough from other sources. Most women can tolerate small amounts of milk, and they should increase their intake of other foods that provide calcium (see Table 9-7). Low-lactose milk is available, or the enzyme lactase (LactAid) can be added to milk.

Nausea and Vomiting of Pregnancy

Morning sickness usually occurs during the first trimester and disappears soon afterward, although some women experience nausea at other times of the day and for longer than 12 weeks. However, most women can consume enough food to maintain nutrition sufficiently. They are often able to manage frequent, small meals better than three large meals. Protein and complex carbohydrates are often tolerated best, but fatty foods increase nausea. Drinking liquids between meals instead of with meals often helps. Taking a bedtime protein snack such as cheese helps maintain glucose levels through the night. Eating a carbohydrate food such as dry toast or crackers before getting out of bed in the morning helps prevent nausea.

Anemia

Anemia is a common concern during pregnancy. A Healthy People 2010 goal is to reduce iron deficiency anemia in females of childbearing age from the 1988 to 1994 baseline of 11% to 7% and reduce anemia in low-income pregnant women in the third trimester from the 1996 baseline of 29% to 20% (U.S. Department of Health and Human Services, 2000).

Although the normal hemoglobin level for nonpregnant women is 13.5 g/dl, hemoglobin values during the second trimester of pregnancy average 11.6 g/dl as a result of the dilution of the blood caused by plasma increases. This increase is often called *physiologic anemia* and is normal (see Chapter 7). During the third trimester, hemoglobin levels generally rise to 12.5 g/dl because of increased absorption of iron from the gastrointestinal tract, even though iron is transferred to the fetus primarily during this time.

Fetal iron stores during the third trimester are sufficient to prevent anemia in the newborn for the first 4 to 6 months after birth. However, if the woman's intake of iron is insufficient, her hemoglobin levels may not rise during the third trimester, nutritional anemia may develop, and transfer of iron to the fetus may be decreased. One large nutritional survey among low-income women showed that more than 37% of women had hemoglobin levels less than 11.0 g/dl (Perry, et al., 1995).

Iron stores may be measured by determining the serum ferritin level of the blood. A ferritin level less than 12 mcg/L indicates anemia caused by iron deficiency. A woman may begin pregnancy with anemia or develop it during pregnancy. Pregnant women are considered anemic if the hemoglobin level is 10.5 g/dl or lower (Duffy, 1999).

Anemic women need help choosing foods high in iron (see Table 9-6). They should take iron supplements because diet alone is unlikely to provide adequate amounts of iron. Iron supplements are best absorbed if taken between meals with a dietary source of vitamin C to increase absorption. Because high intakes of iron inhibit use of zinc and copper, anemic women may also need to take these minerals.

Abnormal Prepregnancy Weight

In addition to teaching about dietary changes, the nurse should be alert for other problems associated with abnormal prepregnancy weight. The woman who is below normal weight may not have enough money for food or may have an eating disorder. In addition, obese woman may have other health problems such as hypertension that may affect the nurse's nutritional counseling plan.

Eating Disorders

Eating disorders include anorexia nervosa (refusal to eat because of a distorted body image and feelings of obesity) and bulimia (overeating sometimes followed by induced vomiting). These conditions can be a threat to pregnancy and fetal development and require close supervision during pregnancy (James, 2000). Some women with these disorders eat normally during pregnancy for the sakes of the fetuses. For others, old fears about obesity may be reactivated by the normal weight gain of pregnancy. They may return to their previous eating patterns during pregnancy or in the early postpartum period when they do not lose weight immediately. These women need a great deal of individual counseling to be sure that they meet the increased nutrient needs of pregnancy and understand normal postpartum weight loss.

Pica

The practice of eating substances not normally considered food is called *pica.* Ice, freezer frost, clay and dirt, solid laundry starch, corn starch, chalk, crushed ice, baking soda, baking powder, burnt matches, and ashes are examples. Pica is more common in the southeastern United States and among African-American women but is not limited to any one socioeconomic group or geographic area.

The cause of pica is unknown, although cultural values may make pica a common practice. Pica may be related to beliefs regarding a material's effects on labor or the baby. For example, some women believe that starch gives the skin a lighter tone or helps the baby to be born more easily. Some women fear that their eating habits are harmful but are unable to ignore the cravings. They may hide their eating practices from caregivers who might disapprove (Cooksey, 1995).

The major concern with pica is that eating nonfood substances decreases the intake of foods and essential nutrients. Iron deficiency was once thought to be a cause of pica but is now considered a result because some substances may bind iron (Abrams & Pickett, 1999). Clay and dirt may decrease absorption of other nutrients such as iron, be contaminated with organisms, and cause intestinal blockage (Grodner, Anderson, & DeYoung, 2000).

CRITICAL THINKING EXERCISE

Joan very hesitantly confides in the nurse that the reason she is not gaining much weight is that she eats large amounts of ice. She buys bags of crushed ice and eats the frost that forms in her freezer. "I know I should be gaining more weight, but I'm just not hungry for anything besides ice," she says.

QUESTIONS:

1. What might happen if Joan believes the nurse disapproves of her actions?
2. How should the nurse handle this situation?

Multiparity and Multifetal Pregnancy

The number and spacing of pregnancies and presence of more than one fetus influence the nutritional requirements. The woman who has had more than five pregnancies may begin a pregnancy with a nutritional deficit. In addition, she may be too busy meeting the needs of her family to be attentive to her own nutritional needs.

Closely spaced pregnancies may not allow a woman to make up any nutritional deficits originating from a previous pregnancy. Thus she begins a new pregnancy with inadequate nutrient stores to maintain both her own needs and fetal requirements. She is not able to draw from those stores as usual during pregnancy and must meet nutritional needs from her daily diet and supplementation alone. The development of morning sickness from a new pregnancy soon after delivery may further interfere with an expectant mother's ability to eat an adequate diet.

The woman with a multifetal pregnancy must provide enough nutrients to meet the needs of each fetus without depleting her own stores. The expectant mother definitely needs more calories to meet her weight gain and energy needs. An additional gain of 4.5 to 9 kg (10 to 20 lb) above that of single pregnancies is suggested for women who are pregnant with twins. Supplementation with calcium, iron, and folic acid also may be necessary.

Substance Abuse

The damaging effects of smoking, alcohol, and drug use on the fetus are discussed in Chapter 24. Substance abuse often accompanies a lifestyle that is unlikely to promote good eating habits. The expense of supporting a substance abuse habit may decrease money available for the purchase of food. Therefore nutrition in pregnant women who abuse substances should be explored fully. Usually, more than one substance is involved. The effects on nutrition of various combinations of substances are not fully understood.

Smoking

Cigarette smoking increases maternal metabolic rate and decreases appetite, which may result in a lower weight gain. Infant birth weight decreases despite an adequate diet as the amount of smoking increases. Smoking causes vasoconstriction that interferes with blood flow through the placenta. The many chemicals found in cigarette smoke may also retard fetal growth. Smokers need more vitamins B_{12} and C, folic acid, iron, zinc, and amino acids because smoking decreases the availability of these nutrients to the pregnant woman and fetus. Vitamin-mineral supplements may help meet their needs during pregnancy. Counseling to help the woman stop smoking or at least decrease the number of cigarettes smoked during pregnancy is important. Infants born to women who stop smoking during pregnancy have higher birth weights than infants of smoking mothers (Groff, et al., 1997).

Caffeine

The effect of caffeine on nutrition during pregnancy is controversial. Most studies show no association between caffeine and preterm labor or congenital defects, although caffeine may be associated with spontaneous abortion. Mothers who consume more than 300 mg per day (3 or 4 cups of coffee) have an increased risk of having infants who are small for gestational age (Andres, 1999). Caffeine also alters calcium, zinc, and iron absorption and excretion. Until more is known about its effects on nutrition and the fetus, caffeine intake should be limited during pregnancy. Because many women think that caffeine is present only in coffee and tea, the nurse should discuss other sources of caffeine. These include chocolate, some carbonated beverages, and some medications.

Alcohol
Because of the association between drinking and fetal alcohol syndrome, women should avoid alcohol completely during pregnancy (see Chapter 24). Alcohol interferes with absorption and use of some nutrients (such as protein, thiamine, folic acid, zinc), impairs metabolism, and often takes the place of food in the diet. Vitamin-mineral supplementation may be necessary for women who had large intakes of alcohol before pregnancy, even if they stop drinking after conception, because their nutrient stores may be depleted.

Drugs
The use of drugs other than those prescribed during pregnancy increases danger to the fetus and may interfere with nutrition. Abusers often use a combination of various drugs. The interaction of various drugs with nutrients is not fully understood.

Marijuana increases appetite, but women may not satisfy their hunger with foods of good nutrient quality. Heroin interferes with insulin response to glucose and metabolism. Cocaine acts as an appetite suppressant, interfering with nutrient intake. Vasoconstriction from cocaine use decreases nutrient flow to the fetus. Cocaine users also tend to drink more caffeine and alcoholic beverages. Amphetamines depress appetite. Women who use amphetamines for dieting should be warned that these drugs should be discontinued during pregnancy.

Other Risk Factors
Women who follow food fads may be at risk for not meeting the requirements for pregnancy. Women who have followed a severely restricted diet for a long time may have depleted nutrient stores. Nurses can help them understand nutrition during pregnancy and the necessary diet changes to help ensure successful pregnancies.

Women with complications of pregnancy such as diabetes, heart disease, and pregnancy-induced hypertension may require dietary alterations. Those with other medical conditions such as extreme obesity, cystic fibrosis, and celiac disease may need nutritional counseling from a dietitian.

Check Your Reading

15. What nutritional problems should the nurse look for and assess when caring for low-income women?
16. What nutritional problems may the adolescent have during pregnancy?
17. What suggestions can the nurse give the vegan about diet during pregnancy?
18. How can lactose-intolerant women increase their intake of calcium?
19. What other conditions present nutritional risk factors during pregnancy?

NUTRITION AFTER BIRTH
Nutritional requirements after birth depend on whether the mother breastfeeds her infant or gives formula. The nurse should review the woman's nutritional knowledge as she returns to her prepregnancy diet and teach the breastfeeding mother ways to adapt her diet to meet the needs of lactation.

Nutrition for the Lactating Mother
The lactating mother must nourish both herself and her baby as she did during pregnancy. Therefore she continues to need a highly nutritious diet. The DRIs for lactating women are increased above pregnancy needs for calories, protein, magnesium, zinc, and vitamins A and C. They are lower for iron and folic acid and remain the same for calcium. They are higher for almost every nutrient compared with the needs of nonpregnant adult women. These recommendations are based on the assumption that the mother produces approximately 750 to 800 ml of breast milk daily. However, the amount of milk produced varies according to the infant's age and whether the infant is taking formula or solid foods with breast milk.

Lactating women with poor diets may have reduced milk levels of selenium, iodine, and some B vitamins (Fagen, 2000). Milk volume is usually adequate even when a mother's diet is less than optimal.

Energy
During the first 6 months of lactation, a woman needs approximately 640 calories per day more than she required before she became pregnant. The RDA during lactation is 500 calories each day in addition to normal needs for women according to age, weight, and height. The other 140 calories per day needed to produce breast milk are drawn from maternal stores, aiding in weight loss over a period of time. For the average adult woman, this represents a total caloric intake of 2700 calories each day. Women who were underweight before pregnancy or those who had inadequate weight gain during pregnancy need more calories. The recommendation for these women is 650 additional calories each day depending on their overall nutritional status.

Protein
The RDA for protein during lactation is 65 g each day, which is 5 g above that needed during pregnancy and 15 to 21 g above that required by nonpregnant women, depending on age. This small increase is easily met. A 5-oz glass of milk supplies the 5 mg of protein needed and also provides calcium.

Vitamins and Minerals
Lactating women may not obtain vitamins and minerals in adequate amounts. One study showed they were not consuming enough calcium, zinc, folic acid, and vitamins E, D, and B_6 (Mackey, et al., 1998). Lactating

women who take in at least 1800 calories (well below the energy intake recommended) probably consume adequate amounts of other essential nutrients to meet the infant's and their own needs. Although the quality of the milk is not affected by the mother's intake of most minerals, the vitamin content may be decreased if her diet is consistently low in vitamins. Nutrient levels in the milk may remain constant because some nutrients such as calcium and folic acid are drawn from the mother's stores if her intake is poor. Routine vitamin-mineral supplements are not necessary unless the diet is considered lacking.

Specific Concerns

Some women have difficulty consuming all required nutrients and need special counseling. This group includes women who are dieting, adolescents, vegans, women who avoid dairy products, and those whose diet is inadequate for other reasons.

Dieting

Women who are concerned about losing weight after pregnancy need special consideration. After the initial losses in the first month, weight gradually decreases as maternal fat is used to meet a portion of the energy needs of lactation. Breastfeeding mothers tend to lose body fat even without dieting (Grodner, 2000). Gradual weight loss is preferable and should be accomplished by a combination of moderate exercise and a diet high in nutrients with at least 1800 calories per day.

Dieting should be postponed for at least 3 weeks after birth to allow the woman to recover fully from childbirth and establish her milk supply if she is breastfeeding. Weight loss of more than 2 kg (about 4.5 lb) per month or intakes below 1500 calories per day are likely to interfere with milk production and the mother's nutrient stores (Institute of Medicine, 1991). Although moderate dieting does not affect the quantity of the milk, the mother should evaluate the infant's apparent satisfaction with feedings. She should not use liquid diet drinks and diets that severely restrict any nutrient because she will not meet her needs. Nursing mothers should avoid appetite suppressants, which may pass into the milk and harm the infant.

Adolescence

The problems of the adolescent diet continue to be of concern during lactation. The adolescent may be deficient in the same nutrients as other mothers during lactation and also lacking in iron. If she dislikes or cannot afford fruits and vegetables, she may have an inadequate vitamin A intake.

Vegan Diet

The milk of the vegan mother may contain inadequate vitamin B_{12}, and she and her infant need supplementation. Vitamin D and calcium may also be low. Vegans can meet their need for other nutrients during lactation by diet alone with careful planning. Those who are not knowledgeable about nutrition need supplementation.

Avoidance of Dairy Products

The recommendation for calcium remains the same for pregnancy and lactation, and the calcium content of breast milk is not affected by maternal intake. However, prolonged lactation with inadequate calcium intake may cause removal of calcium from the mother's bones. Women who do not eat dairy products should obtain calcium from other sources (see Table 9-7) or take a calcium supplement. Unless they consume foods fortified with vitamin D or are exposed to sunlight, they may also require vitamin D supplementation, which is necessary for calcium absorption.

Inadequate Diet

Women with cultural and other food prohibitions may need help choosing a diet adequate for lactation. Those with inadequate income may need referral to agencies such as WIC. If the mother must take medications that interfere with absorption of certain nutrients, her diet should be high in foods containing those nutrients.

Alcohol

Alcohol intake during lactation is another concern. Although the relaxing effect of alcohol was once considered helpful to the nursing mother, the damaging effects of alcohol are too important to consider this suggestion appropriate today. An occasional single glass of an alcoholic beverage may not be harmful, but larger amounts may interfere with the milk-ejection reflex and be harmful to the infant.

Caffeine

Foods high in caffeine should also be limited. The mother should restrict her caffeine intake to two cups of coffee or the equivalent each day. Caffeine in excessive amounts can make the infant irritable and may decrease the iron content of the milk.

Fluids

Nursing mothers should drink fluids sufficient to relieve thirst, which often increases in the early breastfeeding period. At least eight glasses of fluids that do not contain caffeine are adequate. Drinking large quantities of fluids, as was once recommended, is not necessary.

Foods to Avoid

Lactating mothers are often concerned about whether they should avoid certain foods that might adversely affect the infant. Except for foods to which the mother is allergic, no specific foods must be restricted in every case. Most mothers find that few foods affect the infant and fussiness is related to other factors. If the family

Breastfeeding Mothers Want to Know

How Can I Tell Which Foods Are Affecting My Baby?

- Keep a list of any foods you eat that are new or different from your usual diet.
- Look for signs that the baby may be reacting to something you ate. Signs include excessive irritability, crying as if in pain, passing gas, diarrhea, and rash. These signs happen for other reasons than a reaction to your diet, so consider other causes as well.
- When your baby has a fussy period, note whether you ate anything new during the previous 8 to 12 hours.
- Watch the baby's reaction after you have eaten any food that sometimes causes problems for infants. These include foods in the cabbage family, onions, foods that are highly allergenic (such as wheat, eggs, cow's milk) or acidic (such as orange juice), spicy foods, garlic, nuts, chocolate, and large amounts of fresh fruits.
- If you think there may be a connection between something you ate and distress in your baby, avoid that food for several days to 1 week. Then try a small amount of the food again. If the baby seems to be affected, eliminate that food from your diet.
- Eat all foods in moderation. Babies often tolerate small amounts of any food in their mother's diet but react to large amounts.

history places the infant at risk for developing allergies, the woman should avoid highly allergic foods including cow's milk, eggs, fish, and nuts (AAP, 2000).

Nutrition for the Nonlactating Mother

The postpartum woman who is not breastfeeding can return to her prepregnancy diet, provided it meets the RDA for the adult woman. She should plan her diet so that it contains enough protein and vitamin C foods to promote healing. If the woman was taking prenatal vitamin-mineral supplements, many nurse practitioners and obstetricians suggest that she continue to take them until her supply is finished. This ensures adequate intake during the time involution occurs and helps renew nutrient stores.

The nurse should assess the mother's understanding of the number of servings she needs from each food group. A review of important nutrient sources for calcium and iron may be relevant. If the woman was anemic during pregnancy, she should continue to take an iron supplement until hemoglobin levels return to normal.

When her baby is born, a woman can expect to lose about 4.5 to 5.5 kg (10 to 12 lb) immediately. She loses approximately another 2.3 to 3.6 kg (5 to 8 lb) during involution and will probably reach her prepregnancy weight within 6 to 12 months if she follows a well-balanced diet. She should consume 300 calories per day less than she did during pregnancy to avoid retaining weight.

Some women are impatient with slow weight loss and disappointed that they do not lose all their pregnancy weight gain soon after the baby is born. New mothers should wait at least 3 weeks to start dieting to lose weight because they need energy to meet the demands of infant care. Suggestions for sensible calorie reduction combined with exercise are appropriate. Women who gain a large amount of weight beyond that recommended during pregnancy may have difficulty losing it after birth and take longer to do so.

Mothers are sometimes so involved with the needs of the infant during the early days that they fail to eat properly. They may snack instead of planning meals for themselves, especially if they are home alone with the baby during the day. The nurse should remind them that snacking often involves high caloric intake without meeting nutritional needs. During postpartum the mother needs to ensure her own good health so that she is able to care for her baby. Therefore meals and snacks should be high in nutrient content.

Check Your Reading

20. How do the nutritional needs of the lactating mother compare with those of the woman who is not lactating? How do they compare with those of the woman who is pregnant?
21. What foods should the breastfeeding woman avoid in her diet?
22. What changes should the woman who is not breastfeeding make after the birth of her baby?

APPLICATION OF THE NURSING PROCESS: NUTRITION FOR CHILDBEARING

The nursing process focuses on determining the factors that might interfere with the woman's ability to meet the nutrient needs of pregnancy, the postpartum period, and lactation and finding solutions to any problems identified. This process primarily involves education of the woman.

Assessment

Interview

The interview provides an opportunity to develop rapport and identify any specific problems affecting dietary intake.

Appetite. The nurse should begin the interview by discussing the woman's appetite. Has it changed during the pregnancy, and in what ways does it compare with her appetite before pregnancy? Determine the severity and duration of nausea and vomiting associated with morning sickness. For some women the discomfort is mild and occurs only during the morning or when they are fatigued. For others, severe nausea continues throughout the day and beyond the first trimester. Hyperemesis gravidarum is the most serious form of this problem and often requires intravenous correction of fluid and electrolyte imbalance and parenteral nutrition (see Chapter 25).

Eating Habits. Assess the usual pattern of meals to discover poor food habits such as skipping breakfast or eating snack foods for lunch. Determine who does the cooking for the family. If a pregnant teenager's mother cooks for her, discuss nutritional needs during pregnancy with the mother. If the woman does the cooking herself, the likes and dislikes of other family members may influence what she serves, especially if she has little understanding of her own needs during pregnancy.

Food Preferences. Ask about her food preferences and dislikes. The woman who dislikes all fruits and vegetables needs another source of vitamins. During pregnancy, some women experience an aversion to certain foods (such as meats) that they do not have at other times. Careful counseling helps work around dislikes and aversions to find ways of obtaining the nutrients needed.

Discussing likes and dislikes provides an opening to ask about food cravings and pica. Cravings may be for nutritional foods or foods low in nutrient density and eaten in amounts that interfere with intake of other foods. Ask about pica in a matter-of-fact way to avoid giving an impression of disapproval. Food items such as ice are included in pica and should be asked about as well. Also ask whether the mother eats large amounts of a particular food or group of foods.

> When assessing for pica the nurse might say "Have you had any cravings for special things to eat during your pregnancy?" This can be followed with "Women sometimes eat things like ice, clay, and starch during pregnancy. What about you?" Some women are willing to substitute foods such as nonfat dry milk powder for nonfood items such as laundry starch.

Psychosocial Influences. Ascertain whether cultural or religious considerations affect the diet. Do these apply only during pregnancy or at all times? Assess whether the woman follows all or only certain restrictions and determine the effect on her nutrient intake.

Identify other factors that interfere with adequate nutrition. Women with low incomes may not know about sources of assistance. Inquire how long the vegetarian has followed her diet and determine her awareness of changes necessary during pregnancy. A woman's smoking, alcohol intake, and other substance abuse may become obvious during the interview. Ask about prescription drugs and determine whether she takes medications that interfere with nutrient absorption. Other questions include the amount of time she has for food preparation and the frequency of eating fast foods.

Ask the woman if she has any special concerns about her diet. This question may bring out fears about excessive weight gain and concerns that specific foods could hurt the fetus. It also allows her to discuss issues that have not yet been addressed.

Diet History

Diet histories provide information about a woman's usual intake of nutrients. Food intake records, food frequency questionnaires, and 24-hour diet histories can form a basis for counseling about any changes required to meet pregnancy needs. They also help the woman become more aware of her eating habits.

A 24-Hour Diet History. Ask the woman to recall what she ate at each meal and snack during the previous 24 hours and answer specific questions about the size of portions, ingredients, food preparation for each individual meal, and beverages and snacks between meals and at bedtime. Determine whether this sample is typical of her usual daily food intake and whether the woman has met the recommendations for specific food groups, calories, and protein. Detailed analysis for individual nutrients is unnecessary because it is time consuming and daily variation in intake occurs.

The food history may be inaccurate if the woman cannot remember what she ate or is mistaken about amounts of food. Models of food items and use of measuring utensils may be helpful. The expectant mother may alter her reported intake to make it appear that she is eating better. She may be embarrassed about her inability to follow the diet prescribed because of lack of money or cooking facilities. The atmosphere created by the nurse is important in helping mothers feel free to be honest.

Food Intake Records. Food intake records are used to report foods eaten during 1 or more days. Ask the woman to list everything she eats throughout the day. The list is more accurate if she writes down each food immediately after eating. Some women eat more nutritious foods during the recording period when they are concentrating on good diet, then go back to a less wholesome diet later.

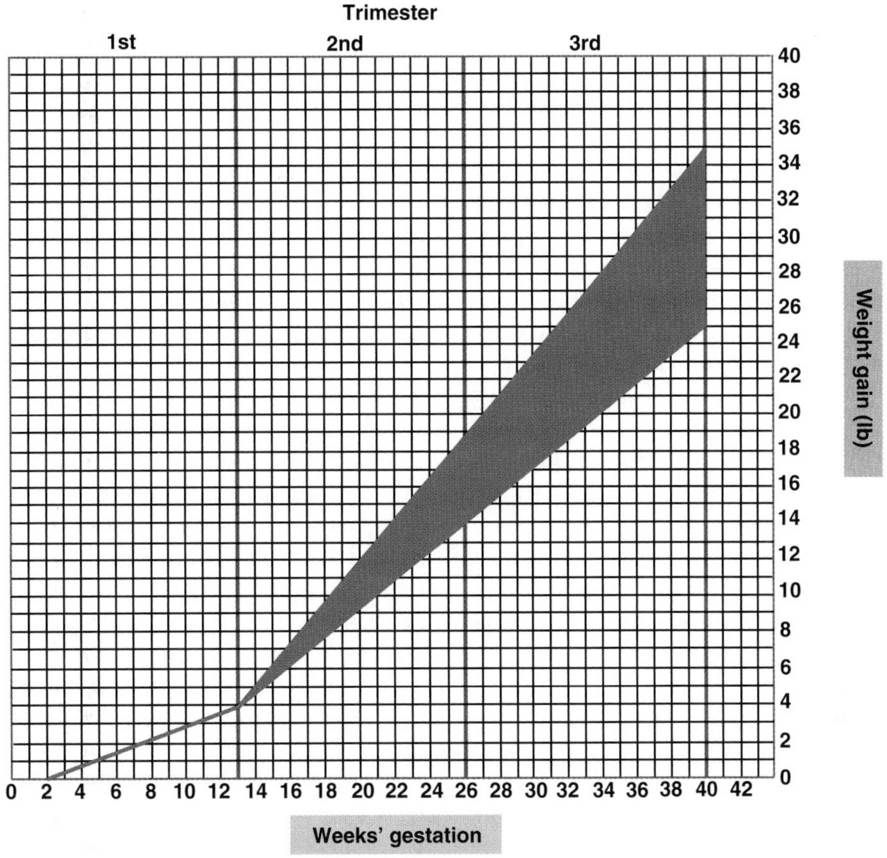

FIGURE 9-4 Weight gain grid for pregnancy. The normal range for weight gain is 11.5 to 16 kg (25 to 35 lb). Adolescents often need to gain in the higher end of the range. Women who are shorter than 157 cm (62 inches) should gain in the lower portion.

Food Frequency Questionnaires. Food frequency questionnaires, which contain lists of common foods, may provide information about diet over a longer time. Review the questionnaire with the woman and ask her how often she eats each food. Foods consumed daily and weekly are her most common source of nutrients. Analyze the list to determine whether foods from each food group are eaten in adequate amounts to meet pregnancy needs and determine whether any major groups are omitted.

Physical Assessment

Information about nutritional status can be obtained during the physical assessment. This assessment includes measurement of weight and examination for signs of nutritional deficiency.

Weight at Initial Visit. The woman's weight at the first prenatal visit can serve as a baseline value for future comparison. Ask her if this is her usual weight or if she has gained or lost weight. Measuring her height without shoes is preferred to asking her for her height because she may not have had an accurate recent measurement. Compare her prepregnancy weight for height to tables of normal values to help draw conclusions about her nutritional condition. If her weight is low for height, nutritional reserves are marginal. If it is high, she may be overweight or obese.

Weight at Subsequent Visits. Assessment of weight gain at each prenatal visit provides an easy method of estimating whether nutrition is adequate and serves as a basis for counseling about nutrition. Weigh the woman at each visit on the same scale with approximately the same amount of clothing. She should remove her shoes and coat to obtain an accurate measurement.

Record the weight on a weight grid at each visit throughout the pregnancy (Figure 9-4). This grid allows examination of the pattern and total gain to date. It also helps keep track of the amount of gain between individual visits.

> Be careful not to overemphasize weight gain. In some instances a woman may be afraid that caregivers will be disapproving if she gains weight and consequently may diet or fast for 1 or 2 days before her prenatal visit.

Signs of Nutrient Deficiency. Other indications of nutritional status include any signs of deficiency. For example, bleeding gums may indicate inadequate intake of vitamin C. However, actual deficiency states are not likely to occur in women in most industrialized countries. Even though intake may not be enough to allow for optimal health and storage of nutrients, most women obtain enough nutrients to avoid signs of deficiency. The most important exception is iron-deficiency anemia, which is common in a mild form. Signs and symptoms include pallor, low hemoglobin level, fatigue, and increased susceptibility to infection.

Laboratory Tests

Laboratory tests are generally impractical for in-depth analysis of nutrient intake. Analysis of specific nutrients is expensive and normal laboratory values during pregnancy have not been determined for all laboratory tests. Hemoglobin, hematocrit, and in some cases serum ferritin tests are most often used to determine anemia, particularly iron-deficiency anemia.

Reassessing Nutritional Status at Each Visit

At each prenatal visit the nurse should (1) reassess the woman's dietary status, (2) ask if she has any questions about her diet and has had any difficulty, (3) check her weight gain to see whether she is within the expected pattern, (4) evaluate her hemoglobin and hematocrit levels to detect anemia, and (5) explain what assessments are being made and why.

Analysis

Although some women consume more calories than necessary during pregnancy and risk obesity as a result, more women are likely to eat fewer nutrients than recommended. The problem may be related to many factors, the most common of which is general lack of knowledge. Therefore the most important nursing diagnosis concerning nutrition is "Altered Nutrition: Less than Body Requirements" related to lack of understanding about the nutrient needs of pregnancy.

Planning

Goals and expected outcomes for this nursing diagnosis include the following:

- The woman will consume a diet meeting the DRIs for nutrients throughout her pregnancy.
- The woman with a normal BMI before pregnancy will gain approximately 1.4 to 1.8 kg (3 to 4 lb) during the first trimester. She will gain 0.44 kg (about 1 lb) per week during the second and third trimesters for a total gain of 11.5 to 16 kg (25 to 35 lb).

Interventions

Identifying Problems

After analyzing food likes and dislikes and taking a 24-hour diet history, identify any obvious areas of potential deficiency and determine the woman's knowledge about the nutrient needs of pregnancy.

Explaining Nutrient Needs

Use the woman's diet history as a basis to introduce information about nutrition during pregnancy. Explain the recommended servings from each food group, help the woman analyze her own diet so that she understands the process and its importance and determine whether she meets the number of servings recommended for each food group. Explain which important nutrients are provided in each food group and why they are necessary for her and the fetus.

Make a rough estimate of calories, protein, iron, and calcium in the diet for a general idea of intake of these nutrients. The usual sources of these major nutrients compared with her diet history and favorite foods can help determine whether the woman eats enough of these foods regularly. Suggest ways to resolve nutrient deficiencies and also remind the woman that adequate nutrition, especially intake of iron and folic acid, is important in reducing the fatigue that is so common during pregnancy and after birth (Lee & Zafke, 1999).

Providing Reinforcement

Give frequent positive reinforcement when the woman is eating appropriately. Assist her in evaluating necessary changes in her diet, and plan ways to overcome weaknesses in her present diet (Figure 9-5). Ask her what problems she foresees in obtaining the nutrients she needs. Explore a variety of options to overcome expected problems and ask about the way these changes will affect the rest of her family. Perhaps the changes she needs to make for her own needs would be beneficial to the entire family.

If the woman can read, give her written materials on nutrition during pregnancy and review them with her. If she can take the information home, she can review it often to ensure that she is eating properly. A small pamphlet with pictures might be placed on the refrigerator to help her remember what foods she needs each day.

Evaluating Weight Gain

Compare the woman's weight to a weight gain grid to ascertain whether she has gained the appropriate amount of weight for this point in her pregnancy. Discuss the importance and expected pattern of weight gain and explain the importance of eating foods high in nutrient density when she is increasing calories. If she is greatly outside of normal ranges, discuss necessary diet modifications with her primary health care provider. For example, an obese woman is expected to gain some weight but the amount must be individualized according to her particular needs.

Although slight variations from the recommended weight gain have little significance, possible reasons for

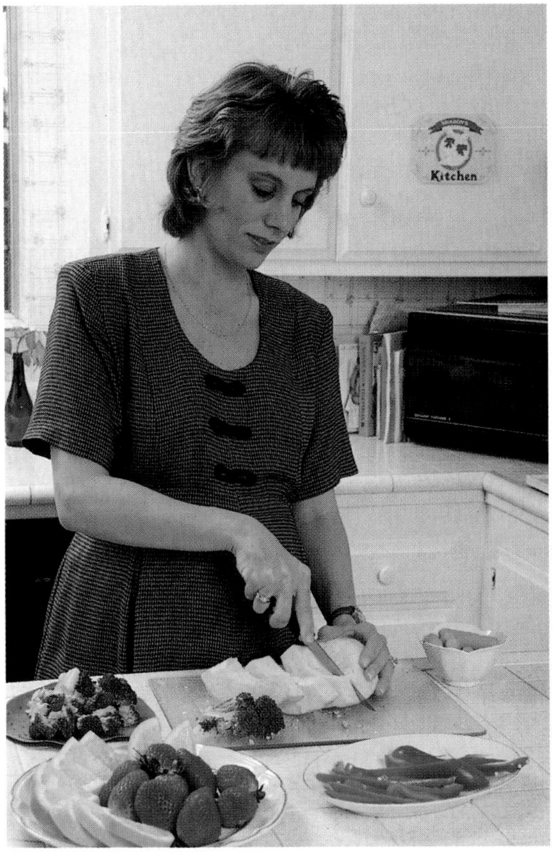

FIGURE 9-5 Women often make changes in their diets for the sakes of their unborn children that they would not consider for themselves alone.

larger differences should be examined carefully. For women of normal weight a monthly gain of less than 1 kg (2.2 lb) should lead to a discussion of diet and possible problems in food intake. A gain of more than 2.9 kg (6.5 lb) per month may signify a serious problem such as pregnancy-induced hypertension (see Chapter 25). However, errors in calculation of gestation may also reflect a pattern of weight gain different from that expected.

Encouraging Supplement Intake

If vitamin-mineral supplements have been prescribed, determine whether she is taking them regularly and, if not, explore reasons and possible solutions. Iron supplements often cause constipation, but dietary changes such as increased intake of fluids and fiber can help prevent this problem (Table 9-12). If the problem is forgetfulness, suggest that she take vitamin-mineral supplements with meals or iron supplements with orange juice at bedtime just before brushing her teeth. If she avoids iron supplements because of side effects such as nausea, she can take them with meals or snacks. Even though taking iron supplements with food decreases the absorption of the iron, it is preferred to not using the supplements at all. Let her know that black stools are a harmless side effect of iron supplements.

Table 9-12
COMMON SOURCES OF DIETARY FIBER

Fruits and vegetables (with skins when possible): apples, strawberries, pears, carrots, corn, potatoes with skins, cabbage, and broccoli
Whole grains and whole grain products: whole wheat bread, bran muffins, bran cereals, oatmeal, brown rice, and whole wheat pasta
Legumes: peas, lentils, kidney beans, lima beans, baked beans, and peanuts

Making Referrals

The nurse can provide nutritional counseling that is more than adequate for most women, but some situations may warrant referral to other sources. Women with health problems that affect nutrition (such as diabetes, celiac disease, extreme weight problems) may need an initial consultation with a dietitian and a follow-up consultation with the nurse. Women with inadequate financial resources to buy food can be referred to public assistance programs such as TANF and WIC. At the next visit, determine whether the woman obtained the help needed and if other assistance is necessary.

Evaluation

Ongoing evaluation of diet and pattern of weight gain throughout the pregnancy determines whether the goals have been met. The woman should meet the RDA for pregnancy by eating the recommended number of servings of each food group. She should gain 1.4 to 1.8 kg (3 to 4 lb) during the first trimester and 0.44 kg (about 1 lb) per week for the second and third trimesters. Total weight gain should fall within 11.5 to 16 kg (25 to 35 lb).

SUMMARY CONCEPTS

- Nutritional education during the childbearing period may have long-term positive effects on the mother, infant, and entire family.
- Weight gain during pregnancy is an important determinant of fetal growth. Poor weight gain in pregnant women is associated with low birth weight in infants, and excessive weight gain may lead to macrosomia and labor complications.
- The recommended weight gain during pregnancy is 11.5 to 16 kg (25 to 35 lb). The amount is greater for women who are underweight or carry more than one fetus and is less for obese women.
- The pattern of weight gain is as important as the total increase in weight. The average should be 1.5 kg (3.5 lb) during the first trimester and 0.44 kg (nearly 1 lb) per week thereafter.

- The recommended increase in energy intake during pregnancy is 300 calories per day. Calorie increases should be attained by choosing foods high in nutrient density to meet other needs of pregnancy.
- Protein should be increased to 60 g daily during pregnancy, which is 10 to 16 g more than nonpregnancy needs.
- Women may not eat enough foods high in vitamins B_6, D, and E and folic acid to meet recommendations. The nurse should encourage clients to eat more foods containing these vitamins.
- Fat-soluble vitamins (A, D, E, K) are stored in the liver. Excess consumption may result in toxicity.
- Daily intake of water-soluble vitamins (B, C) is necessary because excesses are not stored but excreted.
- Minerals most likely to be consumed below recommended amounts in pregnancy are iron, calcium, zinc, and magnesium. Iron is often added as a supplement, whereas calcium is added for women with low intake. The nurse can suggest foods high in iron and calcium.
- Vitamin-mineral supplements must be used carefully to prevent excessive intake and toxicity. Increased intake of some nutrients interferes with use of others and may result in deficiencies.
- Pregnant women should drink at least eight 8-oz glasses of fluids each day. They should eat at least seven servings of whole grains, five servings of fruits and vegetables, three servings of dairy products, and the equivalent of seven 1-oz servings of protein foods.
- Culture can influence diet during pregnancy. The nurse should learn whether a woman follows traditional dietary practices and whether her food practices are consistent with good nutrition.
- Both Southeast Asian and Latino dietary practices include the importance of balancing yin and yang (cold and hot). The nurse must know which foods are acceptable at what times.
- Low-income women may not have enough money or knowledge to meet the nutrient needs of pregnancy. Nurses should refer them for financial assistance and nutritional counseling.
- Adolescents may skip meals and eat snacks and fast foods of low nutrient density, and they are subject to peer pressure that may decrease their nutritional intake.
- Pregnant vegetarians may need help choosing an adequate diet that includes nonanimal sources of energy, protein, iron, calcium, vitamin B_{12}, and other nutrients. They may need vitamin-mineral supplements during pregnancy.
- Lactose-intolerant women should increase calcium intake from foods other than milk such as calcium-rich vegetables.
- Abnormal prepregnancy weight, anemia, eating disorders, pica, multiparity, substance abuse, closely spaced pregnancies, and multifetal pregnancies are all nutritional risk factors that warrant adaptations of diet during pregnancy.
- Lactating women need more of almost every nutrient than women who are not lactating. The increased calories needed for milk production can be met by an added intake of 500 calories, and the remainder comes from maternal fat stores.
- Lactating women should avoid alcohol, caffeine, and foods that seem to cause distress in the infant.
- The postpartum woman who does not breastfeed should decrease her calorie intake by 300 calories but should eat a well-balanced diet to enhance recovery from childbirth. Weight loss should be accomplished slowly and sensibly.

ANSWERS TO CRITICAL THINKING QUESTIONS

1. If Joan feels the nurse is disapproving of her actions, she is unlikely to trust the nurse with further confidences. Because she will probably not end her pica, especially without help, a disapproving nurse will cause her to withdraw and continue to practice it in secret.
2. Being accepting and nonjudgmental is important when responding to Joan. The nurse should use therapeutic communication to explore Joan's feelings about her cravings. The nurse should determine the amount of ice Joan eats each day, whether she has other cravings, and how these affect her intake of important nutrients. Joan and the nurse can work together to find acceptable ways to modify the diet to include more of the food groups that are lacking. Joan should be referred to a dietitian for further counseling. The nurse should continue to discuss the diet at each prenatal visit.

REFERENCES & READINGS

Abrams, B., & Pickett, K.E. (1999). Maternal nutrition. In R.K. Creasy & R. Resnik (Eds.), *Maternal-fetal medicine: Principles and practice* (4th ed., pp. 122-131). Philadelphia: W.B. Saunders.

American Academy of Pediatrics (AAP) Committee on Nutrition. (2000). Hypoallergenic infant formulas. *Pediatrics*, 106(2), 346-349.

American Dietetic Association. (1994). Position of the American Dietetic Association: Nutrition care for pregnant adolescents. *Journal of the American Dietetic Association*, 94(4), 449-450.

Andres, R.L. (1999). Social and illicit drug use in pregnancy. In R.K. Creasy & R. Resnik (Eds.), *Maternal-fetal medicine: Principles and practice* (4th ed., pp. 145-164). Philadelphia: W.B. Saunders.

Andrews, M.M., & Boyle, J.S. (1995). *Transcultural concepts in nursing care* (2nd ed.). Philadelphia: J.B. Lippincott.

Brooks, S.L., Mitchell, A., & Steffenson, N. (2000). Mothers, infants, and DHA: Implications for nursing practice. *MCN: American Journal of Maternal/Child Nursing*, 25(2), 71-75.

Brown, H.L., Watkins, K., & Hiett, A.K. (1996). The impact of the Women, Infants and Children Food Supplement Program on birth outcome. *American Journal of Obstetrics and Gynecology*, 174(4), 1279-1283.

Bronner, Y.L., & Auerback, K.G. (1999). Maternal nutrition during lactation. In J. Riordan & K. Auerback, *Breastfeeding and human lactation* (2nd ed., pp. 515-539). Boston: Jones & Barlett.

Callister, L.C. (1998). Giving birth: Guatemalan women's voices. *Journal of Obstetric, Gynecologic, and Neonatal Nursing*, 27(3), 289-295.

Choudhry, U.K. (1997). Traditional practices of women from India: Pregnancy, childbirth, and newborn care. *Journal of Obstetric, Gynecologic, and Neonatal Nursing*, 26(5), 533-539.

Cooksey, N.R. (1995). Pica and olfactory craving of pregnancy: How deep are the secrets? *Birth*, 23(1), 129-137.

Cunningham, F.G., MacDonald, P.C., Gant, N.F., Leveno, K.J., Gilstrap, L.C., Hankins, G.D.V., & Clark, S.L. (1997). *Williams obstetrics* (20th ed.). Norwalk, CT: Appleton & Lange.

Davis, J., & Sherer, K. (1994). *Applied nutrition and diet therapy for nurses* (2nd ed.). Philadelphia: W.B. Saunders.

Duffy, T.P. (1999). Hematologic aspects of pregnancy. In G.N. Burrow & T.F. Ferris (Eds.), *Medical complications during pregnancy* (5th ed., pp. 79-95). Philadelphia: W.B. Saunders.

Fagen, C. (2000). Nutrition during pregnancy and lactation. In L.K. Mahan & S. Escott-Stump, *Krause's food, nutrition, and diet therapy* (10th ed., pp. 167-195). Philadelphia: W.B. Saunders.

Grodner, M., Anderson, S.L., & DeYoung, S. (2000). *Nutrition, a nursing approach* (2nd ed.). St. Louis: Mosby.

Groff, J.Y., Mullen, P.D., Mongoven, M., & Burau, K. (1997). Prenatal weight gain patterns and infant birth weight associated with maternal smoking. *Birth,* 24(4), 234-239.

Horswill, L.J. & Yap, C. (1999). Consumption of foods from the WIC food packages of Chinese prenatal patients on the U.S. west coast. *Journal of the American Dietetic Association,* 99(12), 1549-1553.

Howse, J.L. (1999). Stopping neural tube defects. *AWHONN Lifelines,* 3(3), 10.

Hutchinson, M.K., & Bazi-Aziz, M. (1994). Nursing care of the childbearing Muslim family. *Journal of Obstetric, Gynecologic, and Neonatal Nursing,* 23(9), 767-771.

Institute of Medicine, Food and Nutrition Board. (1998). *Dietary reference intakes for thiamin, riboflavin, niacin, vitamin B_6, folate, vitamin B_{12}, pantothenic acid, biotin, and choline.* Washington, D.C.: National Academy Press.

Institute of Medicine, Food and Nutrition Board. (1997). *Dietary reference intakes for calcium, phosphorus, magnesium, vitamin D, and* fluoride. Washington, D.C.: National Acad-emy Press.

Institute of Medicine, Food and Nutrition Board. (2000). *Dietary reference intakes for vitamin C, vitamin E, selenium, and carotenoids.* Washington, D.C.: National Academy Press.

Institute of Medicine, National Academy of Sciences, Food and Nutrition Board. (1990). *Nutrition during pregnancy. Part I:* Weight gain. Part II: *Nutrient supplements.* Washington, D.C.: National Academy Press.

Institute of Medicine, National Academy of Sciences, Food and Nutrition Board. (1991). *Nutrition during lactation.* Washington, D.C.: National Academy Press.

Institute of Medicine, National Academy of Sciences, Subcommittee for a Clinical Application Guide. (1992). *Nutrition during pregnancy and lactation, an implementation guide.* Washington, D.C.: National Academy Press.

James, D.C. (2000). Eating disorders in pregnancy: Challenges to nursing care. *Mother Baby Journal,* 5(4), 37-41.

Johnson, J.W.C., Longmate, J.A., & Frentzen, B. (1992). Excessive maternal weight gain and pregnancy outcome. *American Journal of Obstetrics and Gynecology,* 174(4), 1279-1283.

Kane, A. (1999). The Women, Infants, and Children Supplemental Food Program (WIC): What you should know. *International Journal of Childbirth Education,* 14(2), 21-23.

Lawrence, R.A., & Lawrence, R.M. (1999). *Breastfeeding: A guide for the medical profession* (5th ed.). St. Louis: Mosby.

Lee, K.A., & Zafke, M.E. (1999). Longitudinal changes in fatigue and energy during pregnancy and the postpartum period. *Journal of Obstetric, Gynecologic, and Neonatal Nursing,* 28(2), 183-191.

LeMone, P. (1999). Vitamins and minerals. *Journal of Obstetric, Gynecologic, and Neonatal Nursing,* 28(5), 520-533.

Lust, K.D., Brown, J.E., & Thomas, W. (1996). Maternal intake of cruciferous vegetables and other foods and colic symptoms in exclusively breastfed infants. *Journal of the American Dietetic Association,* 96(1), 46-48.

Mackey, A.D., Picciano, M.F., Mitchell, D.C., & Smiciklas-Wright, H. (1998). Self-selected diets of lactating women often fail to meet dietary recommendations. *Journal of the American Dietetic Association,* 98(3), 297-302.

Mattson, S. (1995). Culturally sensitive perinatal care for Southeast Asians. *Journal of Obstetric, Gynecologic, and Neonatal Nursing,* 24(4), 335-341.

Monga, M. (1999). Cardiovascular and renal adaptation to pregnancy. In R.K. Creasy & R. Resnik, *Maternal-fetal medicine: Principles and practice* (4th ed., pp. 783-792). Philadelphia: W.B. Saunders.

Morin, K.H. (1998). Perinatal outcomes of obese women: A review of the literature. *Journal of Obstetric, Gynecologic, and Neonatal Nursing,* 27(4), 431-440.

National Research Council. (1989). *Recommended dietary allowances* (10th ed.). Washington, D.C.: National Academy Press.

Peckenpaugh, N.J., & Poleman, C.M. (1999). *Nutrition essentials and diet therapy* (8th ed.). Philadelphia: W.B. Saunders.

Perry, G.S., Yip, R., & Zyrkowski, C. (1995). Nutritional risk factors among low-income pregnant U.S. women: The Centers for Disease Control and Prevention (CDC) pregnancy nutrition surveillance system 1979 through 1993. *Seminars in Perinatology,* 19(3), 211-221.

Purfield, P., & Morin, K. (1995). Excessive weight gain in primigravidas with low-risk pregnancy: Selected obstetric consequences. *Journal of Obstetric, Gynecologic, and Neonatal Nursing,* 24(5), 434-439.

Rainville, A.J. (1998). Pica practices of pregnant women are associated with lower maternal hemoglobin level at delivery. *Journal of the American Dietetic Association,* 98(3), 293-296.

Reifsnider, E. & Gill, S.L. (2000). Nutrition for the childbearing years. *Journal of Obstetric, Gynecologic, and Neonatal Nursing,* 29(1), 43-55.

Scholl, T.O., & Hediger, M.L. (1995). Weight gain, nutrition, and pregnancy outcome: Findings from the Camden study of teenage and minority gravidas. *Seminars in Perinatology,* 19(3), 171-181.

Seidman, R.Y., Jacobson, S., Primeaux, M., Burns, P., & Weatherby, F. (1996). Assessing American Indian families. *MCN: American Journal of Maternal/Child Nursing,* 21(6), 274-279.

Spear, B.A. (2000). Nutrition in adolescence. In L.K. Mahan, & S. Escott-Stump. *Krause's food, nutrition, and diet therapy* (10th ed., pp. 257-270). Philadelphia: W.B. Saunders.

Strychar, I.M., Chabot, C., Champagne, F., Ghadirian, P., Leduc, L., Lemonnier, M., & Raynauld, P. (2000). Psychosocial & lifestyle factors associated with insufficient and excessive maternal weight gain during pregnancy. *Journal of the American Dietetic Association,* 100(3), 353-356.

Tulman, L., Morin, K.H., & Fawcett, J. (1998). Prepregnant weight and weight gain during pregnancy: Relationship to functional status, symptoms, and energy. *Journal of Obstetric, Gynecologic, and Neonatal Nursing,* 27(6), 629-634.

U.S. Department of Agriculture. (1992). USDA's food guide pyramid. *Home and Garden Bulletin,* April (249).

U.S. Department of Agriculture, & U.S. Department of Health and Human Services. (1990). Nutrition and your health: Dietary guidelines for Americans (3rd ed.). *Home and Garden Bulletin,* November (232).

U.S. Department of Health and Human Services. (2000). *Healthy People 2010* (Conference ed., 2 volumes). Washington, D.C.: Author.

Williams, S.R. (1999). *Essentials of nutrition and diet therapy* (7th ed.). St. Louis: Mosby.

Williams, S.R. (1997). Nutrition assessment and guidance in prenatal care. In B. Worthington-Roberts & S.R. Williams (Eds.), *Nutrition in pregnancy and lactation* (6th ed.). Madison, WI: Brown & Benchmark.

Wilkerson, N.N. (2000). Nutrition. In F.H. Nichols & S.S. Humenick. *Childbirth education: Practice, research, & theory,* Philadelphia: W.B. Saunders.

Worthington-Roberts, B.S. (1997a). Energy and vitamin needs during pregnancy. In B. Worthington-Roberts & S.R. Williams (Eds.), *Nutrition in pregnancy and lactation* (6th ed.). Madison, WI: Brown & Benchmark.

Worthington-Roberts, B.S. (1997b). Mineral needs during pregnancy. In B. Worthington-Roberts & S.R. Williams (Eds.), *Nutrition in pregnancy and lactation* (6th ed.). Madison, WI: Brown & Benchmark.

Worthington-Roberts, B.S. (1997c). Nutrition, fertility, and family planning. In B. Worthington-Roberts & S.R. Williams (Eds.), *Nutrition in pregnancy and lactation* (6th ed.). Madison, WI: Brown & Benchmark.

Worthington-Roberts, B.S., & Rees, J.M. (1997). The pregnant adolescent. Special concerns. In B. Worthington-Roberts & S.R. Williams (Eds.), *Nutrition in pregnancy and lactation* (6th ed.). Madison, WI: Brown & Benchmark.

10 Antepartal Fetal Assessment

OBJECTIVES

1. Identify indications for fetal diagnostic procedures.
2. Discuss the purpose, procedure, advantages, and risks of specific diagnostic procedures:
   - Fetal ultrasonography
   - Doppler ultrasound blood flow assessment
   - Alpha-fetoprotein testing
   - Triple-marker screening
   - Chorionic villus sampling
   - Amniocentesis
   - Percutaneous umbilical blood sampling
   - Fetal surveillance techniques (such as nonstress test, vibroacoustic stimulation test, contraction stress test, biophysical profile)
   - Maternal assessment of fetal movement
3. Provide information for common questions that clients may have about antepartal fetal assessment procedures.
4. Apply the nursing process to care of clients having antepartal fetal assessment procedures.

DEFINITIONS

Alpha-Fetoprotein Plasma protein produced by the fetus.

Amniocentesis Transabdominal puncture of the amniotic sac to obtain a sample of amniotic fluid that contains fetal cells and biochemical substances for laboratory examination.

Amniotic Fluid Index (AFI) An ultrasound examination in which the vertical depth of the largest fluid pocket in each of the four quadrants of the uterus is measured and totaled.

Biophysical Profile Method for evaluating fetal status during the antepartum period based on five variables originating with the fetus: fetal heart rate, breathing movements, gross body movements, muscle tone, and amniotic fluid volume.

Baseline Risk The risk, usually in reference to birth defects or spontaneous abortion, of the general population of pregnant women who have no identified high-risk factors or invasive procedures.

Chorionic Villus Sampling Transcervical or transabdominal procedure to obtain a sample of chorionic villi (projections of the outer fetal membrane) for analysis of fetal cells.

DEFINITIONS—cont'd

Contraction Stress Test Method for evaluating fetal status during the antepartum period by observing response of the fetal heart to the stress of uterine contractions that may induce recurrent episodes of fetal hypoxia.

Δ OD$_{450}$ A test used to measure the change (delta, or Δ) in optical density of the amniotic fluid caused by staining with bilirubin.

Karyotype A display of a cell's chromosomes, arranged from largest to smallest pairs.

Late Deceleration The slowing of the fetal heart rate after the onset of a uterine contraction and persisting after the contraction ends.

Lecithin/Sphingomyelin Ratio (L/S Ratio) Ratio of two phospholipids in amniotic fluid that is used to determine fetal lung maturity; greater than 2:1 usually indicates fetal lung maturity.

Neural Tube Defect A congenital defect in closure of the bony encasement of the spinal cord or skull. Includes defects such as anencephaly, spina bifida, meningocele, myelomeningocele, and others.

Nonstress Test A method for evaluating fetal status during the antepartum period by observing the response of the fetal heart rate to fetal movement.

Percutaneous Umbilical Blood Sampling (PUBS) Procedure for obtaining fetal blood through ultrasound-guided puncture of an umbilical cord vessel to detect fetal problems such as inherited blood disorders, acidosis, or infection; also called *cordocentesis.*

Phosphatidylglycerol A major phospholipid of surfactant whose presence in amniotic fluid indicates fetal lung maturity.

Phosphatidylinositol A phospholipid of surfactant that is produced and secreted in increasing amounts as the fetal lungs mature.

Placenta Previa Abnormal implantation of the placenta in the lower uterus located at or very near the cervical os.

Surfactant Combination of lipoproteins produced by the lungs of the mature fetus to reduce surface tension in the alveoli, thus promoting lung expansion after birth.

Triple-Marker Screening Analysis of maternal serum for abnormal levels of alpha-fetoprotein, human chorionic gonadotropin, and estriols that may predict chromosomal abnormalities of the fetus.

Ultrasonography Technique for visualizing deep structures of the body by recording the reflections (echoes) of high-frequency sound waves directed into the tissue.

Uteroplacental Insufficiency Inability of the placenta to exchange oxygen, carbon dioxide, nutrients, and waste products properly between the maternal and fetal circulations.

Vibroacoustic Stimulation Use of sound stimulation to elicit fetal movement and acceleration (speeding up) of the fetal heart rate.

Until relatively recently, only nonspecific methods were available to assess the condition of the fetus. Fundal height was measured to estimate fetal growth, the fetal heart rate was auscultated, and the mother's perception of fetal movements was noted. The development of many sophisticated methods has allowed the detection of physical abnormalities in the fetus and greater accuracy in the monitoring of the fetal condition.

Antepartal fetal assessments offer reassurance for most expectant parents. If no fetal anomalies are found and the fetus appears to be in good condition, relief and reduced anxiety are usually immediate. If fetal health is uncertain, the woman often faces decisions about further testing. She may experience anxiety throughout the pregnancy if tests continue to question the well-being of the fetus. If tests identify fetal anomalies, the woman may face the choice of whether to continue the pregnancy. This decision also can create emotional conflict as well as ethical dilemmas that impose a great deal of stress on the family.

INDICATIONS FOR FETAL DIAGNOSTIC TESTS

Most fetal diagnostic procedures are reserved for pregnancies in which reason exists to believe the fetus may experience developmental or physical problems. However, many physicians believe that some screening tests such as ultrasonography and maternal serum screening should be offered to all women.

Two broad reasons exist for antepartal fetal assessment testing: (1) to detect congenital anomalies and (2) to evaluate the condition of the fetus. Some procedures such as amniocentesis and ultrasonography may be used for both purposes.

Many factors increase the risk for the fetus during pregnancy. These include maternal medical conditions such as diabetes and hypertension, demographic factors such as age and poverty, and obstetric factors such as previous birth of an infant who was stillborn or had congenital anomalies (Table 10-1).

No antepartal testing or antepartal surveillance procedure can guarantee the birth of a perfect infant. The woman and her support person must be counseled that prenatal diagnostic tests cannot detect all congenital defects. A baseline risk remains for congenital defects in every pregnancy.

The nurse should remember the woman's right to refuse antepartal testing even though she may have an increased risk for a baby with a birth defect that can be

Table 10-1

INDICATIONS FOR FETAL DIAGNOSIS PROCEDURES

MEDICAL CONDITIONS	**OBSTETRIC FACTORS**
Preexisting diabetes mellitus or gestational diabetes	History of low-birth-weight infant (<2500 g)
Hypertension (chronic or pregnancy-induced)	Multifetal pregnancy
Cyanotic heart disease	Malpresentation (breech, shoulder)
Renal disease	Previous fetal loss or birth of infant with congenital anomaly
Chronic infections (such as pyelonephritis)	Previous infant >4000 g at birth
Sexually transmissible diseases	Hydramnios (>2000 ml at term)
Anemia	Rh or other sensitization
Hyperthyroidism	Oligohydramnios (<500 ml at term)
Antiphospholipid syndrome	Decrease or absence in fetal movements
Systemic lupus erythematosus	Uncertainty about gestational age
Parents carry or exhibit genetic disorder (such as sickle cell anemia, cystic fibrosis)	Intrauterine growth restriction
	Postterm pregnancy (>42 weeks)
DEMOGRAPHIC FACTORS	Preterm labor (>20 weeks and <38 weeks of gestation)
Maternal age <16 or >35 years	Grand multiparity (>5 pregnancies)
Poverty	**CONCURRENT MATERNAL FACTORS**
Nonwhite (twice the risk of neonatal or infant death)	Less than ideal-weight-for-height at conception
Inadequate prenatal care (initial visit after 20 weeks of gestation or fewer than 5 prenatal visits to physician or nurse-midwife)	More than 20% above ideal-weight-for-height at conception
	Inadequate weight gain or poor pattern of weight gain
	Excessive weight gain
	Use of drugs, alcohol, and tobacco

diagnosed with one of these tests. If a screening test suggests an abnormality that requires further testing to determine whether the abnormality is actually present, the woman has the right to accept or refuse further testing. Nurses must respect the woman's personal decisions.

ULTRASONOGRAPHY

When high-frequency sound waves of an ultrasonic beam are aimed at body tissues, they are deflected by tissues in their path and returned as echoes. The amount of energy returned as an echo depends on the properties of the tissues in the path of the ultrasonic beam and the angle and strength of the beam. In obstetrics, the ultrasonic beam emitted by a transducer is directed through tissues of the abdomen or vagina to provide two-dimensional images showing structures of different densities (Figure 10-1).

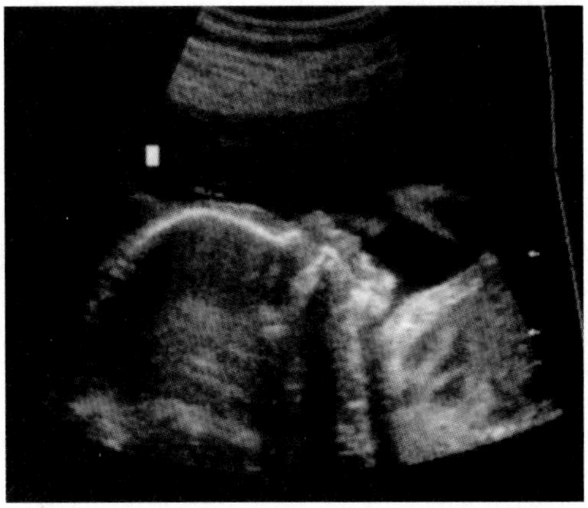

FIGURE 10-1 Two-dimensional sonogram showing profile of fetal facial structures. (Courtesy Karin Buxton, Newport Beach, Calif.)

Technologic and software advances can refine the ultrasound data, producing a three-dimensional image with greater clarity and visual depth than the two-dimensional image. Three-dimensional ultrasound images are useful in confirming normal features and identifying congenital abnormalities, particularly those of surface features such as facial clefts. They provide more accurate identification of the extent and size of abnormalities. Both parents and professionals are better able to understand ultrasound images in three dimensions because they are far more realistic than two-dimensional flat images (Figure 10-2). The ultrasound data can be stored on optical and magnetic media, allowing images to be manipulated and displayed in many views for best clarity and archived for later review or sharing with specialists (Platt, et al., 1998; Pretorius, Nelson, & Lev-Toaff, 2000).

Today's procedures use real-time scanning, showing movement as it happens. Real-time ultrasound allows the observer to see fetal heart motion, fetal breathing activity, and fetal body movement. Real-time scanning also allows the observer to distinguish between moving tissues of the fetus and relatively fixed maternal tissues. Ultrasonography may be used during any trimester, but the procedure and the reasons for its use vary. Ultrasonography is also used in gynecology and infertility care.

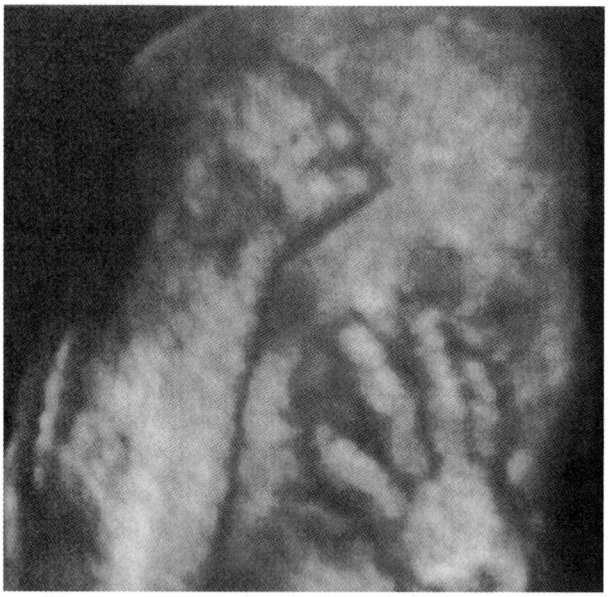

FIGURE 10-2 Three-dimensional ultrasound image of a 30-week fetus holding normal hands in front of the face. (From Callan, P.W. [2000]. *Ultrasonography in obstetrics and gynecology.* Philadelphia: W.B. Saunders.)

Emotional Responses

In some countries a basic ultrasound scan is routine in all pregnancies, but ultrasonography is not considered a routine part of care in the United States, primarily because a major trial failed to show a significant improvement in perinatal outcome when routine ultrasound was used for screening during pregnancy (Manning, 1999b; National Institutes of Health, 1984). However, in actual practice, 65% of women who had a live birth in 1998 had at least one ultrasound scan during pregnancy (National Center for Health Statistics, 2000). The procedure is so common that many women expect to have an ultrasound scan at some time during pregnancy.

Parents' responses to ultrasonography vary widely. Some expectant parents are excited and report feelings of love and protectiveness when they view the fetus. Others report increased anxiety about the fetus and fear that something will be found wrong. Undoubtedly, all parents breathe sighs of relief when scans show normal results. Sometimes the presence of one or more "markers," findings that might indicate a problem, fails to give parents the expected reassurance and puts them on a path to other difficult choices they must make about their baby.

Both parents are usually fascinated by the quality of today's ultrasound images that allow them to see their unborn baby with such clarity. Many couples want to know the gender of the fetus. Others do not want to know the gender, even if it is obvious, and prefer to wait and "be surprised." The sonographer often provides parents with still images and sometimes a short videotape of their fetus. These images are strictly keepsakes and are not used for medical diagnostics. Other views are archived for medical documentation purposes.

Table 10-2

INDICATIONS FOR A LIMITED ULTRASOUND SCAN

Determine placental location
Detect presence or absence of fetal cardiac activity
Assess volume of amniotic fluid
Determine fetal presenting part
Guide delivery of the second twin in a vaginal birth
Assist with amniocentesis and external cephalic version
Assess fetal well-being (such as a biophysical profile)

Levels of Obstetric Ultrasound

Three levels of obstetric ultrasound examination are as follows (Menihan, 2000):

- Basic—The basic scan includes a general survey of the fetus, placenta, and amniotic fluid quantity and should be performed by a sonographer.
- Comprehensive—The comprehensive scan is ordered if abnormalities are found during the basic scan. A maternal-fetal medicine physician often consults with the woman's primary provider when the comprehensive scan is required. The comprehensive scan targets the questionable finding to obtain greater detail and information than that found with the basic scan.
- Limited—Because nonsonographers such as nurses in labor units and emergency departments may need to quickly determine information during pregnancy, the American College of Obstetricians and Gynecologists has recognized limited ultrasound. The Association of Women's Health, Obstetric, and Neonatal Nurses provides specific guidelines for didactic and clinical training. The limited ultrasound scan is less detailed than a basic scan but is appropriate for gathering specific information and emergency circumstances (Table 10-2).

First-Trimester Ultrasonography

During the first trimester, transvaginal ultrasonography allows clear visibility of the uterus, gestational sac, embryo, and deep pelvic structures such as the ovaries and fallopian tubes.

Purposes

During the first trimester, ultrasonography is most frequently used to do the following:

- Confirm pregnancy
- Verify the location of the pregnancy (such as uterine, ectopic)

- Detect multifetal gestations
- Determine gestational age
- Confirm fetal viability
- Identify markers that suggest major anomalies such as Down syndrome (trisomy 21)
- Determine the position of the uterus, cervix, and area of placental formation for transcervical chorionic villus sampling
- Guide the needle insertion for transabdominal chorionic villus sampling

During the first trimester, gestational age is based on the appearance of the gestational sac, which can be seen as early as 25 days after the last menstrual period. At this time the crown-to-rump length of the embryo is the most reliable indicator of gestational age. Fetal viability is confirmed by observation of fetal heartbeat, which is visible as early as 38 days after the last normal menstrual period (Manning, 1999b). Maternal structures and abnormalities such as uterine fibroids, ovarian cysts, and bicornuate uteri also can be seen.

Procedure

The woman is placed in a lithotomy position for transvaginal ultrasonography. A transvaginal probe, which is encased in a disposable cover and coated with a gel that provides lubrication and promotes conductivity, is inserted into the vagina. The woman may feel more comfortable if she inserts the probe herself. The procedure takes about 10 to 15 minutes.

Second- and Third-Trimester Ultrasonography

Transabdominal ultrasonography is most often used during the second and third trimesters because the uterus extends out of the pelvis, allowing clear views of the fetus and placenta, which are no longer obstructed by pelvic bones.

Purposes

Ultrasonography is used throughout the second and third trimesters to do the following:

- Confirm fetal viability
- Evaluate fetal anatomy, including the umbilical cord, its vessels, and the insertion site
- Determine gestational age
- Assess serial fetal growth over several scans
- Compare growth of fetuses in multifetal gestations and evaluate quantity of fluid in each amniotic sac
- Evaluate amniotic fluid volume (see also "Biophysical Profile," p. 234)
- Locate the placenta when placenta previa is suspected
- Determine fetal presentation
- Guide needle placement when amniocentesis or percutaneous umbilical blood sampling is necessary

Gestational age determination by ultrasonography is increasingly less accurate after the first trimester because the combination of individual growth potential and intrauterine environment cause greater variations among fetuses. Two methods improve accuracy of gestational age determination in later pregnancy:

- Multiple variables are measured, such as fetal head biparietal diameter, head circumference, abdominal circumference, and femur length.
- If the woman is between 24 and 32 weeks' gestation, two or three ultrasound measures may be taken 2 weeks apart to compare against standard fetal growth curves

Estimating fetal age by ultrasonography after 32 weeks' is subject to major error. At this time the fetus may be evaluated for other signs of well being or compromise (Manning, 1999b).

Gestational age must be determined accurately when screening for maternal serum alpha-fetoprotein (MSAFP), which is altered by fetal age. Accurate gestational age is also important if intrauterine growth restriction is suspected or the expected date of delivery is questioned.

A comprehensive ultrasound in the second trimester is used to evaluate the fetus when risk factors are present or the basic examination shows abnormal findings. Examples include prior birth of an infant with anomalies or abnormal clinical findings such as hydramnios (excessive amniotic fluid), oligohydramnios (insufficient amniotic fluid), or abnormal levels of MSAFP. Fetal anatomy is carefully and systematically examined to identify major system and organ anomalies. Anomalies that can be detected with comprehensive ultrasonography include most neural tube defects such as myelomeningocele and anencephaly, abdominal wall defects such as gastroschisis and omphalocele, malformed kidneys, hydrocephalus, obstruction in fetal bowel and urinary systems, cleft lip and palate, and limb abnormalities.

Procedure

The woman is positioned on her back with the head and knees supported. If she desires, a display panel can be positioned so that she (and her support person) can see the images on the screen. Her head should be elevated, and she should be turned slightly to one side to prevent supine hypotension, which may be caused by compression of the vena cava and aorta by the gravid uterus. A wedge or rolled blanket is placed under one hip to help her maintain this position comfortably. Warm mineral oil or transmission gel is spread over her abdomen, and the sonographer slowly moves a transducer over the abdomen to obtain a picture (Figure 10-3). The procedure takes 10 to 30 minutes.

During the second trimester a full bladder may displace the gas-filled intestines and elevate the uterus for

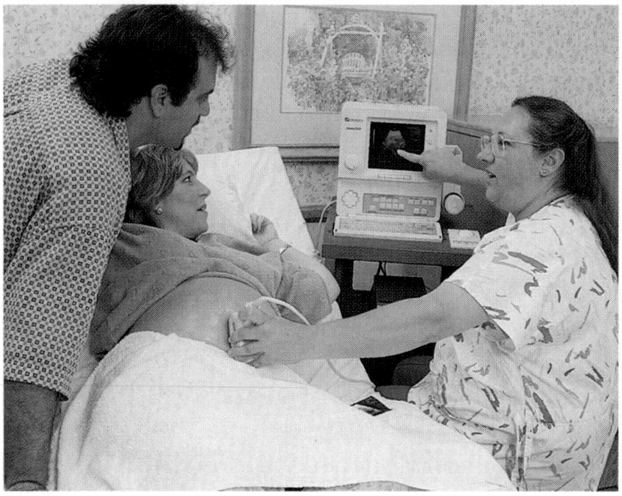

FIGURE 10-3 The sonographer provides information while moving an ultrasound transducer over the mother's abdomen to obtain an image.

better image quality. If a full bladder is necessary, the woman should be instructed to drink several glasses of clear fluid 1 hour before the examination and not void until after the examination. She may experience some discomfort as the transducer is moved over her distended bladder.

Advantages

Ultrasonography allows clear visibility of the fetus and surrounding structures and is safe. No clinically significant adverse effects have been reported (Manning, 1999b). Ultrasonography is noninvasive and relatively comfortable. In addition, results are obtained immediately. It is widely available and portable.

Disadvantages

The cost of ultrasonography can be a problem for women who do not have health insurance. Women who do not have access to prenatal care in the first trimester of pregnancy, including those with uncertain gestation, will not obtain all potential benefits from ultrasonography. Ultrasound cannot identify all structural abnormalities and defects not affecting fetal structures.

The high quality of ultrasound images enables clinicians to identify several structural markers in the fetal anatomy that may predict a serious problem. For example, nuchal translucency, an area at the back of the fetal neck that does not return ultrasound echoes, has been studied as a way to predict chromosome abnormalities. At this time, the predictive value of this finding, as with other ultrasound markers for possible chromosome defects, is not certain (ACOG, 1999b). However, the physician must discuss all scan findings with the expectant mother, including any markers found. The woman and her support person are likely to be very anxious because the exact significance of some markers is not yet known. The woman may have to base decisions about further, possibly invasive, testing on information that is still investigational.

DOPPLER ULTRASOUND BLOOD FLOW ASSESSMENT

When an ultrasound wave is directed at an acute angle to a moving target, as with blood flowing through a vessel, the frequency of echoes changes as the cardiac cycle goes through systole and diastole. This change, referred to as the *Doppler shift,* indicates forward movement of blood within a vessel.

Purpose

Pregnancies complicated by hypertension or fetal growth restriction may have Doppler ultrasound assessment of blood flow through the umbilical artery to identify abnormalities in the diastolic flow. In severe cases, diastolic flow may be absent or even reversed (Opipari & Johnson, 2000). No benefit has been demonstrated for conditions other than intrauterine growth restriction, therefore general use of the test in all pregnancies is not recommended (ACOG, 1999a).

Color Doppler

The direction and velocity of the Doppler shift can be imaged in color depending on the direction of the flow to or from the transducer (Figure 10-4).

Check Your Reading

1. What are the major indications for ultrasonography during the first trimester? During the second and third trimesters?
2. How does the procedure for first-trimester ultrasonography differ from that performed during the second trimester?
3. What are the major advantages and disadvantages of ultrasonography?

ALPHA-FETOPROTEIN SCREENING

Alpha-fetoprotein (AFP) is the predominant protein in fetal plasma and is synthesized by the embryonic yolk sac, developing fetal liver, and gastrointestinal tract. AFP diffuses from fetal plasma into fetal urine and is excreted into the amniotic fluid. Although a portion of the AFP in amniotic fluid is swallowed and digested by the fetus, the remainder crosses placental membranes into the maternal circulation. Therefore AFP can be measured in MSAFP and amniotic fluid (AFAFP). Abnormal

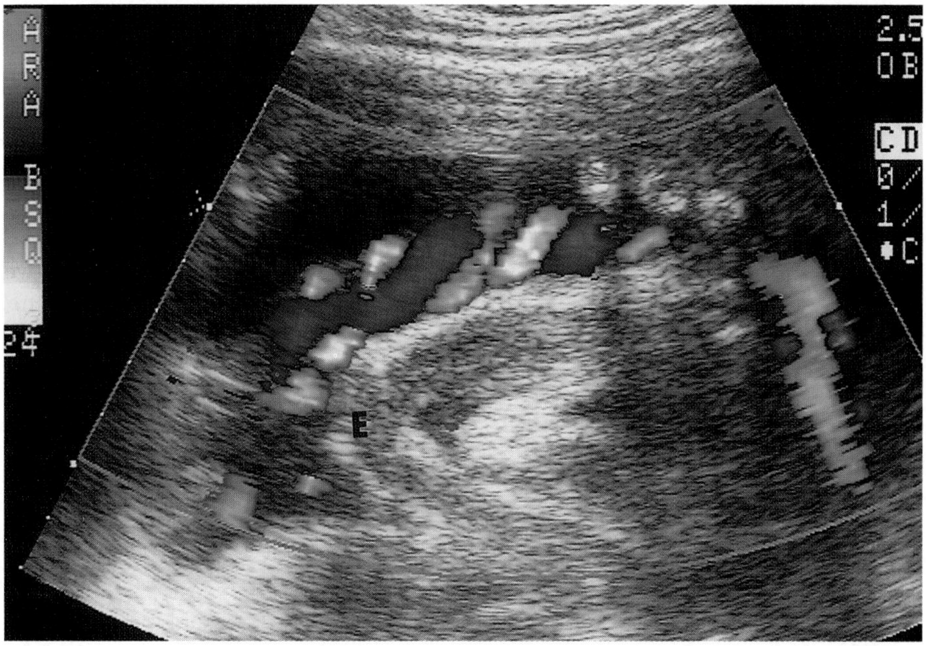

FIGURE 10-4 Color Doppler imaging of the umbilical vein and two arteries. Blood flow toward the transducer is shown as blue and the flow away is shown as red. Three fetal fingers can be seen to grasp and press the cord against the other wrist. (From DuBose, T.J. [1996]. *Fetal sonography.* Philadelphia: W.B. Saunders. Sonogram courtesy T.J. DuBose, MS, RDMS.)

Table 10-3

CONDITIONS ASSOCIATED WITH ABNORMAL MATERNAL SERUM ALPHA-FETOPROTEIN LEVELS

ELEVATED LEVELS OF AFP
Open neural tube defects
Esophageal obstruction
Abdominal wall defects (omphalocele, gastroschisis)
Increased amount leaked by fetal kidney (hydronephrosis)
Threatened abortion
Undetected fetal demise
Normal fetus in conjunction with one or more of the following:
Amniotic fluid contaminated with fetal blood
Underestimation of fetal age
Multifetal gestation
Decreased maternal weight
Maternal insulin-dependent diabetes
LOW LEVELS OF AFP
Chromosomal trisomies (such as Down syndrome)
Gestational trophoblastic disease
Normal fetus in conjunction with:
Overestimation of gestational age
Increased maternal weight

concentrations of AFP are associated with serious fetal anomalies (Table 10-3).

Purpose

Low levels of MSAFP suggest chromosomal abnormalities such as trisomy 21. Elevated MSAFP levels are associated with open neural tube defects and body wall defects. These anomalies leave internal tissues exposed to amniotic fluid, allowing large quantities of AFP to seep into amniotic fluid and enter maternal serum.

The most common open neural tube defects are:

- Anencephaly, in which the cranial vault is absent and most of the brain is undeveloped
- Spina bifida, including meningocele and myelomeningocele. In meningocele the meninges protrude from the spinal canal. In myelomeningocele, the spinal cord and meninges protrude through the defect and extensive nerve damage may be expected.

Spina bifida occulta is not an open neural tube defect and usually causes no problems. Open neural tube defects are fairly common, with anencephaly occurring 10.3 and spina bifida 21.8 per 100,000 live births, respectively, in 1998 (National Center for Health Statistics, 2000).

Procedure

Initial screening is offered to all women between 15 and 18 weeks' gestation (ideally 16 weeks'), when blood may be drawn to evaluate the concentration of MSAFP (AAP & ACOG, 1997). Gestational age, maternal weight, multifetal pregnancy, race, and maternal diabetes can affect MSAFP and must be considered when evaluating the levels. The mother is informed that MSAFP is a screening test rather than a diagnostic test and that further tests will be offered to explain abnormal concentrations (Figure 10-5). If MSAFP levels are elevated, basic ultra-

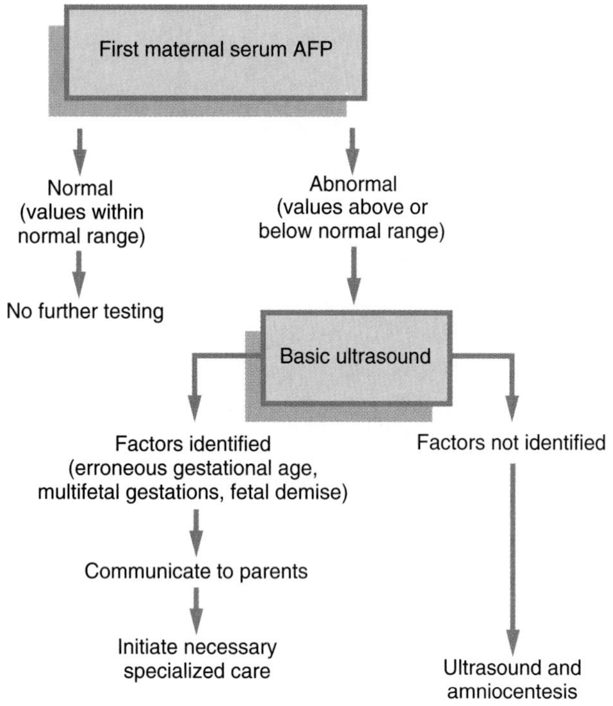

FIGURE 10-5 Abnormal levels of maternal serum alpha-fetoprotein (MSAFP) indicate the need for further testing to identify the cause.

sonography is offered to determine whether the abnormal concentration results from inaccurate gestational age, multifetal gestation, or fetal demise.

If ultrasonography fails to explain the abnormal levels of AFP, amniocentesis is the next step. Amniotic fluid is analyzed for elevated levels of AFP and acetylcholinesterase (AChE). AChE is a neural tissue–specific enzyme that helps distinguish neural tube defects from other causes of elevated AFP (Yankowitz & Williamson, 1999).

Advantages

Maternal serum AFP evaluation has several advantages:

- It is a simple procedure that requires only a sample of maternal blood.
- It is a noninvasive procedure to screen for open neural tube defects and other open defects.
- With addition of other tests (see "Triple Marker Screening"), AFP is useful as a screening test for chromosome defects as well.
- Screening at about 16 weeks' allows time for more comprehensive testing if results for MSAFP are abnormal.

Limitations

Some major limitations of MSAFP are the following:

- Maternal serum AFP evaluation is a screening test only and must be viewed as the first step in a series of potential decisions about diagnostic procedures if abnormal concentrations are found.
- Because conditions such as inaccurate estimation of gestational age can result in apparently abnormal levels in a healthy fetus, the parents may experience a great deal of anxiety and expense if they choose to pursue follow-up testing.
- Timing also imposes some limits. Maternal serum AFP evaluation is performed between the fifteenth and eighteenth weeks of pregnancy, but many women do not seek prenatal care until after the eighteenth week and therefore miss the opportunity for MSAFP screening.
- Because closed neural tube and other defects do not produce elevated levels of AFP, normal levels of AFP do not guarantee a perfect baby.

TRIPLE-MARKER SCREENING

In 1983 a chance association revealed that lower than normal MSAFP levels were more common in infants with trisomy 21 (Evans & Johnson, 2000). Trisomy 21, or Down syndrome, is a common birth defect that occurred in 43.7 per 100,000 births in 1998 (National Center for Health Statistics, 2000). Although the *risk* for having a baby with trisomy 21 rises when a woman is 35 years or older, 80% of infants with trisomy 21 are born to women younger than 35 (Sciosia, 1999). Thus a low-cost, noninvasive screening test for this chromosome abnormality is very desirable.

Human chorionic gonadotropin (hCG) levels tend to be higher and unconjugated estriol levels lower in maternal serum with a fetus with trisomy 21. Adding these two tests—especially hCG, which is about twice normal levels in the fetus with trisomy 21—yields a higher detection rate and a lower false-positive rate than MSAFP screening alone (Yankowitz & Williamson, 1999; Sciosia, 1999). The three markers have also been found to increase the detection of other trisomies such as trisomy 18.

Check Your Reading

4. Why is MSAFP considered a screening test?
5. What are possible causes for elevated levels of AFP?
6. What are possible causes of low levels of AFP?
7. What is triple-marker screening? Why is it performed?

CHORIONIC VILLUS SAMPLING

Purpose

Chorionic villus sampling (CVS) is a first-trimester alternative to amniocentesis for prenatal diagnosis of conditions that can be diagnosed by analysis of fetal cells. Chorionic villi are microscopic projections from

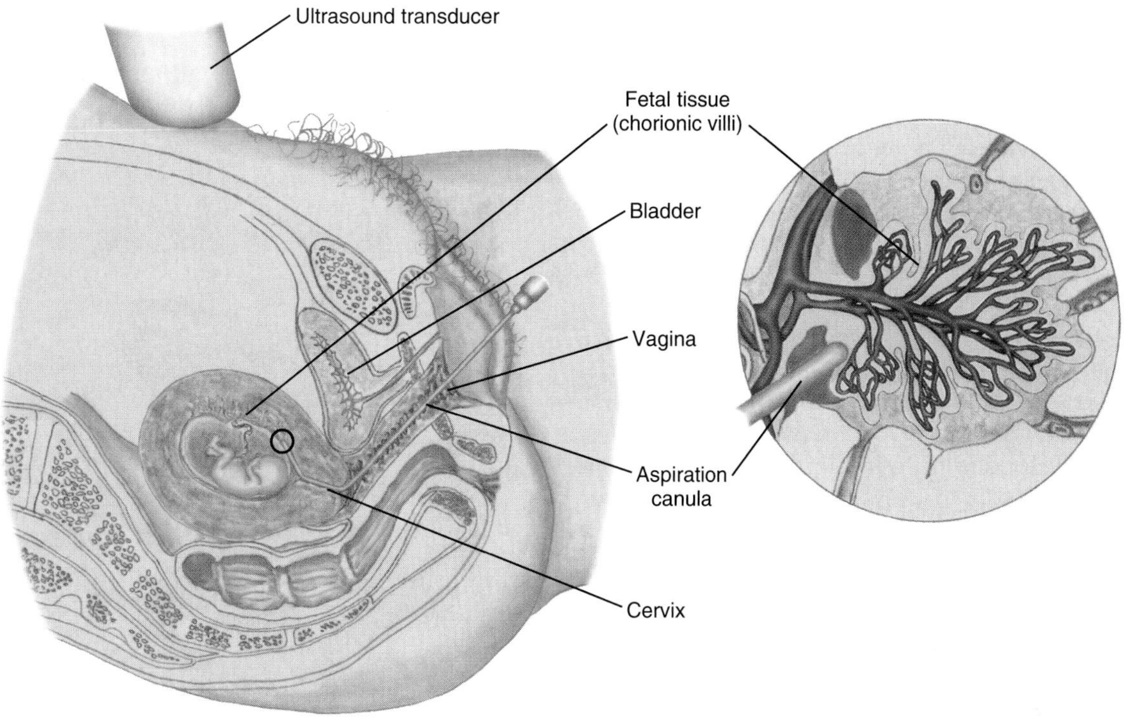

FIGURE 10-6 Transcervical chorionic villus sampling (CVS). Tissue is aspirated to detect the presence of genetic defects in the fetus. Transabdominal aspiration is an alternative method.

the outer membrane (chorion) that develop and burrow into endometrial tissue as the placenta is formed. The villi are fetal tissues and reflect the chromosomal and genetic makeup of the fetus. CVS is usually performed between 10 and 12 weeks of gestation (ACOG, 1997; Beall, 2000).

Indications

CVS is performed to determine fetal karyotype or other DNA studies in the first trimester. Abnormal number and structure of chromosomes are readily identified from the karyotype (see Chapter 5). Because amniotic fluid is not obtained in CVS, alpha-fetoprotein cannot be tested.

Procedure

As with all diagnostic procedures, the woman should receive counseling about both the procedure itself and genetic counseling about the specific defect for which CVS is being performed. The risks and benefits of the procedure should be carefully explained and a signed consent should be obtained.

CVS can be performed by a transcervical or transabdominal approach. Neither method has proven superior (Beall, 2000; Jenkins & Wapner, 1999). The transcervical approach is usually more comfortable for the woman, but it often results in minor post-procedure bleeding. The approach providing the easiest, most direct access is usually chosen (Jenkins & Wapner, 1999).

For transcervical aspiration the woman is placed in the lithotomy position. A full bladder may straighten the angle between the cervix and uterus. The vagina and cervix are washed with an antiseptic germicidal agent before the procedure, and strict aseptic technique is observed to decrease the chance of infection. Some centers require cultures for infections such as gonorrhea, chlamydia, and group B streptococcus before CVS. Under direct ultrasonographic guidance a flexible catheter is inserted through the cervix, and a sample of chorionic villi is aspirated through the catheter into a syringe containing culture medium (Figure 10-6).

Transabdominal CVS is performed with the woman in a supine position. Ultrasound examination first determines the best entry position and angle of passage of the sampling needle. An area on the abdomen is cleansed with antiseptic solution. With ultrasound guidance the clinician inserts a needle through the abdominal wall and myometrium, and the tip is advanced to the placenta. A sample of chorionic villi is withdrawn into the syringe containing culture medium.

After CVS, fetal heart activity is often documented to confirm viability. Maternal vital signs are assessed, and the woman is allowed to void. Rh_O(D) immune globulin (RhoGAM) is given to women who are Rh-negative because CVS increases the risk of Rh sensitization (see Chapter 25, "Drug Guide"). A small amount of vaginal spotting may occur, but heavy bleeding or the passage of amniotic fluid, clots, and tissue should be reported. The woman needs to rest at home for 1 day after the procedure. Sexual intercourse may be restricted for a few days.

Advantages

CVS is performed between 10 and 12 weeks of gestation, so results are known even earlier than early amniocentesis. As a result, CVS offers prenatal diagnosis to women who find later procedures unacceptable. Furthermore, if results are abnormal and the woman chooses abortion, she may consider the earlier abortion less physically and emotionally traumatic than a later procedure.

Risks

Although CVS is now considered a safe and effective technique for first-trimester prenatal diagnosis, the rate of pregnancy loss varies from 0.5% to 1%, which is slightly higher than that of amniocentesis (Beall, 2000). Fetal loss appears to be less frequent in centers that perform many CVS procedures. More than two attempts and bleeding during the week before the procedure increases the risk for fetal loss. Reports of limb reduction defects (LRD) associated with CVS performed before 10 weeks of gestation appeared in the early 1990s. Present data appear to confirm the safety of CVS at the gestational age of 10 to 12 weeks, but the risk for LRD must be shared with the parents (Sciosia, 1999; Beall, 2000, Jenkins & Wapner, 1999).

A disadvantage is that CVS is more expensive than amniocentesis. The laboratory must carefully dissect the tissue to separate maternal and fetal tissue before culture, making the procedure labor intensive. As a result, some insurers are reluctant to pay for CVS without special indications (Beall, 2000).

Karyotypes from CVS were once available almost immediately because the villi cells were rapidly dividing, giving very rapid results. However, these rapid or direct karyotypes were found to be unreliable and villi cells are now usually cultured like amniotic fluid cells with results available in about 7 days (Jenkins & Wapner, 1999). Tests other than karyotyping, such as those for metabolic disorders, may still be available very quickly, however. Karyotypes from CVS are more likely to be questionable because they are from placental cells and require follow-up testing with cells obtained by amniocentesis, adding unexpected expense and invasiveness to the prenatal diagnosis process.

Check Your Reading

8. What is the major advantage of CVS compared with amniocentesis?
9. What are the major risks associated with CVS?

AMNIOCENTESIS

Amniocentesis is the aspiration of amniotic fluid from the amniotic sac for examination (Figure 10-7). The procedure has been traditionally performed at 15 to 16 weeks of gestation. Current techniques allow early amniocentesis at 13 to 14 weeks' gestation.

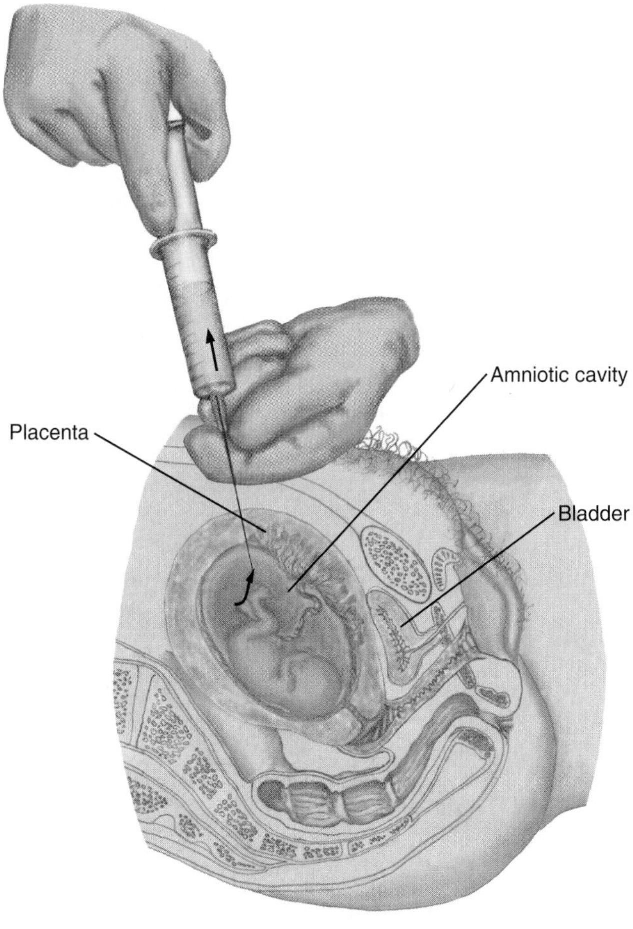

FIGURE 10-7 In amniocentesis a needle is inserted through the expectant mother's abdomen to aspirate fluid from the amniotic sac. The fluid can then be tested to determine fetal maturity, chromosomal abnormalities, and other possible problems.

Purposes

Midtrimester

The most common purpose for midtrimester amniocentesis is to examine fetal cells present in amniotic fluid to identify chromosome abnormalities. Other methods of genetic analysis, such as those for metabolic defects in the fetus, may be performed on the cells as well.

In addition to detecting chromosomal abnormalities, amniocentesis is used to evaluate the fetal condition when the woman is sensitized to Rh-positive blood, diagnose intrauterine infections, and investigate amniotic fluid AFP and AChE when MSAFP is elevated (Table 10-4).

Third Trimester

The most common indications for amniocentesis during the third trimester are to determine fetal lung maturity and evaluate the fetal condition when the woman has Rh isoimmunization. Although several types of

Table 10-4
INDICATIONS FOR SECOND-TRIMESTER AMNIOCENTESIS

Maternal age 35 years or more
Chromosomal abnormality in close family member
Sex determination for maternal carrier of X-linked disorder (such as hemophilia, Duchenne's muscular dystrophy)
Birth of previous infant with chromosomal abnormalities or neural tube defect
Pregnancy after three or more spontaneous abortions
Elevated levels of maternal serum alpha-fetoprotein
Maternal Rh sensitization

maternal-fetal blood incompatibilities exist, Rh incompatibility is most severe (see Chapter 25).

Tests to Determine Fetal Lung Maturity. A test for fetal lung maturity is recommended when delivery is considered before 38 weeks of gestation. Surfactant, a surface-active substance composed primarily of phospholipids, reduces the surface tension on the inner walls of the alveoli, allowing them to stay open slightly when the infant exhales. Without adequate surfactant, the walls adhere to each other, making it difficult to inflate the alveoli with the next breath. Each breath requires greater effort to open the collapsed alveoli and the infant soon tires.

The lecithin/sphingomyelin (L/S) ratio is a test for estimating fetal lung maturity. Lecithin is a phospholipid component of fetal lung fluid and surfactant, and sphingomyelin is a general amniotic membrane lipid. Lecithin and sphingomyelin are present in approximately equal amounts until about 30 weeks of gestation. At this time the level of sphingomyelin plateaus while lecithin continues to rise. An L/S ratio of at least 2:1 generally indicates adequate surfactant and mature fetal lungs. However, an L/S ratio of 2:1 may not indicate lung maturity in some conditions such as maternal diabetes. Therefore amniotic fluid is usually tested for the presence of phosphatidylglycerol (PG) and phosphatidylinositol (PI), two other components of surfactant. The presence of the PG and PI phospholipids supports the likelihood that the fetal lungs are mature. The accuracy of the L/S ratio may be affected by presence of blood and meconium in the amniotic fluid, but these substances are less likely to affect the accuracy of the PG and PI tests.

PG is also useful in evaluating the maturity of the fetal lungs from a sample of amniotic fluid taken from a vaginal pool when the membranes have ruptured prematurely. Although this test is not invasive as amniocentesis, the fluid sample will also be contaminated by numerous substances that may interfere with accuracy, such as mucus, blood, and bacteria (Lenke & Ashwood, 2000).

A newer assay measures the proportion of the phospholipids in surfactant to albumin. This assay assumes that albumin remains constant during pregnancy while the levels of phospholipids rise with increasing pulmonary maturation. Blood and meconium can also interfere with interpretation, as with the L/S ratio (Lenke & Ashwood, 2000).

Test for Fetal Hemolytic Disease. Amniocentesis is also performed to determine fetal bilirubin concentration with a $\Delta\ OD_{450}$ if the mother is Rh negative and is sensitized or isoimmunized to Rh-positive blood. Antibodies of the isoimmunized woman can destroy Rh-positive blood of the fetus, leaving the fetus vulnerable to erythroblastosis fetalis and hydrops fetalis (see Chapter 25).

Erythroblastosis is marked by excessive destruction of mature erythrocytes capable of carrying oxygen and the proliferation of immature erythroblasts incapable of carrying oxygen. Bilirubin, which is released from erythrocyte breakdown, increases. The fetus becomes anemic, jaundiced, and edematous (hydrops fetalis) as the heart fails.

Procedure

Before the examination the woman is placed in a supine position and draped with her abdomen exposed. A rolled towel is placed under her right buttock to shift the weight of the uterus slightly to the side and off the vena cava and aorta. Maternal blood pressure and fetal heart rate (FHR) are assessed for baseline levels.

Ultrasonography is used to locate the fetus and placenta and identify the largest pockets of amniotic fluid that can safely be sampled. When Rh isommunization is the problem, the placenta is avoided using real-time ultrasound guidance during the procedure to prevent worsening the hemolytic disease by possibly mixing fetal Rh-positive blood with maternal Rh-negative blood (Bowman, 1999). The skin is prepared with antiseptic solution. A small amount of local anesthetic may be injected into the skin. The woman may feel pressure as the needle is inserted and mild cramping as the needle enters the myometrium.

A 3.5-inch, 20- or 22-gauge spinal needle is inserted into the pocket of fluid. After discarding the first few milliliters of fluid, approximately 20 to 30 ml of fluid are removed for analysis. An adhesive bandage is applied to the puncture site. The woman rests quietly for observation and ultrasound documentation of the FHR. She may then resume quiet activities. Strenuous exercise such as jogging and other aerobic exercises should be deferred for 1 or 2 days (Evans, Johnson, & Drugan, 2000). She should report persistent uterine contractions, vaginal bleeding, leakage of amniotic fluid, and fever.

As with CVS, $Rh_0(D)$ immune globulin is administered to prevent sensitization in nonsensitized Rh-negative women after amniocentesis.

Advantages

Amniocentesis has several advantages:

- It is a simple, safe procedure that permits the diagnosis of many fetal anomalies and confirms fetal maturity.
- It is a relatively painless procedure that takes only a short time.
- It has been performed for many years with few reported complications and is familiar to most obstetricians.

Disadvantages

Timing has been a major disadvantage of amniocentesis for genetic studies. Until recently, the procedure was performed at approximately 15 to 16 weeks of gestation when the uterus is readily accessible and the volume of amniotic fluid permits removal of at least 20 ml. Analysis of the fluid may add 1 to 2 weeks to the date of the amniocentesis, depending on the test.

Chromosomal study requires the active division of cells. Prepared cells from amniotic fluid are allowed to grow in culture medium until a sufficient number are produced for karyotyping. About 7 to 14 days are required for chromosome analysis from cultured cells. DNA probes allow diagnosis of several common chromosome abnormalities without the requirement for cell culture, making results available in 1 to 3 days. However, DNA probes are not always informative and must be regarded as a screening test for chromosome abnormalities rather than a replacement for conventional karyotyping (Jenkins & Wapner, 1999; Sciosia, 1999).

Abnormal results from amniocentesis usually are known in time to give the woman the choice of pregnancy termination before 20 weeks of gestation. However, this time frame is unacceptable to many women who have felt movements and whose pregnancies are apparent to others. The reluctance of women to undergo procedures so late in the pregnancy has focused interest on alternatives such as CVS, early amniocentesis, improved culture techniques, and DNA

Therapeutic Communication

RESPONDING TO ANXIETY RELATED TO FETAL TESTING

Margaret Kitchner is a 35-year-old primigravida. She has postponed pregnancy to complete her education and establish a law practice. She has been referred for possible amniocentesis at 14 weeks because the risk for chromosome abnormalities increases beginning at age 35. Counseling has already been provided by a specialist in genetics, and the risks and benefits of the amniocentesis have been discussed. The genetic counselor has also discussed the option of triple-marker screening and ultrasound rather than amniocentesis with Margaret and her husband. Together with ultrasound examination to look for signs associated with chromosome defects and the factor of Margaret's age, triple-marker screening can establish a percentage probability for having a child with a chromosome abnormality but cannot definitely diagnose or exclude it.

Margaret: I'm here, but I'm not thrilled to be here.

Nurse: You wish you were somewhere else?

(Clarifying without attempting to lead.)

Margaret: The place isn't the problem really, but what about this test?

Nurse: You have some questions you'd like to ask about the amniocentesis?

(Seeking information, staying with the woman's comments by paraphrasing.)

Margaret: Well, my mother believes that if one thinks bad thoughts, bad things will come to pass.

Nurse: Bad thoughts?

(Knowing that the intergenerational belief system is powerful, the nurse focuses and seeks clarification.)

Margaret: Yes, you know, if we think something could be wrong with the baby, it's more likely to be true.

Nurse: I'd like to hear more.

("I" statement conveys interest and invites more discussion.)

Margaret: Well, my mother is not familiar with the tests, and she's just afraid that the test could hurt the baby.

Nurse: She must be very anxious about this test. How do you feel?

(The nurse notes that Margaret identifies her mother as the person who is concerned and avoids her own feelings. Acknowledging mother's feeling; focusing on woman's feeling by open-ended question.)

Margaret: She's anxious, and to tell you the truth, I'm anxious too.

Nurse: You would rather not be having the test.

(This makes an assumption; she said only that she was anxious. Saying "Tell me more about that" might be more therapeutic.)

Margaret: No, I want the test. I'm glad there is an option to having an amniocentesis for those who want to go that way. But having more choices also makes me worry even more about whether I'm making the right decision. I want this baby so much and I've waited a long time.

Nurse: So the anxiety is really about whether the decision you made is the right one.

(The nurse "hears" the anxiety that Margaret didn't put into words; summarizes concerns and helps the woman identify and focus on what seems unclear to her.)

Margaret: That's for sure. It will be so hard to wait for the results, and I don't know what I would do if the news is bad or if something happens to the baby because of the test.

Nurse: Waiting is difficult, but chances are that the news will be good.

(Acknowledging the difficulty is therapeutic, but offering reassurance blocks the interaction instead of focusing on the uncertainty expressed. The nurse might have said instead: "And it's very hard to imagine something is wrong with the baby." This response would have kept the interaction going and focused on the patient's feelings. Instead the blocking comment ended the interaction without allowing a full expression of feelings.)

Margaret: You think so? I hope so.

analysis not requiring cell culture. Efforts are ongoing to find early, reliable prenatal diagnostic methods for serious birth defects so that women can be given information as early in pregnancy as possible.

Risks

The risks of amniocentesis include a pregnancy loss rate of 0.2% to 0.5% above the baseline risk for fetal loss at 16 weeks' gestation. Several studies have shown a higher fetal loss rate with early amniocentesis than with later amniocentesis (Evans, Johnson, & Drugan, 2000; Sciosia, 1999). Fetal hemorrhage can result from perforation of the placenta and vessels in the umbilical cord but is unlikely when ultrasonography is used to guide needle insertion. Accidental transfer of fetal blood to maternal circulation may also occur, resulting in sensitization of the Rh-negative woman carrying an Rh-positive fetus. $Rh_O(D)$ immune globulin is administered to prevent sensitization in nonsensitized Rh-negative women after amniocentesis.

EARLY AMNIOCENTESIS

Because of the expense and inability to assess amniotic fluid AFP in CVS and the desire of women for earlier diagnostic procedures, early amniocentesis has become more popular. Better techniques for ultrasound imaging and culture of the fetal cells in amniotic fluid now allow amniocentesis as early as 10 weeks. Most are performed between 13 and 14 weeks because some early research showed an increased risk for talipes equinovarus (clubfoot) in infants when procedures were done before 13 weeks (Sciosia, 1999; Evans & Johnson, 1999; Beall, 2000).

Procedure

The technique for early amniocentesis is similar to that of traditional amniocentesis except that a smaller volume of fluid (about 1 ml per week of gestation) is withdrawn. Adequate fluid may be difficult to obtain because of a smaller total volume and the tendency of the membranes to "tent" as the needle is inserted, rather than the needle piercing the membranes cleanly as it enters the amniotic sac.

Risks

Risks for early amniocentesis are similar to those for traditional amniocentesis.

Check Your Reading

10. What factors make a pregnant woman a candidate for amniocentesis?
11. How is fetal lung maturity confirmed?
12. Why is bilirubin in amniotic fluid evaluated?
13. Why is early amniocentesis sometimes chosen over standard amniocentesis for prenatal diagnosis of genetic disorders?

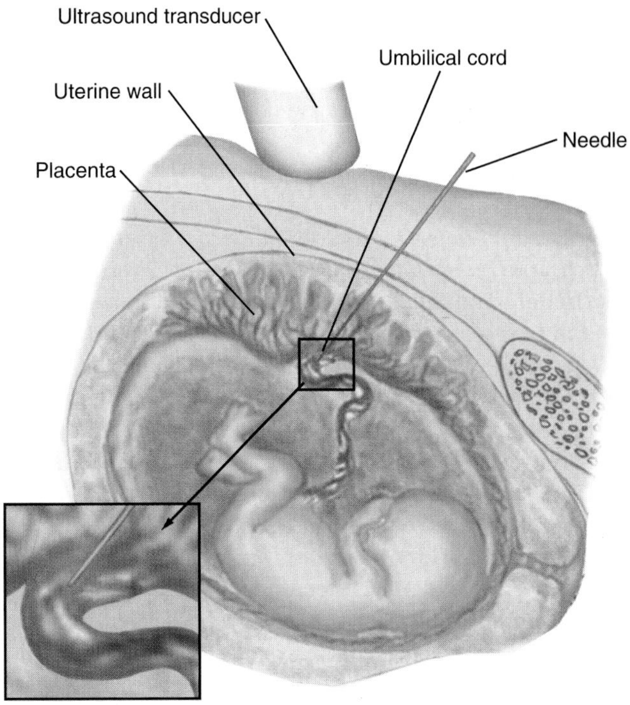

FIGURE 10-8 In percutaneous umbilical blood sampling (cordocentesis) a needle is inserted through the expectant mother's abdomen and into an umbilical vessel (vein or artery) to withdraw a sample of fetal blood.

PERCUTANEOUS UMBILICAL BLOOD SAMPLING

Percutaneous umbilical blood sampling (PUBS), also called *cordocentesis,* involves the aspiration of fetal blood from the umbilical cord for prenatal diagnosis or therapy (Figure 10-8). Major indications for PUBS include management of Rh disease, genetic studies, diagnosis of abnormal blood clotting factors, and acid-base status of the fetus. The same technique can be used to treat blood diseases and deliver therapeutic drugs that cannot be delivered to the fetus in another way.

Procedure

High-resolution ultrasound is used to locate the fetus, placenta, and umbilical cord and guide needle insertion. The needle is inserted into the umbilical cord near the site at which the cord meets the placenta, which affords more cord stability. The umbilical vein is used more commonly than the umbilical arteries because it is larger and less likely to constrict during the procedure. Knowing which vessel (umbilical vein or artery) was sampled is important when testing fetal acid-base parameters. Blood from the umbilical vein contains oxygenated blood and has a lower carbon dioxide content than blood from an umbilical artery that comes directly from the fetus.

After needle withdrawal, the duration of bleeding from the umbilical cord is usually short and can be monitored by ultrasound examination. The fetal heart is monitored electronically for 30 to 60 minutes (Harman, 1999). The Rh-negative woman is given RhoGAM to prevent sensitization by any Rh-positive fetal blood that may have entered her circulation.

Risks

PUBS can occasionally result in a variety of life-threatening complications for the fetus. Therefore the perinatal team must be prepared for emergencies with a plan based on the indication for the sampling and fetal gestational age. This plan must be determined ahead of time and shared with the expectant woman and her support person.

Fetal bradycardia is the most common complication and is usually brief and has no long-term consequence. More severe bradycardia is associated with puncture of the umbilical artery (Harman, 1999). Other complications include prolonged bleeding, cord laceration, cord hematoma, thrombosis, thromboembolism, premature labor, and premature rupture of membranes. Maternal blood sensitization, usually to the Rh factor, may occur if a fetal-to-maternal bleed exceeds 10 ml and inadequate RhoGAM is given for prevention. Sensitization to other blood factors may also occur.

ANTEPARTUM FETAL SURVEILLANCE

Antepartum fetal surveillance has three goals: (1) to prevent perinatal morbidity and mortality, (2) to evaluate the probability of fetal health and compromise, and (3) to determine whether and when intervention by the obstetric team is appropriate. The three most common methods of fetal surveillance are the nonstress test, contraction stress test, and biophysical profile. A fourth method, maternal assessment of fetal movement, provides a way for the expectant mother to alert her health care provider to possible problems in her fetus. These methods are not expected to predict compromise caused by acute events such as abruptio placentae (premature separation of the placenta).

Nonstress Test

Purpose

The nonstress test (NST) identifies whether an increase in the FHR occurs when the fetus moves, indicating adequate oxygenation, a healthy neural pathway from the fetal central nervous system to the fetal heart, and the ability of the fetal heart to respond to stimuli. FHR accelerations without fetal movement are also considered a reassuring sign of adequate fetal oxygenation. If the fetal heart does not accelerate with movement, however, fetal hypoxemia and acidosis are concerns. In those cases, an additional test such as the contraction stress test or biophysical profile is necessary to evaluate the metabolic condition of the fetus. The test may be used as a screening for intraamniotic infection when the membranes have ruptured prematurely (Garite, 1999).

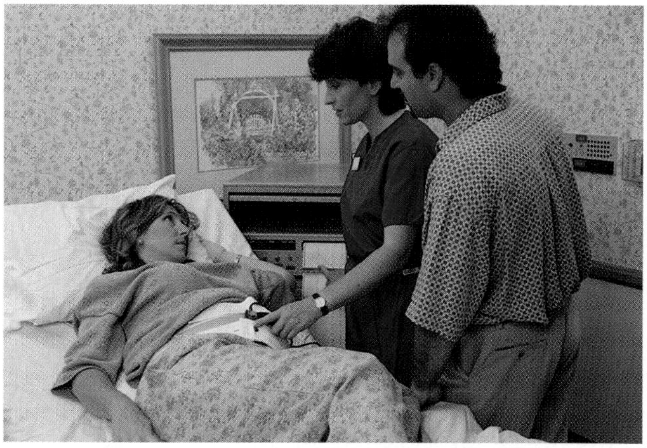

FIGURE 10-9 A nonstress test is a noninvasive test that measures the response of the fetal heart to fetal movements. Here the nurse reassures the parents by pointing to fetal heart accelerations detected by the external fetal monitor.

Procedure

The nonstress test takes about 40 minutes, allowing for most fetal sleep-wake cycles. A nurse with special preparation conducts the test in a hospital or an obstetrician's office. Before the test, the nurse discusses the test with the woman and explains why it is recommended. The test is termed *nonstress* because it consists of monitoring only. The fetus is not challenged or stressed by uterine contractions to obtain the necessary data.

For greatest accuracy the woman should not have smoked recently. The woman sits in a reclining chair or lies in a semi-reclining position in bed with lateral tilting to avoid supine hypotension. One study of 108 women found that nonstress test results were more likely to be reactive if women were in sitting positions rather than lying on their left sides (Nathan, et al., 2000). The woman's blood pressure is checked before the test and every 10 to 15 minutes throughout the test. If hypotension occurs, she should change her position to maintain the baseline pressure.

The nurse applies external electronic monitoring equipment. An ultrasound transducer to record fetal heart activity is secured on the woman's abdomen, where the fetal heart is heard most clearly. Next, a tocotransducer, which detects uterine activity and fetal movement, is secured to the maternal abdomen (Figure 10-9). The woman is given an event marker to press each time she senses movement, or the nurse may palpate and record each movement. Fetal heart activity and movements are recorded on a moving strip of paper or an electronic strip in computerized systems (see Chapter 14).

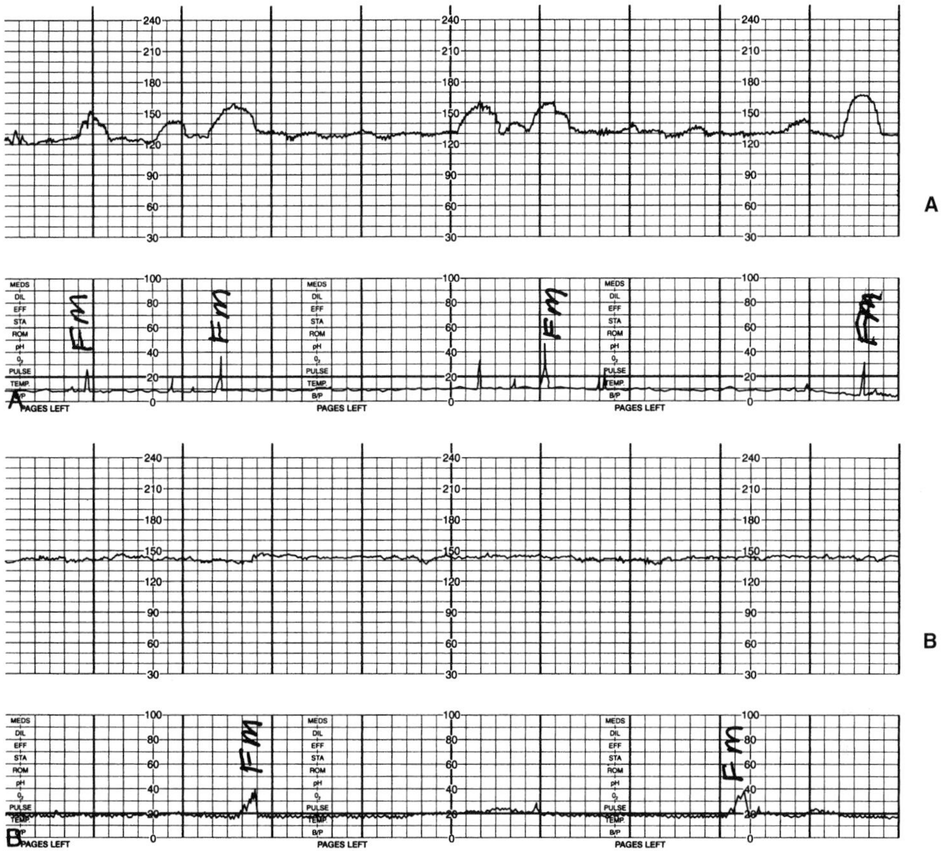

FIGURE 10-10 **A,** In this recording of a reactive nonstress test, the fetal heart rate accelerates by 25 to 30 beats per minute (BPM) for at least 15 seconds in response to fetal movement. Accelerations without fetal movement are also reassuring if the fetal heart rate increases by at least 15 BPM for at least 15 seconds. **B,** In this recording of a nonreactive nonstress test, accelerations are absent following fetal movement (FM). (Courtesy Graphic Controls, Buffalo, New York.)

Interpretation

Physicians must review and interpret nonstress test results although the nurse performs most nonstress tests. Results are classified as reactive (reassuring) or nonreactive (nonreassuring) (AAP & ACOG, 1997).

- Reactive (reassuring)—At least two fetal heart accelerations, with or without fetal movement detected by the woman, occur within a 20-minute period, peak at least 15 beats per minute (BPM) above the baseline, and last 15 seconds from baseline to baseline (Figure 10-10). Acoustic stimulation that elicits similar rate accelerations is also reassuring.
- Nonreactive (nonreassuring)—Tracing does not demonstrate the required characteristics of a reactive tracing within a 40-minute period.

Fetal heart reactivity develops with maturation of the fetal autonomic nervous system. The nonstress test of the healthy preterm fetus is more likely to be nonreactive. Between 24 and 28 weeks of gestation, up to 50% of nonstress tests may be nonreactive, and from 28 to 32 weeks of gestation, 15% of nonstress tests are nonreactive (ACOG, 1999a).

Advantages

The nonstress test is noninvasive and painless and believed to be without risk to mother or fetus. Consequently, it is the primary means of fetal surveillance in pregnancies at increased risk for uteroplacental insufficiency and consequent fetal hypoxia. The nonstress test is easy to administer and often is repeated weekly and even daily if necessary. In addition, results are available immediately. It offers a high confidence estimate of 99.8% that the uteroplacental unit is likely to continue functioning for another week (ACOG, 1999a).

Disadvantages

A major disadvantage is the large number (80%) of nonreactive findings considered false-positive (Parer, 1999). In a false-positive test result a well-oxygenated fetus does not have accelerations that meet the minimum of 15 BPM. Because of the high false-positive rate, many women undergo additional testing even though the fetus is actually healthy. Follow-up testing to a nonreactive nonstress test is usually a contraction stress test or biophysical profile.

Sleep is the usual reason for lack of fetal movement. Fetal sleep cycles average 20 to 40 minutes but may last twice this long (Parer, 1999). Several techniques have been attempted to wake the baby, such as giving the mother juice to raise her glucose level, shaking or jiggling her abdomen, and even playing music with the speakers placed on the abdomen. However, only vibroacoustic stimulation has reliably induced reactivity in the sleeping fetus (Parer, 1999; Richardson & Gagnon, 1999; ACOG, 1999a).

Vibroacoustic Stimulation

Purpose and Procedure

In recent years, vibroacoustic stimulation has been used to confirm nonreactive nonstress test findings and shorten the time required to obtain quality nonstress test data. Reactive test results obtained with vibroacoustic stimulation appear to predict fetal well-being without interfering with detection of the compromised fetus. Vibroacoustic stimulation can be used in intrapartum monitoring to verify questionable findings (see Chapter 14).

The procedure for vibroacoustic stimulation is as follows: A nonstress test is started as usual. Then an artificial larynx or vibroacoustic stimulator is applied to the maternal abdomen over the area of the fetal head for 1 to 2 seconds. The fetus is stimulated by the sound emitted and the vibration created. This may be repeated up to three times for progressively longer durations lasting up to 3 seconds (ACOG, 1999a). The acceleration usually occurs within 10 seconds and may last as long as 5 to 10 minutes (Devoe, 2000).

Fetal Responses

The sound of vibroacoustic stimulation does not appear to damage hearing in the fetus. Temporary changes in fetal body movements, breathing movements, and heart rate have been described. Fetuses near term show an increase in the number of gross (large and easily visible or felt) body movements to vibroacoustic stimulation, whereas fetuses between 26 and 32 weeks of gestation show no response. This suggests maturational change in response to vibroacoustic stimulation. Likewise, near-term fetuses appear to have fewer and more irregular breathing movements after vibroacoustic stimulation. The fetus may have a delayed fetal heart rate response to vibroacoustic stimulation, and persistent fetal tachycardia lasting up to 1.5 hours may sometimes occur. The fetus younger than 32 weeks of gestation often does not respond to vibroacoustic stimulation, which again suggests that the fetal responses change with maturation (Richardson & Gagnon, 1999).

Risks

Vibroacoustic stimulation appears to be safe for the fetus in terms of hearing, although long-term studies are lacking (Devoe, 2000). The amniotic fluid and maternal tissues surrounding the fetus softens the sound of the larynx.

Check Your Reading

14. What is a nonstress test, and why is it so named?
15. What is vibroacoustic stimulation and what is its expected result?

Contraction Stress Test

Purpose

A contraction stress test may be performed initially or if nonstress test findings are nonreactive. Uterine contractions compress the arteries that supply the placenta with oxygenated maternal blood, causing a recurrent decrease in fetal oxygen levels. The contraction stress test records the response of the FHR to stress induced by uterine contractions, identifying the fetus whose oxygen reserves are insufficient to tolerate the recurrent mild hypoxia of uterine contractions.

The fetus with adequate oxygen reserves can tolerate the temporary hypoxia induced by uterine contractions, so the FHR remains unchanged. However, if the fetus has inadequate reserves and substantial hypoxia has led to anaerobic metabolism, fetal acidosis results. This is likely to be manifested in nonreassuring fetal monitoring patterns.

Because contractions are induced, the contraction stress test is contraindicated in some situations (ACOG, 1999a):

- Preterm labor or women who have a high risk for preterm labor
- Preterm membrane rupture
- History of extensive uterine surgery or classical uterine incision for cesarean birth (see Chapter 16)
- Placenta previa (see Chapter 26)

Procedure

The nurse is responsible for administering the test and protecting the safety of the mother and fetus throughout the testing period. The woman is positioned as for a nonstress test, and external electronic fetal monitoring devices are applied to record uterine activity and FHR. An initial recording is taken to determine if the woman is having at least three spontaneous contractions, each with a duration of 40 seconds or longer. If spontaneous uterine contractions are adequate to interpret the test, no method to stimulate contractions is needed. If adequate uterine contractions are not present, two methods are used to achieve adequate contractions for interpretation of the test.

The *breast self-stimulation test* is based on the knowledge that stimulation of the nipples causes the re-

Negative	No late decelerations	Reassuring that the fetus can tolerate labor

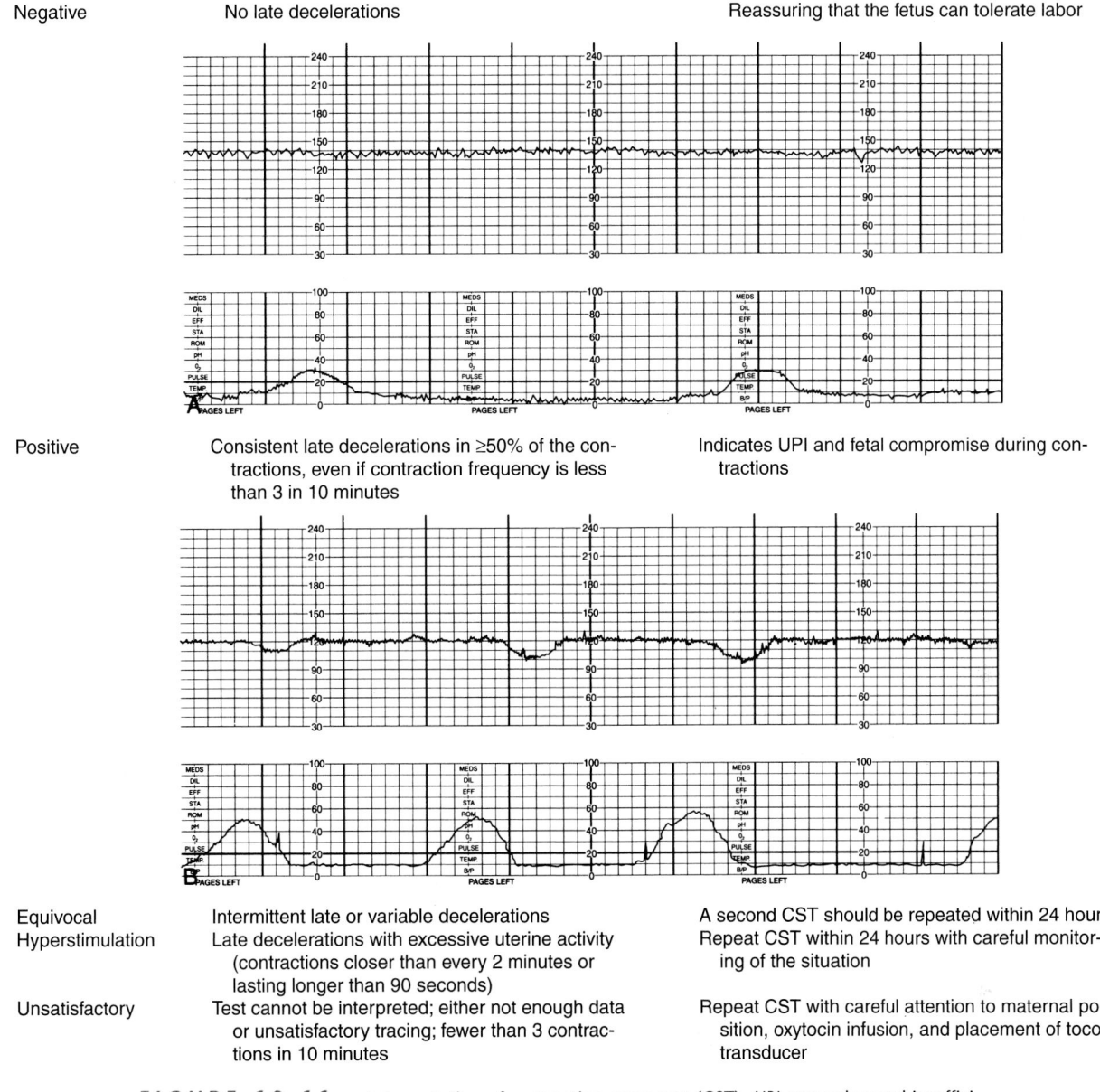

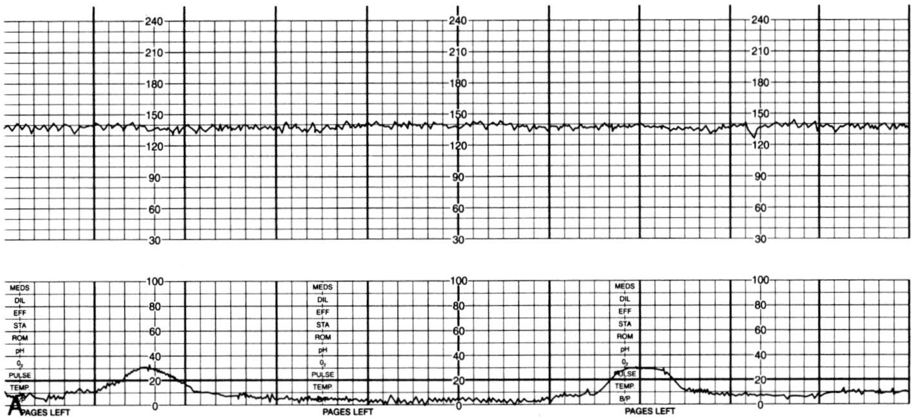

Positive	Consistent late decelerations in ≥50% of the contractions, even if contraction frequency is less than 3 in 10 minutes	Indicates UPI and fetal compromise during contractions

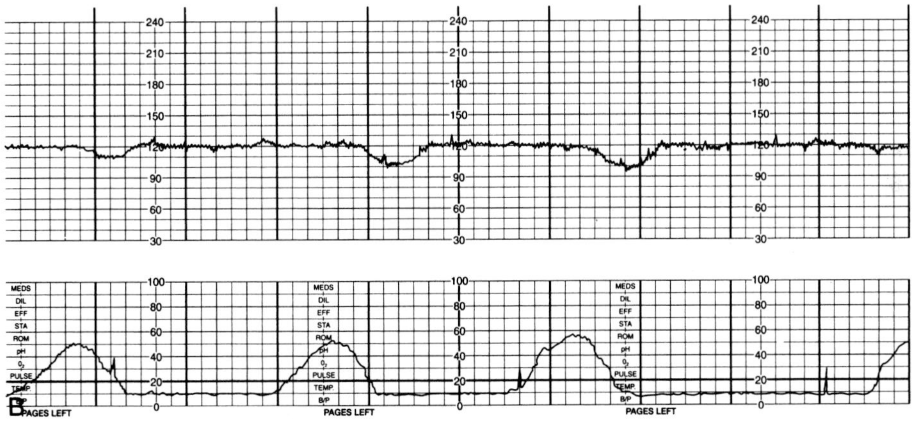

Equivocal	Intermittent late or variable decelerations	A second CST should be repeated within 24 hours
Hyperstimulation	Late decelerations with excessive uterine activity (contractions closer than every 2 minutes or lasting longer than 90 seconds)	Repeat CST within 24 hours with careful monitoring of the situation
Unsatisfactory	Test cannot be interpreted; either not enough data or unsatisfactory tracing; fewer than 3 contractions in 10 minutes	Repeat CST with careful attention to maternal position, oxytocin infusion, and placement of tocotransducer

FIGURE 10-11 Interpretation of contraction stress test (CST). *UPI,* uteroplacental insufficiency. (Courtesy Graphic Controls; Buffalo, New York.)

lease of oxytocin from the posterior pituitary, which can cause uterine contractions. The woman brushes her palm across one nipple through her clothing for 2 minutes, stopping if a contraction begins. The nipple stimulation continues after a 5-minute rest period. This cycle is repeated until an adequate contraction pattern is attained.

The *oxytocin challenge test* involves the intravenous infusion of dilute oxytocin to stimulate uterine contractions. This method is used if the breast self-stimulation test does not effectively stimulate contractions or if the health care provider prefers this method. The nurse conducting the test inserts a primary intravenous line carrying fluid with no additive and a long secondary (piggyback) line for administration of oxytocin. The initial rate is low (0.5 to 1.0 mU/min) and increases every 15 to 20 minutes (AAP & ACOG, 1997; ACOG, 1999a).

Interpretation

Contraction stress test results may be interpreted as negative (normal), positive (abnormal), equivocal, or unsatisfactory (ACOG, 1999a) (Figure 10-11).

- Negative (normal)—No late decelerations (decreases in the FHR persisting after the contraction ends) although the fetus was stressed by three contractions of at least 40 seconds' duration in a 10-minute period
- Positive (abnormal)—Late decelerations accompanying at least 50% of contractions even when fewer than three contractions occur in 10 minutes

- Equivocal (suspicious)—Intermittent late decelerations and significant variable decelerations (sudden decreases in the fetal heart rate that quickly return to the baseline)
- Equivocal (hyperstimulation)—FHR decelerations occurring in the presence of contractions that are closer than every 2 minutes or last longer than 90 seconds
- Unsatisfactory—Fewer than three contractions in 10 minutes or a tracing that cannot be interpreted

Advantages
Contraction stress testing has several advantages:

- The test provides a minimally invasive follow-up of a nonreactive nonstress test result.
- If findings are negative, contraction stress test offers more than 99% reassurance that the uteroplacental unit is likely to support life for at least 1 more week (ACOG, 1999a).
- A positive contraction stress test result allows the physician to analyze available options for further testing and make plans for the birth of an infant who may be compromised because of decreased placental functioning during labor.

Disadvantages
The contraction stress test has three major disadvantages:
- The test is more time consuming than the nonstress test.
- The contraction stress test requires precision, necessitating either the participation of the woman in breast self-stimulation or careful infusion of oxytocin to obtain an adequate contraction pattern without causing hyperstimulation of the uterus.
- The cost is higher than the nonstress test, particularly if the oxytocin challenge test is used. It is usually performed in a hospital setting with a per-hour charge. Equipment and supplies such as IV lines, oxytocin, and infusion pumps add to the cost.

Check Your Reading

16. Why is initiating contractions necessary in a contraction stress test?
17. In a contraction stress test, what do late decelerations of FHR indicate?

Biophysical Profile
The condition of the fetus can be most accurately predicted if several parameters are evaluated. Unlike the nonstress test and contraction stress test, which assess only fetal heart activity, the biophysical profile assesses five parameters of fetal status: FHR, fetal breathing movements, gross fetal movements, fetal muscle tone, and amniotic fluid volume.

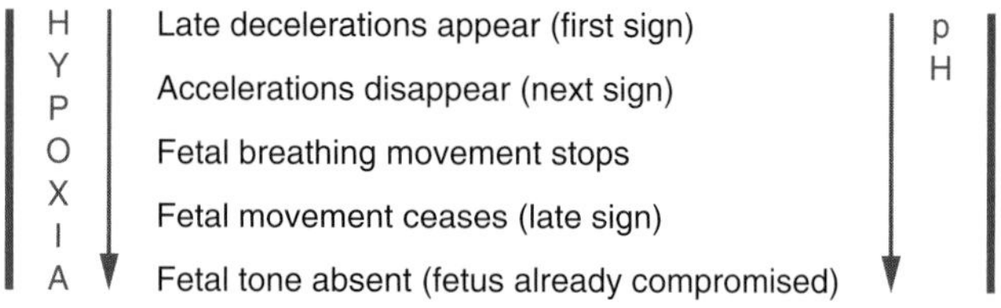

FIGURE 10-12 Cascade effect of gradual hypoxia.

Purpose
The individual components of the examination are a combination of acute and chronic markers of fetal well-being. The acute or short-term markers are the FHR reactivity, fetal breathing movements, gross fetal movements, and fetal tone. The major chronic or long-term marker is the amount of amniotic fluid.

The acute markers are controlled by different central nervous system control centers that develop at different stages in gestation. Fetal tone is the earliest to develop, then fetal movements, then regular breathing movements. Fetal heart rate reactivity develops last at the end of the second trimester or beginning of the third trimester.

The fetal central nervous system centers that control each individual parameter of the biophysical profile react differently to hypoxemia. The control centers that develop later require higher oxygen levels than those developing earlier. Therefore FHR reactivity disappears first. Fetal breathing movements are affected next, and fetal movement and fetal tone are the last areas affected. Thus absence of fetal tone indicates advanced asphyxia and acidosis. This progression has been termed the *gradual hypoxia concept* (Figure 10-12).

The amount of amniotic fluid provides information about chronic hypoxia. During periods of hypoxemia the fetus shunts blood from areas not critical to fetal life, such as the kidneys and lungs, to vital organs such as the heart, brain, and placenta. If hypoxemia is prolonged, blood flow to the fetal kidneys and lungs, which produce much of the amniotic fluid, may virtually cease. Therefore oligohydramnios indicates prolonged fetal hypoxia and is a strong indication of fetal compromise.

Procedure and Interpretation
Fetal heart rate reactivity is interpreted from a nonstress test. The other four parameters are measured by real-time ultrasonography. A scoring technique is used to interpret the data with each parameter contributing either 0 or 2 points. A score of 10 is perfect; a score of 0 is the worst possible score. A total score of 8 to 10 is considered normal unless oligohydramnios

Table 10-5
SCORING THE BIOPHYSICAL PROFILE

Criterion	Points Present (2 Points)	None or Absent (0 Points)
NONSTRESS TEST	Reactive nonstress test: ≥2 FHR accelerations peaking at least 15 BPM above baseline within a 20-minute period with a duration of ≥5 seconds each	Nonreactive nonstress test: absence of the required characteristics of a reactive tracing within a 40-minute period
FETAL BREATHING MOVEMENTS (FBM)	≥1 episode of rhythmic FBM of ≥30 seconds within 30 minutes	Absent FBM or none that meet the criteria listed for "Present"
GROSS BODY MOVEMENTS	≥3 body or limb movements in 30 minutes	≤2 body or limb movements in 30 minutes
FETAL TONE	At least one episode of extension with return to flexion	Slow extension with return to partial flexion, movement of limb in full extension, or absent fetal movement
AMNIOTIC FLUID VOLUME	At least one pocket of fluid that measures at least 1 cm in two perpendicular planes	Volume of amniotic fluid does not meet this criterion

8 to 10 points, Normal/low risk for chronic asphyxia if amniotic fluid volume is adequate; 6 points, suspected chronic asphyxia (consider retesting in 4 to 6 hours or delivery if oligohydramnios is present); 4 points, nonreassuring, suspected chronic asphyxia (base management on gestational age and further evaluation); 0 to 2 points, strong suspicion of chronic asphyxia (base management on gestational age) (ACOG, 1997; Manning, 1999a).

is present (Table 10-5). Oligohydramnios may indicate chronic fetal hypoxia and requires further evaluation (ACOG, 1999a).

Modified Biophysical Profile

Some physicians now assess the fetus only by ultrasonography and omit the nonstress test if all other parameters are normal (ACOG, 1999a). This shortens testing time without significantly compromising accuracy. In other medical centers the test is modified to include only two parameters, an amniotic fluid index (AFI) and a nonstress test. Some physicians now add a sixth parameter, placental grading, but this has not gained widespread acceptance (Manning, 1999).

Advantages

The modified biophysical profile is noninvasive and less costly than some tests because it can be done on an outpatient basis. Results are immediately available and may decrease the number of false-positive nonstress test findings. The biophysical profile allows conservative treatment of high-risk patients because delivery can be delayed if fetal well-being is indicated. The biophysical profile helps identify the presence and severity of hypoxia and acidemia because it measures multiple variables.

The biophysical profile may be used when membranes rupture prematurely and the risk for fetal infection increases. Abnormal biophysical profile results correlate positively with fetal infection (Lettieri, Vintzileos, & Nochimson, 2000; Garite, 1999).

Disadvantages

The biophysical profile is a relatively new test, and additional research is needed to refine interpretation of the test. For example, each variable is given equal weight although some variables may be more important than others. The predictive accuracy of the biophysical profile is best at the extremes, meaning that scores of 0 and 10 are highly predictive of the presence and absence of fetal acidosis, respectively. Scores toward the middle have less predictive accuracy.

Because perinatal asphyxia is a possible cause of cerebral palsy, antepartal surveillance techniques may allow fetal hypoxia to be identified and treated before it reaches critical levels. Early data indicate the biophysical profile may affect the cerebral palsy rate. This data awaits confirmation by other researchers (Manning, 1999).

Check Your Reading

18. What is the relationship between loss of fetal tone and hypoxia?
19. Why is amniotic fluid volume an important parameter in the biophysical profile?

MATERNAL ASSESSMENT OF FETAL MOVEMENT

Fetal movements detected by the mother are often called *kick counts.* The well-oxygenated fetus moves frequently. The fetus with a compromised oxygen supply conserves energy with fewer movements. Daily evaluation of these movements provides a way to evaluate the fetus.

Procedure

Numerous protocols exist for assessing kick counts. The woman lies on her side, places her hands on the largest part of her abdomen, and concentrates on fetal movements. She uses a clock or timer and records the number of movements felt during that time. Examples of kick count protocols include the following:

- Count fetal movements for 30 minutes three times per day (Figure 10-13). Further evaluation is recommended for fewer than four movements in 30 minutes.
- Count fetal movements daily for 1 hour. If fewer than 10 movements are felt, continue counting for another hour. Fewer than 10 movements in a 2-hour period should be reported to the health care provider.
- The Cardiff count-to-10 method entails counting the first 10 movements and noting the time of day when the tenth movement is felt. The health care provider should be notified if the tenth movement occurs later in the day or fewer than 10 movements occur in 12 hours.
- Count fetal movements for 30 minutes in the morning and evening to establish a baseline. If a 50% decrease or no fetal movement occurs, extend the counting period for 30 minutes. If no improvement occurs the woman should report to the hospital or clinic (Devoe, 2000).

Advantages

Counting fetal movement has obvious advantages:

- It is inexpensive.
- It is noninvasive.
- It is convenient for the client and encourages her participation in her care.

Disadvantages

Many variables make interpretation of fetal movement counts difficult:

- Fetal resting state decreases movements.
- Maternal perception of movement may vary. The ability of women to perceive fetal movement varies considerably, even in the same woman at different times.
- The time of day may affect fetal movement (lower in the morning, higher in the evening).
- Drugs taken by the mother (such as methadone, heroin, cocaine, alcohol, tobacco) may affect fetal activity.

APPLICATION OF THE NURSING PROCESS: DIAGNOSTIC TESTING

Many perinatal nurses with special education are actively involved in fetal diagnostic procedures. Nurses perform nonstress tests and contraction stress tests. With additional education, nurses may perform limited ultrasound examinations. Basic ultrasound examinations, which usually occur in an office or a clinical setting, require education beyond that for limited ultrasound. Nurses explain testing procedures and the information that can be determined from the tests. Nurses also reduce anxiety by providing emotional support when decisions about repeated testing or a series of procedures becomes necessary.

Dates: 11/14/01 to 11/20/01

Time of day	Sunday	Monday	Tuesday	Wednesday	Thursday	Friday	Saturday
Morning 8-9 AM	卌 卌	卌 ||	卌 |||				
Afternoon 1-2 PM	卌 |	卌 |||	卌				
Evening 9-10 PM	卌 || 卌	卌 ||||					
Total	28	24					

FIGURE 10-13 Daily fetal movement record in use. The mother counts the number of fetal movements (kicks) within a specified period several times per day and indicates each movement on a chart. She reports any abnormality to her health care provider.

Assessment

Collect as much information as possible about the woman and her reasons for having the tests. The information may be helpful when conducting the tests and interpreting the results. Necessary information includes the following:

- Gravida, para, living children, gestation (in weeks)
- Maternal health problems (such as hypertension, diabetes, heart disease)
- Current obstetric problems (such as vaginal bleeding, decreased fetal movement, multifetal gestation, intrauterine growth restriction, malpresentation, hydramnios, oligohydramnios)
- Prior obstetric problems (such as birth of a stillborn infant or an infant with congenital anomalies, birth of a low-birth-weight infant or a large-for-gestational age infant)
- History of substance abuse, including alcohol and tobacco
- Knowledge of reasons for the test and the procedure to be performed: "Do you have any questions before we start the test?"
- Knowledge of surveillance regimen if additional testing is necessary: "Do you have questions about the need to repeat the test every week?" "Do you understand why it is important to count your baby's movements three times each day?"
- Emotional response to the tests: "What are your major concerns?" "What can we do to make the tests easier for you?"
- Expectations of the diagnostic tests and awareness of the risks of testing, the meaning of the results, and the remaining baseline risk

Analysis

Women at increased risk for problems during pregnancy require fetal diagnostic procedures. Clients' responses vary depending on their levels of knowledge and their usual responses to stressful situations. Many women are concerned with both the test and the condition of the fetus. The relevant nursing diagnosis is "Anxiety related to lack of knowledge of diagnostic procedures and the uncertain condition of the fetus."

Planning

Goals and expected outcomes for this nursing diagnosis are that the woman (and her support person) will do the following:

- Describe how, when, and why she is to be tested before testing procedures are initiated.
- Verbalize concerns about the condition of the fetus and seek information from her health care team at each appointment.

Interventions

Providing Information

Even nurses who do not work in antepartum testing must understand reasons for the tests and should be able to describe them in general terms. Many parents want to know about the safety of the tests and the amount of discomfort the woman will experience. The website of the March of Dimes includes fact sheets for some antepartal tests discussed in this chapter, which may be useful for clients who want general knowledge about testing (www.modimes.org/HealthLibrary2/FactSheets/Default.htm)

Parents often want to know why some tests must be repeated. Many parents become very concerned when screening test results are abnormal, such as an MSAFP assessment. The nurse may need to remind them that other factors may cause abnormal results, which do not necessarily indicate a problem. In addition, nurses often need to interpret technical information that parents receive from physicians because it may be confusing and cause the parents undue anxiety.

Provide simple, clear explanations of what the tests measure and the purpose and frequency of the tests. Describe the procedure, including its usual length of time, to minimize anxiety caused by lack of knowledge. The woman is less likely to forget important information if she is given verbal and written instructions about follow-up care and events that should be reported to the physician.

Providing Support

Identify and respond to feelings expressed by expectant parents when antepartum testing procedures are recommended or fetal problems are confirmed. The woman often experiences frustration with the discomfort, limitations, and time-consuming demands of pregnancy and regimen of fetal testing. Skill in therapeutic communication is never more important than during counseling about fetal diagnostic tests.

Active listening conveys interest and concern. Paraphrasing allows for interpretation because it expresses in different words what concerns the family. The art of reflecting back to the family what they convey about feelings helps them "hear" their feelings. Clarifying helps the woman "see" the issues and available options. Comforting measures such as touch, if culturally acceptable to the woman, convey empathic concern and are especially important during difficult procedures.

Although nurses offer caring concern and careful reflection of feelings, they do not offer advice. The woman, along with her primary support person and other chosen persons, must make decisions about antepartal assessment. Nurses frequently help the family contact persons (such as a clergy member or close relative) to whom they turn in troubled times, such as when abnormal test results are verified.

Helping Clients Set Realistic Goals

Women benefit from knowing that compliance with an antepartal surveillance regimen is beneficial for the fetus. Although the repeated tests may seem tedious, they often offer the best chance for the fetus to be delivered at the best possible time. Explain to the woman that testing helps the perinatal team decide whether intervention is needed and choose the best possible intervention under the circumstances.

If the woman is having testing to identify fetal abnormalities, help her understand that a baseline risk for abnormalities remains when tests show the fetus is normal. Even if performing all diagnostic tests for birth defects on a woman were possible, the background risk would remain.

Supporting the Woman's Decision

Prenatal genetic diagnosis sometimes leads a woman to choose pregnancy termination, often during the second trimester. The woman also has the right to indicated prenatal genetic diagnostic procedures even if she would not terminate her pregnancy for an abnormal fetus. Nurses must examine their own ethical beliefs before becoming involved in fetal diagnostic testing. They must be prepared to support whatever decision a family makes, even if it is not one they would make. A woman who decides to continue or terminate a pregnancy is entitled to compassionate care regardless of the nurse's personal views about her decision.

Evaluation

The goals and expected outcomes are successful if the woman verbalizes knowledge of why tests are recommended and how and when they will be performed. The second goal and expected outcome is met if the woman and family verbalize any concerns about the fetus and seek additional information from the perinatal team as needed.

SUMMARY CONCEPTS

- Ultrasonography is widely used during pregnancy to determine a variety of fetal and placental conditions and aid in the performance of other tests such as amniocentesis and percutaneous umbilical blood sampling. It is also used in gynecology and infertility care.
- AFP assessment is performed on maternal serum or amniotic fluid with the primary goal of detecting open body wall defects such as neural tube defects. Additional tests are required if AFP levels are abnormal. Two other markers, human chorionic gonadotropin and estriol, are usually assessed with MSAFP to screen for chromosomal anomalies such as trisomy 21.
- CVS is performed at 10 to 12 weeks of gestation to provide parents with information about chromosomal and other congenital defects in the first trimester of pregnancy. CVS does not provide a sample of amniotic fluid for AFP testing.
- Amniocentesis is usually performed in the second or third trimester to identify chromosomal defects and evaluate fetal maturity and Rh incompatibility problems. Standard amniocentesis is performed at 15 to 16 weeks of gestation. Early amniocentesis (13 to 14 weeks) allows earlier diagnosis of genetic problems.
- Percutaneous umbilical blood sampling involves aspiration of blood from umbilical vessels to detect blood disorders, acid-base balance, or fetal disease. Therapeutic medications and blood products can also be injected by the same route. Fetal bradycardia is the most common complication.
- The nonstress test determines whether the fetal heart rate accelerates when the fetus moves. Accelerations of the heart rate, regardless of fetal movement, are a reassuring sign because they are associated with adequate fetal oxygenation and an intact neural pathway from the fetal brain to the heart. The healthy fetus younger than 32 weeks of gestation may not have accelerations that meet the criteria for a reactive nonstress test.
- Contraction stress tests evaluate the response of the fetal heart to recurrent short interruptions in placental blood flow and oxygen supply that occur with uterine contractions.
- Maternal assessment of fetal movement ("kick counts") is an inexpensive and noninvasive method of evaluating the fetus. The poorly oxygenated fetus usually moves less than the well-oxygenated fetus. The woman may be advised to follow any of several protocols because no standard protocol exists.
- All perinatal nurses must be prepared to offer clear explanations of diagnostic procedures and provide support for the family requiring fetal diagnostic tests.

REFERENCES & READINGS

American Academy of Pediatrics (AAP), & American College of Obstetricians and Gynecologists (ACOG). (1997). *Guidelines for perinatal care* (4th ed.). Elk Grove Village, IL: Author.

ACOG. (1999a). *Antepartum fetal surveillance,* Practice Bulletin No. 9. Washington, D.C.: Author.

ACOG. (1995). *Chorionic villus sampling,* Committee Opinion, No. 160. Washington, D.C.: Author.

ACOG. (1999b). *First-trimester screening for fetal anomalies with nuchal translucency,* Committee Opinion, No. 223. Washington, D.C.: Author.

Association of Women's Health, Obstetric, and Neonatal Nurses. (1998). *Clinical competencies and education guide: Antepartum and intrapartum fetal heart rate monitoring.* Washington, D.C.: Author.

Anthony, A. (1996). Biological effects and safety. In T.J. Dubose (Ed.), *Fetal sonography* (pp. 27-44). Philadelphia: W.B. Saunders.

Berman, M. (1996). History of fetal sonography. In T.J. DuBose (Ed.), *Fetal sonography* (pp. 11-26). Philadelphia: W.B. Saunders.

Beall, M.H. (2000). Chorionic villus sampling for prenatal diagnosis. In E.J. Quilligan and F.P. Zuspan (Eds.), *Current therapy in obstetrics and gynecology* (5th ed., pp. 736-767). Philadelphia: W.B. Saunders.

Blaas, H. (1998). In-vivo three-dimensional ultrasound reconstructions of embryos and early fetuses. *Lancet* (Oct. 10, 1998): 1182.

Bowman, J.M. (1999). Hemolytic disease (erythroblastosis fetalis). In R.K. Creasy & R. Resnik (Eds.), *Maternal-fetal medicine: Principles and practice* (4th ed., pp. 341-363). Philadelphia: W.B. Saunders.

Calhoun, S. (2000). Focus on fluids: Examining maternal hydration and amniotic fluid volume. *AWHONN Lifelines,* 3(6), 20-24.

Cartier, M.S. (1996). Fetal Doppler. In T.J. DuBose (Ed.), *Fetal sonography* (pp. 275-303). Philadelphia: W.B. Saunders.

Covington, C., Gielghem, P., Board, F., Madison, K., Nedd, D., & Miller, L. (1996). Family care related to alpha-fetoprotein screening. *Journal of Obstetric, Gynecologic, and Neonatal Nursing,* 25(2), 125-130.

Cunningham, F.G., MacDonald, P.C., Gant, N.F., Leveno, K.J., Gilstrap, L.C., Hankins, G.D.V., et al. (1997). *Williams obstetrics* (20th ed.). Norwalk, CT: Appleton & Lange.

Curtin, S.C., & Mathews, T.J. (2000). U.S. obstetric procedures, 1998. *Birth,* 27(2), 136-138.

Devoe, L.D. (2000). Antepartum fetal surveillance. In E.J. Quilligan and F.P. Zuspan (Eds.), *Current therapy in obstetrics and gynecology* (5th ed., pp. 372-376). Philadelphia: W.B. Saunders.

DuBose, T.J. (1996). First trimester. In T.J. DuBose, *Fetal sonography* (pp. 389-425). Philadelphia: W.B. Saunders.

DuBose, T.J. (1996). Second and third trimester. In T.J. DuBose, *Fetal sonography* (pp. 427-471). Philadelphia: W.B. Saunders.

Eganhouse, D.J., & Petersen, L.A. (1998). Fetal surveillance in multifetal pregnancy. *Journal of Obstetric, Gynecologic, and Neonatal Nursing,* 27(3), 312-321.

Evans, M.I., & Johnson, M.P. (2000). Genetic counseling, screening, & diagnosis. In S.B. Ransom, M.P. Dombrowski, S.G. McNeeley, K.S. Moghissi, & A.R. Munkarah (Eds.), *Practical strategies in obstetrics & gynecology* (pp. 215-223). Philadelphia: W.B. Saunders.

Evans, M.I., Johnson, M.P., & Drugan, A. (2000). Amniocentesis for antenatal diagnosis of genetic disorders. In E.J. Quilligan and F.P. Zuspan (Eds.), *Current therapy in obstetrics and gynecology* (5th ed., pp. 226-232). Philadelphia: W.B. Saunders.

Farkouh, L.J., & Hobbins, J.C. (2000). Percutaneous umbilical blood sampling. In E.J. Quilligan and F.P. Zuspan (Eds.), *Current therapy in obstetrics and gynecology* (5th ed., pp. 427-429). Philadelphia: W.B. Saunders.

Filly, R.A. (2000). Obstetrical sonography: The best way to terrify a pregnant woman. *Journal of Ultrasound in Medicine,* 19(1), 1-5.

Garite, T.J. (1999). Premature rupture of the membranes. In R.K. Creasy & R. Resnik (Eds.), *Maternal-fetal medicine: Principles and practice* (4th ed., pp. 644-658). Philadelphia: W.B. Saunders.

Harman, C.R. (1999a). Percutaneous fetal blood sampling. In R.K. Creasy & R. Resnik (Eds.), *Maternal-fetal medicine: Principles and practice* (4th ed., pp. 341-363). Philadelphia: W.B. Saunders.

Harman, C.R. (1999b). The routine obstetric ultrasound scan. In D.K. James, P.J. Steer, C.P. Weiner, & B. Gonik (Eds.), *High-risk pregnancy: Management options* (pp. 171-206). Philadelphia: W.B. Saunders.

Harman, C.R., Menticoglou, S., & Manning, F.A. (1999). Assessing fetal health. In D.K. James, P.J. Steer, C.P. Weiner, & B. Gonik (Eds.), *High-risk pregnancy: Management options* (pp. 249-289). Philadelphia: W.B. Saunders.

Holzgreve, W., & Miny, P. (1999). Chorionic villus sampling and placental biopsy. In D.K. James, P.J. Steer, C.P. Weiner, & B. Gonik (Eds.), *High-risk pregnancy: Management options* (pp. 207-214). Philadelphia: W.B. Saunders.

Jasper, M.L. (2000). Antepartum fetal assessment. In S. Mattson & J.E. Smith (Eds.), *Core curriculum for maternal-newborn nursing* (2nd ed., pp. 127). Philadelphia: W.B. Saunders.

Jenkins, T.M., & Wapner, R.J. (1999). First trimester prenatal diagnosis: Chorionic villus sampling. *Seminars in Perinatology,* 23(5), 403-413.

Jobe, A.H. (1999). Fetal lung development, tests for maturation, induction of maturation, and treatment. In R.K. Creasy & R. Resnik (Eds.), *Maternal-fetal medicine: Principles and practice* (4th ed., pp. 404-422). Philadelphia: W.B. Saunders.

Johnson, D.D., & VanDorsten, J.P. (2000). Second-trimester ultrasonography. In S.B. Ransom, M.P. Dombrowski, S.G. McNeeley, K.S. Moghissi, & A.R. Munkarah (Eds.), *Practical strategies in obstetrics & gynecology* (pp. 239-248). Philadelphia: W.B. Saunders.

Kellner, L.H., Weiss, R.R., Weiner, Z., et al. (1995). The advantages of using triple-marker screening for chromosomal abnormalities. *American Journal of Obstetrics and Gynecology,* 172(3), 831-836.

Kocun, C.C., Harrigan, J.T., Canterino, J.C., Feld, S.M., & Fernandez, C.O. (2000). Changing trends in patient decisions concerning genetic amniocentesis. *American Journal of Obstetrics and Gynecology,* 182(5), 1018-1020.

Lenke, R., & Ashwood, E. (2000). Lung maturity testing. In E.J. Quilligan & F.P. Zuspan (Eds.), *Current therapy in obstetrics and gynecology* (5th ed., pp. 418-420). Philadelphia: W.B. Saunders.

Lettieri, L., Vintzileos, A.M., & Nochimson, D.J. (2000). Biophysical profile. In E.J. Quilligan & F.P. Zuspan (Eds.), *Current therapy in obstetrics and gynecology* (5th ed., pp. 376-380). Philadelphia: W.B. Saunders.

Manning, F.A. (1999a). Fetal assessment by evaluation of biophysical variables: Fetal biophysical profile score. In R.K. Creasy & R. Resnik (Eds.), *Maternal-fetal medicine: Principles and practice* (4th ed., pp. 169-206). Philadelphia: W.B. Saunders.

Manning, F.A. (1999b). General principles and applications of ultrasonography. In R.K. Creasy & R. Resnik (Eds.), *Maternal-fetal medicine: Principles and practice* (4th ed., pp. 169-206). Philadelphia: W.B. Saunders.

McCarthy, K.E., & Narrigan, D. (1995). Is there scientific support for the use of juice to facilitate the nonstress test? *Journal of Obstetric, Gynecologic, and Neonatal Nursing,* 24(4), 303-306.

McRae, M.J. (1999). Fetal surveillance and monitoring: Legal issues revisited. *Journal of Obstetric, Gynecologic, and Neonatal Nursing,* 28(3), 310-319.

Menihan, C.A. (2000). Limited obstetric ultrasound in nursing practice. *Journal of Obstetric, Gynecologic, and Neonatal Nursing,* 29(3), 325-330.

Miller, D.A., & Paul, R. (1999). Antepartum-intrapartum fetal monitoring. In J.R. Scott, P.J. DiSaia, C.B. Hammond, & W.N. Spellacy (Eds.), *Danforth's Obstetrics and Gynecology* (8th ed., pp. 243-256). Philadelphia: Lippincott.

Murray, M. (1997). *Antepartal and intrapartal fetal monitoring* (2nd ed.). Albuquerque, NM: Learning Resources International, Inc.

Nathan, E.B., Haberman, S., Burgess, T., & Minkoff, H. (2000). The relationship of maternal position to the results of brief nonstress tests: A randomized clinical trial. *American Journal of Obstetrics and Gynecology,* 182(5), 1070-1072.

National Center for Health Statistics. (2000). *Births: Final data for 1998,* 48(3).

National Institutes of Health. (1984). *Diagnostic ultrasound imaging in pregnancy: NIH consensus statement online 1984 Feb 6-8;* 5(1):1-16. Retrieved 6/22/2000 from http://text/nlm.nih.gov/nih/cdc/www/41txt.html.

Opipari, A.W., & Johnson, T.R.B. (2000). Fetal assessment. In S.B. Ransom, M.P. Dombrowski, S.G. McNeeley, K.S. Moghissi, & A.R. Munkarah (Eds.), *Practical strategies in obstetrics & gynecology* (pp. 224-233). Philadelphia: W.B. Saunders.

Overton, T.G., & Fisk, N.M. (1999). Amniocentesis. In D.K. James, P.J. Steer, C.P. Weiner, & B. Gonik (Eds.), *High-risk pregnancy: Management options* (pp. 215-223). Philadelphia: W.B. Saunders.

Parer, J.T. (1999). Fetal heart rate. In R.K. Creasy & R. Resnik (Eds.), *Maternal-fetal medicine: Principles and practice* (4th ed., pp. 270-299). Philadelphia: W.B. Saunders.

Platt, L.D., Santulli, T., Carlson, D.E., Greene, N., & Walla, C.A. (1998). Three-dimensional ultrasonography in obstetrics and gynecology: Preliminary experience. *American Journal of Obstetrics and Gynecology,* 178(6), 1199-1206.

Pretorius, D.H., Nelson, T.R., & Lev-Toaff, A.S. (2000). Three-dimensional ultrasound in obstetrics and gynecology. In P.W. Callen (Ed.), *Ultrasonography in obstetrics and gynecology,* (4th ed., pp. 747-762). Philadelphia: W.B. Saunders.

Queenan, J.T. (2000). Rh and other blood group immunizations. In E.J. Quilligan and F.P. Zuspan (Eds.), *Current therapy in obstetrics and gynecology* (5th ed., pp. 429-432). Philadelphia: W.B. Saunders.

Raines, D.A. (1996). Fetal surveillance: Issues and implications. *Journal of Obstetric, Gynecologic, and Neonatal Nursing,* 25(7), 559-564.

Rayburn, W.F. (2000). Fetal movement charting. In E.J. Quilligan and F.P. Zuspan (Eds.), *Current therapy in obstetrics and gynecology* (5th ed., pp. 401-404). Philadelphia: W.B. Saunders.

Richardson, B.S., & Gagnon, R. (1999). Fetal breathing and body movements. In R.K. Creasy & R. Resnik (Eds.), *Maternal-fetal medicine: Principles and practice* (4th ed., pp. 231-247). Philadelphia: W.B. Saunders.

Santalahti, P., Latikka, A.M., Ryynänen, M., & Hemminki, E. (1996). Women's experiences of perinatal serum screening. *Birth,* 23(2), 101-107.

Sciosia, A.L. (1999). Prenatal genetic diagnosis. In R.K. Creasy & R. Resnik (Eds.), *Maternal-fetal medicine: Principles and practice* (4th ed., pp. 40-62). Philadelphia: W.B. Saunders.

Sohaey, R., & Branch, D.W. (1999). Ultrasound in obstetrics. In J.R. Scott, P.J. DiSaia, C.B. Hammond, & W.N. Spellacy (Eds.), *Danforth's obstetrics and gynecology* (8th ed., pp. 213-242). Philadelphia: Lippincott.

Soothill, P.W. (1999). Fetal blood sampling before labor. In D.K. James, P.J. Steer, C.P. Weiner, & B. Gonik (Eds.), *High-risk pregnancy: Management options* (pp. 225-233). Philadelphia: W.B. Saunders.

Treadwell, M.C. (2000). First-trimester ultrasonography. In S.B. Ransom, M.P. Dombrowski, S.G. McNeeley, K.S. Moghissi, & A.R. Munkarah (Eds.), *Practical strategies in obstetrics & gynecology* (pp. 234-238). Philadelphia: W.B. Saunders.

Treanor, C. (1998). Exploring nurses' roles in limited ultrasound. *AWHONN Lifelines,* 2(2), 13.

Trudinger, B. (1999). Doppler ultrasound assessment of blood flow. In R.K. Creasy & R. Resnik (Eds.), *Maternal-fetal medicine: Principles and practice* (4th ed., pp. 216-229). Philadelphia: W.B. Saunders.

Uçkan, E.M., & Townsend, N.S. (1999). Fetal adaptation. In L.K. Mandeville & N.H. Troiano (Eds.), *AWHONN's high-risk & critical care intrapartum nursing* (2nd ed., pp. 32-50). Philadelphia: Lippincott.

Weiner, C.P., & Baschat, A.A. (1999). Fetal growth restriction: Evaluation and management. Abnormalities of alphafetoprotein and other biochemical tests. In D.K. James, P.J. Steer, C.P. Weiner, & B. Gonik (Eds.), *High-risk pregnancy: Management options* (pp. 291-305). Philadelphia: W.B. Saunders.

Wenstrom, K.D., Owen, J., Boots, L., & Ethier, M. (1995). The influence of maternal weight on human chorionic gonadotropin in the multiple-marker screening test for fetal Down syndrome. *American Journal of Obstetrics and Gynecology,* 173(4), 1297-1300.

Yankowitz, J., & Williamson, R.A. (1999). Abnormalities of alpha-fetoprotein and other biochemical tests. In D.K. James, P.J. Steer, C.P. Weiner, & B. Gonik (Eds.), *High-risk pregnancy: Management options* (pp. 153-170). Philadelphia: W.B. Saunders.

11

PERINATAL EDUCATION

OBJECTIVES

1. List the goals of perinatal education.
2. Explain choices in childbearing and the effects of education on these choices.
3. Describe the various types of education for childbearing families.
4. Describe techniques for pain relief taught in Lamaze childbirth classes.
5. Describe the support person's role in helping women during labor and birth.
6. Explain the components frequently included in a birth plan.

DEFINITIONS

BIRTH PLAN A plan describing a couple's preferences for their birth experience (also called a *family preference plan*).

EFFLEURAGE Massage of the abdomen or another body part performed during labor contractions.

HABITUATION Decreased response to a repeated stimulus.

PSYCHOPROPHYLAXIS Method of prepared childbirth that emphasizes mental concentration and relaxation to increase pain tolerance.

Perinatal education has become increasingly important in helping couples learn about pregnancy, birth, and parenting. Many classes not only focus on preparation for childbirth but also include information formerly received during the birth facility stay. Prenatal classes are often included in perinatal clinical pathways (see Figure 7-12).

GOALS OF PERINATAL EDUCATION

The goals of perinatal education are to help parents become knowledgeable consumers, take an active role in maintaining health during pregnancy and birth, and learn coping techniques to deal with pregnancy, childbirth, and parenting. Meeting these goals increases parents' abilities to make decisions regarding childbirth and parenting with confidence and satisfaction. A national goal of Healthy People 2010 is to increase the proportion of women who attend a series of prepared childbirth classes (U.S. Department of Health and Human Services, 2000).

PROVIDERS OF EDUCATION

Although most perinatal education classes are taught by registered nurses, physical therapists or others who have taken special courses also may become perinatal educators. Many instructors are certified by organizations such as the American Society for Psychoprophylaxis in Obstetrics (ASPO) and International Childbirth Education Association (ICEA). Certification ensures that the instructors have received special preparation to provide sound education adhering to the certifying organization's general philosophy. The Association of Women's Health, Obstetric, and Neonatal Nurses (AWHONN) has published guidelines for educator competencies and class curricula (AWHONN, 2000). Teachers must be versed in adult education theory and techniques and skillful in handling groups of people from diverse backgrounds.

Classes may be sponsored by community agencies such as schools, health departments, and civic organizations and health care providers such as medical groups and hospitals. Teachers may be employed by a sponsoring agency or self-employed. Classes may also occur in less traditional sites. For example, some companies offer employees free prenatal classes at the work site. Teaching women ways to reduce risk factors for complications is a way for employers to reduce costs associated with prematurity and low birth weight.

Education may be presented formally in classrooms. Nurses in offices, clinics, and birth sites also educate women informally. Teaching may occur in waiting rooms of clinics before women are called for their appointments or as part of routine care.

CLASS PARTICIPANTS

Participants in classes about childbearing have traditionally been middle-income couples who are older and better educated than those who do not take classes. Low-income women may not have money to pay for classes and transportation to get there. Although inexpensive or free classes are available in some areas, women with little or no prenatal care may not know about them. Classes in languages other than English have become more readily available in areas where they are needed.

People take classes for a variety of reasons. Many have a strong desire to participate actively in all aspects of childbearing. For these people, making decisions about what happens to them is important, and they want the education to help them decide wisely. Others are looking for coping strategies for their fears of childbirth and pain.

Women and their partners report a greater sense of control during labor and delivery when they have taken prepared childbirth classes (Hart & Foster, 1997). When women feel that they are informed and have some control over what happens to them, they are more likely to expect birth to be satisfying and fulfilling and experience it as such.

CHOICES FOR CHILDBEARING

Many changes in childbearing practices during the last 40 years have occurred in response to consumer desire for more input and control over the birth experience. The family-centered approach, designed to make birth less institutional and more personal, is one response to this consumer movement. Choices about the setting and interventions used and inclusion of the father and other support people have resulted from the work of concerned consumers and health care providers.

One purpose of perinatal education is to help parents learn what options are available so that they can make appropriate choices. Parents learn that many ways of birthing are possible and no one "right" method exists. Knowledgeable parents can communicate assertively with their health care providers about their needs and desires.

Health Care Professional

Women contemplating pregnancy and birth may choose a certified nurse-midwife (CNM), nurse practitioner (NP), obstetrician, or family practice physician to be their health care providers. They need to know what to expect from each of these practitioners.

A CNM cares for women at low risk for complications and refers them to a backup physician if problems develop. CNMs, NPs, and physicians treat women during pregnancy and the postpartum period, but NPs do not usually perform deliveries. A CNM, NP, or family practice physician may also care for the newborn. A physician generally arrives for the birth near the end of labor, whereas the CNM is often present through most of labor and birth. Some couples visit several different care providers to discuss their plans for birth before choosing the one they feel is best for them.

Setting

The woman and her partner must choose a birth setting and select a care provider who practices in that setting. Hospitals are the most frequent setting for birth in North America. Hospitals may have birthing suites that provide a homelike atmosphere or traditional labor and delivery rooms. A freestanding birth center provides an atmosphere that is less institutional than the hospital. Home birth allows the woman to give birth in her own surroundings with delivery managed by a nurse-midwife (see Chapter 1, "Current Settings for Childbirth").

Support Person

During labor the woman needs to have someone with her to help her through the experience. The support person is most often the father of her baby, but a relative or friend may also take this role (Figure 11-1).

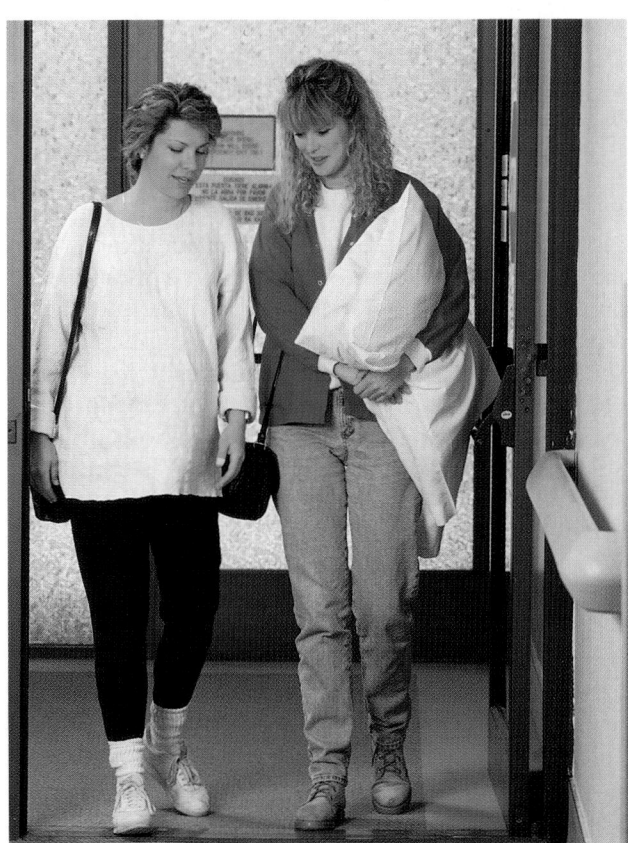

FIGURE 11-1 Often an expectant mother will ask a sister or close female friend to be her labor partner and attend classes with her.

Some women wish to share the birth experience with several relatives and close friends. If the birth setting is traditional, only one person is permitted to be present. In less traditional settings, more support people are usually allowed. Some women hire a support person such as a doula to provide support during labor.

Siblings

The presence of children at birth is controversial. Some believe that children become closer to their new siblings when they are present at birth. Others believe that the sights of the birth process, blood, and their mothers in pain may be too frightening for children. Some debate centers on the age of the child attending the birth.

Children who participate in the birth of a sibling may attend all or part of the labor and birth or may join the parents just after the birth to participate in the immediate celebration. An adult support person stays with the child throughout the experience. The support person should have no role other than attending to the child. This role includes gauging the child's response, providing explanations and reassurance, and taking the child out of the room as needed.

Education

Expectant mothers must also decide on prenatal education classes. Their decisions are based on the classes available in the area, costs, and types of information needed. Some areas have a vast array of classes from which to choose. In other areas, the selection is limited to childbirth preparation classes only.

Small classes of a few women and their partners are ideal but may be too expensive or unavailable. If the class includes more than 10 couples, the teacher should have an assistant to help with individual instruction. The teacher is usually a registered nurse who has experience in maternity nursing and is certified by a nationally known organization.

Prepared childbirth classes based in birth facilities include detailed information on what to expect in that particular setting but may not cover options that are unavailable at that agency. Hospital classes have sometimes been criticized for teaching clients to be "good" and compliant patients. A woman may wish to talk to the instructor before taking a class to ask about class size and the teacher's philosophy, background, and teaching methods.

Check Your Reading

1. What are the goals of perinatal education?
2. What major decisions must couples make in preparation for childbirth?

Table 11-1
TOPICS COVERED IN EARLY PREGNANCY CLASSES

- Pregnancy
  - Anatomy and physiology
  - Physiologic and psychological changes
  - Fetal development
  - Hazards to the mother and fetus (such as drugs, alcohol, smoking, environmental)
  - Medical care (such as importance, what to expect at each visit)
  - Communication with the provider
  - Prenatal screening tests
- Self-care
  - Hygiene
  - Nutrition
  - Exercise and body mechanics
  - Discomforts of pregnancy
  - Danger signs
  - Sexuality
  - Work and pregnancy
- Infant care
  - Selection of a pediatrician
  - Infant development and care
  - Infant feeding
  - Preparation for breastfeeding
- Birth
  - Birth options (such as birth plan, costs)
  - Preterm labor

Types of Classes Available

Although most people think of perinatal education primarily as preparation for the birth experience, classes are available in all areas of pregnancy, childbirth, and parenting.

Preconception Classes

Classes for couples who are thinking about having a baby are designed to help them have a healthy pregnancy from the beginning. Information about nutrition before conception, signs of pregnancy, healthy lifestyle, and selection of a caregiver are presented. The effects of pregnancy and childbirth on a woman's relationships and career are discussed. Preconception classes emphasize ways to reduce risk factors and early and regular prenatal care.

Early Pregnancy Classes

Early pregnancy classes focus on the first two trimesters (Table 11-1). First-trimester classes are sometimes called *early bird* or *right start classes.* They cover information on adapting to pregnancy, dealing with early discomforts such as morning sickness and fatigue, and understanding what to expect in the months ahead. Emphasis is placed on ways to have a healthy pregnancy by obtaining prenatal care and avoiding hazards to the fetus.

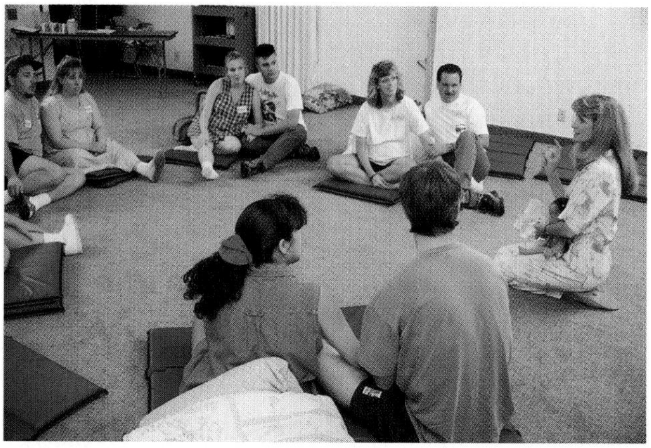

FIGURE 11-2 The nurse teaching this class discusses movement of the fetus through the pelvis.

Second-trimester classes focus on changes that occur during middle pregnancy and preparation for birth. Information on body mechanics in relation to an enlarging abdomen, work during pregnancy, and what to expect during the third trimester are included. Teachers discuss childbirth choices and information to help students become more knowledgeable consumers.

Parents may begin to learn about the needs of the mother and infant after birth in these classes or attend other classes to meet this need. This information is especially important because of the short length of stay in the birth facility.

Exercise Classes

Exercise classes help women keep fit and healthy during pregnancy. Some classes also continue into the postpartum period. Written consent from the primary caregiver may be required to ensure that the woman can participate safely. The instructor should understand the special needs of pregnancy and teach low-impact exercises preceded by warm-up routines. Women should avoid excessive heart rate elevation to prevent diversion of blood away from the uterus.

Childbirth Preparation Classes

Women and their support persons learn self-help measures and what to expect for labor and birth in childbirth preparation classes (Figure 11-2). Although once referred to as "natural childbirth classes," they are now called *prepared childbirth classes* to denote the woman's preparation for all aspects of childbirth, including complications. Couples learn coping methods to help them approach childbirth in a positive manner. Teachers do not promise prevention of all pain in labor. However, the increased confidence gained in prepared childbirth classes is associated with decreased perception and increased tolerance of pain during labor and lower use of drugs for labor pain (Lowe, 1996).

Table 11-2
TOPICS COVERED IN PREPARED CHILDBIRTH CLASSES

Pregnancy	Comfort measures
Physical and psychological changes of the last trimester	Labor rehearsals
Common discomforts and concerns	Pain relief (both pharmacologic and nonpharmacologic)
Nutrition	Complications
Exercise and body mechanics	Danger signs
Sexuality	High-risk pregnancy
Antepartum testing	Cesarean birth
Common third trimester tests	Support person
Labor and birth	Role of the labor partner
Anatomy and physiology of labor	Techniques for support
Plans for the birth (such as consumerism, options, birth plan)	Postpartum
Signs of labor and when to go to the hospital	Physiologic and psychological changes
Hospital admission and procedures	Birth agency stay and early discharge
Physical and emotional aspects of labor	Role adaptation and postpartum blues
Labor variations (such as back labor, inductions)	Family planning
Birthing process	Normal newborn
Recovery	Characteristics
Tour of maternity unit	General care and safety
Coping techniques for labor	Feeding (breast and formula)
Relaxation and breathing techniques	

Classes include tours of birth settings and information about labor and pharmacologic and nonpharmacologic methods of pain relief. Supervised practice of relaxation and coping strategies in "labor rehearsals" is part of every class (Figure 11-3). Films assist women to develop a realistic picture of the birth process (Table 11-2).

The teacher describes advantages and disadvantages of various options in birthing. For example, couples may learn that epidural anesthesia, which is almost routine in many areas, usually removes most pain but may increase the length of labor, cause less effective pushing, and make catheterization and administration of oxytocin more likely. On the other hand, use of relaxation techniques avoids the disadvantages of analgesic drugs and anesthesia but does not remove all discomfort. When women have balanced views of their options, they are able to discuss them intelligently with caregivers and make better decisions.

In recent years, many women have chosen to have epidural anesthesia during childbirth. However, even women who plan to have an epidural as soon as possible should learn and practice methods of pain relief. Birth facilities may not admit women into the labor unit and administer anesthesia until active labor begins. This makes nonpharmacologic pain relief measures necessary until the woman can receive anesthesia.

Class series range from four to nine meetings depending on the content included. Because these may be the only classes a woman attends, information about the third trimester of pregnancy is often presented. Some classes also include discussion of the postpartum period, breastfeeding, and infant care.

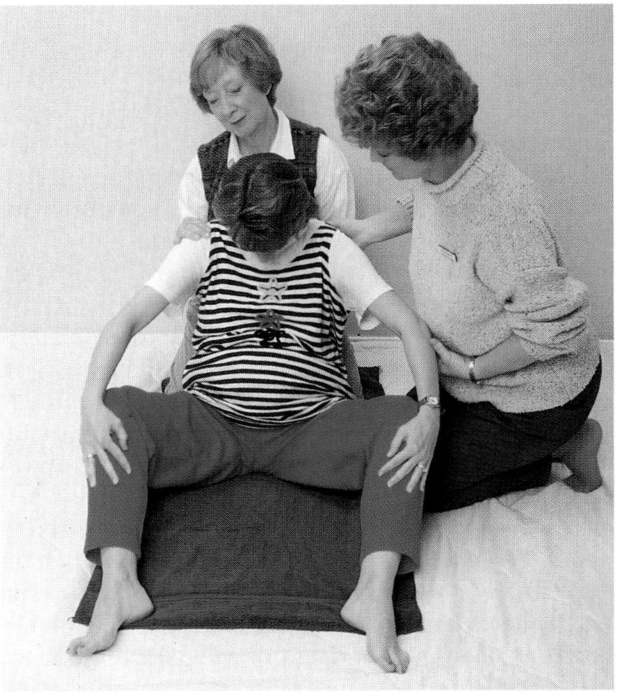

FIGURE 11-3 The teacher helps each couple, individually and together, with pushing during a labor rehearsal.

Refresher Courses

Women whose last prepared childbirth was more than 2 or 3 years ago often take a refresher class for an update of current practices and a review of techniques. Classes consist of one to three sessions in which supervised practice is the major focus. Courses also

Table 11-3

TOPICS COVERED IN CESAREAN BIRTH CLASSES

Indications
Prenatal tests
Preparation (such as NPO, shave, Foley catheter)
Anesthesia
Surgical procedure
Role of support person during surgery
Options
Postsurgical care and pain relief
Relaxation techniques
Postpartum course
Future birth options

CRITICAL THINKING EXERCISE

QUESTION:

Liz, gravida 2, para 1, tells you that she does not plan to attend prepared childbirth classes because she took classes before her son, Danny, was born 5 years ago. What should you discuss with her?

include discussion of role changes in the family and sibling adjustment.

Cesarean Birth Preparation Classes

Education about cesarean birth may take place in general childbirth classes or be conducted separately for those expecting a cesarean birth (Table 11-3).

General Cesarean Classes

More than one of five births are by cesarean delivery, and women need preparation for this possibility (Guyer, et al., 1999). Cesarean birth is usually discussed briefly during general prepared childbirth classes. Topics include indications, options, surgical procedure, and postoperative course.

Reasons for cesarean births should be discussed in detail. A woman might view the terms *failed induction* and *failure to progress* as casting blame on her. She may believe that if she had used relaxation techniques better or been more tolerant of pain, she might have avoided the need for surgery. Teachers often point out that the causes of cesarean births are conditions over which the woman has no control.

> Couples are sometimes inattentive during discussions about cesarean birth because they think "it can't happen to me." Teachers can gain their attention by pointing out the number of couples in the class who may have cesarean births based on the 1998 rate of 21.2% (National Center for Health Statistics, 2000). Written materials may be helpful for later review if the need for surgery develops.

Planned Cesarean Birth Classes

Women who know they will have a cesarean birth may attend planned cesarean birth classes. The class offers those who have had a previous cesarean birth an opportunity to share experiences and feelings and clarify misconceptions. Often these women remember little preparation for the procedure because they were frightened and exhausted. Couples anticipating their first cesarean birth may appreciate hearing from others who have had the experience.

Class content includes indications for cesarean births, care the woman will receive, and possible options. A woman who wishes to go into labor to ensure maturity of the fetus and experience labor should discuss this decision with her caregiver. Class discussion helps couples feel that they have some control over events and provides a basis for discussion with caregivers.

Vaginal Birth after Cesarean Birth

Some women choose to have a vaginal birth after a previous cesarean birth. They may take a vaginal birth after cesarean (VBAC) class. This is also called a *trial of labor after cesarean (TLAC)*. Content includes explanations of when a VBAC is possible, the extra precautions taken and their reasons, what to expect during labor and birth, and coping techniques. Although the focus is on positive expectations, situations that might necessitate another cesarean birth are also covered. Discussion also includes the emotional aspects of a "failed VBAC."

Breastfeeding Classes

Prenatal breastfeeding education is increasingly important because of the short time available to help breastfeeding mothers in the birth facility after birth. Classes help increase a woman's confidence in her ability to breastfeed successfully and provide her with resources if she encounters difficulties. Women who attend prenatal classes that include breastfeeding information are more likely to breastfeed their infants and do so for longer than 6 months compared with women who do not attend classes (Piper & Parks, 1996).

Breastfeeding classes include information on physiology of lactation, feeding techniques, establishment of a milk supply, and solutions to common problems (Table 11-4). Partners who attend learn methods of providing support during breastfeeding. Some teachers hold additional sessions after the birth to provide ongoing counseling at a time when mothers may experience unexpected problems. These sessions allow discussion of problems as they occur.

Parenting Classes

Instruction on parenting and newborn care may be included in prepared childbirth classes or provided separately. Content typically includes infant safety, general care, and common concerns such as infant crying and

Table 11-4
TOPICS COVERED IN BREASTFEEDING CLASSES

Anatomy and physiology
Preparation for breastfeeding
Positioning
Establishment of milk supply
Problems and prevention: engorgement, sore nipples, nipple confusion, insufficient milk supply, and mastitis
Nutrition
Use of bottles and storage of breast milk
Breast pumps
Work and breastfeeding
Weaning

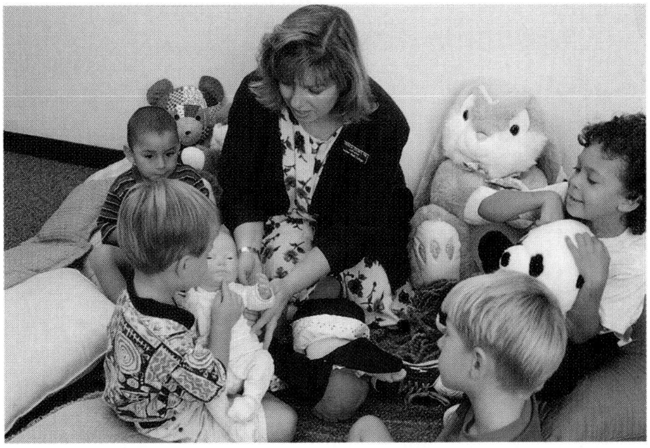

FIGURE 11-4 During sibling classes, children learn about the new babies coming into their lives.

Table 11-5
TOPICS COVERED IN PARENTING CLASSES

Normal newborn characteristics: marks, rashes, normal behavior
General care: diapering, cord care, circumcision care, bathing
Feeding methods and problems, schedules, colic
Other concerns: crying, sleeping through the night
Safety: car seats, "baby proofing" the home
Baby equipment
Early growth and development: expectations, infant stimulation, immunization
Illness: signs of common conditions, taking a temperature, calling the physician
Infant cardiopulmonary resuscitation (CPR)

advantages and disadvantages of circumcision (Table 11-5). Women who receive information about infant communication during the prenatal period may have more positive mother-infant interactions after the infant is born (Leitch, 1999). Baby equipment such as infant car seats are often displayed. Practice with dolls may also be included. Classes may continue after the birth of the infant.

Postpartum Classes

Although the postpartum period is discussed in prepared childbirth classes, the mother can also attend classes after birth. Content includes the physiologic and psychological changes of the postpartum period, role transition, sexuality, and nutrition. Some classes are informal support groups led by a knowledgeable professional. Other classes focus primarily on exercise for the postpartum period. Because many women return to work soon after childbirth, sessions are often held at night and on weekends and include the concerns of working mothers.

Classes for Other Family Members

Siblings

Sibling classes are for children aged 2 to 10 years. The classes help them learn about newborn characteristics and help decrease anxiety about the approaching birth (Figure 11-4).

Many young children have never seen a newborn and are expecting an older child to be a playmate. A tour of the nursery or visit with a newborn infant allows them to see newborns at close range and learn to be safe helpers. Videos and stories promote discussion about normal feelings of jealousy and anger. Emphasis is placed on the important role of big brothers and sisters and the fact that a baby could not replace them in their parents' affection.

A separate parent discussion provides suggestions for further preparation and ways to cope with the transition after birth. Concerns about sibling rivalry and meeting the needs of more than one child are common topics (see Chapter 18). Sibling visitation during hospitalization to help decrease the child's anxiety is also discussed.

Special sibling classes may be held for children who will be present at the birth. These help prepare the child for the sights and sounds of birth. The child's support person also attends the class.

Grandparents

Classes for grandparents provide updates about recent developments in childbirth and parenting practices. Grandparents compare parenting in the past and present in a supportive environment with others in similar situations. Topics generally focus on family-centered childbirth and infant care. Discussions review current views of care, feeding, early growth and development, and accident prevention. The art of grandparenting and the importance of grandparents are particularly emphasized.

Check Your Reading

3. How are early pregnancy classes different from later pregnancy classes?
4. Why should all women learn about cesarean childbirth?
5. Why are sibling and grandparent classes important?

EDUCATION FOR CHILDBIRTH

Many studies have attempted to determine whether education for childbirth affects the outcome with regard to client satisfaction, pain relief, length of labor, and frequency of complications. The results of these studies vary. Some report shorter labors with fewer complications and less need for pharmacologic pain relief measures, whereas others report no difference between prepared and unprepared women. Most studies agree that couples receiving prenatal preparation for childbirth are more satisfied with their birth experiences and have greater feelings of control, even when unexpected complications occur.

Methods of Pain Management

Education

One of the most important aspects of any childbirth preparation class is education to increase the woman's confidence in her ability to cope with birth. Women who are confident about their coping abilities report less pain during labor than those who lack confidence (Lowe, 1996). Confidence may be increased with classes that provide detailed information about childbirth, vicarious experiences such as films and reports of others' births, and techniques to increase coping ability during labor.

By learning what to expect during labor and birth, women and their support persons are able to rehearse the experience in their minds in preparation for the actual event. They practice coping techniques during simulated contractions. Realistic, valid class information and discussion of possible variations are essential so that couples are adequately prepared.

Relaxation

Tension and anxiety during labor cause tightening of abdominal muscles, impeding contractions and increasing pain by stimulation of nerve endings that heighten awareness of pain. Prolonged muscle tension causes fatigue and increased pain perception. When anxiety and tension are high, uterine contractions are less effective and the length of labor increases. A woman who is able to remain relaxed is likely to have more efficient and less painful labor and have increased ability to use other techniques to help herself. A number of different techniques are taught to enhance relaxation during labor.

Conditioning

Many techniques for prepared childbirth are based partially on theories of conditioned response, in which certain responses to stimuli become automatic through frequent association. Women learn to associate uterine contractions with relaxation by practicing relaxation techniques with mental images of contractions. Because effective conditioning requires a great deal of practice, women are encouraged to practice their techniques daily. For some women, the intensity of real uterine contractions is surprisingly different from their experiences during practice sessions. They may have difficulty with relaxation as a result and need to use other methods along with conditioning.

METHODS OF CHILDBIRTH EDUCATION

Although all methods of prepared childbirth education use some combination of pain management techniques, each method has its unique aspects. Some differences exist in types of classes and class content, depending on geographic area. Many classes have an holistic approach, providing a variety of techniques from many sources from which couples can choose those that work best for them.

Dick-Read Childbirth Education

Grantly Dick-Read was an English physician who was one of the first to use education and relaxation techniques to help women through childbirth. His theory was that fear of childbirth results in tension and pain. To prevent the fear-tension-pain cycle, he developed a method of slow abdominal breathing in early labor and rapid chest breathing in advanced labor. His methods were the first to be called *natural childbirth.*

Bradley Childbirth Education

The Bradley method was the first to include the father as a support person for "husband-coached childbirth." Abdominal breathing to increase relaxation and breath control is taught in these classes, which usually last for 12 weeks. The Bradley method also emphasizes avoidance of all medication and other interventions.

LeBoyer Method of Childbirth

LeBoyer childbirth, sometimes called "birth without violence," views birth as a traumatic experience for the newborn. To decrease the trauma at birth, lights are dimmed and noise is decreased to help the newborn adapt to extrauterine life more easily. The infant receives a warm bath immediately after birth to help relaxation.

Lamaze Childbirth Education

The Lamaze method is often called *psychoprophylaxis* because it uses the mind to prevent pain. It involves concentration and conditioning to help the woman respond to contractions with relaxation and various techniques to decrease pain. The Lamaze method is the most popular method used today. Although a variety of techniques are taught, women should feel free to choose those that they feel work best for them. Women should not be taught that there is only one right way of breathing and relaxing in labor.

Class Content

The content of specific Lamaze classes may differ, but most follow a similar pattern. Although the focus is on the childbirth experience, other topics such as the postpartum period and infant care are often included. Techniques for coping with labor include education to prevent fear of the unknown and activities that promote relaxation during labor.

Lamaze teachers acknowledge that labor is painful and do not promise these techniques will produce a pain-free birth. Instead, the techniques are used to increase the woman's ability to cope with pain by relieving some of the accompanying distress.

Exercises

Women learn toning and conditioning exercises to prepare for childbirth and help prevent discomfort in late pregnancy. Because the classes are taken during the third trimester of pregnancy, the instructor must consider the changes in center of gravity and joint stability that occur at that time when selecting exercises (see Chapter 7 for exercises for pregnancy).

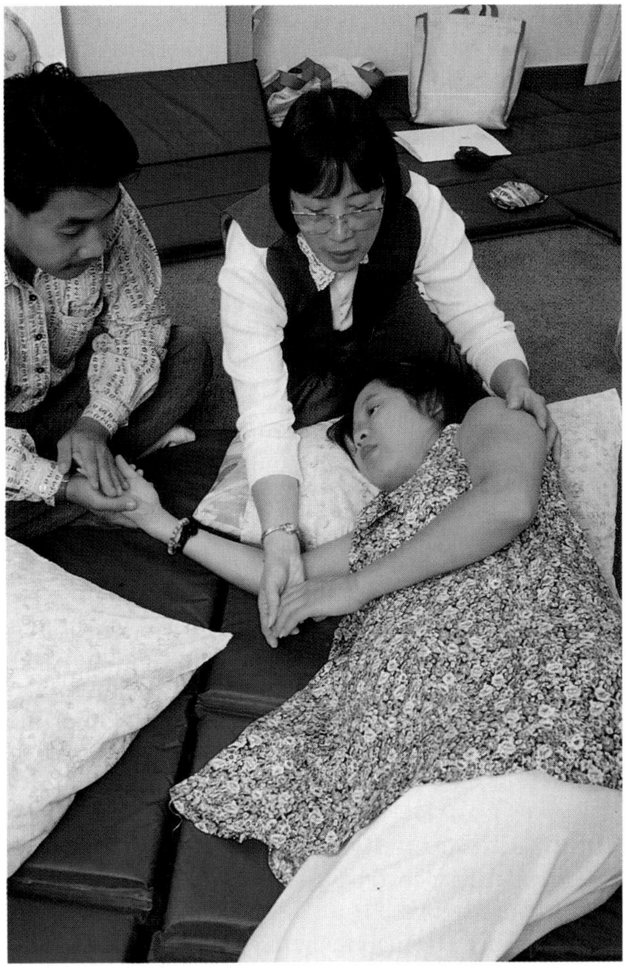

FIGURE 11-5 As the woman practices relaxation techniques for labor, the partner massages her hand and the nurse checks for muscle tension.

Relaxation Techniques

The ability to relax during labor is one of the most important components for coping effectively with childbirth. Relaxation conserves energy, decreases oxygen use, and enhances other pain relief techniques. Women learn various exercises to help them recognize and release tension. The labor partner assists the woman by providing feedback during exercise sessions and labor. The labor partner is alert to ways in which the woman shows tension. For example, she may tighten her shoulders, frown, or jiggle her foot when stressed. The partner helps her focus on areas that she finds difficult to relax. Positive feedback from the partner and teacher encourages women to increase relaxation.

Relaxation exercises must be practiced frequently to be useful during labor. Couples begin practice sessions in a quiet, comfortable setting. Later, they practice in other places that simulate the noise and unfamiliar setting of the hospital. Relaxation exercises may also be combined with other techniques such as imagery and massage (Figure 11-5).

Progressive Relaxation. Progressive relaxation involves contracting and then consciously releasing different muscle groups. The exercise is repeated throughout the body until all voluntary muscles are relaxed. The woman learns to differentiate between the feelings of tense and relaxed muscles. With this knowledge, she can systematically assess and then release muscle tension throughout her body.

Neuromuscular Dissociation. Neuromuscular dissociation (also called *differential relaxation*) helps the woman learn to relax her body even when one group of muscles is strongly contracted. This process helps prepare her to relax during the powerful uterine contractions of labor. The woman contracts an area such as an arm or a leg and then concentrates on releasing tension from the rest of her body. After a short time of contracting one area, she relaxes it and moves on to another. Her partner checks for unrecognized tension by gently moving areas to see that they are limp.

Touch Relaxation. The purpose of touch relaxation is to help the woman learn to loosen taut muscles when they are touched by her partner. The woman tenses an area and then relaxes it as her partner strokes and massages it. With frequent practice of this exercise, the woman becomes conditioned to respond to touch with relaxation. During labor, her partner's touch is a signal for release of tension.

Relaxation against Pain. Because first-time mothers have difficulty imagining the pain and strength of labor contractions, they may occasionally practice use of relaxation against pain. The pain is caused by her partner, who exerts pressure against a tendon or large muscle of the arm or leg. The pressure is applied gradually to simulate the gradual increase, peak, and decrease of a uterine contraction. Sometimes ice is applied as another type of discomfort to simulate contractions.

Other Techniques

Other techniques to aid the woman in relaxation include cutaneous and mental stimulation. Touch stimulates large-diameter sensory nerve fibers and interferes with transmission of pain impulses to the brain through small-diameter sensory nerve fibers. Mental focusing and distraction also interfere with pain messages reaching the brain.

Cutaneous Stimulation Techniques

Effleurage. Effleurage is the massage of the abdomen during contractions (Figure 11-6). Women learn to perform effleurage using both hands in a circular motion. If fetal monitor belts cover the abdomen during labor, the woman can massage between the belts. When she lies on her side, she uses only one hand to massage her abdomen. In the sidelying position, she may be more comfortable making smaller movements on her abdomen and massaging her thigh so that her arm and shoulder remain relaxed.

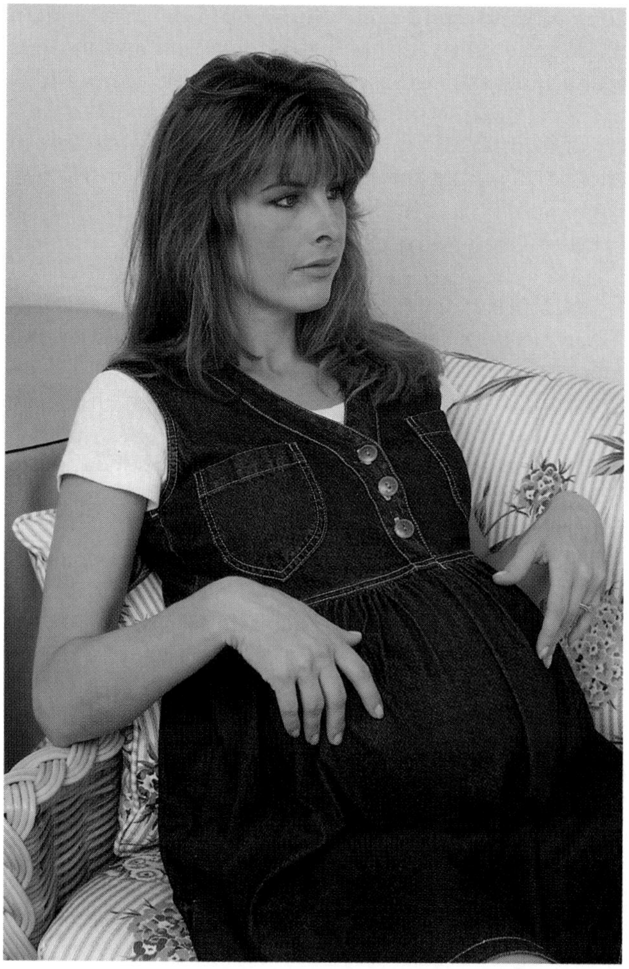

FIGURE 11-6 The woman begins effleurage with the hands at the symphysis and then slowly moves around the sides and down the center toward the symphysis again. As an alternative, she can go up the center of the abdomen and around the sides.

Massage and pressure on the palms and fingertips stimulate large-diameter nerve fibers. Relief is temporary because stimulation of these fibers results in habituation, a decreased response to stimuli. When habituation occurs, pain is more readily perceived. Periodically changing the type and area of stimulation increases effectiveness.

The woman and her partner may alternate effleurage to provide more variety in sensory input and decrease habituation. The woman can massage her thigh instead of her abdomen and use her fingertips to trace circles and figure-eight patterns on the bed. The use of specific patterns of effleurage provide sources of concentration and increased input to the brain. This exercise may also interfere with transmission of pain impulses.

Other Massage. Massage of the temples and shoulders by the labor partner may help relax these areas. The palms and soles of the feet are particularly sensitive to touch, and firm massage of these areas may be helpful. Types of stimuli should be changed whenever they no longer seem effective, generally every 15 to 30 minutes.

Sacral Pressure. Firm pressure against the sacral area may help relieve strain on the sacroiliac joint from a fetal occiput posterior position (Simkin, 1995). The partner begins to increase pressure on the sacrum as soon as the contraction begins. If a fetal monitor is in place, the partner can watch the line depicting the contraction to determine when to begin and end the pressure. The hand may be moved slowly over the area or remain positioned directly over the sacrum, but pressure should be continuous and firm throughout the contraction.

The partner should place the other hand over the woman's hip and steady her during sacral pressure. Care should be taken not to jiggle the woman, which

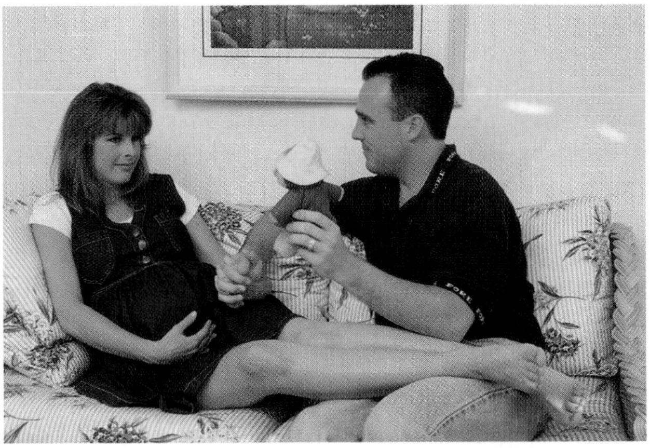

FIGURE 11-7 A stuffed toy or any other object can serve as a focal point on which the expectant mother can fix her attention during labor.

may be irritating. Between contractions the woman gives her partner feedback about hand placement. Often, moving the hands a fraction of an inch increases effectiveness. This technique can be combined with thermal stimulation to increase effectiveness. Tennis balls may also be used to apply pressure to the back.

Thermal Stimulation. Application of heat and cold stimulates thermoreceptors and may decrease pain sensation. Cool cloths used to wipe the woman's face, ice chips offered to the woman for eating, and ice in a glove covered with a washcloth applied to the woman's lower back may be effective. Alternating cold with heat over the back prevents habituation. In early labor, a whirlpool bath or shower with warm water directed against the back may be soothing. A warm bath blanket or glove filled with warm water can be held against the sacrum for pressure and warmth. Heat and cold should never be applied to any anesthetized area because injury could result.

Positioning. Position changes during labor also provide cutaneous stimulation. Women are taught to practice their techniques using a variety of positions and to change positions frequently during labor. Ambulation and an upright position make contractions more efficient and less painful. Position changes approximately every 30 to 60 minutes increase comfort and decrease muscle fatigue.

Mental Stimulation Techniques

Various methods decrease pain by increasing mental concentration. They may modify pain perception as a result of interference with pain impulses in the spinal cord or in the brain itself.

Focal Point. A focal point is an object on which the woman centers her attention during contractions (Figure 11-7). It helps her direct her thoughts away from the contractions. During the contraction, she looks at the focal point and thinks about its shape, size, and gradations of colors. Women often use pictures of infants and restful scenic landscapes as focal points. If a video player is available during labor, a video tape of scenery, perhaps combined with music, may increase interest in the focal point.

Women who do not bring focal points to the birth setting may use anything in their lines of vision, such as a pattern on the wallpaper or the support person's face. Because the fetal monitor is directly next to the bed, many women focus on it. Watching the contraction pattern on the monitor usually is not soothing and tends to increase attention to the strength of the contraction. Focusing on a button or knob may be more helpful.

Women who are familiar with meditation techniques may prefer closing their eyes and using an internal focal point during contractions. This allows them to shut out light and movement around them and focus on a mental picture.

Imagery. Another technique to enhance relaxation is imagery. During imagery exercises, childbirth educators often talk about a pleasant scene or experience while the woman imagines herself in that setting. A walk through a garden is portrayed by describing the flowers, the warmth of the sun, the sound of birds, and a feeling of peacefulness. Couples are encouraged to practice imagery with scenes of their own choosing. While practicing breathing techniques, the woman can picture oxygen entering her body to nourish her baby every time she inhales and tension leaving each time she exhales.

Other imagery suggestions are given for use during labor. The woman might picture a flower bud opening into full bloom to simulate the opening of the cervix. She can imagine the cervix pulling over the infant's head and the infant moving lower in the pelvis with each contraction. Teachers usually advise women to save images of cervical dilation and childbirth until labor actually begins because such images might begin labor.

Music. Some women find that music and other sounds, like rainfall and waves at the seashore, help them relax. They may use tapes and CDs during practice and bring them with headphones when they are in labor and come to the birth setting. Headphones have the added benefit of obscuring surrounding noise. The rhythm of the music may assist the woman in pacing her breathing. Music is often used with other techniques such as imagery to increase relaxation.

Special Techniques

Special techniques may be discussed briefly in classes. Some techniques require further preparation elsewhere. Acupressure is pressure over acupuncture points, which may raise endorphin levels to reduce pain. Biofeedback may lower pain by reducing tension of abdominal muscles. Some women find transcutaneous electrical nerve stimulation helpful. This process provides pain relief through the use of electrodes on the lower back to deliver low-intensity, high-frequency electrical stimulation of the nerves. Aromatherapy, the use of special fragrances, is also sometimes used.

In hydrotherapy the woman is immersed in a tub of water, sometimes with whirlpool jets. The water helps the woman relax, decreases muscle tension and pressure on the abdomen, and helps labor progress more quickly. A tub bath after rupture of membranes does not seem to increase infection (Simkin, 1995).

Breathing Techniques

As with other coping strategies, the primary purpose of breathing techniques is to enhance relaxation and decrease the number of pain impulses recognized by the brain. Although no research proves that breathing techniques decrease pain perception, many women believe that learning the techniques is important and helpful during labor (Hodnett, 1996). As with other techniques, the woman should use breathing as one of many tools to help her cope with labor (see the discussion of breathing techniques in Chapter 15).

The woman and her partner must practice the techniques frequently to gain comfort with them. If they become too complicated or the woman has not practiced, they may not be helpful during labor. In labor, breathing techniques should not be used until they are actually needed, which is usually when the woman can no longer walk and talk during a contraction. If breathing techniques are used too early, the woman tends to move through the different techniques too quickly, and she may stop using them. In addition, use of the more complex breathing patterns in latent labor may increase fatigue (Pugh, et al., 1998).

Check Your Reading

6. How can education, relaxation, and conditioning decrease pain?
7. How do cutaneous stimulation and imagery help reduce pain?
8. What is the purpose of breathing methods in labor?

THE LABOR PARTNER

Almost all methods of childbirth preparation encourage the participation of someone who remains with the woman throughout labor. This person may be called a *labor partner, support person, coach,* or *labor companion.* The presence of a labor partner may help the woman cope more effectively and decrease her distress during labor and result in greater satisfaction with the childbirth experience.

The person who takes on this role may be the father of the baby, a friend or relative, or a doula. A doula is a trained labor support person employed by the mother and her partner to provide continuous labor support. She helps the woman with physical support such as relaxation and massage and provides emotional support and advocacy throughout labor. Some doulas also help during the postpartum period. Continuous support by trained support persons may result in a shorter labor and the need for fewer obstetric interventions (Kennell & Klaus, 1998).

The labor partner generally attends classes with the mother to learn about labor, birth, and techniques to assist during labor. By practicing together, the woman and her partner learn to work smoothly as a team during labor. Classes may increase confidence for support persons, who learn specific techniques to use during labor. When the labor partner is the father, communication and a sense of closeness between the expectant parents may be enhanced.

Role of the Labor Partner

Not all labor partners play identical roles during labor. Some take a major part in assisting the mother with relaxation and breathing techniques, but others provide support in less active ways. They may confine their support to giving verbal encouragement and physical care such as back rubs when requested. Others feel more comfortable with passive support persons who are present but not actively participating. Even with education, the support person may feel somewhat helpless and look to others to provide help to the laboring woman. Expectant fathers often are concerned about the health of the baby and safety of the mother during labor and may feel more comfortable when others provide support (White, 1998).

Some men and women believe that active involvement in labor is not an acceptable role for men, perhaps because of cultural values. For example, Latino couples often expect the partner to offer support by being present and encouraging the woman during labor rather than taking a more active role (Khazoyan & Anderson, 1994).

Encourage couples to think about the support person's labor role before labor begins and then support the partner in whatever role is chosen (Nursing Care Plan 11-1).

Labor partners should not feel responsible for more than is included in the role. Teachers should discuss the duties of the labor nurse and encourage labor partners to seek assistance when they are uncertain. The labor nurse may have helpful suggestions and adaptations of techniques. Class discussion of complications

NURSING CARE PLAN 11-1

Planning for Childbirth

Assessment: Carmen Sanchez, age 19, is 4 months pregnant with her first baby. She and her husband, Ramon, "want to be the best parents possible." Carmen works as a teacher's aide in a primary school. Ramon, age 26, manages a small restaurant. Both Carmen and Ramon are the youngest in their families and have little actual experience with infants. Carmen plans to have her baby at the local hospital in a labor, delivery, and recovery room.

Carmen tells the nurse that Ramon tends to favor the "old ways" and is unsure whether he should be involved during childbirth. She is most anxious for him to participate during her labor. Ramon seems embarrassed and says "Having a baby is for women." He seems very loving toward Carmen and later says "I want to help Carmen, but I don't know anything about these things. I'd just be in the way."

Nursing Diagnosis: Decisional Conflict related to father's ambivalence toward his anticipated role in childbirth.

Critical Thinking: Is this an appropriate use of a nursing diagnosis? If Carmen is the client, should the nurse make a nursing diagnosis that focuses on her husband?

Answer: Although Carmen is the primary client, family-centered nursing involves care of all family members, especially when their needs affect those of the primary client. If the nurse can help Carmen and Ramon resolve this problem, Carmen will be able to focus more positively on preparing for the birth of their baby.

Goals/Expected Outcomes:

Ramon will do the following:

1. Explore various options regarding his role during Carmen's labor and the birth of his baby.
2. Make a decision about his role during childbirth by 1 month before the baby is expected.

Intervention	Rationale
1. Explore Ramon's concerns before beginning discussion of educational opportunities with Carmen.	1. In some cultures the man is the head of the family and makes many of the decisions. Showing respect for his authority is important if health teaching is to be accepted.
2. Use therapeutic communication techniques (such as reflection, paraphrasing) to help Ramon discuss his feelings about participating in childbirth.	2. Use of therapeutic communication shows that the nurse is willing to listen and thinks that the client's feelings are important.
3. Ask Ramon how he views childbirth and the role of the support person during labor and birth.	3. Asking the partner about his perception of his role during birth helps the nurse adapt teaching to his needs.
4. Explain various labor support roles. Include the options of acting as "coach" or merely being present for the labor, birth, both, or neither.	4. The nurse must encourage and accept whatever role the support person chooses.
5. Ask Ramon to consider the advantages and disadvantages of each role. Clarify misinformation and discuss additional advantages and disadvantages if necessary.	5. Participation increases learning.
6. Present all information in a nonjudgmental atmosphere.	6. If the nurse remains nonjudgmental, the client does not feel pressured to make a particular decision.
7. Encourage Ramon to discuss this new information with Carmen, his friends, and family. If possible, refer him to other men who have played various roles during labor and birth.	7. Discussion with family and friends is important when making decisions and provides sources for other viewpoints.
8. Suggest that Ramon think about his options and make a decision at a later date. Provide written information for Ramon and Carmen to review at home.	8. Processing new information and making decisions takes time. Written information provides a readily available source for review.
9. Include Carmen in the discussion.	9. A couple may be unaware of each other's concerns and feelings. Hearing the partner talk about them helps each understand the other's point of view.

Evaluation: Ramon reports 2 months later that he has decided to go with Carmen to classes to learn more about childbirth. He is unsure about his degree of participation during labor and birth and says that he will decide when the time arrives. Carmen says that she feels comfortable with Ramon's decision and is glad he will go to prepared childbirth classes with her.

should include the role of the support person. For example, partners should understand circumstances that would allow and preclude their presence during a cesarean birth.

Support Techniques

Knowledge of specific, practical measures to assist the woman in labor often helps labor partners feel more comfortable in the birth setting. They learn ways to time contractions at home and work with the fetal monitor in the birth setting. Telling the woman when the monitor shows the peak of the contraction is over can be particularly helpful. If the woman is sleeping between contractions, the monitor may show a contraction beginning before she feels it. The labor partner can alert her to begin her breathing techniques before the contraction becomes strong.

The partner suggests ways to make the environment less stressful, such as listening to tapes and CDs with headphones to obscure surrounding noise and turning down the lights to promote rest between contractions.

Labor partners often learn a "panic technique" or "take-charge routine" to use when the woman is having particular difficulty coping with labor. This technique includes making eye contact and breathing along with her to help pace the breathing, helping her move to a more advanced level of breathing, and remaining calm. Having some direction if the woman loses control may make the support person feel more secure.

Providing comfort measures is an important role of the support person. These measures include offering ice chips, wiping the woman's face with a cold cloth, using cold and warm packs, and helping her change positions. The partner applies sacral pressure and gives back rubs and other types of massage. Partners learn ways to provide feedback about breathing and relaxation and make suggestions during practice sessions and labor. They learn the importance of encouraging the woman and giving directions in a positive manner.

The woman and her support person may pack a bag of items that may help comfort the expectant mother during labor (Table 11-6). As labor progresses, the couples use each article as it seems appropriate.

Check Your Reading

9. How does having someone with her help the woman in labor?
10. What are the various roles that the support person might take?
11. What specific techniques do labor partners learn to help the woman in labor?

Table 11-6

ITEMS TO BE INCLUDED IN THE LABOR BAG

Focal point
Lotion and powder to make massage more comfortable
Warm socks for cold feet
Several colored washcloths for washing face (white ones might be lost)
Hand-held fan
Rubber bands and clips for hair
Tennis balls in a sock for sacral pressure
Sugarless sour lollipop for dry mouth
Mouthwash
Lip balm, unflavored
Instruction sheets or reminder checklists
Paper and pencil
Playing cards or simple games for early labor
Camera
Snack for labor partner
Tape or CD player with headphones
Change and telephone numbers for calls after birth
Pillows (use colored pillowcases to prevent loss)

APPLICATION OF THE NURSING PROCESS: EDUCATION FOR CHILDBIRTH

The nursing process focuses on assisting the woman and her partner to obtain the knowledge necessary to plan for a birth experience that is realistic and meets their individual needs. Preparation helps each family progress through the childbearing experience as knowledgeable consumers and full participants in their own health care.

Assessment

Assess the educational needs of the woman and her partner. Some couples are quite knowledgeable about available prenatal classes and childbirth options, but others need direction in choosing classes that are right for them. The couple may come to the nurse with a birth plan already made or may need help in thinking through their expectations and desires.

Determine whether special factors require adaptation of the usual educational approaches. Examples are the pregnant adolescent and the woman with a high-risk pregnancy. Cultural factors may be very influential in determining individual educational needs.

Next, assess the needs of support persons and the degree of participation they wish to have in the birth. They may have concerns about their role, especially during labor and birth. These must be addressed to decrease their anxiety and help them be more effective in supporting their partner.

PARENTS WANT TO KNOW What Options Should We Consider for Our Birth Plan?

Whether the following options are available may depend on the policies of the birth facility and health care provider. Discuss them with your provider to learn more about the options available to you.

Monitoring—Do you have strong feelings about using electronic fetal monitoring? Some women find it reassuring because it provides continuous information about the fetus. Others believe that it interferes with their ability to remain active during labor. Intermittent use of monitoring and auscultation may be possible if no complications occur.

IV fluids—Some health care professionals consider IV fluids necessary to replace fluids lost during labor and give pain medications and emergency drugs. Some women find them painful and intrusive, whereas others do not mind them. Alternatives include waiting until active labor to begin IV fluids, avoiding them unless complications occur, and using a saline lock so that you can move about more freely.

Food and oral fluids—Other than ice chips, food and fluids often are not allowed during active labor because of decreased gastric motility, vomiting, and the possibility of aspiration if general anesthesia is suddenly needed. Clear fluids may be an option.

Enemas—A very small volume enema may or may not be routine. An enema may stimulate contractions, but many women dislike them and have loose stools in early labor.

Position—You may prefer to walk, shower or bathe, and remain active rather than staying in bed throughout labor. Some women wish to squat, kneel, or lie on their sides for birth. A birthing bed or chair may allow a comfortable and effective delivery position.

Episiotomy—Although an episiotomy is frequently performed, you may wish to avoid it unless absolutely necessary. Discuss the use of episiotomy with your birth attendant.

Pain relief—You may plan to avoid medication for pain relief completely, use it only if absolutely necessary, or wish to take it as soon as possible to avoid pain. You may expect to use relaxation techniques throughout labor or only until you can receive anesthesia. Specific ideas about available types of pain relief should also be considered.

Support person—You may wish only the infant's father, a relative or close friend, or a doula to be with you during labor and birth, or you may prefer a number of people present for some or all of the experience.

Breastfeeding—Many women want to begin breastfeeding immediately after birth or within the first hour. You may prefer that no water or formula be given to your baby unless a problem develops. Some mothers ask that the nursery staff feed the baby during the night.

Siblings—You may want your other children to be present at the birth or visit you while you are in the hospital.

Care of the newborn—Having your baby stay with you at all times to promote bonding may be possible. To get more rest, you may prefer to care for the baby only during the day and evening hours. The infant may spend the night in the nursery or return to you for night feedings.

Discharge—Your insurance coverage may influence your discharge time. Mothers usually go home within 48 hours after a vaginal birth or 96 hours after a cesarean birth. You may prefer earlier discharge with follow-up visits from a home visit nurse, in a clinic, or in your provider's office. Or you may wish a longer stay to rest before assuming full care of the newborn along with other responsibilities.

Analysis

The nursing diagnosis pertaining to the couple who is not unusually anxious about childbirth but desires more information is "Health-Seeking Behaviors related to desire for education about pregnancy, childbirth, and/or parenting."

Planning

The goals and expected outcomes for this nursing diagnosis are that the woman and her partner will do the following:

- Write a birth plan that is realistically based on available options and meets their needs.
- Verbalize a plan for obtaining education for pregnancy, childbirth, and parenting.
- Report feelings of increased confidence in their ability to cope with pregnancy, childbirth, and parenting after educational preparation is completed.

Interventions

Making a Birth Plan

Help couples write a plan for their birth experience if they so wish. The birth plan, sometimes called a *family preference plan*, helps women and their partners examine their options and take an active part in planning their birth experience. The plan is a tool for expanding communication with health professionals. It ensures that the couple's wishes are known before labor begins. The plan may help the couple choose a provider, a setting, and classes that are most conducive to meeting specific needs.

Help the couple learn about locally available choices and explain any restrictions. For example, insurance coverage may dictate which facility a woman must use. Those without insurance are concerned about the cost of various options. In addition, the health care provider or birth agency may have set policies on certain issues. Complications during labor and birth may necessitate changes in the plan.

Some couples interview several physicians or nurse-midwives to learn about the provider's usual practices and possible exceptions. With discussion, the couple and provider can create a plan that is satisfactory to all.

Choosing Classes

Help the woman and her partner find classes suited to their educational needs. Give them a list and description of classes in the community and suggest that they talk with others who have taken various classes. They may wish to interview teachers to learn about their preparation and philosophies. Some couples want classes that consider avoidance of medication a primary goal of childbirth. Many prefer those that consider a variety of tools, including medication, for coping with pain.

Suggesting Classes for Special Needs

Women with special needs need referral to specific courses. If none are available, suggest ways to adapt the information presented in regular classes to their own situations.

Adolescents. Although adolescents may attend regular prenatal classes, those designed especially to meet their needs are most effective. High schools with programs for school-aged mothers, hospitals, clinics, and community agencies may offer courses. Teens may find that separate classes for adolescents are more comfortable because they learn with peers with similar problems and concerns. Fathers and other support persons may also attend.

Education for pregnant adolescents is similar to that for adults, but it focuses on the teenager's perceptions of childbearing. Clarification of misconceptions in a nonjudgmental manner makes classes more meaningful. Young women need information about the importance of prenatal care, nutrition, weight gain, body image, contraception, labor, and birth. The effects of substance abuse and sexually transmissible diseases on pregnancy and the fetus are important topics for discussion.

Although the decision about whether to keep the infant is usually made before classes begin, options may be discussed. Because of their lack of experience and unrealistic expectations of infants, adolescents have a greater need for information about infant care than do older mothers. Provide an opportunity for discussion of ways in which the infant will affect the adolescent's life, future goals, and schooling.

Teenagers with academic problems may have difficulty reading material and understanding abstract concepts. The use of concrete terms and simple language can ensure understanding. Models, videos, and presentations by those who have previously taken classes make the course more relevant.

Older Women. Women older than age 35 feel "different" from the younger women in their prenatal class and isolated from their friends who have completed childbearing. Because delayed parenthood is quite common today, classes for older mothers may provide opportunities for these women to make friends with others with similar backgrounds. Older couples may want more sophisticated information than that usually included in regular prenatal classes, and they have many questions about the chances of complications related to age. Offer realistic reassurance and direct them to books and articles that meet their need for in-depth information.

Women with High-Risk Pregnancies. The woman with a high-risk pregnancy may be restricted as to activity and not able to attend regular perinatal classes. If possible, help her arrange for individual instruction. Audio and video tapes, written materials, and phone contact with an instructor are ways for her to learn and practice techniques without attending classes.

Women Who Must Make Cultural Adaptations. Women from other cultures, especially those who do not speak English, are at a disadvantage when they enter birth settings in the United States. Classes in other languages are often available in communities in which large groups with this need exist. They contain the same basic information as the English versions, but the content and process are adapted to meet the cultural needs of the students. The teacher usually has the same cultural background as the students. This cultural match ensures fluency in their language and understanding of their needs, increasing the likelihood that the instructor is accepted.

The instructor discusses childbirth in the United States and compares it with that in the couples' countries of origin. Students learn the importance of prenatal care, which may not have been emphasized in their own cultures. They discuss expectations of health care providers and the birthing experience. Misconceptions about needs and care throughout the childbearing period are clarified.

Women with Other Needs. If necessary, refer the woman and her support person to classes that address other needs. Classes for adoptive couples and women with multifetal pregnancies and disabilities may be available. Women who are concerned about continuing their careers after birth may enroll in courses for working mothers to help them choose child care and learn to balance the needs of family and work. Classes for fathers may provide a comfortable environment for discussions of fathering, sexuality, and roles during labor and birth, breastfeeding, and the postpartum period in the company of other men with similar concerns.

Evaluation

If goals have been achieved, the woman and her partner will do the following:

- Write a realistic birth plan and attend classes that are appropriate for their needs.
- Discuss their plan to obtain education for pregnancy, childbirth, and parenting.
- Verbalize increased confidence in coping with pregnancy, childbirth, and parenting.

SUMMARY CONCEPTS

- Education for childbearing helps couples become knowledgeable consumers and active participants in pregnancy and childbirth.
- Women must make many decisions about childbirth, including choosing a birth attendant, birth setting, support person for labor, and type of educational classes to attend.
- Many classes are available for pregnant women and their support persons. Early pregnancy classes emphasize ways to have a healthy pregnancy. Classes conducted in later pregnancy focus on preparation for childbirth, breastfeeding, and early parenting.
- Because more than 20% of all births are cesarean, women in all prepared childbirth classes should be made aware of this possibility and learn about the procedure.
- Classes for siblings and grandparents help all family members prepare for the birth.
- Education, relaxation, and conditioning are used to increase coping ability for childbirth. Other techniques act to decrease transmission of pain impulses from the spinal cord to the brain.
- Exercises in relaxation help women recognize and learn to reduce tension during labor.
- Cutaneous and mental stimulation techniques act to reduce pain perception. Techniques need to be varied to prevent habituation.
- Women learn a variety of breathing techniques for labor with the purpose of increasing relaxation.
- Having a support person increases a woman's satisfaction with childbirth. The educated support person may find labor less stressful and feel increased confidence.
- The support person may participate in labor actively, minimally, or only by being present. The nurse should accept all roles taken by the support person.
- Specific support techniques include assisting with relaxation and breathing, encouraging the woman, and using sacral pressure, massage, and comfort measures.

ANSWERS TO CRITICAL THINKING EXERCISE

Women and their support people should attend classes before each birth because they may have forgotten some information they learned during a previous childbirth class. Birthing care and options may have changed since the last birth. Couples often have concerns and questions about their last experience, and the nurse can discuss these issues and help them feel more positive about the pending birth. The needs of other children can also be addressed, including practical suggestions about easing the transition.

REFERENCES & READINGS

Association of Women's Health, Obstetric, & Neonatal Nurses (AWHONN). (2000). *Nurse providers of perinatal education: Competencies and program guide.* Washington, D.C.: Author.

AWHONN. (1998). *Standards and guidelines for professional nursing practice in the care of women and newborns* (5th ed.). Washington, D.C.: Author.

Bartlett, L., & McGrath, J.M. (1999). Children's responses to the birth of a sibling: Interventions to assist the family in transition. *Mother Baby Journal,* 4(4), 19-25.

Behnke, A. (1999). Sibling classes: Fun or frenzy? *International Journal of Childbirth Education,* 14(3), 9-11.

Bridgwater, N., & Wiman, B. (1998). Childbirth education options: Exploring one-day classes. *Lifelines,* 2(2), 49-52.

Capik, L.K. (1998). The health promotion model applied to family-centered perinatal education, *Journal of Perinatal Education,* 7(1), 9-17.

Cook, A., & Wilcox, G. (1997). Pressuring pain. *AWHONN Lifelines,* 1(2), 36-41.

Creehan, P.A. (1996). Pain relief and comfort measures during labor. In K.R. Simpson & P.A. Creehan (Eds.), *AWHONN's perinatal nursing.* Philadelphia: J.B. Lippincott.

Dick-Read, G. (1959). *Childbirth without fear.* New York: Harper & Row.

Ellerbee, S.M., & Spangler, A.K. (2000). Childbirth education primer. *Mother Baby Journal,* 5(1), 36-39.

Freedman, L.H. (2000). Honoring childbirth: Birth as a healing experience. *Lifelines,* 4(32), 70-72.

Farrell, M., Bushnell, D.D., Haag-Heitman, B. (1998). Theory and practice for teaching the childbearing couple. *Journal of Obstetric, Gynecologic, and Neonatal Nursing,* 27(6), 613-618.

Grotbo, A.C. (1999). Giving your patients some time out. *American Journal of Nursing,* 99(7), 24HH-26HH.

Guyer, B., Hoyert, D.L., Martin, J.A., Ventura, S.J., MacDorman, M.F., & Strobino, D.M. (1999). Annual summary of vital statistics: 1998. *Pediatrics,* 104(6), 1229-1245.

Harris, K.T. (1999). Hydrotherapy: An alternative method for relieving labor pain. *Mother Baby Journal,* 4(5), 15-20.

Hart, M.A., & Foster, S.N. (1997). Couples' attitudes toward childbirth participation: Relationship to evaluation of labor and delivery. *Journal of Perinatal and Neonatal Nursing,* 11(1), 10-20.

Hodnett, E. (1996). Nursing support of the laboring woman. *Journal of Obstetric, Gynecologic, and Neonatal Nursing,* 25(3), 257-264.

Humenick, S.S. (1996). Commentary: Childbirth education groups should collaborate more to inform parents about birth alternatives. *Birth,* 23(4), 204-205.

Humenick, S.S., Shrock, P., & Libresco, M.M. (2000). Relaxation. In F.H. Nichols & S.S. Humenick. *Childbirth education: Practice, research, and theory* (2nd ed., pp. 179-199). Philadelphia: W.B. Saunders.

International Childbirth Education Association (ICEA). (1999). *ICEA position paper: The role of the childbirth educator and the scope of childbirth education.* Minneapolis, MN: Author.

ICEA. (1999). *ICEA position paper: The role and scope of the doula.* Minneapolis, MN: Author.

Jimenez, S.L. (2000). Comfort and pain management. In F.H. Nichols & S.S. Humenick (Eds.). *Childbirth education: Practice, research, and theory* (2nd ed., pp 157-177). Philadelphia: W.B. Saunders.

Jimenez, S. L. (1998). Pain and comfort—Assessment: The key to effective pain management. *Journal of Perinatal Education,* 7(1), 35-38.

Keenan, P. (2000). Benefits of massage therapy and use of a doula during labor and childbirth. *Alternative Therapies,* 6(1), 66-74.

Kennell, J.H., & Klaus, M.H. (1998). Bonding: Recent observations that alter perinatal care. *Pediatrics in Review,* 19(1), 4-12.

Khazoyan, C.M., & Anderson, N.L.R. (1994). Latinas' expectations for their partners during childbirth. *American Journal of Maternal/Child Nursing,* 19(4), 226-229.

Klaus, M.H., Kennell, J.H., & Klaus, P.H. (1993). *Mothering the mother.* New York: Addison-Wesley.

Leitch, D.B. (1999). Mother-infant interaction: Achieving synchrony. *Nursing Research,* 48(1), 55-58.

Lothian, J.A. (1998). Culturally competent childbirth education. *Journal of Perinatal Education,* 7(1), x-xii.

Lowe, M., Millea, D., & Simpson, K.R. (1996). Discharge planning. In K.R. Simpson & P.A. Creehan (Eds.), *AWHONN's perinatal nursing.* Philadelphia: J.B. Lippincott.

Lowe, N.K. (1996). The pain and discomfort of labor and birth. *Journal of Obstetric, Gynecologic, and Neonatal Nursing,* 25(1), 82-92.

Monto, M.A. (1996). Lamaze and Bradley childbirth classes: Contrasting perspectives toward the medical model of birth. *Birth,* 23(4), 193-201.

Mullaly, L.M. (2000). Psychology of pregnancy. In Mattson, S., & Smith, J.E. (Eds.) *Core curriculum for maternal-newborn nursing* (2nd ed., pp. 101-114). Philadelphia: W.B. Saunders.

Piper, S., & Parks, P. (1996). Predicting the duration of lactation: Evidence from a national survey. *Birth,* 23(1), 7-12.

Pugh, L.C., Milligan, R.A., Gray, S., & Strickland, O.L. (1998). First stage labor management: An examination of patterned breathing and fatigue. *Birth,* 25(4), 241-245.

Redman, B.K. (2001). *The practice of patient education* (9th ed.) St. Louis: Mosby.

Shilling, T. (2000). Cultural perspectives on childbearing. In F.H. Nichols & S.S. Humenick. *Childbirth education: Practice, research, and theory* (2nd ed., pp. 138-154.) Philadelphia: W.B. Saunders.

Simkin, P. (1995). Reducing pain and enhancing progress in labor: A guide to nonpharmacologic methods for maternity caregivers. *Birth,* 22(3), 161-171.

Simkin, P. (1999). Labor support: Where has it been and where is it going? *International Journal of Childbirth Education,* 14(4), 22-23.

Sippert, G. (1998). Attachment and bonding: The doula's role. *International Journal of Childbirth Education,* 13(4), 26-27.

Steffes, S.A. (2000). Relaxation: Imagery. In F.H. Nichols & S.S. Humenick (Eds.). *Childbirth education: Practice, research, and theory* (2nd ed., pp. 227-252). Philadelphia: W.B. Saunders.

U.S. Department of Health and Human Services (2000). *Healthy people 2010.* (Conference ed., in two volumes). Washington, D.C.: Author.

Ventura, S.J., Martin, J.A., Curtin, S.C., Mathews, T.J., & Park, M.M. (2000). Births: Final data for 1998. *National vital statistics reports,* 48(3). Hyattsville, MD: National Center for Health Statistics.

Wallace, K.E. (2000). The Bradley method. *International Journal of Childbirth Education,* 15(1), 9-10.

White, M.B. (1998). Men's concerns during pregnancy, part 1: Reevaluating the role of the expectant father. *International Journal of Childbirth Education,* 13(2), 14-17.

Zwelling, E. (1996). Childbirth education in the 1990s and beyond. *Journal of Obstetric, Gynecologic, and Neonatal Nursing,* 25(5), 425-432.

12 PROCESSES OF BIRTH

OBJECTIVES

1. Describe the woman's physiologic and psychological responses to labor.
2. Describe fetal responses to labor.
3. Explain the ways each component of the birth process affects the course of labor and birth and the interrelation of these components.
4. Relate the mechanisms of labor to the process of vaginal birth.
5. Explain premonitory signs of labor.
6. Compare true labor with false labor.
7. Describe common differences in the labors of nulliparous and parous women.
8. Compare each stage of labor and the phases within the first stage.

DEFINITIONS

ACME Peak, or period of greatest strength, of a uterine contraction.

ATTITUDE Relationship of fetal body parts to one another.

BLOODY SHOW Mixture of cervical mucus and blood from ruptured capillaries in the cervix; often precedes labor and increases with cervical dilation.

BRAXTON-HICKS CONTRACTIONS Irregular, mild uterine contractions that occur throughout pregnancy and become stronger in the last trimester.

DECREMENT Period of decreasing strength of a uterine contraction.

DURATION Period from the beginning of a uterine contraction to the end of the same contraction.

ENGAGEMENT Descent of the widest diameter of the fetal presenting part to at least a zero station (the level of the ischial spines in the maternal pelvis).

FONTANELLE Space at the intersection of sutures connecting fetal or infant skull bones.

FREQUENCY Period from the beginning of one uterine contraction to the beginning of the next.

INCREMENT Period of increasing strength of a uterine contraction.

INTENSITY Strength of a uterine contraction.

INTERVAL Period between the end of one uterine contraction and the beginning of the next.

LIE Relationship of the long axis of the fetus to the long axis of the mother.

LIGHTENING Descent of the fetus toward the pelvic inlet before labor.

LOCHIA Vaginal drainage after birth.

MOLDING Shaping of the fetal head during movement through the birth canal.

NULLIPARA A woman who has not completed a pregnancy to at least 20 weeks' gestation.

PARA A woman who has given birth after a pregnancy of at least 20 weeks' gestation; also designates the number of pregnancies that end after at least 20 weeks' gestation (considered multifetal gestation such as twins as one birth when calculating parity).

DEFINITIONS—cont'd

POSITION Relation of a fixed reference point on the fetus to the quadrants of the maternal pelvis.

PRESENTATION Fetal part that enters the pelvic inlet, or the presenting part.

RIPENING Softening of the cervix as labor nears as the result of an increase in water content and the effects of relaxin on its connective tissue.

STATION Measurement of fetal descent in relation to the ischial spines of the maternal pelvis (see also *engagement*).

SUTURES Narrow areas of flexible tissue that connect fetal skull bones, permitting slight movement during labor.

VBAC Acronym for *vaginal birth after cesarean.*

Understanding the physiologic and psychological components of the birth process helps the nurse provide safe and effective care for the childbearing family during the intrapartum period. Awareness of expected changes allows the nurse to support the laboring woman when these changes occur and provides a basis for identifying abnormal occurrences. This chapter focuses on the changes that occur during normal birth.

PHYSIOLOGIC EFFECTS OF THE BIRTH PROCESS

The birth process affects the physiologic systems of the mother and fetus. The maternal reproductive system and systems related to fetal and neonatal oxygenation are most obviously affected.

Maternal Response

The most obvious changes of pregnancy and birth occur in the woman's reproductive system, but her other systems also respond in various ways. Significant changes occur during labor in her cardiovascular, respiratory, gastrointestinal, urinary, and hematopoietic systems.

Reproductive System

Characteristics of Contractions

Normal labor contractions are coordinated, involuntary, and intermittent.

Coordinated. The uterus can contract and relax in a coordinated way, like the heart and other smooth muscles. Contractions during pregnancy are of low intensity and uncoordinated. As the woman approaches full term, contractions become organized and gradually assume a regular pattern of increasing frequency, duration, and intensity during labor. Coordinated labor contractions begin in the uterine fundus and spread downward toward the cervix to propel the fetus through the pelvis.

Involuntary. Uterine contractions are involuntary in that they are not under conscious control, unlike movement of skeletal muscles. The mother cannot cause labor to start and stop by conscious effort. However, walking and other activities may stimulate existing labor contractions. Anxiety and excessive stress can diminish them, whereas relaxation can facilitate natural processes.

Intermittent. Labor contractions are intermittent rather than sustained, allowing relaxation of the uterine muscle and resumption of blood flow to and from the placenta to permit gas, nutrient, and waste exchange for the fetus.

Contraction Cycle

Each contraction consists of three phases (Figure 12-1). The increment occurs as the contraction begins in the fundus and spreads throughout the uterus. The peak, or acme, is the period during which the contraction is most intense. The decrement is the period of decreasing intensity as the uterus relaxes.

The contraction cycle and pattern of contractions are also described in terms of frequency, duration, and intensity. Frequency is the period from the beginning of one uterine contraction to the beginning of the next. It is expressed in minutes and fractions of minutes (such as "contractions are 3½ to 4 minutes apart").

Duration is the length of each contraction from beginning to end. It is usually expressed in seconds. For example, the nurse might say "Her contractions last 55 to 65 seconds."

Intensity is the strength of the contractions. The terms *mild, moderate,* and *strong* describe contraction intensity as palpated by the nurse. Additional descriptions of intensity apply when an internal fetal monitor is used to record contractions (see Chapter 14).

The interval is the period between the end of one contraction and the beginning of the next. Most fetal exchange of oxygen, nutrients, and waste products occurs at this time.

Uterine Body

Uterine activity during labor is characterized by opposing features. The upper two thirds of the uterus contracts actively to push the fetus down. The lower third of the uterus remains less active, promoting downward passage of the fetus. The cervix is similar to the lower uterine segment in that it is also passive. The net effect of labor contractions is enhanced because the downward push from the upper uterus is accompanied by reduced resistance to fetal descent in the lower uterus.

Myometrial (pertaining to the uterine muscle) cells in the upper uterus remain shorter at the end of each contraction rather than returning to their original length. In contrast, myometrial cells in the lower uterus become longer with each contraction. These two characteristics enable the upper uterus to maintain tension be-

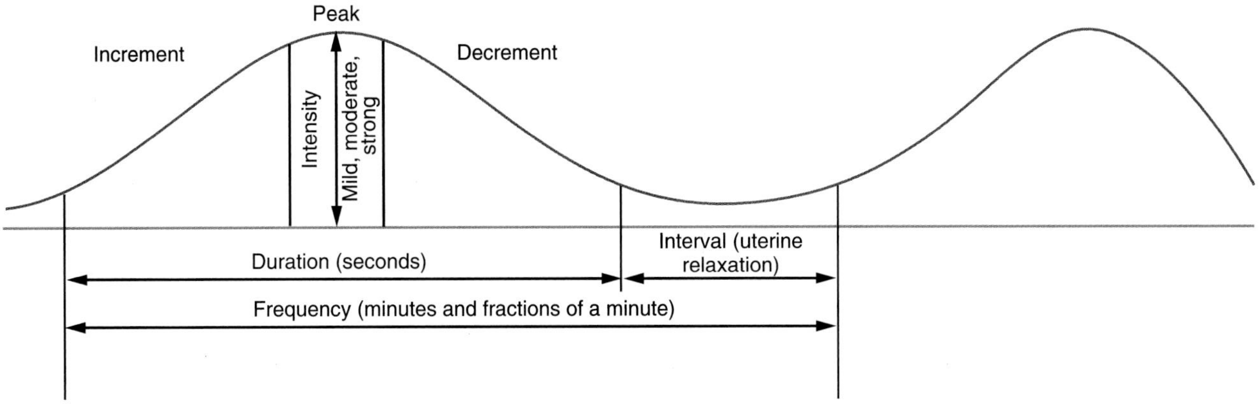
Peak
Increment
Decrement
Intensity
Mild, moderate, strong
Duration (seconds)
Interval (uterine relaxation)
Frequency (minutes and fractions of a minute)

FIGURE 12-1 Contraction cycle.

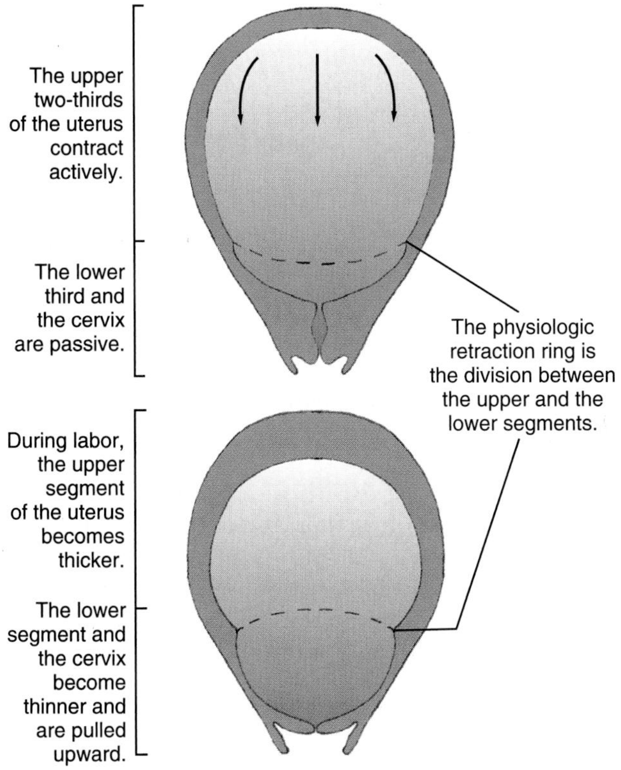
The upper two-thirds of the uterus contract actively.
The lower third and the cervix are passive.
The physiologic retraction ring is the division between the upper and the lower segments.
During labor, the upper segment of the uterus becomes thicker.
The lower segment and the cervix become thinner and are pulled upward.

FIGURE 12-2 Opposing characteristics of uterine contraction in the upper and lower segments of the uterus.

tween contractions to preserve the cervical changes and downward fetal progress made with each contraction.

The opposing characteristics of myometrial contraction in the upper and lower uterine segments cause changes in the thickness of the uterine wall during labor. The upper uterus becomes thicker while the lower uterus becomes thinner and is pulled upward during labor. The physiologic retraction ring marks the division between the upper and lower segments of the uterus (Figure 12-2).

Opposing characteristics of contractions in the upper and lower uterine segments change the shape of the uterine cavity, which becomes more elongated and narrow as labor progresses. This change in uterine shape straightens the fetal body and efficiently directs it downward in the pelvis.

Cervical Changes

Effacement (thinning and shortening) and dilation (opening) are the major cervical changes during labor. Effacement and dilation occur concurrently during labor but at different rates. The nullipara completes most cervical effacement early in the process of cervical dilation. In contrast, the cervix of a parous woman's cervix is usually thicker than that of a nullipara at any point during labor.

Effacement. Before labor the cervix is a cylindric structure about 2 cm long at the lower end of the uterus. Labor contractions push the fetus downward against the cervix while pulling the cervix upward. If the membranes are intact, hydrostatic (fluid) pressure of the amniotic sac adds to the force of the presenting part on the cervix. The cervix becomes shorter and thinner as it is drawn over the fetus and amniotic sac (Figure 12-3). The cervix merges with the thinning lower uterus rather than remaining a distinct cylindric structure. Effacement is estimated as a percentage of the original cervical length. A fully thinned cervix is 100% effaced. Effacement also may be documented as the cervical length estimated during vaginal examination.

Dilation. As the cervix is pulled upward and the fetus is pushed downward, the cervix dilates. Dilation is expressed in centimeters. Full dilation is approximately 10 cm, large enough to allow passage of the average-sized term fetus. The action during effacement and dilation can be likened to pushing a ball out the cuff of a sock.

Cardiovascular System

During each uterine contraction, blood flow to the placenta gradually decreases, causing a relative increase in the woman's blood volume. This temporary change increases her blood pressure slightly and slows her

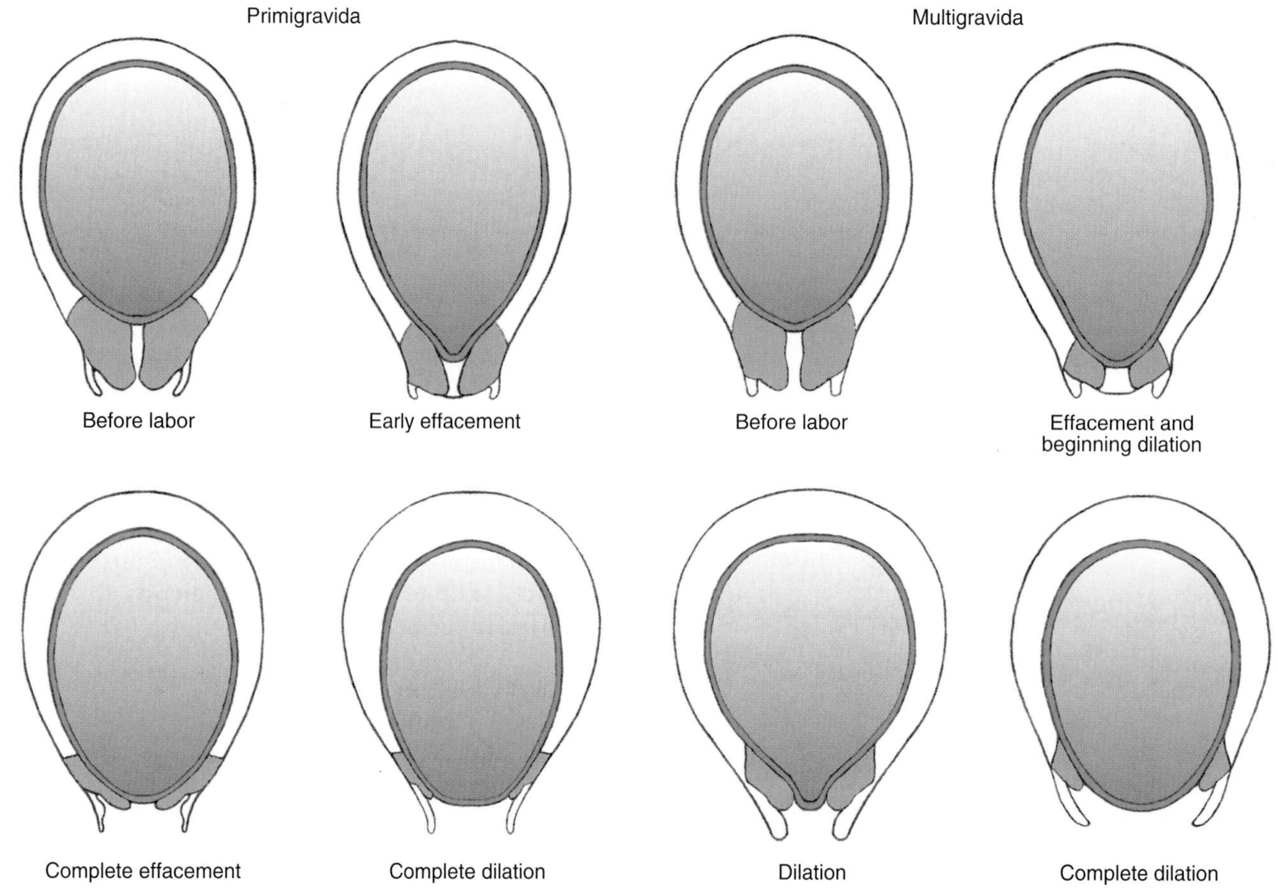

FIGURE 12-3 Cervical dilation and effacement. During labor the cervix of the multipara remains thicker than that of the nullipara.

pulse. Therefore the woman's vital signs are best assessed during the interval between contractions because slight alterations in her blood pressure and pulse may occur during a contraction. Supine hypotension (see p. 124) may occur during labor if the woman lies on her back. The woman should be encouraged to rest in positions other than the supine to promote blood return to her heart and therefore enhance blood flow to the placenta and promote fetal oxygenation.

Respiratory System

The depth and rate of respirations increase, especially if the woman is anxious or in pain. A woman who breathes rapidly and deeply may experience symptoms of hyperventilation if respiratory alkalosis occurs as she exhales too much carbon dioxide. She may feel tingling of her hands and feet, numbness, and dizziness. The nurse should help her slow her breathing and breathe into a paper bag or her cupped hands to restore normal blood levels of carbon dioxide and relieve these symptoms.

Gastrointestinal System

Gastric motility is reduced during labor to varying degrees, which can result in nausea and vomiting. Most women are not hungry but are thirsty and have dry mouths. Ice chips are commonly provided, and small amounts of other clear liquids and juices, popsicles, and hard candy on a stick may be permitted. Solid food is usually withheld in case general anesthesia is required to prevent vomiting and aspiration of undigested food (see Chapter 15).

Urinary System

The most common change in the urinary system during labor is a reduced sensation of a full bladder. Because of intense contractions and the effects of regional anesthesia, the woman may be unaware that her bladder is full, yet it may contribute to discomfort, especially that which persists after regional anesthesia. A full bladder can inhibit fetal descent because it occupies space in the pelvis.

The normal hypervolemia of pregnancy is reversed during the first 5 days postpartum, and large quantities of urine are excreted. The bladder may fill rapidly during the first few days after birth, even if the woman has not had an intravenous infusion during labor.

Hematopoietic System

Most authorities recognize 500 ml as the maximum normal blood loss during vaginal birth. Women usually tolerate this loss well because the blood volume increases during pregnancy by 1 to 2 L (Guyton & Hall,

2000). A woman who is anemic at the beginning of labor has less reserve for normal blood loss and a poor tolerance for excess bleeding. A hemoglobin level of 10.5 g/dl and a hematocrit of 33% or higher give most women an adequate margin of safety for blood loss associated with normal birth (Duffy, 1999). The leukocyte count averages 14,000 to 16,000/mm^3 but may be as high as 25,000 to 30,000/mm^3 during active labor with no other evidence of infection (Cunningham, et al., 1997; Blackburn & Loper, 1992).

Levels of several clotting factors, especially fibrinogen, are elevated during pregnancy and continue to be higher during labor and after delivery. The greater number of clotting factors provides protection from hemorrhage but also increases the mother's risk for a venous thrombosis during pregnancy and after birth.

Fetal Response

Responses to labor are most notable in the placental circulation, cardiovascular system, and pulmonary system.

Placental Circulation

The exchange of oxygen, nutrients, and waste products between the mother and fetus occurs in the intervillous spaces without the mixing of maternal and fetal blood (see Chapter 6). During strong labor contractions, the maternal blood supply to the placenta decreases and eventually stops temporarily as the spiral arteries supplying the intervillous spaces are compressed by the uterine muscle. Therefore most placental exchange occurs during the interval between contractions. The placental circulation usually has enough reserve compared with fetal basal needs to tolerate the periodic interruption of blood flow.

Fetal protective mechanisms include the following:

- Fetal hemoglobin, which more readily takes on oxygen and releases carbon dioxide
- High hemoglobin and hematocrit levels that can carry 20% to 50% more oxygen than adult hemoglobin. The fetal hemoglobin level averages 14.5 to 22.5 gm/dl and the hematocrit is approximately 48% to 69%.
- A high cardiac output of 250 ml/kg/min

The fetus may not tolerate labor contractions well in conditions associated with reduced placental function, such as maternal diabetes and hypertension, and conditions associated with reduced fetal oxygen-carrying capacity, such as fetal anemia.

Cardiovascular System

The fetal cardiovascular system reacts quickly to events during labor. Alterations in the rate and rhythm of the fetal heart may result from normal labor effects or suggest fetal intolerance to the stress of labor. The fetal heart rate is rapid and ranges from 110 to 160 beats per minute (BPM) at term (Menihan, 1996; Harvey, 1997; Feinstein, Sprague, & Trépanier, 2000). The preterm fetus usually has a rate in the higher end of this range.

Pulmonary System

The fetal lungs produce fluid to allow normal development of the airways. Lung fluid must be cleared to allow normal air breathing after birth. As term nears, production of fetal lung fluid decreases to about 65% of its maximum production and its absorption into the interstitium of the lungs increases. Labor speeds the absorption of lung fluid, so about 35% of the maximum amount remains in the airways at birth. Some fluid is expelled from the upper airways as the fetal head and thorax are compressed during passage through the birth canal. Most remaining lung fluid is absorbed into the interstitial spaces of the newborn's lungs and then into the circulatory system. A small amount is cleared by the lymphatic circulation (Jobe, 1999; Cunningham, et al., 1997).

Catecholamines (primarily epinephrine and norepinephrine) produced by the fetal adrenal glands in response to the stress of labor appear to contribute to the infant's adaptation to extrauterine life. They stimulate cardiac contraction and breathing, quicken the clearance of remaining lung fluid, and aid in temperature regulation. Infants born by cesarean birth not preceded by labor are more likely to have transient breathing difficulty (see p. 842).

Check Your Reading

1. How do labor contractions cause the cervix to efface and dilate? How do they cause fetal descent?
2. What differences in effacement are expected in the parous woman compared with the woman who has not previously given birth?
3. What changes occur in the maternal cardiovascular, respiratory, gastrointestinal, renal, and hematopoietic systems during labor?
4. Why are intermittent rather than sustained uterine contractions important?
5. How does the normal process of vaginal birth benefit the newborn after birth?

COMPONENTS OF THE BIRTH PROCESS

Four major factors interact during normal childbirth. These factors are often called the *four Ps:* powers, passage, passenger, and psyche.

Powers

Uterine Contractions. During the first stage of labor (onset to full cervical dilation), uterine contractions are the primary force that moves the fetus through the maternal pelvis.

Maternal Pushing Efforts. During the second stage of labor (full cervical dilation to birth of the baby), uterine contractions continue to propel the fetus through the pelvis. In addition, the woman feels an urge to push and bear down as the fetus distends her vagina and puts pressure on her rectum. She adds her voluntary pushing efforts to the force of uterine contractions in second-stage labor.

Passage

The birth passage consists of the maternal pelvis and soft tissues. The bony pelvis is usually more important to the outcome of labor than the soft tissue because the bones and joints do not readily yield to the forces of labor. However, softening of the cartilage linking the pelvic bones occurs at term because of increased levels of the hormone relaxin.

The linea terminalis (pelvic brim) divides the bony pelvis into the false pelvis (top) and true pelvis (bottom) (see Chapter 4). The true pelvis is most important in childbirth. The true pelvis has three subdivisions: (1) the inlet, or upper pelvic opening; (2) the midpelvis, or pelvic cavity; and (3) the outlet, or lower pelvic opening. During birth, the true pelvis functions like a curved cylinder with different dimensions at different levels (Figure 12-4).

Passenger

The passenger is the fetus, membranes, and placenta. Several fetal anatomic and positional variables influence the course of labor.

Fetal Head

The fetus enters the birth canal in the cephalic presentation 96% of the time. The fetal shoulders are also important because of their width, but they usually can be moved to adapt to the pelvis.

Bones, Sutures, and Fontanelles. The bones of the fetal head involved in the birth process are the two frontal bones on the forehead, two parietal bones at the crown of the head, and occipital bone at the back of the head (Figure 12-5). The five major bones are not fused but are connected by sutures composed of strong but flexible fibrous tissue. The fontanelles are wider spaces at the intersections of the sutures.

The anterior fontanelle has a diamond shape formed by the intersection of four sutures: the two coronal, frontal, and sagittal, which connect the two frontal and two parietal bones. The posterior fontanelle has a triangular shape formed by the intersection of three sutures, one sagittal and two lambdoid, which connect the two parietal bones and occipital bone. The posterior fontanelle is very small and often looks more like a slight indentation in the skull. The sutures and fontanelles allow the bones to move slightly, changing the shape of the fetal head so that it can adapt to the size and shape of the pelvis by molding. The sutures and different shapes of the fontanelles provide important landmarks to determine fetal position and head flexion during vaginal examination.

Fetal Head Diameters. Most fetuses enter the pelvis in the cephalic presentation, but several variations are possible. The major transverse diameter of the fetal head is the biparietal, measured between the two parietal bones. The biparietal diameter averages 9.5 cm in a term fetus.

The anteroposterior diameter of the head varies with the degree of flexion. In the most favorable situation, the head becomes fully flexed during labor and the anteroposterior diameter is suboccipitobregmatic, averaging 9.5 cm (see Figure 12-5, *B*).

Variations in the Passenger

Fetal Lie

The orientation of the long axis of the fetus to the long axis of the woman is called the *fetal lie* (Figure 12-6). In more than 99% of pregnancies, the lie is longitudinal and parallel to the long axis of the woman. In the longitudinal lie, either the head or the buttocks of the fetus enters the pelvis first. A transverse lie exists when the long axis of the fetus is at a right angle to the woman's long axis. This occurs in fewer than 1% of pregnancies. An oblique lie is at some angle between the longitudinal and transverse lie.

Attitude

The relation of fetal body parts to each other is the attitude of the fetus (Figure 12-7). The normal fetal attitude is one of flexion, with the head flexed toward the chest and the arms and legs flexed over the thorax. The back is curved in a convex C shape. Flexion remains a characteristic feature of the term newborn.

Presentation

The fetal part that first enters the pelvis is termed the *presenting part.* Presentation falls into three categories: (1) cephalic, (2) breech, and (3) shoulder. The cephalic presentation with the fetal head flexed is the most common (Figure 12-8). Other presentations are associated with prolonged labor and other problems and are more likely to require cesarean birth.

Cephalic Presentation. The cephalic presentation is more favorable than others for several reasons:

- The fetal head is the largest single fetal part, although the breech (buttocks), with the legs and feet flexed on the abdomen, is collectively larger than the head. After the head is born, the smaller parts follow easily as the extremities unfold.
- During labor, the fetal head can gradually change shape, molding to adapt to the size and shape of the maternal pelvis.

Text continued on p. 268

INLET

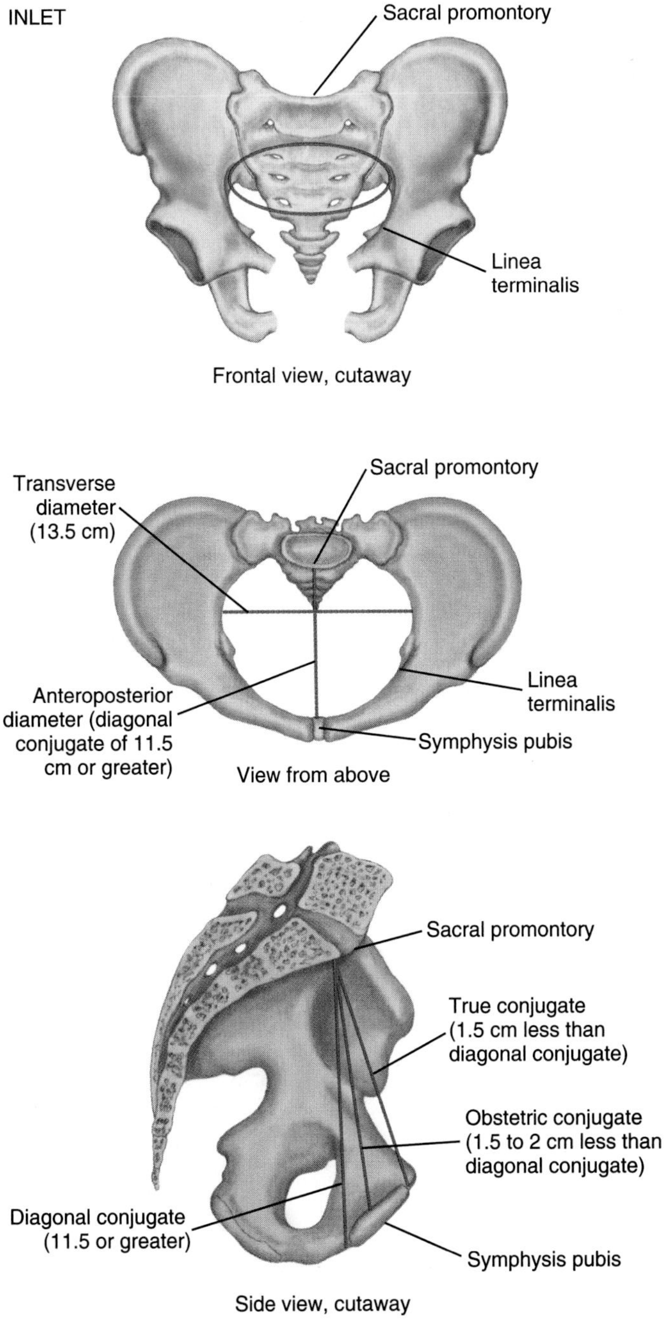

The boundaries of the inlet are the symphysis pubis anteriorly, the sacral promontory posteriorly, and the linea terminalis on the sides. The inlet is slightly wider in its transverse diameter (13.5 cm) than in its anteroposterior (diagonal conjugate) diameter (11.5 cm or greater).

The diagonal conjugate is slightly larger than both the obstetric and true conjugates. The obstetric conjugate is the narrowest of the three conjugate diameters but cannot be measured directly. The obstetric conjugate is estimated by first measuring the diagonal conjugate and then subtracting 1.5 to 2 cm.

If the inlet is small, the fetal head may not be able to enter it. Because it is almost entirely surrounded by bone, except for cartilage at the sacroiliac joint and symphysis pubis, the inlet cannot enlarge much to accommodate the fetus. The bony measurements are essentially fixed.

MIDPELVIS

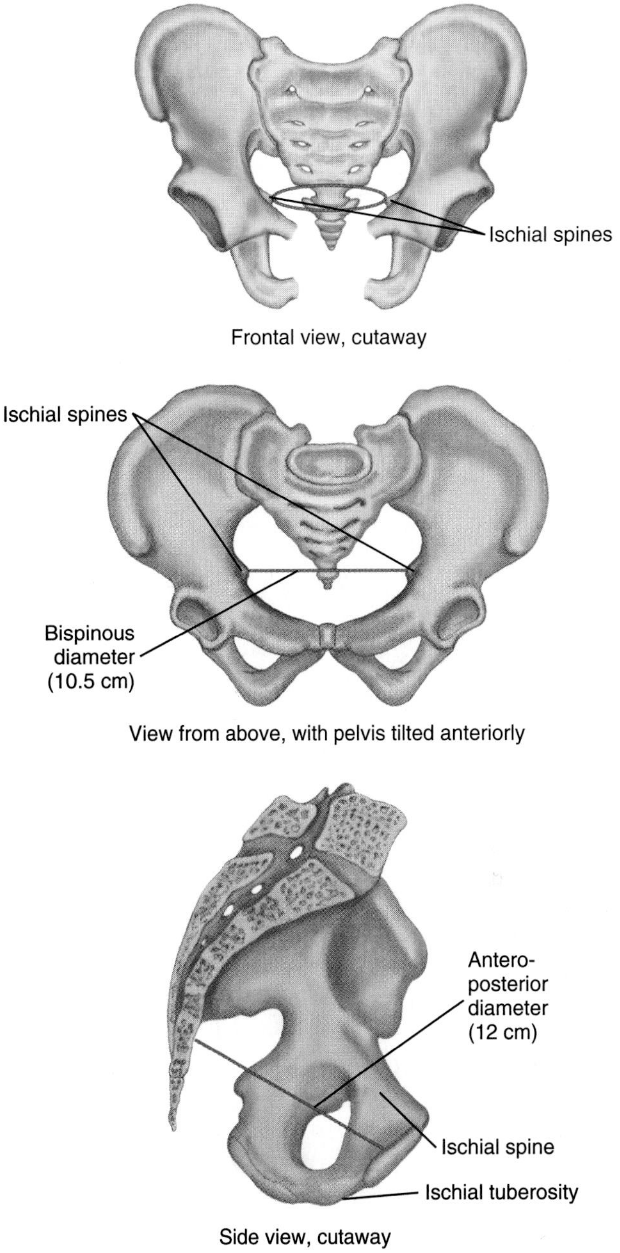

The midpelvis, or pelvic cavity, is the narrowest part of the pelvis through which the fetus must pass during birth. Midpelvic diameters are measured at the level of the ischial spines. The anteroposterior diameter averages 12 cm.

The transverse diameter (bispinous or interspinous) averages 10.5 cm. Prominent ischial spines that project into the midpelvis can reduce the bispinous diameter.

FIGURE 12-4 Pelvic divisions and measurements.

Continued

OUTLET

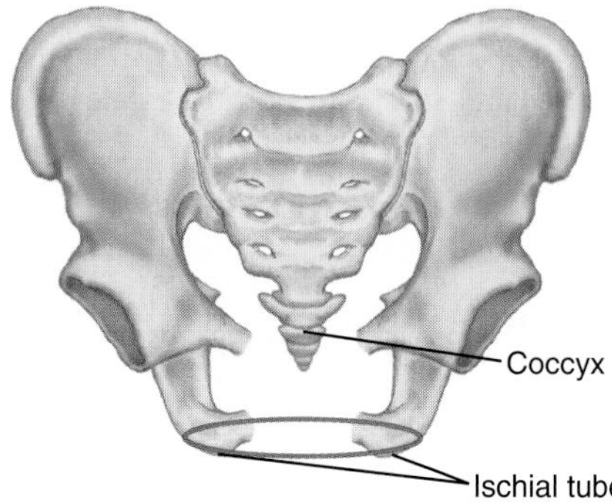

Frontal view, cutaway

Three important diameters of the pelvic outlet are (1) the anteroposterior, (2) the transverse (bi-ischial or intertuberous), and (3) the posterior sagittal. The angle of the pubic arch is also an important pelvic outlet measure.

The anteroposterior diameter ranges from 9.5 to 11.5 cm, varying with the curve between the sacrococcygeal joint and the tip of the coccyx. The anteroposterior diameter can increase if the coccyx is easily movable.

The transverse diameter is the bi-ischial, or intertuberous, diameter. This is the distance between the ischial tuberosities ("sit bones"). It averages 11 cm.

The posterior sagittal diameter is normally at least 7.5 cm. It is a measure of the posterior pelvis. The posterior sagittal diameter measures the distance from the sacrococcygeal joint to the middle of the transverse (bi-ischial) diameter.

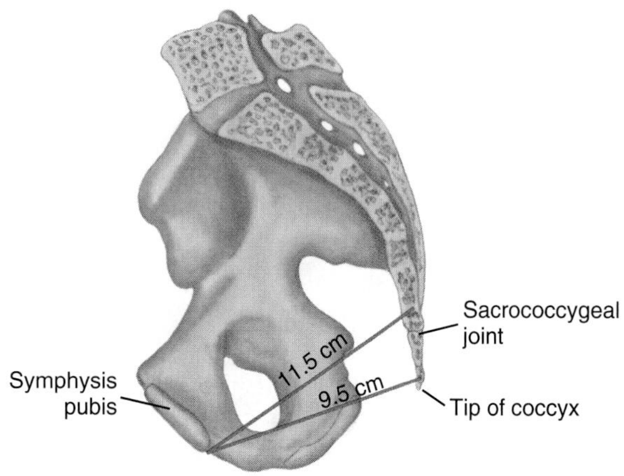

Side view, cutaway

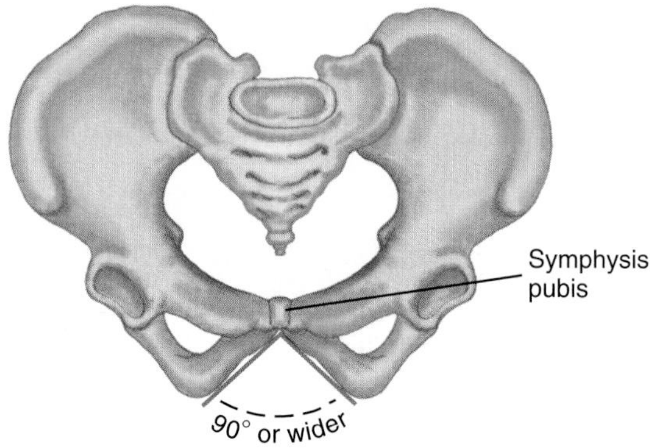

Frontal view, with pelvis tilted anteriorly

The angle of the pubic arch is important because it must be wide enough for the fetus to pass under it. The angle of the pubic arch should be at least 90 degrees. A narrow pubic arch displaces the fetus posteriorly toward the coccyx as it tries to pass under the arch.

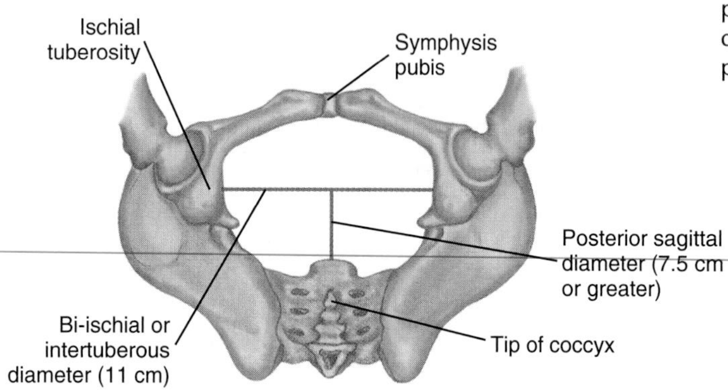

View from below (woman is in lithotomy position)

FIGURE 12-4, cont'd Pelvic divisions and measurements.

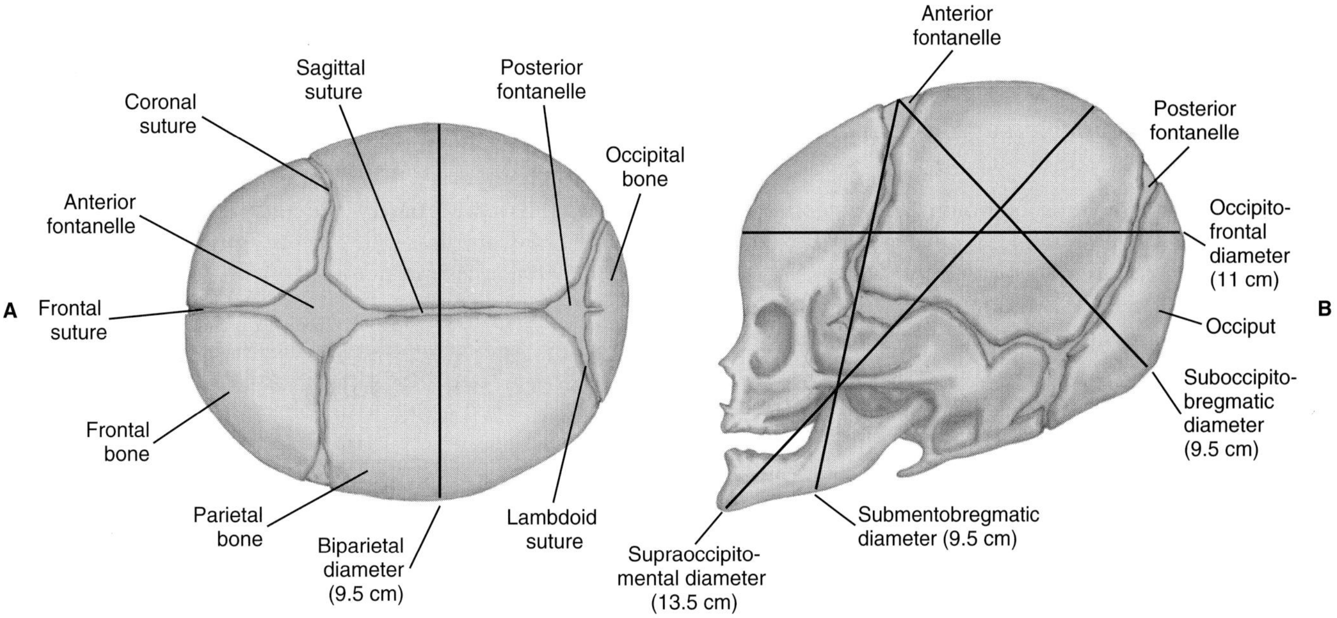

FIGURE 12-5 **A,** Bones, sutures, and fontanelles of the fetal head. Note that the anterior fontanelle has a diamond shape, whereas the posterior fontanelle is triangular. **B,** Lateral view of the fetal head demonstrating that anteroposterior diameters vary with the amount of flexion and extension.

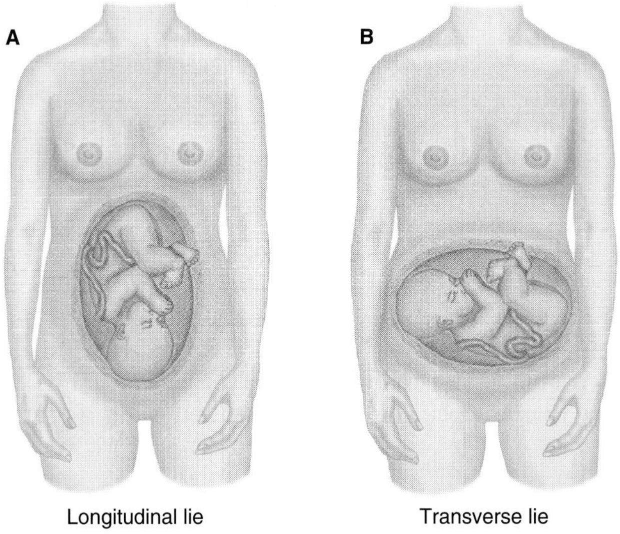

FIGURE 12-6 **A,** Fetal lie. In a longitudinal lie, the long axis of the fetus is parallel to the long axis of the woman. **B,** In a transverse lie, the long axis of the fetus is at right angles to the long axis of the mother. The woman's abdomen has a wide, short appearance.

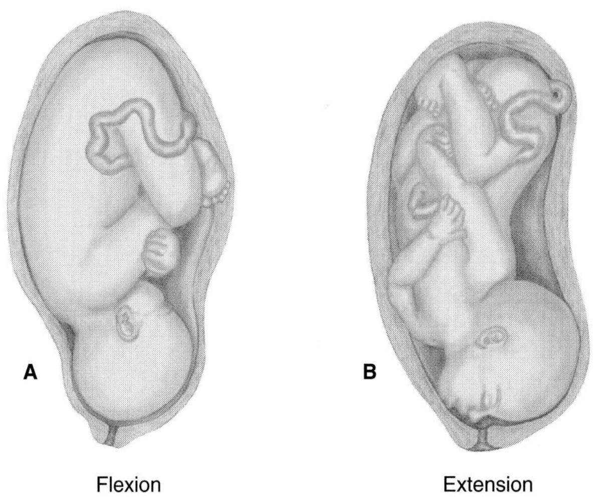

FIGURE 12-7 **A,** Attitude. The fetus is in the normal attitude of flexion, with the head, arms, and legs are flexed tightly against the trunk. **B,** The fetus is in an abnormal attitude of extension. The head is extended, and the right arm is extended. A face presentation is illustrated.

- The fetal head is smooth, round, and hard, making it a more effective part to dilate the cervix, which is also round.

Cephalic presentation has four variations (Figure 12-8):

Vertex—This is the most common type of cephalic presentation, in which the fetal head is fully flexed. It is called a *vertex* or an *occiput presentation* in everyday usage. This presentation is the most favorable for normal progress of labor because the smallest suboccipitobregmatic diameter is presenting.

Military—The head is in a neutral position, neither flexed nor extended. The longer occipitofrontal diameter is presenting.

Brow—The fetal head is partly extended. The brow presentation is unstable, usually converting to a vertex presentation if the head flexes or a face presentation if it extends. The longest supraoccipitomental diameter is presenting.

Face—The head is extended, and the fetal occiput is near the fetal spine. The submentobregmatic diameter is presenting.

Breech Presentation. A breech presentation occurs when the fetal buttocks enter the pelvis first, which happens in about 3% of births. Breech presentation is more common in preterm births and when a fetal abnormality such as hydrocephalus (enlargement of the head with fluid) prevents the head from entering the pelvis. Breech presentation is also more likely to occur with abnormalities of the maternal uterus and pelvis and with placenta previa (placenta in the lower uterus).

Breech presentations are associated with several disadvantages:

- The buttocks are not smooth and firm like the head and are less effective at dilating the cervix.
- The fetal head is the last part to be born. By the time the fetal head is deep in the pelvis, the umbilical cord is outside the mother's body and is subject to compression between the head and maternal pelvis.
- Because the umbilical cord can be compressed after the fetal chest is born, the head must be delivered quickly to allow the infant to breathe. This does not permit gradual molding of the fetal head as it passes through the pelvis.

The breech presentation has three variations, depending on the relationship of the legs to the body (Figure 12-9):

Frank breech—This is the most common variation, occurring when the fetal legs are extended across the abdomen toward the shoulders.

Full (complete) breech—This is a reversal of the usual cephalic presentation. The head, knees, and hips are flexed, but the buttocks are presenting.

Footling breech—This occurs when one or both feet are presenting.

Shoulder Presentation. The shoulder presentation is a transverse lie and accounts for only 0.2% of births (Cunningham, et al., 1997). It occurs more often with preterm birth, high parity, prematurely ruptured membranes, hydramnios, and placenta previa. A cesarean birth is almost always necessary.

Check Your Reading

6. What are the two powers of labor?
7. What are the three divisions of the true pelvis?
8. Why is the vertex presentation best during birth?

Position

Fetal position describes the location of a fixed reference point on the presenting part in relation to the four quadrants of the maternal pelvis (Figure 12-10). The four quadrants are the right and left anterior and right and left posterior. The fetal position is not fixed but changes during labor as the fetus moves downward and adapts to the pelvic contours. Abbreviations indicate the relationship between the fetal presenting part and maternal pelvis.

Right (R) or Left (L). The first letter of the abbreviation describes whether the fetal reference point is to the right or left of the mother's pelvis. If the fetal point is neither to the right nor the left of the pelvis, this letter is omitted.

Occiput (O), Mentum (M), or Sacrum (S). The second letter of the abbreviation refers to the fixed fetal reference point, which varies with the presentation. The occiput is used in a vertex presentation. The chin, or mentum, is the reference point in a face presentation. The sacrum is used for breech presentations. Letters may also designate the less common brow (F for fronto) and shoulder (Sc for scapula) presentations.

Anterior (A), Posterior (P), or Transverse (T). These letters describe whether the fetal reference point is in the anterior or posterior quadrant of the mother's pelvis. If the fetal reference point is in neither the anterior nor the posterior quadrant, it is described as transverse. If the fetal occiput is located in the left anterior quadrant of the mother's pelvis, the position is described as left occiput anterior (LOA). If the occiput is in the mother's anterior pelvis, neither to the right nor to the left, it is described as occiput anterior (OA). If the fetal sacrum is located in the mother's right posterior pelvis, the abbreviation is R (right) S (sacrum) P (posterior) (Figure 12-11).

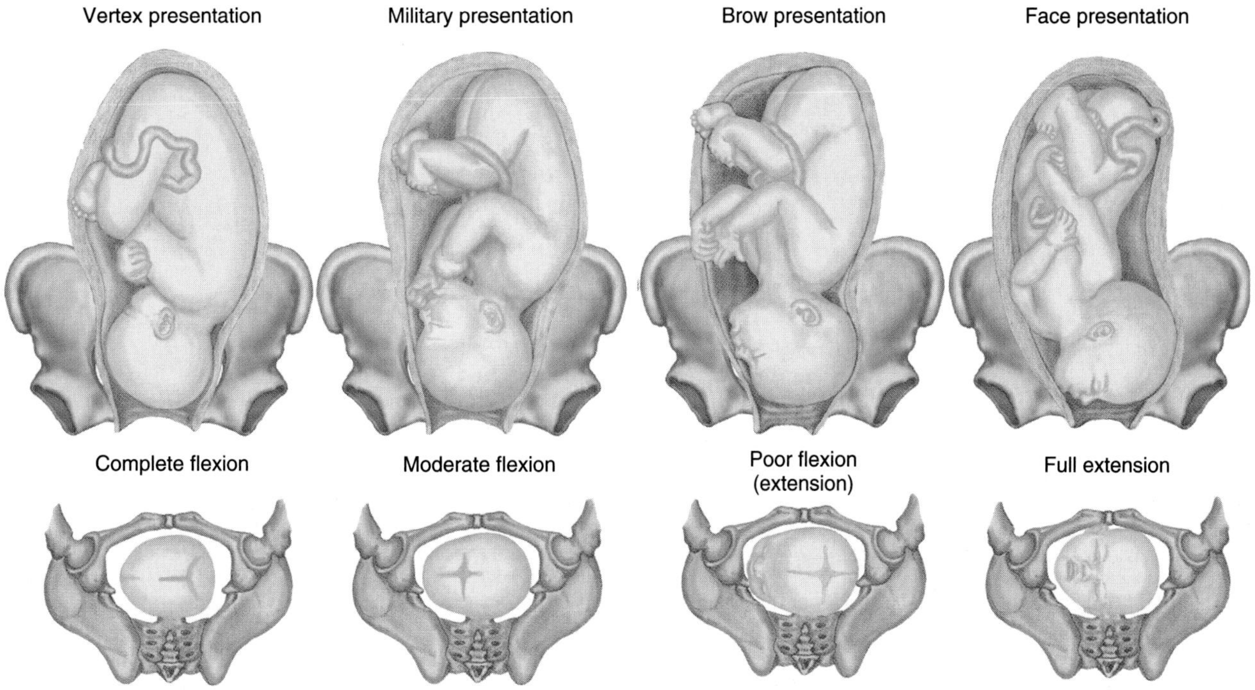

FIGURE 12-8 Four types of cephalic presentation. The vertex presentation is normal. Note positional changes of the anterior and posterior fontanelles in relation to the maternal pelvis.

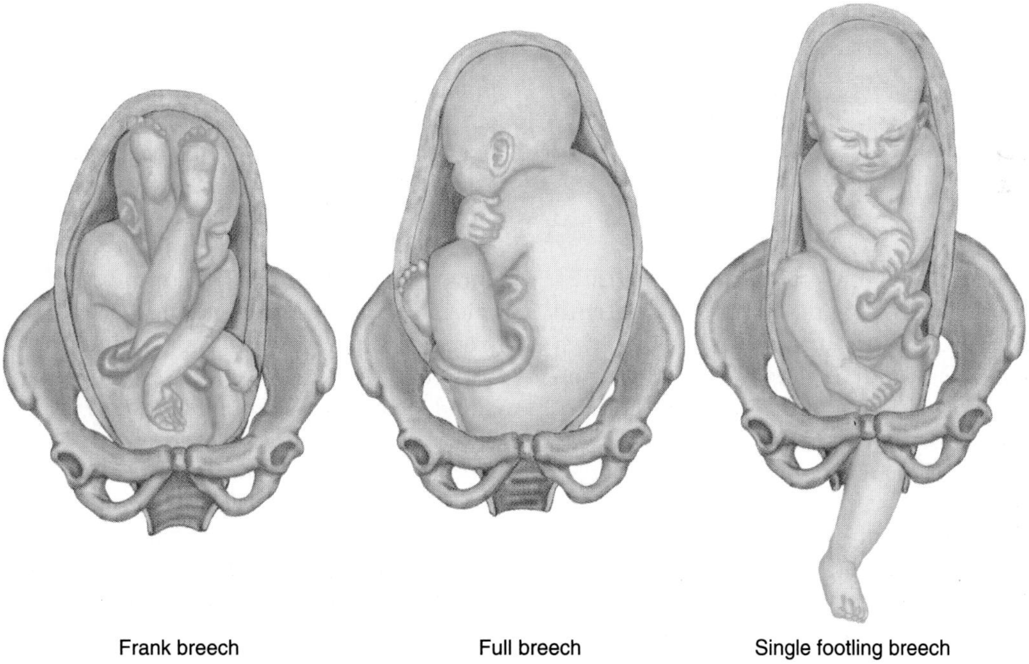

FIGURE 12-9 Three variations of a breech presentation. Frank breech is the most common variation. Footling breeches may be single or double.

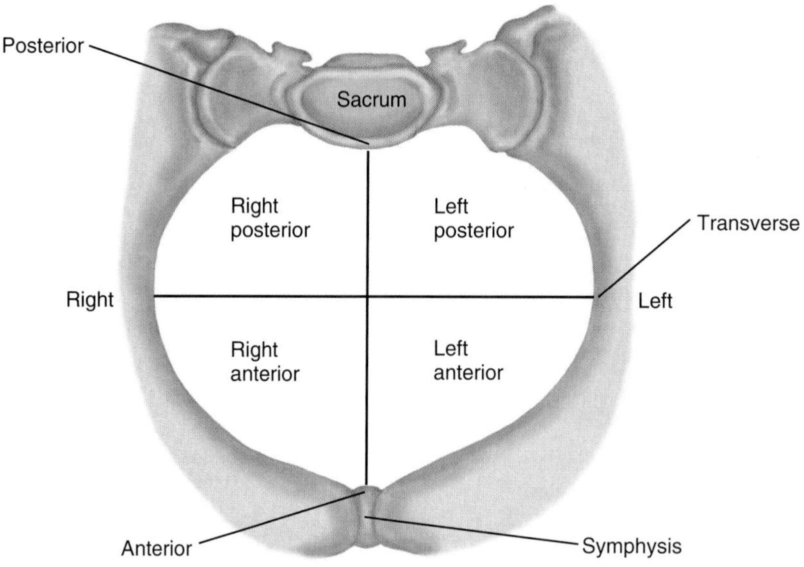

FIGURE 12-10 Four quadrants of the maternal pelvis, which are used to describe fetal position.

Check Your Reading

9. For each fetal position listed, describe the fetal landmark. Where is this landmark located in relation to the mother's pelvis: ROP? OA? RSA? LMA?
10. If the fetus is in a face presentation, why is using the occiput to determine position within the pelvis not possible?

Psyche

The psyche is a crucial part of childbirth. Marked anxiety and fear decrease a woman's ability to cope with pain in labor. Maternal catecholamines secreted in response to anxiety and fear can inhibit uterine contractility and placental blood flow. In contrast, relaxation augments the natural process of labor. Preparation for childbirth can enhance a woman's ability to work with her body's efforts rather than resist the natural forces. Much of the nurse's care during labor involves promoting relaxation and reducing anxiety and fear. Information and a positive sense of control and mastery over the birth increases the woman's sense of satisfaction with her birth experience (Nichols & Gennaro, 2000).

Individual and Cultural Values

A woman in childbirth is more than a physical being. She is a blend of her experiences, present status, and future expectations. She is an individual, a member of a family and cultural group, and a part of her larger society.

A woman's culture affects her views of birth and the practices surrounding it. Culture shapes the values that people hold, their expectations of birth experiences, and their responses to birth. A woman's culture influences her reaction to labor and her expectations of interaction with her newborn. If the woman, her family, and her caregivers have similar viewpoints, little conflict in their values and expectations is likely. However, if these individuals hold markedly different viewpoints, confusion may result because each expects something different of the other. Cultural differences are most obvious when newly immigrated women give birth. After time and exposure to other cultural groups, the distinctive cultural practices and values often become blurred.

Within a culture, a childbearing woman is an individual. The nurse's familiarity with a group's cultural values and practices related to birth provides a foundation for culturally competent care. Cultural knowledge provides a framework to assess and care for the woman and her family as individuals. However, the nurse must assess the personal expectations and values of each woman and her support person related to birth within this general framework. Cultural assessment questions for the intrapartum period might include the following:

- How long have the woman and her family been in the area? Are they recent immigrants, or have their relatives and friends lived in the area for generations?
- What is the primary language used? Do the woman and her support person speak the same language or

Text continued on p. 272

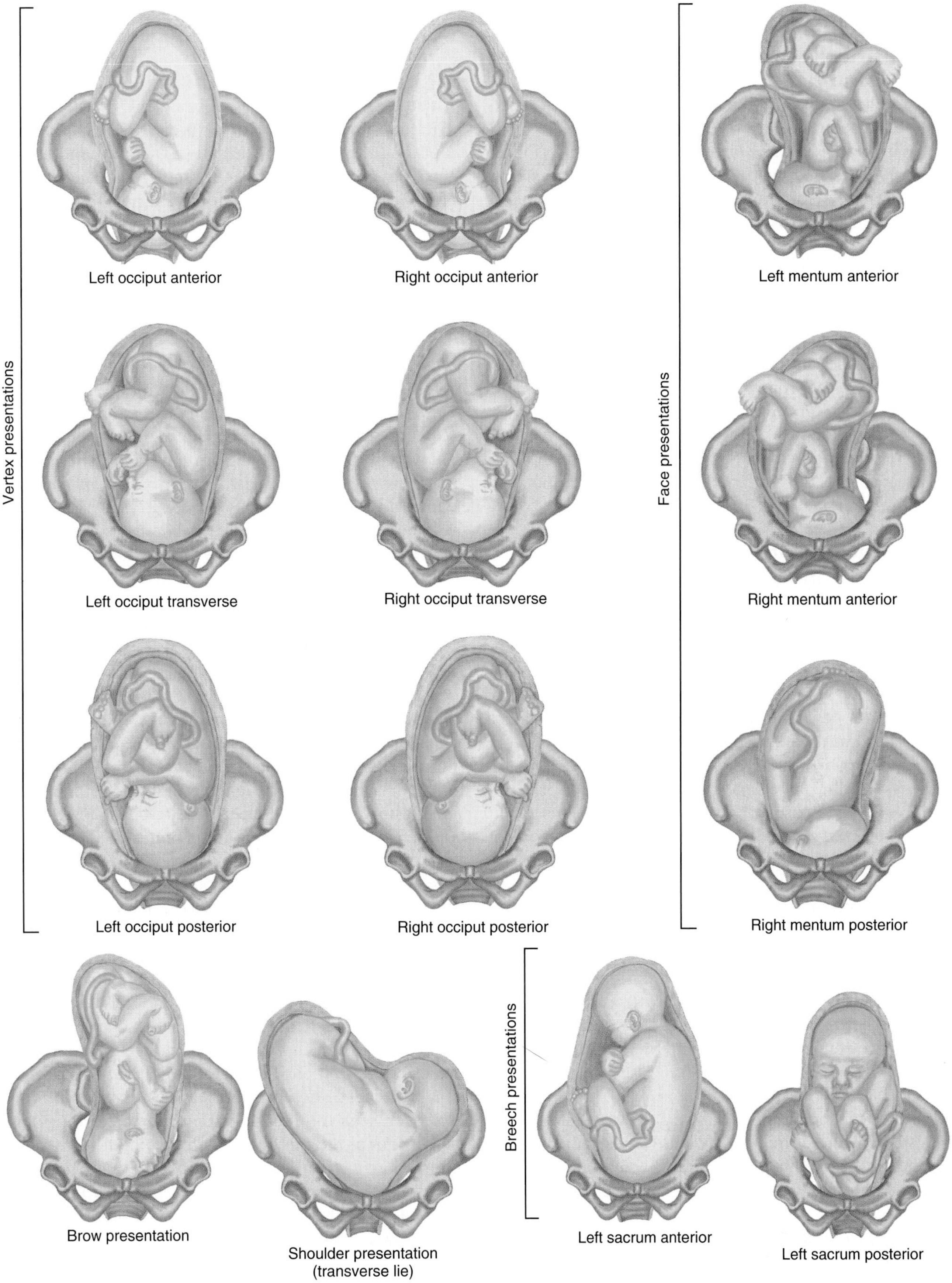

FIGURE 12-11 Fetal presentations and positions.

does only one of them speak the dominant language? Are they relatively comfortable communicating in the nurse's language if that is not their usual language? If an interpreter is needed, what people would the woman or her family consider to be unacceptable interpreters?
- Who is the woman's primary support person for labor? What is that person's role? How extensively will that person interact with the laboring woman? Who will be present at the birth?
- Who is the decision maker in the family, or who must be consulted about important decisions?
- Will another relative (such as a grandmother) assume primary care for the infant?
- Is a professional caregiver (such as a nurse or physician) of the same gender and cultural group essential?
- What are the woman's feelings about touch? Is she comfortable telling the nurse when she does not welcome touch?
- Are specific symbols, practices, and ceremonies used during the birth period? Who will conduct any ceremonies?

Other cultural assessments are needed as labor progresses and birth occurs (see Chapters 15 and 17).

Birth as an Experience

Childbirth is a physical and an emotional experience. It is an irrevocable event that forever changes a woman and a family. Families describe the births of their children as they describe other pivotal events in life, such as marriages, anniversaries, religious events, and even deaths. They do not talk about childbirth as they might discuss an illness or surgery. With the prevalence of smaller families, parents have greater expectations about the experience of childbirth than in the past. A woman who has more realistic expectations about the birth is more likely to have a positive experience. Nursing measures that increase the woman's sense of control and mastery during birth help her perceive the birth as a positive event. The nurse must attend to the psychological and emotional needs of the woman during birth to promote a positive birth experience for the woman.

A number of variables influence the meaning of the birth experience for the woman (Nichols & Gennaro, 2000):

- Relatively constant variables such as the woman's cultural and ethnic beliefs and values, spiritual beliefs, personal history (including whether this is her first baby), and age, education, and socioeconomic class
- Variables that the health care team can influence, such as anxiety and fear, pharmacologic pain management, the birthing environment, labor support, and promotion of the woman's confidence, sense of mastery and control, and self-esteem
- Variables that the health care team may influence in some situations, including obstetric risk factors and the type of birth

Impact of Technology

The goal of maternity care is to protect the health of the mother, fetus, and newborn and to support and enrich the woman's birth experience. Technology helps caregivers identify problems and intervene quickly to protect the health of the mother and fetus. However, extensive use of sophisticated technology may make maternity care seem impersonal. Women may feel that their feelings are less important than data from the monitors and infusion pumps attached to them for normal childbirth. Technology may make some nurses feel less necessary to the well-being of the woman. The nurse must guard against "nursing the machines" and internal feelings of being unnecessary to the woman's birth experience. Most nurses become intrapartum nurses because they enjoy helping women giving birth. If the nurse can keep the focus on the woman as the childbearer and the machine as a tool, frustration for all concerned is less likely.

Uncomplicated birth is a natural process that does not demand routine use of complex technology. Indeed, interventions during birth can lead to other interventions that may inhibit the natural process. For example, epidural analgesia is now almost routine in births. Although epidural analgesia can provide dramatic pain relief, it also requires infusion of large amounts of intravenous fluids and usually confines the woman to bed. Her bladder fills quickly, but she may not feel the urge to void, leading to urinary catheterization. Bed confinement removes some of her choices for labor positions, including many upright positions such as walking and standing.

Another example is electronic fetal monitoring. In 1998, 84% of births in the United States used electronic fetal monitoring (Curtin & Mathews, 2000). Intermittent auscultation would likely have been equally valid and safe for many of these women. The nurse must remember that electronic fetal monitoring is a tool for fetal assessment, but the knowledge, skills, and intuition required to interpret the baby's health are inside the nurse's head.

Although normal labor and birth do not require routine use of sophisticated technology, many women subordinate their preferences for low-intervention birth experiences to their desires for what they perceive offers maximal safety for their babies. They may accept and even seek interventions that they believe best assure them of having healthy children. Other women simply have not thought of a low-technology birth. Regardless, the intrapartum nurse can be the bridge between the technology and humanity of the birth experience. The nurse must continue to provide support and reassurance even if the woman has minimal pain because of an epidural block. The nature of nursing support is simply different in this case than if the woman was not using medication. The nurse must maintain the nursing focus on the woman, fetus, and support person rather than the technology.

Interrelationships of Components

The four Ps have been described separately but are actually an interrelated whole. For instance, a woman with a small pelvis (passage) and a large fetus (passenger) can have a normal labor and birth if the fetus is ideally positioned and the uterine contractions and maternal bearing-down efforts (powers) are vigorous. The nurse's supportive attitude strengthens positive psychological elements (psyche) and enhances the processes of birth. The nurse can act as an advocate for the laboring woman and her support person to increase their sense of control and mastery of labor, which often reduces anxiety and fear and helps them achieve their desired birth experience.

NORMAL LABOR

Theories of Onset

Despite continuing research, the exact mechanisms that initiate labor remain unknown. Labor normally starts when the fetus is mature enough to adjust easily to extrauterine life but before it grows so large that vaginal birth is impossible. This stage (term gestation) occurs between 38 and 42 weeks after the first day of the woman's last menstrual period.

Labor begins when forces favoring continuation of pregnancy are offset by forces favoring its end. Research is ongoing in this area because this knowledge is essential to developing effective measures to treat preterm labor. Factors that appear to have a role in starting labor include the following:

- The ratio of maternal estrogen to progesterone changes so that estrogen levels are higher than progesterone levels. Progesterone, a hormone that relaxes the uterus, remains stable in the blood while the estrogen levels rise (Challis, 1999; Cunningham, et al., 1997). Higher estrogen levels enhance uterine sensitivity to substances that stimulate uterine contractions, such as prostaglandins from the fetal membranes and oxytocin from the maternal posterior pituitary gland. Estrogens also increase the number of gap junctions, connections allowing the individual muscle cells of the uterus to contract as a coordinated unit (Guyton & Hall, 2000).
- One theory is that progesterone levels fall as labor approaches, but this has not been proved on a systemic level. However, progesterone levels may be lower at the local level of the uterus.
- An increase in prostaglandins produced by the decidua and the membranes may have a role in preparing the uterus for stimulation by oxytocin at term. Prostaglandins are secreted from the lower area of the fetal membranes (forebag) during labor and may reflect inflammation caused by contact with microorganisms from the woman's vagina.
- Increased secretion of oxytocin appears to maintain labor once it has begun. Oxytocin does not appear to start labor but may play a part in labor's initiation in conjunction with other substances. Evidence of fetal oxytocin secretion also exists (Challis, 1999; Cunningham, et al., 1997).
- Oxytocin receptors increase markedly as labor begins; the increase continues during labor and peaks at delivery. Oxytocin will have little effect on the uterine muscle if the receptors have not developed.
- A fetal role in the initiation of labor appears likely. The fetal membranes release prostaglandin in high concentrations during labor. In addition to fetal oxytocin secretion, large quantities of cortisol are secreted by the fetal adrenal, possibly acting as a uterine stimulant (Guyton & Hall, 2000).
- Stretching, pressure, and irritation of the uterus and cervix increase as the fetus reaches term size. During the rest of pregnancy, the uterus has not reacted to stretching by contracting as smooth muscle normally does. A feedback loop is probably responsible for labor contractions at term—the fetal head stretches the cervix, causing the fundus of the uterus to contract, pushing the fetal head against the cervix, and causing more fundal contractions. Cervical stretching also causes secretion of oxytocin (Guyton & Hall, 2000).

Premonitory Signs

Braxton Hicks Contractions

Contractions occurring throughout pregnancy are irregular and mild. As term approaches, contractions become more noticeable and even painful. Parous women often describe more uterine activity preceding labor than do nulliparous women.

Increased perception of Braxton Hicks contractions often makes sleep difficult at the end of pregnancy. The contractions may become regular at times, only to decrease spontaneously. Because contractions are often uncomfortable but sometimes regular, the woman may be confused about whether labor has really begun.

Lightening

As the fetus descends toward the pelvic inlet ("dropping"), the woman notices that she breathes more easily because upward pressure on her diaphragm is reduced. However, increased pressure on her bladder causes her to urinate more frequently. Pressure of the fetal head in the pelvis also may cause leg cramps and edema. Lightening is most noticeable in nulliparas and occurs about 2 to 3 weeks before the onset of labor.

Increased Vaginal Mucous Secretions

An increase in clear and nonirritating vaginal secretions occurs as fetal pressure causes congestion of the vaginal mucosa. The woman may need to wear a perineal pad because of the quantity of mucus.

Cervical Ripening and Bloody Show

As full term nears, the cervix softens because of the effects of the hormone relaxin and increased water content. These changes (ripening) allow the cervix to yield more easily to the forces of labor contractions. As the fetal head descends with lightening, it puts pressure on the cervix, starting the process of effacement and dilation. Effacement and dilation cause expulsion of the mucus plug that sealed the cervix during pregnancy, rupturing small cervical capillaries in the process. Bloody show is a mixture of thick mucus and pink or dark brown blood. It may begin several days to a few weeks before the onset of labor, especially in the nulliparous woman, or it may not begin until labor starts.

CRITICAL THINKING EXERCISE

Alan Lindsey phones you as you are working in the birth unit of your hospital one night. He says, "My wife's baby is due. Heather has been having some contractions off and on all day, keeping her awake now. Should we come to the hospital?"

QUESTIONS:

1. Do you need any other information? If so, what information do you need? (Assume that your hospital has a protocol for telephone triage that allows nurses to answer and document similar phone inquiries.)
2. What should you tell Heather about her symptoms? What advice can you give her?

A recent vaginal examination or sexual intercourse also may result in small amounts of bloody show because it disrupts these small vessels. Bloody show increases during labor as the cervix completes dilation and effacement. Women who have previously had a vaginal birth often have less bloody show than nulliparas.

Energy Spurt

Some women have a sudden increase in energy, which is called "nesting." They should be cautioned to conserve their energy so that they are not exhausted when labor actually begins.

Weight Loss

A small weight loss of 1 to 3 lb may occur because the altered estrogen and progesterone ratio causes excretion of some of the extra fluid that accumulates during pregnancy.

True Labor and False Labor

False labor, also called *prodromal labor,* is common because the exact time of labor's onset is rarely known and usually is a gradual process. False labor often causes women to go to the birth center, thinking that labor has started, only to be disappointed when it has not. The term *false labor* is discouraging to women because they do not realize that these "false" contractions are preparation for true labor.

Several characteristics distinguish true labor from false labor: contractions, discomfort, and cervical change. The best distinction between true and false labor is that contractions of true labor cause progressive change in the cervix. An increase in effacement and dilation occurs with true labor contractions.

Some women experience membrane rupture as the first sign of labor's onset. If this occurs, the woman should go to the birth center for evaluation. Infection and compression of the fetal umbilical cord are possible complications.

Mechanisms of Labor

The mechanisms (cardinal movements) of labor occur as the fetus is moved through the pelvis during birth. The fetus undergoes several positional changes to adapt to the size and shape of the mother's pelvis at different levels (Figure 12-12). Although the mechanisms of labor are described separately in Figure 12-12, some occur concurrently. In a vertex presentation, the mechanisms include the following:

- Descent of the fetal presenting part through the true pelvis
- Engagement of the fetal presenting part as its widest diameter reaches the level of the ischial spines of the mother's pelvis
- Flexion of the fetal head so that the smallest head diameters pass through the pelvis
- Internal rotation to allow the largest fetal head diameters to match the largest maternal pelvic diameters
- Extension of the fetal head as the head passes beneath the mother's symphysis pubis
- External rotation of the fetal head, allowing the shoulders to rotate internally to best fit the mother's pelvis
- Expulsion of the fetal shoulders and fetal body

The mechanisms of labor are different in presentations other than the vertex, but the reason is the same: to effectively use the available space in the maternal pelvis.

Check Your Reading

11. What are some signs and symptoms that a woman might experience before labor begins?
12. What are the differences between true and false labor? Which difference is the most significant?
13. Why does the fetus enter the pelvis with the sagittal suture aligned with the transverse diameter of the woman's pelvic inlet?
14. Why does the fetal head turn during labor until the sagittal suture aligns with the anteroposterior diameter of the mother's pelvic outlet?

WOMEN WANT TO KNOW *How to Know Whether Labor Is "Real"*

True labor differs from false labor in three categories.

False Labor	True Labor
CONTRACTIONS	
Are inconsistent in frequency, duration, and intensity	Usually have a consistent pattern of increasing frequency, duration, and intensity
Do not change or may decrease with activity (such as walking)	Tend to increase with walking
DISCOMFORT	
Is felt in the abdomen and groin	Begins in lower back and gradually sweeps around to lower abdomen
May be more annoying than truly painful	May persist as back pain in some women; often resembles menstrual cramps during early labor
CERVIX	
Does not significantly change in effacement or dilation	Includes progressive effacement and dilation (most important characteristic)

Stages and Phases of Labor

Labor is divided into four stages. Each stage has its unique qualities (Table 12-1). This chapter describes typical physiologic characteristics and maternal behaviors in the average woman. Individual women vary in their labor patterns and responses to labor. The woman who chooses an epidural block is likely to behave differently because of this method of pain management.

First Stage

Cervical effacement and dilation occur in the first stage, or stage of dilation. It begins with the onset of true labor contractions and ends with complete dilation (10 cm) and effacement (100%) of the cervix.

CRITICAL THINKING EXERCISE

After examining a woman in labor with her first baby, the nurse-midwife gives you the following information:

"Carmelita Saenz is 2 to 3 cm, 75%, and 0. The baby is vertex and ROP."

QUESTIONS:

What is the correct interpretation of this information? What behaviors would be expected for Mrs. Saenz at this time? What behaviors should suggest to you that she has begun making very rapid labor progress?

The first stage of labor is the longest for both nulliparous and parous women (Ross & Hobel, 1998; Bachman & Kendrick, 1996; Kilpatrick & Laros, 1989). The duration of first-stage labor averages 8 to 10 hours (range of 6 to 18 hours) for the nullipara and 6 to 7 hours (range of 2 to 10 hours) for the parous woman. The rate of labor progress is also important. When the active phase begins, the cervix of the nullipara usually dilates about 1.2 cm per hour and that of the multipara dilates about 1.5 cm per hour. Labor progress is often plotted on a labor progress graph called a *Friedman curve* (Figure 12-13).

First-stage labor differs from the other stages because it has three phases: latent (early), active, and transition. Each phase is characterized by changing maternal behaviors. These behaviors vary with the woman's preparation, use of coping skills, and use of medication.

Latent Phase. The latent phase is the first 3 cm of cervical dilation. Its length varies among women but averages 8.6 hours for the nullipara and 5.3 hours for the multipara (Bachman & Kendrick, 1996). Latent labor may be quite long and much of it may pass unnoticed by the pregnant woman. Cervical effacement and fetal positional change occur during latent phase, preparing for the more rapid changes of active labor.

Contractions gradually increase in frequency, duration, and intensity. The interval between contractions shortens until contractions are about 5 minutes apart as the woman progresses to the active phase. Duration increases to 30 to 40 seconds by the end of the latent phase. Intensity begins with mild contractions, during which the contracting uterus can be easily indented with the fingertips, and progresses to moderate contractions, during which the uterine muscle is indented with more difficulty. The contractions gradually build to their peak intensity and remain at the peak briefly before diminishing.

During latent labor the woman may notice discomfort in her back with each contraction. As labor progresses, back discomfort encircles the lower abdomen with each contraction. Many women describe the dis-

Text continued on p. 278

DESCENT, ENGAGEMENT, AND FLEXION

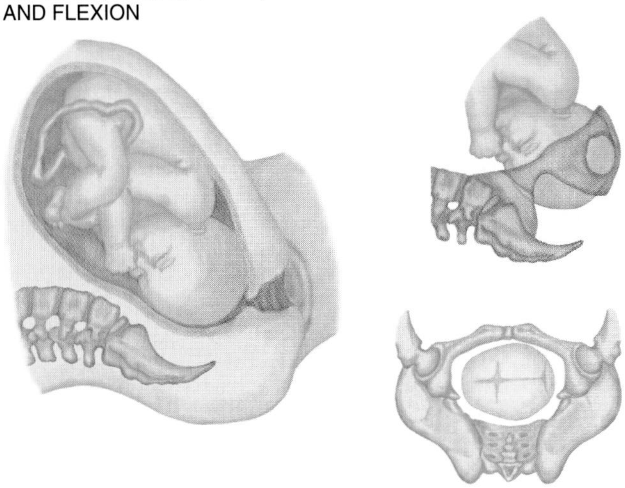

Descent of the fetus is a mechanism of labor that accompanies all the others. Without descent, none of the mechanisms will occur.

STATION

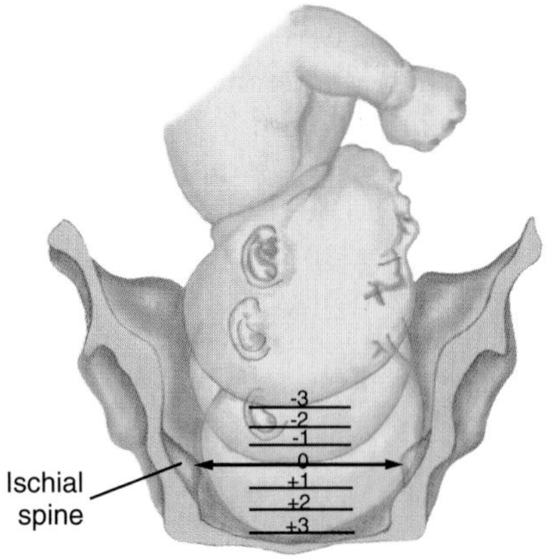

Station describes the descent of the fetal presenting part in relation to the level of the ischial spines. The level of the ischial spines is a zero station. Other stations are described with numbers representing the approximate number of centimeters above (negative numbers) or below (positive numbers) the ischial spines. As the fetus descends through the pelvis, the station changes from higher negative numbers (–3, –2, –1) to zero to higher positive numbers (+1, +2, +3, etc.) Sometimes the terms *floating* or *ballottable* may describe a fetal presenting part that is so high that it is easily displaced upward during abdominal or vaginal examination, similar to tossing a ball upward.

Engagement

Engagement occurs when the largest diameter of the fetal presenting part (normally the head) has passed the pelvic inlet and entered the pelvic cavity. Engagement is presumed to have occurred when the station of the presenting part is zero or lower. Engagement often takes place before onset of labor in nulliparous women. In many parous women and in some nulliparas, it does not occur until after labor begins.

Flexion

As the fetus descends, the fetal head is flexed further as it meets resistance from the soft tissues of the pelvis. Head flexion presents the smallest anteroposterior diameter (suboccipito-bregmatic) to the pelvis.

INTERNAL ROTATION

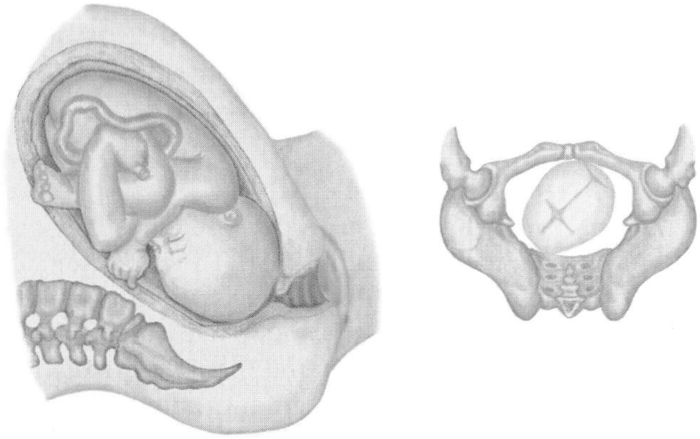

The fetus enters the pelvic inlet with the sagittal suture in a transverse or oblique orientation to the maternal pelvis because that is the widest inlet diameter. Internal rotation allows the longest fetal head diameter (the anteroposterior) to conform to the longest diameter of the maternal pelvis as the fetus descends.

The longest pelvic outlet diameter is the anteroposterior. As the head descends to the level of the ischial spines, it gradually turns so that the fetal occiput is in the anterior of the pelvis (OA position, directly under the maternal symphysis pubis). When internal rotation is complete, the sagittal suture is oriented in the anteroposterior pelvic diameter (OA). Less commonly, the head may turn posteriorly so that the occiput is directed toward the mother's sacrum (OP).

FIGURE 12-12 Mechanisms (cardinal movements) of labor.

EXTENSION

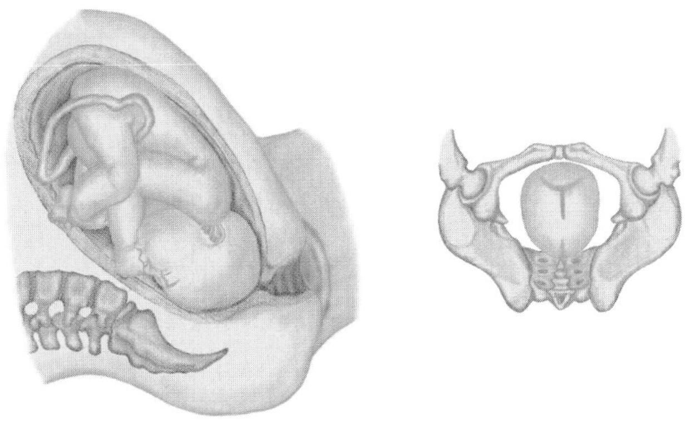

Extension beginning (internal rotation complete)

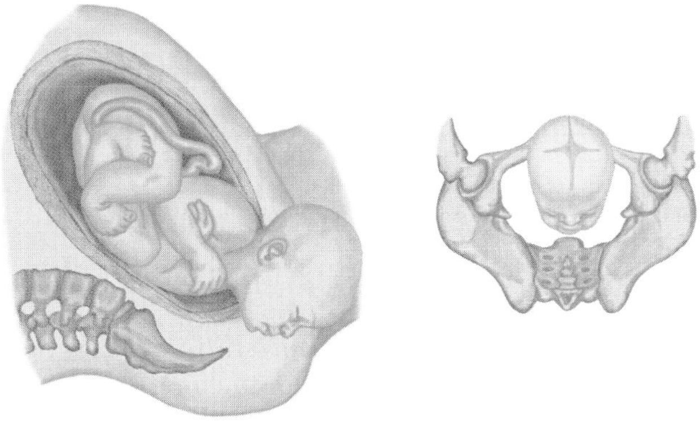

Extension complete

Because the true pelvis is shaped like a curved cylinder, the fetal head is directed posteriorly toward the rectum as it begins its descent. To negotiate the curve of the pelvis, the fetal head must change from an attitude of flexion to one of extension.

While still in flexion, the fetal head meets resistance from the tissues of the pelvic floor. At the same time, the fetal neck stops under the symphysis, which acts as a pivot. The combination of resistance from the pelvic floor and the pivoting action of the symphysis causes the fetal head to swing anteriorly, or extend, with each maternal pushing effort. The head is born in extension, with the occiput sliding under the symphysis and the face directed toward the rectum. The fetal brow, nose, and chin slide over the perineum as the head is born.

EXTERNAL ROTATION

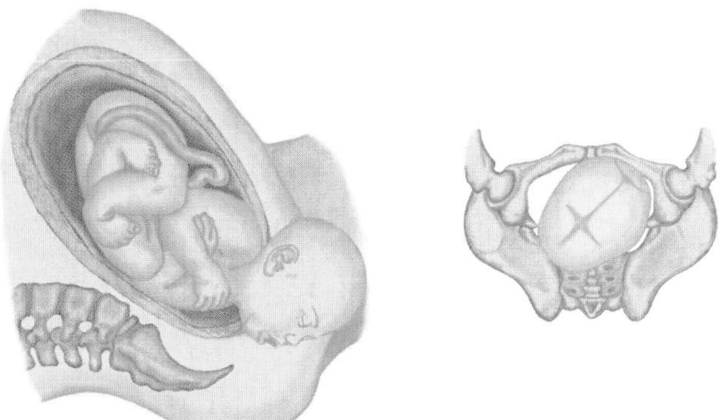

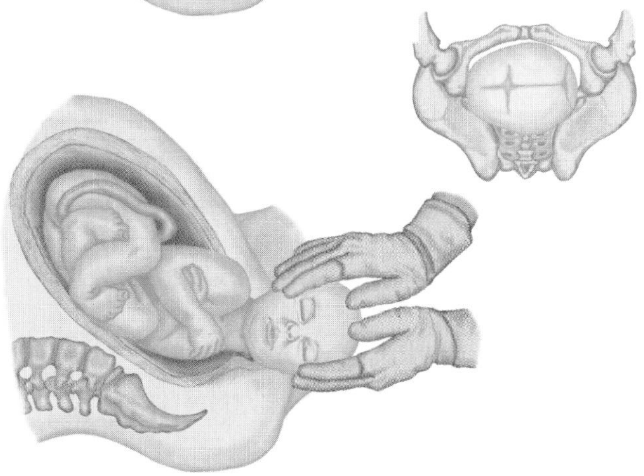

When the head is born with the occiput directed anteriorly, the shoulders must rotate internally so that they align with the anteroposterior diameter of the pelvis.

After the head is born, it spontaneously turns to the same side as it was in utero as it realigns with the shoulders and back (through a process called *restitution*). The head then turns further to that side in external rotation as the shoulders internally rotate and are positioned with their transverse diameter in the anteroposterior diameter of the pelvic outlet. External rotation of the head accompanies internal rotation of the shoulders.

EXPULSION

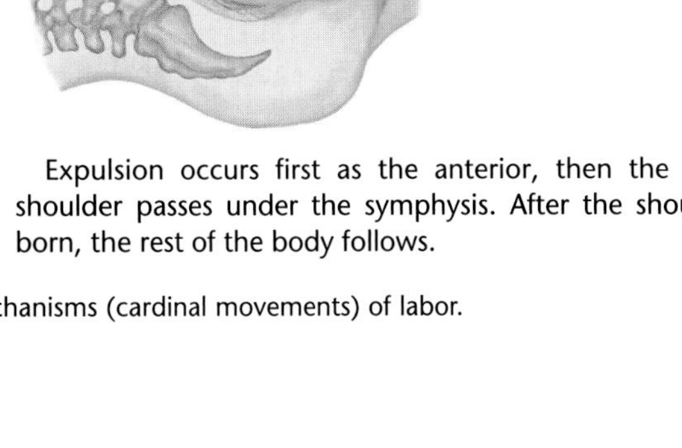

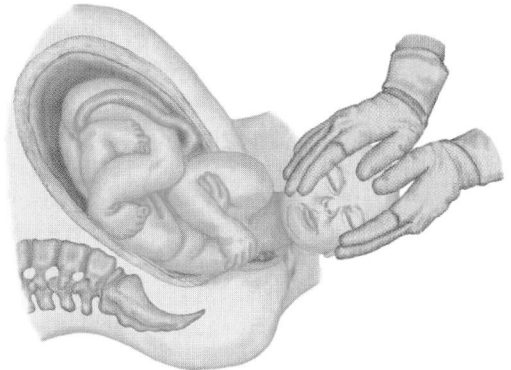

Expulsion occurs first as the anterior, then the posterior, shoulder passes under the symphysis. After the shoulders are born, the rest of the body follows.

FIGURE 12-12, cont'd Mechanisms (cardinal movements) of labor.

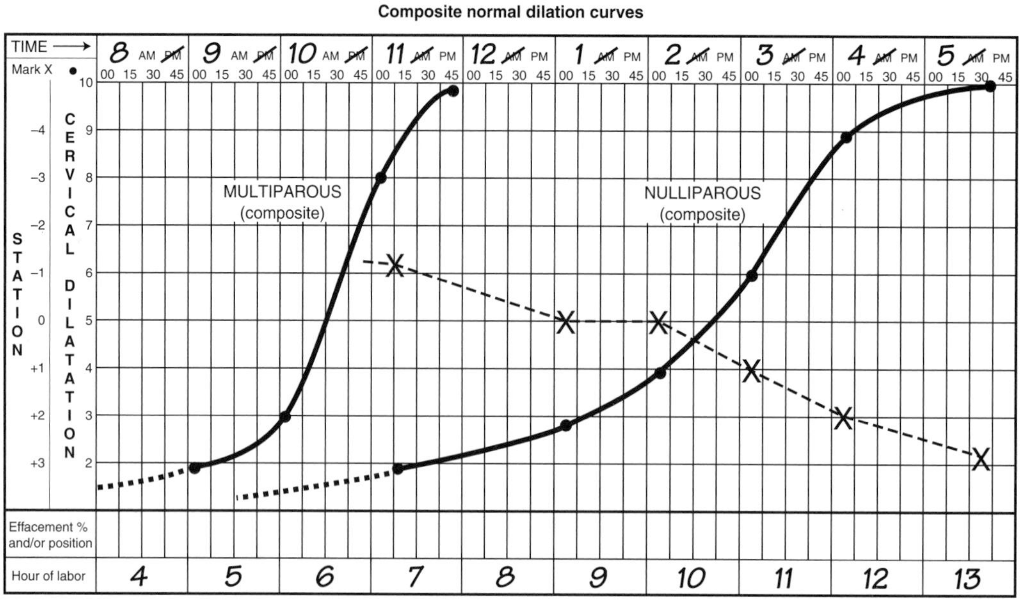

FIGURE 12-13 A labor curve, often called a *Friedman curve,* may be used to identify whether a woman's cervical dilation is progressing at the expected rate. The symbol for station *(X)* is added to the right curve.

comfort as similar to menstrual cramps, especially during early labor.

The woman is usually sociable, excited, and cooperative. She is anxious as she realizes that these contractions are not Braxton-Hicks contractions but the "real thing," yet she is usually relieved that her pregnancy is finally about to end.

Active Phase. The active phase of labor is so named because the pace of labor increases. The cervix dilates from 4 to 7 cm and at a more rapid rate than in the latent phase. The duration averages 4.6 hours for the nullipara and 2.4 hours for the multipara (Bachman & Kendrick, 1996). Effacement of the cervix is completed. The fetus descends in the pelvis, and internal rotation begins.

Contractions average 2 to 5 minutes apart, with a duration of about 40 to 60 seconds, and ranging from moderate to strong intensity. Active labor contractions reach their peak intensity quickly and stay at the peak longer than during the latent phase.

As contractions intensify, discomfort also increases. The site of discomfort during the active phase is similar to that of the latent phase.

The woman's behavior changes. She becomes more anxious and may feel helpless as the contractions intensify. The sociability that characterized early labor is gone and is replaced with a serious, inward focus. She is unlikely to initiate interactions unless she has specific requests. Her behaviors are typical of a person concentrating intently on a demanding task. Women who choose to take pain medication and regional analgesia usually do so during this phase. The nurse helps the woman maintain her concentration, supports her coping techniques, and helps her find alternatives for methods that do not work for her.

Transition Phase. The cervix dilates from 8 to 10 cm, and the fetus descends further into the pelvis. Bloody show often increases with the completion of cervical dilation. Transition is a short but intense phase, averaging 3.6 hours in the nullipara and having a variable length in the multipara (Bachman & Kendrick, 1996).

Contractions are very strong. They may be as frequent as 1.5 to 2 minutes apart, and their duration is 60 to 90 seconds. Strong contractions combined with fetal descent may cause the woman to have an urge to push and bear down during contractions. If she pushes before cervical dilation is complete, the cervix may swell and labor may be prolonged. Leg tremors, nausea, and vomiting are common.

The woman who does not choose epidural analgesia often finds the transition phase to be the most difficult part of her labor. She may be irritable and lose control. Her partner may be confused because actions that were helpful just a short time ago now bother her. The nurse can encourage the woman and her support person that the end of labor is near and help them use coping techniques most effectively. If premature bearing down is a problem, the nurse can help her blow outward with each breath until the urge passes.

Second Stage

The second stage (expulsion) begins with complete (10 cm) dilation and full (100%) effacement of the cervix and ends with the birth of the baby. The duration averages 30 minutes to 3 hours in nulliparas and 5 to 30 minutes in parous women.

Contractions may diminish slightly or even pause briefly as the second stage begins. They are still strong, about 2 to 3 minutes apart, with a duration of 40 to 60 seconds.

As the fetus descends, pressure of the presenting part on the rectum and the pelvic floor causes an involuntary pushing response in the mother. She may say that she needs to have a bowel movement or say "the baby's coming" or "I have to push." Her voluntary pushing efforts augment involuntary uterine contractions. As the fetus descends low in the pelvis and the vulva distends with the crowning of the fetal head, she may feel a sensation of stretching or splitting even if no trauma occurs.

The woman often regains a feeling of control during the second stage of labor. Contractions are strong, but she may feel more in control and know that she is doing something to complete the process by pushing with them. The word *labor* aptly describes the second stage. The woman exerts intense physical effort to push her baby out. Between contractions, she may be oblivious to her surroundings and appear asleep. She feels tremendous relief and excitement as the second stage ends with the birth of the baby.

Third Stage

The third (placental) stage begins with the birth of the baby and ends with the expulsion of the placenta (Figure 12-14). This stage is the shortest, lasting up to 30 minutes, with an average length of 5 to 10 minutes. No difference in duration exists between nulliparas and parous women.

When the infant is born, the uterine cavity becomes much smaller. The reduced size decreases the size of the placenta site, causing it to separate from the uterine wall. Four signs suggest placenta separation:

- The uterus has a spheric shape.
- The uterus rises upward in the abdomen as the placenta descends into the vagina and pushes the fundus upward.
- The cord descends further from the vagina.
- A gush of blood appears as blood trapped behind the placenta is released.

The placenta may be expelled in one of two ways. In the more common Schultze mechanism, the placenta is expelled with the shiny fetal side presenting first (see Figure 12-14, *B*). In the Duncan mechanism, which is less common, the rough maternal side is presenting (see Figure 12-14, *A*).

The uterus must contract firmly and remain contracted after the placenta is expelled to compress open vessels at the implantation site. Inadequate uterine contraction after birth may result in hemorrhage.

Pain during the third stage of labor results from uterine contractions and brief stretching of the cervix as the placenta passes through it.

Fourth Stage

The fourth stage of labor is the stage of physical recovery for the mother and infant. It lasts from the delivery of the placenta through the first 1 to 4 hours after birth.

Immediately after birth, the firmly contracted uterus can be palpated through the abdominal wall as a firm, rounded mass about 10 to 15 cm (4 to 6 inches) in diameter at or below the level of the umbilicus. Uterine size varies with the size of the infant and parity of the mother and is larger when the infant is large or the mother is a multipara. A full bladder or blood clot in the uterus interferes with uterine contraction, increasing blood loss. A soft (boggy) uterus and increasing uterine size are associated with postpartum hemorrhage because large blood vessels at the placenta site are not compressed (see Chapter 28).

The vaginal drainage after childbirth is called *lochia.* The three stages are lochia rubra, lochia serosa, and lochia alba (see p. 427). Lochia rubra, consisting mostly of blood, is present in the fourth stage of labor.

Many women are chilled after birth. The cause of this reaction is unknown but probably relates to the sudden decrease in effort, loss of the heat produced by the fetus, decrease in intraabdominal pressure, and fetal blood cells entering the maternal circulation. The chill lasts for about 20 minutes and subsides spontaneously. A warm blanket, a hot drink, or soup may help shorten the chill and make the woman more comfortable.

Discomfort during the fourth stage usually results from birth trauma and afterpains. Localized discomfort from birth trauma such as lacerations, an episiotomy, edema, or a hematoma is evident as the effects of local and regional anesthetics diminish. Ice packs on the perineum limit this edema and hematoma formation.

Afterpains are intermittent uterine contractions occurring after birth as the uterus begins to return to the prepregnancy state. The discomfort is similar to menstrual cramps. Afterpains are more common in multiparas, women who breastfeed, women who have large babies or other uterine overdistention during pregnancy, and cases involving interference with uterine contraction because of a full bladder or blood clot that remains in the uterus.

The mother is simultaneously excited and tired after birth. She may be exhausted but too excited to rest. The fourth stage of labor is an ideal time for bonding of the new family because the interest of both the parents and the newborn is high. It is the best time to initiate breastfeeding if no maternal and infant problems are present. The baby is alert and seeks eye contact with the new parents, giving powerful reinforcement for the parents' attachment to their newborn.

Table 12-1
CHARACTERISTICS OF NORMAL LABOR

	First Stage	Second Stage	Third Stage	Fourth Stage
WORK ACCOMPLISHED				
	Effacement and dilation of cervix	Expulsion of fetus	Separation of placenta	Physical recovery and bonding with newborn
FORCES				
	Uterine contractions	Uterine contractions and voluntary bearing-down efforts	Uterine contractions	Uterine contraction to control bleeding from placenta site
AVERAGE DURATION				
• NULLIPARA	8- to 10-hour total duration (range of 6 to 18 hours); average 1 cm/hr dilation	Average of 50 minutes (range of 30 minutes to 3 hours)	Average of 5 to 10 minutes or up to 30 minutes for unassisted placental separation	1 to 4 hours after birth
• MULTIPARA	6 to 7 hours (range of 2 to 10 hours); average of 1.2 cm/hr dilation	Average of 20 minutes (range of 5 to 30 minutes)	Same as for nullipara	Same as for nullipara
CERVICAL DILATION				
	Latent phase: 0 to 3 cm; active phase: 4 to 7 cm; transition phase: 8 to 10 cm	10 cm (complete dilation)	Not applicable	Not applicable
UTERINE CONTRACTIONS				
	Latent phase: initially mild and infrequent contractions, progression to moderate strength every 5 minutes with a regular pattern, 30 to 40 seconds' duration by end of latent phase Active phase: increase in frequency, duration, and intensity until every 2 to 5 minutes, 40 to 60 seconds, and moderate to strong intensity Transition phase: strong contractions every 1.5 to 2 minutes, 60 seconds	Strong contractions every 2 to 3 minutes with 40 to 60 seconds' duration; slightly less intensity than during transition phase of first stage; possible brief pause as second stage begins	Firmly contracted	Firmly contracted, approximately at or just below the umbilicus
DISCOMFORT				
	Often beginning with a low backache and sensations similar to those of menstrual cramps; gradual sweep of back discomfort to the lower abdomen, intensification as labor progresses	Urge to push or bear down with contractions, which becomes stronger as fetus descends; stretching or splitting sensation because of distention of vagina and vulva unless epidural block modifies this sensation	Little discomfort; sometimes slight cramp as placenta is passed	Variable discomfort; afterpains common in multigravidas and women with large babies; noticeable perineal discomfort as anesthesia wears off
MATERNAL BEHAVIORS				
	Sociable, excited, and somewhat anxious feelings during early labor; inward focused as labor intensifies; possible loss of control during transition	Intense concentration on pushing with contractions; oblivion to surroundings and appearance of dozing between contractions	Excitement and relief after baby's birth; great fatigue and possible crying	Fatigue and possible difficulty resting because of excitement; eagerness to become acquainted with her newborn

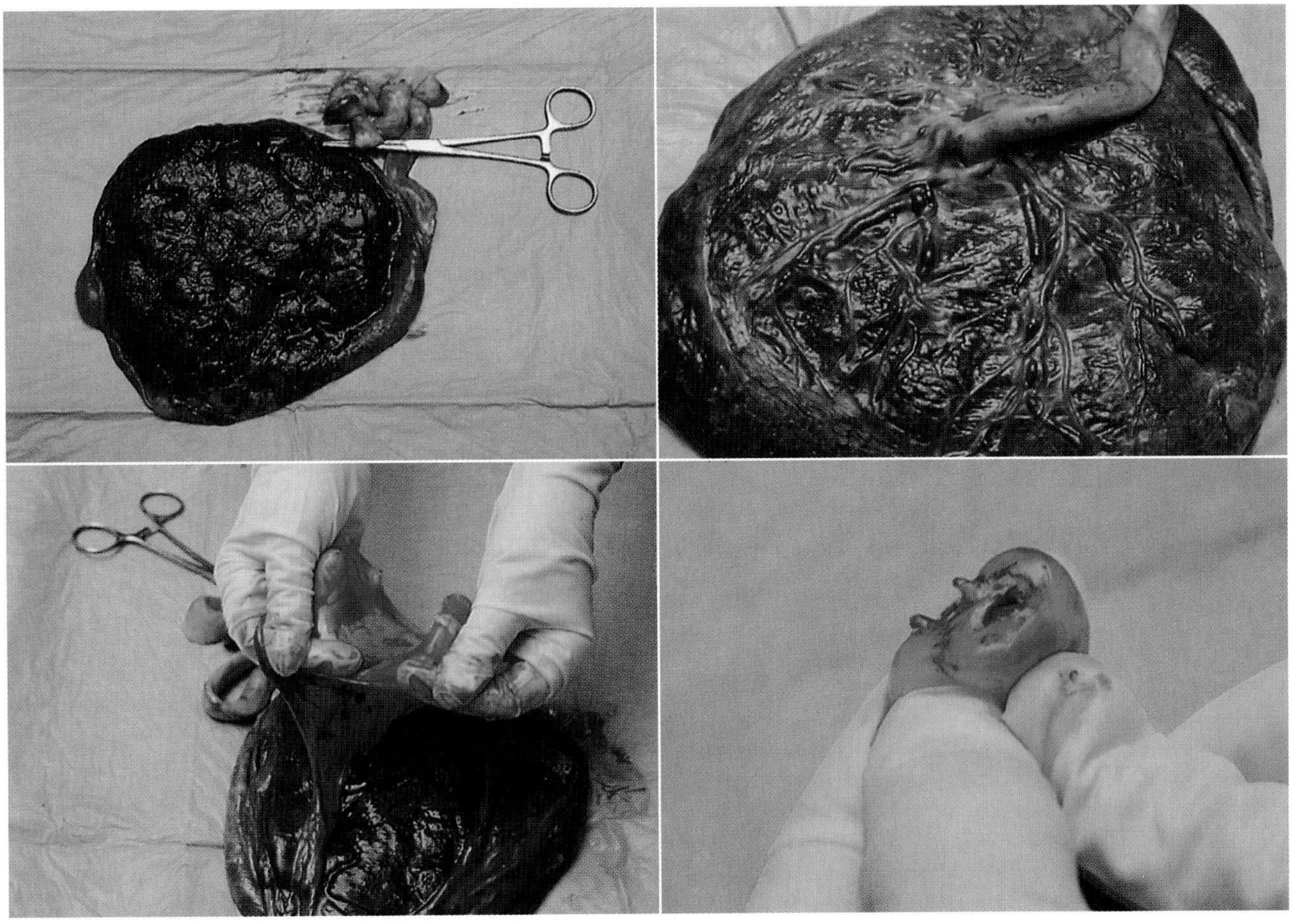

FIGURE 12-14 **A,** Maternal side of the placenta. **B,** Fetal side of the placenta. **C,** Separating membranes. **D,** Umbilical cord vessels, two arteries, and one vein.

Check Your Reading

15. How do maternal behaviors change during each phase of first-stage labor and the second stage?
16. What are typical characteristics of contractions during each phase of first-stage and second-stage labor?
17. What four signs may indicate that the placenta has separated?
18. What complications may occur if the uterus does not contract firmly and remain contracted after the placenta is expelled?

Duration of Labor

The total duration of labor is significantly different for women who have never given birth and those who have previously given birth vaginally. The parous woman usually delivers more quickly than the nulliparous woman. However, women are individuals. Some nulliparas progress through labor quickly, whereas labor for some parous women resembles that of women who have never given birth. A woman who experienced a long labor with her first child may not have a long labor with every baby. If she has a history of rapid labor, however, later births are often rapid as well.

Because vaginal birth after cesarean (VBAC) is common, a parous woman may have had no vaginal births. In this situation, the woman is likely to have a labor more like that of the nullipara, particularly if she did not labor before her previous cesarean birth.

SUMMARY CONCEPTS

- Labor contractions are intermittent, which allows oxygen, nutrients, and waste products to be exchanged between maternal and fetal circulations during the interval between contractions.
- The upper uterus contracts actively during labor, maintaining tension to pull the more passive lower uterus and cervix over the fetal presenting part. These actions bring about cervical effacement and dilation.

- Maternal vital signs are best assessed between contractions because slight alterations in the woman's blood pressure and pulse may occur during a contraction.
- Hyperventilation may occur if the woman breathes deeply and rapidly. Its manifestations include tingling of the hands and feet, numbness, and dizziness.
- The fetal heart rate and rhythm respond rapidly to events occurring during labor.
- Several occurrences during late pregnancy and labor aid the newborn in making adaptations to extrauterine life: reduced production of fetal lung fluid and increased absorption of lung fluid into the interstitium of the fetal lungs, expulsion of fluid from upper airways during the compression forces of labor, and increased catecholamine secretion by the fetal adrenals to stimulate cardiac contraction and breathing, speed clearance of remaining lung fluid, and aid in temperature regulation.
- Four interrelated components affecting the process of birth are the powers, passage, passenger, and psyche. Presentation and position further describe the relation of the fetus (passenger) to the maternal pelvis.
- The mechanisms of labor favor the most efficient passage of the fetus through the mother's pelvis.
- The exact reasons for the beginning of labor are unknown, but several maternal and fetal factors seem to have a role. These include fetal adrenal gland production of cortisol, changes in the ratio of estrogen to progesterone production so that estrogen is higher than progesterone, increased uterine oxytocin receptors and gap junctions, and stretching of the uterus and cervix.
- As labor approaches, the woman may notice one or more premonitory signs preceding its onset: increase in frequency and intensity of Braxton Hicks contractions, lightening, increased vaginal secretions, bloody show, a spurt of energy, and weight loss.
- The conclusive difference between true labor and false labor is that progressive effacement and dilation of the cervix occurs with true labor.
- The four stages and phases of labor are characterized by different physiologic events and maternal behaviors: first stage, cervical dilation and effacement; second stage, expulsion of the fetus; third stage, expulsion of the placenta; and fourth stage, maternal physiologic stabilization and parent-infant bonding.
- Normal labor is characterized by consistent progression of uterine contractions, cervical dilation and effacement, and fetal descent.

ANSWERS TO CRITICAL THINKING EXERCISE, P. 274

1. You need to speak directly to Heather rather than Alan because she is the one who is pregnant and having the symptoms. You need to know which baby this is for her (gravida and para), her due date, whether her membranes have ruptured, and the characteristics of her contractions (for example, frequency, duration, intensity, and effect of activity). After you gather assessment data, you learn that Heather's first baby is due the following week, she has had no leaking of fluid from her vagina, and her baby has been normally active. She says, "My contractions are coming every 2 to 10 minutes, and most of them last about 30 seconds. They didn't bother me much until I tried to go to sleep, but now they are keeping me awake. I'm so tired of all this!"
2. Heather's symptoms sound like those of false labor: irregular contractions that are mild, fairly short, and more annoying than truly painful. Although not harmful, these frequent contractions in late pregnancy interrupt the woman's rest. You should tell Heather that these contractions do not sound like true labor, then review with her the typical signs and symptoms of true labor. Advise her to come to the hospital if her contractions intensify and become more consistent, her "water breaks," the baby seems to move less, or she has vaginal bleeding other than bloody show. Remind her that labor cannot be diagnosed over the phone, and tell her to come to the hospital if she has any continuing concerns.

ANSWERS TO CRITICAL THINKING EXERCISE, P. 275

Mrs. Saenz's cervix is about 2 to 3 cm dilated and has effaced to about one fourth of its original length (now about 0.5 cm long, or 75% effaced). The widest part of the fetal head (the biparietal diameter) is at the level of the ischial spines (0 station) and has passed the pelvic inlet.

The vertex presentation means that the fetal head is well flexed, which is most favorable because it presents the smallest anteroposterior diameter to the maternal pelvis. ROP means that the fetal occiput is in Mrs. Saenz's right posterior pelvic quadrant.

During the early part of first-stage labor (latent phase), you would expect Mrs. Saenz to be relatively comfortable. She may be visiting with her husband and other family members and friends. Although rapid progress is unlikely with the first baby, be alert to behaviors such as sudden grunting and bearing down (usually accompanied by a marked increase in bloody show), crying out "the baby's coming" or "I've got to push," and inability to maintain control with techniques that have previously been helpful. Summon an experienced nurse or her nurse-midwife by using the call signal at once if any of these behaviors occur. Do not leave her unattended in case the baby arrives unexpectedly.

REFERENCES & READINGS

Albers, L.L., Schiff, M., & Gorwoda, J.G. (1996). The length of active labor in normal pregnancies. *Obstetrics and Gynecology,* 87(3), 355-359.

American Academy of Pediatrics (AAP) & American College of Obstetricians and Gynecologists (ACOG). (1997). *Guidelines for perinatal care* (4th ed.). Elk Grove Village, IL: Author.

Association of Women's Health, Obstetric, and Neonatal Nurses (AWHONN). (1997). *Fetal heart monitoring: Principles & practices.* Dubuque, IA: Kendall/Hunt Publishing.

Bachman, J., & Kendrick, J.M. (1996). Childbirth. In K.R. Simpson & P.A. Creehan, *AWHONN'S perinatal nursing* (pp. 151-186). Philadelphia: J.B. Lippincott.

Blackburn, S.T., & Loper, D.L. (1992). *Maternal, fetal, and neonatal physiology: A clinical perspective.* Philadelphia: W.B. Saunders.

Bernstein, D. (2000). The fetal to neonatal circulatory transition. In R.E. Behrman, R.M. Kliegman, & H.B. Jenson (Eds.), *Nelson textbook of pediatrics* (16th ed., pp.1341-1343). Philadelphia: W.B. Saunders.

Bowes, W.A. (1999). Clinical aspects of normal and abnormal labor. In R.K. Creasy & R. Resnik (Eds.), *Maternal-fetal medicine: Principles and practice* (4th ed., pp. 541-568). Philadelphia: W.B. Saunders.

Cady, R.F. (1999). Telephone triage and the office nurse. In D.M. Rostant & R.F. Cady (Eds.) *Liability issues in perinatal nursing* (pp. 149-155). Philadelphia: Lippincott.

Challis, J.R.G. (1999). Characteristics of parturition. In R.K. Creasy & R. Resnik (Eds.), *Maternal-fetal medicine: Principles and practice* (4th ed., pp. 484-497). Philadelphia: W.B. Saunders.

Creehan, P.A. (1996). Pain relief and comfort measures during labor. In K.R. Simpson & P.A. Creehan, *AWHONN'S perinatal nursing* (pp. 227-245). Philadelphia: J.B. Lippincott.

Cunningham, F.G., MacDonald, P.C., Gant, N.F., Leveno, K.J., Gilstrap, L.C., Hankins, G.D.V., & Clark, S.L. (1997). *Williams obstetrics* (20th ed.). Norwalk, CT: Appleton & Lange.

Curtin, S.C., & Mathews, T.J. (2000). U.S. obstetric procedures, 1998. *Birth, 27*(2), 136-138.

Duffy, T.P. (1999). Hematologic aspects of pregnancy. In G.N. Burrow and T.P. Duffy (Eds.), *Medical complications during pregnancy* (5th ed., pp. 79-95). Philadelphia: W.B. Saunders.

Farrington, P.F. & Ward, K. (1999). Normal labor, delivery, and puerperium. In *Danforth's obstetrics and gynecology* (8th ed., pp. 91-109). Philadelphia: Lippincott Williams & Wilkins.

Feinstein, N.F., Sprague, A., & Trépanier, M.J. (2000). *Fetal heart rate auscultation.* Washington, D.C.: Association of Women's Health, Obstetric, and Gynecologic Nurses.

Feinstein, N.F. (2000). Fetal heart rate auscultation: Current and future practice. *Journal of Obstetric, Gynecologic, & Neonatal Nursing, 29*(3), 306-315.

Guyton, A.C., & Hall, J.C. (2000). *Textbook of medical physiology* (10th ed.). Philadelphia: W.B. Saunders.

Haddad, G.G., & Pérez Fontán, J.J. (2000). Development of the respiratory system. In R.E. Behrman, R.M. Kliegman, & H.B. Jenson (Eds.), *Nelson textbook of pediatrics* (16th ed., pp. 1235-1237). Philadelphia: W.B. Saunders.

Hayashi, R.H., & Bashore, R.A. (1998). Gap junctions, uterine contractility, and dystocia. In N.F. Hacker & J.G. Moore (Eds.). *Essentials of obstetrics and gynecology* (3rd ed., pp. 301-311). Philadelphia: W.B. Saunders.

Jobe, A.H. (1999). Fetal lung development, tests for maturation, induction of maturation, and treatment. In R.K. Creasy & R. Resnik (Eds.), *Maternal-fetal medicine: Principles and practice* (4th ed., pp. 404-422). Philadelphia: W.B. Saunders.

Kilpatrick, S.J., & Laros, R.K. (1989). Characteristics of normal labor. *Obstetrics and Gynecology, 74*(1), 85-87.

Lavender, T., Walkinshaw, & Walton, I. (1999). A prospective study of women's views of factors contributing to a positive birth experience. *Midwifery,* 15(1), 40-46.

Leveno, K.J. (2000). Normal and abnormal labor. In S.B. Ransom, M.P. Dombrowski, S.G. McNeeley, K.S. Moghissi, & A.R. Munkarah (Eds.), *Practical strategies in obstetrics and gynecology* (pp. 267-275). Philadelphia: W.B. Saunders.

Manogin, T.W., Bechtel, G.A., & Rami, J.S. (2000). Caring behaviors by nurses: Women's perceptions during childbirth. *Journal of Obstetric, Gynecologic, & Neonatal Nursing,* 29(2), 153-157.

Mayberry, L.J., Wood, S.H., Strange, L.B., Lee, L., Heisler, D.R., & Nielsen-Smith, K. (2000). *AWHONN Symposium: Second stage labor management: Promotion of evidence-based practice and a collaborative approach to patient care.* Washington, D.C.: AWHONN.

Menihan, C.A. (1996). Intrapartum fetal monitoring. In K.R. Simpson & P.A. Creehan, *AWHONN'S perinatal nursing* (pp. 187-225). Philadelphia: J.B. Lippincott.

Murray, M. (1997). *Antepartal and intrapartal fetal monitoring.* Albuquerque, NM: Learning Resources, Inc.

National Institute of Child Health and Human Development Research Planning Workshop. (1977). Electronic fetal heart rate monitoring: Research guidelines for interpretation. *Journal of Obstetric, Gynecologic, & Neonatal Nursing,* 26(6), 635-640.

Nichols, F.H., & Gennaro, S. (2000). The childbirth experience. In F.H. Nichols & S.S. Humenick (Eds.), *Childbirth education: Practice, research and theory* (2nd ed., pp. 66-83). Philadelphia: W.B. Saunders.

Parer, J.T. (1999). Fetal heart rate. In R.K. Creasy & R. Resnik (Eds.), *Maternal-fetal medicine: Principles and practice* (4th ed., pp. 270-299). Philadelphia: W.B. Saunders.

Resnik, R. (1999). Anatomic alterations in the reproductive tract. In R.K. Creasy & R. Resnik (Eds.), *Maternal-fetal medicine: Principles and practice* (4th ed., pp. 90-94). Philadelphia: W.B. Saunders.

Ross, M.G., & Hobel, C.J. (1998). Normal labor, delivery, and the puerperium. In N.F. Hacker & J.G. Moore (Eds.), *Essentials of obstetrics and gynecology* (3rd ed., pp. 150-167). Philadelphia: W.B. Saunders.

Sandelowski, M. (2000). Retrofitting technology to nursing: The case of electronic fetal monitoring. *Journal of Obstetric, Gynecologic, & Neonatal Nursing,* 29(3), 316-324.

Simpson, K.R. (1999). Routine care during labor and birth: Is this really how we want to practice perinatal nursing, or are we ready to advocate for childbearing women and insist on evidence-based care? *Mother-Baby Journal,* 4(4), 5-7.

Stables, D. (1999). *Physiology in childbearing.* Edinburgh: Baillière Tindall.

Steer, P.J., & Danielian, P.J. (1999). Fetal distress in labor. In D.K. James, P.J. Steer, C.P. Weiner, & B. Gonik (Eds.), *High risk pregnancy: Management options* (pp. 1121-1149). London: W.B. Saunders Ltd.

Stoll, B.J., & Kliegman, R.M. (2000). Delivery room emergencies. In R.E. Behrman, R.M. Kliegman, & H.B. Jenson (Eds.), *Nelson textbook of pediatrics* (16th ed., pp. 495-496). Philadelphia: W.B. Saunders.

VanDinter, M.C. (2000). Telephone triage: The rules are changing. *MCN: American Journal of Maternal/Child Nursing,* 25(4), 187-191.

VandeVusse, L. (1999). The essential forces of labor revisited: 13 Ps reported in womens' stories. *American Journal of Maternal/Child Nursing,* 24(4), 176-189.

Winslow, E.H., & Crenshaw, J. (2000). Managing labor: Does walking help or hurt? *American Journal of Nursing,* 100(3), 50-51.

The Childbirth Story

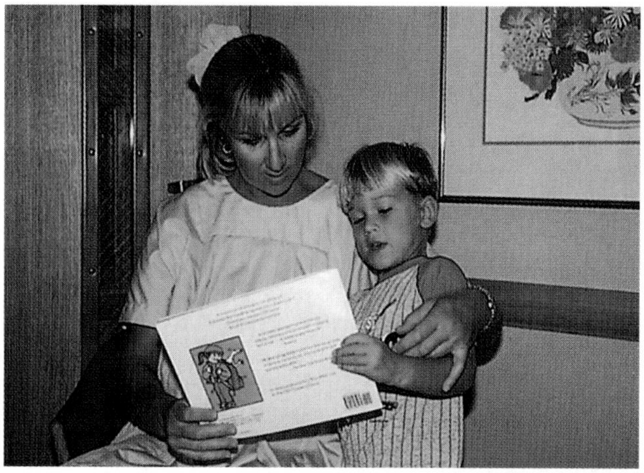

1. Shari, in early labor with her second child, spends time with her 5-year-old son, Adam, in the labor-delivery-recovery room.

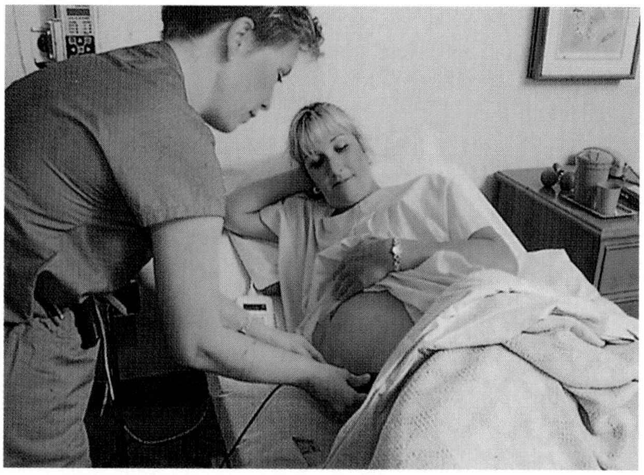

2. The nurse frequently assesses the condition of both the mother and the fetus. Here she listens to the fetal heart rate.

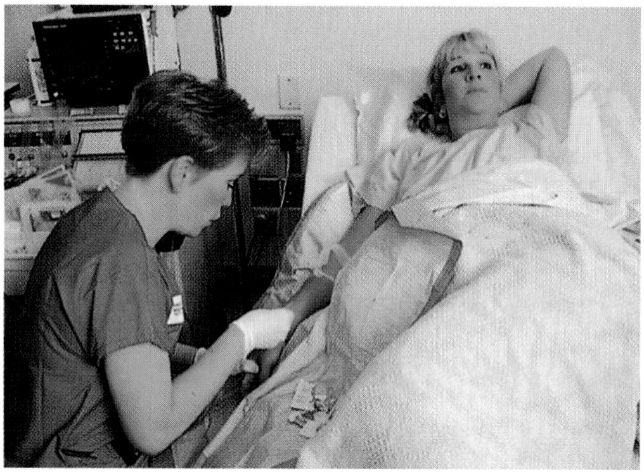

3. Although IV fluids are not always necessary, most physicians order them to prevent dehydration and for access to a vein in case an emergency develops.

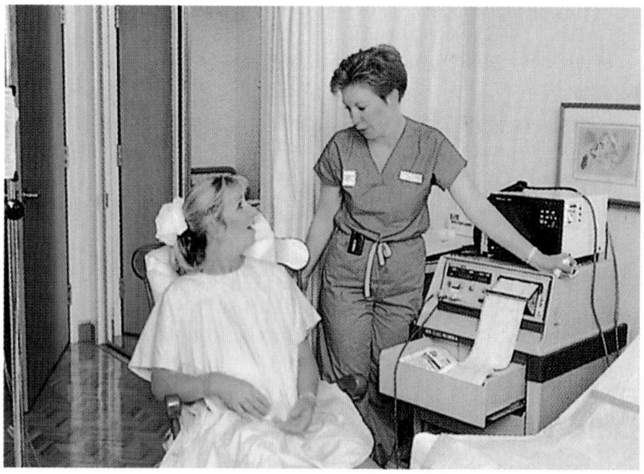

4. The nurse establishes a relationship of trust by assisting Shari into a comfortable position and explaining information obtained by electronic fetal monitoring.

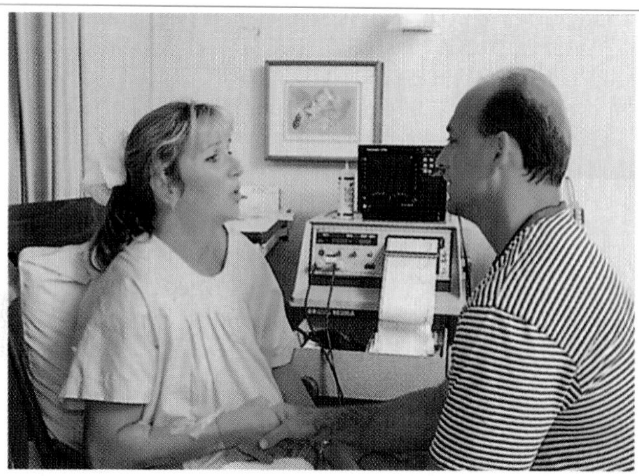

5. Shari plans a childbirth without anesthesia. Darren, the father, uses skills learned in childbirth education classes to help her cope with discomfort.

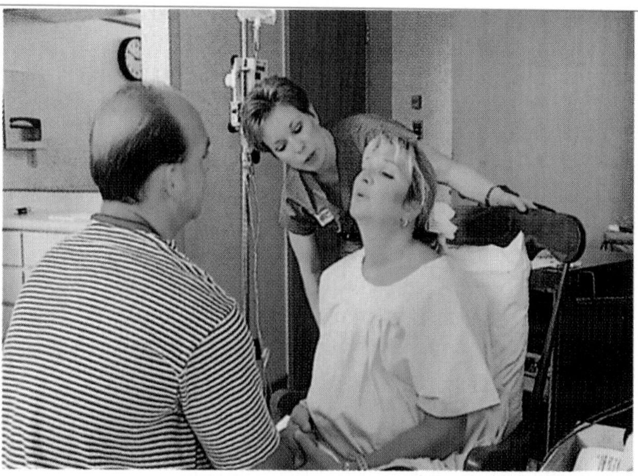

6. Maintaining control is more difficult for Shari as the contractions become stronger. The nurse praises the couple's efforts and reviews measures to reduce discomfort.

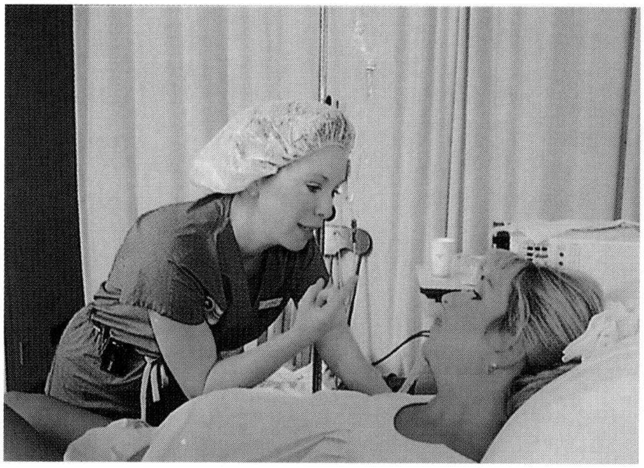

7. During transition, often the most difficult phase of labor, the nurse remains in close contact with Shari and assists her through each contraction.

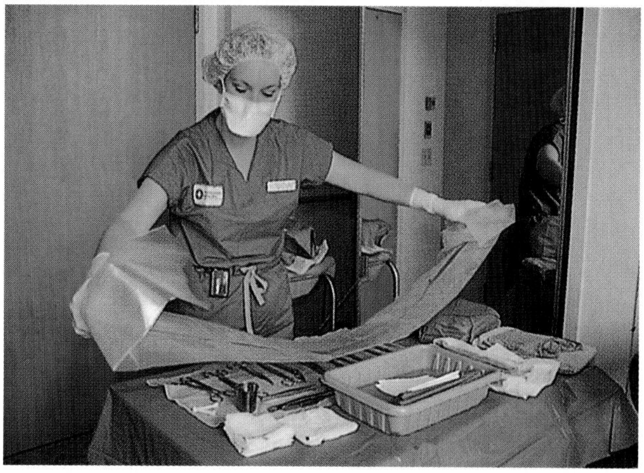

8. The nurse prepares the sterile instruments that will be used during the birth.

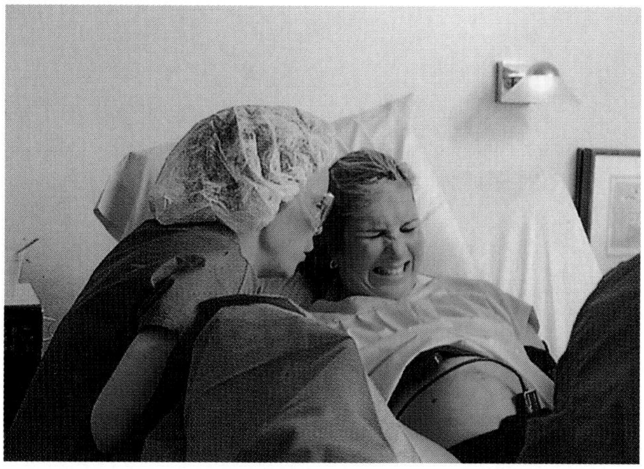

9. As birth approaches, the nurse positions Shari and assists her to push with each contraction. Note that the nurse now wears protective glasses.

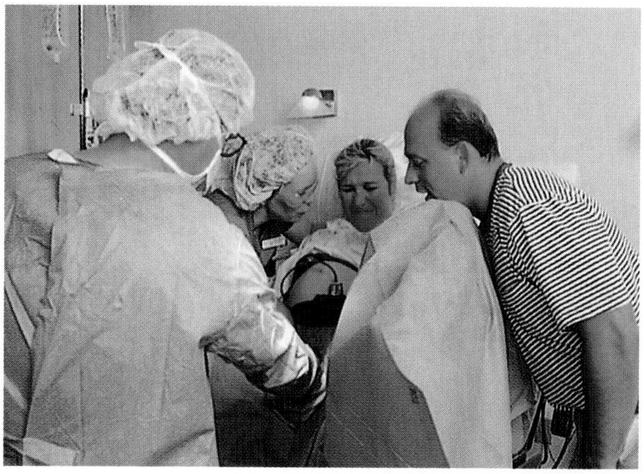

10. The nurse also encourages Darren to remain in close contact with the mother and continue to participate in the birth.

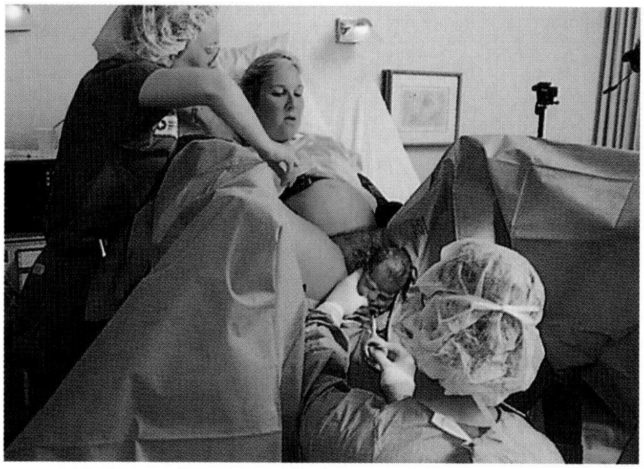

11. The physician suctions secretions from the nose and mouth of the infant when the head is delivered.

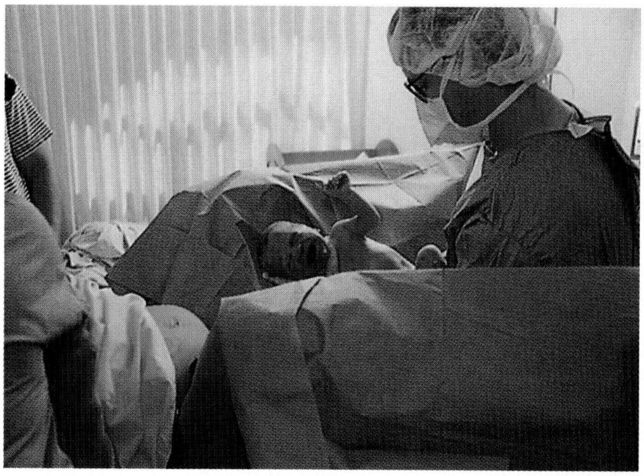

12. The physician holds the infant so that the parents can get their first look at their newborn son.

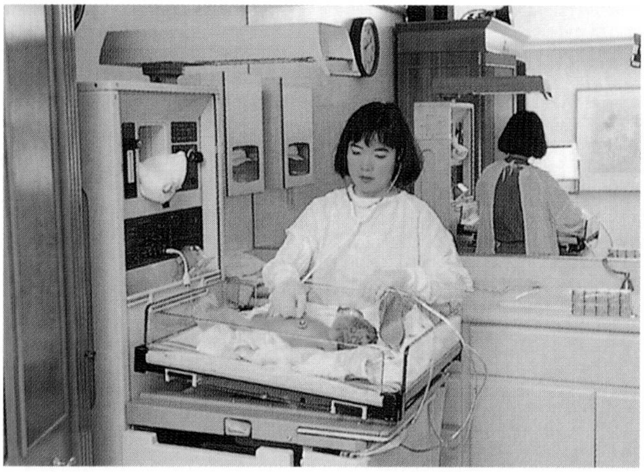

13. A nurse counts the apical pulse and observes the newborn's pink color, which makes the administration of oxygen unnecessary.

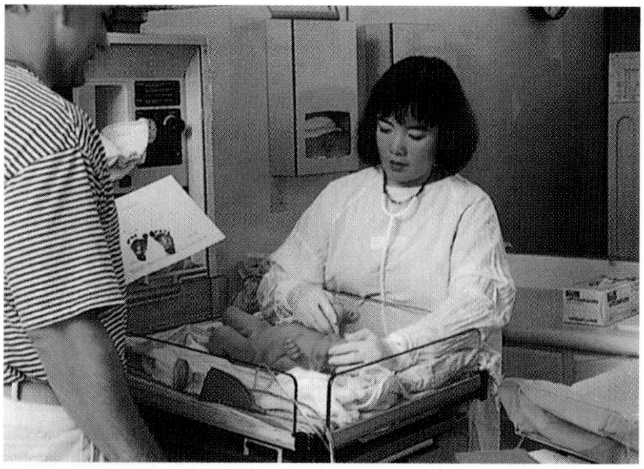

14. The father observes as the nurse suctions secretions from the newborn's nose and mouth and completes identification procedures such as footprinting.

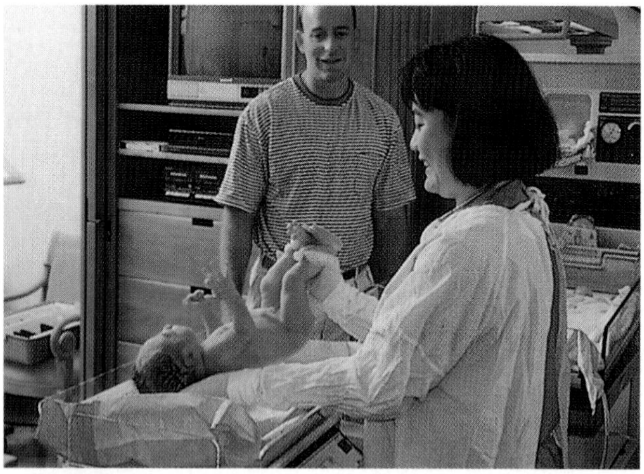

15. Darren is an interested observer as the nurse weighs and measures the newborn.

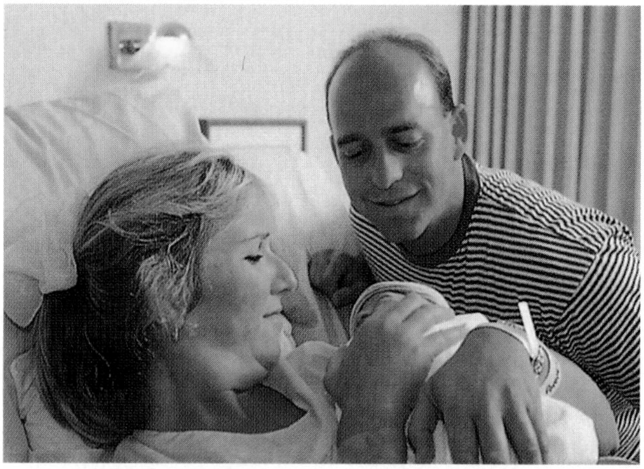

16. Nurses are aware of the importance of early contact, and as soon as possible after birth, the mother, father, and newborn are brought together.

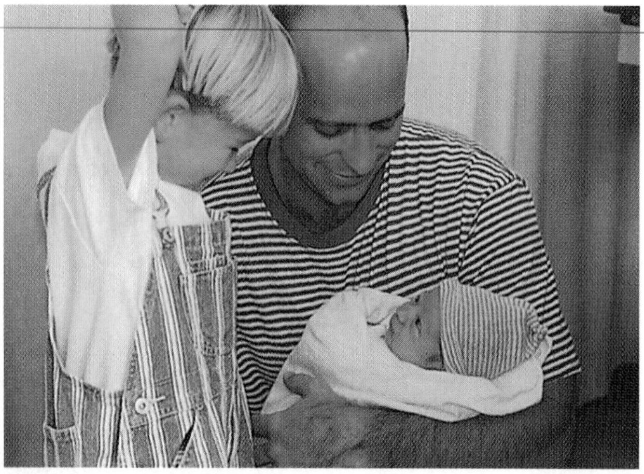

17. Although Adam was not present at the birth, within a short time he meets the wide-eyed baby who gazes intently at his older brother.

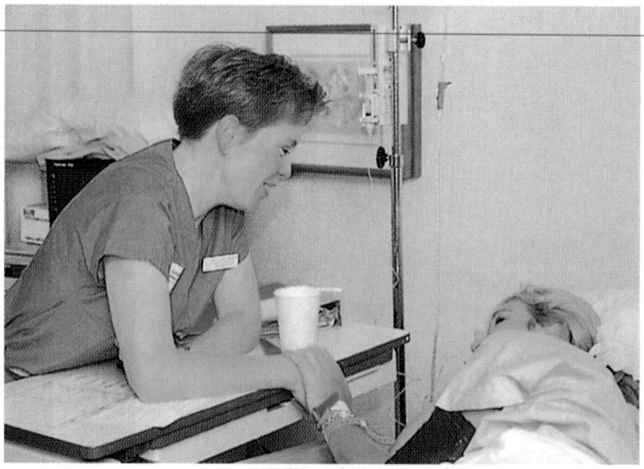

18. Shari and the nurse demonstrate the mutual regard that developed as they shared the intense experience of labor and birth.

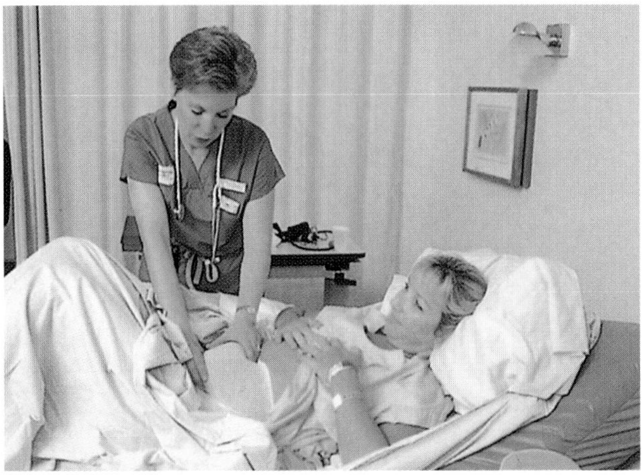

19. The nurse palpates the fundus frequently during the first hour after childbirth to confirm that the uterus is firmly contracted and thus prevent excessive bleeding.

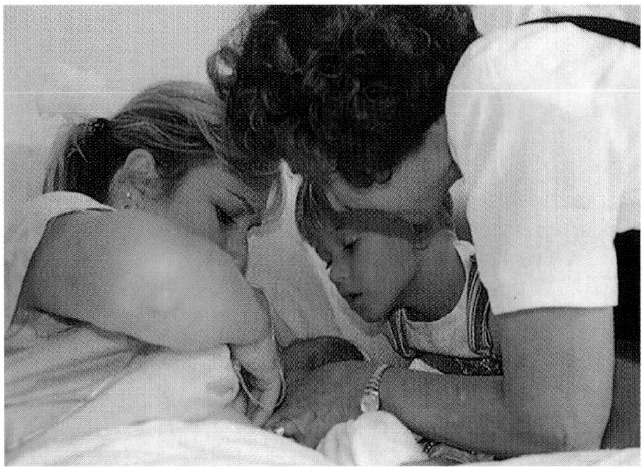

20. Adam watches intently as his mother and grandmother put the baby to breast for the first time.

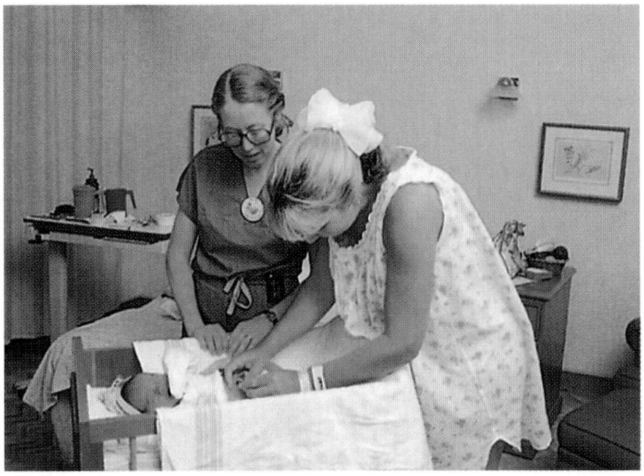

21. Nurse must teach mothers how to care for themselves and their infants within a very short time. Here the nurse instructs Shari in cord care.

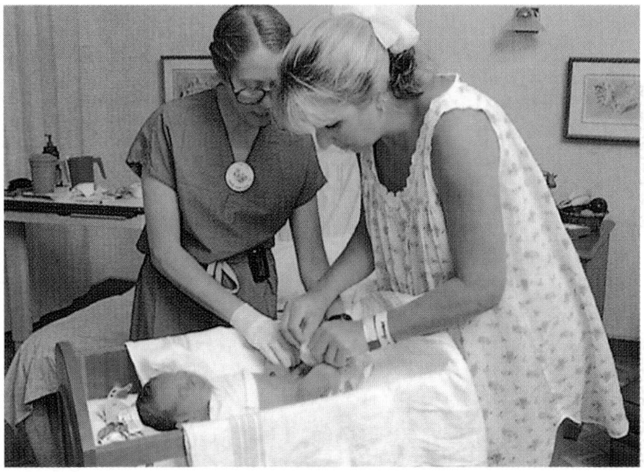

22. Shari gains confidence in circumcision care when the nurse allows for a return demonstration.

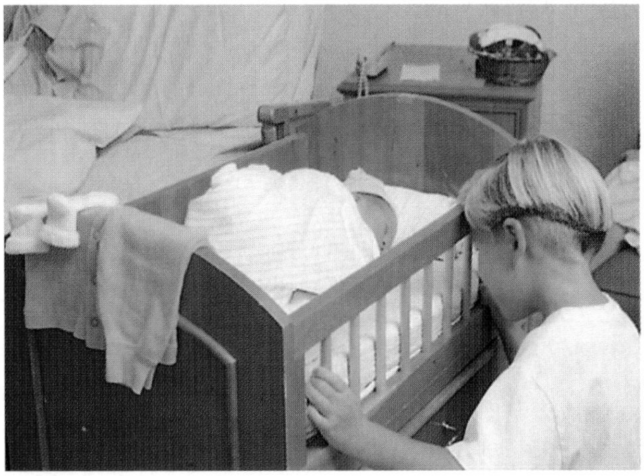

23. Adam peeks at his baby brother while the family receives additional instructions.

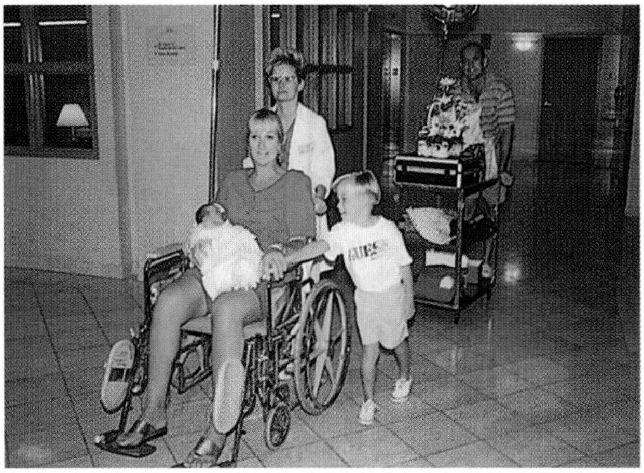

24. Twenty-four hours after her admission, Shari and the infant are discharged from the postpartum unit.

13

Nursing Care during Labor and Birth

OBJECTIVES

1. Analyze issues that may face the new nurse who cares for women during the intrapartum period.
2. Explain teaching guidelines for going to the hospital or birth center.
3. Describe admission and continuing intrapartum nursing assessments.
4. Describe common nursing procedures used when caring for women during the intrapartum period.
5. Identify nursing priorities when assisting the woman to give birth under emergency circumstances.
6. Relate therapeutic communication skills to care of the intrapartum woman and her significant others.
7. Apply the nursing process to care of the woman experiencing false labor.
8. Apply the nursing process to care of the woman and her significant others during the intrapartum period.

DEFINITIONS

Abortion A pregnancy that ends before 20 weeks' gestation, either spontaneously (miscarriage) or electively.

Amniotomy Artificial rupture of the membranes (amniotic sac).

Caput Succedaneum Area of edema over the presenting part of the fetus or newborn that results from pressure against the cervix (usually called *caput*).

Crowning Appearance of the fetal scalp or presenting part at the vaginal opening.

EDD Abbreviation for estimated date of delivery; also may be abbreviated *EDB* (estimated date of birth).

Episiotomy Surgical incision of the perineum to enlarge the vaginal opening.

DEFINITIONS—cont'd

FERNING Microscopic appearance of amniotic fluid resembling fern leaves when the fluid is allowed to dry on a microscope slide; also called *fern test.*

GRAVIDA A pregnant woman; also refers to a woman's total number of pregnancies, including the one in progress, if applicable.

MULTIPARA A woman who has given birth after two or more pregnancies of at least 20 weeks' gestation; also informally used to describe a pregnant woman before the birth of her second child.

NITRAZINE PAPER Paper used to test pH; helps determine whether the amniotic sac has ruptured.

NUCHAL CORD Umbilical cord around the fetal neck.

NULLIPARA A woman who has not completed a pregnancy to at least 20 weeks' gestation.

PARA A woman who has given birth after a pregnancy of at least 20 weeks' gestation; also designates the number of a woman's pregnancies that have ended after at least 20 weeks' gestation.

PRIMIPARA A woman who has given birth after a pregnancy of at least 20 weeks' gestation; also used informally to describe a pregnant woman before the birth of her first child.

Care of the woman and her family during labor and birth is a rewarding yet demanding specialty within nursing. The birth of a baby is more than a physical event. Birth has deep personal and social significance for the family, whose roles and relationships are forever altered by this event.

The nurse must support natural physical processes, promote a meaningful experience for the family, and be alert for complications. Additionally, the nurse cares for two clients, one of whom—the fetus—cannot be observed directly.

The intrapartum area is typically a happy place, and good outcomes for mothers and infants are usual. Most women have accepted their pregnancies and look forward to meeting their infants. Yet some women have had stressful pregnancies because of physical and substance abuse, economic hardship, unsupportive personal relationships, and other problems (see Chapter 24).

ISSUES FOR NEW NURSES

New nurses and nursing students often approach care of laboring women with apprehension. They may face several common issues when caring for families during birth.

Pain Associated with Birth

Working with people in pain is difficult, and most nurses feel compelled to relieve pain promptly. Yet pain is expected in labor and cannot always be eliminated. Some women choose to have unmedicated births. Helping the woman manage the pain of birth is a critical part of nursing care, and many nurses find this to be the most creative aspect of their roles.

Inexperience and Negative Experiences

The nurse who has never given birth may feel inadequate to care for laboring women, even though the same nurse rarely thinks that experiencing a fracture is necessary to care for someone with that problem. Nursing skills needed by the intrapartum nurse are basic: observation, critical thinking, problem solving, therapeutic communication, comfort promotion, empathy, and common sense.

Nurses also may be anxious because of their own difficult experiences during birth. They must be careful not to convey negative attitudes to the laboring woman and her significant other.

Unpredictability

Birth follows its own timetable, even with efforts to "manage" it. Some nurses find the uncertain nature of an intrapartum area troubling, whereas others find it exciting. Some occurrences cannot be predicted or explained. In addition, the number of women needing care and the levels of care they require can change quickly.

Intimacy

The intimate nature of intrapartum care and its sexual overtones make some nurses uncomfortable. They may feel that they are intruding on a private time.

The male nurse often is anxious about this aspect of intrapartum care. Although he may have cared for other female clients, his care rarely has been so focused on the reproductive system. He often wonders whether a woman's male partner will accept him as a care provider.

Both male nurses and female nurses should maintain professional conduct and take cues from the couple. If the couple wants privacy, the nurse should intervene only as needed to assess the woman and fetus. In more advanced labor, both partners often welcome the presence of a competent, caring nurse of either gender.

ADMISSION TO THE BIRTH CENTER

The Decision to Go to the Hospital or Birth Center

During the last trimester, the woman needs to know when she should go to the hospital or birth center. Factors to consider include:

- Number and duration of any previous labors
- Distance from the hospital
- Available transportation
- Child care needs

Women Want to Know: When to Go to the Hospital or Birth Center

These are guidelines for providing individualized instruction to women about when to enter the hospital or birth center.

Contractions—A pattern of increasing regularity, frequency, duration, and intensity.

- Nullipara—Regular contractions, 5 minutes apart, for 1 hour
- Multipara—Regular contractions, 10 minutes apart, for 1 hour

Ruptured membranes—A gush or trickle of fluid from the vagina should be evaluated, regardless of whether contractions are occurring.

Bleeding—Bright-red bleeding should be evaluated promptly. Normal bloody show is thicker, pink or dark red, and mixed with mucus.

Decreased fetal movement—If you notice a substantial decrease in the baby's movement, notify your physician or nurse-midwife or come to the labor unit.

Other concerns—These guidelines cannot cover all situations and do not replace specific instructions given to you by your birth attendant. Therefore please go to the hospital for evaluation of any concerns and feelings that something may be wrong.

Therapeutic Communication

Establishing a Therapeutic Relationship

Sandra Hall is a nursing student assigned to the intrapartum unit. A woman walks toward Sandra. The woman is leaning on a man and breathing rapidly. She says to Sandra, "I think I'm in labor, and my water broke on the way to the hospital."

Sandra: It sounds like today's the day! Let's find you a room.

Sandra asks the woman's name (Amy James) and that of her birth attendant (Donna Moore, CNM, a nurse-midwife) as they walk to a room.

Sandra: I'm Sandra Hall, a nursing student. What names do you want us to call each of you? *(Questioning for information. Shows respect by not assuming how the couple wants to be addressed.)*

Amy: I'm Amy, and my husband is Jeff.

Sandra: Is this your first baby, Amy, or have you had others? *(Questioning in a way that avoids yes or no answers.)*

Amy: It's my second, and the first took forever! I've been having contractions off and on since midnight, but they didn't get regular till about 6:00 this morning. They are coming every 3 minutes now and starting to hurt a lot.

Sandra helps Amy put a gown on and applies the external fetal monitor while they wait for the RN. She does not follow up on Amy's implied concern about having a long labor, however.

Amy: Oh no . . . the monitor . . .

Sandra: You have a problem about the monitor? *(Clarifying the nonspecific remark that Amy made about the monitor.)*

Amy: I hated having that thing on with my last baby. I had to lie the same way all the time or they couldn't hear the baby. I know it's best for the baby, though.

Sandra: You seem to have mixed feelings about the monitor. *(Reflecting what Amy seems to be feeling.)*

Amy: Yes, I didn't like it, but I do feel better knowing the baby's OK.

Sandra: We can usually find ways so it doesn't bother you so much. We don't want you to feel tied down because that will make you more uncomfortable. *(Giving information without promising that Amy will be totally comfortable with the external fetal monitor.)*

Sandra observes that Amy's contractions are every 3 minutes and strong. She finds an experienced nurse to help evaluate Amy. Sandra used critical thinking and wisely sought help from an experienced nurse because Amy seems to be in active labor and this is her second baby. The fact that Amy's first labor "took forever" does not necessarily mean that this labor will be long.

Nurses instruct women to distinguish between false and true labor. Nurses teach guidelines for going to the birth center and reinforce those given by the physician or nurse-midwife (Women Want to Know: When to Go to the Hospital or Birth Center). Not everyone has a typical labor, so a woman should be encouraged to go to the birth center if she is uncertain or has other concerns.

Nursing Responsibilities during Admission

The two nursing priorities when the woman arrives at the birth center are to: (1) establish a therapeutic relationship and (2) assess the condition of the mother and fetus.

Establishing a Therapeutic Relationship

The nurse must quickly establish a therapeutic relationship with the woman and her significant other. The woman's first impression influences her perception of the quality of her entire birth experience.

Making the Family Feel Welcome

A warm greeting makes the woman and her significant other feel valued. Even if the unit is busy, the nurse should communicate interest, friendliness, caring, and competence. People understand if the nurse is busy, but they do not understand rudeness and insensitivity to their needs.

When caring for a woman who has not had prenatal care or childbirth classes, which are behaviors that most nurses value, the nurse must not be judgmental in either words or actions. The woman's priorities and values may be different from those of the nurse, but she deserves the same respect, support, and care as the woman who made every preparation for her baby's birth.

Nurses often encounter women who speak a language other than English. Arranging for a culturally acceptable interpreter who is fluent in the woman's language makes the woman and her family feel welcome and promotes safety because it enhances understanding among the woman, her family, and the nurse.

Determining Family Expectations about Birth

Regardless of their number of children, women and their partners have expectations about the birth experience. The partners may have studied their options extensively and planned a birth that best fits their ideals. Those who have not made specific plans also have expectations shaped by contact with relatives and friends and previous birth experiences. A couple may want to repeat a previous satisfying experience or avoid repeating a poor experience. Sometimes one part of a past birth has negatively influenced the couple's impression of the entire experience.

Conveying Confidence

From the first encounter, the nurse should convey confidence and optimism in the woman's ability to give birth and the ability of her significant other to support her. Women having their first baby may be overwhelmed by the power of normal labor contractions. The nurse can reassure these women that intense contractions are normal in active labor while helping them manage contractions and watching for true problems.

Think about the different perspectives implied by the phrases *give birth* and *be delivered.* The woman who gives birth is an active and able participant; she is the principal action figure. However, the language of *be delivered* implies that the woman is passive. The nurse might ask "Who will attend you as you give birth?" rather than "Who will deliver your baby?"

Assigning a Primary Nurse

Having one nurse give care during all of labor is ideal but often unrealistic. However, changes in caregivers should be as limited as possible. The woman should know the name of and what to expect from each caregiver. For example, the primary nurse might explain the role of a nursing student in the woman's care. Common roles of nursing students in the intrapartum area include promoting comfort, giving emotional support, and helping the primary nurse observe for maternal and fetal problems.

Using Touch for Comfort

Touch can communicate acceptance and reassurance and provide physical and emotional comfort to many laboring women. Women who usually do not welcome touch may appreciate it during labor. Cultural norms and personal history influence a woman's comfort with touch from an unrelated person. The nurse should not assume that the woman desires touch but instead ask her if she welcomes or benefits from touch. As labor progresses, the woman's desire for touch may change, and touch may become irritating rather than comforting.

Respecting Cultural Values

Cultural beliefs and practices give structure, meaning, and richness to the birth experience. They influence the behavior of both the childbearing family and the professional staff. Most cultural groups have specific practices related to childbearing. The nurse should incorporate a family's beneficial and neutral cultural practices into care as much as possible.

People naturally believe that their own cultural values are best. The nurse should avoid using an attitude that is superior or diminishes the validity of another person's cultural beliefs. Trust in technology is a common value of many caregivers in the United States, but such reliance on technology is considered unnecessary, odd, and even harmful by many other cultures.

Check Your Reading

1. What communication skills can the nurse use to establish a therapeutic relationship when the woman and her family enter the hospital or birth center?
2. How can the nurse incorporate a couple's cultural practices into intrapartum care?

Making Assessments at the Time of Admission

A paper or computerized record of prenatal care is sent to the center where the woman plans to give birth and added to her chart when she is admitted. Admission information can be obtained from the prenatal record and verified or updated as needed. Women who have not had prenatal care need more extensive assessment by the nurse and physician (Table 13-1).

Focus Assessment

A focus assessment is performed before the broader database assessment in the intrapartum unit, opposite of the usual order. Assessment priorities are to deter-

Text continued on p. 298

Table 13-1

INTRAPARTUM ASSESSMENT GUIDE

Women who have had prenatal care have much of this information available on their prenatal records. The nurse must verify or update it on admission.

Assessment and Method (Selected Rationales)	Common Findings	Significant Findings and Nursing Action
INTERVIEW		
Purpose: To obtain information about the woman's pregnancy, labor, and conditions that may affect her care Is curtailed if she seems to be in advanced labor.		
Introduction: Introduce yourself and ask the woman how she wants to be addressed. Ask her which persons she wants to stay during the interview and assessment. (This maintains privacy while giving her control over those she wants to remain with her.)	Many women prefer to be addressed by their first names during labor, but checking with her is respectful.	The surname (family name) precedes the given name in some cultures. Clarify which name is used to properly address the woman and identify the mother and newborn.
Culture/language: If she is from another culture, identify her preferred language and what language(s) she speaks, reads, and verbally understands. (This enables the most accurate data collection.)	Common non-English languages of women in the United States are Spanish and Asian dialects. French is common in parts of Canada. The most common non-English language varies with location.	Try to secure an interpreter fluent in the woman's primary language. Determine whether some persons are not acceptable as interpreters (such as males, those from a group in conflict with her ethnic group). Note that family members may interpret selectively, adding or subtracting information as they see fit.
Communication: Ask the woman to tell you when she has a contraction, and pause during the interview and physical assessment. (This shows that the nurse is sensitive to her comfort and allows her to concentrate more fully on the information the nurse requests.)	Women in active labor have difficulty answering questions and cooperating with physical examinations while they are having contractions.	If contractions are very frequent, assess the woman's labor status promptly rather than continuing the interview. Ask only the most critical questions.
Nonverbal cues: Observe the woman's behaviors and interactions with her family and the nurse. (This permits estimation of her level of anxiety and identifies behaviors indicating that she should have a vaginal examination to determine whether birth is imminent.)	*Latent phase:* The woman is sociable and mildly anxious. *Active phase:* The woman concentrates intently with contractions and often uses prepared childbirth techniques. *Transition phase:* The woman may lose control or indicate that the baby is coming.	The unprepared or extremely anxious woman may breathe deeply and rapidly, displaying a tense facial and body posture during and between contractions. These behaviors suggest that birth is imminent: 1. Stating "the baby is coming" 2. Grunting 3. Bearing down with contractions 4. Sitting on one buttock Euphoria, combativeness, and sedation suggest recent illicit drug ingestion.
Reason for admission: "What brings you to the hospital/birth center today?" (An open-ended question promotes a more complete answer.)	Labor contractions at term are the usual reason. Observation for false labor is another common reason for admission.	Bleeding, preterm labor, and pain other than labor contractions should be reported to the physician or nurse-midwife promptly with other assessments.
Prenatal care: "Did you see a doctor or nurse-midwife during your pregnancy?" "Who is your doctor or nurse-midwife?" "How far along were you in your pregnancy when you saw the physician or nurse-midwife?" "When did you last see the physician or nurse-midwife?" (These questions enables location of prenatal record.)	Early and regular prenatal care promotes maternal and fetal health and early identification of complications at their most treatable stage.	No prenatal care or care that was irregular or begun in late pregnancy means that complications may not have been identified.

Table 13-1
INTRAPARTUM ASSESSMENT GUIDE—cont'd

Assessment and Method (Selected Rationales)	Common Findings	Significant Findings and Nursing Action
Estimated date of delivery (EDD): "When is your baby due?" (This determines if gestation is term.) "When did your last menstrual period begin?" (This estimates the EDD if the woman did not have prenatal care.)	*Term gestation (38 to 42 weeks):* The woman's gestation may have been confirmed or adjusted during pregnancy with an ultrasound or other clinical examination.	Gestations earlier than 38 weeks (preterm) or later than the end of the 42nd week (postterm) are associated with more fetal and neonatal problems.
Gravidity, parity, abortions: "How many times have you been pregnant?" "How many babies have you had?" "Were they full-term or premature?" "How many children are now living?" "Have you had any miscarriages or abortions?" "Were there any problems with your babies after they were born?" (These questions help estimate probable speed of labor and anticipate neonatal problems.)	Labor may be faster for the parous woman than for the nullipara. *Miscarriage* is a good word for the nurse to use to describe spontaneous abortion because lay people associate *abortion* with induced abortions.	Parity of 5 or more (grand multiparity) may be associated with placenta previa (placenta in lower uterus) and postpartum hemorrhage. Women who have had several spontaneous abortions or given birth to infants with abnormalities may face a higher risk for infants with birth defects.
Pregnancy history (identifies problems that may affect this birth)		
Present pregnancy: "Have you had any problems during this pregnancy, such as high blood pressure, diabetes, or bleeding?"	Complications are not expected.	Women with diabetes and hypertension may have poor placental blood flow, possibly resulting in fetal compromise. Some complications of past pregnancies, such as diabetes, may recur in another pregnancy.
Past pregnancies: "Were there any problems with your other pregnancy(ies)?" "Were your other babies born vaginally or by cesarean birth?"	Women who had previous cesarean birth(s) often have a trial of labor and vaginal birth (VBAC).	A woman who previously had a difficult labor may be more anxious than one who had an uncomplicated labor and birth.
Other: "Is there anything else you think we should know so that we can better care for you?"	This open-ended question gives the woman a chance to share information that may not be elicited by other questions.	
Labor status: "When did your contractions become regular?" "What time did you begin to think you might be in labor?" (These questions facilitate a more accurate estimation of the time labor began.)	Answers vary among women. Many women go to the birth facility when contractions first begin. Others wait until they are reasonably sure that they are really in labor.	Women who say they have been "in labor" for an unusual length of time ("for two days") probably had false labor. These women may be very tired from the annoying contractions.
Contractions: "How often are your contractions coming?" "How long do they last?" "Are they getting stronger?" "Tell me if you have a contraction while we are talking." (These questions allow the nurse to obtain the woman's subjective evaluation of her contractions and alert the nurse to palpate contractions that occur during the interview.)	Answers vary according to her stage and phase of labor. Labor contractions are usually regular and show a pattern of increasing frequency, duration, and intensity.	Irregular contractions and those that do not increase in frequency, duration, and intensity are more likely to represent false labor. Contractions occurring more frequently than every 2 minutes, with durations longer than 90 seconds, and with intervals of full uterine relaxation shorter than 60 seconds can reduce placental blood flow.
Membrane status: "Has your water broken?" "What time did it break?" "What did the fluid look like?" "About how much fluid did you lose—was it a big gush or a trickle?" (These questions alert the nurse of the need to verify whether the membranes have ruptured if it is not obvious and identify possible prolonged rupture of membranes.)	Most women go to the birth facility for evaluation soon after their membranes rupture. If a woman is not already in labor, contractions usually begin within a few hours after the membranes rupture at term.	If the woman's membranes have ruptured and she is not in labor or not at term, a vaginal examination may be deferred. Labor may be induced if she is at term with ruptured membranes.

Table 13-1
INTRAPARTUM ASSESSMENT GUIDE—cont'd

Assessment and Method (Selected Rationales)	Common Findings	Significant Findings and Nursing Action
Allergies: "Are you allergic to any foods or medicines?" "What kind of reaction do you have?" "Have you ever had a problem with anesthesia when you had dental work?" (These questions determine possible sensitivity to drugs that may be used.)	Record any known allergies to food and medication. As needed, describe their effects on the woman.	Allergy to seafood, iodized salt, and x-ray contrast media may indicate iodine allergy. Because iodine is used in many "prep" solutions, alternative solutions should be used. Allergy to dental anesthetics may indicate possible allergy to the drugs used for local and regional anesthetics. These drugs usually end in the suffix *-caine.*
Food intake: "When was the last time you had something to eat or drink?" "What did you have?" (These questions help evaluate the risk for regurgitation and aspiration of stomach contents.)	Record the time of the woman's last food intake and what she ate. Include both liquids and solids.	If the woman says she has not had intake for an unusual length of time, question her more closely: "Is there any food you may have forgotten, such as a snack or drink of water?"
Recent illness: "Have you been ill recently?" "What was the problem?" "What did you do for it?" "Have you been around anyone with a contagious illness recently?"	Most pregnant women are healthy. An occasional woman may have had a minor illness such as an upper respiratory infection.	Untreated urinary tract infections are associated with preterm labor. The woman who has had contact with someone having a communicable disease may become ill and possibly infect others in the facility.
Medications: "What drugs do you take that your doctor or nurse-midwife has prescribed?" "Do you use any over-the-counter drugs, including vitamins?" "Do you use any herbal or botanical medicines?" "What are the purposes of these drugs?" "I know this is uncomfortable for you to discuss, but we need to know about any illegal substances that you use to more safely care for you and your baby." (These questions permit evaluation of the woman's drug intake and encourage her to disclose nonprescribed use.)	Prenatal vitamins and iron are commonly prescribed. People often do not consider herbal and botanical substances to be drugs because they are "natural" and may not reveal that they use them unless specifically asked. Record all drugs the woman takes, including time and amount of last ingestion. Women who use illegal substances often conceal or diminish the extent of their use because they fear reprisals.	Drugs may interact with other medications given during labor, especially analgesics and anesthetics. Substance abuse is associated with complications for the mother and infant (see Chapter 24). If the woman discloses that she uses illegal drugs, ask her what kind and the last time she ingested them (the last time she "used"). A nonjudgmental approach is more likely to result in honest information.
Tobacco and alcohol: "Do you smoke or use tobacco in any other form? About how many cigarettes a day?" "Do you use alcohol? About how many drinks do you have each day (or week)?" (These questions evaluate use of these legal but harmful substances.)	As with substance abuse, women may underreport the extent of their uses of tobacco and alcohol.	Infants of heavy smokers are often smaller and may have reduced placental blood flow during labor. Infants of women who use alcohol may show fetal alcohol effects (see Chapter 24).
Birth plans (shows respect for the woman and her family as individuals and promotes achievement of their expectations; enables more culturally appropriate care)	A birth plan allows the woman and her significant other to put into words the elements that are most important to them in making the birth the experience they desire.	If the woman or couple has elements of their birth plan that are not compatible with the facility in some way, negotiation may be necessary to provide them with the most satisfactory service.
Coach or primary support person: "Who is the main person you want to be with you during labor? Ask how to address the support person, such as "Mr. Smith" or "Bob" or "Laura."	This person is usually the woman's husband or baby's father but may be her mother, sister, or a friend, especially if she is single.	The woman who has little or no support from significant others needs more nursing support during labor and after the birth. These clients may have problems with parent-infant attachment.
Other support: "Is there anyone else you would like to be present during labor?"	Women often want another support person to be present.	

Table 13-1

INTRAPARTUM ASSESSMENT GUIDE—cont'd

Assessment and Method (Selected Rationales)	Common Findings	Significant Findings and Nursing Action
Preparation for childbirth: "Did you attend prepared childbirth classes?" "Did someone go with you?"	Ideally, the woman and a partner have had some preparation in classes or self-study. Women who attended classes during previous pregnancies do not always repeat the classes during subsequent pregnancies.	The unprepared woman may need more support with simple relaxation and breathing techniques during labor. Her support person may need to learn techniques to assist her.
Preferences: "Do you have any special plans for this birth?" "Is there anything you want to avoid?" "Did you plan to record the birth with pictures or video?" (Videotaping the birth is restricted at many facilities.)	Some women and couples have strong feelings regarding certain interventions. Common ones are: (1) analgesia or anesthesia, (2) IV lines, (3) fetal monitoring, (4) shave prep or enema, and (5) use of episiotomy or forceps.	Conflict may arise if the woman has not previously discussed her preferences with her physician or nurse-midwife or is unaware of available services at the birth facility.
Cultural needs: "Do you plan any special cultural practices when you have your baby?" "How can we best help you to fulfill these practices?"	Women from Asian and Hispanic cultures often subscribe to the "hot/cold" theory of illness and want specific foods after birth, such as soft-boiled eggs. They may not want their water iced.	Try to incorporate all positive or neutral cultural practices. If a practice is harmful, explain why and try to find a way to work around it if the family does not want to give it up.
FETAL EVALUATION		
Purpose: To determine if the fetus seems to be healthy and tolerating labor well.		
Fetal heart rate (FHR): Assess by intermittent auscultation, or apply an external fetal monitor (most common in the United States). Document FHR at least this often for the fetus at low risk for complications: 1. Every hour during the latent phase 2. Every 30 minutes during active and transition phases 3. Every 15 minutes during the second stage	Average at term is a lower limit of 110 to 120 BPM and an upper limit of 150 to 160 BPM. Reassuring signs are a regular rhythm, accelerations, and absence of decelerations (see Chapter 14).	The nursery should be notified if a fetus has meconium-stained fluid and other amniotic fluid abnormalities, postterm gestation, and nonreassuring FHR characteristics.
LABOR STATUS		
Purpose: To identify whether the woman is in labor and birth is imminent. If she displays signs of imminent birth, this assessment is done as soon as she is admitted.		
Contractions (Yields objective information about labor status): In addition to asking the woman about her contraction pattern, assess the contractions by palpation with the fingertips of one hand with the same frequency as FHR evaluations.	See "Interview."	See "Interview." Women who have intense contractions or are making rapid progress need to be assessed more frequently.
Vaginal examination (Determines cervical dilation and effacement; fetal presentation, position, and station; bloody show; and status of the membranes)	Results vary according to the stage and phase of labor. Determining fetal position by vaginal examination may not be possible when membranes are intact and bulging over the presenting part.	A vaginal examination is not performed if the woman reports or has evidence of active bleeding (not bloody show).

Table 13-1
INTRAPARTUM ASSESSMENT GUIDE—cont'd

Assessment and Method (Selected Rationales)	Common Findings	Significant Findings and Nursing Action
Status of membranes: During a vaginal examination, a flow of fluid suggests ruptured membranes. A Nitrazine test, fern test, or both may be done. Other tests for fetal lung maturity may be done if the woman is not at term. (The test is needed only if membrane rupture is not obvious.)	Amniotic fluid should be clear and possibly contain flecks of white vernix. Its odor is distinctive but not offensive. Nitrazine test with a color change to blue-green to dark blue (pH >6.5) suggests true rupture of the membranes but is not conclusive. The fern test is more diagnostic of true rupture of membranes.	Meconium-stained fluid is associated with fetal compromise, postterm gestation, or both. Meconium respiratory compromise after birth may occur, especially if thick ("pea-soup"). Thick green-black meconium may be passed normally by the fetus in a breech presentation. Cloudy, yellowish, and strong or foul-smelling fluid suggests infection. Bloody fluid may indicate partial placental separation (p. 673).
Leopold's maneuvers: Identifies fetal presentation and position. Helps identify the best location for external FHR (most accurate when combined with information from vaginal examination).	A cephalic presentation with the head well flexed (vertex) is normal. The fetal head often is easily displaced upward ("floating") if the woman is not in labor. When the head is engaged, it cannot be displaced upward with Leopold's maneuvers.	A hard, round, freely movable object in the fundus suggests a fetal head, meaning the fetus is in a breech presentation. Less commonly, the fetus may be crosswise in the uterus (transverse lie).
Pain: Note discomfort during and between contractions. Note tenderness when palpating contractions. (This distinguishes between normal labor pain and abnormal pain that may be associated with a complication.)	Verbal or nonverbal evidence of pain may occur with contractions, but the woman should be relatively comfortable between contractions. The skin around the umbilicus often is sensitive.	Constant pain or a tender, rigid uterus suggests a complication such as abruptio placentae (prematurely separated placenta) (see p. 673) or less commonly, uterine rupture (see p. 748).
PHYSICAL EXAMINATION		
Purpose: To evaluate the woman's general health and identify conditions that may affect her intrapartum and postpartum care.		
General appearance: Observe skin color and texture, nutritional state, and appearance of rest or fatigue. Examine the woman's face, fingers, and lower extremities for edema. Ask her if she can take her rings off.	Women are often fatigued if their sleep has been interrupted by Braxton Hicks contractions, fetal activity, and frequent urination. Mild edema of the lower extremities is common in late pregnancy.	Pallor suggests anemia. Edema of the face and fingers or extreme (pitting) edema of the lower extremities is associated with pregnancy-induced hypertension (see p. 682).
Vital signs: Take the woman's temperature, pulse, respirations, and blood pressure on admission and by facility policy. A guideline for reassessment of vital signs is • Temperature every 4 hours (every 2 hours if membranes rupture or if elevated) • Blood pressure, pulse, and respirations every hour	*Temperature:* 36.2° to 37.6° C (98° to 99.6° F). Pulse: 60 to 90/min *Respirations:* 12-20/min, even and unlabored. Blood pressure should be near baseline levels established during pregnancy. Transient elevations of blood pressure are common on admission, but they return to baseline levels within about 30 minutes.	Report abnormalities to the physician or nurse-midwife. Temperature of 38° C (100.4° F) or higher, especially with elevated pulse and respirations, suggests infection. Pulse and blood pressure may be elevated if the woman is anxious or in pain. A blood pressure of 140/90 or higher is considered hypertensive. For women who did not have prenatal care, no baseline blood pressure exists to compare.

Table 13-1

INTRAPARTUM ASSESSMENT GUIDE—cont'd

Assessment and Method (Selected Rationales)	Common Findings	Significant Findings and Nursing Action
Heart and lung sounds: Auscultate all areas with a stethoscope.	Heart sounds should be clear with a distinct S_1 and S_2. A physiologic murmur is common because of the increased blood volume and cardiac output. Breath sounds should be clear with even and unlabored respirations.	The woman who is breathing rapidly and deeply may have symptoms of hyperventilation, such as tingling and spasm of the fingers and numbness around the lips.
Breasts: Palpate for a dominant mass.	Breasts are full and nodular. Areolas are darker, especially in dark-skinned women. Breasts may leak colostrum (clear, sticky, straw-colored fluid).	Report a dominant mass to the physician or nurse-midwife.
Abdomen: Observe for scars while assessing Leopold's maneuvers and the FHR. Assessing the fundal height by observing its relation to the xiphoid process usually is sufficient. Measure the fundal height (see Chapter 7) if the fetus seems small for gestation.	Striae (stretch marks) are common. If scars are noted, ask the woman about previous surgeries. The fundus at term usually is slightly below the xiphoid process.	Report a previous cesarean birth to the physician or nurse-midwife. Transverse uterine scars are least likely to rupture if the woman is in labor, but the skin incision does not always match the uterine incision (see p. 411).
Deep tendon reflexes: Assess patellar reflex (see p. 687). Upper-extremity, deep tendon reflexes should be used after epidural block analgesia.	Brisk knee jerk without spasm or sustained muscle contraction is usual. Some women normally have slightly hypoactive reflexes.	Report absent and hyperactive reflexes. Hyperactive reflexes and clonus (repeated tapping when the foot is dorsiflexed) are associated with pregnancy-induced hypertension and often precede a seizure (see p. 748).
Midstream urine specimen: Assess protein and glucose levels with a dipstick if that is routine on the unit. Follow instructions on the package for waiting times. Send for urinalysis if ordered.	Negative or trace of protein; negative glucose.	Proteinuria is associated with pregnancy-induced hypertension but may also be associated with urinary tract infections or a specimen contaminated with vaginal secretions. Glucosuria is associated with diabetes.
Laboratory tests: Women who have had prenatal care may not need additional tests. Common tests include		
Complete blood count (or hematocrit done on unit)	Hemoglobin levels should be at least 10.5 g/dl, and hematocrit should be at least 33%.	Values lower than these reduce maternal reserve for normal blood loss at birth.
Platelet count	This is done to identify clotting abnormalities before epidural analgesia. Normal range averages 150,000 to 400,000/mm^3.	A rapid fall in platelets may occur in women with severe pregnancy-induced hypertension and could contraindicate epidural analgesia.
Blood type and Rh factor	The woman who is Rh negative usually has received Rh immune globulin (RhoGAM) at about 28 weeks' gestation to prevent formation of anti-Rh antibodies	Rh-negative mothers should receive Rh immune globulin within 72 hours postpartum if their infants are Rh positive.
Serologic tests for syphilis	Negative test results are ideal.	A positive test may indicate that the baby is infected and needs treatment after birth. The mother should be treated if she has not been treated already.

mine the condition of the mother and fetus and whether birth is imminent.

Fetal Heart Rate. For assessment of a term fetus using intermittent auscultation, the following fetal heart rate (FHR) guidelines are considered reassuring (Feinstein, Sprague, & Trépanier, 2000):

- A lower limit of 110 to 120 beats per minute (BPM) and an upper limit of 150 to 160 BPM
- Regular rhythm
- Presence of accelerations in the FHR
- Absence of decelerations from the baseline

These findings also would be reassuring in an electronically monitored fetus (see Chapter 14).

Maternal Vital Signs. Maternal vital signs are assessed to identify signs of hypertension and infection. Hypertension during pregnancy is defined as a sustained blood pressure increase to 140 mm Hg systolic or 90 mm Hg diastolic. An elevation of 30 mm Hg systolic or 15 mm Hg diastolic from second-trimester levels is no longer considered diagnostic of hypertension (ACOG, 1996). A temperature of 38° C (100.4° F) or higher suggests infection.

Impending Birth. Grunting sounds, bearing down, sitting on one buttock, and saying urgently "The baby's coming" suggest imminent birth. The nurse abbreviates the initial assessment and collects other information after birth. While caring for the mother, the following minimal information can be quickly gathered if birth is imminent:

- Names of mother and support person(s)
- Name of her physician or nurse-midwife if she had prenatal care
- Number of pregnancies and prior births, including whether the birth was vaginal or cesarean
- Status of membranes
- Estimated date of delivery
- Any problems during this or other pregnancies
- Allergies to medications
- Time and type of last oral intake
- Maternal vital signs and FHR

If focus assessments of mother and fetus are normal and birth is not imminent, a more complete admission assessment is taken. If the initial assessments show that birth is near or another urgent condition is identified, the physician or nurse-midwife is notified promptly with essential assessment information.

Check Your Reading

3. What are the two assessment priorities when a woman comes to the intrapartum unit?
4. What FHR characteristics (when auscultated) are reassuring?
5. What observations suggest that a woman is about to give birth very soon? What should the nurse do in that case?

Database Assessment

In addition to the focus assessment, the nurse should assess the mother, fetus, and available maternal support persons.

CRITICAL THINKING EXERCISE

During a labor admission assessment, a woman quickly denies her use of drugs and herbal preparations other than her prescribed prenatal vitamins. She becomes quiet, answering the nurse's questions in a terse manner.

QUESTIONS:
What might explain the woman's change in behavior? Should the nurse alter the assessment interview?

Basic Information. Intrapartum admission forms guide the nurse to obtain required information. Typical information includes the following:

- The woman's reason for coming to the hospital or birth center (such as contractions, rupture of membranes)
- Prenatal care: when it began, her most recent visit, and her physician or nurse-midwife's name
- Her estimated date of delivery
- Number of pregnancies, births, and abortions
- Medical, surgical, and pregnancy history
- Allergies: medications, botanical and herbal preparations, and foods
- Food intake: what food and when it was eaten
- Recent illness, including treatment
- Medications, including prescription and over-the-counter drugs, vitamins, and herbal and botanical preparations and their purposes
- Complementary/alternative therapy in addition to herbal and botanical preparations and its purpose
- Use of tobacco, alcohol, and illicit substances
- Her subjective evaluation of her labor
- Birth plans, including planned pain management methods
- Support persons: who they are and the role of each
- Potential domestic violence (ask only when the woman is alone)

Women often bring several people with them to the birthing room and want them to stay during admission. However, be careful about asking for sensitive information, such as prior pregnancies and births and potential abuse, when others are present. A woman may have had an abortion or relinquished a baby for adoption, and her family may not know about it. Even if her partner knows about previous pregnancies, her family or friends may not. Asking about domestic violence when the abuser is present will result in a quick denial and can be dangerous for the woman. Delay asking sensitive information until the woman is alone for confidentiality, safety, and accuracy.

Fetal Assessments. The fetal presentation and position are assessed using a combination of vaginal exam and Leopold's maneuvers (Figure 13-1, Procedure 13-1). The FHR is assessed by intermittent auscultation and electronic monitoring (see Chapter 14). The nurse documents the color of the amniotic fluid and the time of rupture if the membranes have ruptured at admission.

Labor Status. The woman's labor status is determined by assessing her contraction pattern, performing vaginal examination if there are no contractions, and determining whether her membranes have ruptured. Contractions are assessed by palpation (Procedure 13-2), the fetal monitor, or both. Cervical dilation and effacement and the fetal station, presentation, and position are evaluated by vaginal examination. The vaginal examination may also reveal whether the membranes have ruptured if fluid is not obviously leaking from the vagina. Vaginal examination is not performed if the woman has active bleeding (other than bloody show) because the procedure can increase bleeding.

Physical Examination. A brief physical examination evaluates the woman's overall health. Other important observations relating to birth include the presence and location of edema, abdominal scars, and height of the fundus.

Check Your Reading

6. Which tests may be done if the nurse is not certain whether the woman's membranes have ruptured? (See Table 13-1.)
7. Which characteristics of contractions may reduce blood flow to the placenta? (See Procedure 13-2.)

Admission Procedures

Notifying the Birth Attendant. After assessment, the nurse notifies the woman's birth attendant to report her status and obtain orders. The nurse includes the following data in the report:

- Gravidity, parity, abortions, and term and preterm births
- Estimated date of delivery (EDD) and fundal height if it conflicts with the EDD
- Contraction pattern
- Results of vaginal examination:
- Fetal presentation and position
  Cervical dilation and effacement; station of the presenting part
  FHR evaluation
- Maternal vital signs
- Any identified abnormalities and concerns about the maternal or fetal condition
- Reactions to labor: use of childbirth class techniques, pain, anxiety, support of coach

If the birth attendant admits the woman, any of several procedures may be performed.

Consent Forms. The woman signs consent for care during labor, anesthesia, vaginal birth, and possible cesarean birth. Consent for newborn care also is usually completed at this time.

Laboratory Tests. Women who had regular prenatal care need laboratory tests only for specific indications, whereas those who did not have prenatal care need more extensive laboratory tests. Simple tests that are often done on the unit include the following:

- Hematocrit obtained by finger stick
- Midstream urine specimen to assess protein and glucose levels—usually obtained before notifying the birth attendant

Intravenous Access. If used, IV access is started with at least an 18-gauge catheter. A saline lock may be used, or the woman may receive continuous infusion of fluids. The lock eases walking during early labor but provides quick access if fluids or drugs are needed. Continuous fluid infusion prevents and relieves dehydration and is necessary if epidural block analgesia is used. IV solutions containing electrolytes, such as lactated Ringer's solution, are most common.

Perineal Preparation. If necessary, hair in the immediate area of an episiotomy is removed by shaving or clipping the hair near the skin with a shaver or disposable scissors.

Enema. A small-volume enema (such as Fleet enema) may be given if stool in the rectum causes the woman discomfort or would interfere with fetal descent. Extra lubricant on the enema tip reduces discomfort from hemorrhoids.

Making Assessments after Admission

The woman is usually observed if whether she is in true labor is unclear after the initial assessment. After 1 or 2 hours, progressive cervical change (effacement, dilation, or both) strongly suggests true labor. The woman and fetus are assessed during the observation period as if in early labor.

After the admission assessment, the woman and fetus need regular assessments based on their risk status and whether they have interventions such as oxytocin stimulation or epidural analgesia. General guidelines for continuing assessments are listed here.

Fetal Assessments

Fetal assessments are performed to identify signs of well-being and those that suggest compromise. The principal fetal assessments include the FHR and patterns and character of the amniotic fluid. Abnormalities

Text continued on p. 306

CARE PATH FOR STAGES OF LABOR 1 & 2

NANDA Problem Number	LOCATION	PREADMIT	ADMISSION	LATENT PHASE (0-4 cm)
IV 5, 8, 9, 16 I 5, 6 III I I	Assessments	High risk screening with referrals prn: – MFM – Homecare – Genetic Counsel – Social Services	T, P, R, BP Deep tendon reflexes / clonus Labor status: – admit for labor per protocol: CRITERIA FOR LABOR: 1. complete effacement; or 2 cm in nullipara 2. cervical change 3. rupture of membranes $\bar{s}$ labor 4. contractions at least 5 min apart – cervix: sterile vaginal exam unless contraindicated – uterine activity (toco / palpation) – membrane status, color, amount, odor of fluid Fetus: – presentation (ultrasound prn) – FHR: 20 min or electronic fetal monitoring strip (continue electronic fetal monitoring if non-reassuring pattern) Urine – dip for protein & ketones Level of childbirth preparation Family interaction Beta-strep risk factors – preterm labor – rupture of membranes < 37 wk – previous baby $\bar{c}$ Beta-strep	P, R, BP $\bar{q}$ 1 hr T $\bar{q}$ 2 hr if rupture of membranes, $\bar{q}$ 4 hr if bag of waters intact BP, P $\bar{q}$ 15 min if epidural anesthetic Bladder status $\bar{q}$ 2 hr Urine protein/ketones dip-stick prn Deep tendon reflexes/clonus prn Fetal monitoring: electronic fetal monitor or electronic fetal monitoring while in bed or intermittent auscultation Labor status: – frequency, duration, strength, resting tone of contractions $\bar{q}$ 1 hr by toco/palpation or intrauterine pressure catheter – membrane status; color, amount and odor of fluid – sterile vaginal exam prn & prior to meds as indicated Fetus: – low risk: FHR $\bar{q}$ 30 min – high risk: FHR $\bar{q}$ 15 min In and out catheterization **Progress to active phase $\bar{c}$ in 6° of admission** verified ________
IV 5, 6	Procedures/ Tests		CBC, VDRL, ABO-Rh stat on admission HBSAG if not on prenatal record	**If intrauterine pressure catheter labor pattern shows > 250 Montevideo unit** verified ________
	Treatments		Initiate Labor Curve Initiate "Active Management of Labor Protocol" if criteria are met. Notify Special Care Nursery of potential problems.	Consider amniotomy for prolonged latent phase. Consider use of intrauterine pressure catheter if inadequate cervical change.
VI 3 XI 5	Medication			PAIN CONTROL: Parenteral analgesia as ordered. (Consider Stadol or Nubain). If inadequate pain control, anesthesia consult, re-evaluate for epidural _______ Narcotic epidural _______ Anesthetic epidural
	Signatures	____ / ________ ____ / ________	____ / ________ ____ / ________	____ / ________ ____ / ________

MED REC NO. ____________________

PATIENT ____________________

PHYSICIAN ____________________

BAYLOR UNIVERSITY MEDICAL CENTER
DALLAS, TEXAS

CARE PATH FOR STAGES OF LABOR 1 & 2

PAGE 1 OF 4

FIGURE 13-1 Care path for labor, stages 1 and 2. *HBSAG,* Hepatitis B surface antigen; *MFM,* Maternal-Fetal Medicine; *VBAC,* vaginal birth after cesarean. (Modified from Baylor University Medical Center, Dallas, Texas.)

CARE PATH FOR STAGES OF LABOR 1 & 2

NANDA Problem Number	LOCATION	PREADMIT	ADMISSION	LATENT PHASE (0-4 cm)
III 11	Elimination			Encourage voiding q̅ 2-3 hr In and out catheterization if unable to void & bladder is distended Bladder remains nondistended
II 7	Nutrition Hydration		Clear liquids/ice chips, hard candy if desired	Clear liquids/ice chips, hard candy if desired IV fluids prn and as ordered for T > 101 on 2 consecutive readings (notify attending MD) IV (18G) or heplock if VBAC Hydration status will be maintained
IV 11	Activity			Bag of waters intact or rupture of membranes with presenting part engaged: encourage up ad lib; chair prn Ambulates frequently
VI 2, 5, 6	PT/Family Education	At 1st OB appt, give info on: – Labor warnings – Kick counts – Prepared childbirth classes – Optional classes: VBAC Baby care Breastfeeding Advise in selection of a pediatrician Goal: By 28 wks, pt identifies when to call the doctor & describes when & how to do kick counts	Ambulation & position changes Electronic Fetal Monitor Breathing & Relaxation (B & R) techniques Analgesia & Anesthesia (A & A) options Labor progress & expectations **Verbalizes understanding** verified ____________	**Appropriate B & R maintained** verified ____________
VIII 7, 8	Psycho Social Emotional		**Support person identified** verified ____________	Support person identified
	Signatures	Initials for these signatures will be found throughout the care path.	____/____ ____/____	____/____ ____/____

MED REC NO. ________________

PATIENT ________________

PHYSICIAN ________________

BAYLOR UNIVERSITY MEDICAL CENTER
DALLAS, TEXAS

CARE PATH FOR STAGES OF LABOR 1 & 2

PAGE 2 OF 4

FIGURE 13-1, cont'd For legend see opposite page.

Continued

CARE PATH FOR STAGES OF LABOR 1 & 2

NANDA Problem Number	LOCATION	ACTIVE PHASE (4-10 cm)	SECOND STAGE (10 cm – Delivery)
IV 5, 8, 9, 16 I 5, 6 III I I	Assessments	T, q̄ 4° if bag of waters intact; q̄ 2° if rupture of membranes BP, P, R, q̄ 1 hr BP, P q̄ 15 min if epidural anesthetic Bladder status q̄ 2 hr Urine protein/ketones dipstick prn Deep tendon reflexes/clonus prn Fetal monitoring: electronic fetal monitoring while in bed, or intermittent auscultation Labor status: – frequency, duration, strength, resting tone of contraction q̄ 1 hr by toco/palpation or intrauterine pressure catheter – membrane status; color, amount and odor of fluid – sterile vaginal exam prn & prior to meds Fetus: – low risk: FHR q̄ 30 min – high risk: FHR q̄ 15 min In and out catheterization **If intrauterine pressure catheter, labor pattern shows > 250 Montevideo units** verified ____________ **Cervix changes at a rate of > 1.2 cm/hr for nullips; > 1.5 cm/hr for multips** verified ____________	T, q̄ 4° if bag of waters intact; q 2° if rupture of membranes BP, P, R, q̄ 1 hr BP, P q̄ 15 min if epidural anesthetic Bladder status q̄ 2 hr Urine protein/ketones dipstick prn Deep tendon reflexes/clonus prn Fetal monitoring: electronic fetal monitoring while in bed, or intermittent auscultation Labor status: – frequency, duration, strength, resting tone of contraction q̄ 1 hr by toco/palpation or intrauterine pressure catheter – membrane status; color, amount and odor of fluid – sterile vaginal exam prn & prior to meds Fetus: – low risk: FHR q̄ 15 min – high risk: FHR q̄ 5 min – VBAC continous electronic fetal monitor or electronic fetal monitoring Effectiveness of expulsive efforts – descent of presenting part – position; document if abnormal presentation – caput
IV 5, 6	Procedures / Tests		
	Treatments	Plot cervical dilation q̄ 2 hours or per exam Consider use of intrauterine pressure catheter if inadequate cervical change	
VI 3 XI 5	Medications	PAIN CONTROL: Parenteral analgesics as ordered. (Consider Stadol or Nubain). Anesthesia consult; epidural prn Oxytocin augmentation, if indicated per protocol If rupture of membranes > 24 hr antibiotics as ordered **Maintains control; utilizes B & R techniques prn** verified ____________	**Maintains control; utilizes B & R techniques prn** verified ____________
	Signatures	___/___ ___/___	___/___ ___/___ ___/___ ___/___

MED REC NO. ________________

PATIENT ________________

PHYSICIAN ________________

BAYLOR UNIVERSITY MEDICAL CENTER
DALLAS, TEXAS

CARE PATH FOR STAGES OF LABOR 1 & 2

PAGE 3 OF 4

FIGURE 13-1, cont'd For legend see p. 300.

CARE PATH FOR STAGES OF LABOR 1 & 2

NANDA Problem Number	LOCATION	ACTIVE PHASE (4-10 cm)	SECOND STAGE
IIII I I	Elimination	Encourage voiding q̄ 2-3 hr In and out catheterization if unable to void & bladder is distended Bladder remains nondistended	Encourage voiding q̄ 2-3 hr In and out catheterization if unable to void & bladder is distended Bladder remains nondistended
II 7	Nutrition Hydration	Clear liquids/ice chips IV fluids prn and as ordered for T > 101 on 2 consecutive readings (notify attending MD) IV (18G) or heplock if VBAC Hydration status will be maintained	Clear liquids/ice chips IV fluids prn: and as ordered for T > 101 on 2 consecutive readings (notify attending MD) IV (18G) or heplock if VBAC Hydration status will be maintained
IV 11	Activity	Bag of waters intact or rupture of membranes with presenting part engaged: encourage up ad lib; chair prn Facilitate frequent position changes (q̄ 1-2 hr) while in bed	Facilitate frequent position changes (q̄ 1-2 hr) while in bed
VI 2, 5, 6	PT/Family Education	**Appropriate B & R maintained** verified ______________	**Appropriate B & R maintained** verified ______________
	Psycho Social Emotional	Support person identified	Support person identified
	Signatures	____/________ ____/________	____/________ ____/________ ____/________ ____/________

MED REC NO. ______________

PATIENT ______________

PHYSICIAN ______________

BILLING NO. ______________

BAYLOR UNIVERSITY MEDICAL CENTER

DALLAS, TEXAS

CARE PATH FOR STAGES OF LABOR 1 & 2

PAGE 4 OF 4

FIGURE 13-1, cont'd For legend see p. 300.

PROCEDURE 13-1

[redacted]

Purpose: To determine presentation and position of the fetus and aid in location of fetal heart sounds.

1. Explain the procedure to the woman and the rationale for each step as it is performed. Tell her what is found at each step. *Gives information, teaches the woman, and reassures her when the assessment findings are normal.*
2. Ask the woman to empty her bladder if she has not done so recently. Have her lie on her back with her knees flexed slightly. Place a small pillow or folded towel under one hip. *Decreases discomfort of a full bladder during palpation and improves ability to feel fetal parts in the suprapubic area. Knee flexion helps the woman relax her abdominal muscles to enhance palpation. Uterine displacement prevents aortocaval compression, which could reduce blood flow to the placenta.*
3. Wash your hands with warm water. Wear gloves if contact with secretions is likely. *Prevents transmission of microorganisms. Warm hands are more comfortable during palpation and prevent tensing of abdominal muscles.*
4. Stand beside the woman, facing her head, with your dominant hand nearest her. *The first three maneuvers are most easily performed in this position.*

First Maneuver

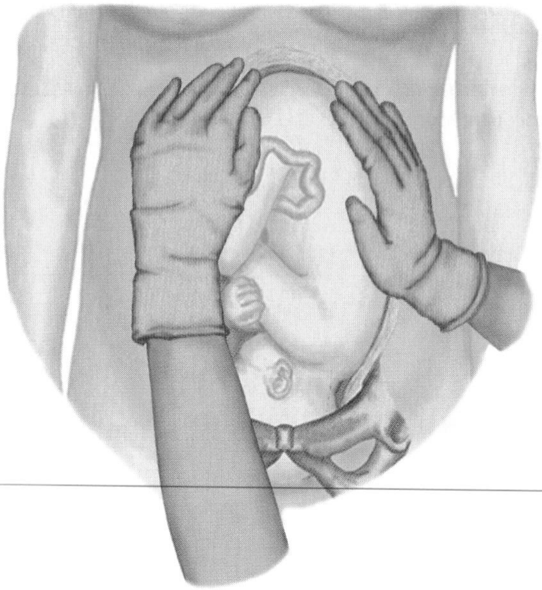

5. Palpate the uterine fundus. The breech (buttocks) is softer and more irregular in shape than the head. Moving the breech also moves the fetal trunk. The head is harder and has a round, uniform shape. The head can be moved without moving the entire fetal trunk. *Distinguishes between a cephalic and breech presentation. If the fetus is in a cephalic presentation, the breech is felt in the fundus. If the presentation is breech, the head is felt in the fundus.*

Second Maneuver

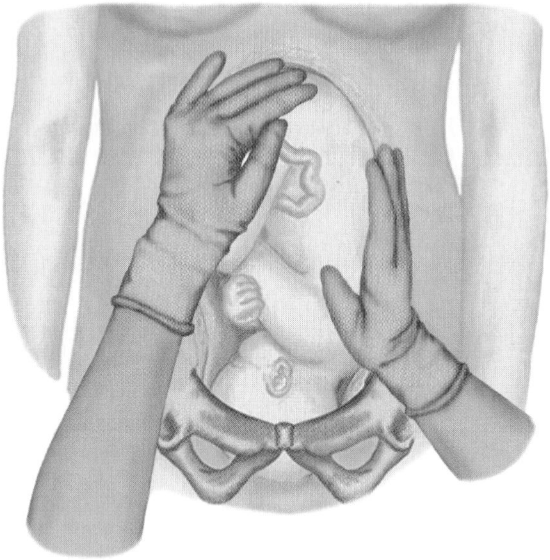

6. Hold the left hand steady on one side of the uterus while palpating the opposite side of the uterus with the right hand. Then hold the right hand steady while palpating the opposite side of the uterus with the left hand. The fetal back is a smooth, convex surface. The fetal arms and legs feel nodular, and the fetus often moves them during palpation. *Determines on which side of the uterus is the back and on which side are the fetal arms and legs ("small parts").*

Third Maneuver

7. Palpate the suprapubic area. If a breech was palpated in the fundus, expect a hard, rounded head in this area. Attempt to grasp the presenting part gently between the thumb and fingers. If the presenting part is not engaged, the grasping movement of the fingers moves it upward in the uterus. *Confirms the presentation determined in the first maneuver. Determines whether the presenting part is engaged (widest diameter at or below a zero station) in the maternal pelvis.*
8. Omit the fourth maneuver if the fetus is in a breech presentation. *Is performed only in cephalic presentations to determine whether the fetal head is flexed.*

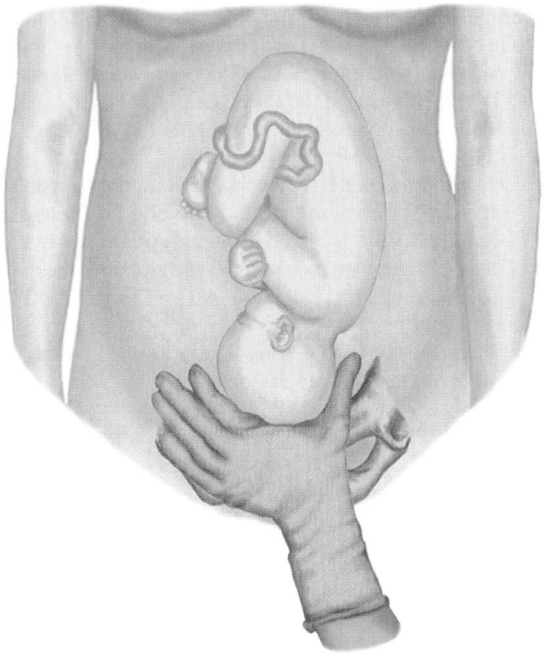

Fourth Maneuver

9. Turn so that you face the woman's feet. *Is most easily performed in this position.*
10. Place your hands on each side of the uterus with fingers pointed toward the pelvic inlet. Slide hands downward on each side of the uterus. On one side, your fingers easily slide to the upper edge of the symphysis. On the other side, your fingers meet an obstruction, the cephalic prominence. *Determines whether the head is flexed (vertex) or extended (face). The vertex presentation is normal. If the head is flexed, the cephalic prominence (the forehead in this case) is felt on the opposite side from the fetal back. If the head is extended, the cephalic prominence (the occiput in this case) is felt on the same side as the fetal back.*

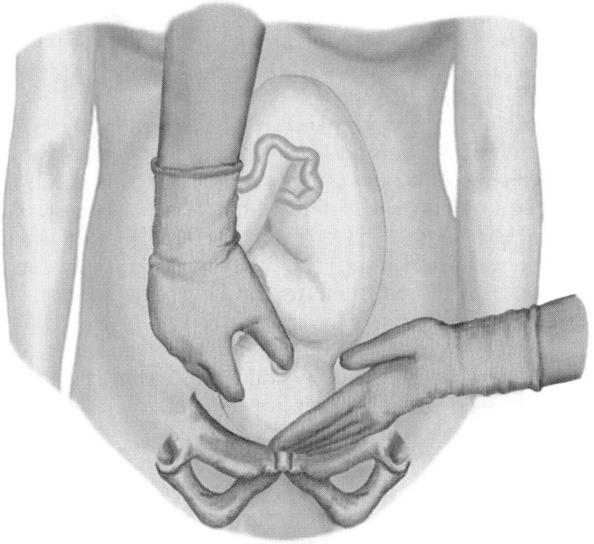

PROCEDURE 13-2
Palpating Contractions

Purpose: To determine whether a contraction pattern is typical of true labor. To identify abnormal contractions that may jeopardize the health of the mother or fetus.

1. Assess at least three contractions in a row at the time the FHR is checked. Guidelines for minimal frequency of assessments are therefore:
   a. Hourly during latent phase
   b. Every 30 minutes during active phase and transition
   c. Every 15 minutes during second stage

   Assess more frequently if abnormalities are identified. *Assessment of at least three sequential contractions permits better evaluation of the pattern. Palpate contractions periodically when an external fetal monitor is used because it is less accurate for intensity as a result of thickness of the abdominal fat pad, maternal position, and fetal position.*
2. Place fingertips of one hand on the uterine fundus, using light pressure. Keep fingertips relatively still rather than moving them over the uterus. The fingertips are more sensitive to the first tightening of the uterus. Contractions usually begin in the fundus, although the mother usually feels them in her lower abdomen and back. Constant moving of the hand over the uterus may stimulate contractions and give an inaccurate assessment of their true pattern.
3. Note the time when each contraction begins and ends.
   a. Determine frequency by noting the average time that elapses from the beginning of one contraction to the beginning of the next one.
   b. Determine duration by noting the average time in seconds from the beginning to the end of each contraction.
   c. Determine interval by noting the average time between the end of one contraction and the beginning of the next one. *Contractions are expected to increase in frequency, duration, and intensity as labor progresses. False labor is usually characterized by contractions that are irregular and do not increase in frequency, duration, and intensity.*
4. Estimate the average intensity of contractions by noting how easily the uterus can be indented during the peak of the contraction:
   a. Mild contractions are easily indented with the fingertips. They feel similar to the tip of the nose.
   b. Moderate contractions can be indented with more difficulty. They feel similar to the chin.
   c. Firm contractions feel "woody" and cannot be readily indented. They feel similar to the forehead. Contractions during labor are expected to intensify progressively. If they do not the woman may not be in true labor or she may be experiencing dysfunctional labor (see Chapter 27).
5. Report hypertonic contractions:
   a. Occurring less than 2 minutes apart
   b. Durations longer than 90 seconds
   c. Intervals shorter than 60 seconds
   d. Incomplete relaxation of the uterus between contractions

   Hypertonic contractions reduce placental blood flow by prolonged compression of the vessels that supply the intervillous spaces.

revealed in these assessments may be associated with impaired fetal gas exchange and infection.

Fetal Heart Rate. The FHR is assessed using either intermittent auscultation or electronic fetal monitoring. Frequency of assessment and documentation depends on the risk status of the mother and fetus.

Amniotic Fluid. A spontaneous rupture of membranes (SROM) may occur, or the birth attendant may perform an amniotomy. The FHR is assessed for at least 1 minute when the membranes rupture. The umbilical cord could be displaced in a large fluid gush, resulting in compression and interruption of blood flow through it (prolapsed cord; see p. 764). Charting related to membrane rupture includes the time, FHR, and character of the fluid.

CRITICAL THINKING EXERCISE

Chloe Green is in labor with her second baby. The baby is in a left occiput anterior (LOA) position, and Chloe's cervix is 5 cm dilated and completely effaced. Her membranes rupture at the end of a strong contraction. You note that the fluid is green and watery.

QUESTIONS:
What nursing actions are most important at this time? Why?

Amniotic fluid should be clear and may include bits of vernix, the creamy white fetal skin lubricant. Cloudy, yellow, and foul-smelling amniotic fluid suggest infection. Green fluid indicates that the fetus passed meconium before birth. Meconium passage may have been in response to transient hypoxia, although the cause is often unknown. The newborn often will need extra respiratory suctioning at birth if the fluid is heavily stained with meconium.

Quantity should be described in approximate terms; for example, at term, a "large" amount is more than 1000 ml, a "moderate" amount is about 500 to 1000 ml, and "scant" amniotic fluid is a trickle, barely enough to detect. If the fetus is well down into the pelvis when the membranes rupture, a small amount of fluid in front of the fetal head may be discharged (forewaters), with the rest lost at birth.

Maternal Assessments

Several maternal assessments also relate to the health of the fetus, such as vital signs and contractions.

Vital Signs. Abnormalities should be reported and the assessment frequency increased (see Table 13-1).

Contractions. Contractions can be assessed by palpitation or with the electronic fetal monitor.

Progress of Labor. A vaginal examination is done periodically to determine cervical dilation and effacement and fetal descent (Figure 13-2). The frequency of vaginal examinations depends on the woman's parity, status of her membranes, and overall speed of her labor. Vaginal examinations are limited to avoid the introduction of microorganisms from the perineal area into the uterus.

Intake and Output. Oral and IV intake and each voiding are recorded. Labor may reduce a woman's urge to void, so her suprapubic area should be checked every 2 hours or more frequently to identify bladder distention if she has received large quantities of IV fluids.

Pressure of the fetal head on the rectum in late labor makes many women feel the need to defecate. The nurse should look at the perineum for crowning of the fetal head if the woman suddenly expresses the need to defecate during a contraction.

Response to Labor. The woman's behavioral responses change as labor intensifies, especially if she has not had epidural analgesia. She withdraws from interactions but needs more nursing presence and reassurance. She may become more anxious because of pain and fear of bodily injury, unknown outcome, loss of control, unresolved psychological issues that influence her readiness to give birth (such as sexual abuse, previous birth experiences), and unexpected occurrences during labor.

Women vary in their ability to handle the pain of labor. The nurse constantly must assess whether additional pain control measures are needed. Behaviors that suggest the woman may want help with pain management include the following:

- Specific requests for medication and other pain control
- Statements that nonpharmacologic measures are ineffective
- Tension of her muscles and arching of her back during contractions
- Persistence of muscle tension between contractions
- A tense facial expression
- Expressions such as "I can't take it anymore"

The Support Person's Response

Labor is stressful for the woman's support person, who often is the baby's father. He may become anxious, fearful, or tired. He feels a responsibility to protect and support the woman but may have limited resources for doing so. Watching the woman he loves in pain is difficult, even if the pain is normal. He may respond to stress in many ways, including being quiet, suffering silently, or reacting with pacing and anger. Some fathers respond by leaving the room frequently or for long periods, whereas others resist even short breaks.

Nurses encourage and value the father's presence during labor and birth. However, this may conflict with a couple's cultural norms dictating that birth is a strictly female activity. The father may be pulled in two directions, wanting to be included but hesitating because men in his culture are not customarily part of birth. The nurse should respect the values of each couple and their wishes about father involvement.

The support person also may be a parent or another relative, a friend of either gender, or a homosexual partner. The nurse must remember that anyone who assists the woman during labor may have feelings of anxiety and helplessness at times. Reassurance and care for the labor partner strengthen the person's ability to support the woman and enhance the likelihood that both will view the birth experience as positive.

Check Your Reading

8. What is the routine frequency for FHR assessment in uncomplicated labor? Why should the FHR be assessed after the membranes rupture?
9. What is the significance of greenish amniotic fluid? Of cloudy, yellowish, or foul-smelling amniotic fluid?
10. Why are frequent vaginal examinations undesirable during labor?
11. What observations suggest that the woman may need additional help with pain management during labor?

APPLICATION OF THE NURSING PROCESS: FALSE OR EARLY LABOR

Assessment

After observation, the nurse may realize that the woman is not in true labor. If findings are normal and the woman's membranes are intact, she is usually discharged. The woman who is in very early labor may be discharged to await active labor, especially if she is a nullipara and lives nearby.

Analysis

A woman may be frustrated because she cannot tell whether labor is real. She may resist returning to the birth center, possibly causing needless delay of care. She often is tired of being pregnant and just wants it to be over. A nursing diagnosis applicable to many women with false labor contractions is "Knowledge Deficit: Characteristics of True Labor."

Planning

A goal or expected outcome for this nursing diagnosis is that before discharge, the woman and her support person will describe reasons for returning to the birth center for evaluation.

Interventions

Providing Reassurance

A woman sent home after observation may feel foolish and frustrated. Reassure her that even professionals cannot always identify true labor and false labor. Also,

Purposes

To determine whether membranes have ruptured.
To determine cervical effacement and dilation.
To determine fetal presentation, position, and station.

Method

Vaginal examination is not performed by the inexperienced nurse except when training for graduate nursing practice in the intrapartum area.

Equipment

Sterile gloves, sterile lubricant. If Nitrazine paper is being used to test for ruptured membranes, lubricant is not used to avoid altering the test paper.

Hand Position

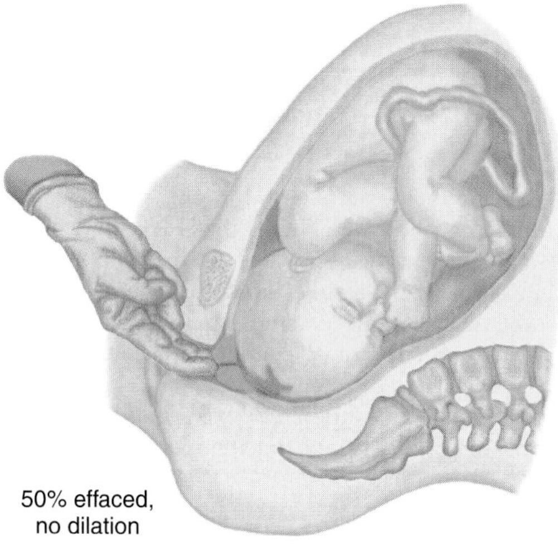

The nurse usually uses the index and middle fingers of the dominant hand for vaginal examination. The thumb and other fingers are kept out of the way to avoid carrying microorganisms into the vagina.

Determining Whether Membranes Have Ruptured

Intact membranes feel like a slippery membrane over the fetal presenting part.

If the membranes are *bulging,* they feel like a slippery, fluid-filled balloon over the presenting part. It may be difficult to feel the fetal presentation clearly if the membranes are bulging tensely.

If the membranes have ruptured, fluid often will drain from the vagina as the nurse manipulates the cervix and presenting part.

Determining Cervical Effacement and Dilation

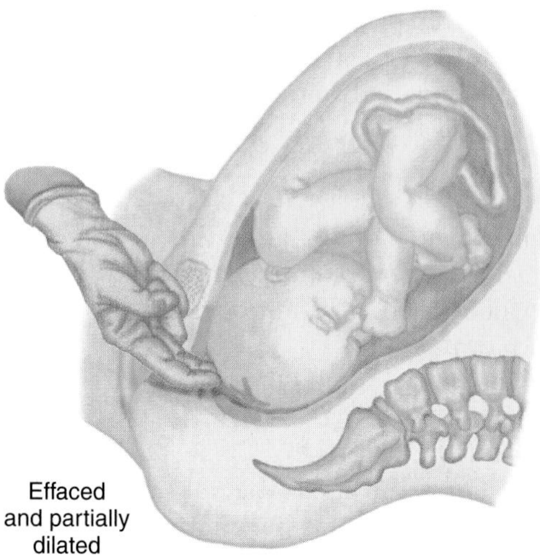

The nurse determines *effacement* by estimating the thickness of the cervix. The uneffaced cervix is about 2 cm long. If it is 50% effaced, it is about 1 cm long. Effacement is expressed as a percentage of 0% to 100%, or it may be described as the length in centimeters.

Dilation is determined by sweeping the fingertips across the cervical opening. The average woman's index finger is about 1.5 cm in diameter.

Determining the Presenting Part

The fetal skull feels smooth, hard, and rounded in a cephalic presentation. The fetal buttocks are softer and more irregular in a breech presentation. If the membranes are ruptured, the fetus in a breech presentation may expel thick, green-black meconium. (Presence of meconium in a breech presentation is *not* necessarily a sign of fetal compromise. The nurse must evaluate other signs of fetal condition.)

Determining the Fetal Position

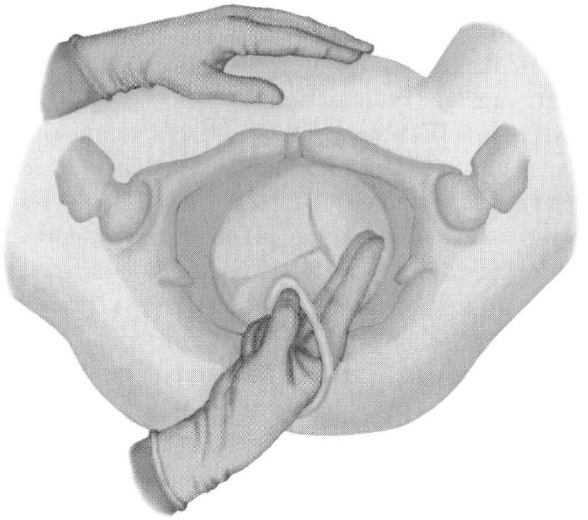

In a cephalic presentation, the nurse feels for the distinctive features of the fetal skull. The posterior fontanelle is usually felt in a vertex presentation and is triangular with three suture lines (two lambdoid and one sagittal) leading into it. The anterior fontanelle is not felt unless the head is poorly flexed or is in the mechanism of extension in late labor. It feels like a diamond-shaped depression with four suture lines (one frontal, two coronal, and one sagittal) leading into it.

Determining the Station

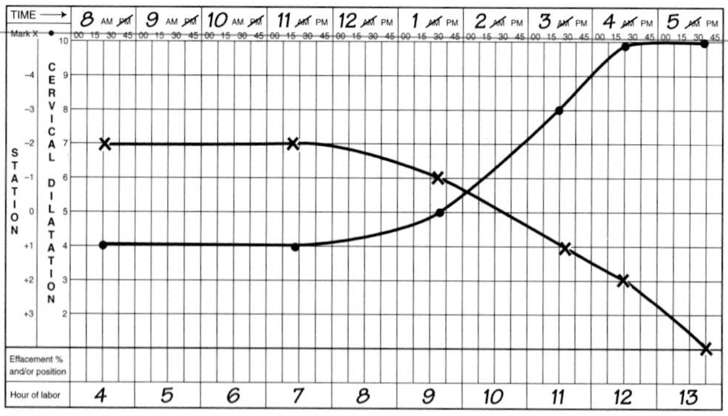

Findings of the vaginal examination may be recorded on a labor flow sheet, narrative, or a graph. The graph may be termed a *Friedman curve*, a *partogram*, or a *labor curve*.

FIGURE 13-2 Vaginal examination during labor.

tell her that important preparation occurs during late pregnancy, such as softening of the cervix, even if obvious progress like cervical dilation has not yet occurred.

Teaching

Review guidelines for returning to the birth center and explain that these are only guidelines and she should return if she has any concerns. Returning with false labor is better than entering in advanced labor or developing complications at home. The woman is not the first and will not be the last in this situation.

Evaluation

The woman and her support person should describe guidelines for returning to the birth center. These include regular contractions, leaking of amniotic fluid, bleeding other than bloody show, and decreased fetal movement.

APPLICATION OF THE NURSING PROCESS: TRUE LABOR

The admission assessment may confirm that the woman is in true labor, or true labor may be evident after observation. Nursing diagnoses and collaborative problems change during labor because the intrapartum period is an active process. Problems covered in this chapter relate to fetal oxygenation, maternal discomfort, and maternal injury.

Nursing diagnoses often interact during labor. For example, high anxiety reduces effectiveness of pain-relief measures by interfering with relaxation. A maternal fluid volume deficit can alter fetal oxygenation because less blood is available to circulate to the placenta.

FETAL OXYGENATION

Assessment

The main assessments related to fetal well-being are the following (see Tables 13-1 and 13-2):

- FHR evaluation
- Amount and character of amniotic fluid and time of rupture
- Maternal vital signs
- Contractions: frequency, duration, intensity, and resting interval

Analysis

Several factors can reduce fetal oxygen, nutrient, and waste exchange, such as maternal hypotension and hypertension, maternal fever, excessively strong and long contractions (tetanic), and compression of the umbilical cord. The healthy fetus usually tolerates labor well, and the nurse simply needs to be alert for problems. Therefore a valid collaborative problem is "Potential Complication: fetal compromise" (see Chapter 14).

Table 13-2
ASSISTING WITH AN EMERGENCY BIRTH

The inexperienced nurse rarely must deliver a baby in the hospital or birth center but occasionally helps the more experienced nurse do so. Unplanned, out-of-hospital births are not common but do occur occasionally.

Nursing Priorities for an Emergency Birth in Any Setting

Avoid or reduce injury to the mother and infant.
Maintain the infant's airway and temperature after birth.

Preparing for an Emergency Birth

Study the delivery sequence in Figures 13-7 and 13-8.
Locate the emergency delivery tray ("precip" tray) on the unit.

During the Birth

Remain with the woman to assist in giving birth. Use the call bell or ask her partner to call for help. Stay calm to reduce anxiety.
Put on gloves (preferably sterile) to prevent contamination with blood and other secretions: Sterile gloves reduce transmission of environmental organisms to the mother and infant.
The nurse will be "catching" the infant in this situation. No invasive procedure is performed, so sterile gloves are not essential. However, the nurse should take precautions against contact with body fluids.

After the Birth

Observe the infant's color and respirations for distress. Suction excess secretions with a bulb syringe, suctioning the mouth before the nose.
Dry and place the infant skin-to-skin with the mother or cover with warmed blankets to maintain warmth.
Put the infant to the mother's breast, and encourage suckling to promote uterine contraction, facilitating expulsion of the placenta and controlling bleeding.

CRITICAL TO REMEMBER

Conditions Associated with Fetal Compromise

- FHR outside the normal range for a term fetus: lower limit of 110 to 120 BPM and upper limit of 150 to 160 BPM
- Meconium-stained (greenish) amniotic fluid
- Cloudy, yellowish, or foul-smelling amniotic fluid (suggests infection)
- Contractions that occur less than 2 minutes apart (may not give placental blood flow time to resume during interval)
- Contractions lasting longer than 90 seconds (reduces placental blood flow)
- Incomplete uterine relaxation and intervals shorter than 60 seconds between contractions (reduces placental blood flow)
- Maternal hypotension (may divert blood flow away from the placenta to ensure adequate perfusion of the maternal brain and heart)
- Maternal hypertension (may be associated with vasospasm in spiral arteries, which supply the intervillous spaces of the placenta)
- Maternal fever (38° C [100.4° F] or higher)

See Chapter 14 for other FHR characteristics associated with fetal compromise.

Planning

Client-centered goals are not made for collaborative problems as they are for nursing diagnoses. Planning includes nursing responsibilities to (1) promote normal placental function and (2) observe for and report problems to the physician or nurse-midwife.

Interventions

Promoting Placental Function

Maternal positioning is the primary measure to promote placental function during normal labor. The supine position should be avoided because it can cause the woman's uterus to compress her aorta and inferior vena cava (aortocaval compression), reducing blood flow to the placenta. If she must be in the supine position for a procedure such as catheterization, a small pillow under one hip shifts her uterus to maintain good placental blood flow.

Observing for Conditions Associated with Fetal Compromise

If conditions associated with fetal compromise are identified (Critical to Remember), assess the fetus more frequently and notify the birth attendant.

Evaluation

Evaluation of client goals and expected outcomes does not apply to a collaborative problem. Throughout labor, compare actual data with the norms for the mother and fetus.

DISCOMFORT

Assessment

See Table 13-1 for continuing assessments of the laboring woman.

Analysis

Women vary in their responses to labor's pain and choices of pain management methods. The woman with choices for pain management and support for her choices has an increased sense of control over her birth experience. The woman who successfully masters the pain and other physical demands of labor is more likely to view her experience as positive. Her support person also is likely to feel more satisfaction with the experience.

Related nursing diagnoses are pain and anxiety. Excess anxiety reduces pain tolerance, and pain worsens anxiety. The nurse clusters assessment data to determine which is the primary problem. For example, several cues suggest that anxiety is primary, such as a previous poor experience during birth and expressions of worry and concern. However, if contractions are intense and labor is progressing quickly, the primary nursing diagnosis would be pain. Of these two options, the nursing diagnosis selected for this discussion is "Pain related to effects of uterine contractions."

Planning

The elimination of labor's pain is not realistic. Although highly effective pharmacologic methods exist, they cannot be implemented until the woman is in established labor. Therefore appropriate goals and expected outcomes related to pain include:

1. During labor, the woman will state that her chosen method or methods of pain management are satisfactory and will notify the nurse if others are needed.
2. By discharge from the birth facility, the woman's support person will express satisfaction with having provided labor support.
3. By discharge from the birth facility, the woman will describe her birth experience as positive.

Interventions

Labor pain management includes measures to promote comfort and specific methods to relieve pain, such as breathing techniques and medication (see Chapters 11 and 15).

Providing Comfort Measures

Ordinary measures reduce irritating surroundings that impair a woman's ability to relax and use coping skills.

Lighting. Soft, indirect lighting is soothing, whereas a bright overhead light is irritating. Bright lights imply a hospital ("sick") atmosphere rather than a normal event like birth. A bright, overhead light should be used only when needed. A small flashlight is handy if the woman wants her room dark.

Temperature. Labor is work and women in labor are often hot and perspiring. Cool, damp washcloths on the woman's face and neck promote comfort (Figure 13-3). Keep an ample supply of damp washcloths available and change them often to keep them cool. The woman should wear socks if her feet are cold. An electric fan circulates air in the labor room and directs a breeze on the woman. Be sure that the fan does not blow on the infant after birth, which might lead to hypothermia.

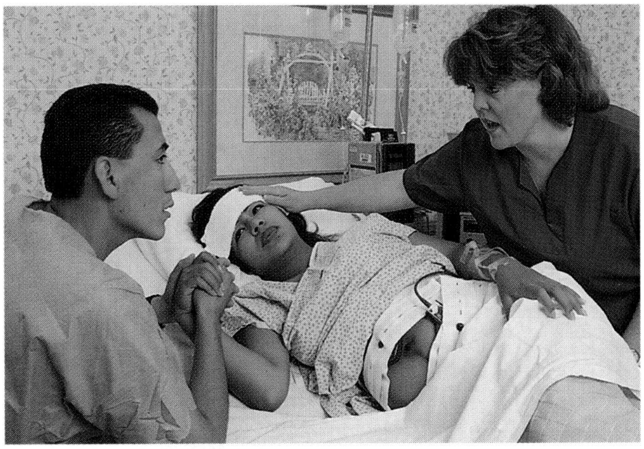

FIGURE 13-3 Cool, damp washcloths placed where the woman finds them most comforting helps her relax during each contraction. Several washcloths should be kept near the area to maintain their cool dampness.

Cleanliness. Bloody show and amniotic fluid leak from the woman's vagina during labor. The nurse should change the sheets and gown as needed to keep her dry and comfortable. Her preferences should be the guide because she may not want to be disturbed during late labor. Change the disposable underpad regularly to reduce microorganisms that may ascend into the vagina. A folded towel absorbs larger quantities of amniotic fluid than the pad alone.

Mouth Care. Ice chips (Figure 13-4), frozen juice bars, and hard candy on a stick reduces the discomfort of a dry mouth. If oral intake is contraindicated, brushing the teeth (without swallowing water) and simply rinsing the mouth is helpful to the woman. Many women appreciate a moist washcloth applied to their lips.

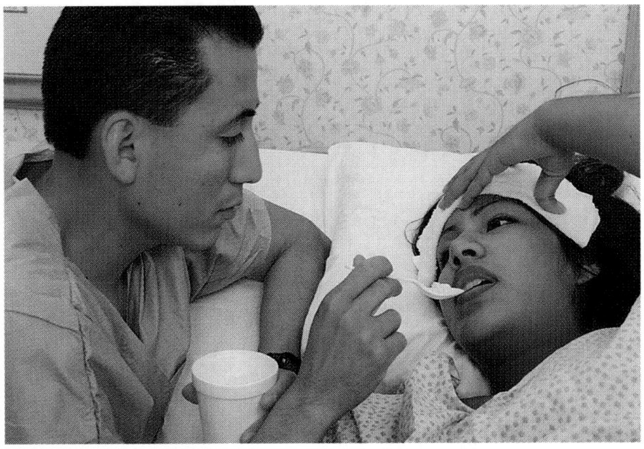

FIGURE 13-4 Most laboring women welcome ice chips to ease their dry mouths.

Bladder. A full bladder intensifies pain during labor and can delay fetal descent. It may cause pain that remains after an epidural is instituted. Remind the woman to empty her bladder at least every 2 hours and check her suprapubic area at least that often or more frequently if she has had large amounts of fluids.

Positioning. Occasionally, a specific maternal position is helpful to reduce discomfort and assist the labor process. Encourage the woman to assume any position she finds comfortable (other than the supine) and change positions frequently (Figure 13-5). Frequent changes reduce discomfort from constant pressure, help the fetus adapt to the pelvic contours, and promote fetal descent.

Upright positions benefit labor by adding the force of gravity to uterine contractions. Women who labor upright often need less analgesia and have more effective contractions. Studies also have shown improved newborn blood gases and pH levels in women who labored upright (Mayberry, Wood, Strange, Lee, Heisler, & Nielsen-Smith, 2000b).

"Back labor" commonly occurs, in which the back of the fetal head puts pressure on the woman's sacral promontory (occiput posterior position). The discomfort of back labor is difficult to relieve with medication alone. Positions that encourage the fetus to move away from the sacral promontory, such as those in which the mother uses the hands-and-knees position or leans forward over a birthing ball (a sturdy ball similar to a beach ball), reduce back pain and enhance the internal rotation mechanism of labor. Smaller versions of the birthing ball are available for use when the mother is sitting and leaning forward.

Water. Water in the form of a shower, tub, or whirlpool is relaxing for many women (see Chapter 15). However, a bath may slow labor if used in latent labor. It should be used in active labor or if persistent, nonproductive contractions during early labor have caused the woman to become very fatigued (Simkin & Frederick, 2000).

Standing

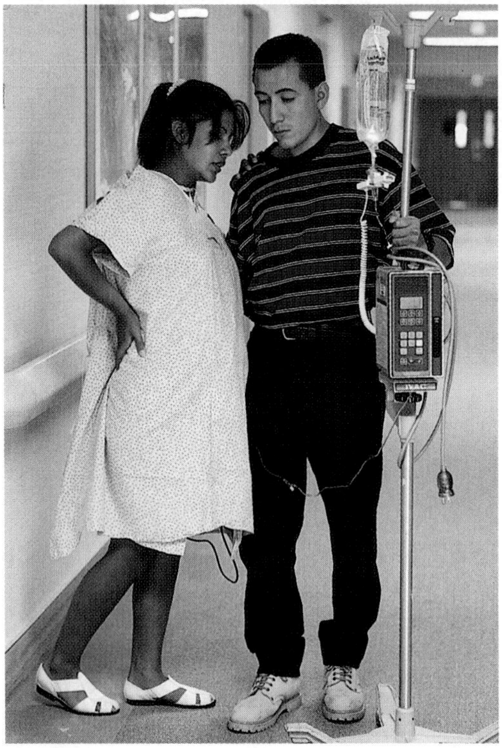

ADVANTAGES

Adds gravity to force of contractions to promote fetal descent.
Contractions are less uncomfortable and more efficient.
Variation: Standing, leaning forward with support reduces back pain because fetus falls forward, away from the sacral promontory.

DISADVANTAGES

Tiring over long periods.
Continuous electronic fetal monitoring is not possible without telemetry.

NURSING IMPLICATIONS

If the woman has intravenous fluid running, give her a rolling pole. Encourage her to alternate walking with other positions whenever she tires or desires to do so.
Remind the woman and her partner when she should return to the labor area for evaluation of the fetal heart rate and her labor status.

Sitting Upright

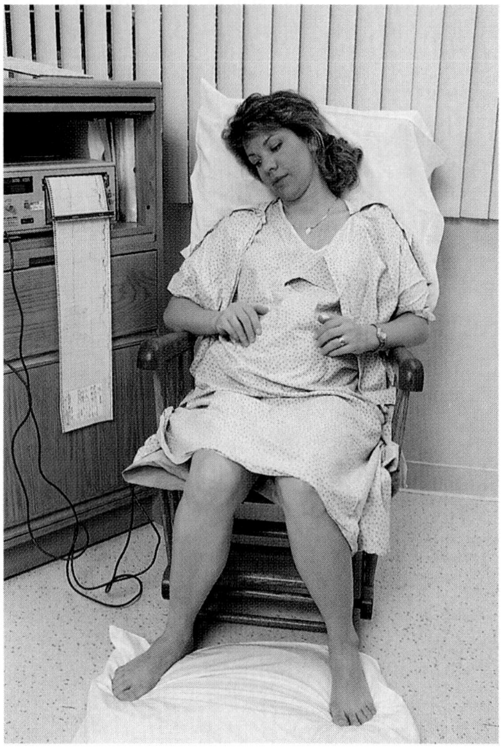

ADVANTAGES

Uses gravity to aid fetal descent.
Can be done when sitting on side of bed, in a chair, or on the toilet.
Can be used with continuous fetal monitoring.
Avoids supine hypotension.

DISADVANTAGES

May increase suprapubic discomfort.
Contractions are the most efficient when the woman alternates sitting with other positions.

NURSING IMPLICATIONS

A rocking chair is soothing.
Place a pillow on a chair with a disposable underpad over the pillow to absorb secretions.
Use pillows or a foot stool to keep the short woman's legs from dangling.
Encourage the woman to alternate positions periodically; for example, she can alternate walking with sitting or sitting with side lying.

FIGURE 13-5 Maternal positions for labor.

Teaching

Teaching the woman in labor is a continuously changing task.

First Stage

Many women become discouraged because several hours are needed to reach 4 or 5 cm of cervical dilation. They believe that the last 5 cm will take as long as the first 5 cm. From a time standpoint, 5 cm is more like two thirds of the way through first-stage labor rather than half of the way because the rate of dilation increases during the active phase.

A woman's urge to push usually occurs when her cervix is fully dilated and effaced and the fetus descends to about a +1 station and internally rotates. However, as she nears the second stage, the fetus may descend enough to give her an urge to push before full cervical dilation. If her cervix, which is usually 8 or 9 cm dilated

Sitting, Leaning Forward with Support

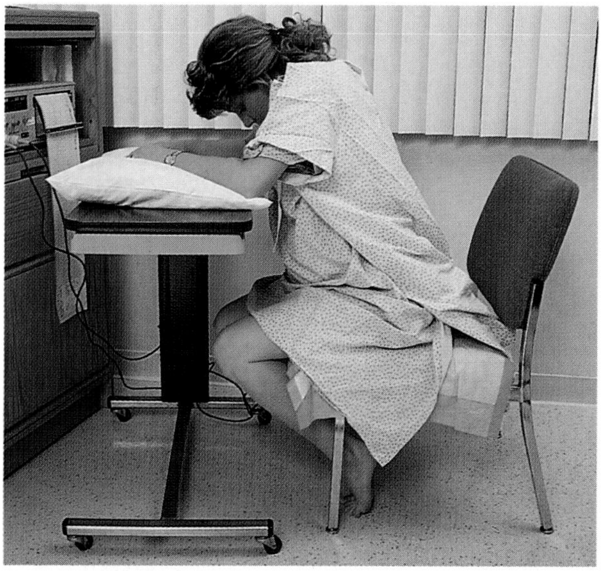

ADVANTAGES

Same as for sitting.
Reduces back pain because fetus falls forward, away from sacral promontory.
Partner or nurse can rub back or give sacral pressure to relieve back pain.

DISADVANTAGES

Same as for sitting.

NURSING IMPLICATIONS

Same as for sitting.

Semi-Sitting

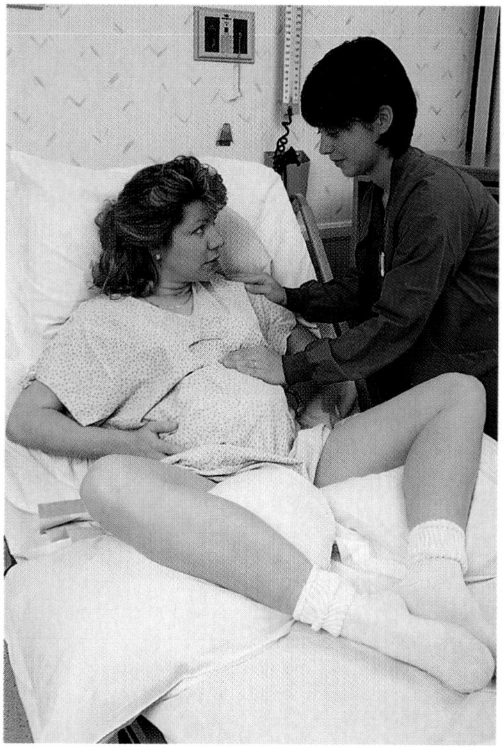

ADVANTAGES

Same as for sitting.
Aligns long axis of uterus with pelvic inlet, which applies contraction force in the most efficient direction through pelvis.

DISADVANTAGES

Same as for sitting.
Does not reduce pain as well as the forward-leaning positions.

NURSING IMPLICATIONS

Same as for sitting.
Raise bed to about a 30- to 45-degree angle.
Encourage the woman to use sitting (leaning forward) or side lying if she has back pain so that the caregiver can rub her back or apply sacral pressure.

FIGURE 13-5, cont'd For legend, see opposite page.

Continued

at this time, yields easily to downward pressure, pushing in response to her spontaneous urge rarely causes problems, especially if this is a second or later birth.

Either of two problems may occur if she pushes against a cervix that does not easily yield to pressure from the fetal presenting part:

- The cervix may become edematous, which can block progress.
- The cervix may be lacerated.

Teach the woman to exhale in short breaths if pushing is likely to injure her cervix or cause cervical edema.

Second Stage

The woman may need help to trust the sensations from her body and push most effectively during second-stage labor.

Time Limit. A 2-hour period was once accepted as the upper limit for the duration of the second stage with little evidence of the benefits of restricting the second stage and even the accuracy of this time limit. A second stage longer than 2 hours is now recognized as safe as long as the mother and fetus show no signs of compromise.

Women push most effectively when they feel the reflex urge to do so. Women having epidural analgesia

Side Lying

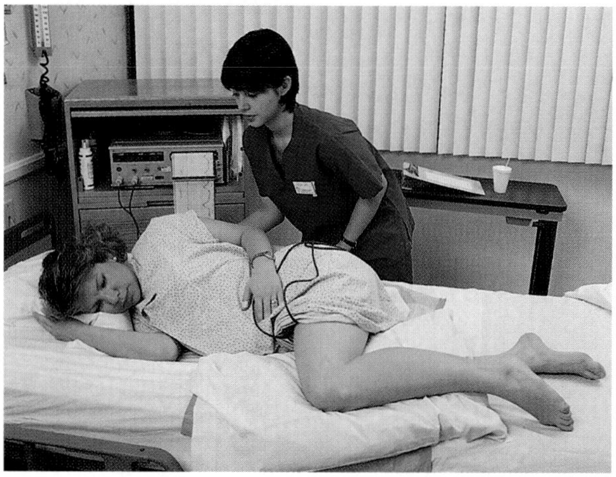

Advantages

Is a restful position.
Prevents supine hypotension and promotes placental blood flow.
Promotes efficient contractions, although they may be less frequent than with other positions.
Can be used with continuous fetal monitoring.

Disadvantages

Does not use gravity to aid fetal descent.

Nursing Implications

Teach the woman and her partner that although the contractions are less frequent, they are more effective.
This position offers a break from more tiring positions.
Use pillows for support and to prevent pressure: at her back, under her superior arm, and between her knees.
Use disposable underpads to protect the pillow between the woman's knees from secretions.
Some women like to put their superior leg on the bed rail; if the woman wants this variation, pad the bed rail; with a blanket to prevent pressure.
If she wants to remain recumbent, she should use this position to promote placental blood flow.

Kneeling, Leaning Forward with Support

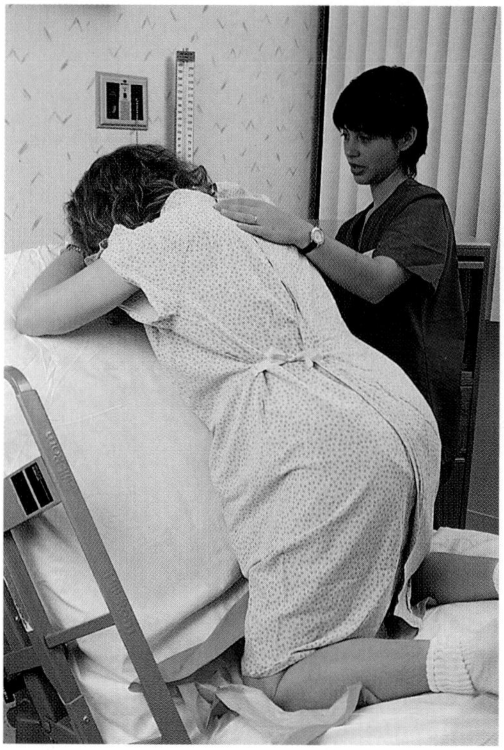

Advantages

Reduces back pain because fetus falls forward, away from sacral promontory.
Adds gravity to force of contractions to promote fetal descent.
Can be used with continuous fetal monitoring.
Caregivers can rub her back or apply sacral pressure.
Promotes normal mechanisms of birth.

Disadvantages

Knees may become tired or uncomfortable.
Tiring if used for long periods.

Nursing Implications

Raise the head of the bed, and have the woman face the head of the bed while she is on her knees.
Another method is for the partner to sit in a chair, with the woman kneeling in front, facing her partner, and leaning forward on him or her for support.
Use pillow under the knees and in front of the woman's chest, as needed, for comfort.
Encourage her to change positions if she becomes tired.

FIGURE 13-5, cont'd For legend, see p. 312.

Continued

Hands and Knees

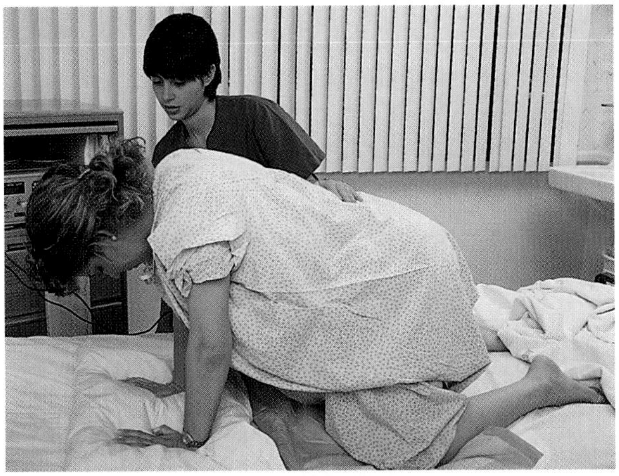

ADVANTAGES

Reduces back pain because the fetus falls forward, away from the sacral promontory.
Promotes normal mechanisms of birth.
The woman can use pelvic rocking to decrease back pain.
Caregivers can rub the woman's back or apply sacral pressure easily.

DISADVANTAGES

The woman's hands (especially wrists) and knees can become uncomfortable.
Tiring when used for a long time.
Some women are embarrassed to use this position.

NURSING IMPLICATIONS

Encourage the woman to change to less tiring positions occasionally.
Ensure privacy when encouraging the reluctant woman to try this position if she has back pain.
A second hospital gown with the opening in front covers her back and hips but may be too warm.

Positions for Pushing in Second-Stage Adaptations of Positions for Pushing

STANDING

This position may be tiring, and access to the woman's perineum is difficult. Because the infant could fall to the ground if birth occurs rapidly, provide padding under the mother's feet. Gravity aids fetal descent.

HANDS AND KNEES

Advantages and disadvantages are similar to those during first-stage labor. In addition, caregivers must reorient themselves because the landmarks are upside down from their usual perspective.
A variation is for the mother to kneel and lean forward against a beanbag or the side of the bed. This variation reduces some of the strain on her wrists and hands.

Squatting

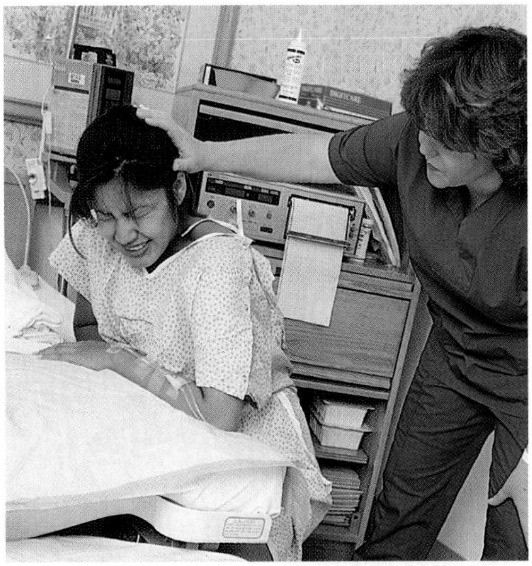

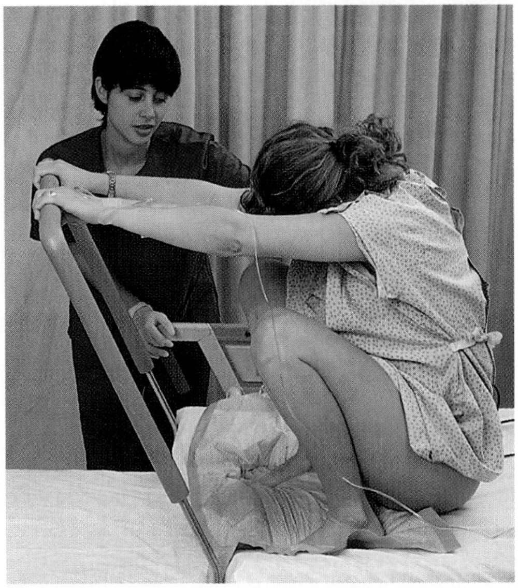

ADVANTAGES

Adds gravity to force of contractions to promote fetal descent.
Straightens the pelvic curve slightly for more direct fetal descent.
Increases dimensions of pelvis slightly.
Promotes effective pushing efforts in the second stage.
Caregivers can rub back or provide sacral pressure.

DISADVANTAGES

Knees and hips may become uncomfortable because of prolonged flexion.
Tiring over a long time.

NURSING IMPLICATIONS

Provide support with a squat bar attached to the bed or by two people standing on each side of the woman.
If she becomes tired, or between contractions, she can lean back into the sitting position.
Variation: Have the woman squat beside the bed as she pushes.

FIGURE 13-5, cont'd For legend, see p. 312.

Continued

Semi-Sitting

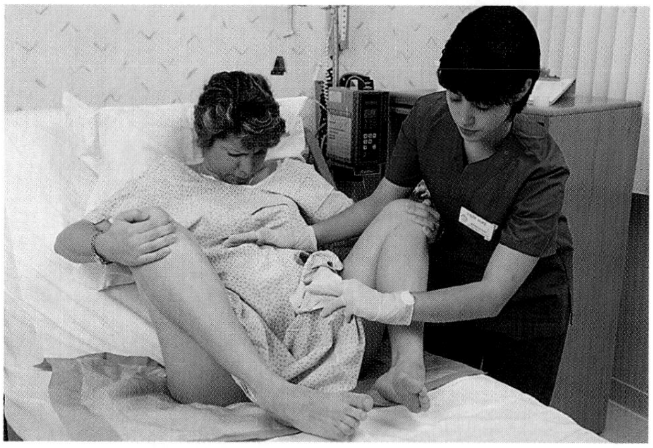

Many woman prefer this because they have the security of a back rest; it is also familiar to caregivers and allows easy observation of the perineum. Elevate the woman's back at least 30 to 45 degrees so that gravity aids fetal descent. The woman pulls on her flexed knees (behind or in front of them) as she pushes. She should keep her head flexed and her sacrum flat on the bed to straighten the pelvic curve.

Side-Lying

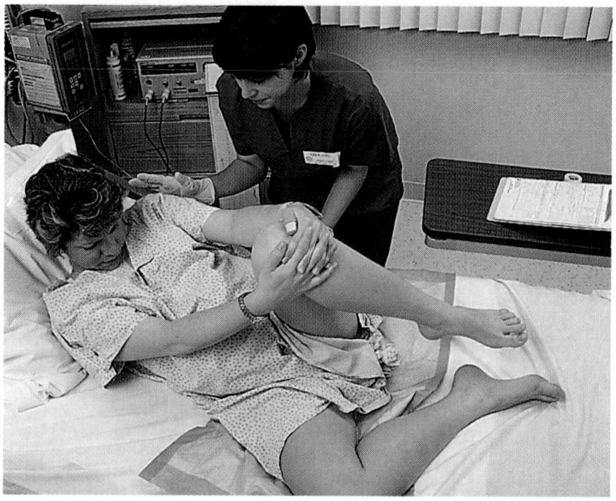

The woman flexes her chin on her chest and curls around her uterus as she pushes. She pulls on her flexed knees or the knee of the superior leg as she pushes.

FIGURE 13-5, cont'd For legend, see p. 312.

with modern techniques usually can detect an urge to push. Many women do not immediately feel the urge to push when the cervix is fully dilated. A brief slowing of contractions often occurs at the beginning of the second stage. Pushing vigorously sooner than the onset of the reflex urge may contribute to birth canal injury because her vaginal tissues are stretched more forcefully and rapidly than if she pushed spontaneously and in response to her body's signals. The mother may be frustrated and uncomfortable because she is asked to do something that does not feel right to her.

The technique of delaying pushing until the reflex urge to push occurs may be called any of several names, including *delayed pushing, laboring down, rest and descend,* and *passive pushing.* Delayed pushing has been shown to have a lower incidence of variable FHR decelerations, less maternal fatigue, and Apgar scores equal to those of women who pushed immediately on full cervical dilation (Mayberry, Wood, Strange, Lee, Heisler, & Nielsen-Smith, 2000).

Positions. Squatting is an ideal position for pushing because it enlarges the pelvic outlet slightly and adds the force of gravity to the mother's efforts, which is an advantage if she has a small pelvis or the fetus is large. Some women push effectively while sitting on the toilet because that is where they are accustomed to giving in to the sensation of rectal pressure. Pushing while sitting on a birthing ball and pulling against a squatting bar on the bed or playing "tug of war" with another person provides a similar gravitational advantage. Women may find that pulling on something from above is efficient. Her upper torso should be in front of her pelvis to allow her coccyx to move backward as the fetus descends deeply into her pelvis. Squatting is not possible for women having epidurals because the block causes leg weakness, although women can gain some of the position's advantages using sitting and semi-sitting positions.

If the mother pushes in a sitting or semi-sitting position, teach her to curve her body around her uterus in a C shape rather than arching her back. For most effectiveness, the woman should pull on her knees, handholds, or a squatting bar while pushing. She should maintain a similar C shape to her upper body if she pushes on her side.

Method and Breathing Pattern. Support the woman's spontaneous pushing techniques if they are effective. The woman should push with her abdominal muscles while relaxing her perineum. If she needs coaching, teach her to begin by taking a breath and exhaling and then take another breath and exhale while pushing for about 4 to 6 seconds at a time. Sustained pushing while holding a breath (Valsalva maneuver or "purple pushing") reduces blood flow to the placenta and is fatiguing. Another deep breath that is more like a sigh helps her relax after the contraction.

A woman who is modest or fears losing control may inhibit her best pushing efforts if she is instructed to push as if she were having a bowel movement, particularly if she is in a bed or chair. An anatomically correct image is to teach the woman to push down and out under her symphysis (pubic bone), following the pelvic curve. Seeing a diagram of the pelvis helps her to visualize the curve.

Providing Encouragement

Success breeds success. Tell the woman when her labor is progressing. If she can see that her efforts are effective, she has more courage to continue. Help her touch or see the baby's head with a mirror as crowning occurs.

Praise the woman and her support person when they use breathing and other coping techniques effectively. This reinforces their actions, gives them a sense of control, and conveys the respect and support of the nurse. If one technique is not helpful after a reasonable trial (at least three to five contractions), encourage them to try other techniques.

Giving of Self

The importance of the nurse's caring presence cannot be overlooked as a component of labor support. Even independent women may become dependent during labor and need human contact. Many times, the woman simply needs reassurance that all is going well and the nurse is there for her. The nurse's presence helps to allay her fears of abandonment and conveys safety, acceptance, support, and comfort.

Although the woman and her support person may have prepared for childbirth, they often welcome suggestions and affirmation from the nurse. They are more likely to use the techniques they learned if the nurse helps them use them. The nurse's presence, gentle coaching, and encouragement help the woman have confidence in her own body and fitness to give birth.

> Labor nursing is a contact sport. Laboring women need the human support of a skilled, empathic, and intuitive nurse at their bedside—coaching them, reassuring them, and most of all, being there for them. This degree of support cannot be matched by the nurse who spends more time observing a fetal monitor at a central nurses' station than in the company of the laboring mother.

Offering Pharmacologic Measures

Birth is usually a normal process, and the prepared woman and labor partner can deliver their infant without medication if they choose to do so. However, many do choose pharmacologic pain management. The nurse must be informative but neutral when explaining about available pain medication.

Some women may have a firm goal of avoiding pain medication during labor. A woman who planned an unmedicated birth may interpret the nurse's information about available medication as pressure for her to take medication. If the woman takes the medication offered, she may later feel that she "gave in" at a "weak moment," thus reducing her sense of mastery over her birth. She may feel disappointed and guilty because she took medication despite her planned nonmedicated birth.

Other women may plan to use a specific method such as epidural analgesia. If something prevents use of a chosen method, the woman may be upset about this unexpected development in her birth experience. In either case, allow the woman to vent her feelings about her experience. Although the event may not be what she wanted, expressing her feelings helps her put it into perspective.

Caring for the Birth Partner

The woman's support person is an integral part of her labor care. Her labor partner can provide care and comfort, which support the woman's ability to give birth. However, do not expect too much of the support person or make assumptions about the type and amount of involvement desired.

Some partners are coaches in the true sense of the word, actively assisting the woman through labor. Others want the woman and nurse to lead them and tell them how to help. They are eager to do what they can but expect instructions about methods and timing. Many couples see the partner's role as encouraging, offering moral support, and simply being there for the woman. In addition, the woman herself may expect her partner's nearness and emotional support rather than active coaching (Chapman, 1992).

Imposing unrealistic expectations of leadership, care, and comfort on the partner makes the birth experience unnecessarily stressful. To ensure a positive experience for both, accept whatever pattern of support the partner is able and willing to provide and is comfortable to the couple. Without taking over or diminishing this role, provide any support that the partner cannot.

Encourage the partner to conserve physical strength, eat, and drink liquids. The partner may have missed sleep during the hours of early labor and need a break. Encouraging the partner to eat a meal or snack may be necessary. Some partners think that they should not eat because the laboring woman is not doing so. However, hypoglycemia has caused more than one support person to faint at the time of birth and miss the main event.

Evaluation

Achievement of the three goals or expected outcomes occurs if the following conditions are met:

1. The woman indicates satisfaction with her method of pain management or requests nursing assistance to find other, more satisfactory methods.
2. The woman's support person expresses satisfaction with having provided labor support by the time of discharge.
3. The woman describes her birth experience as positive by the time of discharge.

The first nursing diagnosis regarding pain management is continually reevaluated throughout labor. The ability of the woman's support person is also continually evaluated. The last nursing diagnosis is evaluated after the woman and her significant other have had time to begin putting the birth experience into perspective.

PREVENTION OF INJURY

Assessment

Nursing assessments of the mother and fetus continue as the woman nears birth. During the second stage, observe the woman's perineum to determine when to make final birth preparations.

The exact time for final birth preparations varies according to the woman's parity, overall speed of labor, and fetal station. Preparations are usually completed when crowning in the nullipara reaches a diameter of about 3 to 4 cm. The multipara is prepared sooner, usually when her cervix is fully dilated and the fetal head is well down in the pelvis but before much crowning has occurred.

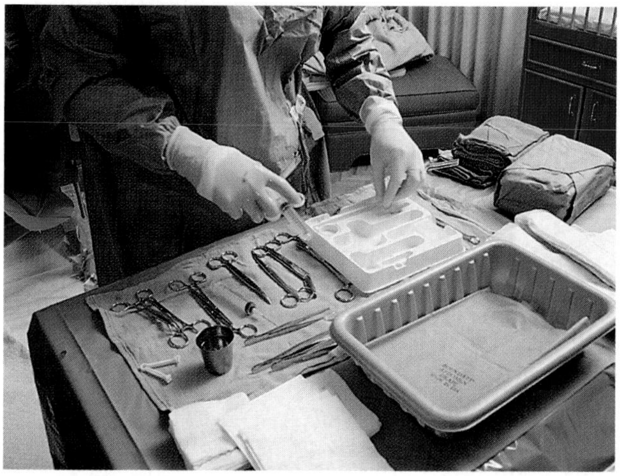

FIGURE 13-6 The nurse makes final preparations for birth. Included on the sterile table are anesthesia trays (if needed), instruments for birth and repair of maternal injury and episiotomy, and infant care materials.

Analysis

The woman is vulnerable to injury immediately before and after birth for several reasons: (1) altered physical sensations such as intense pressure and effects of medication, (2) positional changes for birth, and (3) unexpectedly rapid progress. The nursing diagnosis selected for the laboring woman near the time of birth is "Risk for Injury (maternal) related to altered sensations and positional or physical changes."

Planning

The nurse's primary objective is to prevent and minimize injuries that can occur during final birth preparations and because of a sudden birth. The goal or expected outcome for this nursing diagnosis is that the woman does not have a preventable injury such as muscle strains, thrombosis, and lacerations during birth.

Interventions

Transfering the woman to the delivery site and positioning her in the birthing bed is the first step in the sequence of events that culminates in the birth of the baby (Figures 13-6 to 13-8). During the period around birth, the nurse reduces factors that contribute to maternal injuries.

Transferring to a Delivery Room

Most births occur in a combination labor, delivery, and recovery room. Occasionally, the woman must be transferred to a separate room for birth. If so, she should be transferred early to avoid rushed, last-minute preparations that cause anxiety for everyone.

Positioning for Birth

Upright positions promote effective pushing and take advantage of gravity. Squatting is a good position for uncomplicated birth but limits accessibility to the woman's perineum and may not be an option for women having epidural analgesia. Squatting, during which the upper body leans forward, promotes expulsive efforts, directs the fetus efficiently toward the pelvic outlet, and increases the diameters of the pelvic outlet.

Other upright positions for the birth include standing and kneeling upright positions. The semirecumbent position limits movement of the coccyx as the fetus descends during birth but maintains some advantages of gravity. Sitting on a birthing bed with a cutout for the perineal area maintains many advantages of squatting and may be less tiring. The hands and knees position may be helpful if the fetus is in the occiput posterior position and to rotate wide fetal shoulders.

Many women and birth attendants are more comfortable using stirrups and foot rests to support the woman's legs and feet and make her perineum more accessible. If she cannot move her legs because of motor block from anesthesia, raise and lower her legs together and do not separate them too widely. Surfaces that contact the popliteal space behind the knee should be padded because of veins near the surface, on which pressure could lead to thrombus formation. The woman's upper body should be in a semi-reclining or sitting rather than a flat position.

Observing the Perineum

The exact time at which a woman is ready to give birth is an educated guess. A woman who has been having a slow labor may suddenly make rapid progress. Birth is near when the fetal head swings anteriorly in the mechanism of extension as the occiput slips under the symphysis pubis. Observe the woman's perineum, especially during late second-stage labor.

As birth nears, perineal massage with warm mineral oil may be useful. This technique is considered to relax the perineum, allowing it to stretch and better ac-

Transfer and Positioning for Birth

Action: When the woman is almost ready to give birth, transfer her to the delivery room or position the birthing bed. The exact time varies with several factors (such as overall speed of labor and rate of fetal descent). Rationale: Rushed, last-moment preparations are anxiety-producing for the woman, her partner, and the nurse. Remaining in the birth position for a long time can be tiring.

Action: Continue observing her perineum while making final preparations for birth. Rationale: Birth may occur unexpectedly, and the nurse should be prepared to "catch" the infant if the attendant (physician or nurse-midwife) is not in the room.

Action: Continue observing the fetal heart rate (FHR) with continuous monitoring or intermittent auscultation. Rationale: Detects changes in fetal condition that may require interventions by the attendant to speed birth.

Action: Elevate the woman's back, shoulders, and head with a wedge (on a delivery table) or by raising the head of the birthing bed. Rationale: Allows more effective maternal pushing and uses gravity to aid fetal descent.

Action: Stirrups or foot rests to support the woman's legs and feet may be used on a birthing bed. Pad the surface. Rationale: Padding reduces pressure, preventing venous stasis and possible thrombus formation.

Action: When placing the woman's legs in stirrups, elevate them and remove them simultaneously. Do not separate her legs widely. Rationale: Reduces strain on muscles and ligaments.

Prepping and Draping

Action: After the woman is in position, cleanse the perineal area with a sterile iodophor and water preparation unless she is allergic. Use warm water to dilute the iodophor scrub. Rationale: Removes secretions and feces from perineal area.

Action: After handwashing, apply sterile gloves for the prep procedure. Take a fresh sponge to begin each new area, and do not return to a clean area with a used sponge. Six sponges are needed. The proper order and motions are as follows:

1. Use a zig-zag motion from clitoris to lower abdomen just above the pubic hairline.

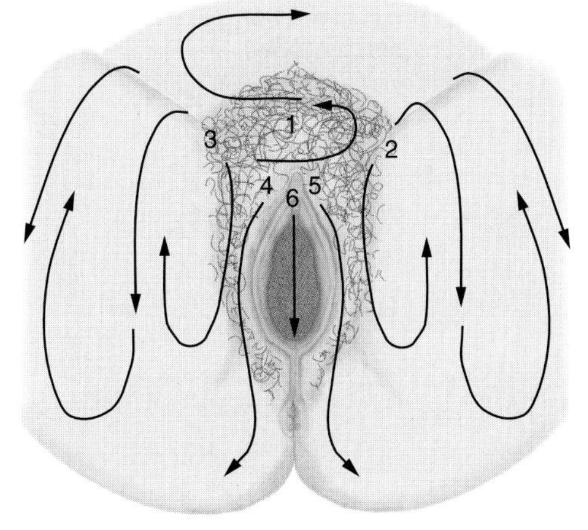

2., 3. Use a zig-zag motion on the inner thigh from the labia majora to about halfway between the hip and knee. Repeat for the other inner thigh.

4., 5. Apply a single stroke on one side from clitoris over labia, perineum, and anus. Repeat for the other side.

6. Use a single stroke in the middle from the clitoris over the vulva and perineum.

Rationale: Prevents cross-contamination or recontamination of an area that is already clean.

Action: The attendant may apply sterile drapes if desired. Rationale: A vaginal birth is a clean procedure rather than a sterile one because the vagina is not sterile. Sterile drapes are unnecessary, but some attendants may prefer to use them.

Birth of the Head

Action: If an episiotomy is needed, the attendant will perform it when the head is well crowned (see Chapter 16). Rationale: Minimizes blood loss from the episiotomy.

Action: As the vaginal orifice encircles the fetal head, the attendant applies gentle pressure to the woman's perineum with one hand while applying counterpressure to the fetal head with the other hand (Ritgen's maneuver). The attendant may ask the mother to blow so that she avoids pushing, or to push gently. Rationale: Controls the exit of the fetal head so that it is born gradually rather than popping out; this minimizes trauma to the maternal tissues.

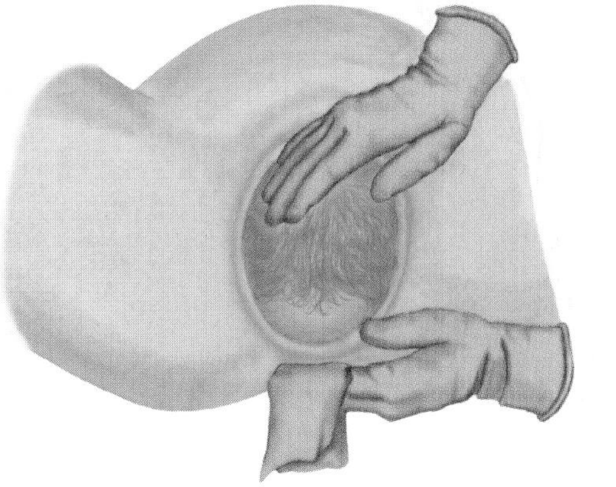

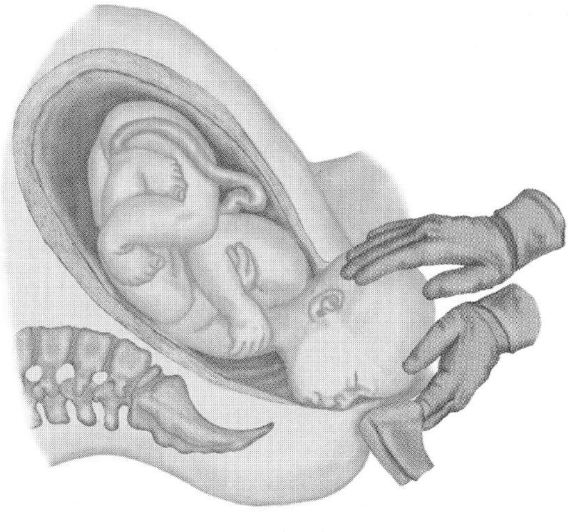

FIGURE 13-7 Sequence for delivery.

Continued

Action: The attendant wipes secretions from the infant's face and suctions the nose and mouth with a bulb syringe. Rationale: Removes blood and secretions, preventing the infant from aspirating them with the first breaths.

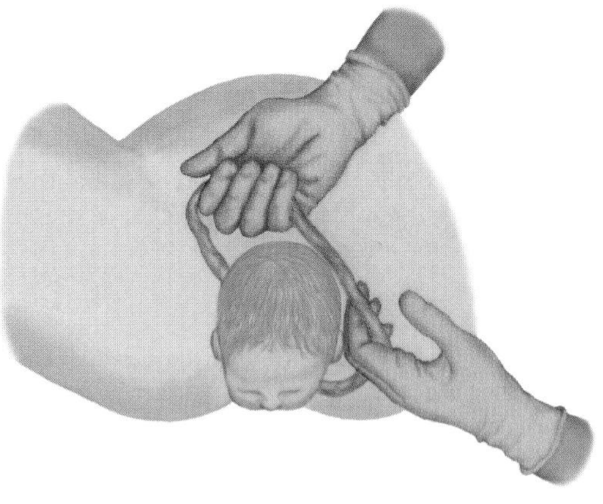

Action: The attendant feels for a cord around the fetal neck (nuchal cord). If it is loose, it is slipped over the head. If tight, it is clamped and cut between two clamps before the rest of the baby is born. Rationale: Allows the rest of the birth to occur and prevents stretching or tearing the cord.

Birth of the Shoulders

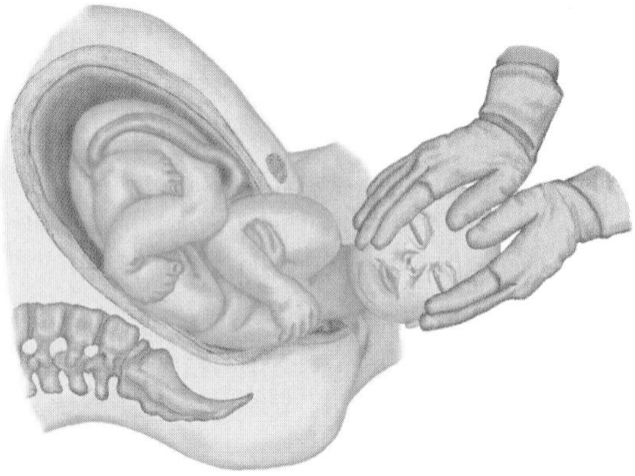

Action: After external rotation, the attendant applies gentle traction on the fetal head in the direction of the mother's perineum. Rationale: External rotation allows the shoulders to rotate internally and aligns their transverse diameter with the anteroposterior diameter of the mother's pelvic outlet. Traction on the head in the direction of her perineum allows the anterior fetal shoulder to slip under the symphysis pubis.

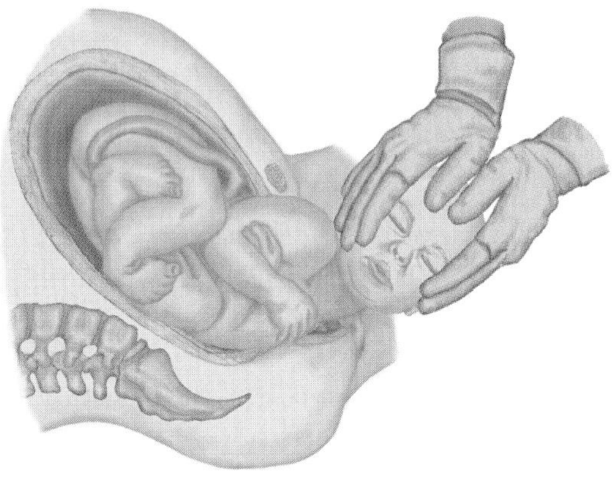

Action: The attendant then lifts the head toward the mother's symphysis pubis. Rationale: Permits the posterior fetal shoulder to be eased over the perineum, minimizing trauma to the maternal tissues.

Action: The rest of the infant's body is born quickly after the shoulders are born. The attendant maintains the infant in a slightly head-dependent position while suctioning excess secretions with a bulb syringe. The infant is often placed on the mother's abdomen. Rationale: Gravity aids spontaneous drainage of secretions and prevents aspiration of oral mucus and secretions.

Action: The attendant clamps the cord. Either the father or the attendant cuts the cord above the clamp. Rationale: Allows parents to interact more freely with their infant. Prevents flow of blood between placenta and infant, which might result in anemia (if infant is higher than placenta) or polycythemia (if infant is below the placenta).

Delivery of the Placenta

Action: After the placenta separates, it usually can be delivered if the mother bears down. The attendant may pull gently on the cord. Rationale: Excess traction on the cord may cause it to break, making the placenta harder to deliver.

Action: The attendant inspects both sides of the placenta. Rationale: Ensures that no fragments remain inside the uterus that might cause hemorrhage and infection.

After the infant and placenta are born, the attendant inspects the birth canal for injuries. If needed, any injuries and the episiotomy (if one was done) are repaired.

FIGURE 13-7, cont'd For legend, see p. 319.

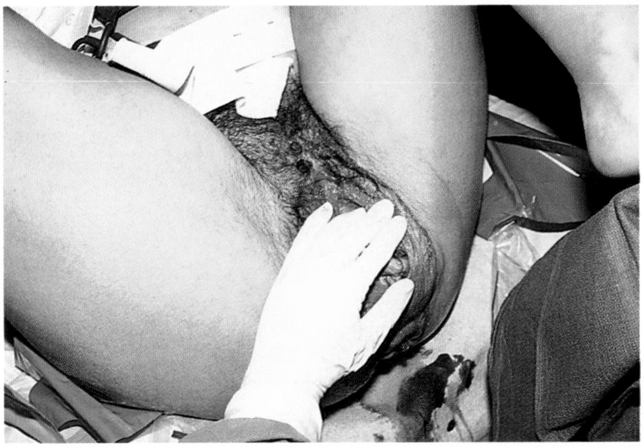

A. Crowning. The fetal head distends the labial and perineal tissues. The anus is stretched wide, and it is not unusual to see the woman's anterior rectal wall at this time. Any feces expelled are wiped posteriorly to avoid contaminating the vulva. The attendant (physician or nurse-midwife) is not holding the fetal head back but rather controlling its exit by using gentle pressure on the fetal occiput.

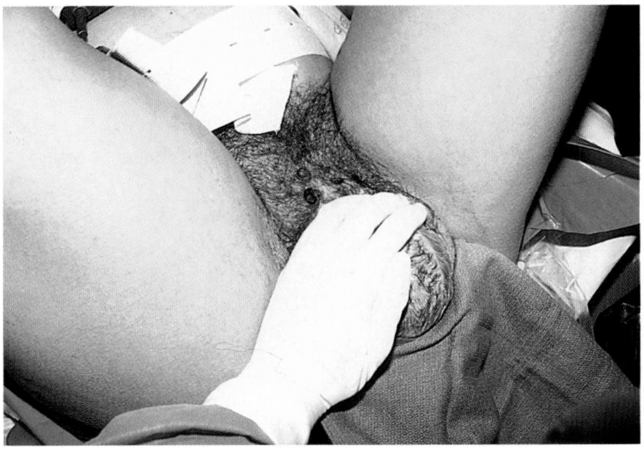

B. Ritgen maneuver. Pressure is applied to the fetal chin through the perineum at the same time pressure is applied to the occiput of the fetal head. This action aids the mechanism of extension as the fetal head comes under the symphysis.

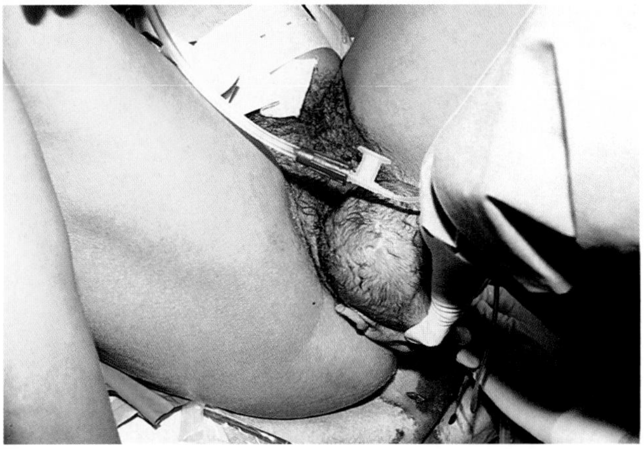

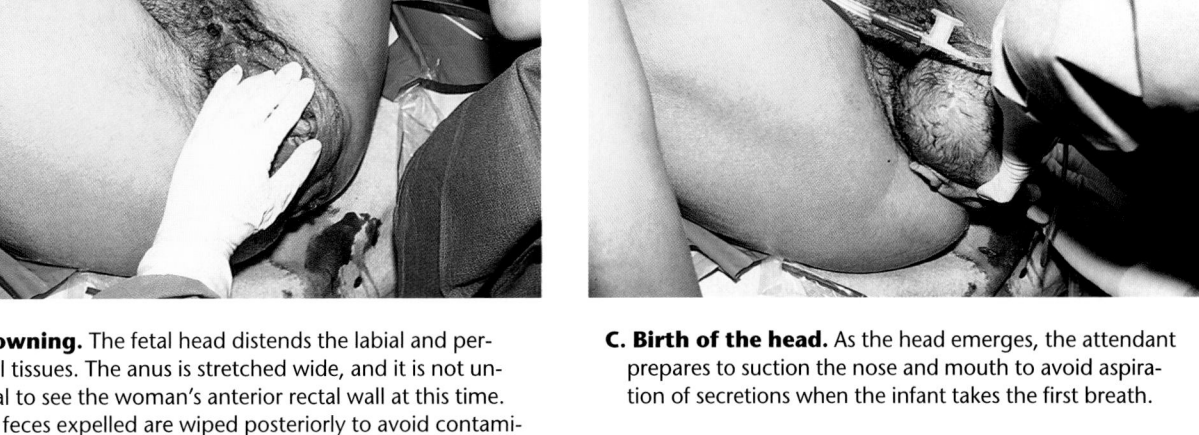

C. Birth of the head. As the head emerges, the attendant prepares to suction the nose and mouth to avoid aspiration of secretions when the infant takes the first breath.

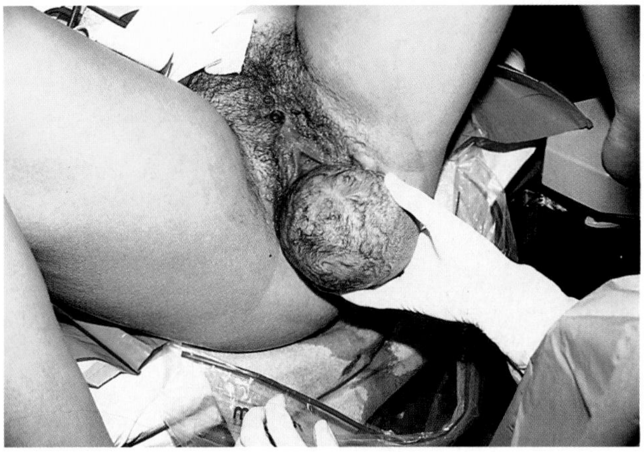

D. Restitution and external rotation. After the head emerges, it realigns with the shoulders (restitution). External rotation occurs as the fetal shoulders internally rotate, aligning their transverse diameter with the anteroposterior diameter of the pelvic outlet.

FIGURE 13-8 Vaginal birth.

Continued

commodate the baby's head during expulsion, minimizing the need for an episiotomy and reducing the risk of a large laceration. However, this benefit has not been proven. In contrast, daily perineal massage and stretching by the woman from about 34 weeks' gestation until birth has been shown to reduce the risk for perineal trauma during birth (Eason, Labrecque, Wells, & Feldman, 2000).

A classic sign of imminent birth is the mother's urgent cry, "The baby's coming!" Look at her perineum, and if the baby will be born before the physician or nurse-midwife arrives, remain calm and support the infant's head and body with gloved hands as it emerges (Figure 13-8). The support person should push the call button to summon help.

Evaluation

The goal or expected outcome for this nursing diagnosis is evaluated throughout the postpartum period because injuries such as muscle strains or thrombus for-

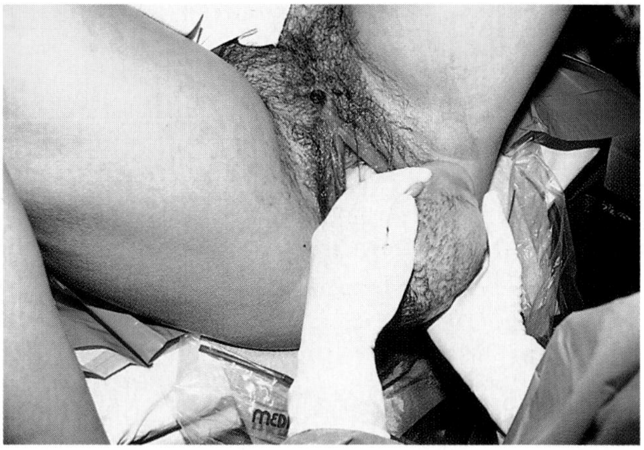

E. Birth of the anterior shoulder. The attendant gently pushes the fetal head toward the woman's perineum to allow the anterior shoulder to slip under her symphysis. The bluish skin color of the fetus is normal at this point; it becomes pink as the infant begins air breathing.

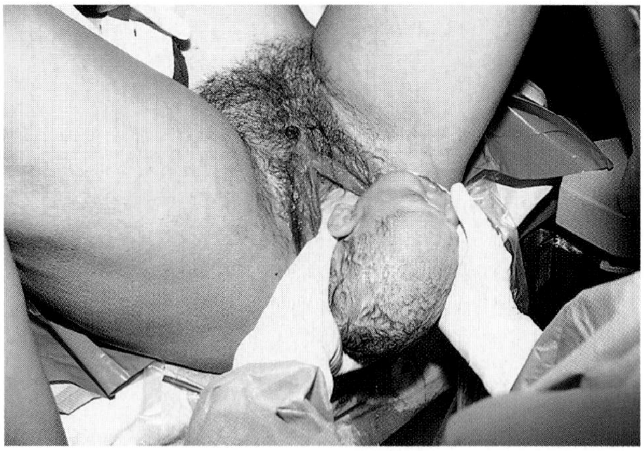

F. Birth of the posterior shoulder. The attendant now pushes the fetal head upward toward the woman's symphysis to allow the posterior shoulder to slip over her per-

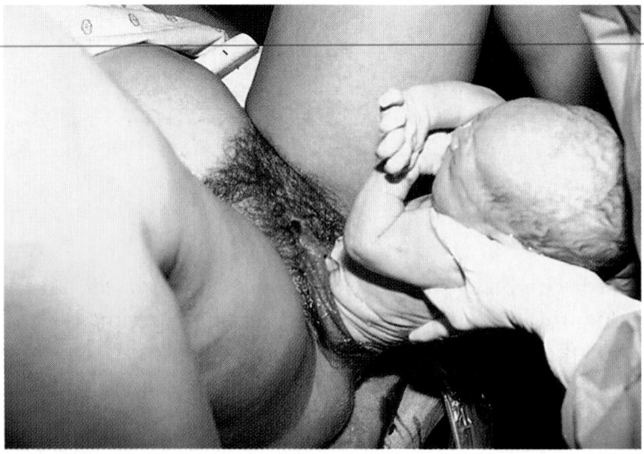

ineum.

G. Completion of the birth. The attendant supports the fetus during expulsion. Note that the fetus has excellent muscle tone, as evidenced by facial grimacing and flexion

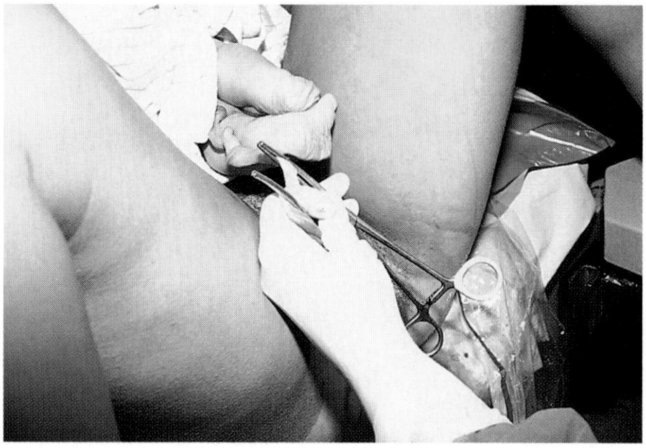

of the arms and hands.

H. Cord clamping. While the infant is in skin-to-skin contact on the mother's abdomen, the attendant doubly clamps the umbilical cord. The cord is then cut between

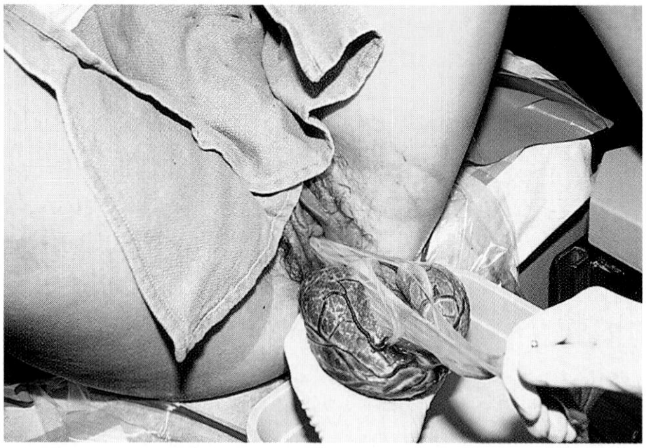

the two clamps. Samples of cord blood are collected after it is cut.

I. Birth of the placenta. The attendant applies gentle traction on the cord to aid expulsion of the placenta. This placenta is expelled in the more common Schultze mechanism, with the shiny fetal surface and membranes emerging. Note the fetal membranes that surrounded the fetus and amniotic fluid during pregnancy. The chorionic vessels that branch from the umbilical cord are readily visible on the fetal surface of the placenta.

FIGURE 13-8, cont'd For legend, see p. 319.

mation are not evident until later (see Chapter 17). The birth attendant notes lacerations after the baby's birth and makes necessary repairs.

Check Your Reading

12. How might maternal hypotension or hypertension affect the fetus?
13. What position should the woman avoid during labor? Why? What if the woman must be in this position temporarily?
14. What general measures can make the woman more comfortable during labor? How can the nurse support the woman's labor partner?
15. Why is watching the perineum as a woman pushes important?
16. How can perineal massage and heat applications reduce the risk for maternal birth injury?

NURSING CARE DURING THE LATE INTRAPARTUM PERIOD

Responsibilities during Birth

The nurse's responsibilities during birth may include the following:

- Preparation of a sterile delivery table with gowns, gloves, drapes, solutions, and instruments (see Figure 13-6)
- Perineal cleansing preparation
- Initial care and assessment of the newborn
- Administration of medications (usually oxytocin) to contract the uterus and to control blood loss (see Drug Guide 16-1). The anesthesiologist or nurse-anesthetist also may give maternal medications.

A nurse from the nursery is usually present if the newborn is at risk for problems such as respiratory depression and if problems occurred during labor. A person certified to provide neonatal resuscitation must be present at all births.

Personal protective equipment, including eye shields, should be worn as protection from fluid splashing and blood spurting as the cord is cut. The newborn is covered with blood, amniotic fluid, vernix, and other body substances. Persons involved in infant care should wear gloves and other needed protective equipment until after the first bath to avoid contact with potentially infectious secretions.

Responsibilities after Birth

Intrapartum nursing care extends through the fourth stage of labor and includes care of the infant, mother, and family unit (for more information, see also Chapters 17 through 23).

Care of the Infant

Nursing care of the newborn includes supporting cardiopulmonary and thermoregulatory function and identifying the infant. In addition, assess the infant for approximate gestational age (see p. 533) and examine for obvious anomalies and birth injuries. A full neonatal assessment may be delayed for about 1 hour to give the family a chance to meet their new member and initiate breastfeeding.

Maintaining Cardiopulmonary Function

Assess the infant's Apgar score (Table 13-3) at 1 and 5 minutes after birth for rapid evaluation of early cardiopulmonary adaptation. If the Apgar score is 8 or higher, no intervention is needed other than promoting normal respiratory efforts. If the infant is obviously in distress—no or low heart rate and respirations, limp muscle tone, lack of response to stimulation, blue or pale color), interventions to correct the problem are instituted immediately rather than waiting for the 1-minute Apgar score.

Place the infant on a prewarmed warmer with the head turned to one side to allow drainage of secretions. After the infant has a vigorous cry and minimal secretions, turn the baby to one side with the head flat or slightly elevated and suction secretions from the infant's mouth and nose with a bulb syringe as needed. Suction with a catheter may be necessary for more copious secretions.

Supporting Thermoregulation

Hypothermia raises the infant's metabolic rate and oxygen consumption, worsening any respiratory problems. Place the infant on a prewarmed warmer and quickly apply warm towels to reduce evaporative heat loss. The head should be dried well because substantial heat loss can occur from the head, which is about one fourth of the neonate's body surface area. The stimulus of drying the skin promotes vigorous crying and lung expansion in most healthy infants.

Skin-to-skin contact with a parent also maintains the infant's temperature and promotes bonding between the infant and parent. Avoid coming between the infant and the radiant heat source in the warmer. The infant should be wrapped in warm blankets when not in the warmer or making skin-to-skin contact. A stockinette cap further reduces heat loss if it is placed on the baby's dry head. A cap is not worn while the infant is in the radiant warmer because the cap slows transfer of heat to the baby.

Identifying the Infant

Bands with matching imprinted numbers and identifying information are the primary means to ensure that

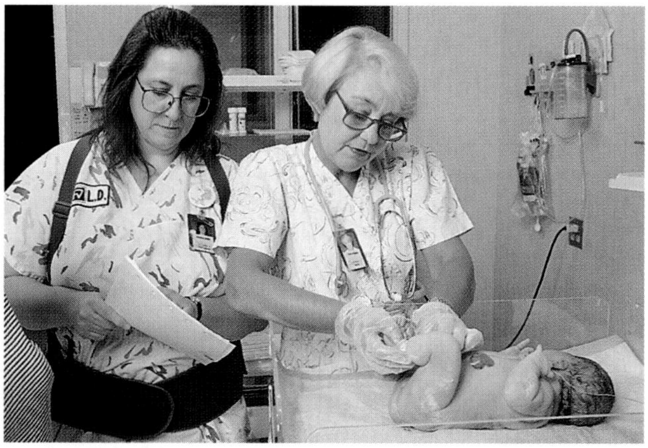

FIGURE 13-9 When the birthing room nurse turns over care of the infant to the nurse who will provide ongoing newborn care, both nurses check the identification bands and record for the same information.

Table 13-3

APGAR SCORE*

Assessment \ Points	0	1	2
Heart Rate	Absent	Below 100/min	100/min or higher
Respiratory Effort	No spontaneous respirations	Slow respirations or weak cry	Spontaneous respirations with a strong, lusty cry
Muscle Tone	Limp	Minimal flexion of extremities, sluggish movement	Flexed body posture, spontaneous and vigorous movement
Reflex Response	No response to suction or gentle slap on soles	Minimal response (grimace) to suction or a gentle slap on the soles	Responds promptly to suction or a gentle slap to the sole with a cry or active movement
Color	Pallor or cyanosis	Bluish hands and feet	Pink (light-skinned) or absence of cyanosis (dark-skinned)

*The Apgar score is a method of rapid evaluation of the infant's cardiorespiratory adaptation after birth. The nurse scores the infant at 1 minute and 5 minutes in each of five areas. The assessments are arranged from most important (heart rate) to least important (color). The infant is assigned a score of 0 to 2 in each of the five areas and the scores are totaled. General guidelines for the infant's care are based on three ranges of 1-minute scores:

0 1 2 3	4 5 6 7	8 9 10
Infant needs resuscitation.	Gently stimulate by rubbing the infant's back while administering oxygen. Determine whether mother received narcotics, which may have depressed infant's respirations. Have naloxone (Narcan) available for administration.	Provide no action other than support of the infant's spontaneous efforts and continued observation.

Note: Neonatal resuscitation measures, if needed, do not await 1-minute Apgar scoring but are instituted at once.

the right baby goes to the right mother after any separation (Figure 13-9). Check that imprinted band numbers and mother's names are identical on each set of bands and have the parent(s) verify this information at the time of banding. Apply two bands on the infant, one on an arm and another on an ankle, or one on each ankle to prevent facial scratching. Infant bands are applied more snugly than those worn by an adult, with about one adult fingerwidth of slack in the bands. Trim the excess band ends and apply the longer band to the mother's wrist. The mother's primary support person usually wears a fourth band. The infant will not be released to any adult who is not wearing a band with a matching name and number. A set of bands is needed

Table 13-4
PROBLEMS DURING THE FOURTH STAGE OF LABOR

Sign	Potential Problem	Immediate Nursing Action
Rising pulse rate, falling blood pressure, or both	These are early signs of hypovolemia because of excessive blood loss (visible or concealed).	Identify the probable cause of the blood loss, which usually is a poorly contracted uterus. Take steps to correct it (see below).
Soft (boggy) uterus	A poorly contracted uterus does not adequately compress large open vessels at the placental site, resulting in hemorrhage.	With one hand securing the uterus just above the symphysis and the other on the fundus, massage the uterus until it is firm. Push downward on the firm uterus to expel any clots. Empty the woman's bladder (by voiding or catheterization) if it is contributing to the uterine atony.
High uterine fundus, often displaced to one side	This suggests a full bladder that can interfere with uterine contraction and result in hemorrhage.	Massage the uterus if it is not firm. Help the woman urinate in the bathroom or bedpan. If she cannot void, catheterize her.
Lochia exceeding one saturated perineal pad per hour during the fourth stage	This suggests hemorrhage; however, consider that perineal pads vary in their absorbency.	Identify cause of hemorrhage, usually uterine atony, which is manifested by a soft uterus. Correct the cause. If lacerations are the suspected cause (excess bleeding, often bright red, with a firm fundus), notify the birth attendant. The woman should not take anything by mouth until the birth attendant evaluates her.
Intense perineal or vaginal pain, poorly relieved with usual analgesics	This suggests hematoma, usually of the vaginal wall or perineum. Signs of hypovolemia may occur with substantial blood loss into tissues.	If the hematoma is visible, apply cold packs to the area to slow bleeding into tissues. Notify the birth attendant, and anticipate possible surgical drainage. The woman should not take anything by mouth.

for each baby in a multiple birth. Some facilities take an early photo of the infant, when the infant is often alert, which serves two purposes: as a keepsake for the parents and identification in the event of abduction.

Care of the Mother

Nursing care of the mother during the fourth stage of labor focuses on observing for hemorrhage and relieving discomfort (Table 13-4).

Observing for Hemorrhage

Important assessments related to hemorrhage are the woman's vital signs, uterine fundus, bladder, lochia, and perineal and labial areas (see Chapter 17).

Vital Signs. Assess the woman's temperature when fourth-stage care begins. Blood pressure, pulse, and respirations should be assessed every 15 minutes during the first hour. A rising pulse is an early sign of excessive blood loss because the heart pumps faster to compensate for reduced blood volume. The blood pressure falls as the blood volume diminishes, but this is a later sign of hypovolemia.

Fundus. The most common reason for excessive postpartum bleeding is that the uterus does not firmly contract and compress open vessels at the placental site. Assess the firmness, height, and positioning of the uterine fundus with each vital sign assessment. The fundus should be firm, in the midline, and below the umbilicus (about the size of a large grapefruit). If the fundus is firm, no massage is needed; if it is soft (boggy), it should be massaged until it is firm. Nipple stimulation from the infant's sucking releases oxytocin from the mother's posterior pituitary gland to maintain firm uterine contraction. Oxytocin in IV solution or intramuscularly has the same effect.

Bladder. A full bladder interferes with contraction of the uterus and may lead to hemorrhage. A full bladder is suspected if the fundus is above the umbilicus or displaced to one side, usually the right. The first two voidings are often measured until it is evident that she voids without difficulty and empties her bladder completely. Each voiding is usually at least 300 to 400 ml if she is emptying her bladder. If no contraindication such as altered sensation occurs, the mother can walk to the bathroom (with assistance the first few times). She should sit on the side of the bed to make sure she is not light headed, move her legs back and forth, and raise her knees to be sure she has adequate strength and movement before ambulation.

Lochia. Assess for lochia with each vital sign and fundal assessment. The amount of lochia seems large to the inexperienced nurse and new mother. Perineal pads vary in their absorbency, but saturation of one standard pad (one that does not contain a cold pack) within the first hour is a guideline for the maximal normal lochia flow. Turn her to check for lochia pooling under the mother's buttocks and back. Small clots may be present, but the presence of large clots is not normal and the physician or nurse-midwife should be notified.

Perineal and Labial Areas. Observe these areas for hematoma formation. Small hematomas usually are easily limited by ice packs that are also applied for comfort. Large and rapidly expanding hematomas may cause significant enlargement of the tissues involved, a bluish color, and pain.

Promoting Comfort

Uterine contractions (afterpains) and perineal trauma are common causes of pain after birth. A postpartum chill often adds to discomfort. Pain usually is mild and readily relieved by simple measures. Notify the birth attendant if pain is intense or does not respond to common relief measures.

Ice Packs. Apply an ice pack to the perineum promptly after birth to reduce edema and limit hematoma formation. Some perineal pads include chemical cold packs. These pads absorb less lochia than ordinary pads, so this should be considered when estimating pad saturation. Ice packed into a glove is cheaper and colder than a chemical cold pack, although it melts quickly.

Analgesics. Afterpains and perineal pain respond well to mild oral analgesics. Regular urination reduces the severity of afterpains because the uterus contracts most effectively. The nurse should encourage the woman to take analgesics on a regular schedule to stay ahead of both perineal and afterpain discomfort.

Warmth. A warm blanket shortens the chill common after birth. A portable radiant warmer provides warmth to both the mother and infant. The mother may enjoy warm drinks initially.

Promoting Early Family Attachment

The first hour after birth is ideal for parent-infant attachment because the healthy neonate is alert and responsive. Provide privacy while unobtrusively observing the parents and infant. The infant can remain in the parent's arms while the nurse takes vital signs and suctions small amounts of secretions. Many newborn admission assessments can be performed while the parent holds the baby. (See Table 13-5 for possible nursing diagnoses for the intrapartum family.)

Assist the mother to nurse during the recovery period if she plans to breastfeed. The infant is usually attentive and nurses briefly. Early nipple stimulation helps initiate milk production and contract the uterus.

When the parents are ready, siblings, other family members, and friends should be allowed to visit. Help siblings see and touch their new brother or sister by putting a stool at the bedside or letting them sit on the bed.

Toddlers are often upset by the separation from their mother and may not be interested in the new baby. With supervision, children of preschool age or older may sit in a chair and hold the baby. School-age chil-

Table 13-5

COMMON NURSING DIAGNOSES FOR INTRAPARTUM FAMILIES

*Anxiety
Fear
Fluid Volume Deficit
Impaired Verbal Communication
Ineffective Family or Individual Coping
*Knowledge Deficit
*Pain
*Risk for Injury
Powerlessness

*Nursing diagnoses explored in this chapter.

NURSING CARE PLAN 13-1

Normal Labor and Birth

Assessment: Cathy Taggart, 17 years old, has been admitted in early labor with her first baby. Her cervix is 3 cm dilated and completely effaced. The fetus is at a 0 station and the membranes are intact. Cathy's husband Tim is with her. They did not attend childbirth classes. Cathy is holding Tim's hand tightly and breathing rapidly with each contraction. She says in a shaky voice, "I'm so scared. I've never been in a hospital before. I just don't know if I can do this."

Critical Thinking: What assumptions and biases must the nurse avoid in this situation?

Answer: The nurse should not assume that a 17-year-old girl is not married to the baby's father. The nurse should not assume that because the parents are young and did not attend childbirth classes, they are not interested in the baby and Cathy will tolerate labor's demands poorly. Cathy's age and nonattendance in childbirth classes should be considered when supporting her during birth, but the nurse should assess her needs individually, as with all clients.

Nursing Diagnosis: Anxiety related to unfamiliar environment and lack of birth preparation.

Critical Thinking: What cues led the nurse to choose this nursing diagnosis?

Answer: Several objective facts relate to the nursing diagnosis: (1) Cathy is having her first baby, (2) she has never been in the hospital, (3) she and Tim did not attend childbirth classes, (4) she is in early labor, (5) she has physical signs of anxiety, including holding tightly to Tim, breathing rapidly, and talking shakily, (6) she says she is "scared," and (7) she expresses doubt about her ability to tolerate labor. Although Cathy is probably having pain with contractions, anxiety is her dominant problem at this time.

Goals/Expected Outcomes

Cathy will do the following:

1. Express less anxiety after admission procedures are completed.
2. Have a relaxed facial and body posture between contractions.

Intervention	Rationale
1. Maintain a calm and confident manner when caring for Cathy. Express confidence in her ability to give birth.	1. This provides nonverbal and verbal reassurance that labor is normal and she has the resources within her to manage it.
2. Adapt therapeutic communication to the changing situation during Cathy's labor, simplifying explanations and directions as labor intensifies.	2. This identifies dominant concerns so that they can be properly addressed. Intense physical sensations reduce the ability to comprehend complex information.
3. Determine if Cathy and Tim have a birth plan and work within it as much as possible.	3. This enhances their sense of control and helps them to have a satisfying birth experience.
4. Maintain regular contact with Cathy and Tim throughout labor.	4. This provides security of human contact and reduces fears of abandonment and also allows Tim to have the degree of labor support he and Cathy desire.
5. Orient Cathy and Tim to the labor room and explain procedures and equipment she will encounter.	5. This reduces fear of the unknown.

Evaluation: Cathy relaxes somewhat after talking with the nurse and slows her breathing. She still holds Tim's hand but not as tightly. Cathy says, "I feel a little better now. I hope I can have my baby before you go home."

Assessment: Cathy's admission vital signs are normal: Temperature 98.8° F, pulse 88, respirations 20, and blood pressure 112/70. The FHR averages 140 to 150. Her contractions are every 4 minutes with a duration of 50 seconds and of moderate intensity.

Potential Complication: Fetal compromise.

Goals/Expected Outcomes:

Goals are not formulated for a potential complication because the nurse cannot independently manage fetal compromise. The nurse will do the following:

1. Take actions to promote normal placental function.
2. Observe for and report signs associated with fetal compromise.

Intervention	Rationale
1. Encourage Cathy to use any position she desires except the supine.	1. The supine position can cause aortocaval compression, reducing blood flow to the placenta.
2. Assess and document the FHR hourly during latent labor, every 30 minutes during active labor, and every 15 minutes during second stage. Report nonreassuring rates and patterns. Assess the FHR more frequently if deviations from normal are identified (see Chapter 14).	2. Cathy does not presently have risk factors and this is the recommended frequency for assessment to identify FHR assessments outside expected limits.
3. When the membranes rupture, observe for a clear color and mild odor and estimate the amount of fluid. Note the time of rupture. If the fluid is abnormal, notify the nursery staff.	3. Meconium-stained fluid may be associated with fetal or newborn compromise and should be reported. A nursery nurse, neonatal nurse-practitioner, or pediatrician often attends the birth when meconium staining is present. Cloudy, yellow, and strong- or foul-smelling fluid suggests infection. Prolonged rupture of membranes increases the risk of infection.
4. Assess contractions when FHR is assessed. Report contraction frequencies closer than every 2 minutes, durations longer than 90 seconds, intervals shorter than 60 seconds, and incomplete uterine relaxation between contractions.	4. Most placental exchange occurs during the interval between contractions. Contractions that are too long and have inadequate intervals decrease the time available for the intervillous spaces of the placenta to eliminate wastes and refill with oxygenated blood and nutrients.
5. Assess Cathy's blood pressure, pulse, and respirations every hour. Assess her temperature every 4 hours until her membranes rupture and then every 2 hours.	5. Maternal hypotension and hypertension can decrease blood flow to the placenta. Maternal fever can increase the fetus' demand for oxygen above the mother's ability to supply it. A rising maternal pulse and FHR may precede the temperature elevation.
6. See Nursing Care Plan 14-1 for additional interventions if signs of fetal compromise occur.	6. This nursing care plan addresses only basic actions to promote fetal oxygenation and identify possible problems.

Evaluation: Because no client goal is established for a potential complication, evaluation is not performed. The FHR remains at approximately the same rate, and no signs of fetal compromise occur. Cathy finds that sitting in a rocking chair is the most comfortable position.

Assessment: In 1.5 hours, Cathy's cervical dilation progresses to 5 cm, and the fetus descends to a +1 station. Her contractions are every 3 minutes, 60 seconds long, and of strong intensity. The FHR remains near its admission level. Cathy is having difficulty relaxing between contractions and is complaining of back pain. She is relieved that her labor is progressing normally.

Nursing Diagnosis: Pain related to effects of uterine contractions.

Goal/Expected Outcome: Cathy will express that she can manage labor pain satisfactorily.

Intervention	Rationale
1. Encourage Cathy to try positions such as standing/sitting and leaning forward, side-lying, leaning over the back of the bed, and hands and knees. Remind her to change positions about every half hour and when she feels the need for a change.	1. These positions shift the weight of the fetus away from the sacral promontory, reducing back pain. Alternating positions relieves strain and constant pressure and also helps the fetus adapt to the pelvis.
2. Teach Tim to rub and apply firm pressure to Cathy's back. Ask her where the best place is and how hard to press. Apply powder to the area rubbed.	2. Back rubs and firm pressure counteract some of the back pain. Powder decreases friction and promotes skin comfort.
3. Teach Cathy simple breathing and relaxation techniques (see Chapters 11 and 15).	3. These techniques provide distraction from pain and give her a sense of control. Relaxation enhances a woman's ability to manage pain and enhances normal labor processes.
4. Observe Cathy's suprapubic area and palpate for a full bladder every 2 hours or more frequently if she has had large amounts of fluid. Remind her to void if she has not done so recently.	4. A full bladder contributes to discomfort and can prolong labor by obstructing fetal descent.
5. Tell Cathy about her progress in labor. Explain that she will probably begin to dilate faster now that she has entered active labor.	5. Encouragement and the knowledge that her efforts are having the desired results increases a woman's willingness to continue.
6. Tell Cathy what pharmacologic pain relief measures are available to her. (This may be done during early labor to give a woman more time to consider her options.)	6. Knowing available options gives the woman a sense of control because she can choose whether she wants these measures.
7. See Nursing Care Plan 15-1 for additional interventions.	7. Nursing Care Plan 15-1 provides guidance about several nonpharmacologic and pharmacologic pain management measures.

Evaluation: Cathy continues to have back pain but says she is more comfortable sitting on the side of the bed with her head on a pillow on the overbed table. Tim rubs her back during contractions. She says she is able to manage the pain and does not want medication yet.

Assessment: After another 2 hours, Cathy is quite uncomfortable and requests pain medication. She is occasionally feeling an urge to push. Cathy cries and says she is "losing it" and "can't take it anymore." Tim asks anxiously, "What's wrong? Is Cathy OK? Why is she acting this way?" The FHR remains near the admission range and shows no signs suggesting fetal compromise. Contractions are every 2 minutes, 70 seconds, and strong.

Critical Thinking: What do these observations suggest? Does the nurse need more data?

Answer: Cathy's behaviors and the characteristics of her contractions suggest that she has entered the transition phase of first-stage labor, but her urge to push could indicate second-stage labor. The nurse usually performs a vaginal examination at this point to determine whether to encourage Cathy's pushing and identify the most appropriate pain-relief methods.

Assessment: A vaginal examination reveals that Cathy's cervix is dilated 8 cm and the station is +1. Butorphanol (Stadol), 0.5 mg IV, gives her enough analgesia to regain control and work with her contractions. She avoids pushing by blowing out at the peak of each contraction.

Cathy is fully dilated in 45 minutes, and the fetal station is +2. While in the squatting position next to the bed, she pushes spontaneously several times with each contraction. The end of the birthing bed is removed and a squatting bar is in place, but Cathy tends to not use the bar with contractions.

Nursing Diagnosis: Knowledge Deficit: Effective pushing techniques.

Goal/Expected Outcome: After instruction in effective pushing techniques, Cathy will use them until the birth occurs.

Intervention	Rationale
1. Observe Cathy's perineum for fetal crowning with each push.	1. A woman having her first baby can still give birth rapidly. Observation permits the nurse to maintain her safety and that of the baby, should rapid birth occur.
2. Encourage Cathy to exhale as she pushes strongly for about 4 to 6 seconds at a time.	2. Prolonged pushing against a closed glottis reduces blood return to the heart and maternal oxygen saturation and decreases placental blood flow.
3. Teach Cathy techniques to make each push more effective: a. Flex head slightly with each push.	3. a. Flexing directs each push downward into the pelvic cavity.
b. Pull against the squatting bar as she pushes down, relaxing her pull as she takes a deep breath.	b. Pulling provides leverage to gain more effective push from abdominal muscles. Squatting enlarges the pelvic outlet slightly.
c. Push toward the vaginal outlet, relaxing the perineum as she pushes.	c. This is an anatomically correct pushing direction. Reduces soft tissue resistance to fetal descent.
d. Keep her upper torso tilted forward and in front of her pelvis	d. This tilting permits backward movement of coccyx to allow easier fetal descent.
4. Do not talk to Cathy unnecessarily between contractions.	4. This allows her to conserve her energy for pushing efforts.

Evaluation: Cathy pushes effectively with the nurse's coaching. In another hour, she gives birth with an intact perineum to a 7-lb, 6-oz (3346 g) boy. The baby's Apgar scores are 9 at both 1 and 5 minutes. The new family gets acquainted during the recovery period. See Chapters 14 and 15 for more detailed nursing care relating to fetal monitoring and pain management.

dren are often fascinated by the new baby and surroundings and ask many questions. Adolescents react in various ways. They may be excited and eager to be a substitute parent, or they may be embarrassed about their parents' obvious sexuality "at their age."

Observe for signs of early parent-infant attachment. Parent behaviors are tentative at first, progressing from fingertip touch to palm touch to enfolding of the infant. Parents usually make eye contact with the infant and talk to the baby in higher-pitched, affectionate tones.

Cultural variations should be considered when assessing early attachment (see Chapter 18). The nurse should be knowledgeable about the typical practices of the populations commonly served. In some cultures, great attention to the newborn is considered unlucky ("evil eye").

SUMMARY CONCEPTS

- Some women do not have symptoms typical of true labor. They should enter the birth center for evaluation if they are uncertain and have concerns other than those listed in the guidelines.
- The childbearing family's first impression on admission to the intrapartum unit is important to promote a therapeutic relationship with caregivers and a positive birth experience.
- Initial intrapartum assessments quickly evaluate maternal and fetal health and labor status.
- The fetus is the more vulnerable of the maternal-fetal pair because of complete dependence on the mother's physiologic systems.
- The normal FHR at term averages 110 to 120 BPM at the lower limit and 150 to 160 BPM at the upper limit. Other reassuring signs include regular rhythm, presence of accelerations, and absence of decelerations.
- Persistent contraction frequencies closer than every 2 minutes, durations of longer than 90 seconds, and intervals shorter than 60 seconds may reduce placental blood flow and fetal oxygen, nutrient, and waste product exchange.
- A maternal supine position can reduce placental blood flow because the uterus compresses the aorta and inferior vena cava.
- General comfort measures promote the woman's ability to relax and cope with labor.
- Regular changes in position during labor promote maternal comfort and help the fetus adapt to the pelvis.
- The nurse must be alert for signs of impending birth: The woman may state "The baby's coming," make grunting sounds, and bear down.
- The priority nursing care of the newborn immediately after birth is to promote normal respirations, maintain normal body temperature, and promote attachment.
- The priority nursing care of the mother after birth is to assess for hemorrhage and promote firm uterine contraction, promote comfort, and promote parent-infant attachment.

ANSWERS TO CRITICAL THINKING EXERCISE, p. 298

The woman's behavior may have changed for several reasons, so the nurse must not make assumptions. For example, she may have felt insulted that the nurse found it necessary to ask her questions about illicit drug use. Or she may use other drugs and herbal preparations (licit or illicit) but prefer not to admit it. However, she may simply have been surprised at the question about drug use. Women often want their family to remain with them during the admission assessment but may not admit substance use and physical abuse in their presence. Nonverbal cues, such as a too-quick denial, avoidance of eye contact, and vague responses, are clues that the woman may not be answering these questions truthfully. The nurse should follow up on maternal behaviors privately to clarify underlying facts. Also, the nurse should delay asking any sensitive questions until alone with the woman.

ANSWERS TO CRITICAL THINKING EXERCISE, p. 306

Assess the fetal heart rate for at least 1 minute to identify any abnormal rate or pattern. Note the time of rupture, odor, and approximate amount of amniotic fluid. Report the findings to the physician or nurse-midwife because green, meconium-stained amniotic fluid may be associated with fetal compromise. A foul or strong odor is associated with infection. The FHR should be assessed more often, and an electronic fetal monitor is usually applied if not already in place.

REFERENCES & READINGS

American Academy of Pediatrics & American College of Obstetricians and Gynecologists (ACOG). (1997). *Guidelines for perinatal care* (4th ed.). Elk Grove Village, IL, & Washington, D.C.: Author.

ACOG. (1995a). *ACOG practice patterns: Vaginal delivery after previous cesarean birth.* Washington, D.C.: Author.

ACOG. (1995b). ACOG technical bulletin number 207: Fetal heart rate patterns: Monitoring, interpretation, and management. Washington, D.C.: Author.

ACOG. (1996). *ACOG technical bulletin number 219: Hypertension in pregnancy.* Washington, D.C.: Author.

Arrabal, P.P., & Nagey, D.A. (1996). Is manual palpation of uterine contractions accurate? *American Journal of Obstetrics and Gynecology,* 174(1, part 1), 217-219.

Bachman, J., & Kendrick, J.M. (1996). Childbirth. In K.R. Rice & P.A. Creehan (Eds.), *Perinatal nursing* (pp. 151-186). Philadelphia: J.B. Lippincott.

Bloom, S.L., McIntire, D.D., Kelly, M.A., Beimer, H.L., Burpo, R.H., Garcia, M.A., & Leveno, K.J. (1998). Lack of effect of walking on labor and delivery. *New England Journal of Medicine,* 339(2), 76-79.

Bowes, W.A. (1999). Clinical aspects of normal and abnormal labor. In R. Creasy & R. Resnik (Eds.), *Maternal-fetal medicine: Principles and practice* (4th ed., pp. 541-568). Philadelphia: W.B. Saunders.

Burian, J. (1995). Helping survivors of sexual abuse through labor. *MCN: American Journal of Maternal/Child Nursing,* 20(5), 252-256.

Callister, L.C. (1995). Cultural meanings of childbirth. *Journal of Obstetric, Gynecologic, and Neonatal Nursing,* 24(4), 327-331.

Chapman, L.L. (1992). Expectant fathers' roles during labor and birth. *Journal of Obstetric, Gynecologic, and Neonatal Nursing,* 21(2), 114-120.

Copeland, D.B., & Douglas, D. (1999). Communication strategies for the intrapartum nurse. *Journal of Obstetric, Gynecologic, and Neonatal Nursing,* 28(6), 579-586.

Creehan, P.A. (1996). Pain relief and comfort measures during labor. In K.R. Rice & P.A. Creehan (Eds.), *Perinatal nursing* (pp. 227-245). Philadelphia: Lippincott.

Cunningham, F.G., MacDonald, P.C., Gant, N.F., Leveno, K.J., Gilstrap, L.C., Hankins, G.D.V., et al. (1997). *Williams obstetrics* (20th ed.). Norwalk, CT: Appleton & Lange.

Eason, E., Labrecque, M., Wells, G., & Feldman, P. (2000). Preventing perineal trauma during childbirth: A systematic review. *Obstetrics and Gynecology,* 95(3), 464-471.

Enkin, M.W., Keirse, M.J., Renfrew, M.J., & Neilson, J.P. (1995). Effective care in pregnancy and childbirth: A synopsis. *Birth,* 22(2), 101-110.

Evans, S., & Jeffrey, J. (1995). Maternal learning needs during labor and delivery. *Journal of Obstetric, Gynecologic, and Neonatal Nursing,* 24(3), 235-240.

Feinstein, N.F., Sprague, A., & Trépanier, M.J. (2000). *AWHONN Symposium: Fetal heart rate auscultation.* Washington, D.C.: Author.

Fowles, E. (1998). Labor concerns of women two months after delivery. *Birth,* 25(4), 235-240.

Gagnon, A.J., Waghorn, K., & Covell, C. (1997). A randomized trial of one-to-one nurse support of women in labor. *Birth,* 24(2), 71-77.

Gagnon, A.J., & Waghorn, K. (1996). Supportive care by maternity nurses: A work sampling study in an intrapartum unit. *Birth* 23(1), 1-6.

Geissler, E.M. (1998). *Mosby's pocket guide: Cultural assessment* (2nd ed.). St. Louis: Mosby.

Goer, H. (1999). Does walking enhance labor progress? *Birth,* 26(2), 127-129.

Hodnett, E. (1997). Commentary: Are nurses effective providers of labor support? Should they be? Can they be? *Birth,* 24(2), 78-80.

Hodnett, E. (1996). Nursing support of the laboring woman. *Journal of Obstetric, Gynecologic, and Neonatal Nursing,* 25(3), 257-264.

Hutchinson, M.K., & BaqiAziz, M. (1994). Nursing care of the childbearing Muslim family. *Journal of Obstetric, Gynecologic, and Neonatal Nursing,* 23(9), 767-771.

Jackson, M.M., & Rymer, T.E. (1995). Nurses: At special risk. *Journal of Obstetric, Gynecologic, and Neonatal Nursing,* 24(6), 533-540.

Khazoyan, C.M., & Anderson, N.L.R. (1994). Latinas' expectations for their partners during childbirth. MCN: *American Journal of Maternal/Child Nursing,* 19(4), 226-229.

Lavender, T., Walkinshaw, & Walton, I. (1999). A prospective study of women's views of factors contributing to a positive birth experience. *Midwifery,* 15(1), 40-46.

Mattson, S. (1995). Culturally sensitive perinatal care for Southeast Asians. *Journal of Obstetric, Gynecologic, and Neonatal Nursing,* 24(4), 335-341.

Mattson, S. (2000). Striving for cultural competence. *AWHONN Lifelines,* 4(3), 48-52.

Mayberry, L.J., Wood, S.H., Strange, L.B., Lee, L., Heisler, D.R., & Nielsen-Smith, K. (2000a). *AWHONN Symposium: Second stage labor management: Promotion of evidence-based practice and a collaborative approach to patient care.* Washington, D.C.: Association of Women's Health, Obstetric, and Neonatal Nurses.

Mayberry, L.J., Wood, S.H., Strange, L.B., Lee, L., Heisler, D.R., & Nielsen-Smith, K. (2000b). Managing second stage labor: Exploring the variables during the second stage. *AWHONN Lifelines,* 3(6), 28-34.

Mayberry, L.J., Hammer, R., Kelly, C., True-Driver, B., & De., A. (1999). Use of delayed pushing with epidural anesthesia: Findings from a randomized, controlled trial. *Journal of Perinatology,* 19(1), 26-30.

McCartney, P.A. (1998). Caring for women with epidurals using the "laboring down" technique. *MCN: American Journal of Maternal/Child Nursing,* 23(5), 274.

Menihan, C.A. (1996). Intrapartum fetal monitoring. In K.R. Rice & P.A. Creehan (Eds.), *Perinatal nursing* (pp. 187-225). Philadelphia: Lippincott.

Murray, M. (1997). *Antepartal and intrapartal fetal monitoring* (2nd ed.). Albuquerque, NM: Learning Resources International.

Perez, P.G., & Herrick, L.M. (1998). Doulas: Exploring their roles with parents, hospitals, and nurses. *AWHONN Lifelines,* 2(2), 54-55.

Petersen, L., & Besuner, P. (1997). Pushing techniques during labor: Issues and controversies. *Journal of Obstetric, Gynecologic, and Neonatal Nursing,* 26(6), 719-726.

Renfrew, M.J., Hannah, W., Albers, L., & Floyd, E. (1998). Practices that minimize trauma to the genital tract in childbirth: A systematic review of the literature. *Birth,* 25(3), 143-160.

Roberts, J., & Woolley, D. (1996). A second look at the second stage of labor. *Journal of Obstetric, Gynecologic, and Neonatal Nursing,* 25(5), 415-423.

Rothman, B.K. (1996). Women, providers, & control. *Journal of Obstetric, Gynecologic, and Neonatal Nursing,* 25(3), 253-256.

Rush, J., Burlock, S., Lambert, K., Loosley-Millman, M., Hutchison, B., & Enkin, M. (1996). The effects of whirlpool baths in labor: A randomized controlled trial. *Birth,* 23(3), 136-143.

Simkin, P. (1996). The experience of maternity in a woman's life. *Journal of Obstetric, Gynecologic, and Neonatal Nursing,* 25(3), 247-252.

Simkin, P., & Frederick, E. (2000). Labor support. In F.H. Nichols & S.S. Humenick (Eds.), *Childbirth education: Practice, research, & theory* (pp. 307-341). Philadelphia: W.B. Saunders.

Simpson, K.R. (2000). Routine care during labor and birth: Is this really how we want to practice perinatal nursing, or are we ready to advocate for childbearing women and insist on evidence-based care? *Mother Baby Journal,* 4(4), 5-7.

Shermer, R.H., & Raines, D.A. (1997). Positioning during the second stage of labor: Moving back to basics. *Journal of Obstetric, Gynecologic, and Neonatal Nursing,* 26(6), 727-734.

Supplee, R.B., & Vezeau, T.M. (1996). Continuous electronic fetal monitoring: Does it belong in low-risk births? *MCN: American Journal of Maternal and Child Nursing,* 21(6), 301-306.

Technical Working Group, World Health Organization. (1997). Care in normal birth: A practical guide. *Birth,* 24(2), 121-123.

Tomlinson, P.S., & Mattson Bryan, A.A. (1996). Family-centered intrapartum care: Revisiting an old concept. *Journal of Obstetric, Gynecologic, and Neonatal Nursing,* 25(4), 331-337.

Tourangeau, A., Carter, N., Tansil, N., McLean, A., & Downer, V. (1999). Intravenous therapy for women in labor: Implementation of a practice change. *Birth,* 26(1), 31-36.

Waymire, V. (1997). A triggering time: Childbirth may recall sexual abuse memories. *Lifelines,* 1(2), 47-50.

Winslow, E.H., & Crenshaw, J. (2000). Managing labor: Does walking help or hurt? *American Journal of Nursing,* 100(3), 50-51.

Woolley, D., & Nelsson-Ryan, S. (2000). Second stage labor. In F.H. Nichols & S.S. Humenick (Eds.), *Childbirth education: Practice, research, & theory* (pp. 342-375). Philadelphia: W.B. Saunders.

INTRAPARTUM FETAL ASSESSMENT

14

OBJECTIVES

1. Identify the purposes of intrapartum fetal assessment.
2. Explain the normal and pathologic mechanisms that influence fetal heart rate.
3. Identify the advantages and limitations of each method of intrapartum fetal surveillance: auscultation and electronic monitoring.
4. Explain the types of equipment used for auscultation and electronic fetal monitoring during labor.
5. Describe the interpretation of intrapartum fetal assessment data.
6. Explain the methods that may be used in addition to electronic fetal monitoring to judge fetal well-being.
7. Describe nursing responses to nonreassuring fetal heart rate patterns.
8. Use the nursing process to plan care for a woman having intrapartum fetal assessment.

DEFINITIONS

Acidosis Condition resulting from accumulation of acid (hydrogen ions) or depletion of base (bicarbonate); acid-base balance measured by pH.

Amnioinfusion Infusion of lactated Ringer's solution or isotonic saline into the uterine cavity during labor to reduce umbilical cord compression; also done to dilute meconium in amniotic fluid, reducing the risk of infant aspiration of thick meconium at birth.

Asphyxia Insufficient oxygen and excess carbon dioxide in the blood and tissues.

Baroreceptors Cells that are sensitive to blood pressure changes.

Chemoreceptors Cells that are sensitive to chemical changes in the blood, specifically changes in oxygen and carbon dioxide levels, and changes in acid-base balance.

Hypercapnia Excess carbon dioxide in the blood, evidenced by an elevated Pco_2.

Hypertonic Contractions Uterine contractions that are too long or too frequent, have too short a resting interval, or have an inadequate relaxation period to allow optimal uteroplacental exchange.

Hypoxemia Reduced oxygenation of the blood, evidenced by a low Po_2.

DEFINITIONS—cont'd

Hypoxia Reduced availability of oxygen to the body tissues.

Intermittent Monitoring Variation of electronic fetal monitoring in which an initial strip is obtained on admission. If patterns are reassuring the woman is remonitored for 15 minutes at regular intervals (such as every 30 to 60 minutes).

Montevideo Unit Method to calculate the intensity of uterine contractions as measured with an intrauterine pressure catheter in mm Hg. The contraction intensity minus the resting tone is multiplied by the number of contractions in 10 minutes.

Nuchal Cord Umbilical cord around the fetal neck.

Telemetry Transmission of electronic fetal monitoring data to the bedside or central monitor unit with radio signals.

Tocolytic Drug that inhibits uterine contractions.

Transducer Device that translates one physical quantity to another, such as fetal heart motion to an electric signal for rate calculation or generation of sound or of a written record.

Uterine Resting Tone Degree of uterine muscle tension when the woman is not in labor or during the interval between labor contractions; may be called *baseline tone.*

Intrapartum fetal assessment is the process of fetal surveillance to identify signs associated with well-being and with compromise. Accurate identification of these signs permits appropriate and timely care to reduce hazards to the fetus. At a minimum, intrapartum fetal assessment includes the fetal heart rate (FHR) and the mother's uterine activity. More comprehensive monitoring adds assessment of fetal activity, fetal response to stimulation, and fetal pulse oximetry.

The purposes of intrapartum fetal assessment are to evaluate how the fetus tolerates labor and to identify hypoxic insult to the fetus during labor. However, no method of fetal assessment can identify every compromised fetus.

Fetal assessment data plays a major role in malpractice claims. These lawsuits may be brought many years, often decades, after the birth of a neurologically handicapped child. The nurse's documentation must prove that the standard of care was met at the time of birth. The nurse should be able to detect signs associated with fetal hypoxia in a timely manner, inform the physician or nurse-midwife promptly, and institute the facility's chain of command if the birth attendant does not respond promptly to the nurse's report of fetal problems. The perinatal nurse must obtain initial competency in fetal assessment that meets standards of care and facility policy and must maintain currency in fetal assessment. Documentation of data must be complete and clear to provide proper communication among professionals and for the best defense in any future lawsuit.

Two basic approaches are taken to intrapartum fetal monitoring: low technology and high technology. Each has advantages and limitations. The nurse may use either or both of these approaches to assess a fetus during labor, depending on the woman's wishes, risk status, and facility policy.

The low-technology approach uses intermittent auscultation (IA) of the FHR and palpation of uterine activity. In the United States, this type of fetal observation is more often used in home births and birth centers. It also may be used during hospital births.

Electronic fetal monitoring (EFM) is the high-technology approach to intrapartum fetal surveillance. In 1998, 84% of live births in the United States were electronically monitored (Curtin & Mathews, 2000). Despite the almost routine use of electronic monitoring, its benefits to the fetus over intermittent auscultation have not been established.

FETAL OXYGENATION

Adequate fetal oxygenation needs five related factors:

- Normal maternal blood flow and volume to the placenta
- Normal oxygen saturation in maternal blood
- Adequate exchange of oxygen and carbon dioxide in the placenta
- An open circulatory path between the placenta and the fetus through vessels in the umbilical cord
- Normal fetal circulatory and oxygen-carrying functions

An understanding of the dynamics of uteroplacental exchange and fetal circulation is critical to the understanding of fetal responses to labor (see Chapter 6.)

Uteroplacental Exchange

Oxygen-rich and nutrient-rich blood from the mother enters the intervillous spaces of the placenta via the spiral arteries (see Figure 6-7). Oxygen and nutrients in the maternal blood pass into the fetal blood that circulates within capillaries inside the chorionic villi in the intervillous spaces. Carbon dioxide and other waste products pass from the fetal blood into the maternal blood at the same time. Maternal blood carrying fetal waste products drains from the intervillous spaces through endometrial veins and returns to the mother's circulation for elimination by her body. Substances pass back and forth between mother and fetus without mixing of maternal and fetal blood.

During labor, contractions gradually compress the spiral arteries, temporarily stopping maternal blood flow into the intervillous spaces at the peak of strong contractions. The fetus depends on the oxygen supply already present in body cells, fetal erythrocytes, and the intervillous spaces during contractions. The oxygen supply in these areas is enough for about 1 to 2 minutes. As each contraction relaxes, fresh oxygenated maternal blood reenters the intervillous spaces and blood containing carbon dioxide and other fetal waste products drains out.

Fetal Circulation

The fetal heart circulates oxygenated blood from the placenta throughout the body and returns deoxygenated blood to the placenta. The umbilical vein carries oxygenated blood to the fetus, and the two umbilical arteries carry deoxygenated blood from the fetus to the placenta (see Figure 6-7).

Regulation of Fetal Heart Rate

Mechanisms that regulate the heart rate are balanced to maintain cardiac output at a level that keeps the fetal heart and brain oxygenated. Fetal cardiac output increase is primarily accomplished by an increase in the heart rate. Conversely, a marked decrease in FHR decreases fetal cardiac output.

Five fetal factors interact to regulate the FHR:

1. Autonomic nervous system
2. Baroreceptors
3. Chemoreceptors
4. Central nervous system
5. Adrenal glands

The balance among forces that increase and those that slow the heart rate result in the characteristic fluctuations in FHR during the latter one third of pregnancy.

Autonomic Nervous System

The sympathetic and parasympathetic branches of the autonomic nervous system are balanced forces that regulate the FHR. Sympathetic stimulation increases the heart rate and strengthens myocardial contractions through release of epinephrine and norepinephrine. The net result of sympathetic stimulation is an increase in cardiac output.

The parasympathetic nervous system, through stimulation of the vagus nerve, reduces the FHR and maintains variability (see p. 344). The parasympathetic branch gradually exerts greater influence as the fetus matures, beginning between 28 and 32 weeks of gestation. Therefore the average FHR in the term fetus is lower than in the preterm fetus.

Baroreceptors

Cells in the carotid arch and major arteries respond to stretching when the fetal blood pressure increases. The baroreceptors stimulate the vagus nerve to slow the FHR and decrease the blood pressure, thus lowering cardiac output.

Chemoreceptors

Cells that respond to changes in oxygen, carbon dioxide, and acid-base levels, or pH, are found in the medulla oblongata and in the aortic and carotid bodies. Decreased oxygen, increased carbon dioxide content, or a lower pH in the blood or cerebrospinal fluid triggers an increase in the heart rate. However, prolonged hypoxia, hypercapnia, and acidosis depress the FHR.

Adrenal Glands

The adrenal medulla secretes epinephrine and norepinephrine in response to stress, causing a sympathetic response that accelerates the FHR. The adrenal cortex responds to a fall in the fetal blood pressure with release of aldosterone and retention of sodium and water, resulting in an increase in the circulating fetal blood volume.

Central Nervous System

The fetal cerebral cortex causes the heart rate to increase during fetal movement and decrease when the fetus is quiet. As the fetus becomes mature enough to have distinct wake and sleep states, the FHR responds with variations in rate. For example, the rate is slower, with little variability during deep fetal sleep, but faster and with greater variability and accelerations when awake.

The hypothalamus coordinates the two branches of the autonomic nervous system, the sympathetic and parasympathetic. The medulla oblongata maintains the balance between stimuli that speed and slow the heart rate.

Pathologic Influences on Fetal Oxygenation

Compromise of fetal oxygenation may occur because of alterations in any of the placental or fetal factors or those of the pregnant woman.

Maternal Cardiopulmonary Alterations

Actual or relative reductions in the mother's circulating blood volume impair perfusion of the intervillous spaces with oxygenated maternal blood. Hemorrhage causes an actual decrease in her blood volume. Relative reductions in maternal circulating volume involve altered distribution of the blood volume without blood loss. For example, epidural block analgesia may cause vasodilation, which increases the capacity of the maternal vascular bed. However, the amount of blood available to fill her vessels is unchanged. Hypotension results, with reduction of placental blood flow.

Aortocaval compression can occur when a pregnant woman lies in the supine position and the weight of the uterus compresses the aorta and inferior vena cava. Aortocaval compression reduces blood return to her heart, lowers her cardiac output (supine hypotension), and can reduce placental perfusion.

Maternal hypertension may reduce blood flow to the placenta because of vasospasm and narrowing of the spiral arteries. Hypertension may be pregnancy in-

Table 14-1

CONDITIONS ASSOCIATED WITH DECREASED FETAL OXYGENATION

Antepartum Period	Intrapartum Period
Maternal history	Maternal problems
Prior stillbirth	Hypotension
Prior cesarean birth	Hypertonic uterine contractions
Chronic diseases, such as cardiac disease, hypertension, and diabetes	Abnormal labor: preterm or dysfunctional
Drug abuse	Prolonged ruptured membranes
	Chorioamnionitis
Problems Identified during Pregnancy	Fever
Fetal growth restriction	Fetal or placental problems
Gestation longer than 42 weeks	Abnormal fetal heart rate
Marked decrease in fetal movement	Meconium-stained amniotic fluid
Multifetal gestation	Abnormal presentation or position
Pregnancy-induced hypertension	Prolapsed cord
Gestational diabetes	Abruptio placentae
Placenta previa	
Maternal severe anemia	
Maternal infection	

duced or chronic or may result from ingestion of drugs such as cocaine.

A lowered oxygen level in the mother's blood reduces the amount available to the fetus. Maternal acid-base alterations that accompany respiratory abnormalities also can compromise exchange in the placenta. A lower maternal oxygen tension may result from respiratory disorders, such as asthma, or from smoking.

Uterine Activity

Hypertonic uterine activity reduces the time available for exchange of oxygen and waste products in the placenta. Contractions may be too long, too frequent, or have too short an interval. The uterus may not fully relax between contractions, applying continuous compression to the spiral arteries and reducing maternal-fetal exchange in the intervillous spaces. Hypertonic uterine activity may occur spontaneously or with uterine stimulants such as oxytocin (Pitocin), prostaglandins, or misoprostol (Cytotec).

Placental Disruptions

Conditions such as abruptio placentae (partial separation before birth) and infarcts reduce the placental surface area available for exchange. The amount and location of placental disruption relate to the degree of impairment in uteroplacental exchange. Large infarcts or separations cause greater impairment than smaller ones. Central infarcts or separations usually cause greater impairment than those on edges of the placenta.

Interruptions in Umbilical Flow

The usual cause of interrupted blood flow through the umbilical cord is compression. Blood flow through the umbilical cord may be reduced by compression between the fetal presenting part and the pelvis, a nuchal cord or one that is wrapped around the fetal body, or a knot in the cord. It may occur with oligohydramnios, because the amount of amniotic fluid is inadequate to cushion the cord. The umbilical cord also may become entangled between fetal body parts or it may have inadequate Wharton's jelly for cushioning.

The thin-walled umbilical vein is compressed initially, resulting in a reduced inflow of more highly oxygenated blood to the fetus. This results in initial hypoxia with hypotension. Baroreceptors and chemoreceptors respond by accelerating the FHR. Flow through the firmer-walled umbilical arteries that carry blood from the fetus to the placenta is reduced as cord compression continues, resulting in hypertension. Baroreceptors respond to hypertension by stimulating the vagus nerve, thus reducing blood pressure and slowing the fetal heart. The FHR again accelerates as pressure is relieved on the arteries and then on the vein.

Fetal Alterations

Fetal cells may be hypoxic despite adequate oxygen supply from the woman and adequate exchange within the placenta. A low circulating fetal blood volume, fetal hypotension, or fetal anemia may result in cellular hypoxia. Central nervous system or cardiac abnormalities may cause an abnormal rate or rhythm. For example, a fetus with complete heart block may not respond to stimuli that would normally cause a rate increase.

A prolonged rate lower than 50 beats per minute (BPM) may reduce fetal cardiac output enough to impair brain and heart perfusion. However, a persistent heart rate faster than 200 BPM also decreases cardiac output, because the ventricles do not have time to refill with oxygenated blood during diastole.

Risk Factors

When conditions associated with reduced fetal oxygenation exist (Table 14-1), assessments by either in-

A

B

C

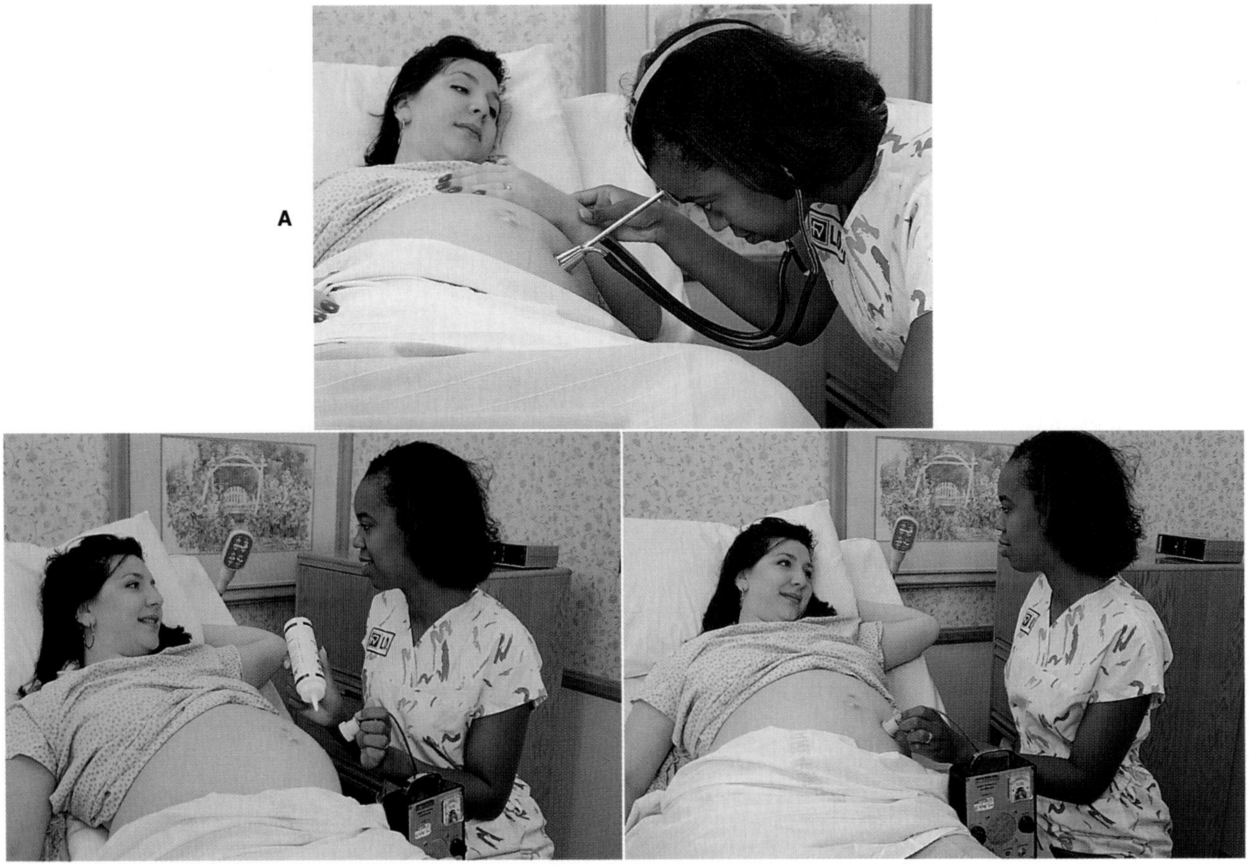

FIGURE 14-1 Low-intervention methods for evaluating the fetal heart rate during labor. **A,** Fetoscope, showing the head attachment to enhance conduction of faint fetal heart sounds. **B,** Transmission gel improves the clarity of the fetal heart movement sensed by the Doppler ultrasound transducer. **C,** The nurse moves the transducer until the sounds representing fetal heart motion are heard clearly. This location is usually over the fetal back, which is most likely to be located in the woman's right or left lower abdomen.

termittent auscultation and palpation or electronic fetal monitoring are done more often. No absolute indications, including the presence of risk factors, require the use of electronic fetal monitoring during labor. Properly performed intermittent auscultation is equivalent to continuous electronic monitoring in assessing fetal condition (ACOG, 1995a).

Check Your Reading

1. What five factors influence fetal oxygenation?
2. What changes in the FHR occur when the umbilical cord is compressed?
3. How is the FHR related to fetal cardiac output?
4. What risk factors indicate that fetal monitoring should be done more frequently? (See Table 14-1.)

AUSCULTATION AND PALPATION

Intermittent auscultation of the FHR can be done using either the nonelectronic fetoscope or Doppler ultrasound fetoscope (Figure 14-1). The nurse's expert fingertips palpate uterine activity (see Procedure 13-2).

Advantages

Mobility is a major advantage of auscultation and palpation for intrapartum fetal assessment. The woman is free to change position and walk around. Nothing restricts her freedom to move and she is likely to change positions more often, which promotes normal labor. The nurse must have regular, close, and frequent personal contact with the woman when performing intermittent auscultation and palpation. Water-based methods of pain management, such as whirlpool baths or showers can be used more freely. The atmosphere is more natural than technologic and less invasive, which is important to some women during their birth experience. Some trials that compared auscultation and palpation with electronic fetal monitoring noted a lower cesarean birth rate in the women having auscultation and palpation during labor (Feinstein, Sprague, & Trépanier, 2000b). The equipment is less costly than electronic fetal monitoring equipment, but staffing to achieve the needed 1:1 nurse-client ratio may offset this cost advantage.

Limitations

A disadvantage of auscultation and palpation as the primary method of fetal assessment is that FHR and uterine activity are assessed for a small percentage of the total labor. The fetus is most stressed during contractions because of normal reduction of blood flow to the placenta at that time. The FHR is assessed during some contractions but is not recorded during every contraction. No continuous printed or computer archived record exists to show the fetal response throughout labor or to identify subtle trends in the response.

Some women find that interruptions for auscultation are distracting. The pressure of the instrument on the abdomen is uncomfortable for some, and it may require several moves to locate the best place for auscultation. Maternal obesity or large amniotic fluid volume may make it difficult to hear the fetal heart sounds.

Intermittent auscultation is more staff-intensive than electronic monitoring, with a 1:1 nurse-client ratio recommended in clinical trials. When this nurse-client ratio cannot be achieved, auscultation may not be a realistic option as the primary method of intrapartum fetal surveillance.

Auscultation Equipment

Two basic types of auscultation equipment are used: a fetoscope and a Doppler ultrasound transducer. When listening with a fetoscope, the listener hears actual fetal heart sounds. The Doppler device senses motion and translates that motion into a sound that represents the cardiac events. An external fetal monitor, which is the same technology as the Doppler transducer, can be used, but the recording must be turned off, including computer archiving, for this to be valid as intermittent auscultation. If the FHR is recorded on a paper or computer monitor strip, the nurse must interpret that added data (Feinstein, Sprague, & Trépanier, 2000b).

Evaluation of Ausculated Fetal Heart Rate Data

Both the fetoscope and Doppler transducer can be used to identify the FHR baseline, rhythm, and changes from the baseline. Because the fetoscope is detecting actual fetal heart sounds, it can also detect dysrhythmias. The Doppler transducer (and external fetal monitor if it is being used for intermittent auscultation) also can be used to detect baseline, rhythm, and changes in the baseline. However, the Doppler transducer or external fetal monitor cannot be used to reliably detect dysrhythmias. (Procedure 14-1 explains auscultation of the FHR with the fetoscope and the Doppler transducer.)

ELECTRONIC FETAL MONITORING

Electronic fetal monitoring may be continuous, starting shortly after the woman is admitted, or intermittent, with a short strip taken at regular intervals during labor, or it may be intermittent during early labor and continuous during late labor.

Advantages

The electronic monitor supplies more data about the fetus than auscultation and archives a permanent record on paper, computer disk, or both (Figure 14-2). Continuous electronic fetal monitoring shows how the fetus responds before, during, and after each contraction rather than occasional contractions.

Many women in the United States expect electronic monitoring and find the constant sound of the fetal heartbeat comforting. Their support person can use the tracing of contractions on the monitor strip to help the woman anticipate the beginning and end of each contraction.

Electronic monitoring allows one nurse to observe two laboring women, primarily during uncomplicated early labor. A 1:1 nurse-client ratio is needed during the second stage, regardless of the monitoring method used. Electronic monitoring can give the nurse more time for teaching and supporting the laboring woman with breathing and relaxation techniques if the nurse maintains the primary focus on the woman not on the machine.

Limitations

Reduced mobility is a limitation of electronic fetal monitoring. Telemetry or intermittent monitoring gives the woman more freedom of movement than continuous electronic monitoring without telemetry. Otherwise the woman is limited to her bed or a nearby chair if electronic fetal monitoring is continuous.

Frequent maternal position changes or an active fetus often requires constant adjustment of equipment. The belts or stockinette band, used to keep sensors positioned properly for external monitoring, are uncomfortable for some women.

The high-tech atmosphere created by the electronic fetal monitor may be objectionable to a woman and her partner.

Electronic fetal monitoring, though used in more than 80% of United States births, has not proven to be

PROCEDURE 14-1

Auscultating Fetal Heart Rate

Purpose: To evaluate the fetal condition and tolerance of labor

1. Explain the procedure, and wash hands with warm water. *This gives information to the woman and partner and reduces transfer of microorganisms. Warm hands are more comfortable.*
2. Use Leopold's maneuvers to identify the fetal back (see Procedure 13-1). Illustrations show approximate locations of the FHR in different presentations and positions. *The FHR is most easily heard through the fetal back because it usually lies closest to the surface of the maternal abdomen.*
3. Assess the FHR with a fetoscope, Doppler transducer, or external fetal heart monitor. Turn the recording off (including computer archiving) if the external fetal monitor is used. *The FHR can be assessed with any of these instruments. The nurse is obligated to fully assess and respond to data recorded on an external fetal monitoring strip so this should not be used for intermittent auscultation (Feinstein, Sprague, & Trépanier, 2000a).*
4. Fetoscope (see Figure 14-1): Place the bell of the fetoscope over the fetal back with the head plate pressed against your forehead. Move the fetoscope until you locate where the sound is loudest. Use your forehead to maintain pressure during auscultation. *The head plate adds bone conduction to the sound coming through the earpieces. The FHR is faint with the fetoscope because sounds pass through several layers of maternal and fetal tissue.*
5. Doppler transducer (see Figure 14-1): Review manufacturer's instructions for operating the Doppler device. Place water-soluble conducting gel over the transducer, and turn it on. Place the transducer over the fetal back, and move it until you clearly hear the double sounds of the fetal heart. *The Doppler transducer uses sound waves reflected off the moving fetal heart to create an audible signal. Gel makes a liquid interface for clear signal transmission.*
6. With one hand, palpate the mother's radial pulse. If her pulse is synchronized with the sounds from the fetoscope or Doppler transducer, try another location for the fetal heart. *The nurse must be sure that the FHR is what is actually heard. Other sounds that may be heard are the funic souffle (blood flowing through the umbilical cord) or uterine souffle (blood flowing through the uterine vessels). The funic souffle is synchronized with the fetal heart; the uterine souffle is synchronized with the mother's pulse.*
7. Assess the FHR for 30 to 60 seconds immediately after a contraction. Note the baseline rate, rhythm, accelerations, and slowing of the rate. *Allows identification of the major components of auscultation. Determines whether findings are reassuring or whether further steps should be taken to clarify data or correct problems.*
8. Note reassuring signs:
   a. Average rate between 110 and 160 BPM at term
   b. Rhythm: regular or irregular
   c. Accelerations from the baseline rate, often occurring with fetal movement
   d. Absence of decreases from the baseline rate
9. Note nonreassuring signs and take corrective actions. Make more frequent intermittent auscultation assessments or consider using electronic fetal monitoring to clarify data. Notify the physician or nurse-midwife. See Procedure 14-2 for corrective actions.

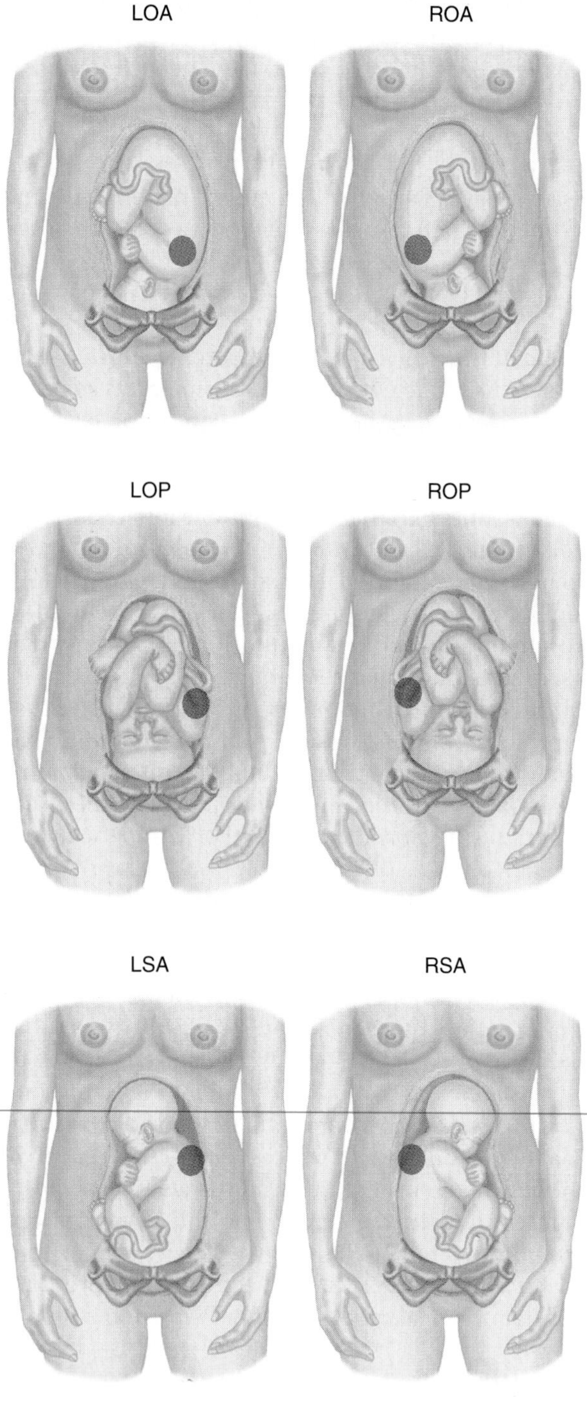

   a. FHR outside normal limits
   b. Irregular rate (slight fluctuations are normal)
   c. Decreases from the baseline rate

If nonreassuring FHR data are found, the priority is to improve fetal oxygenation with appropriate measures and notify the birth attendant for further instructions.

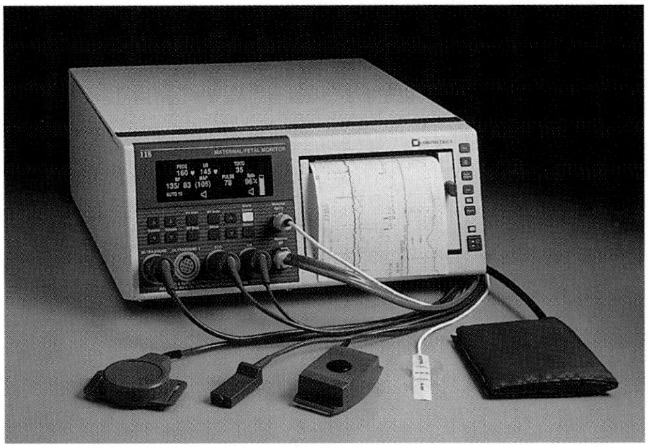

FIGURE 14-2 Bedside unit for electronic fetal monitoring. In addition to fetal heart rate and uterine activity, the unit can help the nurse evaluate the woman's pulse, blood pressure, and saturation of oxygen in her blood. Both fetuses in a twin gestation can be assessed. (Courtesy Corometrics Medical Systems, Inc., Wallingford, Conn.)

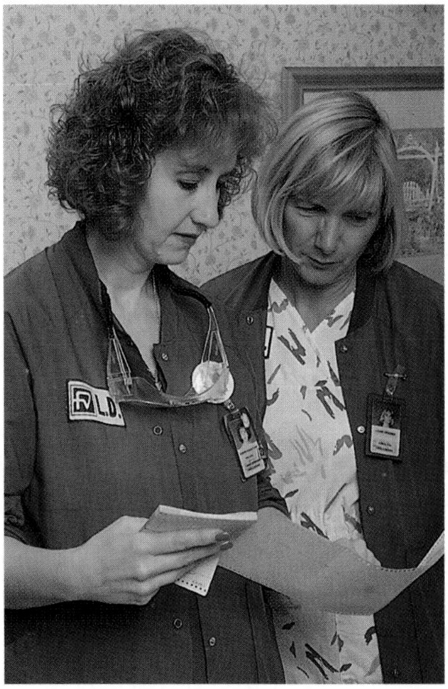

FIGURE 14-3 Electronic fetal monitoring can be continuous and provides nurses with monitor strips on which uterine activity and fetal heart rate are permanently recorded. Some "strips" are on computer monitor screens rather than paper.

consistently reliable at identifying the fetus who is truly in trouble. Electronic fetal monitoring best identifies the well-oxygenated fetus, but it does not as reliably identify the compromised fetus. Thus electronic fetal monitoring must be considered to be a screening rather than a diagnostic tool.

ELECTRONIC FETAL MONITORING EQUIPMENT

Electronic fetal monitoring equipment consists of the bedside monitor unit and sensors for FHR and uterine activity. Sensors for each function may be either internal or external. Additional equipment may include data entry devices, remote screens, and computer interfaces.

Bedside Monitor Unit

The bedside monitor unit receives information about the FHR and uterine activity from the sensors. It processes the information and provides output in the form of a numeric display and a printed strip (Figure 14-3). Current units can record rates for both fetuses in a twin pregnancy and have inputs for maternal blood pressure, pulse, blood oxygen saturation. (The maternal blood pressure may be signified on the strip by the abbreviation *NIBP,* which means noninvasive blood pressure.)

Paper Strip

Data about the FHR and uterine activity are printed on a paper strip having a horizontal grid for the FHR and another for the uterine activity (Figure 14-4). Segments of paper between perforations are numbered for identification and reassembly of a multi-part strip. The FHR is recorded on the upper strip. The range of rates is from 30 to 240 BPM. Other countries may use a strip with a slightly different configuration and paper speed.

Uterine activity is recorded on the lower grid as bell-shaped curves. Contraction intensity and uterine resting tone from 0 to 100 mm Hg are recorded on the lower grid.

Vertical lines on both upper and lower grids are time divisions. At a paper speed of 3 cm/minute, dark vertical lines are 1 minute apart. Lighter lines subdivide the 1-minute divisions into six 10-second segments. The vertical lines are used to time contraction frequency and duration and to identify the fetal response in relation to the contractions.

Sometimes the "paper" is a computer's monitor screen with the same appearance as the paper strip. The strip may not be routinely printed on paper at all. The nurse moves backward or forward through the strip on the screen using keyboard arrows or a pointing device, such as a mouse.

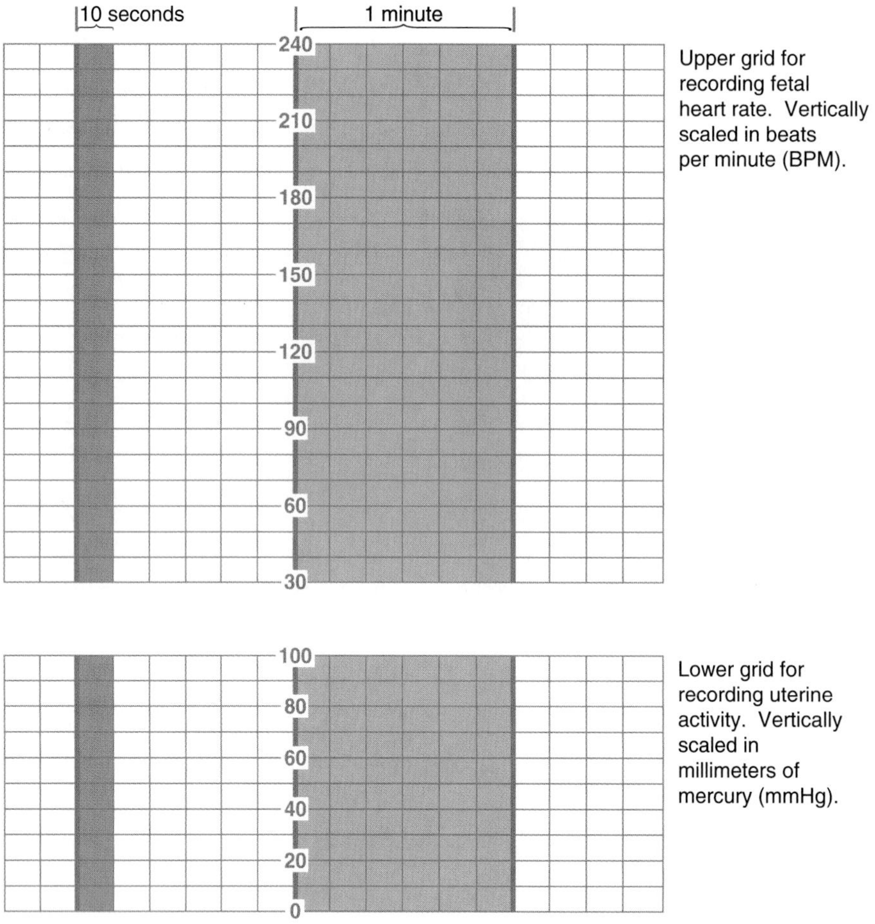

FIGURE 14-4 Paper strip for recording electronic fetal monitoring data. Each dark vertical line represents 1 minute, and each lighter vertical line represents 10 seconds.

Data Entry Devices and Computer Software

Monitors print some notations automatically, such as the date, time, paper speed, and the type of device being used to detect the FHR and uterine activity. Most also have data entry devices, allowing entry of data to be printed on the strip. Computer software is commonly used to archive fetal monitoring information plus other information relating to the care of mother and fetus. The software may extend beyond the intrapartum stay and be used for documentation in the postpartum and newborn periods.

Computer-assisted analysis of EFM data uses software to interpret patterns the nurse sees on the electronic fetal monitor. Automated analysis is likely to become a common adjunct in the review of EFM data and in suggesting possible interventions for problems. The professional person—nurse, nurse-midwife, or physician—chooses whether to accept the software analysis.

Remote Surveillance

Many facilities have display units at the nursing station or other locations to allow surveillance when the nurse is not at the bedside. These units display the tracing on a screen and have settings for alerts, such as upper and lower limits for the heart rate, decelerations, and end of the paper.

Devices for External Fetal Monitoring

Both the FHR and uterine activity can be monitored by external sensors, or transducers. External devices are secured on the mother's abdomen by elastic straps, a tube of wide stockinette, or an adhesive ring (Figure 14-5). External devices are somewhat less accurate than internal ones but are noninvasive; they do not require ruptured membranes or cervical dilation. (Procedure 14-2 contains instructions for using the external electronic fetal monitor.)

Fetal Heart Rate Monitoring with an Ultrasound Transducer

The Doppler ultrasound device detects movements other than fetal heart motion, such as fetal or maternal activity or blood flow through the umbilical cord and the woman's aorta. Most monitors today ignore these extraneous sounds to provide a clean tracing.

PROCEDURE 14-2

External Fetal Monitor

Purpose: To properly apply the external electronic fetal monitor. To perform a basic evaluation of the fetal heart rate (FHR) and uterine activity patterns.

1. Read instruction manual for equipment. *Become familiar with proper operation of the equipment and identify equipment.*
2. Perform a function test following manufacturer's instructions. Press TEST button and observe for result. Common correct test results are the following:
   a. Fetal heart rate: The monitor prints a line at 120, 150, or 200 BPM, depending on the model.
   b. Uterine activity: The monitor adds 50 to uterine activity display.

A correct function test ensures that the bedside monitor unit is calibrated properly so that caregivers are assured of accurate data to interpret. Each manufacturer sets standards for indicators of proper function.

3. Explain the basic procedure of electronic fetal monitoring to the woman and her partner or family. Vary instructions according to equipment being used and hospital protocols. A sample is:
   a. Using the electronic fetal monitor is the way we normally assess the baby's response to labor contractions.
   b. Two belts go around your abdomen, one for the fetal heart rate sensor and one for contractions.
   c. Feel free to move with the monitor on. If the tracing is poor, we can adjust the sensors.

Knowledge decreases the woman's fear of the unknown. Teaching her that she can move with the monitor in place enhances her comfort and promotes normal labor.

4. Apply belts or stockinette if an adhesive ring is not used:
   a. Slide both belts under the woman's back without the sensors attached. Be sure to keep the belts smooth under her back.
   b. Cut a length of stockinette tubing about 15 to 18 inches long for the average-sized woman. Cut a longer length of wide stockinette for a heavier woman. Slide the stockinette up from her feet to her abdomen.

Smooth application of straps or stockinette enhances a woman's comfort and improves contact of external sensors with her abdomen. Good contact improves the quality of the tracing and may reduce the number of adjustments needed.

5. Use Leopold's maneuvers (see Procedure 13-1) to locate the fetal back as in Intermittent Auscultation, Procedure 14-1.
6. Apply ultrasound gel to the Doppler ultrasound transducer and place it on the woman's abdomen at the approximate location of the fetus' back. Move the transducer until a clear signal is heard. Most bedside units have a green light or flashing heart shape to indicate a good signal. *Gel improves transmission and reception of the ultrasound waves to provide more accurate data.*
7. Place the uterine activity sensor in the fundal area or the area where contractions feel the strongest when palpated. This is often near the umbilicus. When the woman has a contraction, observe the tracing for the bell shape. The line for uterine activity is jagged because it also senses the rise and fall of the abdomen with breathing. Fetal or maternal movement, coughing, or sneezing causes a spike in the line. Observe through several contractions. *The external uterine activity monitor senses the change in the abdominal contour as the uterus rotates forward with each contraction. Contractions are usually strongest in the fundus of the uterus. Observation of the uterine activity line (on the lower paper grid) through several contractions verifies correct placement and identifies needed changes in placement of the sensor.*
8. Observe the strip for baseline FHR, presence of variability, periodic changes, and uterine activity (contraction duration, and frequency). Palpate contractions for intensity and relaxation between contractions. Notify the physician or nurse-midwife of nonreassuring patterns. *Identifies reassuring and nonreassuring FHR patterns (see Table 14-2). Contractions having a frequency greater than every 2 minutes, duration longer than 90 seconds, a resting interval shorter than 60 seconds, or incomplete uterine relaxation between contractions may reduce maternal blood flow into the intervillous spaces and impair exchange of oxygen and waste products. The external uterine activity sensor is useful only for contraction frequency and duration. It is not accurate for actual intensity or uterine resting tone.*

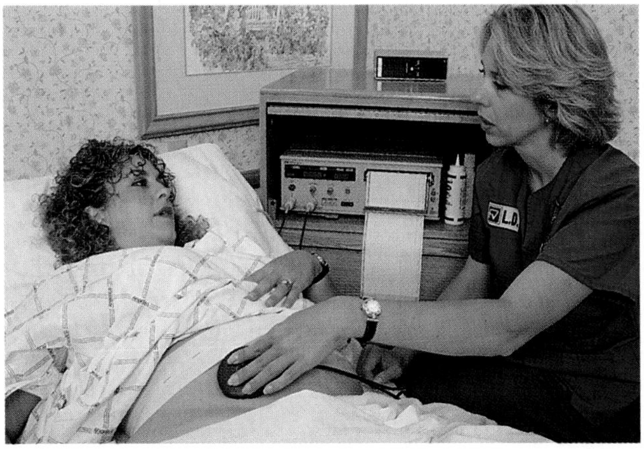

FIGURE 14-5 The nurse applies the uterine activity transducer on the woman's upper abdomen, in the fundal area. The Doppler transducer for sensing the fetal heart rate is usually placed on her lower abdomen when the fetus is in the cephalic presentation.

The Doppler transducer produces a two-part muffled sound, resembling galloping horses. The two closely linked sounds represent closure of the heart valves during systole (mitral and tricuspid valves) and diastole (aortic and pulmonic valves). Fetal or maternal activity produces a rough, erratic sound rather than the crisp, rhythmic sound characteristic of the fetal heart.

Uterine Activity Monitoring with a Tocotransducer

A tocotransducer (also called a *tocodynamometer* or simply a "toco") with a pressure-sensitive area detects changes in abdominal contour to measure uterine activity. The uterus pushes outward against the mother's anterior abdominal wall with each contraction. The monitor calculates changes in this signal and prints them as bell shapes on the lower grid of the strip.

Movement other than uterine activity also registers on the monitor. For example, maternal respirations cause the uterine activity line to have a zigzag appearance. Other fetal or maternal movements appear as spikes on the uterine activity tracing.

Uterine activity is sensed through the woman's abdomen and is therefore useful for observing the frequency and duration of contractions. It does not reliably measure actual contraction intensity and uterine resting tone. Several factors affect apparent intensity as printed on the strip.

- Fetal size—The uterus will not push firmly against the abdominal wall with each contraction when the fetus is small, making contractions appear less intense.
- Abdominal fat thickness—A thick layer of abdominal fat absorbs energy from uterine contractions, reducing their apparent intensity on the printed strip. The uterine activity recording of a thin woman whose uterus rotates sharply forward with each contraction may appear to be more intense than it actually is.
- Maternal position—Different maternal positions may increase or decrease the pressure against the transducer, changing the apparent intensity of contractions on the tracing.
- Location of the transducer—Uterine activity is best detected where it is strongest and where the fetus lies close to the uterine wall. This is usually over the fundus. Changes during contractions may not be detectable if the transducer is located elsewhere.

Devices for Internal Fetal Monitoring

Accuracy is the main advantage of using internal devices for electronic fetal monitoring. However, their use requires ruptured membranes and about 2 cm of cervical dilation. The devices are invasive, and the risk of infection is slightly increased.

Fetal Heart Rate Monitoring with a Scalp Electrode

The fetal scalp electrode (or spiral electrode) detects electric signals from the fetal heart (Figure 14-6). Fetal or maternal movement does not interfere with accuracy because the rate is calculated from electrical events in the fetal heart. The monitor unit generates a beeping sound with each fetal heartbeat, but this sound can be silenced as can sounds from the Doppler transducer.

Although called a *fetal scalp electrode,* the device may be applied to the buttocks in a breech presentation. Areas to avoid for electrode application are the fetal face, fontanelles, and genitals. The electrode wire protrudes from the mother's vagina and is attached to a leg plate on the woman's thigh. A cord from the leg plate connects to the bedside unit.

Because it barely penetrates the fetal skin (about 1 mm), the electrode is easily displaced. The tracing then becomes erratic or stops if the electrode is fully detached. Secure attachment of the electrode is often difficult if the fetus has thick hair. The electrode is removed by turning it counterclockwise about one and one half turns until it detaches.

Uterine Activity Monitoring with an Intrauterine Pressure Catheter

Two kinds of intrauterine pressure catheters (IUPC) can be used to measure uterine activity, including contraction intensity and resting tone:

- A solid catheter with a pressure transducer in its tip (Figure 14-7), which may have an additional lumen for amnioinfusion
- A hollow, fluid-filled catheter that connects to a pressure transducer on the bedside monitor unit

Both types sense intrauterine pressure and increases in intraabdominal pressure, such as with coughing or vomiting.

The solid catheter is not affected by height because its transducer is in the catheter. However, the sensor in its tip measures hydrostatic pressure from the amniotic fluid above the fetal presenting part as well as the pressure from uterine activity. Therefore recorded intrauterine pressures from the solid catheter are higher than those from the fluid-filled catheter, and the nurse must consider this fact when assessing whether uterine activity is normal or hypertonic.

The tip of the fluid-filled catheter in the uterus should be at the level of the transducer on the outside for best accuracy. If the tip is lower than the transducer, the recorded pressure is lower than the actual intrauterine pressure. If the tip is higher, the recorded pressure may be artificially high. Changes in the mother's position may alter the height of the catheter tip, requiring adjustment of the transducer's height.

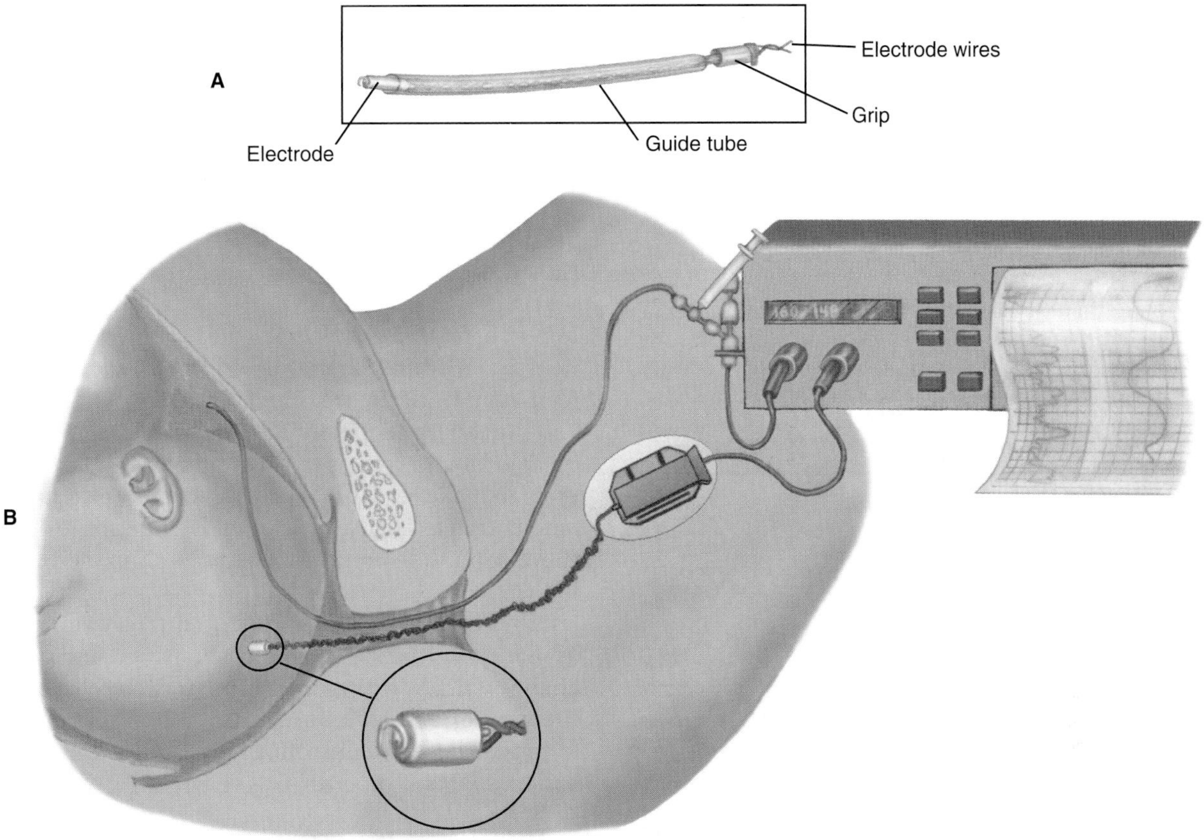

FIGURE 14-6 Internal spiral electrode and intrauterine pressure catheter. **A,** Parts of the fetal scalp electrode before it is applied. **B,** Fetal scalp electrode and intrauterine pressure catheter in place and connected to the bedside monitor unit.

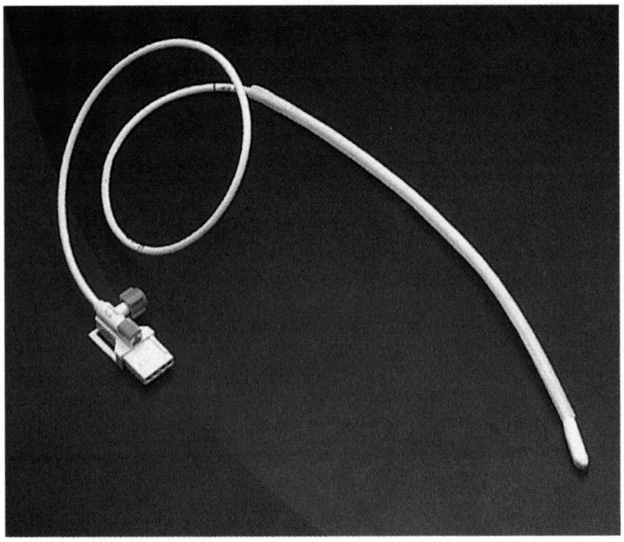

FIGURE 14-7 Solid intrauterine pressure catheter with transducer in its tip. This model also has a lumen for amnioinfusion and is shown with its introducer over the catheter. (Courtesy Utah Medical Products, Midvale, Utah.)

Check Your Reading

5. What are the advantages and limitations of each fetal monitoring method?
6. Which grid on the paper strip of the electronic fetal monitor is used to record the FHR? Uterine activity? What other information may be recorded on the monitor strip?
7. Which electronic fetal monitoring sensor uses heart motion to measure FHR?
8. What are some variables that can affect the accuracy of the external uterine activity sensor?
9. What are the two types of internal uterine activity catheters? Which one tends to record higher intrauterine pressures? Which one is affected by its height in relation to the mother's position?

EVALUATING INTERMITTENT AUSCULTATION AND PALPATION DATA

Data about FHR and uterine activity obtained by intermittent auscultation of the FHR and palpation of uterine activity should be evaluated in an orderly way to identify reassuring and nonreassuring signs. Some characteristics of FHR data obtained by intermittent auscultation are also evaluated when the data are obtained by electronic fetal monitoring. However, characteristics unique to electronic fetal monitoring strips, such as variability or deceleration patterns, should not be evaluated when intermittent auscultation is used (Feinstein, 2000).

The baseline FHR is evaluated for the following:

- Rate
- Regularity of rhythm
- Absence of decrease from the baseline

A reassuring rate is between 110 and 160 BPM and regular. If the rate is within normal limits but has changed significantly from the previous assessment, a longer listening period or more frequent assessments may clarify whether the rate is a change in the baseline. Accelerations in the rate may be heard and are a reassuring sign. An abrupt decrease in rate from the baseline rate is not reassuring and should be followed with other measures to clarify the fetal condition.

Contractions are palpated for frequency, duration, intensity, and resting interval and resting tone. If the fetus begins labor well oxygenated, contractions that are no more frequent than every 2 minutes, 90 seconds or less in duration, and have a resting interval of at least 60 seconds will allow adequate reoxygenation for the next contraction. Also, the uterus must fully relax for the intervillous spaces to refill with maternal oxygenated blood.

EVALUATION OF ELECTRONIC FETAL MONITORING STRIPS

The nurse evaluates the FHR tracing for baseline rate, variability, and presence of periodic changes. Uterine activity is evaluated by determining the frequency, duration, and intensity of contractions and by assessing uterine resting, or baseline, tone. Fetal heart rate and uterine activity patterns must be evaluated together.

Between 1995 and 1996, a series of workshops was held to clarify and standardize definitions for electronic fetal monitoring data (National Institute of Child Health and Human Development Research Planning Workshop, 1997). A major purpose was to have standard definitions to make research data that was more comparable among studies. Many health care facilities have adopted these definitions in their policies. A simplified version is used here.

Other data are relevant to strip interpretation, such as maternal vital signs, maternal position and position changes, drug or oxygen administration, character of the amniotic fluid, labor status, and procedures performed. These are customarily recorded on the strip and in the labor record.

Fetal Heart Rate Baseline

The FHR baseline is the average heart rate, rounded to 5 beats per minute (BPM), measured over a 10-minute segment when the uterus is at rest (Figure 14-8). The baseline excludes instances of periodic changes (see p. 346), periods of marked FHR variability, or segments of the baseline that differ by more than 25 BPM. The baseline rate is classified as follows (Harvey, 1997; Murray, 1997; Menihan, 1996; National Institute of Child Health and Human Development Research Planning Workshop, 1997):

- Normal—For the term fetus, a lower limit of 110 to 120 BPM and an upper limit of 150 to 160 BPM
- Bradycardia—Less than 110 BPM, persisting at least 10 minutes
- Tachycardia—Greater than 160 BPM, persisting at least 10 minutes

Some healthy term fetuses have bradycardia between 100 and 110 BPM with no other signs of compromise. A normal preterm fetus may have a baseline rate at the higher end of this range because the parasympathetic nervous system is immature.

Baseline Fetal Heart Rate Variability

Variability denotes the fluctuations in the baseline FHR that cause the printed line to have an irregular rather than a smooth appearance (Figure 14-9). Two types of variability, short-term and long-term, are often described, but the NIH consensus does not distinguish between the two types because they occur to-

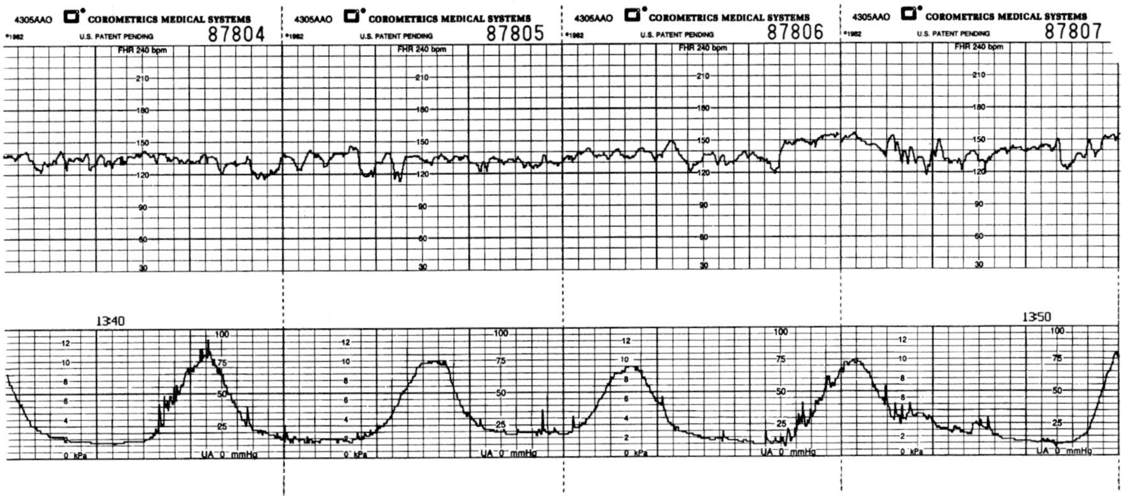

FIGURE 14-8 Electronic fetal monitor strip showing a reassuring pattern of fetal heart rate (FHR) and uterine activity. The FHR baseline is 130 to 140 beats per minute (BPM), variability is about 10 BPM. There are no periodic changes in this strip. Contraction frequency is approximately every 2 to 3 minutes, duration is about 50 to 60 seconds, intensity is 75 to 90 mmHg with the internal spiral electrode, and uterine resting tone is approximately 10 mmHg. (Courtesy Corometrics Medical Systems, Inc., Wallingford, Conn. Redrawn with permission.)

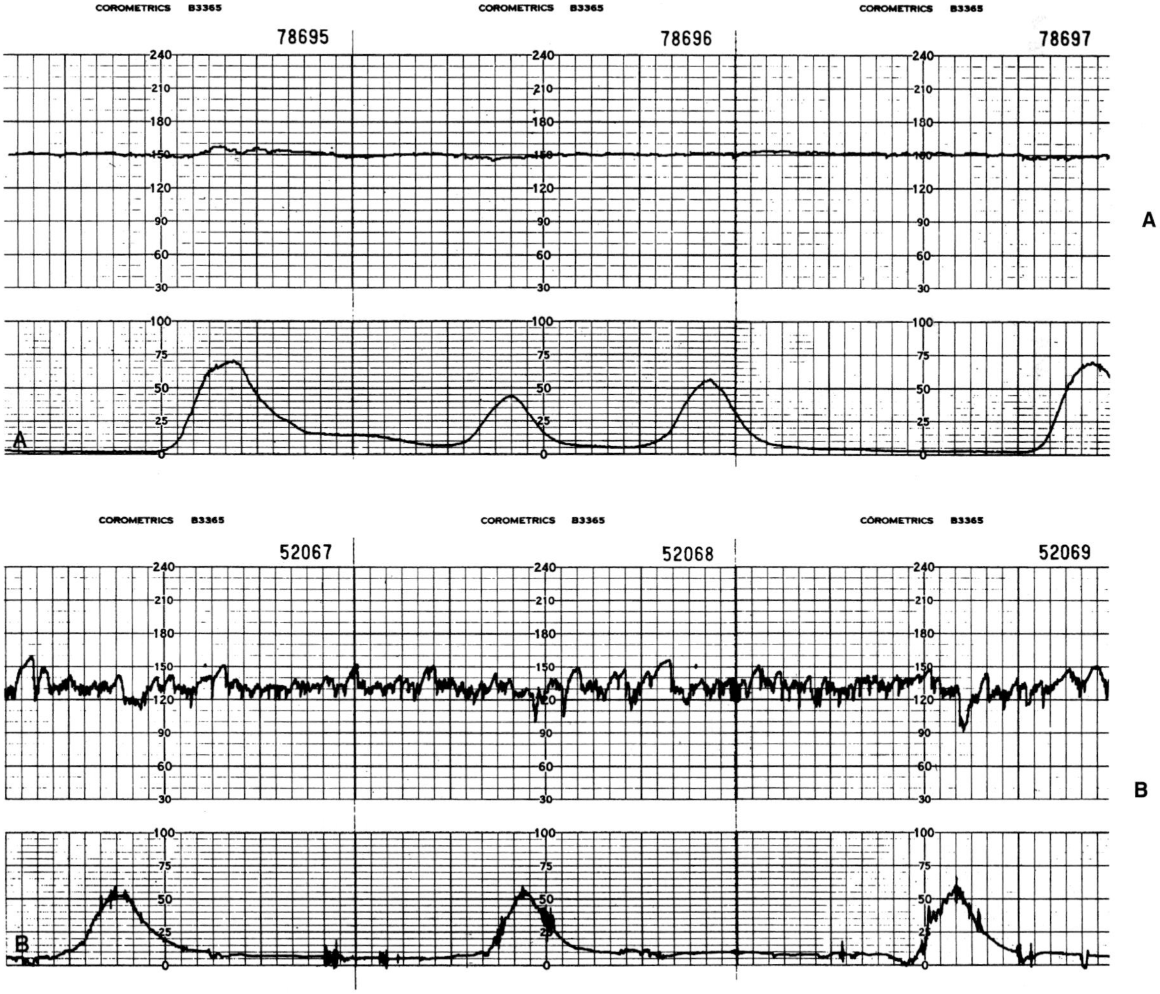

FIGURE 14-9 Contrasts in fetal heart rate variability. A fetal scalp electrode is being used. **A,** Minimal variability (less than 3 BPM). Note the smooth, flat line in the FHR channel. **B,** Moderate variability (about 20 BPM). Note the marked zigzag appearance of the fetal heart rate line. (Courtesy Corometrics Medical Systems, Inc., Wallingford, Conn. Redrawn with permission.)

gether. Some facilities may continue to distinguish between the two types.

Variability occurs because multiple factors constantly speed and slow the fetal heart in a push-and-pull manner. Evaluation of variability helps to clarify how a fetus is tolerating the stress of labor, including factors that cause hypoxia. Variability is a significant component of the FHR tracing on the electronic monitor for two reasons:

- Adequate oxygenation promotes normal function of the autonomic nervous system and helps the fetus adapt to the stress of labor.
- Variability evaluates the function of the fetal autonomic nervous system, especially the parasympathetic branch.

Variability may be decreased by both nonpathologic and pathologic factors, such as the following:

- Narcotics or other sedative drugs given to the woman, including those given with epidural analgesia
- Tachycardia
- Prematurity
- Decreased oxygenation of the fetal central nervous system
- Abnormalities of the central nervous system, heart, or both
- Fetal sleep, with variability being reduced as the fetus sleeps (about 20 to 30 minutes at a time) and increasing when the fetus awakens

The following descriptions classify variability in BPM:

- Absent—Undetectable
- Minimal—Undetectable to ≤5 BPM
- Moderate—6 to 25 BPM
- Marked—>25 BPM

Periodic Patterns in the Fetal Heart Rate

Periodic patterns are transient and recurrent changes from the baseline rate associated with uterine contractions. They include accelerations and decelerations. Periodic patterns are evaluated with baseline characteristics (rate and variability).

Accelerations

An acceleration is an abrupt, temporary increase in the FHR that peaks at least 15 BPM above the baseline and lasts at least 15 seconds (Figure 14-10). Accelerations often occur with fetal movement. They may be nonperiodic (having no relation to contractions) as well as periodic. They may occur with vaginal examinations, uterine contractions, and mild cord compression and when the fetus is in a breech presentation. Accelerations are usually a reassuring sign, reflecting a responsive, nonacidotic fetus.

The healthy preterm fetus may have FHR accelerations less than 15 BPM. Before 32 weeks of gestation, an abrupt increase in the FHR that peaks at least 10 BPM above the baseline and lasts at least 10 seconds is considered an acceleration.

Accelerations lasting longer than 2 minutes but less than 10 minutes are prolonged accelerations. Accelerations that last longer than 10 minutes are a change in the baseline rate.

Decelerations

Periodic decelerations are classified into three types based on their shape and relationship to uterine contractions.

Early Decelerations. Fetal head compression briefly increases intracranial pressure, causing the vagus nerve to slow the heart rate. Early decelerations are not associated with fetal compromise and require no intervention. They occur during contractions as the fetal head is pressed against the woman's pelvis or soft tissues, such as the cervix.

Early decelerations have a gradual, rather than abrupt, decrease from the baseline. They have a consistent appearance in that one early deceleration looks similar to others. The early decelerations mirror the contraction, beginning near its onset and returning to the baseline by the end of the contraction, with the low point of the deceleration occurring near the contraction's peak (Figure 14-11). The rate at the lowest point of the deceleration usually remains above 100 BPM.

Late Decelerations. Deficient exchange of oxygen and waste products in the placenta (uteroplacental insufficiency) may result in a pattern of late (delayed) decelerations. This nonreassuring pattern suggests that the fetus has reduced reserve to tolerate the recurrent reductions in oxygen supply that occur with contractions. The cause of uteroplacental insufficiency may be acute, such as maternal hypotension. It may also occur with chronic conditions that impair placental exchange, such as maternal hypertension or diabetes.

Late decelerations are gradual decelerations that look similar to early decelerations but are shifted to the right in relation to the contraction. They often begin after the peak of the contraction. The FHR returns to the baseline *after* the contraction ends (Figure 14-12). They have a consistent appearance. The FHR may remain in the normal range and may not fall much below its baseline level. The amount of rate decrease from the baseline is not related to the amount of uteroplacental insufficiency.

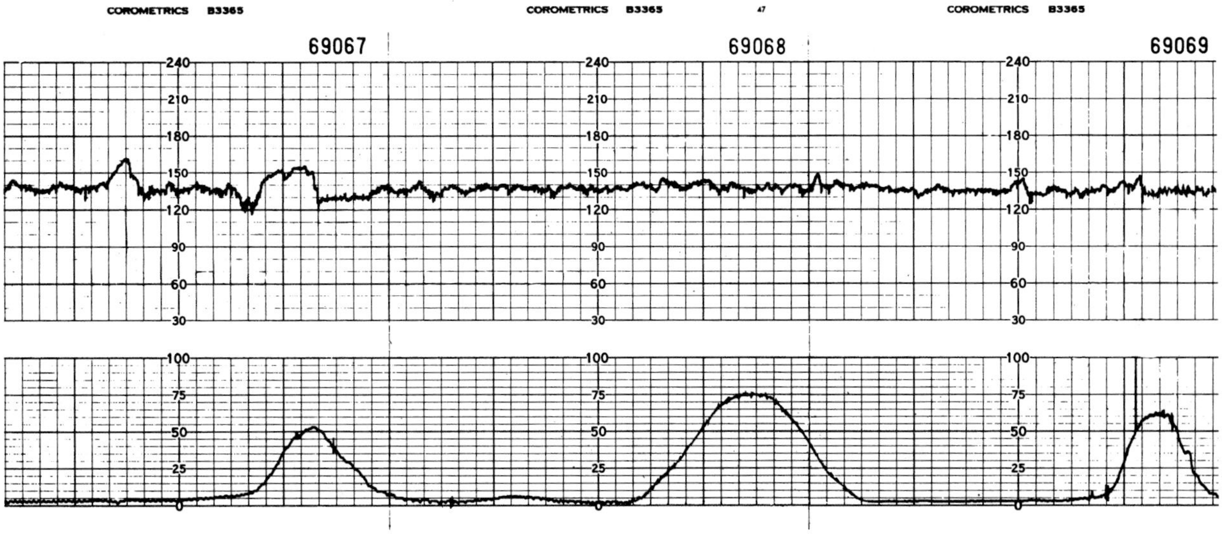

FIGURE 14-10 Acceleration of the fetal heart rate. (Courtesy Corometrics Medical Systems, Inc., Wallingford, Conn. Redrawn with permission.)

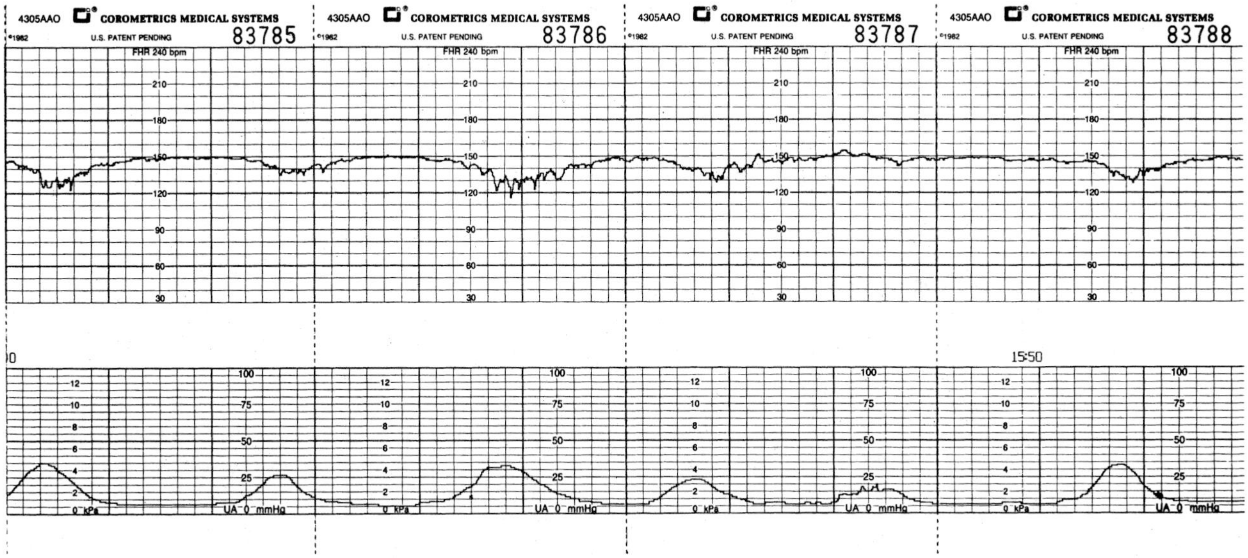

FIGURE 14-11 Early decelerations. Note that the slowing of the fetal heart rate mirrors the contraction. It begins near the beginning of the contraction and returns to the baseline by the end of the contraction. Cause: fetal head compression. (Courtesy Corometrics Medical Systems, Inc., Wallingford, Conn.)

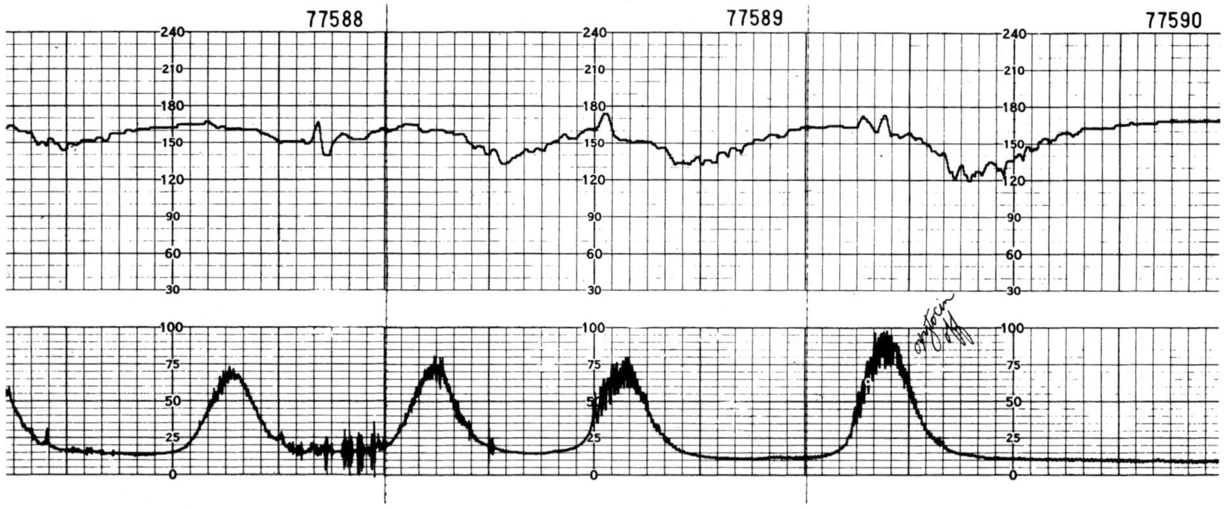

FIGURE 14-12 Late decelerations. Note that the decelerations look similar to early decelerations but are offset to the right. They begin at about the peak of the contraction and do not return to the baseline until after the contraction ends. Cause: uteroplacental insufficiency. (Courtesy Corometrics Medical Systems, Inc., Wallingford, Conn. Redrawn with permission.)

CRITICAL TO REMEMBER

Differences between Early and Late Decelerations

Early decelerations

Occur only during contractions as the fetal head is compressed

Return to the baseline fetal heart rate by the end of the contraction

Are mirror images of the contraction (fetal heart rate line goes down as contraction line goes up)

Are not associated with fetal compromise and require no added interventions

Late decelerations

Look similar to early decelerations but begin well after the contraction begins (often near the peak)

Return to baseline after the contraction ends

Reflect impaired placental exchange (uteroplacental insufficiency)

The degree of fall in rate from baseline is unrelated to the amount of uteroplacental insufficiency

Should be addressed by nursing interventions to improve placental blood flow and fetal oxygen supply

Variable Decelerations. Conditions that restrict flow through the umbilical cord may result in variable decelerations. These decelerations do not have the uniform appearance of early and late decelerations. Their shape, duration, and degree of fall below baseline rate are variable. They fall and rise abruptly with the onset and relief of cord compression, unlike the gradual fall and rise of early and late decelerations (Figure 14-13). Variable decelerations also may be nonperiodic, occurring at times unrelated to contractions.

Several methods are used to classify variable decelerations according to depth and duration, but no uniform agreement exists. One guideline suggests that variable decelerations are significant when the FHR repeatedly decreases to less than 70 BPM and persists at that level for at least 60 seconds before returning to the baseline (ACOG, 1995a). Baseline rate and variability are also considered when evaluating variable decelerations.

Uterine Activity

Assessment of uterine activity has four components: frequency, duration, and intensity of the contractions, and uterine resting tone. Contraction frequency may be measured with the electronic monitor the same way as with palpation (beginning of one contraction to beginning of the next) or from peak to peak. Duration is calculated from the beginning to end of each contraction.

Palpation is used to estimate contraction intensity and uterine resting tone when an external uterine activity monitor is used (see Procedure 13-2). Contraction intensity is described as mild, moderate, or strong.

With either type of intrauterine pressure catheter, the scale on the paper is used to describe intensity and resting tone. Intensity increases as labor progresses. Uterine contraction intensity with the intrauterine pressure catheter is about 50 to 75 mmHg during labor, although it may reach 110 mmHg with pushing during the second stage. Average resting tone is 5 to 15 mmHg.

Montevideo units (MVU) may be used to describe contraction intensity when an intrauterine pressure catheter is used. The MVU is calculated by noting the contraction intensity in mmHg above the resting tone and multiplying by the number of contractions in

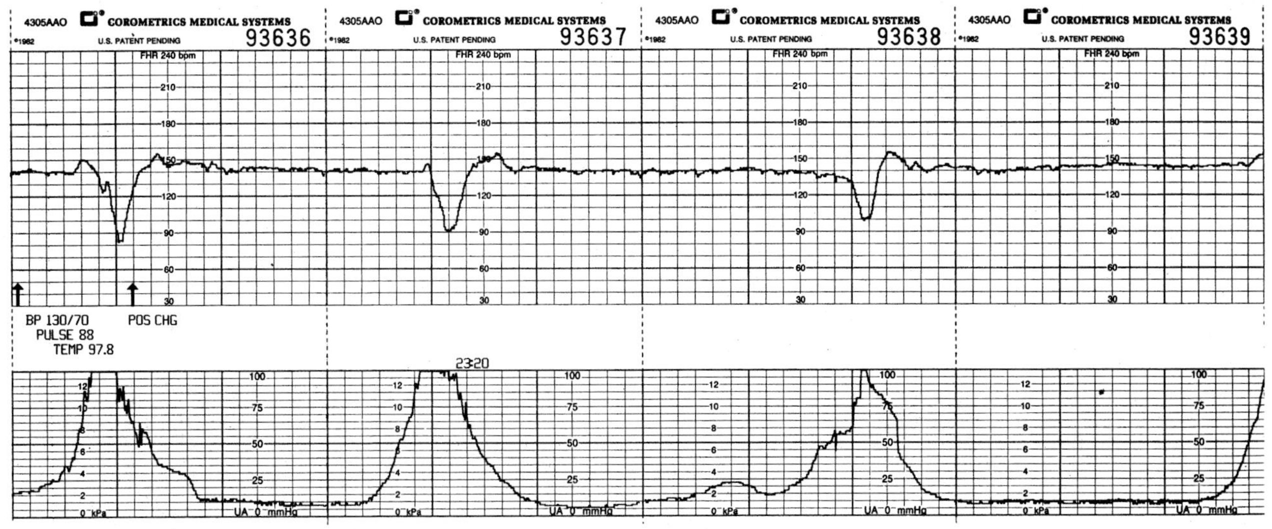

FIGURE 14-13 Variable decelerations. The decelerations are sharp in onset and offset. Note slight rate accelerations (shoulders) after each variable deceleration. Cause: umbilical cord compression. (Courtesy Corometrics Medical Systems, Inc., Wallingford, Conn. Redrawn with permission.)

10 minutes. For example, if a woman has three contractions in 10 minutes, each of which has an intensity 50 mmHg higher than the resting tone, the Montevideo units are 150. A maximum of 280 MVU is normal for active spontaneous labor (Parer, 1997).

CRITICAL THINKING EXERCISE

Nancy Joe is having her labor induced with oxytocin and is having internal electronic fetal monitoring. Her contractions average 2.5 minutes apart, are 90 seconds in duration, and reach 75 mmHg on the scale for the intrauterine pressure catheter. Uterine resting tone between contractions is 20 mmHg. The baseline fetal heart rate is 135 to 145 BPM with about 7 BPM variability.

Her nurse, Jackie Brown, notes a pattern of uniform decelerations that begin at the peak of each contraction. The rate falls to 125 BPM before returning to the previous baseline about 30 seconds after the contraction ends.

QUESTIONS:

1. What pattern does this describe?
2. What is the most appropriate nursing response?

Check Your Reading

10. What is the significance of FHR accelerations?
11. What are the differences between early and late decelerations? Which pattern is nonreassuring?
12. What do variable decelerations look like? What is their cause?

SIGNIFICANCE OF FETAL HEART RATE PATTERNS

As with intermittent auscultation, fetal heart rate patterns on the electronic monitor are classified as either "reassuring" or "nonreassuring." Between these two classifications are patterns that are "equivocal," neither clearly reassuring nor clearly nonreassuring. For equivocal (ambiguous) patterns or for questionable intermittent auscultation data, several methods may be used to further evaluate the fetal condition. Table 14-2 summarizes reassuring and nonreassuring patterns.

Reassuring Patterns

Reassuring patterns, such as accelerations with fetal movement, are associated with fetal well-being. No intervention is required because the pattern suggests that the fetus has adequate reserves to tolerate intrapartum stressors.

Nonreassuring Patterns

Nonreassuring patterns occur if favorable signs are absent or if signs that are associated with fetal hypoxia or acidosis are present. Nonreassuring patterns do not necessarily indicate that fetal hypoxia or acidosis has occurred. They indicate that steps should be taken to identify possible causes for the nonreassuring patterns and correct those causes.

Nonreassuring patterns are more significant if they occur together and are persistent. For example, bradycardia with short-term variability of less than 3 BPM and late decelerations suggests greater fetal stress than bradycardia alone. The healthy fetus may demonstrate occasional late decelerations, but a persistent pattern

Table 14-2

REASSURING AND NONREASSURING FETAL HEART RATE PATTERNS

Reassuring Patterns

Baseline rate: Stable, with a lower limit of 110-120 BPM and an upper limit of 150-160 BPM at term
Variability of 6 to 25 BPM
Accelerations with fetal movement: Increases that peak at least 15 BPM above the baseline and last for at least 15 seconds
Uterine activity:

- Contraction frequency: no more frequent than every 2 minutes
- Contraction duration: no longer than 90 seconds
- Interval between contractions: at least 60 seconds
- Uterine resting tone: uterus relaxed between contractions (with external monitor); maximum uterine resting tone < 20 mmHg (with intrauterine pressure catheter)
- Montevideo units: maximum of 280 in active labor

Nonreassuring Patterns

Pattern and Description	Possible Causes
Tachycardia Baseline FHR > 160 BPM for at least 10 minutes Mild: 161 to 180 BPM Severe: > 181 BPM	Maternal fever (fetal tachycardia may precede maternal fever) Maternal dehydration Maternal or fetal hypoxia Fetal acidosis Maternal or fetal hypovolemia Fetal cardiac arrhythmias Maternal severe anemia Maternal hyperthyroidism Drugs administered to mother (such as terbutaline)
Bradycardia Baseline FHR < 110 BPM for at least 10 minutes Baseline rates between 100 and 110 BPM in the term fetus are usually not associated with fetal compromise if there are no nonreassuring patterns	Fetal head compression Fetal hypoxia Fetal acidosis Fetal heart block Umbilical cord compression Second stage labor with maternal pushing
Absent or Minimal Variability FHR baseline has a smooth, flat appearance	Fetal sleep (usually lasts no longer than 30 minutes at a time in the absence of CNS depressants) Fetal hypoxia with acidosis Drug effects: • CNS depressants • Local anesthetic agents
Late Decelerations Recurrent decelerations with a uniform appearance and a consistent relation to the contraction; begin after the contraction starts (usually at the peak) and do not return to baseline until after the contraction ends	Uteroplacental insufficiency, which may be secondary to the following: Maternal hypotension Excess uterine activity Placental interruption, such as abruptio placentae or placenta previa Pregnancy-induced or chronic hypertension Maternal diabetes Maternal severe anemia Maternal cardiac disease
Variable Decelerations Sharp in onset and offset Appearance and relationship to contractions is not consistent, may occur as a nonperiodic pattern (randomly) or may occur regularly with contractions (periodic)	Umbilical cord compression, which may be secondary to the following: Prolapsed cord Nuchal cord (around fetal neck) Oligohydramnios (abnormally small amount of amniotic fluid) Cord between fetus and mother's uterus or pelvis, without obvious prolapse Cord between fetal body parts Knot in cord

BPM, Beats per minute; *FHR,* fetal heart rate.

of late decelerations is more likely to represent compromise in a fetus, especially if it is combined with other nonreassuring patterns. Nonreassuring patterns include but are not limited to the following:

- Tachycardia
- Bradycardia
- Absent or minimal variability
- Late decelerations
- Variable decelerations falling to less than 70 BPM for longer than 60 seconds
- Prolonged decelerations
- Hypertonic uterine activity

Nonreassuring patterns do not always indicate that labor should end immediately. Several interventions may be used to clarify the fetal condition and to determine the best course of action. Other interventions can increase fetal oxygenation.

Clarification of Data

Several methods may clarify data to better understand the fetal condition. Two methods are used during the intrapartum period: vibroacoustic stimulation and fetal scalp stimulation. Fetal scalp blood sampling is less common. A fourth method, analysis of umbilical cord blood gases and pH, is used immediately after birth.

In addition to these methods, fetal oxygen saturation monitoring, similar to pulse oximetry used in adult and pediatric care, is a new method that is being added to the fetal monitoring units of many intrapartum facilities.

Vibroacoustic Stimulation. Vibroacoustic, or simply acoustic (or sound), stimulation (VAS) may be used by the nurse, physician, or nurse-midwife as the initial method to stimulate the fetus, to supplement fetal scalp stimulation, or used if scalp stimulation is contraindicated.

An artificial larynx or vibroacoustic stimulator is applied to the mother's lower abdomen, and it is turned on for up to 3 seconds. A reassuring response is an acceleration that peaks at 15 BPM for 15 seconds or more. An absent response, however, does not necessarily mean that the fetus is suffering from hypoxia or acidosis.

Fetal Scalp Stimulation. Scalp stimulation evaluates the fetus' response to tactile stimulation (Figure 14-14). The nurse, physician, or nurse-midwife may perform this procedure. The examiner applies pressure to the scalp (or other presenting part) with a gloved finger or fingers and sweeps the fingers in a circular motion. An FHR acceleration, as in VAS, is a reassuring response that suggests the fetus is in normal oxygen and acid-base balance. The acceleration may be delayed as much as 10 minutes rather than immediate (Miller, 2000).

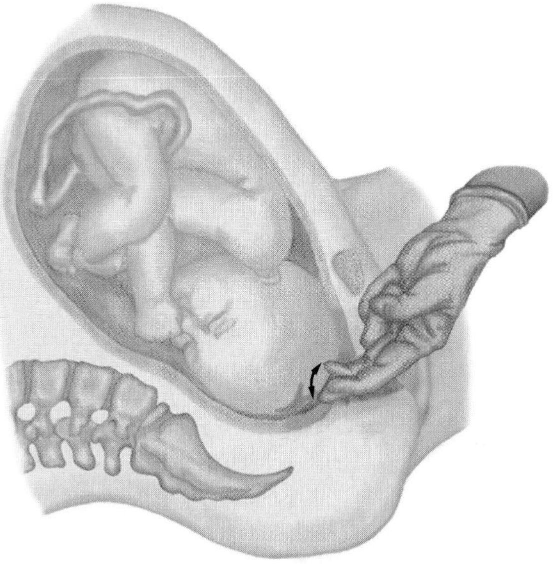

FIGURE 14-14 Fetal scalp stimulation helps identify whether the fetus responds to gentle massage. An acceleration in the FHR peaking 15 BPM above the baseline and lasting for 15 seconds suggests that the fetus is in normal oxygen and acid-base balance.

Fetal scalp stimulation is not done in some cases:

- Preterm fetus (may cause contractions)
- Prolonged rupture of membranes (higher risk of infection)
- Chorioamnionitis (intrauterine infection)
- Placenta previa (placenta overlies the cervix and hemorrhage is likely)
- Maternal fever of unknown origin (possibility of introducing microorganisms into the uterus)

Fetal Scalp Blood Sample. Occasionally, the physician may obtain a sample of fetal scalp blood to evaluate the pH. Normal scalp pH is 7.25 to 7.35. Scalp sampling is less common because it is invasive and the results are not available immediately.

Fetal Oxygen Saturation Monitor. This type of fetal surveillance, also called fetal pulse oximetry, is relatively new in the United States. Ideally, fetal pulse oximetry will help caregivers make better judgments about whether a nonreassuring fetal heart rate pattern is one that requires immediate operative intervention (cesarean or forceps birth) or if labor can safely continue (Seelbach-Göbel, Heupel, Kühnert, & Butterwegge, 1999; Simpson, 1998a & 1998b).

The technique is similar to that used for the mother's pulse oximetry. A special sensor is placed alongside the fetal cheek or temple area to pick up the fetal pulse for calculation of oxygen saturation (Figure 14-15). An oxygen saturation of 30% to 70% is considered normal

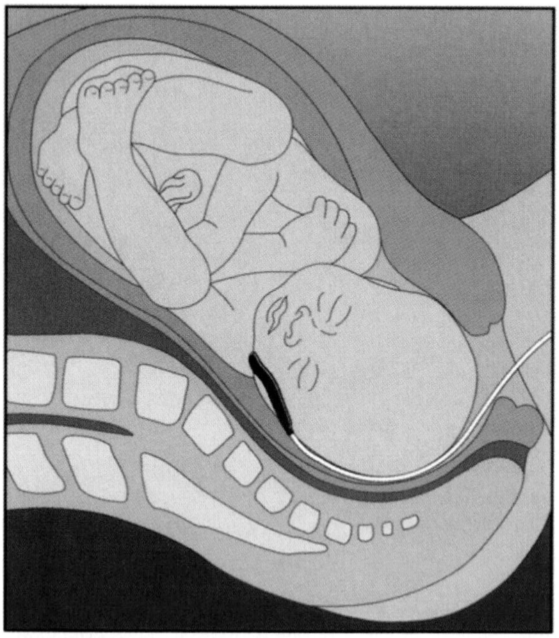

FIGURE 14-15 The sensor for the fetal pulse oximeter is inserted vaginally so that it lies against the fetal cheek or temple. The sensor is held in place by the wall of the uterus. (Courtesy Oxifirst.)

for fetuses because of their high hemoglobin and hematocrit (compared with a normal of 95% to 100% oxygen saturation for an adult). Technical difficulties have included the normally faint pulses of a fetus, interference of vernix and other debris between fetal skin and the sensor, and displacement of the sensor.

Cord Blood Gases and pH. Umbilical cord blood analysis is used to assess the infant's oxygenation and acid-base balance immediately after birth. The samples are analyzed for pH, PCO_2, PO_2, and bicarbonate and for base deficit. This information helps identify whether acidosis exists and whether it is respiratory (short-term), metabolic (prolonged), or mixed. Normal cord blood gases and pH can confirm that the fetus was adjusting normally to the stresses of labor even though the fetal monitoring pattern may have been nonreassuring.

The cord is promptly double clamped (within 20 to 30 seconds of birth) and cut to isolate a 10 to 20 cm (4 to 8 inches) segment. Blood samples from an umbilical artery provide the most accurate information about the newborn's acid-base status. The sample can also be obtained from a fetal artery on the surface of the placenta. Blood is drawn into heparinized syringes to prevent coagulation, and the syringes are capped to avoid altering values by exposure to room air (Figure 14-16). Samples kept at room temperature are reliable for 30 to 60 minutes (ACOG, 1995b). Samples should be kept in ice if there is a delay beyond this time.

Interventions for Nonreassuring Patterns

Any of several nursing or medical interventions, or both, may be indicated if a nonreassuring FHR pattern is present. All are directed toward identifying the cause of the nonreassuring pattern and improving fetal oxygenation.

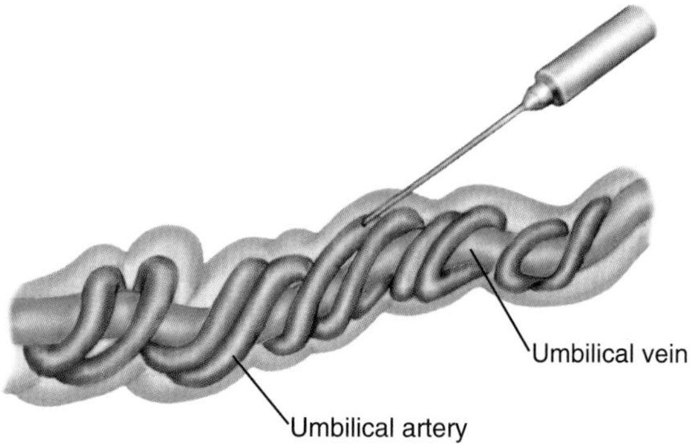

FIGURE 14-16 Obtaining a blood sample for umbilical cord blood gases and pH after birth. Samples are drawn from the umbilical artery, vein, or both. The samples in capped syringes may be kept for up to 60 minutes at room temperature and 3 hours on ice.

CRITICAL TO REMEMBER

Nursing Responses to Nonreassuring Fetal Heart Rate Patterns

1. Identify the cause of the nonreassuring pattern to plan the best interventions:
   a. Evaluate the pattern to determine its probable cause (late or variable decelerations, bradycardia or tachycardia, absent variability).
   b. Evaluate maternal vital signs to identify hypotension, hypertension, or fever.
   c. Perform vaginal examination to identify a prolapsed umbilical cord.
2. Stop oxytocin infusion if the drug is being administered.
3. Reposition the woman, avoiding the supine position, for patterns associated with cord compression; repositioning may improve other nonreassuring patterns as well.
4. Increase the rate of a nonadditive intravenous fluid to expand the mother's blood volume and improve placental perfusion.
5. Administer oxygen by face mask at 8 to 10 L per minute to increase her blood oxygen saturation, making more oxygen available to the fetus.
6. Initiate electronic fetal monitoring if intermittent auscultation data are questionable.
7. Initiate continuous electronic fetal monitoring with internal devices if no contraindication exists.
8. Notify physician or nurse-midwife as soon as possible. Report and document the following:
   a. The pattern that was identified
   b. Nursing interventions taken in response to the pattern
   c. The fetal response after nursing interventions
   d. The response of the physician or nurse-midwife (orders, other response)
9. If the nonreassuring pattern is severe, other staff members should begin preparing for immediate delivery (usually cesarean birth unless vaginal birth is imminent).

Identifying the Cause of a Nonreassuring Pattern. Careful examination of the strip may suggest a cause for the nonreassuring FHR pattern and direct the most appropriate interventions. For example, a pattern of late decelerations suggests uteroplacental insufficiency. However, uteroplacental insufficiency may be secondary to a variety of causes, such as maternal hypotension or excessive uterine activity. Different causes require different corrective interventions. Checking the mother's vital signs identifies hypotension, hypertension, and fever. Maternal medications such as opioids may be a benign cause of decreased variability.

A vaginal examination may identify a prolapsed cord, which may cause variable decelerations, bradycardia, or both, as it is compressed. A vaginal examination also evaluates the woman's labor status, which helps the birth attendant decide if labor should continue. For example, labor may be allowed to continue, or it may be ended with forceps or a vacuum extractor if a nonreassuring pattern occurs during late labor. If the same nonreassuring pattern persisted during early labor despite interventions to correct it, a cesarean birth would be more likely.

Internal monitoring is often chosen for greater accuracy if a nonreassuring pattern develops when external devices are used. The fetal scalp electrode gives a clear picture of variability, and the intrauterine pressure catheter allows the most precise determination of actual contraction intensity and resting tone.

CRITICAL THINKING EXERCISE

LaShonda Blair is in active labor and is having intermittent auscultation for fetal assessment. Her baseline FHR has been 130 to 140 BPM. LaShonda has not had medication, and her labor has been normal so far. Her membranes ruptured about 1 hour ago, and the amniotic fluid was clear. Contractions are every 3 minutes, 60 seconds in duration, and of moderate intensity. Her uterus fully relaxes between each contraction.

The nurse who is caring for LaShonda notes abrupt slowing of the fetal heart rate to about 90 BPM during a routine auscultation. The nurse continues listening and the FHR remains at 90 BPM for 15 seconds then rapidly returns to the previous level of 140 BPM with a regular rhythm.

QUESTIONS:

1. Are any nursing actions needed?
2. If nursing actions are needed, what are they and in what order should they be done?

Increasing Placental Perfusion. The woman is placed in a nonsupine position to eliminate aortocaval compression, which can reduce placental blood flow. Increasing nonadditive intravenous fluids such as lactated Ringer's solution increases the maternal blood volume to better perfuse the placenta if maternal hypotension is the problem.

Uterine activity reduces blood flow into the intervillous spaces, and a fetus with little reserve for stress may be unable to tolerate even normal contractions. Persistent hypertonic uterine activity may compromise a fetus with normal reserves. If a woman is receiving oxytocin, it is discontinued, or its rate may be slowed so that uterine activity is not stimulated. A tocolytic drug, such as terbutaline (0.125 to 0.25 mg intravenously or 0.25 mg subcutaneously), may be given to reduce uterine activity.

Increasing Maternal Blood Oxygen Saturation. Administration of 100% oxygen through a snug face mask makes more oxygen available for transfer to the fetus. A commonly suggested rate is 8 to 10 L per minute.

Reducing Cord Compression. If cord compression is suspected, the woman is repositioned. She may be turned from side to side, or her hips may be elevated to shift the fetal presenting part toward her diaphragm. A hands-and-knees position may reduce compression on the cord that is entrapped behind the fetus. Several position changes may be required before the pattern improves or resolves.

Amnioinfusion increases the fluid around the fetus and cushions the cord. Lactated Ringer's solution or normal saline is infused into the uterus through an intrauterine pressure catheter. The underpads must be changed regularly because fluid leaks out constantly. Possible complications include overdistention of the uterus and increased uterine resting tone. These complications are relieved by releasing some of the fluid. Amnioinfusion also may be used to wash out and dilute fluid that contains thick meconium so that the infant does not aspirate it at birth.

Check Your Reading

13. What is the rationale for performing fetal scalp stimulation or vibroacoustic stimulation? What is the expected fetal response to these actions?
14. What is the purpose of blood gas and pH determinations on cord blood samples?
15. What nursing actions are appropriate for a nonreassuring FHR pattern? Why are they performed?
16. How can a tocolytic drug increase oxygen supply to the fetus?
17. What are the two purposes of amnioinfusion?

APPLICATION OF THE NURSING PROCESS: INTERMITTENT AUSCULTATION AND ELECTRONIC FETAL MONITORING

Assessment of the fetus using either intermittent auscultation or electronic fetal monitoring requires additional education after entering the intrapartum nursing specialty. The novice nurse or student usually provides care in the form of applying the external monitor,

Enhancing Comfort

Nursing care involves finding ways to make the mother comfortable and the monitor as nonintrusive as possible. Teach the woman ways to improve comfort while still obtaining an adequate tracing.

Explain that staying in one position not only is uncomfortable but also does not promote normal labor. The woman may assume any position except supine in most cases. She can sit in a chair, stand beside the bed, and assume most positions in the labor bed. She should find her most comfortable position, then the nurse can adjust the external devices to best detect contractions and the fetal heartbeat. Internal devices may be an option if external devices cannot be adjusted to provide useful data.

If the woman finds the sound produced by the electronic fetal monitor distracting or inconsistent with the atmosphere she wants, turn the sound off. The auditory cues for rate accelerations and decelerations are absent if the sound is muted.

If no other contraindications to walking exist, the woman may go to the bathroom to urinate or defecate. Unplug the sensors at the machine, let her walk to the bathroom, and reconnect and adjust the sensors when she returns. Alternatively, roll the machine to the door of the bathroom; the cords are usually long enough to remain connected. Document ambulation and any interruption in monitoring on the strip. If the fetus has a nonreassuring pattern, it is preferable not to interrupt the recording.

Evaluation

The evaluation of knowledge is continuous because most women think of questions after initial explanations and as conditions change. Achievement of the goal or expected outcome is evident if the partners indicate their understanding after each explanation. Their understanding may be accompanied by a decrease in anxiety signs as well.

FETAL OXYGENATION

Assessment

Evaluate the fetal monitoring strip systematically for the elements noted previously. Assessment and documentation intervals recommended are the same as those for intermittent auscultation:

- Low-risk women—Every 30 minutes during the active phase and every 15 minutes during the second stage
- High-risk women—Every 15 minutes during the active phase and every 5 minutes during the second stage

Take the woman's temperature every 4 hours (every 2 hours after membranes rupture). Maternal fever increases the fetal temperature and fetal oxygen requirements. The nurse should assess the woman's pulse, respirations, and blood pressure hourly. Hypotension or hypertension may reduce maternal blood flow to the intervillous spaces.

Assessment of mother and fetus is continuous during the dynamic process of labor. Compare data about FHR patterns, uterine activity, and maternal vital signs with baseline data and normal ranges. Observe for subtle trends in the data; and distinguish between patterns having similar appearances, such as early and late decelerations.

Vaginal examination may be performed to evaluate specific FHR patterns, for example, to check for a prolapsed cord if a pattern of variable decelerations occurs (see p. 348).

Analysis

The collaborative problem "Potential Complication: Fetal Compromise" is selected for nursing care related to fetal oxygenation when electronic fetal monitoring is used.

Planning

Because the nurse does not manage fetal compromise independently, client (fetal) goals are not made. The nurse's responsibility includes planning to do the following:

- Promote adequate fetal oxygenation.
- Take corrective actions to increase fetal oxygenation if nonreassuring patterns are identified.
- Report nonreassuring patterns to the physician or nurse-midwife.
- Support the woman and her partner if a complication develops.
- Document assessments and care.

Interventions

Measures to promote fetal oxygenation are also discussed with the care of the woman in normal labor (see Chapter 13) and the woman having an epidural or subarachnoid block (see Chapter 15).

Taking Corrective Actions

The priority of nursing care is to improve fetal oxygenation. If a nonreassuring pattern is noted, identify its cause and improve fetal oxygenation (see p. 352). Birth facilities have protocols to give nurses a framework for steps to take if nonreassuring patterns develop. Nursing interventions may include both independent nursing actions and delegated medical actions.

Reassuring Parents

Parents understandably become anxious when a nonreassuring pattern occurs. Remain at the bedside and

Table 14-3
DOCUMENTING ELECTRONIC FETAL MONITORING

DOCUMENTATION WHEN MONITORING INITIATED **Monitor Strip** Woman's name Physician's or nurse-midwife's name Date and time of admission Date and time electronic monitoring is begun (verify date and time if this information is automatically printed by monitor) Gravidity, parity, abortions, living children Gestation in weeks Presence of identified risk factors Character of amniotic fluid (if membranes are ruptured) Function test of monitor accuracy Initial mode of monitoring (external or internal devices) **Labor Record** Same information as on monitor strip First panel number when strip is begun **CONTINUING DOCUMENTATION** **Monitor Strip** Maternal vital signs Vaginal examinations, including cervical dilation and effacement and fetal station Rupture of membranes (spontaneously or artificially)	Color, quantity, and character (such as foul odor or cloudiness) of amniotic fluid Maternal position changes Maternal or fetal movement Maternal vomiting, coughing, or other movement that affects tracing Adjustment of equipment Medication and anesthesia, including related interventions Changes of equipment mode (such as external to internal device) Interventions for nonreassuring patterns Temporary interruptions in strip, such as woman walking **Labor Record** Same information as on monitor strip Periodic summary of the baseline rate, variability, periodic changes, and uterine activity (frequency, duration, and intensity of contractions and uterine resting tone) Communications with physician or nurse-midwife, including their response to reports of problems Actions taken in chain of command if the physician or nurse-midwife fails to respond appropriately to the nurse's report of a problem

remain calm to avoid increasing their anxiety. The call bell can be used to summon other nurses to help with corrective actions and to notify the physician or nurse-midwife if it is impossible to leave.

Explain any problems and the reason for corrective actions in simple, concise language. Severe anxiety reduces the parents' ability to understand information. Inform them if the FHR returns to a reassuring pattern. Some corrective actions, such as oxygen administration and positioning, may continue after a reassuring pattern returns. Tell the woman she may talk while wearing the oxygen mask. Document parental reassurance and their response.

Nonreassuring Patterns

Notify the birth attendant of nonreassuring patterns as soon as possible after taking corrective actions. In addition, document the time and content of all consultations with the physician or nurse-midwife about the mother or fetus and the birth attendant's response.

Documenting Assessments and Care

Record data related to fetal well-being in both the labor record and on the monitor strip if that is facility policy. Table 14-3 shows guidelines for documentation on the monitor strip and labor record. Documentation can demonstrate good nursing care and show that the standard of care has been met.

Write the woman's name, the date, and the time on the strip when electronic fetal monitoring begins. If a break in the strip occurs, such as to change paper, label the new strip with the woman's name, the date, and the time. Record the last panel number of the previous strip on the new strip so that the entire record can be reassembled sequentially.

Continue documenting the heart rate and maternal observations until vaginal birth occurs. If a cesarean birth is needed, continue monitoring by auscultation or electronic means as long as practical while preparing the woman for surgery. Remove internal devices before securing her legs to the operating table with a strap. Document the time at which monitoring is stopped and the time of abdominal incision.

Evaluation

Client-centered goals are not formulated for a collaborative problem. Compare data with established standards to determine whether they are within normal limits. If nonreassuring patterns are identified, the following steps are necessary:

- Take measures to increase fetal oxygenation
- Notify the physician or nurse-midwife of nonreassuring patterns
- Document all relevant data

NURSING CARE PLAN 14-1

Intrapartum Fetal Compromise

Assessment: Glenda Brown is a 30-year-old African-American woman. She is a gravida II, para I and has a 7-year-old son. Glenda had early and regular prenatal care. She had a biophysical profile during her pregnancy because of a slight blood pressure elevation. Glenda's labor is being induced with oxytocin (Pitocin) at 37 weeks' gestation because of pregnancy-induced hypertension. Her admission blood pressure was 148/94, and repeat assessments have been about the same level. Glenda's fetus will be monitored with electronic fetal monitoring. Glenda is accompanied by her husband, Paul. Glenda said they did not take classes because they felt that they remembered enough from their prior labor. Chris Lowe is Glenda's intrapartum nurse.

Critical Thinking: What nursing diagnosis is appropriate at this time? Should the nurse include Paul when considering the initial nursing diagnosis?

Answer: Although the Browns have had one successful pregnancy, the nurse should not assume that they know about the use of fetal monitoring in labor, especially because their son was born 7 years ago. The fact that they did not attend classes also increases the likelihood that they need teaching about the electronic fetal monitor.

Nursing Diagnosis: Knowledge deficit: Electronic fetal monitoring.

Goals/Expected Outcomes: Glenda and Paul will state that they understand the reason for electronic monitoring, related equipment and procedures, and the data that are expected.

Intervention	Rationale
1. Assess the parents' present knowledge about electronic fetal monitoring.	1. This builds on existing accurate knowledge and correct misunderstandings.
2. Explain information about the monitor to Glenda and Paul:	2. Explain that the use of the electronic fetal monitor does not mean something is wrong with Glenda or the baby.
a. Purposes: To record the fetal response to labor and guide interventions if nonreassuring patterns are identified	a. This provides a realistic explanation of how the monitor is used.
b. Safety: The monitoring sensors are electrically isolated from the wall current. The fetal scalp electrode (if used) penetrates the outer layer of skin, about a dime's thickness. The intrauterine pressure catheter lies between the baby and the wall of the uterus.	b. This answers possible safety concerns of parents.
c. Encourage Glenda to call for assistance if she is concerned about anything related to the monitor, such as being unable to hear the fetal heartbeat. Tell her that a nurse will adjust her monitor as needed.	c. Sensors, especially external devices, are easily displaced. Preparing Glenda and Paul for this possibility reduces their fears if they should stop hearing the fetal heartbeat.
d. Encourage Glenda to move about freely. Explain that she should urinate at least every 2 hours and that the nurse can help her roll the monitor to the bathroom door or temporarily disconnect the sensors.	d. Maternal movement and regular urination enhance normal labor processes. A woman is likely to become anxious and uncomfortable if she concentrates more on maintaining data from the monitor than on coping with labor.

Evaluation: Glenda and Paul say they expected electronic fetal monitoring during labor and are familiar with the external monitor because it was used for the biophysical profile. Glenda agrees to have internal monitoring if needed, saying that she understands that greater accuracy is important because of her higher risk status.

Assessment: Chris applies the external fetal monitor, which shows irregular spontaneous contractions. The fetal heart rate (FHR) baseline averages 125 to 135 BPM with accelerations. The nurse begins an oxytocin infusion to induce labor. Glenda's blood pressure is 160/96, pulse 76, respirations 18.

Critical Thinking: Does the nurse need other data at this point?

Answer: Added information would help clarify whether the elevation in Glenda's blood pressure is in response to anxiety or pain or is a part of her pregnancy-induced hypertension. The nurse should assess Glenda for hyperactive reflexes and edema, particularly of her face and fingers (see Chapters 13 and 26).

Potential Complication: Fetal compromise.

Goals/Expected Outcomes:

Client goals for the fetus are inappropriate because nurses cannot independently manage fetal compromise. Chris's planning for Glenda should reflect the need to do the following:

1. Compare FHR and uterine activity data with baseline levels before oxytocin induction.
2. Promote normal fetal oxygenation.
3. Take corrective actions for nonreassuring patterns.
4. Notify Glenda's physician if nonreassuring patterns develop.

Intervention	Rationale
1. Identify relevant risk factors for fetal compromise.	1. The development of pregnancy-induced hypertension is a risk factor that means Glenda should have increased frequency of fetal assessments.
2. Encourage Glenda to assume any comfortable position other than the supine position. Encourage her to change positions regularly, about every half hour.	2. The supine position can reduce blood return to the heart by compressing the inferior vena cava. Compression of the aorta and reduced cardiac output reduce placental perfusion. Regular changes of position promote normal labor progress and comfort.
3. Evaluate the tracing at the following times, signing or initialing the strip, or using computer documentation, each time. Document a summary of the evaluation on the labor record.	3. Documents that assessment was done. Documenting on both strip and labor record allows each to stand alone (if that is facility policy).
a. Every 15 minutes during the first stage and every 5 minutes during the second stage.	a. This situation describes a high-risk pregnancy, and the fetus should be evaluated by those guidelines.
b. Before and after procedures such as amniotomy, medications, epidural anesthesia.	b. Rupture of membranes (spontaneously or by amniotomy) may result in cord compression. Medications may alter the rate or variability of the fetal heartbeat. Epidural anesthesia may cause hypotension, which can decrease uteroplacental perfusion.
c. With changes of activity, such as urination and repositioning.	c. Changes in activity or position could alter the uterine or umbilical cord blood flow. Sensors may slip and need adjustment with activity.
4. Use a four-step approach to evaluate the strip:	4. Systematic framework allows evaluation of the fetal response to labor.
a. Baseline FHR	a. Tachycardia may be an early response to hypoxia. Bradycardia may occur in response to vagal stimulation or prolonged hypoxia.
b. Variability (if fetal scalp electrode is used)	b. Normal variability suggests that the fetus is well oxygenated and not in acidosis.
c. Periodic changes: Accelerations, decelerations (Note relationship of periodic changes to fetal movement, contractions, and the woman's status and activity. Note nonperiodic [random] accelerations or variable decelerations.)	c. Accelerations are a reassuring sign of fetal well-being. Early decelerations are a response to head compression. Late (uteroplacental insufficiency) and variable (umbilical cord compression) decelerations are nonreassuring. The nurse should attempt to identify their cause, correct it if possible, and take steps to improve fetal oxygenation.
d. Uterine activity (Evaluate frequency and duration using either external or internal devices. When external uterine activity monitoring is done, palpate three or more contractions. Note whether the uterus relaxes between contractions for at least 60 seconds. If an intrauterine pressure catheter is used, read contraction intensity and uterine resting tone from scale on strip. Calculate Montevideo units (MVU) if that is the policy in facility.)	d. Contractions that are too long (more than 90 seconds duration) or too frequent (closer than every 2 minutes), a resting interval of less than 60 seconds, or baseline (resting) intrauterine pressure of more than 20 mmHg reduces the time available for normal uteroplacental exchange. Because of diabetes and pregnancy-induced hypertension, uteroplacental exchange may be reduced before labor begins. Oxytocin stimulates uterine activity and adds to risk.
5. For a fetal pulse oximeter, evaluate for a reassuring reading of 30% to 70%.	5. Pulse oximeter readings between 30% and 70% are considered normal for the fetus because of their high hemoglobin and hematocrit.
6. If nonreassuring patterns develop, take appropriate corrective actions such as discontinuing the oxytocin, increasing the rate of the nonadditive intravenous solution, repositioning Glenda, and administering oxygen. Notify physician of nonreassuring patterns, corrective actions taken, and the fetal response. Document response and any orders.	6. The first priority is to identify the cause of the nonreassuring pattern and improve fetal oxygenation. The physician should be notified of the maternal-fetal status for needed medical orders or interventions as soon as possible.

Evaluation: Goals are not established for collaborative problems. Chris compared data from the fetal monitor and other nursing evaluations with the baseline data before Glenda started receiving oxytocin to start contractions. For the first 4 hours of the oxytocin induction, the FHR continued near its baseline of 125 to 135 RPM, with variability averaging 10 BPM. Fetal heart rate accelerations continue. No nonreassuring patterns or fetal pulse oximeter readings were noted.

Assessment: The physician ruptures Glenda's membranes and inserts internal devices for the FHR and uterine activity. Glenda's blood pressure is 145/90, and her oxytocin infusion continues. She is having contractions every 4 minutes; they are of 50 seconds' duration and 50 mm Hg intensity, and she has a uterine resting tone of 10 mm Hg. One hour after Glenda's membranes are ruptured, Chris notes that the baseline FHR has risen to approximately 145 to 150 BPM with variability averaging 3 BPM. A pattern of repeated late decelerations develops. The fetal pulse oximeter readings remain in the reassuring range, however. Chris stops the oxytocin infusion and increases the rate of Ringer's lactate intravenous fluid, positions Glenda on her left side, and administers 100% oxygen at 10 L per minute with a snug face mask. The physician is notified. Baseline variability improves to 5 BPM, but repeated late decelerations continue. Glenda is holding Paul's hand tightly and breathing rapidly. Her vital signs are blood pressure, 158/96; pulse, 90; respirations, 32. Uterine activity is unchanged.

Critical Thinking: What new nursing diagnosis or collaborative problem seems apparent based on the latest assessment data? Why?

Answer: Glenda displays several behaviors typical of anxiety: rapid pulse and respiratory rates and gripping her husband's hand. The rise in her blood pressure could be due to anxiety or to the disease process. Because of added complications and the minimal improvement in fetal status superimposed on her higher-risk status, anxiety seems appropriate. Helping her control her anxiety can promote a more normal labor as well as make her more comfortable.

Nursing Diagnosis: Anxiety related to unexpected development of complications.

Goals/Expected Outcomes:
1. Glenda will have a reduced respiratory rate (12-20/min) after interventions.
2. Glenda will have a more relaxed face and body posture after interventions.

Intervention	Rationale
1. Maintain calm behavior while performing corrective actions and notifying the physician.	1. Calm behavior nonverbally communicates competence to parents. Anxious behavior on the part of caregivers tends to increase the parents' anxiety.
2. Use simple, concise language for all explanations.	2. High anxiety or intense physical sensations impair a person's ability to comprehend explanations.
3. Explain the following to Glenda and Paul: a. The problem that was identified b. The usual cause of the problem c. Reasons for corrective actions d. Expected results e. That Glenda can talk with oxygen mask on	3. If Glenda and Paul understand what is happening and why the corrective actions are taken, they are more likely to comply with the care. Knowledge decreases fear of the unknown. Assuring Glenda that she can talk with the oxygen mask on allows her to ask questions and express feelings to reduce anxiety and fear.
4. Inform Glenda and Paul if the pattern improves or is resolved. For example, tell them when baseline variability improves and that the fetal pulse oximetry readings remain normal.	4. This decreases anxiety about the fetus's condition.
5. Allow Glenda and Paul to express their feelings about the labor and birth during the postpartum period. Explain any gaps in their understanding about what happened.	5. This helps the couple accept and put unexpected occurrences in perspective. It decreases the possibility that one or both parents feel like "a failure" if emergency intervention (cesarean birth) becomes necessary.

Evaluation: Over the next hour, the FHR pattern gradually improves. The baseline rate slows (130 to 140 BPM), and late decelerations are sporadic. Baseline short-term variability improves to about 8 BPM and fetal pulse oximetry readings remain in the normal range. Glenda gradually relaxes her grip on Paul's hand and her body relaxes. Her respiratory rate slows to 20 breaths per minute. Glenda requires a cesarean birth because her cervix does not dilate to greater than 7 cm, despite adequate contractions.

SUMMARY CONCEPTS

- The purpose of intrapartum fetal assessment is to identify fetal well-being and to identify the fetus who may be having hypoxic stress beyond the ability to compensate for it.
- The two approaches to intrapartum fetal assessment are intermittent auscultation with palpation of uterine activity and electronic fetal monitoring. Each type has advantages and limitations.
- Fetal oxygenation depends on a normal flow of oxygenated maternal blood into the placenta, normal exchange within the placenta, patent umbilical cord vessels, and normal fetal circulatory and oxygen-carrying function.
- Stimulation of the sympathetic nervous system increases the FHR and strengthens the heart contraction. Stimulation of the parasympathetic nervous system slows the heart rate and maintains short-term variability. The parasympathetic nervous system matures later than the sympathetic, beginning about 28 to 32 weeks of gestation.
- An advantage of the fetoscope over Doppler ultrasound devices is that the fetoscope assesses actual fetal heart sounds and thus can identify fetal cardiac dysrhythmias. Doppler devices sense cardiac motion and convert the motion into sound that represents the cardiac activity.
- External electronic fetal monitoring is less accurate for FHR and uterine activity patterns than internal monitoring, but it is noninvasive.
- Greater accuracy is the main advantage of internal electronic fetal monitoring devices.
- Nursing responsibilities related to intrapartum fetal monitoring include promoting fetal oxygenation, identifying and reporting nonreassuring findings, supporting parents, communicating with the physician or nurse-midwife, and documenting all care.

ANSWERS TO CRITICAL THINKING EXERCISE, p. 349

The pattern described is one of late decelerations, probably caused by excess uterine activity secondary to the use of oxytocin. Jackie's initial action should be to stop the oxytocin infusion and increase the rate of Nancy's nonadditive IV fluid. Oxygen should be given through a snug face mask at about 8 to 10 L per minute. Nancy should be placed on her side, if she is not already in this position, to increase placental blood flow. After the immediate corrective actions are completed, Jackie should contact Nancy's physician or nurse-midwife, documenting her interventions and the content of the call.

ANSWERS TO CRITICAL THINKING EXERCISE, p. 353

A change of position may relieve cord compression. These changes include turning from side to side or a hands-and-knees position to release the cord from its entrapped position. Positioning LaShonda with her hips higher than her head may also relieve pressure on the cord. Although the auscultated findings are similar to a variable deceleration, it is not possible to accurately determine this pattern with intermittent auscultation. One option is to apply an external fetal monitor to clarify whether a variable deceleration pattern truly exists or if what was heard was an isolated dip in the rate. Another option is to increase the frequency of auscultation to determine if the decreases in FHR are repetitive or if the decrease was an isolated one.

LaShonda's oxygenation and hydration should be considered as well. Oxygen at 8 to 10 L/min by face mask and increasing the plain IV fluid can correct inadequacies in these areas.

REFERENCES & READINGS

American Academy of Pediatrics & American College of Obstetricians and Gynecologists. (1997). *Guidelines for perinatal care* (4th ed.). Elk Grove Village, IL: Author.

American College of Obstetricians and Gynecologists (ACOG). (1995a). *ACOG technical bulletin,* No. 207. Fetal heart rate patterns: Monitoring, interpretation, & management. Washington, DC: Author.

ACOG. (1995b). *ACOG technical bulletin,* No. 216. Umbilical artery blood acid-base analysis. Washington, DC: Author.

Arikan, G.M., Haeusler, M.C.H., Deutsch, M.T., Greimel, E.R., & Dorfer, M. (1998). Maternal perceptions of labor with fetal monitoring by pulse oximetry in a research setting. *Birth,* 25(3), 182-189.

Bloom, S.L., Swindle, R.G., McIntire, D.D., & Leveno, K.J. (1999). Fetal pulse oximetry: Duration of desaturation and intrapartum outcome. *Obstetrics and Gynecology,* 93, 1036-1040.

Brown, C.E. (1998). Intrapartal tocolysis: An option for acute intrapartal fetal crisis. *Journal of Obstetric, Gynecologic, and Neonatal Nursing,* 28(4), 257-260.

Committee on Obstetric Practice and A.P. Committee on Fetus and Newborn. (1996). ACOG Committee opinion number 174: Use and abuse of the Apgar score. *International Journal of Gynecology and Obstetrics,* 54, 303-305.

Cunningham, F.G., MacDonald, P.C., Gant, N.F., Leveno, K.J., Gilstrap, L.C., Hankins, G.D.V., et al. (1997). *Williams obstetrics* (20th ed.). Norwalk, CT: Appleton & Lange.

Curtin, S.C., & Mathews, T.J. (2000). U.S. Obstetric procedures, 1998. *Birth,* 27(2), 136-138.

Eganhouse, D.J., & Petersen, L.A. (1998). Fetal surveillance in multifetal pregnancy. *Journal of Obstetric, Gynecologic, and Neonatal Nursing,* 27(3), 312-321.

Feinstein, N.F. (2000). Fetal heart rate auscultation: Current and future practice. *Journal of Obstetric, Gynecologic, and Neonatal Nursing,* 29(3), 306-315.

Feinstein, N., & McCartney, P. (Eds.). (1997). *AWHONN'S fetal heart monitoring: Principles and practices.* (2nd ed.). Dubuque, IA: Kendall/Hunt Publishing.

Feinstein, N.F., Sprague, A., & Trépanier, M.J. (2000a). *AWHONN Symposium: Fetal heart rate auscultation.* Washington, DC: Author.

Feinstein, N.F., Sprague, A., & Trépanier, M.J. (2000b). Fetal heart rate auscultation. *AWHONN Lifelines,* 4(3), 35-44.

Folsom, M.S. (1997). Amnioinfusion for meconium: Does it help? *MCN: American Journal of Maternal-Child Nursing,* 22(2), 74-79.

Garite, T.J., Dildy, G.A., McNamara, H., Nageotte, M.P., Boehm, F.H., Dellinger, E.H., Knuppel, R.A., Porreco, R.P., Miller, H.S., Sunderji, S., Varner, M.W., & Swedlow, D.B. (2000). A multicenter controlled trial of fetal pulse oximetry in the intrapartum management of nonreassuring fetal heart rate patterns. *American Journal of Obstetrics and Gynecology,* 183(5), 1049-1058.

Gilstrap, L.C. (1999). Fetal acid-base balance. In R. Creasy & R. Resnik (Eds.), *Maternal-fetal medicine: Principles and practice* (4th ed., pp. 331-340). Philadelphia: W.B. Saunders.

Glantz, J.C., & Woods, J.R. (1999). Significance of amniotic fluid meconium. In R. Creasy & R. Resnik (Eds.), *Maternal-fetal medicine: Principles and practice* (4th ed., pp. 393-403). Philadelphia: W.B. Saunders.

Haggerty, L.A. (1999). Continuous electronic fetal monitoring: Contradictions between practice and research. *Journal of Obstetric, Gynecologic, and Neonatal Nursing, 28*(4), 409-416.

Harvey, C.J. (1997). A look at the new terms: Electronic fetal monitoring update. *AWHONN Lifelines, 1*(6), 49-51.

Helwig, J.T., Parer, J.T., Kilpatrick, S.J., & Laros, R.K. (1996). Umbilical cord blood acid-base state: What is normal? *American Journal of Obstetrics and Gynecology, 174*(6), 1807-1814.

Jackson, D. (2000). Fetal distress in the intrapartum period. In F. Zuspan & E. Quilligan (Eds.), *Current therapy in obstetrics and gynecology, 5* (pp. 398-401). Philadelphia:W.B. Saunders.

McRae, M.J. (1999). Fetal surveillance and monitoring: Legal issues revisited. *Journal of Obstetric, Gynecologic, and Neonatal Nursing, 28*(3), 310-319.

Menihan, C.A. (1996). Intrapartum fetal monitoring. In K.R. Simpson & P.A. Creehan (Eds.), *AWHONN perinatal nursing* (pp. 187-225). Philadelphia: Lippincott.

Miller, F. (2000). Fetal scalp stimulation. In F. Zuspan & E. Quilligan (Eds.), *Current therapy in obstetrics and gynecology, 5* (pp. 404-405). Philadelphia: W.B. Saunders.

Murray, M. (1997). *Antepartal and intrapartal fetal monitoring* (2nd ed.). Albuquerque, NM: Learning Resources International.

National Institute of Child Health and Human Development Research Planning Workshop. (1997). Electronic fetal monitoring: Research guidelines for interpretation. *Journal of Obstetric, Gynecologic, and Neonatal Nursing, 26*(6), 635-640.

Parer, J. (1999). Fetal heart rate. In R. Creasy & R. Resnik (Eds.), *Maternal-fetal medicine: Principles and practice* (4th ed., pp. 270-299). Philadelphia: W.B. Saunders.

Parer, J. (1997). *Handbook of fetal heart rate monitoring* (2nd ed.). Philadelphia: W.B. Saunders.

Pierce, J. (2000). Intrapartum amnioinfusion for meconium-stained fluid: Meta-analysis of prospective clinical trials. *Obstetrics and Gynecology, 95*(6), Part 2, 1051-1056.

Phelan, J.P., & Kim, J.O. (2000). Fetal heart rate observations in the brain-damaged infant. *Seminars in Perinatology, 24*(3), 221-229.

Pschirrer, E.R., & Yeomans, E.R. (2000). Does asphyxia cause cerebral palsy? *Seminars in Perinatology, 24*(3), 215-220.

Rostant, D.M., & Murray, M.L. Fetal heart rate monitoring and interpretation. In D.M. Miller & R.F. Cady (Eds.), *AWHONN's liability issues in perinatal nursing* (pp. 105-117). Philadelphia: Lippincott.

Sandelowski, M. (2000). Retrofitting technology to nursing: The case of electronic fetal monitoring. *Journal of Obstetric, Gynecologic, and Neonatal Nursing, 29*(3), 316-324.

Schmidt, J. (1997). Fluid check: Making the case for intrapartum amnioinfusion. *AWHONN Lifelines, 1*(5), 47-51.

Schmidt, J.V., & McCartney, P.R. (2000). History and development of fetal heart assessment. *Journal of Obstetric, Gynecologic, and Neonatal Nursing, 29*(3), 295-305.

Seelbach-Göbel, B., Heupel, M., Kühnert, M., & Butterwegge, M. (1999). The prediction of fetal acidosis by means of intrapartum fetal pulse oximetry. *American Journal of Obstetrics and Gynecology, 180*, 73-81.

Simpson, K.R. (1998a). Fetal oxygen saturation monitoring during labor. *Journal of Perinatal and Neonatal Nursing, 12*(3), 26-37.

Simpson, K.R. (1998b). Intrapartum fetal oxygen saturation monitoring: Ongoing clinical research explores partnering new method with EFM. *AWHONN Lifelines, 2*(6), 21-24.

Sprague, A., & Trépanier, M.J. (1999). Charting in record time: Setting guidelines for documenting FHR enhances care for laboring women. *AWHONN Lifelines, 3*(5), 25-30.

Supplee, R.B., & Vezeau, T.M. (1996). Continuous electronic fetal monitoring: Does it belong in low-risk births? *MCN: American Journal of Maternal/Child Nursing, 21*(6), 301-306.

15

Pain Management during Childbirth

OBJECTIVES

1. Compare childbirth pain with other types of pain.
2. Describe the way excessive pain can affect the laboring woman and her fetus.
3. Examine how physical and psychological forces interact in the laboring woman's pain experience.
4. Describe use of nonpharmacologic pain management techniques in labor.
5. Describe the way medications may affect a pregnant woman and the fetus or neonate.
6. Identify benefits and risks of specific pharmacologic pain control methods.
7. Explain nursing care related to different types of intrapartum pain management, both nonpharmacologic and pharmacologic.

DEFINITIONS

Agonist Substance causing a physiologic effect.

Analgesic Systemic agent that relieves pain without loss of consciousness.

Anesthesia Loss of sensation, especially to pain, with or without loss of consciousness.

Anesthesiologist Physician who specializes in administration of anesthesia.

Antagonist Drug that blocks the action of another drug or of body secretions.

Aspiration Pneumonitis Chemical injury to the lungs that may occur with regurgitation and aspiration of acidic gastric secretions.

Endorphin Substance similar to opioids, which occurs naturally in the central nervous system and modifies pain sensations; related to enkephalins.

Enkephalin Substance similar to opioids, which occurs naturally in the central nervous system and modifies pain sensations; related to endorphins.

Epidural Space Area outside the dura, between the dura mater and the vertebral canal.

Gate Control Theory A theory about pain based on the premise that a gating mechanism in the dorsal horn of the spinal cord can open or close a "gate" for transmission of pain impulses to the brain.

General Anesthesia Systemic loss of sensation with loss of consciousness.

Motor Block Loss of voluntary movement caused by regional anesthesia.

DEFINITIONS—cont'd

Nurse Anesthetist A registered nurse who has advanced education and certification in administration of anesthetics; also, certified registered nurse anesthetist (CRNA).

Pain Threshold (or Pain Perception) The lowest level of stimulus one perceives as painful; relatively constant under different conditions.

Pain Tolerance Maximum pain one is willing to endure. Pain tolerance may increase or decrease under different conditions.

Regional Anesthesia Anesthesia that blocks pain impulses in a localized area without loss of consciousness.

Sensory Block Loss of sensation caused by regional anesthesia.

Subarachnoid Space Space between the arachnoid mater and the pia mater containing cerebrospinal fluid.

Each woman has unique expectations about birth, including expectations about pain and her ability to manage it. The woman who successfully deals with the pain of labor is more likely to view her experience as a positive life event. A woman's experience with labor pain varies with several physical and psychological elements, and each woman responds differently. Nonpharmacologic and pharmacologic methods offer a selection of pain management techniques from which the laboring woman may choose.

UNIQUE NATURE OF PAIN DURING BIRTH

Pain is a universal experience but is difficult to define. It is an unpleasant sensation of distress resulting from stimulation of sensory nerves. Pain involves two components:

- A physiologic component including reception by sensory nerves and transmission to the central nervous system
- A psychological component, which involves recognizing the sensation, interpreting it as painful, and reacting to the interpretation

Pain is subjective and personal. No one can feel another's pain. Evidence of pain is a person's reaction to it. Childbirth pain, however, differs from other pain in several important respects:

- *It is part of a normal process.* Childbirth pain is part of a normal process, whereas other types of pain are connected with injury or illness. Pain may lead a woman to assume different positions in labor, favoring descent of the fetus through her pelvis.
- *Preparation time exists.* The pregnant woman has several months to prepare for labor, including acquiring skills to help manage pain. Realistic preparation and knowledge about the birth process help her develop skills to cope with labor pain.
- *It is self-limiting.* Labor pain has a foreseeable end. Although it is intense, a woman can expect her labor to end in hours, rather than days, weeks, or months. Other kinds of pain may also be brief, but the baby's birth brings a rapid decrease in pain.
- *Labor pain is not constant but intermittent.* A woman may describe little discomfort with contractions during early labor. Even during late labor, a woman may be relatively comfortable between contractions.
- *Labor ends with the birth of a baby.* The emotional significance of her child's birth cannot be ignored when trying to understand a woman's response to pain. Care about her fetus often motivates a woman to tolerate more pain during labor than she otherwise might be willing to endure.

ADVERSE EFFECTS OF EXCESSIVE PAIN

Although expected during labor, pain that exceeds a woman's tolerance can have harmful effects on her and the fetus.

Physiologic Effects

Excessive pain can heighten a woman's fear and anxiety, which stimulates sympathetic nervous system activity and results in increased secretion of catecholamines (epinephrine and norepinephrine). Catecholamines stimulate alpha and beta receptors, causing effects on the blood vessels and uterine muscles. Epinephrine stimulates both alpha and beta receptors, whereas norepinephrine stimulates primarily alpha receptors.

Stimulation of the alpha receptors causes uterine and generalized vasoconstriction and an increase in the uterine muscle tone. These effects reduce uterine blood flow as they raise the maternal blood pressure.

Stimulation of the beta receptors relaxes the uterine muscle and causes vasodilation. However, uterine vessels are already dilated in pregnancy, so dilation of other maternal vessels allows her blood to pool in them. The pooling of blood reduces the amount of blood available to perfuse the placenta.

The combined effects of excessive catecholamine secretion are therefore the following:

- Reduced blood flow to and from the placenta, restricting fetal oxygen supply and waste removal
- Reduced effectiveness of uterine contractions, slowing labor progress

Labor increases a woman's metabolic rate and her demand for oxygen. Pain and anxiety increase her already high metabolic rate. She breathes fast to obtain more oxygen, exhaling too much carbon dioxide in the process. Significant changes, more than those expected during labor, can occur in the woman's PaO_2 and $PaCO_2$ and in her arterial pH. These maternal respiratory and metabolic changes alter placental exchange. The fetus may have less oxygen available for uptake and have less ability to unload carbon dioxide to the mother. The net result is that the fetus shifts to anaerobic metabolism, with buildup of hydrogen ions (acidosis). This type of acidosis is metabolic and does not resolve as quickly after birth as respiratory acidosis, which results from shorter periods of hypoxia.

Psychological Effects

Poorly relieved pain lessens the pleasure of this extraordinary life event for both partners. The mother may find it difficult to interact with her infant because she is depleted from a painful labor. Unpleasant memories of the birth may affect her response to sexual activity or another labor. Her support person may feel inadequate during birth. The woman's partner may feel helpless and frustrated when her pain is unrelieved.

Check Your Reading

1. How does the pain of childbirth differ from other kinds of pain?
2. How can excessive pain adversely affect a laboring woman and her fetus?

VARIABLES IN CHILDBIRTH PAIN

A variety of physical and psychosocial factors contribute to a woman's pain response during labor. These factors provide possibilities for nursing interventions for pain relief.

Physical Factors

Childbirth pain is of two types—visceral and somatic. Visceral pain is a slow, deep, poorly localized pain that is often described as dull or aching. Visceral pain dominates during first-stage labor as the uterus contracts and the cervix dilates.

Somatic pain is a quick, sharp pain that can be precisely localized. Somatic pain is most prominent during late first-stage labor and during second-stage labor as the descending fetus puts direct pressure on maternal tissues.

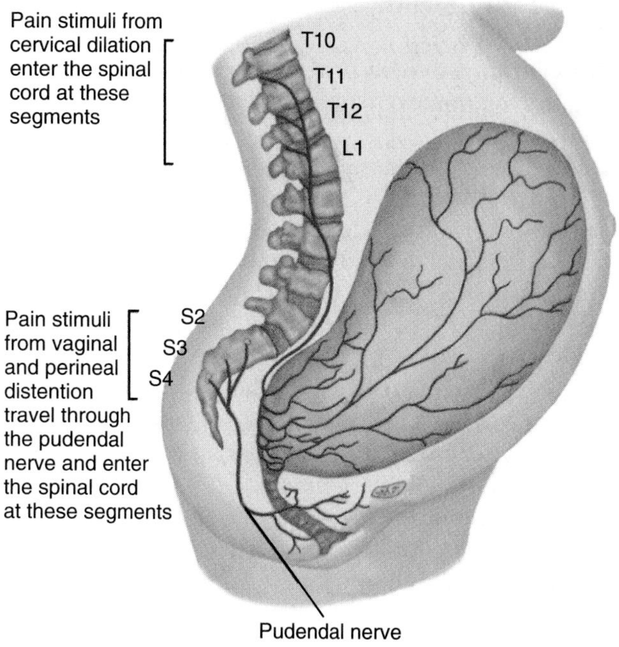

Pain stimuli from cervical dilation enter the spinal cord at these segments
T10
T11
T12
L1
Pain stimuli from vaginal and perineal distention travel through the pudendal nerve and enter the spinal cord at these segments
S2
S3
S4
Pudendal nerve

FIGURE 15-1 Pathways of pain transmission during labor.

Sources of Pain

Four sources of labor pain exist in most labors. Other physical factors may modify labor pain, increasing or decreasing it.

Tissue Ischemia. The blood supply to the uterus decreases during contractions, leading to tissue hypoxia and anaerobic metabolism. Ischemic uterine pain has been likened to ischemic heart pain.

Cervical Dilation. Dilation and stretching of the cervix and lower uterus are a major source of pain. Pain stimuli from cervical dilation travel through the hypogastric plexus, entering the spinal cord at the T10, T11, T12, and L1 levels (Figure 15-1).

Pressure and Pulling on Pelvic Structures. Some pain results from pressure and pulling on pelvic structures, such as ligaments, fallopian tubes, ovaries, bladder, and peritoneum. The pain is a visceral pain; a woman may feel it as referred pain in her back and legs.

Distention of the Vagina and Perineum. Marked distention of the vagina and perineum occurs with fetal descent, especially during the second stage. The woman may describe a sensation of burning, tearing, or splitting (somatic pain). Pain from vaginal and perineal distention and pressure and pulling on adjacent structures enters the spinal cord at the S2, S3, and S4 levels (see Figure 15-1).

Factors Influencing Perception or Tolerance of Pain

Although physiologic processes cause labor pain, a woman's tolerance of pain is affected by other physical influences.

Intensity of Labor. The woman who has a short, intense labor may complain of severe pain because each contraction does so much work (effacement, dilation, and fetal descent). A rapid labor may limit her options for pharmacologic pain relief as well.

Cervical Readiness. If prelabor cervical changes (softening, with some dilation and effacement) are incomplete, the cervix does not open as easily as it does when it is soft and dilation and effacement has begun. More contractions are needed to achieve dilation and effacement, resulting in a longer labor and greater fatigue in the laboring woman.

Fetal Position. Labor is likely to be longer and more uncomfortable when the fetus is in an unfavorable position. An occiput posterior position is a common variant seen in otherwise normal labors. In this position, each contraction pushes the fetal occiput against the woman's sacrum. She experiences intense back discomfort *(back labor)* that persists between contractions. A woman may not be able to deliver her baby until it rotates to the occiput anterior position. The fetal head must therefore rotate a wider arc before the mechanisms of extension and expulsion occur, so labor is often longer (see Figure 12-12). Back pain may decrease dramatically when a fetus rotates into the more favorable position. The rate of labor progress usually increases as well.

Characteristics of the Pelvis. The size and shape of a woman's pelvis influence the course and length of her labor. Abnormalities may cause a difficult and longer labor and may contribute to fetal malpresentation or malposition.

Fatigue and Hunger. Fatigue reduces a woman's ability to tolerate pain and to use coping skills she has learned. She may be unable to focus on techniques that would otherwise help her tolerate labor. An extremely fatigued woman may have an exaggerated response to contractions, or she may be unable to respond to sensations of labor such as the urge to push. Because oral intake is limited, her energy reserves are also likely to be depleted in a long labor.

Many women find that sleep is difficult during the last weeks of pregnancy. A woman's shortness of breath when lying down, frequent urination, and fetal activity interrupt sleep so that she often begins labor with a sleep deficit. If labor begins late in the evening, she may have been awake more than 24 hours by the time she gives birth. Even if a woman begins labor well rested, slow progress may exhaust her.

Intervention of Caregivers. Although they may be appropriate for the well-being of a woman and fetus, some interventions add discomfort to the natural pain of labor.

IV lines cause pain when inserted and remain noticeable to many women during labor. Fetal monitoring equipment is uncomfortable to some women. Both may hamper a woman's mobility, which she might use to assume a more comfortable position.

A woman whose labor is induced or augmented often reports more pain and increased difficulty coping with it because contractions reach peak intensity quickly. Vaginal examinations, amniotomy, and insertion of internal fetal monitoring devices also increase a woman's discomfort briefly because of vaginal and cervical stretching. Vaginal manipulation often stimulates a contraction because of a reflex known as Ferguson's reflex.

Psychosocial Factors

Several psychosocial variables influence a woman's experience of pain.

Culture

A woman's sociocultural roots influence how she perceives, interprets, and responds to pain during childbirth. Some cultures encourage loud and vigorous expression of pain, whereas others value self-control. However, women are individuals within their cultural groups. The experience of pain is personal, and caregivers should not make assumptions about how a woman will behave during labor.

Women should be encouraged to express themselves in any way they find comforting, and the diversity of their expressions must be respected. Accepting a woman's individual response to labor and pain promotes a therapeutic relationship.

CRITICAL THINKING EXERCISE

Truc Pham is a Vietnamese-American in labor with her first baby. Her cervix is dilated 6 cm, effacement is 100%, and the fetus is at a +1 station. Truc's contractions are every 3 minutes, 50 to 60 seconds, and of strong intensity. She smiles at the nurse each time the nurse talks to her but does not talk much herself. Truc stiffens her body during contractions and interacts little with her husband or the nurse at those times.

QUESTIONS:

1. How should the nurse interpret Truc's assessment and behavior?
2. Does the nurse need additional data?
3. What nursing actions are appropriate?

The nurse should avoid praising some behaviors (such as stoicism) while belittling others (such as noisy expression). This restraint is difficult because noisy women are challenging to work with and may disturb others.

The unique nature of childbirth pain and women's diverse responses to it make nursing management complex. The nurse can miss important cues if the woman is either stoic or outspoken about her pain. With either extreme, the nurse may not readily identify critical information such as impending birth or symptoms of a complication.

Anxiety and Fear

Mild or moderate anxiety can enhance attention and learning. However, high anxiety and fear magnify sensitivity to pain and impair a woman's ability to tolerate it. They consume energy she needs to cope with the birth process, including its painful aspects.

Anxiety and fear increase muscle tension, diverting oxygenated blood to the brain and skeletal muscles. Tension in pelvic muscles counters the expulsive forces of uterine contractions and the laboring woman's pushing. Prolonged tension results in general fatigue, increased pain perception, and reduced ability to use skills to cope with pain.

If a previous pregnancy had a poor outcome, such as a stillborn infant or one with abnormalities, a woman is probably more anxious during labor and for a time after birth. She is likely to examine and reexamine her infant to assure herself that this baby is normal.

Previous Experiences with Pain

Early in life a child learns that pain means bodily injury. Consequently, fear and withdrawal are a woman's natural reactions to pain during labor. Learning about the normal sensations of labor, including pain, helps a woman suppress her natural reactions of fear and withdrawal, allowing her body to do the work of birth.

A woman who has given birth previously has a different perspective. If she has had a vaginal delivery, she is probably aware of normal labor sensations and is less likely to associate them with injury or abnormality. Also, time has a way of blunting the memory of painful experiences.

A woman who had a child by cesarean birth and has never experienced labor may be particularly anxious. The experience of cesarean birth is known to her, whereas labor is unknown. A repeat cesarean birth may seem to be the quicker and less painful option. She may have difficulty yielding to the normal forces of birth.

A woman with a previous long and difficult labor is more likely to be anxious about the outcome of the present one. If she had a cesarean birth following the difficult labor, she may doubt her ability to give birth vaginally. Her anxiety often intensifies when she reaches the point at which her prior labor ended with the cesarean birth.

Previous experiences may positively affect a woman's ability to deal with pain. She may have learned ways to cope with pain during other episodes of pain or during other births and use these skills adaptively during labor.

Preparation for Childbirth

Preparation for childbirth does not ensure a pain-free labor. A woman should be prepared for pain realistically, including reasonable expectations about analgesia and anesthesia. She may feel unexpected events during labor may invalidate her childbirth preparation.

Preparation reduces anxiety and fear of the unknown. It allows a woman to rehearse for labor and learn a variety of skills to master pain as labor progresses. She and her partner learn about expected behavioral changes during labor, and their knowledge decreases their anxiety when those changes occur.

Support System

An anxious partner is less able to provide the support and reassurance that the woman needs during labor. In addition, anxiety in others can be contagious, increasing her anxiety. She may assume that if others are worried, something is wrong.

The birth experiences of a woman's family and friends cannot be ignored. Those individuals can be an important source of support if they express realistic information about labor pain and its control. If they describe labor as intolerable, however, she may have needless distress. Hearing that labor is painless is equally detrimental. No two labors are alike, even in the same woman.

Check Your Reading

3. How may physical and psychological factors interact in a woman's labor pain experience?
4. What four sources of pain are present in most labors?
5. How can each of these physical factors influence the pain a woman experiences during childbirth: (a) Labor intensity? (b) Cervical readiness? (c) Fetal position? (d) Maternal pelvis? (e) Fatigue?
6. How do psychosocial factors influence a woman's experience with labor pain?

STANDARDS FOR PAIN MANAGEMENT

The Joint Commission on Accreditation of Healthcare Organizations (JCAHO) has recognized that pain management is an essential part of the care of all clients in health care settings. The organization has added a number of explicit pain management standards to its accreditation manuals and will begin scoring these standards for compliance during accreditation visits in 2001. The JCAHO standards relate to the following:

- The rights of all patients to appropriate assessment, reassessment, management, and follow-up of pain
- Staff competency in pain assessment and management
- Establishment of policies and procedures that support prescribing of appropriate pain medications
- Education of patients and families about effective pain management
- Discharge planning related to pain management

NONPHARMACOLOGIC PAIN MANAGEMENT

The nurse who cares for women in labor and birth can offer many nonpharmacologic and pharmacologic pain management methods. Education about nonpharmacologic pain management is the foundation of prepared childbirth classes. Most women use these methods to complement pharmacologic methods, although some use them as their only pain management techniques.

The intrapartum nurse should know methods that are taught in local childbirth classes to be most helpful to women and their labor partners. Teaching techniques during labor that conflict with what a woman learned and practiced may confuse her. Other techniques can be reserved for use if a woman finds learned techniques ineffective.

Advantages

Nonpharmacologic methods have several advantages over pharmacologic methods if pain control is adequate. They do not slow labor and have no side effects or risk of allergy.

The woman who chooses analgesia needs alternate pain management until it is given, usually after labor is established. Also, some pharmacologic methods may not eliminate labor pain, and a woman needs these techniques to control the pain that remains.

Nonpharmacologic methods may be the only realistic option for a woman who enters the hospital in advanced, rapid labor. Drugs might not have enough time to take effect, and the newborn might have respiratory depression if a systemic opioid reaches its peak action about the time of birth.

Limitations

Nonpharmacologic methods also have limitations, especially as the sole method of pain control. Women do not always achieve their desired level of pain control using these methods alone. Because of the many variables in labor, even a well-prepared and highly motivated woman may have a difficult labor and need analgesia or anesthesia.

Gate Control Theory

A discussion of nonpharmacologic pain management techniques would not be complete without discussing the gate control theory of pain. According to this theory, transmission of nerve impulses is controlled by a neural mechanism in the dorsal horn of the spinal cord that acts like a gate to control impulses transmitted to the brain. Transmission is affected by stimulation of large- or small-diameter sensory nerve fibers and descending impulses from the brain. This mechanism opens or closes the "gate" to pain sensation by allowing or preventing some impulses from reaching the brain, where they are recognized as pain.

Pain is transmitted through small-diameter sensory nerve fibers. Stimulation of large-diameter fibers in the skin blocks conduction of pain through small-diameter fibers, thus "closing the gate" and decreasing the amount of pain felt. Examples of this stimulation would be tactile stimulation such as massage, thermal stimulation, or hydrotherapy.

Impulses from the brain have a similar ability to impede transmission through the dorsal horn using visual and auditory stimulation techniques. Examples of visual or auditory stimulation include use of a focal point or breathing techniques.

Memory and cognitive processes affect the perception of stimuli as painful. Education and support during labor are used to increase the woman's relaxation, confidence, and feeling of control. Although these methods may not completely prevent pain, they may decrease the severity of perceived pain (Creehan, 1996).

Preparation for Pain Management

The ideal time to prepare for nonpharmacologic pain control is before labor. During the last few weeks of pregnancy, the woman learns about labor, including its painful aspects, in childbirth classes. She can prepare to confront the pain, learning a variety of skills to use during labor. Her support person learns specific methods to encourage and support her. After admission, the nurse can review and reinforce what the partners learned in class.

The nurse can teach the unprepared woman and her support person nonpharmacologic techniques. The latent phase of labor is the best time for intrapartum teaching because the woman is usually anxious enough to be attentive and interested, yet comfortable enough to understand. The nurse must usually teach one contraction at a time during late labor because the woman's focus is very narrow.

No one method or combination of methods helps every woman. Most methods may become less effective (habituation) after prolonged use, and changing tech-

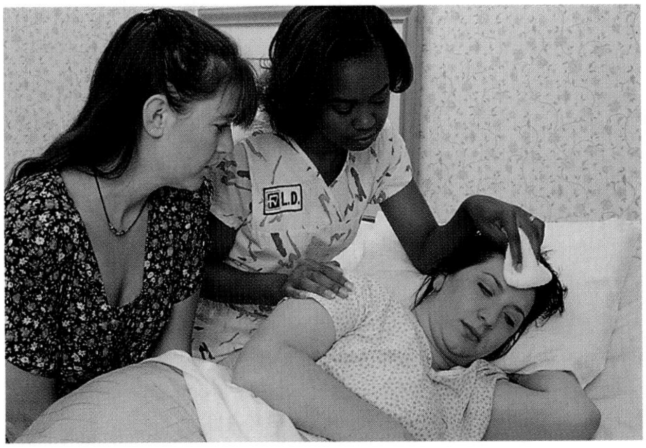

FIGURE 15-2 General comfort measures such as the nurse's reassuring presence or a cool cloth to the face supplement other methods of nonpharmacologic and pharmacologic pain control.

niques counters this problem. Knowing a variety of methods gives the nurse a selection.

Application of Nonpharmacologic Techniques

Techniques that can be applied during labor include relaxation, cutaneous stimulation, hydrotherapy, mental stimulation, and breathing techniques (see Chapter 13).

Relaxation

Promoting relaxation is a basis for all other methods, both nonpharmacologic and pharmacologic, because it does the following:

- Promotes uterine blood flow, improving fetal oxygenation
- Promotes efficient uterine contractions
- Reduces tension that increases pain perception and decreases pain tolerance
- Reduces tension that can inhibit fetal descent

Environmental Comfort. Comfortable surroundings support relaxation. The nurse can reduce irritants such as bright lights and uncomfortable temperature and change soiled underpads.

Music masks outside noise and provides a background for use of imagery and breathing techniques. This distraction shifts the woman's attention from pain perception. Television has a similar effect for some women.

General Comfort. Promoting the woman's personal comfort helps her focus on using pain management techniques during labor (Figure 15-2). This includes actions to increase comfort and reduce the effect of irritants.

Reducing Anxiety and Fear. The nurse may reduce a woman's anxiety and increase her self-control by providing accurate information and focusing on birth as a normal process. Simple nursing actions keep the focus on the normality of childbirth. For example, calling the woman by her name rather than calling her a "patient" (meaning "sick") helps her to see birth as a normal process. Empowering the woman by giving her choices whenever possible helps her to see herself as competent and capable of giving birth.

Implementing Specific Relaxation Techniques. Many techniques discussed in Chapter 11 are most successful if practiced before labor. However, during labor, caregivers can watch a woman for signs of tension and help her focus on relaxing tense muscles. Her partner often recognizes subtle signs of tension and can be guided to massage the area or call attention to the tension, thus helping the laboring woman to release it. Pillows provide support for extremities so that they are positioned for minimal tension.

Cutaneous Stimulation

Cutaneous stimulation has several variations that are often combined with each other or with other techniques.

Self-Massage. The woman may rub her abdomen, legs, or back during labor (effleurage) to counteract discomfort. Some women find abdominal touch irritating, especially near the umbilicus. Women in labor may find firm stroking more helpful than light stroking (see Figure 11-6).

Some women benefit from firm palm or sole stimulation during labor. They may like someone to rub their palms vigorously or to independently rub their hands or feet together or bang their palms on, or grip, a cool surface. They may hold another's hand tightly during a contraction. The nurse should determine if these actions indicate excess pain or if they are a woman's way of countering pain and therefore useful.

Massage by Others. Massage increases circulation and reduces muscle tension. The support person or nurse can rub the woman's back, shoulders, legs, or any area where she finds massage helpful. Body powder on the skin reduces friction during massage. Powder should be kept away from the nose and mouth of the newborn.

Counterpressure. Sacral pressure may help when the woman has back pain, usually most intense when her fetus is in an occiput posterior position. Sacral pressure may be applied, using the palm of the hand, the fist or fists, or a firm object such as two tennis balls in a sock (Figure 15-3). A variation of sacral pressure is a double hip squeeze, in which the palms are placed on the woman's hips and pressed down and inward toward

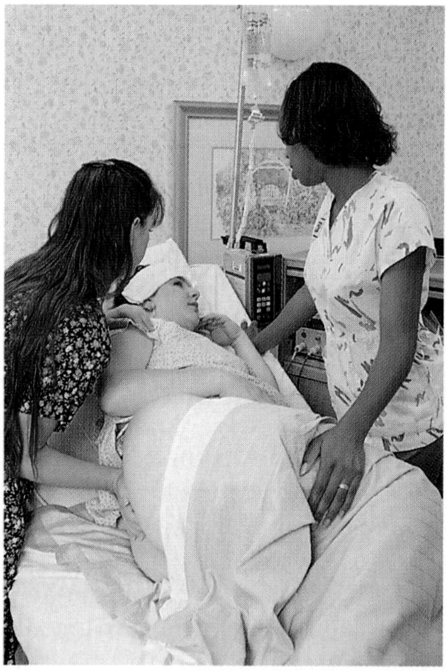

FIGURE 15-3 The coach applies sacral pressure to counter back pain common during labor.

the symphysis (Simkin & Frederick, 2000). When using pressure, the woman should guide the support person as to the exact location and amount of pressure.

Touch. Nonclinical touch by the nurse is a powerful tool if the woman does not object to it. Holding her hand, stroking her hair, or similar actions convey caring, comfort, affirmation, and reassurance at this vulnerable time.

Thermal Stimulation. Many women appreciate warmth to their back, abdomen, or perineum during labor. Warmth increases local blood flow, relaxes muscles, and raises the pain threshold. Massage is often more comfortable to a tense woman after her skin is warmed (Simkin & Frederick, 2000). Caution must be used when placing warm compresses over areas with reduced sensation (such as those affected by epidural block) to avoid burning the skin.

Laboring women often feel hot when the room is cool. Damp washcloths provide comforting coolness. She may put them on her head, throat, abdomen, or any place she wants. She also may want to put them in her mouth to relieve dryness. Ice chips cool the mouth and provide hydration.

Hydrotherapy

A shower, tub bath, or whirlpool bath is relaxing and provides thermal stimulation. Several studies have shown benefits of water therapy during labor, including immersion in a tub or whirlpool (jet hydrotherapy, or jacuzzi). The major concern about immersion therapy has been newborn and postpartum maternal infections caused by microorganisms in the water. The organisms may be from ascending vaginal organisms or organisms from previous births if the tub has not been cleaned properly between births. However, several studies have not found a significant association between newborn or postpartum maternal infections and use of immersion hydrotherapy with proper cleaning (Kabler, 2000; Teschendorf & Evans, 2000). More research is needed to clarify both the benefits and the concerns about hydrotherapy (Table 15-1). Facility policies should be written to outline specific guidelines based on most recent evidence for use of hydrotherapy.

Mental Stimulation

Mental techniques occupy the woman's mind and compete with pain stimuli. They also aid relaxation by providing a tranquil imaginary atmosphere.

Imagery. If the woman has not practiced a specific imagery technique, the nurse can help her create a relaxing mental scene. Most women find images of warmth, softness, security, and total relaxation most comforting.

Imagery can help the woman dissociate herself from the painful aspects of labor. For example, the nurse can help her visualize the work of labor: the cervix opening with each contraction or the fetus moving down toward the outlet each time she pushes. This technique is like visualizing success or movement toward a goal with each contraction. The nurse can help the woman visualize being in a pleasant and relaxing place.

Focal Point. When using nonpharmacologic techniques, a woman may prefer to close her eyes or may want to concentrate on an external focal point. She may bring a picture of a relaxing scene or an object to use as a focal point and to aid in the use of imagery. She can use any point in her room as a focal point.

Check Your Reading

7. How does the gate control theory of pain relate to nonpharmacologic methods of pain control?
8. What are some nursing actions to encourage relaxation during labor?
9. How can the nurse reduce a laboring woman's anxiety or fear?
10. How might each of these cutaneous stimulation techniques be used to aid relaxation during labor: Self-massage? Massage by others? Counterpressure? Warmth or cold?
11. Why are these cautions needed related when hydrotherapy is used during labor: Adequate maternal hydration? Control of water temperature?

Table 15-1
BENEFITS AND CAUTIONS RELATED TO HYDROTHERAPY DURING LABOR

BENEFITS Promotes relaxation; reduces muscle spasms and cramps Reduces stress resulting in catecholamine secretion Promotes a sense of well-being Reduces pain by increasing pain threshold Reduces pressure of abdominal muscles on uterus, reducing pain Upright position favors fetal descent Buoyancy allows greater freedom of movement Nipple stimulation promotes oxytocin stimulation from the posterior pituitary Reduces blood pressure by causing diuresis **CAUTIONS** Hydrotherapy may slow labor if used during the latent phase but is useful if the woman needs rest and relaxation. During active labor, nipple stimulation from whirlpool bubbles or shower spray causes natural oxytocin secretion that can stimulate contractions. If contractions become hypertonic, remove nipples from the stimulating water.	Water temperature should be maintained between 95° and 100° F (35° to 37.8° C) to avoid maternal hyperthermia or hypothermia, each of which could increase her metabolic rate, reducing fetal oxygen supply and increasing glucose demand. The woman should have generous hydration to prevent dehydration from the diuresis that occurs with water immersion. A nurse or support person should remain with the woman while she is in the tub. Underwater birth may not be planned in the facility, but labor could proceed rapidly with relaxation and pain relief. If birth occurs, bring the infant immediately, but gently, to the surface. Cut the cord outside the water. Have a shower chair available to the woman if she uses a shower. Clean tubs with hospital-approved germicide between uses, including circulating through whirlpool jets and filters. Culture equipment periodically.

From Kabler, J. (2000). Water immersion during labor and birth. In *Childbirth education: Practice, research, and theory* (2nd ed., pp. 284-294). Philadelphia: W.B. Saunders; and Teschendorf, M.E., & Evans, C.P. (2000). Hydrotherapy during labor: An example of developing a practice policy. *MCN: American Journal of Maternal/Child Nursing,* 25(4), 198-203.

Breathing Techniques

Breathing techniques give a woman a different focus during contractions, interfering with pain sensory transmission (Figure 15-4). They begin with simple patterns and progress to more complex as greater distraction is needed. No universal right time exists to change patterns during labor. However, complex patterns are fatiguing to use for a long time.

For best results, the woman and her partner must practice the techniques frequently. If patterns are too complicated or if the woman has not practiced, they may not be helpful during labor. Breathing techniques should be used only when needed, usually when the woman can no longer walk or talk during a contraction. The woman should not change from a simpler technique to the next, more complex, technique until necessary so that use of the most complex techniques is limited to the shortest time possible.

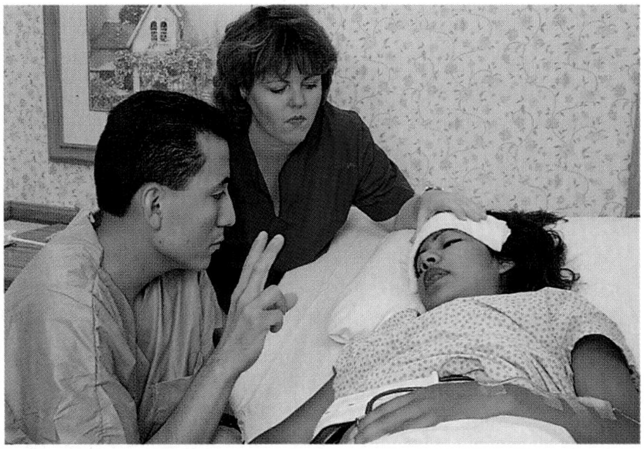

FIGURE 15-4 A woman and her partner who are prepared for labor have learned a variety of skills to master pain as labor progresses. The coach uses hand signals to tell the woman how to change her pattern of paced breathing.

First-Stage Breathing

Breathing in the first stage of labor consists of a cleansing breath and progressively more complex techniques of paced breathing.

Taking a Cleansing Breath. Each contraction begins and ends with a deep inspiration and expiration known as the cleansing breath. Like a sigh, a cleansing breath helps the woman release tension. It provides oxygen to help reduce myometrial hypoxia, one cause of pain in labor. The cleansing breath also helps the woman clear her mind to focus on relaxing and signals her labor partner that the contraction is beginning or ending. The woman may inhale through the nose and exhale through the mouth or take her cleansing breath in any way comfortable for her. When electronic monitors are used, a partner may help ease the discomfort of rapid contractions by watching for the rise in the lower part of the strip that signals the beginning of the contraction and tell the woman to take a cleansing breath.

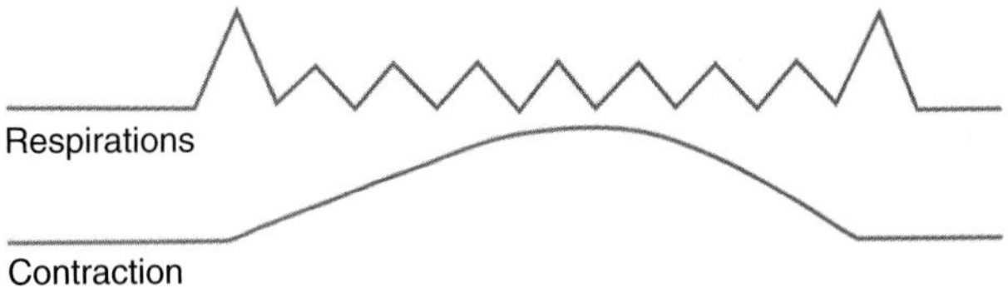

FIGURE 15-5 Slow-paced breathing. Although a specific rate may or may not be used, slow-paced breathing should be *no slower than half* the woman's usual respiratory rate to ensure adequate oxygenation. This pace is generally about six to nine breaths per minute.

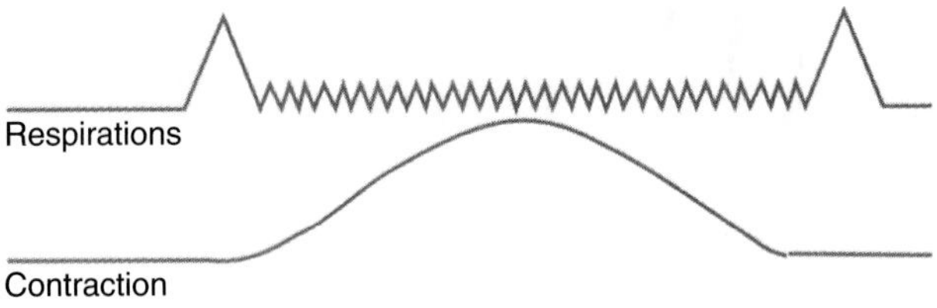

FIGURE 15-6 Modified-paced breathing. The pattern for modified-paced breathing should be comfortable to the woman and *no faster than twice* her normal respiratory rate to prevent hyperventilation or interference with relaxation.

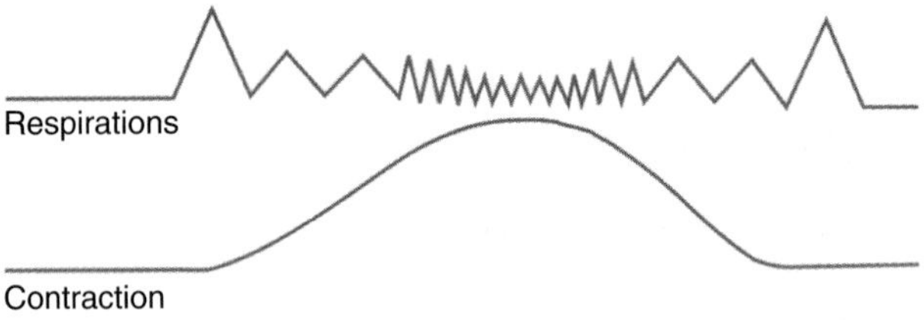

FIGURE 15-7 Combining techniques. Slow and modified-paced breathing can be combined by using the slower breathing at the beginning and end of the contraction and the more rapid breathing over the peak of the contraction.

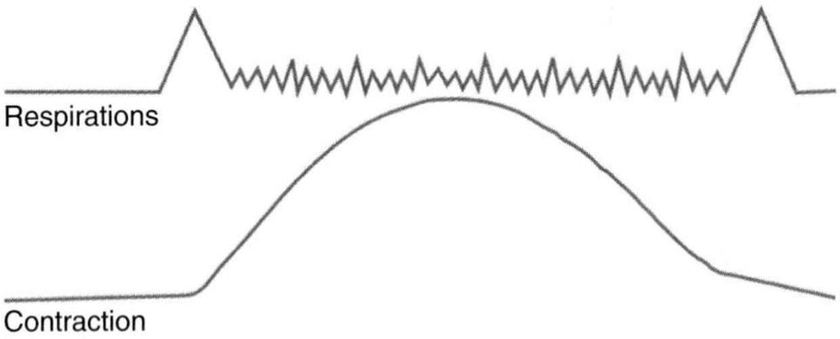

FIGURE 15-8 Patterned-paced breathing. Patterned-paced breathing adds a slight emphasis or "blow" on the exhalation in a pattern. The diagram shows the emphasis after every third inhalation.

Slow-Paced Breathing. The first breathing is slow-paced breathing, a slow, deep breathing that increases relaxation (Figure 15-5). The woman should concentrate on relaxing her body rather than on regulating the rate of her breathing. Relaxation naturally brings about slower breathing, similar to that during sleep. She can use nose, mouth, or a combination, depending on which is most comfortable.

Slow-paced breathing should be used as long as possible during labor because it promotes relaxation and oxygenation. Labor nurses often teach the technique to women who enter labor unprepared. It is easy to learn between contractions and, with the support of the nurse, helps even a frightened woman become calm and able to work with her contractions.

As with all techniques, variety prevents habituation. Adding other pain-relief approaches such as effleurage may help prolong the effectiveness of slow-paced breathing. Using another type of breathing for a short time may allow the woman to return to slower breathing again later.

Modified-Paced Breathing. When slow-paced breathing is no longer effective, the woman begins modified-paced breathing (Figure 15-6). This chest breathing at a faster rate matches the natural tendency to use more rapid breathing during stress or physical work, such as labor. Although modified-paced breathing is more shallow than slow-paced breathing, the faster rate allows oxygen intake to remain about the same. As with slow-paced breathing, the focus is on release of tension rather than on the actual number of breaths taken.

Women sometimes learn to combine slow and modified-paced breathing during a contraction (Figure 15-7). They begin slowly and use shallow, faster breathing over the peak of the contraction. During labor, women often do this naturally. The most important concern is that the breathing not interfere with relaxation but enhance it.

Patterned-Paced Breathing. Patterned-paced breathing (sometimes called *pant blow breathing*) involves focusing on the pattern of breathing (Figure 15-8). It is similar to modified-paced breathing. After a certain number of breaths, however, the woman exhales with a slight emphasis or blow and then begins the modified-paced breathing again. This addition causes her to focus more on her breathing and reduces habituation. The mouth should remain relaxed, and the woman should not try to make specific sounds that would tighten her vocal cords. Relaxation of her entire body is the goal.

The number of breaths before the blow may remain constant (usually between two and six) or may change in a pattern. Variations include a set pattern such as "3-1, 5-1, 3-1" or a decreasing, "stair-step," pattern such as "6-1, 5-1, 4-1, 3-1." Some couples use a random pattern determined by the coach, who uses hand signals to show the number of breaths the woman should take before each blow. The coach holds up fingers to show the total breaths to be taken or a single finger for each breath. Use of the random pattern, however, may be ineffective without sufficient practice to enable the two to work together well.

Breathing to Prevent Pushing. If a woman pushes strenuously before the cervix is completely dilated, she risks injury to the cervix and the fetal head. Blowing prevents closure of the glottis and breath holding, helping to overcome the urge to push strenuously. The woman blows repeatedly using short puffs when the urge to push is strong. The support person may learn to blow along with her to help the woman concentrate. Some women vary the blowing by using one short breath and one blow.

Overcoming Common Problems. Hyperventilation and mouth dryness are common when breathing techniques are used. Hyperventilation is due to rapid deep breathing that causes excessive loss of carbon dioxide, resulting in respiratory alkalosis. The woman may feel dizzy or lightheaded and have impaired thinking. Vasoconstriction leads to tingling and numbness in fingers and lips. If hyperventilation continues, tetany resulting from decreased calcium in tissues and blood may result in stiffness of the face and lips and carpopedal spasm.

Women are taught to blow into a paper bag or their own cupped hands if they begin to feel dizzy. This kind of blowing increases the carbon dioxide levels by having the woman rebreathe her exhaled air. The woman should slow her rate of breathing to reduce the loss of carbon dioxide.

The woman's mouth becomes dry with prolonged mouth breathing. To avoid dryness, she can place her tongue gently against the roof of her mouth to moisturize entering air. The support person can offer ice, mouthwash, sugarless suckers, or liquids if they are allowed.

Second-Stage Breathing

Many women find some relief when they begin pushing during the second stage (see Chapter 13). Some professionals promote vigorous pushing as soon as the woman's cervix is completely dilated. In this technique, the woman uses closed-glottis pushing (Valsalva's maneuver) usually for as long as she can hold her breath, which raises intrathoracic pressure and reduces her cardiac output and blood pressure. Over time, this type of pushing is fatiguing for the mother and can reduce fetal oxygenation.

A more physiologic pushing method is to wait for the woman's spontaneous urge to push or for fetal descent to a +1 to +2 station if epidural analgesia reduces her sensation of this urge. If pushing in response to her own sensations, the woman usually pushes in short bursts initially, as the fetal head exerts pressure on her perineal tissues. As the fetus descends and pressure increases, her pushes become longer, about 4 to 6 seconds each, and she may make groaning or guttural sounds, as if lifting a heavy weight. If the woman cannot feel the urge to push even with fetal descent, the nurse may have to direct her pushing and should try to mimic this physiologic process. Points to remember about physiologic pushing are as follows (AWHONN, 2000):

- Push with an open glottis, about 4 to 6 seconds at a time
- Avoid prolonged breath-holding longer than 6 to 8 seconds
- Avoid more than four pushing efforts per contraction

Check Your Reading

12. Why is it important to avoid advancing to more complex breathing techniques sooner than needed?
13. What is the purpose of a cleansing breath?

PHARMACOLOGIC PAIN MANAGEMENT

Most laboring women want pharmacologic pain relief, even if they use nonpharmacologic methods. Pharmacologic methods for pain management include systemic drugs, regional pain management techniques, and general anesthesia.

Special Considerations for Medicating a Pregnant Woman

Medicating a woman when she is pregnant is not as simple as before pregnancy, for the following reasons:

- Any drug taken by the woman is likely to affect her fetus.
- Drugs may have effects in pregnancy that they do not have in the nonpregnant person.
- Drugs can affect the course and length of labor.
- Pregnancy complications may limit the choice of pharmacologic pain management methods.
- Women who require other therapeutic drugs, use herbal or botanical preparations, or who practice substance abuse may have fewer safe choices for pain relief.

Effects on the Fetus

Effects on the fetus of drugs given to the mother may be direct, resulting from passage of the drug or its metabolites across the placenta to the fetus. An example of a direct effect on the fetus is decreased fetal heart rate (FHR) variability following administration of an analgesic to the woman.

Effects on the fetus may be indirect, or secondary to drug effects in the mother. For example, if a drug causes maternal hypotension, blood flow to the placenta is reduced. Fetal hypoxia and acidosis may result.

Maternal Physiologic Alterations

Normal pregnancy changes in four body systems have the greatest implications for pharmacologic pain management methods.

Cardiovascular Changes. Compression of the aorta and inferior vena cava by the uterus can occur when a woman lies in the supine position (aortocaval compression). If the woman must be in the supine position temporarily, the uterus is displaced to one side with the hands or with a small wedge or towel roll under one hip. Displacement is often to the left (left uterine displacement, or LUD).

Respiratory Changes. A pregnant woman's full uterus reduces her respiratory capacity. To compensate, she breathes more rapidly and deeply. As a result, she is more vulnerable to reduced arterial oxygenation during induction of general anesthesia and is more sensitive to inhalational anesthetic agents. The normal edema of pregnancy is also present in her upper airways and may present difficulty if she must be intubated for general anesthesia.

Gastrointestinal Changes. A pregnant woman's stomach is displaced upward by her large uterus and has a higher internal pressure. Progesterone slows peristalsis and reduces the tone of the sphincter at the junction of the stomach and esophagus. These changes make a pregnant woman vulnerable to regurgitation and aspiration of gastric contents during general anesthesia.

Nervous System Changes. During pregnancy and labor, circulating levels of endorphins and enkephalins, natural substances with analgesic properties, are high. These substances modify pain perception and reduce requirements for analgesia and anesthesia.

The epidural and subarachnoid spaces are smaller during pregnancy, enhancing the spread of anesthetic agents used for epidural or subarachnoid blocks. Cerebrospinal fluid (CSF) pressure is higher during a contraction and when the woman is pushing. Nerve fibers are more sensitive to local anesthetic agents. High intraabdominal pressure causes engorgement of the epidural veins, increasing the risk for intravascular injection of anesthetic agents. The net result of these changes is that a reduced volume of local anesthetic is needed to achieve satisfactory epidural or subarachnoid block.

Effects on the Course of Labor

Ideally, analgesics are given when labor is well established to avoid slowing progress. However, caregivers must consider the adverse effects of excessive pain on labor progress, regardless of the cervical dilation. Regional analgesia, primarily the epidural block, can slow progress during the second stage by impairing the laboring woman's natural urge to push.

Effects of Complications

Complications during pregnancy may limit the choices of analgesia or anesthesia. For example, infusion of large volumes of IV fluids is done to prevent hypotension with regional analgesia and anesthesia. If a pregnant woman has heart disease, this fluid load could be detrimental. Yet without it, she is vulnerable to hypotension.

Interactions with Other Substances

A woman who ingests drugs (therapeutic, over-the-counter, or illicit), herbal or botanical preparations, or other substances may have fewer options because of interactions between these substances and analgesics or anesthetics. For example, recent alcohol use increases the depressant effects of opioid analgesics, making both the mother and newborn susceptible to respiratory depression.

Check Your Reading

14. How can drugs taken by the expectant mother affect the fetus?
15. How do changes in these maternal body systems affect pharmacologic pain management: (a) Cardiovascular? (b) Respiratory? (c) Gastrointestinal? (d) Nervous system?
16. Why is it important to know about a woman's intake of drugs, botanical medicines, legal substances (such as alcohol), and illegal drugs?

Systemic Drugs for Labor

Systemic drugs have effects on multiple systems because they are distributed throughout the body. These intrapartum drugs include opioid analgesics and adjunctive drugs. Although general anesthesia is also systemic, it is discussed separately because it is used only at birth and causes loss of consciousness.

Parenteral Analgesia

Opioid analgesics are the most common parenteral medications given to reduce perception of pain without loss of consciousness. Analgesics that may be used for labor are meperidine (Demerol), fentanyl (Sublimaze), butorphanol (Stadol) (Drug Guide), and nalbuphine (Nubain) (Table 15-2).

Meperidine and fentanyl are pure opioid agonists, but butorphanol and nalbuphine have mixed opioid agonist and antagonist effects. A women who is dependent on

DRUG GUIDE: BUTORPHANOL (STADOL)

Classification: Opioid analgesic

Action: Opioid analgesic with some agonist-antagonist effects; exact mechanism of action unknown; produces respiratory depression that does not increase markedly with larger doses

Indications: Systemic pain relief during labor

Dosage and Route: Intravenous: 1 mg every 3 to 4 hours; range 0.5 to 2 mg; may be given undiluted

Absorption: Onset of analgesia almost immediate with IV administration, peaks about 30 minutes, and lasts about 3 hours; faster onset and shorter duration of action than meperidine or morphine

Excretion: Excreted in urine; crosses placental barrier; secreted in breast milk

Contraindications and Precautions: Contraindicated in persons who are hypersensitive; not used in opiate-dependent persons because antagonist activity of the drug may cause withdrawal symptoms in the woman or newborn; cautiously used during birth of preterm infant; drug actions potentiated (enhanced) by barbiturates, phenothiazines, cimetidine, and other tranquilizers

Adverse Reactions: Respiratory depression or apnea (woman or newborn), anaphylaxis; dizziness, lightheadedness, sedation, lethargy, headache, euphoria, mental clouding, fainting, restlessness, excitement, tremors, delirium, insomnia; nausea, vomiting, constipation, increased biliary pressure, dry mouth, anorexia; flushing, altered heart rate and blood pressure, circulatory collapse; urinary retention; sensitivity to cold

Nursing Considerations: Assess for allergies and opiate dependence. Observe vital signs and respiratory function in woman (12 per minute or more) and newborn (30 per minute or more). Have naloxone and resuscitation equipment available for respiratory depression in woman and neonate. Report nausea or vomiting to the birth attendant for a possible order for an antiemetic. Antiemetics or other central nervous system depressants may enhance the respiratory depressant effects of butorphanol.

Table 15-2
DRUGS COMMONLY USED FOR INTRAPARTUM PAIN MANAGEMENT

Drug/Dose	Comments
OPIOID ANALGESICS	
Meperidine (Demerol) 12.5-50 mg every 2-4 hr IV; may also be given by PCA	Respiratory depression (primarily in the neonate) is the main side effect.
Fentanyl (Sublimaze) 50-100 mcg; may be repeated every hour; may also be given PCA	Onset is quick (5 min for IV administration). Less nausea, vomiting, and respiratory depression occurs than with meperidine.
Adjunct to epidural analgesia during labor (dose individualized)	Epidural use may cause pruritus.
Butorphanol (Stadol) 1 mg every 3-4 hr; range 0.5-2 mg IV; may also be given by PCA	Has some narcotic antagonist effects; should not be given to the opiate-dependent woman (may precipitate withdrawal) or after other narcotics such as meperidine (may reverse their analgesic effects); also a respiratory depressant.
Nalbuphine (Nubain) 10 mg every 3-6 hr IV; may also be given by PCA	Same as butorphanol.
ADJUNCTIVE DRUGS	
Promethazine (Phenergan) 12.5-25 mg every 4-6 hr IV	Duration of action is longer than most narcotics; enhances respiratory depressant effects of narcotics.
Diphenhydramine (Benadryl) 10-50 mg every 4-6 hr IV	Given to relieve pruritus from epidural narcotics.
Hydroxyzine (Atarax, Vistaril) 25-100 mg IM Z-track only	See promethazine.
NARCOTIC ANTAGONISTS	
Naloxone (Narcan) Adult: 0.4-2 mg IV	Action shorter than most narcotics it reverses; must observe for recurrent respiratory depression and be prepared to give additional doses.
To reverse pruritus from epidural opioids: 0.04-0.2 mg IV or IV infusion 5-10 mcg/kg/hr	Will reduce some analgesic effect when given for pruritus.
Neonate: 0.1 mg/kg IV (umbilical vein) or intratracheal	Neonatal resuscitation dose.
Naltrexone (Trexan): 3-6 mg p.o. × 1 dose	Long-acting drug to relieve pruritus from epidural narcotics (investigational when used for this purpose). Will reduce some analgesic effect when given for pruritus.

IV, Intravenously; *p.o.,* orally; *IM,* intramuscularly.

opiates (such as heroin) should avoid agonist-antagonist drugs, because they may cause withdrawal effects in her and the newborn. They should not be given if the woman has already received a pure opioid, because some analgesic effect of the first drug will be reversed. Agonist-antagonist drugs have a "ceiling effect" on the amount of analgesia they provide and are unsuitable for the increasing pain of the entire labor for many women (Britt & Pasero, 1999).

Although commonly used in labor because of its rapid onset, meperidine has a number of undesirable effects. These effects include CNS irritability such as twitching, jerking, restlessness, tremors, shakiness, and delirium (Pasero, Portenoy, & McCaffery, 1999). If these occur, her birth attendant should be notified for a change in pain relief method.

The primary side effect of opioids is respiratory depression, which is more likely to affect the newborn. Timing of administration is important to reduce neonatal respiratory depression. An infant who is born at the peak of the drug's action is more likely to have respiratory depression than if born earlier or later. Meperidine's metabolite, normeperidine, is active for a long time in the newborn and can cause delayed respiratory depression.

Opioid analgesics are given in small, frequent doses by the IV route during labor to provide a rapid onset of analgesia and a predictable duration of action. A woman benefits from rapid pain control, with less likelihood of neonatal respiratory depression. Starting the injection at the beginning of the contraction, when blood flow to the placenta is normally reduced, limits transfer to the fetus. When placental blood flow resumes, much of the drug is in maternal tissues. The drugs also may be delivered by patient-controlled analgesia (PCA) pump.

Opioid Antagonists

Naloxone (Narcan) reverses opioid-induced respiratory depression. Naloxone does not reverse respiratory depression from other causes, such as barbiturates, anesthetics, nonopioid drugs, or pathologic conditions. Naloxone has a shorter duration of action than most of the opioids it reverses and respiratory depression may recur. In an opiate-dependent woman or newborn, naloxone can induce withdrawal symptoms. Naloxone is used with other measures as needed to support cardiopulmonary function (see Chapter 30).

Naloxone is most often given to the neonate. The recommended neonatal route for administration is IV or intratracheal. The neonatal resuscitation dose is 0.1 mg/kg by the IV or intratracheal route (American Academy of Pediatrics & American College of Obstetricians and Gynecologists, 1997). IV naloxone is given to the neonate through the umbilical vein. The adult dose is 0.4 to 2 mg.

Small doses of naloxone may be given to relieve the pruritus occurring with intrathecal or epidural narcotics. Naltrexone (Trexan), another opioid antagonist, and diphenhydramine (Benadryl), an antihistamine, may also be given for relief of pruritus.

Adjunctive Drugs

Adjunctive drugs during the intrapartum period include those with antiemetic and tranquilizing effects and sedatives. These drugs are given to reduce nausea and anxiety and to promote rest (see Table 15-2).

Promethazine (Phenergan) relieves nausea and vomiting, which may occur when opioid drugs are given. Promethazine may be given by either the intramuscular or IV route. Promethazine does not potentiate the opioid's analgesic effects but can add to the opioid's respiratory depressant effects.

Hydroxyzine (Atarax, Vistaril) is also an antihistamine with antiemetic effects. Parenteral hydroxyzine can be given only into a large muscle with a deep Z-track technique. *Hydroxyzine is not given by the IV route.*

Sedatives

Sedatives such as barbiturates are not routinely given because they have prolonged depressant effects on the neonate. However, a small dose of a short-acting barbiturate may be given to promote rest if a woman is fatigued from false labor or a prolonged latent phase.

Check Your Reading

17. What is the primary adverse effect of opioid administration? How can this effect be reduced?
18. What should the nurse watch for after birth in the infant who received naloxone?

Regional Pain Management Techniques

Regional pain control methods may be used for intrapartum analgesia, anesthesia, or both. These methods provide pain relief without loss of consciousness. Depending on the specific technique, it may be used for only labor or the birth, or both labor and birth.

Epidural block provides pain control during much of labor and for the birth itself. Intrathecal opioids are used for pain control during labor; additional measures are needed during late labor and for the birth. Regional anesthetics that are used only during the birth include the local, pudendal, and subarachnoid blocks.

The major advantage of regional pain management methods is that the woman can participate in birth yet have good pain control. The woman usually feels some pressure and discomfort, although these sensations are greatly reduced. She does not lose her protective airway reflexes, as can happen with general anesthesia. Disadvantages depend on the specific technique. The ef-

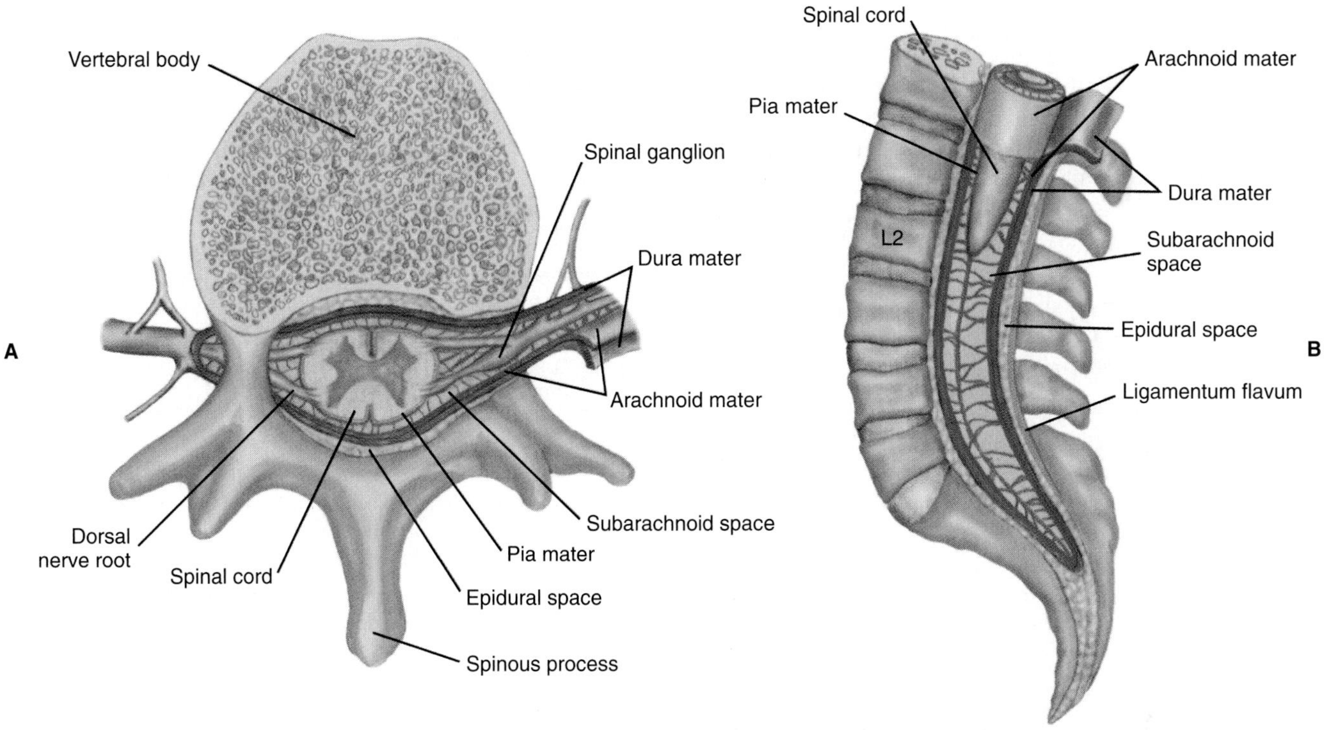

FIGURE 15-9 **A,** Cross section of spinal cord, meninges, and protective vertebra. The dura and arachnoid lie close together. The pia mater is the innermost of the meninges and covers the brain and spinal cord. The subarachnoid space is between the arachnoid and pia mater. **B,** Sagittal section of spinal cord, meninges, and vertebrae. The epidural and subarachnoid spaces are illustrated. Note that the spinal cord ends at the L2 vertebra.

fects on the fetus depend primarily on how the woman responds rather than on direct drug effects.

Epidural Block

The lumbar epidural block is a popular regional block that provides analgesia and anesthesia for labor and birth without sedation of the woman and fetus. It is used for both vaginal and cesarean births. Epidural blocks are started and maintained by an anesthesiologist or nurse-anesthetist. The obstetrician may do this, but this is becoming less common.

The epidural space is outside the dura mater, between the dura and the spinal canal. It is loosely filled with fat, connective tissue, and epidural veins that are dilated during pregnancy (Figure 15-9).

An epidural block is done by injecting local anesthetic agent, usually combined with an opioid, into the tiny epidural space. It provides substantial relief of pain from contractions and birth canal distention. The level of the epidural block can be extended upward to provide anesthesia for a cesarean birth or tubal ligation after birth. Analgesia, rather than full anesthesia that results in complete loss of movement and sensation, is preferred for labor. Therefore lower concentrations of the anesthetic agent and an epidural opioid will provide adequate pain relief without complete motor block for most women. Higher concentrations of the anesthetic agent used for abdominal surgery result in greater loss of both motor and sensory functions.

Technique. The exact time to begin an epidural block is individualized. It is started just before a scheduled cesarean birth. For labor, the best time to start the block is when the woman is in active labor to avoid slowing progress. A number of ways to customize the epidural block for different pain management exist, however. If she is in early labor and needs pain relief, the woman may be given parenteral opioids until her labor is more active. Or she may be given an epidural opioid via the epidural catheter, with the local anesthetic agent added later, when her labor becomes more active. In this way, she obtains pain relief and relaxation in early labor with less likelihood of slowing labor progress resulting from the epidural.

The epidural space is entered at about the L3-L4 interspace (below the end of the spinal cord), and a catheter is passed through the needle into the epidural space (Figure 15-10). The catheter allows continuous infusion or intermittent injection of medication to maintain pain relief during labor and vaginal or cesarean birth. The infusion of epidural medication may also be regulated by a patient-controlled epidural analgesia (PCEA) pump.

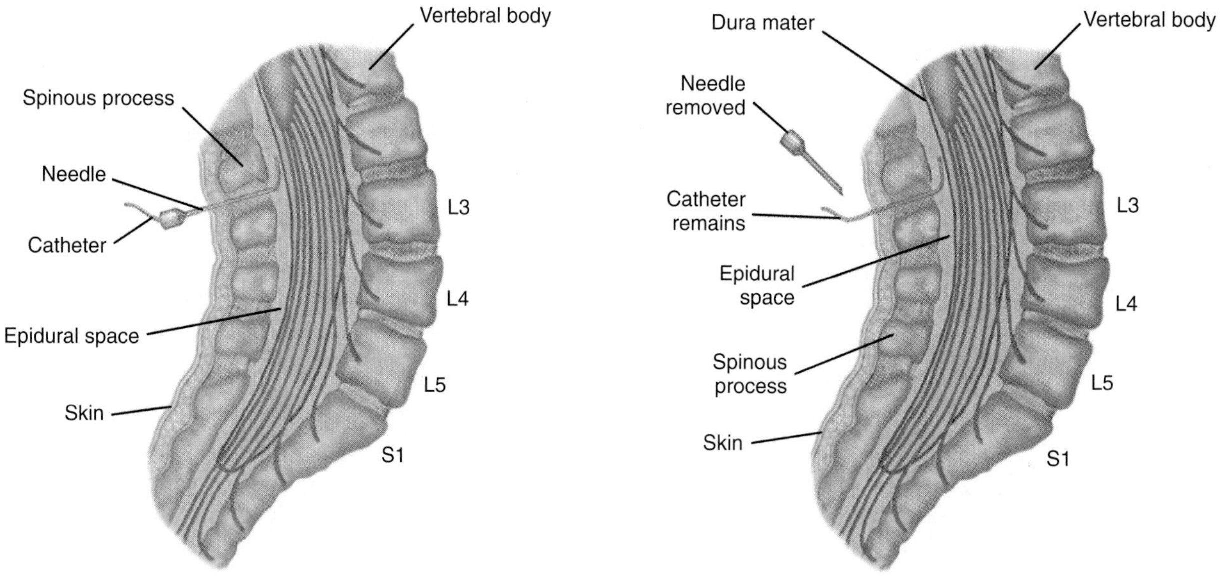

The epidural space is entered with a needle below where the spinal cord ends. A fine catheter is threaded through the needle.

After the catheter is threaded into the epidural space, the needle is removed. Medication can then be injected into the epidural space intermittently or by continuous infusion for pain relief during labor and birth.

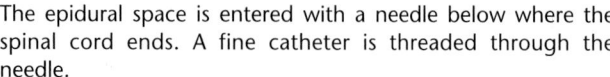

FIGURE 15-10 Technique for epidural block.

Epidural block requires a larger volume of anesthetic agent than the subarachnoid block because it is outside the meninges. A test dose is given to determine if the epidural catheter has inadvertently punctured a blood vessel or the dura before giving the full epidural dose. Several regimens for test doses have been proposed, but one is to give 7.5 mg bupivacaine with 15 mcg of epinephrine through the epidural catheter. If the catheter is in the subarachnoid space instead of the epidural space, the woman experiences rapid, intense motor and sensory block. Numbness of the tongue and lips, lightheadedness, dizziness, and tinnitus may occur with intravascular injection. Epinephrine in the test dose produces tachycardia if injected intravascularly, although the tachycardia can have other causes, such as pain.

Epidural opioids used during labor include fentanyl (Sublimaze), sufentanyl (Sufenta), and morphine (Duramorph, Astramorph). *All drugs injected into the epidural or subarachnoid spaces must be preservative free.* The combination of local anesthetic and epidural opioid provides quicker and longer-lasting pain relief for labor with a lower total dose of local anesthetic and less motor block.

A single dose of a long-acting epidural analgesic such as morphine (Duramorph, Astramorph) is often given after cesarean birth before removing the epidural catheter to provide long-acting pain relief with a low dose of opiate. The mother is comfortable enough to interact with her infant and family. She may require no added analgesics for almost 24 hours, or oral ones may be sufficient.

For vaginal birth, the anesthetized area is usually from the T10 to the S5 level (Cunningham, et al., 1997). For cesarean birth, a higher block is needed, up to T4 to T6 (Zuspan, 2000a).

Dural Puncture. Because the tough dura and the fragile weblike arachnoid membranes lie close together, dural puncture also punctures the arachnoid. If the dura is unintentionally punctured with the needle used to introduce the epidural catheter, leakage of CSF can occur, which may result in a postdural puncture ("spinal") headache (see p. 381). Dural puncture and headache also can occur without obvious CSF leakage.

Contraindications and Precautions. Epidural block is not suitable for all laboring women and some refuse the block. Contraindications include coagulation defects, uncorrected hypovolemia, an infection in the area of insertion or a severe systemic infection, allergy, or a fetal condition that demands immediate birth.

Adverse Effects of Epidural Block. Epidural block has several adverse effects. The causes of some possible adverse effects have not been conclusively determined.

Maternal Hypotension. Sympathetic nerves are blocked along with pain nerves, which may result in vasodilation and hypotension. Before the epidural, expanding the woman's blood volume by infusing 500 to 1000 ml of warmed IV solution such as lactated Ringer's solution offsets vasodilation by filling her vascular system. If hypotension occurs, additional fluids are infused. IV ephedrine in 5- to 10-mg increments may be required to cause vasoconstriction and raise her blood pressure.

Bladder Distention. A woman's bladder fills quickly because of the large quantity of IV solution, yet her sensation to void is reduced. Bladder distention may cause pain that remains after initiation of the block.

Prolonged Second Stage. The urge to push may be less intense than if a woman does not have an epidural block, particularly if she has an intense motor block. The pelvic muscles may be relaxed, which can interfere with the mechanism of internal rotation (see Figure 12-12). These factors increase the chance of forceps- and vacuum extractor-assisted births.

Catheter Migration. After accurate placement, the catheter may move. A woman may then have symptoms of intravascular injection, an intense block or one that is too high, absence of anesthesia, or a unilateral block. The anesthesia professional should be notified of any question about catheter placement.

Cesarean Births. Results of research have been mixed on whether epidural analgesia is associated with an increase in cesarean births. Reasons for cesarean birth are often complex and interrelated. For example, abnormal labor may result in a cesarean birth but also cause more severe pain that requires epidural block.

Maternal Fever. For reasons that are not totally clear, fever after epidural analgesia during labor is common. The fever associated with epidural analgesia is not usually caused by infection but may be due to the reduced hyperventilation and decreased heat dissipation, such as reduced sweating, that occur when the woman's pain is relieved. Also, women who are having prolonged labors may be more likely to have epidural block analgesia. However, maternal fever increases the fetal temperature and the fetal demand for oxygen, which can lead to fetal hypoxia and acidosis.

Fever is also a marker for infection. To avoid needless administration of antibiotics and sepsis evaluations in the newborn, other indicators for infection should be identified as well, such as the amniotic fluid for a cloudy or yellow color and a foul or strong odor and for fetal tachycardia. One study found that a maternal temperature of more than 101° F (38.3° C) was associated with the need for infant resuscitation at birth and 1-minute Apgar scores less than 7 (Lieberman, et al., 2000).

Adverse Effects of Epidural Opioids. Adverse effects associated with epidural opioids may include nausea and vomiting, pruritus, and delayed maternal respiratory depression.

Nausea and Vomiting. Adjunctive drugs such as promethazine (Phenergan) reduce nausea and vomiting that can occur with epidural opioids.

Pruritus. Itching of the face and neck is an annoying side effect that may occur with epidural opioids. Although she may not specifically complain of itching, a woman may rub or scratch her face and neck. Diphenhydramine (Benadryl), naloxone (Narcan), or naltrexone (Trexan) may relieve pruritus (see Table 15-2). Naloxone or naltrexone will also reduce some analgesic effect.

Delayed Respiratory Depression. The possibility of late respiratory depression exists for up to 24 hours after the administration of an epidural opioid, depending on the duration of action of the drug used.

Nursing Care. The nurse's role is to identify maternal or fetal risk factors that may impact the choice of pain relief method, assist the woman while the anesthesia clinician performs the block, and monitor the woman for signs of complications after the block is initiated (see Application of the Nursing Process). Additional care relates to the effects of the epidural on labor.

Facility protocols and the maternal-fetal risk status should guide the frequency of maternal vital signs and fetal assessments. Pulse oximetry is commonly used to check maternal blood oxygenation. If an epidural opioid is given after a cesarean birth, maternal respiratory monitoring may continue for up to 24 hours after birth, depending on the duration of action for the opioid given.

If she does not have an indwelling catheter, the woman's bladder must be assessed frequently because of the large IV fluid load and her reduced sensation to void. She should be observed for persistent pain, which may indicate a full bladder. The nurse should observe for signs associated with catheter migration from the epidural space and for adverse effects, such as nausea and vomiting and pruritus. The woman may need help to push if she cannot feel the urge to push and the fetus has descended to a +1 to +2 station.

Intrathecal Opioid Analgesics

Intrathecal injection of an opioid analgesic provides another option for pain management without sedation. The drug is injected into the subarachnoid space, where it binds to opiate receptors, allowing much smaller doses than would be adequate if given systemically. The woman can feel her contractions but not the pain they would otherwise cause.

Advantages of intrathecal analgesics include the following:

- Rapid onset of pain relief without sedation
- No motor block, enabling the woman to ambulate during labor
- No sympathetic block, with its hypotensive effects

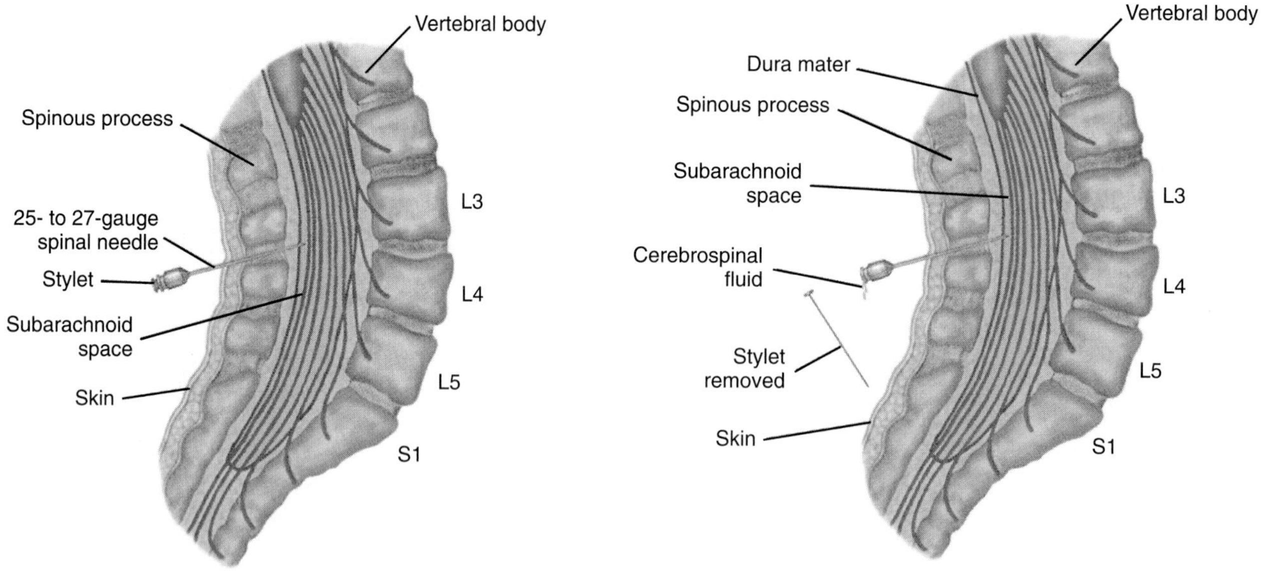

A 25- to 27-gauge spinal needle with a stylet occluding its lumen is passed into the subarachnoid space below where the spinal cord ends.

The stylet is removed, and one or more drops of clear cerebrospinal fluid at needle hub confirm correct needle placement. Medication is then injected, and the needle is removed.

FIGURE 15-11 Technique for subarachnoid block.

Disadvantages may include the following:

- Limited duration of action, possibly requiring another procedure for continued pain relief
- Inadequate pain relief for late labor and the birth, requiring added measures to manage pain at that time

Use of intrathecal opioids may also be combined with epidural block in a combined spinal-epidural (CSE). The woman would receive the intrathecal opioids for early pain relief, with placement of an epidural catheter at that time. She would later receive an epidural drug combination as described previously. This method is somewhat controversial, because it has the potential of allowing epidural medications to enter the dural puncture site (Paull, 2000).

Technique. The subarachnoid space is entered with a spinal needle, as in the subarachnoid block. A preservative-free opioid analgesic is then injected.

The drug chosen depends on the expected duration of labor at the time it is given. Drugs that may be used by this route include fentanyl, sufentanyl, and morphine. Fentanyl and sufentanyl have a rapid onset of action and last up to 3 hours. Morphine has a slightly longer onset but lasts longer.

Adverse Effects of Intrathecal Opioids. As with epidural opioids, nausea, vomiting, and pruritus may occur. Delayed maternal respiratory depression may occur, depending on the drug used.

Nursing Care. Vital signs and fetal heart rate are taken at the usual intervals for the woman's stage of labor. Side effects, such as nausea and vomiting or pruritus, are reported and managed similarly to those occurring with the epidural block. Reduced effectiveness suggests that the drug's duration of action is ending or that the woman is in late labor. Other pain management methods may be needed for the remainder of labor and for birth.

Subarachnoid (Spinal) Block

A subarachnoid block (SAB) is a simpler procedure than the epidural block and may be done when a quick cesarean birth is necessary and an epidural catheter is not in place. It is similar to local infiltration and pudendal block. SAB is performed just before birth, providing no pain relief during most of labor.

The physician or nurse-anesthetist injects local anesthetic into the subarachnoid space in a single dose. The woman loses both sensory and motor function below the level of the subarachnoid block, with complete relief of pain from contractions.

Technique. A 25- to 27-gauge spinal needle is placed in the subarachnoid space. Appearance of CSF at the needle hub assures correct placement, and the local anesthetic is injected (Figure 15-11).

The level of anesthesia for both epidural and subarachnoid blocks is determined by the volume, concentration, and density of the drug (Figure 15-12).

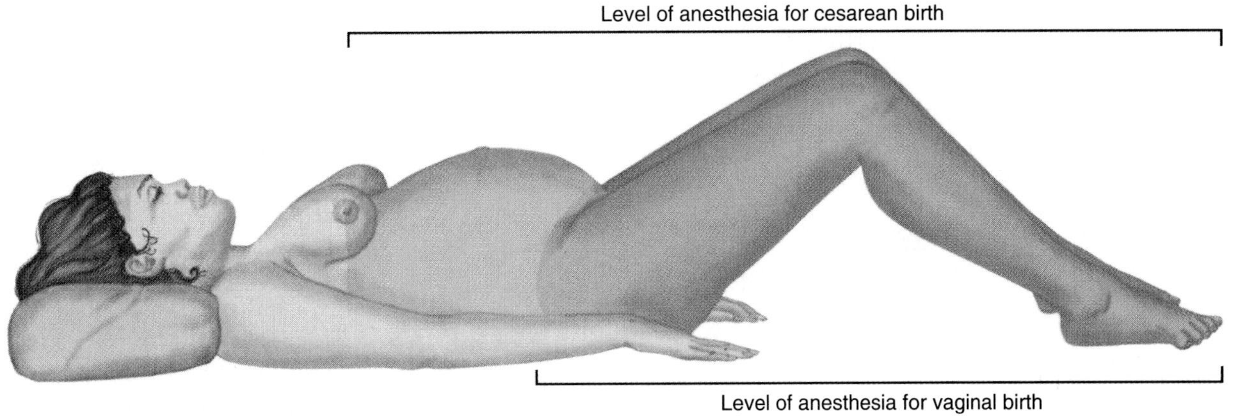

FIGURE 15-12 Levels of anesthesia for epidural and subarachnoid blocks. A level of T10 through S5 is adequate for vaginal birth. A higher level to T4 to T6 is needed for cesarean birth.

Contraindications and Precautions. Contraindications and precautions are similar to those for epidural block: the woman's refusal, coagulation defects, uncorrected hypovolemia, infection in the area of insertion, systemic infection, and allergy. Subarachnoid block can be done more quickly than an epidural block if prompt birth is necessary.

Adverse Effects. Three adverse effects of a subarachnoid block are maternal hypotension, bladder distention, and postdural puncture headache. Hypotension is more likely with the subarachnoid block than with the epidural block and is treated the same.

Postdural Puncture Headache. Postdural puncture headache may occur after subarachnoid block in some women because of CSF leakage at the site of dural puncture. A spinal headache is postural. It is worse when a woman is upright and may disappear when she is lying flat. Headache is less likely if a small-gauge needle is used.

Bedrest with oral or IV hydration helps relieve the postdural puncture headache. A blood patch often gives dramatic, definitive relief. The blood patch is done by injecting 10 to 15 ml of the woman's blood (obtained with sterile technique) into the epidural space. The blood forms a gelatinous seal over the hole in the dura, stopping spinal fluid leakage (Figure 15-13). The blood patch can be repeated if needed. Epidural injection of sterile saline also has had some success.

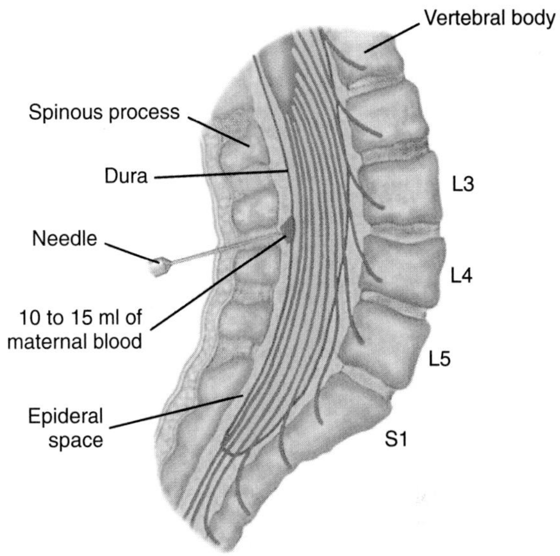

FIGURE 15-13 Blood patch for relief of spinal headache. 10 to 15 ml of the woman's blood is injected into the epidural space to seal a dural puncture.

Local Infiltration Anesthesia

Infiltration of the perineum with a local anesthetic is done by the physician or nurse-midwife just before performing an episiotomy or suturing a laceration (Figure 15-14). Local infiltration does not alter pain from uterine contractions or distention of the vagina. The local agent provides anesthesia in the immediate area of the episiotomy or laceration. A short delay occurs between anesthetic injection and onset of numbness, and the drug burns before its anesthetic action begins. Local infiltration rarely has adverse effects on either mother or infant.

Pudendal Block

A pudendal block anesthetizes the lower vagina and part of the perineum to provide anesthesia for an episiotomy and vaginal birth, using low forceps if needed. A pudendal block does not block pain from uterine contractions, and the mother feels pressure.

The physician or nurse-midwife injects the pudendal nerves near each ischial spine with about 10 ml of local anesthetic (Figure 15-15). The perineum is infiltrated with local anesthetic because the pudendal block does not fully anesthetize this area. As in local infiltration, a delay occurs between injection and onset of numbness.

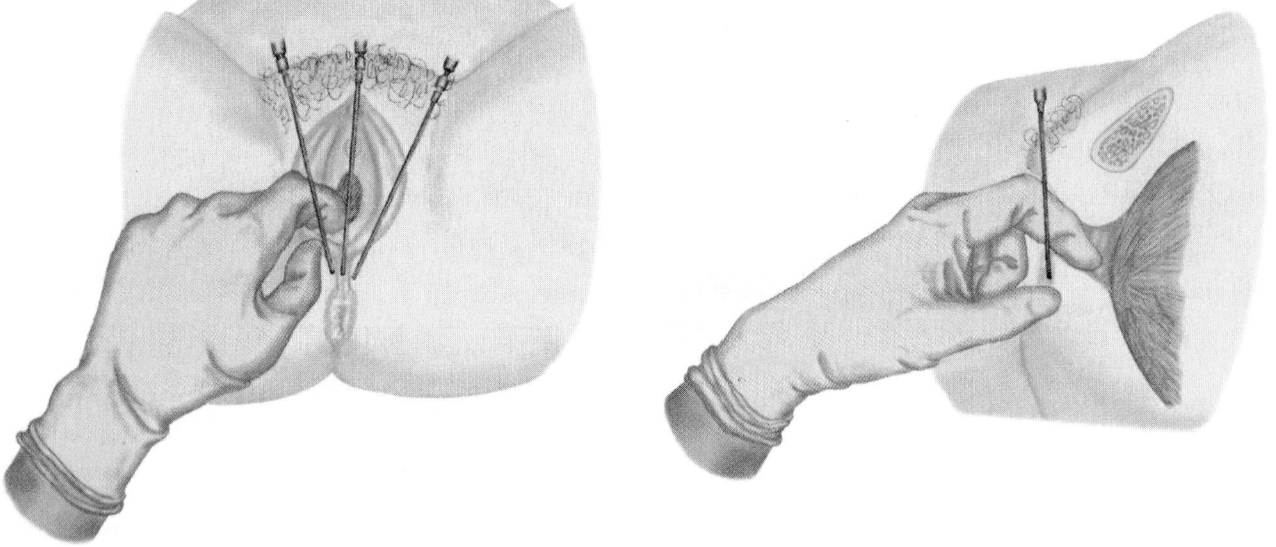

FIGURE 15-14 Local infiltration anesthesia numbs the perineum just before birth for an episiotomy or after birth for suturing of a laceration. The birth attendant protects the fetal head by placing a finger inside the vagina while injecting the perineum in a fan-like pattern.

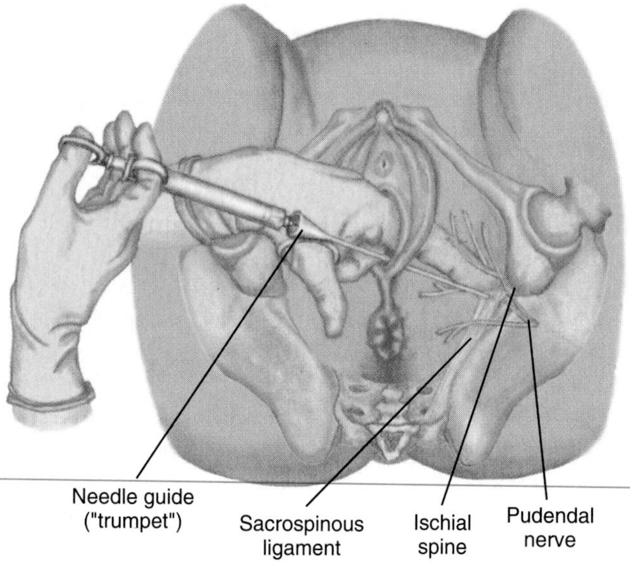

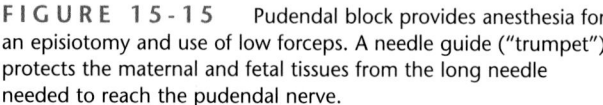

FIGURE 15-15 Pudendal block provides anesthesia for an episiotomy and use of low forceps. A needle guide ("trumpet") protects the maternal and fetal tissues from the long needle needed to reach the pudendal nerve.

Possible maternal complications include a toxic reaction to the anesthetic, rectal puncture, hematoma, and sciatic nerve block. If maternal toxicity is avoided, the fetus is usually not affected.

General Anesthesia

General anesthesia is systemic pain control that involves loss of consciousness. It is rarely used for vaginal births, but it still has a place in cesarean birth. Some women either refuse or are not good candidates for epidural or subarachnoid block for cesarean or their blocks failed. In other cases, a cesarean birth may be necessary so quickly that no time is available to establish either type of regional block. Any laboring woman may need general anesthesia unexpectedly and quickly.

Technique. Before induction of anesthesia, a woman breathes oxygen for 3 to 5 minutes, or at least four deep breaths, to increase her oxygen stores and those of her fetus for the short period of apnea during rapid anesthesia induction. The woman has a wedge under her right side (or the operating table is tilted toward her left

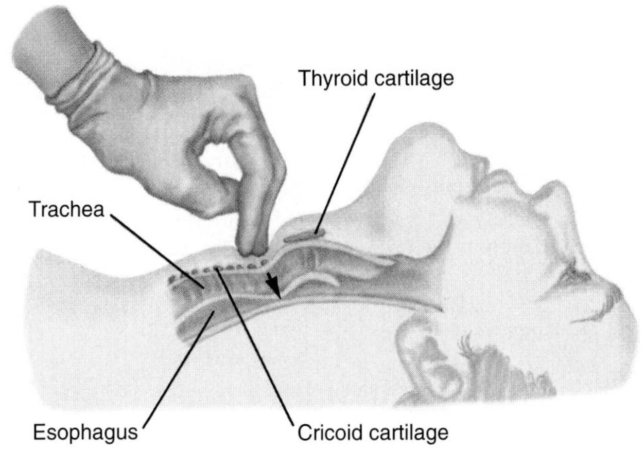

FIGURE 15-16 Sellick's maneuver to prevent vomitus from entering the woman's trachea while she is being intubated for general anesthesia. An assistant applies pressure to the cricoid cartilage to obstruct the esophagus. Once the woman is successfully intubated with a cuffed endotracheal tube, gastric secretions cannot enter the trachea.

side) to reduce aortocaval compression and increase placental blood flow.

Adverse Effects. Major adverse effects are possible with the use of general anesthesia.

Maternal Aspiration of Gastric Contents. Regurgitation with aspiration of acidic gastric contents is a potentially fatal complication of general anesthesia. Aspiration of food particles may result in airway obstruction. Aspiration of acidic secretions results in a chemical injury to the airways—aspiration pneumonitis. Infection often occurs after the initial lung injury.

Respiratory Depression. Respiratory depression may occur in either the mother or the infant but is more likely in the baby. This is more likely to occur if the interval between induction of anesthesia and cord clamping is long.

Uterine Relaxation. Some inhalational anesthetics may cause uterine relaxation. This characteristic is desirable for some complications, such as replacing an inverted uterus (see p. 768). However, postpartum hemorrhage may occur if the uterus relaxes after birth.

Methods to Minimize Adverse Effects. Measures to reduce the risk of maternal aspiration or to limit lung injury if aspiration occurs include the following:

- Restricting intake to clear fluids or nothing by mouth if surgery is anticipated
- Administering a clear non-particulate antacid, such as sodium citrate (Bicitra, Alka-Seltzer Gold)
- Administering an H_2-receptor antagonist, such as ranitidine (Zantac), cimetidine (Tagamet), or famotidine (Pepcid), to increase the gastric pH
- Administering drugs to reduce secretions, such as glycopyrrolate (Robinul) or omeprazole (Prilosec)
- Administering drugs to speed gastric emptying, such as metoclopramide (Reglan)
- Use of cricoid pressure (Sellick's maneuver) to block the esophagus by pressing the rigid trachea against it (Figure 15-16)

Neonatal respiratory depression may be prevented by doing the following:

- Reducing the time from induction of anesthesia until the umbilical cord is clamped
- Keeping the anesthesia level as light as possible until the cord is clamped

To reduce the time from induction of anesthesia to cord clamping, the woman is prepared and draped and the physicians are ready before anesthesia is begun. The anesthesia is kept light until the infant is born and the woman may move slightly on the table, although she usually has no memory of the experience. The anesthesia level is deepened as soon as the cord is clamped.

Check Your Reading

19. What are two major advantages of using regional pain management techniques during childbirth?
20. What is the major adverse effect of the epidural or subarachnoid block? How can the fetus be affected? How may this effect be reduced?
21. What are common side effects of epidural or intrathecal opioid analgesics, and how are these managed?
22. What are the major adverse effects of general anesthesia? What measures reduce the risks?

APPLICATION OF THE NURSING PROCESS: PAIN MANAGEMENT

Nursing care related to pain management should be combined with support for normal labor and any complications that arise. Care of the fetus remains important (see Chapter 14). Two problems that affect many women are pain and care related to epidural analgesia (Nursing Care Plan 15-1).

NURSING CARE PLAN 15-1

Intrapartum Pain Management

Assessment: Beth Anderson is a 28-year-old primigravida who was admitted 1 hour ago in early labor. Beth is 3 cm dilated and 100% effaced, and the fetal station is −2. Her membranes are intact. Contractions are every 3 minutes, last 40 to 50 seconds, and are of moderate intensity. The fetal heart rate averages 135 to 145 beats per minute and has no abnormal patterns on the monitor. Although relatively comfortable when admitted, Beth is becoming more uncomfortable because of back pain. Beth and her husband, Sam, are using breathing techniques they learned in childbirth class.

Nursing Diagnosis: Pain related to effects of uterine contractions and pressure on pelvic structures.

Goals/Expected Outcomes:
During labor, Beth will do the following:
1. Continue to use techniques she learned in prepared childbirth classes.
2. Have a relaxed facial and body posture between contractions.

Critical Thinking: At this time, what methods for pain management are most appropriate to suggest, nonpharmacologic or pharmacologic?

Answer: If no one has already done so, the nurse should explore Beth's preferences for pain relief with her before labor becomes more intense. Nonpharmacologic methods are ideal in early labor if they provide adequate pain management. Walking or other upright positions often ease back discomfort and aid fetal descent. However, Beth's ability to use these would be less if she receives some pharmacologic methods of pain control, such as systemic analgesics. Her labor pattern is normal, membranes are intact, and the fetal heart rate is stable and within normal limits, so walking is not contraindicated.

Intervention	Rationale
1. Adjust the environment for comfort: a. Adjust room thermostat. b. Add warm blankets and socks for warmth. c. Offer small electric fan or hand fan if Beth is hot.	1. A comfortable environment is conducive to relaxation. Relaxation underlies all other interventions because it increases a woman's ability to use her coping skills to tolerate discomfort.
2. Reduce unwanted distractions: a. Reduced outside noise. b. Offer music of Beth's choice to mask noise and promote relaxation. c. Do not stand in front of her focal point. d. Try to delay assessments and interventions until after a contraction is over.	2. Unwanted distractions interfere with use of the skills for pain management Beth and Sam learned and practiced in prepared childbirth classes. Distractions interfere with focused relaxation.
3. Reduce irritating stimulants. a. Keep sheets and underpads dry. b. Dim lights as Beth desires. Use bright lights only when necessary. c. Do all procedures and nursing interventions as gently as possible. d. Avoid bumping the bed.	3. Irritating stimulants reduce ability to relax and add to discomfort.
4. Check for bladder distention hourly, and encourage Beth to void at least every 2 hours. With an order, catheterize her if her bladder is full and she cannot void.	4. The sensation to void may be decreased during labor. A full bladder contributes to overall discomfort and may impede fetal descent and prolong labor.
5. If permitted, give Beth small amounts of clear fluids such as ice chips. If oral intake is prohibited, moisten her mouth with a damp washcloth or have her rinse her mouth with water.	5. Women often use mouth breathing during labor, resulting in a dry mouth. These methods may relieve discomfort of a dry mouth. Clear liquids limit the risk of aspiration if general anesthesia is needed.
6. Assist Beth and Sam with use of the breathing techniques they learned in their prepared childbirth class, breathing with Beth during a contraction if she is having a problem using the technique. Help her change techniques if one is not working well.	6. This refreshes the couple's skills and increases their effectiveness. Breathing through a contraction with Beth makes her focus on the technique as she uses it. If one technique becomes ineffective, another breathing technique may be more effective.

7. Offer a back rub or firm, constant sacral pressure. Ask Beth where and how firm pressure should be. Use baby powder when providing massage. Instruct her to tell caregivers if this technique becomes uncomfortable or if the location on her back needs to be changed. If Sam is rubbing her back, offer to relieve him occasionally and encourage him to take a break.	7. Back rubs or sacral counterpressure may reduce discomfort associated with back labor by stimulating large-diameter fibers and interfering with transmission of the pain impulse to the brain. As labor continues, back rubs may become less effective or even uncomfortable. Powder reduces friction, which could be another source of discomfort. The support person needs a break to conserve energy and better help the woman in later labor.
8. Keep Beth and Sam informed about the progress of labor and their baby's condition.	8. This reduces anxiety and fear of the unknown. Anxiety and fear increase pain perception and reduce pain tolerance.

Evaluation: Beth uses her breathing techniques with each contraction but says she can relax between contractions. About 2 hours later she begins to have greater difficulty coping with labor. Interventions are revised to include those for pharmacologic pain management.

Assessment: Four hours after admission, Beth's cervix is 4 cm dilated and 100% effaced, and the fetal station is −1. Membranes have ruptured and the amniotic fluid is clear. Contractions are every 2 to 3 minutes, last 50 seconds, and are firm. Fetal heart rate and monitor patterns are essentially unchanged. Beth's back pain is worse, and she is having difficulty relaxing between contractions, despite using a variety of nonpharmacologic techniques with the nurse's help. She is discouraged that labor is not progressing as quickly as she expected. Beth requests an epidural block, which will be given by continuous infusion.

Critical Thinking: At this point, what are some advantages and disadvantages of having an epidural? Are added measures needed to safeguard the fetus because of an epidural block?

Answer: An epidural may slow labor if performed earlier than this, but labor progress may benefit from the relief of pain and tension if done at this point or later. A disadvantage of the epidural block is that her activity is more restricted, reducing her options for positions that might improve fetal descent and rotation through the pelvis.

To safeguard the fetus, the nurse gives Beth a preload of at least 500 ml of ordered IV solution before the block begins, which offsets its hypotensive effects. Fetal monitoring, usually by continuous electronic means, helps identify nonreassuring patterns that may occur. Beth is kept in a position that avoids aortocaval compression.

Nursing Diagnosis: Risk for injury related to altered sensation in her lower extremities.

Goals/Expected Outcomes:
1. Beth will not fall or suffer other injury while experiencing the effects of epidural block.
2. The fetus will not be born in an uncontrolled manner.

Intervention	Rationale
1. Assist Beth to change positions regularly. Keep Beth in bed as long as she has any motor block.	1. Changing positions reduces constant pressure on one area, reduces muscle strain, and promotes normal labor. Ambulation is contraindicated as long as motor and sensory functions are impaired to avoid falls.
2. Observe for signs of labor progress: a. Contractions increase in frequency, duration, and intensity b. Increase in bloody show c. Statement or behavior (such as grunting) reflecting urge to push (may *not* be present)	2. Labor may progress quickly when pain is relieved. Sensation is altered to varying extent with an epidural, and rectal pressure associated with fetal descent may or may not be felt as fetus descends. The fetus could be born unattended because of reduced sensation.
3. If fetus descends to a +1 to +2 station during second stage labor and Beth cannot feel the urge to push, assist her to push with each contraction.	3. Epidural block may alter the reflex urge to push. Coaching about when to push aids fetal descent.
4. Check for return of movement and sensation prior to ambulating after birth. Have an assistant help with the first ambulation.	4. This prevents falls resulting from weakness and inability to sense location of her feet. Having assistance prevents injury if a woman is unexpectedly weak when she ambulates.

Evaluation: Beth is satisfied with her pain relief after the epidural block. She has little motor block. Her blood pressure and the fetal heart rate remain within expected limits. Vaginal dilation progresses to 10 cm (complete) without injury to Beth or her fetus. However, despite her vigorous pushing efforts, the fetal station remains at 0. Beth has a cesarean birth, delivering an 8-pound, 10-ounce girl.

PAIN

Assessment

Pain assessment begins at admission and continues throughout labor (see Table 13-1). Pain-related assessments include the following:

- Preferences for pain management
- Maternal vital signs
- Fetal heart rate and electronic fetal monitor patterns
- Allergies, focusing especially on allergy to opioid analgesics, dental anesthetics, and iodine (used in most prep solutions)
- Oral intake—Time and type of last intake
- Evidence of pain—Verbal statement, requests for pain relief measures, crying, moaning, and tense, guarded posture or facial expression
- Labor status

In addition to these routine assessments, ask the woman if she needs help with pain management. A stoic woman may give little evidence of pain yet may say she wants medication or other pain control if asked.

When assessing pain, clarify the words a woman uses. When asked if she has "pain," the woman may deny it. Yet changing the word used to "discomfort," "cramping," "aching," "pressure," or other words that may describe labor pain may bring a different response. Do not assume that everyone uses the same words to describe their pain. Pain is an individual experience and so is the expression of pain.

Asking a woman to rate her pain on a scale of 0 to 10 (or your facility's standard scale) helps clarify her pain's intensity. A 0 represents no pain, whereas 10 is the worst possible pain. Ask the woman to rate her pain on this scale before and after pain relief measures to evaluate their effectiveness. Multilingual and picture scales are available for those who do not speak the dominant language.

Body language gives a clue to comfort level. Moaning, crying, thrashing, and an inability to use nonpharmacologic techniques are obvious indicators that a woman needs help with pain control, including pharmacologic pain relief. However, more subtle clues such as remaining tense between contractions also suggest difficulty coping with pain.

Evaluate the woman's labor status to help her choose the most appropriate method of pain control. Inform her if she has reached a mandatory decision point in labor to use or not use a specific pharmacologic method. No standard time or amount of cervical dilation serves as a guideline for this critical point. This is estimated based on projected time of birth, amount of time needed to establish a specific method, and the pharmacology of the drug or drugs.

Avoid making assumptions about a woman's pain based on her rate of labor progress, cervical dilation, or apparent intensity of contractions. Do not assume that a woman whose cervix is 2 cm dilated has little pain and that a woman whose cervix is dilated 8 cm has intense pain. An obese woman's contractions may be strong, but they may seem mild if they are assessed by palpation or an external monitor because of her thick abdominal fat pad. *Labor progress or contraction intensity cannot be equated with a woman's pain perception or tolerance.*

A woman's need for pain relief should not be based only on her outward expression. A quiet woman may need medication but may be reluctant to ask, whereas the expressive woman may be satisfied with only nonpharmacologic measures. Because women who do not speak the prevailing language may not know what is available, seek an interpreter to communicate effectively.

Observe for and report pain that is not typical of normal labor. Although labor pain is often intense, it should come and go with each contraction. The uterus should not be tender or boardlike between contractions.

Analysis

Pain is expected in normal childbirth, and most laboring women have nursing needs that relate to its management. The nursing diagnosis is: Pain related to effects of uterine contractions and fetal descent.

Planning

Because pain is a subjective experience and expected in labor, two goals or expected outcomes are realistic. The woman will do the following:

1. Describe pain relief measures, both nonpharmacologic and pharmacologic, as satisfactory during labor.
2. Effectively use breathing and relaxation techniques learned in childbirth class or from nurse during labor.

Interventions

Nursing care related to intrapartum pain management focuses on reducing factors that hinder the woman's pain control and enhancing those that benefit it (see Chapter 13).

Promoting Relaxation

Simple attention to details promotes relaxation. Make the environment more comfortable. If noise is a problem, suggest music or television to mask it. A warm blanket, a cool cloth, or hot pack provides tangible comfort and conveys the nurse's caring attitude. Change the linens or underpads as needed to keep the woman reasonably clean and dry.

Offer the woman a warm shower or bath, especially if she is tense and if no contraindications exist (see Table 15-1). In general, walking is good during early labor, and water therapy is better during active labor. The mild nipple stimulation that occurs in a whirlpool or shower may intensify contractions in a woman whose labor has slowed, causing her posterior pituitary gland to secrete oxytocin.

Reduce intrusions as much as possible. For example, wait until a contraction is over before asking questions or doing a procedure. Longer assessments and procedures may span several contractions, but try to stop during each contraction if possible.

Reducing Outside Sources of Discomfort

Anesthetize the IV site with lidocaine (Xylocaine) before inserting the line if the woman is not allergic and if policy permits. Normal saline infiltration of the site has a similar effect. Remind her to change position regularly to reduce tension and discomfort from constant pressure. Support her with pillows.

Observe the woman's bladder for distention hourly, and encourage her to void every 2 hours or more often if she has received a large quantity of IV fluids. Most intrapartum orders include one for catheterization if she cannot void and her bladder is full. An indwelling catheter is sometimes inserted for women who have an epidural to reduce repeated catheterizations.

Reducing Anxiety and Fear

Accurate information reduces the negative psychological impact of the unknown. Tell the woman about her labor and its progress. You cannot predict when she will give birth, but tell her if labor progress is or is not on course. Sometimes she needs only the reassurance from an experienced nurse that her intense contractions are indeed normal. The woman may be willing to endure more discomfort than she otherwise would if she is making progress.

Be honest if problems do occur. A woman usually knows if a problem exists and is more anxious if she does not know what it is. Explain all measures taken to correct the problem, and inform her of the results.

Helping the Woman Use Nonpharmacologic Techniques

If the nonpharmacologic method is safe for the woman and fetus and if it is effective, do not interfere with its use. Try not to distract the woman from whatever technique she is using.

Massage. Fetal monitor belts hinder abdominal effleurage. Encourage the woman to do effleurage on uncovered areas of her abdomen or to stroke her thighs. Consider using intermittent auscultation or intermittent electronic fetal monitoring (see Chapter 14).

Use powder to avoid friction and seek feedback from the woman about the best location and amount of pressure to use for sacral pressure or other massage. Because this information may change during labor or massage may become uncomfortable rather than helpful, seek the woman's feedback regularly.

Mental Stimulation. Use a low, soothing voice when helping a woman use imagery. Speaking close to her ear is often helpful when trying to create a tranquil imaginary scene or to calm her. Use of a low, soothing voice during an emergency has a calming effect as well. Music can enhance mental stimulation techniques.

Breathing. Women often modify the techniques they learn in class or invent some of their own during labor. Encourage the woman to change techniques when she needs to, but save the complex ones for later labor. If she has trouble maintaining her concentration, the nurse or her support person may try to make eye contact (if culturally appropriate) and breathe the pattern with her.

Symptoms of hyperventilation (dizziness, tingling and numbness of the fingers and lips, carpopedal spasm) are likely if a woman breathes fast and deep. If she hyperventilates, she should breathe into her cupped hands, a paper bag, or a washcloth placed over her nose and mouth. Talk to her gently to slow her breathing.

Teach breathing techniques to the unprepared woman when she is admitted. Review them when she seems to need a different method. If she makes up a breathing technique that works, leave it alone.

When teaching the unprepared woman who is in advanced labor pain management techniques, follow these guidelines:

- Teach one method at a time.
- Demonstrate the method between contractions.
- Use breathing techniques with the woman while maintaining eye contact.
- Give her control over her labor: who is present, what technique she will use, and the like.
- Speak in a soft, calm tone of voice

Incorporating Pharmacologic Methods

All pharmacologic methods require collaboration with medical personnel for orders. Tell the woman soon after admission what medication is available if she needs it. This is not intended to undermine her self-confidence but allow her to make an informed choice about medication when necessary. Analgesia is most effective if it is given before pain is severe.

Tell her that her preferences about pain relief methods will be honored if possible, but predicting the course of her labor is impossible. Her preferred method of pain management may be inappropriate if labor has unexpected developments. Assure her that no pharmacologic method will be given without her understanding and consent (Parents Want to Know: How Will This Medicine Affect Our Baby?).

If a woman finds nonpharmacologic methods inadequate, help her try other ones or offer her available medication. When contacting the birth attendant for medication orders, report the fetal and maternal status and vital signs, labor status, and her request for medication. If she has a continuous epidural block, contact the person who inserted it if problems occur. Observe special nursing considerations associated with the method used (Table 15-3).

Text continued on p. 390

Table 15-3
PHARMACOLOGIC METHODS OF INTRAPARTUM PAIN MANAGEMENT

Method and Uses	Nursing Considerations
OPIOID ANALGESICS	
Systemic analgesia during labor and for postoperative pain after cesarean birth; may be combined with adjunctive drug such as promethazine to reduce nausea and vomiting that sometimes occur with narcotic use	Assess the woman for drug use at admission. Women who are opiate-dependent should not receive analgesics having mixed agonist and antagonist actions (butorphanol and nalbuphine). Observe neonate for respiratory depression, especially if the mother had narcotics within 4 hours of birth: • Delay in initiating or sustaining respirations • Rate <30/min • Poor muscle tone: limp, floppy • Use of adjunctive drugs, such as promethazine, enhances respiratory depressant effects. • Have naloxone available. Observe for recurrent respiratory depression after administration of naloxone. Repeat at 20- to 60-minute intervals as needed.
EPIDURAL OPIOIDS	
Labor: Mixed with a local anesthetic agent to give better pain relief with less motor block. *Postoperatively:* Gives long-acting analgesia without sedation, allowing the mother and infant to interact more easily.	*Labor:* Observe same nursing implications as with epidural block. *Postoperatively:* 1. Do not give additional opioids or other CNS depressants except as ordered by the anesthesia clinician. 2. Respiratory depression may be delayed up to 24 hr. Observe respiratory rate, depth, and arousability hourly for 24 hr or as ordered. Notify anesthesia clinician for rate <12/min, oxygen saturation <95% on pulse oximeter, reduced respiratory effort, or difficulty arousing. Cyanosis is a late sign. 3. Have naloxone, 0.4 mg, readily available. 4. Observe for pruritus or rubbing of the face and neck. Notify anesthesia clinician for relief measures. 5. Urinary retention may occur. Observe for adequate voiding if the woman does not have a catheter. 6. Notify anesthesia clinician for relief of nausea or vomiting. 7. Assess sensation and mobility before allowing ambulation.
INTRATHECAL OPIOID ANALGESICS	
Provides analgesia for most of first-stage labor without maternal sedation Small dose of the drug needed because it is injected very near the spinal cord where sensory fibers enter Usually not adequate for late labor or the birth itself May be combined with epidural analgesia in the combined spinal epidural analgesia.	1. Observe for the common side effects of nausea, vomiting, and pruritus. Notify the anesthesia clinician if these occur, and have an antagonist such as naloxone or naltrexone available. 2. Observe for delayed respiratory depression, depending on the drug given. Use a pulse oximeter as indicated.
LOCAL INFILTRATION ANESTHESIA	
Numbs perineum for episiotomy or repair of laceration at vaginal birth; no relief of labor pain; not adequate for forceps-assisted birth	1. Assess for drug allergies, especially to dental anesthetics because they are related to those used in maternity care. 2. Apply ice to perineum immediately after birth to reduce edema and hematoma formation and to increase comfort.
PUDENDAL BLOCK	
Numbs the lower vagina and perineum for vaginal birth No relief of labor pain because performed just before birth Provides adequate anesthesia for many forceps-assisted births	1. Same as local infiltration. A woman may be alarmed by the long needle (about 6 inches). Teach her that it must be long to reach the pudendal nerve and that it will be inserted only about 0.5 inch into her tissue and is shielded by a guide to avoid damaging her or her fetus' tissue.

CNS, Central nervous system; *BP,* blood pressure; *FHR,* fetal heart rate; *IV,* intravenous.

Table 15-3

PHARMACOLOGIC METHODS OF INTRAPARTUM PAIN MANAGEMENT—cont'd

Method and Uses	Nursing Considerations
Epidural Block	
Labor: Insertion of catheter provides pain relief for labor and vaginal birth (T10-S5 levels) *Cesarean birth:* If epidural was used during labor, level of block can be extended upward (T4-T6 level). Also used for planned cesarean birth and post-birth tubal ligation.	1. Prehydrate the woman with warmed nonglucose crystalloid solution such as Ringer's lactate. Common amounts: 500-1000 ml for labor and vaginal birth; 1500-2000 ml for cesarean birth. 2. Displace uterus to left manually or with a pillow under woman's hip to enhance placental perfusion. Avoid aortocaval compression throughout labor. 3. Assess for hypotension every 2-3 minutes, or by facility policy, after block is begun until vital signs are stable. Report to anesthesia clinician: systolic BP <100 mmHg or a fall of 20% or more from baseline levels; FHR decelerations. 4. Assess FHR for signs of impaired placental perfusion and report to anesthesia clinician and nurse-midwife: Tachycardia (>150–160/min); bradycardia (<110–120/min); late decelerations. 5. If hypotension or signs of impaired placental perfusion occur: increase rate of nonadditive IV fluid; turn woman to her left side, administer oxygen by face mask 8-10 L/minute. Have ephedrine available for use (5-10 mg IV). 6. Observe for bladder distention. Get an order to catheterize woman if she cannot void. 7. Change woman's position to promote labor progress and distribute anesthetic medication evenly. 8. If block is being given by intermittent injection, notify anesthesia clinician for re-injection when pain recurs. 9. Observe progress of labor. Assist woman to push if she cannot feel the urge during second stage if her fetus reaches a station of +1 to +2. 10. Observe for signs of catheter migration: unilateral or absent pain relief, too intense motor and sensory block, signs of intravascular injection (numbness of tongue and lips, lightheadedness, dizziness, and tinnitus). 11. Transfer carefully because the woman may not have full use of her legs. Assess for return of sensation and movement before ambulation.
Subarachnoid Block	
Cesarean birth. Is simpler and can be established more quickly than epidural block May rarely be used for complicated vaginal birth Is a shorter-acting pain relief method than the epidural	1. See Epidural Block for these interventions: a. IV prehydration b. Uterine displacement c. Observation of blood pressure and FHR d. Care for hypotension or signs of impaired placental perfusion e. Bladder distention f. Transfer and ambulation precautions 2. Observe for post-spinal headache: a headache that is worse when woman is upright and that may disappear when she is lying flat. Notify anesthesia clinician if it occurs (a blood patch may be done). 3. Nursing interventions for postdural puncture headache: bedrest, increase oral fluids if not contraindicated, oral caffeine, and give analgesics as ordered.

Continued

Table 15-3
PHARMACOLOGIC METHODS OF INTRAPARTUM PAIN MANAGEMENT—cont'd

Method and Uses	Nursing Considerations
General Anesthesia	
Cesarean birth if epidural or spinal block is not possible or if the woman refuses regional anesthesia May be required for emergency procedures such as replacement of inverted uterus	1. Determine type and time of last food intake on admission. 2. Restrict oral intake to clear liquids or as ordered. Consult with physician or nurse-midwife if surgical intervention is likely. 3. Report to anesthesia clinician: oral intake before and during labor, vomiting. 4. Displace uterus (see Epidural Block). 5. Give ordered drugs such as clear antacid. 6. Maintain cricoid pressure (Sellick's maneuver) during intubation. 7. Maintain in a side-lying position (after surgery) until protective (gag) reflexes have returned. 8. Interventions for postoperative respiratory depression: give oxygen by face mask; observe oxygen saturation with pulse oximeter until woman is awake and alert; have woman take several deep breaths if oxygen saturation falls below 95%.

CNS, Central nervous system; *BP,* blood pressure; *FHR,* fetal heart rate; *IV,* intravenous.

Evaluation

Labor is not expected to be painless, even with the most effective pharmacologic methods. The first goal or expected outcome is achieved if the woman is satisfied with her ability to manage her pain. Many women have occasional difficulty using breathing or other techniques, even if they have practiced faithfully. They achieve the second goal/expected outcome if they use coping skills somewhat consistently during labor.

EPIDURAL ANALGESIA

Many women choose epidural analgesia for pain relief during labor because of its effectiveness without sedation. Epidural block analgesia requires a number of specific nursing assessments and interventions.

Assessment

The admission assessment focuses on possible allergies to local anesthetics or opioid drugs that might be used in the block. Determine baseline maternal vital signs and the fetal heart rate and pattern. Assess for any skin infection in the area of the back where the epidural will be inserted.

Analysis

The primary risks associated with epidural analgesia are maternal hypotension and injury. These result in a collaborative problem and a nursing diagnosis:

- Potential complication—maternal hypotension with secondary fetal hypoxia
- Risk for Injury related to reduced sensation and movement secondary to anesthetic effects

Planning

Goals or expected outcomes are not appropriate for collaborative problems such as the potential complication of hypotension. The nurse's responsibility is to observe for hypotension and report its occurrence to the professional who is in charge of the anesthetic for definitive treatment. However, a goal/expected outcome is appropriate for the risk for injury nursing diagnosis: The woman does not suffer a treatment-related injury while her sensation and mobility are reduced.

Interventions

Maternal Hypotension

Maternal hypotension reduces blood supply to the placenta, decreasing fetal oxygen and nutrient supply and waste removal. Birth facilities will have policies that provide specific guidelines for care when women receive epidural block. Infuse the prescribed warmed IV solution, at least 500 to 1000 ml before the block's initiation. If the woman has not received the full amount when the block is begun, notify the anesthesia professional.

The epidural may be placed with the woman in a sitting or side-lying position. If she is in a sitting position, hugging a pillow or a small-size birth ball helps her hold the correct position. Tell the anesthesia clinician when the woman is having a contraction. She may feel a brief "electric shock" sensation as the catheter is passed. After the epidural is initiated, maintain her position so that aortocaval compression is avoided, such as by placing a pillow under her right hip.

Take the woman's blood pressure and pulse (usually done with an automatic cuff) every 2 to 3 minutes, or according to the facility's protocol, for 15 to 20 minutes after the initial injection of medication, comparing it to her baseline pressure. Maintain continuous electronic fetal monitoring. A significant blood pressure decrease is a 20% fall from her baseline or a fall to 100 mm Hg systolic. Hypotension of any degree accompanied by FHR decelerations is significant. If hypotension occurs, increase the rate of her IV fluid, keeping her positioned to avoid aortocaval compression. Ephedrine, 5 to 10 mg, is ordered if hypotension is significant and a fluid increase does not quickly improve it. When the blood pressure is stable, assess it every 15 minutes. Pulse oximetry identifies a fall in maternal oxygenation status to below 95%.

Continue observing the FHR. Signs of reduced placental perfusion may be evident before the woman shows signs of hypotension. These include fetal tachycardia (more than 150 to 160 BPM) or bradycardia (less than 110 to 120 BPM) and late decelerations (see Chapter 14). Take the mother's temperature to identify elevations that may also contribute to fetal tachycardia.

Avoidance of Injury

Epidural block reduces lower extremity sensation and movement to varying degrees. Some women have such a light motor block that theirs is called a "walking epidural." However, to prevent falls, these women should not walk alone. Most women must remain in bed or sometimes a nearby chair, after their epidural is begun because of reduced sensation.

Assess the degree of motor block and sensation hourly. If a distinct increase or change is noted, report it to the anesthesia clinician because this may indicate catheter migration or another complication.

Table 15-4
NURSING DIAGNOSES RELATED TO PAIN MANAGEMENT DURING BIRTH

Anxiety
*Pain
Powerlessness
Risk for aspiration
*Risk for injury
Situational low self-esteem
Urinary retention

*Nursing diagnoses explored in this chapter.

A woman who has reduced mobility and sensation should be moved so that she maintains an anatomic position. Avoid prolonged pressure on one area. Remember that changing position often improves labor progress, even if the woman does not need to change positions for comfort. If surgery is needed, pad bony prominences to reduce pressure on those areas.

Before any ambulation, such as urination after birth, test the woman's ability to raise and move her legs. Have her push her legs against your hands to determine her leg strength. When ambulating, accompany her, observing for her ability to move and her strength the entire time until the epidural's effects have worn off (Table 15-4).

Evaluation

The collaborative problem is not evaluated, but the nurse compares the woman's baseline blood pressure and fetal heart rate to those after the block is begun to identify any significant changes. The goal/expected outcome related to injury is achieved if the woman does not have an injury related to her altered sensation and mobility while the epidural block is exerting its effects.

PARENTS WANT TO KNOW *How Will This Medicine Affect Our Baby?*

Women and their support persons often ask whether pain medication or anesthesia will harm the baby. The nurse can help parents to choose wisely from available options by providing honest information.

- Pain that is beyond your ability to tolerate is not good for you or your baby, and it reduces the joy of this special event.
- Some risk is associated with every type of pain medication or anesthesia, but careful selection and use of preventive measures minimize this risk. If complications occur, corrective measures can reduce the risk to you and your baby.
- Some pain relievers can cause your baby to be slow to breathe at birth, but carefully controlling the timing and dose of the medication reduces the likelihood that this will occur. We can use another medication to reverse this effect if needed.
- Epidural or spinal anesthesia can cause your blood pressure to fall, which can reduce the blood flow to your baby. However, we give you lots of IV fluids to reduce this effect. We have other medications to increase your blood pressure if the fluids are not enough.
- General anesthesia can cause your baby to be slow to breathe at birth. To reduce this risk, the anesthesia will not be started until everything is ready for the surgery, and the doctors will clamp the baby's umbilical cord as quickly as possible.

SUMMARY CONCEPTS

- Childbirth pain is unique because it is normal and self-limiting, can be prepared for, and ends with a baby's birth.
- Excess or poorly relieved pain may be harmful to the mother and fetus.
- Pain is a complex physical and psychological experience. It is subjective and personal.
- Four sources of pain are present in most labors, but other physical and psychological factors may increase or decrease the pain felt from these sources. These sources are cervical dilation, uterine ischemia, pressure and pulling on pelvic structures, and distention of the vagina and perineum.
- Relaxation enhances all other pain management techniques.
- Several nonpharmacologic pain management techniques supplement relaxation—cutaneous stimulation, hydrotherapy, mental stimulation, and breathing techniques.
- Physiologic alterations of pregnancy may affect a woman's response to medications.
- Any drug that the expectant mother takes, whether therapeutic or abused, including herbal or botanical preparations, also may affect the fetus. Fetal effects may be direct or indirect.
- The nurse should observe for respiratory depression, primarily in the newborn, when the mother has received opioid analgesics during labor.
- The major advantages of regional pain management methods are that the woman can participate in the birth and that she retains her protective airway reflexes.
- The nurse should observe for and take actions to prevent maternal hypotension with the epidural or subarachnoid block.
- The nurse should observe for fetal heart rate changes associated with impaired placental perfusion if the woman receives a regional technique that has the risk for maternal hypotension.
- The main nursing observations for the woman who receives epidural or intrathecal opioids are for nausea and vomiting, pruritus, and delayed respiratory depression.
- Regurgitation with aspiration of acidic gastric contents is the greatest risk for a woman who receives general anesthesia.

ANSWERS TO CRITICAL THINKING QUESTIONS

1. Truc's labor progress and pattern of contractions and her tension suggest that she needs assistance with pain management. However, the nurse should not assume that she needs or wants medication, either. Truc may prefer nonpharmacologic measures and these may also complement medication.

   The nurse cannot make assumptions about Truc's needs for pain relief based on her behavior. Asian women often value stoicism and are concerned with harmonious relationships. Truc may be smiling to please the nurse rather than because she is comfortable.
2. The nurse needs additional data about Truc's real needs and preferences for pain management.
3. The nurse can share observations about Truc's body posture during contractions. If Truc does not speak English well, an interpreter or picture-type pain scale may improve assessment of her need for pain relief. The nurse might demonstrate simple breathing and relaxation techniques, offer hydrotherapy in the form of a shower, tub, or whirlpool, and suggest position changes or ambulation.

REFERENCES & READINGS

American Academy of Pediatrics & American College of Obstetricians and Gynecologists. (1997). *Guidelines for perinatal care* (4th ed.) Washington, D.C.: Author.

Association of Women's Health, Obstetric, and Neonatal Nurses (AWHONN). (1996a). Clinical commentary: Obstetric epidural analgesia and the role of the professional registered nurse. *AWHONN Voice,* 4(8).

Association of Women's Health, Obstetric, and Neonatal Nurses (AWHONN). (1996b). *Position statement: Role of the registered nurse (RN) in the management of the patient receiving analgesia by catheter techniques (epidural, intrathecal, intrapleural, or peripheral nerve catheters).* Washington, D.C.: Author.

Association of Women's Health, Obstetric, and Neonatal Nurses (AWHONN). (2000). *Symposium: Second stage labor management: Promotion of evidence-based practice and a collaborative approach to patient care.* Washington, D.C.: Author.

Baram, D.A. (1995). Hypnosis in reproductive health care: A review and case reports. *Birth,* 22(1), 37-42.

Biribo, M.A. (2000). General anesthesia for cesarean section. In D.J. Birnbach, S.P. Gatt, S. Datta (Eds.), *Textbook of obstetric anesthesia* (pp. 245-266). New York: Churchill Livingstone.

Britt, R., & Pasero, C. (1999). Pregnancy, childbirth, postpartum, and breastfeeding: Use of analgesics. In M. McCaffery & C. Pasero (Eds.), *Pain: Clinical manual* (2nd ed., pp. 608-625). St. Louis: Mosby.

Chapman, L.L. (2000). Expectant fathers and labor epidurals. *MCN: American Journal of Maternal/Child Nursing,* 25(3), 133-138.

Cheek, T.G., & Gutsche, B.B. (1997). Analgesia for labor. In D.M. Dewan & D.D. Hood (Eds.), *Practical obstetric anesthesia* (pp. 95-124). Philadelphia: W.B. Saunders.

Cheek, T.G., Gutsche, B.B., & Gaiser, R.R. (1999). The pain of childbirth and its effect on the mother and fetus. In D.H. Chestnut (Ed.), *Obstetric anesthesia: Principles and practice* (2nd ed., pp. 320-335). St. Louis: Mosby.

Chestnut, D.H. (1999a). Alternative regional anesthetic techniques: Paracervical block, lumbar sympathetic block, pudendal block, and perineal infiltration. In D.H. Chestnut (Ed.), *Obstetric anesthesia: Principles and practice* (2nd ed., pp. 427-437). St. Louis: Mosby.

Chestnut, D.H. (1999b). Epidural and spinal analgesia/anesthesia: Section III: Effect on the progress of labor and method of delivery. In D.H. Chestnut (Ed.), *Obstetric anesthesia: Principles and practice* (2nd ed., pp. 408-426). St. Louis: Mosby.

Conklin, K.A. (1998). Obstetric analgesia and anesthesia. In N.F. Hacker & J.G. Moore (Eds.), *Essentials of obstetrics and gynecology* (3rd ed., pp. 168-180). Philadelphia: W.B. Saunders.

Cook, A., & Wilcox, G. (1997). Pressuring pain. *Lifelines,* 1(2), 35-41.

Creehan, P.A. (1996). Pain relief and comfort measures during labor. In K.R. Simpson & P.A. Creehan (Eds.), *AWHONN'S perinatal nursing* (pp. 227-245). Philadelphia: J.B. Lippincott.

Cunningham, F.G., MacDonald, P.C., Gant, N.F., Leveno, K.J., Gilstrap, L.C., Hankins, G.D.V., et al. (1997). *Williams obstetrics* (20th ed.). Norwalk, CT: Appleton & Lange.

Dargie, C. & Marsh, H.M. (2000). Obstetric anesthesia. In S.B. Ransom, M.P. Dombrowski, S.G. McNeeley, K.S. Moghissi, & A.R. Munkarah (Eds.), *Practical strategies in obstetrics and gynecology* (pp. 276-289). Philadelphia: W.B. Saunders.

Dewan, D.M., & Hood, D.D. (1997). *Practical obstetric anesthesia.* Philadelphia: W.B. Saunders.

Dick, M.J. (1995). Assessment and measurement of acute pain. *Journal of Obstetric, Gynecologic, and Neonatal Nursing,* 24(9), 843-848.

Faucher, M.A. & M.C. Brucker. (2000). Intrapartum pain: Pharmacologic management. *Journal of Obstetric, Gynecologic, and Neonatal Nursing,* 29(2), 169-180.

Fehder, W.P., & Gennaro, S. (1998). Immune alterations associated with epidural analgesia for labor and delivery. *MCN: American Journal of Maternal/Child Nursing,* 23(6), 292-299.

Fishburne, J.I. (1999). Obstetric analgesia and anesthesia. In J.R. Scott, P.J. Di Saia, D.B. Hammond, & W.N. Spellacy (Eds.) *Danforth's obstetrics and gynecology* (8th ed., pp. 111-129). Philadelphia: Lippincott Williams & Wilkins.

Glosten, B. (1999). Epidural and spinal analgesia/anesthesia: Section I: Local anesthetic techniques. In D.H. Chestnut (Ed.), *Obstetric anesthesia: Principles and practice* (2nd ed., pp. 360-386). St. Louis: Mosby.

Goldberg, A.B., Cohen, A., & Lieberman, E. (1999). Nulliparas' preferences for epidural analgesia: Their effects on actual use in labor. *Birth,* 26(3), 139-143.

Grabowska, C. (2000). Alternative therapies for pain relief. In M. Yerby (Ed.), *Pain in childbearing,* pp. 93-109. Edinburgh: Baillière Tindall.

Halpern, S.H., Leighton, B.L., Ohlsson, A., Barrett, J.F.R., & Rice, A. (1998). Effect of epidural vs parenteral opioid analgesia on the progress of labor: A meta-analysis. *Journal of the American Medical Association,* 280(24), 2105-2110.

Holden, D.L. (1997). Anesthesia for Cesarean section. In D.M. Dewan & D.D. Hood (Eds.), *Practical obstetric anesthesia* (pp. 125-137) Philadelphia: W.B. Saunders.

Hurley, R.J. (2000). Continuous spinal anesthesia techniques for labor and delivery. In D.J. Birnbach, S.P. Gatt, S. Datta (Eds.), *Textbook of obstetric anesthesia* (pp. 183-188). New York: Churchill Livingstone.

Joint Commission on Accreditation of Healthcare Organizations. (1999). Patient rights and organization ethics chapter. *Comprehensive accreditation manual for hospitals: The official handbook.* Retrieved July 30, 2000 from http://www.jcaho.org/standard/pm_mpfrm.html.

Kabler, J. (2000). Water immersion during labor and birth. In *Childbirth education: Practice, research, and theory* (2nd ed., pp. 284-294). Philadelphia: W.B. Saunders.

Lieberman, E., Lang, J., Richardson, D.K., Frigoletto, F.D., Heffner, L.J., & Cohen, A. (1999). Epidurals and cesareans: The jury is still out. *Birth,* 26(3), 196-198.

Lieberman, E., Lang, J., Richardson, D.K., Frigoletto, F.D., Heffner, L.J., & Cohen, A. (2000). Intrapartum maternal fever and neonatal outcome. *Pediatrics,* 105(1), 8-13.

Lowe, N.K. (1996). The pain and discomfort of labor and birth. *Journal of Obstetric, Gynecologic, and Neonatal Nursing,* 25(1), 82-92.

Manning, J. (1996). Intrathecal narcotics: New approach for labor analgesia. *Journal of Obstetric, Gynecologic, and Neonatal Nursing,* 25(3), 221-224.

Minnich, M.E. (1999). Childbirth preparation and nonpharmacologic analgesia. In D.H. Chestnut (Ed.), *Obstetric anesthesia: Principles and practice* (2nd ed., pp. 336-345). St. Louis: Mosby.

Mussell, S. (1998). Narcotic analgesia during labor and birth: Maternal and newborn effects. *Mother Baby Journal,* 3(6), 19-23.

Newton, E.R., Schroeder, B.C., Knape, K.G., & Bennett, B.L. (1995). Epidural analgesia and uterine function. *Obstetrics and Gynecology,* 85(5), 749-755.

Paech, M. (2000). Patient-controlled epidural analgesia. In D.J. Birnbach, S.P. Gatt, S. Datta (Eds.), *Textbook of obstetric anesthesia* (pp. 189-202). New York: Churchill Livingstone.

Pasero, C., Portenoy, R.K., & McCaffery, M. (1999). Opioid analgesics. In M. McCaffery & C. Pasero (Eds.) *Pain: Clinical manual* (2nd ed., pp. 161-299). St. Louis: Mosby.

Paull, J. (2000). Epidural analgesia for labor. In D.J. Birnbach, S.P. Gatt, S. Datta (Eds.), *Textbook of obstetric anesthesia* (pp. 145-156). New York: Churchill Livingstone.

Petrou, S., Coyle, D., Fraser, W.D. (2000). Cost-effectiveness of a delayed pushing policy for patients with epidural anesthesia. *American Journal of Obstetrics and Gynecology,* 182, 1158-1164.

Rawal, N., Holmström, Björn, Van Zundert, A., & Crowhurst, J.A. (2000). The combined spinal-epidural technique. In D.J. Birnbach, S.P. Gatt, S. Datta (Eds.), *Textbook of obstetric anesthesia* (pp. 157-182). New York: Churchill Livingstone.

Riley, E.T., & Ross, B.K. (1999). Epidural and spinal analgesia/anesthesia: Section II: Opioid techniques. In D.H. Chestnut (Ed.), *Obstetric anesthesia: Principles and practice* (2nd ed., pp. 386-408). St. Louis: Mosby.

Riquelme, J., & Lacassie, H.J. (2000). Nonpharmacologic alternatives for obstetric analgesia. In D.J. Birnbach, S.P. Gatt, S. Datta (Eds.), *Textbook of obstetric anesthesia* (pp. 203-205). New York: Churchill Livingstone.

Robinson, J.N., Norwitz, E.R., Cohen, A.P., McElrath, T.F., & Lieberman, E.S. (2000). Epidural analgesia and third- or fourth-degree lacerations in nulliparas. *Obstetrics and Gynecology,* 94, 259-262.

Rout, C.C. (2000). Regional anesthesia for cesarean section. In D.J. Birnbach, S.P. Gatt, S. Datta (Eds.), *Textbook of Obstetric Anesthesia* (pp. 245-266). New York: Churchill Livingstone.

Rowe, T.F. (1997). Acute gastric aspiration: Prevention and treatment. *Seminars in Perinatology,* 21(4), 313-319.

Segal, S., Carp, H., & Chestnut, D.H. (1999). Fever and infection. In D.H. Chestnut (Ed.), *Obstetric anesthesia: Principles and practice* (2nd ed., pp. 711-724). St. Louis: Mosby.

Sharma, S.K., Sidawi, J.E., Ramin, S.M., Lucas, M.J., Leveno, K.J., & Cunningham, F.G. (1997). Cesarean delivery: A randomized trial of epidural versus patient-controlled meperidine analgesia during labor. *Anesthesiology,* 87(3), 487-494.

Simkin, P., & Frederick, E. (2000). Labor support. In *Childbirth education: Practice, research, and theory* (2nd ed., pp. 307-341). Philadelphia: W.B. Saunders.

Simkin, P. (1995). Reducing pain and enhancing progress in labor: A guide to nonpharmacologic methods for maternity caregivers. *Birth,* 22(3), 161-171.

Sinatra, R.S., & Ayoub, C.M. (1999). Postoperative analgesia: Epidural and spinal techniques. In D.H. Chestnut (Ed.), *Obstetric anesthesia: Principles and practice* (2nd ed., pp. 521-555). St. Louis: Mosby.

Stem, J. (1997). Flirting with disaster. *Lifelines,* 1(1), 31-35.

Teschendorf, M.E., & Evans, C.P. (2000). Hydrotherapy during labor: An example of developing a practice policy. *MCN: American Journal of Maternal/Child Nursing,* 25(4), 198-203.

Thorp, J., & Breedlove, G. (1996). Epidural analgesia in labor: An evaluation of risks and benefits. *Birth,* 23(2), 63-83.

Visalyaputra, S. (2000). Systemic analgesia for labor. In D.J. Birnbach, S.P. Gatt, S. Datta (Eds.), *Textbook of obstetric anesthesia* (pp. 209-227). New York: Churchill Livingstone.

Wakefield, M.L. (1999). Systemic analgesia: Parenteral and inhalational agents. In D.H. Chestnut (Ed.), *Obstetric anesthesia: Principles and practice* (2nd ed., pp. 346-359). St. Louis: Mosby.

Ward, M.E., & Cousins, M.J. (2000). Pain mechanisms in labor. In D.J. Birnbach, S.P. Gatt, S. Datta (Eds.), *Textbook of obstetric anesthesia* (pp. 3-30). New York: Churchill Livingstone.

Weber, S.E. (1996). Cultural aspects of pain in childbearing women. *Journal of Obstetric, Gynecologic, and Neonatal Nursing,* 25(1), 67-72.

Woolley, D., & Nelsson-Ryan, S. (2000). Second-stage labor. Labor support. In *Childbirth education: Practice, research, and theory* (2nd ed., pp. 342-375).

Youngstrom, P.C., Baker, S.W., & Miller, J.L. (1996). Epidurals redefined in analgesia and anesthesia: A distinction with a difference. *Journal of Obstetric, Gynecologic, and Neonatal Nursing,* 25(4), 350-354.

Zuspan, K. (2000a). Anesthesia for obstetrics. In E.J. Quilligan & F.P. Zuspan (Eds.), *Current therapy in obstetrics and gynecology* (pp. 236-242). Philadelphia: W.B. Saunders.

Zuspan, K. (2000b). Control of postpartum pain. In E.J. Quilligan & F.P. Zuspan (Eds.), *Current therapy in obstetrics and gynecology* (pp. 261-262). Philadelphia: W.B. Saunders.

16

Nursing Care during Obstetric Procedures

OBJECTIVES

1. Identify clinical situations in which specific obstetric procedures are appropriate.
2. Explain risks, precautions, and contraindications for each procedure.
3. Identify nursing considerations for each procedure.
4. Identify methods to provide effective emotional support to the woman having an obstetric procedure.
5. Apply the nursing process to care for the woman having a cesarean birth.

DEFINITIONS

Abruptio Placentae Premature separation of a normally implanted placenta.

Amniotomy Artificial rupture of the amniotic sac (fetal membranes).

Augmentation of Labor Artificial stimulation of uterine contractions that have become ineffective.

Cephalopelvic Disproportion Fetal head size that is too large to fit through the maternal pelvis at birth (also called *fetopelvic disproportion*).

Cesarean Birth Surgical birth of the fetus through an incision in the abdominal wall and uterus.

Chignon Newborn scalp edema created by a vacuum extractor.

Chorioamnionitis Inflammation of the amniotic sac (fetal membranes); usually caused by bacterial and viral infections (also called *amnionitis*).

Dystocia Difficult or prolonged labor; often associated with abnormal uterine activity and cephalopelvic disproportion.

Episiotomy Surgical incision of the perineum to enlarge the vaginal opening.

DEFINITIONS—cont'd

Hydramnios Excessive volume of amniotic fluid, more than about 2000 ml at term (also called *polyhydramnios*).

Iatrogenic An adverse condition resulting from treatment.

Induction of Labor Artificial initiation of labor.

Montevideo Unit A method to calculate the intensity of uterine contractions in mmHg as measured with an intrauterine pressure catheter: the contraction intensity minus the resting tone multiplied by the number of contractions in 10 minutes.

Nuchal Cord Umbilical cord around the fetal neck.

Oligohydramnios Abnormally small quantity of amniotic fluid, less than about 500 ml at term.

Placenta Previa Abnormal implantation of the placenta in the lower uterus.

Premature Rupture of the Membranes Spontaneous rupture of the membranes before the onset of labor (term, preterm, or postterm gestation).

Version Turning the fetus from one presentation to another before birth, usually from breech to cephalic.

Although labor is a normal process, some women require special procedures to help them and their fetuses. A physician or nurse-midwife performs these procedures. Nursing considerations for each are addressed in this chapter.

AMNIOTOMY

Indications

Amniotomy is usually performed in conjunction with induction and augmentation of labor and to allow internal electronic fetal monitoring (see Chapter 14). Amniotomy is not often used as the sole means to induce and augment labor, and more data are needed to determine its effectiveness when used in this way (Simpson & Poole, 1998). Amniotomy also is associated with several risks that must be considered by the birth attendant before performing the procedure.

Risks

Amniotomy is performed by the physician or nurse-midwife. The nurse must observe for three risks associated with amniotomy and assist in emergency procedures.

Prolapse of the Umbilical Cord. The primary risk is that the umbilical cord will slip down in the gush of fluid. The cord can be compressed between the fetal presenting part and the woman's pelvis, obstructing blood flow to and from the placenta and reducing fetal gas exchange.

Infection. With interruption of the membrane barrier, vaginal organisms have free access to the uterine cavity and may cause chorioamnionitis. The risk is low at first but increases as the interval between membrane rupture and birth increases. Birth within 24 hours of membrane rupture is desirable, although infection does not occur at any absolute time.

Abruptio Placentae. Abruptio placentae can occur if the uterus is distended with excessive amniotic fluid when the membranes rupture. As the uterus collapses with discharge of the amniotic fluid, the area of placental attachment shrinks. The placenta then no longer fits its implantation site and partially separates. A large area of placental disruption can significantly reduce fetal oxygenation, nutrition, and waste disposal.

Technique

A disposable plastic hook (such as Amnihook) is commonly used to perforate the amniotic sac (Figure 16-1). The birth attendant performs a vaginal examination to determine cervical dilation and effacement, fetal station, and fetal presenting part. Amniotomy is often deferred if the fetal presenting part is high or the presentation is not cephalic. The risk of a prolapsed cord is higher in these situations because more room is available for the cord to slip down.

The hook is passed through the cervix, snagging the membranes. The hole is enlarged with the finger, allowing fluid to drain.

Nursing Considerations

Obtaining Baseline Information

The fetal heart rate (FHR) is assessed with electronic monitoring and auscultation to verify a reassuring rate and pattern before amniotomy is performed. The initial fetal assessment provides a baseline to compare with later assessments. A minimum of 20 to 30 minutes is needed for adequate baseline fetal evaluation.

Assisting with Amniotomy

Before amniotomy, two or three underpads should be placed under the woman's buttocks to absorb the fluid and overlapped to extend from her waist to her knees. A folded bath towel under the buttocks absorbs more amniotic fluid.

Other supplies needed are a disposable plastic hook, sterile glove for the birth attendant, and packet of sterile lubricant. The nurse should partly open the package containing the plastic hook at the handle end and hold back the package until the birth attendant takes the hook with a sterile, gloved hand.

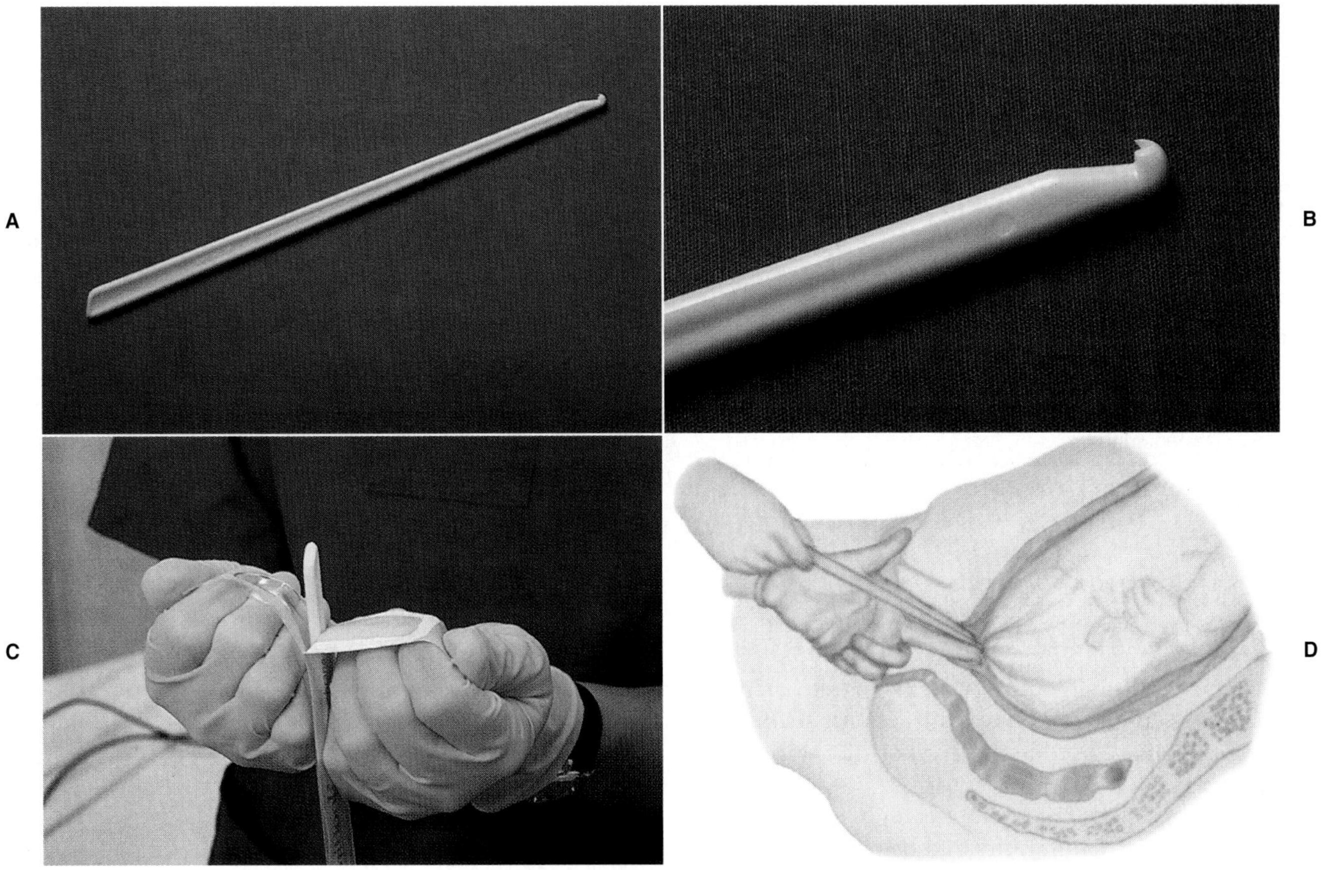

FIGURE 16-1 **A,** Disposable plastic membrane perforator. **B,** Closeup of hook end of plastic membrane perforator. **C,** Correct method to open the package. **D,** Technique for artificial rupture of membranes.

CRITICAL THINKING EXERCISE

A physician performs an amniotomy on a laboring woman whose cervix is dilated to 5 cm. The amniotic fluid is pale yellow and moderate in amount, and it has a strong odor. The FHR is 164 and accelerates when the fetus moves. Maternal vital signs are temperature 37.6° C (99.7° F), pulse 92, respirations 22, blood pressure 116/80. Contractions are moderate to firm intensity, every 3 to 4 minutes, with a duration of 50 to 60 seconds and complete uterine relaxation between contractions.

QUESTIONS:
1. Which of these observations should the nurse regard as normal? Which factors are abnormal?
2. Should the nurse modify routine labor care based on the postamniotomy assessments?

Providing Care after Amniotomy

Nursing care after amniotomy is the same as that following spontaneous membrane rupture.

Identifying Complications. The FHR is assessed for at least 1 full minute after amniotomy. Nonreassuring monitor patterns or significant changes from previous assessments are reported promptly to the birth attendant. Cord compression is usually accompanied by a rate less than 100 beats per minute (BPM), which further falls during contractions.

The quantity, color, and odor of the amniotic fluid are charted. The fluid should be clear (often with bits of vernix) and have a mild odor. A large amount of vernix in the fluid suggests that the fetus may be preterm. Greenish, meconium-stained fluid may be seen in postterm gestation or placental insufficiency. Fluid with a foul or strong odor, cloudy appearance, or yellow color suggests chorioamnionitis. Hydramnios is associated with some fetal abnormalities. Oligohydramnios may be associated with placental insufficiency or fetal urinary tract abnormalities.

Adequate amniotic fluid is necessary for lung development. The fetus with prolonged oligohydramnios may have respiratory problems after birth because the lungs cannot expand normally.

The woman's temperature should be assessed every 2 to 4 hours after the membranes rupture. Elevations above 38° C (100.4° F) should be reported. A rising FHR and fetal tachycardia (above 160 BPM) may precede maternal fever.

Promoting Comfort. Amniotic fluid continues to leak from the woman's vagina. Regularly changed underpads keep her drier and reduce the moist environment that favors bacterial growth.

Check Your Reading

1. What are three risks associated with amniotomy?
2. Why is the FHR assessed before and after the membranes rupture?
3. What is the significance of green amniotic fluid?
4. What maternal and fetal signs are associated with chorioamnionitis?

INDUCTION AND AUGMENTATION OF LABOR

Induction and augmentation of labor use artificial methods to stimulate uterine contractions. Techniques and nursing care are similar for both induction and augmentation.

Induction of labor is an increasingly common procedure in intrapartum units and has more than doubled in just over a decade. In 1989, 9% of live births were induced compared with 19.2% in 1998 (Curtin & Mathews, 2000).

Indications

Induction of labor is performed when a continued pregnancy may jeopardize the health of the woman or fetus and labor and vaginal birth are considered safe. Labor induction is not done if the fetus must be delivered more quickly than the process permits, in which case a cesarean birth is performed. Induction is indicated in these conditions (ACOG, 1999a):

- Pregnancy-induced hypertension, which is associated with reduced placental blood flow
- Spontaneous rupture of the membranes at or near term without onset of labor, also called *premature rupture of the membranes (PROM)*
- Chorioamnionitis (inflammation of the amniotic sac)
- Maternal medical conditions that worsen with continuation of the pregnancy (such as diabetes, renal disease, pulmonary disease, heart disease)
- Conditions in which the intrauterine environment is hostile to fetal well-being (intrauterine fetal growth restriction, postterm gestation, maternal-fetal blood incompatibility)
- Abruptio placentae
- Fetal death

Induction solely for convenience is not recommended. However, factors such as having a history of rapid labors and living a long distance from the hospital are valid reasons to induce labor because of the real possibility that the baby would be born in uncontrolled circumstances. Considerations such as maternity leave also may be valid.

Prenatal diagnosis sometimes identifies a fetal anomaly that will require specialized neonatal care at a distant facility. The mother may be transported to that facility for labor induction with needed equipment and specialists to care for the newborn.

Augmentation of labor with oxytocin is considered when labor has begun spontaneously but progress has slowed or stopped because of poor contractions (dystocia).

Contraindications

Any contraindication to labor and vaginal birth is a contraindication to induction or augmentation of labor. Possible contraindications and cautions to induction include the following (ACOG, 1999a):

- Complete placenta previa, which would result in hemorrhage during labor
- Umbilical cord prolapse
- Abnormal fetal presentation for which vaginal birth is often more hazardous (fetus may turn to normal position before spontaneous labor occurs)
- Fetal presenting part above the pelvic inlet, which may be associated with cephalopelvic disproportion or a preterm fetus
- Active genital herpes infection, which can cause serious consequences if the fetus acquires it during passage through the birth canal
- Previous surgery in the upper uterus, such as a previous classical cesarean incision
- One or more previous low-transverse cesarean deliveries (a caution but not a contraindication)
- Conditions in which the uterus is overdistended, such as a multifetal pregnancy and hydramnios, because the risk of uterine rupture is higher
- Severe maternal conditions such as heart disease and severe hypertension
- Nonreassuring FHR patterns because the added stress of stimulated contractions will reduce placental perfusion

Risks

Induction and augmentation of labor, like spontaneous labor, are associated with risks:

- Hypertonic (excessive) uterine activity that can reduce placental perfusion and fetal oxygenation
- Uterine rupture
- Maternal water intoxication, which is more likely if a dextrose and water intravenous solution is used to dilute the oxytocin and with rates greater than 20 mU per minute (Cunningham, et al., 1997).

Table 16-1
BISHOP SCORING SYSTEM* TO EVALUATE THE CERVIX

Factor	Score 0	1	2	3
DILATION	0 cm	1 to 2 cm	3 to 4 cm	5 to 6 cm
EFFACEMENT	0% to 30%	40% to 50%	60% to 70%	80% or more
STATION	−3	−2	−1 or 0	+1 or +2
CERVICAL CONSISTENCY	Firm	Medium	Soft	
CERVICAL POSITION	Posterior	Middle	Anterior	

Adapted from Bishop, E.H. (1964). Pelvic scoring for elective induction. *Obstetrics and Gynecology,* 24(2), 266-268.
*This system is used to estimate how easily a woman's labor can be induced. Higher scores are associated with a greater likelihood of successful induction because her cervix has undergone prelabor changes, often called *ripening.* A woman who previously has given birth usually has a successful induction when her Bishop score is 5 or higher. A woman who is having her first baby is most successfully induced if her score is 7 or higher.

Two studies of more than 2500 births found that the risk for cesarean birth doubled when a woman was induced (Maslow & Sweeny, 2000; Seyb, et al., 1999). The increased risk for cesarean birth was present regardless of whether the woman's induction was medically indicated or elective, having no medical indication. Total hospitalization costs also were higher for the induction group.

Technique

Surgical and medical methods may be used for labor induction and augmentation. Amniotomy is the method of surgical induction and augmentation because rupturing membranes stimulates uterine contractions and occasionally may be adequate in itself if the cervix is very favorable. Medical methods for induction and augmentation use drugs such as prostaglandins, intravenous oxytocin (Pitocin), or both to stimulate contractions.

Determining Whether Induction Is Indicated

The birth attendant evaluates whether the benefits of ending the pregnancy outweigh those of continuing it for the woman and fetus. Labor is not induced if the fetus is younger than 39 weeks unless a compelling reason exists. Also, induction is more likely to be successful at term because prelabor cervical changes favor dilation.

Cervical assessment estimates whether the cervix is favorable for induction. The Bishop scoring system (Table 16-1) is used to estimate cervical readiness for labor with five factors: cervical dilation, effacement, consistency, position, and fetal station. Induction is likely to be successful with a Bishop score higher than six.

The Bishop score is subjective and depends on the experience of the examiner. A more objective method to evaluate a woman's readiness for induction of labor is assessment of fetal fibronectin (fFN) in the cervical and vaginal secretions. fFN is a protein concentrated at the junction of the decidua and chorion. It is found in the vaginal secretions in decreasing amounts until about 20 weeks' gestation but then reappears in these secretions about 2 weeks before the onset of term labor (Garite, 2000; Parsons & Spellacy, 1999). fFN appears promising in the determination of which women will have the most successful induction, particularly if induction is not urgent.

Cervical Ripening

Procedures to ripen (soften) the cervix and make it more likely to dilate with the forces of labor are a common adjunct to induction. Most are done the day before the scheduled induction.

Chemical Methods. Prostaglandin is a drug that may be used to cause cervical ripening. Prostaglandin E_2 (PGE_2) preparations may be given as an intravaginal gel, an intracervical gel, and a timed-release vaginal insert (Table 16-2).

Misoprostol (Cytotec) is a prostaglandin E_1 (PGE_1) analog usually given for gastric ulcers. Misoprostol can be used for both cervical ripening and induction of labor. Misoprostol currently is not approved by the U.S. Food and Drug Administration for these purposes. In addition to its effectiveness, misoprostol is attractive for its low cost (about $0.36 to $1.20) and stability at room temperature (ACOG, 1999a). However, it should not be given to a woman who has had a previous cesarean birth.

Misoprostol is available in 100- and 200-mcg tablets. The usual dose is 25 mcg, one quarter of the already tiny, unscored 100-mcg tablet. The quarter-tablet is placed high in the vagina.

The major adverse reaction to prostaglandins is hyperstimulation of uterine contractions. Prostaglandins are administered in a setting in which fetal monitoring

Table 16-2
PROSTAGLANDIN E_2 PREPARATIONS FOR CERVICAL RIPENING

Hospital-Prepared Gel	Commercially Prepared Gel (Prepidil)	Commercially Prepared Vaginal Insert (Cervidil)
DOSAGE		
For vaginal application: up to 5 mg For intracervical application: 0.5 mg (Repeat up to three times in 24 hr at 4 to 6-hr intervals.)	For intracervical application: 0.5 mg. Repeat up to three times in 24 hr at 6-hr intervals.	10 mg in a time-released vaginal insert. Rate of release is 0.3 mg/hr. Remove at onset of active labor or 12 hr after insertion.
ACTIONS FOR UTERINE HYPERSTIMULATION		
Side-lying position Oxygen by face mask at 8 to 10 L/min Tocolytic drug such as terbutaline or magnesium sulfate	Same as for hospital-prepared gel	Remove insert. Implement actions as for hospital-prepared gel if necessary.
WHEN OXYTOCIN FOR INDUCTION MAY BEGIN		
4 hr after last dose	At least 6 hr after last dose	30 min after removal of insert

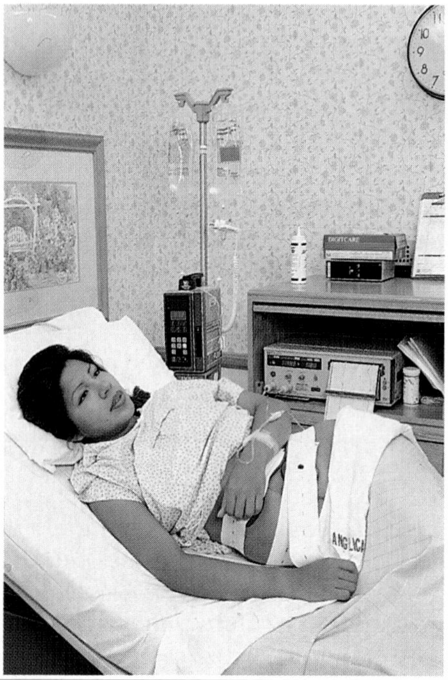

FIGURE 16-2 IV oxytocin setup for induction or augmentation of labor. The primary line (nonadditive, or maintenance line) on the left side of the pole contains no medication. The secondary line with the orange "medication added" label contains oxytocin. The secondary oxytocin line is regulated by the infusion pump and is inserted into the lowest port in the primary fluid line. An external fetal monitor is used to assess the fetal response to oxytocin-stimulated contractions. The woman lies on her side to promote uterine blood flow.

and emergency care are immediately available. Prostaglandin should be given cautiously to women who have asthma, glaucoma, and pulmonary, hepatic, and renal disease. The woman should lie flat for 15 to 20 minutes after the gel is inserted to reduce leakage. The FHR should be monitored for at least 30 minutes for changes, and the uterus should be assessed for excessive contractions.

Mechanical Methods. The most common mechanical method for cervical ripening involves placing hydrophilic (moisture-attracting) inserts into the cervical canal, where they absorb water and swell, gradually dilating the cervix. Examples of these dilators are the following:

- Dilapan—a synthetic material
- Lamicel—a synthetic sponge containing 450 mg of magnesium sulfate
- Laminaria tents—sterile, cone-shaped preparations of dried seaweed

Oxytocin Adminstration

Oxytocin is the most common drug given for induction and augmentation of labor (Drug Guide). Oxytocin is a powerful drug, and predicting a woman's response to it is impossible. Several precautions reduce the chance of adverse reactions in the mother and fetus.

- Oxytocin is diluted in a physiologic, electrolyte-containing fluid and given as a secondary (piggyback) infusion so that it can be stopped quickly if complications develop (Figure 16-2).
- The oxytocin line is inserted into the primary (nonadditive or maintenance) IV line as close as possible to the venipuncture site (the proximal port) to limit the amount of drug infused after changing to the nonadditive fluid.
- Oxytocin is started slowly, increased gradually, and regulated with an infusion pump.
- Uterine activity and FHR and patterns are monitored when oxytocin is given.

DRUG GUIDE: Oxytocin (Pitocin)

Classification: Oxytocic.

Action: Synthetic compound identical to the natural hormone from the posterior pituitary. Stimulates uterine smooth muscle, resulting in increased strength, duration, and frequency of uterine contractions. Uterine sensitivity to oxytocin increases gradually during gestation. Has vasoactive and antidiuretic properties.

Indications: Induction or augmentation of labor at or near term. Maintenance of firm uterine contraction after birth to control postpartum bleeding. Management of inevitable or incomplete abortion.

Dosage and Route: *Induction or augmentation of labor:*

1. IV infusion via a secondary (piggyback) line. Dilute 10 units (1 ml) of oxytocin in 1000 ml of a balanced electrolyte solution such as lactated Ringer's solution, resulting in a concentration of 10 milliunits (mU) of oxytocin per milliliter. Other mixtures of oxytocin and solution may be used, such as 15 units of oxytocin (1.5 ml) with 250 ml IV solution, resulting in a concentration of 60 mU/ml. Oxytocin infusion is controlled with a pump. The drug also may be given in 10-minute pulsed infusions rather than continuously to better simulate spontaneous labor.
2. Administration protocols vary, but a guideline from the American College of Obstetricians and Gynecologists (1999a) provides examples of two protocols: a low-dose and high-dose protocol.
   Low-dose protocol—(a) starting dosages of 0.5 to 1 mU/minute and (b) increasing dosage by 1 mU/minute increments every 30 to 40 minutes.
   High-dose protocol—(a) starting dosages of about 6 mU/minute and (b) increasing dosage by either 6-, 3-, or 1-mU/minute increments every 20 to 40 minutes.
   The actual oxytocin dose is based on uterine response and absence of adverse effects. Shorter intervals between dose increases may result in uterine hyperstimulation. A lower starting dose usually is required to augment labor.
3. After an adequate contraction pattern is established and the cervix is dilated 5 to 6 cm, the oxytocin may be reduced by similar increments.

Control of postpartum bleeding: IV infusion—Dilute 10 to 40 units in 1000 ml of IV solution. The rate of infusion must control uterine atony. Begin at a rate of 20 to 40 mU/minute, increasing or decreasing rate according to uterine response and rate of postpartum bleeding.

Intramuscular injection—10 units after delivery of placenta

Inevitable or incomplete abortion: Dilute 10 units in 500 ml of intravenous solution, and infuse at 10 to 20 mU/minute

Absorption: Intravenous, immediate; intramuscular, 3 to 5 minutes

Excretion: Liver and urine

Contraindications and Precautions: Include but are not limited to placenta previa, vasa previa, nonreassuring FHR patterns, abnormal fetal presentation, prolapsed umbilical cord, presenting part above the pelvic inlet, previous classic uterine incision, active genital herpes infection, pelvic structural deformities, and invasive cervical carcinoma

Adverse Reactions: Most result from hypersensitivity to drug or excessive dosage. Adverse reactions include hypertonic uterine activity, impaired uterine blood flow, uterine rupture, and abruptio placentae. Uterine hypertonicity may result in fetal bradycardia, tachycardia, reduced FHR variability, and late decelerations. Fetal asphyxia may occur with diminished uterine blood flow. Fetal trauma, maternal trauma, or both may occur from rapid birth. Prolonged administration may cause maternal fluid retention, leading to water intoxication. Hypotension (seen with rapid IV injection), tachycardia, cardiac dysrhythmias, and subarachnoid hemorrhage are rare adverse reactions.

Nursing Considerations:

Intrapartum: Assess FHR for at least 20 minutes before induction to identify reassuring or nonreassuring patterns. Perform Leopold's maneuvers, a vaginal examination, or both to identify fetal presentation. Do not begin induction and notify physician if nonreassuring FHR patterns are identified or fetal presentation is other than cephalic.

Observe uterine activity for establishment of effective labor pattern: contraction frequency every 2 to 3 minutes, duration 40 to 90 seconds, and intensity 50 to 80 mm Hg (using intrauterine pressure catheter). Observe for hypertonic uterine activity: contractions less than 2 minutes apart, rest interval shorter than 60 seconds, duration longer than 90 seconds, an elevated resting tone greater than 20 mm Hg with an intrauterine pressure catheter, and Montevideo units exceeding 250. Observe FHR for nonreassuring patterns such as tachycardia, bradycardia, decreased variability, and late decelerations.

If uterine hypertonicity or a nonreassuring FHR pattern occurs, intervene to reduce uterine activity and increase fetal oxygenation: stop oxytocin infusion; increase rate of nonadditive solution; position woman in side-lying position; and administer oxygen by snug face mask at 8 to 10 L/minute. Notify physician of adverse reactions, nursing interventions, and response to interventions. Record maternal blood pressure every 30 to 60 minutes or with each dosage increase. Record intake and output.

Postpartum: Observe uterus for firmness, height, and deviation. Massage until firm if uterus is soft (boggy). Observe lochia for color, quantity, and presence of clots. Notify birth attendant if uterus fails to remain contracted or if lochia is bright red or contains large clots. Assess for cramping. Assess vital signs every 15 minutes or according to protocol. Monitor intake and output to identify fluid retention or bladder distention.

Inevitable or incomplete abortion: Observe for cramping, vaginal bleeding, clots, and passage of products of conception. Observe maternal vital signs, intake, and output as noted under postpartum nursing implications.

The woman's uterus becomes more sensitive to oxytocin as labor progresses. Therefore the rate of oxytocin infusion may be gradually reduced when she is in the active phase of labor (about 5 to 6 cm of cervical dilation). It may be stopped or reduced after her membranes rupture. When labor is augmented with oxytocin, a lower total dose usually is needed to achieve adequate contractions.

Serial Induction of Labor

Serial induction of labor is an occasional variation that may be encountered. Serial induction may be performed when the woman's cervix is not favorable and she has an indication for induction, but same-day birth is not imperative. For example, serial induction may be performed for postdate pregnancy (gestation past the expected delivery date).

Oxytocin solution is given over a 2- to 3-day period for about 8 to 10 hours each day. If the woman's labor has not made progress during the day, the oxytocin is stopped, she is given a light meal, and the infusion is resumed the next morning. At the end of the third day, the woman is reevaluated if she is not yet in labor.

Active Management of Labor

Active management of labor is a protocol for labor augmentation that first was used in Ireland. It applies only to nulliparous women in spontaneous labor at term and is aimed at reducing the cesarean birth rate in this group. The goal of active labor management is to achieve birth within 12 hours of admission. Criteria for diagnosing labor and defining abnormal labor progress are strict.

If the membranes remain intact, amniotomy is performed within 1 hour of admission. Oxytocin augmentation is begun if the rate of progress is less than 1 cm per hour after amniotomy. Oxytocin dosages given by the Irish protocol are higher than those typical in the United States. Cesarean delivery may be performed 12 hours after admission if birth is not imminent.

Nursing Considerations

When providing care during cervical ripening and labor induction or augmentation, the nurse observes the woman and fetus for complications and takes corrective actions if abnormalities are noted. The nurse has a great responsibility when administering uterine stimulants to a pregnant woman. The nurse must decide when to start, change, and stop an oxytocin infusion using the facility's protocols and medical orders. This responsibility requires additional education and refinement of the nurse's critical thinking skills.

Observing the Fetal Response

Oxytocin stimulates uterine contractions, and they may become too strong or hypertonic (hyperstimulation). Uterine hyperstimulation can reduce placental blood flow (uteroplacental insufficiency), which decreases exchange of fetal oxygen and waste products. Before induction and augmentation of labor, the nurse determines whether the FHR and patterns are reassuring. The FHR is charted in the labor record at least every 30 minutes during first-stage labor and every 15 minutes during second-stage labor. If risk factors are present, the interval is reduced to every 15 minutes during first-stage labor and every 5 minutes during second-stage labor (see Chapters 13 and 14).

The nurse remains alert for fetal heart patterns suggesting reduced placental exchange secondary to hypertonic contractions. Examples are fetal bradycardia (rate <110 to 120 BPM at term), tachycardia (rate >150 to 160 BPM at term), late decelerations (after the peak of the contraction and persisting after the contraction ends), and decreased FHR variability (reduced rate fluctuations). Reduced placental exchange also may have causes other than excess uterine activity, such as maternal hypotension. The nurse must assess the woman and fetus carefully to identify the most likely cause of the problem and institute corrective actions.

CRITICAL THINKING EXERCISE

A woman is having labor induced with oxytocin. Her cervix is 4 cm dilated and fully effaced, and the fetal head is at station 0. The nurse notes that the FHR (internal monitor) is near its baseline of 120 to 130 BPM, with a variability of 10 BPM. Contractions are firm, occur every 2 to 2.5 minutes, and typically last 95 to 100 seconds. Montevideo units average 260.

QUESTIONS:

1. What is the correct interpretation of these assessments?
2. What are appropriate nursing actions in this situation, and why are they done?

If nonreassuring patterns occur or contractions are hypertonic, the nurse takes steps to reduce uterine activity and increase fetal oxygenation.

1. Reduce or stop the oxytocin infusion and increase the rate of the primary nonadditive infusion.
2. Keep the woman in a nonsupine position (usually sidelying) to prevent aortocaval compression and increase placental blood flow.
3. Give 100% by face mask at 8 to 10 L/min to increase the woman's oxygen saturation, making more available for the fetus.

The physician may order a drug to reduce uterine activity, such as terbutaline (Brethine) and magnesium sulfate.

Observing the Mother's Response

If the woman who had a cervical ripening procedure is discharged overnight, the signs of labor's onset should

CRITICAL TO REMEMBER

Signs of Hypertonic Uterine Activity

- Contraction duration longer than 90 seconds
- Contractions occurring less than 2 minutes apart or relaxation of less than 60 seconds between contractions
- Uterine resting tone above 20 mmHg (with intrauterine pressure catheter)
- Peak pressure higher than 90 mmHg during first-stage labor (with intrauterine pressure catheter)
- Montevideo units exceeding 250
- A FHR pattern of late decelerations accompanying hypertonic uterine activity

Nursing Actions for Hypertonic Uterine Activity

- Reduce or stop the oxytocin infusion
- Increase the rate of the primary nonadditive infusion
- Keep the laboring woman in a lateral position
- Give oxygen by face mask, 8 to 10 L/min
- Notify the physician or nurse-midwife

be reviewed (see p. 273) and she should be instructed to return to the birth facility if they occur or she has other concerns.

Uterine activity must be assessed for hypertonus that may reduce fetal oxygenation and contribute to uterine rupture. Contractions are assessed for frequency, duration, and intensity, and uterine resting tone is assessed for relaxation of at least 60 seconds between contractions. A maximal value of 250 is commonly used for Montevideo units when oxytocin is being administered, although they may reach slightly higher maximal values in spontaneous labor. Uterine activity observations are charted at the same intervals as the FHR. Corrective actions for hypertonic uterine activity are the same as those listed in the discussion of the fetal response.

If the oxytocin must be discontinued, the decision about resuming it is individualized. The oxytocin infusion may be restarted at the same or lower dose if the contractions are no longer hypertonic and the FHR is reassuring. If the oxytocin has been discontinued for as long as 40 minutes, the drug that was in the woman's system has been metabolized. Therefore it should be restarted at the beginning dose ordered and advanced more slowly to prevent a recurrence of uterine hyperstimulation and nonreassuring FHR patterns.

The woman's blood pressure and pulse are taken every 30 to 60 minutes or with each oxytocin dose change increase to identify changes from her baseline. Her temperature is checked every 2 to 4 hours to identify infection that can occur with ruptured membranes.

The woman may need to use pharmacologic and nonpharmacologic pain management techniques sooner. Although the goal of induced and augmented labor is to mimic natural labor, stimulated contractions often increase in intensity more quickly.

Recording intake and output identifies fluid retention, which may precede water intoxication. Signs and symptoms of water intoxication include headache, blurred vision, behavioral changes, increased blood pressure and respirations, decreased pulse, rales, wheezing, and coughing. Water intoxication is more likely when larger doses of oxytocin are given, such as a multiday serial induction and higher infusion rates.

After birth, the mother is observed for postpartum hemorrhage caused by uterine relaxation, similar to the mother who had spontaneous labor. Postpartum uterine atony is more likely if she has received oxytocin for a long time because the uterine muscle becomes fatigued and does not contract effectively to compress vessels at the placental site. It is manifested by a soft uterine fundus and excess amounts of lochia, usually with large clots. Hypovolemic shock may occur with hemorrhage.

Check Your Reading

5. What precautions are taken to enhance the safety of oxytocin administration for the woman and fetus?
6. How may oxytocin administration differ if labor is being augmented rather than induced?
7. What signs may indicate an abnormal fetal response to oxytocin?
8. What are the signs of hypertonic uterine activity?
9. How can induction of labor with oxytocin contribute to postpartum hemorrhage?

VERSION

Either of two methods may be used to change fetal presentation: external cephalic and internal version. Each has different indications and technique. External cephalic version is much more common.

Indications

External Cephalic Version. The fetus may be changed from breech, shoulder (transverse lie), and oblique presentations to a cephalic presentation using external version. Successful version may allow the woman to avoid a cesarean birth. A review of 20 studies showed that an average of 58% of versions successfully turned the fetus from the breech to cephalic presentation (ACOG, 2000). Another study had almost a 63% success rate (Regalia, et al., 2000).

Internal Version. Malpresentation in twin gestations is usually managed by cesarean birth, but internal version is sometimes used for the vaginal birth of the second twin.

Contraindications

External cephalic version is not done if a woman is unlikely to have vaginal birth, which is the goal of the procedure. Contraindications are similar for internal and external procedures. Maternal and fetal conditions that may contraindicate external cephalic version and reduce its success include the following:

- Uterine malformations that limit the room available to perform the version and may be the reason for the abnormal fetal presentation
- Previous cesarean birth with a vertical uterine incision—Manipulation of the fetus within the uterus may strain and rupture the old incision.
- Disproportion between fetal size and maternal pelvic size
- Placenta previa—Manipulation of the fetus within the uterus may cause hemorrhage, endangering both mother and fetus. Placenta previa other than marginal is an indication for cesarean birth.
- Multifetal gestation, which reduces available room to turn the fetus or fetuses. External cephalic version may be attempted after the first twin is born vaginally.
- Oligohydramnios, ruptured membranes, and a cord around the fetal body or neck (nuchal cord) —These conditions limit the room to turn the fetus and may lead to cord compression and fetal hypoxia.
- Uteroplacental insufficiency—Uterine contractions occurring during the version and labor may worsen the insufficiency and cause fetal compromise.
- Engagement of the fetal head into the pelvis

Risks

Few risks to the woman are present. The principal risk is that the fetus may become entangled in the umbilical cord, compressing its vessels and resulting in hypoxia. Abruptio placentae also may occur if fetal manipulation disrupts the placental site. Fetal and maternal blood could become mixed because of small breaks in placental vessels, possibly resulting in maternal sensitization to the fetal blood type. Cesarean birth may be needed for fetal compromise at the time of the external version or later if the fetus returns to an abnormal presentation.

Technique

External Cephalic Version. External cephalic version is performed at a location and time to allow emergency cesarean delivery if necessary. A nonstress test or biophysical profile (see Chapter 10) is done before the procedure to evaluate fetal health and placental function. If nonreassuring fetal signs are present, the version is not performed. External cephalic version would add stress to the fetus, who already is functioning with reduced physiologic reserve. An ultrasound examination confirms fetal gestational age and presentation and identifies adequacy of amniotic fluid.

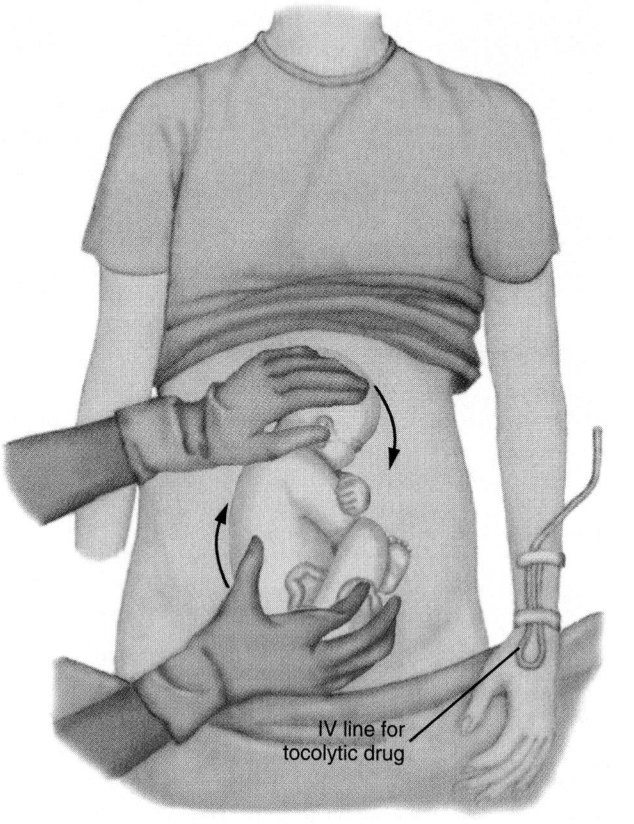

FIGURE 16-3 External cephalic version.

External cephalic version usually is attempted after 37 weeks' gestation but before the woman is in labor for the following reasons:

- As term nears, the fetus may spontaneously turn to a cephalic presentation.
- The fetus is more likely to return to an abnormal presentation if version is attempted before 37 weeks' gestation.
- If fetal compromise and onset of labor occur, a fetus born after 37 weeks' gestation is not likely to have major problems associated with preterm birth, such as respiratory distress syndrome.

The woman often is given a tocolytic drug such as terbutaline to relax the uterus while the version is performed. Some physicians use epidural and subarachnoid block analgesia and IV sedation to reduce discomfort during the procedure. Other physicians avoid these pain-relief methods because they feel that the mother's discomfort is an important guide to knowing if they have manipulated the uterus excessively during the procedure (Asrat & Quilligan, 2000).

Real-time ultrasonography guides fetal manipulations during external cephalic version and monitors the FHR about every 2 minutes. The physician gently pushes the breech out of the pelvis in a forward or backward roll (Figure 16-3).

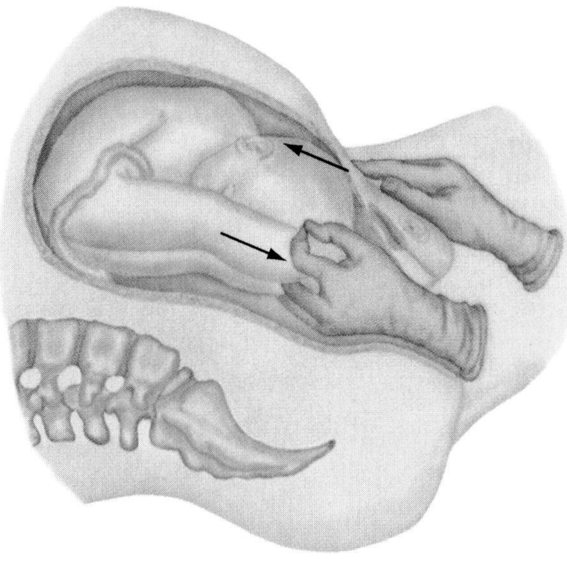

FIGURE 16-4 Internal version for vaginal birth of a second twin.

If indicated, Rh immunoglobulin (RhoGAM) is given to the Rh-negative woman after external version to prevent Rh sensitization.

Internal Version. Internal version is an unexpected procedure. The physician reaches into the uterus with one hand and with the other hand on the maternal abdomen, maneuvers the fetus into a longitudinal lie (cephalic or breech) (Figure 16-4) to allow delivery.

Nursing Considerations

When caring for the woman having external version, the nurse provides information, assesses the woman and fetus, and helps reduce her anxiety.

Providing Information

The birth attendant explains the indications and risks for external cephalic version to the woman before she signs an informed consent. The nurse verifies the woman's understanding of the purposes, risks, and limitations of the procedure.

The purposes and side effects of any planned tocolytic drug are reviewed. Tachycardia and tremors are common side effects of tocolytics such as terbutaline and stop shortly after the medication is discontinued at the end of the procedure.

Promoting Maternal and Fetal Health

Admission information is collected as if the woman were in labor or having a cesarean birth because the need for operative intervention may arise suddenly. The woman should have nothing by mouth during this short procedure. An IV line is placed.

Maternal vital signs are assessed, and fetal monitoring is begun to obtain baseline values and evaluate the initial nonstress test or biophysical profile. Abnormalities and nonreassuring FHR patterns should be reported promptly. Fetal bradycardia may occur during the procedure, but the FHR usually returns to normal when manipulation ends. The nurse administers the tocolytic drug. The blood pressure and pulse are checked every 5 minutes.

After the version, the tocolytic drug is discontinued if given by IV infusion. The mother and fetus are observed for at least 1 hour after the procedure for a return of their vital signs to baseline values. Reassuring fetal signs are a heart rate about the same range as on admission, resolution of any bradycardia, and the presence of FHR accelerations.

Maternal vital signs are taken every 15 minutes until they return to their baseline level. The presence of regular contractions suggests onset of labor. Spontaneous rupture of membranes sometimes occurs, with leakage of fluid from the mother's vagina. RhoGAM is given if indicated.

Discomfort should diminish quickly after the version. Persistent and continuous pain suggests a complication such as abruptio placentae.

Because the woman having external cephalic version is near term, the nurse should review the signs of true labor with her and explain guidelines for returning to the hospital (see Chapter 13).

Reducing Anxiety

The woman may be anxious before version because its success is not certain and complications may require emergency cesarean delivery. Afterwards, she still may be anxious because the fetus can return to its previous position. The nurse should keep her informed about what is occurring during the version to reduce her fear of the unknown.

The expectant mother and her partner are probably concerned about the fetal condition. The nurse can point out reassuring fetal monitor patterns such as a normal rate and rate accelerations to help reduce anxiety about the baby. If problems develop, such as bradycardia, the nurse should explain what has happened, what steps are being done to relieve it, and the result of these interventions.

Check Your Reading

10. Why is observing the FHR important during and after external cephalic version?
11. Why should the uterine activity be monitored after external cephalic version?

FORCEPS AND VACUUM EXTRACTION

The physician may use forceps or vacuum extraction to apply traction to the fetal head during birth, aiding the woman's expulsive efforts. Both techniques assist

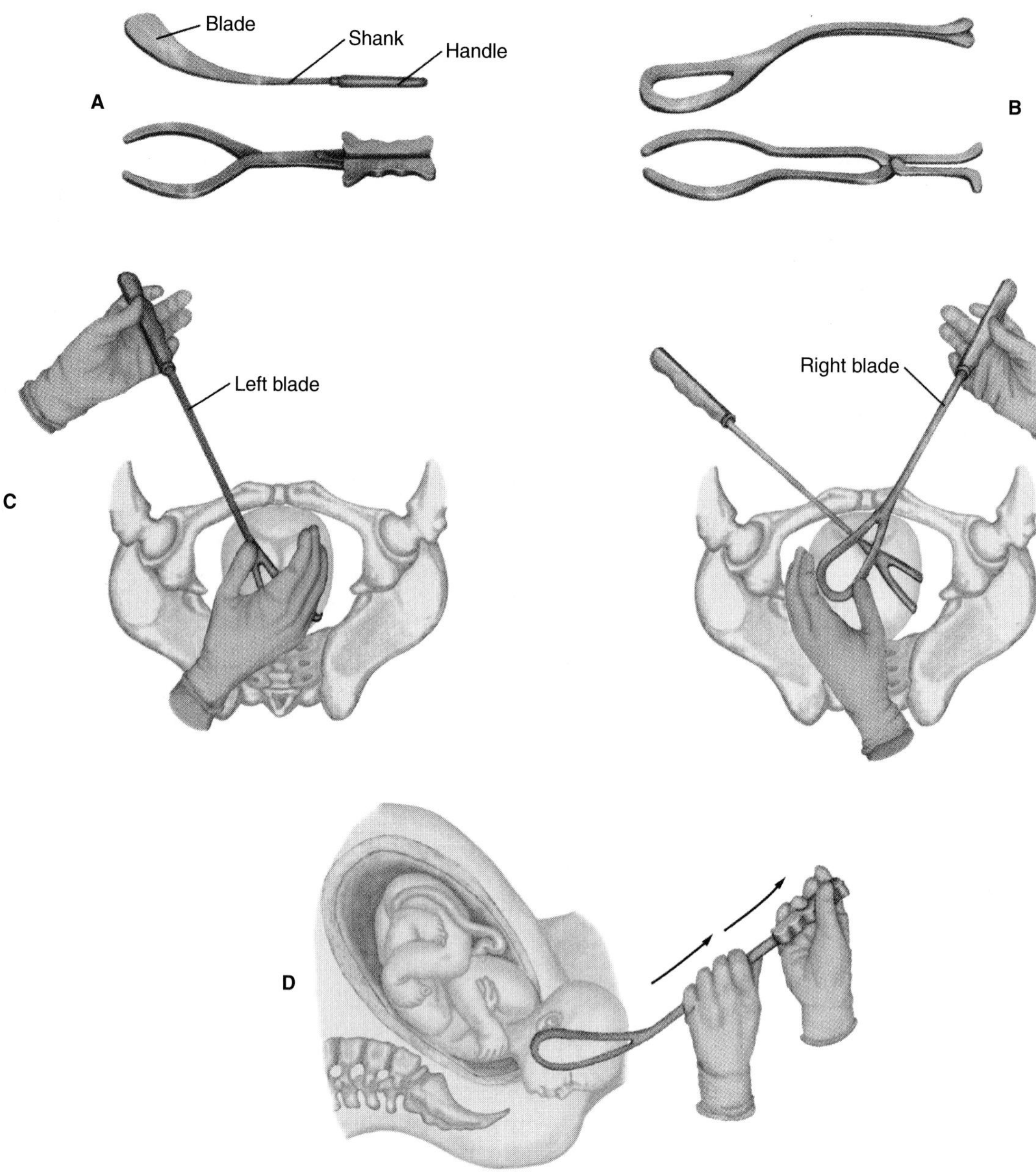

FIGURE 16-5 Obstetric forceps and their application. **A,** Solid blade Tucker-McLean forceps. **B,** Piper forceps, used to deliver the head when the fetus is in a breech presentation. **C,** Application of forceps with an open (fenestrated) blade. **D,** Direction of traction in a forceps-assisted birth.

descent only or both descent and rotation of the fetal head from an occiput posterior or occiput transverse position to the occiput anterior position.

Forceps are curved, metal instruments with two curved blades that can be locked in the center. Many styles are available for different needs. The blades may be closed or open and are shaped to grasp the fetal head (Figure 16-5). Disposable foam pads are available to cushion the fetal head from the blades. Piper forceps are a special type used to assist birth of the head as it is born last in a vaginal breech birth. Forceps and a vacuum extractor also may be used during cesarean birth.

A vacuum extractor uses suction to grasp the fetal head while traction is applied (Figure 16-6). The vacuum extractor was used more than twice as frequently as forceps for births in 1998 (Curtin & Mathews, 2000). It is not used to deliver the fetus in a nonvertex presentation such as breech or face; otherwise, its use is similar to that of forceps. It also is not used for the very preterm fetus because the suction is more likely to injure the head, scalp, and intracranial vessels (Newnham & Hobel, 1998).

Indications

Forceps or vacuum extraction is considered if the second stage should be shortened for the well-being of the woman, fetus, or both and if vaginal birth can be accomplished quickly without undue trauma. Maternal

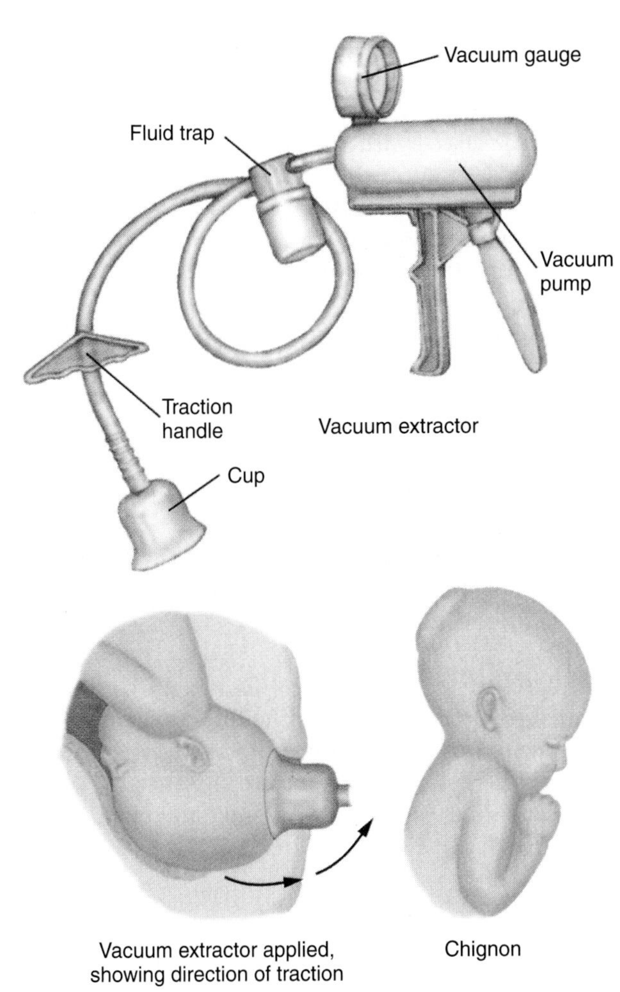

FIGURE 16-6 Birth assisted with a vacuum extractor. The chignon is scalp edema that often forms under the suction cup when the vacuum extractor is used.

indications may include exhaustion, inability to push effectively, and cardiac and pulmonary disease. Fetal indications may include nonreassuring FHR patterns or failure of the fetal presenting part to fully rotate and descend in the pelvis.

Contraindications

Cesarean birth is preferable if the maternal and fetal conditions mandate a more rapid birth than can be accomplished with forceps or vacuum extraction and if the procedure would be too traumatic. Examples of these conditions are severe fetal compromise, acute maternal conditions such as congestive heart failure and pulmonary edema, a high fetal station, and disproportion between the size of the fetus and maternal pelvis.

Risks

The main risk of forceps and vacuum extraction is trauma to maternal and fetal tissues. Because of the relative safety of cesarean birth, the attempt at an instrumental birth usually is abandoned if the fetal head does not descend easily.

Maternal risks include laceration and hematoma of the vagina. The infant may have ecchymoses, facial and scalp lacerations and abrasions, facial nerve injury, cephalhematoma, subgaleal hemorrhage, and intracranial hemorrhage. A vacuum extractor may create scalp edema called a *chignon* at the application area (see Figure 16-6).

Technique

Preparation for forceps or vacuum extraction is similar to that for any vaginal birth. The presentation, position, and station of the fetal presenting part are verified. The woman is catheterized to provide more room in the pelvis and limit bladder trauma. Membranes must be ruptured and the cervix completely dilated for forceps or vacuum extraction birth. The woman needs adequate anesthesia, usually a regional block such as an epidural.

Forceps and vacuum extractor–assisted births are classified according to the extent of descent of the fetal head into the pelvis during the procedure and necessary degree of rotation for the fetal head to be born (AAP & ACOG, 1997).

Outlet. The fetal head is at or on the perineum, and the scalp is visible at the vaginal opening without separating the labia. The fetal skull has reached the pelvic floor. The position is OA, ROA, LOA, or OP.

Low. The leading edge of the fetal skull is at station +2 (about 2 cm below the level of the mother's ischial spines) or lower and not on the pelvic floor.

Midforceps. The leading edge of the fetal skull is between a 0 (at the level of the ischial spines) and +2 station.

The physician determines the presentation, position, and station of the fetal head and amount of cervical dilation. When correctly applied, the long axis of the blades lies over the fetal cheeks and parietal bones. After checking for proper application, the physician locks the two blades in the center and pulls gently, following the curve of the pelvis. An episiotomy is usually performed as the fetal head distends the perineum. The physician may keep the forceps on until the head is born or may remove the blades just before expulsion. The rest of the fetus is born in the usual way.

For vacuum extraction, the cup is connected to a machine that creates a vacuum to hold the cup on the fetal head in the midline of the occiput. The physician may apply traction intermittently, as in forceps birth, or maintain traction between contraction to avoid losing fetal head descent.

The advantage of vacuum extraction is that the vacuum cup does not take up space on either side of the fetal head, unlike forceps. Also, use of excessive force to deliver a fetus is more difficult because the cup will dislodge if too much traction is applied. However, the preterm infant is more likely to be injured by the vacuum because the tissues are more delicate.

Nursing Considerations

When a forceps or vacuum extraction birth is anticipated, a catheter is added to the instrument table for the birth unless the woman has an indwelling catheter. The physician specifies the type of forceps and vacuum cup. If the nurse must apply the suction to the cup, suction should not go outside the green zone on the suction indicator. FHR should be assessed and any rate lower than 100 BPM reported.

After birth, the mother and infant are observed for trauma. The mother may have vaginal wall lacerations or hematoma. Vaginal wall lacerations bleed brighter red than normal lochia and somewhat continuously. The fundus usually is firm unless uterine atony also is present. Women with vaginal wall hematomas complain of severe and unrelenting pain and may have edema and discoloration of the labia and perineum. Cold applications for the first 12 hours reduce pain by numbing the area and limit bruising and edema of the tissues. Heat applications after 12 hours aid resolution of the edema and bruising.

The infant often has reddening and mild bruising of the skin where the forceps were applied. These areas do not need treatment. Cold treatment is not done for an infant because of hypothermia. Skin breaks that allow entry of microorganisms should be noted and kept clean. Facial asymmetry, which is most obvious when the infant cries, suggests facial nerve injury.

> After a forceps birth a parent may ask why the baby's cheeks are reddened or bruised. A good response is to explain that the pressure of the forceps on the baby's delicate skin may cause minor bruising that usually resolves without treatment. Point out improvement in the area during the postpartum stay.

Episiotomy

Episiotomy is the most common operation in women and is performed on 70% of primiparas and 30% of multiparas (Newton, 2000). Routine performance of an episiotomy remains controversial. However, the decision about whether to do an episiotomy must be made just before birth, and indications are not always clear.

Indications

Fetal indications for episiotomy are similar to those for forceps and vacuum extraction. Episiotomy may be done to reduce pressure on the head when a small, preterm infant is born.

Maternal benefits are less clear. Episiotomy was once thought to limit perineal trauma and reduce relaxation of pelvic floor muscles. Pelvic floor relaxation is associated with uterine prolapse and stress incontinence. Better-controlled studies have questioned these benefits, however. Although an episiotomy provides some control over the direction and extent of any opening in the perineum, a midline episiotomy, the most common kind, is associated with a higher incidence of the more severe third- and fourth-degree lacerations extending from the episiotomy. Other studies also showed that episiotomies did not exert a protective effect in preventing stress incontinence (Newton, 2000). However, the episiotomy has clean edges rather than irregular edges like a laceration, making for simpler repair.

Risks

Infection is the main risk of episiotomy. Perineal pain occurs with both episiotomy and spontaneous tears. However, perineal pain may last longer with episiotomy, mainly because of its tendency to extend into deeper lacerations. Prolonged perineal pain impairs resumption of sexual intercourse and makes it uncomfortable for the woman.

Technique

An episiotomy is done when the fetal presenting part has crowned to a diameter of about 3 to 4 cm. The two types of episiotomies have different advantages and disadvantages: median (midline) and mediolateral (Figure 16-7).

Nursing Considerations

An episiotomy sometimes can be avoided or limited in length with nursing measures. An upright position while pushing promotes gradual stretching of the woman's perineum. Daily perineal massage and stretching by the woman from about 34 weeks' gestation until birth has been shown to reduce the risk for perineal trauma during birth (Eason, Labrecque, Wells, & Feldman, 2000). The birth attendant must promote this action on the woman's part.

Nursing interventions during the recovery and postpartum periods are similar for episiotomy and perineal laceration. The perineum should be observed for hematoma and edema. As with use of forceps, perineal cold applications are done for at least the first 12 hours and followed by perineal heat.

Check Your Reading

12. What are the similarities in the uses of forceps and vacuum extractors? What are the differences?
13. Why should the nurse add a urinary catheter to the instrument table if a forceps-assisted birth is expected?
14. A woman has a forceps birth with a median episiotomy. What nursing interventions can make her more comfortable?
15. What injury is suggested by an asymmetric facial appearance when the infant cries?

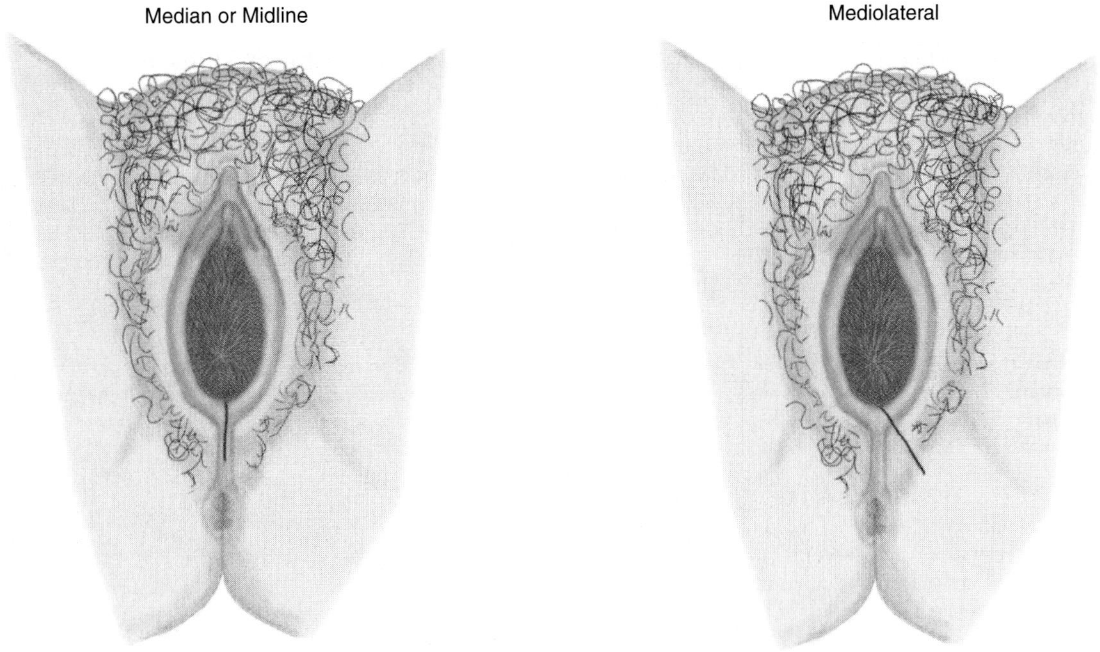

Median or Midline: Advantages	Median or Midline: Disadvantages	Mediolateral: Advantages	Mediolateral: Disadvantages
Minimal blood loss Neat healing with little scarring Less postpartum pain than the mediolateral episiotomy	An added laceration may extend the median episiotomy into the anal sphincter Limited enlargement of the vaginal opening because perineal length is limited by the anal sphincter	More enlargement of the vaginal opening Little risk that the episiotomy will extend into the anus	More blood loss Increased postpartum pain More scarring and irregularity in the healed scar Prolonged dyspareunia (painful intercourse)

FIGURE 16-7 Types of episiotomies.

CESAREAN BIRTH

In 1965 the cesarean birth rate in the United States was 4.5% of all births, rising to 24% in the late 1980s. The 1999 rate was 21.7% of all births. Of these cesareans, 14.9% were primary or first cesarean births (Curtin & Mathews, 2000). Preliminary data for 1999 shows a 22% cesarean birth rate (Curtin & Martin, 2000).

Many factors contributed to the rise in the national cesarean birth rate, some of which include the following:

- Relative safety of the surgery for the woman because of better choices in anesthesia such as the epidural block
- Use of cesarean to deliver most term and near-term fetuses in the breech presentation
- Use of cesarean to protect the fragile head of the immature preterm fetus from the forces of labor
- Smaller families and high consumer expectations of a perfect outcome for the birth
- Multimillion-dollar legal settlements if birth outcomes are not good

A national goal for the Healthy People 2010 initiative is to reduce the rate of first-time cesarean births in low-risk women to no more than 15.5% and reduce the percentage of repeat cesarean deliveries from the 1997 rate of 71% to 63% (U.S. Department of Health and Human Services, 2000). Efforts to accomplish the goal include (1) promotion of vaginal birth after cesarean (VBAC) (Table 16-3), (2) careful evaluation of dystocia, and (3) selection of some women to deliver their infants in the breech presentation. Because previous cesarean birth and dystocia contribute substantially to the current rate, promotion of VBAC and critical evaluation of dystocia can reduce the total rate. The American College of Obstetricians and Gynecologists noted that the continuous presence and support of educated individuals such as nurses also may help reduce the rates (ACOG, 2000b).

Experience with electronic fetal monitoring has improved knowledge of normal fetal responses to labor, promoting interventions for fetal benefit that may avoid cesarean delivery. Labor professionals increasingly recognize that simple interventions such as walking and squatting during the second stage may promote normal labor progress. However, epidural analgesia, the most popular choice, limits use of these measures.

Table 16-3

VAGINAL BIRTH AFTER CESAREAN BIRTH (VBAC)

General Information

- Between 60% and 80% of women with one low transverse uterine incision from a previous cesarean birth have successful VBACs.
- Women whose previous cesarean births were done for nonrecurring reasons such as a breech presentation or a nonreassuring FHR appear to have more success with VBAC than if primary cesarean birth were for dystocia or cephalopelvic disproportion.
- A woman who has had a previous vaginal birth before or after her cesarean birth is more likely to have a successful VBAC.
- Women who attempt VBAC and are unsuccessful have an increased risk for infection. Their infants also have an increased risk for neonatal infection.

Candidates for VBAC Include the Following:

- Most women with one previous cesarean birth with a low transverse uterine incision may be offered a trial of labor.
- A woman who has two previous low transverse uterine incisions and no contraindications and wishes to attempt VBAC should be advised that the risk for uterine rupture increases as the number of cesarean births increases.
- Epidural analgesia and anesthesia may be used when a woman is having VBAC.

Contraindications to VBAC Include the Following:

- A previous classic uterine incision or other uterine incision extending into the uterine fundus.
- A contracted pelvis that is too small for the fetus.
- Medical or obstetric complication that contraindicates vaginal birth.
- Inadequate facility or personnel resources to perform an emergency cesarean birth in a reasonable time.
- Use of oxytocin or prostaglandin gel for VBAC—requires close client monitoring.

Data from American College of Obstetricians and Gynecologists (ACOG). (1999). Vaginal birth after previous cesarean delivery. *ACOG practice bulletin, no. 5.* Washington, D.C.: Author.

One group of researchers found that regular exercise during pregnancy (at least 3 times per week) was associated with a lower risk for cesarean birth in nulliparas when compared with those who were sedentary (Bungum, Peaslee, Jackson, & Perez, 2000). The two groups were similar for length of labor, newborn birth weight, maternal weight gain, and length of gestation. Vaginal birth occurred in 84% of active women but only 72% of sedentary women. The most common type of exercise reported was vigorous walking.

Controversy exists about the wisdom of setting a numerical goal for cesarean births, and the issue is complex (Sachs, Kobelin, Castro, & Frigoletto, 1999; Young, 1999; ACOG, 1999c). One part of the plan to achieve the Healthy People 2010 cesarean birth target is to promote VBAC when appropriate. Recent evidence has shown that maternal and newborn complications are more frequent if VBAC is not successful. Also, some women do not want to attempt VBAC but prefer an elective repeat cesarean birth. For these reasons, some physicians argue against any target percentage set by the government and managed care.

Indications

Cesarean birth is performed when awaiting vaginal birth would compromise the mother, fetus, or both. Possible indications for cesarean birth include but are not limited to the following:

- Dystocia
- Cephalopelvic (fetopelvic) disproportion
- Pregnancy-induced hypertension if prompt delivery is necessary
- Maternal diseases such as diabetes, heart disease, or cervical cancer if labor is not advisable
- Active genital herpes
- Some previous uterine surgical procedures such as a classic cesarean incision
- Persistent nonreassuring FHR patterns
- Prolapsed umbilical cord
- Fetal malpresentations such as breech or transverse lie
- Hemorrhagic conditions such as abruptio placentae or placenta previa

Contraindications

Few absolute contraindications exist, but cesarean birth in some conditions is not desirable because the risks to the woman are too great compared with the potential benefits to the woman and fetus. These conditions include fetal death, a fetus that is too immature to survive, and maternal coagulation defects.

Risks

Cesarean birth is one of the safest major surgical procedures; however, it poses greater risk for the mother than vaginal birth. Maternal risks include the following:

- Infection
- Hemorrhage
- Urinary tract trauma
- Thrombophlebitis
- Paralytic ileus
- Atelectasis
- Anesthesia complications such as aspiration of gastric contents

Cesarean delivery poses added risks to the infant, which may include the following:

- Inadvertent preterm birth
- Transient tachypnea of the newborn caused by delayed absorption of lung fluid (see p. 842)
- Persistent pulmonary hypertension of the newborn (see p. 846)
- Injury such as laceration, bruising, and other trauma

Lung immaturity is the greatest risk if the fetus is delivered preterm. Therefore tests for fetal lung maturity (see Chapter 10) are done if elective cesarean birth is planned.

Technique

Preparation

Regional anesthesia such as an epidural block is commonly used for cesarean birth. However, general anesthesia, with its risk for vomiting and aspiration of gastric contents, may be needed unexpectedly. Placement of the regional block may not be possible, and an inadequate block may require supplemental general anesthesia. Therefore the woman receives nothing by mouth. A drug such as famotidine (Pepcid) and sodium citrate (Bicitra) is given to reduce gastric acidity before surgery. The woman does not have routine premedication other than drugs to control gastric and respiratory secretions.

The fetus is monitored for at least 20 to 30 minutes after admission if the woman is having a scheduled cesarean birth. If electronic fetal monitoring is being used when a cesarean birth becomes necessary, it continues as long as possible before the surgery. A fetal scalp electrode should be removed before birth so that it is not pulled from the vagina through the uterus as the infant is delivered. A wedge under one hip and a tilted operating table avoid aortocaval compression and promote placental blood flow.

Routine laboratory studies vary with the mother's condition and type of anesthesia but often include complete blood count, clotting studies such as prothrombin and activated partial thromboplastin times, and blood typing and screening. The physician may order one or more units of blood typed and crossmatched to be available for transfusion if the woman's hemoglobin and hematocrit values are low and she is at greater risk for hemorrhage, such as grand multiparity (five or more births).

A single IV dose of a prophylactic antibiotic often is ordered. Additional antibiotic doses are given to a woman who has an increased risk for infection, such as one who has had prolonged rupture of membranes.

If a Pfannenstiel (transverse or bikini) skin incision is planned, the woman's abdomen is shaved from about 3 inches above the pubic hairline to the mons pubis, about where her legs come together. For a vertical skin incision, the upper border of the shave is just above the umbilicus. Some units shave the larger abdominal area for all skin incisions.

An indwelling catheter inserted before the surgery keeps the bladder away from the operative area, reducing the risk for injury. The catheter allows accurate observation of urine output during and after surgery, which helps evaluate maternal circulatory status. To reduce discomfort, insertion may be delayed until an epidural block has taken effect.

Preoperative preparations are completed before a general anesthetic is begun to reduce neonatal exposure to anesthesia. The team scrubs, puts on gowns and gloves, and drapes the woman before general anesthesia is induced.

An abdominal scrub is done just before sterile draping. As in other surgical skin preparations, the direction is circular from the center of the operative area outward.

Incisions

Two incisions are made, one in the abdominal wall (skin incision) and the other in the uterine wall. Either of two skin incisions are used: a midline vertical incision between the umbilicus and the symphysis or a Pfannenstiel incision just above the symphysis (Figure 16-8).

Three types of uterine incisions are possible, each with different indications and limitations: (1) low transverse, (2) low vertical, and (3) classic, a vertical incision into the upper uterus (Figure 16-9). The low transverse uterine incision is preferred. The uterine incision does not always match the skin incision. For example, a woman may have a vertical skin incision and a low transverse uterine incision.

The low transverse uterine incision may not be suitable if the fetus is very large. The length of this incision is limited because the uterine artery and vein enter the uterus at its lower right and left sides. The low transverse incision may not be large enough to deliver a large fetus without tearing these large vessels. Sometimes a vertical uterine incision must be added to a transverse one (making an inverted T) to deliver a very large baby.

A classic uterine incision occasionally must be used when the other two incisions are not possible, such as when a placenta previa is located in the lower anterior uterus. The vertical uterine incision, especially the classic one, is more likely to rupture during later pregnancies.

Sequence of Events in a Cesarean Birth

The sequence of events in cesarean birth is similar to that in a vaginal birth. When the woman is anesthetized and draped, the physician makes the skin incision. If general anesthesia is used, the level is very light until the fetus is delivered and is deepened after the umbilical cord is clamped.

The bladder is separated from the uterine wall and held downward with a wide bladder retractor. The uterus is incised, usually in a low transverse incision. If the membranes are intact, they are ruptured with a sharp instrument and amniotic fluid is suctioned from the operative field. As in vaginal births, the color, odor,

Vertical

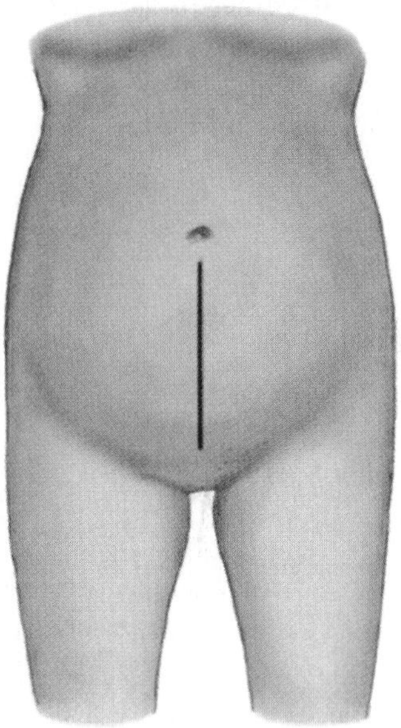

Advantages
Quicker to perform
Better visualization of the uterus
Can quickly extend upward for greater visualization if needed
Often more appropriate for obese women

Disadvantages
Easily visible when healed
Greater chance of dehiscence and hernia formation

Pfannenstiel

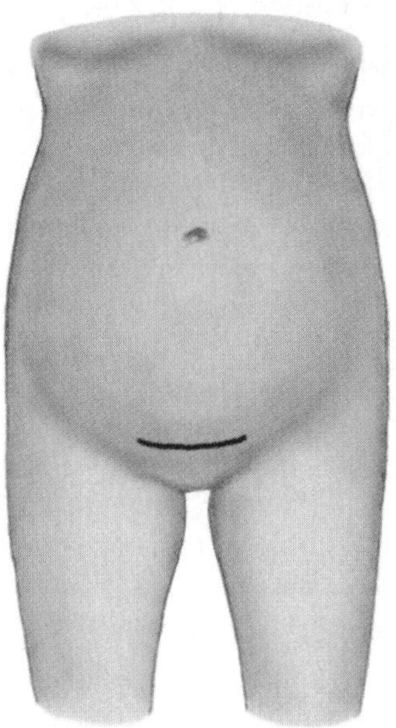

Advantages
Less visibility when healed and the pubic hair grows back
Less chance of dehiscence or formation of a hernia

Disadvantages
Less visualization of the uterus
Cannot be done as quickly, which may be important in an emergency cesarean birth
Cannot easily be extended to give greater operative exposure
Re-entry at a subsequent cesarean birth may require more time

FIGURE 16-8 Skin (abdominal wall) incisions for cesarean birth.

Low Transverse

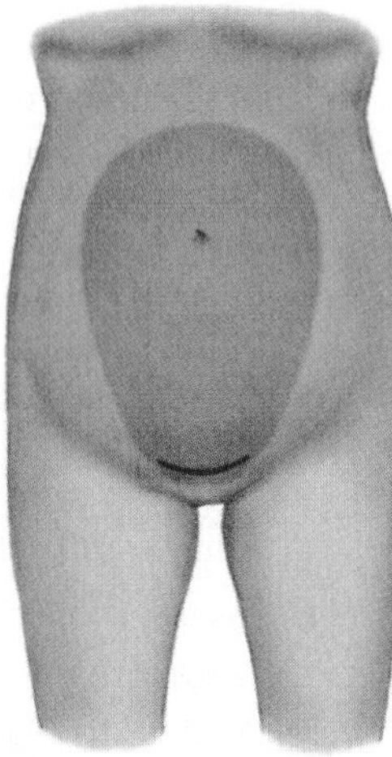

Low Vertical

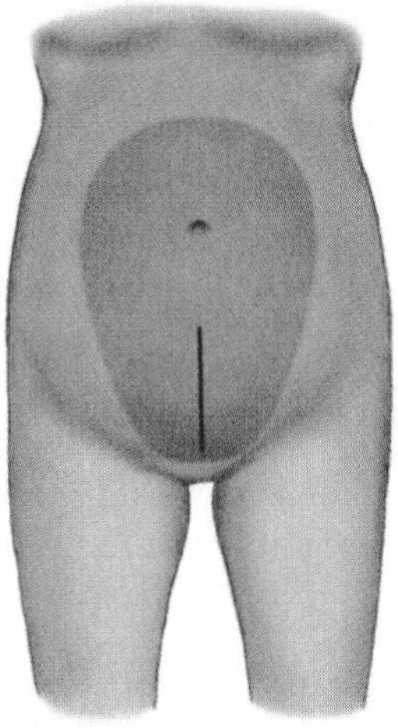

Classic

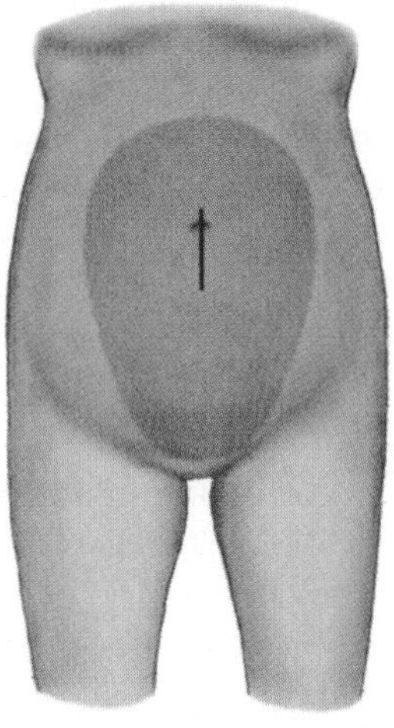

Advantages
Unlikely to rupture during a subsequent birth
Makes VBAC possible for subsequent pregnancy
Less blood loss
Easier to repair
Less adhesion formation

Disadvantage
Limited ability to extend laterally to enlarge the incision

Advantage
Can be extended upward to make a larger incision if needed

Disadvantages
Slightly more likely to rupture during a subsequent birth
A tear may extend the incision downward into the cervix

Advantage
May be the only choice in these situations:
Implantation of a placenta previa on the lower anterior uterine wall
Presence of dense adhesions from previous surgery
Transverse lie of a large fetus with the shoulder impacted in the mother's pelvis

Disadvantages
Most likely of the uterine incisions to rupture during a subsequent birth
Eliminates VBAC as an option for birth of a subsequent infant

FIGURE 16-9 Uterine incisions for cesarean birth. The abdominal and uterine incisions do not always match. *VBAC,* Vaginal birth after cesarean.

Table 16-4
SUMMARY OF NURSING CARE FOR A WOMAN HAVING CESAREAN BIRTH

Before the Cesarean Birth	During the Recovery Period
• Assess time of last oral intake and what was eaten. • Assess for allergies. • Have the woman sign informed consent form (verify that she has discussed the risks, benefits, and alternate treatments with her physician and understands these; the nurse is a witness to her signature only). • Obtain ordered laboratory work. • Do preoperative teaching: what to expect in the operating and recovery rooms. • Start ordered intravenous infusion. • Do abdominal shave. • Insert an indwelling catheter. • Administer ordered medication to control gastric secretions or other preoperative medications. • Assist woman to operating table, positioning her with a wedge under her hip (or tilt table) and securing her legs with a strap. • Apply grounding pad for electrocautery. • Do cleansing prep of abdomen.	• Begin anesthesia-related interventions: pulse oximeter, oxygen administration, cardiac monitor. a. Assess for return of sensation and movement if regional anesthesia was used. b. Assess level of consciousness if general anesthesia was used. • Do routine assessments every 15 minutes for the first hour, every 30 minutes for the second hour, and hourly until she is transferred to the postpartum unit. a. Vital signs b. Uterine fundus for firmness, height, and deviation—Massage if poorly contracted c. Lochia for color, quantity, and presence of large clots d. Urine output for color, quantity, and patency of the catheter and tubing e. Abdominal dressing for drainage • Assess need for analgesia and administer as ordered. • Change position hourly if no contraindication exists. Have her breathe deeply and cough at each routine assessment time. Provide a small pillow to support her incision when coughing or turning.

and quantity of the amniotic fluid are noted and the time of rupture is recorded.

The physician lifts the fetal presenting part through the uterine incision. An assistant may push on the uterine fundus to help deliver the fetus through the abdominal incision. A vacuum extractor or forceps may be needed to facilitate birth of the fetal head.

The infant's face is wiped, and the mouth and nose are suctioned to remove secretions that would impair breathing. The cord is quickly clamped and cut. The physician collects cord blood for analysis.

After the infant's birth, the physician removes the placenta. Oxytocin is given IV to contract the uterus firmly. The physician then closes the uterine and abdominal incisions, approximating each layer separately. Some physicians flush the operative area with saline or antibiotic solution before abdominal closure.

Nursing care for the infant is similar to that after vaginal birth. Resuscitation equipment should be readied for use. Professional personnel who care for the infant born by cesarean vary with the baby's anticipated condition and facility policy. A pediatrician, neonatal nurse-practitioner, or neonatal nurse (often more than one) usually attends the infant at the time of cesarean birth.

Nursing Considerations

Nursing care for a woman who has a cesarean birth varies according to the situation. She may be planning a cesarean birth, or a surgical birth may be unexpected. Even within these two situations, women differ. For example, is the planned cesarean her first, or has she had a cesarean birth before? Was her previous cesarean planned? An unplanned cesarean birth may occur after hours of unsuccessful labor or be needed quickly in an emergency.

Nursing care is similar for women having cesarean childbirth, but the approach in each situation is different (Table 16-4). For example, although preoperative teaching is important, it must be abbreviated or even omitted in a true emergency.

Providing Emotional Support

Emotional support may begin before and extend after the birth. A mother who has had a previous cesarean birth may harbor unresolved feelings of grief, guilt, and inadequacy because she perceives that she somehow failed in her expected birth experience. Therapeutic communication techniques help identify stressors and misunderstandings to promote a positive childbirth experience.

> The nurse in the prenatal setting can open the subject of a woman's previous cesarean birth with a broad lead such as "Tell me about your experience with the birth of your other baby."

Anxiety is an expected and normal reaction to surgery and is useful within limits. For example, mild to moderate anxiety may prompt the woman who expects a cesarean birth to learn more about her upcoming experience. However, high anxiety inhibits concentration. The woman who has an emergency cesarean birth is more likely to have high levels of anxiety, but the woman who expects the surgery also is vulnerable.

Table 16-5

NURSING DIAGNOSES FOR THE WOMAN HAVING AN OPERATIVE OBSTETRIC PROCEDURE

* Anxiety
Fear
Pain
Risk for Altered Respiratory Function (mother or newborn)
* Risk for Aspiration
* Risk for Injury
Hypothermia (mother or newborn)
Family Coping: Potential for Growth

*Nursing diagnoses explored in this chapter.

The staff's behavior can either reduce or increase the woman's anxiety. A calm and confident manner helps her feel that she is being cared for by competent professionals. A quiet, low voice is calming. Shouting is unnecessary, even in an emergency.

The nurse and the woman's significant others are important sources of emotional support. The nurse should remain with her and let her express her fears. Therapeutic communication helps clarify her concerns, so explanations to reduce her fear of the unknown can be most effective.

Her support person should be encouraged to remain with her during surgery if she has regional anesthesia. In some hospitals, the support person may come into the operating room after the woman is intubated for general anesthesia to foster attachment with the infant and help the mother integrate her birth experience afterward.

Nurses also support a woman's partner and significant others during the cesarean birth. The partner may be as anxious as the woman but afraid to express it because she needs so much support. The partner may be physically exhausted after hours of labor coaching. The staff should not expect more support from partners than can be reasonably provided.

> Although cesarean births are routine in the intrapartum unit they are not routine to women who undergo them and their families. Avoid belittling their fears by telling women and their families not to worry and that everything will be all right.

After birth, visiting the mother and her family allows the nurse to answer questions about the surgery and fill in any gaps in their understanding. This helps them understand the experience and promotes a positive perception of the birth (Nursing Care Plan 16-1).

Teaching

Knowledge reduces fear of the unknown and increases a woman's sense of control over her infant's birth. The nurse cannot assume that a woman who had a previous cesarean birth already knows what will happen and why. If her previous surgery was done after a long labor or in an emergency, she may recall only parts and not understand those parts she does remember. Teaching should be given in simple language and include her support person.

The nurse explains preoperative procedures and their purposes, such as the abdominal shave, indwelling catheter, intravenous lines, and dressings. The catheter and IV lines usually remain in place no longer than 24 hours after birth. The nurse may need to reinforce information provided by others, such as an anesthesiologist.

Women who have regional anesthesia, such as an epidural or a subarachnoid block, often fear that they will feel pain during surgery. They do feel pressure and pulling, but these sensations do not mean that the anesthesia is wearing off. The nurse reassures her that her pain management is regularly assessed by the anesthesiologist.

If a woman is having general anesthesia, the nurse explains why operative preparations are completed before she is anesthetized. She should be reassured that her surgery will not begin until she is asleep and she will not wake up during the procedure.

The nurse describes the operating room and everyone who will be present to make it less intimidating to her. The operating room is very cool, and the surgery table is narrow. Her labor nurse often is the circulating nurse during surgery and reassures her with a familiar face and voice.

The support person should be told when to expect to come into the operating room. If it is not already in place, an epidural block often is established after the woman goes to the operating room. The partner may not be brought in until the regional block and other preparations such as the indwelling catheter are complete. These preparations may take 30 to 45 minutes if no rush exists. Support persons should be told that they will not be forgotten and that apparent delays do not indicate problems.

The recovery room and any equipment that will be used, such as a pulse oximeter and automatic blood pressure cuff, are explained to the couple. The nurse reviews routine assessments and interventions such as fundus and lochia checks, coughing, and deep breathing. The woman is taught simple exercises to promote normal circulation. The nurse reassures her that every effort will be made to promote her comfort with medication, positioning, and other interventions.

Promoting Safety

The woman's food intake is assessed for type and time on admission because general anesthesia occasionally is necessary. Oral intake and emesis during labor are recorded and reported to the anesthesia clinician. Oral intake other than ordered medications should be discontinued if a cesarean birth becomes very likely. Drugs to control gastric and respiratory secretions are administered as ordered.

NURSING CARE PLAN 16-1

Cesarean Birth

Assessment: Christina Cole is 22 years old and expecting her first baby. Her due date is 1 week from today. She is in early labor, has mild contractions, and will have a cesarean birth because her baby is in a complete (full) breech presentation. Although her physician has discussed cesarean birth with her, Christina is anxious and has many questions about what will happen to her and her baby. She says she is very nervous about the upcoming surgery. She has never been a patient in a hospital before this time. Christina's mother and husband Bruce are with her.

Nursing Diagnosis: Anxiety related to unfamiliarity with the setting and procedures for cesarean birth.

Goals/Expected Outcomes:
After interventions, Christina will do the following:
1. State that she feels less apprehensive.
2. Verbalize understanding of preoperative and postoperative care.
3. Demonstrate postoperative techniques for coughing and deep breathing.

Intervention	Rationale
1. Assess Christina's level of anxiety. Mild to moderate levels of anxiety are expected.	1. Assessment enables the nurse to approach preoperative care of the woman in the most appropriate manner. Mild to moderate anxiety may facilitate learning, but higher levels impair learning.
2. Remain with Christina as much as possible. Allow her to express her fears. Encourage her mother and Bruce to remain with her.	2. This provides support from significant others and a caring nurse and enables the nurse to answer the woman's concerns specifically.
3. Elicit Christina's feelings about surgery by using broad leads such as "What were your thoughts when you found out you might have your baby by cesarean?"	3. This identifies expectations of the birth experience so that actions can be taken to make it a positive one. If a woman's expected and actual experience closely match, she is likely to be more satisfied with it. Identifies misunderstandings and possible feelings of inadequacy and anger.
4. Explain the following preoperative preparations using simple language, verifying Christina's understanding and giving her the opportunity to ask questions. a. The anesthesiologist or nurse-anesthetist visits her to explain anesthesia. The epidural anesthetic will be given in the operating room. b. Shave prep (a Pfannenstiel incision is planned): from about 3 inches above the pubic hair to the level where the thighs meet. Other preparation if ordered, such as cleansing enema. c. Indwelling urinary catheter, which is usually inserted after shave prep and epidural anesthesia is begun. d. Operating room: appearance, narrow table, wedge under one hip (or tilted table), cool temperature, equipment. e. People who will be in the operating room: circulating nurse, scrub nurse, surgeon's assistant, neonatal nurse, pediatrician, any others.	4. Knowledge decreases anxiety and fear of the unknown. Simple language facilitates understanding when a woman's attention is narrowed from anxiety. These interventions show respect and give the woman a greater sense of control.
5. Explain what to expect postoperatively, demonstrating as needed. a. Oxygen mask will be used briefly. b. Pulse oximeter on finger. Automatic blood pressure cuff. c. Frequent checks of her vital signs, fundus, lochia, and anesthesia-related assessments. Emphasize that nurses will be as gentle as possible when palpating her fundus. d. Catheter usually remains in place up to 24 hours. e. She will be kept as comfortable as possible with analgesics and should tell the nurse if she needs pain medication before pain is too bad for greatest effectiveness. f. She will be asked to move and change position several times. g. Demonstrate effective coughing (splinting the abdomen with a pillow) and deep breathing techniques; have Christina demonstrate each.	5. Explanations reduce anxiety and fear of the unknown and promote understanding and acceptance that care will be painful while providing reassurance of pain control. Return demonstration verifies learning and identifies the need for additional teaching. Analgesics are most effective if given before pain is severe.

Continued

6. Reduce unnecessary stimulation: a. Keep lights low and noise to a minimum. b. Limit unnecessary visitors and staff. c. Plan operative preparations so that they are done efficiently. d. Maintain calm and friendly behavior.	6. These measures avoid adding to her anxiety and emphasize that a cesarean delivery is a birth, not just a surgical procedure.

Evaluation: Christina says she believes that a cesarean birth is best for her baby, although she would have preferred to have her baby "naturally." She asks a few other questions and then states that she understands preoperative and postoperative care. She demonstrates effective coughing and deep breathing techniques.

Assessment: Christina had soup and a sandwich about 2 hours before admission. She will have epidural anesthesia for her birth. Her vital signs are temperature 37.2° C (99° F), pulse 88 BPM, respirations 20 breaths per minute, blood pressure 122/70. The FHR is 130 to 140 BPM and accelerates with fetal movement.

Critical Thinking: Does this assessment suggest another nursing diagnosis? What interventions should the nurse institute for the nursing diagnosis?

Answer: Risk for Aspiration would apply during the intraoperative period because general anesthesia might be needed unexpectedly and Christina has food in her stomach that might be vomited and aspirated. The woman is given nothing by mouth if general anesthesia is a possibility. The nurse should expect orders for a drug to reduce gastric acidity.

Assessment: Christina is transferred to the operating room, and epidural anesthesia is begun. She gives birth to an 8-lb, 8-oz (3856 g) baby. Christina is transferred to the recovery room for postoperative care.

Nursing Diagnosis: Risk for injury related to altered sensation from epidural anesthesia and use of electrical equipment during surgery.

Goals/Expected Outcomes:
Christina will not have injury such as pressure areas, muscle strains, and electrical injury during the perioperative period.

Intervention	Rationale
1. Pad the operating table carefully, particularly under bony prominences. Avoid obstructing her popliteal area.	1. Padding reduces potential for tissue damage caused by pressure and venous stasis with possible thrombus formation.
2. Transfer Christina to and from the operating table carefully, using enough staff members to keep her body in alignment. Brace the bed and operating table to keep them from separating.	2. These measures reduce the risk of fall and muscle strains for both Christina and the staff.
3. After anesthesia is begun, position Christina on the operating table and secure her legs with a safety strap. She should have a wedge under one hip, or the table should be tilted.	3. Securing her legs prevents falls or displacement of legs that have lost sensation. A hip wedge or tilting the table reduces aortocaval compression, which might reduce placental blood flow.
4. Apply grounding pad if electrocautery is to be used.	4. A grounding pad avoids electrical shock or burn.

Evaluation: During surgery, Christina's body was secured in proper alignment with proper padding of all her bony prominences. The grounding pad ensured electrical safety for electrocautery. Christina was transferred to the recovery room without incident. During the recovery period, she showed no signs of pressure, electrical, or musculoskeletal injury.

The woman is transferred and positioned carefully to prevent injury, especially if she has received regional anesthesia that reduces motor control and sensation. Her bony prominences are well padded. A safety strap placed across her thighs secures her on the narrow operating table. A wedge under one hip or a tilted operating table avoids aortocaval compression and reduced placental blood flow. During positioning, the drain tube of the indwelling catheter should be routed under her leg to promote drainage and keep the tube away from the operative area. The catheter bag is placed near the head of the table so that the anesthesia clinician can monitor urine output, an important measure of fluid balance.

The nurse verifies proper function of machines such as suction devices, monitors, and electrocautery. Leads for the cardiac monitor and pulse oximeter are placed to observe heart and respiratory functions. A grounding pad permits safe use of an electrocautery.

After the surgery, the incision area is cleansed with sterile water and a sterile dressing is applied. Blood and amniotic fluid are cleaned from the woman's abdomen, buttocks, and back before she is transferred to a bed. Smooth transfers reduce pain and hypotension.

Providing Postoperative Care

Postoperative care for the mother who has had a cesarean birth is similar to that for one who has had a vaginal birth, with added interventions. Her temperature is assessed on admission and according to protocol thereafter. If her condition is stable, other assessments are done every 15 minutes during the first 1 to 2 hours and progress to every 30 minutes to 1 hour until she is transferred to her postpartum room. In addition to temperature, routine postoperative assessments include the following:

- Return of motion and sensation if a regional block was given
- Level of consciousness, particularly if general anesthesia and sedating drugs were given
- Vital signs, respiratory character, and oxygen saturation
- Abdominal dressing
- Uterine firmness and position (midline or deviated)
- Lochia
- Urine output (such as quantity, color, other characteristics)
- IV infusion
- Pain relief needs

The nurse observes for return of motion and sensation if the woman had epidural or subarachnoid block anesthesia. The level of consciousness and respiratory status (skin and mucous membrane color, rate and quality of respirations, pulse oximeter readings) are important observations if she had general anesthesia. Respiratory observations also are important if the woman received epidural opioid narcotics, which can cause delayed respiratory depression. Naloxone (Narcan) should be available to reverse opioid-induced respiratory depression (see Chapter 15).

The pulse, respirations, and blood pressure provide important clues to the woman's circulatory and respiratory status. If oxygen saturation falls below 95%, it usually can be raised with several deep breaths. A persistent respiratory rate of less than 12 breaths per minute suggests respiratory depression. Deep breathing and coughing move secretions out of the lungs. A small pillow to support her incision reduces pain when she coughs. Position changes every 2 hours improve ventilation, reduce pooling of lung secretions, and decrease discomfort from constant pressure.

As with vaginal birth, the fundus is assessed for height, firmness, and position. This examination is painful after regional anesthesia wears off, but the postcesarean mother also can have uterine atony. To relax her abdominal muscles and thus reduce pain from fundus checks, she should flex her knees and take slow, deep breaths. The nurse can gently "walk" the fingers toward the fundus to determine uterine firmness. The woman who has a Pfannenstiel skin incision usually has less pain with fundus checks than the woman with a vertical skin incision. A firm fundus does not need massage. The dressing is checked for drainage with each fundus check.

The nurse assesses the lochia and urine output with other assessments. Lochia may pool under the mother's buttocks and lower back. Urine may be bloody temporarily if the cesarean delivery was done after a long labor or an attempted forceps delivery. The urine drain tubing should be observed for gradual clearing of the blood. Urine should drain freely to prevent bladder distention, which worsens pain and increases the risk for postpartum hemorrhage. The nurse must remember that falling urine output is an early sign of hypovolemia.

The woman's needs for pain relief should be regularly assessed. The woman who received an epidural opioid may not need other analgesia during the early postpartum period. If she needs added pain relief while the epidural opioid is still in effect, the dose ordered often is lower than if she had not had that form of analgesia. If she did not receive an epidural opioid, analgesia usually is given by patient-controlled analgesia pump. Oral analgesics usually replace parenteral ones the day after surgery.

Having a Vaginal Birth after Cesarean

The decision about whether to have a VBAC has never been more difficult than at present. At one time, the dictum "once a cesarean, always a cesarean" was accepted without question. For many years, the only women who had VBACs were those who entered the hospital in such advanced labor that no time was available to perform a repeat cesarean.

As low transverse uterine incisions became the norm for almost all women having cesarean births, the safety of a trial of labor became established. Gradually, VBAC became accepted as a way to lower the overall cesarean birth rate (ACOG, 1999c).

Recent studies have found that VBAC is associated with a small but significant risk of uterine rupture resulting in a poor outcome for the mother and infant. An unsuccessful trial of labor resulting in a cesarean birth also is associated with more maternal and infant complications (ACOG, 1999c). For these reasons, many obstetricians now are more conservative when recommending VBAC.

Women may be anxious about attempting vaginal birth in a later pregnancy. They may know that they are a good candidate for VBAC but find it impossible to disregard even small risks. Scheduling a repeat cesarean seems safer, simpler, and something on which they can count. The prospect of laboring and perhaps still needing a cesarean birth is worrisome as well.

The physician discusses VBAC during prenatal care, and the nurse reinforces these explanations and identifies misunderstandings. If the woman chooses VBAC, the nurse should reinforce the appropriateness of attempting VBAC and advantages of a vaginal birth, such as fewer overall complications. VBAC should be presented in a positive way, yet the possibility of cesarean delivery should be acknowledged.

Check Your Reading

16. Why is the low transverse uterine incision preferred for cesarean birth?
17. What should a woman who expects a cesarean birth be taught about the operating room? The recovery room?
18. How should the nurse modify recovery room care of the mother who had a cesarean birth from that of the mother who had a vaginal delivery?

SUMMARY CONCEPTS

- Prolapse and compression of the umbilical cord are the primary risks of amniotomy. As the fluid gushes out, the cord can become compressed between the fetal presenting part and the expectant woman's pelvis.
- Infection is more likely to occur when membranes have been ruptured for a long time (such as 24 hours).
- Induction of labor may be done if continuing the pregnancy is more hazardous to the maternal and fetal health than the induction. It is not done if a maternal or fetal contraindication exists to labor and vaginal birth.
- Oxytocin-stimulated uterine contractions may be hypertonic, decreasing placental perfusion.
- External cephalic version is done to promote vaginal birth by changing the fetal presentation from a breech or transverse lie to a cephalic presentation. Internal version sometimes is used to change presentation of a second twin after the birth of the first twin.
- Trauma to maternal and fetal tissue is the primary risk associated with use of forceps and vacuum extraction. Possible trauma to the mother includes vaginal wall laceration and hematoma. Trauma to the infant may include ecchymoses, lacerations, abrasions, facial nerve injury, and intracranial hemorrhage.
- The median episiotomy is less painful but more likely to extend into the rectum than the mediolateral episiotomy.
- The preferred uterine incision for cesarean birth is the low transverse incision because it is least likely to rupture in a subsequent pregnancy. The skin incision does not always match the uterine incision and is unrelated to the risk of later uterine rupture.
- Some women have feelings of guilt and inadequacy if they have a cesarean birth. Therapeutic communication and sensitive, family-centered care are essential to help them achieve a positive perception of their birth experience.

ANSWERS TO CRITICAL THINKING EXERCISE, p. 397

1. The amount of amniotic fluid is normal, but the pale yellow color and strong odor suggest chorioamnionitis, or infection of the amniotic sac. The risk for chorioamnionitis increases as the duration of ruptured membranes increases, but it can be apparent at any time, including at initial rupture. The FHR is slightly elevated from the normal maximal rate at term of 160 BPM. Accelerations with fetal movement are a reassuring sign. The maternal temperature, pulse, and respirations are slightly elevated. Accurately interpreting these values is difficult because the baseline values are not stated. The contractions are typical for a woman entering the active phase of first-stage labor.
2. The nurse should continue to assess the fetus for tachycardia, which often precedes maternal fever. Assess the woman's temperature at least every 2 hours for temperature of 38° C (100.4° F) or higher. Report abnormalities to the physician. Also observe for fetal tachycardia and signs of fetal compromise that may occur with maternal infection.

ANSWERS TO CRITICAL THINKING EXERCISE

1. The woman is having hypertonic uterine activity because the duration of contractions is longer than 90 seconds and the rest interval is no longer than 55 seconds. Montevideo units also are high for a stimulated labor, although they may reach this level in spontaneous labor. Oxytocin stimulation is the probable cause of the excessive contractions. The normal FHR suggests that the fetus is now tolerating the excessive contractions.
2. Fetal oxygenation may be compromised if the excessive contractions continue. Reduce or stop the oxytocin infusion to decrease uterine stimulation. Increase the primary (nonadditive) intravenous infusion as needed to maintain adequate circulating volume and ensure maximum uterine blood flow. Keep the woman in a lateral position to reduce aortocaval compression and increase placental blood flow. Oxygen at 8 to 10 L/min with a snug face mask increases her blood oxygen saturation, making more available to the fetus (see Chapter 14).

REFERENCES & READINGS

American Academy of Pediatrics (AAP) & American College of Obstetricians and Gynecologists (ACOG). (1997). *Guidelines for perinatal care* (4th ed.). Elk Grove Village, IL: Author.

ACOG. (2000a). External cephalic version. *ACOG practice bulletin no. 13.* Washington, D.C.: Author.

ACOG. (2000b). ACOG News Release: OB-Gyns issue recommendations on cesarean delivery rates. Retrieved August 14, 2000 from http://www.acog.org/from home/publications/press releases/m08-09-00.htm.

ACOG. (1999a). Induction of labor. *ACOG practice bulletin no. 10.* Washington, D.C.: Author.

ACOG. (1999b). Induction of labor with misoprostol. *ACOG committee opinion no. 228.* Washington, D.C.: Author.

ACOG. (2000c). Operative vaginal delivery. *ACOG practice bulletin no. 17.* Washington, D.C.: Author.

ACOG. (1999c). Vaginal birth after previous cesarean delivery. *ACOG practice bulletin no. 5.* Washington, D.C.: Author.

Asrat, T., & Quilligan, E.J. (2000). Breech delivery. In E.J. Quilligan and F.P. Zuspan (Eds.), *Current therapy in obstetrics and gynecology* (5th ed., pp. 248-249). Philadelphia: W.B. Saunders.

Bachman, J., & Kendrick, J.M. (1996). Childbirth. In K.R. Simpson & P.A. Creehan (Eds.), *AWHONN's perinatal nursing* (pp. 151-245). Philadelphia: Lippincott.

Bishop, E.H. (1964). Pelvic scoring for elective abortion. *Obstetrics and Gynecology,* 24(2), 266-268.

Bowes, W.A. (1999). Clinical aspects of normal and abnormal labor. In R. Creasy & R. Resnik (Eds.), *Maternal-fetal medicine: Principles and practice* (4th ed., pp. 541-568). Philadelphia: W.B. Saunders.

Brisson-Carroll, G., Fraser, W., Bréart, G., Krauss, I., & Thornton, J. (1996). The effect of routine early amniotomy on spontaneous labor: A meta-analysis. *Obstetrics and Gynecology, 87*(5): Part 2, 891-896.

Bungum, T.J., Peaslee, D.L., Jackson, A.W., & Perez, M.A. (2000). Exercise during pregnancy and type of delivery in nulliparae. *Journal of Obstetric, Gynecologic, and Neonatal Nursing, 29*(3), 258-264.

Busowski, J.D., & Parsons, M.T. (1995). Amniotomy to induce labor. *Clinical Obstetrics and Gynecology, 38*(2), 246-258.

Clayworth, S. (2000). The nurse's role during oxytocin administration. *MCN: American Journal of Maternal/Child Nursing, 25*(2), 80-84.

Cunningham, F.G., MacDonald, P.C., Gant, N.F., Leveno, K.J., Gilstrap, L.C., Hankins, G.D.V., et al. (1997). *Williams obstetrics* (20th ed.). Norwalk, CT: Appleton & Lange.

Curtin, S.C., & Martin, J.A. (2000). *Births: Preliminary data for 1999.* Hyattsville, MD: National Center for Health Statistics.

Curtin, S.C., & Mathews, T.J. (2000). U.S. obstetric procedures, 1998. *Birth, 27*(2), 136-140.

Davis, L.J., Okuboye, S., & Ferguson, S.L. (2000). Healthy People 2010: Examining a decade of maternal & infant health. *AWHONN Lifelines, 4*(3), 26-33.

Dudley, D.J. (1999). Complications of labor. In J.R. Scott, P.J. Di Saia, C.B. Hammond, W.N. Spellacy (Eds.), *Danforth's obstetrics and gynecology* (8th ed., pp. 437-455). Philadelphia: Lippincott, Williams-Wilkins.

Eason, E., & Feldman, P. (2000). Clinical commentary: Much ado about a little cut: Is episiotomy worthwhile? *Obstetrics and Gynecology, 95*(4), 616-618.

Eason, E., Labrecque, M., Wells, G., & Feldman, P. (2000). Preventing perineal trauma during childbirth: A systematic review. *Obstetrics and Gynecology, 95*(3), 464-471.

Flamm, B.L., Berwick, D.M., & Kabcenell, A. (1998). Reducing cesarean section rates safely: Lessons from a "breakthrough series" collaborative. *Birth, 25*(2), 117-124.

Gagnon, A.J., & Waghorn, K. (1999). One-to-one nurse labor support of nulliparous women stimulated with oxytocin. *Journal of Obstetric, Gynecologic, and Neonatal Nursing, 28*(4), 371-376.

Garite, T.J. (2000). Fetal fibronectin: Its role in obstetrics. In E.J. Quilligan and F.P. Zuspan (Eds.), *Current therapy in obstetrics and gynecology* (5th ed., pp. 277-279). Philadelphia: W.B. Saunders.

Hannah, M.E., Huh, C., Hewson, S.A., & Hannah, W.J. (1996). Post-term pregnancy: Putting the merits of a policy of induction of labor into perspective. *Birth, 23*(1), 13-19.

Kramer, M.S., Demissie, K., Yang, H., Platt, R.W., Sauvé, R., & Liston, R. (2000). The contribution of mild and moderate preterm birth to infant mortality. *Journal of the American Medical Association, 284*, 843-849.

Labreque, M., Eason, E., Marcoux, S., Lemeux, F., Penault, J., Feldman, P., & Laperrière, L. (1999). Randomized controlled trial of prevention of perineal trauma by perineal massage during pregnancy. *American Journal of Obstetrics and Gynecology, 180*, 593-600.

Maier, J.S., & Maloni, J.A. (1997). Nurse advocacy for selective versus routine episiotomy. *Journal of Obstetric, Gynecologic, and Neonatal Nursing, 26*(2), 155-161.

Mancuso, K.M., Yancey, M.K., Murphy, J.A., & Markenson, G.R. (2000). Epidural analgesia for cephalic version: A randomized trial. *Obstetrics and Gynecology, 95*(5), 648-651.

Maslow, A.S., & Sweeny, A.L. (2000). Elective induction of labor as a risk factor for cesarean delivery among low-risk women at term. *Obstetrics and Gynecology, 95*(6), 917-922.

McNiven, P.S., Williams, J.I., Hodnett, E., Kaufman, K., & Hannah, M.E. (1998). An early labor assessment program: A randomized, controlled trial. *Birth, 25*(1), 5-10.

Menihan, C.A. (1996). Intrapartum fetal monitoring. In K.R. Simpson & P.A. Creehan (Eds.), *AWHONN's perinatal nursing* (pp. 187-225). Philadelphia: Lippincott.

Newnham, J.P., & Hobel, C.J. (1998). Forceps delivery, vacuum extraction, and cesarean section. In N.F. Hacker and J.G. Moore (Eds.), *Essentials of obstetrics and gynecology* (3rd ed., pp. 352-359). Philadelphia: W.B. Saunders.

Newton, E. (2000). Genital tract trauma. In E.J. Quilligan and F.P. Zuspan (Eds.), *Current therapy in obstetrics and gynecology* (5th ed., pp. 283-286). Philadelphia: W.B. Saunders.

Parsons, M.T., & Spellacy, W.N. (1999). Preterm labor. In J.R. Scott, P.J. Di Saia, C.B. Hammond, W.N. Spellacy (Eds.), *Danforth's obstetrics and gynecology* (8th ed., pp. 257-267). Philadelphia: Lippincott, Williams-Wilkins.

Paul, R.H., & Miller, D.A. (1995). Cesarean birth: How to reduce the rate. *American Journal of Obstetrics and Gynecology, 172*(6), 1903-1911.

Porreco, R.P., & Thorp, J.A. (1996). The cesarean birth epidemic: Trends, causes, and solutions. *American Journal of Obstetrics and Gynecology, 175*(2), 369-374.

Radabaugh, S., & Everhart, A. (1999). Cesarean births: Reducing incidence while improving outcomes. *AWHONN Lifelines, 3*(1), 28-34.

Rayburn, W.F. (2000). Prostaglandin E_2 for cervical ripening. In E.J. Quilligan and F.P. Zuspan (Eds.), *Current therapy in obstetrics and gynecology* (5th ed., pp. 334-337). Philadelphia: W.B. Saunders.

Regalia, A.L., & Curiel, P., Natale, N., Galluzzi, A., Spinelli, G., Ghezzi, G.V.L., Tampieri, A., & Terzian, E. (2000). Routine use of external cephalic version in three hospitals. *Birth, 27*(1), 19-24.

Robinson, J.N., Norwitz, E.R., Cohen, A.P., & Lieberman, E. (2000). Predictors of episiotomy use at first spontaneous vaginal delivery. *Obstetrics and Gynecology, 96*(2), 214-218.

Ross, M.G., & Hobel, C.J. (1998). Normal labor, delivery, and the puerperium. In N.F. Hacker and J.G. Moore (Eds.), *Essentials of obstetrics and gynecology* (3rd ed., pp. 150-167). Philadelphia: W.B. Saunders.

Sachs, B.P., Kobelin, C., Castro, M.A., & Frigoletto, F. (1999). The risks of lowering the cesarean delivery rate. *New England Journal of Medicine, 340*, 54-57.

Seyb, S.T., Berka, R.J., Socol, & Dooley, S.L. (1999). Risk of cesarean delivery with elective induction of labor at term in nulliparous women. *Obstetrics and Gynecology, 94*(4), 600-607.

Scott, J.R. (1999). Cesarean delivery. In J.R. Scott, P.J. Di Saia, C.B. Hammond, W.N. Spellacy (Eds.), *Danforth's obstetrics and gynecology* (8th ed., pp. 457-470). Philadelphia: Lippincott, Williams-Wilkins.

Simpson, K.R., & Poole, J.H. (1998). *Practice resource: Cervical ripening and induction and augmentation of labor.* Washington, D.C.: Association of Women's Health, Obstetric and Neonatal Nurses.

U.S. Department of Health and Human Services. (2000). Healthy People 2010 Website. Retrieved August 14, 2000, from http://www.health.gov/healthypeople/default.htm.

Young, D. (1999). Whither cesareans in the new millennium? *Birth, 26*(2), 67-70.

The Cesarean Birth Story

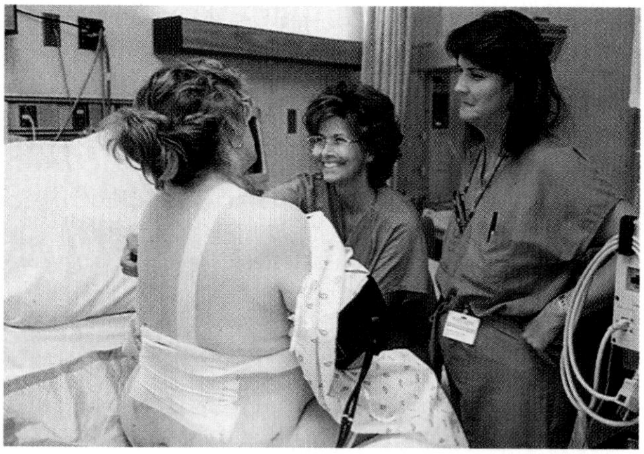

1. Vicky is in active labor. An epidural catheter allows injection of medications to provide analgesia during labor. Additional epidural medications can be used to provide anesthesia if surgery becomes necessary. An intravenous infusion precedes placement of the epidural block to offset the tendency of the block to cause hypotension.

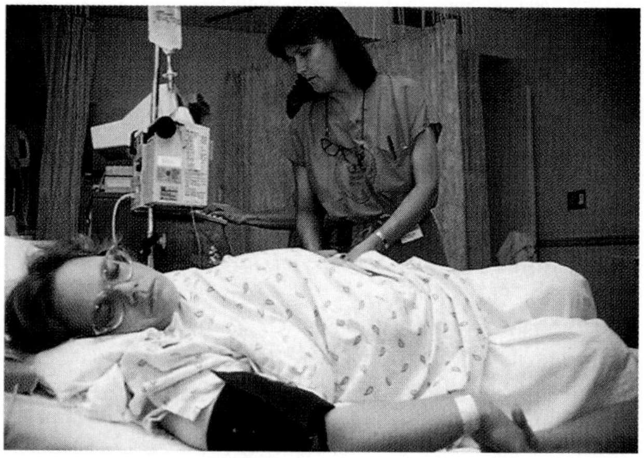

2. Support under her left hip displaces Vicky's uterus, thus avoiding pressure on her inferior vena cava and aorta and enhancing placental circulation. An automatic blood pressure cuff helps keep up with the frequent blood pressure assessments that are necessary when an epidural block is first begun.

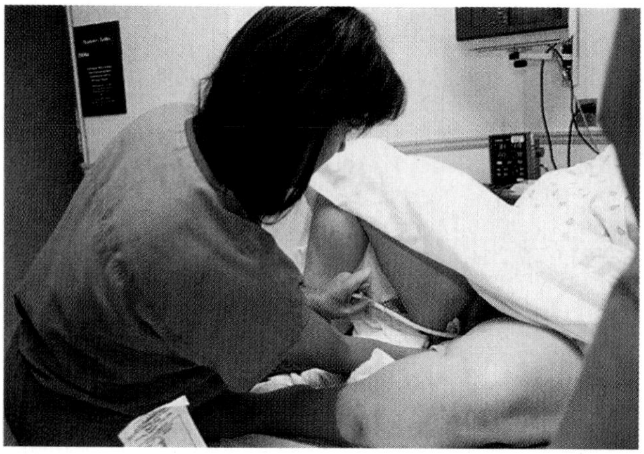

3. After rupturing the membranes, the nurse-midwife applies a spiral electrode to the fetal scalp to improve the accuracy of the fetal heart tracing on the monitor.

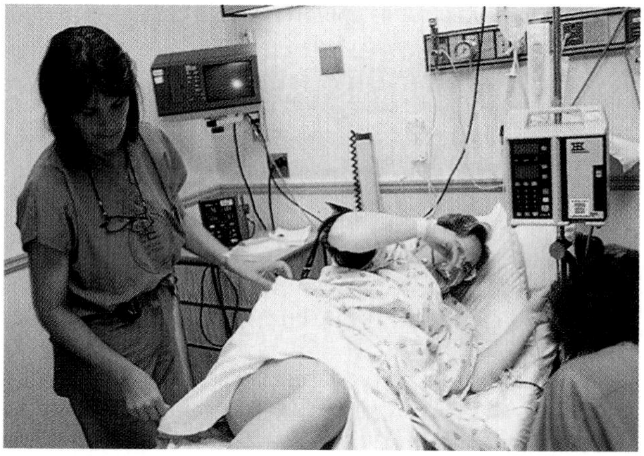

4. Because the fetal monitor shows patterns suggesting fetal compromise, Vicky will need a cesarean birth. Monitors for her blood pressure, pulse, and cardiac rhythm help identify maternal factors contributing to the fetal heart rate patterns. She receives oxygen by face mask to provide the maximal amount to her fetus.

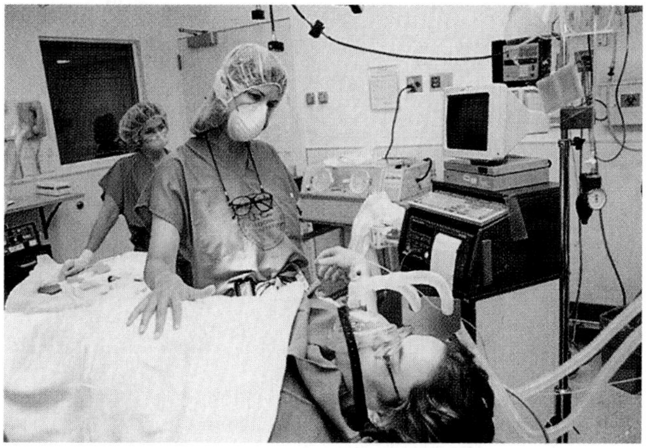

5. While Vicky is prepared for surgery, fetal monitoring and maternal oxygen administration continue. If possible, the same nurses accompany the woman to the operating room so that she has a continuing relationship during the cesarean birth, as she would have for most vaginal births.

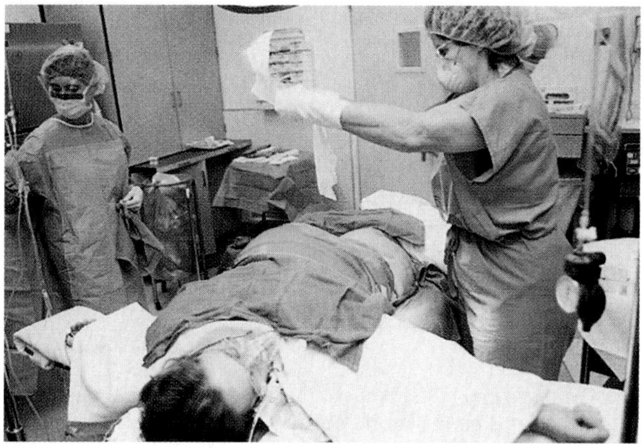

6. Vicky's abdomen is shaved to prepare for the surgery and then is cleansed with an antimicrobial prep solution. Shaving extends from just above the umbilicus to the point where the legs come together if a vertical incision is expected. If a Pfannenstiel (transverse) incision is expected, the top border can be about 3 inches above the upper pubic hairline.

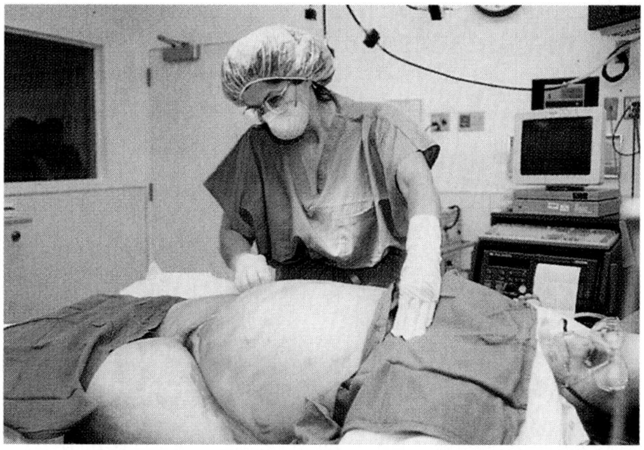

7. An iodine-based prep solution is used to cleanse the abdomen using a circular motion beginning at the incisional area and extending outward. The cleansing sponge should not be returned toward the center. During preparations for surgery, Vicky's trunk is tilted slightly toward her left side by a wedge under her right hip to promote circulation to the placenta. The internal fetal scalp electrode is removed before the incision is made so that it is not brought from the unsterile vagina through the incision as the baby is born.

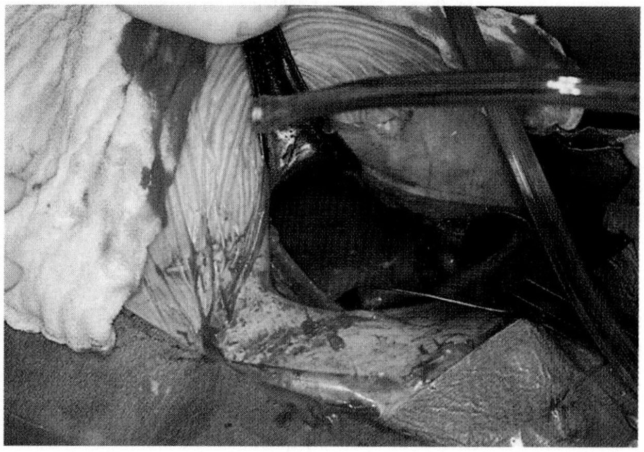

8. After making a Pfannenstiel skin incision, the physician separates the layers until the uterus is reached. The uterus is then opened in a low transverse incision. Wide retractors hold the mother's tissues back to expose an area large enough to allow the fetus to emerge. A suction device is available to suction blood and amniotic fluid from the uterus when it is incised.

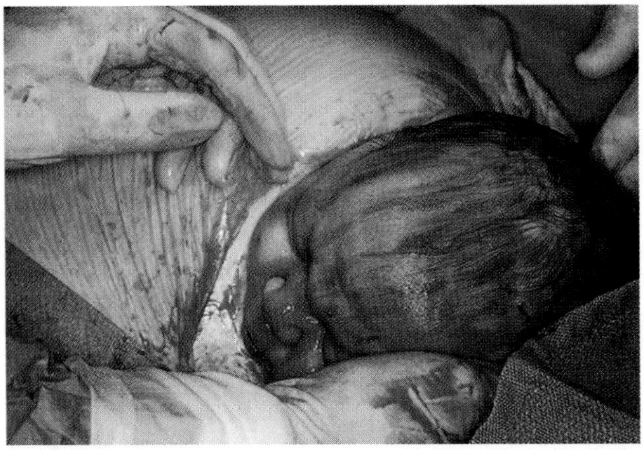

9. The fetal head is first brought through the incision. The bluish skin color is normal at this point.

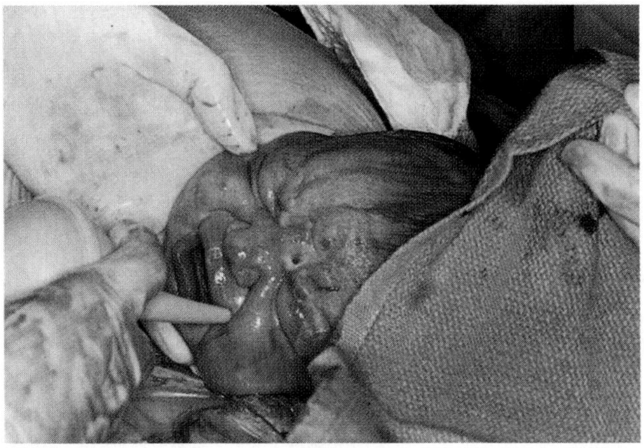

10. After birth of the head, the mouth and nose are suctioned to remove blood and other secretions before the infant takes his first breath. This baby is grimacing with the suction, which usually is associated with adequate oxygenation.

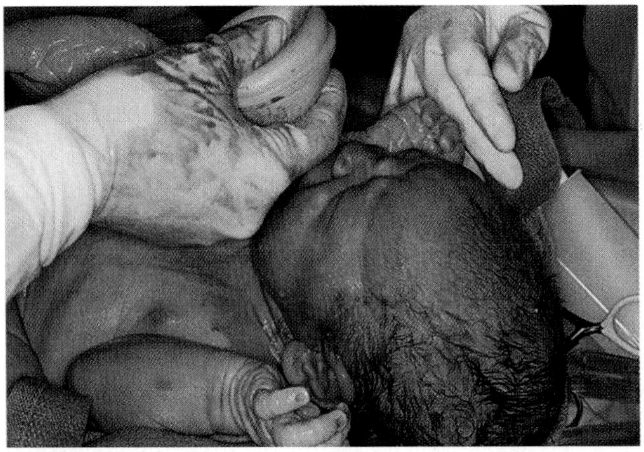

11. Further infant suctioning is done after the baby emerges.

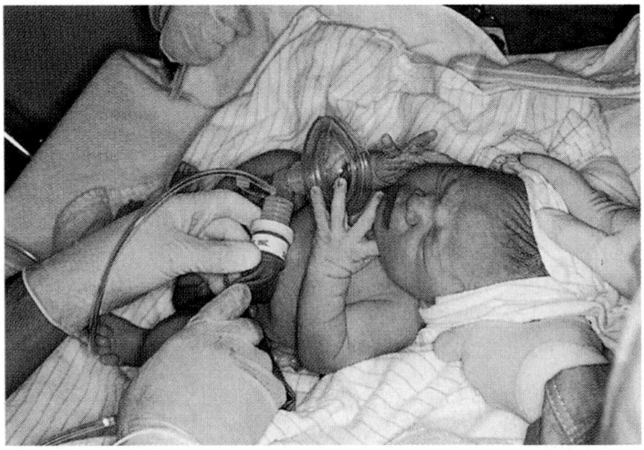

12. The infant is briefly given supplemental oxygen by face mask. His color is becoming pinker than it was immediately after birth because he has a larger proportion of oxygenated hemoglobin. At the same time, another nurse dries the baby to prevent cold stress, which could increase his oxygen needs. Note that nurses handling the baby wear gloves to protect them from blood and other secretions.

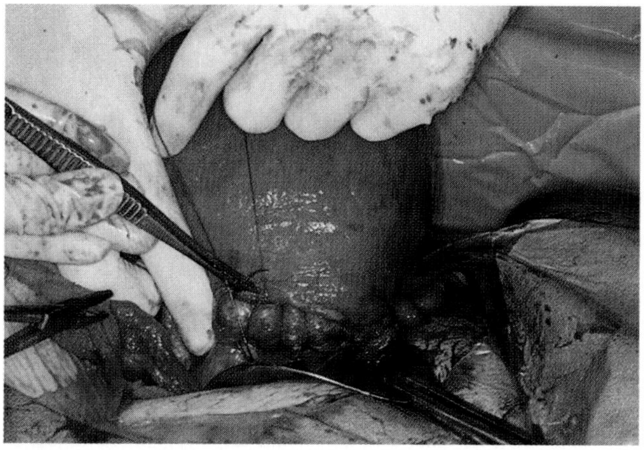

13. Heavy sutures are used to close the muscular layers of the transverse uterine incision.

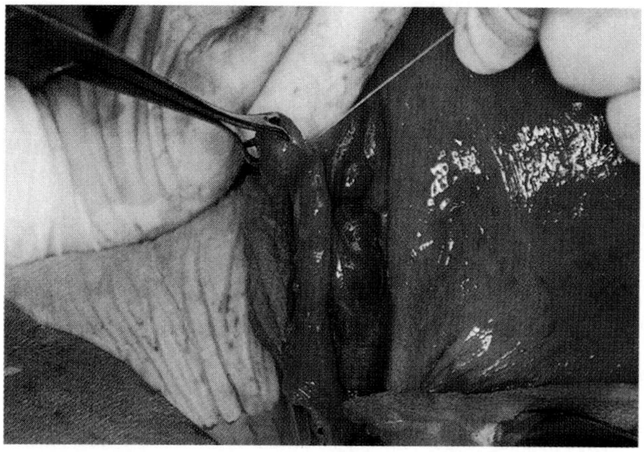

14. Vicky is having a bilateral tubal ligation for sterilization. One fallopian tube is identified by its connection to the uterus to distinguish it from her ureter. It then is doubly tied, and a segment of the tube is cut away and sent to the pathology laboratory for analysis.

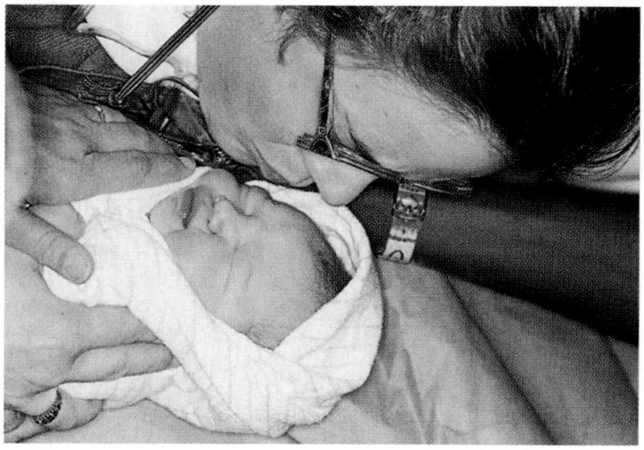

15. As her surgery continues and the infant's condition is stable, Vicky sees her baby up close for the first time.

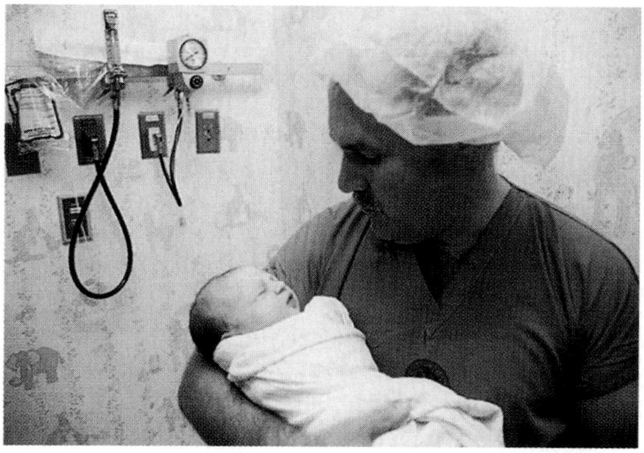

16. Vicky's husband, Greg, holds his newborn son shortly after birth.

17 Postpartum Physiologic Adaptations

OBJECTIVES

1. Explain the physiologic changes that occur during the postpartum period.
2. Identify the purpose of clinical pathways in postpartum care.
3. Describe nursing assessments and nursing care during the postpartum period.
4. Recount expected outcomes and interventions for the most common nursing diagnoses.
5. Discuss the role of the nurse in health education, and identify important areas of teaching.
6. Describe postpartum home and community care in terms of criteria for discharge, common problems, and available health care services.
7. Compare cesarean birth and vaginal birth in terms of nursing assessments and care.
8. Use critical thinking exercises to improve selected nursing care plans.

DEFINITIONS

Afterpains Cramping pain after childbirth caused by alternate relaxation and contraction of uterine muscles.

Atony Absence or lack of usual muscle tone.

Catabolism Destructive process that converts living cells into simpler compounds; process involved in involution (changes) of the uterus after childbirth.

Decidua Name applied to the endometrium during pregnancy; all except the deepest layer is shed after childbirth.

Diastasis Recti Separation of the longitudinal muscles of the abdomen (rectus abdominis) during pregnancy.

Dyspareunia Difficult or painful coitus in women.

Engorgement Swelling of the breasts resulting from increased blood flow, edema, and presence of milk.

Episiotomy Surgical incision of the perineum to enlarge the vaginal opening.

Fundus Part of the uterus that is farthest from the cervix, above the openings of the fallopian tubes.

DEFINITIONS—cont'd

INVOLUTION Retrogressive changes that return the reproductive organs, particularly the uterus, to their nonpregnant size and condition.

KEGEL EXERCISES Alternate contracting and relaxing of the pelvic muscles; these movements strengthen the pubococcygeal muscle, which surrounds the urinary meatus and vagina.

LACTATION Secretion of milk from the breasts; also describes the time when a child is breastfed.

LOCHIA ALBA White or cream-colored vaginal discharge that follows lochia serosa; occurs when the amount of blood is decreased and the number of leukocytes is increased.

LOCHIA RUBRA Reddish vaginal discharge that occurs immediately after childbirth; composed mostly of blood.

LOCHIA SEROSA Pink or brown-tinged vaginal discharge that follows lochia rubra and precedes lochia alba; composed largely of serous exudate, blood, and leukocytes.

MILK-EJECTION REFLEX Release of milk from the alveoli into the ducts; also known as the *letdown reflex.*

OXYTOCIN Posterior pituitary gland hormone that stimulates uterine contractions and the milk-ejection reflex; also prepared synthetically.

PROLACTIN Anterior pituitary hormone that promotes growth of breast tissue and stimulates production of milk.

PUERPERIUM Period from the end of childbirth until involution of the uterus is complete; approximately 6 weeks.

REEDA Acronym for redness, ecchymosis, edema, discharge, and approximation; useful for assessing wound healing or the presence of inflammation or infection.

SUBINVOLUTION Delayed return of the uterus to its nonpregnant size and consistency.

The first 6 weeks after the birth of an infant are known as the *postpartum period,* or puerperium. During this time, mothers experience numerous physiologic and psychosocial changes. Physiologic and psychosocial changes and their implications are presented in separate chapters, although in actual practice they occur at the same time. (See Appendix D, "Keys to Clinical Practice," for a summary of postpartum assessment and care.)

Many of the physiologic changes are retrogressive in nature; that is, changes that occurred in body systems during pregnancy are reversed as the body returns to the nonpregnancy state. Progressive changes also occur, most obviously in the initiation of lactation.

REPRODUCTIVE SYSTEM

Involution of the Uterus

Involution includes the changes the reproductive organs, particularly the uterus, undergo after childbirth to return to their nonpregnant size and condition. Involution depends on three processes: (1) contraction of muscle fibers, (2) catabolism, and (3) regeneration of uterine epithelium. Involution begins immediately after delivery of the placenta, when uterine muscle fibers contract firmly around maternal blood vessels at the area where the placenta was attached. This contraction controls bleeding from the area left denuded when the placenta separated. The uterus decreases in size when muscle fibers, which have been stretched for many months, contract and gradually regain their former contour and size.

Although the total number of cells remains unchanged, the enlarged muscle cells of the uterus undergo catabolic changes in protein cytoplasm that cause a reduction in individual cell size. The products of the catabolic process are absorbed by the bloodstream and excreted in urine as nitrogenous waste.

Regeneration of the uterine epithelial lining begins soon after childbirth. The outer portion of the endometrial layer is expelled with the placenta. Within 2 to 3 days, the remaining decidua separates into two layers. The first layer is superficial and shed in lochia. The basal layer remains intact and is the source of new endometrium. Regeneration of the endometrium, except at the site of placental attachment, occurs by 2 to 3 weeks.

The placental site, which is about 7 cm (2.7 in) in diameter, heals by a process of *exfoliation* (dead tissue scales off). New endometrium is generated at the site from glands and tissue that remain in the lower layer of the decidua after separation of the placenta (Cunningham, et al., 1997). This process leaves the endometrial layer smooth and spongy, as it was before pregnancy, and leaves the uterine lining free of scar tissue, which would interfere with implantation of future pregnancies. Healing at the placental site occurs more slowly and requires approximately 6 to 7 weeks.

Descent of the Uterine Fundus

The location of the uterine fundus helps determine whether involution is progressing normally. Immediately after delivery, the uterus is about the size of a large grapefruit or softball, and the fundus can be palpated midway between the symphysis pubis and umbilicus. Within a few hours, the fundus rises to the level of the umbilicus and should remain at this level for about 24 hours. Although individual differences occur, the uterus now weighs approximately 1000 g (2 lb, 4 oz).

After 24 hours, the fundus begins to descend by approximately 1 cm, or one fingerbreadth, per day. By the tenth to fourteenth day, the fundus is in the pelvic cavity and cannot be palpated abdominally. Descent is

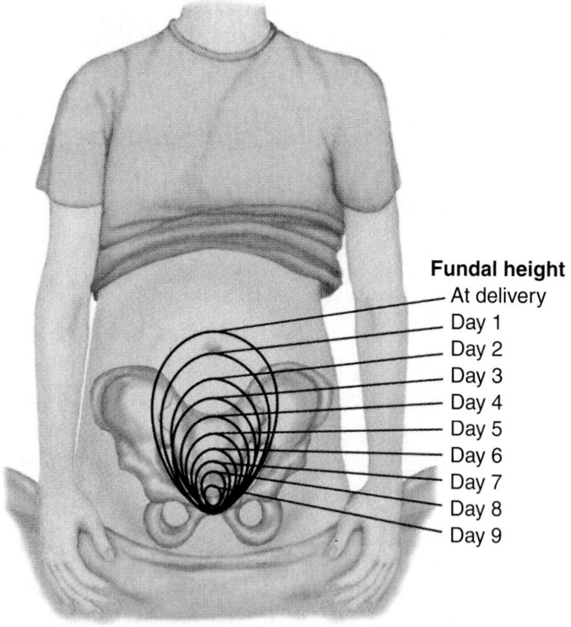

FIGURE 17-1 Involution of the uterus. Height of the uterine fundus decreases by approximately 1 cm per day.

documented in relation to the umbilicus. For instance, *U-1* indicates that the fundus is palpable one fingerbreadth below the umbilicus. Within a week, the weight of the uterus decreases to about 500 g (1 lb); at 6 weeks, the uterus weighs 60 g (2 oz), which is roughly the prepregnancy weight (Figure 17-1).

This process is normally slower when the uterus was distended during pregnancy with more than one pregnancy, a large fetus, or hydramnios (excessive amniotic fluid). When the process of involution does not occur properly, subinvolution occurs. Subinvolution can cause postpartum hemorrhage (see Chapter 28).

Afterpains

Intermittent contractions, known as *afterpains,* are a source of discomfort for many women. The discomfort is more acute for multiparas because repeated stretching of muscle fibers leads to loss of muscle tone that results in alternate contraction and relaxation of the uterus. The uterus of a primipara tends to remain contracted, but she also may experience severe afterpains if her uterus has been overdistended or blood clots are retained.

Severity. Afterpains are particularly severe during breastfeeding. Oxytocin, released from the posterior pituitary to stimulate the milk-ejection reflex, stimulates strong contractions of uterine muscles.

Nursing Considerations. Analgesics frequently are used to lessen the discomfort of afterpains. Medication that a breastfeeding mother takes just before nursing the infant may not reach the milk for 30 minutes or more. Many breastfeeding mothers are reluctant to take medication for fear that the infant will be harmed by the medication in breast milk. However, health care experts generally agree that analgesics may be used for short-term pain relief without harm to the infant. The benefits of pain relief, such as comfort and relaxation that facilitate the milk-ejection reflex, usually outweigh the negligible effects of the medication on the infant.

Some mothers also find that lying in a prone position, with a small pillow or folded blanket under the abdomen, helps keep the uterus contracted and provides relief. The nurse can reassure the mother that afterpains are self-limiting and decrease rapidly after 48 hours.

Lochia

Changes in the color and amount of lochia also provide information about whether involution is progressing normally.

Changes in Color. For the first 3 days after childbirth, lochia consists almost entirely of blood, with small particles of decidua and mucus. It is called *lochia rubra* because of its red color. The amount of blood decreases by about the fourth day, when leukocytes begin to invade the area, as they do any healing surface. The color of lochia then changes from red to pink or brown-tinged *(lochia serosa).* Lochia serosa is composed of serous exudate, erythrocytes, leukocytes, and cervical mucus. By about the eleventh day, the erythrocyte component decreases. The discharge becomes white or cream colored *(lochia alba).* Lochia alba contains leukocytes, decidual cells, epithelial cells, fat, cervical mucus, and bacteria. It is present in most women until the third week after childbirth but may persist for 6 weeks.

Amount. Because estimating the amount of lochia on a peripad (perineal pad) is difficult, nurses frequently document lochia in terms that are difficult to quantify, such as *scant, moderate,* and *heavy.* Agreement on the meanings of terms in an agency is important to make charting accurate. The following terms and descriptions for the amount of lochia in 1 hour provide an example.

Scant—Less than a 1-inch (2.5-cm) stain on the peripad
Light—1- to 4-inch (2.5- to 10-cm) stain
Moderate—4- to 6-inch (10- to 15-cm) stain
Large—Saturated peripad in 1 hour
Excessive—Saturated peripad in 15 minutes (Scoggin, 2000)

Determining the amount of time the woman has been wearing a peripad is important. What appears to be a moderate amount of lochia may be only a light flow if the peripad has been in use for more than an hour (Figure 17-2). The amount of lochia absorbed by a peripad varies according to the brand used.

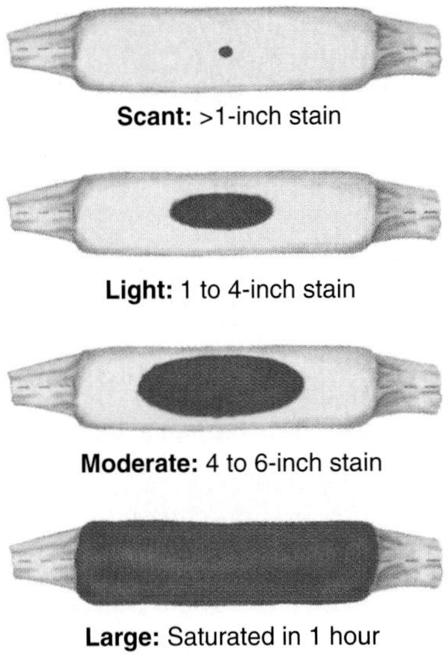

FIGURE 17-2 Guidelines for assessing the amount of lochia on the perineal pad.

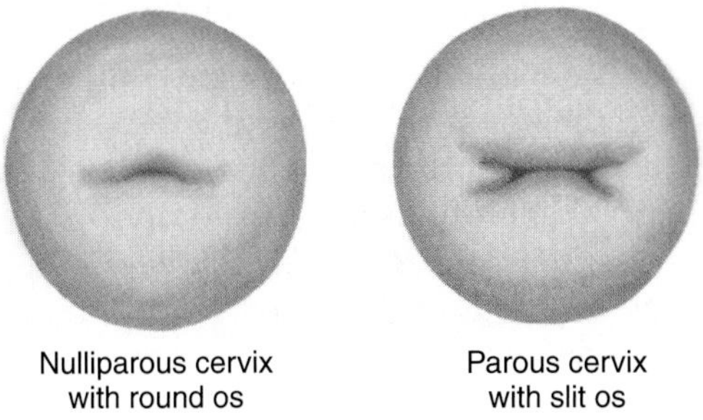

FIGURE 17-3 A permanent change occurs in the cervical os after childbirth.

Table 17-1
CHARACTERISTICS OF LOCHIA

Time and Type	Normal Discharge	Abnormal Discharge
Days 1-3: lochia rubra	Bloody; small clots; fleshy, earthy odor	Large clots; saturated perineal pads; foul odor
Days 4-10: lochia serosa	Decreased amount; serosanguineous; pink or brown	Excessive amount; foul smell; continued or recurrent reddish color
Days 11-21: lochia alba	Creamy, yellowish color; decreasing amounts	Persistent lochia serosa; return to lochia rubra, foul odor; discharge continuing

The time between delivery and assessment of lochia also is important. Lochia flow will be greater immediately after delivery, but will gradually decrease. It is less after cesarean birth because of removal of some endometrial lining during surgery. The lochia of the cesarean mother will go through the same phases as that of the woman who had a vaginal birth, even though the amount may be reduced.

Lochia flow often is heavier when the new mother first gets out of bed after birth or after sleeping because gravity allows blood that pooled in the vagina during the hours of rest to flow freely when she stands. (Table 17-1 summarizes the characteristics of normal and abnormal lochial discharge.)

Cervix

Immediately after childbirth, the cervix is formless, flabby, and open wide enough to admit the entire hand. This allows manual extraction of the placenta, if necessary, and manual examination of the uterus. Small tears or lacerations may be present, and the cervix is often edematous. Rapid healing takes place, and by the end of the first week the cervix feels firm and the external os is the width of a pencil. The internal os closes as before pregnancy, but the shape of the external os is permanently changed. It remains slightly open and appears slit-like rather than round, as in the nulliparous woman (Figure 17-3).

Table 17-2

LACERATIONS OF THE BIRTH CANAL

PERINEUM

Perineal lacerations are classified in degrees to describe the amount of tissue involved. Some physicians or nurse-midwives also use degrees to describe the extent of midline episiotomies.

First-degree: Involves the superficial vaginal mucosa or perineal skin.

Second-degree: Involves the vaginal mucosa, perineal skin, and deeper tissues, which may include muscles of the perineum.

Third-degree: Same as second-degree lacerations but involves the anal sphincter.

Fourth-degree: Extends through the anal sphincter into the rectal mucosa.

PERIURETHRAL AREA

A laceration in the area of the urethra may cause women to have difficulty urinating after birth. They may require an indwelling catheter for a day or two.

VAGINAL WALL

A laceration involving the mucosa of the vaginal wall.

CERVIX

Tears in the cervix may be a source of significant bleeding after birth.

Vagina

The vagina and vaginal introitus are greatly stretched during birth to allow passage of the fetus. Soon after childbirth, the vaginal walls appear edematous, and multiple small lacerations may be present. Very few vaginal rugae (folds) are present. The hymen is permanently torn and heals with small, irregular tags of tissue visible at the vaginal introitus.

Although the vaginal mucosa heals and rugae are regained by 3 weeks, the entire postpartum period (6 weeks) is needed for the vagina to complete involution and to gain approximately the same size and contour it had before pregnancy. The vagina does not entirely regain the nulliparous size, however.

During the postpartum period, vaginal mucosa becomes atrophic and vaginal walls do not regain their thickness until estrogen production by the ovaries is reestablished. Because ovarian function, and therefore estrogen production, is not well established during lactation, breastfeeding mothers are likely to experience vaginal dryness and may experience discomfort during intercourse (dyspareunia) for 4 to 6 months.

Perineum

The muscles of the pelvic floor stretch and thin greatly during the second stage of labor, when the fetal head applies pressure as it descends, rotates, and then extends to be delivered. After childbirth, the perineum may be edematous and bruised. In the United States, many women who give birth also have a surgical incision (episiotomy) of the perineal area.

Generally, the episiotomy is median or midline, extending straight back from the lower edge of the introitus toward the anus. Occasionally, mediolateral incisions, begun at the introitus and directed laterally and downward away from the rectum to either the right or the left side, are made to provide additional room for birth of the infant.

Lacerations of the perineum may also occur during delivery. Lacerations and episiotomies are classified according to tissue involved (Table 17-2). (See Chapters 13 and 16 for further discussion of episiotomy and lacerations.)

Discomfort

Although the episiotomy is relatively small, the muscles of the perineum are involved in many activities (for example, walking, sitting, stooping, squatting, bending, defecating). An incision in this area can cause a great deal of discomfort. In addition, many pregnant women are affected by hemorrhoids (distended rectal veins), which are pushed out of the rectum during the second stage of labor.

Nursing Considerations

Hemorrhoids, as well as perineal trauma, episiotomy, or lacerations, can make physical activity or bowel elimination difficult during the postpartum period. Relief of perineal discomfort is a nursing priority that includes teaching self-care measures such as sitz baths, perineal care, topical anesthesia, and ordered analgesics.

Check Your Reading

1. Which three processes are involved in involution?
2. How is the fundus expected to descend after childbirth?
3. Which mothers are most likely to experience afterpains? How are they treated?
4. What are the differences between lochia rubra, lochia serosa, and lochia alba in appearance and expected duration?

CARDIOVASCULAR SYSTEM

Hypervolemia, which produces a 45% increase in blood volume at term, allows the woman to tolerate a substantial blood loss during childbirth without ill effect. On average, 500 ml of blood is lost in vaginal deliveries and 1000 ml is lost in cesarean births (Cunningham, et al., 1997).

Cardiac Output

Despite the blood loss, a transient increase in maternal cardiac output occurs after childbirth. This increase is caused by increased flow of blood back to the heart when blood from the uteroplacental unit returns to the central circulation, as well as mobilization of excess extracellular fluid into the vascular compartment.

The rise in cardiac output persists for at least 48 hours after childbirth (Resnik, 1999). It is caused by an increase in stroke volume and results in bradycardia during the early postpartum period. Bradycardia is defined as a pulse rate of 50 to 60 beats per minute. Gradually, cardiac output decreases and returns to normal levels by 12 weeks after childbirth.

Plasma Volume

The body rids itself of excess plasma volume, which was necessary during pregnancy, by two methods: diuresis and diaphoresis.

- Diuresis (increased excretion of urine) is facilitated by a decline in the adrenal hormone aldosterone, which is increased during pregnancy to counteract the salt-wasting effect of progesterone. As aldosterone production decreases, sodium retention declines and fluid excretion accelerates. A decrease in oxytocin, which promotes reabsorption of fluid, also contributes to diuresis. A urinary output of 3000 ml per day is common for the first few days of the postpartum period.
- Diaphoresis (profuse perspiration) also rids the body of excess fluid. Although not clinically significant, diaphoresis can be uncomfortable and unsettling for the mother who is not prepared for it. Explanations of the cause and comfort measures, such as showers and dry clothing, are generally sufficient.

Coagulation

Significant changes that occur during pregnancy also affect the body's ability to coagulate blood and form clots. During pregnancy, plasma fibrinogen (necessary for coagulation) increases as a protection against postpartum hemorrhage. As a result, the mother's body has a greater ability to form clots and thus prevent excessive bleeding. She does not, however, have an increased ability to eliminate clots because plasminogen (necessary for lysis of clots) remains the same. The result is that during pregnancy and the postpartum period, she is at risk for thrombus (clot) formation.

Although the incidence of thrombophlebitis has declined greatly in recent years, probably as a result of early postpartum ambulation, new mothers are still at increased risk for thrombus formation. Women who have varicose veins, have a history of thrombophlebitis, or have experienced a cesarean birth are at further risk, and the lower extremities should be monitored closely. Antiembolism hosiery may be applied before a cesarean birth or if the mother is at particular risk because of a history of previous phlebitis or the presence of varicosities (see Chapter 28).

Blood Values

Besides clotting factors, other components of the blood change during the postpartum period. Marked leukocytosis occurs, with the white blood cell count increasing from the nonpregnancy normal range of 5000 to $10,000/mm^3$ up to $30,000/mm^3$ (Cunningham, et al., 1997). The average increase is to 14,000 to $16,000/mm^3$ (Scoggin, 2000).

Neutrophils, which increase in response to inflammation, pain, and stress to protect against invading organisms, account for the major increase in white blood cells.

Maternal hemoglobin and hematocrit values are difficult to interpret during the first few days after birth because of the remobilization and rapid excretion of excess body fluid. The hematocrit is low when plasma (the liquid part of blood) increases and dilutes the concentration of blood cells and other substances carried by the plasma. As excess fluid is excreted, the dilution gradually is reduced. Hematocrit should return to normal limits within 3 to 7 days unless excessive blood loss has occurred.

GASTROINTESTINAL SYSTEM

Soon after childbirth, digestion begins to be active. The new mother usually is hungry because of the energy expended in labor. She usually is thirsty because of the decreased oral intake during labor, the fluid loss from exertion, mouth breathing, and early diaphoresis. Nurses anticipate the mother's needs and provide food and fluids soon after childbirth.

Constipation is a common problem during the postpartum period for a variety of reasons. Bowel tone, which was diminished during pregnancy as a result of progesterone, remains sluggish for several days. Restricted food and fluid intake during labor often results in small, hard stools. Perineal trauma, episiotomy, and hemorrhoids cause discomfort and interfere with effective bowel elimination. In addition, many women anticipate pain when they attempt to defecate and are unwilling to exert pressure on the perineum. Women who are taking iron have an added cause of constipation.

Temporary constipation is not harmful, although it can cause a feeling of abdominal fullness and flatulence. Many

Table 17-3
COMMONLY RECOMMENDED LAXATIVES FOR THE POSTPARTUM PERIOD

Types	Examples	Comments
Fecal wetting agents	Docusate calcium (Surfak) Docusate sodium (Colace)	Detergent-like action, permit easier mixing of fats and fluids with fecal mass; produce softer, more easily passed stools
Saline laxatives	Milk of magnesia	Work by osmotic action, drawing water through the intestinal wall to soften stool
Stimulant laxatives	Bisacodyl (Dulcolax)	Should not be taken within 1 hour of taking antacid or milk products
Suppositories	Glycerine, bisacodyl	Chill and moisten with cold water before insertion

Data from Hodgson, B.B. & Kizior, R.J. (2000). *Saunders nursing drug handbook 2000.* Philadelphia: W.B. Saunders.

women become extremely concerned about constipation, and stool softeners and laxatives frequently are prescribed to prevent or treat constipation (Table 17-3).

URINARY SYSTEM

Physical Changes

The kidneys return to normal function by 4 weeks after delivery. Both protein and acetone may be present in the urine in the first few postpartum days. Acetone suggests dehydration that often occurs during the exertion of labor. Mild proteinuria usually is the result of the catabolic processes involved in uterine involution. Sugar in the form of lactose also is sometimes present.

Changes during pregnancy cause the bladder of the postpartum woman to have increased capacity and decreased muscle tone. During childbirth, the urethra, bladder, and tissue around the urinary meatus may become edematous and traumatized as the fetal head passes beneath the bladder. This often results in diminished sensitivity to fluid pressure, and many mothers have no sensation of needing to void even when the bladder is distended.

The bladder fills rapidly because of the diuresis that follows childbirth. As a consequence, the mother is at risk for overdistention of the bladder, incomplete emptying of the bladder, and retention of residual urine. Women who have received regional anesthesia are at particular risk for bladder distention and difficulty in voiding until feeling returns.

Urinary retention and overdistention of the bladder may cause two complications: urinary tract infection and postpartum hemorrhage. Urinary tract infection occurs when urinary stasis allows time for bacteria to multiply. Risk of postpartum hemorrhage increases because uterine ligaments, which were stretched during pregnancy, allow the uterus to be displaced upward and laterally by the full bladder (Figure 17-4). The displacement results in an inability of the uterine muscles to contract (uterine atony), a primary cause of excessive bleeding.

Stress incontinence occuring during pregnancy usually improves after birth, but some women state that bladder function is worse after birth than it was before pregnancy (Thorp, et al., 1999). For some, the problem will resolve with exercises (for example, Kegel) and time for healing. Others have continued problems (see Chapter 33).

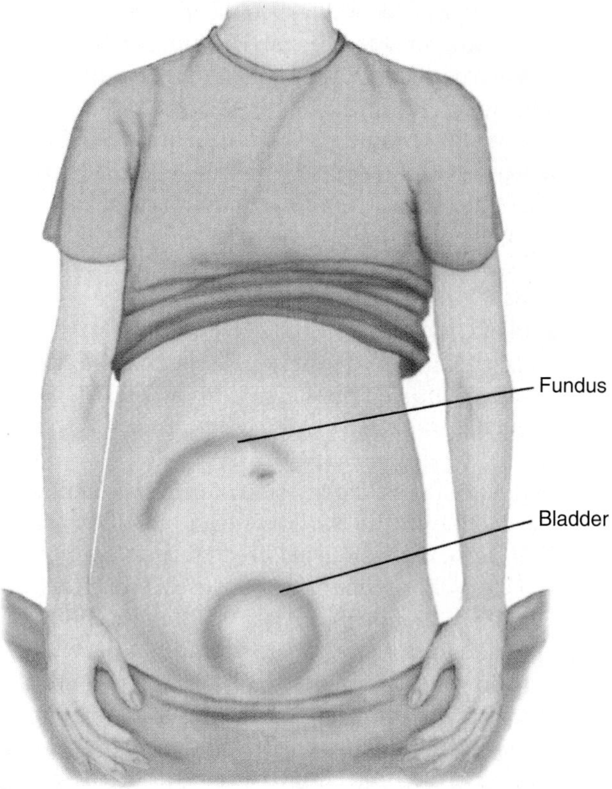

FIGURE 17-4 A full bladder displaces and prevents contraction of the uterus.

MUSCULOSKELETAL SYSTEM

Muscles and Joints

In the first 1 to 2 days after childbirth, many women experience muscle fatigue and aches, particularly of the shoulders, neck, and arms because of exertion during labor. Warmth and gentle massage increase circulation to the area and provide comfort and relaxation.

During the first few days, levels of the hormone relaxin gradually subside, and ligaments and cartilage of the pelvis begin to return to their prepregnancy posi-

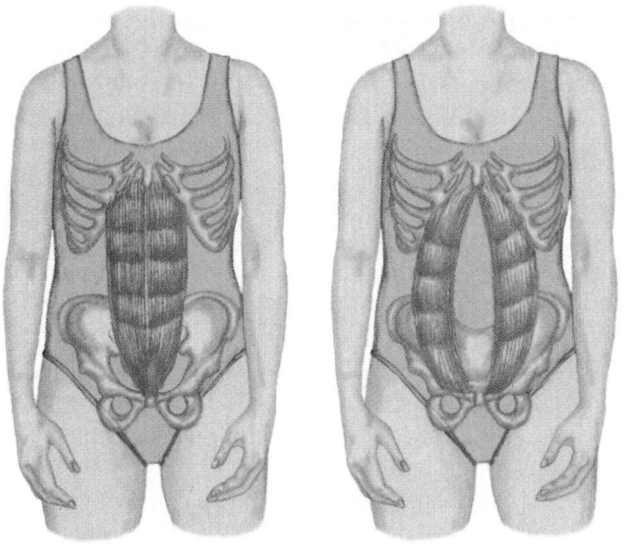

FIGURE 17-5 Diastasis recti occurs when the longitudinal muscles of the abdomen separate during pregnancy.

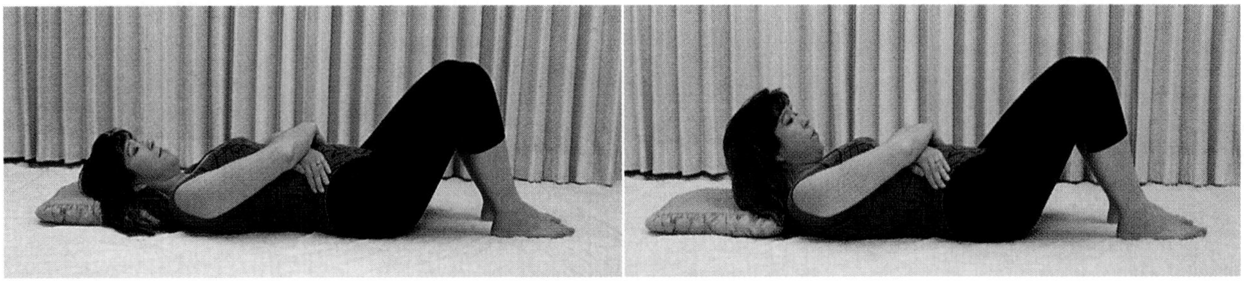

FIGURE 17-6 Abdominal exercises for diastasis recti. **A,** The woman inhales and supports the abdominal wall firmly with her hands. **B,** Exhaling, the woman raises her head as she pulls the abdominal muscles together.

tions. These changes can cause hip and joint pain that interferes with ambulation and exercise. The mother should be told that the discomfort is temporary and does not indicate a medical problem. Good body mechanics and correct posture are extremely important during this time to prevent low back pain and injury to the joints (see Figures 7-13 and 7-14).

Abdominal Wall

During pregnancy, the abdominal walls stretch to accommodate the growing fetus, and muscle tone is diminished. Many women, expecting that the abdominal muscles will return to the prepregnancy condition immediately after childbirth, are dismayed to find the abdominal muscles weak, soft, and flabby.

The longitudinal muscles of the abdomen may also separate (diastasis recti) during pregnancy (Figure 17-5). The separation may be minimal or severe. The mother can determine the amount of separation by placing the fingertips at the umbilicus and raising the head and shoulders while in a supine position. She may benefit from special exercises to strengthen the abdominal wall if there is a separation of three fingerbreadths or more (Figure 17-6).

INTEGUMENTARY SYSTEM

Many skin changes that occur during pregnancy are caused by an increase in hormones. When the hormone levels decline after childbirth, the skin gradually reverts to the prepregnancy state. For example, levels of melanocyte-stimulating hormone, which caused hyperpigmentation during pregnancy, decrease rapidly after childbirth, and pigmentation begins to recede. This change is particularly noticeable when the "mask of pregnancy" (chloasma or melasma) and linea nigra disappear. In addition, spider nevi and palmar erythema, which may develop during pregnancy as a result of increased estrogen levels, gradually disappear.

Striae gravidarum (stretch marks), which develop during pregnancy when connective tissues in the abdomen and breasts are stretched, gradually fade to silvery lines but do not disappear. Increased loss of hair may especially concern the woman. This is a normal response to the hormonal changes that caused decreased hair loss during pregnancy. Hair loss may last as long as 3 to 4 months but regrowth generally occurs by 9 months after birth (Cunningham, et al., 1997).

NEUROLOGIC SYSTEM

Anesthesia or analgesia may produce temporary neurologic changes such as lack of feeling in the legs and dizziness. During this time, prevention of injury from falling is a priority.

Complaints of headache require careful assessment. Although they are uncommon, postpuncture headaches after regional anesthesia may occur. They may be most severe when the woman is in an upright position and are relieved by a supine position. They should be reported to the appropriate health care provider, usually an anesthesiologist. Headache, along with blurred vision, photophobia, and abdominal pain, also may indicate development or worsening of pregnancy-induced hypertension (see Chapter 25).

ENDOCRINE SYSTEM

After expulsion of the placenta, a fairly rapid decline occurs in placental hormones such as estrogen, progesterone, human placental lactogen, and human chorionic gonadotropin. Adrenal hormones such as aldosterone return to prepregnancy levels. If the mother is not breastfeeding, the pituitary hormone prolactin, which stimulates milk secretion, disappears in about 2 weeks.

Resumption of Ovulation and Menstruation

The average time for nonnursing mothers to resume menstruation is 7 to 9 weeks after childbirth, although this varies (Resnik, 1999). Breastfeeding delays return of both ovulation and menstruation. The length of the delay depends on the frequency of breastfeeding and the duration of lactation. Women who breastfeed six or more times daily are likely to ovulate and menstruate later than women who breastfeed less often (Kennedy, 1999).

The longer the period of lactation, the longer the average time to the first menstrual period. Women who breastfeed for less than 28 days ovulate at approximately the same time as nonnursing mothers. Menses while lactating may resume as early as 12 weeks or as late as 18 months (Scoggin, 2000). Menses and ovulation are increasingly likely after the infant is 6 months old. Although the first few cycles for both lactating women and nonlactating women are often anovulatory, ovulation may occur before the first menses. Breastfeeding is not an effective form of contraception.

Lactation

During pregnancy, estrogen and progesterone prepare the breasts for lactation. Although prolactin levels also rise during pregnancy, lactation is inhibited at this time by the high levels of estrogen and progesterone. After expulsion of the placenta, levels of estrogen and progesterone decline rapidly, and prolactin initiates milk production within 2 to 3 days after childbirth. Once milk production is established, it continues because of frequent removal of milk from the breast. That is, the more the infant nurses, the more milk the mother produces.

Whereas prolactin is essential for initiating milk production, oxytocin is necessary for milk ejection or "let down." Oxytocin, a hormone from the posterior pituitary gland, causes milk to be expressed from the alveoli into the lactiferous ducts during suckling (see Chapter 22).

Weight Loss

Approximately 4.5 to 5.5 kg (10 to 12 lb) are lost during childbirth. This includes the weight of the fetus, placenta, and amniotic fluid and blood lost during the birth. An additional 2.3 to 3.6 kg (5 to 8 lb) are lost as a result of duresis in the early postpartum days and as the reproductive organs undergo the process of involution (Scoggin, 2000).

Adipose (fatty) tissue that was gained during pregnancy to meet the energy requirements of breastfeeding is not lost initially, and the usual rate of loss is slow. Most women approach their prepregnancy weight about 6 months after childbirth, but it may be a year before all weight is lost. Many mothers are frustrated during this time because they desire an immediate return to prepregnancy weight. Nurses must be prepared to provide information about diet and exercise that will produce an acceptable weight loss but does not deplete the energy or impair the health of the mother.

Check Your Reading

5. Why is the mother at risk for urinary retention? Which two complications may result?
6. Why does hyperpigmentation decrease after childbirth?
7. How does breastfeeding affect the resumption of ovulation and menstruation?
8. Should the nurse be concerned if a woman who delivered a baby yesterday has a WBC of 14,000? Why or why not?
9. When should a woman who is formula feeding her infant expect her menses to resume? The woman who is breastfeeding?
10. How much weight will the woman lose during childbirth? How much can she expect to lose by 6 weeks after childbirth?

POSTPARTUM ASSESSMENTS

Providing essential, cost-effective postpartum care to new families is a challenge for maternity nurses. Legislation allows women and their health care providers to determine the length of stay and provides for insurance payments for covered care. This allows most women to stay in the birth facility for 48 hours after an uncomplicated vaginal birth and 96 hours after a cesarean birth. Many women, however, choose to leave at an earlier time.

Although the length of stay is short, the family's need for care and information remains the same. This need causes nurses a great deal of concern for families who are discharged without adequate preparation or support. Nurses are actively involved in developing ways to provide continuing care in the home. They use measures such as clinical pathways to structure assessments, care, and teaching during the birth facility stay.

Clinical Pathways

Many institutions use clinical pathways (also called *critical pathways, care maps,* or *multidisciplinary action plans*) to provide necessary care while reducing the LOS. Clinical pathways identify expected outcomes and establish time frames for specific assessments and interventions that prepare the mother and infant for discharge. The clinical pathway is a guideline and documentation tool (Figure 17-7).

Initial Assessments

Caring for postpartum clients exposes the nurse to the risk of coming into contact with body fluids such as colostrum, breast milk, amniotic fluid, and lochia from the mother as well as urine, stool, and blood from the infant. Therefore the recommendations of the Centers for Disease Control and Prevention for standard blood and body fluid precautions must be maintained diligently (see Appendix A).

Postpartum assessments begin during the fourth stage of labor (1 to 2 hours after childbirth). The mother is examined to determine whether she is physically stable. Initial assessments include the following:

- Vital signs
- Skin color
- Location and firmness of the fundus
- Amount and color of lochia
- Perineum (edema, episiotomy, lacerations, hematoma)
- Presence and location of pain
- IV infusions: type of fluid and rate, added medications (type and amount), and patency of the IV line; site for redness, pain, or edema
- Urinary output: Time of last void or presence of catheter; color, character, and amount of urine
- Status of abdominal incision, if present
- Level of feeling and ability to move the legs if regional anesthesia was administered

Chart Review

When the initial assessments confirm that the mother's physical condition is stable, nurses should review the chart to obtain pertinent information and determine whether factors are present that increase the risk of complications during the postpartum period. Relevant information includes the following:

- Gravida, parity
- Time and type of delivery (use of forceps, vacuum extractor)
- Anesthesia or medications administered during labor
- Significant medical and surgical history, such as diabetes, heart disease, and hypertension
- Medications routinely taken and reasons for their use
- Food and drug allergies
- Chosen method of infant feeding
- Condition of the baby

Laboratory data also are examined. Of particular interest are the prenatal hemoglobin and hematocrit values, blood type and Rh factor, hepatitis B surface antigen, syphilis screen, and group B streptococcus status (see Chapter 26).

Need for Rh_0(D) Immune Globulin

Prenatal and neonatal records are checked to determine whether Rh_0(D) immune globulin (RhoGAM) should be administered. Rh_0(D) immune globulin may be necessary if the mother is Rh-negative, the newborn is Rh-positive, and the mother is not already sensitized. Rh_0(D) immune globulin should be administered within 72 hours after childbirth to prevent the development of maternal antibodies that would affect subsequent pregnancies (see Chapter 25 for maternal Rh incompatibility and Rh_0[D] immune globulin drug guide).

Need for Rubella Vaccine

A prenatal rubella antibody screen is performed on each pregnant woman to determine whether she is immune to rubella. If she is not immune, rubella vaccine is offered after childbirth to prevent her from acquiring rubella during subsequent pregnancies, when it can cause serious fetal anomalies. Although defects in infants born to mothers who received rubella vaccine during pregnancy have not been reported, the vaccine is a live virus and defects might occur in the fetus if the mother becomes pregnant soon after it is administered (Duerbeck & Reed, 1998).

Before administration, the mother usually is asked to give written permission to receive the vaccine. Some agencies require that she sign a statement indicating she understands the risks of becoming pregnant again within 3 months after the injection. If a written statement from the mother is not required, the nurse should document in the chart that the risk has been explained and that the parents verbalize their understanding (see Drug Guide).

Risk Factors for Hemorrhage and Infection

Nurses must be aware of conditions that increase the risk of hemorrhage and infection, the two most common complications of the puerperium.

Text continued on p. 438

Date:

CARE PATH FOR POSTPARTUM VAGINAL DELIVERY

Problem Number	LOCATION	2 TO 8 HR p̄ DELIVERY	8 TO 16 HR p̄ DELIVERY	16 TO 24 HR p̄ DELIVERY
I 5 II 7,8 IV 16	Assessments	q̄ 4 hr: TPR, BP PP check (fundus–location & tone; lochia–amount, color, odor, clots) Bladder status q̄ shift Perineum–epis, ± hematoma, ± edema Homan's sign, redness, swelling, tenderness of calf Lungs, breasts Bowel sounds, abd distention If tubal, incision site Bladder checks × 3: time ______, ______ amount of void ______, ______ fundus @ ______, ______ bladder ______, ______ (NP–nonpalpable; P–palpable)	q̄ 4 hr: TPR, BP PP check Bladder status q̄ shift Perineum–epis, ± hematoma, ± edema Homan's sign, redness, swelling, tenderness of calf Lungs, breasts Bowel sounds, abd distention If tubal, incision site time ______, ______ amount of void ______, ______ fundus @ ______, ______ bladder ______, ______ (NP–nonpalpable; P–palpable)	q̄ 4 hr: TPR, BP PP check Bladder status q̄ shift Perineum–epis, ± hematoma, ± edema Homan's sign, redness, swelling, tenderness of calf Lungs, breasts Bowel sounds, abd distention ± BM If tubal, incision site
		Fundus firm @ U or lower **Lochia min to mod s̄ clots, odor** **Bladder nonpalpable p̄ void × 3** **Perineum intact s̄ hematoma** verified ______________	**Fundus firm @ U or lower** **Bladder nonpalpable p̄ void** **Perineum intact s̄ hematoma** verified ______________	**Fundus firm @ U or lower** **Bladder nonpalpable p̄ void** **Perineum intact s̄ hematoma** verified ______________
	Procedures/ Tests	HCT the AM p̄ delivery	HCT the AM p̄ delivery result ______________	
I 5,7,21	Treatments	Ice to perineum Fundal massage prn to maintain uterine tone Pericare q̄ void Performs self peri care Assist c̄ breastfeeding	Ice to perineum Fundal massage prn to maintain uterine tone Pericare q̄ void Assist c̄ breastfeeding	Sitz bath prn Fundal massage prn to maintain uterine tone Pericare q̄ void Assist c̄ breastfeeding
VI 3 XI 5	Activity	**Up c̄ assistance × 1 then ad lib** verified ______________	**Ad lib** verified ______________	**Ad lib** verified ______________
	Signatures	____/____ ____/____ ____/____ ____/____ ____/____	____/____ ____/____ ____/____ ____/____ ____/____	____/____ ____/____ ____/____ ____/____ ____/____

MED REC NO. ______________

PATIENT ______________

PHYSICIAN ______________

BILLING NO. ______________

BAYLOR UNIVERSITY MEDICAL CENTER
DALLAS, TEXAS

CARE PATH FOR POSTPARTUM VAGINAL DELIVERY

PAGE 1 OF 4

FIGURE 17-7 Clinical pathway for uncomplicated vaginal birth. (Copyrighted by and courtesy Baylor University Medical Center, Dallas, Texas.)

Date:

CARE PATH FOR POSTPARTUM VAGINAL DELIVERY

Problem Number	LOCATION	2 TO 8 HR p̄ DELIVERY	8 TO 16 HR p̄ DELIVERY	16 TO 24 HR p̄ DELIVERY
VI 3 III 1	Meds/IV's	Analgesics: For ____________ pain Pain level ________ on pain scale ____ Lortab 1-2 q̄ 3-4 hr prn Time ____ Time ____ ____ Darvocet N 100 1-2 po q̄ 4-6 hr prn Time ____ Time ____ ____ Tylenol __ Tabs Time ____ Local anesthetics ____ Epifoam tid prn ____ Proctofoam tid prn Stool softener ____ Doxidan 1 hs prn ____ Senokot 1 hs prn ____ Dulcolax supp. 1 pr prn	Analgesics: For ____________ pain Pain level ________ on pain scale ____ Lortab 1-2 q̄ 3-4 hr prn Time ____ Time ____ ____ Darvocet N 100 1-2 po q̄ 4-6 hr prn Time ____ Time ____ ____ Tylenol __ Tabs Time ____ Local anesthetics ____ Epifoam tid prn ____ Proctofoam tid prn Stool softener ____ Doxidan 1 hs prn ____ Senokot 1 hs prn ____ Dulcolax supp. 1 pr prn	Analgesics: For ____________ pain Pain level ________ on pain scale ____ Lortab 1-2 q̄ 3-4 hr prn Time ____ Time ____ ____ Darvocet N 100 1-2 po q̄ 4-6 hr prn Time ____ Time ____ ____ Tylenol __ Tabs Time ____ Local anesthetics ____ Epifoam tid prn ____ Proctofoam tid prn Stool softener ____ Doxidan 1 hs prn ____ Senokot 1 hs prn ____ Dulcolax supp. 1 pr prn Rhogam ____ given ____ na verified ____
		Comfort maintained @ ≤2 on pain scale verified ____________	**Comfort maintained @ ≤2 on pain scale** verified ____________	**Comfort maintained @ ≤2 on pain scale** verified ____________
	Nutrition	General diet **Tolerates** verified ________	General diet **Tolerates** verified ________	General diet **Tolerates** verified ________
VI 2 I 4	PT/Family Education	Assess current knowledge; teach/reinforce: Postpartum routine Safety (assistance c̄ 1st time out of bed, infant security) Bladder checks Postpartum checks Fundal massage Breast feeding Pain control/comfort measures Pericare	Assess current knowledge; teach/reinforce: All previous teaching +: Breasts/nipple care Nutrition Elimination Uterine regression Lochia changes	Assess current knowledge; teach/reinforce: All previous teaching +: Kegel exercises S&S of illness/complications Activity/exercise Contraception Nothing in vagina FU MD visit Take home meds
		Demonstrates/verbalizes understanding verified ____________	**Demonstrates/verbalizes understanding** verified ____________	**Demonstrates/verbalizes understanding** verified ____________
	Discharge Planning	**Baseline educational needs identified by pt & nurse** verified ____________	Discuss homecare needs	Provide c̄ written discharge instructions
		Initiate SW consult if inidicated ____________	Pastoral care visit	
VIII 2,7	Psycho-Social Emotional Spiritual	**Parents will demonstrate + interactions c̄ infant (hold, establish eye contact)** verified ____________ **Identifies support person/system** verified ____________	**Parents will demonstrate + interactions c̄ infant (hold, establish eye contact)** verified ____________	**Parents will demonstrate + interactions c̄ infant (hold, establish eye contact)** verified ____________
	Signatures	____/________ ____/________	____/________ ____/________	____/________ ____/________

MED REC NO. ____________________

PATIENT ____________________

PHYSICIAN ____________________

BILLING NO. ____________________

BAYLOR UNIVERSITY MEDICAL CENTER
DALLAS, TEXAS

CARE PATH FOR POSTPARTUM VAGINAL DELIVERY

PAGE 2 OF 4

FIGURE 17-7, cont'd For legend see opposite page.

Continued

Date:

CARE PATH FOR POSTPARTUM VAGINAL DELIVERY

Problem Number	LOCATION	24 TO 32 HR p̄ DELIVERY	32 TO 40 HR p̄ DELIVERY	40 TO 48 HR p̄ DELIVERY	DC CRITERIA
I 5 II 7,8 IV 16	Assessments	q̄ 8 hr: TPR, BP PP check Bladder status q̄ shift Perineum–epis, ± hematoma, ± edema Homan's sign, redness, swelling, tenderness of calf Lungs Breasts Bowel sounds, abd distention ± BM If tubal, incision site	q̄ 8 hr: TPR, BP PP check Bbladder status q̄ shift Perineum–epis, ± hematoma, ± edema Homan's sign, redness, swelling, tenderness of calf Lungs Breasts Bowel sounds, abd distention ± BM If tubal, incision site	q̄ 8 hr: TPR, BP PP check Bladder status q̄ shift Perineum–epis, ± hematoma, ± edema Homan's sign, redness, swelling, tenderness of calf Lungs Breasts Bowel sounds, abd distention ± BM If tubal, incision site	VSS, Temp ≤ 100.4 **Verified** __________ Fundus firm, at U or lower **Verified** __________ Lochia minimal to moderate s̄ clots **Verified** __________ Emptying bladder s̄ difficulty + Bowel sounds + Flatus **Verified** __________
		Fundus firm @ U or lower **Bladder nondistend p̄ void** **Perineum intact s̄ hematoma** verified __________	**Fundus firm @ U or lower** **Bladder nondistend p̄ void** **Perineum intact s̄ hematoma** verified __________	**Fundus firm @ U or lower** **Bladder nondistend p̄ void** **Perineum intact s̄ hematoma** verified __________	
	Procedures/ Tests				
I 5,7,21	Treatments	Sitz bath prn Fundal massage prn to maintain uterine tone Pericare q̄ void Assist c̄ breastfeeding	Sitz bath prn Fundal massage prn to maintain uterine tone Pericare q̄ void Assist c̄ breastfeeding	Sitz bath prn Fundal massage prn to maintain uterine tone Pericare q̄ void Assist c̄ breastfeeding	
IV 2	Activity	**Ad lib** verified __________	**Ad lib** verified __________	**Ad lib** verified __________	**Able to perform self & infant care** verified __________
	Signatures	___/___ ___/___ ___/___ ___/___ ___/___	___/___ ___/___ ___/___ ___/___ ___/___	___/___ ___/___ ___/___ ___/___ ___/___	___/___ ___/___ ___/___ ___/___ ___/___

MED REC NO. ____________________

PATIENT ____________________

PHYSICIAN ____________________

BILLING NO. ____________________

BAYLOR UNIVERSITY MEDICAL CENTER

DALLAS, TEXAS

CARE PATH FOR POSTPARTUM VAGINAL DELIVERY

PAGE 3 OF 4

FIGURE 17-7, cont'd For legend see p. 434.

Date:

CARE PATH FOR POSTPARTUM VAGINAL DELIVERY

Problem Number	LOCATION	24 TO 32 HR p̄ DELIVERY	32 TO 40 HR p̄ DELIVERY	40 TO 48 HR p̄ DELIVERY	DC CRITERIA
VI 3 III 1	Meds/IV's	Analgesics: For ________ pain Pain level ___ on pain scale ____ Lortab 1-2 q̄ 3-4 hr prn Time ____ Time ____ ____ Darvocet N 100 1-2 po q̄ 4-6 hr prn Time ____ Time ____ __ Tylenol __ Tabs Time __ Local anesthetics ____ Epifoam tid prn ____ Proctofoam tid prn Stool softener ____ Doxidan 1 hs prn ____ Senokot 1 hs prn ____ Dulcolax supp. 1 pr prn	Analgesics: For ________ pain Pain level ___ on pain scale ____ Lortab 1-2 q̄ 3-4 hr prn Time ____ Time ____ ____ Darvocet N 100 1-2 po q̄ 4-6 hr prn Time ____ Time ____ __ Tylenol __ Tabs Time __ Local anesthetics ____ Epifoam tid prn ____ Proctofoam tid prn Stool softener ____ Doxidan 1 hs prn ____ Senokot 1 hs prn ____ Dulcolax supp. 1 pr prn	Analgesics: For ________ pain Pain level ___ on pain scale ____ Lortab 1-2 q̄ 3-4 hr prn Time ____ Time ____ ____ Darvocet N 100 1-2 po q̄ 4-6 hr prn Time ____ Time ____ __ Tylenol __ Tabs Time __ Local anesthetics ____ Epifoam tid prn ____ Proctofoam tid prn Stool softener ____ Doxidan 1 hs prn ____ Senokot 1 hs prn ____ Dulcolax supp. 1 pr prn Rubella____given ____na **verified** ____________	
		Comfort maintained @ ≤ 2 on pain scale verified ____________	**Comfort maintained @ ≤ 2 on pain scale** verified ____________	**Comfort maintained @ ≤ 2 on pain scale** verified ____________	
	Nutrition	General diet	General diet	General diet	Tolerates general diet
		Tolerates verified ________	**Tolerates** verified ________	**Tolerates** verified ________	
VI 2 I 4	PT/Family Education	Assess current knowledge; teach/reinforce: All previous teaching +: Kegel exercises S&S of illness/ complications Activity/exercise Contraception Nothing in vagina FU MD visit Take home meds	Assess current knowledge; teach/reinforce: All previous teaching +: Kegel exercises S&S of illness/ complications Activity/exercise Contraception Nothing in vagina FU MD visit Take home meds	Assess current knowledge; teach/reinforce: All previous teaching +: Kegel exercises S&S of illness/ complications Activity/exercise Contraception Nothing in vagina FU MD visit Take home meds	Verbalizes/demonstrates knowledge of self care: Breast/nipple care Breastfeeding Activity/exercise Elimination Diet S&S of comps
		Demonstrates/verbalizes understanding verified ____________	**Demonstrates/verbalizes understanding** verified ____________	**Demonstrates/verbalizes understanding** verified ____________	**Verbalizes/demonstrates knowledge of infant care—see infant discharge teaching.** verified ____________
	Discharge Planning	Provide c̄ written discharge instructions	Provide c̄ written discharge instructions	Provide c̄ written discharge instructions	Expresses confidence in ability to care for self & infant. Identities FU appt date. **verified** ____________
VIII 2,7	Psycho-Social Emotional Spiritual	**Parents will demonstrate + interactions c̄ infant (hold, establish eye contact)** verified ____________	**Parents will demonstrate + interactions c̄ infant (hold, establish eye contact)** verified ____________	**Parents will demonstrate + interactions c̄ infant (hold, establish eye contact)** verified ____________	**Identifies at least 1 person or service to assist with self and infant care at home** verified ____________
	Signatures	____/____ ____/____	____/____ ____/____	____/____ ____/____	____/____ ____/____

MED REC NO. ____________________

PATIENT ____________________

PHYSICIAN ____________________

BILLING NO. ____________________

BAYLOR UNIVERSITY MEDICAL CENTER
DALLAS, TEXAS

CARE PATH FOR POSTPARTUM VAGINAL DELIVERY

PAGE 4 OF 4

FIGURE 17-7, cont'd For legend see p. 434.

DRUG GUIDE: Rubella Vaccine

Classification: Attenuated live virus vaccine

Action: Produces a modified rubella infection that is not communicable, causing the formation of antibodies against rubella virus

Indications: The vaccine is administered after childbirth or abortion to women whose antibody screen is less than 1:8, showing they are not immune to rubella (German measles). This prevents rubella infection and possible severe congenital defects in the fetus during a subsequent pregnancy.

Dosage and Route: The entire reconstituted volume of a single dose vial or 0.5 ml from a multiple dose vial. Inject subcutaneously in the upper outer aspect of the upper arm.

Absorption: Well absorbed

Contraindications and Precautions: The vaccine is contraindicated in women who have a respiratory or febrile infection, active untreated tuberculosis, or conditions that affect the bone marrow or lymphatic systems or are immunosuppressed, pregnant, or sensitive to neomycin or eggs. The attenuated virus may appear in breast milk, but is not a contraindication to vaccination of lactating women. It should be deferred for 3 months in clients receiving immune serum globulin or blood transfusions.

Adverse Reactions: Transient stinging at site, lymphadenopathy, rash, urticaria, fever, malaise, sore throat, headache, dizziness, nausea, vomiting, arthralgia, arthritis. Arthralgia or arthritis is frequent 2 to 4 weeks after administration.

Nursing Implications: Adverse fetal effects have been identified during early pregnancy, so the mother and her partner must be warned to avoid pregnancy for at least 3 months after vaccination because of the possibility that a fetus might be affected by the live virus in the vaccine. Signed informed consent is usually required.

Vials should be refrigerated. Reconstitute only with diluent supplied with the vial. Use immediately after reconstitution and discard if not used within 8 hours. Protect from light. Do not give at the same time as immune globulin.

CRITICAL TO REMEMBER

Postpartum High-Risk Factors

Hemorrhage

Multiparity (greater than three)
Overdistention of the uterus (large baby, twins, hydramnios)
Precipitous labor (less than 3 hours)
Prolonged labor
Retained placenta
Placenta previa or abruptio placentae
Induction or augmentation of labor
Administration of tocolytics to stop uterine contractions
Operative procedures (vacuum extraction, forceps, cesarean birth)

Infection

Operative procedures (cesarean birth, vacuum extraction, forceps)
Multiple cervical examinations
Prolonged labor (more than 24 hours)
Prolonged rupture of membranes
Manual extraction of placenta
Diabetes
Indwelling catheter
Anemia (hemoglobin less than 10.5 mg/dl)

Focus Assessments after Vaginal Birth

Nurses perform postpartum assessments according to facility protocol or as follows:

- First hour: every 15 minutes
- Second hour: every 30 minutes
- First 24 hours: every 4 hours
- After 24 hours: every 8 hours (Scoggin, 2000)

Although assessments vary depending on the particular problems experienced by the mother, in general a focus assessment for a vaginal delivery includes the vital signs, fundus, lochia, perineum, bladder elimination, breasts, and lower extremities. The assessment for women whose infants were born vaginally differs from that performed for postcesarean mothers (see p. 446).

Vital Signs

Blood Pressure. Blood pressure varies with position, and to obtain accurate results it should be measured with the mother in the same position each time. Therefore nurses must document both the mother's position when taking blood pressure and the pressure obtained. Postpartum blood pressure should be compared with that of the predelivery period so that deviations from what is normal for the mother can be quickly identified. An increase from the baseline suggests pregnancy-induced hypertension. A decrease may indicate dehydration or hypovolemia resulting from excessive bleeding.

Orthostatic Hypotension. After birth, a rapid decrease in intraabdominal pressure results in dilation of blood vessels supplying the viscera. The resulting engorgement of abdominal blood vessels contributes to a rapid fall in blood pressure of 15 to 20 mm Hg when the woman moves from a recumbent to a sitting position. As a result of the sudden drop in blood pressure, mothers often say that they feel dizzy or lightheaded, or they faint when they stand. The nursing diagnosis "Risk for Injury" applies to women with orthostatic hypotension (Nursing Care Plan 17-1).

Hypotension also may indicate hypovolemia. Careful assessments for hemorrhage (location and firmness of the fundus, amount of lochia, pulse rate for tachycardia) should be made if the postpartum blood pressure

NURSING CARE PLAN 17-1

Postpartum Hypotension, Fatigue, and Pain

Assessment: Jacqueline Tilden, gravida II, para II, gave birth to a baby girl weighing 3400 g (7.5 lb) 4 hours ago. She became weak and dizzy and said, "Everything is going black" when she attempted to ambulate the first time. Her gait was unsteady, and the nurse had to lower her back to bed to prevent her from fainting. Her color was pale, and her pulse was rapid.

Nursing Diagnosis: Risk for Injury related to physiologic effects of orthostatic hypotension

Critical Thinking: Does the nurse have enough data to make this diagnosis? If not, what other data are necessary? Why?

Answer: Although dizziness and feeling faint may indicate orthostatic hypotension, they may also indicate hypovolemia. The nurse must also assess Jacqueline for signs of excessive blood loss, such as the location and firmness of the uterine fundus, the amount of lochia, the pulse rate at rest, and hemoglobin and hematocrit levels. If these data are within expected levels, a diagnosis of "Risk for Injury related to the effects of orthostatic hypotension" is appropriate.

Expected Outcome:
Jacqueline will remain free of injury caused by fainting and falling during the postpartum period.

Intervention	Rationale
1. Check the mother's blood pressure using the same arm while she is in a supine position and in a sitting position.	1. A decrease of 20 mm Hg in systolic pressure in the upright position indicates orthostatic hypotension. Measuring from the same arm provides more accurate information because the reading may differ slightly in each arm.
2. Instruct the mother in measures to overcome the sudden drop in blood pressure: a. Elevate the head of the bed for a few minutes before she attempts to stand. b. Help her sit on the side of the bed for several minutes before standing, and help her to stand slowly.	2. This allows time for blood pressure to stabilize before she is fully upright, thus maintaining circulation to the brain.
3. Instruct the mother to move her feet constantly when she first stands.	3. Moving the feet increases venous return from the lower extremities to maintain cardiac output and increase cerebral circulation.
4. Suggest that she take brief, tepid (not hot) showers and that she bend her knees and "march" during the shower.	4. Hot water dilates peripheral blood vessels, allowing additional blood to remain in the vessels of the legs. Moving the feet and legs increases blood return from the legs and increases blood to the brain.
5. Initiate measures to prevent injuries that could be sustained if she fainted: a. Stay with the mother when she ambulates, and be prepared to assist her in sitting down or to lower her gently to the floor if she becomes faint. b. Call for assistance before attempting to return her to bed. c. Remind her to call for assistance before trying to ambulate. Check to see that the call light is conveniently located.	5. Gravity increases blood flow to the brain when the head is lowered and thus prevents fainting. Adequate assistance prevents falling and possible injury during a fainting episode.

Evaluation: Jacqueline has participated in self-care and has sustained no injury during her hospital stay.

Assessment: Jacqueline demonstrates skill in breastfeeding but wonders how she will be able to care for the baby and her 18-month-old boy when she gets home. She states he "is busy every minute." She has a third-degree episiotomy and asks what can be done to prevent the pain she experienced during intercourse for several months after the last child was born.

Nursing Diagnosis: Anxiety related to anticipated fatigue and discomfort

Critical Thinking: What assumption is the nurse making? How might the nurse validate the assumption? Can you identify another diagnosis that is more specific?

Answer: The nurse assumes the client is anxious. Neither signs nor symptoms of anxiety are part of the assessment data. The nurse can validate the assumption by asking Jacqueline if she is anxious. "Anxiety" is a very broad diagnostic category. Based on data available, a more specific and therefore more helpful nursing diagnosis might be "Risk for Altered Sexuality Patterns related to fatigue and pain."

Continued

Expected Outcomes:
The couple will do the following:
1. Verbalize measures to promote comfort during sexual activity by (date)
2. Verbalize a plan to reduce fatigue, which interferes with interest in and energy for sexual activity by (date)

Intervention	Rationale
1. Recommend that the parents postpone vaginal intercourse until the perineum is healed, usually about 3 weeks. Suggest that the mother continue perineal care, sitz baths, and the use of topical agents until the perineum is healed.	1. These measures promote rapid healing and reduce pain or fear of pain when sexual activity is resumed.
2. Suggest the use of a water-soluble vaginal lubricant (KY Jelly, Lubrin, Replens) if the mother is planning to breastfeed for longer than 6 weeks.	2. Breastfeeding delays the resumption of ovarian hormones, including estrogen, which may result in vaginal dryness that is most noticeable after 6 weeks of breastfeeding.
3. Prior to vaginal intercourse, as part of foreplay, suggest that one finger be inserted into the vaginal introitus to determine areas of tenderness or pain.	3. Locating areas of discomfort and stretching the perineal scar gently help increase comfort.
4. Suggest that the woman assume the superior position during intercourse.	4. In the superior position, the woman controls the depth and location of penetration and can reduce her discomfort.
5. Explain that sexual arousal may be slower because of decreased hormones and fatigue. More stimulation may be required before the mother is sexually aroused.	5. Knowledge of the physiologic changes reduces the anxiety and tension that occur if the parents are unprepared for them.
6. Remind the mother to perform Kegel exercises until she can comfortably do 30 contraction-relaxation cycles each day.	6. Kegel exercises strengthen the muscles around the vagina and promote increased sexual satisfaction.
7. Suggest that the infant be breastfed just before initiating sexual activity.	7. Feeding the infant before lovemaking reduces the chance of leaking milk, which interferes with sexual pleasure for some couples and helps prevent interruptions.
8. Suggest measures that may lessen fatigue: a. Recommend a 30-minute nap for each partner during the day or evening. b. Suggest that sexual activity be resumed in the morning or afternoon rather than at the end of a tiring day. c. Suggest that parents rest when the infant sleeps and that they postpone major projects until the infant is sleeping through the night.	8. Fatigue is a major cause of decreased interest in sexual activity after childbirth for both mothers and fathers.
9. Encourage frank communication between partners about measures that reduce discomfort and specific concerns and needs.	9. Communication facilitates understanding and fosters a feeling of closeness that can enhance sexual interest.

Evaluation: The couple expresses interest in learning measures that reduce fatigue and discomfort; they verbalize a plan to use the instructions provided.

is significantly less than the prenatal baseline blood pressure.

Pulse. Bradycardia, defined as a pulse rate of 50 to 60 beats per minute, may occur although the average range is 60 to 90 beats per minute. The lower pulse rate reflects the large amount of blood that returns to the central circulation after delivery of the placenta. The increase in central circulation results in increased stroke volume and allows a slower heart rate to provide adequate maternal circulation.

Tachycardia may indicate excitement, fatigue, dehydration, hypovolemia, pain, or infection. If tachycardia is noted, additional assessments should include blood pressure, location and firmness of the uterus, amount of lochia, estimated blood loss at delivery, hemoglobin, and hematocrit values. The objective of the additional assessments is to rule out excessive bleeding and intervene at once if hemorrhage is suspected.

Respirations. A normal respiratory rate of 12 to 20 per minute should be maintained. Assessing breath sounds is not necessary if the mother has had a normal vaginal delivery, is ambulatory, and is without signs of respiratory problems. Breath sounds always should be auscultated if the birth has been cesarean or if the mother is a smoker, has a history of frequent or recent upper respiratory infections, or has a history of asthma.

Temperature. A temperature of 38° C (100.4° F) is common during the first 24 hours after childbirth and may be caused by dehydration or normal postpartum leukocytosis. If the elevated temperature persists for

PROCEDURE 17-1

Assessing the Uterine Fundus

Purpose: To determine the location and firmness of the uterus

1. Explain the procedure and rationale for each step before beginning the procedure. *This reduces anxiety and elicits cooperation.*
2. Ask the mother to empty her bladder if she has not voided recently. *A distended bladder lifts and displaces the uterus.*
3. Place the mother flat in a supine position with her knees slightly flexed. *This relaxes the abdominal muscles and permits accurate location of the fundus.*
4. Put on clean gloves and lower the perineal pads to observe lochia as the fundus is palpated. *Gloves are recommended whenever the possibility exists of coming into contact with body fluids.*
5. Place your nondominant hand above the woman's symphysis pubis. *This supports and anchors the lower uterine segment during palpation or massage of the fundus.*

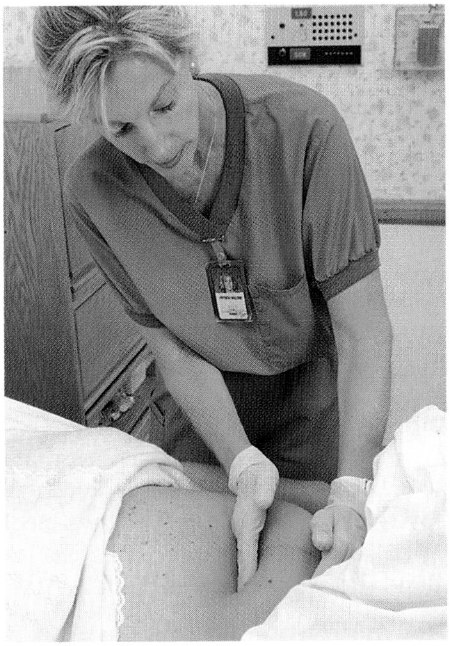

6. Use the flat part of your fingers (not the fingertips) for palpation (see illustration). *The larger surface provides more comfort. Palpation may be painful, particularly for the mother who had a cesarean birth.*
7. Begin palpation at the umbilicus, and palpate gently until the fundus is located. The hand "cups" the uterus to determine firmness and location of the fundus. *The fundus should be firm, in the midline, and approximately at the level of the umbilicus. Locating the fundus is more difficult if the woman is obese or if the abdomen is distended.*
8. If the fundus is difficult to locate or is soft or "boggy," keep the nondominant hand above the woman's symphysis pubis and massage the fundus with the dominant hand until the fundus is firm. *The nondominant hand anchors the lower segment of the uterus and prevents trauma while the uterus is massaged. The uterus contracts in response to tactile stimulation and this helps control excessive bleeding.*
9. After massaging a boggy fundus until it is firm, press firmly to expel clots. Keep one hand pressed firmly just above the symphysis (over the lower uterine segment) during the entire time. *Removing clots allows the uterus to contract properly. Providing pressure over the lower uterine segment prevents uterine inversion.*
10. If the fundus is above or below the umbilicus, use your fingers to determine the number of fingerbreadths between the fundus and the umbilicus. *Using the fingers to measure allows an approximation of the number of centimeters.*
11. Document the consistency and location of the fundus. Consistency is recorded as "fundus firm," "firm with massage," or "boggy." Fundal height is recorded in fingerbreadths above or below the umbilicus. For example, "fundus firm, midline, U–2" (two fingerbreadths below umbilicus). As another example, "fundus firm with light massage, U+2 (two fingerbreadths above umbilicus), displaced to right." *This promotes accurate communication and identifies deviations from expected so that potential problems can be identified early.*

longer than 24 hours or if it exceeds 38° C, infection is possible and the fever is reported to the physician or nurse-midwife.

Pain. Pain is considered the fifth vital sign and should be assessed along with vital signs to determine the type, location, and severity on a pain scale. Pain medication and other measures should be used as needed.

Fundus

The fundus should be assessed for consistency and location (Procedure 17-1). It should be firmly contracted and at or near the level of the umbilicus. If the uterus is above the expected level or shifted from the midline position (usually to the right), the bladder may be distended. The location of the fundus should be rechecked after the woman has emptied her bladder. If the fundus is difficult to locate or is soft or "boggy," the nurse stimulates the uterine muscle to contract by gently massaging the uterus. The nondominant hand must support and anchor the lower uterine segment if massaging an uncontracted uterus is necessary. Uterine massage is not necessary if the uterus is firmly contracted.

The uterus can contract only if it is free of intrauterine clots. To expel clots, the nurse must support the lower uterine segment to prevent inversion of the uterus (turning inside out) when the nurse applies firm

Table 17-4
OBSERVATIONS OF THE UTERINE FUNDUS REQUIRING NURSING ACTIONS

Normal Findings	Abnormal Findings	Nursing Actions
Fundus firmly contracted	Fundus soft, "boggy," uncontracted, or difficult to locate	Support lower uterine segment. Massage until firm.
Fundus remains contracted when massage is discontinued	Fundus becomes soft and uncontracted when massage is stopped	Continue to support the lower uterine segment. Massage until firm and apply pressure to the fundus to express clots that may be accumulating in uterus. Notify the health care provider and begin oxytocin administration, as prescribed, to maintain a firm fundus.
Fundus located at the level of the umbilicus and midline	Fundus above the umbilicus and/or displaced from the midline	Assess bladder elimination. Assist the mother in urinating or catheterize, if necessary.

pressure downward toward the vagina. This expresses clots that have collected in the uterus. Nurses should observe the perineum for the number and size of clots expelled. (Table 17-4 describes normal and abnormal findings of the uterine fundus and includes follow-up nursing actions for abnormal findings.)

CRITICAL THINKING EXERCISE

Linda Welker, a 22-year-old multipara, was admitted from the labor, delivery, and recovery unit 2 hours after the birth of an 8 lb (3600 g) baby boy. An hour later, her fundus is boggy, located three fingerbreadths above the umbilicus, and displaced to the right. Her perineal pads, which were changed just before transfer, are saturated.

QUESTIONS:

1. What do these data suggest? Why?
2. What nursing action should be taken first? What follow-up assessments are necessary?
3. Why is it necessary to remind and assist Linda to void?

Drugs sometimes are needed to maintain contraction of the uterus and thus prevent postpartum hemorrhage. The most commonly used drugs are methylergonovine (Methergine) and oxytocin (Pitocin) (Table 17-5). In addition, a drug guide for methylergonovine is presented on p. 777 and for oxytocin on p. 401.

Lochia

Important assessments include the amount, color, and odor of lochia. Nurses observe the amount and color of lochia on peripads and while checking the perineum. They also watch vaginal discharge while palpating or massaging the fundus so that the amount of lochia and the number and size of any clots expressed during these procedures can be observed. Note these important guidelines:

- A constant trickle of lochia indicates excessive bleeding and requires immediate attention.
- Excessive lochia in the presence of a contracted uterus suggests lacerations of the birth canal. The health care provider must be notified so that the laceration can be located and repaired.

The odor of lochia is usually described as fleshy, earthy, and musty. A foul odor suggests endometrial infection, and assessments should be made for additional signs of infection. These signs include maternal fever, tachycardia, and uterine tenderness and pain.

Absence of lochia, like the presence of a foul odor, also may indicate infection. Lochia may be scant, particularly if the birth was cesarean when the cavity of the uterus was wiped by sponges, removing some of the endometrial lining. Lochia should not be entirely absent, however.

Perineum

The acronym *REEDA* is used as a reminder that the site of an episiotomy or a perineal laceration should be assessed for five signs: redness, edema, ecchymosis (bruising), discharge, and approximation (the edges of the wound should be close, as though stuck or glued together).

Redness of the wound may indicate the usual inflammatory response to injury. If accompanied by excessive pain or tenderness, however, it may indicate the beginning of localized infection. Ecchymosis or edema indicates soft tissue damage that can delay healing. No discharge should come from the wound. Rapid healing necessitates that the edges of the wound be closely approximated. (Procedure 17-2 describes the perineal examination.)

Bladder Elimination

Because the mother may not experience the urge to void even if the bladder is full, nurses must rely on physical assessment to determine whether the bladder is distended. Bladder distention often produces an obvious or palpable bulge that feels like a soft, movable mass above the symphysis pubis. Other signs include an upward and lateral displacement of the uterine fun-

Table 17-5

COMMONLY USED DRUGS DURING THE POSTPARTUM PERIOD

Indications	Usual Dosage	Nursing Considerations
METHYLERGONOVINE MALEATE (METHERGINE)		
Prevention and treatment of hemorrhage resulting from uterine atony	0.2 mg IM or p.o. q 6-8 hr	Monitor and record the woman's blood pressure, pulse rate, and uterine response. Report any sudden change in vital signs, continued uterine relaxation, or excessive lochia.
OXYTOCIN (PITOCIN, SYNTOCINON)		
Reduction of bleeding after expulsion of the placenta	10 to 40 units in 1000 ml Ringers lactate or normal saline solution IV at a rate to control bleeding (usually 20 to 40 mU/minute), or 10 units IM	Administer by infusion, not by bolus (a concentrated mass). Monitor and record the woman's uterine contraction, heart rate, and blood pressure every 15 minutes. Assess and record the amount of lochia.
SIMETHICONE (MYLICON)		
Flatulence, abdominal distention	40 to 80 mg chewable tablets after each meal and at bedtime	Assess for bowel activity, relief of distention.
IBUPROFEN (MOTRIN, ADVIL)		
Mild to moderate pain	400 to 600 mg p.o. q 4-6 hr	Assess for nausea, vomiting, diarrhea.
ACETAMINOPHEN (TYLENOL, PANADOL)		
Mild to moderate pain	325 to 650 mg p.o. q 4-6 hr	Side effects are rare; assess for allergic reaction, such as skin rash.
TYLENOL WITH CODEINE #3 (325 MG ACETAMINOPHEN WITH 30 MG CODEINE)		
Moderate pain	Tylenol #3, two tablets q 3-4 hr	Determine sensitivity to acetaminophen or codeine.
PERCOCET (325 MG ACETAMINOPHEN AND 5 MG OXYCODONE) **TYLOX (500 MG ACETAMINOPHEN AND 5 MG OXYCODONE)**		
Moderate pain	1-2 tablets p.o. q 4 hr	Determine sensitivity to acetaminophen or oxycodone. Observe for signs of respiratory depression. Watch for nausea, vomiting, vertigo. Do not administer with sedatives.
LORTAB (2.5, 5, OR 7.5 MG HYDROCODONE AND 500 MG ACETAMINOPHEN) **VICODIN (5 MG HYDROCODONE AND 500 MG ACETAMINOPHEN)** **VICODIN ES (7.5 MG HYDROCODONE AND 750 MG ACETAMINOPHEN)**		
Moderate to moderately severe pain	1 to 2 tablets p.o. q 4-6 hr	Determine sensitivity to acetaminophen or hydrocodone. Observe for signs of respiratory depression. Watch for nausea, vomiting, vertigo. Do not administer with sedatives.
RH_0(D) IMMUNE GLOBULIN (RHOGAM, GAMULIN RH, HYPRHOD)		
Prevention of sensitization to Rh factor in Rh-negative mothers who gave birth to Rh-positive infants	One vial (one standard dose) IM within 72 hr after childbirth	Confirm that administration is necessary. Check with second licensed personnel that medication is cross matched for the specific woman. Record lot number, expiration date, and manufacturer.
RUBELLA VIRUS VACCINE, LIVE (MERUVAX II)		
See drug guide, p. 434		

q, Every; *p.o.*, orally (per os); *IM*, intramuscularly; *IV*, intravenously; *mU*, milliunit; *SC*, subcutaneously.
Data from Hodgson, B.B. & Kizior, R.J. (2000). *Saunders nursing drug handbook 2000.* Philadelphia: W.B. Saunders.

PROCEDURE 17-2
Assessing the Perineum

Purpose: To observe perineal trauma and the state of healing

1. Provide privacy, and explain the purpose of the procedure. *This elicits cooperation and reduces anxiety about the procedure.*
2. Put on clean gloves. *Implement standard precautions to provide protection from possible contact with body fluids.*

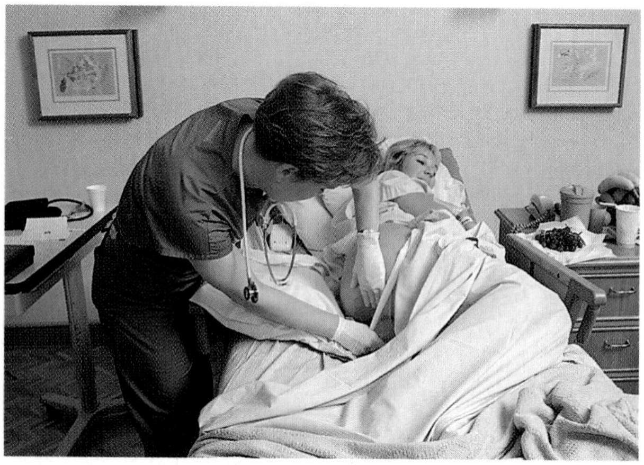

3. Ask the mother to assume a Sims (side) position and flex her upper leg. Lower the perineal pads and lift her superior buttock. If necessary, use a flashlight to inspect the perineal area. *Position provides an unobstructed view of the perineum; light allows better visualization.*
4. Note the extent and location of edema or bruising. *Extensive bruising or asymmetric edema may indicate formation of a hematoma (see Chapter 28).*
5. Examine the episiotomy or laceration for redness, ecchymosis, edema, discharge, and approximation (REEDA). *Redness, edema, or discharge may indicate infection of the wound; extensive bruising may delay healing; wound edges must be in direct contact for uncomplicated healing to occur.*
6. Note the number and size of hemorrhoids. *Swollen, painful hemorrhoids interfere with activity and bowel elimination.*

dus and increased lochia. Frequent voidings of less than 150 ml suggest urinary retention with overflow. Signs of an empty bladder include a firm fundus in the midline and a nonpalpable bladder.

CRITICAL TO REMEMBER

Signs of a Distended Bladder

Location of fundus above *baseline* level, which is obtained when the bladder is empty
Fundus displaced from midline
Excessive lochia
Bladder discomfort
Bulge of bladder above symphysis
Frequent voidings of less than 150 ml of urine, which indicates urinary retention with overflow

Some facilities measure the first two to three voidings to determine whether normal bladder function has returned. When the mother can void at least 300 to 400 ml, the bladder usually is empty. Regardless of the amount voided, however, the fundus must be assessed to confirm that the bladder is empty. Subjective symptoms of urgency, frequency, and dysuria suggest urinary tract infection and should be reported to the health care provider.

Breasts

For the first day or two after delivery, the breasts should be soft and nontender. After that, breast changes depend largely on whether the mother is breastfeeding or taking measures to prevent lactation. The breasts should be examined even if she chooses formula feeding because the breasts may become engorged despite preventive measures. The size, symmetry, and shape of the breasts should be observed. Some mothers need reassurance that breast size has no relationship to successful breastfeeding. The skin should be inspected for dimpling or thickening, which, although rare, can indicate breast tumor.

The areola and nipple should be carefully examined for potential problems such as flat or retracted nipples, which may make breastfeeding more difficult. Signs of nipple trauma (redness, blisters, or fissures) often are noted during the first days of breastfeeding, especially if the mother needs assistance in positioning the infant correctly (see Chapter 22).

The breasts should be palpated for firmness and tenderness, which indicate increased vascular and lymphatic circulation that may precede milk production. The breasts may feel "lumpy" as various lobes begin to produce milk.

The breast assessment is an excellent opportunity to provide information or reassurance about breast care and breastfeeding techniques.

Lower Extremities

The legs are examined for varicosities and signs and symptoms of thrombophlebitis. Indications of thrombophlebitis include localized areas of redness, heat, edema, and tenderness. Pedal pulses may be obstructed

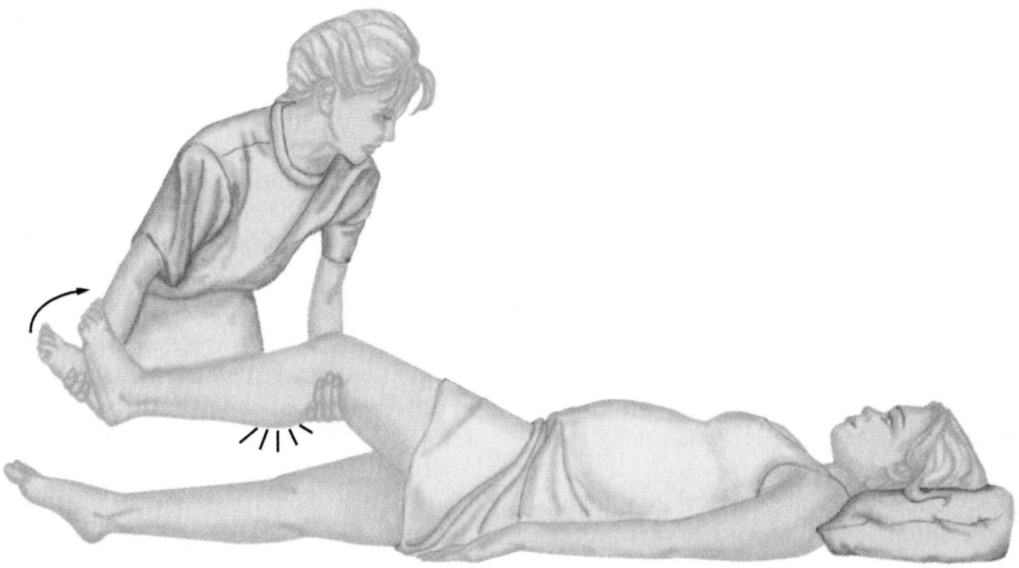

FIGURE 17-8 Homans' sign is positive when the mother experiences discomfort in the calf on sharp dorsiflexion of the foot.

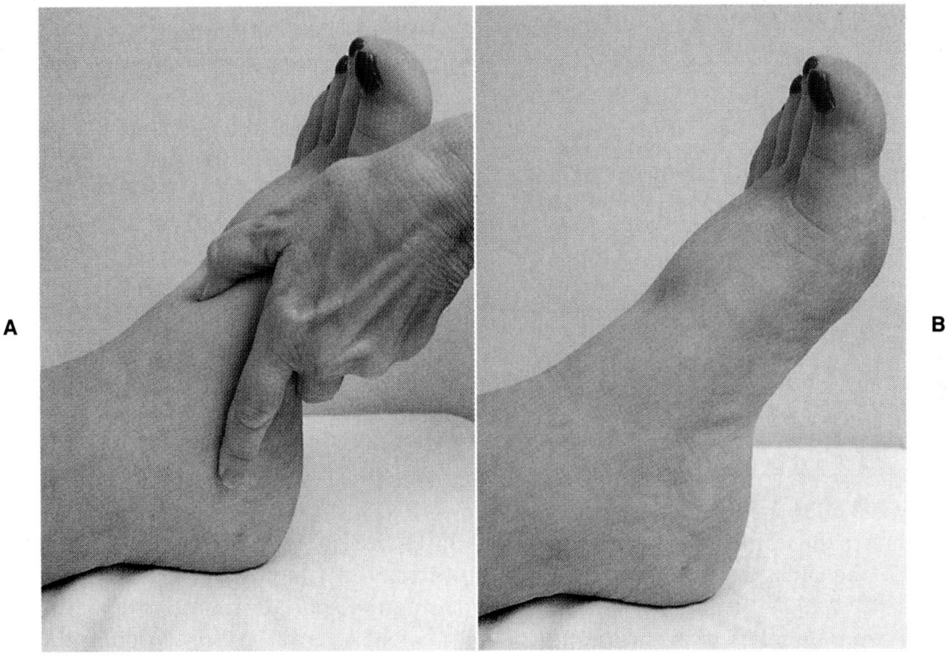

FIGURE 17-9 Pedal edema. **A,** Apply pressure to foot. **B,** "Pit" appears when fluid moves into adjacent tissue and away from point of pressure.

by thrombophlebitis and should be palpated with each assessment (see Chapter 28).

Homans' Sign

Discomfort in the calf with sharp dorsiflexion of the foot (Figure 17-8) may indicate deep vein thrombosis. A negative Homans' sign indicates the absence of discomfort. A positive Homans' sign indicates the presence of discomfort and should be reported to the physician or nurse-midwife. Homans' sign is of limited value in assessment of the lower extremities (Cunningham, et al., 1997). Confusion arises because a deep venous thrombosis may not produce pain with dorsiflexion. In addition, the woman may report pain that is caused by strained muscles from positioning and pushing during delivery.

Edema and Deep Tendon Reflexes

Pedal or pretibial edema may be present for the first day or two, until excess interstitial fluid is remobilized and excreted. (Figure 17-9 shows how to assess for pitting edema.)

Deep tendon reflexes should be 1+ to 2+. Report brisker-than-average and hyperactive reflexes (3+ to 4+), which suggest pregnancy-induced hypertension (see p. 687 for a description of assessing deep tendon reflexes).

Comfort Level

Comfort is essential to postpartum recovery, but some new mothers are too excited by the birth of their child to complain of discomfort. Others don't want to "bother the nurse" or may come from cultures in which complaining is not acceptable. Nurses must remain alert to covert signs of afterpains, perineal discomfort, and breast tenderness. Signs of discomfort include an inability to relax or sleep, a change in vital signs, restlessness, irritability, and facial grimaces. Women should be encouraged to take prescribed medications for afterpains and perineal discomfort.

Check Your Reading

11. What additional assessments are necessary when tachycardia is noted? Why?
12. What are the typical cause, onset, and symptoms experienced by the mother with orthostatic hypotension?
13. When is uterine massage necessary? How is the uterus supported during massage?
14. What does excessive bleeding suggest when the uterus is firmly contracted?

CARE IN THE IMMEDIATE POSTPARTUM PERIOD

The postpartum period often is divided into three periods. The first 24 hours is the immediate postpartum period, the first week is the early postpartum period, and the second to the sixth week is the late period. Care of the mother during the immediate postpartum period focuses on the following:

- Maintaining physiologic safety of the mother through frequent assessments
- Providing comfort measures
- Establishing bladder elimination
- Providing health education

Providing Comfort Measures

Ice Packs

Both cold and warmth are used to alleviate perineal pain after childbirth. Ice causes vasoconstriction and is most effective if applied soon after the birth to prevent edema and to numb the area. Chemical ice packs and plastic bags filled with ice often are used during the first 12 hours after a vaginal birth. The ice pack is wrapped in paper before applying it to the perineum. It should be left in place until the ice melts. It then is removed for 10 minutes before a fresh pack is applied. Some peripads have cold packs incorporated in them, but they do not absorb as much lochia as other peripads.

Some women have varicosities of the vulva and wish to use ice packs at home. An inexpensive way for women to apply cold to the perineum is to freeze a wash cloth placed in a plastic bag and wrap it in a paper towel before applying to the perineum.

Perineal Care

Perineal care consists of squirting warm water over the perineum after each voiding or bowel movement. Perineal care cleanses, provides comfort, and prevents infection of an area that often has an episiotomy or lacerations. The perineum is gently patted rather than wiped to dry.

Topical Medications

Anesthetic sprays decrease surface discomfort and allow more comfortable ambulation. The mother is instructed to hold the nozzle of a benzocaine spray such as Americaine, Dermoplast, or Epifoam 6 to 12 inches from her body and direct it toward the perineum. The spray should be used after perineal care and before clean pads are applied.

Sitting Measures

The mother should be advised to squeeze her buttocks together before sitting and lower her weight slowly onto her buttocks. This measure prevents stretching of the perineal tissue and avoids sharp impact on the traumatized area.

Sitz Baths

Sitz baths, which provide continuous circulation of water, cleanse and comfort the traumatized perineum. They also increase circulation to the area to help healing. Cool water reduces pain caused by edema and may be most effective within the first 24 hours. Warm water increases circulation, promotes healing, and may be most effective after 24 hours. Nurses must be sure that the emergency bell is within easy reach in case the mother feels faint during the sitz bath. If the sitz bath is used by more than one client, it must be thoroughly cleaned after each use.

Sitz baths are offered two to three times a day and women are instructed about ways to continue the procedure at home. Women often are given disposable sitz baths to take home. If the woman plans to use her tub at home for sitz baths, she should be instructed to clean it well before using it.

Analgesics

Analgesics such as acetaminophen (Tylenol) and nonsteroidal antiinflammatory drugs such as ibuprofen (Motrin, Advil) frequently are prescribed to provide relief for mild to moderate discomfort. Acetaminophen with codeine (Tylenol No. 3), acetaminophen and oxycodone (Percocet), and hydrocodone and acetaminophen (Vicodin) often are prescribed for more severe discomfort (see Table 17-5).

In some agencies, women receive self-medication kits for use during their postpartum stays. The kit may include routine stool softeners and nonnarcotic or narcotic (limited supply) pain medications. Women are instructed on ways to take their medications and given a log to record each dose. This allows them to receive pain medication quickly when they need it and helps them develop an understanding of the medications available for them.

CRITICAL THINKING EXERCISE

Elizabeth Brown has made good progress since she delivered her first baby yesterday by cesarean. Her foley catheter was removed three hours ago and she was medicated with two Percocet (325 mg acetaminophen and 5 mg oxycodone) tablets for pain 1 hour ago. Now she is wincing and moaning with pain and asking for more pain medication. She says she got up to the bathroom a short time after her catheter was removed and urinated but did not measure it. Her fundus is slightly above the umbilicus and slightly to the right. A thick pressure dressing covers the lower abdomen making it difficult to palpate the bladder. Elizabeth says she doesn't have to urinate.

QUESTIONS:

1. What other assessments should the nurse make?
2. What should the nurse do?
3. What are possible causes of Elizabeth's pain?

Promoting Bladder Elimination

Many new mothers have difficulty voiding because of edema and trauma of the perineum and diminished sensitivity to fluid pressure in the bladder. As soon as they are able to ambulate safely, mothers should be assisted to the bathroom. Providing privacy and allowing adequate time for the first voiding is important. Common measures to promote relaxation of the perineal muscles and stimulate the sensation of needing to void include the following:

- Running water, placing the mother's hands in water, and pouring water over the vulva
- Medicating the woman for pain to help her relax
- Encouraging urination in the shower or sitz bath
- Providing hot tea or fluids of choice.
- Asking the mother to blow bubbles through a straw

A nonpalpable bladder and firm fundus at or below the level of the umbilicus and in the midline confirm that the bladder is empty and rule out urinary retention with overflow.

A distended bladder lifts and displaces the uterus, making it difficult for the uterus to remain contracted. Thus urinary retention is a major cause of uterine atony (loss of tone), which permits excessive bleeding. In addition, stasis of urine in the bladder predisposes the woman to urinary tract infection. Therefore the mother must be catheterized if

- She is unable to void.
- The amount voided is less than 150 ml and the bladder can be palpated.
- The fundus is elevated or displaced from the midline.

Repeated catheterizations increase the chance of urinary tract infection because bacteria may be pushed into the bladder despite scrupulous aseptic technique. To decrease the risk of infection, an indwelling catheter often is inserted for 24 hours if catheterization is necessary more than once.

Providing Fluid and Food

Adequate fluids help restore the balance altered by fluid loss during labor and the birth process. Women should be encouraged to drink approximately 2500 ml of fluids each day. Offering warm fluids may be more culturally appropriate for some women. They may prefer hot or room-temperature water to ice water.

If a woman is unable to tolerate oral fluids, IV administration may be necessary. Women usually are able to have ice chips soon after cesarean birth, and, although protocols vary, most are able to progress to a regular diet after passing flatus.

Women generally have a hearty appetite after normal childbirth, and nurses should encourage healthy food choices with respect for ethnic background. Meals and snacks should be available at all times.

Preventing Thrombophlebitis

The mother should be encouraged to ambulate early after childbirth to prevent the development of thrombi. Frequent trips to the bathroom will help accomplish this.

NURSING CARE AFTER CESAREAN BIRTH

Many facilities have developed clinical pathways or care maps for cesarean births that are similar to those used for uncomplicated vaginal births. The clinical pathway identifies outcomes and establishes a time frame for assessments and interventions for post-cesarean mothers and their infants (Figure 17-10).

YORK HEALTH SYSTEM
YORK, PENNSYLVANIA

CLINICAL PATHWAY
Cesarean Delivery

CLINICAL PATH DAY		EXPECTED PATIENT FAMILY OUTCOMES	INTERDISCIPLINARY ASSESSMENT	TESTS	CONSULT
Day 1 (Surgery)	Date	N D E ☐☐☐ Achieves desired level of pain relief [1] ☐☐☐ > 50 cc/hr urine ouput [4] ☐☐☐ Incision site w/o complication [4] ☐☐☐ Postpartum parameters stable [4]	T, P, R, B/P, q4° × 6 Fundus, lochia, incision, breath sounds q4° × 3 Bowel sounds qs Fluid balance qs Level of comfort		
Day 2	Date	☐☐☐ Achieves desired level of pain relief [1] ☐☐☐ > 50 cc/hr urinary output [4] ☐☐☐ Incision site w/o complication [4] ☐☐☐ Postpartum parameters stable [4] ☐☐☐ Ambulates tid with assistance [4] ☐☐☐ Adequate home support system identified [6]	TPR B/P q4° × 6, then bid Breasts, lochia, fundus, incision, breath sounds, bowel sounds qs WA Fluid balance qs Level of comfort Home support system Readiness to learn Knowledge of self & newborn care	WCBC	
Day 3	Date	☐☐☐ Achieves desired level of pain relief [1] ☐☐☐ Voiding qs [4] ☐☐☐ Postpartum parameters stable [4] ☐☐☐ Cares for self and infant ☐☐☐ Incision site w/o complication [4] ☐☐☐ Verbalizes probable D/C plan [3] ☐☐☐ Referral made for potential or identified risk (physical/psychosocial)	T, P, R, BP bid Breasts, fundus, lochia, bladder, bowel sounds, incision qs WA Level of comfort Readiness to learn Knowledge of self & newborn care		
Day 4/Discharge	Date	☐☐☐ Achieves desired level of pain relief [1] ☐☐☐ V.S. & postpartum physiologic parameters within D/C guidelines [4] ☐☐☐ Incision site without complications [4] ☐ Pt/SO/family verbalization of D/C instructions [3] ☐ Discharged within 4 days after delivery ☐ Postpartum Home Visit not needed based on Interqual Criteria	T, P, R, BP bid Breasts, fundus, lochia, incision, bowel functions qs WA Level of comfort Readiness to learn Pt/SO/family knowledge of self & newborn care		

NAME	INT.	NAME	INT.	NAME	INT

Note: Each patient requires an individual assessment & treatment plan. This Clinical Path is a recommendation for the average patient which requires modification when necessary by the professional staff.

FIGURE 17-10 Clinical pathway for cesarean birth. Figure shows only the postpartum aspects of care although the pathway begins during the prenatal period. (Courtesy York Health System, York, Pennsylvania, with adaptations.)

INTERVENTIONS/ACTIVITIES	MEDICATIONS	NUTRITION	EDUCATION AND DISCHARGE PLANNING
Foley CT & DB, leg exercises q2° I & O Dangle, assist OOB × 1 Assist with hygiene	Analgesia prn IV with pitocin	Sips & chips to clear liquids	N D E ☐ ☐ ☐ Continue post-op teaching ☐ ☐ ☐ Initiate/continue maternal newborn education record, D/C booklet
D/C foley D/C IV Dressing removed Assist OOB to ambulate Assist with bath/shower	Analgesia prn	Adv to diet as tolerated	☐ ☐ ☐ Continue maternal newborn education record
OOB ad lib Shower	Analgesia prn	Regular diet	☐ ☐ ☐ Reinforce maternal newborn education record
OOB ad lib Shower	Analgesia prn ☐ Rhogam, when indicated ☐ Rubella, when indicated	Regular diet	☐ Completion of maternal newborn education record ☐ Physician D/C instruction ☐ Support services in community: ☐ Breast Feeding Support/Supplies ☐ Perinatal Coaching ☐ City/State Health ☐ Other ____________ ☐ D/C after Pt/family review instructions

Discharge Date	Discharge Time	Discharged To	Accompanied By
____________	____________	____________	☐ W/C ☐ Ambulate

COMORBIDITIES

__ 1. Cardiac Disease
__ 2. Chronic Hypertension
__ 3. IDDM–Class:
__ 4. Renal Disease
__ 5. Thyroid Disease
__ 6. Seizure Disorder
__ 7. Multiple Gestation
__ 8. Hemoglobinopathy
__ 9. Asthma
__ 10. Thromboembolic Disorder
__ 11. Recurring Infections
__ 12. Developmental Delay
__ 13. ____________
__ 14. ____________
__ 15. ____________

DOCUMENTATION CODES

Initial = Meets Standard
★ = Exception on pathway identified
C = Chronic problems
N = Not applicable
D = Deferred

PATIENT/FAMILY PROBLEMS

1. Pain r/t childbirth
2. Anxiety r/t childbirth and/or parenting
3. Knowledge deficit r/t childbirth and/or parenting
4. Potential alteration maternal/fetal homeostasis
5. Potential for ineffective parenting
6. ____________
7. ____________

FIGURE 17-10, cont'd For legend see opposite page.

Pathways or care maps are guidelines only. A problem, sometimes called a *variance,* mandates additional assessments and interventions.

Assessment

In addition to the usual postpartum assessments, the postcesarean mother must be assessed like any other postoperative patient.

Pain Relief

Assessment of pain relief is important to nursing care. Postcesarean clients differ from typical postoperative clients in three important ways. First, they often are eager to be alert so that they can interact with their newborn infants. Second, they are concerned that the analgesics they receive may pass into their breast milk and potentially harm their infants. Third, compared with other postoperative patients, postcesarean clients want to have more input and control of their care.

Intramuscular injection of narcotics for postcesarean pain was the most common pain relief method in the past. This regimen causes discomfort from intramuscular injections, drowsiness that interferes with the mother's ability to care for the infant, and side effects such as nausea and vomiting.

Some institutions use patient-controlled analgesia (PCA), administered by continuous IV infusion of a low-concentration narcotic solution using a pump specifically designed for that purpose. If analgesia is insufficient, the woman can self-administer intermittent small doses of narcotic from the infusion pump. The machine is programmed to administer only a certain amount of the narcotic within a specified time interval to prevent an overdose. This allows the woman to have pain relief immediately when she needs it without waiting for a nurse to administer it. Side effects include respiratory depression, itching (pruritus), nausea and vomiting, and urinary retention.

A single dose of narcotic (often preservative-free morphine) injected into the epidural or subarachnoid space immediately after surgery provides 18 to 24 hours of postcesarean analgesia. Itching is a major side effect with an incidence as high as 84%. Other side effects are the same as for PCA use (Zuspan, 2000). Oral analgesics usually are effective if women need additional pain relief measures.

Respirations

When mothers receive epidural narcotics for postoperative pain relief, respirations must be assessed frequently because narcotics depress the respiratory center. In some facilities, an apnea monitor is used for 18 to 24 hours to detect a decreased respiratory rate. A pulse oximeter also may be used. Both will emit an alarm if respirations decrease. If an apnea monitor or oximeter is not used, the respiratory rate and depth should be checked every 15 minutes for the first hour, every 30 minutes for 3 to 6 hours, and every 30 to 60 minutes for the remainder of the first 24 hours.

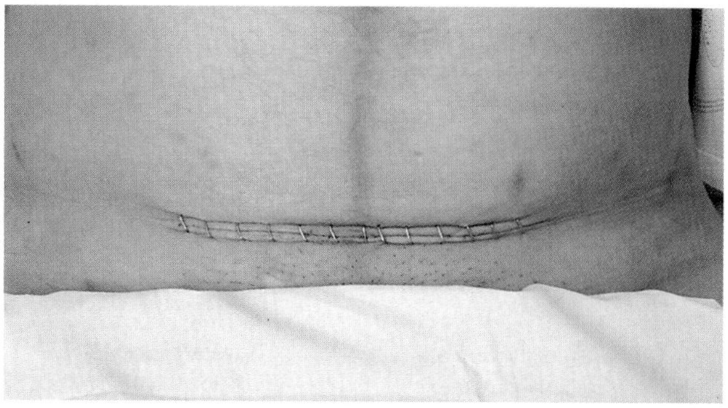

FIGURE 17-11 The incision after cesarean birth is closed with staples. Note the absence of all signs of infection, such as redness, edema, bruising (ecchymosis), discharge, and loss of approximation.

In addition to observing respiratory rate and depth, the mother's breath sounds should be auscultated because depressed respirations and a longer period of immobility allow secretions to pool in the bronchioles.

Abdomen

Nurses assess gastrointestinal function by auscultating for bowel sounds until normal peristalsis is noted in all abdominal quadrants. Although paralytic ileus (lack of movement in the bowel) is rare after cesarean birth, nurses must be aware of the signs, which include abdominal distention, absent or decreased bowel sounds, and no passage of flatus or stool.

The surgical dressing should be observed for intactness and discharge. When the dressing is removed, nurses observe the incision, which should be approximated, and use the acronym REEDA to assess for signs of infection such as redness and edema (Figure 17-11).

The fundus must be palpated gently because of increased discomfort caused by the uterine incision.

Intake and Output

The IV infusion should be monitored for the rate of flow and the condition of the IV site. Any signs of infiltration such as edema and coolness at the site and signs of infection such as edema, redness, and pain should be reported. The amount, color, and clarity of urine should be monitored.

Interventions

The First 24 Hours

The mother who gave birth by cesarean is cared for as one would care for other postoperative clients.

Providing Pain Relief. The nurse should offer pain medication on a regular basis if the woman is not using a PCA. Relief of pain increases the woman's ability to increase her activity, helps prevent thrombophlebitis, and promotes healing. For women with epidural or spinal opioids, the nurse should continue to assess the respiratory status. If the respiratory rate begins to decline or is less than 12 per minute, the nurse should do the following:

- Notify the anesthesiologist immediately
- Elevate the head of the bed to facilitate lung expansion and have the woman breathe deeply
- Administer oxygen and apply a pulse oximeter (if not already in place) to measure oxygen saturation
- Follow facility protocol to administer narcotic antagonists, such as naloxone hydrochloride (Narcan)
- Observe for recurrence of respiratory depression because the duration of naloxone is only approximately 30 minutes
- Recognize that naloxone reduces the level of pain relief

Overcoming Effects of Immobility. The new mother is on bedrest for the first 8 to 12 hours. To prevent pooling of secretions in the airway, she must be helped every 2 hours to turn, cough, and to expand the lungs by breathing deeply. Incentive spirometers also are used to expand the lungs and thus prevent hypostatic pneumonia that can result from immobility and shallow, slow respirations.

Splinting the abdomen with a small pillow reduces incisional discomfort when the woman coughs. She should be encouraged to flex her legs and move her feet and legs frequently to improve peripheral circulation. She needs assistance to sit and dangle her feet for the first few times. She should be helped to get out of bed and walk a short distance within 24 hours to help prevent thrombophlebitis.

Providing Comfort. Placing a pillow behind her back and one between her knees prevents strain and discomfort in a side-lying position. Excellent physical care (such as oral hygiene, perineal care, a sponge bath, clean linen) comforts and refreshes her.

After 24 Hours

Reinstating Normal Activities. After 24 hours, several normal functions return as postcesarean women are able to participate more actively in their own care:

- Both the indwelling catheter and IV infusion usually are discontinued.
- The dressing usually is removed, and often staples or clamps also are removed. Steri-Strips or a small nonstick dressing may be used to cover the incision.
- Mothers usually are helped to ambulate by the first postpartum day and are comfortable sitting in a chair for brief periods of time.
- Clear liquids may be changed to a soft diet once the mother is passing flatus. If abdominal distention is minimal, the diet then progresses to a regular regimen.

Nurses must encourage the mother to increase her activity and ambulation each postpartum day. By the second day, she usually is allowed to shower, if she wishes. Some health care providers request that the incision be covered with plastic; others permit showering without covering the incision.

Assisting the Mother with Infant Feeding. Helping the mother find a comfortable position for holding and feeding her infant is important. A side-lying position may be most comfortable. Some mothers prefer sitting with a pillow on the lap to protect the incisional area. The football hold often is the most comfortable position for breastfeeding because the infant is not on the lap and thus does not cause incisional discomfort (see Chapter 22).

Preventing Abdominal Distention. Abdominal distention is a major source of discomfort. Measures to prevent and minimize it include the following:

- Early, frequent ambulation
- Pelvic lifts—Lying supine with her knees bent, the woman lifts her pelvis from the bed and repeats the exercise up to 10 times, several times each day
- Tightening and relaxing the abdominal muscles
- Avoiding carbonated beverages and the use of straws, which increase the accumulation of intestinal gas
- Simithecone to disperse upper gastrointestinal flatulence
- Rectal suppositories to help stimulate peristalsis and passage of flatus

Check Your Reading

15. What additional assessments are necessary for the post cesarean mother?
16. How can hypostatic pneumonia be prevented?
17. Which measures are used to prevent or minimize abdominal distention?

APPLICATION OF THE NURSING PROCESS: KNOWLEDGE OF SELF-CARE

Assessment

Nurses are responsible for providing health education about a long list of subjects before the family is discharged from the birth facility. This task causes concern because so much must be taught during this short time, which is not ideal for teaching mothers who are not fully recovered from the birth process.

Table 17-6

COMMON NURSING DIAGNOSES FOR POSTPARTUM WOMEN

* Risk for Altered Health Maintenance
* Risk for Altered Sexuality Patterns
* Risk for Injury
Alterations in Nutrition More (or less) Than Body Requirements
Altered Urinary Elimination
Constipation
Health-Seeking Behaviors
Ineffective Breastfeeding
Parental Role Conflict

*Nursing diagnoses discussed in this chapter.

Before beginning teaching, determine the learning needs and the major concerns of each family. Multiparas remember some aspects of self-care but often benefit from a review. Primiparas may be anxious about self-care measures and all aspects of infant care. They require more thorough teaching and practice. Identify the most common barriers to learning: age and developmental level, cultural factors, and difficulty understanding the language.

Analysis

In general, mothers adapt to the physiologic changes after childbirth, and most nursing care is wellness oriented. Some new mothers, however, lack knowledge of self-care and thus are at risk for a disruption in health. Because of the need for health education, a nursing diagnosis that applies to many women and forms the basis for nursing interventions is "Risk for Altered Health Maintenance related to insufficient knowledge of self-care, signs of complications, and preventive measures." (The diagnoses "Risk for Injury" and "Altered Sexuality Patterns" appear in Nursing Care Plan 17-1. Common nursing diagnoses are listed in Table 17-6.)

Planning

Goals and expected outcomes for the nursing diagnosis "Risk for Altered Health Maintenance" related to insufficient knowledge of self-care, signs of complications, and preventive measures are that the mother will:

- Verbalize or demonstrate understanding of self-care instructions by (date).
- Verbalize understanding of practices that promote maternal health by discharge.
- Describe plans for follow-up care and signs and symptoms that should be reported to the physician, nurse-midwife, or nurse practitioner by discharge.

Interventions

Determining Teaching Topics

Make a teaching plan with the mother to include topics most important to her. The mother's perceptions of what is most important may differ from those of the nurse. One study found nurses focused more on infant care, whereas mothers were more concerned about their own care during the first few days after birth (Ruchala, 2000). Determining the mother's educational needs ensures her interest in the subjects selected and makes best use of the short time available. Topics of less interest may require just a brief review. The review may elicit questions from the mother and interest in more in-depth information.

Teaching the Process of Involution

The woman will need basic information about involution, including how to assess lochia and how to locate and palpate the fundus. This information allows her to recognize abnormal signs such as prolonged lochia, reappearance of bright-red lochia after lochia rubra has ended, and uterine tenderness, which should be reported to the health care provider. If the mother is a very young adolescent, another family member also may need the information.

Therapeutic Communication

TEACHING SELF-CARE MEASURES

Clare Beauchamp gave birth to a baby boy 48 hours ago. Terry Meyer is a nurse preparing to teach Clare self-care measures before discharge from the birth facility.

Clare: Look at me! I still look pregnant, and my husband calls me Tubby.

Terry: You were looking forward to your abdomen being flat after the baby was born.

This clarifies the woman's concern by reflecting content.

Clare: Well, I was always so flat. I'm really disappointed.

Terry: Remember it took 9 months for those muscles to stretch. You can't expect them to snap back in a few days.

This blocks communication by ignoring the feeling expressed. A more helpful response would be to acknowledge the disappointment and to delay giving information until feelings have been expressed. For example: "It is upsetting! When you are ready, we can discuss some exercises that will help."

Teaching Self-Care

Hand Washing. Emphasize the importance of thoroughly washing her hands before the woman touches her breasts, after diaper changes, after bladder and bowel elimination, and always before handling the infant. This also is emphasized to parents when they see nurses performing careful hand washing.

Breast Care for Lactating Mothers. Instruct the breastfeeding mother to wash her nipples with clear water and to avoid soaps that remove the natural lubrication secreted by Montgomery's glands. Keeping the nipples dry between feedings helps prevent tissue damage, and wearing a good bra provides necessary support as breast size increases (see Chapter 22).

Measures to Suppress Lactation. If the mother chooses not to breastfeed, measures should be initiated to suppress lactation. The safest method is to prevent breast distention by either binding the breasts or having the mother wear a tight-fitting bra 24 hours per day until the breasts become soft. Discomfort usually can be managed by application of ice, which reduces vasocongestion, and administration of analgesics. The woman should be advised to refrain from doing anything to stimulate milk production, such as allowing warm water to fall on the breasts during showers and pumping or massaging the breasts.

Perineal Care. Information about cleansing the perineum is important. The most common method is to fill a squeeze bottle with warm water and spray the perineal area from the front toward the back. Warm water alone or with a small amount of cleansing solution added is used. Remind the new mother not to separate the labia during this procedure because that would allow water to enter the vagina. If a commercial product that includes a nozzle attached to the faucet is used, teach the mother that the nozzle should not touch the perineum during use.

Moist antiseptic towelettes or toilet paper are used in a patting motion to dry the perineum. Teach the mother to dry from front to back to prevent fecal contamination of the vaginal introitus from the anal area. She should perform perineal cleansing after each voiding or defecation, and she should change peripads at the same time.

Many women do not use peripads for menstrual protection and must be taught to use them correctly. Mesh panties or adhering peripads are used in most facilities. Careful handling of the pads is important to prevent localized perineal infection.

- Thorough hand washing is required before and after changing pads.
- Unused pads should be stored inside their packages.
- Pads should be applied without touching the side that contacts the perineum.
- The pads should be applied and removed in a front-to-back direction to prevent contamination of the vagina and perineum.
- Used pads must be disposed of properly.

Kegel Exercises. All women should become familiar with Kegel exercises. These movements strengthen the pubococcygeal muscle, which surrounds the vagina and urinary meatus. This exercise helps prevent the loss of muscle tone that can occur after childbirth and sometimes leads to urinary incontinence.

The exercise, which may be started in the postpartum period, involves contracting muscles around the vagina (as though stopping the flow of urine), holding tightly for 10 seconds, and then relaxing for 10 seconds. Each contraction should be of moderate to near maximum intensity and a full 10 seconds should be allowed for relaxation between each contraction. The woman should work up to 30 contraction-relaxation cycles each day.

Promoting Rest and Sleep

Many women experience fatigue after childbirth. They appear worn out and lethargic and often verbalize a generalized decrease in energy and strength. The extreme fatigue they feel has many causes. They often are tired when they begin the postpartum period. Many pregnant women do not sleep well during the third trimester, and they are further exhausted by the exertion of labor. Feelings of excitement and euphoria after childbirth interfere with their ability to rest. Numerous visitors and phone calls during the first few days, hospital routines, and an unfamiliar environment interrupt rest. In addition, afterpains, discomfort from an episiotomy or incision, muscle aches, and breast engorgement may contribute to a woman's discomfort and inability to sleep.

Most mothers are discharged from the facility within 24 to 48 hours after vaginal birth or 72 to 96 hours after cesarean birth, and most go home with a tremendous deficit in sleep and energy. Yet new parents may be unprepared for the conflict between their need for sleep and the infant's need for care and attention. The joys of parenting can be easily overshadowed by the exhaustion and frustration that result. Women who have had cesarean births often state they are still concerned about incisional discomfort and that their need for sleep and rest is unmet at 10 to 14 days after discharge (Eakes & Brown, 1998).

Rest at the Birth Facility. Hospital routines continue around the clock, making uninterrupted rest difficult and increasing the probability that the mother is fatigued when she is discharged. Make every attempt to allow the mother adequate time for uninterrupted rest periods. Group assessments and care, and try to correlate them with times when the mother would be awake, such as just before or after meals, infant feeding times, and visiting hours. If the room is shared, providing care for both women at the same time also reduces activities that interrupt sleep.

Try to persuade the mother to select a time when phone calls and visitors are restricted so that she can use this time for napping. A quiet, softly lit environment also promotes sleep.

Rest at Home. Help the mother understand the impact that her physical discomfort and the demands of the newborn will have on her energy during the first few weeks. Teach measures that conserve energy, including the following:

- Maintaining a relaxed, flexible routine that focuses on care of the mother and infant
- Napping when the infant sleeps, if possible

- Planning simple meals and flexible meal times
- Accepting assistance with food shopping and meal preparation
- Postponing major household projects
- Involving friends and family to provide care for other children

Explain to the mother that she should delay her return to employment, if possible, until the infant sleeps through the night (usually by 4 months). Advise all mothers to restrict coffee, tea, colas, and chocolate, which contain the stimulant caffeine, or use caffeine-free versions for the first few weeks. Suggest rest whenever the infant sleeps rather than using that time to catch up on housecleaning tasks. Total relaxation exercises (lying quietly, alternately tightening and relaxing the muscles of the neck, shoulders, arms, legs, and feet) are helpful when a nap is not possible.

Emphasize to the mother the importance of asking for help when she begins to feel exhausted or overwhelmed. Encourage her to share these feelings with family, friends, and other new mothers.

Infant Sleep and Feeding Schedules. Many families require information about infant sleep cycles, frequency of feeding, and probable crying episodes during the first weeks. Although newborns sleep 16 to 20 hours per day, they may awaken every 2 to 3 hours for feeding (see Chapter 22 regarding infant feeding and Chapter 23 regarding parenting during the first weeks).

Providing Nourishment and Nutrition Counseling

Food Supply. Determining the amount and type of food that is available to the mother and her family sometimes is appropriate. This is particularly true for families of low socioeconomic status, who might benefit from referral to government-sponsored programs, such as food stamps or the Special Supplemental Food Program for Women, Infants, and Children (WIC). Determining the facilities available for cooking and storing food also may be necessary. Sometimes the new family must be referred to a social worker so that the best solutions for their unique problems can be found.

Diet. Although many women are not satisfied with the slow rate of weight loss, severe restriction of caloric intake can leave the mother feeling tired, lower her immunity, and may interfere with the ability to synthesize milk (Lawrence & Lawrence, 1999). Advise the mother to select foods that provide adequate calories to meet her energy needs, taking into account the time and energy required to care for a newborn. A balanced, low-fat diet with adequate protein, complex carbohydrates, fruits, and vegetables provides the energy needed (see Chapter 9).

Promoting Regular Bowel Elimination

Progressive exercise, adequate fluid, and dietary fiber are effective means of preventing constipation. Walking perhaps is the best exercise, and the distance can be increased as strength and endurance increase. Drinking at least eight glasses of water daily helps maintain normal bowel elimination. Fruits and vegetables, particularly when they are unpeeled, provide dietary fiber. Prunes act as a natural laxative. Additional fiber is found in whole grain cereals, bread, and pasta.

A regular schedule of bowel elimination also is important in overcoming constipation. For instance, bowel elimination after breakfast allows the mother to take advantage of the gastrocolic reflex (stimulation of peristalsis induced in the colon when food is consumed on an empty stomach). In addition, measures that reduce perineal and hemorrhoidal pain, such as sitz baths, prepackaged witch hazel astringent compresses, and ointments facilitate bowel elimination.

Promoting Good Body Mechanics

Exercise. Exercise has been shown to have beneficial physical and psychological effects during the postpartum period. Vigorous exercise is associated with greater weight loss, greater satisfaction with motherhood, and more confidence in mothering tasks (Sampselle, et al., 1999).

Teach exercises in the early postpartum period to strengthen the abdominal muscles and firm the waist (Figure 17-12). The exercises can be started soon after childbirth. At first, each exercise should be repeated five times, twice each day. Gradually, the number of exercises is increased as the mother gains strength.

Postcesarean mothers should follow the instructions of their health care provider. They may need to avoid a vigorous exercise program for 4 to 6 weeks but can participate in less strenuous activities such as walking.

Prevention of Back Strain. Back strain often can be prevented if the mother and father find a location for infant care, such as a kitchen table or bathroom counter, that does not require bending and leaning forward. For lifting objects, teach parents to hold the back straight as they squat and use the legs rather than bending at the waist (see Figure 7-14).

Counseling About Sexual Activity

The couple may have concerns about the resumption of sexual intercourse and contraceptive choices. Fatigue, perineal pain, fear of pregnancy, concerns about the baby, and a feeling of unattractiveness may interfere with a woman's sexual desire. Cultural or religious convictions may restrict the choice of contraceptive method for some couples, whereas availability of health care or inadequate finances may dictate the choice for others. Discuss previous experience with contraceptives and the satisfaction with that method. Some women choose to have a tubal ligation before discharge after birth (see Chapter 31).

Many new parents are reluctant to ask about when to resume sexual activity and potential alterations in sexuality resulting from pregnancy and childbirth. Nurses must be sensitive to unasked questions and should try to provide anticipatory guidance.

> If couples do not indicate such concerns, introduce the topic in a general, nonspecific manner, such as "You have an episiotomy that may cause some discomfort with intercourse until it is completely healed" or "Sometimes couples are not aware that some vaginal dryness occurs as a result of breastfeeding." Such broad opening statements permit the couple to pursue the topic as they desire.

Nursing Care Plan 17-1 (see p. 439) describes interventions for the nursing diagnosis "Risk for Altered Sexuality Patterns related to perineal discomfort, dryness of vaginal mucosa, or fatigue."

Instructing About Follow-Up Appointments

Remind the new mother to make an appointment with her physician or nurse-midwife for a postpartum examination at the time suggested by her provider. This is often at 2 weeks and 6 weeks after childbirth. Emphasize that examination at those times allows early identification and treatment of problems that may be developing.

Teaching About Signs and Symptoms That Should Be Reported

Teach new mothers and at least one member of the family which physical signs and symptoms should be reported to the health care provider right away. These signs and symptoms include the following:

- Fever
- Localized area of redness, swelling, or pain in either breast that is not relieved by support or analgesics
- Persistent abdominal tenderness
- Feelings of pelvic fullness or pelvic pressure
- Persistent perineal pain
- Frequency, urgency, or burning on urination
- Change in character of lochia (increased amount, resumption of bright red color, passage of clots, foul odor)
- Localized tenderness, redness, swelling, or warmth of the legs
- Swelling, redness, drainage from, or separation of an abdominal incision

Ensuring a Thorough Education

Although mothers often prefer individual teaching (Beger & Cook, 1998), group instruction and hospital classes, such as those that demonstrate infant care and provide breastfeeding instructions, make more efficient use of the nurse's time. Nurses streamline and organize information so that it can be presented in the time available. In some agencies, women are given some information pertaining to postpartum self-care during the prenatal period. During the hospital stay, the nurse reviews and rechecks the mother's understanding of previous teaching.

Table 17-7
POSTPARTUM DISCHARGE TEACHING TOPICS

Uterine massage
Lochia norms
Involution
Episiotomy care
Care of abdominal incisions
Breast care for lactating and nonlactating women
Bowel function
Urinary function
Nutrition
Rest
Exercise
Contraception
Sexual activity
Postpartum danger signs
Follow-up care
Medications
Emotional responses
Infant care and feeding
Family adjustment
Available resources

Documentation is an important aspect of teaching, just as it is for other aspects of nursing care. Documentation that discharge teaching was performed and the client indicates comprehension of teaching is required by accrediting agencies. To prevent omissions, many hospitals use teaching checklists to record topics that must be taught (Table 17-7) (see Chapter 21 for teaching about infant care).

Evaluation

- The mother's demonstration of correct breast and perineal hygiene provides evidence of her ability to perform self-care measures.
- The mother's ability to discuss practices that promote health in the areas of diet, exercise, rest, and sleep confirm understanding of these measures.
- Her ability to describe a plan for future appointments with the health care provider for examinations or follow-up of complications increases the likelihood that she will experience an uncomplicated recovery.

Postpartum Home and Community-Based Care

Criteria for Discharge

Most women must leave the hospital when they are just beginning to recover from giving birth and to learn to care for themselves and their infants. The American Academy of Pediatrics and the American College of

ABDOMINAL BREATHING

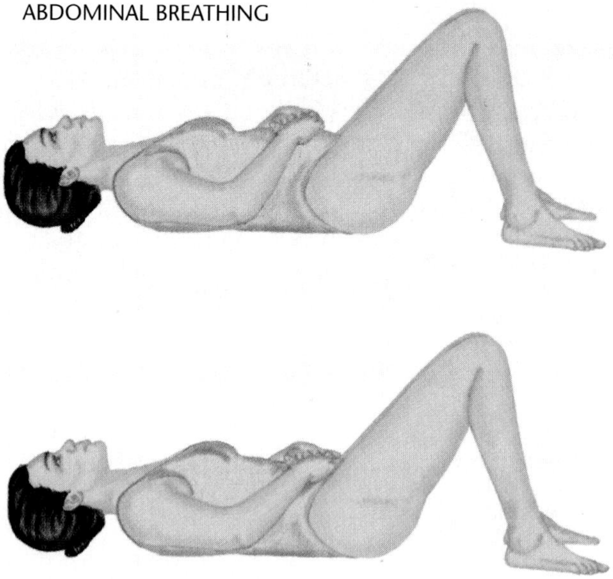

This is one of the simplest exercises and can be started on the first postpartum day. The woman assumes a supine position with knees bent. She inhales through the nose, keeps the rib cage as stationary as possible, and allows the abdomen to expand. She then contracts the abdominal muscles as she exhales slowly through the mouth.

HEAD LIFT

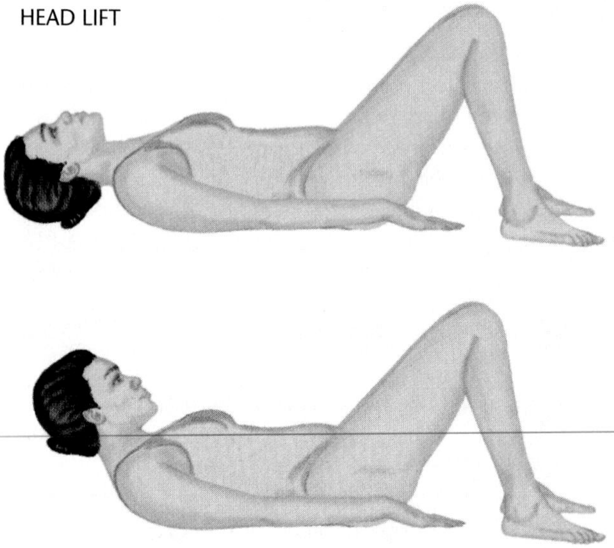

This exercise can be started within a few days after childbirth. The mother is supine with knees bent and arms outstretched at her side. She inhales deeply to begin, then exhales while lifting the head slowly; she holds the position for a few seconds and relaxes.

MODIFIED SIT-UPS

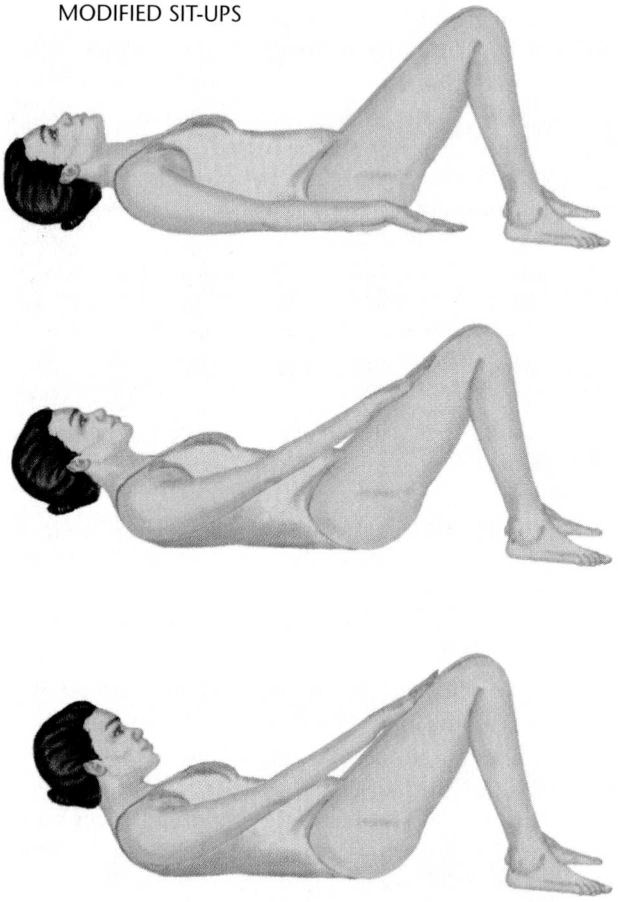

Head lifts may progress to modified sit-ups with the approval of the health care provider; the mother should follow the advice of the health care provider about the number of repetitions.

The exercise begins with the mother supine with arms outstretched and the knees bent. She raises her head and shoulders as her hands reach for her knees. She raises the shoulders only as far as the back will bend; her waist remains on the floor.

FIGURE 17-12 Postpartum exercises. Exercises should be approved by the woman's physician, nurse-midwife, or nurse practitioner before she begins them.

KNEE AND LEG ROLLS

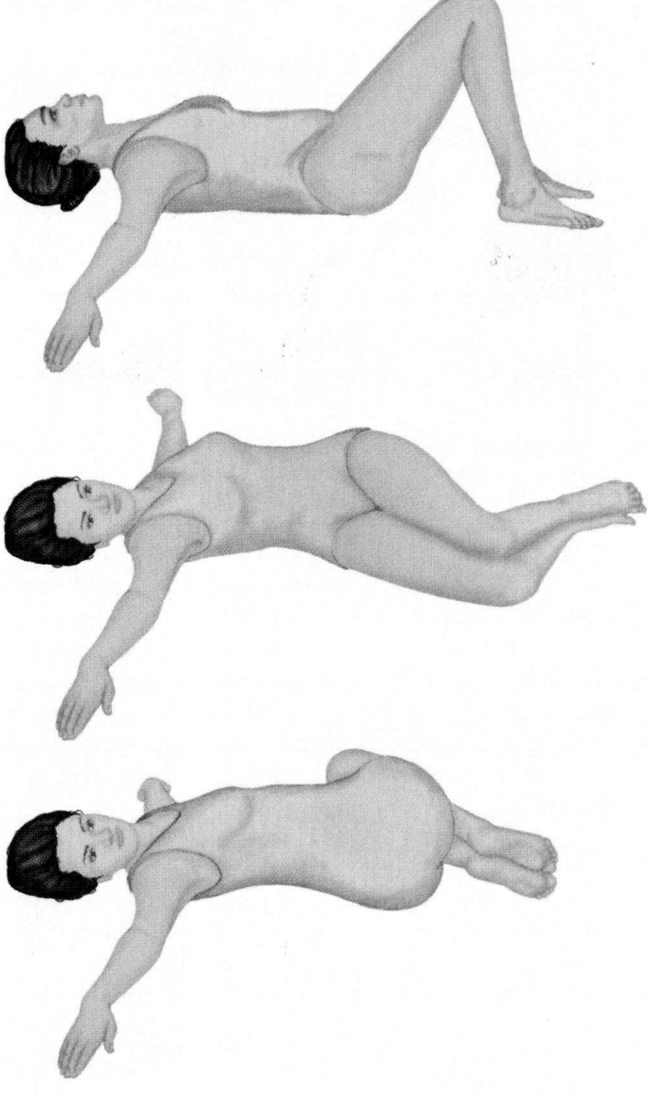

This is an excellent exercise to begin firming the waist. The mother lies flat on her back with knees bent and feet flat on the floor or bed; she keeps the shoulders and feet stationary and rolls the knees to touch first one side of the bed, then the other. She maintains a smooth motion as the exercise is repeated five times. Later, as flexibility increases, the exercise can be varied by the rolling of one knee only. The mother rolls her left knee to touch the right side of the bed, returns to center, and rolls the right knee to touch the left side of the bed.

CHEST EXERCISES

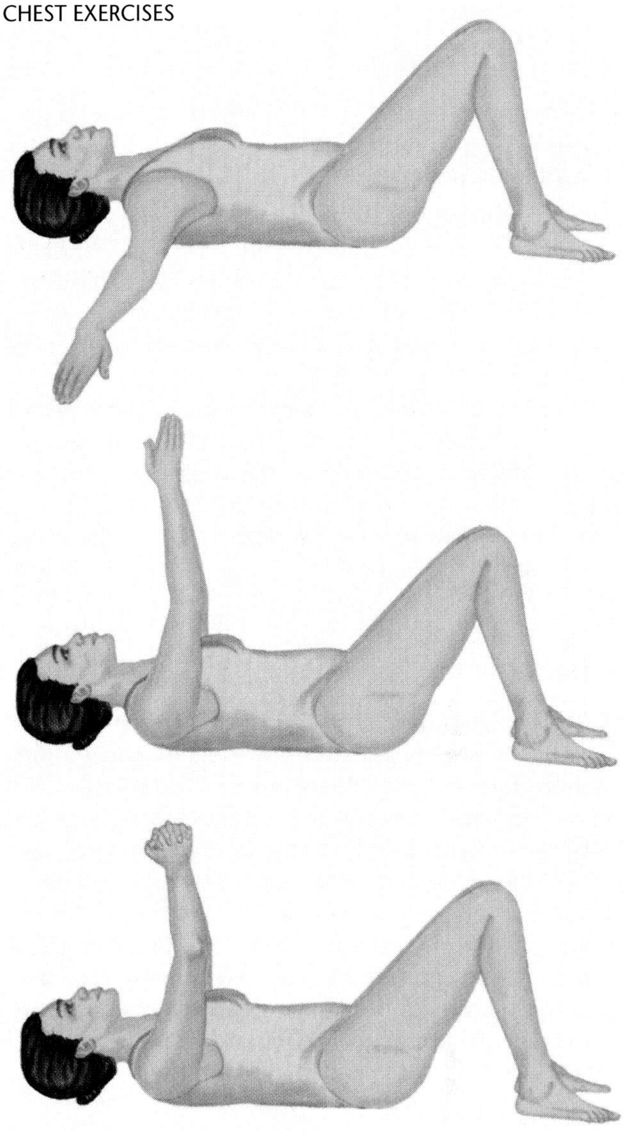

This is an excellent exercise to strengthen the chest muscles. The mother lies flat with arms extended straight out to the side; she brings the hands together above the chest while keeping the arms straight; she holds for a few seconds and returns to the starting position. She repeats the exercise five times initially and follows the advice of the health care provider for increasing the number of repetitions.

Isometric exercises also increase strength and tone; the mother bends her elbows, clasps her hands together above her chest, and presses her hands together for a few seconds. This is repeated at least five times.

FIGURE 17-12, cont'd For legend see opposite page.

Obstetricians and Gynecologists developed criteria for discharge of mothers (1997):

- The mother has no complications and assessments are normal (including vital signs, lochia, fundus, urinary output, incisions, ambulation, ability to eat and drink and emotional status).
- Pertinent laboratory data have been reviewed and immune globulin has been administered, if necessary.
- The mother has received instructions on self-care, deviations from normal, and proper response to danger signs and symptoms.
- The mother demonstrates readiness to care for herself and her baby.
- The mother has received instructions on postpartum activity, exercises, and relief measures for common postpartum discomforts.
- Arrangements have been made for postpartum care.
- Family members or other support persons are available to the mother for the first few days after discharge.

Common Problems of the Postpartum Period

When new mothers go home, they often experience continued perineal, incisional, and nipple pain and uterine cramping. They also may have problems with fatigue, constipation, and breastfeeding. In one study, more than 78% of postpartum women had concerns great enough that they called a health care provider within 2 weeks of delivery (Fishbein & Burggraf, 1998). They may be apprehensive about assuming additional responsibilities. Women who have had a cesarean birth often have concerns about the need for assistance with housekeeping chores and infant care (Eakes & Brown, 1998).

Home Care Services

New parents must be made aware of the services available for home care in their area. These services may include information lines, follow-up telephone calls, home visits, and nurse-managed postpartum outpatient clinics. In addition, some facilities offer breastfeeding and parenting classes, "baby and me" walks, exercise sessions, and postpartum support groups (see Chapter 23 for information about community care).

Information Lines. Ideally, information lines should be open 24 hours a day, 7 days a week. They should be staffed by qualified nurses who use agency protocols to respond to the family's questions. These nurses must be prepared to "triage." That is, they must be skilled at soliciting information to identify problems and to determine the priority of the problems identified. For instance, does the information obtained indicate that the family should come to the office or clinic for a more thorough assessment by their health care provider? Should they come now or can they wait? Can their problem be solved by information or advice?

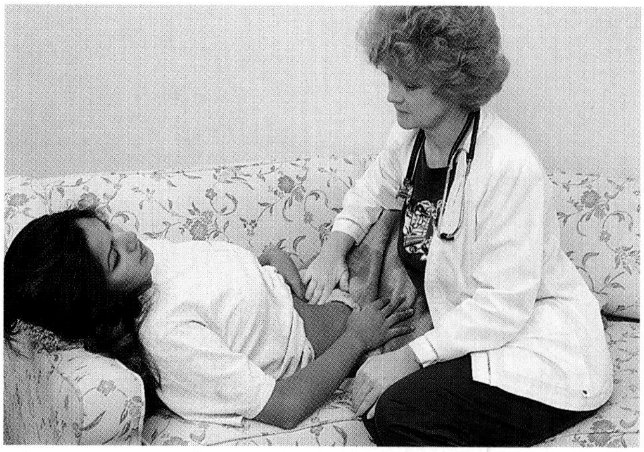

FIGURE 17-13 Postpartum home visits include assessments and health education. Here the nurse evaluates involution while teaching the mother how to palpate her fundus.

Legal liability is a concern for all agencies and personnel who identify problems, set priorities, and provide information by telephone. The staff must be educated and evaluated for the task. Protocols must be devised, a documentation system must be developed, and adequate consultation or "backup" support must be available.

A major disadvantage of information lines is that they rely on families to initiate a request for assistance. Not all families recognize when a problem begins to develop and, as a result, may delay in seeking information.

Telephone Calls. Some facilities initiate telephone interviews to assess new families and provide information to families at home. The calls usually are made 1 to 3 days after discharge. As with information lines, a qualified nurse, following the facility protocol, conducts a systematic assessment of the mother and infant. The nurse solicits questions and reinforces important information. Telephone calls are relatively inexpensive. The major disadvantage is that the nurse cannot confirm data but must rely on observations made by the family.

Home Visits. Home visits allow physical examination of the mother and infant and assessment of family adaptation and the home environment. Maternal assessment should include the breasts, fundus, lochia, perineum, abdominal incision (if applicable), and psychosocial status (Figure 17-13). If possible, nurses should allow time to observe breastfeeding and provide encouragement and reassurance that is badly needed during the first days before lactation is well established.

The newborn's weight, color, elimination pattern, and feeding history are important parts of the home visit. Ample time should be allowed to reinforce previous learning, answer questions, and introduce new topics.

Although home visits are expensive, some agencies believe that they are less expensive than readmission of the mother or infant to the hospital or outpatient treatment for problems that could be prevented by follow-up care.

Outpatient Clinics. Nurse-managed outpatient clinics offer another option for postpartum care. Although transportation is a problem for some families, clinic visits are less costly for the agency than home visits and more clients can be seen in a day than with home visits. Clinic visits may be used either to replace or supplement home visits. Like home care, clinic visits include an examination of the mother and infant. Adequate time is provided to answer questions about maternal self-care, provide assistance with infant feeding, and deal with special concerns such as care of the umbilical cord or circumcision. Visits have been found to reduce infant morbidity and increase maternal satisfaction with care (Lieu, et al., 1998).

Check Your Reading

18. How is lactation suppressed when the mother elects not to breastfeed?
19. What is the major challenge that early discharge presents for the nurse? How do clinical pathways affect nursing care?
20. What are the criteria for discharge of the mother?
21. What are the advantages and disadvantages of information lines, telephone calls, home visits, and nurse-managed outpatient clinics?

SUMMARY CONCEPTS

- After childbirth, the uterus returns to its nonpregnant size and condition by involution, which involves contraction of stretched muscle fibers, catabolic processes that reduce enlarged muscle cells, and regeneration of uterine epithelium.
- The site of placental attachment heals by a process of exfoliation, which leaves the endometrium smooth and without scars.
- Involution can be evaluated by measuring the descent of the fundus (about 1 cm/day). By the tenth to fourteenth day after childbirth, the fundus should be located in the pelvic cavity and should no longer be palpable abdominally.
- Afterpains, or intermittent uterine contractions, cause discomfort for many women, particularly multiparas who breastfeed.
- Vaginal discharge (lochia) progresses from lochia rubra (mostly blood) to lochia serosa (serous exudate, blood, and leukocytes) to lochia alba (increased amounts of leukocytes and decidual cells) in a predictable time frame. Lochia should be assessed for volume, type, and odor. Foul odor suggests endometrial infection.
- Although vaginal mucosa heals within 3 weeks, it takes 6 weeks for the vagina to regain its nonpregnant size and contour.
- Hemorrhoids and perineal trauma, including edema, bruising, episiotomy, and lacerations, can cause a great deal of discomfort and interfere with bladder and bowel elimination.
- As blood from the uteroplacental unit returns to central circulation and extracellular fluid is mobilized into the vascular compartment, the cardiac output increases and excess fluid is excreted by diuresis and diaphoresis.
- Increased clotting factors predispose the postpartum woman to thrombus formation. Early, frequent ambulation is the best method for preventing thrombophlebitis.
- Constipation may occur as a result of inadequate fluid intake during labor, reduced activity, decreased muscle tone, and fear of pain during defecation.
- Increased bladder capacity and decreased sensitivity to fluid pressure may result in urinary retention. Stasis of urine allows time for bacteria to grow and can lead to urinary tract infection.
- A distended bladder lifts and displaces the uterus and can interfere with uterine contraction and cause excessive bleeding.
- Exercises to strengthen the abdominal muscles and good posture and body mechanics may reduce musculoskeletal discomfort.
- As hormone levels decline, the skin gradually reverts to its prepregnancy state.
- Breastfeeding may delay the return of ovulation and menstruation but is not a reliable method of family planning. Both lactating and nonlactating mothers need information about family planning.
- Breastfeeding mothers are more likely to experience dyspareunia as a result of vaginal dryness that results from inadequate estrogen.
- Lactation may be suppressed by wearing a snug bra, binding the breasts, and avoiding stimulation of the breasts.
- The postpartum woman should be afebrile but her temperature may be higher during the first 24 hours after delivery because of exertion, dehydration, and leukocytosis.
- Bradycardia is expected. Tachycardia may be caused by excitement, infection, dehydration, pain, and hypovolemia. Additional assessments (for example, lochia, fundus) are required to determine whether excessive bleeding is the cause.
- Orthostatic hypotension occurs when the mother goes from a supine to standing position quickly. It may result in injury if precautions to protect her are not initiated.
- The common practice of early discharge challenges nurses to streamline information and develop a plan for teaching self-care and infant care in a short amount of time.
- The postcesarean woman requires postoperative and postpartum assessments and care. She is at increased risk for problems associated with immobility and discomfort.

ANSWERS TO CRITICAL THINKING EXERCISE, p. 442

1. The birth of a large infant increases the risk of postpartum hemorrhage. Saturation of pads in a short time suggests excessive bleeding. Location of the fundus above the umbilicus and displaced to the side indicates that the cause of excessive bleeding might be a distended bladder.

2. Assisting the mother to void is the most appropriate nursing action. If, after voiding, the fundus is located at the level of the umbilicus and firmly contracted, the nurse can be relatively certain that the cause of the bleeding was a distended bladder, which made it difficult for the uterus to contract firmly. The location and consistency of the uterus, amount of lochia, blood pressure, and pulse should be assessed frequently so that further excessive bleeding can be promptly identified and controlled.
3. Linda does not experience the urge to void because the bladder has not regained the muscle tone lost during pregnancy and the sensitivity to pressure is decreased.

ANSWERS TO CRITICAL THINKING EXERCISE, p. 447

1. Any time a client has more pain than would be expected, further assessment is necessary to determine the cause. Ask Elizabeth whether she urinated a large or small amount. Ask her to rate her pain. Exactly where is the pain located? What type of pain is it? Burning, pressure, dull ache? How much lochia does she have compared with previous assessments?
2. Regardless of the amount she thinks she voided previously, assist Elizabeth to the bathroom to see if she can void. If she voids, measure the amount to see if it is adequate (approximately 300 ml) and determine if she feels relief after voiding. If she is unable to void and an order exists, catheterize her. If no order exists, call the health care provider to obtain an order.
3. The client may have a very low pain tolerance. She may need a different kind of analgesic. In this case, however, Elizabeth had surgery yesterday and has received pain medication since that time. A low pain tolerance or a drug that was ineffective for her would already have been noted. Some surgical complication may exist. If the pain continues, refer the problem to the provider.

REFERENCES & READINGS

Alteneder, R.R. & Hartzell, D. (1997). Addressing couples' sexuality concerns during the childbearing period: Use of the PLISSIT model. *Journal of Obstetric, Gynecologic, and Neonatal Nursing* 26(6), 651-658.

American Academy of Pediatrics & American College of Obstetricians and Gynecologists. (1997). *Guidelines for perinatal care.* (4th ed.). Elk Grove Village, IL: Author.

AWHONN (1998). *Standards & guidelines for professional nursing practice in the care of women and newborns.* (5th ed.). Washington, D.C.: Author.

Beger, D. & Cook. C.A.L. (1998). Postpartum teaching priorities: The viewpoints of nurses and mothers. *Journal of Obstetric, Gynecologic, and Neonatal Nursing* 27(2), 161-168.

Blackburn, S.T., & Loper, D.L. (1992). *Maternal, fetal, and neonatal physiology: A clinical perspective.* Philadelphia: W.B. Saunders.

Britt, R. & Pasero, C. (1999) Pregnancy, Childbirth, Postpartum, and Breastfeeding: Use of analgesics. In M. McCaffery & C. Pasero, *Pain: Clinical manual* (2nd ed., 608-625). St. Louis: Mosby.

Britton, J. R. (1998). Postpartum early hospital discharge and follow-up practices in Canada and the United States. *Birth,* 25(3), 161-168.

Brooten, B., Knapp, H., Jacobsen, B., & Arnold, L. (1996). Early discharge after unplanned cesarean birth: Nursing care time. *Journal of Obstetric, Gynecologic, and Neonatal Nursing,* 25(7), 595-600.

Burton, J. (1999). When your patient is postpartum: Are you confident in your skills? *American Journal of Nursing,* 99(2), 64-70.

Carpenter, J.A. (1998). Shortening the short stay. *AWHONN Lifelines,* 2(1), 29-34.

Cunningham, F.G., MacDonald, P.C., Gant, N.F., Leveno, K.J., Gilstrap, L.C., Hankins, G.D.V., et al. (1997). *Williams obstetrics* (20th ed.). Norwalk, CT: Appleton & Lange.

Duerbeck, N.B., & Reed, K.L. (1998). Pregnancy and lactation. In L.A. Wallis (Ed.). *Textbook of women's health* (pp. 663-674). Philadelphia: Lippincott.

Eakes, M., & Brown, H. (1998) Home alone: Meeting the needs of mothers after cesarean birth. *Lifelines,* 2(1), 37-40.

Ewy-Edwards, D. (2000). Transition to parenthood. In F.H. Nichols & S.S. Humenick. Childbirth education: Practice, research, and theory. (2nd ed., pp. 84-113). Philadelphia: W.B. Saunders.

Farrington, P.F., & Ward, K. (1999). Normal labor, delivery, and puerperium. In J.R. Scott, P.J. Disaia, C.B. Hammond, & W.N. Spellacy (Eds.), *Danforth's obstetrics and gynecology* (8th ed., pp. 91-109). Philadelphia: Lippincott, Williams & Wilkins.

Fishbein, E.G., & Burggraf, E. (1998). Early postpartum discharge: How are mothers managing? *Journal of Obstetric, Gynecologic, and Neonatal Nursing,* 27(2), 142-148.

Gennaro, S., Fehder, W.P., York, R., & Douglas, S.D. (1997). Weight, nutrition, and immune status in postpartal women. *Nursing Research,* 46(1), 20-25.

Gorczyca, J. (1999). Risky business: Legal issues in perinatal discharge. *Mother Baby Journal,* 4(5), 25-30.

Grohar, J. (1996). Postpartum care. In K.R. Simpson & P.A. Creehan (Eds.). *AWHONN perinatal nursing.* Philadelphia: Lippincott-Raven Publishers.

Gupton, A., & McKay, M. (1995). The Canadian perspective on postpartum home care. *Journal of Obstetric, Gynecologic, and Neonatal Nursing,* 24(2), 173-179.

Hayashi, R.H., & Zettelmaier, M.A. (2000). Postpartum management. In S.B. Ransom, M.P. Dombrowski, S.G. McNeeley, K.S. Moghissi, & A.R. Munkarah (Eds.), *Practical strategies in obstetrics and gynecology* (pp. 321-325). Philadelphia: W.B. Saunders.

Jacobson, B.B., Brock, K.A., & Keppler, A.B. (1999). The post birth partnership: Washington state's comprehensive approach to improve follow-up care. *Journal of Perinatal Neonatal Nursing,* 13(1), 43-52.

Kennedy, K.I. (1999). Fertility, sexuality, & contraception during lactation. In J. Riordan & K.C. Auerbach (Eds.), *Breastfeeding and human lactation* (2nd ed., pp. 675-705). Boston: Jones & Bartlett.

Keppler, A.B., & Roudebush, J.L. (1999). Postpartum follow-up care in a hospital-based clinic: An update on an expanded program. *Journal of Perinatal Neonatal Nursing,* 13(1), 1-14.

Lawrence, R.A., & Lawrence, R.M. (1999). *Breastfeeding: A guide for the medical profession* (5th ed.). St. Louis: Mosby.

Lieu, T.A., Braveman, P.A., Escobar, G.J., Fischer, A.F., Jensvold, N.G., & Capra, A.M. (2000). A randomized comparison of home and clinic follow-up visits after early postpartum hospital discharge. *Pediatrics,* 105(5), 1058-1065.

Lieu, T.A., Wikler, C., Capra, A.M., Martin, K.E., Escobar, G.J., & Braveman, P. (1998). A. Clinical outcomes and maternal perceptions of an updated model of perinatal care. *Pediatrics,* 102(6), 1437-1444.

Mason, L., Glenn, S. Walton, I., & Appleton, C. (1999). The experience of stress incontinence after childbirth. *Birth,* 26(3), 164-171.

Martell, L.K. (2000). The hospital and the postpartum experience: A historical analysis. *Journal of Obstetric, Gynecologic, and Neonatal Nursing,* 29(1), 65-72.

Resnik, R. (1999). The puerperium. In R.K. Creasy & R. Resnik (Eds.), *Maternal-fetal medicine* (4th ed., pp. 102-105). Philadelphia: W.B. Saunders.

Ruchala, P.L. (2000). Teaching new mothers: Priorities of nurses and postpartum women. *Journal of Obstetric, Gynecologic, and Neonatal Nursing,* 29(3), 265-273.

Sampselle, C.M., Burns. P.A., Dougherty, M.C., Newman, D.K., Thomas, K.K., & Wyman, J.F. (1997). Continence for women: Evidence-based practice. *Journal of Obstetric, Gynecologic, and Neonatal Nursing,* 26(4), 375-385.

Scoggin, J. (2000). Physical and psychological changes. In S. Mattson & J.E. Smith (Eds.), *Core curriculum for maternal-newborn nursing* (2nd ed., pp. 302-316). Philadelphia: W.B. Saunders.

Stables, D. (1999). *Physiology in childbearing.* Edinburgh: Bailliere Tindall.

Thorp, J.M., Norton, P.A., Wall, L.L., Kuller, J.A., Eucker, B., & Wells, E. (1999). Urinary incontinence in pregnancy and the puerperium: A prospective study. *American Journal of Obstetrics & Gynecology,* 181(2), 266-273.

Valaitis, R., Tuff, K., & Swanson, L. (1996). Meeting parents' postpartal needs with a telephone information line. *MCN: The American Journal of Maternal Child Nursing,* 21(2), 90-95.

Weber, S.E. (1996). Cultural aspects of pain in childbearing women. *Journal of Obstetric, Gynecologic, and Neonatal Nursing,* 25(1), 67-72.

Wilkerson, N.N. & Shrock, P. (2000). Sexuality in the perinatal period. In F.H. Nichols & S.S. Humenick (Eds.), *Childbirth education: Practice, research, and theory* (2nd ed., pp. 48-65). Philadelphia: W.B. Saunders.

Williams, L.R., & Cooper, M.K. (1996). A new paradigm for postpartum care. *Journal of Obstetric, Gynecologic, and Neonatal Nursing,* 25(9), 745-749.

Zuspan, K. (2000). Control of postpartum pain. In F.P. Zuspan & E.J. Quilligan (Eds.), *Current therapy in obstetrics and gynecology* (5th ed., pp. 261-263). Philadelphia: W.B. Saunders.

18

Postpartum Psychosocial Adaptations

OBJECTIVES

1. Explain the process of bonding and attachment, including maternal touch and verbal interactions.
2. Describe the progressive phases of maternal adaptation to childbirth and the stages of maternal role attainment.
3. Identify maternal concerns and the way they change over time.
4. Discuss the cause, manifestations, and interventions related to postpartum blues.
5. Describe the processes of family adaptation to the birth of a baby.
6. Explain factors that affect family adaptation.
7. Discuss cultural influences on family adaptation.
8. Describe assessments and interventions related to postpartum psychosocial adaptations.
9. Discuss the need for additional care after discharge of the mother and infant from the birth facility.

DEFINITIONS

Attachment Development of strong affectional ties as a result of interaction between an infant and a significant other.

Bonding Development of a strong emotional tie of a parent to a newborn; also called *claiming* or *binding in.*

En Face Position that allows eye-to-eye contact between the newborn and a parent.

Engrossment Intense fascination and close face-to-face observation between the father and newborn.

Entrainment Newborn movement in rhythm to adult speech, particularly high-pitched tones, which are more easily heard.

Fingertipping First tactile (touch) experience between the mother and newborn in which the mother explores the infant's body, mainly with her fingertips.

Fourth Trimester First 12 weeks after birth; a time of transition for parents and siblings.

DEFINITIONS—cont'd

Letting-Go A phase of maternal adaptation that involves relinquishment of previous roles and assumption of a new role as a parent.

Postpartum Blues Temporary, self-limited period of weepiness experienced by many new mothers within the first few days after childbirth.

Reciprocal Bonding Behaviors Repertoire of infant behaviors that promote attachment between the parent and newborn.

Sibling Rivalry Feelings of jealousy and fear of replacement when a young child must share the attention of the parents with a newborn infant.

Taking-Hold Second phase of maternal adaptation during which the mother assumes control of her own care and initiates care of the infant.

Taking-In First phase of maternal adaptation during which the mother passively accepts care, comfort, and details about the newborn.

Perhaps no other event requires such rapid change in family structure and function as the birth of a baby. The mother progresses through restorative phases to replenish the energy lost during labor and childbirth and gain confidence in her role as mother. Both the mother and the father begin the process of attachment with the newborn. Siblings must adapt to a new standing in the family structure and deal with feelings of jealousy and rivalry that may result from the birth of an infant. Numerous factors such as previous experience and the availability of a strong support system influence family adaptation. In addition, culture is among the most significant variables that influence a family's perception of childbearing.

The role of maternity nurses has gradually expanded from the care of the mother-infant dyad to include the well-being of the entire family. Nurses are concerned with the family's adjustment to childbearing, not only during the hospital stay but also during the early weeks at home as the family makes the transition to parenthood.

THE PROCESS OF BECOMING ACQUAINTED

Nursing literature has described the way parents and newborns become acquainted and progress to develop feelings of love, concern, and deep devotion that last throughout life. The terms *bonding* and *attachment* are commonly used to describe the initial steps. Although the terms are sometimes used interchangeably, their meanings do differ.

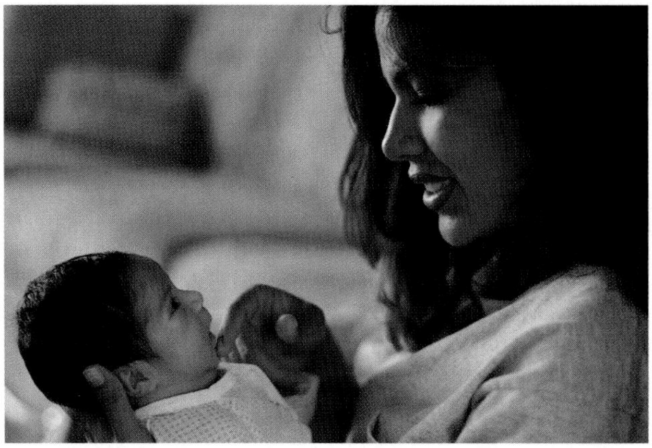

FIGURE 18-1 The infant is quiet and alert during the initial sensitive period. The newborn gazes at the mother and responds to her voice and touch.

Bonding

Bonding describes the rapid process of attachment that occurs soon after childbirth, the initial attraction felt by parents. It is unidirectional, from parent to child, and is enhanced when parents and infants are permitted to touch and interact during a so-called *sensitive period* extending through the first 30 to 60 minutes after birth. During this time the infant is in a quiet, alert state and seems to gaze directly at the parents (Figure 18-1).

Nurses frequently delay procedures that would interfere with this time between parents and newborns. Instillation of prophylactic eye medication, administration of vitamin K injections, and measurements are often postponed so that the parents can have this time with their newborn baby.

The concept of a sensitive period can be misinterpreted by parents and health care workers, who may believe it is the only time for the process of attachment to begin. Early and sustained contact between the parents and infant can enhance bonding and attachment. However, if early contact between parent and infant is limited because of an obstetric emergency or neonatal illness, bonding and attachment can still occur.

Attachment

Attachment is the process by which an enduring bond to a child is developed through pleasurable, satisfying parent-child interaction. The process begins in pregnancy and extends for many months after childbirth. The infant receives warmth, food, and security from the parent. The parent, usually the mother, accepts responsibility for the infant's care and places the child's needs above her own for years to come. In return, she receives enjoyment and establishes her identity as a mother. Both benefit from the formation of irreplaceable links that continue long after the child ceases to be dependent.

The process of attachment follows a progressive or developmental course that changes over time. It is rarely instantaneous. Attachment behaviors of inexperienced or first-time mothers do not differ significantly from those of experienced mothers (Mercer & Ferketich, 1994b).

Attachment occurs through mutually satisfying experiences. Therefore if the newly delivered mother is in severe pain or physically exhausted, she needs pain relief, assistance, or both to be able to enjoy the early experiences with the baby.

Unlike bonding, attachment is reciprocal—it occurs in both directions between parent and infant. It is facilitated by positive feedback, either real or perceived, from the infant. Alert infants have a repertoire of responses called *reciprocal attachment behaviors.* An infant's grasp reflex around a parent's finger means "I love you" to the parent. These behaviors represent the infant's part in the process of early attachment that progresses to lifelong, mutual devotion.

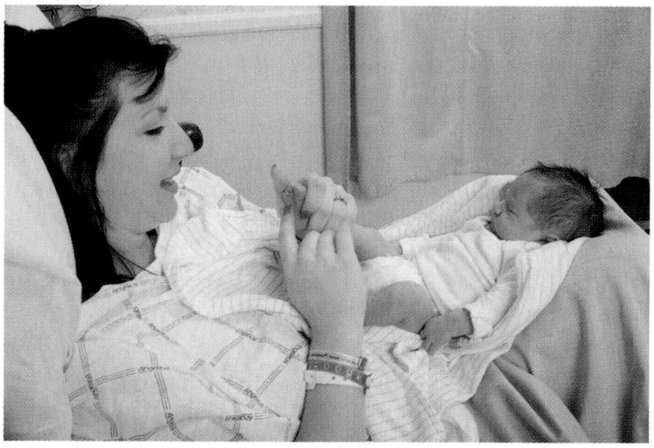

FIGURE 18-2 The mother's initial touch includes fingertipping, whereby she becomes acquainted with her infant by touching only with her fingertips.

CRITICAL TO REMEMBER

Reciprocal Attachment Behaviors

Newborn infants have the ability to do the following:
- Make eye contact and engage in prolonged, intense, mutual gazing
- Move their eyes and attempt to "track" the parent's face
- Grasp and hold on to the parent's finger
- Move synchronously in response to rhythms and patterns of the parent's voice (called *entrainment*)
- Root, latch on to the breast, and suckle
- Be comforted by the parent's voice or touch

Maternal Touch

Maternal behavior, particularly maternal touch, changes rapidly as the mother progresses through a discovery phase with her infant. Initially, the mother may not reach for the infant, but if the infant is placed in her arms, she holds the baby in an *en face* position with the infant's face in the same vertical plane as her own. When the infant is awake, the two engage in prolonged, mutual gazing (see Figure 18-1).

The mother needs time to get acquainted with the tiny stranger. She may gently explore the infant's face, fingers, and toes with her fingertips only. This exploration, called *fingertipping,* is common during the early minutes (Figure 18-2).

After fingertipping the infant, the mother begins to stroke the baby's chest and legs with the palm. Next, she uses her entire hand to enfold the infant and to bring her baby close to her body (Figure 18-3). She holds the newborn closer, strokes the baby's hair, presses her cheek against the infant's cheek, and finally feels comfortable enough to engage in a full range of consoling behaviors.

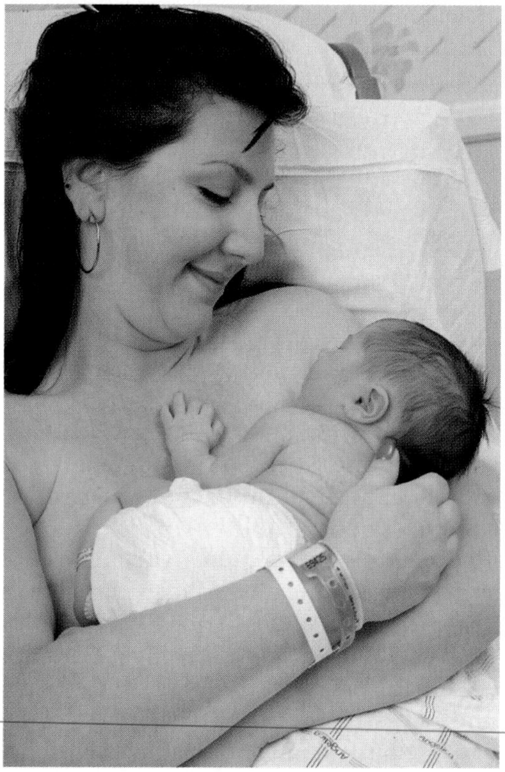

FIGURE 18-3 Mothers progress from exploratory touching to enfolding the infant. Their pleasure is enhanced by skin-to-skin contact.

The mother next begins to identify specific features of the newborn: "Look at his little pink mouth." Then she begins to relate features to family members: "He has his father's chin and nose" (Figure 18-4). This identification process has been termed *claiming* or *binding-in* (Rubin, 1977).

Verbal Behaviors

Verbal behaviors are important indicators of maternal attachment. Most mothers speak to the infant in a high-

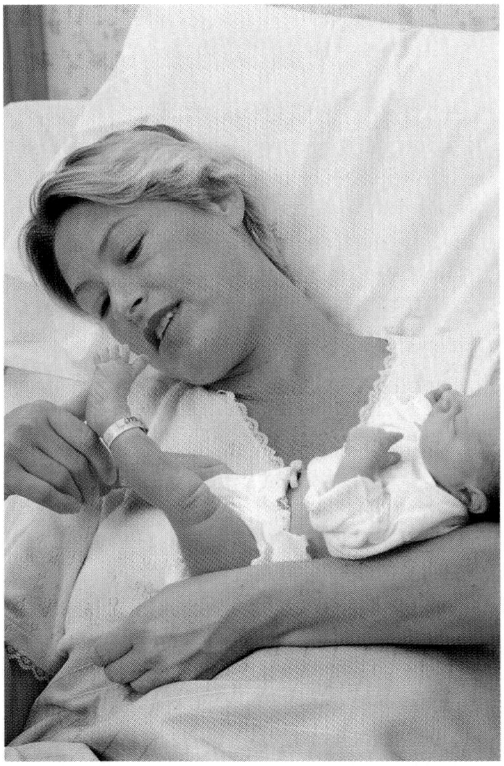

FIGURE 18-4 During the binding-in or claiming process, the mother identifies her baby's specific features and relates them to other family members. This mother states, "His long toes are exactly like mine."

pitched voice and progress from calling the baby "it" to "he or she" and then to using the given name. "I cannot believe it is here" rapidly becomes "Michele is such a good girl." Verbal behaviors may provide clues to a mother's early psychological relationship to her infant. Nurses are in a position to observe interactions of mothers and their infants and, if necessary, teach and model interactions that foster early attachment between them.

Check Your Reading

1. How do bonding and attachment differ?
2. How does maternal touch change over time?
3. How does verbal interaction change over time?

THE PROCESS OF MATERNAL ADAPTATION

Puerperal Phases

In the early 1960s, Rubin identified restorative phases that the mother must go through to replenish the energy lost during labor and attain comfort in the role of mother. The puerperal phases are called *taking-in*, *taking-hold*, and *letting-go* and provide a useful method to observe progressive change in maternal behavior. Although they should not be used as strict guidelines for maternal assessment, the phases can help the nurse anticipate maternal needs and intervene to meet those needs.

Taking-In Phase

During the taking-in phase, the mother is focused primarily on her own need for fluid, food, and deep, restorative sleep. Inexperienced nurses may be puzzled by the mother's passive, dependent behavior as she receives, or takes in, attention and physical care. She also takes in every detail of the neonate but seems content to allow others to make decisions.

A major task for the mother during this time is to integrate her birth experience into reality. To do this, she recounts the details of her labor and delivery many times. She may spend a great deal of time on the telephone describing her labor and the birth. She repeats her experiences for visitors and attempts to piece together all the details from those who were involved in the birth. This process helps the mother realize that the pregnancy is over and the newborn is now a separate individual.

Although Rubin believed that the taking-in phase lasted for approximately 2 days, less time is probably involved today. The taking-in phase may be prolonged when a cesarean birth, especially an emergency cesarean delivery, has been necessary. These women may have difficulty assimilating the unfamiliar and intrusive procedures that occurred in rapid succession and have negative perceptions of the birth experience. Women who have had cesarean births need continued attention and sensitive care that takes into account their special needs for pain relief and assistance with care of their newborns.

Taking-Hold Phase

The mother becomes more independent during the taking-hold phase. She exhibits concern about managing her own body functions and assumes responsibility for her own self-care. When she feels more comfortable and in control of her body, she shifts her attention from her own needs to the performance of the infant. She compares her infant with other infants to validate wellness and wholeness. She welcomes information about the wide variety of behaviors exhibited by newborns.

During the taking-hold phase, the mother may verbalize a great deal of anxiety about her competence as a mother. She may compare her caretaking skills unfavorably with those of the nurse.

Nurses must be careful not to assume the mothering role but instead allow the mother to perform as much of the caretaking as possible and praise each attempt, even if the mother's early care is awkwardly performed.

The taking-hold phase, which extends over several days, has been called the "teachable, reachable, referable moment." Nurses who provide home or clinic care can take advantage of this ideal time to review previously taught material and provide additional instructions and demonstrations.

Therapeutic Communication

Anxiety about Caretaking Skills

Fawn Jackson is a nurse in the postpartum unit. When she enters the room of Tamara Bradley, a new mother, she finds the woman crying.

Tamara (crying): I can't do anything right. The pediatrician just asked me a bunch of questions, and I couldn't answer any of them.

Fawn: Actually, you are doing a lot right, but it's distressing when you feel you don't have all the answers. *(Offering reassurance and acknowledging feelings.)*

Tamara: He just fired the questions at me and I couldn't think so fast.

Fawn: You feel that you're not measuring up because you couldn't answer the questions. *(Paraphrasing and focusing on Tamara's feelings.)*

Tamara: Well, I want to be a good mother, but I'm so worried that I won't know what to do.

Fawn: You have some concerns. *(Reflecting feelings without leading.)*

Tamara: There is just so much to caring for a baby. I don't know where to start.

Fawn: It can be overwhelming when you're unsure about how to take care of the baby. What concerns you most? *(Reflecting feelings and inviting the mother to describe specific concerns. By allowing Tamara to express her feelings, Fawn has helped dissipate the feelings and set the stage for effective teaching.)*

Letting-Go Phase

The letting-go phase is a time of relinquishment for the mother and often for the father. If this child is their first, the couple must give up their previous role as a childless couple and acknowledge the loss of a carefree lifestyle. Many mothers also must give up idealized expectations of the birth experience. For example, they may have planned to have a vaginal birth with minimal or no anesthesia, but instead they required a cesarean birth or regional anesthesia.

In addition, some mothers and fathers are disappointed in the size, gender, and characteristics of the infant who does not "match up" with the fantasy baby of pregnancy. They must relinquish the infant of their fantasies and accept the real infant.

These losses often provoke subtle feelings of grief that may be unexamined or unacknowledged. However, both parents may benefit if given the opportunity to verbalize unexpected feelings and realize that these feelings are common. If the mother is very young or the pregnancy was unplanned, the feelings of loss and grief may be acute.

Maternal Role Attainment

Role attainment is a process in which the mother achieves confidence in her ability to care for her infant and becomes comfortable with her identity as a mother. The process begins during pregnancy and continues for several months after childbirth.

The transition to the maternal or paternal role includes four stages (Mercer, 1995b):

1. The anticipatory stage begins during the pregnancy when the pregnant woman chooses a physician or nurse-midwife and a location for the infant's birth. Many women attend childbirth classes to be prepared and have some control over the birth experience. Expectant mothers seek role models to help them learn the role of a mother.
2. The formal stage begins with the birth of the infant and continues for approximately 4 to 6 weeks (Mercer, 1995a). During this stage, parents' behaviors are largely guided by others such as health professionals, close friends, and parents. A major task during this stage is for mothers and fathers to become acquainted with their infants so that they can mesh their parenting activities with cues from their infants.
3. The informal stage may overlap with the formal stage. It begins once the woman has learned appropriate responses to her infant's cues and signals. The mother begins to respond according to the unique needs of the infant and develops the maternal role to fit herself rather than following the directives of textbooks or health professionals.
4. The personal stage is attained when the woman feels a sense of harmony in the role, enjoys the infant, sees the infant as a central person in her life, and has internalized the parental role. The mother or father accepts the role of parent and feels comfortable in this role. The range of time for achieving the parental role is highly variable, with some parents reaching that point in the first month and others taking much longer.

Women from other cultures may go through many of the same steps but with variations that are particular to their cultures. For example, Gichia (2000) found in a small study that African-American women progressed through four stages as part of maternal role integration: preparing, checking, becoming, and evaluating. Preparing for the maternal role begins very early in life where a young girl cares for younger relatives. Checking occurs in adolescence when the girl compares her ideas of mothering with those of others. Becoming begins before pregnancy and continues through the early phase of parenting as the woman learns to care for her own infant. Evaluating begins when the woman takes over care of her infant and works to become a good mother.

Redefined Roles

The mother is particularly concerned with redefining roles and focuses on maintaining a strong, adaptive relationship with her partner. She observes him carefully for any change in behavior and is acutely sensitive to his interaction with the infant. From the father's perspective, anxieties about succeeding in his new role put added pressure on the family. Conflicting demands between work and home, feelings of exclusion, and concerns about his relationship with his partner present additional challenges.

The new parents may need to agree on a division of tasks and responsibilities that was not necessary before the birth of the infant. This process is accomplished quickly and with very little discord in some families. Role assignment in other families is much less flexible, and any change can be a source of tension and frustration.

Although nurses are not actively involved in redefining family roles, they can use their communication skills to assist the family in expressing their feelings and concerns so that the changes can be accomplished with minimal stress.

Role Conflict

Role conflict occurs when a person's perception of role responsibilities differs significantly from reality. For example, if the mother perceives her responsibility as providing the majority of care for the infant, but reality dictates that she must place the infant with another caregiver and return to full-time employment, role conflict may occur. More than 9 million women with children under age 6 are employed in the United States (Chadwick & Heaton, 1999). When they return to work after giving birth, many experience feelings of guilt for leaving their infants and experience intense "separation grief" when they first leave infants with caregivers. Some report feeling jealous of the caregiver, whom they fear will supplant them in the infant's affection.

The nurse may help by acknowledging these feelings and reassuring the mother that her emotions are normal. The mother also needs time to reestablish feelings of closeness when she comes home from work, and she needs to develop a schedule that allows maximal time with the infant when she is at home. She may have to negotiate with another family member to take over some of the household tasks until she feels more comfortable with the situation (Nursing Care Plan 18-1).

NURSING CARE PLAN 18-1

Adaptation of the Working Mother

Assessment: Rebecca Sanders, a 30-year-old single mother, gave birth to a baby boy, Derrek, by cesarean delivery 5 days ago. Breastfeeding is going well. During her visit at a nurse-managed postpartum clinic, Rebecca discusses her need to return to work as a sales executive in 6 weeks. She states that she does not want to leave the baby with someone else while she works. "I've always wanted to stay home when I had a baby, but it is impossible. How can I be a mother and work full time?"

Nursing Diagnosis: Anticipatory Grieving related to inability to perform role of mother as she wishes because of the need to return to full-time employment.

Critical Thinking: Grieving is related to loss. What has Rebecca lost or what must she give up?

Answer: Rebecca must give up her idealized picture of motherhood. She also must give up mothering tasks and time with the infant to another caregiver. She will have to modify her self-concept based on the perception of these losses.

Expected Outcomes:
Rebecca will do the following:
1. Describe the concerns and feelings that result from her need to leave her infant with a secondary caregiver by (specific date).
2. Verbalize plans to achieve maximal satisfaction in her role as mother by the time she returns to work.

Intervention	Rationale
1. Allow Rebecca to describe her perception of her role as a mother and express concerns about the way employment will interfere with her ability to fulfill this role.	1. Role conflict, stress, and grief can result when a mother, who envisions her role as the primary caregiver, must leave the infant with another caregiver and return to her job.
2. Suggest free expression of feelings of anxiety, guilt, and jealousy to significant others and the care provider.	2. Candid expression of feelings helps to resolve them and allows for a discussion of measures that will help to overcome the intense feelings that cause conflict.
3. Acknowledge the feelings Rebecca expresses, and reassure her that the feelings are common.	3. Knowledge that the feelings are not trivial and are common reinforces their validity and importance.

Continued

4. Help Rebecca develop a schedule that allows her maximal time with the infant:
   a. Make a list of errands and supplies needed to avoid frequent stops that delay getting home from work.
   b. Double the recipe when cooking, and freeze half for future use.
   c. Pick up nutritious takeout meals to avoid cooking each evening.
   d. Schedule appointments on the same day when possible.
   e. Include the baby in daily walks, exercise, and social visits.

   4. Feelings of frustration and stress can be alleviated if the mother has a plan that allows her long periods of uninterrupted time with the infant.

5. Recommend that Rebecca allow 30 to 45 minutes when she first gets home to hold the infant. Delay all other activities until this need is satisfied for both mother and infant.

   5. Time is needed to reestablish feelings of closeness, comfort, and attachment.

6. Suggest that Rebecca delay her return to employment, if possible, until the infant is at least 16 weeks old.

   6. By 16 weeks, most infants are able to sleep through the night, reducing the sleep deprivation that often adds to the stress of working and infant care.

7. Recommend that Rebecca investigate several daycare providers before choosing. She should check references, make unannounced visits, see required licenses and certification, discuss the number and ages of children cared for and the daily schedule, determine the provider's philosophy of infant care, determine if the care provider is trained in emergency measures, and know what emergency plans are in place.

   7. A great deal of stress is eliminated if parents feel confident that a competent and nurturing daycare provider has been found.

8. Suggest that Rebecca leave the infant with the chosen daycare provider for 2 to 3 days before resuming full-time employment.

   8. Allowing both mother and infant to "practice separating" while their schedules still are somewhat flexible helps ease the transition.

9. Recommend that Rebecca pump her breasts and feed the infant by bottle at least once per day before returning to work.

   9. Becoming proficient at pumping the breasts and introducing the infant to bottle feeding prepares both the mother and infant for all-day separation.

Evaluation: Rebecca freely expressed her feelings of guilt, anxiety, and concern about leaving her infant. She has organized a plan to investigate daycare in her area and discussed plans to reorganize her work and social schedule so that she can spend more time with her son.

Major Maternal Concerns

Nurses must plan follow-up care based on the knowledge that mothers' major concerns change over time after childbirth. For instance, during the first month, primary concerns are about feeding, infant behavior, and physical care of the infant. Maternal concerns related to the self include discomfort and fatigue. Concerns about family relationships include having less time with older children. In later months, concerns focus on issues with work or school, childcare, finances, sleep, and the mother's own needs (Horowitz & Damato 1999).

Body Image

As the woman gains confidence in her ability to care for the infant and her physical discomfort decreases, emotional concerns related to the self become more intense. In particular, women express concern about regaining their normal figures. Some mothers have unrealistic expectations about weight loss and the time it takes for the body to regain its nonpregnant shape.

Nurses must emphasize that weight loss should be gradual and about 6 to 12 months is usually required to lose most weight gained during pregnancy. Rigid restriction of calories can lead to depleted energy, decreased immunity, and decreased production of milk.

In addition, nurses should teach the importance of safe activities such as walking and graduated exercises to regain muscle tone. Mothers should seek the advice of a health care professional before initiating a rigorous exercise program (see Chapter 17).

Postpartum Blues

Mild depression, also known as *postpartum blues* or *maternity blues,* is a frequently expressed concern. This mild, transient condition affects 50% to 70% of American women who have just given birth. The condition begins 3 to 4 days after childbirth, peaks on the fourth to fifth days, and resolves within 2 weeks. It may reoccur with future pregnancies (Stewart & Robinson, 1998). It is characterized by insomnia, fatigue, tearfulness, mood instability, and anxiety. The symptoms are usually unrelated to events, and the condition does not seriously affect the ability of the mother to care for the infant.

Although the direct cause is unknown, postpartum blues generally is considered related to the wide hormonal fluctuations that occur during labor, delivery, and the immediate postpartum period. Postpartum blues is self-limiting, but mothers benefit greatly when unsolicited empathy and support are freely given by the family and the health care team. The mother is encouraged to rest, take some time for herself, and discuss her feelings.

Postpartum blues must be distinguished from postpartum depression and postpartum psychosis (see Chapter 28). These separate entities are disabling and require therapeutic management for full recovery. Nurses should teach women to call their providers if depression becomes severe or lasts longer than expected.

Check Your Reading

4. How do maternal behaviors in the taking-in phase differ from those in the taking-hold phase?
5. What does the mother (and the father) relinquish in the letting-go phase?
6. How do the parents progress through the stages of role attainment?
7. What causes postpartum blues? How can nurses intervene for this common emotional response?

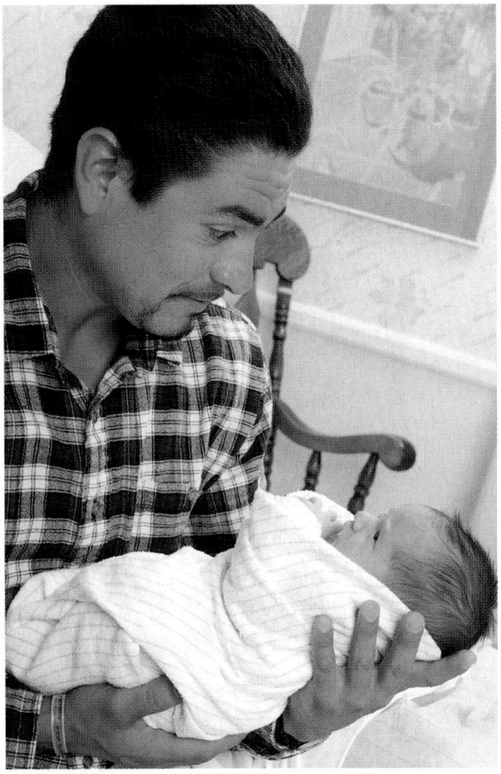

FIGURE 18-5 Fathers' behaviors during initial contact with their infants often correspond with maternal behaviors. The intense fascination that fathers exhibit is called *engrossment.* Note eye-to-eye contact between the father and infant.

THE PROCESS OF FAMILY ADAPTATION

The birth of an infant requires the reorganization of roles and relationships within the family. The previously childless couple now must integrate a new member into the family unit. Fathers learn new skills and often adjust to new roles. Siblings must adapt to a new standing in the family structure. Expectations and involvement of grandparents vary widely.

Fathers

The father's developing bond to his newborn is called *engrossment.* It is characterized by intense interest in the ways the infant looks and responds, along with a desire to touch and hold the baby. Many fathers comment on the baby's distinctive features and view the baby as perfect. They experience strong attraction to the infant and express elation after the baby's birth. Attachment behaviors of the father increase when the infant is awake, makes eye contact, and responds to the father's voice (Figure 18-5).

Fathers who were active participants in the birth have been thought to experience early bonding and develop stronger ties to the newborn. Research indicates, however, that other factors such as the relationship with his own parents, previous experiences with children, and the relationship with the mother are more important variables (Ferketich & Mercer, 1995b).

Many fathers eagerly look forward to coparenting with their mates. However, they may lack confidence in providing infant care and are sensitive to exclusion from instructions and demonstrations of infant care. They may feel that others expect them only to support the mother.

Although fathers may attend prenatal classes about parenting, they often do not know what to expect from infants and need more information about normal growth and development during infancy. A review of information about childcare presented in the prenatal period is helpful after the child is born, at which time the information is relevant and the father is ready to learn.

Siblings

Sibling response to the birth of a new brother or sister depends on age and developmental level. Toddlers usually are not completely aware of the impending birth. They may view the infant as competition or fear that they will be replaced in the parents' affection. Negative behaviors may surface and indicate the degree of stress experienced by the youngster. These behaviors include sleep problems, an increase in attention-seeking efforts, and regression to more infantile behaviors such as renewed bedwetting and thumbsucking. Some may exhibit hostile behaviors toward the mother, particularly when she holds or feeds the newborn. These behaviors are manifestations of the jealousy and frustration that young children feel as they observe the mother's attention being given to another. Parents must find opportunities to affirm their continued love and affection for the very vulnerable sibling.

Preschool siblings may engage in more looking than touching. Most spend at least some time in proximity

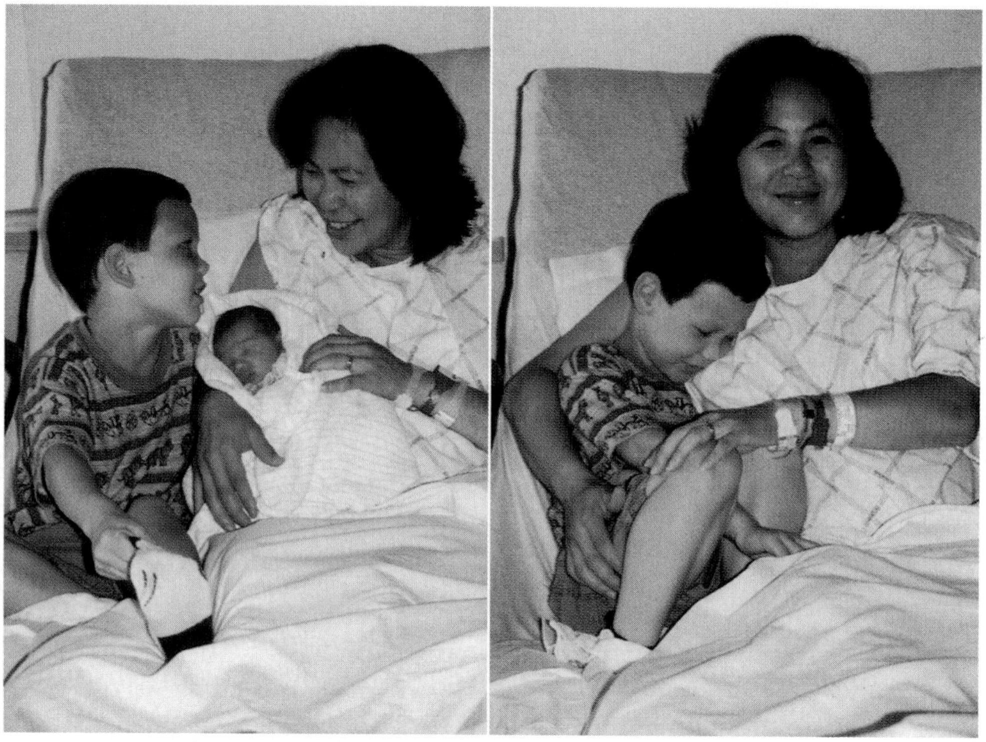

FIGURE 18-6 **A,** Although they may hesitate to touch the infant, children often want to be close. **B,** This boy's relief and joy are obvious as he reclaims a favorite spot.

to the infant and talk to the mother about the infant (Figure 18-6). Older children may adapt more easily. All siblings need extra attention from the parents and reassurance that they are loved and important.

Sibling classes, available in many agencies, may help ease the transition (see Chapter 11). Siblings often visit the mother and new baby in the birth agency.

At home, a relaxed approach without time constraints may facilitate interactions between young children and infants. Special care must be taken by the parents, visitors, and nurses to pay as much attention to the sibling as to the new baby. Parents can emphasize the advantages of being an older sibling and allow siblings to participate in age-appropriate aspects of infant care.

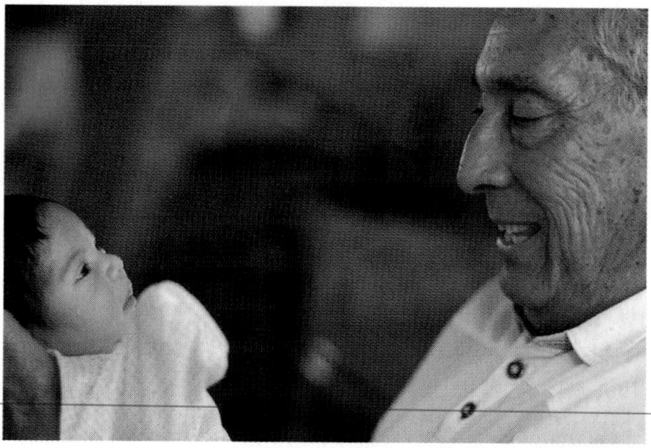

FIGURE 18-7 Grandfathers may develop strong bonds with grandchildren.

Grandparents

The involvement of grandparents with grandchildren depends on many factors, especially proximity. Grandparents who live near enough to see the child frequently develop strong attachment that evolves into unconditional love and a special relationship bringing joy to the grandparents and an added sense of security to the grandchildren.

When grandparents live many miles from grandchildren and have sporadic contact, forming a close attachment is more difficult. Grandparents must devise ways to foster a relationship with grandchildren they seldom see.

Expectations of the role of grandparents are also a factor in the adaptation of the grandparents to the birth of a grandchild. Many grandparents strive to be fully involved in the care and upbringing of the child, but others desire less involvement. This may cause some conflict with parents, or it may be a comfortable arrangement for both families.

Grandparents often are a major part of the support system that new parents need. Grandmothers in particular provide assistance with household tasks and infant care, which allows the mother to recover from childbirth and make the transition to parenthood. Grandfathers who were very busy providing for their own children may enjoy the opportunity to nurture their grandchildren (Figure 18-7).

FACTORS AFFECTING FAMILY ADAPTATION

Numerous factors influence the family's adjustment. Some, such as discomfort and chronic fatigue, can be anticipated because they are so common. Additional factors include knowledge of infant needs, expectations of the infant, previous experience, age of the parents, and temperaments of the mother and infant. Unanticipated events such as cesarean birth, birth of a preterm or ill infant, and birth of multiple infants also affect the ease and speed with which the family adjusts.

Discomfort and Fatigue

Normally, discomfort associated with childbirth, such as perineal pain and afterpains, resolve within the first days after the birth. However, discomfort may make focusing on the needs of the newborn difficult. Fatigue often remains a problem during the first few weeks, during which the infant's schedule is erratic and the chance for uninterrupted sleep is minimal. When the infant begins to sleep through the night (at about 16 weeks), the parents usually can reestablish familiar patterns, and fatigue often becomes less of a factor. Persistent fatigue, however, has been found to be present in women as long as 18 months after delivery (Parks, et al., 1999).

CRITICAL TO REMEMBER

Factors That Affect Adaptation

- Lingering discomfort or pain
- Chronic fatigue
- Knowledge of infant needs
- Available support system
- Expectations of the newborn
- Previous experience with infants
- Maternal temperament
- Infant characteristics
- Unanticipated events: cesarean birth, preterm or ill infant, or birth of more than one infant (such as twins)

Knowledge of Infant Needs

Parents experience powerful feelings of protectiveness when they discover that they can console their infant and the infant responds to their care. First-time parents, however, often are unsure of the way to care for a newborn and become very anxious if they are unable to console a crying infant. In addition, many are concerned about nutrition and specific procedures such as care of the umbilical cord and circumcision. Breast-feeding benefits both the mother and the infant but may add to the stress initially experienced by parents who lack sufficient knowledge (see Chapters 22 and 23 for breastfeeding information and early parenting, respectively).

Some parents have concerns about spoiling the infant. They are particularly concerned about responding each time the infant cries and may believe that this causes the child to cry to get attention. Reminding parents that infants cry to indicate needs such as hunger, cold, wetness, cuddling, and gentle stimulation may be necessary, and responding to crying does not spoil the child. Prompt, gentle response to crying helps the infant develop trust in the world as a safe, secure place. Trust is a basic developmental task of infancy and depends on the child's learning that caregivers respond consistently and gently.

Previous Experience

Previous experience with newborns also may affect family adjustment. Multiparas are more comfortable with infants and exhibit attachment behaviors earlier than primiparas, who may spend many more hours in the early, discovery phase of attachment. Mothers who previously have given birth to infants with anomalies or infants that did not survive may need more time to feel comfortable with this infant.

Expectations for the Newborn

Unrealistic expectations of the infant also may influence adjustment. Parents who have little experience with newborns may be disappointed at the way a newborn looks. They are unprepared for the normal characteristics of newborns, such as cranial molding, blotchy skin, and blue hands and feet. Nurses must teach normal growth and development and assist parents in working through misconceptions about normal infant behavior. For instance, the capacity of an infant's stomach is small, and the infant must be fed frequently. Also, infants are neurologically unable to sleep through the night for several weeks.

Some mothers may be very disappointed in the gender of their infants or sense that their partners are disappointed. These feelings must be acknowledged and resolved before attachment can take place. For example, a mother of four sons might be so disappointed that the fifth child is a boy that she cries and refuses to pick out a boy's name at first. Later, when she holds the baby and begins to observe differences between this infant and her other sons, she can begin her discovery period with this unique child.

Maternal Age

Adjustment to parenthood is a challenge for teenagers who have not achieved strong senses of their own identities. In general, teenagers tend to talk less, respond less, appear more passive, and sometimes appear less affectionate with their children than adult parents. Clearly, teenage mothers and fathers need special assistance to develop necessary parenting skills that promote optimal development of the infant (see Chapter 24 regarding adolescent parenting).

Maternal Temperament

Maternal personality traits greatly influence attachment. Mothers who are calm, secure in their abilities to learn, and free from unnecessary anxiety adjust more easily to the demands of motherhood. Conversely, mothers who are excitable, insecure, and anxious have more difficulty.

NURSING CARE PLAN 18-2

Adaptation to the Birth of Twins

Assessment: Maureen Parry, a 32-year-old primipara, gave birth to twin girls 22 hours ago. Her labor began at 39 weeks, and she delivered vaginally.

Both she and her husband are inexperienced in caring for infants. They attended breastfeeding and parenting classes during her pregnancy. Both infants are in the room, and she moves anxiously from one to the other. She has examined both infants but has not had individual time with each infant. She touches the infants cautiously and asks, "How in the world will I be able to care for two babies?"

Nursing Diagnosis: Risk for Altered Parent-Infant Attachment related to inadequate time with individual infants and lack of confidence in ability to provide care for two infants.

Critical Thinking: What data (behaviors) led to this diagnosis? What other data would confirm the diagnosis?

Answer: A common belief is that parents can become attached to only one child at a time, and Maureen has not had time with each child individually. Observing the way she touches and interacts verbally with each child and noting that names have not been selected might confirm the diagnosis.

Goals/Expected Outcomes:

Maureen will do the following:

1. Demonstrate progressive bonding behaviors with each infant before discharge.
2. Collaborate with nursing staff and her husband to devise a plan for caring for the infants during the early weeks at home.
3. Verbalize increased confidence in her ability to care for the infants before discharge.

Intervention	Rationale
1. Promote bonding and attachment with individual infants by allowing separate time with each infant and pointing out the unique characteristics of each child.	1. Parents attach more easily to one infant at a time. They must go through the getting-acquainted phases separately.
2. Make sure that the parents have contact with the infant who is awake and responsive.	2. The infant must respond to the parent by some signal, such as eye contact or gazing, for attachment to occur.
3. Foster a relaxed atmosphere that permits unlimited contact between the parents and twins. Model behaviors such as holding, consoling, and talking to the infants.	3. A relaxed atmosphere and prolonged contact with the twins enhance interaction that promotes bonding. Modeling is a very effective teaching strategy for demonstrating appropriate interactions.
4. Encourage participation in infant care. Model infant care, and praise all maternal efforts to provide care.	4. Caring for the infant or successfully consoling a crying infant elicits feelings of nurturing and greatly increases feelings of confidence and competence.
5. Assist Maureen in making a plan for caring for the twins. a. Provide instruction on breastfeeding twins and refer parents to a lactation educator for continuing support. b. Suggest that the parents keep a record of care for each baby for the first few days at home so that they do not become confused. c. Reassure parents that a bath every day is unnecessary. Suggest bathing every other day because the face, neck, and buttocks are bathed as necessary.	5. During the time that breastfeeding is being established, the mother needs information and encouragement. Collaborating on a plan for providing and recording care increases the parents' confidence in their ability to care for the infants. This is particularly true when the parents receive reassurance that care does not have to be on a strict schedule.
6. Emphasize the importance of obtaining adequate rest. Suggest that the mother sleep when the infants sleep and the parents take turns caring for the infants. Recommend that they accept assistance with household tasks from family and friends so that they can concentrate on care of the twins.	6. Sleep deprivation and chronic fatigue can interfere with the joys of parenting unless the parents anticipate the problem and make plans to deal with it.

Evaluation: Maureen progressed from fingertipping to enfolding her baby girls and selected names for them. By discharge on the second postpartum day, she stated she was feeling more confident with breastfeeding and caring for the infants but would need continued help. Both parents participated in infant care and identified family members who would assist them during the early weeks at home.

Assessment: During discharge teaching, Maureen states that she does not work outside the home and always has assumed total responsibility for household tasks. She reveals that a perfectly maintained home is important to her and especially to her husband. She wonders about his possible reaction to the disruption that the twins will create.

Nursing Diagnosis: Risk for Altered Family Processes related to the impact of the twins on family functioning.

Goals/Expected Outcomes:
The couple will do the following:
1. Share concerns with each other and identify family strengths by (specific date).
2. Identify measures that reduce stress and promote family adjustment to the birth of twins by discharge.
3. Renegotiate responsibilities for the first few weeks at home by (specific date).

Intervention	Rationale
1. Determine whether Maureen has shared her concerns with her husband. If she has not, suggest that she tell him she is worried about the effect of the twins on their normal life.	1. Open communication is the first step in identifying stressors and clarifying feelings.
2. Attempt to determine overlooked resources, such as the ability to afford hired help with the housework for a few weeks. Discuss what available family members or others might do to help.	2. Many families develop a higher level of functioning during times of stress, and individual members participate actively. Many families overlook community resources such as neighbors and friends.
3. Assist the family in identifying measures to reduce stress that may occur when family patterns are disrupted: a. Recommend simple meals that are easy to prepare and use of disposable dishes for a few weeks. b. Emphasize the importance of good nutrition and daily exercise. c. Review measures to obtain rest, but point out that fatigue is likely to persist until the twins sleep through the night. d. Recommend that both parents continue to participate in activities that provide recreation and relaxation.	3. During times of stress, many parents overlook the benefits of good nutrition, exercise, and recreation. Even short periods of recreation can refresh spirits and replenish energy.
4. Suggest that the couple negotiate sharing household tasks such as meal preparation during first few weeks, even though this is not part of their usual roles.	4. Sharing tasks reduces fatigue and helps prevent frustration and arguments during this time of stress.

Evaluation: Maureen discussed her concerns about the effect of the twins on the usual pattern of family life with her husband and was surprised to learn that he was very willing to assume many of the household tasks while the infants require so much care. Maureen's mother is available to babysit, so the couple can have some time for exercise and recreation.

Temperament of the Infant

The infant's temperament is important. Infants who are calm, are easily consoled, and enjoy cuddling increase parental confidence and feelings of competence. Conversely, irritable infants who are difficult to console and do not need or respond to cuddling increase parental frustration and interfere with attachment.

Availability of a Strong Support System

A strong, consistent support system is a major factor in the adjustment of the new mother. She needs assistance with household tasks such as meal preparation, laundry, and shopping. In addition, she needs encouragement, praise, and reassurance that she is a good mother. That others see the baby as special and demonstrate love and affection is very important to the new mother. Support may be needed for an extended period of time after childbirth. Satisfaction with social support has been found to decrease during the first 6 months after the birth of the baby (McVeigh, 2000).

Unanticipated Events

Cesarean Birth

Unanticipated events can make parental adjustment more difficult. For example, an unplanned cesarean birth may result in financial strain, a longer recovery time for the mother, additional discomfort, and increased stress for the family. Birth of a preterm or ill infant creates additional concern about the condition of the infant and may cause prolonged separation of parents and the child. This separation may delay the process of attachment and create stress on the normally functioning family.

Birth of Multiple Infants

Even if expected, the birth of more than one infant may present problems of attachment. The process of attachment is structured so that the parents become attached to only one infant at a time. Therefore parents should be encouraged to interact with each child individually, especially in the early, getting-acquainted period. Nurses must help the parents relate to each infant as an individual rather than part of a unit by pointing out the individual responses and uniqueness of each infant.

Early, frequent contacts or rooming-in helps the parents gain confidence in caretaking and facilitates the attachment process. Mothers sometimes are overwhelmed at the prospect of breastfeeding multiple infants. They need reassurance that they will produce an ample supply of milk for each infant because supply increases with demand (see Nursing Care Plan 18-2 and Chapter 22 regarding breastfeeding after multiple birth).

Check Your Reading

8. What does a father mean when he says he feels "out of place"?
9. What feelings may siblings experience when a new baby is born into the family?
10. How does the birth of multiple infants affect parental attachment?

CULTURAL INFLUENCES ON ADAPTATION

A major goal of nursing practice in the postpartum period is to provide nursing care that is culture specific; that is, it fits the health beliefs, values, and practices of a particular culture. This is difficult because of the increasing ethnic diversity in countries such as the United States and Canada. A major challenge for nurses is to be aware of cultural beliefs and acknowledge their importance in family adaptation. Postpartum often is thought to be a time of vulnerability for the woman and infant (Mattson, 2000). Many cultural factors relevant to the postpartum period can be grouped into communication, dietary practices, and health beliefs.

Communication

Verbal communication may be difficult because of the numerous dialects and languages spoken. An interpreter should be fluent in the language, of the same religion, and of the same country of origin, if possible. This compatibility is particularly important for Middle Eastern families, whose religious orientation may vary widely and who have long-standing social and religious conflicts with some other groups.

Respect of the privacy and modesty of all people is important, but modesty is especially important to Latinas (ancestry from Mexico, Central America, and South America) and Middle Eastern and Asian women. If a private room is not possible, privacy screens or curtains should be used. Laws of modesty require that Muslim women cover their hair, bodies, arms to the wrists, and legs to the ankles.

Health care workers often place a premium on efficiency and come directly to the point, but they must remember that tactfulness and warmth are important. Direct communication can be distressing, particularly for Latinas and Native Americans, who tend to approach a subject only after exchanging polite and gracious comments.

> When the nurse and family speak different primary languages, verifying the family's understanding is important. An affirmative nod may be a sign of courtesy rather than understanding or agreement. To be certain the message has been received, the nurse should ask the family to repeat in their own words what they have been told.

Dietary Practices

Some dietary practices that must be considered center on the hot-cold theory of health and diet. This theory concerns intrinsic properties of certain foods, not temperature. For example, Southeast Asians (such as Cambodians, Vietnamese, Hmong, Laotians) believe that after childbirth, the woman should eat only "hot" foods such as eggs, chicken, and rice. They believe these foods help replace blood that was lost during childbirth (Mattson, 1995).

Some Chinese women believe that a combination of yin and yang maintains balance. Yin foods include bean sprouts, broccoli, carrots, and cauliflower. Yang foods include broiled meat, chicken, soup, and eggs. Women from India eat special foods to regain a state of balance after childbirth. Dried ginger often is eaten to control postpartum bleeding and cleanse the uterus (Choudhry, 1997).

Health Beliefs

Cultural beliefs and practices provide a sense of security for new mothers. For example, Muslims believe that the first sounds a child hears should be from the Koran in praise and supplication to God (Allah), and parents want to say a prayer in the newly born child's ears at the time of birth. Facilitating this practice goes a long way toward building trust in the relationship with the family.

Many Middle Eastern families believe that compliments should be directed to Allah rather than the newborn. The compliment thus is converted into a blessing so that mistrust or jealousy does not occur. Some Southeast Asians believe the spirit resides in the head and are troubled if someone pats or rubs the head of the newborn.

Health beliefs relating to hygiene and breastfeeding cause the most conflict in the postpartum period. Southeast Asians and Latinas believe that the mother should be kept warm to avoid upsetting the balance of hot and cold. Some women do not wish to take baths and wash their hair during the postpartum period. This practice is upsetting for nurses who are concerned about hygiene. A great deal of tact and sensitivity is required to find a compromise.

Many Southeast Asian women believe that colostrum is "unclean" and they should not breastfeed until the milk comes in. Guatemalan women also believe that colostrum is "bad" for the baby (Callister, 1998). This belief conflicts with the theory that breastfeeding should start as soon after birth as possible. Determining when the woman believes the milk comes in and the way the infant will be fed until the supply of breast milk is adequate may be helpful.

Specific religious practices should be accepted and supported. For instance, Muslim mothers are exempted from their obligation to pray while they are bleeding. However, the father and other family members kneel, place their heads on the floor, and pray five times per day. If possible, a clean, quiet room should be provided so that this obligation can be fulfilled without having to leave the birthing center.

Complementary/Alternative Therapy

Incorporating cultural beliefs regarding health into health services shows respect and may increase client interest in receiving care. For example, nurses working with Native Hawaiian, Filipino, and Japanese women in Hawaii may use a "talkstory" approach to teaching that is based on reciprocal storytelling. Nurses may discuss finding a cultural name identity for the new infant to incorporate cultural traditions and rituals into the plan of care. The woman may be referred to a therapist for lomilomi massage, which is believed to be beneficial during pregnancy and postpartum. Massages may be combined with talkstories about health promotional topics (Mayberry, et al., 1998).

HOME AND COMMUNITY-BASED CARE

Because many mothers and infants are discharged from the birth facility soon after childbirth, most assessments and interventions described in this chapter occur in the home or clinic setting. Mothers may leave the birth facility while still in the taking-in phase. Many still have discomfort and are not fully recovered from the childbirth experience. Consequently, most psychosocial concerns such as family adaptation and postpartum blues surface later, when support from health care professionals is not as available.

Many methods currently are used to provide care for mothers and infants who leave the birth facility within hours after childbirth. These methods include telephone calls, nurse-managed postpartum clinics, home visits, and "baby lines" staffed by nurses who provide information and guidance for callers (see Chapters 1 and 17). All methods have advantages and disadvantages.

The overlap between nursing care in the birth facility and home makes communication among nurses extremely important. Nurses in the birth facility, who perform the initial assessments, should make information such as nursing diagnoses available to nurses who give follow-up care.

APPLICATION OF THE NURSING PROCESS: MATERNAL ADAPTATION

Assessment

Several factors such as the mother's progression through the puerperal phases, her mood, her interaction with the infant, and unanticipated events affect maternal adaptation to the birth (Table 18-1).

Analysis

Parenting involves the ability of the parents to create an environment that nurtures the growth and development of the infant. Parenting may be altered when one or more caregivers experience difficulty creating or continuing a nurturing environment. This difficulty occurs most often when factors such as maternal discomfort, fatigue, and lack of knowledge or confidence in infant care come into play. Therefore a common nursing diagnosis is "Risk for Altered Parenting related to multiple factors such as fatigue, discomfort, and lack of knowledge of infant care" (Table 18-2).

Planning

Expected outcomes for this nursing diagnosis are that the mother will do the following:

- Verbalize feelings of comfort and support as she progresses through the phases of recovery.
- Demonstrate progressive attachment behaviors by (specific date).
- Participate in care of the newborn by discharge.

Interventions

Assisting the Mother through Recovery Phases

"Mother" the Mother. The early, taking-in phase is a time to mother the mother so that she can move on to more complex tasks of maternal adjustment. During the first few hours after childbirth, she has a great need for physical care and comfort. Provide ample fluids and favorite foods. Keep linens dry, tuck warm blankets around her until chilling has stopped, and use warm water for perineal care.

Monitor and Protect. The new mother is dependent on nurses to monitor and protect her. Remind her of the need to void and assist her to ambulate. Assess her level of comfort and offer analgesia before discomfort is severe and analgesia is less effective. Tell her not to delay requesting analgesia because it is more effective and the postpartum course is smoother if her pain stays well controlled. At the first signs of fatigue, encourage her to sleep.

Listen to the Birth Experience. Be prepared to listen to details of the birth experience and offer sincere praise for her efforts during labor.

> Many mothers spend so much time on the telephone that completing assessments and care is difficult. Nurses may be reluctant to interrupt, but the mother's physical safety is a priority. Offering a choice is often helpful: "Excuse me for a moment. I will need to check you soon. I can do it now or come back in 5 minutes."

Fostering Independence

As the mother becomes more independent, allow her to schedule her care as much as possible. Collaborate with

Table 18-1
ASSESSING MATERNAL ADAPTATION

Assessments	Nursing Considerations
PROGRESSION THROUGH PUERPERAL PHASES	
Taking-in (passive, dependent) Taking-hold (autonomous, seeks information) Letting-go (relinquishes fantasy baby, begins to see self as mother)	Consider the mother's need to rest, her need to tell the details of her labor and childbirth, and her readiness to learn infant care and assume control of her own care.
MATERNAL MOOD	
Mood and energy level, eye contact, posture, and comfort	Tense body posture, crying, or anxiety (may indicate the beginning of postpartum blues, fatigue, or discomfort)
FACTORS THAT AFFECT MATERNAL ADAPTATION	
Age of mother	May need additional support if under 18 years of age
Previous experience	Slow progression through puerperal phases for primaparas, who may need more assistance; for multiparas, more experience and knowledge but may be delayed in cases of previous birth of a child with problems or infant death
Maternal/infant temperament	Less assistance required for mothers who are calm, secure, and free from anxiety; more teaching necessary for parents of infants who are difficult to console
Unanticipated events	Increased discomfort and longer recovery with cesarean birth; attachment problems with birth of an ill infant or multiple infants
INTERACTION WITH INFANT	
Maternal touch	Progression from "fingertipping" to enfolding and a variety of comforting behaviors
Verbal interaction	Mother may call infant "it" initially but progresses quickly to using given name and identifying specific characteristics.
Response to infant cues or signals	Prompt, gentle, consistent response indicates progressive adaptation to parenting role.
PREPARATION FOR PARENTING	
Classes in breastfeeding, parenting, and infant care	Many mothers feel more prepared after completing classes and participate in care sooner.

Table 18-2
COMMON NURSING DIAGNOSES FOR POSTPARTUM

* Altered Family Processes
* Altered Parenting
* Anticipatory Grieving
Altered Parent-Infant Attachment
Altered Role Performance
Anxiety
Body Image Disturbance
Diversional Activity Deficit
Health-Seeking Behaviors
Parental Role Conflict

* Nursing diagnoses discussed in this chapter.

her to plan procedures such as sitz baths. Encourage her to assume responsibility for self-care, and emphasize that the nurse's role at this point is to assist and teach.

Promoting Bonding and Attachment

Early, unlimited contact between parents and infants is of primary importance to facilitate the attachment process. In many birth facilities, infants remain in the room with the parents all or most of the time, unless complications intervene. This arrangement may be called *mother-baby care, couplet care,* or *dyad care.*

In mother-baby care, one nurse cares for both the mother and the baby and is able to provide teaching and help with bonding as part of ongoing nursing care (Figure 18-8). The mother participates as she is able. If she does not feel well for a short period or is too tired to care for the infant, the nurse cares for the infant in the mother's room. Mother-baby care reduces fragmentation of care and helps the parents to be more prepared for discharge (Phillips, 1997).

Prolonged contact between mothers and infants leads to more touching and caring for infants as they learn their infants' characteristics and needs. Nursing measures to promote bonding and attachment include:

- Assist the parents in unwrapping the baby to inspect the toes, fingers, and body. Inspection fosters identification and allows the parents to become acquainted with the "real" baby, which must replace

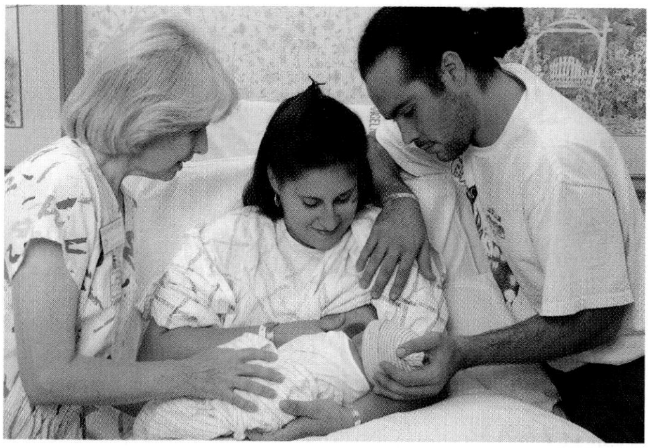

FIGURE 18-8 By teaching about the newborn and family, the nurse helps parents develop confidence in their ability to provide care for the infant.

the fantasy baby that many parents imagined during the pregnancy.

- Position the infant in an *en face* position and discuss the infant's ability to see the parent's face. Face-to-face and eye-to-eye contact helps establish mutual interaction between the infant and parent.
- Point out the reciprocal bonding activities of the infant: "Look how she holds your finger." "He has not taken his eyes off you."
- Allow the infant to remain with the parents as long as they wish so that they can progress at their own speed through the getting-acquainted phase.
- Assist the mother in putting the infant to the breast if she plans to breastfeed. If necessary, reassure her that many infants do not latch on to the breast right away. If she is using formula, assist her in positioning the infant securely and reassure her that holding and cuddling the infant provides comfort and security.
- Model behaviors by holding the infant close and speaking in high-pitched, soothing tones.
- Point out the positive characteristics of the infant: "She has the tiniest pink ears and such a lot of dark hair."
- Provide comfort and ample time for rest because the mother must replenish her energy and be relatively free of discomfort before she can progress to initiating care of the infant.

Involving Parents in Infant Care

Providing care for the infant fosters feelings of responsibility and nurturing and is an important component of attachment. In addition, it allows parents to develop confidence in their ability to care for an infant before they go home.

Although teaching begins during pregnancy, review information and repeat demonstrations if time allows. Demonstrate first the simpler tasks such as care of the cord and progress to more complicated procedures such as bathing. When the parents receive positive reinforcement for the simple tasks, they are more willing to try the more complicated ones (see Chapters 21 and 23).

Agreement among the entire staff on the way to teach basic care is important. Mothers seek confirmation of information, and they become confused and lose faith in the credibility of the staff if information varies. Allow time for practice and repeated encouragement. Parents become easily discouraged if they have difficulty with early attempts at care.

> Suggestions for care must be tactfully phrased to avoid the implication that the parents are inept. "You burped that baby like a professional. There are a couple of little hints I can share about diapering."

Evaluation

- Independent self-care confirms the mother's progression through the phases of recovery.
- Progressive attachment behaviors include enfolding the infant, calling the infant by name, and responding gently when the infant cries.
- Participation in infant care includes diapering, feeding, and care of the umbilical cord and circumcision.

APPLICATION OF THE NURSING PROCESS: FAMILY ADAPTATION

Assessment

Fathers

The father's emotional status and interaction with the infant are particularly important because he usually serves as the mother's primary support person. Is the father involved with the mother and infant? How does he interact with the infant? How much information does he have about infant characteristics and care? What are his expectations about his partner's recovery? Unrealistic expectations of the infant (will sleep through the night, smile, be easily consoled) may lead to problems. In addition, if he expects the mother to recover her energy and libido rapidly, he may become resentful if her recovery takes longer than anticipated.

Siblings

Noting the ages of siblings and their reactions to the newborn is important. Are they interested and helpful? Are they hostile and aggressive? How do the parents react to sibling behaviors?

Support System

Family members often provide a powerful support system, and their involvement is important to the adaptation of the family. Are grandparents available and involved? Do sisters and brothers live nearby? Are they available to help the new parents? If the family is unavailable, who provides support? What arrangements have been made for assistance?

Table 18-3
ASSESSING FAMILY ADAPTATION

Assessment	Nursing Considerations
CHARACTERISTICS OF INFANT THAT MAY AFFECT FAMILY ADAPTATION	
Sex and size of infant	The sex of an infant may be very important for some families. Disappointment in the sex or concern about the small size may interfere with bonding.
Unexpected characteristics (cephalhematoma, jaundice, cranial molding, newborn rash)	Be prepared to explain unexpected appearance or behavior in language the parents can comprehend.
Infant behavior (is irritable, is easily consoled, cuddles)	An easily consoled, cuddly infant increases bonding and attachment.
PATERNAL ADAPTATION	
Response to the mother and infant	The father often provides the most important support for the mother. His involvement with the infant indicates acceptance of the parenting role.
Knowledge of infant care	Is useful in planning teaching that includes the father.
Response to infant cues or signals (crying, fussing)	Many fathers feel awkward handling the infant but want to become proficient in infant care so that they can coparent.
AGES AND DEVELOPMENTAL LEVELS OF SIBLINGS	
Reaction of siblings	Young children often fear that the newborn will replace them in the affection of parents. The parents may need anticipatory guidance about sibling rivalry.
SUPPORT SYSTEM	
Interest and availability of family or friends to assist during early weeks	Families may need assistance in identifying available support.
Plans for first few days at home	Suggest parents plan for support and rest. Provide resources such as telephone "hot lines."
Follow-up plans	Appointments are generally scheduled at 2 weeks and 6 weeks with clinic or health care provider.
CULTURAL FACTORS	
Cultural beliefs and practices that may affect nursing care	Culture-specific care can be planned for hygiene, dietary preferences, usual care and feeding of infants, and role of mate and family in child care.
Expectations of health care team	

Nonverbal Behavior

Nonverbal behavior is equally important. Are the parents' words congruent with their actions? For example, does the mother verbalize satisfaction with her infant's characteristics but respond slowly to infant signals?

> Validate impressions and conclusions arrived at during a psychosocial assessment. One of the best ways to do this is to ask questions such as "How much experience have you had with newborns?" "You really thought you were having a girl and a boy is a big surprise?" "How are newborns fed in Vietnam until the mother's milk comes in?" "What are your plans when you go home? How long can your mother stay?"

Analysis

Family assessment will identify family strengths and areas in which nursing interventions could promote family adaptation or prevent disruptions in family functioning (Table 18-3). Sometimes a family that usually functions effectively is unable to cope because of a specific event. In this case, the event is the birth of a baby and the necessity of the family to integrate a newborn into the existing family structure. Therefore a common nursing diagnosis is "Altered Family Processes related to lack of knowledge of infant needs and behaviors, stress during the early weeks at home, and sibling rivalry."

Planning

Goals and expected outcomes for this nursing diagnosis may overlap with care after discharge because they often cannot be evaluated before the family leaves the birth facility.

By (specific date) the family will:

- Verbalize understanding of infant needs and behaviors.
- Identify methods for reducing stress during the early weeks at home.
- Describe measures to reduce sibling rivalry.
- Identify external resources and support system.

Interventions

Teaching the Family about the Newborn

Infant Needs. Some new parents have unrealistic expectations of the newborn, and nurses must provide information about what the infant is capable of doing and needs to thrive. For example, parents sometimes are surprised to hear that infants sleep 16 to 20 hours per day but must be fed every 2 to 4 hours and will not sleep through the night for 12 to 16 weeks.

Infant Signals. Discuss the importance of responding promptly and gently to cues such as crying and fussing that indicate the infant needs attention. Reassure parents that responding to cues does not "spoil" their child but helps the child learn to trust the world as a safe, secure place.

Help parents recognize signals that indicate when their infant has had enough and wants to avoid further stimulation. The so-called *avoidance cues,* including looking away, splaying the fingers, arching the back, and acting fussy, indicate that the infant is ready for a quiet time.

Helping the Family Adapt

Providing Anticipatory Guidance about Stress Reduction. Nurses can help the family adjust to the demands of a newborn by providing anticipatory guidance about the first weeks at home. This is a time when the need for rest is great but the opportunity for uninterrupted sleep is minimal. As a result, fatigue is a common problem. The nurse can assist as follows:

- Emphasize that the priority during the first 4 to 6 weeks should be caring for mother and baby.
- Recommend that mothers establish a relaxed home atmosphere and flexible meal schedule because attempts to maintain a rigid schedule or meticulous environment increase tension within the family.
- Recommend that the mother sleep when the infant sleeps and conserve her energy for care of the baby.
- Encourage family members to let friends and relatives know sleep and nap times and request that they telephone and visit at other times. Adequate rest is necessary for mental and physical restoration and integration of new information into the memory.
- Advise parents to place a "Do Not Disturb" sign on the door and an answering machine on the telephone.
- Instruct the family about the need to restrict coffee, tea, colas, and chocolate because they contain the stimulant caffeine.
- Teach breathing exercises and progressive relaxation to reduce stress and energize, especially when a nap is not possible.
- Encourage both parents to delay tiring projects until the infant is older. Remind them that although schedules are chaotic for a while, the infant's behavior is generally more predictable by 12 to 16 weeks of age.
- Encourage open expression of feelings between parents as a first step in coping with stress.
- Remind parents of the need for healthy nutrition and recreation. Fatigue and tension easily can overwhelm the anticipated joys of parenting if no respite is available from constant care.
- Suggest that new parents enlist grandparents, other relatives, and friends to help with meal preparation and shopping.

CRITICAL THINKING EXERCISE

Carol, a 35-year-old primipara, had an infant daughter by cesarean birth after failure to progress in labor. Carol is very tired, although she is relatively comfortable. Her husband was present during the labor and birth and is excited about being a father. He has no experience with children, and his job requires almost constant travel. Carol has never taken care of a newborn.

On the day of delivery, Carol readily accepts assistance with hygiene. She passively follows the nurse's suggestions to turn, cough, and breathe deeply. She discusses the details of her labor and wonders why the physician did not proceed with a cesarean birth earlier. She examines her baby girl closely and touches the face and hands gently with her fingertips. She remarks that she plans to breastfeed and is surprised that the infant sleeps so much.

QUESTIONS:

1. What are Carol's priority needs at this time?
2. What phase of recovery is she manifesting? Why does she "fingertip" the infant?

The first postoperative day, Carol's indwelling catheter is removed and IV fluids are discontinued. Carol ambulates with minimal assistance and is pleased to be able to urinate without difficulty. She asks about bowel function and requests the prescribed stool softener. She spends a great deal of time getting the baby to breastfeed. She is very frustrated that the infant does not breastfeed well and asks for assistance from the lactation educator.

QUESTIONS:

3. What are Carol's priority needs now?
4. How have her behaviors changed?

Before discharge, Carol is breastfeeding well. The infant latches on and nurses for 10 to 15 minutes, and Carol's nipples are free of tenderness and signs of trauma. Carol has no relatives in the area, and her husband is home for the weekend only. She states that she will just have to get along by herself after that.

QUESTIONS:

5. What anticipatory guidance should Carol receive before she goes home?
6. What further nursing interventions would be most helpful to her and the baby?

Providing Ways to Reduce Sibling Rivalry. Suggest that parents plan time alone with older children and praise and reassure the children frequently of their places in the family. The parents should try to offer frequent expressions of love and affection. Visitors and family also can help by not focusing exclusively on the infant and including older children in their gift giving and exclamations about the newborn.

Emphasize the importance of responding calmly and with understanding when a child regresses to more infantile behaviors or expresses hostility toward the infant. Acknowledging the child's feelings and offering prompt reassurance of continued love are most valuable actions.

Some children, particularly those older than 3 years of age, enjoy being a big brother or sister and respond well when they are included in infant care. This participation may not be possible with younger children, and setting aside separate time to participate in a favorite activity may be more worthwhile for the parents.

Identifying Resources. In many homes, women assume the major responsibilities of day-to-day homemaking. With the birth of an infant, this task becomes more difficult. A division of labor must be negotiated to prevent undue stress and fatigue. This division of labor is particularly important when the needs of other children for time, attention, and comfort also must be met.

The mother's primary support often is the father of the baby, but extended family members, particularly grandmothers and sisters, also provide valuable support. Community resources such as daycare centers, parenting classes, and breastfeeding support are available in many areas. In addition, close friends and neighbors often share solutions to specific problems. Remind the mother that resources are available when she begins to feel isolated and exhausted.

Evaluation

A prompt, gentle response to infant crying and fussing indicates a parent's understanding of the infant's need. Devising a plan for obtaining rest and lessening anxiety in siblings is a first step in reducing stress. Identifying external resources in the family, neighborhood, and community may help the family function to meet its needs during the early weeks at home.

SUMMARY CONCEPTS

- Bonding and attachment are gradual processes that begin before childbirth and progress to feelings of love and deep devotion lasting all through life. Nurses foster bonding and attachment by providing early, unlimited contact between the parents and infant and modeling attachment behaviors.
- For bonding and attachment to occur, interaction between parents and the infant is required. Contact is particularly important when the infant is awake, alert, and able to interact with the parents. Nurses often delay care that can be postponed so that the parents and infant can have this time together.
- Maternal touch changes over time as many mothers progress from exploratory "fingertipping" to enfolding and finally demonstrating a full range of comforting behaviors.
- Verbal behaviors are important indicators of maternal attachment as mothers progress from referring to the infant as "it" to calling the infant by name and identifying unique characteristics. Nurses often model the way to speak to the infant and point out the infant's response to the verbal stimulation.
- Maternal adjustment to parenthood is a gradual process involving restorative phases that allow the mother to replenish her energy, relinquish her role as a woman without a child, and develop attachment to the infant. Nurses play a valuable role in the process by first "mothering the mother" and fostering independence as the mother becomes ready.
- Postpartum blues, a temporary, self-limiting period of weepiness, often is ignored by the health care team. Explanations and support are generally all that are required to assist the mother through this distressing episode.
- Mothers (and fathers) usually progress through four stages of role attainment—anticipatory, formal, informal, and personal—before they attain a sense of comfort and structure their parenting behaviors to mesh with the unique needs of their children.
- Many women experience role conflict when they must leave the infant with a caregiver and return to work. Nurses can offer anticipatory guidance that makes the conflict less difficult.
- The birth of a baby necessitates reorganization of family structure and renegotiation of family responsibilities. Nurses can ease the process by assisting the father in coparenting the infant and helping the new parents identify family resources.
- Siblings feel jealousy and fear that they will be replaced by the newborn in the affection of the parents. Nurses can reduce the negative feelings by providing information about ways to reduce sibling rivalry.
- Nurses recognize that families leave the birth facility with unmet needs and nursing care in the facility overlaps with follow-up care provided in the home.

ANSWERS TO CRITICAL THINKING EXERCISE

1. Carol's priority needs are for physical care and comfort. She also needs to make the experience of childbirth part of her reality and does this by recounting the details of the birth and trying to fill in the missing pieces about the cesarean birth.
2. Carol is in the taking-in phase. She is getting acquainted with her "real" baby by exploring with her fingertips. This usually is the first maternal touch observed.
3. Carol's priorities are to assume control of her own body functions and manage her care so that she can "take hold" and assume care of the baby.
4. Carol has become more independent and now initiates breastfeeding. She demonstrates readiness to learn by requesting the assistance of the lactation educator.
5. Anticipatory guidance should focus on ways she can manage the care of the infant while still getting adequate rest and nutrition. Keeping a flexible schedule, resting while the infant rests, and preparing easy meals are some of the most important items to emphasize.
6. Assisting her in identifying friends and neighbors who could provide some support while her husband is away would be

most helpful. If this is not possible, she should have telephone numbers for community resources such as the hospital "baby line." A follow-up home visit, visit to a postpartum clinic, or telephone call initiated by the nurse would be very helpful. The nurse could assess the mother and infant, reinforce teaching, and provide encouragement.

REFERENCES & READINGS

Affonso, D.D., Mayberry, L., Inaba, A., Matsuno, R., & Robinson, E. (1996). Hawaiian-style "talkstory": Psychosocial assessment and intervention during and after pregnancy. *Journal of Obstetric, Gynecologic, and Neonatal Nursing,* 25(9), 737-742.

American College of Obstetricians and Gynecologists (ACOG). (1998). Cultural competency in health care. (ACOG Committee Opinion 201). Author.

Ament, L.A. (1990). Maternal tasks of the puerperium reidentified. *Journal of Obstetric, Gynecologic, and Neonatal Nursing,* 19(4), 330-335.

Bajo, K., Hager, J., & Smith, J. (1998). Keeping moms and babies together. *AWHONN Lifelines,* 2(2), 44-48.

Bartlett, L., & McGrath, J.M. (1999). Children's responses to the birth of a sibling: Interventions to assist the family in transition. *Mother Baby Journal,* 4(4), 19-25.

Britton, J.R., Britton, H.L., & Gronwaldt, V. (1999). Early perinatal hospital discharge and parenting during infancy. *Pediatrics,* 104(5), 1070-1076.

Callister, L.C. (1995). Cultural meanings of childbirth. *Journal of Obstetric, Gynecologic, and Neonatal Nursing,* 24(4), 327-334.

Callister, L.C. (1998). Giving birth: Guatemalan women's voices. *Journal of Obstetric, Gynecologic, and Neonatal Nursing,* 27(3), 289-295.

Chadwick, G.A., & Heaton, T.B. (1999). *Statistical handbook on the American family* (2nd ed.). Phoenix, AZ: Oryx Press.

Choudhry, U.K. (1997). Traditional practices of women from India: Pregnancy, childbirth, and newborn care. *Journal of Obstetric, Gynecologic, and Neonatal Nursing* 26(5), 533-539.

Ewy-Edwards, D. (2000). Transition to parenthood. In F.H. Nichols & S.S. Humenick. *Childbirth education: Practice, research, and theory* (2nd ed., pp. 84-113). Philadelphia: W.B. Saunders.

Ferketich, S.L., & Mercer, R.T. (1995a). Predictors of role competence for experienced and inexperienced fathers. *Nursing Research,* 44(2), 89-95.

Ferketich, S.L., & Mercer, R.T. (1995b). Paternal-infant attachment of experienced and inexperienced fathers during infancy. *Nursing Research,* 44(1), 31-37.

Geissler, E.M. (1998). *Pocket guide to cultural assessment* (2nd ed.). St. Louis: Mosby.

Gichia, J.E.U. (2000). African-American women's preparation for motherhood. *MCN: The American Journal of Maternal Child Nursing,* 25(2), 86-91.

Hayashi, R.H., & Zettelmaier, M.A. (2000). Postpartum management. In S.B. Ransom, M.P. Dombrowski, S.G. McNeeley, K.S. Moghissi, & A.R. Munkarah. *Practical strategies in obstetrics-gynecology* (pp. 321-325). Philadelphia: W.B. Saunders.

Horowitz, J.A., & Damato, E.G. (1999). Mothers' perceptions of postpartum stress and satisfaction. *Journal of Obstetric, Gynecologic, and Neonatal Nursing,* 28(6), 595-605.

Lee, K.A., & Zafke, M.E. (1999). Longitudinal changes in fatigue and energy during pregnancy and the postpartum period. *Journal of Obstetric, Gynecologic, and Neonatal Nursing,* 28(2), 183-191.

Lipson, J.G., Dibble, S.L., & Minarik, P.A. (1996). *Culture & nursing care: A pocket guide.* San Francisco: University of California San Francisco Nursing Press.

Logsdon, M.C. (2000). *Social support for pregnant and postpartum women.* Washington, D.C.: AWHONN.

Martell, L.K. (1996). Is Rubin's "taking-in" and "taking-hold" a useful paradigm? *Health Care for Women International,* 17(1), 1-13.

Martell, L.K., & Mitchell, S.K. (1984). Rubin's puerperal change reconsidered. *Journal of Obstetric, Gynecologic, and Neonatal Nursing,* 13(3), 145-148.

Mattson, S. (1995). Culturally sensitive perinatal care for Southeast Asians. *Journal of Obstetric, Gynecologic, and Neonatal Nursing,* 24(4), 335-341.

Mattson, S. (2000). Ethnocultural considerations in the childbearing period. In S. Mattson & J.E. Smith (Eds.), *Core curriculum for maternal-newborn nursing* (2nd ed., pp. 70-84). Philadelphia: W.B. Saunders.

Mayberry, L.J., Affonso, D.D., Shibuya, J., & Clemmens, D. (1998). Integrating cultural values, beliefs, and customs into pregnancy and postpartum care: Lessons learned from a Hawaiian public health nursing project. *Journal of Perinatal Neonatal Nursing,* 13(1), 15-26.

McVeigh, C.A. (2000). Investigating the relationship between satisfaction with social support and functional status after childbirth. *MCN: The American Journal of Maternal/Child Nursing,* 25(1), 25-30.

Mercer, R.T. (1986). Predictors of maternal role attainment at one year postbirth. *Western Journal of Nursing Research,* 8(1), 932.

Mercer, R.T. (1990). *Parents at risk.* New York: Springer.

Mercer, R.T. (1995a). *Becoming a mother: Research on maternal identity from Rubin to the present.* New York: Springer.

Mercer, R.T. (1995b). Predictors of maternal role attainment. *Nursing Research,* 34(4), 198-204.

Mercer, R.T., & Ferketich, S.L. (1990). Predictors of parental attachment during early parenthood. *Journal of Advanced Nursing,* 15, 268-280.

Parks, P.L., Lenz, E.R., Milligan, R.A., & Han, H. (1999). What happens when fatigue lingers for 18 months after delivery? *Journal of Obstetric, Gynecologic, and Neonatal Nursing,* 28(1), 87-93.

Phillips, C.R. (1997). *Mother-baby nursing.* Washington D.C.: Association of Women's Health, Obstetric and Neonatal Nurses.

Podkolinski, J. (1998). Women's experience of postnatal support. In S. Clement. *Psychological perspectives on pregnancy and childbirth* (pp. 205-225). Edinburgh: Churchill Livingstone.

Rubin, R. (1961). Puerperal change. *Nursing Outlook,* 9(12), 743-755.

Rubin, R. (1977). Binding-in in the postpartum period. *MCN: The American Journal of Maternal/Child Nursing,* 6(1), 65-75.

Rubin, R. (1984). *Maternal identity and the maternal experience.* New York: Springer.

Scoggin, J. (2000). Physical and psychological changes. In S. Mattson & J.E. Smith (Eds.), *Core curriculum for maternal-newborn nursing* (2nd ed., pp. 302-316). Philadelphia: W.B. Saunders.

Stark, M.A. (2000). Is it difficult to concentrate during the third trimester and postpartum? *Journal of Obstetric, Gynecologic, and Neonatal Nursing, 29*(4), 378-389.

Stewart, D.E., & Robinson, G.E. (1998). Postpartum depression. In L.A. Wallis (Ed.), *Textbook of women's health* (pp. 675-677). Philadelphia: Lippincott.

Sullivan-Lyons, L. (1998). Men becoming fathers: "Sometimes I wonder how I'll cope." In S. Clement, *Psychological perspectives on pregnancy and childbirth* (pp. 227-243). Edinburgh: Churchill Livingstone.

Waldenström, U., Borg, I.M., Olsson, B., Sköld, M., & Wall, S. (1996). The childbirth experience: A study of 295 new mothers. *Birth, 23*(3), 144-153.

Willis, W.O. (1999). Culturally competent nursing care during the perinatal period. *Journal of Perinatal Neonatal Nursing, 13*(1), 45-58.

Wood, A.F., Thomas, S.P., Droppleman, P.G., & Meighan, M. (1997). The downward spiral of postpartum depression. *MCN: The American Journal of Maternal/Child Nursing, 22*(6), 308-316.

19

NORMAL NEWBORN: PROCESSES OF ADAPTATION

OBJECTIVES

1. Explain the physiologic changes that occur in the respiratory and cardiovascular systems during the transition from fetal to neonatal life.
2. Describe thermoregulation in the newborn.
3. Compare gastrointestinal functioning in the newborn and adult.
4. Explain the causes and effects of hypoglycemia.
5. Describe the steps in normal bilirubin excretion and the development of physiologic, pathologic, and breast milk jaundice.
6. Describe kidney functioning in the newborn.
7. Explain the functioning of the newborn's immune system.
8. Describe the periods of reactivity and the six behavioral states of the newborn.

DEFINITIONS

ASPHYXIA Insufficient oxygen and excess carbon dioxide in the blood and tissues.

BILIRUBIN Unusable component of hemolyzed erythrocytes.

BROWN FAT (OR BROWN ADIPOSE TISSUE [BAT]) Highly vascular specialized fat found in the newborn that provides more heat than other fat when metabolized.

FETAL LUNG FLUID Fluid that fills the fetal lungs, expanding the alveoli and promoting lung development.

FIRST PERIOD OF REACTIVITY Period beginning at birth in which newborns are active and alert. It ends when the infant first falls asleep.

HYPERBILIRUBINEMIA Excessive amount of bilirubin in the blood.

JAUNDICE Yellow discoloration of the skin and sclera caused by excessive bilirubin in the blood.

NEUTRAL THERMAL ENVIRONMENT Environment in which body temperature is maintained without an increase in metabolic rate or oxygen use.

DEFINITIONS—cont'd

Nonshivering Thermogenesis Process of heat production, without shivering, by oxidation of brown fat.

Polycythemia Abnormally high number of erythrocytes.

Second Period of Reactivity Period of 4 to 6 hours after the first sleep following birth when the newborn may have an elevated pulse and respiratory rate and excessive mucus.

Surfactant Combination of lipoproteins produced by the lungs of the mature fetus to reduce surface tension in the alveoli, thus promoting lung expansion after birth.

Thermogenesis Heat production.

Thermoregulation Maintenance of body temperature.

At birth, neonates must make profound physiologic changes to adapt to extrauterine life and meet their own respiratory, digestive, and regulatory needs. This chapter focuses on these changes and will assist nurses to identify behaviors signifying problems or abnormalities. It provides a foundation for discussion of nursing assessment and care related to those changes detailed in Chapters 20 and 21.

INITIATION OF RESPIRATIONS

The first vital task the newborn must accomplish is the initiation of respirations. Forces occurring throughout pregnancy and during birth bring about this change.

Development of the Lungs

During fetal life, the respiratory tract produces a fluid within the lungs. Fetal lung fluid expands the alveoli and is essential for normal development of the lungs. Some of the fluid empties from the lungs into the amniotic fluid. As the fetus nears term, changes in chloride and sodium secretion in the lungs and increased oncotic pressure cause the lung fluid to begin to move into the interstitial spaces. The fluid shift continues during normal labor and after birth. This helps reduce the pulmonary resistance to blood flow that was present before birth and enhances the advent of air breathing (Lowe & Reiss, 1996).

As the lungs mature, they begin to produce surfactant, a slippery, detergent-like lipoprotein. Surfactant reduces surface tension within the alveoli. This allows them to remain partially open when the infant begins to breathe at birth. Without surfactant, the alveoli collapse as the infant exhales and must be reopened with each breath. This greatly increases the work of breathing. Sufficient surfactant is usually produced between 34 and 36 weeks of gestation for most infants born at that time to breathe without difficulty.

Causes of Respirations

At birth, the infant's first breath must force fetal lung fluid into the interstitial spaces around the alveoli so that air can enter the respiratory tract. This requires a much larger negative pressure (suction) for the first breath than for subsequent breathing. Breathing is initiated by chemical, thermal, and mechanical factors that stimulate the respiratory center in the medulla of the brain and trigger respirations (Figure 19-1).

Chemical Factors

Chemoreceptors in the carotid arteries and the aorta respond to changes in blood chemistry brought about by the hypoxia that occurs with normal birth. A decrease in the blood oxygen level (PO_2) and the pH of the blood and an increased blood carbon dioxide level (PCO_2) cause impulses from these receptors to stimulate the respiratory center in the medulla. In addition, occlusion of the vessels in the cord may end flow of a chemical from the placenta that inhibits respirations (Lowe & Reiss, 1996). A forceful contraction of the diaphragm results, causing air to enter the lungs. However, stimulation of the respiratory center and breathing do not occur if prolonged hypoxia causes central nervous system depression.

Thermal Factors

The temperature change that occurs with birth is an important stimulus to the initiation of respirations. At birth, the infant moves from the warm, fluid-filled uterus into an environment where the temperature is more than 20° F cooler. Sensors in the skin respond to this sudden change in temperature by sending impulses to the brain that stimulate the respiratory center and breathing.

Mechanical Factors

During a vaginal birth, the narrow birth canal compresses the fetal chest. A small amount of the fetal lung fluid is forced out of the lungs into the upper air passages during birth. The fluid passes out of the mouth or nose or is suctioned as the head emerges from the vagina. When the pressure against the chest is released, it recoils, drawing a small amount of air into the lungs.

Tactile stimuli that occur during birth stimulate skin sensors. Nurses hold, dry, and wrap infants in blankets, providing further stimulation to skin sensors. The stimulation of the sounds and lights at delivery may also aid in initiating respirations.

Continuation of Respirations

Once the alveoli expand, surfactant acts to keep them partially open between respirations. About half of the air from the first breath remains in the lungs to become the functional residual capacity. Because the alveoli remain partially expanded with this residual air, subse-

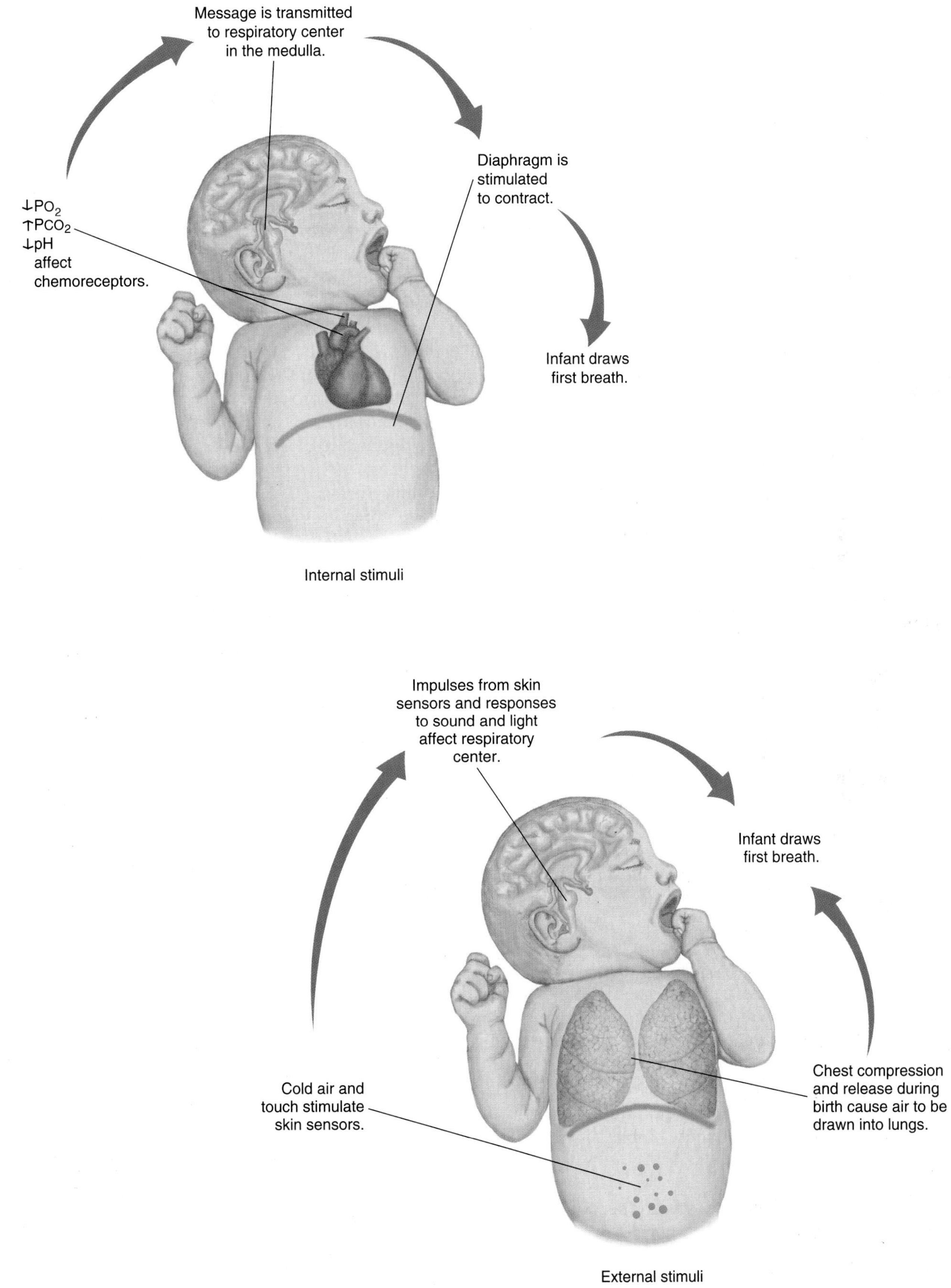
Message is transmitted to respiratory center in the medulla.
Diaphragm is stimulated to contract.
↓PO_2
↑PCO_2
↓pH
affect chemoreceptors.
Infant draws first breath.
Internal stimuli
Impulses from skin sensors and responses to sound and light affect respiratory center.
Infant draws first breath.
Cold air and touch stimulate skin sensors.
Chest compression and release during birth cause air to be drawn into lungs.
External stimuli

FIGURE 19-1 Internal causes of the initiation of respirations are the chemical changes that take place at birth. External causes of respirations include thermal and mechanical factors.

quent breaths require much less effort than the first one. With each of the first few respirations, more alveoli are opened.

The remaining fetal lung fluid moves into the interstitial spaces, where it is absorbed by the circulatory and lymphatic systems. Absorption is accelerated by the process of labor and may be delayed after cesarean birth. Although most fluid is absorbed within a few hours, complete absorption may take as long as 24 hours. This explains why the lungs may sound moist when first auscultated but become clear a short time later.

Check Your Reading

1. How do hypoxia during birth, a cool delivery room, and handling at birth stimulate the newborn to breathe?
2. Why is surfactant important to the newborn's ability to breathe easily?
3. How is fetal lung fluid removed before and after birth?

CARDIOVASCULAR ADAPTATION: TRANSITION FROM FETAL TO NEONATAL CIRCULATION

During fetal life, most of the fetal blood flow bypasses the nonfunctional lungs and liver. Three structures cause this: the ductus arteriosus, foramen ovale, and ductus venosus, which shunt blood away from the lungs and liver. It also results from high pressures within the lungs that permit only a small amount of blood flow into the pulmonary vessels. At birth, the infant's blood must begin to circulate to the lungs for oxygenation and to the liver for filtration (see Chapter 6, pp. 115-116).

For these changes to occur after birth, the shunts must close and the pulmonary vessels must dilate. This occurs in response to increases in the blood oxygen level, shifts in pressure within the heart and pulmonary and systemic circulations, and the end of blood flow through the umbilical vessels. The changes necessary for transition from fetal to neonatal circulation occur simultaneously within the first few minutes after birth. They are discussed separately here (Table 19-1).

Ductus Arteriosus

In the fetus, the ductus arteriosus connects the pulmonary artery and the descending aorta. Prostaglandin E_2 from the placenta and low blood oxygen levels keep the ductus arteriosus widely dilated during fetal life. The vessel directs most of the blood that enters the pulmonary artery into the aorta. This causes the majority of blood flow to bypass the nonfunctioning lungs.

As the newborn takes the first breaths at birth, the ductus arteriosus, which responds to a rise in oxygen by constricting, begins to close. At the same time, resistance within the pulmonary circulation decreases and resistance throughout the systemic circulation increases. This change in resistance, along with the constriction of the ductus arteriosus, causes blood to flow from the pulmonary artery into the lungs for oxygenation.

The ductus arteriosus closes gradually as the flow of prostaglandin E2 from the placenta ends and oxygenation improves. Functional closure occurs within 15 to 24 hours. Until closure is complete, the blood that does flow through the vessel reverses, moving from the aorta to the pulmonary artery and increasing blood flow to the lungs. This is because pressure in the aorta is now higher than that in the pulmonary artery. A murmur may be heard as a result of blood flow through the partially open vessel.

The ductus arteriosus closes permanently by 3 to 4 weeks (Lott, 1998). Once closed, it is called the ligamentum arteriosum. Until permanent closure occurs, low levels of oxygen in the blood may cause the ductus arteriosus to dilate and the pulmonary vessels to constrict. This may cause a return to fetal blood flow patterns and is a serious complication. A patent ductus arteriosus may occur in the infant who experiences asphyxia at birth, becomes hypoxic, or is preterm (see Chapter 30, p. 863).

Pulmonary Blood Vessels

The blood vessels in the lungs must be able to accommodate the large increase in blood flow they receive once the ductus arteriosus closes. They can do this because the vessels dilate in response to the increased oxygenation that occurs when the neonate begins to breathe. At the same time, fetal lung fluid is shifting into the interstitial spaces and is removed by the blood and lymph systems, allowing more room for dilation of the pulmonary blood vessels. This decreases pulmonary vascular resistance and allows the vessels within the lungs to expand to hold the suddenly increased blood flow from the pulmonary artery.

Foramen Ovale

The foramen ovale is a flap in the septum between the right and the left atria of the fetal heart. As blood returns to the heart, most of the oxygenated blood from the inferior vena cava enters the right atrium and crosses the foramen ovale to the left side of the heart. Little mixing occurs with the less oxygenated blood that enters from the superior vena cava and continues to the right ventricle. Blood flows through the foramen ovale, into the left atrium and the left ventricle and through the aorta. About two thirds of the blood in the ascending aorta flows to the brain and upper extremities. Thus most of the better-oxygenated blood bypasses the nonfunctioning lungs before birth.

Table 19-1

CIRCULATORY CHANGES AT BIRTH

Structure	Purpose in Fetal Life	Change at Birth	Cause of Change at Birth	Results of Change at Birth	Time of Functional and Permanent Change
Ductus Arteriosus	Is widely dilated; carries blood from PA to aorta and avoids nonfunctioning lungs.	Reversal of blood flow and constriction.	Pressure in aorta and oxygen level in blood increase.	Blood in PA directed to lungs for oxygenation.	Functional: beginning within minutes after birth. Complete closure in 15 to 24 hr. Permanent in 3 to 4 weeks. Becomes ligamentum arteriosum.
Pulmonary Blood Vessels	Narrowed vessels increase resistance in lungs to blood flow.	Dilation of all vessels in lungs.	Elevated blood oxygen level and removal of fetal lung fluid.	Decreased pulmonary resistance allows blood to enter freely to be oxygenated.	Beginning with first breath.
Foramen Ovale	Provides opening between RA and LA so that blood can avoid nonfunctioning lungs and go directly to LV and aorta. Opens only in R to L direction because of high RA pressure and low LA pressure.	Closes when pressure in LA becomes higher than pressure in RA.	Cord occlusion elevates systemic resistance. Blood returns from PV to LA. Both increase L heart pressure. Decreased pulmonary resistance allows free flow of blood into lungs and decreased pressure in RA.	Blood entering RA can no longer pass through to LA; instead, it goes to RV and through PA to the lungs.	Functional: within minutes Permanent: 3 months. Becomes fossa ovale.
Ductus Venosus	Shunts 50% of blood from umbilical vein to inferior vena cava and away from immature liver.	Blood flow occluded with end of umbilical circulation.	Occlusion of cord stops flow of blood from placenta through umbilical vein to ductus venosus.	Blood travels through liver to be filtered as in adult circulation.	Functional: when cord is occluded. Permanent: 1 week. Becomes ligamentum venosum.

R, Right; *L,* left; *PA,* pulmonary artery; *PV,* pulmonary veins; *RV,* right ventricle; *LV,* left ventricle; *RA,* right atrium; *LA,* left atrium.

The foramen ovale opens only from right to left. The right-to-left shunting of blood through the foramen ovale operates because the pressure in the right atrium is higher than that in the left atrium. Resistance to blood flow through the constricted pulmonary artery and pulmonary blood vessels causes the elevated pressure in the right side of the heart. Pressure is low on the left side of the heart because little resistance exists to blood leaving the left ventricle. Blood from the left ventricle travels to the rest of the body and into the placental vessels, which are widely dilated. This ensures adequate blood flow into the intervillous spaces during fetal life.

CRITICAL THINKING EXERCISE

Understanding the changes that occur during the transition from fetal to neonatal circulation helps in predicting the effect on blood flow of various defects in the heart.

QUESTION:
What would be the effect on neonatal blood flow of an opening in the septum of the atria of the heart?

At birth, pressures are reversed between the right and the left atria. Blood flows freely from the right ventricle to the dilated vessels of the lungs. Blood return to the right atrium decreases after occlusion of the umbilical vessels. These two events combine to decrease pressure in the right side of the heart.

Pressure in the left side of the heart builds as blood enters the left atrium from the pulmonary veins. When blood flow to the placenta ceases, the resistance to blood leaving the left ventricle increases, further elevating the pressure in the left side of the heart. In addition, cooling of the skin causes vasoconstriction of the peripheral vessels, further increasing the systemic vascular resistance. Because the foramen ovale opens only from right to left, it closes when the pressure in the left heart is higher than that in the right heart.

Closure of the foramen ovale prevents blood flow from the right to the left atrium and forces the blood into the right ventricle and pulmonary artery. Because the ductus arteriosus is also closing, the blood continues into the lungs for oxygenation and returns to the left atrium through the pulmonary veins. It enters the left ventricle and leaves through the aorta to circulate to the rest of the body. Thus blood flow through the heart and lungs changes from fetal to neonatal circulation and is similar to that in the normal adult (see Figure 6-9, p. 114-115, and Table 19-1).

The foramen ovale is functionally closed soon after birth because the pressure changes within the heart prevent it from opening. However, conditions such as asphyxia may reverse the pressures in the heart and cause the foramen ovale to reopen. The foramen ovale becomes permanently closed several months after birth. It is then called the *fossa ovale.*

Ductus Venosus

During fetal life, the liver does not have to filter the blood as it does after the infant is born. The ductus venosus directs about half of the blood flow from the umbilical vein away from the liver and directly to the inferior vena cava. Once the vessels in the umbilical cord are occluded, little blood enters the ductus venosus. Fibrosis of the ductus venosus occurs by the end of the first week of life and it then is called the *ligamentum venosum.*

Check Your Reading

4. What brings about the closure of the ductus arteriosus, foramen ovale, and ductus venosus at birth?
5. What causes the pulmonary blood vessels to dilate?

NEUROLOGIC ADAPTATION: THERMOREGULATION

At birth the infant must assume thermoregulation, the maintenance of body temperature. Although the fetus produces heat in utero, the consistently warm temperature of the amniotic fluid makes thermoregulation unnecessary. However, the temperature of the delivery room may be more than 20° F lower than that of the uterus. Neonates must produce and maintain enough heat to prevent cold stress, which can have serious and even fatal effects.

Newborn Characteristics Leading to Heat Loss

Some characteristics of newborns predispose them to lose heat. The skin is thin, and blood vessels are close to the surface. Little subcutaneous fat exists to serve as a barrier to heat loss. Heat is readily transferred from the warmer internal areas of the body to the cooler skin surfaces and then to the surrounding air. Newborns have three times more surface area to body mass than the adult, which provides more area for heat loss. They lose heat at a rate four times greater than adults do (Stoll & Kliegman, 2000).

To conserve heat, the healthy full-term infant remains in a position of flexion. This reduces the amount of skin surface exposed to the surrounding temperatures and decreases heat loss. This is not the case for the sick or preterm infant, who has decreased muscle tone and does not maintain a flexed position. Preterm infants also have thinner skin and less subcutaneous fat than the full-term infant. Thus they are at increased risk for cold stress (see Chapter 29).

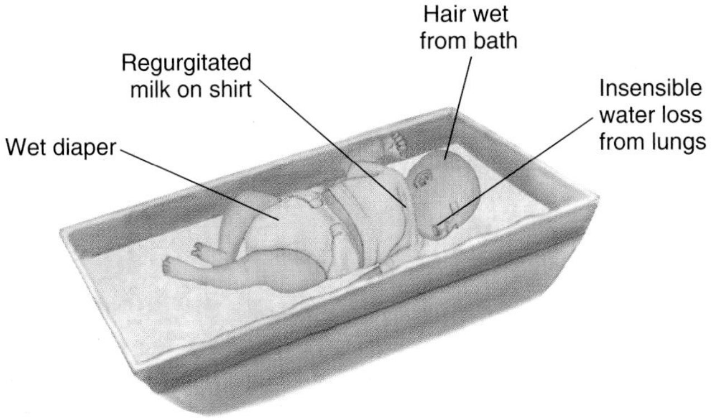

Evaporation can occur during birth or bathing from moisture on skin, as a result of wet linens or clothes, and from insensible loss.

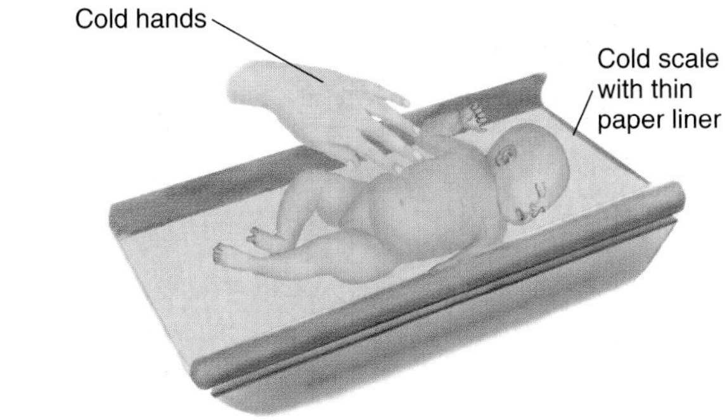

Conduction occurs when the infant comes in contact with cold objects or surfaces such as a scale, a circumcision restraint board, cold hands, or a stethoscope.

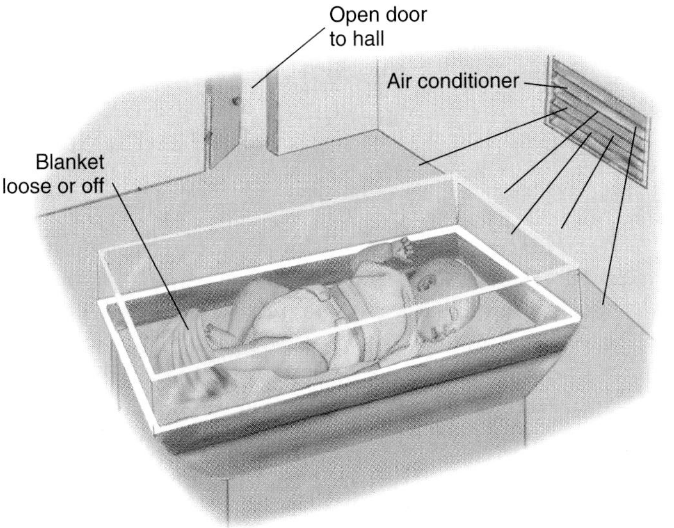

Convection occurs when drafts come from open doors, air conditioning, or even air currents created by people moving about.

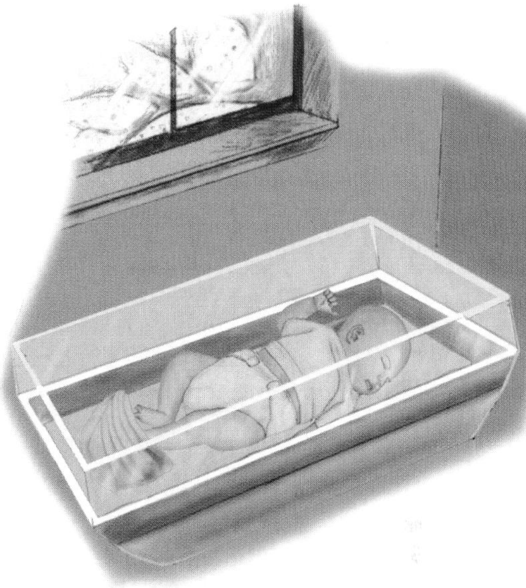

Heat is lost by radiation when the infant is near cold surfaces. Thus heat is lost from the infant's body to the sides of the crib or incubator and to the outside walls and windows.

FIGURE 19-2 Methods of heat loss.

Methods of Heat Loss

Heat is lost in four ways in the neonate: evaporation, conduction, convection, and radiation (Figure 19-2). The nurse can prevent heat loss by each method and must be watchful for situations in which intervention is needed.

Evaporation. Evaporation occurs when wet surfaces are exposed to air. As the surfaces dry, heat is lost. At birth, the infant loses heat when amniotic fluid on the skin evaporates. Evaporation also occurs during bathing. Drying the infant as quickly as possible at birth and after bathing helps prevent excessive heat loss. Insensible water loss from the skin and respiratory tract increases heat loss by evaporation.

Conduction. Conduction of heat away from the body occurs when newborns come in direct contact with objects that are cooler than their skin. Placing infants on cold surfaces such as scales or circumcision restraint boards or touching them with cold hands or a cold stethoscope causes this type of heat loss. The reverse is also true. That is, wrapping newborns in warm blankets or placing them against the mothers' skin can warm them.

Convection. Convection occurs when heat is transferred to air surrounding the infant. Air currents from air conditioning or people moving around increase the loss of heat. Keeping the newborn out of drafts and maintaining warm environmental temperatures help prevent

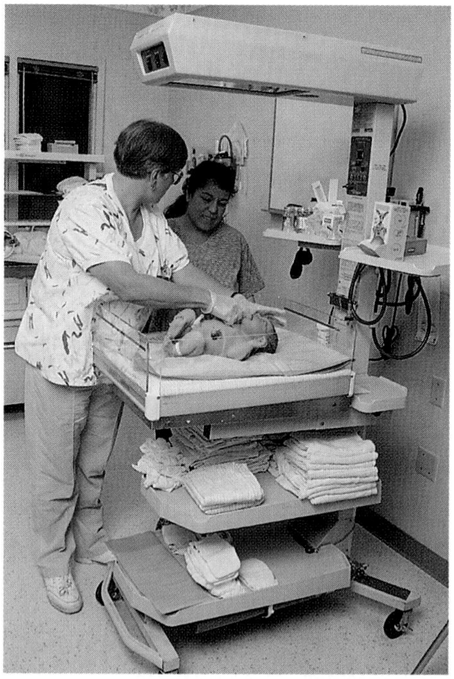

FIGURE 19-3 Radiant warmers allow easy access to the infant without increasing heat loss due to exposure. The nurse should be careful not to come between the infant and the overhead source of heat when caring for the infant.

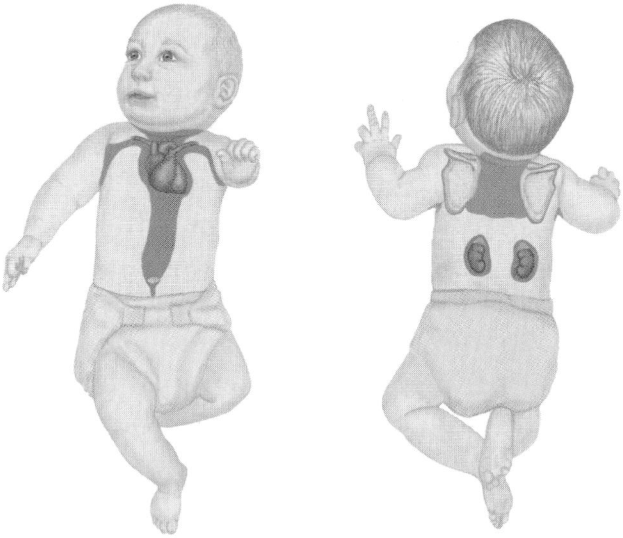

FIGURE 19-4 Sites of brown fat in the neonate.

this type of heat loss. Oxygen should be warmed before administration.

Radiation. Radiation is the transfer of heat to cooler objects that are not in direct contact with the infant. For example, infants placed near cold windows lose heat by radiation. Infants in incubators transfer heat to the walls of the incubator. If the walls of the incubator are cold, the infant is cooled, even when the temperature of the air inside the incubator is warm. Incubators often have double walls to combat this problem. Cribs and incubators should be kept away from windows and outside walls to minimize radiant heat loss.

Newborns can gain heat by radiation, too. They are often placed under radiant warmers for a short time after birth and warmed by radiant heat (Figure 19-3).

Nonshivering Thermogenesis

When adults are cold, they shiver, increasing muscle activity to produce heat. Newborns rarely shiver except at low temperatures (Bruck, 1998). Instead they become restless. Their increased activity and flexion helps generate some warmth and reduces the loss of heat from exposed surface areas of the body.

Exposure to cool temperatures also results in vasoconstriction of the vessels of the skin and decreased flow of warm blood to the skin. This helps prevent heat loss from the skin and causes the skin to feel cool to the touch. In addition, infants increase body metabolism.

The primary method of heat production in infants is nonshivering thermogenesis, the metabolism of brown fat to produce heat. Brown fat (also called brown adipose tissue or BAT) is a special kind of highly vascular fat found only in newborns. It contains an abundant supply of blood vessels, which cause the brown color. Brown fat is located primarily around the back of the neck; in the axillae; around the kidneys, adrenals, and sternum; between the scapula; and along the abdominal aorta (Figure 19-4).

Nonshivering thermogenesis begins when thermal receptors in the skin detect a drop in skin temperature. Thermal receptor stimulation causes release of norepinephrine, which begins metabolism of brown fat.

As brown fat is metabolized, it generates more heat than other fats. Blood passing through brown fat is warmed and carries heat to the rest of the body.

Nonshivering thermogenesis goes into effect even before a change occurs in core or interior body temperature, as measured with a rectal thermometer. Activating thermogenesis before core temperature decreases allows the body to maintain internal heat at an even level. Therefore nonshivering thermogenesis may begin in an infant when skin temperature is cool, even though a core temperature taken rectally shows a normal reading.

Some infants have inadequate brown fat stores. The preterm infant may have been born before stores of brown fat could accumulate. Newborns with intrauterine growth restriction may have depleted brown fat stores before birth. The fat may be consumed in newborns exposed to prolonged cold stress. These infants are not able to raise their body temperature if they are

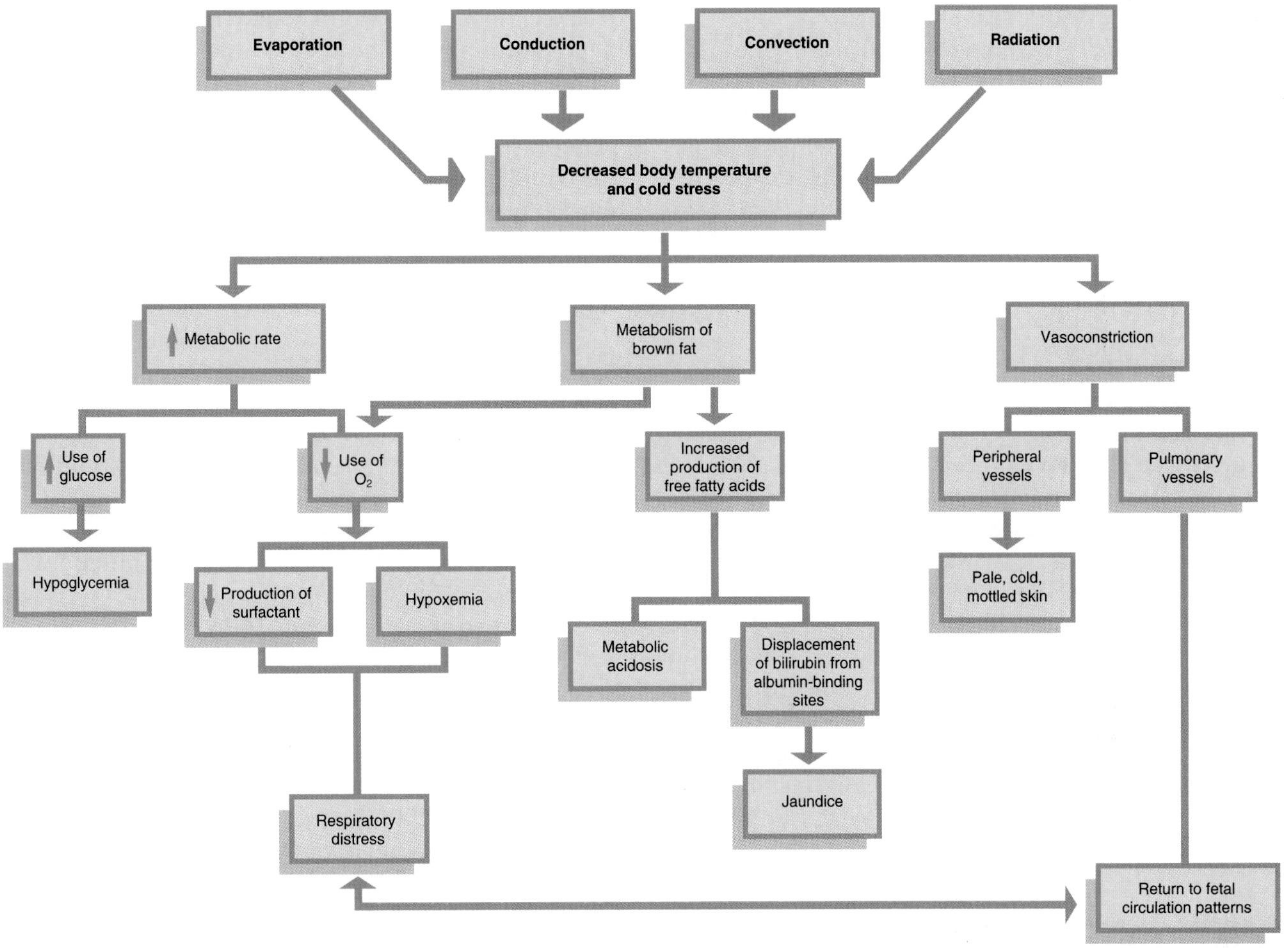

FIGURE 19-5 Effects of cold stress.

subjected to further episodes of cold stress and may have serious complications. Brown fat is used up during the early weeks after birth and is not present in the older infant.

Effects of Cold Stress

The metabolism of brown fat increases the need for oxygen (Figure 19-5). A small increase in metabolic rate can lead to a significant rise in the need for oxygen. Cold stress also causes a decrease in surfactant production, which impedes the expansion of the lungs. Prolonged cold stress can cause respiratory difficulty even in a healthy full-term infant. Mild respiratory distress can become severe hypoxia if oxygen must be used for heat production.

Glucose is also necessary in larger amounts for the increased metabolism that results from cold stress. When the infant's temperature drops, glycogen stores are converted to glucose. The stores may be quickly depleted, causing hypoglycemia. Metabolism of glucose in the presence of insufficient oxygen causes increased production of acids. Infants who must use glucose for temperature maintenance have less available for growth.

Metabolism of brown fat also releases fatty acids. This can cause metabolic acidosis, which can be a life-threatening condition. Elevated free fatty acids in the bloodstream interfere with transport of bilirubin to the liver, increasing the risk of jaundice.

CRITICAL TO REMEMBER

Hazards of Cold Stress

Increased oxygen need
Decreased surfactant production
Respiratory distress
Hypoglycemia
Metabolic acidosis
Jaundice

As the infant's body attempts to conserve heat, vasoconstriction of the peripheral blood vessels occurs to reduce heat loss from the skin's surface. However, decreased oxygen levels in the blood may also cause vasoconstriction of the pulmonary vessels and a return to fetal circulation patterns, further increasing respiratory distress.

Neutral Thermal Environment

A neutral thermal environment helps prevent heat loss in newborns. This is an environment in which the infant can maintain a stable body temperature without an increase in oxygen or metabolic rate. The range of environmental temperature that allows this is called the thermoneutral zone. In healthy, unclothed, full-term newborns, an environmental temperature of 32° to 35° C (89.6° to 95° F) provides a thermoneutral zone (Bruck, 1998).

Hyperthermia

Infants also respond poorly to hyperthermia. With an elevated temperature, the metabolic rate rises, causing an increased need for oxygen and glucose. In addition, vasodilation leads to increased insensible fluid losses. Sweating may occur but is often delayed because sweat glands are immature.

The most frequent cause of hyperthermia in newborns is overheating by poorly regulated equipment designed to keep them warm. When infants are under radiant warmers, warming lights, or in warmed incubators, the temperature mechanism must be set to vary the heat according to the infant's skin temperature and thus prevent heat that is too high or too low. Alarms to signify that the infant's temperature is too high or too low should be functioning properly.

Check Your Reading

6. Why are neonates more prone to heat loss than older children or adults?
7. What are the effects of low temperature in newborns?

HEMATOLOGIC ADAPTATION

Factors Affecting the Blood

In the newborn, the volume of the blood depends partially on whether clamping of the cord occurs immediately after birth or is delayed. It also depends on the position of the infant just before the cord is clamped. The average blood volume of the newborn is 80 to 85 ml/kg. The placenta contains approximately 100 ml of fetal blood, which can enter the infant's circulation at birth before the cord is clamped. If the cord is not clamped for a few minutes, the infant may have a 75 ml increase in blood volume (Guyton & Hall, 2000). Holding the infant below the level of the placenta before the cord is clamped also increases the blood volume. The extra blood volume increases the workload of the heart excessively. In addition, as the added red blood cells break down, bilirubin is released, increasing the risk of jaundice.

The various components found in the blood also depend on the time of cord clamping and the site from which the blood is drawn. The erythrocyte count and the hemoglobin level are higher after a delay in cord clamping. Blood samples drawn from the heel, where the circulation is sluggish, indicate higher levels of hemoglobin and hematocrit than samples taken from central areas. Venous blood samples are more accurate and are taken when precise measurement is essential. (See Appendix B for specific laboratory values.)

Blood Values

Erythrocytes and Hemoglobin

At birth, the infant has comparatively more erythrocytes (red blood cells) and higher hemoglobin and hematocrit levels than the adult. This is necessary because the partial pressure of oxygen of fetal blood in the umbilical vein is only about 30 mm Hg, much lower than the normal adult level (Guyton & Hall, 2000). The large number of erythrocytes (4 to 6.6 million/mm^3) and higher hemoglobin level (14.5 to 22.5 g/dl) enable the fetal cells to receive enough oxygen (Nicholson & Pesce, 2000). Adequate oxygenation to the cells is also possible because fetal hemoglobin (hemoglobin F) carries 20% to 50% more oxygen than adult hemoglobin (Guyton & Hall, 2000).

Erythrocytes in the newborn have a shorter life span than those of the adult and break down soon after birth. When this happens, hemoglobin is broken down, releasing bilirubin. Excess bilirubin resulting from the hemolysis of large numbers of red blood cells may lead to jaundice.

Hematocrit

The hematocrit level in the normal infant is 48% to 69% from peripheral sites during the first day and ranges from 44% to 72% by the third day (Nicholson & Pesce, 2000). A level above 65% from a central site indicates polycythemia, an abnormally high erythrocyte count. Polycythemia increases the risk of jaundice and damage to the brain and other organs as a result of blood stasis. Respiratory distress and hypoglycemia are more common in these infants.

Leukocytes

The leukocyte count in the newborn is 9000 to 30,000/mm^3. In newborns, an elevated white blood cell count does not necessarily indicate infection. In fact, the white blood cell count may decrease in infections. Increased numbers of immature leukocytes are a sign of infection or sepsis in the neonate. Platelets may also decrease as a result of infections.

Risk of Clotting Deficiency

Newborns are at risk for clotting deficiency during the first few days of life because they lack vitamin K, which is necessary to activate several of the clotting factors (Factors II, VII, IX, and X). Vitamin K is synthesized in the intestines, but food and normal intestinal flora are necessary for this process. At birth, the intestines are sterile and therefore unable to produce vitamin K. To decrease the risk of hemorrhagic disease of the newborn, vitamin K is administered intramuscularly to most infants during the initial assessment and care. Drugs such as phenytoin (Dilantin), phenobarbital, and aspirin taken by the mother during pregnancy interfere with clotting ability in the infant after birth.

GASTROINTESTINAL SYSTEM

Newborns must begin to take in, digest, and absorb food after birth because the placenta no longer performs these functions for them.

Stomach

The newborn's stomach capacity is about 6 ml/kg at birth (Blackburn & Loper, 1992) but expands to about 90 ml within the first few days of life. The stomach begins to empty during feeding and is completely empty within 2 to 4 hours. Peristalsis is rapid and is increased by feeding. The gastrocolic reflex is stimulated when the stomach fills, causing increased intestinal peristalsis. Infants frequently pass a stool during or after a feeding. The cardiac sphincter between the esophagus and the stomach is relaxed in the newborn, which explains the tendency to regurgitate feedings easily.

Intestines

The intestines of the newborn are long in proportion to the infant's size and compared with those of the adult. The added length allows more surface area for absorption. However, it makes infants more prone to water loss should diarrhea develop. Air enters the gastrointestinal tract soon after birth, and bowel sounds are present within the first hour. Once the infant is exposed to the external environment and begins to take in fluids, bacteria enter the gastrointestinal tract. Normal intestinal flora is established within the first few days of life.

Digestive Enzymes

Maturation of the ability to digest and absorb occurs at different rates for various nutrients. Pancreatic amylase is deficient for the first 4 to 6 months after birth (Vanderhoof, Zach, & Adrian, 1999). As a result, the newborn cannot digest complex carbohydrates such as those in cereals. Amylase is also produced by the salivary glands. However, saliva is not secreted in adequate amounts until about the third month of life.

The newborn is also deficient in pancreatic lipase, limiting fat absorption significantly. Lipase in breast milk may make it more digestible for the newborn than formula. Protein and lactose, the major carbohydrate in the infant's milk diet, are both well digested.

Stools

Meconium is the first stool excreted by the newborn. It consists of particles from amniotic fluid such as skin cells and hair, along with cells shed from the intestinal tract, bile, and other intestinal secretions. Meconium, which is greenish black with a thick, sticky, tarlike consistency, accumulates in the fetus's intestines throughout gestation. The first meconium stool is usually passed within the first 12 hours of life and 99% of neonates have passed meconium within 48 hours (Stoll & Kliegman, 2000). Failure to pass meconium within that time leads to suspicion of obstruction.

The second type of stool excreted by the newborn is called *transitional stool.* It is greenish brown and of a looser consistency than meconium. These stools are a combination of meconium and milk stools. They are followed by the stool characteristic of the type of food the infant eats.

The stools of infants fed with breast milk are seedy, the color and consistency of mustard with a sweet-sour smell. The breastfed infant generally has more frequent stools than the infant who is formula fed. Breastfed newborns excrete as many as 10 small stools each day, although some older infants pass only one stool every 2 to 3 days. The normal breastfed newborn should have at least four stools daily.

The formula-fed infant excretes pale yellow to light brown stools. They are firmer in consistency than those of the breastfed infant. The infant may excrete several stools daily, or only one or two. The stools have the characteristic odor of feces.

Check Your Reading

8. Why do newborns have higher levels of erythrocytes, hemoglobin, and hematocrit than adults?
9. How do the stools change over the first few days after birth?

HEPATIC SYSTEM

The liver assumes many different functions after birth. Some of the most important include maintenance of blood glucose levels, conjugation of bilirubin, production of factors necessary for blood coagulation, storage of iron, and metabolism of drugs.

Blood Glucose Maintenance

Throughout gestation, glucose is supplied to the fetus by the placenta. During the last 4 to 8 weeks of pregnancy,

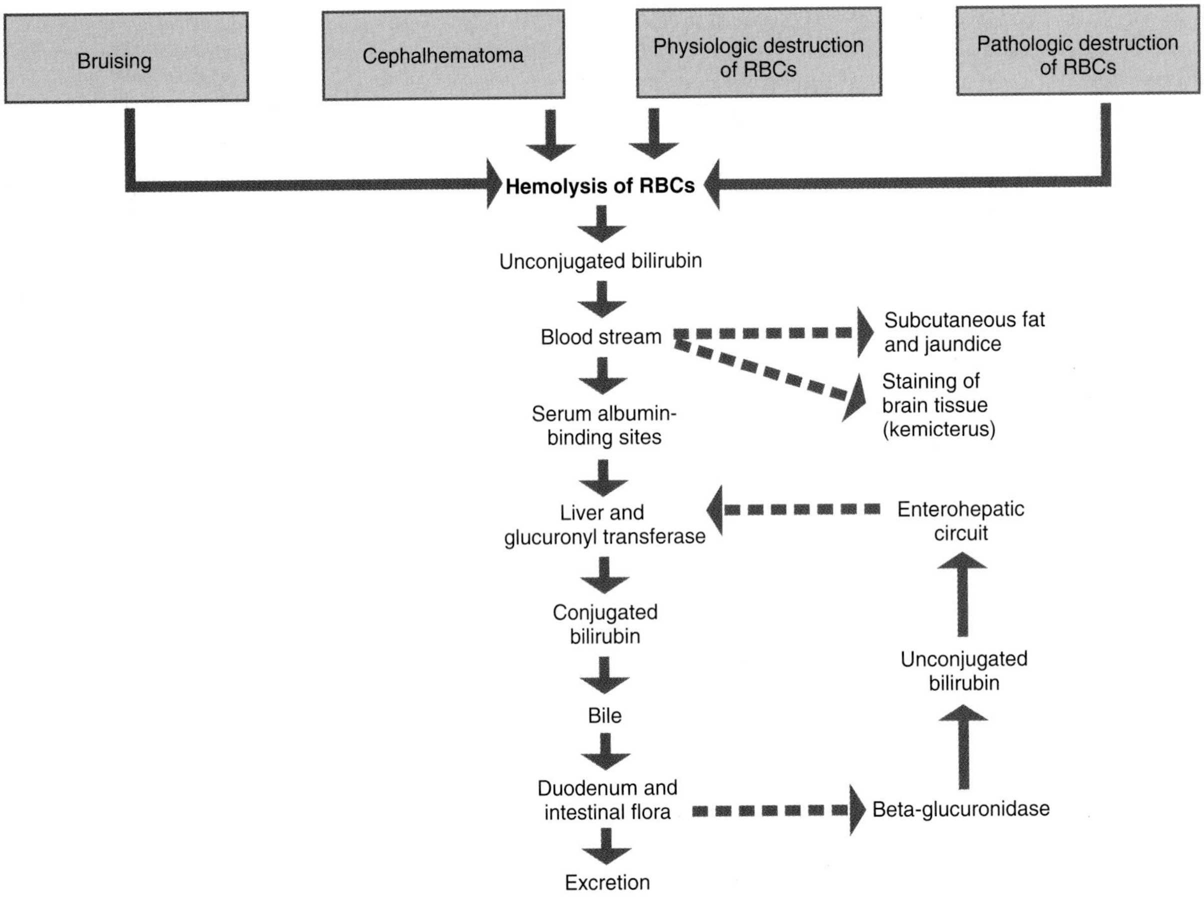

FIGURE 19-6 Sources of bilirubin and how it is removed from the body.

glucose is stored in the fetal liver as glycogen for use after birth. Glucose is used more rapidly in the newborn than in the fetus because energy is needed during the stresses of delivery and for breathing, heat production, movement against gravity, and activation of all the functions that the neonate must take on at birth. In addition, glucose must be readily available for use by the brain, which needs a constant supply. Without adequate glucose, the brain may be damaged. Therefore the liver's ability to convert glycogen to glucose is essential.

Until newborns begin regular feedings and their intake is adequate to meet energy requirements, the glucose that is present in the body is used. As the blood glucose level falls, the liver begins to convert glycogen to glucose, which is made available for the rest of the body. In the term infant, glucose levels should be 40 to 60 mg/dl on the first day and 50 to 90 thereafter (Nicholson & Pesce, 2000). A blood glucose level below 40 mg/dl in the term infant is considered hypoglycemia. For screening tests on capillary blood, a glucose level below 40 to 45 mg/dl is used in some agencies as an indicator for hypoglycemia because screening tests are less accurate.

Many newborns are at increased risk for hypoglycemia. In the preterm and small-for-gestational age infant, adequate stores of glycogen or even fat for metabolism may not have accumulated. Stores of glycogen may be used up before birth in the postterm infant because of poor intrauterine nourishment from a deteriorating placenta.

Large-for-gestational age newborns may produce excessive insulin that consumes available glucose quickly. This is particularly true if the mother is diabetic. Infants of diabetic mothers receive large amounts of glucose from the mother throughout pregnancy and must produce enough insulin to use the glucose. Although the supply of glucose is cut off at birth, the infants may continue to produce more insulin than needed, which results in hypoglycemia soon after birth (see Chapter 29 for discussion of the infant of a diabetic mother).

When infants are exposed to such stressors as asphyxia or infection, the glycogen in the liver may quickly be exhausted, and signs of hypoglycemia appear. In newborns who are not kept warm, available glucose may be depleted to increase metabolism and raise body temperature (see Critical to Remember: Signs of Hypoglycemia, p. 516).

Conjugation of Bilirubin

A major function of the liver is the conjugation of bilirubin (Figure 19-6). Although the newborn's liver is able to perform this function, it may not be mature enough to prevent the development of jaundice during the first week of life. Jaundice occurs in 60% of term newborns and 80% of preterm infants (Stoll & Kliegman, 2000).

Source and Effect of Bilirubin

The principal source of bilirubin is the hemolysis of erythrocytes. This is a normal occurrence after birth, when fewer erythrocytes are needed than during fetal life. The breakdown of red blood cells releases their components into the bloodstream to be reused by the body. Only bilirubin remains as an unusable residue in the blood. This substance is toxic to the body and must be excreted.

Bilirubin is released in an unconjugated form. Unconjugated bilirubin, also called *indirect bilirubin,* is soluble in fat but not in water. The liver must change it to a water-soluble form by a process called conjugation before excretion can occur. The bilirubin is then known as *conjugated* or *direct bilirubin.*

Because unconjugated bilirubin is fat soluble, it may be absorbed by the subcutaneous fat, causing the yellowish discoloration of the skin called jaundice. If enough unconjugated bilirubin accumulates in the blood, staining of the tissues in the brain occurs, called *kernicterus.* This may result in bilirubin encephalopathy, which may cause severe brain damage.

Normal Conjugation

When unconjugated bilirubin is released into the bloodstream, it attaches to binding sites on albumin in the plasma and is carried to the liver. There it binds to ligandin and other proteins and is changed to the conjugated form by the enzyme glucuronyl transferase in the smooth endoplasmic reticulum of the liver cells. Conjugated bilirubin is excreted into the bile and then into the duodenum. In the intestines, the normal flora acts on bilirubin to reduce it to urobilinogen and stercobilin, which are excreted in the stools. A small amount of urobilinogen is also excreted by the kidneys.

A small percentage of conjugated bilirubin may be deconjugated or converted back to the unconjugated state by the intestinal enzyme beta glucuronidase. This enzyme is important in fetal life because bilirubin is transported to the placenta for conjugation by the mother's liver. The placenta can clear only unconjugated bilirubin. In the newborn, deconjugated bilirubin in the intestines is reabsorbed into the portal circulation and carried directly back to the liver, where it again undergoes the conjugation process. This recirculation of bilirubin is called the *enterohepatic circuit.* It creates additional work for the liver.

Blood tests for bilirubin measure total bilirubin and direct (conjugated) bilirubin in the serum. Total bilirubin is a combination of indirect (unconjugated) and direct bilirubin.

Factors in Increased Bilirubin

A number of factors lead to the production of excessive amounts of bilirubin or interfere with the normal process of conjugation, resulting in an increased incidence of jaundice in the first week of life.

Excess Production. Bilirubin is produced in infants during the first 2 weeks of life at a rate twice that in adults (Maisels, 1999). Newborns have more red blood cells per kilogram of weight than adults. This is because oxygen levels are low during fetal life and more erythrocytes are needed to carry enough oxygen to the cells.

Red Blood Cell Life. Fetal red blood cells break down more quickly than adult erythrocytes. They last only two thirds as long as adult erythrocytes before hemolysis occurs (70 to 90 days in the neonate; 120 days in the adult [Watson, 1999]). For their size, neonates have more red blood cells breaking down faster and producing greater amounts of bilirubin to excrete than adults.

Liver Immaturity. The newborn's immature liver produces less than 0.1 % of the glucuronyl transferase of the adult during the first 10 days of life but then increases production rapidly reaching adult levels by 6 to 14 weeks of age (Maisels, 1999). Insufficient availability of this enzyme limits the amount of bilirubin that can be conjugated. This problem may be increased for the preterm and low-birth-weight infant.

Intestinal Factors. At birth, the intestines of the newborn are sterile. Conjugated bilirubin cannot be reduced to urobilinogen or stercobilin for excretion without the action of intestinal flora. In addition, the newborn intestines have a large amount of the enzyme beta glucuronidase, which changes bilirubin back to the unconjugated state. These two factors may result in high levels of unconjugated bilirubin, which is reabsorbed into the blood circulation.

Delayed Feeding. Feeding the newborn helps establish the normal intestinal flora and promotes passage of meconium, which is high in bilirubin. When feeding is delayed or stools are not passed, exposure to beta glucuronidase is longer, increasing the chance of conversion of conjugated bilirubin to the unconjugated state and absorption into the blood.

Trauma. Trauma during birth may result in increased hemolysis of red blood cells. This is particularly true in cases of bruising, which may be caused by use of a vacuum extractor. The infant born in a breech position may also have bruising. A cephalhematoma contains a large number of erythrocytes. As the red blood cells in the bruised areas break down, they add to the bilirubin load.

Fatty Acids. Free fatty acids have a greater affinity than bilirubin for the binding sites on albumin and bind to albumin in place of bilirubin. Fatty acids are released when brown fat is used to increase heat during cold stress. During asphyxia, anaerobic metabolism also produces free fatty acids. Thus in infants who suffer cold stress or asphyxia, unbound unconjugated bilirubin is in the circulation and jaundice may develop.

Other Factors. Bilirubin levels are more likely to be elevated in infants who are East Asian or Native American, preterm, male, or whose mothers have diabetes, or siblings have also had the problem. Maternal intake of sulfonamides and aspirin during pregnancy or oxytocin used during labor also increase jaundice. Swallowing blood during birth causes more breakdown of erythrocytes and increased bilirubin.

Hyperbilirubinemia

Physiologic Jaundice

Physiologic jaundice is due to the transient hyperbilirubinemia that occurs for any of the reasons already discussed. It is not present during the first 24 hours of life in term infants but appears on the second or third day after birth and is considered a normal phenomenon in newborns. Jaundice of the face occurs when the bilirubin level reaches 5 to 7 mg/dl, the midabdomen at about 15 mg/dl, and about 20 when it reaches the soles of the feet (Stoll & Kliegman, 2000). Physiologic jaundice may have some positive effects. Bilirubin is an antioxidant and may act to prevent damage to membranes from free-radicals (Maisels, 1999).

CRITICAL TO REMEMBER

Factors That Increase Hyperbilirubinemia

Hemolysis of excessive erythrocytes
Short red blood cell life
Liver immaturity
Lack of intestinal flora
Delayed feeding
Trauma resulting in bruising or cephalhematoma
Fatty acids from cold stress or asphyxia

The rate at which bilirubin in the blood rises and falls is important because it helps determine whether the rate for a particular infant is following the expected curve for age and birth weight. Cord blood has an average bilirubin level of less than 2 mg/dl. In physiologic jaundice, the indirect bilirubin rises rapidly, peaking at 5 to 6 mg/dl between the second and fourth day of life. The bilirubin then begins to fall, declining below 2 mg/dl by the end of the first week. For preterm infants jaundice begins at the same time or slightly later and lasts longer. Peak levels of 8 to 12 mg/dl occur on the fifth to seventh day and may last until 10 days after birth (Stoll & Kliegman, 2000).

Physiologic jaundice may be treated with phototherapy when the bilirubin levels rise faster or to higher levels than expected. Because preterm and low-birth-weight infants are more susceptible to kernicterus at lower bilirubin levels, phototherapy may be used earlier than in the full-term infant (see p. 847).

Pathologic Jaundice

Pathologic jaundice occurs during the first 24 hours after birth, whereas physiologic jaundice begins after the first 24 hours (Smith, 2000). Any of the following bilirubin levels may indicate a nonphysiologic cause (Stoll & Kliegman, 2000):

1. A direct bilirubin level above 2 mg/dl
2. A total bilirubin concentration that increases by more than 5 mg/dl per day or is higher than 12 mg/dl in a full-term infant or 10 to 14 mg/dl in a preterm infant
3. The above bilirubin level persisting after 10 to 14 days of life

Pathologic jaundice is most commonly a result of abnormalities causing excessive destruction of erythrocytes. These include incompatibilities between the mother's and infant's blood types (see p. 693), infection, and metabolic disorders (see discussion of pathologic jaundice, p. 846). When jaundice begins after the third day but during the first week, the cause is likely to be infection resulting in hemolysis or liver damage (Stoll & Kliegman, 2000).

Breast Milk Jaundice

Breastfed infants are three times more likely than formula-fed infants to have total bilirubin levels above 12 mg/dl (Maisels, 1999). Jaundice may be of early or late onset.

Early Onset Breast Milk Jaundice. The most common cause of jaundice in breastfed infants is insufficient intake. It is called *early onset breast milk jaundice* or *breastfeeding jaundice,* begins 2 to 5 days after birth, and usually lasts about 10 days. Peak bilirubin levels are 15 mg/dl or less (Lawrence & Lawrence, 1999).

Infants who are sleepy, have a poor suck, or who nurse on an infrequent schedule may not receive enough colostrum, the substance that precedes true breast milk, to take advantage of its normal laxative effect. This delays the elimination of meconium, which is high in bilirubin. When meconium is not eliminated, the bilirubin may be deconjugated by beta glucuronidase in the intestine, absorbed, and recirculated to the liver for conjugation again.

Lack of adequate suckling also depresses production of breast milk and increases the problem further. Helping the mother with breastfeeding to increase the infant's intake and to stimulate milk production may be the most important treatment.

True Breast Milk Jaundice. Approximately 1% to 2% of breastfed infants develop true breast milk jaundice (Frank, 1998). In true breast milk jaundice, also called *late onset breast milk jaundice,* the jaundice occurs 5 to 10 days after birth and lasts more than a month. Levels may be higher than 20 mg/dl (Lawrence & Lawrence, 1999).

The exact cause of breast milk jaundice is unknown. Substances in the breast milk such as pregnanediol and free fatty acids may interfere with conjugation, and beta glucuronidase may be present to increase deconjugation and absorption of bilirubin from the intestine. However, no proven cause is known.

Treatment of breast milk jaundice includes close monitoring of bilirubin levels in the blood and at least 8 to 10 feedings each 24 hours. Although the levels are higher and last longer than in physiologic jaundice, reported cases of bilirubin encephalopathy from this type of jaundice are unusual (Stoll & Kliegman, 2000). If bilirubin levels become too high, phototherapy is begun. Breastfeeding may be continued or discontinued for 24 to 48 hours. Temporarily switching to formula causes a rapid drop in bilirubin. The level may rise again when breastfeeding is resumed but generally not high enough to interfere with further breastfeeding.

Blood Coagulation

Prothrombin and coagulation factors II, VII, IX, and X are produced by the liver and activated by vitamin K, which is deficient in the newborn. This is discussed under hematologic adaptation (p. 488).

Iron Storage

Iron is stored in the liver during the last weeks of pregnancy. The full-term infant whose mother's diet was adequate in iron has enough stored iron to prevent anemia during the early months, when the diet is poor in iron. By 4 to 6 months, the iron supply may be depleted and the infant should begin iron-containing foods or an iron supplement. Infants with inadequate prenatal stores need iron-fortified formula.

Metabolism of Drugs

The liver metabolizes drugs inefficiently in the newborn. This must be considered when drugs are given to the neonate. In addition, a breastfeeding mother should alert her primary caregiver before taking medications, as harmful amounts may be transferred to the infant via the breast milk.

Check Your Reading

10. Why is hypoglycemia a problem for the newborn?
11. Why are infants more likely to become jaundiced than adults?
12. What are the differences among physiologic, pathologic, and breast milk jaundice?

URINARY SYSTEM

Kidney Development

The kidneys begin to produce urine at about the twelfth week of gestation. Fetal urine is not actually a waste product because the placenta eliminates wastes for the fetus. The kidneys become the major source of amniotic fluid by the second half of pregnancy. Failure to produce urine causes oligohydramnios, or lack of sufficient amniotic fluid.

The kidneys are completely developed at 35 weeks of gestation. Full kidney function does not occur until after birth, however, when the kidneys take over the elimination of wastes from the blood. Blood flow to the kidneys increases after birth because of decreased resistance in the renal vessels. The improved perfusion results in a steady improvement in kidney function during the first few days of life.

Kidney Function

Although the formation of nephrons is complete by birth, kidney function is immature compared with that of the adult. The ability of the glomeruli to filter and the renal tubules to reabsorb is considerably less than in adults. The glomerular filtration rate doubles during the first weeks of life but does not reach adult levels until 1 to 2 years of age (Bonilla-Felix, Brannan, & Portman, 1998). Therefore infants have a decreased ability to filter waste products from the blood.

Substances such as glucose and protein may escape into the urine of the neonate. They disappear within the first 3 days of life as kidney function improves. Urate crystals may give a pink color to the urine that is sometimes mistaken for blood.

The first voiding occurs within 24 hours of birth in most newborns. Failure to void in that time may be due to hypovolemia from inadequate intake of fluids. Absence of kidneys or anomalies that interfere with excretion of urine are usually discovered before birth because lack of urine excretion causes oligohydramnios, a deficiency of amniotic fluid. This generally prompts investigation into the cause during pregnancy. Only two to six voidings may occur during the first 2 days of life. Then the infant voids at least once after every feeding, which is at least six times a day (Brion, Bernstein, & Spitzer, 1997).

Fluid Balance

Newborns have a lower tolerance for changes in total volume of body fluid than do older infants. This is because of the location of water within the newborn's body and the inability of the kidneys to adapt to large changes in body fluids. In addition, the fluid turnover rate is greater than that in adults. To maintain fluid balance, newborns need 65 ml/kg (30 ml/lb) daily during the first 2 days of life and then 100 to 150 ml/kg (45 to 68 ml/lb) a day (Tsang, DeMarini, & Rath,

Table 19-2
DISTRIBUTION OF WATER IN NEWBORNS AND ADULTS

	Newborn	Adult
Total body water	78%	55% to 60%
Extracellular water	44%	20%
Intracellular water	34%	40%

Comparison of distribution of body water in newborns and adults as a percent of body weight.

CRITICAL TO REMEMBER

Intake and Output in the Newborn

First 2 days of life
- Intake: 65 ml/kg (30 ml/lb) a day
- Output: 2 to 6 voids

After the first 2 days
- Intake: 100 to 150 ml/kg (45 to 68 ml/lb) a day
- Output: At least 6 a day

1998). For example, an infant who weighs 3.4 kg (7.5 lb) on the third day of life needs 340 to 510 ml of fluid each day.

Water Distribution

A large percentage of the infant's body is composed of water, which is distributed differently than it is in the adult (Table 19-2). Water constitutes 78% of the newborn's body weight. Body fluid decreases to the adult level of 55% to 60% of body weight by 1 year of age (Adelman & Solhaug, 2000).

In the newborn, 44% of body weight is composed of extracellular water located in the interstitial or intravascular spaces (Bell & Oh, 1999). This is more than twice as high as the extracellular water in adults, which is 20% of body weight. Although fluid within the cells is relatively stable, extracellular water is easily lost from the body. Because infants have more fluid for their size than adults, and because a larger proportion of it is located outside the cells, total body water is easily depleted. Conditions such as vomiting and diarrhea can quickly result in life-threatening dehydration.

Insensible Water Loss

Water lost from the skin and respiratory tract contributes to insensible water loss. Insensible water losses are increased in the newborn because of the large surface area of the body and the rapid respiratory rate. Fluid losses increase greatly when infants are placed under radiant heaters, which accelerate evaporation from the skin. An elevated respiratory rate or low humidity in the air surrounding the infant raises insensible water losses even further.

Urine Dilution and Concentration

The ability of a newborn's kidneys to dilute urine is relatively good, to a specific gravity of 1.001 to 1.005 (Bonilla-Felix, Brannan, & Portman, 1998). However, a newborn's kidneys cannot handle large increases in fluids, which result in fluid overload. This is most likely to happen when infants receive too much intravenous fluid. Normal urine output is 1 to 3 ml/kg per hour (Brion, Bernstein, & Spitzer, 1997).

Newborns have more difficulty preventing loss of fluid in the urine than do adults because they have only about half the adult's ability to concentrate urine (Guyton & Hall, 2000). Neonates can concentrate urine only to a specific gravity of 1.015 to 1.020 (Bonilla-Felix, Brannan, & Portman, 1998), compared with the adult level of 1.040. It takes 3 to 6 months for urine concentrations to reach adult levels. When abnormal conditions such as diarrhea cause excessive loss of fluid, the newborn's limited ability to conserve water may result in dehydration more quickly than in the older infant or child.

Acid-Base and Electrolyte Balance

The maintenance of acid-base and electrolyte balance is a primary function of the kidneys and may be precarious in neonates. Newborns tend to lose bicarbonate at lower levels than adults, increasing their risk for acidosis. The excretion of solutes is less efficient in newborns as well. Although newborns conserve needed sodium well, they are less able to excrete sodium efficiently if they receive excessive amounts (Brion, Satlin, & Edelmann, 1999).

IMMUNE SYSTEM

The neonate is less effective in fighting off infection than the older infant or child. The various white blood cells respond slowly and inefficiently when the body is invaded by organisms. Leukocytes are delayed in moving to the site of invasion and are not efficient in destroying the invader. Fever and leukocytosis, which normally occur during infection of the older child, are often not present in the newborn with infection. This is because the hypothalamus and inflammatory responses are immature.

Full-term newborns received antibodies from the mother during the last trimester of pregnancy. The mother continues to give the infant antibodies in her milk, if she chooses to breastfeed. This transfers passive immunity to the infant. Immunoglobulins (serum globulins with antibody activity) help protect the newborn from infection. The major immunoglobulins are IgG, IgM, and IgA. Each immunoglobulin performs a different function.

IgG

IgG crosses the placenta readily and provides the fetus with passive temporary immunity to bacteria and viruses to which the mother has developed immunity. IgG also protects the fetus from bacterial toxins. It begins to cross the placenta during the first trimester, but most of the transfer occurs in the third trimester. At birth the infant's IgG levels equal that of the mother.

Although the fetus begins to make its own IgG before birth, very little is produced until 3 to 4 weeks after birth. The infant gradually produces larger quantities of the immunoglobulin to replace IgG from the mother, which is being catabolized. The passive immunity lasts for varying amounts of time. It disappears about 6 to 8 months of age, but some last longer (Buckley, 2000). Administration of measles vaccine is delayed until about 12 to 15 months so that the passive immunity does not interfere with the infant's ability to form active immunity to measles.

IgM

IgM is the first immunoglobulin produced by the body when the newborn is challenged. This immunoglobulin helps protect against gram-negative bacteria. Small amounts of IgM are produced beginning at 20 weeks of gestation. It is rapidly produced beginning a few days after birth and rises to adult levels by 1 year of age. IgM cannot cross the placenta because the molecules are too large. If IgM is found in larger than normal amounts, exposure to infection in utero is probable.

IgA

IgA does not cross the placenta and must be produced by the infant. Because IgA is important in protection of the gastrointestinal and respiratory systems, newborns are particularly susceptible to infections of those systems. A form of IgA is included in colostrum and breast milk. Therefore breastfed infants receive protection that formula-fed infants do not.

Check Your Reading

13. How does the distribution of fluid in the newborn compare with that in the adult?
14. Why are IgG, IgM, and IgA important to the newborn?

PSYCHOSOCIAL ADAPTATION

Periods of Reactivity

In the early hours after birth, the infant goes through changes called the periods of reactivity. The two periods of reactivity are separated by a period of sleep.

First Period of Reactivity

The first period of reactivity begins at birth. Infants are active at this time and appear awake, alert, and interested in their surroundings. Parents enjoy watching the infant gaze directly at them when held in the en face (face-to-face) position. Infants move their arms and legs energetically, root, and appear hungry. If allowed to nurse, many infants latch on to the nipple and suck well.

Respirations during the first period of reactivity may be as high as 80 breaths per minute. The heart rate may be elevated to 180 beats per minute. Crackles, retractions, nasal flaring, and increased mucous secretions may be present. The pulse and respirations gradually slow, and the infant becomes sleepy after about 30 minutes.

Period of Sleep

After the first period of reactivity, infants become quiet and eventually fall into a deep sleep, which lasts 2 to 4 hours. During this time, the pulse and respirations drop to the normal range but the temperature may be low.

Second Period of Reactivity

When infants waken from the period of sleep, they enter the second period of reactivity. Infants are alert, and parents may enjoy the opportunity to get to know them at this time. Infants become interested in feeding and may pass meconium. The pulse and respiratory rates may increase, and some infants become cyanotic or have periods of apnea. Mucous secretions increase, and infants may gag or regurgitate.

The second period of reactivity may last 4 to 6 hours, although individual variation is great. Many infants pass through all stages within 8 hours. Once the second period of reactivity is over, the infant is usually stable.

Behavioral States

Six gradations in the behavioral state of the infant have been identified, ranging from deep sleep to crying. The amount of time infants spend in the different sleep-wake states varies and is a key to their individuality. Infants tend to move from one state to the next in the following sequence.

Quiet Sleep State

During the quiet sleep state, the infant is in a deep sleep with closed eyes and no eye movements. Respirations are quiet, regular, and slower than in the other states. Although startles occur at intervals, the infant's body is quiet. Little or no response to noise or stimuli occurs, and the infant returns to deep sleep quickly if not disturbed.

Active Sleep State

In the active sleep state, infants move their extremities, stretch, change facial expressions, and may fuss briefly. During this period, respirations tend to be more rapid and irregular and rapid eye movements (REM) occur. Infants are more likely to startle from noise or disturbances and may return to sleep or move to an awake state.

Drowsy State

The drowsy state is a transitional period between sleep and waking similar to that experienced by adults as they awake. The eyes may remain closed or, if open, appear glazed and unfocused. Infants startle and move their extremities slowly. They may go back to sleep or, with gentle stimulation, gradually awaken.

Quiet Alert State

Parents should learn to identify the quiet alert state (also called *alert inactivity*), which is an excellent time for bonding. Infants focus on objects or people, respond to the parents with intense gazing, and seem bright and interested in their surroundings. Body movements are minimal; infants seem to concentrate on the environment.

Active Alert State

In the active alert state infants are often fussy. They seem restless, have faster and more irregular respirations, and seem more aware of feelings of discomfort from hunger or cold. Although their eyes are open, infants seem less focused on visual stimuli than during the quiet alert state.

Crying State

The crying state may quickly follow the active alert state if no intervention occurs to comfort the infant. The cries are continuous and lusty, active body movement occurs, and the infant does not respond positively to stimulation. It may take a period of comforting to move the infant to a state in which feeding or other activities can be accomplished.

Check Your Reading

15. What are newborns like during the first and second periods of reactivity?
16. How do infant behavioral states vary?

SUMMARY CONCEPT

- Chemical, thermal, and mechanical factors combine to stimulate the respiratory center in the brain and initiate respirations at birth.
- Surfactant lines the alveoli and reduces surface tension to keep the alveoli open. Fetal lung fluid moves into the interstitial spaces before, during, and after birth and is absorbed by the lymphatic and vascular systems.
- Increases in blood oxygen levels, shifts in pressure in the heart and lungs, and closing of the umbilical vessels cause closure of the ductus arteriosus, foramen ovale, and ductus venosus at birth.
- Infants are predisposed to heat loss because they have thin skin with little subcutaneous fat, blood vessels close to the surface, and a large skin surface area. They lose heat by evaporation, conduction, convection, and radiation.
- Heat is produced in newborns by an increased activity and flexion, vasoconstriction, and nonshivering thermogenesis. These factors increase oxygen and glucose consumption and may cause respiratory distress, hypoglycemia, acidosis, and jaundice.
- Laboratory values for erythrocytes, hemoglobin, and hematocrit are higher for newborns than for adults because oxygen available to them in fetal life was less than after birth.
- After birth, the stools progress from thick, greenish-black meconium to loose, greenish-brown transitional stools to milk stools. Stools of breastfed infants are frequent, soft, seedy, and mustard-colored, whereas those of formula-fed infants are pale yellow to light brown, firmer, and less frequent.
- The neonate uses glucose rapidly and is at risk for hypoglycemia.
- Physiologic jaundice occurs in normal newborns after the first 24 hours of life as a result of hemolysis of red blood cells and immaturity of the liver. Pathologic jaundice is abnormal, begins within the first 24 hours, and often requires treatment with phototherapy. Breast milk jaundice begins later than physiologic jaundice and may be due to substances in the milk.
- The newborn's kidneys filter, reabsorb, and monitor fluid and electrolyte balance less efficiently than the adult's kidneys. The newborn's body is composed of a greater percentage of water, with more located in the extracellular compartment, than in the adult.
- Newborns receive passive immunity when IgG crosses the placenta in utero. After birth, IgM and IgA are produced to protect against infection.
- During the first and second periods of reactivity, newborns are active and alert and may be interested in feeding. Their pulse and respiratory rates may be elevated, and they may show some transient signs of respiratory distress.
- Newborns progress through six behavioral states: quiet sleep, active sleep, drowsy, quiet alert, active alert, and crying.

ANSWERS TO CRITICAL THINKING EXERCISE

If an opening existed between the right and left atria after birth, blood would flow from the left atrium, where pressures are high, into the right atrium, where pressures are low. This is the reverse of the blood flow through the foramen ovale during fetal life. The blood would then flow to the right ventricle, the pulmonary artery, and to the lungs. This would cause an increased workload on the lungs and could lead to serious complications.

REFERENCES & READINGS

Adelman, R.D., & Solhaug, M.J. (2000). Pathophysiology of body fluids and fluid therapy. In R.E. Behrman, R.M. Kliegman, & H.B. Jenson (Eds.) *Nelson textbook of pediatrics* (16th ed., pp. 189-227). Philadelphia: W.B. Saunders.

American Academy of Pediatrics & American College of Obstetricians and Gynecologists (1997). *Guidelines for perinatal care* (4th ed.). Elk Grove, IL: American Academy of Pediatrics.

Amlung, S.R. (1998). Neonatal thermoregulation. In C. Kenner, J.W. Lott, & A.A. Flandermeyer (Eds.), *Comprehensive neonatal nursing, a physiologic perspective* (2nd ed., pp. 207-219). Philadelphia: W.B. Saunders.

Anderson, S. (2000). Thermoregulation. In *Core curriculum for neonatal intensive care nursing* (2nd ed., pp. 63-73). Philadelphia: W.B. Saunders.

Association of Women's Health, Obstetric, and Neonatal Nurses (AWHONN). (1996). *Physiologic assessment of the healthy newborn.* Washington, D.C.: Author.

Bell, E.F., & Oh, W. (1999). Fluid and electrolyte management. In G.B. Avery, M.A. Fletcher, & M.G. MacDonald (Eds.), *Neonatology: Pathophysiology and management of the newborn* (5th ed., pp. 345-361). Philadelphia: Lippincott.

Berkowitz, C.D. (2000). *Pediatrics: A primary care approach* (2nd ed.). Philadelphia: W.B. Saunders.

Blackburn, S.T. (1998). Assessment and management of neonatal neurobehavioral development. In C. Kenner, J.W. Lott, & A.A. Flandermeyer (Eds.), *Comprehensive neonatal nursing, a physiologic perspective* (2nd ed., pp. 564-607). Philadelphia: W.B. Saunders.

Blackburn, S.T., & Loper, D.L. (1992). *Maternal, fetal, and neonatal physiology: A clinical perspective.* Philadelphia: W.B. Saunders.

Blake, W.W., & Murray, J.A. (1998). Heat balance. In G.B. Merenstein & S.L. Gardner (Eds.), *Handbook of neonatal intensive care* (4th ed., pp. 100-115). St. Louis: Mosby.

Bonilla-Felix, M., Brannan, P., & Portman, R. (1998). Neonatal nephrology. In G.B. Merenstein & S.L. Gardner (Eds.), *Handbook of neonatal intensive care* (4th ed., pp. 535-570). St. Louis: Mosby.

Bowden, V.R., Dickey, S.B., & Greenberg, C.S. (1998). *Children and their families: The continuum of care.* Philadelphia: W.B. Saunders.

Brazelton, T.B. (1999). Behavioral competence. In G.B. Avery, M.A. Fletcher, & M.G. MacDonald (Eds.), *Neonatology: Pathophysiology and management of the newborn* (5th ed., pp. 321-332). Philadelphia: Lippincott.

Brion, L.P., Bernstein, J., & Spitzer, A. (1997). Kidney and urinary tract. In Fanaroff, A.A. & Martin, R.J. (1997). *Neonatal-perinatal medicine* (Vol. 2, 6th ed., pp. 1564-1636). St. Louis: Mosby.

Brion, L.P., Satlin, L.M., & Edelmann, C.M. (1999). Renal disease. In G.B. Avery, M.A. Fletcher, & M.G. MacDonald (Eds.), *Neonatology: Pathophysiology and management of the newborn* (5th ed., pp. 887-973). Philadelphia: Lippincott.

Brooks, C. (1997). Neonatal hypoglycemia. *Neonatal Network,* 16(2), 15-21.

Bruck, K. (1998). Neonatal thermal regulation. In R.A. Polin & W.W. Fox (Eds.), *Fetal and neonatal physiology* (Vol. 1, 2nd ed., pp. 676-702). Philadelphia: W.B. Saunders.

Buckley, R.H. (2000). T-, B-, and NK-Cell systems. In R.E. Behrman, R.M. Kliegman, & H.B. Jenson (Eds.), *Nelson textbook of pediatrics* (16th ed., pp. 590-596). Philadelphia: W.B. Saunders.

Dodd, V. (1996). Gestational age assessment. *Neonatal Network,* 15(1), 27-36.

Fletcher, M.A. (1999). Physical assessment and classification. In G.B. Avery, M.A. Fletcher, & M.G. MacDonald (Eds.), *Neonatology: Pathophysiology and management of the newborn* (5th ed., pp. 301-320). Philadelphia: Lippincott.

Gomella, T.L., Cunningham, M.D., Eyal, F.G., & Zenk, K.E. (Eds.) (1999). *Neonatology* (4th ed.). Norwalk, CT: Appleton & Lange.

Guyton, A.C., & Hall, J.E. (2000). *Textbook of medical physiology* (10th ed.). Philadelphia: W.B. Saunders.

Hagedorn, M.I., Gardner, S.L., & Abman, S.H. (1998). Respiratory diseases. In G.B. Merenstein & S.L. Gardner (Eds.), *Handbook of neonatal intensive care* (4th ed., pp. 437-497). St. Louis: Mosby.

Halamek, L.P. & Stevenson, D.K. (1997). Neonatal jaundice and liver disease. In A.A. Fanaroff & R.J. Martin (Eds.), *Neonatal—perinatal medicine* (Vol. 2, 6th ed., pp. 1345-1389). St. Louis: Mosby.

Hernandez, J.A., Zabloudil, C. & Hernandez, P.W. (1999). Adaptation to extrauterine life and management during transition. In P.J. Thureen, J. Deacon, P. O'Neil, & J. Hernandez (Eds.), *Assessment and care of the well newborn* (pp. 83-100). Philadelphia: W.B. Saunders.

Howard-Glenn, L. (2000). Adaptation to extrauterine life and immediate nursing care. In *Core curriculum for maternal-newborn nursing* (2nd ed., pp. 346-359). Philadelphia: W.B. Saunders.

Howard-Glenn, L. (2000). Newborn biological/behavioral characteristics and psychosocial adaptations. In *Core curriculum for maternal-newborn nursing* (2nd ed., pp. 360-373). Philadelphia: W.B. Saunders.

Johnson, C.B. (1996). Head, eyes, ears, nose, mouth, and neck assessment. In E.P. Tappero & M.E. Honeyfield (Eds), *Physical Assessment of the newborn* (2nd ed., pp. 53-66). Petaluma, CA: NICU Ink.

Lawrence, R.A. & Lawrence, R.M. (1999). *Breastfeeding: A guide for the medical profession* (5th ed.). St. Louis: Mosby.

Leick-Rude, M.K. & Bloom, L.F. (1998). A comparison of temperature-taking methods in neonates. *Neonatal Network,* 17(5), 21-37.

Lepley, C.J., Gardner, S.L., & Lubchenco, L.O. (1998). Initial nursery care. In G.B. Merenstein & S.L. Gardner (Eds.), *Handbook of neonatal intensive care* (4th ed., pp. 70-99). St. Louis: Mosby.

Lott, J.W. (1998). Assessment and management of cardiovascular dysfunction. In C. Kenner, A. Brueggemeyer, & L.P. Gunderson (Eds.), *Comprehensive neonatal nursing: A physiologic perspective* (2nd ed., pp. 306-335). Philadelphia: W.B. Saunders.

Lowe, N.K., & Reiss, R. (1996). Parturition and fetal adaptation. *Journal of Obstetric, Gynecologic, and Neonatal Nursing,* 25(4), 339-349.

MacMahon, J.R., Stevenson, D.K., & Oski, F.A. (1998). Physiologic jaundice. In H.W. Taeusch & R.A. Ballard (Eds.), *Avery's diseases of the newborn* (7th ed., pp. 1003-1007). Philadelphia: W.B. Saunders.

Maisels, M.J. (1999). Jaundice. In G.B. Avery, M.A. Fletcher, & M.G. MacDonald (Eds.), Neonatology: *Pathophysiology and management of the newborn* (5th ed., pp. 765-819). Philadelphia: Lippincott.

Meehan, R.M. (1998). Heelsticks in neonates for capillary blood sampling. *Neonatal Network,* 17(1), 17-24.

Miklos, A.B., & Creehan, P.A. (1996). Newborn physical assessment. In K.R. Simpson & P.A. Creehan (Eds.), *AWHONN's perinatal nursing* (pp. 307-335). Philadelphia: Lippincott.

National Association of Neonatal Nurses. (1997). *Neonatal thermoregulation: Guidelines for practice.* Petaluma, CA: Author.

Nelson, N. (1999). The onset of respirations. In G.B. Avery, M.A. Fletcher, & M.G. MacDonald (Eds.), *Neonatology, pathophysiology and management of the newborn* (5th ed., pp. 257-278). Philadelphia: Lippincott.

Nicholson, J.F., & Pesce, M.A. (2000). Reference ranges for laboratory tests and procedures. In R.E. Behrman, R.M. Kliegman, & H.B. Jenson (Eds.), *Nelson textbook of pediatrics* (16th ed., pp. 2181-2229). Philadelphia: W.B. Saunders.

Philip, A. (1996). *Neonatology, a practical guide* (4th ed.) Philadelphia: W.B. Saunders.

Pressler, J.L. & Hepworth, J.T. (1997). Newborn neurologic screening using NBAS reflexes. *Neonatal Network,* 16(6), 33-46.

Reimann, D., & Coughlin, M. (1996). Newborn adaptation to extrauterine life. In K.R. Simpson & P.A. Creehan (Eds.), *AWHONN's perinatal nursing* (pp. 289-306). Philadelphia: Lippincott-Raven.

Sansoucie, D.A., & Cavaliere, T.A. (1997). Transition from fetal to extrauterine circulation. *Neonatal Network,* 16(2), 5-12.

Smith, J. E. (2000). Hyperbilirubinemia. In *Core curriculum for maternal-newborn nursing* (2nd ed., pp. 705-715). Philadelphia: W.B. Saunders.

Smith, J.B., Ley, S.J., Curley, M.A.Q., Elixson, E.M., & Dodds, K.M. (1996). Tissue perfusion. In M.A.Q. Curley, J.B. Smith, & P.A. Moloney-Harmon (Eds.), *Critical care of infants and children* (pp. 155-248). Philadelphia: W.B. Saunders.

Sperling, M.A. (2000). Hypoglycemia. In R.E. Behrman, R.M. Kliegman, & H.B. Jenson (Eds.), *Nelson textbook of pediatrics* (16th ed., pp. 439-450). Philadelphia: W.B. Saunders.

Stoll, B.J. & Kliegman, R.M. (2000). The newborn infant. In R.E. Behrman, R.M. Kliegman, & H.B. Jenson (Eds.), *Nelson textbook of pediatrics* (16th ed., pp. 454-460). Philadelphia: W.B. Saunders.

Taeusch, H.W. & Sniderman, S. (1998). Initial evaluation: History and physical examination. In H.W. Taeusch & R.A. Ballard (Eds.), *Avery's diseases of the newborn* (7th ed., pp. 334-353). Philadelphia: W.B. Saunders.

Tsang, R.C., DeMarini, S., Rath, L.L. (1998). Fluids, electrolytes, vitamins, and trace minerals: Basis of ingestion, digestion, elimination, and metabolism. In C. Kenner, J.W. Lott, & A.A. Flandermeyer (Eds.), *Comprehensive neonatal nursing, a physiologic perspective* (2nd ed., pp. 336-353). Philadelphia: W.B. Saunders.

Vanderhoof, J.A., Zach, T.L., & Adrian, T.E. (1999). Gastrointestinal disease. In G.B. Avery, M.A. Fletcher, & M.G. MacDonald (Eds.), *Neonatology: pathophysiology and management of the newborn* (5th ed., pp. 739-763). Philadelphia: Lippincott.

Vargo, L. (1996). Cardiovascular assessment of the newborn. In E.P. Tappero & M.E. Honeyfield (Eds.), *Physical assessment of the newborn* (2nd ed., pp. 77-92). Petaluma, Calif.: NICU INK.

Watson, R.L. (1999). Gastrointestinal disorders. In J. Deacon & P. O'Neill. *Core curriculum for neonatal intensive care nursing* (2nd ed., pp. 254-293). Philadelphia: W.B. Saunders.

20 ASSESSMENT OF THE NORMAL NEWBORN

OBJECTIVES

1. Describe initial assessments of the newborn.
2. Explain the nurse's responsibilities in cardiorespiratory and thermoregulatory assessments.
3. Describe nursing assessments of body systems.
4. Explain the importance and components of gestational age assessment.
5. Describe newborn behavior, including periods of reactivity and behavior states.

DEFINITIONS

ACROCYANOSIS Bluish discoloration of the hands and feet because of reduced peripheral circulation.

CAFÉ-AU-LAIT SPOTS Light-brown birthmarks.

CAPUT SUCCEDANEUM Area of edema over the presenting part of the fetus or newborn resulting from pressure against the cervix; often called simply *caput.*

CEPHALHEMATOMA Bleeding between the periosteum and skull from pressure during birth; does not cross suture lines.

CHOANAL ATRESIA Abnormality of the nasal septum that obstructs one of both nasal passages.

CRANIOSYNOSTOSIS Premature closure of the sutures of the infant's head.

CRYPTORCHIDISM Failure of one or both testes to descend into the scrotum.

EPISPADIAS Abnormal placement of the urinary meatus on the dorsal side of the penis.

ERYTHEMA TOXICUM Benign rash of unknown cause in newborns, with blotchy red areas that may have white or yellow papules and vesicles in the center.

HYPOSPADIAS Abnormal placement of the urinary meatus on the ventral side of the penis.

LANUGO Fine, soft hair covering the fetus.

MILIA White cysts, 1 to 2 mm in size, from distended sebaceous glands.

MOLDING Shaping of the fetal head during movement through the birth canal.

MONGOLIAN SPOTS Bruise-like marks that occur mostly in newborns with dark skin tones.

NEVUS FLAMMEUS Permanent purple birthmark; also called *port wine stain.*

NEVUS VASCULOSUS Rough, red collection of capillaries with a raised surface that disappears with time.

DEFINITIONS—cont'd

Periodic Breathing Cessation of breathing lasting 5 to 10 seconds without changes in color or heart rate.

Point of Maximum Impulse (PMI) Area of the chest in which the heart sounds are loudest when auscultated.

Polydactyly More than 10 digits on the hands or feet.

Pseudomenstruation Vaginal bleeding in the newborn, resulting from withdrawal of placental hormones.

Strabismus A turning inward (crossing) or outward of the eyes because of poor muscle tone.

Syndactyly Webbing between fingers or toes.

Tachypnea Respiratory rate above 60 breaths per minute in the newborn after the first hour of life.

Telangiectatic Nevi Flat, pink areas on the nape of the neck and over the eyelids resulting from dilation of the capillaries; also called *stork bites* or *nevus simplex.*

Vernix Caseosa Thick, white substance that protects the skin of the fetus.

A very important role of the nurse is assessing the newborn to identify abnormalities and problems in adapting to life outside the uterus. The first complete assessment of the newborn often is called an *admission assessment.* Subsequent assessments are less detailed (Table 20-1). "Keys to Clinical Practice" (Appendix D) describes the order of initial assessments and care.

Early Assessments

Assessment for Anomalies

Immediately after birth, the infant is quickly examined for respiratory problems and obvious anomalies. The nurse determines whether resuscitation (p. 841) and other immediate interventions are necessary. When the infant is stable and oxygenating well, a more thorough assessment can be performed.

> The nurse should wear gloves when handling newborns until they are bathed and all blood is removed from the skin and hair. Wearing gloves helps protect the nurse from blood-borne infections.

If major abnormalities are present at birth, the nurse must maintain a calm, quiet demeanor to avoid frightening the parents. The physician should be alerted quietly and will explain the condition and possible plan of treatment to the parents.

Head

The newborn's head constitutes one fourth of the body size (Lepley, Gardner & Lubchenco, 1998). It is much larger in proportion to the rest of the body than in the adult. The head is palpated to assess the shape and identify abnormalities. The newborn who was in a breech position or delivered by cesarean not preceded by labor usually has a round head, whereas the infant born vaginally usually has some molding. The degree of molding, size of the fontanelles, and presence of caput succedaneum or later development of a cephalhematoma are noted.

The hair should be fine with a consistent hair pattern. Abnormal hair growth patterns may indicate genetic abnormalities. The nurse separates the hair, if necessary, to display bruises, rashes, and other marks on the scalp. A small, red mark is apparent if a fetal monitor electrode was inserted into the skin of the scalp. Later, a small scab forms. Occasionally, this area becomes infected.

Molding. The term *molding* refers to changes in the shape of the head that allow it to pass through the birth canal. It is caused by overriding of the cranial bones at the sutures and is common, especially after a long second stage of labor. The parietal bones often override the occipital and frontal bones, and a ridge can be felt at those areas. The condition generally resolves within a few days to 1 week after birth. Often, dramatic improvement is seen by the end of the first day of life. Parents may need reassurance that the infant's head is normal.

All suture lines should be palpated. Separation of more than 1 cm may indicate increased intracranial pressure (Johnson, 1996). If no space is found between suture lines, it may be the result of molding and overriding of the bones. However, lack of space between suture lines may indicate premature closure. This condition, called *craniosynostosis,* may impair brain growth and the shape of the head and requires surgery.

Fontanelles. The fontanelles are the areas of the head where sutures between the bones meet. In the newborn, the areas are not calcified but are covered by membrane. This allows space for the brain to grow.

The anterior fontanelle is a diamond-shaped area where the frontal and parietal bones meet (see Figure 12-5). It measures 1 to 4 cm and varies because of molding and individual differences. The fontanelle closes between 12 and 18 months of age. The posterior fontanelle is a triangular area where the occipital and parietal bones meet. It is much smaller than the anterior fontanelle, measuring 0.5 to 1 cm. This fontanelle closes by the time the infant is 2 to 3 months of age.

The nurse palpates the fontanelles and notes the position in relation to the other bones of the skull (Figure 20-1). Each fontanelle should be flat or level with the surrounding bones and feel soft. When the anterior fontanelle is palpated, the infant's head is elevated for accurate assessment. The infant can be placed in a

Text continued on p. 510

Table 20-1

SUMMARY OF NEWBORN ASSESSMENT

Normal	Abnormal (Possible Causes)	Nursing Considerations
INITIAL ASSESSMENT		
Assess for obvious problems first. If infant is stable and has no problems that require immediate attention, continue with the complete assessment.		
VITAL SIGNS		
Temperature		
36.5 to 37.5° C (97.7 to 99.5° F) axillary, 36.5 to 37.6° C (97.7 to 99.7° F) rectal. Axilla is preferred site.	Decreased (hypoglycemia, CNS problem, infection, cold environment). Increased (infection, environment too warm).	*Decreased:* Institute warming measures and check in 30 min. Check blood glucose. *Increased:* Remove excessive clothing. Check for dehydration. *Decreased or increased:* Look for signs of infection. Check radiant warmer or incubator temperature setting. Check thermometer for accuracy if skin is warm or cool to touch. Report abnormals to physician.
Pulses		
Heart rate 120 to 160 BPM (100 sleeping, 180 crying). Rhythm regular. Point of maximum impulse (PMI) at third to fourth intercostal space, slightly to left of midclavicular line, may be visible. Brachial, femoral, and pedal pulses present and equal bilaterally.	Tachycardia (respiratory problems, anemia, infection, cardiac conditions). Bradycardia (asphyxia, increased intracranial pressure). PMI to right (dextrocardia, pneumothorax). Murmurs (functional or congenital heart defects) and arrhythmias should be assessed by skilled practitioners. Absent or unequal pulses (coarctation of the aorta).	Note location of murmurs. Refer abnormal rates, rhythms, sounds, and pulses.
Respirations		
Rate 30 to 60 (average 40) per min. Respirations irregular, shallow, unlabored. Chest movements symmetric. Breath sounds present and clear bilaterally.	Tachypnea especially after the first hour. Slow respirations (maternal medications). Nasal flaring. Grunting (respiratory distress syndrome). Gasping (respiratory depression). Periods of apnea more than 20 seconds or with change in heart rate or color (respiratory depression, sepsis, cold stress). Asymmetry or decreased chest expansion (pneumothorax). Intercostal, xiphoid, subcostal, or supraclavicular retractions or seesaw respirations (respiratory distress). Moist, coarse breath sounds (rales, crackles, rhonchi) (fluid in lungs). Bowel sounds in chest (diaphragmatic hernia).	Mild variations require continued monitoring and usually clear in early hours after birth. If persistent or more than mild, suction, give oxygen, call physician, and initiate more intensive care.
Blood Pressure		
Average 65 to 95 mm Hg systolic and 30 to 60 mm Hg diastolic. Varies with activity, gestational age, and size.	Hypotension (hypovolemia, shock, sepsis). Difference of 20 mm Hg between arms and legs (coarctation of the aorta).	Refer abnormal blood pressures. Prepare for intensive care if very low.
MEASUREMENTS		
Weight		
Weight 2500 to 4000 g (5 lb, 8 oz to 8 lb, 13 oz). Weight loss up to 10% in early days.	Above normal range (LGA, maternal diabetes). Below normal range (SGA, preterm, multifetal pregnancy, medical conditions in mother that affect intrauterine growth). Weight loss above 10% (dehydration, feeding problems).	Determine cause. Monitor for complications common to cause.

CNS, Central nervous system; *BPM,* beats per minute; *LGA,* large for gestational age; *SGA,* small for gestational age.

Continued

Table 20-1
SUMMARY OF NEWBORN ASSESSMENT—cont'd

Normal	Abnormal (Possible Causes)	Nursing Considerations
Length		
48 to 53 cm (19 to 21 inches).	Below normal range (SGA, congenital dwarfism). Above normal range (LGA, maternal diabetes).	Determine cause. Monitor for complications common to cause.
Head Circumference		
33 to 35.5 cm (13 to 14 inches). Head approximately one fourth of infant's length.	Small (SGA, microcephaly, anencephaly). Large (LGA, hydrocephalus, increased intracranial pressure).	Determine cause. Monitor for complications common to cause.
Chest Circumference		
30.5 to 33 cm (12 to 13 inches). Generally 2 to 3 cm less than head circumference.	Large (LGA). Small (SGA).	Determine cause. Monitor for complications common to cause.
POSTURE		
Flexed extremities resist extension, return quickly to flexed state. Hands usually clenched. Movements symmetric. Slight tremors on crying. Breech extended, stiff legs. "Molds" body to caretaker's when held, responds by quieting when needs met.	Limp, flaccid, "floppy," or rigid extremities (preterm, hypoxia, medications, CNS trauma). Hypertonic (neonatal abstinence syndrome, CNS damage). Jitteriness or tremors (low glucose or calcium level). Opisthotonus, seizures, stiff when held (CNS damage).	Seek cause, refer abnormalities.
CRY		
Lusty, strong.	High pitched (increased intracranial pressure). Weak, absent, irritable, catlike "mewing" (neurologic problems). Hoarse or crowing (laryngeal irritation).	Observe for changes, report abnormalities.
SKIN		
Color pink or tan (according to race) with acrocyanosis. Vernix caseosa in creases. Small amounts of lanugo over shoulders, sides of face or forehead, and upper back. Skin turgor good with quick recoil. Some cracking and peeling of skin. Normal variations: Milia. Erythema toxicum (flea bite rash). Puncture on scalp (from electrode). Mongolian spots. Telangiectatic nevi (nevus simplex or "stork bites").	Color: Cyanosis of mouth and central areas (hypoxia). Pallor (anemia, hypoxia). Gray (hypoxia, hypotension). Red, sticky, translucent skin (very preterm). Ruddy (polycythemia). Greenish brown discoloration of skin, nails, cord (possible fetal compromise, postterm). Harlequin color (normal or cardiac problems, sepsis). Mottling (normal or cold stress, hypovolemia, sepsis). Yellow vernix (blood incompatibilities). Jaundice (pathologic if first 24 hours). Thick vernix (preterm). Delivery marks: Bruises on body (pressure), scalp (vacuum extractor), or face (cord around neck). Petechiae (pressure, low platelets, infection). Forceps marks. Birthmarks: Nevus flammeus (port wine stain). Nevus vasculosus (strawberry hemangioma). Café-au-lait spots (>6 or spots >13 cm, neurofibromatosis). Other: Excessive lanugo (preterm). Excessive peeling, cracking (postterm). Skin tags. Pustules or other rashes (infection). "Tenting" of skin (dehydration).	Differentiate facial bruising from cyanosis. Central cyanosis requires suction, oxygen, and further treatment. Refer jaundice in first 24 hr. Watch for respiratory problems in infants with meconium staining. Look for other signs and complications of preterm or postterm birth. Record location, size, shape, color, type of rashes, and marks. Check for facial movement with forceps marks. Watch for jaundice with bruising and ruddy color. Point out and explain normal skin variations to parents.

CNS, Central nervous system; *BPM,* beats per minute; *LGA,* large for gestational age; *SGA,* small for gestational age.

Table 20-1
SUMMARY OF NEWBORN ASSESSMENT—cont'd

Normal	Abnormal (Possible Causes)	Nursing Considerations
HEAD		
Sutures palpable with small separation between each. Anterior fontanelle diamond shaped, 1 to 4 cm across, soft and flat. May bulge slightly with crying. Posterior fontanelle triangular, 0.5 to 1 cm in size. Hair silky and soft with individual hair strands and consistent pattern. Normal variations: Overriding sutures (molding). Caput succedaneum or cephalhematoma (pressure during birth).	Head large (hydrocephalus, increased intracranial pressure) or small (microcephaly). Widely separated sutures (hydrocephalus) or sutures not palpable (craniosynostosis). Anterior fontanelle depressed (dehydration, molding), full or bulging at rest (hydrocephalus, increased intracranial pressure). Woolly, bunchy hair (preterm). Unusual hair pattern (genetic abnormalities).	Seek cause of variations. Observe for signs of dehydration with depressed fontanelle, increased intracranial pressure with bulging of fontanelle and wide separation of sutures. Refer for treatment. Differentiate caput succedaneum from cephalhematoma and reassure parents of normal outcome. Observe for jaundice with cephalhematoma.
EARS		
Ears well formed and complete. Area where upper ear meets head even with imaginary line drawn from inner to outer canthus of eye. Startle response to loud noises. Alerts to high-pitched voices.	Low-set ears (chromosomal disorders). Skin tags, preauricular sinuses, dimples, malformations (kidney anomalies). No response to sound (deafness).	Check voiding if ears abnormal. Look for signs of chromosomal abnormality if position abnormal. Refer for evaluation if no response to sound.
FACE		
Symmetric in appearance and movement. Parts proportional and appropriately placed.	Asymmetry of jaw (pressure and position in utero). Drooping of mouth or one side of face, "one-sided cry" (facial nerve damage). Abnormal appearance (chromosomal abnormalities).	Seek cause of variations. Check delivery history for possible cause of damage to facial nerve.
EYES		
Symmetric. Eyes clear. Transient strabismus. Scant or absent tears. Pupils equal, react to light. Alerts to interesting sights. Follows objects across midline. Doll's eye sign present. Red reflex present. May have subconjunctival hemorrhage or edema of eyelids from pressure during delivery.	Inflammation or drainage (chemical or infectious conjunctivitis). Constant tearing (plugged lacrimal duct). Unequal pupils. Failure to follow objects (blindness). White areas over pupils (cataracts). Setting-sun sign (hydrocephalus). Yellow sclera (jaundice). Blue sclera osteogenesis imperfecta.	Clean and monitor any drainage; seek cause. Reassure parents that subconjunctival hemorrhage and edema will clear. Refer other abnormalities.
NOSE		
Both nostrils open to air flow. May have slight flattening from pressure during birth.	Blockage of one or both nasal passages (choanal atresia). Malformations (congenital conditions). Flaring, mucus (respiratory distress).	Observe for respiratory distress; report malformations.
MOUTH		
Mouth, gums, tongue pink. Tongue normal in size and movement. Lips and palate intact. Sucking pads. Sucking, rooting, swallowing, gag reflexes present. Normal variations: precocious teeth, Epstein's pearls.	Cyanosis (hypoxia). White patches on cheeks or tongue (candidiasis). Protruding tongue (Down syndrome). Diminished movement of tongue, drooping mouth (facial nerve paralysis). Unilateral or bilateral cleft lip or palate, or both. Absent or weak reflexes (preterm, neurologic problem). Excessive drooling (tracheoesophageal fistula, esophageal atresia).	Oxygen for cyanosis. Expect loose teeth to be removed. Obtain order for nystatin medication for candidiasis. Check mother for vaginal or breast infection. Refer anomalies.

Continued

Table 20-1
SUMMARY OF NEWBORN ASSESSMENT—cont'd

Normal	Abnormal (Possible Causes)	Nursing Considerations
Feeding		
Good suck/swallow coordination. Retains feedings.	Poorly coordinated suck and swallow. Duskiness or cyanosis during feeding (cardiac defects). Choking, gagging, excessive drooling (tracheoesophageal fistula, esophageal atresia).	Feed slowly. Stop frequently if difficulty occurs. Suction and stimulate if necessary. Refer infants with continued difficulty for further investigation.
Neck/Clavicles		
Short neck turns head easily side to side. Infant raises head when prone. Clavicles intact.	Weakness, contractures, or rigidity (muscle abnormalities). Webbing of neck or large fat pad at back of neck (chromosomal disorders). Crepitus, lump, or crying when clavicle palpated, with diminished or absent movement of arm on that side (fractured clavicle).	Fracture of clavicle occurs especially in large infants with shoulder dystocia at birth. Immobilize arm. Look for other injuries. Refer abnormalities.
Chest		
Cylinder or barrel shape. Xiphoid process may be prominent. Symmetric. Nipples present and located properly. May have engorgement, white nipple discharge (maternal hormone withdrawal).	Asymmetry (diaphragmatic hernia, pneumothorax). Supernumerary nipples. Redness (infection).	Report abnormalities.
Abdomen		
Rounded, soft. Bowel sounds present soon after birth. Liver palpable 1 to 3 cm below costal margin. Skin intact. Three vessels in cord. Clamp tight and cord drying. Meconium passed within 12 to 48 hr. Urine passed within 12 to 24 hr. Normal variation: Brick dust staining of diaper (urate crystals).	Sunken abdomen (diaphragmatic hernia). Distended abdomen or loops of bowel visible (obstruction, infection, enlarged organs). Absent bowel sounds after first hr (paralytic ileus). Masses palpated (kidney tumors, distended bladder). Enlarged liver (infection, heart failure, hemolytic disease). Abdominal wall defects (umbilical or inguinal hernia, omphalocele, gastroschisis, extrophy of bladder). Two vessels in cord (other anomalies). Bleeding (loose clamp). Redness, drainage from cord (infection). No passage of meconium (imperforate anus, obstruction). Lack of urinary output (kidney problems) or inadequate amounts (dehydration).	Refer abnormalities. Look for other anomalies if only two vessels in cord. Tighten or replace loose cord clamp. If stool and urine output abnormal, check to see whether a void or stool was not recorded, increase feedings, report.
Genitals		
Female		
Labia majora dark, cover clitoris and labia minora. Small amount of white mucous vaginal discharge. Urinary meatus and vagina present. Normal variations: Vaginal bleeding (pseudomenstruation). Hymenal tags.	Clitoris and labia minora larger than labia majora (preterm). Large clitoris (ambiguous genitalia). Edematous labia (breech birth).	Check gestational age for immature genitalia. Refer anomalies.

CNS, Central nervous system; *BPM,* beats per minute; *LGA,* large for gestational age; *SGA,* small for gestational age.

Table 20-1
SUMMARY OF NEWBORN ASSESSMENT—cont'd

Normal	Abnormal (Possible Causes)	Nursing Considerations
GENITALS—CONT'D		
Male		
Testes within scrotal sac, rugae on scrotum, prepuce nonretractable. Meatus at tip of penis.	Testes in inguinal canal or abdomen (preterm, cryptorchidism). Lack of rugae on scrotum (preterm). Edema of scrotum (pressure in breech birth). Enlarged scrotal sac (hydrocele). Small penis, scrotum (preterm, ambiguous genitalia). Urinary meatus located on upper side of penis (epispadias), underside of penis (hypospadias), or perineum.	Check gestational age for immature genitalia. Refer anomalies. Explain to parents why circumcision cannot be performed with abnormal placement of meatus.
EXTREMITIES		
Upper and Lower Extremities		
Equal and bilateral movement of extremities. Correct number and formation of fingers and toes. Nails to ends of digits or slightly beyond. Flexion, good muscle tone.	Crepitus, redness, lumps, swelling (fracture). Diminished or lack of movement, especially during Moro reflex (fracture, nerve damage, paralysis). Polydactyly (note presence or absence of bone in extra digits). Syndactyly (webbing) or fused or absent digits. Poor muscle tone (preterm, neurologic damage, hypoglycemia, hypoxia).	Refer all anomalies, look for others.
Upper Extremities		
Two transverse palm creases.	Simian crease (single transverse palm crease) (Down syndrome). Diminished movement of arm with extension and forearm prone (Erb-Duchenne paralysis).	Refer all anomalies, look for others.
Lower Extremities		
Legs equal in length, abduct equally, gluteal and thigh creases and knee height equal, no hip "clunk." Normal position of feet.	Resistance when one leg is abducted, unequal thigh or gluteal creases, abnormal Ortolani and Barlow tests, unequal leg length (developmental dysplasia of the hip). Malposition of feet, which may or may not be manually manipulated into normal position (position in utero, talipes equinovarus).	Refer all anomalies, look for others.
BACK: VERTEBRAL COLUMN		
No openings observed or felt. Anus patent. Pilonidal dimple.	Failure of vertebra to close (spina bifida), with or without sac with spinal fluid and meninges (meningocele) and/or cord (myelomeningocele) enclosed. Tuft of hair over spina bifida occulta. Pilonidal dimple with sinus. Imperforate anus.	Refer abnormalities. Observe for movement below level of defect. If sac, cover with sterile dressings wet with sterile saline. Protect from injury.
REFLEXES		
Moro, palmar and plantar grasp, rooting, sucking, swallowing, tonic neck, Babinski, Galant, and stepping reflexes present (see Table 20-2).	Absent, asymmetric, or weak reflexes.	Observe for signs of fractures, nerve damage, or injury to CNS.

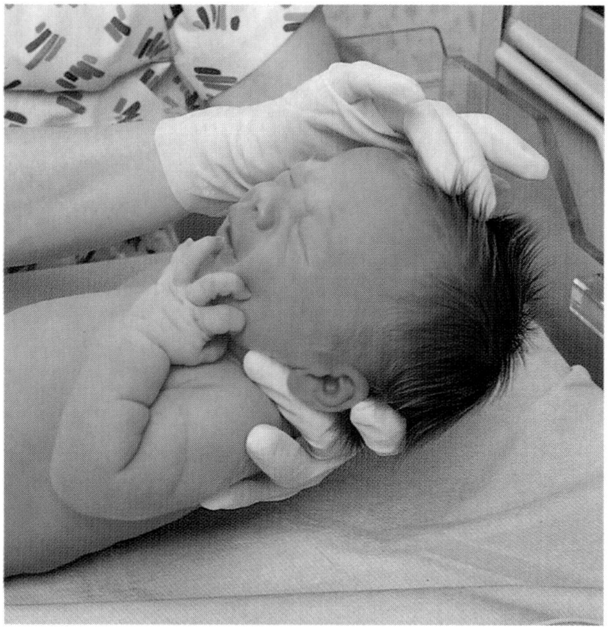

FIGURE 20-1 Palpation of the anterior fontanelle. Note elevation of the head.

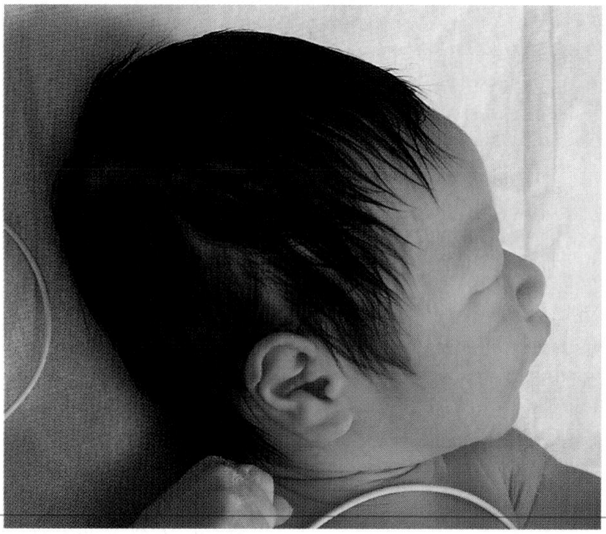

FIGURE 20-2 Caput succedaneum is an edematous area on the head from pressure against the cervix. It may cross suture lines.

semi-sitting position or held in an upright position. The fontanelle should be palpated when the infant is quiet because vigorous crying may cause it to protrude.

Although the anterior fontanelle may bulge slightly when the infant cries, bulging at rest may indicate increased intracranial pressure. A fontanelle that is between flat and bulging is termed *full.* A larger-than-normal fontanelle may be a sign of increased pressure within the skull. A depressed fontanelle is unusual in a newborn unless it is the result of molding. After molding resolves, a depressed fontanelle is a sign of dehydration. Abnormal signs are reported to the primary care provider.

Molding may complicate the identification of the posterior fontanelle because the overlapping bones impinge on that space. The posterior fontanelle feels like a dimple at the juncture of the occipital and parietal bones. Careful palpation is necessary.

Caput Succedaneum. A caput succedaneum often appears over the vertex of the newborn's head as a result of pressure against the mother's cervix during labor (Figure 20-2). The pressure interferes with blood flow from the area, causing localized edema at birth. The edematous area crosses suture lines, is soft, and varies in size. It resolves quickly and disappears within 12 hours to several days after birth. Caput also may occur when a vacuum extractor is used to hasten second stage labor. When a vacuum is used, the caput corresponds to the area where the extractor was placed on the skull. The amount of edema and presence of bruising are assessed.

Cephalhematoma. In a cephalhematoma, bleeding occurs between the periosteum and skull as a result of pressure during birth (Figure 20-3). It occurs on one or both sides of the head over the parietal bones, although it occasionally forms over the occipital bone. The firm swelling is not present at birth but develops within the first 24 to 48 hours.

The area is carefully palpated to determine whether the swelling crosses suture lines. A cephalhematoma has clear edges that end at the suture lines. It does not cross the suture lines, unlike a caput succedaneum, because the bleeding is held between the bone and its covering, which is the periosteum. A cephalhematoma reabsorbs slowly and is generally gone within a few weeks after birth. Because of the breakdown of the red blood cells within the hematoma, affected infants are at greater risk for jaundice.

Both caput succedaneum and cephalhematoma may be frightening to parents. During the assessment, the nurse can reassure parents that the conditions are not harmful to the infant. Even if parents do not ask, they need information about the causes and length of time required for the areas to resolve.

Face. The face is examined for symmetry, positioning of the facial features, movement, and expression. A transient asymmetry from intrauterine pressure may occur, lasting a few weeks or months. Irregularities of the facial features should be reported.

Neck and Clavicles

The nurse assesses the infant's neck visually and notes the infant's ability to turn the head easily from side to side. The neck is very short. Webbing may indicate Turner's syndrome. An unusually large fat pad between

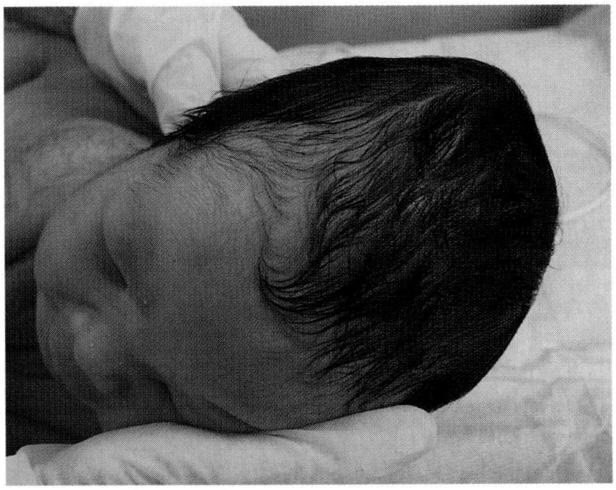

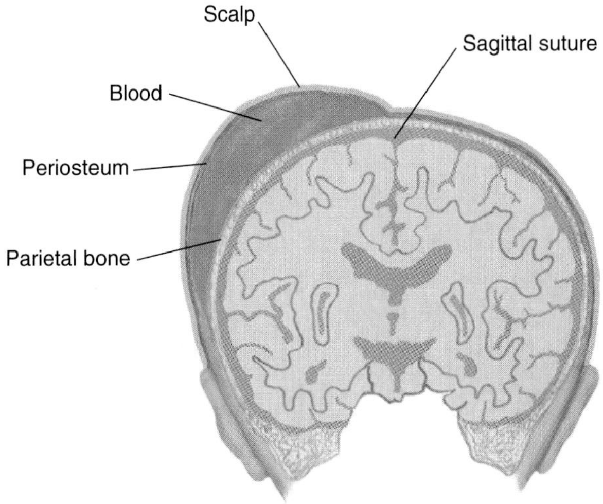

FIGURE 20-3 A cephalhematoma is characterized by bleeding between the bone and its covering, the periosteum. It may occur on one or both sides and does not cross suture lines.

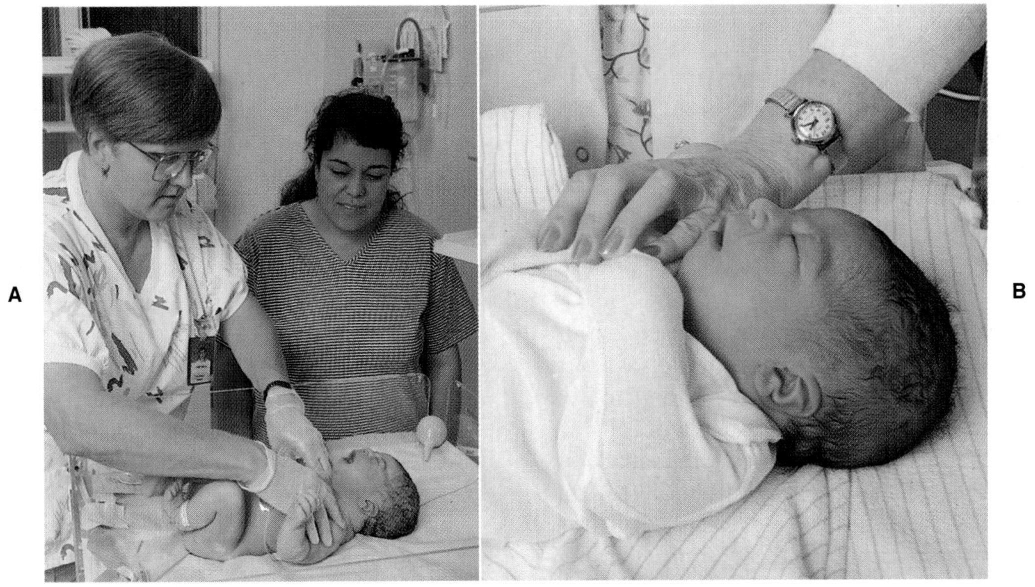

FIGURE 20-4 **A,** The nurse palpates the clavicles to identify fractures. A fracture of the left clavicle is present. **B,** The arm on the side of the fractured clavicle is immobilized by pinning the sleeve to the shirt.

the occiput and the shoulders may indicate Down syndrome. When lying in a prone position, the newborn should be able to raise the head briefly and turn it to the other side.

Fractures of the clavicle are more likely to occur in large infants, especially when shoulder dystocia occurred. If a fracture is present, a lump or tenderness over the area of the fracture may be observed. Crepitus (grating of the bone) and movement of the bone may be felt during palpation. Swelling of the area and decreased movement of the arm on the affected side also may occur. A difference in the movement of the arms is especially noticeable when the Moro reflex is elicited. Damage to the brachial plexus may cause paralysis of the arm on the side of the fracture. Treatment of a fractured clavicle includes immobilization of the affected arm (Figure 20-4).

Cord

The umbilical cord should contain three vessels. The two arteries are small and may stand up at the cut end. The single vein is larger than the arteries and resembles a slit because its walls are more easily compressed. If only one artery is present, the infant is carefully assessed for other anomalies. A two-vessel cord is associated with chromosomal, renal, and gastrointestinal de-

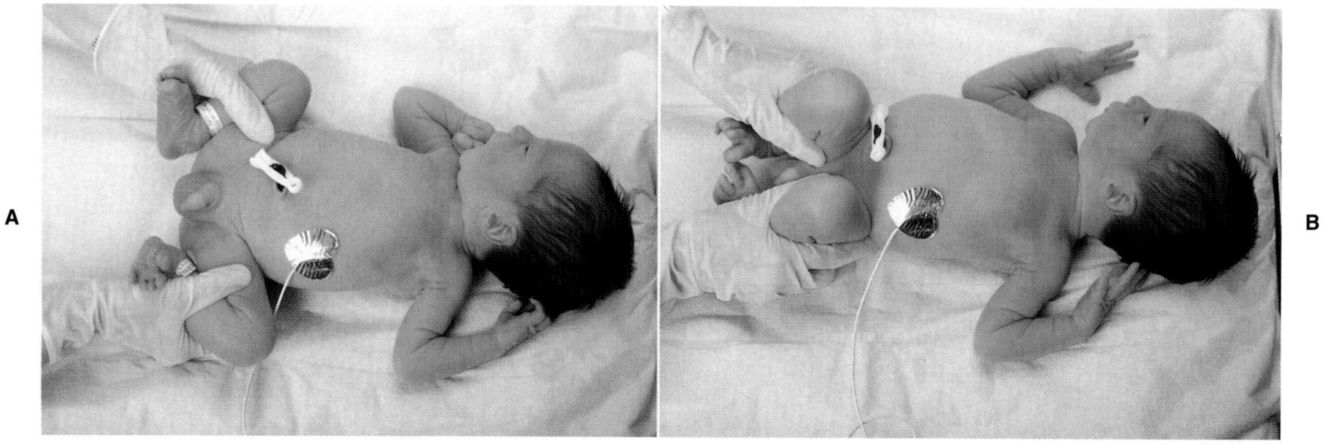

FIGURE 20-5 Assessment of the hips. Place the fingers over the infant's greater trochanter and thumbs over the femur. Bend the knees and hips at a 90-degree angle. **A,** Ortolani test: Abduct the thighs, and apply gentle pressure forward over the greater trochanter. A "clunking" sensation indicates a dislocated femoral head moving into the acetabulum. A hip click may be felt or heard but is usually normal. **B,** Barlow test: Adduct the hips and apply gentle pressure down and back with the thumbs. In hip dysplasia, the examiner can feel the femoral head move out of the acetabulum.

fects. The amount of Wharton's jelly in the cord is noted. If the cord appears thin, the infant may have been poorly nourished in utero. A yellow-brown or green tinge to the cord indicates that meconium was released at some time before birth, perhaps as a result of fetal compromise.

Extremities

The normal infant should actively move the extremities equally in a random manner. The extremities of a term infant should remain sharply flexed and resist extension during examination. Poor muscle tone results in a limp or "floppy" infant, which may be the result of inadequate oxygen during birth but should resolve within a few minutes as oxygen intake increases. Continued poor muscle tone may result from prematurity or neurologic damage. Infants with previously good muscle tone may show decreased flexion if they become hypoglycemic or experience respiratory difficulty.

All extremities are examined for signs of fractures such as crepitus, redness, lumps or swelling, and lack of use. Independent movement of each extremity should be determined to identify possible damage to nerves that may occur with or without fractures.

Injury to the brachial nerve plexus may result in Erb's palsy (Erb-Duchenne paralysis), paralysis of the shoulder and arm muscles. Instead of the usual flexed position, the affected arm is extended at the infant's side with the forearm prone. Movement of this arm is diminished during the Moro reflex. The condition is treated by exercise, splinting, or both.

Hands and Feet. The fingers and toes are examined for extra digits (polydactyly) and webbing between digits (syndactyly). Extra digits often are small and may not have bones. Tying the extra digits with sutures causes them to atrophy. Presence of a bone in the extra digit requires surgical removal. Webbed fingers or toes may be corrected by surgery. Nails in a term infant should extend to the end of the fingers or slightly beyond.

The creases in the hands also are examined. Normally, two long transverse creases extend most of the way across the palm. A single crease that crosses the palm without a break parallel with the base of the fingers is called a *simian crease* or *line.* It may be seen with an incurving of the little finger in Down syndrome. The simian line alone is not diagnostic of Down syndrome, however, and may occur in normal infants, usually on one hand only.

The feet are assessed for talipes equinovarus, or clubfoot, a common malformation of the feet. If a foot looks abnormal, it should be gently manipulated. If it moves to a normal position, the abnormality is probably temporary, resulting from the position of the infant in the uterus. In true clubfoot, the foot turns inward and cannot be moved to a midline position. Casting is the usual treatment, but sometimes surgery is necessary.

Hips. The hips are examined for developmental dysplasia of the hip. This is a condition where instability of the hip joint occurs and the femur can be moved in and out of the acetabulum. Partial dislocation and inadequate development of the acetabulum may occur. The condition occurs more often in breech presentation and if prolonged oligohydramnios prevented normal movement. Identifying a hip problem early is important to prevent permanent damage to the joint.

Ortolani and Barlow tests are methods of assessing for hip instability in the newborn period (Figure 20-5). Both legs should abduct equally in normal infants.

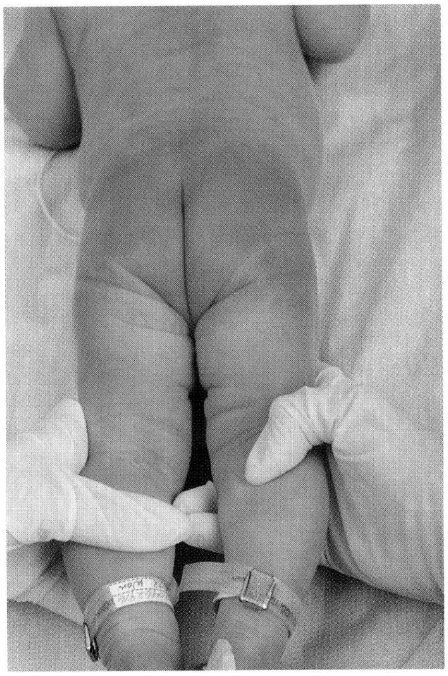

FIGURE 20-6 Note the symmetry of gluteal and thigh creases.

Abducting the affected hip may be difficult. A hip click may be felt or heard but is usually normal and different from the "clunk" of hip dysplasia (Thompson & Scoles, 2000).

The infant's knees should be bent with the feet flat on the bed to compare the height of the knees. If the hip is dislocated, the knee on the affected side is lower. The legs are extended while the infant is in a prone position to determine whether they are equal in length and thigh and gluteal creases are symmetric (Figure 20-6). If the hip is dislocated, the leg on the affected side is shorter and the creases are asymmetric. Because the hip may be unstable but not yet dislocated, these signs are not always present at birth.

Treatment of developmental dysplasia of the hip involves immobilizing the leg in a flexed, abducted position, usually with a harness. Early identification and treatment is essential to provide the best results in correcting the problem. Treatment may involve surgery and casting if the condition is not discovered early.

Vertebral Column

The nurse palpates the entire length of the newborn's vertebral column to discover any defects in the vertebrae. An indentation is a sign of spina bifida occulta (failed closing of a vertebra). The defect is not obvious on visual inspection because it is covered with skin, but sometimes a tuft of hair grows over the area. Other, more obvious neural tube defects include meningoceles and myelomeningoceles, which are protrusions of nerves, the spinal cord, or both through the defect in the vertebrae. They appear as a sac on the back and may be covered by skin or only the meninges. The tissue should be covered with moist, sterile, saline dressings immediately after birth (p. 865). A pilonidal dimple may be present at the base of the spine. It should be examined for a sinus and the depth noted.

Measurements

Measurements provide information about the infant's growth in utero. The weight, length, and head and chest circumference are part of the initial assessment (Procedure 20-1). The measurements are compared with the norms for the infant's gestational age. When a difference is noted between the expected and actual values, expanded assessments are necessary. For example, a newborn may be larger or smaller than expected because of an error in calculating the length of the pregnancy.

Weight

The newborn's weight ranges between 2500 and 4000 g (5 pounds, 8 ounces and 8 pounds, 13 ounces) (Howard-Glenn, 2000). The average weight of a full-term newborn is 3400 g (7.5 pounds). If the infant's weight is outside the average range, possible causes are assessed. Factors affecting weight include gestational age, placental functioning, maternal diabetes, and genetic factors such as race and parental size.

Infants are weighed each day they are in the birth facility and at follow-up visits. They can be expected to lose between 5% and 10% of their birth weight during the first few days of life (Bell & Oh, 1999). This weight loss is because of excretion of meconium from the bowel and normal loss of extracellular fluid. In addition, newborns generally do not consume enough calories to maintain their weight during this period. Infants normally regain birth weight by the tenth day of life. Thereafter they gain about 20 g (⅔ oz) per day until the middle of the first year (Bowden, Dickey, & Greenberg, 1998).

Length

The infant's length is measured from the top of the head to the end of the outstretched leg. The average length of a full-term newborn is 48 to 53 cm (19 to 21 inches) (Howard-Glenn, 2000). Some agencies also record the crown-to-rump measurement, which is approximately equal to the head circumference.

Head and Chest Circumference

The diameter of the head is measured around the occiput and just above the eyebrows. The average head circumference of the term newborn is 33 to 35.5 cm (13 to 14 inches) (Howard-Glenn, 2000). The measurement may be affected by molding of the skull during the birth process. If a large amount of molding occurred, the head is remeasured when it regains its normal shape. An abnormally small head may indicate poor brain growth and microcephaly. A very large head may be a sign of hydrocephalus.

PROCEDURE 20-1

Weighing and Measuring the Newborn

Purpose: To obtain accurate measurements of the newborn

Weight

1. Cover the scale with a blanket. Place a paper cover over the blanket if desired. *Prevents conductive heat loss from contact between the infant and a cold surface, helps prevent cross-contamination, and makes cleaning easier.*
2. Balance or adjust the scale to zero after the covering is placed. Electronic scale: push the "on" button and check to see that the digital readout is at zero. The electronic scale is usually self adjusting. Balance scale: Adjust until the balance arm is horizontal. *Results in accurate weighing of the infant without including weight of the scale covering.*
3. Place the infant in supine position on the scale. Keep one hand just above the infant and watch the infant carefully throughout the procedure. *Infants often are upset when first placed on the scale, and the startle or Moro reflex may occur. They may be in danger of sliding off the scale.*

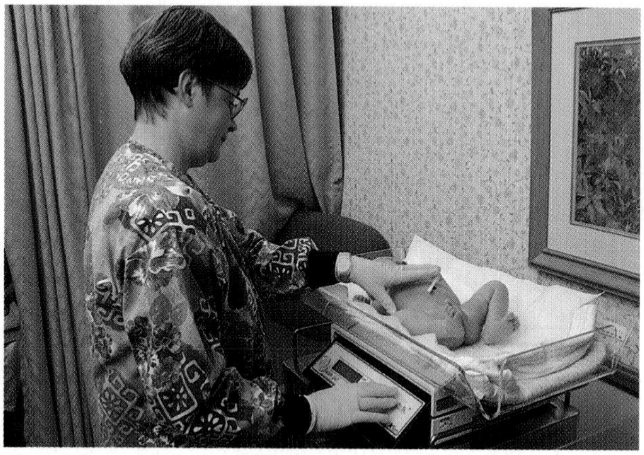

4. Wait until the infant is somewhat quiet. The electronic scale displays weight in pounds and ounces or in grams. Some electronic scales display "stable" when an accurate weight has been obtained. For a balance scale, move weights slowly until the arm is level. *Waiting until the infant is quiet increases accuracy.*
5. Write the numbers down immediately. If the scale is covered with paper, the weight can be written on the paper and taken with the infant to the warmer. Write it on the nurses' notes when the infant is safely settled. *Prevents forgetting the weight.*
6. Compare weight with the normal range for term infants: 2500 to 4000 g (5 lb, 8 oz to 8 lb, 13 oz). *Shows whether the infant is within expected range.*

Length

Ruler Printed on Scale or Crib

1. Place the infant in supine position with his or her head at the upper edge of the ruler. *Places the infant in the proper position.*
2. While holding the infant with one hand so that the head does not move, use the other hand to fully extend the infant's leg along the ruler. Note the length at the bottom of the heel. *Holding the infant firmly ensures safety and allows an accurate measurement.*

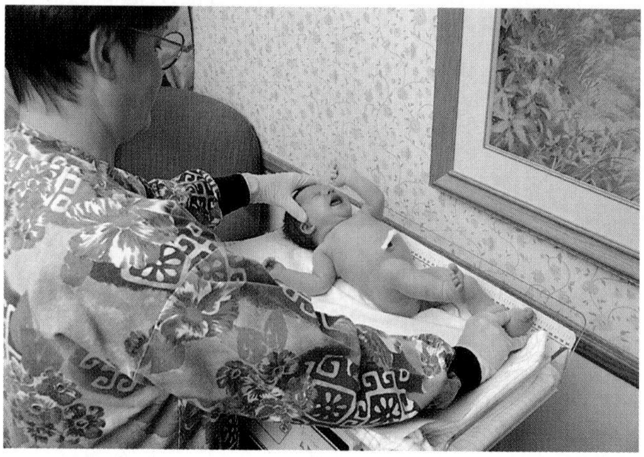

Tape Measure

1. When using a paper tape, be sure that it has no partial tears in it. *A torn measuring tape would give an inaccurate measurement.*
2. Place tape beside the infant, with the upper end at the top of the head. Tuck it beneath the shoulder, and extend it down to the feet. *Prevents movement of the tape and helps ensure accurate measurements.*
3. Hold the tape straight alongside the infant's body while extending one leg full length. Be sure that the tape has not moved from the top of the head. *Careful attention to tape placement ensures accurate measurement.*

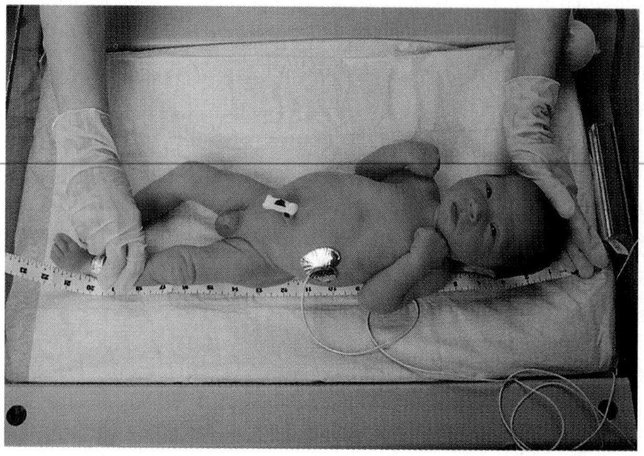

4. Another method is to mark the paper on which the infant is lying at the top of the head and the end of the extended leg. Then measure the distance between the two marks. *(Makes measuring more accurate when the infant is very active.)*
5. Compare with normal range of 48 to 53 cm (19 to 21 in). *Helps determine abnormalities.*

Head and Chest Circumference

1. Measure around the fullest part of the head with the tape placed around the occiput and just over the eyebrows. *Allows measurement of the largest diameter of the head.*

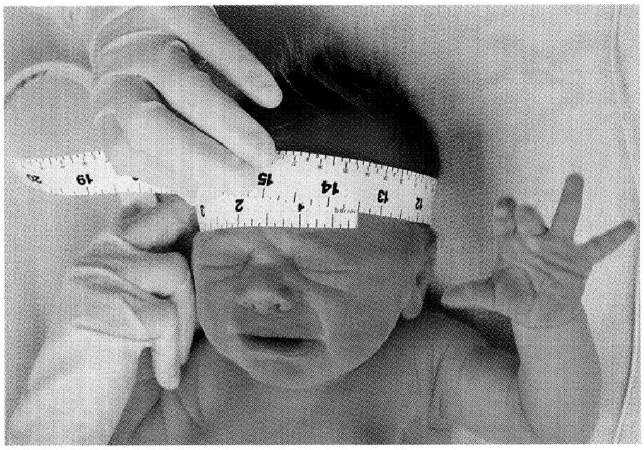

2. Move tape down to measure the chest at the level of the nipples. Be sure that the tape is even and taut. *Ensures accurate measurement.*

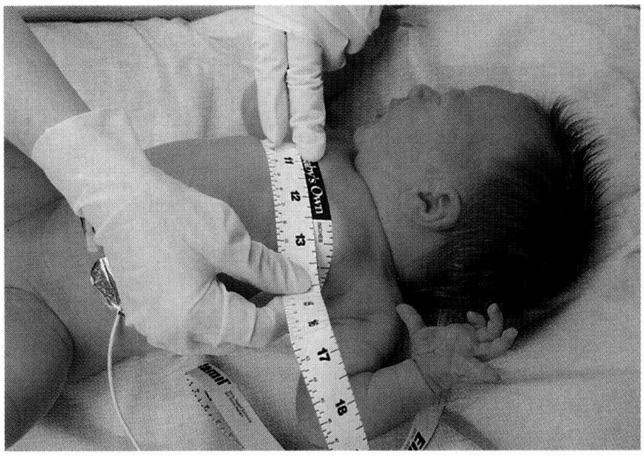

3. Remove tape by lifting or rolling the infant instead of pulling the tape. *Pulling tape can cut the infant's skin.*
4. Compare measurements with normal range. Head: 33 to 35.5 cm (13 to 14 in). Chest: 30.5 to 33 cm (12 to 13 in). *Determines whether the infant's measurements are normal.*

The chest is measured at the level of the nipples. It usually is 2 to 3 cm smaller than the head. The average circumference of the chest is 30.5 to 33 cm (12 to 13 inches) (Howard-Glenn, 2000). If molding of the head is present, the head and chest measurement may be equal at birth.

Check Your Reading

1. What are the differences among molding, caput succedaneum, and cephalhematoma?
2. What is the purpose of the quick initial assessment of the infant after birth?
3. Why are measurements of the neonate important?

ASSESSMENT OF CARDIORESPIRATORY STATUS

Assessments of respiratory and cardiovascular status are performed together because transitional changes take place in both systems at birth. Problems of adaptation in one system likely will result in problems in the other system.

History

Information about the pregnancy, labor, and delivery is important in assessing the infant's cardiovascular and respiratory status and likelihood of problems at birth. For example, if the mother received narcotic analgesics late in labor, depression of the fetal central nervous system may interfere with initiation of respirations in the neonate. Preterm infants may not produce adequate amounts of surfactant, and atelectasis may occur because the alveoli do not remain open.

CRITICAL TO REMEMBER

Normal Vital Signs in the Newborn

- Temperature: 36.5 to 37.5° C (97.7 to 99.5° F) axillary, 36.5 to 37.6° C (97.7 to 99.7° F) rectal
- Apical pulse: 120 to 160/BPM (100 sleeping, 180 crying)
- Respirations: 30 to 60 breaths/minute (average 40/minute)

Airway

During birth, some fetal lung fluid is forced into the upper airway. Excessive fluid and mucus in the infant's respiratory passages may cause respiratory difficulty for several hours after birth.

Respiratory Rate

The nurse assesses respirations at least once every 30 minutes until the infant has been stable for 2 hours after birth (AAP/ACOG, 1997). If abnormalities are noted, respirations are assessed more often. The nor-

PROCEDURE 20-2

Assessing Vital Signs in the Newborn

Purpose: To obtain an accurate measurement of newborn vital signs.

Respirations

1. Assess respirations when the infant is quiet or sleeping and before disturbing the infant for other assessments, if possible. *Allows the lung sounds to be heard more clearly.*
2. Assess respirations by observing and auscultating the chest and abdomen. *The rapid, shallow, irregular respirations can be confused with other movements in an active infant. A combination of methods increases accuracy of the assessment.*
3. Lift the infant's blanket and shirt to visualize the chest and abdomen. Observe the pattern of respirations before beginning to count. *Respirations are often irregular, but a basic pattern exists. Observation of the pattern makes it easier to count the rate.*
4. To auscultate respirations, place a stethoscope on the right side of the infant's chest. *Allows the sounds of the lungs to be heard with less interference from heart sounds.*
5. If desired, place a hand lightly over the infant's chest or abdomen to feel the movement. *Palpation helps keep track of the rate.*
6. Count for a full minute. *Respirations are normally irregular in the newborn. Counting for a full minute increases accuracy.*
7. If the infant is crying, continue to count and note it on the chart. Allow the infant to suck on a pacifier or gloved finger. *Although respirations are most easily assessed on a quiet infant, they can be counted when the infant is crying. Sucking may quiet the infant. Respirations may be faster on a crying infant.*
8. Expect the respiratory rate to be 30 to 60 breaths/minute (average 40) when the infant is at rest. Observe for signs of respiratory distress, including tachypnea, retractions, flaring, cyanosis, grunting, seesawing, apneic periods, and asymmetry of chest movements. *Allows identification and follow-up of abnormalities.*

Pulse

1. Listen to the apical pulse before disturbing the infant for other assessments. *The heart sounds are heard more clearly on a quiet or sleeping infant.*
2. Use a pediatric head on the stethoscope to listen to apical pulse. *Although a larger head may be used if necessary, the small head allows better contact between the stethoscope and the chest wall and eliminates some of the sounds from the lungs and intestines.*
3. If the infant is crying, insert a pacifier or a gloved finger into his or her mouth. *Sucking often quiets infants.*
4. If the infant cannot be quieted, increase concentration and time spent listening. *Helps separate the sounds heard and to focus in on the heart beat.*
5. Listen briefly before beginning to count. Tapping a finger in rhythm with the beat may be helpful. Count for a full minute. Expect the heart rate to be 120 to 160 BPM at rest. *Listening to the pattern allows time to get used to the rapid heart beat before counting. Counting for a full minute increases chances of identifying abnormalities.*
6. Move stethoscope over the entire heart area to listen to all sounds. Assess for arrhythmias, murmurs, or other abnormal sounds. Refer any abnormal sounds. *Listening over the entire area increases chances of hearing abnormal sounds. Reporting abnormalities to the pediatrician allows further investigation.*

Temperature

Axillary

1. Place the thermometer vertically along the chest wall in the center of the axillary space with the infant's arm held firmly over it. *If the thermometer is held horizontally, it may protrude behind the axilla and give an inaccurate reading. Holding the arm keeps the thermometer positioned correctly and prevents accidental injury if the infant moves unexpectedly.*
2. Read the thermometer at the proper time: electronic or digital, when indicator sounds; plastic strip, 1 to 1.5 minutes (with a 10-second wait before reading) or according to manufacturer's direction; glass, 5 minutes. Normal range: 36.5 to 37.5° C (97.7 to 99.5° F). *Ensures an accurate reading.*

Rectal

1. Avoid taking a rectal temperature if possible. Take a rectal temperature only when necessary and according to birth facility policy. Use the axillary method whenever possible. *Rectal and axillary readings are very similar. Rectal temperature involves the potential risk of perforation of the rectum, which can be life threatening.*
2. Lubricate the tip of the thermometer with water-soluble lubricant. *Allows the thermometer to be inserted without irritation to the sphincter. Water-soluble lubricant dissolves and washes away.*
3. Place the infant in a supine position and hold the ankles firmly in one hand. Bend the infant's knees against the abdomen and raise the legs to expose the anus. Or place the infant prone or on the side and separate the buttocks. *Provides visualization and prevents excessive movement that might dislodge the thermometer or cause it to break (if glass) or insert too far, resulting in injury to delicate tissues.*
4. Insert the thermometer carefully and gently no more than 0.5 inch into the rectum. *The rectum turns to the right 1 inch from the sphincter. Inserting the thermometer farther may cause perforation.*
5. Do not force the thermometer if it does not insert easily. *An obstruction may be preventing insertion of the thermometer.*
6. Hold the thermometer securely throughout the time it remains in the rectum. *Maintains control to avoid inserting the thermometer too far and prevents injury if the infant moves.*
7. Read the thermometer at the proper time: electronic or digital, when indicator sounds; glass, 5 minutes. Normal range: 36.5 to 37.6° C (97.7 to 99.7° F). *Ensures accurate reading.*

mal respiratory rate is 30 to 60 breaths per minute, with an average rate of 40 breaths per minute. The infant may breathe faster immediately after birth, during crying, and during the first and second periods of reactivity. Respirations should not be labored, and the chest movements should be symmetric. Because the pattern and depth of respirations are irregular, they must be counted for 1 full minute for accuracy.

Counting the rapid, shallow, irregular respirations of a newborn can be difficult at first. Differentiating between the respirations and other movements may be difficult while observing the infant's chest. Observation, auscultation, or palpation, alone or in combination, may be used to obtain an accurate respiratory rate (Procedure 20-2).

The nurse observes for periodic breathing, which are pauses in breathing lasting 5 to 10 seconds without other changes. This occurs is some full-term infants during the first few days but most often in preterm infants. Apnea lasting longer than 20 seconds or accompanied by cyanosis, heart rate changes, or other signs of difficult breathing is abnormal (Hagedorn, Gardner, & Abman, 1998).

Breath Sounds

The entire anterior and posterior lung fields are auscultated for breath sounds, which should be present equally throughout. Breath sounds should be clear over most areas. However, hearing sounds of moisture in the lungs during the first hour or two after birth is not unusual because fetal lung fluid has not been completely absorbed. Infants born by cesarean birth may not experience the changes that occur in the lungs during labor and birth and are more likely to have coarse breath sounds.

When the listener is not experienced in assessing the lungs of a newborn, distinguishing between clear breath sounds and coarse or moist sounds is less difficult than trying to describe crackles or wheezes. Abnormal and diminished sounds always should be reported to the primary care provider if they continue. They may indicate a pneumothorax. Bowel sounds in the chest may be a sign of diaphragmatic hernia.

Signs of Respiratory Distress

Throughout the assessment, the nurse must be alert for signs of respiratory distress, which may be present at birth or develop later. They include tachypnea, retractions, flaring nares, central cyanosis, grunting, moaning, and seesaw respirations. Whenever one sign of labored breathing is present, the assessment must be carefully expanded to identify others.

Tachypnea. Tachypnea, a respiratory rate above 60 breaths per minute, is the most common sign of respiratory distress. It is not unusual during the first hour after birth and during the second period of reactivity, but continued tachypnea is abnormal.

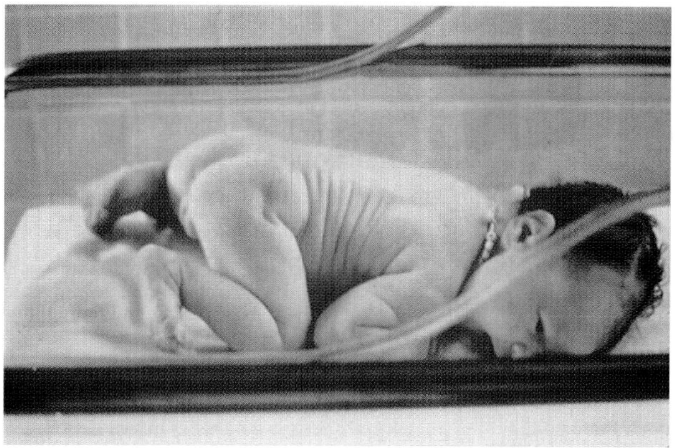

FIGURE 20-7 Acrocyanosis. (Courtesy Jane Deacon, The Children's Hospital, Denver, Colorado.)

Retractions. When the infant's weak chest wall muscles are used to help draw air into the lungs, retractions result. The soft tissue around the bones of the chest is drawn in with the effort of pulling air into the lungs. Xiphoid (substernal) retractions occur when the area under the sternum retracts each time the infant inhales. When the muscles between the ribs are pulled in so that each rib is outlined, intercostal retractions are present. The muscles above the sternum and around the clavicles also may be used to aid in respirations (supraclavicular retractions). Retractions may be mild or severe, depending on the degree of respiratory difficulty. Occasional mild retractions are common immediately after birth but should not continue after the first hour.

Flaring of the Nares. A reflex widening of the nostrils occurs when the infant is receiving insufficient oxygen. This helps to decrease airway resistance and increase the amount of air entering the lungs. Intermittent flaring may occur in the first hour after birth. Continued flaring indicates a more serious respiratory problem.

Cyanosis. Cyanosis is a purplish blue discoloration indicating that the infant is not getting enough oxygen. It may be preceded by a dusky or gray hue to the skin. Central cyanosis involves the lips, tongue, and trunk and indicates true hypoxia. It indicates that not enough oxygen is reaching the vital organs and requires immediate attention. Central cyanosis must be differentiated from peripheral cyanosis (acrocyanosis), which involves only the extremities. Acrocyanosis is normal in the first few hours after birth and if the infant becomes cold. It results from poor perfusion of blood to the periphery of the body (Figure 20-7).

Cyanosis may be present at birth or become apparent later. It is not unusual to see a purplish blue discoloration at birth that quickly turns pink as the infant begins to breathe. Cyanosis occurs whenever the infant's breathing is impaired. It may occur during feedings because of difficulty in coordinating sucking, swallowing, and breathing. Infants who become cyanotic on exertion or crying may have a congenital heart defect.

Grunting. *Grunting* describes a noise made on expiration when pressure is increased within the alveoli to help keep them open. Grunting may be very mild and heard only with a stethoscope or loud enough to hear unaided in an infant having severe respiratory difficulty. Persistent grunting is a common sign of respiratory distress syndrome and necessitates expanded assessment and referral for treatment.

Seesaw Respirations. Normally, the chest and abdomen rise and fall together during respiration. In the infant with severe respiratory difficulty, the chest falls when the abdomen rises and the chest rises when the abdomen falls, causing a seesaw effect. This is a sign of severe respiratory difficulty.

Asymmetry. Chest expansion should be equal on both sides. Asymmetry or decreased movement on one side may indicate the collapse of a lung (pneumothorax).

Choanal Atresia

Assessment for choanal atresia is important because newborns are obligate nose breathers for approximately the first 3 weeks of life. This means that they breathe mostly through the nose except when crying. In choanal atresia, one or both nasal passages are blocked by an abnormality of the septum.

Bilateral choanal atresia causes severe respiratory distress and requires surgery. Blockage of one side puts the infant at risk for respiratory distress if the other side becomes occluded by mucus or edema.

The nurse can assess for choanal atresia by closing the infant's mouth and occluding one nostril at a time. The infant is observed for breathing, and breath sounds are auscultated while each nostril is occluded. Another method of assessment for choanal atresia is to pass a catheter (No. 5 to 8 French) through each nostril to check for patency. Infants with choanal atresia may become cyanotic when quiet but pink when crying because air is then drawn in through the mouth.

Color

In addition to cyanosis, the nurse assesses for pallor and ruddiness.

Pallor. Some infants have a pale skin color. Pallor can indicate that the infant is slightly hypoxic or anemic. The physician may order a laboratory examination of hemoglobin and hematocrit or a complete blood count.

Ruddy Color. In contrast to pallor, a ruddy color (plethora) occurs in some infants. This reddish color of the skin may indicate polycythemia, an excessive number of red blood cells. A hematocrit determination confirms polycythemia. Infants with elevated hematocrits are at increased risk for jaundice from the normal destruction of excessive red blood cells that occurs after birth. Jaundice may occur in infants with hematocrits above 65%.

Heart Sounds

The heart is auscultated for rate, rhythm, and the presence of murmurs or abnormal sounds. The nurse should count the apical pulse for 1 full minute for accuracy and listen for abnormalities. The rate should range between 120 and 160 beats per minute (BPM) with normal activity. It may elevate to 180 BPM when infants are crying or drop as low as 100 BPM when they are in deep sleep.

If no problems exist at birth, the heart rate should be recorded at least once every 30 minutes until the infant has been stable for 2 hours after birth (AAP/ACOG, 1997). Monitoring is more frequent if abnormalities are present. Once stable, the heart rate is checked once every 8 hours unless a reason for more frequent assessment exists.

Position. An experienced examiner can determine the position of the heart in the chest by the location of heart sounds and the point of maximum impulse. The apex of the heart is located at the point of maximum impulse, where the pulse is most easily felt and the sound is loudest. This is at the third or fourth intercostal space, slightly left of the midclavicular line (a line drawn from the middle of the left clavicle). It may be slightly lower in some newborns and at the fifth intercostal space (Vargo, 1996). Conditions that affect the position of the heart include pneumothorax and dextrocardia (a right-to-left reversal of the heart position from normal).

Rhythm and Murmurs. The rhythm of the heart should be regular, and the first and second sounds (lub and dub) should be heard clearly. Abnormalities in rhythm and sounds such as murmurs should be noted. Murmurs are sounds of abnormal blood flow through the heart and may indicate openings in the septum of the heart or problems with blood flow through the valves. Most murmurs in the newborn are temporary and result from incomplete transition from fetal to neonatal circulation. A murmur is not uncommon until the ductus arteriosus is functionally closed. Although it may be a "normal" or functional murmur, any abnormal sounds

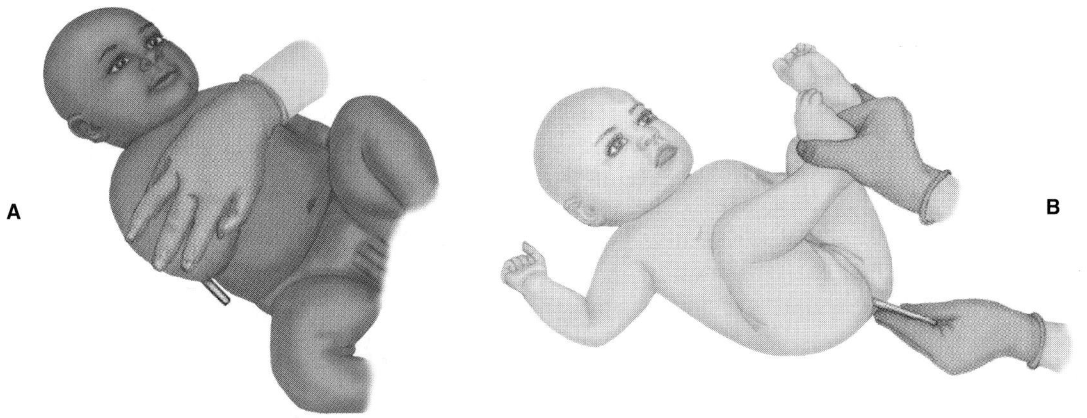

FIGURE 20-8 An axillary (A) or a rectal (B) temperature may be taken. The infant is held securely to prevent injury and obtain an accurate reading.

of the heart are investigated because they may be signs of cardiac defects.

Brachial and Femoral Pulses

The brachial and femoral pulses should be present and equal bilaterally. The brachial pulse is located over the antecubital space, and the femoral pulse is located at the groin. Differences between the brachial and femoral pulses may result from impaired blood flow in coarctation of the aorta, a congenital heart defect. In this condition, a narrowed area of the aorta impedes blood flow to the lower part of the body and causes weaker pulses in the lower extremities.

Blood Pressure

Measurement of blood pressure is not a necessary part of a routine assessment of the newborn, according to the American Academy of Pediatrics (AAP/ACOG, 1997). However, the blood pressure is taken on all extremities if the infant shows signs such as unequal pulses or murmurs. Doppler ultrasonography and other electronic measurement (such as Dynamap) make obtaining an accurate blood pressure easier. To ensure accurate measurement, the infant should be quiet when the blood pressure is taken because crying elevates blood pressure. The width of the blood pressure cuff should be 20% greater than the diameter of the extremity, which would extend around about 40% of the extremity. The bladder of the cuff should cover two thirds of the upper arm or thigh (Smith, Ley, Curley, Elixson, & Dodds, 1996). A cuff that is too narrow gives a false high reading, whereas a cuff that is too wide gives a false low reading.

The average blood pressure for full-term newborns is 65 to 95 mm Hg systolic and 30 to 60 mm Hg diastolic, although variation exists according to the infant's weight (Hernandez, Zabloudil & Hernandez, 1999). It normally is lower in smaller babies. Hypotension may occur in the sick infant. The blood pressure of the lower extremities should be the same as or slightly higher than that of the upper extremities. If a difference of as much as 20 mm Hg exists, coarctation of the aorta may be present.

ASSESSMENT OF THERMOREGULATION

The neonate's temperature is taken soon after birth while the infant is being held by the mother or placed in a radiant warmer with a skin probe attached to the abdomen. The probe allows the warmer to measure and display the infant's temperature continuously. The temperature control is set to regulate the amount of heat produced according to the infant's skin temperature. The temperature should be assessed at least once every 30 minutes until the infant has been stable for 2 hours after birth (AAP/ACOG, 1997). It often is checked again at 4 hours and then once every 8 hours as long as it remains stable.

The most common method of taking the neonate's temperature is axillary (Figure 20-8, Procedure 20-2). Axillary temperatures provide readings very close to rectal measurements and avoid hazards associated with rectal measurement. The normal range for axillary temperature is 36.5 to 37.5° C (97.7 to 99.5° F) (Blake & Murray, 1998).

In some agencies, the first temperature is taken rectally to provide information about the neonate's core temperature and patency of the anus. The nurse should insert the thermometer no more than 0.5 inch into the anus when taking a rectal temperature. The colon turns at a sharp right angle approximately 1 inch from the anal sphincter. Farther insertion of the thermometer might result in potentially fatal perforation of the intestinal wall. A thermometer should never be forced into the rectum because of the possibility of an imperforate (closed) anus. The normal range of rectal temperature is 36.5 to 37.6° C (97.7 to 99.7° F).

Temperatures can be measured with an electronic, digital, or glass thermometer or a disposable plastic strip. Glass thermometers are no longer used in some agencies because of concerns about the dangers of mercury if the thermometer breaks. Digital thermometers used while the infant is in the hospital sometimes are given to the parents for home use. Disposable plastic strips change color to indicate temperature change. Tympanic thermometers generally are not used because they are considered less accurate in newborns.

ASSESSMENT OF HEPATIC FUNCTION

The major early assessments of the hepatic system are related to blood glucose and bilirubin conjugation.

Blood Glucose

The nurse must be alert for newborns at increased risk for hypoglycemia, which can cause brain damage. Factors that might have caused the infant to deplete available glucose are noted. A quick estimate to determine whether the newborn appears to be near term and of appropriate size for gestational age is performed at birth.

Observing for signs of hypoglycemia is necessary throughout routine assessment and care. Early signs include jitteriness and other central nervous systems signs and signs of respiratory difficulty, a decrease in temperature, and poor feeding. Some infants with hypoglycemia show no signs at all.

CRITICAL TO REMEMBER

Risk Factors for Hypoglycemia

- Prematurity
- Postmaturity
- Intrauterine growth restriction
- Large or small for gestational age
- Asphyxia
- Cold stress
- Maternal diabetes
- Maternal intake of terbutaline or ritodrine

In some facilities, all infants are screened for hypoglycemia shortly after birth. However, the American Academy of Pediatrics states that screening for the blood glucose level is necessary only for infants in risk categories and those showing early signs of hypoglycemia (AAP/ACOG, 1997). Normal blood glucose during the first day of life is 40 to 60 mg/dl (Nicholson & Pesce, 2000) and 50 to 90 mg/dl thereafter. Because capillary blood is used in screening tests, these tests are less accurate than laboratory tests using venous blood. Therefore a laboratory analysis (per agency policy) often is used to verify readings of 40 to 45 mg/dl or below. Infants are usually fed if the reading is 40 to 45 mg/dl, especially if the infant shows signs of hypoglycemia, to prevent a further decrease in glucose.

CRITICAL TO REMEMBER

Signs of Neonatal Hypoglycemia

- Jitteriness
- Poor muscle tone
- Diaphoresis
- Poor suck
- Tachypnea
- Dyspnea
- Cyanosis
- Apnea
- Low temperature
- High-pitched cry
- Irritability
- Lethargy
- Seizures, coma
- Some infants may be asymptomatic

Avoiding injuries to the infant's foot is important when taking blood from the heel (Procedure 20-3). If the lancet goes into the calcaneus bone, osteomyelitis may result. The skin should be punctured to a depth of less than 2 mm to avoid piercing the bone for the full-term infant and less than 1.5 mm for the preterm infant (Meehan, 1998). Commercial devices for heel puncture are designed to puncture the heel to the proper depth. The chosen site must avoid damage to major nerves and arteries in the area. Other complications include cellulitis, abscess, scarring, bruising, and pain.

Bilirubin

The nurse assesses for jaundice and watches for its development, particularly in infants at risk. Pressing the infant's skin over a firm surface, such as the end of the nose or the sternum, helps identify jaundice. The skin blanches as the blood is pressed out of the tissues, making it easier to see the yellow color that remains. Because jaundice begins at the head and moves down the body, the severity of the problem can be roughly estimated. A rough estimate of bilirubin level can be made by noting the areas of the body involved. Jaundice of the face occurs when the bilirubin level reaches 5 to 7 mg/dl, the midabdomen at about 15 mg/dl, and the soles of the feet at about 20 mg/dl (Stoll & Kliegman, 2000).

PROCEDURE 20-3

Obtaining Blood Samples from the Newborn by Heel Puncture

Purpose: To obtain infant blood sample by heel puncture for analysis of blood glucose, newborn screening tests, or other tests.

1. Wash hands. *Helps prevent spread of infection.*
2. Bathe the infant or wash the area before puncturing the skin. *Avoids contamination of the puncture site with maternal blood on the infant's skin. This is especially important should the mother have a known or unknown infection such as hepatitis B or human immunodeficiency virus.*
3. Gather supplies needed. Common supplies may include: gloves, alcohol wipe, 2 × 2- inch gauze, lancet or commercial lancing device, adhesive bandage, cotton balls, pipette, cloth or commercial warming pack to warm heel, blood collecting devices (glucometer, glucose screening reagent strips, blotting paper for PKU tests, capillary tubes). *Having all supplies ready allows efficient performance of the procedure.*
4. If using a glucometer, calibrate or program it and use quality control measures according to the manufacturer's guidelines. *Ensures proper functioning of the machine.*
5. Warm the infant's foot for a few minutes if it is cold or if blood is needed for several tests. Dampen a cloth with warm water and fasten it over the heel, or use a heel warming pack according to directions. Use caution to prevent burning the infant's skin! *Warming causes vasodilation and allows blood to flow more easily. This avoids having to make more than one puncture because of insufficient blood flow. Hot packs can cause burns to the infant's delicate skin.*
6. Apply gloves. *Prevents contamination of the hands with blood and is part of standard precautions.*
7. Hold the heel in one hand. Palpate the bone of the heel and place the thumb or finger over the walking surface. Choose a site for the puncture. *Stabilizes the heel to prevent movement and inadvertent injury from the lancet. Locating the bone helps avoid puncturing the calcaneus bone, which could result in osteomyelitis. Covering the walking surface avoids damage to nerves and arteries of this area.*

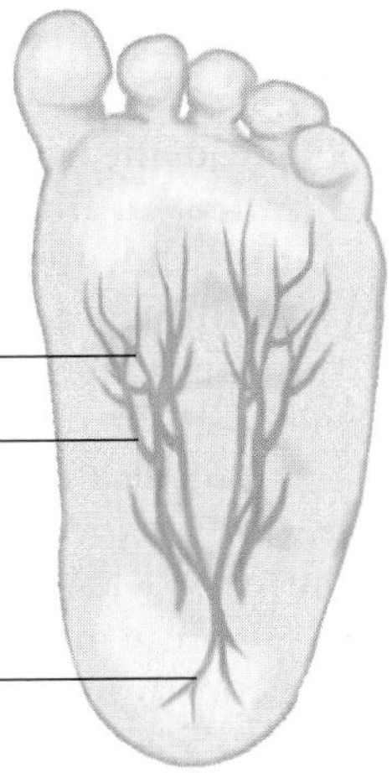

8. Clean the lateral heel with alcohol. Wipe dry with sterile gauze. *Alcohol reduces contaminants. Drying prevents diluting the specimen with alcohol and increases accuracy of results.*
9. Puncture side of heel with a lancet that punctures to a depth of <2.0 mm for full-term infants and <1.5 mm for preterm infants. Place lancet in a sharps container immediately. *Proper depth avoids injury to the infant and ensures blood flow so that further punctures are unnecessary. Proper disposal prevents injury to the infant and injury or unnecessary exposure of the nurse and others to the infant's blood.*

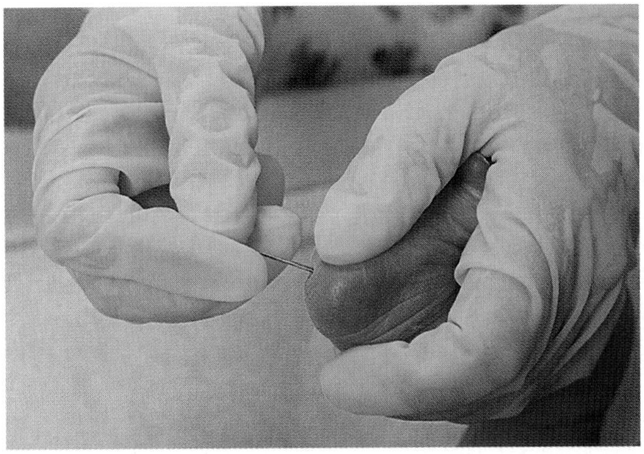

10. If automatic puncture device is used, place over appropriate site and activate according to manufacturer's directions. *Ensures proper use of device.*
11. Follow agency policy or manufacturer's direction about whether to wipe away the first drop of blood, how to collect sample, amount of blood to collect, proper handling, and reading of results. *Correct procedure promotes accuracy of test results.*
12. Avoid excessive squeezing of the foot. Apply gentle pressure at a point higher than the puncture site if necessary. *Excessive squeezing causes bruising and dilution of the sample with fluid from the tissues.*
13. Apply adhesive bandage. Check site frequently. *A bandage helps prevent bleeding and infection of the site. Checking ensures no further bleeding has occurred. Remove the bandage when the bleeding stops.*
14. Document the procedure and results. Send specimens to the laboratory as appropriate. Report abnormal readings and follow up according to agency policy. *Helps ensure proper handling of specimens and proper care of the infant for abnormal results.*

CRITICAL TO REMEMBER

Common Risk Factors for Hyperbilirubinemia

- Prematurity
- Cephalhematoma
- Bruising
- Delayed or poor intake
- Cold stress
- Asphyxia
- Rh incompatibility
- ABO incompatibility
- Sepsis
- Sibling with jaundice
- Breastfeeding

In physiologic jaundice, the bilirubin level peaks at 5 to 6 mg/dl between the second and fourth days of life and then begins to drop. Jaundice appearing before the second day of life may indicate that the bilirubin is rising more quickly and to higher levels than normal and may not be physiologic. The physician or nurse practitioner may order laboratory determinations of the bilirubin level based on the nurse's assessment. If serial bilirubin assays are ordered, the nurse notes changes from one reading to the next and correlates the results with the infant's age.

Check Your Reading

4. What is included in assessment of the newborn's cardiovascular status?
5. Why is taking a rectal temperature dangerous in an infant?
6. What are some signs of hypoglycemia?
7. Why is using the correct site for heel punctures to obtain blood samples important?

ASSESSMENT OF BODY SYSTEMS

Neurologic System

Reflexes

Assessment of the presence and strength of the reflexes is important to determine the health of the newborn's central nervous system. The nurse notes the strength of the reflexes and whether both sides of the body respond symmetrically (Figure 20-9). A diminished overall response occurs in preterm and ill infants. Absence of reflexes may indicate a serious neurologic problem. Asymmetric responses may indicate that trauma during birth caused nerve damage, paralysis, or fracture. For example, trauma to the facial nerve from forceps or pressure during birth may cause drooping of the mouth. The infant may appear to have a one-sided cry and have no rooting reflex on the affected side. Some newborn reflexes gradually weaken and disappear during the early months (Table 20-2).

CRITICAL THINKING EXERCISE

QUESTION:
What might be the effect on normal development if reflexes are retained beyond the age when they should disappear?

Sensory Assessment

Ears. The ears are assessed for placement, overall appearance, and maturity. An imaginary line drawn from the inner to outer canthus of the eye should be even with the area where the upper ear joins the head (Figure 20-10). Low-set ears may indicate chromosomal abnormalities.

The nurse examines the ears for skin tags and preauricular sinuses and dimples. Abnormalities of the ear may indicate chromosomal abnormalities, mental retardation, hearing problems, and kidney defects. The stiffness of the cartilage and degree of incurving of the pinna are checked as part of the gestational age assessment.

Infants can hear by the last trimester of pregnancy, and their hearing is very good after birth. Hearing is assessed by noting the infant's reaction to sudden loud noises, which should cause a startle response. The infant should respond to the sound of voices, particularly if it is a high-pitched tone of voice or the sound of the mother's voice.

Eyes. The eyes should be symmetric and of the same size. The usual slate gray–blue color gradually changes to the true color by 3 to 12 months of age. Infants with dark skin may have brown eyes. The eyes are examined for abnormalities and signs of inflammation. Edema of the eyelids and subconjunctival hemorrhages (reddened areas of the sclera) result from pressure on the head during birth, which causes capillary rupture in the sclera. The edema diminishes in a few days, and the hemorrhages resolve in 1 or 2 weeks.

Conjunctivitis may result from infection and chemical reaction to medications. *Staphylococcus, Chlamydia,* and *Neisseria gonorrhoeae* are common organisms that cause infection. Gonorrhea in the mother can cause infection of the infant during birth. The resulting ophthalmia neonatorum may cause blindness. To prevent this condition, all infants are treated prophylactically with antibiotics to the eyes. Any discharge from the eyes is reported for possible culture and treatment.

The sclera should be white. A yellow color indicates jaundice. A blue color occurs in osteogenesis imperfecta, a congenital bone condition.

Transient strabismus (crossed eyes) is common for the first 3 to 4 months after birth because infants have poor control of their eye muscles. The doll's-eye sign is

Text continued on p. 527

Table 20-2
SUMMARY OF NEONATAL REFLEXES

Reflex	Method of Testing	Expected Response	Abnormal Response/Possible Cause	Time Reflex Disappears
Babinski	Stroke lateral sole of foot from heel to across base of toes.	Toes flare with dorsiflexion of the big toe.	No response Bilateral: CNS deficit. Unilateral: Local nerve damage.	12 months.
Galant (trunk incurvation)	Lightly stroke the back lateral to the vertebral column.	Entire trunk flexes toward side stimulated.	No response: CNS deficit.	1 month.
Grasp reflex (palmar and plantar)	Press finger against base of fingers or toes.	Fingers curl tightly; toes curl forward.	Weak or absent: Neurologic deficit or muscle damage.	Palmar grasp lessens 3 to 4 months, disappears by 5 to 6 months. Plantar grasp disappears by 8 to 9 months.
Moro	Let infant's head drop back approximately 30 degrees.	Sharp extension and abduction of arms with thumbs and forefingers in C position. Followed by flexion and adduction to "embrace" position. Legs follow similar pattern.	Absent: CNS dysfunction. Asymmetry: Brachial plexus injury, paralysis, or fractured extremity. Exaggerated: Maternal drug use.	6 months.
Rooting	Touch or stroke from the corner of the mouth toward the cheek.	Infant turns to side touched. Difficult to elicit if infant sleeping or just fed.	Weak or absent: Prematurity, neurologic deficit, depression from maternal drug use.	3 to 4 months.
Startle	Make a loud noise.	Similar to Moro but hands remain clenched,	Weak or absent: Neurologic damage, deafness.	4 months.
Stepping	Hold infant so that feet touch solid surface.	Infant lifts alternate feet as if walking.	Asymmetry: Fracture of extremity, neurologic deficit.	3 to 4 months.
Sucking	Place nipple or finger in mouth, rub against palate.	Infant begins to suck. Weak if recently fed.	Weak or absent: Prematurity, neurologic deficit, maternal drug use.	Disappears by 1 yr.
Swallowing	Place fluid on the back of the tongue.	Infant swallows fluid. Should be coordinated with sucking.	Coughing, gagging, choking, cyanosis: Tracheoesophageal fistula, esophageal atresia, neurologic deficit.	Present throughout life.
Tonic neck reflex	Gently turn head to one side while infant is supine.	Extension of extremities on side to which head turned, with flexion on opposite side.	Prolonged period of time in position: Neurologic deficit.	Disappears by 6 to 7 months.

CNS, Central nervous system.

A. **Moro reflex.**
The Moro reflex is the most dramatic reflex. It occurs when the infant's head and trunk are allowed to drop back 30 degrees when the infant is in a slightly raised position. The infant's arms and legs extend and abduct, with the fingers fanning open and thumbs and forefingers forming a C position. The arms then return to their normally flexed state with an embracing motion. The legs may also extend and then flex.

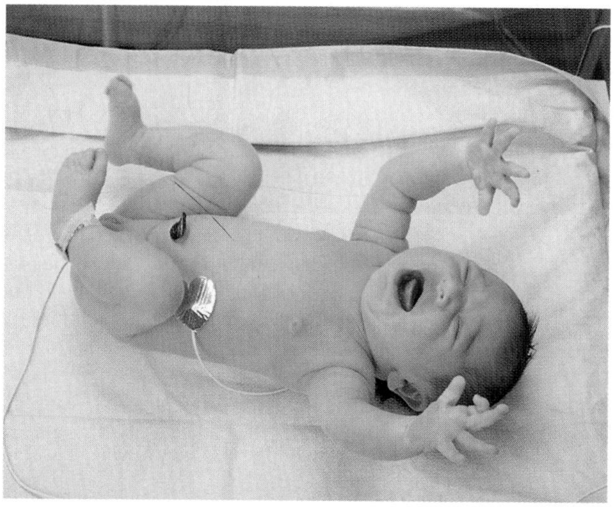

B. **Palmar grasp reflex.**
The palmar grasp reflex occurs when the infant's palm is touched near the base of the fingers. The hand closes into a tight fist. The grasp reflex may be weak or absent if the infant has damage to the nerves of the arms.

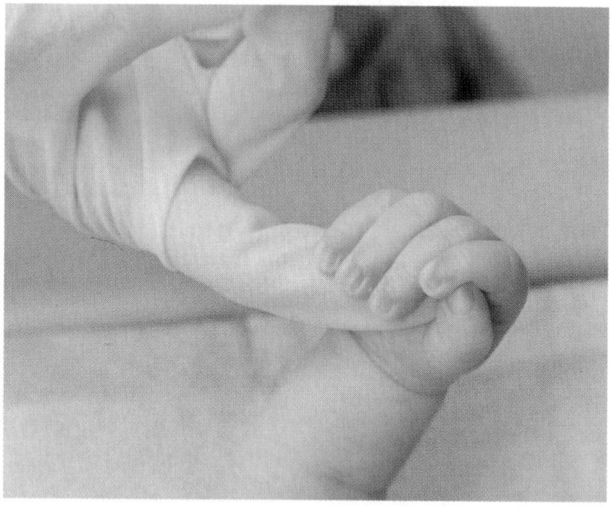

C. **Plantar grasp reflex.**
The plantar grasp reflex is similar to the palmar grasp reflex. When the area below the toes is touched, the infant's toes curl over the nurse's finger.

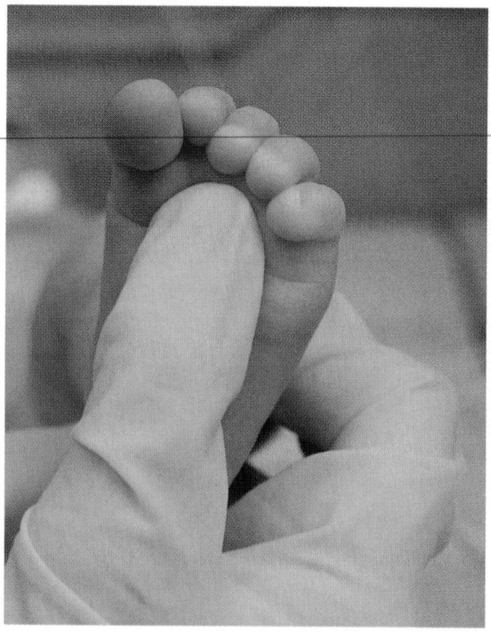

FIGURE 20-9 Reflexes.

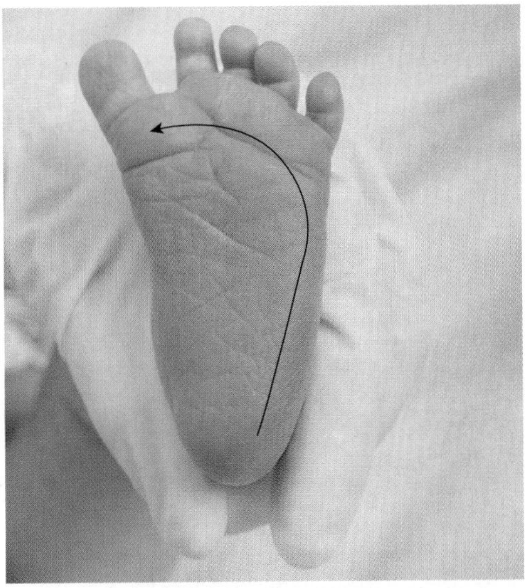

D. **Babinski reflex.**
The Babinski reflex is elicited by stroking the lateral sole of the infant's foot from the heel forward and across the ball of the foot. This causes the toes to flare outward and the big toe to dorsiflex.

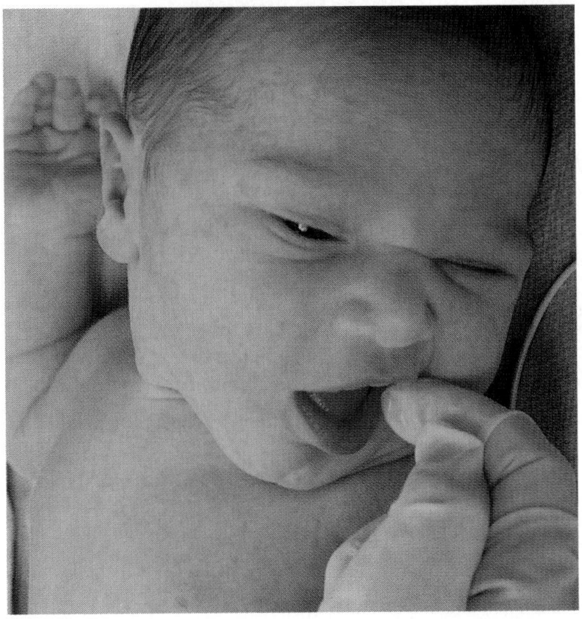

E. **Rooting reflex.**
The rooting reflex is important in feeding and is most often demonstrated when the infant is hungry. When the infant's cheek is touched near the mouth, the head turns toward the side that has been stroked. This helps the infant find the nipple for feeding. The reflex occurs when either side of the mouth is touched. Touching the cheeks on both sides at the same time confuses the infant.

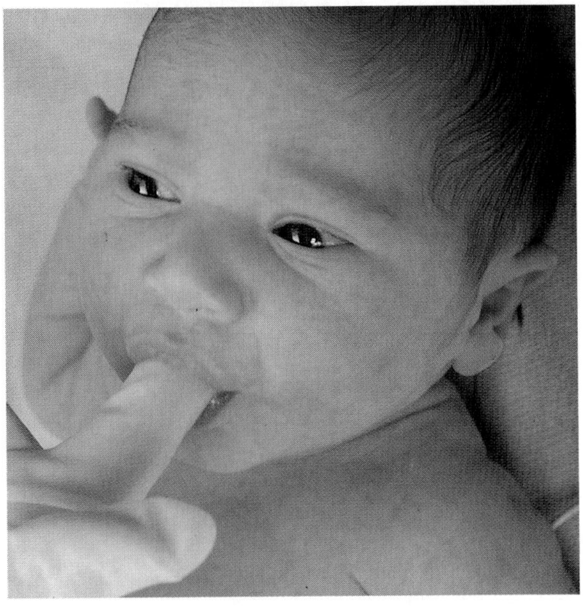

F. **Sucking reflex.**
The sucking reflex is essential to normal life. When the mouth or palate is touched by the nipple or a finger, the infant begins to suck. The sucking reflex is assessed for its presence and strength. Feeding difficulties may be related to problems in the infant's ability to suck and to coordinate sucking with swallowing.

FIGURE 20-9, cont'd For legend see opposite page.

Continued

G. **Tonic neck reflex.**
The tonic neck reflex refers to the posture assumed by newborns when in a supine position. The infant extends the arm and leg on the side to which the head is turned and flexes the extremities on the other side. This is sometimes referred to as the "fencing reflex" because the infant's position is similar to that of a person engaged in a fencing match.

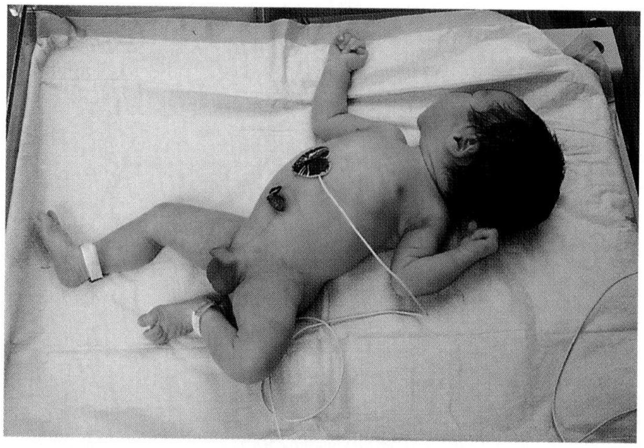

H. **Stepping reflex.**
The stepping reflex occurs when infants are held upright with their feet touching a solid surface. They lift one foot and then the other, giving the appearance that they are trying to walk.

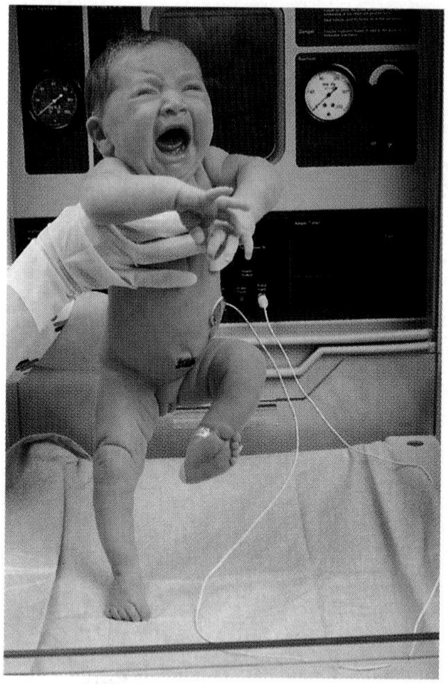

FIGURE 20-9, cont'd For legend see p. 520.

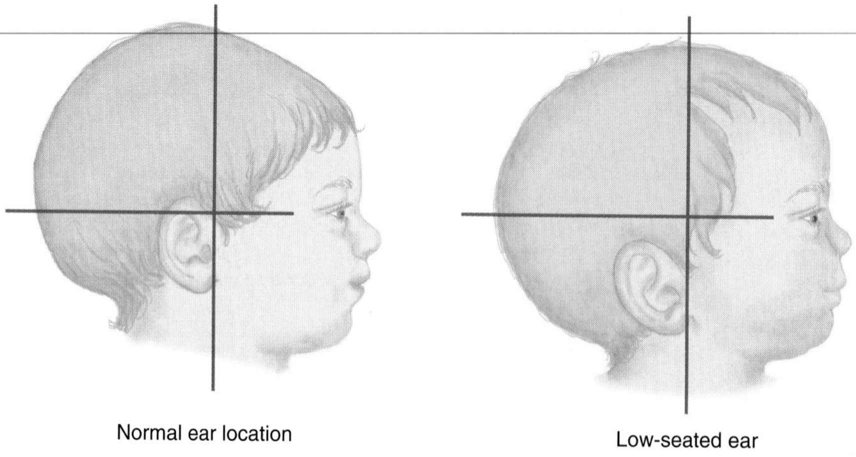

FIGURE 20-10 An imaginary line is drawn from the inner to the outer canthus of the eye and then to the ear. The line should intersect with the area where the upper ear joins the head.

a normal finding in the newborn: When the head is turned quickly to one side, the eyes move toward the other side. The setting-sun sign, during which the iris appears low in the eye and part of the sclera can be seen above the iris, may be an indication of hydrocephalus.

The pupils should be equal in size and react to light. Cataracts (opacities of the lens) appear as white areas over the pupils. They may develop in infants of mothers who had rubella or other infections during the pregnancy. When a light is directed into the eyes, the normal red reflex may not be seen if large cataracts are present. Tears are scant or absent for the first 2 to 4 weeks of life. Excessive tearing may indicate a plugged lacrimal duct, which is treated with massage or surgery.

Although visual acuity is not well developed and the eyes cannot accommodate for distance, newborns should show a visual response to the environment. They should make eye contact when held in a cradle position during a period of alertness and focus on objects that are 20 to 30 cm (8 to 12 in) away. Newborns can follow interesting objects horizontally across midline and vertically. They should respond well to human faces and geometric patterns of black and white or medium bright colors but show little interest in pastel colors.

Newborns should blink or close their eyes in response to bright lights. Any infant who does not respond to visual stimuli should be reported to the physician or nurse practitioner for further investigation.

Sense of Smell. Newborns have a good sense of smell, and discrimination develops quickly. They can identify the odor of the mother's breast milk within 5 days after birth (Brazelton, 1999). The ability of infants to distinguish taste is shown by their increased suck when given sweet liquids and rejection of sour, salty, and bitter liquids.

Other Neurologic Signs

The newborn is assessed for jitteriness and tremors. If jitteriness is present, the blood glucose level should be checked because hypoglycemia is the most common cause. If blood glucose is within normal range, the cause may be low calcium levels or prenatal exposure to drugs. Tremors increase each time the infant is touched or moved but stop briefly if the extremity is flexed and held firmly.

CRITICAL TO REMEMBER

Differentiating Jitteriness and Seizures

Jitteriness or Tremors
- Stop when the extremities are held firmly in a flexed position
- Commonly caused by low glucose or calcium levels

Seizures
- Continue even if extremities are held
- May have abnormal mouth or eye movements
- Indicate central nervous system abnormality

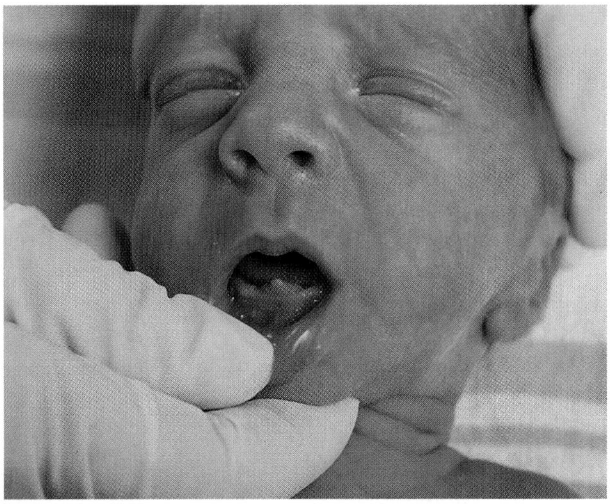

FIGURE 20-11 A precocious tooth.

Seizures indicate central nervous system abnormality. To differentiate between jitteriness and seizures, the infant's extremities are held in a flexed position. This causes tremors to stop, whereas a seizure continues. Seizure activity also may include abnormal movements of the eyes and mouth and other subtle signs. Any infant thought to be having seizures is referred for further assessment and treatment.

The pitch of the cry is important. Cries that are shrill, high-pitched, hoarse, and catlike (mewing) are abnormal. These cries may indicate a neurologic disorder or other problem.

Normal infants are quiet and appear content when their needs are met. Infants should respond to soothing, gentle touch and holding. Rocking motions often are effective in quieting an irritable infant. Most infants "mold" their bodies to those of the people holding them, making them easy to hold and cuddle. The neonate who stiffens the body, seems to pull away from contact, and arches the back when held displays signs of central nervous system damage. Infants should react to painful stimuli with crying and an increase in vital signs. Excessive irritability and a high-pitched cry also may be signs of damage to the central nervous system. All such abnormal signs are reported for further neurologic assessment.

Gastrointestinal System

The initial assessment of the gastrointestinal tract occurs during the first hours after birth, when the nurse visualizes the parts that can be seen and the infant takes the initial feeding. Abnormalities and normal variations in structure and function are identified.

Mouth

The mouth is inspected visually and by palpation. Some infants are born with precocious teeth, usually incisors (Figure 20-11). If the teeth are loose, the physician usually removes them to prevent aspiration. Epstein's pearls may be present on the hard palate and gums. These small, white, hard, inclusion cysts are accumulations of epithelial cells and disappear without treatment. They are similar to milia.

The nurse examines the tongue for size and movement. A large, protruding tongue is present in some chromosomal disorders such as Down syndrome. Paralysis of the facial nerve causes drooping of the mouth and affects the movement of the tongue. The tongue may appear to be tongue tied because of the short frenulum, but this is normal and usually has no effect on the infant's ability to feed. Clipping of the frenulum seldom is practiced because of the potential for infection.

Although candidiasis (thrush) is not apparent in the mouth immediately after birth, it may appear a day or two later. The lesions resemble milk curds on the tongue and cheeks that bleed if attempts are made to wipe them away. Newborns may become infected with *Candida albicans* during passage through the birth canal if the mother has a candidal vaginal infection. The infant is treated with nystatin suspension.

A cleft lip or palate results if the lip or palate fails to close. Cleft palate may involve the hard palate, soft palate, or both and may appear alone or with a cleft lip. The palate is inspected when the infant cries. A gloved finger is inserted into the mouth to palpate the hard and soft palates. A very small cleft of the soft palate may be missed if only a visual examination is done (see p. 864).

Suck

The normal full-term infant should have a strong suck reflex, which is elicited when the lips or palate are stimulated. The reflex is weaker in the neonate who is preterm, ill, or has just been fed. The newborn's cheeks have well-developed muscles and sucking pads that enhance the ability to suck. These fatty sucking pads last until late in infancy, when sucking is no longer essential. Blisters may be present on the newborn's hands or arms because of strong sucking before birth.

Abdomen

The abdomen should be rounded and protrude slightly but not be distended. The stomach may be distended by mucus, blood, and amniotic fluid swallowed during birth. Fluid may be emptied through a feeding tube, if necessary. An abdomen so distended that the skin is stretched and shiny may indicate obstruction. Loops of bowel should not be visible through the abdominal wall. Visible bowel could indicate that air, meconium, or both are not passing through the intestines normally.

A sunken or scaphoid appearance of the abdomen occurs in diaphragmatic hernia, in which the intestines are located in the chest cavity instead of the abdomen. This condition interferes with development of the lungs, resulting in respiratory difficulty at birth. The nurse listens over the abdomen for bowel sounds, which usually appear within the first hour after birth. Bowel sounds heard in the chest may indicate diaphragmatic hernia.

An umbilical hernia occurs when the intestinal muscles fail to close around the umbilicus, allowing the intestines to protrude through the weak area. The condition is more common in African-American infants. By the time the infant is walking well, the muscles are usually strong enough that the hernia no longer is present. Some umbilical hernias require surgical repair.

Palpating the abdomen is easiest when the infant is relaxed and quiet. The abdomen should feel soft because the muscles are not yet well developed. Masses may indicate tumors of the kidneys. Palpation of the liver and kidneys generally is not part of routine nursing assessment of the abdomen. When palpated, the liver normally is felt no more than 1 to 3 cm below the right costal margin. If the organ seems large, it should be reported to the physician or nurse practitioner because it may be a sign of congestive heart failure or congenital infection.

Initial Feeding

The initial feeding is an opportunity to further assess the newborn. If the mother is breastfeeding, the nurse can observe the infant's response unobtrusively while assisting the mother to position the infant. A LATCH score should be given to all breastfeeding infants to identify problems with feeding (see Chapter 22, p. 583). To decrease regurgitation from overdistention of the stomach, an initial formula feeding should be no more than 1 oz.

Whether the infant is breastfeeding or formula feeding, the nurse evaluates the infant's ability to suck, swallow, and breathe in a coordinated manner. Although the fetus sucks and swallows in utero, these acts may not have been performed together. The addition of breathing to sucking and swallowing is a new experience. Choking, coughing, or experiencing cyanosis may indicate a connection between the trachea and esophagus, such as tracheoesophageal fistula.

Some newborns choke or gag during the first feeding. Others may become dusky or cyanotic because they become apneic while they are feeding. In either case, the nurse should stop the feeding immediately, suction if necessary, and stimulate the infant to cry by rubbing the back.

Most infants learn to coordinate sucking, swallowing, and breathing by the time the first feeding is finished. Neonates who continue to have difficulty may have a cardiac anomaly, tracheoesophageal fistula, or esophageal atresia (see p. 864). Infants with tracheoesophageal fistula or esophageal atresia also may drool excessively. Further assessment and referral are necessary.

Stools

Observe stools for normal color and consistency. Meconium stools are dark greenish–black. They are soft but thick and tend to adhere to the skin. The infant may pass meconium at delivery, when a rectal temperature is taken, or after the initial feeding. Meconium stools are followed by transitional loose, greenish-brown stools.

CRITICAL THINKING EXERCISE

You are caring for an infant who was born 20 hours ago and you hear on report that the infant has not passed meconium yet.

QUESTION:
What should you do?

Breastfed infants pass very soft, seedy, mustard-yellow stools after transitional stools. Formula-fed infants excrete stools that are more solid and pale yellow to light brown. A "water ring" should never occur around the solid part of any stool. This indicates diarrhea, with the watery part absorbed into the diaper.

The nurse should be aware of when the infant's last stool occurred and whether any stools have been passed after birth. Neonates usually pass the first meconium stool within 12 hours of birth and 99% have the first stool within 48 hours (Stoll & Kliegman, 2000). If a question exists about whether the infant has excreted a stool, the nurse must investigate further. Feeding may cause the infant to have a stool. Although rectal temperatures are not recommended, a thermometer may be gently inserted into the rectum to determine patency and stimulate stool passage.

Check Your Reading

8. Why is assessment of newborn reflexes important?
9. Why is it important for the nurse to observe the first feeding carefully?
10. When do newborns pass the first stool? What can be done to stimulate stool passage?

Genitourinary System

Kidney Palpation

Palpation of the kidneys is not usually part of the routine nursing assessment of the newborn. However, the kidneys may be felt 1 to 2 cm above the level of the umbilicus on each side of the abdomen during the first hours after birth. Abdominal masses may indicate enlargement or tumors of the kidneys.

Anomalies of the kidney may accompany other defects. For example, infants with only one umbilical artery and defects involving the ears may have renal anomalies. The nurse should observe carefully for urinary output in these infants to determine whether the kidneys are functioning.

Urine

Most newborns void within 12 hours of birth, and 95% void by 24 hours (Stoll & Kliegman, 2000). Because absence of urine output during this time may indicate anomalies, the time of the first void is recorded on the chart. The newborn's bladder empties as little as two to six times during the first 2 days, and the first void may be missed. Sometimes it occurs in the delivery room but goes unnoticed because attention is focused on the infant's overall condition.

If concern exists about whether the newborn has urinated, the delivery notes should be carefully read to see if the infant voided at birth. The nurse should ask the mother if she has changed a wet diaper. Increasing the infant's fluid intake often can initiate urination. If no void occurs in the expected time, the physician or nurse practitioner is alerted.

After the first 2 days of life, the newborn's bladder empties at least once after every feeding (Brion, Bernstein, & Spitzer, 1997). Thus at least six wet diapers would be expected each day. Each void is recorded in the infant's chart, including the number of diapers changed by the mother. The total number is correlated with that appropriate for the age of the infant. Mothers should be taught that approximately 6 to 10 wet diapers after the first 2 days indicate the infant is taking adequate fluid.

If an infant is having feeding difficulties, noting the number of wet diapers is especially important. Disposable diapers are very absorbent, and determining whether the diaper is wet is sometimes difficult. The pale color of the newborn's urine may cause very little color change on the diaper. Wet diapers generally feel heavier than dry ones. If necessary, the nurse can put on gloves and take the diaper apart to examine it. The absorbent inner lining is damp if urine is present. Cotton balls and tissue placed in the diaper also may be used to increase visibility of small amounts of urine.

The newborn's urine may contain urate crystals that cause a reddish or pink stain on the diaper. This is known as "brick dust staining" and may be frightening to parents, who may think the infant is bleeding. It does not continue beyond the first few days as the kidneys mature.

Genitalia

The nurse examines the newborn's genitalia for size, maturation, and presence of any abnormalities.

Female. In the full-term female infant, the labia majora should be large and completely cover the clitoris and labia minora. The labia may be darker than the surrounding skin, especially in infants with dark skin tones. This pigmentation is a normal response to exposure to the mother's hormones before birth. Edema of the labia and white mucous vaginal discharge are normal. A small amount of vaginal bleeding, known

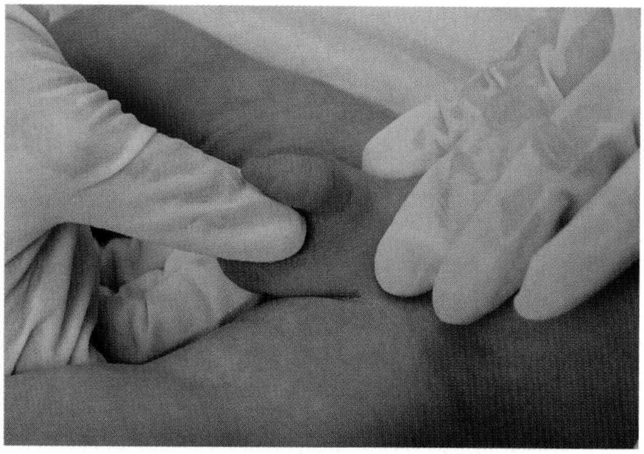

FIGURE 20-12 The testes are palpated from front to back with the thumb and forefinger. Placing a finger over the inguinal canal holds the testes in place for palpation.

as *pseudomenstruation,* may occur from the sudden withdrawal of the mother's hormones at birth. Hymenal (vaginal) tags are small pieces of tissue at the vaginal orifice. These are normal and disappear in a few weeks. The urinary meatus and vagina should be present.

Male. The scrotum should be pendulous at term and may be dark brown from maternal hormones. Pressure during a breech delivery may cause it to be edematous. Rugae (creases in the scrotum) are deep and cover the entire scrotum in the full-term infant.

Enlargement of one or both sides of the scrotum may result from a hydrocele. This collection of fluid around the testes may make palpating the testes difficult. Placing a flashlight against the sac may outline the testes. Parents should be told that hydroceles are not painful and often reabsorb within 1 year. Some require later surgery.

The testes begin to descend through the inguinal canal at about 30 weeks of gestation and should be within the scrotal sac at 36 weeks. Palpation of the scrotum determines whether the testes have descended (Figure 20-12). Testes feel like small, round, movable objects that "slip" between the fingers. If the testes are not present in the scrotal sac, they may be felt in the inguinal canal. An empty scrotal sac appears smaller than one with testes. Undescended testis (cryptorchidism) occurs on one or both sides in approximately 3.4% of full-term and about 30% of preterm newborn boys. Most undescended testes will descend within 3 months. If the testes do not descend within 6 months, the condition must be treated surgically to preserve fertility (Elder, 2000).

The meatus should be at the tip of the glans penis. It may be abnormally located on the underside of the penis (hypospadias), on the upper side (epispadias), or on the perineum. The prepuce or foreskin of the penis covers the glans and is adherent to it. Attempts to retract it in the newborn are unnecessary and can cause damage. Abnormal placement of the meatus may not be visible because it is covered by the prepuce, but often the prepuce in these infants is incompletely formed. Hypospadias may be accompanied by chordee, a condition in which fibrotic tissue causes the penis to curve downward. These abnormalities are later corrected by surgery.

Parents are very concerned about any abnormalities of the genitalia. If the meatus is abnormally positioned, they need an explanation of the condition and why the infant should not be circumcised. The foreskin may be needed for later plastic surgery to repair the defect.

Integumentary System

Skin

The skin of the newborn is fragile and easily shows marks, especially in infants with fair coloring. Because the skin is so sensitive, reddened areas and rashes may develop during the early days of life. The nurse must examine every inch of skin surface carefully during the initial assessment and at the beginning of each shift.

Color. The color of the newborn's skin should be pink or tan. Red, thin skin occurs in preterm infants. Redness in the full-term infant may indicate polycythemia. Acrocyanosis is common during the first day or two as a result of poor peripheral circulation. The infant's mouth and central body areas should not be cyanotic at any time. Blanching the skin over the nose or chest shows the presence of jaundice. Jaundice is abnormal during the first day of life but common during the first week.

A greenish-brown discoloration of the skin, nails, and cord results if meconium was passed before birth. This may indicate that the infant was compromised at some time before birth, and it is more common in the postterm infant. These infants must be watched for other complications such as respiratory difficulty.

Harlequin coloration is a clear color division over the body from the head to the abdomen with one half deep pink or red and the other half pale or of normal color. The cause is unknown and it is usually transient and benign. It may indicate shunting of blood with cardiac problems or sepsis. Redness may occur on the lower side when the infant lies on the side.

Mottling (cutis marmorata) is a lacy, red pattern from dilated blood vessels under the skin. It is usually normal but may be a sign of cold stress, hypovolemia, or sepsis. If persistent, it may indicate a chromosomal abnormality.

Vernix Caseosa. Vernix, a thick, white substance, resembles cream cheese and provides a protective covering for the fetal skin in utero. The full-term infant has little vernix left on the body except small amounts in the creases. A thick covering of vernix may indicate a preterm infant, but a postterm infant may have none at all. Most vernix is removed when the infant is dried at

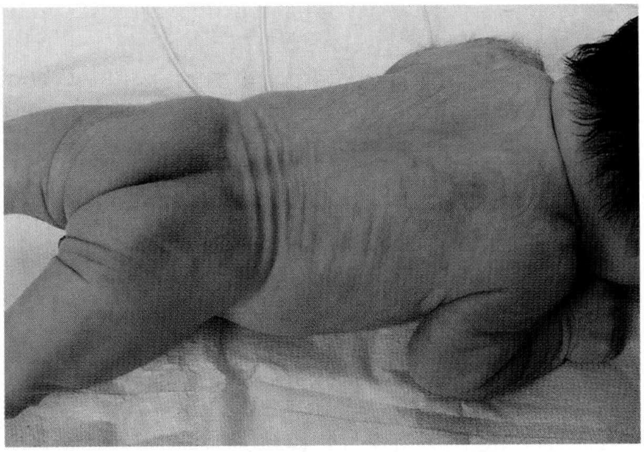

FIGURE 20-13 Lanugo is abundant on this slightly preterm infant.

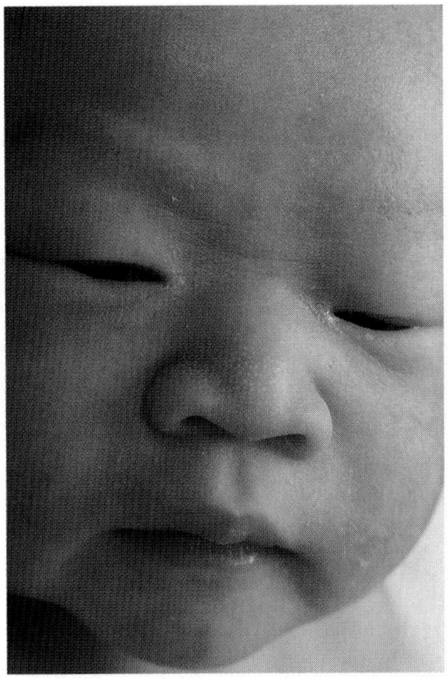

FIGURE 20-14 Milia.

birth or during the first bath. The remaining vernix is absorbed by the skin. Yellow-tinged vernix may indicate elevated bilirubin levels in utero, and green-tinged vernix is the result of meconium staining.

Lanugo. Lanugo is fine hair that covers the fetus during intrauterine life (Figure 20-13). As the fetus nears term, the lanugo becomes thinner. The term infant may have a small amount of lanugo on the shoulders, forehead, sides of the face, and upper back. Dark-skinned infants have more lanugo than infants with lighter coloring, and their darker hair is more visible.

Milia. Milia are white cysts, 1 to 2 mm in size, resulting from distention of sebaceous glands (oil glands) that are not yet functioning properly. They occur on the face over the forehead, nose, and chin and disappear within 2 months without treatment (Figure 20-14).

Erythema Toxicum. The nurse notes the presence of erythema toxicum, which are red, blotchy areas that may have white or yellow papules or vesicles in the center (Figure 20-15). It is commonly called "flea bite" rash or *newborn rash* and resembles small bites or acne. The rash appears during the first 24 to 48 hours after birth, although occasionally not until 1 to 2 weeks. It is most common over the back, shoulders, and chest. The condition does not result from infection but should be differentiated from a pustular rash caused by staphylococcal infection or vesicles from herpes simplex. The cause of erythema toxicum is unknown, and it disappears within hours or up to 10 days.

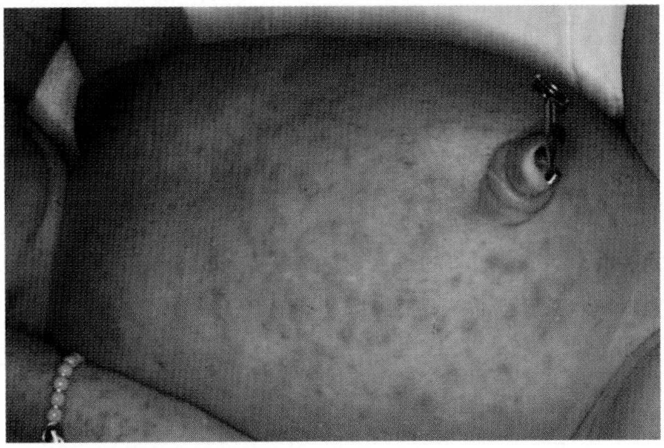

FIGURE 20-15 Erythema toxicum. (From Hurwitz, S. [1993]. *Clinical pediatric dermatology* [2nd ed., p. 13]. Philadelphia: W.B. Saunders.)

Birthmarks. The size and location of all birthmarks should be carefully documented. Some more common birthmarks are listed here.

- Mongolian spots are bluish-black marks that resemble bruises (Figure 20-16). They usually occur in the sacral area but may appear on the buttocks, arms, shoulders, and other areas. Mongolian spots occur most frequently in newborns with dark skin and usually disappear after the first few years of life. Some continue into adulthood.
- A telangiectatic nevus is sometimes called *nevus simplex* or "stork bite" (Figure 20-17). It is a flat, pink or reddish discoloration from dilated capillaries that occur over the eyelids, above the bridge of the nose, or at the nape of the neck. The color

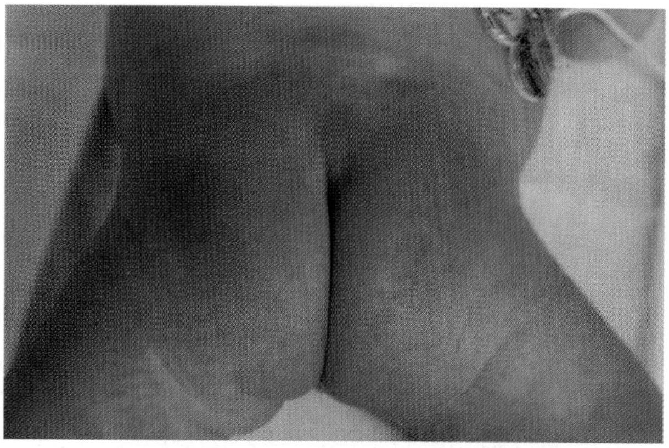

FIGURE 20-16 Mongolian spots.

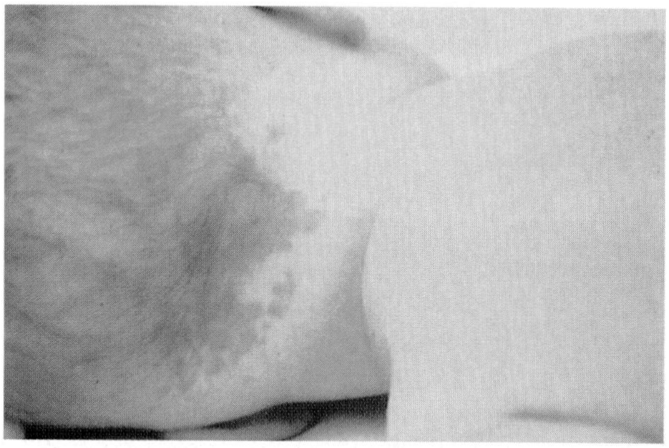

FIGURE 20-17 Stork bite. (Courtesy Jane Deacon, The Children's Hospital, Denver, Colorado.)

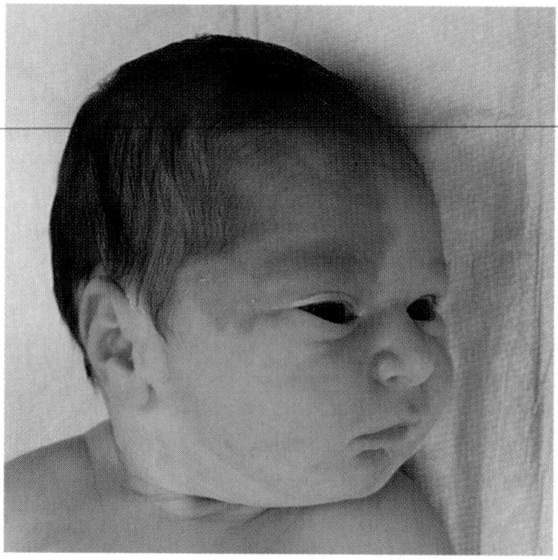

FIGURE 20-18 Port wine stain.

blanches when pressed and is more prominent during crying. Stork bites disappear by 2 years of age, although those at the nape of the neck may persist.

- Nevus flammeus (port wine stain) is a permanent, flat, dark, reddish-purple mark (Figure 20-18). It varies in size and location and does not blanch with pressure. If it is large and in a visible area, it can be removed by laser surgery.
- Nevus vasculosus (strawberry hemangioma) consists of enlarged capillaries in the outer layers of skin. It is dark red and raised with a rough surface, giving a strawberry-like appearance. The hemangioma usually is located on the head. It may grow larger for 5 to 6 months but usually disappears by the early school years. No treatment is necessary.
- Café-au-lait spots are permanent, light-brown areas that may occur anywhere on the body. Although they are harmless, the number and size are important. More than six spots or spots larger than 3 cm are associated with neurofibromatosis, a genetic condition of neural tissue.

Marks from Delivery. The infant is inspected for marks that may have occurred from injury or pressure during labor or delivery.

- Bruises may occur on any part of the body where pressure occurred during delivery. This is especially true when second-stage labor was difficult. Bruising of the face may be present if the cord was wrapped around the neck during birth. Bruising on the head may occur from use of a vacuum extractor.
- Petechiae, pinpoint bruises that resemble a rash, may appear over areas such as the back and face. They result from increased intravascular pressure during the birth process, such as occurs with a nuchal cord (cord around the neck) during delivery. Widespread or continued formation of petechiae may indicate infection or a low platelet count.
- A small puncture mark is present on the newborn's head if a fetal monitor scalp electrode was attached. The area should scab and heal normally but should be observed for signs of infection.
- Forceps marks occur over the cheeks and ears where the instruments were applied. Their size, color, and location are carefully documented. Lack of movement or symmetry of the face may indicate damage to the facial nerve.

Other Aspects. Other aspects of the skin that may indicate abnormalities should be recorded. Localized edema may be caused by trauma of delivery. Generalized edema indicates more serious conditions such as heart failure. Peeling of the skin is normal in full-term newborns. Excessive amounts of peeling may indicate a postterm infant.

Breasts

The nurse notes the placement of the nipples and looks for extra (supernumerary) nipples, which may appear on the chest or in the axilla. Occasionally, the breasts become engorged 2 or 3 days after birth and secrete a small amount of white fluid (sometimes called "witch's milk") a few days later. This condition results from maternal hormones and resolves within a few weeks without treatment. The breasts should not be expressed or manipulated, as this could cause infection.

Hair and Nails

The hair on the full-term infant should be silky and soft, whereas that on the preterm infant is woolly or fuzzy. The nails come to the end of the fingers or beyond. Very long nails may indicate a postterm infant.

Documentation

All marks, bruises, rashes, and other abnormalities of the skin must be recorded in the nurses' notes. The location, size, color, elevation, and texture of each mark are described. Subsequent changes in appearance from previous descriptions also are noted on the chart.

The nurse may not always know the proper name for each type of mark on the infant's skin. Most agencies have books with pictures of the common skin variations.

> When in doubt about the name of a mark, a description is sufficient. For example, a stork bite (telangiectatic nevus) might be described as a "flat, reddened area 1 × 2 cm in size over right eyelid that blanches with pressure."

ASSESSMENT OF GESTATIONAL AGE

The gestational age assessment is an examination of the newborn's physical and neurologic characteristics to determine the number of weeks from conception to birth. It is important because neonates born before or after term and those whose sizes are not appropriate for gestational age are at increased risk for complications. Although the gestational age often is calculated from the mother's last menstrual period and by ultrasonography during the pregnancy, the date of the last menstrual period is not always accurate, and ultrasonography is not always performed.

Because the times of development for various fetal characteristics are known, the presence or absence of these characteristics can help estimate gestational age. The estimated age then can be compared with the newborn's weight, length, and head circumference to determine whether the neonate is large, appropriate (average), or small in size for gestational age. It is important to understand that the total score of all assessed characteristics determines the gestational age. One or two characteristics alone cannot be used to assign a gestational age.

Assessment Tools

Several different tools are used to assess gestational age. The Dubowitz scoring system is an in-depth, detailed assessment tool that includes examination of physical, neurologic, and behavioral characteristics. The New Ballard Score (Figure 20-19) is a simplified adaptation of the Dubowitz tool that has been revised to include characteristics of very preterm infants. It can be performed quickly yet provides accurate information within 1 week when performed by an experienced examiner (Fletcher, 1999). The Ballard tool focuses on physical and neuromuscular characteristics, eliminating the behavioral characteristics. With each tool, a score is given to each assessment, and the total score is used to determine the gestational age of the infant. The New Ballard Score is described in the following section.

Neuromuscular Characteristics

Posture

The posture and degree of flexion of the extremities are scored before disturbing the quiet infant to perform the remainder of the examination (Figure 20-20). Preterm neonates have immature flexor muscles and little energy or muscle tone. Therefore they have extended, limp arms and legs that offer little resistance to movement by the examiner. Full-term infants hold their arms close to the body with the elbows sharply flexed. The legs should be flexed at the hips, knees, and ankles. Posture is scored from zero (0) for a limp, flaccid posture to 4 if the newborn demonstrates good flexion of all extremities.

Square Window

The square window sign is elicited by bending the hand at the wrist until the palm is as flat against the forearm as possible with gentle pressure (Figure 20-21). The angle between the palm and forearm is measured. If the palm bends only 90 degrees (the extent of flexion of the adult wrist and looks like a square window), the score is 0. The gestational age of the infant is probably 32 weeks or less. The more mature the neonate, the smaller the angle until the palm folds flat against the forearm at term.

Arm Recoil

In testing for arm recoil, the nurse holds the neonate's arms fully flexed at the elbows for 5 seconds, then pulls the hands straight down to the sides (Figure 20-22). The hands are quickly released and the degree of flexion is measured as the arms return to their normally flexed position. Preterm infants

NEWBORN MATURITY RATING & CLASSIFICATION

ESTIMATION OF GESTATIONAL AGE BY MATURITY RATING

Symbols: X - 1st Exam O - 2nd Exam

Gestation by Dates________________wks

Birth Date__________Hour__________am/pm

APGAR__________1 min__________5 min

NEUROMUSCULAR MATURITY

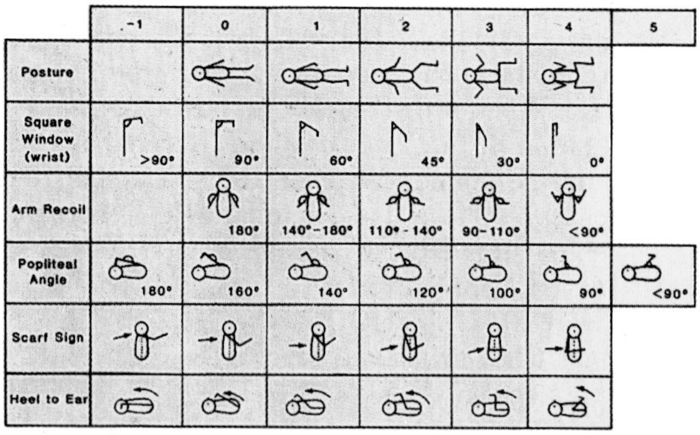

-1
0
1
2
3
4
5
Posture
Square Window (wrist)
>90°
90°
60°
45°
30°
0°
Arm Recoil
180°
140°-180°
110°-140°
90-110°
<90°
Popliteal Angle
180°
160°
140°
120°
100°
90°
<90°
Scarf Sign
Heel to Ear

PHYSICAL MATURITY

Skin	sticky friable transparent	gelatinous red, translucent	smooth pink, visible veins	superficial peeling &/or rash. few veins	cracking pale areas rare veins	parchment deep cracking no vessels	leathery cracked wrinkled
Lanugo	none	sparse	abundant	thinning	bald areas	mostly bald	
Plantar Surface	heel-toe 40-50 mm: -1 <40 mm: -2	>50mm no crease	faint red marks	anterior transverse crease only	creases ant. 2/3	creases over entire sole	
Breast	imperceptible	barely perceptible	flat areola no bud	stippled areola 1-2mm bud	raised areola 3-4mm bud	full areola 5-10mm bud	
Eye/Ear	lids fused loosely:-1 tightly:-2	lids open pinna flat stays folded	sl. curved pinna; soft; slow recoil	well-curved pinna; soft but ready recoil	formed &firm instant recoil	thick cartilage ear stiff	
Genitals male	scrotum flat, smooth	scrotum empty faint rugae	testes in upper canal rare rugae	testes descending few rugae	testes down good rugae	testes pendulous deep rugae	
Genitals female	clitoris prominent labia flat	prominent clitoris small labia minora	prominent clitoris enlarging minora	majora & minora equally prominent	majora large minora small	majora cover clitoris & minora	

MATURITY RATING

score	weeks
-10	20
-5	22
0	24
5	26
10	28
15	30
20	32
25	34
30	36
35	38
40	40
45	42
50	44

SCORING SECTION

	1st Exam=X	2nd Exam=O
Estimating Gest Age by Maturity Rating	______Weeks	______Weeks
Time of Exam	Date______ Hour______am/pm	Date______ Hour______am/pm
Age at Exam	______Hours	______Hours
Signature of Examiner	______ M.D.	______ M.D.

FIGURE 20-19 New Ballard score. (Courtesy Bristol-Myers Company, Evansville, Indiana. From Ballard, J.L., Khoury, J.C., Wedig, K., Wang, L., Eilers-Walsman, B.L., & Lipp, R. [1991]. New Ballard score, expanded to include extremely premature infants. *Journal of Pediatrics,* 19[3], 417-423.)

A 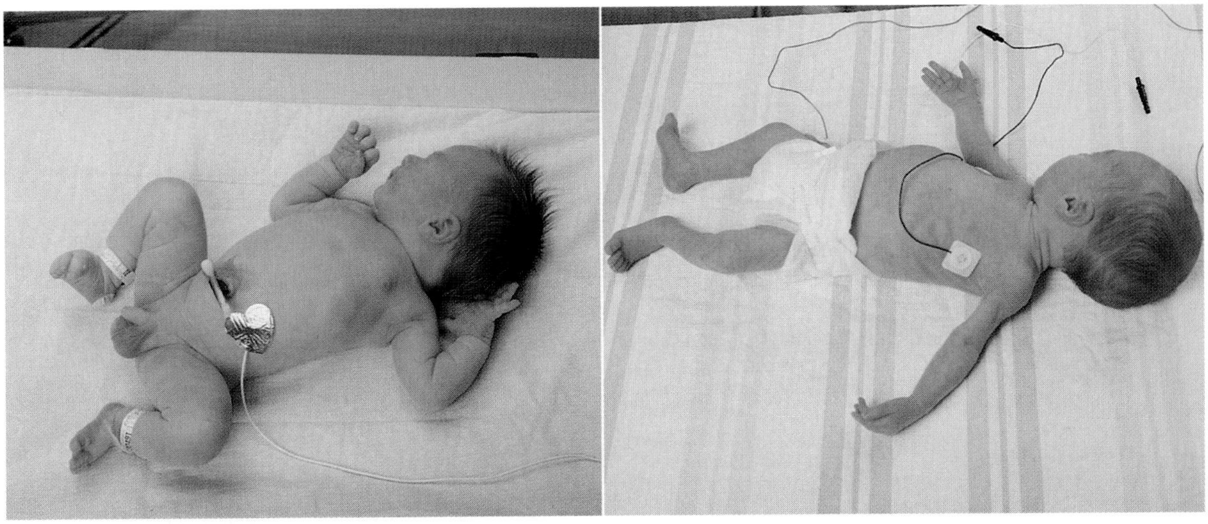 B

FIGURE 20-20 Posture in newborns. **A,** The healthy full-term infant remains in a strongly flexed position. **B,** The preterm infant's extremities are extended.

A 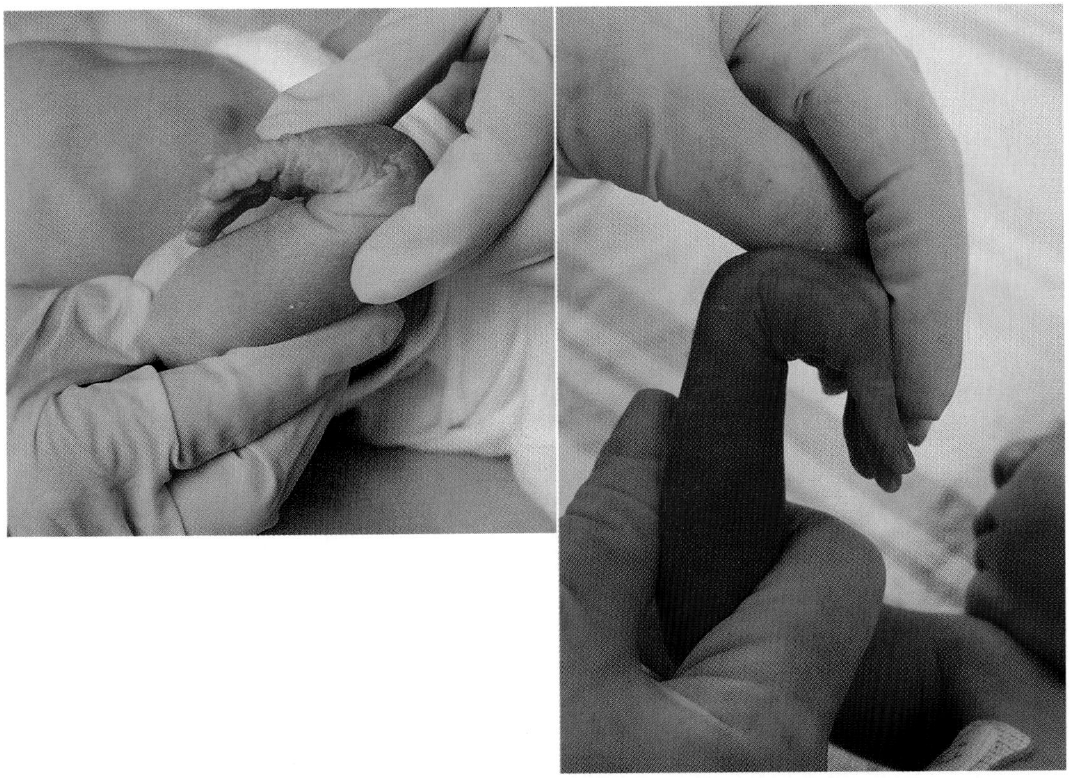 B

FIGURE 20-21 The square window sign is performed on the arm without the identification bracelet. The nurse bends the wrist and measures the angle. **A,** Infant near full term. **B,** Preterm infant.

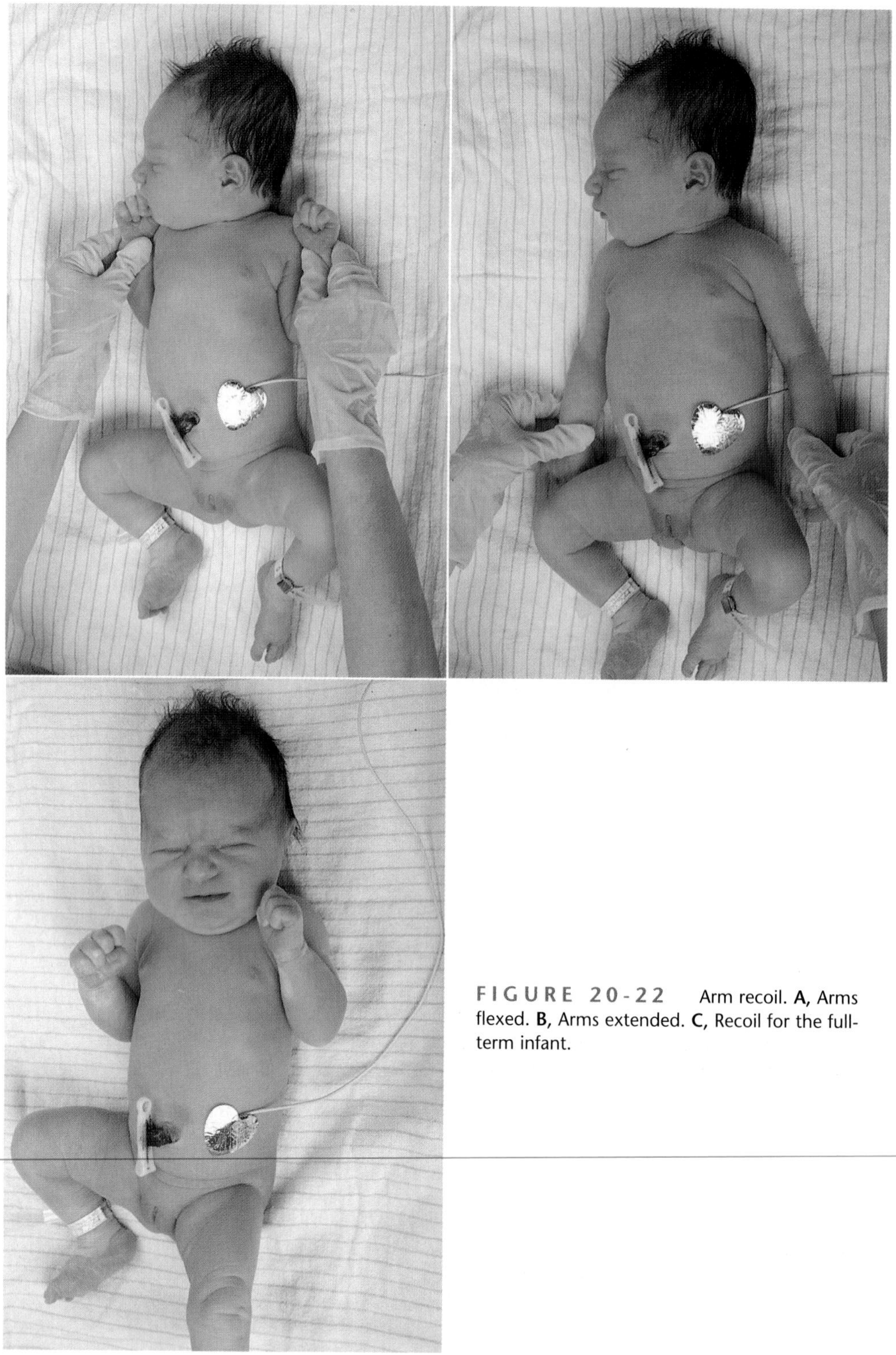

FIGURE 20-22 Arm recoil. **A,** Arms flexed. **B,** Arms extended. **C,** Recoil for the full-term infant.

may not move the arms at all and receive a score of 0. Somewhat older infants have a sluggish recoil, with only partial return to flexion. If the arms move briskly to an angle of less than 90 degrees at the elbows, the score is 4.

Popliteal Angle

To measure the popliteal angle, the newborn's lower leg is folded against the thigh, with the thigh on the abdomen (Figure 20-23). The infant's hips must remain flat on the bed. With the thigh still flexed on the abdomen, the lower leg is straightened just until resistance is met. Continued pressure causes the infant to further extend the leg and results in an inaccurate score. The angle at the popliteal space when resistance is first felt is scored, with a range of 1 if the leg can be fully extended to a score of 5 if the angle at the popliteal space is less than 90 degrees.

A 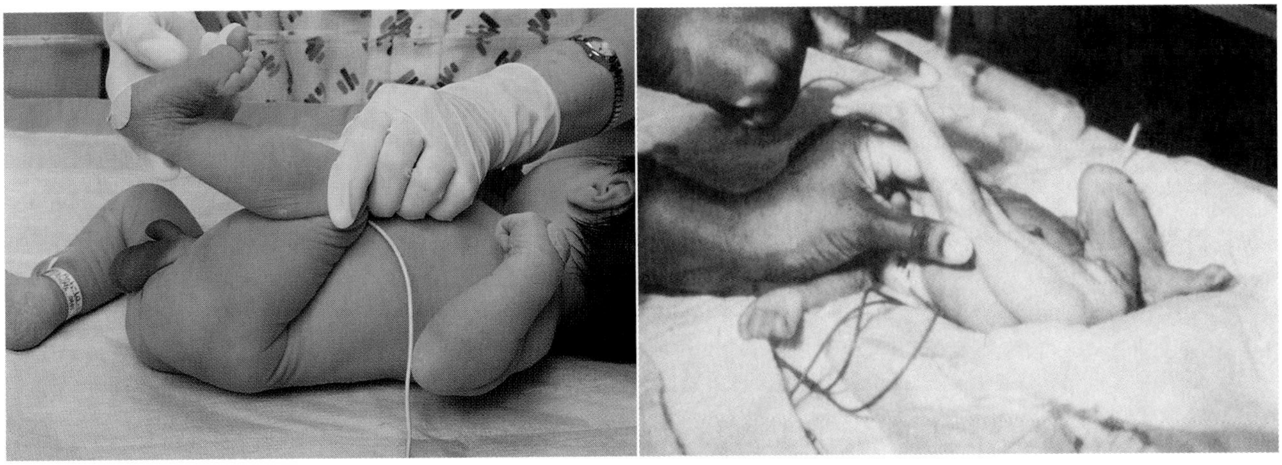 B

FIGURE 20-23 The popliteal angle is measured by flexing the thigh against the abdomen and extending the lower leg to the point of resistance. **A,** Full-term infant. **B,** Preterm infant.

A 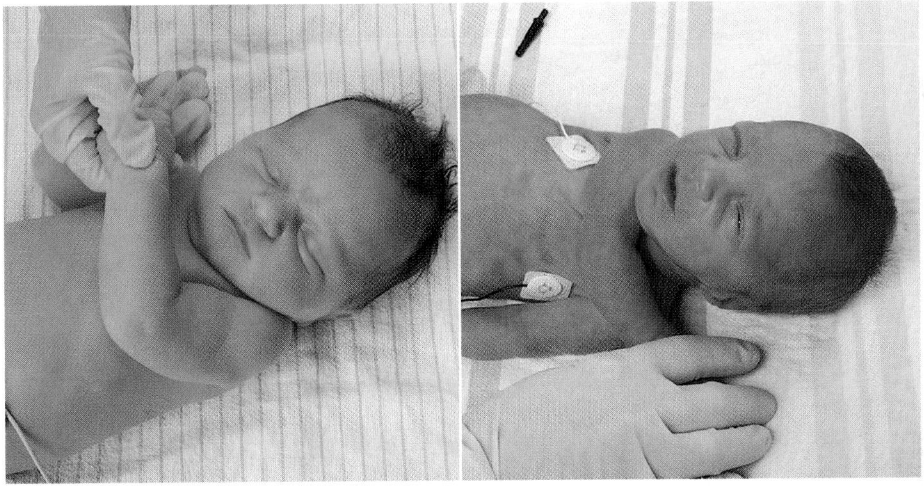 B

FIGURE 20-24 Scarf sign. The nurse determines how far the arm will move across the chest and observes the position of the elbow when resistance is felt. **A,** Full-term infant. **B,** Preterm infant. (Note the many visible veins in the preterm infant and the absence of visible veins in the full-term infant.)

Scarf Sign

For the scarf sign, the nurse grasps the infant's hand and brings the arm across the body to the opposite side (Figure 20-24). The shoulder should not be lifted from the surface on which the infant is lying. The position of the elbow in relation to the midline of the infant's body is noted. The infant receives a score of 1 if muscle tone is so poor that the arm wraps across the body like a scarf with the elbow beyond the edge of the body. A full score (4) shows that the elbow fails to reach near to midline.

Heel to Ear

The heel-to-ear assessment is similar to the measurement of the popliteal angle. However, in this case, the nurse grasps the infant's foot and pulls it straight up toward the ears while the hips remain flat on the surface of the bed (Figure 20-25). When resistance is felt, the position of the foot in relation to the head and the amount of flexion of the leg are compared with the diagrams. The more resistance and flexion, the more mature the infant.

Record the position when resistance is first felt because the neonate may relax the leg if pressure continues. This assessment may be inaccurate in infants who were in a breech position at delivery because they may lie with the legs extended toward the head. It may be necessary to omit this part of the examination until later or estimate the score temporarily.

Physical Characteristics

Skin

The skin is assessed for color, visibility of veins, and peeling and cracking. The very preterm infant's skin is translucent because it is thin and has little subcutaneous fat beneath the surface. The skin is red, sticky,

A

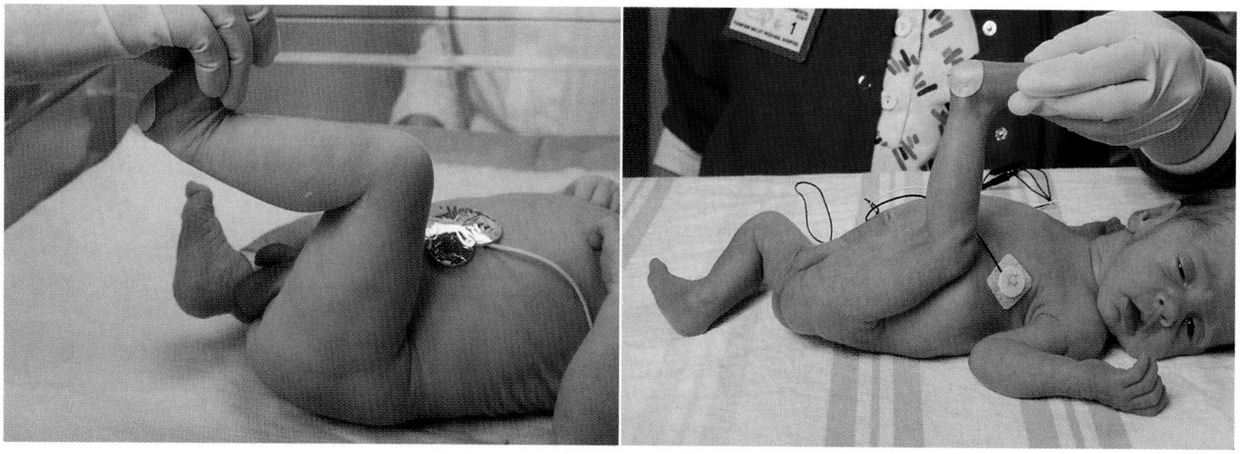

B

FIGURE 20-25 Heel to ear. The nurse grasps the foot and brings it up toward the ear, keeping the hips flat. The score is recorded when resistance is felt. **A**, Full-term infant. **B**, Preterm infant.

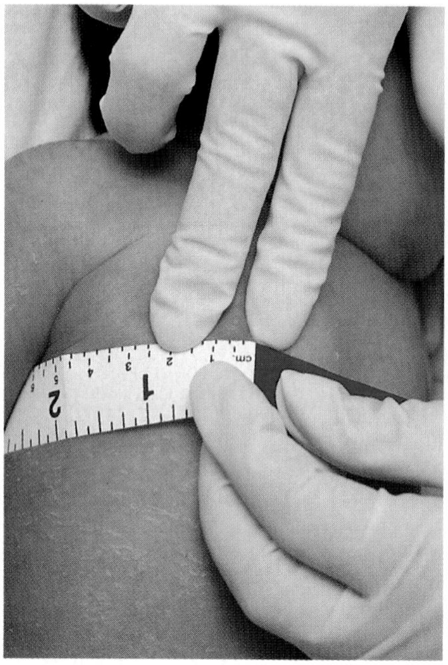

FIGURE 20-26 The nurse places a finger on either side of the breast bud tissue and measures the size. In the full-term infant, breast tissue is raised and the nipple is easily distinguished from surrounding skin. (Note the peeling skin.)

and fragile, with easily visible veins. In the mature newborn, the skin color is paler and few veins are visible, usually over the chest and abdomen (see Figure 20-24). At term, vernix is present only in the creases.

The full-term infant exhibits some peeling and cracking of the skin, especially around areas with creases, such as the ankles and feet. The postmature infant has deeply cracked skin that appears as dry and thick as leather. Peeling becomes even more apparent during the hours after birth as the skin loses moisture (Figure 20-26).

Lanugo

Lanugo appears at 20 weeks of gestation and increases in amount until 28 to 30 weeks' (see Figure 20-13). At that time, it begins to disappear until little is left at term. A small amount may remain over the upper back, shoulders, and over the ears or on the sides of the forehead. Newborns with dark coloring may have more lanugo (which is dark and more easily noticed) than infants with fair skin and very light hair, even though they are the same gestational age. The infant receives a score based on the amount of lanugo present.

Plantar Surface

Plantar creases begin to appear at 32 weeks of gestation (Figure 20-27). Although the creases are only red lines near the toes at first, they gradually spread down toward the heel and become deeper. At 37 weeks of gestation, creases cover the anterior two thirds of the sole. By 40 weeks of gestation, the entire sole is covered with deep creases. The plantar creases must be assessed during the early hours after birth because creases appear more prominent as the infant's skin begins to dry. For the very preterm infant, the length of the foot is measured to help determine gestational age.

Breasts

The nipples, areolae, and subcutaneous fat pads (breast buds) are assessed and scored. In very preterm infants, the structures are not visible. Gradually, they grow larger and the areolae become raised above the chest wall. The fat pads or buds enlarge until they are approximately 1 cm at term. To determine their size, the nurse places a finger on each side and measures the diameter. Use of the thumb and forefinger may cause excess tissue to be drawn together, resulting in an inaccurate score (see Figure 20-26).

Eyes and Ears

In the very preterm infant, the eyelids are fused. They open at 26 to 28 weeks of gestation. At about 33 to 34 weeks of gestation, the upper pinnae, which have been

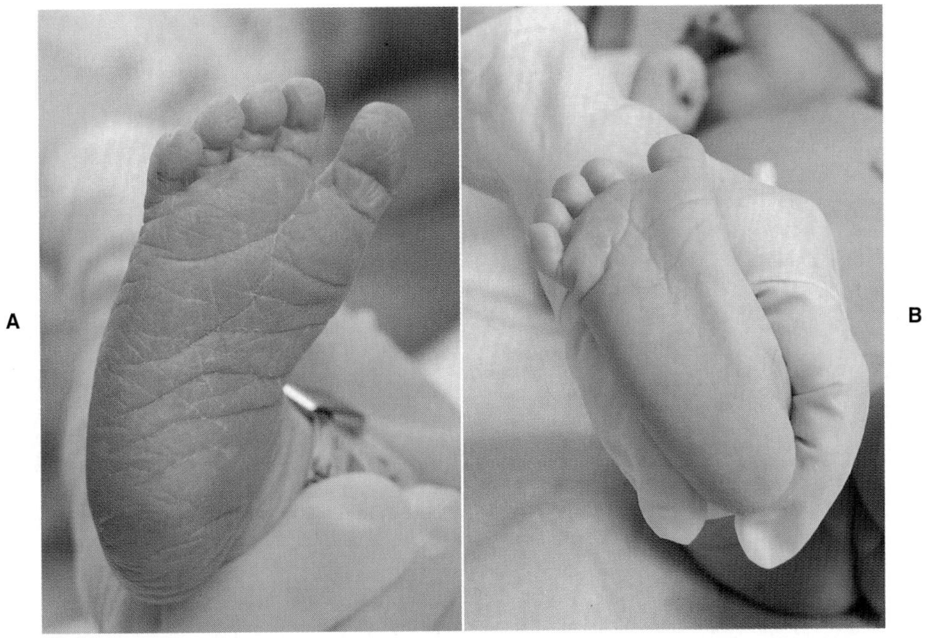

FIGURE 20-27 Plantar creases begin to develop at the base of the toes and extend to the heel. **A,** The postterm infant has deep creases. **B,** The preterm infant has few creases on the entire foot.

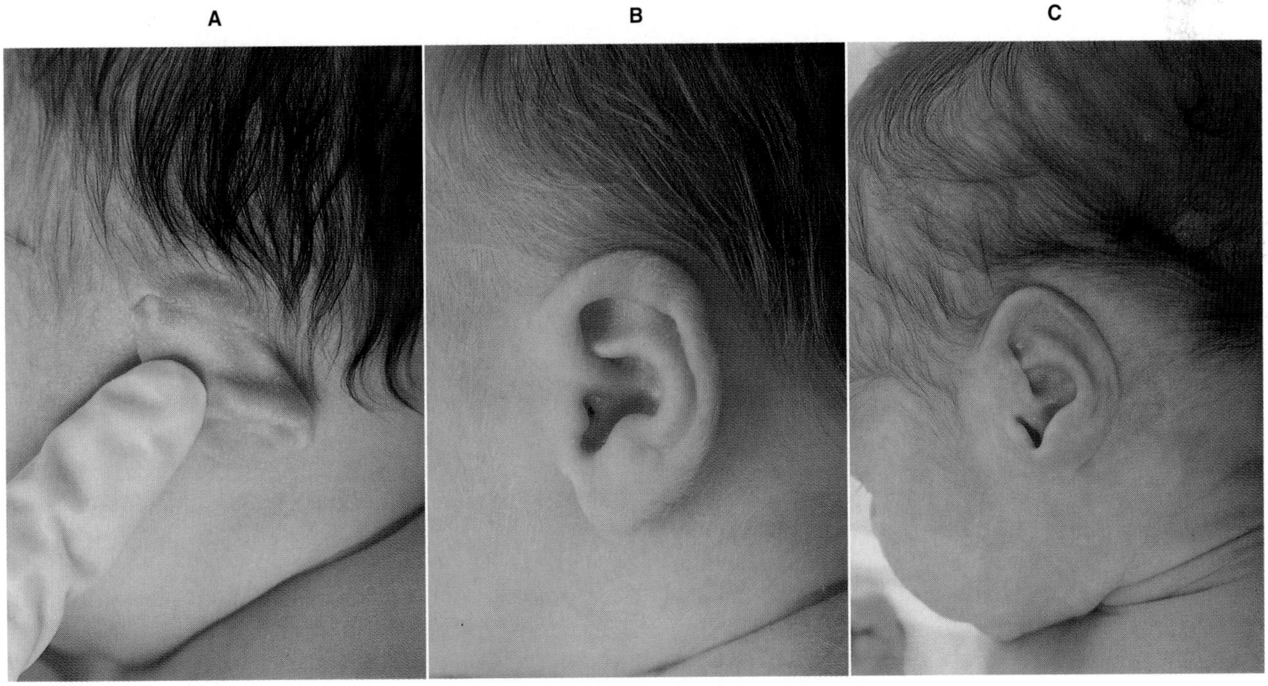

FIGURE 20-28 Ear maturation. **A,** The nurse folds the ears and notes the quickness with which they return to position. **B,** Ears in the full-term infant are well formed and have instant recoil. **C,** In the preterm infant, ears show less curving of the pinna and recoil slowly or not at all.

flat, begin to curve over. The incurving continues around the ear until it reaches near the earlobe at 39 to 40 weeks' gestation. The amount of cartilage present in the ears is a more accurate guide to gestational age than the curving of the pinnae because of individual differences in ear shape. As cartilage is deposited in the pinnae, the ears become stiff and stand away from the head.

In assessing the ear, the incurving and thickness of each pinna are rated (Figure 20-28). The ear is folded longitudinally and horizontally to assess the resistance and speed with which the ear returns to its original state. In infants less than 32 weeks' gestation, the ear has little cartilage to keep it stiff. When folded, it remains folded over or returns slowly. In the term neonate, the ear springs back to its original position immediately.

A 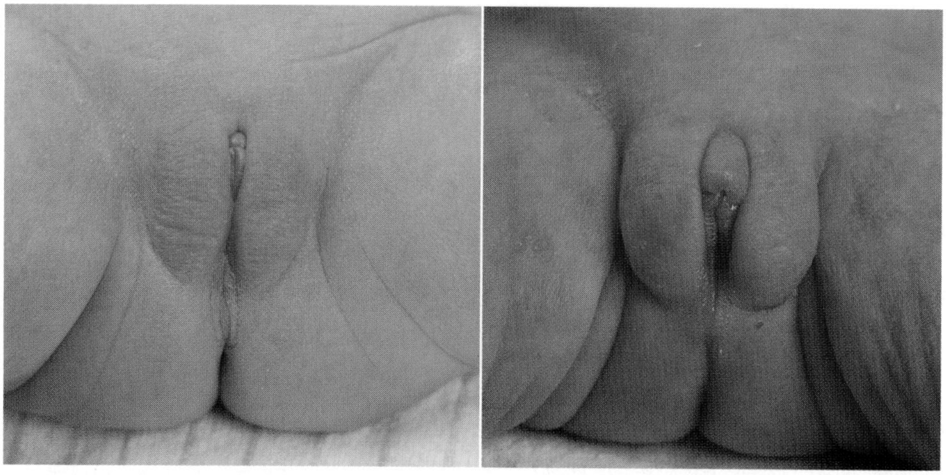 B

FIGURE 20-29 Female genitals. As the female matures, the labia majora cover the labia minora and clitoris completely; in the preterm infant, these structures are not covered. **A,** Near-term infant. **B,** Preterm infant.

A 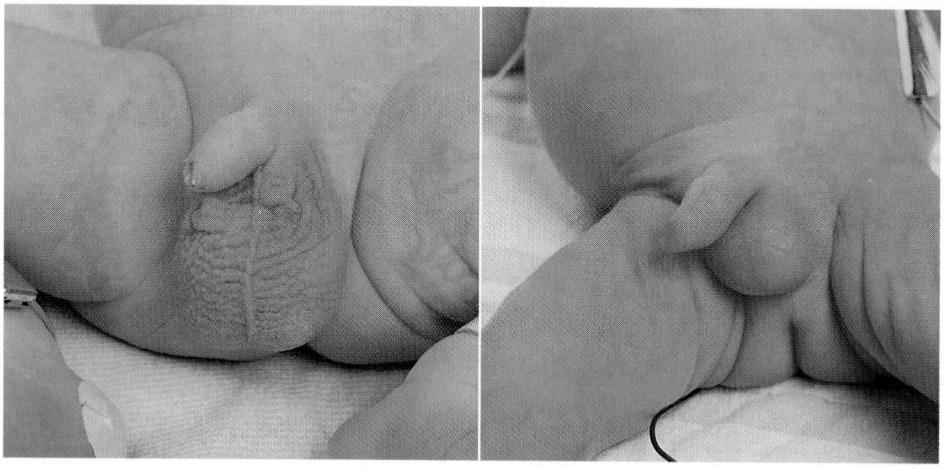 B

FIGURE 20-30 Male genitals. **A,** The full-term infant has a pendulous scrotum with deep rugae. **B,** In the preterm infant, the testes may not be descended and rugae are few.

Genitals

In the female infant, the relationship in size of the clitoris, labia minora, and labia majora is noted (Figure 20-29). In the preterm infant, the labia majora are small and separated, whereas the clitoris and labia minora are large by comparison. As the infant nears term, the labia majora enlarge until the clitoris and labia minora are completely covered. Because the size of the labia majora is affected by the amount of fat deposited, the infant who is malnourished in utero may have genitalia with an immature appearance.

In the male infant, the location of the testes and the rugae on the scrotum are assessed (Figure 20-30). The testes originate in the abdominal cavity but move down into the inguinal canal at 30 weeks of gestation. By 37 weeks' gestation, they are located high in the scrotal sac, and they are generally completely descended by term. Rugae form on the surface of the scrotum beginning at about 36 weeks' and cover the sac by 40 weeks' gestation. Once the testes are completely down into the scrotum, the scrotum appears large and pendulous.

Scoring

As each part of the assessment is performed, the infant's response is matched with the diagrams and explanations on the assessment tool. The total score is compared with the corresponding gestational age. Although slight differences in the scores may be obtained by different examiners, a difference of 2.5 points is necessary to change the gestational age by 1 week. Therefore slight differences in the scores of different examiners are not likely to cause significant differences in the outcome of the examination.

Gestational Age and Infant Size

The appropriateness of the neonate's size for gestational age is determined by plotting the gestational age, weight, length, and head circumference on a graph of intrauterine development (Figure 20-31). This score

CLASSIFICATION OF NEWBORNS – BASED ON MATURITY AND INTRAUTERINE GROWTH

Symbols: X-1st Exam O-2nd Exam

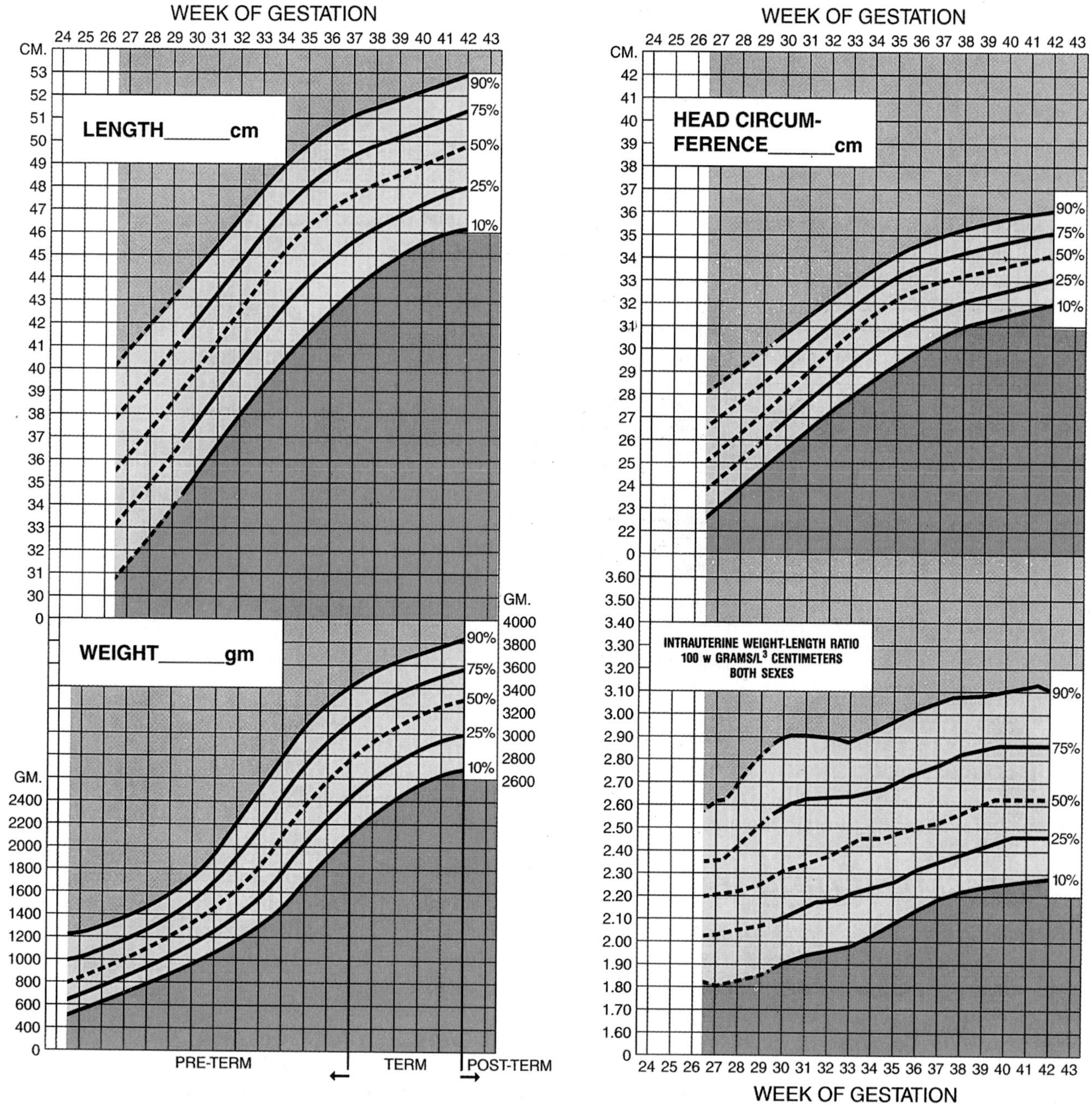

	1st Exam (X)	2nd Exam (O)
LARGE FOR GESTATIONAL AGE **(LGA)**		
APPROPRIATE FOR GESTATIONAL AGE **(AGA)**		
SMALL FOR GESTATIONAL AGE **(SGA)**		
Age at Exam	hrs	hrs
Signature of Examiner	M.D.	M.D.

FIGURE 20-31 Intrauterine growth grids. (Courtesy Bristol-Myers Company, Evansville, Indiana. Adapted from Lubchenko, L.C., Hansman, C, & Boyd, E. [1966]. *Pediatrics,* 37, 403 and from Battaglia, F.C., & Lubchenko, L.C. [1967]. *Journal of Pediatrics,* 71, 159.)

determines how well the infant has grown for the amount of time spent in the uterus. An infant may be small, large, or appropriate for gestational age. The infant who is appropriate for gestational age falls between the 10th and 90th percentile on the graph. The large-for-gestational age (LGA) infant is above the 90th percentile, whereas the small-for-gestational age (SGA) infant is below the 10th percentile.

Although people sometimes think that the SGA infant is always preterm, SGA infants can also be full term or postterm. Similarly, the LGA infant can be born before term, at term, or beyond term. For example, an infant born at 28 weeks of gestation may have measurements that correspond to the 92nd percentile on the intrauterine growth curve chart. The infant would be LGA even though he or she is preterm. An infant judged to be 43 weeks' gestational age may have measurements that correspond to the 7th percentile on the growth curve. The infant would be SGA.

Further Assessments

When an infant's gestational age or measurements fall outside the expected range, the nurse monitors for complications. Specific complications are common to preterm, postterm, SGA, and LGA infants. For example, pregnancy complications may cause a poorly functioning placenta and an SGA infant. These infants are more prone to hypoglycemia, thermoregulation, and respiratory problems.

The most common causes of an LGA infant are diabetes in the mother and very large parents. The nurse monitors these infants especially carefully for hypoglycemia and birth injuries because of the difficulty of the large infant passing through the birth canal.

ASSESSMENT OF BEHAVIOR

Assessment of the infant's behavior helps determine intactness of the central nervous system and provides information about the infant's ability to respond to caretaking activities. Because behavior differs at various times after birth, the nurse should be aware of the periods of reactivity and the six different states of behavior so that nursing care can be adapted appropriately.

Periods of Reactivity

During the first and second periods of reactivity (see Chapter 19), newborns may have elevated pulse and respiratory rates, low temperatures, and excessive respiratory secretions. Careful observation of infants is important during this time, but assessment can usually be done unobtrusively so that parents can continue to enjoy their newborn. During the sleep period between the first and second periods of reactivity, newborns cannot be awakened easily and are not interested in feeding. Infants in the sleep phase have relaxed muscle tone that may affect the score on a gestational age assessment.

Behavioral Changes

Nurses assess the infant's behavior and alert the physician of abnormalities. Assessment includes the six different behavioral states: deep sleep, active sleep, drowsy, quiet alert, active alert, and crying. Movement between states should be smooth and not abrupt. The Brazelton Neonatal Behavioral Assessment Scale often is used when detailed knowledge about the infant is needed. In addition to assessing behavioral states, the scale analyzes other aspects of the newborn's behavior, such as orientation, habituation, self-consoling behaviors, social behaviors, and the appropriateness of the amount of time in each of these activities.

Orientation

The nurse notes the infant's orientation (ability to pay attention) to interesting visual or auditory stimuli. It is most prominent during the quiet alert state. Infants focus their eyes and turn their heads toward a stimulus in an attempt to prolong contact with it. Preterm and ill neonates have less ability to orient to stimuli. Attempts to stimulate these newborns may result in overfatigue.

Habituation

The infant's response to a visual, auditory, or tactile stimulus is an important assessment. Generally, the first response of a healthy newborn to an interesting stimulus, such as a brightly colored object or bell, is a period of alertness. If the stimulus is disturbing, like a bright light flashed in the eyes or a pinprick to the foot, the infant startles and attempts to escape by averting the eyes or pulling the foot away.

Infants gradually stop responding to continued noxious stimuli. This allows them to ignore the stimuli and save energy for physiologic needs. Newborns may go into a dull, drowsy state or fall into a deep sleep. Those who seem unresponsive in a bright, noisy nursery may be in a state of habituation. The preterm infant or one with damage to the central nervous system may not be able to habituate.

Self-Consoling Activities

Normal newborns are able to console themselves for short periods of time. Self-consoling activities include attempting to bring their hands to the mouth, sucking on their fists, and watching objects in the environment. Infants who are ill, preterm, or exposed to drugs prenatally have less ability to console themselves.

Parents' Response

The parents' growing ability to respond to the infant's behavioral cues should be noted. The nurse can point out the infant's behavioral changes to facilitate bonding and help the parents learn to interpret the infant's cues. The methods which the parents use to meet the infant's needs during different behavior states also are noted.

Check Your Reading

11. When should the first voiding occur? How often do infants void?
12. What is the nurse's responsibility regarding marks on the newborn's skin?
13. Why is the gestational age assessment important?
14. How do the periods of reactivity affect nursing care?

SUMMARY CONCEPTS

- Nurses assess newborns immediately after birth to detect serious abnormalities. If no problems are detected with a quick assessment, a more comprehensive examination is performed.
- Molding of the head is normal during birth and may cause the head to appear misshaped. Caput succedaneum (localized swelling from pressure against the cervix) or a cephalhematoma (bleeding between the periosteum and the bone) may occur.
- Measurements are an important way to learn about growth before birth. Abnormal measurements alert the nurse that complications may occur.
- Assessment of cardiorespiratory status includes history, airway, color, heart sounds, pulses, and blood pressure.
- Axillary temperatures are preferred to rectal temperatures because they are safer and provide accurate measurement.
- Hypoglycemia can cause damage to the brain. Early signs of hypoglycemia include jitteriness, poor muscle tone, respiratory distress, perspiration, low temperature, and poor suck.
- In performing heel sticks for blood glucose, the nurse must choose the site carefully to avoid damage to the bone, nerves, and blood vessels of the heel.
- Reflexes are an indication of the health of the central nervous system. Asymmetry or retention of reflexes beyond the time when they should disappear is abnormal.
- The initial feeding provides information about the neonate's tolerance to feeding and ability to coordinate sucking, swallowing, and breathing.
- Newborns pass the first stool within 12 to 48 hours of birth. Feeding and inserting a rectal thermometer may stimulate stool passage.
- The newborn's first void occurs within 12 to 24 hours. Infants void two to six times the first two days and then at least 6 times daily.
- Marks on the skin should be documented, including location, size, color, elevation, and texture. Because marks can be upsetting, they should be explained to the parents.
- The gestational age assessment provides an estimate of the infant's age from conception.
- During the first and second periods of reactivity, the infant may have a low temperature, elevated pulse and respirations, and excessive respiratory secretions. Between these periods, the infant is in a deep sleep with relaxed muscle tone and no interest in feeding.

ANSWERS TO CRITICAL THINKING EXERCISE, p. 522

Failure of the reflexes to fade on schedule may interfere with normal development. For example, the palmar grasp reflex must disappear so that the infant can learn to grasp voluntarily and later to release objects at will. Persistence of the plantar reflex would interfere with walking. Retention of reflexes beyond the age when they should disappear indicates pathology and should prompt further investigation.

ANSWERS TO CRITICAL THINKING EXERCISE, p. 529

Begin by expanding your assessment of the facts. First, check through the chart to be sure that no stool is recorded. Did the infant pass meconium at delivery? Check the delivery notes. Ask the mother if she has changed a diaper with stool in it. Instruct her to inform the nurse if she does. If the first temperature performed on the infant was rectal, the anus is patent. If whether a rectal temperature was done is not clear, take one to check patency. Taking a rectal temperature may stimulate peristalsis and passage of meconium. However, even with a patent anus, obstruction of the intestine above the anus is possible.

Consider the infant's intake. How often is the infant feeding and how well are feedings being taken? If the infant has been sleepy and has fed poorly, increase the feedings. Asking the nursing mother to feed more often or offering the neonate extra formula may make the difference.

Alert other caregivers to watch for a stool and let the mother know that the infant is being watched for stools without alarming her. Although some infants do not have a stool until near 48 hours after birth, the primary caregiver may wish to know about the situation at 24 hours.

REFERENCES & READINGS

American Academy of Pediatrics & American College of Obstetricians and Gynecologists (1997). *Guidelines for perinatal care* (4th ed.). Elk Grove, IL: American Academy of Pediatrics.

American Academy of Pediatrics (AAP). (2000). Clinical practice guideline: Early detection of developmental dysplasia of the hip. *Pediatrics,* 105(4), 896-905.

Association of Women's Health, Obstetric, and Neonatal Nurses (AWHONN). (1996). *Physiologic assessment of the healthy newborn.* Washington, D.C.: Author.

Ballard, J.L., Khoury, J.C., Wedig, K., Wang, L., Eilers-Walsman, B.L., & Lipp, R. (1991). New Ballard score, expanded to include extremely premature infants. *Journal of Pediatrics,* 19(3), 417-423.

Bell, E.F., & Oh, W. (1999). Fluid and electrolyte management. In G.B. Avery, M.A. Fletcher, & M.G. MacDonald (Eds.), *Neonatology: Pathophysiology and management of the newborn* (5th ed., pp. 345-361). Philadelphia: Lippincott.

Berkowitz, C.D. (1996). *Pediatrics: A primary care approach.* Philadelphia: W.B. Saunders.

Blackburn, S.T. (1998). Assessment and management of neonatal neurobehavioral development. In C. Kenner, J.W. Lott, & A.A. Flandermeyer (Eds.), *Comprehensive neonatal nursing, a physiologic perspective* (2nd ed., pp. 564-607). Philadelphia: W.B. Saunders.

Blake, W.W., & Murray, J.A. (1998). Heat balance. In G.B. Merenstein & S.L. Gardner (Eds.), *Handbook of neonatal intensive care* (4th ed., pp. 100-115). St. Louis: Mosby.

Bowden, V.R., Dickey, S.B., & Greenberg, C.S. (1998). *Children and their families: The continuum of care.* Philadelphia: W.B. Saunders.

Brazelton, T.B. (1999). Behavioral competence. In G.B. Avery, M.A. Fletcher, & M.G. MacDonald (Eds.), *Neonatology: Pathophysiology and management of the newborn* (5th ed., pp. 321-332). Philadelphia: Lippincott.

Buschbach, D. (2000). Physical assessment of the newborn infant. In *Core curriculum for neonatal intensive care nursing* (2nd ed., pp. 74-100). Philadelphia: W.B. Saunders.

Dodd, V. (1996). Gestational age assessment. *Neonatal Network,* 15(1), 27-36.

Dubowitz, L., & Dubowitz, V. (1977). *Gestational age of the newborn.* Reading, MA: Addison-Wesley.

Elder, J.S. (2000). Urologic disorders in infants and children. In R.E. Behrman, R.M. Kliegman, & H.B. Jenson (Eds.). *Nelson textbook of pediatrics* (16th ed., pp. 1650-1654). Philadelphia: W.B. Saunders.

Fletcher, M.A. (1999). Physical assessment and classification. In G.B. Avery, M.A. Fletcher, & M.G. MacDonald (Eds.), *Neonatology: Pathophysiology and management of the newborn* (5th ed., pp. 301-320). Philadelphia: J.B. Lippincott.

Gomella, T.L., Cunningham, M.D., Eyal, F.G. & Zenk, K.E. (Eds.). (1999). *Neonatology* (4th ed.). Norwalk, CT: Appleton & Lange.

Hagedorn, M.I.E., Gardner, S.L., & Abman, S.H. (1998). Respiratory diseases. In G.B. Merenstein & S.L. Gardner (Eds.), *Handbook of neonatal intensive care* (4th ed., pp. 437-497). St. Louis: Mosby.

Hagedorn, M.I.E., & Gardner, S.L. (1999). Hypoglycemia in the newborn, part I: Pathology and nursing management. *Mother Baby Journal,* 4(1), 15-21.

Hernandez, J.A., Zabloudil, C., & Hernandez, P.W. (1999). Adaptation to extrauterine life and management during transition. In P.J. Thureen, J. Deacon, P. O'Neil, & J. Hernandez. *Assessment and care of the well newborn* (pp. 83-100). Philadelphia: W.B. Saunders.

Howard-Glenn, L. (2000). Adaptation to extrauterine life and immediate nursing care. In *Core curriculum for maternal-newborn nursing* (2nd ed., pp. 346-359). Philadelphia: W.B. Saunders.

Howard-Glenn, L. (2000). Newborn biological/behavioral characteristics and psychosocial adaptations. In *Core curriculum for maternal-newborn nursing* (2nd ed., pp. 360-373). Philadelphia: W.B. Saunders.

Johnson, C.B. (1996). Head, eyes, ears, nose, mouth, and neck assessment. In E.P. Tappero & M.E. Honeyfield (Eds.). *Physical assessment of the newborn* (2nd ed.). Petaluma, CA: NICU INK.

Katz, K., & Nishioka, E. (1998). Neonatal assessment. In C. Kenner, J.W. Lott, & A.A. Flandermeyer (Eds.), *Comprehensive neonatal nursing, a physiologic perspective* (2nd ed., pp. 223-251). Philadelphia: W.B. Saunders.

Leick-Rude, M.K., & Bloom, L.F. (1998). A comparison of temperature-taking methods in neonates. *Neonatal Network,* 17(5), 21-37.

Lepley, C.J., Gardner, S.L., & Lubchenco, L.O. (1998). Initial nursery care. In G.B. Merenstein & S.L. Gardner (Eds.), *Handbook of neonatal intensive care* (4th ed., pp 70-99). St. Louis: Mosby.

Meehan, R.M. (1998). Heelsticks in neonates for capillary blood sampling. *Neonatal Network,* 17(1), 17-24.

Miklos, A.B., & Creehan, P.A. (1996). Newborn physical assessment. In K.R. Simpson & P.A. Creehan (Eds.), *AWHONN's perinatal nursing.* Philadelphia: Lippincott-Raven.

Nicholson, J.F., & Pesce, M.A. (2000). Reference ranges for laboratory tests and procedures. In R.E. Behrman, R.M. Kliegman, & H.B. Jenson (Eds.). *Nelson textbook of pediatrics* (16th ed., pp. 2181-2229). Philadelphia: W.B. Saunders.

Philip, A. (1996). *Neonatology, a practical guide* (4th ed.). Philadelphia: W.B. Saunders.

Sganga, A., Wallace, R., Kiehl, E., Irving, T., & Witter, L. (2000). A comparison of four methods of normal newborn temperature measurement. *MCN: The American Journal of Maternal/Child Nursing,* 25(2), 76-79.

Sifuentes, M. (2000). Neonatal examination and nursery visit. In C.D. Berkowitz (Ed.), *Pediatrics: A primary care approach* (2nd ed., pp. 20-23). Philadelphia: W.B. Saunders.

Smith, J.B., Ley, S.J., Curley, M.A.Q., Elixson, E.M., & Dodds, K.M. (1996). Tissue perfusion. In M.A.Q. Curley, J.B. Smith, & P.A. Moloney-Harmon, *Critical care of infants and children.* Philadelphia: W.B. Saunders.

Stoll, B.J., & Kliegman, R.M. (2000). The newborn infant. In R.E. Behrman, R.M. Kliegman, & H.B. Jenson (Eds.). *Nelson textbook of pediatrics* (16th ed., pp. 454-460). Philadelphia: W.B. Saunders.

Taeusch, H.W. & Sniderman, S. (1998). Initial evaluation: History and physical examination. In H.W. Taeusch & R.A. Ballard (Eds.), *Avery's diseases of the newborn* (7th ed., pp. 334-353). Philadelphia: W.B. Saunders.

Thompson, G.H., & Scoles, P.V. (2000). Orthopedic problems. In R.E. Behrman, R.M. Kliegman, & H.B. Jenson (Eds.), *Nelson textbook of pediatrics* (16th ed., pp. 2055-2098). Philadelphia: W.B. Saunders.

Vargo, L. (1996). Cardiovascular assessment of the newborn. In E.P. Tappero & M.E. Honeyfield (Eds.), *Physical assessment of the newborn* (2nd ed., pp. 77-92). Petaluma, CA: NICU INK.

21

CARE OF THE NORMAL NEWBORN

OBJECTIVES

1. Describe the purpose and use of routine prophylactic medications for the normal newborn.
2. Explain the nurse's responsibility in cardiorespiratory and thermoregulatory assessments and care.
3. Describe collaborative interventions for hypoglycemia.
4. Discuss prevention and parent teaching for jaundice.
5. Explain the risks and benefits of circumcision.
6. Describe the care of circumcised and uncircumcised male infants.
7. Describe ongoing nursing assessments and care of the newborn.
8. Describe methods of protecting newborns by proper identification.
9. Explain how nurses can help prevent infant abductions.
10. Describe methods of preventing infections in newborns.
11. Discuss important considerations in parent teaching.
12. Explain the importance of newborn screening tests.

The role of the nurse in ongoing assessments and care of the newborn is to help the newborn and parents have a successful transition after birth. The nurse identifies changes in the condition of newborns as they adapt to life outside the uterus, keeps infants safe, and teaches parents how to provide care.

CLINICAL PATHWAYS

Using clinical pathways assists parents and infants to reach the goal of successful transition after childbirth. Birth facilities develop these guides to ensure that mothers and infants are adequately prepared for discharge and that they meet criteria for discharge. Figure 21-1 provides one example of a clinical pathway for newborns. Pathways are individualized by each institution based on protocols to meet clients' needs.

EARLY CARE

Early care after birth involves assessment and stabilization of the infant as necessary (see discussion of immediate care on p. 323 and infant resuscitation, p. 843). Prophylactic medications are given within the first hour. They are vitamin K, to prevent hemorrhagic disease of the newborn, and erythromycin, to prevent ophthalmia neonatorum.

Administering Vitamin K

Vitamin K is given to the neonate within the first hour after birth (Procedure 21-1 and Drug Guide: Vitamin K_1 [Phytonadione]). Although vitamin K is available in oral form, current recommendations are for intramuscular administration (AAP/ACOG, 1997). Because infants cannot synthesize vitamin K in the intestines without bacterial flora they are deficient in clotting factors. One dose of vitamin K prevents bleeding problems until the infant is able to produce it adequately.

Providing Eye Treatment

All infants receive prophylactic treatment to prevent ophthalmia neonatorum in case the mother is infected with gonorrhea or Chlamydia. Currently the most common medication for eye prophylaxis is erythromycin ointment (Figure 21-2 and Drug Guide: Erythromycin Ophthalmic Ointment), although tetracycline or silver nitrate are used in some areas.

Some infants develop a mild inflammation a few hours after prophylactic treatment. However, any discharge from the eyes, especially if it is purulent, should alert the nurse to the possibility of infection. Drainage should be removed with sterile saline and cotton. If the mother is infected, the infant needs additional antibiotics because routine prophylactic treatment may not completely prevent infection.

Because the ointment may temporarily blur the infant's vision, parents may wish to delay treatment for a short time during initial bonding. It may be delayed for as long as an hour after birth without adverse effects.

APPLICATION OF THE NURSING PROCESS: CARDIORESPIRATORY STATUS

In the early newborn period, problems of transition may include temporary problems in cardiorespiratory status. If identified and managed promptly, most resolve within a short time.

Assessment

Assess the newborn for signs of difficult transition to newborn life. Note the rate and character of the heart rate, respirations, pulse, and breath sounds. Look for

Text continued on p. 552

DRUG GUIDE: VITAMIN K_1 (PHYTONADIONE)

Classification: Fat-soluble vitamin

Other Names: Phytonadione, AquaMEPHYTON, Konakion

Action: Promotes the formation of Factors II (prothrombin), VII, IX, and X by the liver for clotting; provides vitamin K, which is not synthesized in the intestines for the first 5 to 8 days after birth because the newborn lacks intestinal flora necessary for vitamin K production

Indication: Prevention or treatment of hemorrhagic disease of the newborn

Neonatal Dosage and Route: 0.5 to 1 mg (0.25 to 0.5 ml) given once intramuscularly within 1 hour of birth for prophylaxis; may be repeated if the infant shows bleeding tendencies

Absorption: Readily absorbed after intramuscular injection; effective within 1 to 2 hours

Adverse Reactions: Pain and edema at site of administration; hemolysis or hyperbilirubinemia, especially in a preterm infant or when large doses are used

Nursing Considerations: Protect the drug from light until just before administration, as it decomposes and loses potency on exposure to light. This drug is incompatible with other drugs. Observe all infants for signs of vitamin K deficiency: ecchymoses or bleeding from any site. Check that the newborn has had vitamin K before a circumcision is performed.

PROCEDURE 21-1

Administering Intramuscular Injections to Newborns

Purpose: To place medication into the muscle without injury.

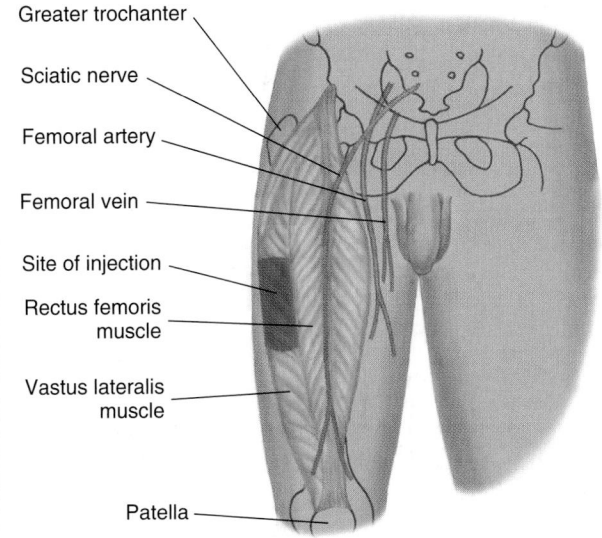

1. Wash the infant's thigh if the bath has not yet been given. *This removes blood from the mother that may be present on the infant's skin to prevent carrying it into the infant's tissues during the needle insertion.*
2. Prepare medication for injection. Use a 1-ml syringe with a ⅝-inch 25-gauge needle. Use a filter needle to draw up medications in glass ampules. Remove the filter needle and replace the original sterile needle to give the injection. *A small needle reaches the newborn's muscle but avoids striking the bone. Use of a filter needle prevents particles of glass from being drawn into the syringe.*
3. Put on gloves. *This protects the nurse from contamination with blood.*
4. Locate the correct site. The best site for intramuscular injections is the infant's vastus lateralis muscle. If necessary, the rectus femoris muscle can be used. Divide the area between the greater trochanter of the femur and the knee into thirds. Give the injection in the middle third of the muscle, lateral to the midline of the anterior thigh. *The large vastus lateralis is located away from the sciatic nerve, and the femoral artery and vein. The rectus femoris muscle is nearer to these structures and poses more of a danger. (Note: The gluteal muscles are never used until a child has been walking for at least a year. These muscles are poorly developed and dangerously near the sciatic nerve.)*

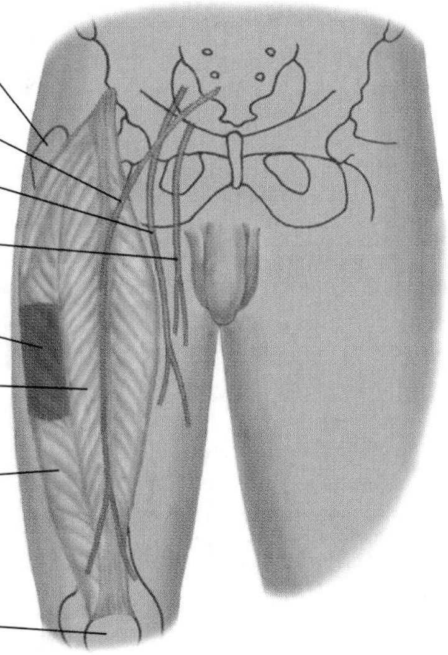

5. Cleanse the area with an alcohol wipe. *This removes organisms and prevents infection.*
6. Stabilize the leg firmly while grasping the thigh between the thumb and fingers. *This prevents sudden movement by the infant and possible injury.*
7. Insert the needle at a 90-degree angle. *This places the medication into the muscle rather than the subcutaneous tissue.*

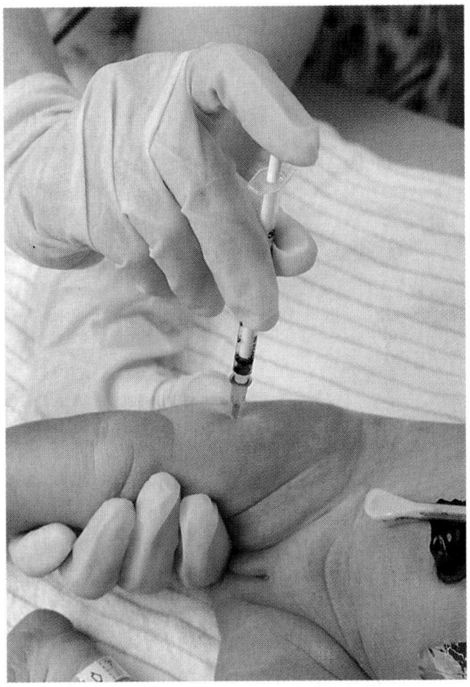

8. Aspirate and inject the medication slowly if no blood returns. If blood returns, withdraw the needle. Discard the medication and syringe and prepare new medication. *Blood return on aspiration indicates that the needle is in a blood vessel. Slow injection reduces discomfort.*
9. Withdraw the needle and massage the site with an alcohol wipe. *Both reduce discomfort. Massage helps absorption of the medication.*

YORK HEALTH SYSTEM
YORK, PENNSYLVANIA
CLINICAL PATHWAY
NEWBORN

CLINICAL PATH DAY		EXPECTED PATIENT FAMILY OUTCOMES	INTERDISCIPLINARY ASSESSMENT	TESTS	CONSULT
Immediate Newborn Care	Date & Time	☐ Apgar score >7 at 5 min [4] ☐ Maintains axillary temp of 36.5° C to 37.2° C while in radiant warmer or in double blankets [1] ☐ Physiologic parameters WNL [4] ☐ Demonstrates proper latch when breastfeeding [2] ☐ ________	Apgar score 1 & 5 min Transitional newborn assessment q 30 min. Suck reflex ________ ________	Hypoglycemia protocol when indicated ________ ________	________ ________
Newborn Admission	Date & Time	☐ Maintains axillary temp of 36.5° C to 37.2° C while in radiant warmer or in double blankets [1] ☐ Physiologic parameters WNL [4] ☐ Tolerates initial feeding [2] ☐ Mother's blood type O/Rh− [4] ☐ ________	Weight Temp q 30 min × 4 Multisystem admission assessment Suck reflex ________ ________	Hypoglycemia protocol when indicated ________ ________	________ ________
0-24 Hours	Date	☐☐☐ Maintains axillary temp of 36.5° C to 37.2° C independent of external heat source [1] ☐☐☐ Parents/family verbalize understanding of safety & security measures [6] ☐☐☐ Physiologic parameters WNL [4] ☐☐☐ Parent(s)/family & infant demonstrate attachment behaviors [3] ☐☐☐ Feeding [2] ☐☐☐ Latch score is 7 or greater for breastfed newborn [2] ☐☐☐ No jaundice [4] ☐☐☐ Infant seen by physician within 12 hours [6] ☐☐☐ ________	Temp, apical pulse, neuro, cardiac, resp., GI, GU, integ. q shift Parent/infant attachment Positioning and LATCH score of breastfed newborn Freq. and amount of bottle-feeding ________ ________	Hypoglycemia protocol when indicated ________ ________	________ ________

NAME	INITIALS	NAME	INITIALS
________	____	________	____
________	____	________	____

Note: Each patient requires an individual assessment & treatment plan. This Clinical Path is a recommendation for the average patient and requires modification when necessary by the professional staff.

FIGURE 21-1 An example of a clinical pathway for the newborn from birth through discharge. This form is printed on both sides and is used by all caregivers to plan and document care. (Courtesy Women and Children Services of the York Health System, York, Pennsylvania. Modified with permission.)

DOCUMENTATION CODES

Initial = Meets Standard

★ = Exception on pathway identified

C = Chronic problems

N = Not applicable

PATIENT/FAMILY PROBLEMS

1. Potential for altered thermoregulation
2. Potential for feeding intolerance, neonate
3. Potential for ineffective parenting
4. Potential for altered newborn metabolism
5. Potential for infection
6. Safety concerns
7. __________
8. __________

INTERVENTIONS/ACTIVITIES	MEDS	NUTR.	EDUC & DC PLANNING
Clamp cord Dry newborn Radiant warmer or double blanket while being held until temp stable ID bands ________ ________	Neonatal eye prophylaxis & Aquamephyton ________	Determine if bottlefeeding or breastfeeding Assist with initial breastfeeding ________	☐ Initiate safety & security measures with parents/family ☐ Teach breastfeeding mother proper latch ☐ ________
Cord care Admission bath ________ ________	HBIG if indicated ________	<u>Initial feeding</u>: ________ ________	☐ ________ ☐ ________
Cord care Circumcision care when indicated ________ ________	________ ________	Breast/bottle feed on demand ________ ________	☐ ☐ ☐ Reinforce safety and security measures w/parents/family ☐ ☐ ☐ Observe & reinforce proper latch and instruct breastfeeding mother/family in alternative positioning ☐ Give and review new pamphlets: –Message to mothers –Newborn screening –Car seat –Health insurance for newborns –Preparing formula –Breastfeeding, A Guide for Success ☐ ☐ ☐ ________ ________

NAME	INITIALS	NAME	INITIALS

FIGURE 21-1, cont'd For legend see opposite page.

Continued

CLINICAL PATH DAY		EXPECTED PATIENT/ FAMILY OUTCOMES	INTERDISCIPLINARY ASSESSMENT	TESTS	CONSULT
24-48 Hours	Date	☐☐☐ Maintains axillary temp of 36.5° C to 37.2° C indep. of external heat source [1] ☐☐☐ Parent(s)/family & newborn demonstrate attachment behaviors [3] ☐☐☐ Physiologic parameters WNL [4] ☐☐☐ Feeding [2] ☐☐☐ LATCH score 7 or greater for breastfed newborn [2] ☐☐☐ No jaundice [4] ☐☐☐ ______	Temp. apical pulse, cardiac, resp., neuro, GI, GU, integ. q 8 hr Weight Parent(s)/family & infant attachment behaviors LATCH score of breastfed newborn Freq. & amt. of bottle feeding ______ ______	______ ______ ______	☐☐☐ Referral made to LC for LATCH score <7 ______ ______ ______
48-72 Hours	Date	☐☐☐ Maintains axillary temp of 36.5° C to 37.2° C indep. of external heat source [1] ☐☐☐ Parent(s)/family & newborn demonstrate attachment behaviors [3] ☐☐☐ Physiologic parameters WNL [4] ☐☐☐ Feeding [2] ☐☐☐ LATCH score 7 or greater for breastfed newborn [2] ☐☐☐ No jaundice [4] ☐☐☐ ______	Temp, apical pulse, cardiac, resp., neuro, GI, GU, integ. q 8 hr Weight Parent(s)/family & infant attachment behaviors LATCH score of breastfed newborn Freq. & amt. of bottle feeding ______ ______	______ ______ ______	☐☐☐ Referral made to LC for LATCH score <7 ______ ______ ______
Day of Discharge	Date	☐ Maintains axillary temp of 36.5° to 37.2° C indep. of external heat source [1] ☐ Parent(s)/family & newborn demonstrate attachment behaviors and appropriate care of newborn [3] ☐ Physiologic parameters WNL [4] ☐ Circumcision w/o bleeding [5] ☐ Voided × 1 [4] ☐ Stooled × 1 [4] ☐ Feeding [2] ☐ LATCH score 7 or greater for breastfed newborn [2] ☐ Parent(s)/family verbalize newborn D/C instr [6] ☐ No jaundice [4] ☐ Physician aware of Coombs results ☐ ______	Temp, apical pulse, cardiac, resp., neuro, GI, GU, integ. q 8 hr Weight Parent(s)/family & infant attachment behaviors LATCH score of breastfed newborn Freq. & amt. of bottle feeding ______ ______	☐ Newborn screening tests prior to D/C ______ ______	☐ Referral made to LC for LATCH score <7 ______ ______ ______

NAME	INITIALS	NAME	INITIALS

Note: Each patient requires an individual assessment & treatment plan. This Clinical Path is a recommendation for the average patient and requires modification when necessary by the professional staff.

FIGURE 21-1, cont'd For legend see p. 548.

TREATMENTS	MEDS	NUTR.	EDUC & DC PLANNING
Cord care Circumcision care when indicated ________ ________	________ ________ ________	Breast/bottle fed on demand ________ ________ ________	☐ ☐ ☐ Observe return demonst. of breastfeeding mother's use of –alternative positioning –infant's suck, swallow ☐ ☐ ☐ Observe parent(s) providing appropriate newborn care; reinforce ☐ ☐ ☐ ________ ________
Cord care Circumcision care when indicated ________ ________ ________	________ ________ ________	Breast/bottle fed on demand ________ ________ ________	☐ ☐ ☐ Observe return demonst. of breastfeeding mother's use of –alternative positioning –infant's suck, swallow ☐ ☐ ☐ Observe parent(s) providing appropriate newborn care; reinforce ☐ ☐ ☐ ________ ________ ☐ ☐ ☐ ________ ________
Cord care Circumcision care when indicated Cord clamp removed prior to D/C ________ ________ ________	☐ Hepatitis B vaccine per order ________ ________ ________	NPO for circumcision when indicated Breast/bottle fed on demand ________ ________ ________	☐ Review D/C instructions with parent(s)/family ☐ Home visit scheduled ☐ D/C to mother's care ________ ________ ________

Discharge Date	Discharge Time	Discharged To	Accompanied By
________	________	________	☐ W/C ☐ Ambulate

FIGURE 21-1, cont'd For legend see p. 548.

DRUG GUIDE: ERYTHROMYCIN OPHTHALMIC OINTMENT

Other Name: Ilotycin

Classification: Antibiotic

Action: Inhibits protein synthesis in bacteria

Indications: Prophylaxis against the organisms *Neisseria gonorrhoeae* and *Chlamydia trachomatis;* prevents ophthalmia neonatorum in infants of mothers infected with gonorrhea and conjunctivitis in infants of mothers infected with *Chlamydia;* prophylaxis against gonorrhea required by law for all infants, whether or not the mother is known to be infected

Neonatal Dosage and Route: A "ribbon" of 0.5% erythromycin ointment, 1 to 2 cm (0.5 to 0.8 inch) long, is applied to the lower conjunctival sac of each eye within 1 hour after birth. It also may be used in drop form.

Adverse Reaction: Irritation may result in chemical conjunctivitis, lasting 24 to 48 hours. Ointment may cause temporary blurred vision.

Nursing Considerations: Cleanse the infant's eyes before application, as needed. Hold the tube in a horizontal rather than a vertical position to prevent injury to the eye from sudden movement. Administer from the inner canthus to the outer canthus. Do not touch the tip of the tube to any part of the eye, as this may spread infectious material from one eye to the other. Do not rinse. Ointment may be wiped from outer eye after 1 minute. Observe for irritation. Use a new tube for each infant to prevent spread of infection. Other medications used for prevention of gonorrhea include tetracycline and silver nitrate solution.

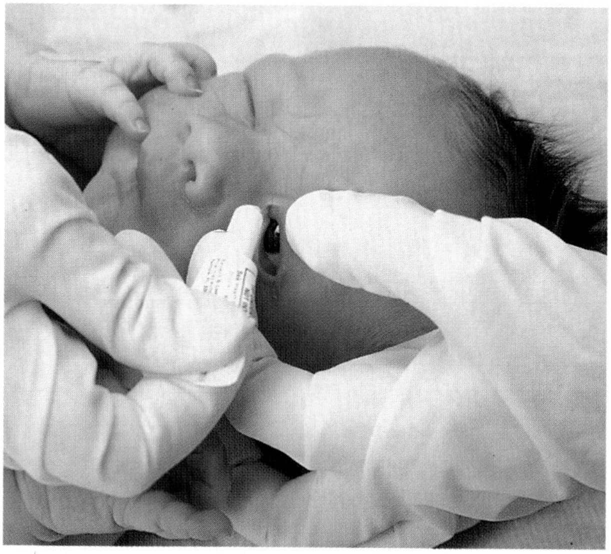

FIGURE 21-2 Administration of ophthalmic ointment. The nurse gently cleans the eyes of blood or vernix using sterile saline. Then, placing a finger and thumb near the edge of each lid, the nurse gently presses against the periorbital ridges to open the eyes, avoiding pressure on the eye. A ribbon of ointment is squeezed into each conjunctival sac.

signs of respiratory distress, including tachypnea, retractions, flaring of the nares, pallor or cyanosis, grunting, seesaw respirations, and asymmetry. Check blood pressure if indicated.

Analysis

Fluid from the lungs must be removed by absorption or drainage from the respiratory passages after birth. This does not happen immediately and may cause a temporary problem during the early hours after birth. The nursing diagnosis "Ineffective Airway Clearance related to excessive secretions in the respiratory passages" addresses this problem.

Planning

The goals/expected outcomes for this nursing diagnosis are that the newborn will

- Maintain a patent airway with a respiratory rate within the normal range of 30 to 60 breaths per minute
- Show no signs of respiratory distress

Interventions

Positioning the Infant

Position the infant with the head slightly lower than the extremities to aid in draining fluid from the respiratory passages immediately after birth. Use this position briefly if the infant has difficulty clearing the airways later, such as during regurgitation. Do not leave the infant in a head-dependent position longer than necessary because pressure from the intestines may interfere with movement of the diaphragm.

Suctioning Secretions

Use the bulb syringe, if necessary, to suction secretions as they drain into the infant's mouth or nose (Procedure 21-2). Suction the mouth first because the infant may gasp when the nose is suctioned, and aspiration could occur if mucus or fluid is in the mouth. Then gently suction the nose if needed, taking care to avoid trauma to the delicate mucous membranes. (Trauma could cause edema and occlude the passages.) Avoid unnecessary suctioning.

Keep the bulb syringe in the crib near the infant's head, where it is available if needed quickly. Teach both

PROCEDURE 21-2

Using a Bulb Syringe

Purpose: To provide an open airway by removing secretions or regurgitated feeding from the infant's mouth and nose

1. Position the infant's head to the side or hold the infant with the head slightly lower than the rest of the body. *This allows for drainage from the mouth.*
2. Compress the bulb before inserting it into the mouth. *This removes the air from the syringe so that it will suction. (Do not compress the bulb while it is in the infant's mouth or secretions in the bulb will be expelled back into the mouth.)*
3. Gently insert the bulb into the side of the infant's mouth between the gum and the cheek. Do not insert it straight to the back of the throat. *Gagging or a vagal response with bradycardia or apnea may result from inserting the bulb to the back of the throat.*
4. Release the bulb slowly while it is in the mouth. Remove and empty it by compressing several times before using again to remove secretions. *Releasing the bulb draws secretions into the bulb. Emptying it prepares it for use again.*
5. Suction the nose, if necessary, after the mouth is suctioned. *Infants often gasp when the nose is suctioned and might aspirate secretions in the mouth if it is not cleared first.*
6. Suction the nose gently and avoid unnecessary suction. *Trauma could cause edema and obstruction of delicate nasal passages. Infants have respiratory difficulty if nasal passages are blocked.*

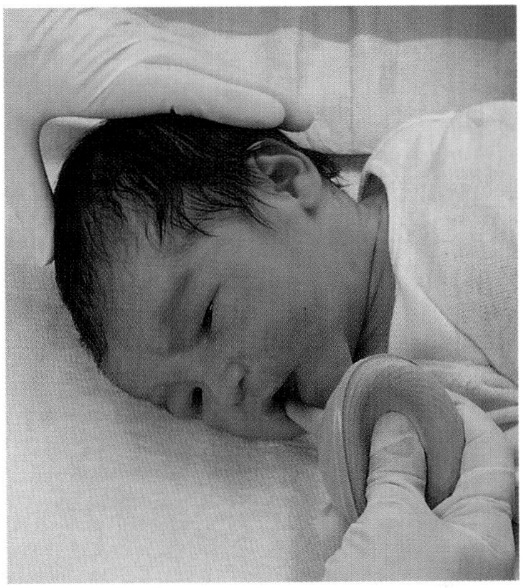

parents how to use the bulb syringe correctly. Send the syringe home with the infant so that the parents can use it if the infant experiences a problem.

If mechanical suctioning is necessary to remove deeper secretions, choose a small catheter to avoid damaging the tissues of the respiratory tract. Suction for no more than 5 seconds at a time, using minimal negative pressure to avoid trauma, laryngospasm, and bradycardia.

Providing Continuing Care

Continue monitoring the infant for problems throughout the stay at the birth facility. By the second period of reactivity, the infant may be alone with the mother. Although nurses know that regurgitation, gagging, and episodes of cyanosis are normal during the first and second periods of reactivity, these may be very frightening to the mother. Teach the appropriate responses to the behaviors common to this phase. Remind the mother to use the bulb syringe and call for help if needed. Check frequently with the mother to see if the infant is having difficulty. Assess her ability to use the bulb syringe and her comfort with its use.

Evaluation

The normal newborn has little difficulty clearing the airway after the first few hours of life. Goals are met if

- The respiratory rate is between 30 and 60 breaths per minute
- The infant shows no signs of respiratory distress

APPLICATION OF THE NURSING PROCESS: THERMOREGULATION

Because any neonate may have difficulty with thermoregulation, the nurse must identify problems and intervene to prevent complications related to this vital function.

Assessment

Assess the newborn's temperature shortly after birth and then according to agency policy. Generally the temperature is assessed every half hour until it has been stable for 2 hours. It is checked again at 4 hours and then every 8 hours. Assess the newborn more often if the temperature is abnormal.

Analysis

Newborns often have temporary difficulty maintaining a stable temperature. Therefore an appropriate nursing diagnosis is "Risk for Ineffective Thermoregulation related to immature compensation for changes in environmental temperature."

Planning

The goal/expected outcome for this diagnosis is that the infant will maintain body temperature within the normal ranges:

- Axillary, 36.5° to 37.5° C (97.7° to 99.5° F)
- Rectal, 36.5° to 37.6° C (97.7° to 99.7° F)

NURSING CARE PLAN 21-1

The Normal Newborn

Assessment: Nicholas, a full-term newborn, was delivered after 18 hours of normal labor. He weighs 7 pounds, 8 ounces and is 20 inches long. His mother, Vicki, is happy and excited about her first baby. Nicholas receives Apgar scores of 8 at 1 minute and 9 at 5 minutes. During the initial assessment, Nicholas has an excessive amount of mucus. His respiratory rate is 62, apical pulse is 164, and breath sounds are slightly moist. He has mild substernal retractions. His color is pink with acrocyanosis.

Critical Thinking: Should the nurse worry about Nicholas, based on the assessment above? What other signs would indicate a serious problem?

Answer: The infant's condition is not unusual immediately after birth. The nurse should be concerned if Nicholas develops central cyanosis, flaring of the nares, grunting, or further increases in pulse and respiratory rate or if signs do not improve during the first hour or two after birth.

Nursing Diagnosis: Risk for Ineffective Airway Clearance related to excessive secretions in airways.

Expected Outcomes:

1. Nicholas will maintain a patent airway and have no signs of respiratory distress throughout birth facility stay as demonstrated by respiratory rate of 30 to 60 breaths per minute, apical pulse 120 to 160, clear breath sounds, and no cyanosis, retractions, flaring, or grunting.
2. Before discharge, Vicki will demonstrate correct use of the bulb syringe and verbalize when it should be used.

Intervention	Rationale
1. Place Nicholas in a side-lying position and observe for the amounts of secretions and any respiratory difficulty.	1. A side-lying position facilitates drainage of secretions from the airways.
2. Use a bulb syringe to gently suction the mouth, if necessary. If the nose also requires suctioning, suction it after suctioning the mouth.	2. Suctioning removes secretions. Suctioning the mouth first prevents aspiration of oral secretions should Nicholas gasp when his nose is suctioned.
3. Change the infant's position frequently.	3. Position changes promote expansion and drainage of all parts of the lungs.
4. Provide reassurance to Vicki.	4. Suctioning and other care may make parents feel something is wrong.
5. Demonstrate and explain use of the bulb syringe to Vicki. Assess her ability and make suggestions as needed during a return demonstration.	5. Demonstration and return demonstration ensure parents learn correct techniques.
6. Continue to observe Nicholas for signs of respiratory distress. Count pulse and respirations every 30 minutes until they have been stable for 2 hours. Once they are stable, assess vital signs every 8 hours, or according to birth facility procedure. Assess more often if there is any sign of abnormality. Observe for other signs of respiratory difficulty, such as cyanosis, retractions, flaring, and grunting.	6. Monitoring should be based on history of excessive mucus, ability to cope with mucus, and other signs of respiratory difficulty, changes in the infant's condition.

Evaluation: Nicholas has clear breath sounds within 3 hours of birth, his apical pulse is 138 to 153, and his respiratory rate is 41 to 53. He has no signs of respiratory difficulty. Vicki uses the bulb syringe to suction Nicholas appropriately.

Assessment: Nicholas's axillary temperature ranges from 36.2° to 36.8° C (97.2° to 98.2° F). Vicki is eager to hold him and frequently unwraps him to admire him. When reminded about the need to keep Nicholas warm, she states, "It seems hot in here to me. Will he get too warm with so many blankets?"

Nursing Diagnosis: Risk for Ineffective Thermoregulation related to parental lack of knowledge of newborn thermoregulation abilities and needs.

Goals/Expected Outcomes:

1. Nicholas will maintain a temperature within the normal range of 36.5° to 37.5° C (97.7° to 99.5° F) axillary throughout his birth facility stay.
2. Vicki will verbalize and practice methods of preventing heat loss by the end of the first day.

Intervention	Rationale
1. Explain why newborns have problems with thermoregulation.	1. When parents understand the reasons behind precautions given to them, they are more likely to practice them.
2. Teach Vicki to dry Nicholas promptly whenever he is wet, such as during bathing and when changing wet diapers or clothing.	2. Heat loss from evaporation occurs when the infant's skin is wet.
3. Instruct Vicki to keep the infant's crib away from cold walls, windows, or drafts from air conditioners and open doors or windows.	3. Heat loss by radiation and convection occurs from exposure to cold objects or air drafts.
4. Point out commonly used objects that may be cold when they touch Nicholas. Explain the effect of this contact, and suggest methods to warm them before use.	4. Heat can be gained or lost by conduction.
5. Assess the infant's axillary temperature every 30 minutes until it has been stable for 2 hours, or according to birth facility procedure. Report Nicholas's progress to Vicki.	5. Continued assessment shows response to interventions. Keeping the parents aware of the infant's progress involves them in his care.
6. Check blood sugar if Nicholas is jittery or lethargic. Feed him if blood sugar is at or below 40 to 45 mg/dl. Help Vicki to breastfeed him if she wishes, or use formula.	6. Nonshivering thermogenesis results in use of glycogen stores. Infants may show tremors or lethargy as a result of hypoglycemia. Feeding provides calories for heat production.
7. Monitor for tachypnea or other signs of respiratory distress. Suction and apply oxygen if needed.	7. Nonshivering thermogenesis requires use of large amounts of oxygen, increases work of the respiratory system, and may lead to hypoxia.
8. If Nicholas is slow to warm, try placing him (wearing only a diaper) next to Vicki's skin.	8. Placing the infant "skin to skin" with the mother uses conduction to help warm the infant with the mother's body heat.
9. If his temperature is still low or has repeated episodes of low temperature, place him in a radiant warmer or an incubator. Alert the physician or nurse practitioner if the problem continues.	9. Radiant heat warms infants and can be adjusted according to their needs. Temperature instability is one sign of infection in newborns. The health care provider may order further tests for continued low temperature.
10. When Nicholas is ready to go into an open crib, warm his clothes before dressing him. Place two warmed blankets, wrapped separately, around him. After he is swaddled, place one or two blankets over him.	10. Warming clothing and blankets keeps Nicholas warm by conduction. Wrapping blankets separately traps air between layers, which acts as an insulating agent.
11. Remove extra blankets according to the infant's temperature.	11. Overheating increases oxygen and glucose consumption.
12. Apply a stockinette or insulated hat to the infants' head.	12. Covering the head decreases heat loss from this large surface area.
13. After transfer to an open crib, monitor the infant's temperature every 30 to 60 minutes until it is stable.	13. Continued monitoring provides prompt identification of problems infants may have in adjusting to changes in environmental temperature.
14. Teach Vicki how to wrap Nicholas and to expose only small areas of the body at a time when bathing or diapering him. Also teach her how to take Nicholas' axillary temperature at home.	14. Teaching increases parents' competence in infant care.

Evaluation: Nicholas's axillary temperature at 3 hours after delivery is 37° C (98.6° F). He has no further problems with temperature instability during his birth facility stay. Vicki is conscientious in using correct measures to keep Nicholas warm.

Interventions

Preventing Heat Loss

Preparing the Environment Before Birth. Begin preventive measures before the infant is born. Prepare a neutral thermal environment with a radiant warmer to use during initial assessments. This ensures that excess oxygen and glucose are not necessary to maintain body temperature. Ensure the radiant warmer is functioning properly before the delivery. Turn it on early enough that the bed is ready and warm for the newborn. Set the servocontrol between 36.0° and 36.5° C (96.8° and 97.7° F). This regulates the amount of heat produced by the warmer to maintain the infant's skin temperature at the normal level.

Providing Immediate Care. Immediately after birth, place the infant on the mother's abdomen to provide skin-to-skin contact for warmth or under the radiant warmer to counteract the cool temperature of the delivery room. Dry the wet infant quickly with warm towels to prevent heat loss by evaporation. Pay particular attention to drying the hair because the head is a large surface area and hair that remains damp increases heat loss. Remove towels or blankets as soon as they become wet and replace them with dry, warmed linens. Cover the infant's head with a cap when the infant is not under a radiant warmer.

If the infant is moved from the mother's abdomen to a radiant warmer, attach a skin probe to the abdomen. The probe allows the warmer to monitor and display the infant's temperature continuously. Check frequently to see that the infant's skin temperature is increasing as expected.

Providing Ongoing Prevention. Warm objects that are cool and will come in contact with the infant to avoid conduction of heat away from the body. Pad cool surfaces such as scales before placing infants on them. Warm stethoscopes and clothing before using them. Before touching the infant, run warm water over your hands if they are cold.

To prevent heat loss by radiation, position the newborn's crib or incubator away from walls or windows that are part of the outside of the building. These sources of heat loss are easily overlooked when the objects and air around the infant seem warm, but infants may lose heat to objects not in close contact with them. Keep this in mind when positioning cribs in mothers' rooms, which are often short of space. Place the crib at the end of the mother's bed or between the beds (in a two-bed room) rather than next to the windows. Avoid areas with a draft. Keep traffic low around radiant warmers because movement increases air currents.

When assessing or caring for newborns, avoid exposing more of their bodies than necessary. Remove clothing and blankets from only the areas being assessed. Keep the upper part of the infant covered when changing diapers. Wrap them in blankets, and use a stockinette or insulated hat to prevent heat loss from the large surface area of the head.

Restoring Thermoregulation

A normal temperature in a newborn may decrease. When this happens, institute nursing measures to assist thermoregulation immediately. If the axillary temperature is low, some agency policies are to check the rectal temperature to determine core temperature. A normal rectal temperature does not mean nonshivering thermogenesis is not already taking place. Core temperature changes indicate that the infant's thermoregulatory resources are exhausted.

First look for obvious causes for the infant's low temperature. Perhaps the infant is unwrapped or is wearing wet diapers or clothing. The mother's room may be cold, or the crib may be placed near the air conditioner. These causes easily can be corrected.

A slight drop in temperature may require only the addition of extra clothing. Put a shirt on the baby upside down by placing the baby's legs in the sleeves for added warmth. Use two blankets, each wrapped separately around the infant, to increase insulation of heat by trapping air between the layers. Place another blanket over the infant in the crib and a hat on the infant's head. Heat linens in a warmer before use if added warmth is desired.

CRITICAL THINKING EXERCISE

You are caring for Nancy Belinsky and her son, Andy, who have both been doing well since Andy was born early this morning. As you enter the room after lunch, Nancy says, "Andy's hands and feet are so cold! But I've heard that all babies have cold hands and feet. Are they always so shaky, too?"

QUESTIONS:

1. What are the nursing priorities in this situation?
2. What expanded assessments are necessary?
3. What interventions are necessary?
4. How will you respond to Nancy?

A greater drop in temperature requires additional measures. Place the infant under a radiant warmer for a short time. For an infant with a markedly decreased temperature, set the temperature control on the warmer slightly above the infant's temperature to warm the infant slowly. Gradually increase the temperature until the infant's temperature is within the normal range. Warming the infant too rapidly increases oxygen consumption and may cause apnea.

Performing Expanded Assessments

Expanded assessments are necessary whenever temperature is decreased in a newborn. Assess the respiratory rate because nonshivering thermogenesis increases the need for oxygen. Observe for signs of respiratory distress brought on by the additional oxygen requirement.

Because the cold infant uses more glucose to produce heat, test the blood glucose level when the temperature is abnormal. A reading of 40 to 45 mg/dl or lower by screening tests requires feeding, especially if the infant shows signs of hypoglycemia. The mother should breastfeed or use warmed formula. Heating the formula helps warm the infant.

Infants who do not respond to these simple measures need additional treatment. Notify the physician or nurse practitioner and keep the infant in an incubator in the nursery for close observation until the temperature stabilizes. Observe for signs of infection, such as low temperature.

Evaluation

When a temperature within the normal range has been maintained for several hours, the infant can be considered stable in thermoregulation. Ongoing monitoring of thermoregulation continues throughout the birth facility stay.

Check Your Reading

1. Why are prophylactic medications given to all newborns?
2. How can nurses prevent heat loss in newborns?

APPLICATION OF THE NURSING PROCESS: HEPATIC FUNCTION

The major early assessments and care of the hepatic system are related to blood glucose levels and bilirubin conjugation.

BLOOD GLUCOSE

Assessment

Assess all infants for risk factors and signs of hypoglycemia. Perform screening tests for blood glucose according to the signs exhibited and the agency's policy.

Analysis

For infants who have glucose levels of 40 mg/dl by laboratory analysis or 40 to 45 mg/dl by screening tests, the collaborative problem "Potential complication: Hypoglycemia" is appropriate.

Planning

Client-centered goals for hypoglycemia are inappropriate because this problem requires collaboration between the nurse and the physician. Planning revolves around the nurse's role, including the following:

- Monitoring for signs of hypoglycemia
- Notifying the physician about signs of hypoglycemia or following agency protocol for infants with hypoglycemia
- Intervening to minimize hypoglycemia

Interventions

Maintaining Safe Glucose Levels

If glucose is not constantly available to the brain, permanent damage may occur. To prevent this, follow agency policy and physician orders regarding feeding infants with low glucose levels. A common practice is to feed the newborn if the glucose screening test shows a level of 40 to 45 mg/dl or less to prevent further depletion of glucose. (Screening tests are less accurate than laboratory analysis, and intervening early treats the problem before hypoglycemia becomes severe.)

If this is the infant's first feeding, provide breast milk or formula. Some agencies give glucose water for the first feeding, but this is not recommended. Although glucose water raises blood glucose, insulin production also increases, causing a rebound drop in blood glucose. Milk provides a longer-lasting supply of glucose because of the other nutrients included.

Assist the breastfeeding mother with the first feeding. If she is unable to nurse the infant immediately (because of pain or exhaustion from delivery), feed the infant formula and help her breastfeed at the next feeding. Help formula-feeding mothers give the bottle to infants.

Repeating Glucose Tests

Closely observe newborns who have shown signs of hypoglycemia until glucose levels are stable. The schedule for retesting varies from one agency to another. It is often performed 30 to 60 minutes after feeding and then before later feedings several times until results are normal. No further testing is performed unless new indications of hypoglycemia develop.

Keep the physician or nurse practitioner aware of the newborn's status. If the blood glucose does not remain at an adequate level, other causative factors are investigated. The infant may be transferred to a nursery for more intensive treatment, including intravenous feedings, until blood glucose is regulated with oral feedings.

Providing Other Care

Watch for signs of other complications. If infants do not have enough glucose, they may experience a drop in temperature that could lead to respiratory distress as oxygen is used for nonshivering thermogenesis. Explain the situation to parents. They will be distressed over the multiple heel sticks their infant must endure. Explain the importance of maintaining adequate blood glucose levels and why the tests and frequent feedings are necessary. Encourage parents to feed the newborn as instructed so that enough glucose is available to meet the infant's needs. Discuss the plans for blood testing and criteria for discontinuing it.

Evaluation

In evaluating collaborative interventions for hypoglycemia, note the presence or absence of continued signs of hypoglycemia and compare blood glucose screening with normal values. The blood glucose should remain above 40 to 45 mg/dl on screening or 40 mg/dl on laboratory analysis.

BILIRUBIN

Because elevated bilirubin levels are common in newborns, be alert to situations that require intervention. Infants who need treatment for hyperbilirubinemia in the birth facility are discussed in Chapter 30. Preventive aspects are discussed here.

Assessment

Assess for jaundice by blanching the infant's skin on the nose or sternum. Determine how far down the body the jaundice extends. When serum bilirubin tests are ordered, compare the results with what is expected for the infant's age and previous results.

Analysis

Hyperbilirubinemia may not occur until after discharge, especially when infants go home early. Teach parents appropriately so that infants with jaundice receive proper treatment. A nursing diagnosis for this situation is "Risk for Injury related to lack of parental knowledge about hyperbilirubinemia."

Planning

The goals/outcomes for this diagnosis are the following:

- Infants with jaundice will be identified early in the birth facility or at home.
- Parents will identify infants with jaundice when at home.
- Parents will identify methods of preventing or reducing jaundice when at home.

Interventions

During assessment and care of newborns, be aware of which infants are at increased risk for hyperbilirubinemia (see Critical to Remember, p. 522). By using extra vigilance in caring for infants at higher risk, nurses can detect jaundice earlier and take measures to decrease it.

Explain to parents the importance of adequate feedings to stimulate passage of stools and help prevent high levels of bilirubin in the infant. When a newborn is feeding poorly, determine the reasons for jaundice and intervene appropriately. Help mothers wake sleepy infants to feed, spend extra time with an infant with a poor suck, or teach the mother the appropriate amount to feed at each feeding. Encourage breastfeeding mothers to nurse within 2 hours after birth and every 2 to 3 hours thereafter. Avoid giving water to jaundiced infants because water does not stimulate stool excretion.

Explain the significance of the color change in the skin and why blood testing is necessary. Answer parents' questions, especially if their infant needs phototherapy (see Nursing Care Plan 30-1).

Before discharge, instruct parents about how to check for jaundice at home and to contact their care provider if it increases. Tell them to call the physician if the infant is not eating every 3 to 4 hours, voiding 6 to 10 times a day, and producing stools appropriately (at least once daily for formula-fed infants, at least four stools daily for breastfed infants).

Continue to check the infant for jaundice during the early home or clinic visits. Use a transcutaneous bilirubinometer (jaundice meter), if available, to verify the level of bilirubin. The meter is placed on the infant's skin to measure the intensity of the skin color, which is correlated with bilirubin levels (Ruchala, Seibold, & Stremsterfer, 1996). Reinforce teaching about identification of jaundice and importance of feedings and stooling. Answer questions parents may have developed since discharge from the birth facility.

If an infant develops true breast milk jaundice, explain it to the parents. The mother who must discontinue breastfeeding for a day or two will be concerned. Reassure her that her milk is adequate and not harmful to the infant. Help her maintain her milk supply by using a manual or electric breast pump during the time the infant is taking formula.

Evaluation

With proper nursing observation and parent teaching, infants with hyperbilirubinemia are identified early to allow for appropriate treatment and prevention of injury. Parents are able to discuss signs, prevention, and management of jaundice at home.

Check Your Reading

3. What should the nurse do for infants with signs of hypoglycemia?
4. What are some interventions for preventing jaundice in newborns?

ONGOING ASSESSMENTS AND CARE

A complete assessment is necessary every 8 hours according to the birth facility's policy, but the nurse should be alert at all times for signs of change in the newborn's condition (see Appendix D for daily nursing activities for meeting newborn needs). Vital signs are assessed once every 8 hours or more often if they are abnormal. The infant is weighed once daily and weight loss or gain noted.

Providing Skin Care

The skin should be assessed for new marks or changes in old ones. Marks on the scalp may not be obvious if covered by abundant hair. To assess skin turgor, the nurse pinches a small area of skin over the chest or abdomen and notes how quickly it returns to its normal position. The return should be immediate in the normal newborn, with no "tenting." Skin that remains "tented" is an indication of dehydration.

Bathing

The infant receives a bath to remove blood and excessive vernix as soon after birth as the temperature is stable. This should be done before performing any invasive procedures that might draw organisms on the skin into the infant's subcutaneous tissues or blood stream. Early bathing decreases exposure to maternal blood and possible blood-borne organisms on the infant's skin, such as hepatitis B and human immunodeficiency virus (HIV). Gloves are worn during all contact with the infant until the bath is completed because of the blood on the infant's skin from birth. After the bath, gloves are necessary only when contact with body fluids is likely.

Studies have shown that infants with stable temperatures can be bathed within 1 hour of birth with no significant drop in temperature when compared to infants bathed 2 to 4 hours after birth (Varda & Behnke, 2000; Penny-MacGillivray, 1996). The temperature at which infants are bathed varies according to agency policy and may range from 36.5° C (97.7° F) to 36.8° C (98.2° F). The bath should be performed quickly and the infant thoroughly dried to prevent heat loss by evaporation.

While shampooing the hair, the nurse combs through it to remove dried blood. Combing the hair hastens drying. After the bath the infant remains under the radiant warmer until the hair is dry and the temperature returns to the previous level. The infant is dressed, wrapped in two blankets, and a cap placed on the head before removal from the radiant warmer. The temperature should be rechecked within an hour to ensure the infant is maintaining thermoregulation adequately.

After the initial bath, the infant may not receive another full bath during the birth facility stay. However, the skin is cleansed at diaper changes and for removal of regurgitated milk. Only clear water or a mild soap solution should be used according to agency policy.

Parents are taught to give sponge baths until the cord is off and the circumcision is healed. Some authors, however, have found that tub baths for newborns do not increase infection and that infants maintain their temperatures better than with sponge baths (Cole, Brissette, & Lunardi, 1999). The practice of giving tub baths to newborns may become more common in the future.

Providing Cord Care

Check the cord for bleeding or oozing during the early hours after birth. The cord clamp must be securely fastened with no skin caught in it. Purulent drainage or redness or edema at the base indicates infection. The cord begins to dry shortly after birth. It becomes brownish black within 2 to 3 days and falls off within approximately 10 to 14 days.

The cord may be treated with a bactericidal substance such as triple dye solution, alcohol or antibiotic ointment. In some facilities, triple dye is applied one or more times and mothers are taught to apply alcohol at home. The cord may also be allowed to dry naturally. In one study, cords allowed to dry naturally separated earlier and did not become infected more often than cords treated with alcohol at each diaper change (Dore et. al., 1998).

Mothers often have concerns about care of the cord, especially in cases of odor or bleeding when the cord separates (Ford & Ritchie, 1999). Parents should be taught that these occurrences are not unusual but that redness at the base of the cord and discharge may indicate infection. If alcohol is used, parents are taught to clean the cord with alcohol at least three times a day until the cord falls off. All parents should be taught to fold the diaper below the cord to keep it dry and free from contamination by urine.

The cord clamp is removed about 24 hours after birth if the end of the cord is dry (Figure 21-3). The base of the cord is still moist, but no danger of bleeding exists if the end is dry and crisp. If the neonate is discharged before the cord is dry enough for the clamp to be removed, it may be tied. In some birth facilities, the nurse removes the clamp during the home visit.

Cleansing the Diaper Area

Wear clean gloves while changing diapers because contact with body fluids is likely. Meconium is thick and sticky and can be difficult to remove from the skin. Plain water or special soap solutions may be used for cleaning the diaper area. Petroleum jelly or baby oil is sometimes used to make cleaning meconium stools easier and to prevent skin irritation.

Assisting with Feedings

Ensure that the infant is eating well and that parents understand their chosen feeding method. Assign a LATCH score for breastfeeding mothers and infants and look for changes in the score (see Chapter 22, p. 583).

Although infants should sleep on the back, positioning them on the right side for a short time after feedings allows gravity to help empty the stomach because the lower end of the stomach is on the right side. The head of the bed may be elevated to help keep stomach contents from flowing into the esophagus through the relaxed cardiac sphincter. The crib should be flat when transporting infants, however, so that it is not dislodged as the crib is moving.

Protecting the Infant

Safeguarding the infant is a major role of the nurse. Primary ways nurses protect newborns are by (1) ensuring that infants always go to the correct parents, (2) taking precautions to prevent infant abductions, and (3) preventing or recognizing early signs of infection.

Identifying the Infant

A method to identify newborns is instituted at birth, before mothers and infants are separated, to ensure that a mother is never given the wrong infant. This type of mistake could result in interference with bonding, exposure to infections, lack of confidence in the reliability of the staff, and lawsuits.

The most common method of identifying infants is the use of identification bands, which are placed on the mother, the infant, and the father or other support person. Information on each band is identical and includes a number that is imprinted on the plastic band. The imprinted number is used to identify the mother and the

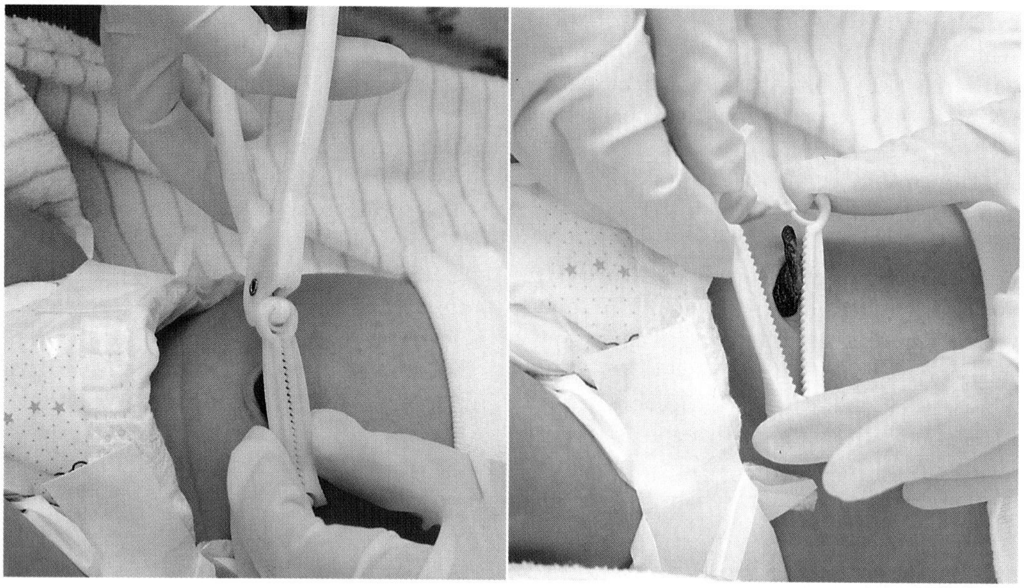

FIGURE 21-3 The cord clamp is removed when the end of the cord is dry and crisp. The clamp is cut **(A)** and separated **(B)**.

PROCEDURE 21-3

Identifying Infants

Purpose: To ensure that each infant is always given to the correct mother

1. Always identify infants and mothers (or support person) with identification (ID) bands when reuniting them, even after a brief separation. *This step ensures that infants are given to correct parents.*
2. When taking infants into mothers' rooms, unwrap the blankets to expose the ID band on the infant's wrist or ankle. Do *not* rely on memory of the number. *This allows visualization of the band number.*
3. Explain the ID procedure and its purpose to the mother. Show her the imprinted ID number on her band and the matching number on the infant's bands. *This ensures the mother's understanding and cooperation.*
4. Look at the number on the infant's band and ask the mother to read off the ID number on her band. Do *not* reverse the process by reading the infant's number to the mother. *If the numbers are read to a mother who does not understand, she might indicate that the numbers are correct when they are not.*
5. An alternative procedure is for the nurse to compare the mother's and the infant's bands visually. *If the mother does not speak English or might have difficulty with the process, the nurse can be certain that the infant is identified correctly.*
6. If the infant is to be released to a support person who is wearing an identification band, follow the same identification procedure. *This ensures that the infant is given to the correct support person.*

infant every time the infant is brought to the mother after a period of separation, however brief (Procedure 21-3 and Figure 21-4). All staff must follow the facility protocol for identification of infants.

Other methods of identifying infants include taking footprints of the infant and a fingerprint of the mother. The infant may be photographed, and a notation of birthmarks or other distinguishing features included in the nurses' notes. Cord blood may be used for DNA analysis in cases of a later need for identification.

Preventing Infant Abduction

An unfortunate but essential role of the nurse is protection of the infant against infant abduction (kidnapping). Between 1983 and 1999, 104 infants were abducted from health care facilities (Rabun, 2000). Precautions include teaching parents how to recognize birth facility personnel, whether by a picture identification badge or by other means. Written and verbal information, including a picture of the special identification badge worn by staff, should be given to parents. Parents must be cautioned never to give their infant to anyone who does not have proper identification (Table 21-1).

Staff who are working temporarily on the unit must have a special means of identification that is recognized by parents and other staff. Temporary identification badges are assigned and monitored each shift so that none can be removed from the premises without alerting the staff.

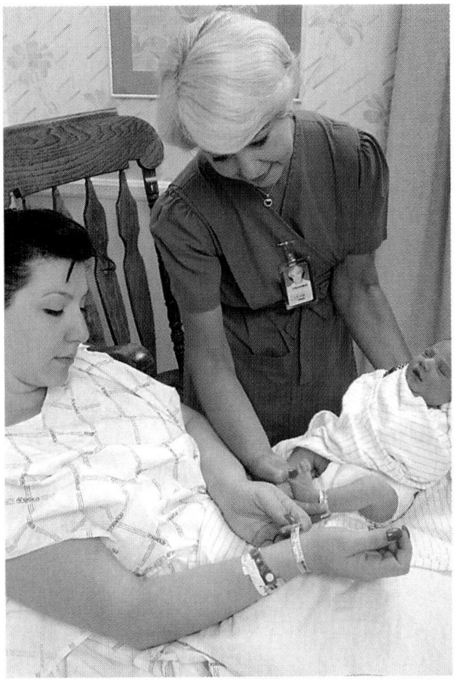

FIGURE 21-4 The nurse checks the infant's identification band with the mother's band.

Table 21-1

PRECAUTIONS TO PREVENT INFANT ABDUCTIONS

All personnel must wear appropriate identification at all times. No one without appropriate identification should handle or transport infants.

Enlist parents' help in preventing kidnapping. Teach them to allow only hospital staff with proper identification to take their infants from them.

Teach parents and staff to transport infants only in their cribs and never by carrying them. Question anyone walking in the hallway carrying an infant.

Question anyone with a newborn near an exit or in an unusual part of the facility.

Be suspicious of anyone who does not seem to be visiting a specific mother or who asks detailed questions about nursery or discharge routines.

Be suspicious of unknown people carrying large bags or packages that could contain an infant.

Respond immediately when an alarm sounds signaling that a remote entrance has been opened or an infant has been taken into an unauthorized area.

Never leave infants unattended at any time. Teach parents that infants must be observed at all times. Suggest that they send the infant to the nursery if they or a family member cannot watch the infant.

Take infants to mothers one at a time. This avoids having an infant in a crib waiting outside in the hall while the nurse is in a room with another mother. Never leave an infant in the hall unsupervised.

When infants are left in mothers' rooms, position the crib away from the doorways.

If entrances to the maternity unit or nurseries are equipped with locks that open to codes or card keys, protect them from others.

Identification bracelets are often given to mothers' support persons so that they can come to the nursery to get the infant. When a parent or family member comes to the nursery, always match the infant and adult identification bracelet numbers. Never give an infant to anyone without the correct identification bracelet or other proper identification.

Alert hospital security when any suspicious activity occurs.

In some agencies, an electronic device is attached to each infant's wrist or ankle. The maternity unit exits are wired so that an alarm is triggered when the device is near.

Entrances to the maternity unit should be in areas where staff can watch those entering and leaving. Unit doors may be locked at all times. Entrance requires knocking on the door or use of a cardkey or a code on the lock (Figure 21-5). Visitors to maternity units may be required to check in with security guards and wear special visitor identification tags.

Remote exits are often locked and equipped with video cameras and alarms. Staff must respond quickly whenever a door alarm sounds. Although alarms usually are triggered accidentally, a kidnapper may be using a remote exit for a quick getaway.

Newborns are usually abducted by women who are familiar with the birth facility and its routines. Abduc-

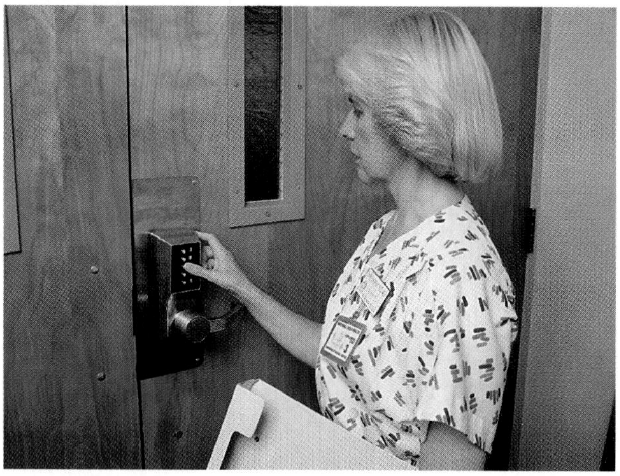

FIGURE 21-5 The nurse uses a code to open the door to the nursery.

tors often live near the birth facility. They usually visit several times to learn the routines so that they can impersonate birth facility staff to gain access to a newborn. They often know the layout of the facility and the locations of exits well.

The abducting woman is often married or involved in a relationship and may want an infant to solidify the relationship. She may have had a previous pregnancy loss or have been unable to have a child of her own. Although the woman plans the kidnapping, she waits for an appropriate opportunity to take any infant that is available.

Preventing Infection

Because the newborn has a limited ability to respond to infection, prevention is of utmost importance throughout the birth facility stay and constitutes a major part of parent teaching.

A number of nursing actions are designed to prevent infection. At the beginning of their shift, nurses wash their hands and arms thoroughly, and, in some agencies, use a scrub brush. Throughout the day, hand washing is important before and after touching any infant. Nurses must not handle one neonate and then another without again washing their hands. Otherwise an infection that develops in one infant could quickly spread to others.

The nurse should encourage parents and visitors to wash their hands before handling infants. Parents should be instructed to discourage visitors with colds or other infections from coming in contact with the mother or newborn at the birth facility or during the early days at home.

Each infant's supplies should be kept separate from those used for other infants to avoid cross-contamination. Supplies in drawers or cupboards of the crib unit belonging to one infant should be used only for that infant because they are likely to be touched by the nurse while giving care. Using them for another neonate could result in the transfer of infectious organisms.

When the mother has an infection, the physician decides whether it is safe for the newborn to remain with her. Although mothers and infants may well share the same organisms, if a mother is acutely ill, her infant may need to stay in the nursery until the mother is no longer contagious and feels able to perform infant care.

Some birth facilities have a policy governing when separation of mother and newborn is necessary. Often the degree of the mother's fever is one of the determining factors. The separation of mother and infant should be as short as possible, of course, to promote attachment.

Nurses must be vigilant for signs of infection during assessment and care of the infant. These signs are often different from those of the older infant or child and may be subtle (see discussion of sepsis and Signs of Infection, pp. 851 and 854). Instead of a fever, temperature may decrease. The infant may feed poorly or be lethargic. Periods of apnea sometimes occur without obvious cause. Any change in behavior that is unexplained should be recorded and investigated. The same holds true, of course, for the more obvious signs of infection such as drainage from the eyes, cord, or circumcision site.

Check Your Reading

5. How can the nurse prevent a parent from getting the wrong baby?
6. What can nurses and parents do to prevent infant abductions?
7. What is the most important method of preventing infection in newborns?

CIRCUMCISION

Circumcision is the most common surgical procedure of the neonate and is performed on approximately 65% of newborns in the United States. It is the removal of the prepuce (foreskin), a fold of skin that covers the glans penis. Although it can be retracted easily for cleaning in the older child, the prepuce usually is not fully retractable until age 3 or older. The prepuce should never be forcibly retracted in any infant because trauma and adhesions can result.

Circumcision is an area of controversy. The American Academy of Pediatrics (AAP) states that although potential benefits exist to the procedure, data is not sufficient to recommend routine neonatal circumcision (AAP, 1999). Not all physicians, however, agree with this position (Schoen, Wiswell, & Moses, 2000). Parents must make an informed choice about whether to have their sons circumcised.

Reasons for Choosing Circumcision

Circumcision may reduce urinary tract infections, which occur in approximately 1% of uncircumcised infants. Cancer of the penis, which is very rare, and some sexually transmissible infections occur more frequently in uncircumcised males. However, other factors, such as poor hygiene and risk-taking behavior are also important causes of infection (Zderic, 1998).

Some parents choose circumcision for religious, cultural, or social reasons. Jewish parents may have their infants circumcised on the eighth day after birth as part of a special ceremony. Muslim culture also includes circumcision. Some parents want their son to look like his circumcised father or peers. Others feel circumcision is an expected part of newborn care, and some do not realize that they have a choice in the matter.

Parents may be concerned that when older, the child might develop phimosis, a tightening of the prepuce that prevents its retraction and requires circumcision. Although the number of such cases is small, surgery after the newborn period involves hospitalization and anesthesia and can be psychologically disturbing to the young child.

Lack of knowledge about the care of the prepuce leads to some circumcisions. Poor hygiene may increase the risk of infections and other problems. Teaching the proper care of the uncircumcised penis to the parents and child can prevent surgery and complications related to inadequate cleanliness.

Reasons for Rejecting Circumcision

Reasons why parents decide against circumcision vary. Some believe that although a few conditions are seen more often in uncircumcised males, the total incidence is too low to make the pain and risk of surgery necessary for every infant. Others believe that having the infant circumcised to look like the father or peers is cosmetic surgery and unnecessary. These parents especially object to subjecting their sons to pain during and after the surgery. Circumcision is uncommon in most European countries and less often practiced by families from Asian, Latino, and Native American cultures.

Parents may be concerned about removing the prepuce, which serves to protect the glans. When unprotected by the prepuce, the glans is more prone to irritation from constant exposure to urine and rubbing against diapers. Many believe that circumcision decreases sexual pleasure later in life because the glans becomes less sensitive.

Complications after circumcision are unusual but most often include bleeding and infection. Other complications include recurrent phimosis, wound separation, unsatisfactory cosmetic result, urinary retention, meatitis, meatal stenosis, chordee, and inclusion cysts (AAP, 1999).

Only healthy newborns should undergo circumcision. The preterm or sick infant should not be circumcised until he is healthy enough to tolerate the procedure. Infants with blood dyscrasias may have excessive bleeding if circumcised. For the repair of anatomic abnormalities of the penis, such as hypospadias or epispadias, an intact prepuce may be needed for use in plastic surgery.

CRITICAL TO REMEMBER

Signs of Complications after Circumcision

Bleeding more than a few drops with first diaper changes
Failure to urinate
Signs of infection: fever or low temperature, purulent or foul-smelling drainage
Displacement of the Plastibell

Pain Relief

Some circumcisions are performed without anesthesia. At one time it was commonly believed that newborns do not feel pain, but it is now known that the fetus is able to perceive pain by the third trimester. During circumcision, newborns show changes in vital signs, oxygen saturation levels, and increased cortisol levels, indicating that they feel pain. Infants may show irritability, more frequent crying, and changes in eating and sleeping behavior during the first day after the procedure. Later in infancy, circumcised boys may show more pain responses than uncircumcised boys when undergoing painful procedures such as vaccinations (Taddio, Katz, Ilersich, & Koren, 1997).

A subcutaneous ring block or a dorsal penile nerve block may be used to safely reduce pain during circumcision. Both involve injection of the penis with an anesthetic such as lidocaine, but the ring block is more effective (Lander, Brady-Fryer, Metcalfe, Nazarali, & Muttitt, 1997). Complications are uncommon but most often include bruising and hematomas. Anesthetic cream (such as EMLA) applied before the procedure may also be used but is less effective and requires a longer waiting period before the surgery can be performed. Acetaminophen may be given before surgery or for postoperative pain relief.

Nonpharmacologic pain relief methods include pacifiers with or without sucrose solution, soothing music, recordings of intrauterine sounds, and talking softly to the infant. All have shown some success in reducing an infant's pain responses to circumcision but are not as effective as anesthetics.

Methods

The Gomco (Yellen) clamp (Figure 21-6) and the Plastibell (Figure 21-7) are two commonly used devices for performing circumcisions. In each method, the prepuce is first separated from the glans with a probe and

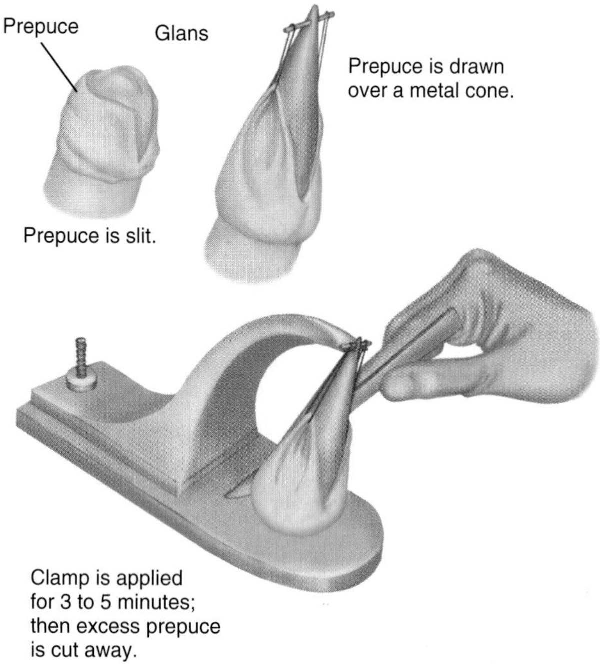
Prepuce
Glans
Prepuce is drawn over a metal cone.
Prepuce is slit.
Clamp is applied for 3 to 5 minutes; then excess prepuce is cut away.

FIGURE 21-6 Circumcision using the Gomco (Yellen) clamp. The physician pulls the prepuce over a cone-shaped device that rests against the glans. A clamp is placed around the cone and prepuce and is tightened to provide enough pressure to crush the blood vessels. This prevents bleeding when the prepuce is removed after 3 to 5 minutes.

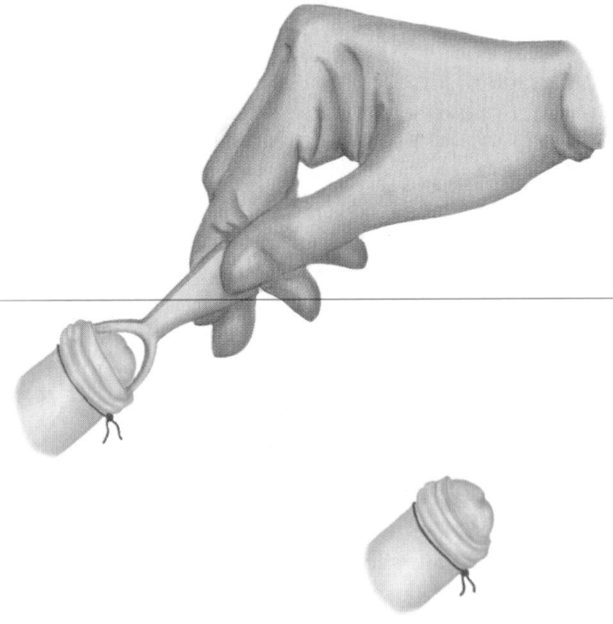

FIGURE 21-7 Circumcision using the Plastibell. The physician places the Plastibell, a plastic ring, over the glans, draws the prepuce over it, and ties a suture around the prepuce and Plastibell. This prevents bleeding when the excess prepuce is removed. The handle is removed, leaving only the ring in place over the glans. The Plastibell falls off in 5 to 8 days.

incised to expose the glans. A Mogan clamp may also be used for circumcisions, especially for ritual circumcisions for Jewish families.

Nursing Considerations

Assisting in Decision Making

Ideally, parents decide about circumcision early in pregnancy on the basis of careful consideration of the risks and benefits. However, this is not always the case. Some parents are not well informed about circumcision. The physician is responsible for explaining the risks and benefits to the parents, but the nurse may be called on to answer questions or clarify misconceptions that the parents may have.

Nurses must be certain that their own biases about circumcision do not interfere with their ability to give objective information to parents. Once the parents come to a decision, the nurse should support it. Although nurses generally teach parents of circumcised infants how to care for the penis, they may not think about providing teaching for parents who decide against circumcision. They should include care of the intact penis in the teaching plan for these parents.

Providing Care During Circumcision

As with any surgical procedure, informed consent is necessary from the parents before a circumcision is performed. The nurse sees that the consent has been signed, that the infant has received vitamin K, and informs the physician of any problems that might impair the infant's ability to withstand circumcision. The infant should be at least 12 hours old so that he has recovered from the stress of birth.

The nurse gathers equipment and supplies before the procedure. To prevent regurgitation, the infant may not be fed for 2 to 4 hours before the procedure. Because he is restrained in a supine position, regurgitation may cause aspiration. A bulb syringe should be placed nearby in case suction is necessary.

When the physician and equipment are ready, the infant is placed on a circumcision board. This is a plastic holder that is molded to fit the infant's body and has restraints for his arms and legs (Figure 21-8). A blanket is placed under the infant and only the diaper is removed. A drape provides warmth and maintains sterility. A heat lamp or radiant warmer helps prevent cold stress.

The nurse should comfort the infant during the procedure, especially if no anesthesia is used. A pacifier, talking to the infant, or soft music or tapes of intrauterine sounds may help distract the infant from pain.

Providing Postprocedure Care

The infant should be removed from the restraints immediately after the circumcision is completed. If a Gomco clamp was used, the nurse squeezes petroleum jelly or antibiotic ointment over the circumcision site to prevent

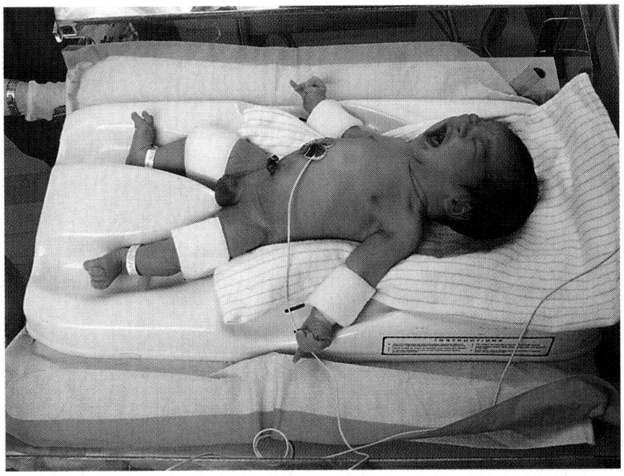

FIGURE 21-8 The infant is placed on the circumcision board just before the procedure is begun.

PARENTS WANT TO KNOW *Caring for the Uncircumcised Penis*

Wash your son's penis daily and when soiled diapers are changed. Retracting the foreskin is not necessary because it is still attached to the glans, or end of the penis. It will gradually separate from the glans, but it may take 3 or more years for complete separation to occur.

Occasionally, you can gently pull back on the foreskin to see how much separation has occurred. However, *never* force the foreskin to retract. This is painful and may cause bleeding, infections, and adhesions.

As your son gets older and takes over his own care, teach him to wash under the foreskin by gently pulling it back only as far as it retracts easily. This should become a part of his daily bath.

PARENTS WANT TO KNOW *How to Care for the Circumcised Site*

Observe the circumcision site at each diaper change. Note the amount of bleeding. Call the physician if more than a few drops of blood are noted during diaper changes the first day or any bleeding thereafter.

Continue to apply petroleum jelly to the penis with each diaper change according to your physician's instructions. If a Plastibell was used, petroleum jelly should not be applied because of possible displacement of the ring.

Keeping the circumcision site clean is important for healing. Squeeze warm water from a clean washcloth over the penis to wash it. Fasten the diaper loosely to prevent rubbing or pressure on the incision site.

Expect a yellow crust to form over the circumcision site. This is a normal part of healing and should not be removed. If a Plastibell was used, the plastic rim will fall off in 5 to 8 days. If it does not fall off by that time, notify your physician. Watch for signs of infection, such as fever or drainage accompanied by a bad odor or pus. *Call your physician if you suspect any abnormalities.* Also call the physician immediately if the plastic rim moves onto the penis. The circumcision site should be fully healed in approximately 10 days.

the diaper from sticking to it. A 2- × 2-inch piece of gauze may be placed over the area. Petroleum jelly should not be used with a Plastibell because it may cause it to slip. The infant should be comforted and returned to his mother, who may be anxious about her son.

The nurse watches carefully for signs of complications following the circumcision. The wound is checked frequently for bleeding during the first few hours after the procedure. If the infant is to be discharged after the circumcision, he should be observed for 2 hours before release.

If excessive bleeding occurs, pressure is applied to the penis with sterile gauze. If bleeding continues, the nurse notifies the physician, who may suture the small blood vessels. A small amount of blood loss may be significant in an infant, who has a small total blood volume.

Noting the first urination after circumcision is important because edema could cause an obstruction. If the infant goes home before voiding, the mother is instructed to call the physician if the baby does not urinate within 6 to 8 hours.

Teaching Parents

Because circumcision is often performed on the day of discharge, the parents take over care of the site. Each time the site is checked for bleeding, the nurse should show the parents the amount of blood on the diaper to help them understand how much to expect. The normal yellowish exudate that forms over the site should be described and differentiated from purulent drainage. Signs of complications should be discussed fully.

Check Your Reading

8. What are the reasons parents decide for or against circumcision?
9. What information do parents need about care of the intact and circumcised penis?

APPLICATION OF THE NURSING PROCESS: PARENTS' KNOWLEDGE OF NEWBORN CARE

New mothers often feel unprepared, physically and emotionally, to take over full care of a newborn and themselves. Mothers dealing with exhaustion and physiologic changes from childbirth may have difficulty remembering all the information they are given about care of themselves and their infants. Therefore finding creative teaching methods is especially important. The nurse must use every contact with the parents as an opportunity for further teaching.

Assessment

Assess parents' changing learning needs throughout the birth facility stay. Consider the mother's and infant's physical conditions and any special concerns that the mother may have.

Determine learning needs for experienced mothers. They may be unaware of information that has changed since the birth of the last infant. For example, mothers who have always placed their infants in the prone position for sleep need to know that this position is no longer recommended because it may be associated with sudden infant death syndrome. Mothers should be taught to use the supine position for sleep (AAP & ACOG, 1997). Differences in physical requirements or temperament between siblings cause concern. Parents may need information about helping other children adjust to the newborn.

Assess the father's learning needs and his plans for involvement with infant care. In some cultures, the father participates little in the care of the young infant. He may become more involved as the child gets older. In other families, fathers actively participate in child care, even during the birth facility stay. They often have many questions and are eager to learn about care of their infant.

Analysis

An appropriate nursing diagnosis for the family with learning needs is "Health Seeking Behaviors related to the desire for information about infant care."

Planning

The primary goals/expected outcomes for the diagnosis of "Health Seeking Behaviors" are that the parents will

- Identify their own information needs and seek assistance from nurses to meet those needs
- Correctly demonstrate infant care before discharge
- Express confidence in their ability to meet their infant's needs

Interventions

Determining Who Teaches

In many agencies, the same nurse is responsible for care of both mother and infant during a shift. This may be called *couplet* or *mother/baby care.* Over a 24-hour period several different nurses will care for the couplet. Teaching must be coordinated so that all concerns are met. Many facilities use a checklist of major teaching topics to ensure that all important areas are covered (Table 21-2).

Setting Priorities

Because of the short time available for teaching, set priorities in determining what to teach. After assessing the parents' individual learning needs, make a teaching plan. Use a topic list to help them point out major concerns regarding infant care. This ensures that precious teaching time is spent most effectively. Begin by discussing their most pressing concerns. This enhances further learning by decreasing their anxiety so that they can concentrate on the information. Then, as time allows, proceed to other subjects.

Table 21-2
MAJOR TEACHING TOPICS

Newborn characteristics and behavior
Use of bulb syringe
Breastfeeding
Frequency, length, positioning, latch on, supply and demand, supplementing, potential problems
Formula feeding
Frequency, amount, positioning, avoiding propping, formula preparation
Burping
Cord care
Care of the penis, uncircumcised or circumcised
Holding/positioning
Sleep patterns
Elimination patterns
Bathing
Clothing
Signs of problems
Taking a temperature
Infant safety
Car seat

Using Various Teaching Methods

Use a variety of teaching methods to increase effectiveness, make the subject more interesting, and increase retention of the material. Use verbal and written methods and demonstrations. Ask the parents to return each demonstration of care skills. Parents benefit from seeing skills performed correctly and then practicing them under supervision while the nurse gives suggestions and makes corrections as needed.

Discuss information with the mother alone or with her family members, roommate, or a group of mothers. Some women learn better with one-to-one teaching, whereas others benefit from watching and listening to others. Group teaching allows nurses to make more efficient use of time.

Use audiovisual materials, including pamphlets, baby magazines, films or videos, and television programs. Highlight the most important areas in written material, watch the videos with the new mother, and clarify information as necessary. This helps reinforce the learning.

An increasing number of parents use the Internet to obtain information about child care. Suggest to those who plan to use this source that they look for those that are accurate, current, and provided by well-known organizations such as health care providers, consumer advocacy groups, or university medical schools. Warn them to be wary of sites with unclear sources of the information or information that seems contrary to generally accepted knowledge. Suggest that they confirm information with their health care provider if they are unsure about it. Commend parents for their interest in obtaining information to increase their parenting skills.

Explain the rationale for each point made during teaching sessions. Understanding the reasons behind the actions increases the likelihood that parents will follow the nurse's instructions.

Modeling Behavior

Modeling by the nurse is an important teaching tool. Mothers watch closely when nurses handle infants. The nurse demonstrates mothering behavior by the way the infant is held and care is given and by talking to the infant. Modeling is particularly important for the mother with no experience in child care.

Use opportunities such as a bath demonstration or general care of the infant to point out infant characteristics and behavior states and to model how to calm crying infants. Teach mothers to use progressive consoling interventions such as talking to the infant, touching or folding the infant's arms across the chest, holding, swaddling, and facilitating sucking of the infant's hands or a pacifier. These actions can help parents learn about their infants' capabilities and identify and intervene appropriately to the infant's behavior cues (Karl, 1999).

Teaching Intermittently

Plan teaching in small segments that are interspersed with the care of the infant. Check the parents' understanding frequently. Encourage them to take over various tasks until they are performing all of the infant's routine care.

Including the Father

Identify fathers who would like to participate in care of their infants but hesitate because of lack of experience. Offer them the same teaching given the inexperienced mother. Give praise liberally to increase confidence and skill when parents practice their new infant care skills.

Documenting Teaching

Document all teaching performed and the parent's abilities to carry out infant care. This record helps other nurses to know what teaching has been completed and

Text continued on p. 570

PARENTS WANT TO KNOW *Techniques for Infant Care*

This guide is written in language that the nurse might use when teaching parents about infant care. Adapt the subjects to meet the needs of individual parents.

Handling the Infant

Head Support

An infant's head is the heaviest part of the body and makes up one fourth of the total body length. Infants are unable to support their heads when held in an upright position. You must place your hand behind the infant's head during carrying and positioning. After the first few months of life, babies' muscles become strong enough to support their head.

Positions

Most mothers hold the infant in the cradle position. In the "football" position, the baby's head is supported in the palm of the hand and the body is held along the arm and supported against your side. This position allows one hand to be free when washing the baby's hair or breastfeeding.

The shoulder hold is good for burping the baby. Or sit the baby on your lap and support the head and chest with one hand while gently patting or rubbing the infant's back with the other hand. This allows you to see the baby's face in case of spit-ups.

Always place your baby on the back for sleep, unless your baby's doctor tells you otherwise. This position is recommended by the American Academy of Pediatrics for all infants. It helps prevent sudden infant death syndrome (SIDS), the sudden unexplained death of an infant. The baby should sleep on a firm mattress to avoid suffocation.

Wrapping

Young infants seem more secure when wrapped firmly in a blanket, which may feel like the small space of the uterus. Fussy babies often respond well to swaddling. To swaddle the infant, turn down one corner of a blanket and position the baby's head over the edge. Fold one side of the blanket over

Continued

PARENTS WANT TO KNOW *Techniques for Infant Care—cont'd*

the body and arm. Bring the lower corner up and fold it over the chest. Then bring the other side around the infant and tuck it underneath snugly.

Normal Body Processes

Breathing

Newborns normally breathe about 30 to 60 times a minute. Their breathing is irregular and may vary from loud to soft. Sometimes breathing is so quiet that mothers wake babies to be sure that they actually are breathing. Sneezing is usually a normal response to lint from new baby clothes rather than a sign of a cold.

Using a Bulb Syringe

Use the bulb syringe if the infant has excessive mucus in the mouth or nose or spits up milk. Squeeze the bulb before you gently insert it into the mouth and aim it to the side of the mouth rather than to the back. Extra mucus is common in the first days of life but is usually not a problem thereafter unless a cold develops. Clean the bulb as necessary with soap and water. Rinse and dry well before using again. Call your physician if the baby's skin becomes blue or if the baby stops breathing for more than 15 seconds, has difficulty breathing, or has yellow or green drainage from the nose.

Regulating Temperature

Newborns have difficulty regulating their temperature. If they become cold, they need more calories and more oxygen than when they are warm enough. A drop in body temperature can be dangerous. Dress your baby as you would like to be dressed. Add a light receiving blanket over the young infant, except in very hot weather.

Using a Thermometer

Check your baby's temperature during illness. Take the temperature under the infant's arm to prevent injury to the rectum. Place the thermometer under the arm so that the bulb does not protrude behind the arm. Hold the arm firmly over the thermometer and read it according to manufacturer's directions. A digital thermometer is easy to read and takes little time. Call your physician if the baby has a temperature higher than 100° F or lower than 97.7° F.

Urine Output

Your baby will have at least 2 to 6 wet diapers a day during the first day or two and 6 to 10 wet diapers a day thereafter. Counting the number of wet diapers helps you know if the baby is getting enough milk. *Call your baby's doctor if the baby has no wet diapers for more than 12 hours.*

Stool Output

Breastfed infants pass soft, seedy stools that have a sweet-sour odor and are mustard yellow. They should have at least four stools a day. Formula-fed infants pass one to several stools each day that are pale yellow to light brown and formed. Babies may appear constipated when they turn red and seem to strain when passing a stool. However, constipated stools are dry with small, hard pieces and are usually fewer stools per day than average. If the movement is soft, you do not need to worry if the baby seems to strain.

Diarrhea

Babies with diarrhea pass an increased number of stools, and the color and consistency change. Because the contents move through the intestines more quickly than normal, the color is greener and the stools are more liquid than usual. You may see a water ring, an area in the diaper where the liquid has absorbed, sometimes around an area of more solid stool. Call your physician for further instructions if the infant passes more than two diarrhea stools.

Skin Care

A number of normal marks occur on the newborn's skin. One is a rash called *erythema toxicum* and resembles small insect bites. Another is small whiteheads called *milia*. These are normal and disappear without treatment. Do not squeeze them or they may become infected and last longer.

Newborns have dry, peeling skin because they were surrounded by water for 9 months and the outer layers of the skin were not shed. After peeling, the baby has soft skin. Lotions or creams are unnecessary and may cause irritation.

Cord

If you have been instructed to use alcohol on the cord, use a cotton swab dipped in alcohol to clean the cord and the crevices at the base of the cord about three times a day. This does not hurt the baby because no nerves are in the cord. If you have been instructed to let the cord dry naturally, do not apply anything to it. Notify your physician if you see bleeding or signs of infection, such as redness at the base of the cord with drainage or a foul odor.

Keep the cord dry by folding the diaper below it so that it is not wet by urine. The cord generally falls off in about 10 to 14 days. It may bleed a few drops when it detaches. Do not start tub baths until the cord is off and the area is well healed.

Diaper Area

Clean the diaper area with each diaper change. For girls, separate the labia (folds) and remove all stool. For boys, wash under the scrotum to help prevent rashes. If the diaper area becomes red, change the diaper more often. Leaving the diaper off to expose the area to air is also helpful. If an ointment is needed, petroleum jelly or a barrier-type ointment may be used. *If redness persists, ask your baby's doctor for suggestions.*

Bathing

Give your baby a sponge bath until the cord and circumcision areas are healed. At that time, tub baths can begin. Because infants are washed as needed after they spit up and with diaper changes, baths are not necessary every day. Fathers often enjoy giving the infant a bath and make this their special time with the baby.

Sponge Baths

Before the bath, gather all the supplies: a container or sink for the warm water, washcloth, towel, baby shampoo, alcohol, cotton or cotton-tipped swabs, and clean clothes. Soap is not necessary for the young infant, but if used, it should be gentle and nonalkaline to protect the natural acids of the infant's skin.

PARENTS WANT TO KNOW Techniques for Infant Care—cont'd

Give the bath in a room that is warm and free of drafts. Bathe the baby on a surface that is comfortable and safe. If you use a counter, pad it with blankets or towels.

Never leave the infant alone on an unprotected surface, even for a minute. Keep one hand on the infant at all times to prevent falls. Taking the phone off the hook during the bath prevents distractions. If you must leave the room, take the baby along or place the baby in the crib.

You can shampoo the head before fully undressing the baby and while holding the baby in a football position. Although the fontanelle or "soft spot" may seem delicate, it is covered with a tough membrane. It is not injured by washing. You may see pulse movements in the fontanelle, but this is normal. Dry the hair well to prevent heat loss.

Keep the baby warm by uncovering only the area you are washing. Wash and dry the baby's body, one part at a time, to prevent chilling. Start by washing the face with clean water. Use a separate clean area of the washcloth to wipe each eye. Use a washcloth to clean in and around the ears, where milk may accumulate. Do not use cotton-tipped swabs in the infant's ears or nose, as injury may occur if the baby moves suddenly. Clean the diaper area last, using the principle of "clean to least clean." For baby girls, wipe the diaper area from front to back. This avoids infections that may occur if stool gets into the vagina or urethra.

To clean the neck folds, put one hand under the baby's shoulders and lift slightly. This causes the head to drop back enough that the creases in the neck can be washed.

Tub Bath

For a tub bath, use a small plastic tub or a clean sink. Pad the bottom with a towel or foam pad to make it more comfortable and prevent the infant from slipping. Place about 3 inches of warm water in the tub. Wash the face and hair before placing the baby in the tub. Keeping the baby dressed until after the hair is washed helps prevent chilling.

It may be easier, at first, to lather your hands with soap and water and then lather the infant's body. Then immerse the baby in the tub for rinsing. Infants may be frightened when they are first put in water. Talk softly and calmly while holding your baby securely to help the baby adjust to this new experience.

Feeding

See Chapter 22 for more information on breastfeeding and formula feeding.

Hold a bottle so that the nipple is filled with milk to prevent the infant from swallowing air. Gently rubbing the palate with the nipple encourages the infant to begin sucking. However, excessive movement of the nipple in the baby's mouth is distracting to the baby.

Burp the baby once midway during the feeding, using the shoulder or the sitting position. After feeding, always place the baby on the side with a rolled blanket behind the back to prevent choking if the baby spits up.

Behavior

Knowing infants' different behavioral states helps you learn about your baby's individual characteristics.

Sleep Phases

During quiet sleep, the infant sleeps soundly with quiet breathing and little movement. Your baby will not be disturbed by noises from appliances or other children at this time. In active sleep, the baby moves or fusses while still asleep. If your baby sleeps in your room, you may have difficulty sleeping because of the baby's noises and movements. During the drowsy state, the baby is beginning to wake but may go back to sleep if not disturbed. However, if it is time for feeding or other activities, talk softly to help the baby awaken.

Awake Phases

The quiet alert state is the one that parents enjoy most because the infant seems so intent on studying objects and people nearby. This is a good time for infant stimulation and "play time." Parents soon learn to recognize the active alert or "fussy" phase in their infants. The infant may be signaling hunger or discomfort from wet and cold diapers. If you do not intervene, the baby soon moves to the crying state. Babies who cry too long may not respond at first to care activities. A few minutes of rocking and holding close may be necessary before the infant settles down.

Socialization

Infants are social beings who enjoy contact with people. They hear voices in the uterus and respond with interest when their parents talk to them after birth. The baby should be part of family life. Use an infant seat or carrier to keep the baby near you and the rest of the family. Infants enjoy watching the human face. Hold your baby close and talk to your baby to provide social stimulation.

Stimulation

Sounds—Play music of different types to provide auditory stimulation. Infants prefer music that is not too loud. Music boxes, tapes, CDs, or a radio can provide a variety of sound.

Sights—Because babies focus their eyes best at a distance of 7 to 12 inches, items such as mobiles should be placed within this range. Infants especially like black and white geometric figures. They enjoy bright colors early but are not particularly interested in pastels.

Variety—Place the baby in an infant seat in the kitchen while you prepare meals to stimulate the senses of sight, hearing, and smell. An infant carrier pack provides the stimulation of motion as well.

Timing—Stimulation is best used during the baby's quiet alert state. Do not try to use stimulation techniques with a fussy infant because it can cause overstimulation. This causes the baby to be irritable and have difficulty going to sleep.

what is still needed. It also provides legal proof that teaching was completed before discharge.

Providing for Follow-Up Care

Provide information about unmet learning needs to the home or clinic nurse who will see the mother and infant. Reinforcement can then be provided at a time when the mother's memory has improved after the stress of birth.

Provide as much information as possible in written form so that parents can refer to it if they have concerns. Also provide telephone numbers for further help. Offer written information in the parents' primary language, if possible. Even if they speak English as a second language, they may prefer to read in their native language.

Remind parents about timing of follow-up care. Suggest that they call early for an appointment so that the infant can receive care on time.

Incorporating Cultural Considerations

Take the family's cultural beliefs about child care into consideration when teaching. For example, some Southeast Asian and Latino women are hesitant to breastfeed in the birth facility and wish to wait until the milk comes in when they are home. Asian parents may be uneasy when caregivers are too complimentary about the baby or casually touch the infant's head. However, Latino parents may prefer that a person who compliments the infant touch the infant's face or head to ward off *mal ojo* or the "evil eye." "Evil eye" or *najar* is also a concern to women from India who place a black dot on the newborn's forehead to ward it off.

Native Hawaiian, Filipino, and Japanese women in Hawaii may use infant massage provided by a lomilomi practitioner to improve their relationship with the infant and to mold the body and spirit of the child (Mayberry, Affonso, Shibuya, & Clemmens, 1998). Parents from these cultures may wish to perform the massage during the birth facility stay.

Ask the parents who will be helping them care for the baby to determine family members who should be included in the teaching. This may vary according to the culture and availability of the traditional caregiver. In addition to the father of the infant, the woman's mother is often the major support person. However, in the Korean culture, the husband's mother is the primary caregiver for the infant and the mother in the early weeks to allow the mother to recover from the birth. If the mother will not be the primary infant caregiver, she may appear uninterested in the nurse's teachings.

Evaluation

Ongoing evaluation of parents' learning is necessary throughout the birth facility stay and during the follow-up home, clinic, or office visits. Determine whether they feel their questions have been answered and they can demonstrate important aspects of infant care safely and correctly. As they learn more caregiving skills, their confidence should increase as well.

Table 21-3
COMMON NURSING DIAGNOSES FOR NEWBORNS

Family Coping: Potential for Growth
*Health Seeking Behaviors
Risk for Altered Parent-Infant Attachment
Risk for Altered Parenting
*Risk for Ineffective Airway Clearance
*Risk for Ineffective Thermoregulation
Risk for Infection
*Risk for Injury

*Nursing diagnoses that are explored in this chapter.

IMMUNIZATION

Hepatitis B is a growing problem in the United States. Immunization for this disease is now included with other routine childhood vaccinations. Infants of mothers with acute or chronic hepatitis B infection (HBsAg positive) may become infected from exposure to the mother's blood at birth. Approximately 70% to 90% of infants infected at birth become chronic carriers unless they are vaccinated against hepatitis B (AAP & ACOG, 1997). Chronic infection may cause later cancer or other serious liver damage.

These infants should receive both the vaccine and hepatitis B immune globulin (HBIG). The immune globulin provides passive immunity to hepatitis to protect infants until they develop their own antibodies and should be given within 12 hours of birth. The vaccine promotes antibody formation to protect infants from further exposure to the disease.

NEWBORN SCREENING TESTS

Two types of screening tests required in many states are hearing screening and blood tests performed for certain inborn errors of metabolism or other genetic disorders. These tests are performed before discharge from the birth facility.

Hearing loss in infants is estimated to be approximately 1 to 3 per 1000 well newborns and 2% to 4% of those with complications requiring intensive care (AAP & ACOG, 1997). Detection before the age of 3 months greatly improves outcomes. Because of this, auditory screening of all newborns is now recommended by the American Academy of Pediatrics and is mandated by law in some states. A goal of Healthy People 2010 is to increase the proportion of newborns who are screened for hearing loss by the age 1 month, have audiologic evaluation by age 3 months, and are enrolled in appro-

DRUG GUIDE: HEPATITIS B VACCINE

Classification: Vaccine

Other Names: Engerix-B, Recombivax HB

Action: Immunization against hepatitis B infection

Indications: Prevention of hepatitis B in exposed and unexposed infants

Neonatal Dosage and Route: Recombivax HB: 5 mcg to infant of infected mother, 2.5 mcg if mother not infected

Engerix-B: 10 mcg (whether or not mother is infected)

For infants of HBsAg-negative mothers the first dose of vaccine is given by 2 months. The second dose is given 1 month after the first dose. The third dose is given at least 2 months after the second dose but not before the infant is 6 months old.

For infants of HBsAg-positive mothers the vaccine is given within 12 hours of birth and at 1 to 2 months and 6 months. Hepatitis B immune globulin (HBIG) is also given within 12 hours of birth at a different site than the vaccine.

If the mother's HbsAg status is unknown, the infant receives the vaccine within 12 hours of birth and the mother is tested. If the HbsAg test is positive, the infant should receive HBIG as soon as possible and by 1 week of age.

Give intramuscularly in the anterolateral thigh.

Absorption: Well absorbed from muscle; not affected by maternal antibodies

Contraindications: Hypersensitivity to yeast

Adverse Reactions: Pain or redness at site, fever

Nursing Considerations: Shake solution well before preparing. Give vaccine within 12 hours of birth to infants of infected mothers. Do not inject intravenously or intradermally. Bathe infants before the injection to remove blood and prevent contamination of the injection site with maternal blood on the infant's skin. Obtain parental consent before administering.

Vaccine with thimerosal, a mercury-containing preservative, should be avoided if possible for infants younger than 2 months of age. Hepatitis B vaccine without thimerosal is now available. If necessary, vaccine with thimerosal should be given to infants born to mothers who are HBsAg-positive rather than risk them becoming infected (CDC, 1999).

DRUG GUIDE: HEPATITIS B IMMUNE GLOBULIN (HBIG)

Classification: Immune globulin

Other Names: BayHep B

Action: Provides antibodies and passive immunity to hepatitis B

Indications: Prophylaxis for infants of hepatitis B surface antigen positive mothers

Neonatal Dosage and Route: 0.5 ml within 12 hours of birth intramuscularly in the anterolateral thigh; should not be given intravenously

Absorption: Well absorbed from muscle

Contraindications: None known

Adverse Reactions: Pain and tenderness at site, urticaria

Nursing Considerations: Bathe infants before the injection to remove blood and prevent contamination of the injection site with maternal blood on the infant's skin. Give at a site separate from one used for hepatitis B vaccine.

priate intervention services by age 6 months (U.S. Department of Health and Human Services, 2000).

To accomplish this goal, a screening test is given infants before discharge from the birth facility and referrals are made for further testing if the infant shows signs of hearing problems. This allows early intervention that will prevent developmental delays and enable the child to communicate better than if hearing loss is found later in childhood. Current tests use evoked otoacoustic emmisions and auditory brainstem response to provide screening. The nurse ensures that infants receive screening if offered at the birth facility and explains the testing to the parents. Parents of infants referred for further testing will need more explanation and emotional support.

Blood tests are performed to detect conditions that result from inborn errors of metabolism or other genetic conditions. Without early treatment, the disorders may cause mental retardation or other serious problems. The tests are easy and inexpensive. More thorough testing is necessary to confirm any abnormal test results. Although each state determines which conditions must be tested, those most commonly included are phenylketonuria (PKU), hypothyroidism, galactosemia, hemoglobinopathies, and certain other conditions.

Screening tests require a blood sample taken from the infant's heel and are usually performed shortly before discharge. Parents may have questions about the purpose of the tests that the nurse will need to answer. Nurses often refer to the tests as "PKU tests," but they should call them screening tests to emphasize that a number of conditions are included in the tests.

Tests performed within the first 24 hours of life are less sensitive than those performed after 24 hours. Infants tested before 24 hours should have repeat tests within 1 to 2 weeks of age so that disorders are not missed because of early testing (AAP & ACOG, 1997). These tests are performed at a home, clinic, or office visit.

Phenylketonuria

Phenylketonuria is a genetic condition in which the infant cannot metabolize the amino acid phenylalanine, which is common in protein foods such as milk. Although some phenylalanine is essential to growth, accumulations of it can result in severe mental retardation. If treatment is begun in the first 2 months of life, retardation can be prevented, in most cases. Phenyl-ketonuria is treated with a special low-phenylalanine diet, in which the amount of the amino acid is carefully regulated.

Hypothyroidism

Hypothyroidism occurs in 1 in 3600 to 1 in 5000 newborns (U.S. Public Health Service, 1995). In this condition, the thyroid does not produce enough of the hormone thyroxine. Thyroid hormones affect the entire body, and the symptoms in an untreated infant include respiratory, feeding, and growth problems as well as irreversible brain damage. Early and consistent treatment with thyroid hormones allows normal growth and development of full intellect.

Galactosemia

Absence of the enzyme necessary for the conversion of the milk sugar galactose to glucose causes galactosemia. The condition results in damage to the liver, brain, and eyes and eventually causes death. Treatment includes elimination of milk from the diet and use of soy milk.

Hemoglobinopathies

Hemoglobinopathies include sickle cell anemia, thalassemia, and other diseases. The diseases are most often found in infants of African, Mediterranean, Asian, or South and Central American background. In sickle cell anemia, erythrocytes may become sickle shaped, resulting in obstruction of blood vessels and erythrocyte destruction. The other hemoglobinopathies cause chronic anemias, sepsis, and other serious conditions.

Other Conditions

Screening may also be performed for maple syrup urine disease, homocystinuria, congenital adrenal hyperplasia, biotinidase deficiency, and other conditions. Knowing which conditions are included in testing allows the nurse to include appropriate information in parent teaching.

Check Your Reading

10. What are some important considerations in planning parent teaching?
11. What immunization may be performed at the birth facility and why?
12. Why is it important to perform screening tests on infants as close to discharge as possible? For which infants is retesting important?

DISCHARGE AND NEWBORN FOLLOW-UP CARE

Discharge

Although state and federal legislation allows women and infants to stay in the birth facility for 48 hours after vaginal birth and 96 hours after cesarean birth, some women choose to go home earlier. The time of discharge varies according to the mother and newborn's needs and wishes and the primary caregivers' assessment of their conditions.

Discharge occurs when term newborns who are appropriate for gestational age have normal physical examination results and show that they are making the transition from fetal to neonatal life without difficulty. Infants should have vital signs within normal limits, have fed successfully at least twice, passed urine and stool, have no excessive bleeding at the circumcision site for at least 2 hours and no significant jaundice in the first 24 hours of life. The mother should show adequate knowledge, ability, and confidence to provide adequate care of the newborn and have support available (AAP & ACOG, 1997).

Follow-Up Care

Follow-up care after discharge from the birth facility is important. The American Academy of Pediatrics recommends that follow-up by a health care professional for all newborns who go home from the birth facility less than 48 hours after birth. This should occur within 48 hours of discharge and can be provided in the home, clinic, or office (AAP & ACOG, 1997). When mothers and infants are seen within 2 days of discharge, maternal satisfaction with care increases and infant morbidity decreases (Lieu, Braveman, Escobar, Fischer, Jensvold, & Capra, 2000).

Follow-up care can be provided in a number of ways. One or more home visits by a nurse are offered as a part of the maternity package in some birth facilities. In other areas, families return to the birth facility, a clinic, or the pediatrician's office to have the newborn checked. Clinics are held in the birth facility in some agencies.

Some birth facilities have "hot lines" or "warm lines" that mothers can call when they have questions about care of their infants or themselves. In many facilities, nurses call mothers during the first few days after discharge to assess the adjustment and health of the mother and baby, clarify information given before discharge, and answer questions. Any identified problems result in the appropriate referrals. This method is less expensive than home visits but does not allow the nurse to perform assessments in person. It may be combined with home visits used only for high-risk families. Follow-up care for newborns is discussed further in Chapter 23, p. 606.

SUMMARY CONCEPTS

- Prophylaxis against hemorrhagic disease of the newborn and ophthalmia neonatorum are necessary shortly after birth. It is provided by an injection of vitamin K and use of erythromycin ophthalmic ointment.
- Newborns may need help in clearing the airway. Positioning, suction, and close observation may be necessary.
- Nurses can prevent heat loss in newborns by keeping them dry and covered, avoiding contact between them and cold objects or surfaces, and keeping them away from drafts and outside windows and walls.
- The nurse must identify actual or potential hypoglycemia and intervene appropriately.
- Important interventions for jaundice are to monitor for its occurrence, to be sure that the infant is feeding well, and to explain the condition to the parents.
- The nurse must prevent mistaken identification of infants by checking the mother and infant identification bands whenever they have been separated.
- Parents and nurses must work together to prevent infant abductions. Parents must know how to identify hospital staff. Nurses should be alert for suspicious behavior.
- Infection can best be prevented by scrupulous hand washing by staff and all who come in contact with newborns.
- Potential benefits of circumcision may include decreased incidence of urinary tract infections, penile cancer, phimosis, and sexually transmissible infections. Other reasons for circumcision include religious dictates, parent preference, and lack of knowledge about care of the foreskin.
- Parents reject circumcision because of belief that the above conditions are too uncommon to necessitate surgery and pain in infants and concerns about bleeding, infection, phimosis, meatitis, meatal stenosis, urinary retention, chordee, and inclusion cysts.
- Parents with uncircumcised sons should be taught not to retract the foreskin until it becomes separate from the glans later in childhood.
- Parents of circumcised infants should be taught signs of complications and how to care for the area.
- Every nursing contact with parents should be used as an opportunity to teach.
- Screening tests are commonly performed to rule out hearing abnormalities, PKU, hypothyroidism, galactosemia, and hemoglobinopathies.

ANSWERS TO CRITICAL THINKING EXERCISE

1. Determine whether Andy is showing signs of hypothermia, hypoglycemia, or both. Reassure and teach Nancy as assessments and interventions are completed.
2. While taking the infant's temperature, assess for skin temperature, jitteriness, and general behavior. Check the blood glucose level if indicated. Also assess the environment for possible causes of heat loss.
3. If the baby's temperature is slightly low, intervene by changing any wet linens, double wrapping, and applying a hat. Recheck the temperature in 30 minutes. If it is still low, place Andy under a radiant warmer. Feed him if the blood glucose level is low. Notify the physician if Andy continues to have difficulty maintaining temperature. (See Nursing Care Plan 21-1 for other interventions.)
4. Praise Nancy for being so observant of her son. If Andy's temperature is normal and he is not jittery, discuss the fact that peripheral circulation is sluggish in newborns and that their hands and feet tend to be cool. If "shakiness" is the Moro reflex or normal newborn behavior, discuss the reflex and the immaturity of the central nervous system. Show Nancy how to wrap Andy so that he stays warm and the Moro reflex is not elicited. Discuss methods of temperature control, and be sure that Nancy knows how to read a thermometer. Explain all interventions.

REFERENCES AND READINGS

American Academy of Pediatrics. (2000). Immunization protects children: 2000 immunization schedule. Retrieved July 17, 2000 from http://www.aap.org/family/parents/immunize.htm.

American Academy of Pediatrics, Task Force on Circumcision. (1999). Circumcision policy statement. *Pediatrics,* 103(3), 686-693.

American Academy of Pediatrics, Task Force on Newborn and Infant Hearing. (1999). Newborn and Infant Hearing Loss: Detection and Intervention. *Pediatrics,* 103(2), 527-530.

American Academy of Pediatrics and American College of Obstetricians and Gynecologists. (1997). *Guidelines for perinatal care* (4th ed.). Elk Grove, IL: American Academy of Pediatrics.

American Academy of Pediatrics & Canadian Paediatric Society. (2000). Prevention and management of pain and stress in the neonate. *Pediatrics,* 105(2), 454-461.

Association of Women's Health, Obstetric, and Neonatal Nurses (AWHONN). (1996). Physiologic assessment of the healthy newborn. Washington, D.C.: Author.

Association of Women's Health, Obstetric and Neonatal Nurses (AWHONN). (1998). *Standards and guidelines for professional nursing practice in the care of women and newborns* (5th ed.). Washington, D.C.: AWHONN.

Carroll, V. (2000). Infant abduction: Lowering the risk. *AWHONN Lifelines,* 3(6), 25-27.

Choi, E.C. (1995). A contrast of mothering behaviors in women from Korea and the United States. *Journal of Obstetric, Gynecologic, and Neonatal Nursing,* 24(4), 363-369.

Cole, J.G., Brissette, N.J., & Lunard:, B. (1999). Tub bath or sponge baths for newborn infants? *Mother Baby Journal,* 4(3), 39-43.

Communicable Disease Center. (1999). Recommendations regarding the use of vaccines that contain thimerosal as a preservative. *Morbidity & Mortality Weekly Report,* 48(43), 996-998.

Corrarino, J.E. (1998). Perinatal hepatitis B: Update and recommendations. *MCN: The American Journal of Maternal/Child Nursing,* 24(3), 151-155.

Corrarino, J.E., Walsh, P.J., & Anselmo, D. (1999). A program to educate women who test positive for the hepatitis B virus during the perinatal period. *MCN: The American Journal of Maternal/Child Nursing,* 24(3), 151-155.

Dore, S., Buchan, D., Coulas, S., Hamber, L., Stewart, M., Cowan, D., & Jamieson, L. (1998). Alcohol versus natural drying for newborn cord care. *Journal of Obstetric, Gynecologic, and Neonatal Nursing,* 27(6), 621-627.

Ewy-Edwards, D. (2000). Transition to parenthood. In F.H. Nichols & S.S. Humenick (Eds.), *Childbirth education: Practice, research, and theory* (2nd ed., pp. 84-113). Philadelphia: W.B. Saunders.

Ford, L.A., & Ritchie, J.A. (1999). Maternal perceptions of newborn umbilical cord treatments and healing. *Journal of Obstetric, Gynecologic, and Neonatal Nursing,* 28(5), 501-506.

Freitag-Koontz, M.J. (1997). Prevention of hepatitis B and C transmission during pregnancy and the first year of life. *Journal of Perinatal and Neonatal Nursing,* 10(2), 40-55.

Glass, S.M. (1999). Routine care. In P.J. Thureen, J. Deacon, P. O'Neil, & J. Hernandez (Eds.), *Assessment and care of the well newborn.* (pp 188-195). Philadelphia: W.B. Saunders.

Hagedorn, M.I.E., & Gardner, S.L. (1999). Hypoglycemia in the newborn, part I: Pathology and nursing management. *Mother Baby Journal,* 4(1), 15-21.

Herschel, M., Khoshnood, B., Ellman, C., Maydew, N., & Mittendorf, R. (1998). Neonatal circumcision: Randomized trial of sucrose pacifier for pain control. *Archived of Pediatric Adolescent Medicine,* 152, 279-284.

Hodgson, B.B., & Kizior, R.J. (2000). *Nursing drug handbook 2000.* Philadelphia: W.B. Saunders.

Howard, C.R., Howard, F.M., Fortune, K., et al. (1999). A randomized, controlled trial of a eutectic mixture of local anesthetic cream (lidocaine and prilocaine) versus penile nerve block for pain relief during circumcision. *American Journal of Obstetrics & Gynecology,* 18(6), 1506-1511.

Howard-Glen, L. (2000). Adaptation to extrauterine life and immediate nursing care. In S. Mattson & J.E. Smith (Eds.). *Core curriculum for maternal-newborn nursing* (2nd ed., pp. 346-359).

Howard-Glen, L. (2000). Newborn biological/behavioral characteristics and psychosocial adaptations. In S. Mattson & J.E. Smith (Eds.), *Core curriculum for maternal-newborn nursing* (2nd ed., pp. 360-373).

Karl, D.J. (1999). The interactive newborn bath: Using infant neurobehavior to connect parents and newborns. *MCN: The American Journal of Maternal/Child Nursing,* 24(6), 280-286.

Kennell, J.H., & Klaus, M.H. (1998). Bonding: Recent observations that alter perinatal care. *Pediatrics in Review,* 19(1), 4-12.

Lamp, J.M., & Howard, P.A. (1999). Guiding parents' use of the Internet for newborn education. *MCN: The American Journal of Maternal/Child Nursing,* 24(1), 33-36.

Lander, J., Brady-Fryer, B., Metcalfe, J.B., et al. (1997). Comparison of ring block, dorsal penile nerve block, and topical anesthesia for neonatal circumcision. *Journal of the American Medical Association,* 278(24), 2157-2162.

Lieu, T.A., Braveman, P.A., Escobar, G.J., Fischer, A.F., Jensvold, N.G., & Capra, A.M. (2000). A randomized comparison of home and clinic follow-up visits after early postpartum hospital discharge. *Pediatrics,* 105(5), 1058-1065.

Lock, M., & Ray., J.G. (1999). Higher neonatal morbidity after routine early hospital discharge: Are we sending newborns home too early? *Canadian Medical Association Journal,* 161(3), 249-253.

Mayberry, L.J., Affonso, D.D., Shibuya, J., & Clemmens, D. (1998). Integrating cultural values, beliefs, and customs into pregnancy and postpartum care: Lessons learned from a Hawaiian public health nursing project. *Journal of Perinatal Neonatal Nursing,* 13(1), 15-26.

McCartney, P.R. (2000). Bulb syringes in newborn care. *MCN: The American Journal of Maternal/Child Nursing,* 25(4), 217.

National Center for Missing & Exploited Children. (2000). *For Healthcare Professionals: Guidelines on Prevention of and Response to Infant Abductions* (6th ed.). Alexandria, VA: Author.

Nelson, T.E. (1999). Safeguarding newborns: Managing the risk. *RN,* 62(3), 67-69.

Pearson, J. (1999). Crying and calming: Important information and effective techniques to teach parents of full-term newborns. *Mother Baby Journal,* 4(5), 39-42.

Peeke, K., Hershberger, M., Kuehn, D., & Levett, J. (1999). Infant sleep position: Nursing practice and knowledge. *MCN: The American Journal of Maternal/Child Nursing,* 24(6), 301-304.

Penny-MacGillivray, T. (1996). A newborn's first bath: When? *Journal of Obstetric, Gynecologic, and Neonatal Nursing,* 25(6), 481-487.

Phillips, C.R. (1997). Mother-Baby Nursing. Washington DC: Association of Women's Health, Obstetric and Neonatal Nurses.

Purdy, I.B. (2000). Newborn auditory follow-up. *Neonatal Network,* 19(2), 25-33.

Rabun, J.B. (2000). *For healthcare professionals: Guidelines on prevention of and response to infant abductions.* Alexandria, VA: National Center for Missing and Exploited Children.

Ruchala, P., Seibold, L., & Stremsterfer, K. (1996). Validating assessment of neonatal jaundice with transcutaneous bilirubin measurement. *Neonatal Network,* 15(4), 33-37.

Schneiderman, J.U. (1996). Postpartum nursing for Korean mothers. *MCN: The American Journal of Maternal/Child Nursing,* 21(3), 155-158.

Schoen, E.J., Wiswell, T.E., & Moses, S. (2000). New policy on circumcision—Cause for concern. *Pediatrics,* 105(3), 620-623.

Simpson, K.R., & Creehan, P.A. (Eds.). (1996). *AWHONN's perinatal nursing.* Philadelphia: Lippincott-Raven.

Taddio, A., Katz, J., Ilersich, A.L., & Koren, G. (1997). Effect of neonatal circumcision pain response during subsequent routine vaccination. *Lancet,* 349, 599-603.

U.S. Department of Health and Human Services. (2000). *Healthy people 2010: Healthy People 2010 (Conference Edition, in Two Volumes).* Washington, D.C.: Author.

Varda, K.E., & Behnke, R.S. (2000). The effect of timing of initial bath on newborn's temperature. *Journal of Obstetric, Gynecologic, and Neonatal Nursing,* 29(1), 24-32.

Zderic, S.A. (1998). Developmental abnormalities of the genitourinary system. In H.W. Taeusch & R.A. Ballard (Eds.), *Avery's diseases of the newborn* (7th ed., pp. 1144-1157). Philadelphia: W.B. Saunders.

22

Infant Feeding

OBJECTIVES

1. Identify the nutritional and fluid needs of the infant.
2. Compare the composition of breast milk with that of formula.
3. Explain important factors in choosing a method of infant feeding.
4. Explain the physiology of lactation.
5. Describe nursing management of initial and continued breastfeeding.
6. Describe nursing assessments and interventions for common problems in breastfeeding.
7. Describe nursing assessments and interventions in formula feeding.

DEFINITIONS

Colostrum Breast fluid secreted during pregnancy and the first week after childbirth.

Engorgement Swelling of the breasts resulting from feedings that are delayed, too short, or not frequent enough.

Foremilk First breast milk received in a feeding.

Hindmilk Breast milk received near the end of a feeding; contains higher fat content than foremilk.

Latch-On Attachment of the infant to the breast.

Let-Down Reflex See *milk-ejection reflex.*

Mastitis Inflammation of the breast, usually caused by stasis of milk in the ducts or infection.

Mature Milk Breast milk that appears after the first 2 weeks of lactation.

Milk-Ejection Reflex Release of milk from the alveoli into the ducts; also known as the let-down reflex.

Nonnutritive Sucking Sucking during which no milk flow is obtained.

Nutritive Suckling (Sucking) Steady, rhythmic suckling at the breast or sucking at a bottle to obtain milk.

Oxytocin Hormone produced by the posterior pituitary gland that stimulates uterine contractions and the milk-ejection reflex; also prepared synthetically.

Prolactin Anterior pituitary hormone that promotes growth of breast tissue and stimulates production of milk.

Suckling Giving or taking nourishment from the breast. Sometimes used interchangeably with sucking, which refers only to drawing into the mouth with a partial vacuum, as with a bottle or pacifier.

Transitional Milk Breast milk that appears between secretion of colostrum and mature milk.

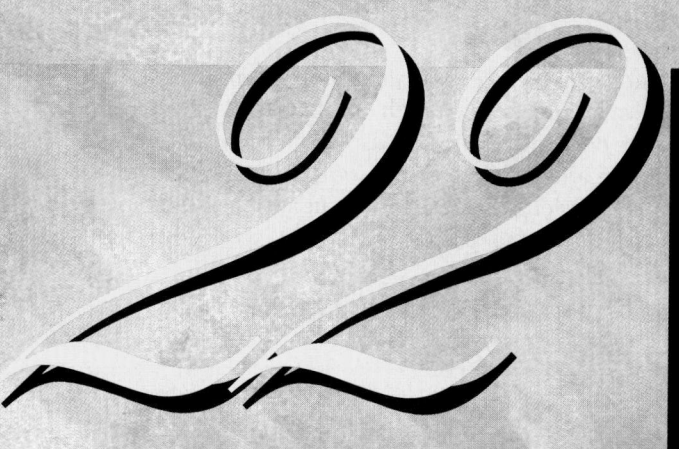

Infant feeding is an important part of parenting, and a woman may derive much satisfaction as a mother from her perception of success with feeding. Helping her choose and feel comfortable with a feeding method requires knowledge of the infant's nutritional needs and the techniques to meet those needs.

NUTRITIONAL NEEDS OF THE NEWBORN

Calories

The full-term newborn needs 110 to 120 kcal/kg (50 to 55 kcal/lb) of body weight each day. The infant must consume sufficient calories to meet energy needs, prevent use of body stores, and provide for growth.

Breast milk and formulas used for the normal newborn contain 20 kcal/oz. The average newborn weighing 3.4 kg (7.5 lb) requires approximately 19 to 21 oz of breast milk or formula each day to meet caloric requirements. This is about 45 to 75 ml (1.5 to 2.5 oz) at each feeding for infants who breastfeed every 2 to 3 hours. Formula-fed infants who feed every 3 to 4 hours need approximately 75 to 105 ml (2.5 to 3.5 oz) at each feeding.

CRITICAL TO REMEMBER

Daily Calorie and Fluid Needs of the Newborn

Calories: 110 to 120 kcal/kg (50 to 55 kcal/lb)
Fluid: 100 to 150 ml/kg (after first 2 days of life)

During the early days after birth, many infants lose 5% to 10% of their birth weight. This is because of normal loss of extracellular water and the fact that they often consume fewer calories than needed. Newborns have a small stomach capacity and may fall asleep before feeding adequately or sleep through feeding times in the early days. Capacity increases rapidly so that many infants take 2 to 3 oz within 3 to 7 days. Infants usually regain the lost weight by 10 days of age. This information should be explained to parents.

Nutrients

Nutrients needed by the newborn are provided by carbohydrates, proteins, and fat in breast milk or formula. Full-term neonates digest simple carbohydrates and proteins well. Fats are less well digested because of the lack of pancreatic lipase in the newborn. Vitamins and minerals are provided by both breast milk and formula.

Water

The newborn needs much larger amounts of fluid in relationship to size than does the adult because infants lose water more easily from the skin, kidneys, and intestines. Infants require fluids equal to 10% to 15% of their body weight each day, whereas adults need only 2% to 4% of their body weight daily (Curran & Barness, 2000). The normal newborn needs approximately 65 ml/kg (30 ml/lb) a day for the first 2 days of life and 100 to 150 ml/kg (45 to 68 ml/lb) a day after the first 2 days of life (Tsang, DeMarini, & Rath, 1998). Breast milk or formula supplies the infant's fluid needs. Additional water is unnecessary.

BREAST MILK AND FORMULA COMPOSITION

Breast Milk

Breast milk is species specific (designed for human infants) and offers many advantages compared with formula. The nutrients in breast milk are proportioned appropriately for the neonate and change to meet the newborn's changing needs. Breast milk provides protection against infection and is easily digested.

Changes in Composition

The composition of breast milk changes in three phases: colostrum, transitional milk, and mature milk, which vary in makeup to meet the newborn's changing nutritional needs.

Colostrum. The major secretion of the breasts during the first week of lactation is colostrum, a thick, yellow substance. Colostrum is higher in protein, fat-soluble vitamins, and minerals than mature milk but lower in calories, fat, and lactose. It is rich in immunoglobulins, especially secretory IgA, which helps protect the infant's gastrointestinal tract from infection. Colostrum helps establish the normal flora in the intestines, and its laxative effect speeds the passage of meconium.

Transitional Milk. Transitional milk appears 7 to 10 days after lactation begins, when the milk changes from colostrum to mature milk. Immunoglobulins and proteins decrease while lactose, fat, and calories increase. The vitamin content is approximately the same as that of mature milk.

Mature Milk. After the first 2 weeks of lactation, mature milk replaces transitional milk. Because breast milk is bluish and not as thick as colostrum, some mothers think their milk is not "rich" enough for their infants. Nurses should explain the normal appearance of breast milk. Mature milk contains approximately 20 kcal/oz and nutrients sufficient to meet the infant's needs. Unless otherwise stated, discussions of breast milk and its contents refer to mature milk.

Nutrients

The nutrients provided in breast milk are present in the amounts and proportions needed by the human infant.

Protein. The concentrations of amino acids in breast milk are suited to the infant's needs and ability to metabolize them. Breast milk contains a high level of taurine, which is important for bile conjugation and brain development. Tyrosine and phenylalanine are low in breast milk to correspond to the infant's low level of enzymes to digest them. The proteins produce a lower solute load for the infant's immature kidneys.

Casein and whey are the proteins in milk. Casein forms a large, insoluble curd that is harder to digest than the curd from whey, which is very soft. Breast milk is easily digested because it has a high ratio of whey to casein. Commercial formulas are adapted to increase the amount of whey so that the curd is more digestible.

The body's immune system recognizes and may react to the protein in cow's milk, making it one of the most common allergens. Allergies develop in approximately 2% to 7% of infants fed cow's milk formula. Because breast milk is species specific (made for human infants), it does not cause allergies (Lawrence & Lawrence, 1999). Long-term follow-up studies have shown a significant decrease in allergic conditions when infants are breastfed exclusively for at least 1 month (Saarinen & Kajosaari, 1995). This is of particular importance when a family history of allergies exists.

Mothers who breastfeed infants at risk for allergies should avoid highly allergenic foods that might affect the breast milk. These include cow's milk, eggs, fish, and nuts (AAP, 2000).

Carbohydrate. Lactose is the carbohydrate in breast milk. Its higher level in breast milk may improve absorption of calcium (Lawrence & Lawrence, 1999). Lactose also promotes growth of the normal bacterial flora in the intestines.

Fat. Between 30% and 55% of the calories in breast milk are from fat. The fat composition of human milk differs greatly from that of cow's milk. The majority is in the form of triglycerides with higher amounts of several essential fatty acids, such as the long-chain polyunsaturated fatty acids, docosahexanoic acid (DHA), and arachidonic acid (AA), that are important for growth of the brain. In addition, the fat in human milk may have antibacterial and antiviral properties (Hamosh, et al., 1999). Cholesterol also is higher in breast milk than in cow's milk. The high level of cholesterol may aid in the development of the central nervous system. The fat in breast milk is more easily digested by the newborn than that in cow's milk.

The amount of fat in breast milk varies during the feeding and between feedings on the same or different days. More fat is present in the hindmilk, the milk produced at the end of the feeding. Hindmilk produces satiety and helps the infant gain weight. Expressed hindmilk is sometimes used to increase caloric intake in preterm infants.

Vitamins. Vitamin C levels in human milk meet the infant's needs if the mother has an adequate intake. Vitamin D may be inadequate if the mother's diet is poor and she or the infant is not exposed to the sun. These infants need supplementation with 400 IU of vitamin D daily. The infant of a vegan mother may need supplementation with vitamin B_{12}.

Minerals. Although iron in breast milk is lower than in formula, approximately 49% is absorbed, compared with only 4% of that in iron-fortified formula (Lawrence & Lawrence, 1999). The increased absorption may result from the higher lactose and vitamin C content in breast milk. The full-term infant who is breastfed exclusively maintains iron stores for the first 6 months of life. The addition of formula or other foods, however, may decrease the absorption of iron, making supplementation necessary.

Sodium, calcium, and phosphorus are higher in cow's milk than in human milk. This could cause an excessively high renal solute load if formula is not diluted properly. The amount of fluoride in breast milk is not influenced by the mother's diet. Fluoride supplements may be given starting at 6 months of age to improve dental health.

Enzymes

Breast milk contains enzymes that aid in digestion. Pancreatic amylase, necessary to digest carbohydrates, is low in the newborn but present in breast milk. Breast milk also contains lipase to increase fat digestion.

Check Your Reading

1. Why do some newborns lose weight after birth?
2. What are the differences among colostrum, transitional milk, and mature breast milk?
3. How does breast milk compare with commercial formulas?

Infection-Preventing Components

Other factors present in human milk help prevent infection in the newborn. Bifidus factor promotes the growth of *Lactobacillus bifidus,* an important part of the intestinal flora that helps produce an acid environment in the gastrointestinal tract. This protects the infant against infection from common intestinal pathogens.

Leukocytes present in breast milk also help protect against infection. Macrophages are most abundant and secrete lysozyme and lactoferrin. Lysozyme is a bacteriolytic enzyme that acts against gram-positive and enteric bacteria. Lactoferrin is a protein that binds iron in iron-dependent bacteria, such as *Staphylococcus* and *Escherichia coli,* preventing their growth. It also acts against *Candida albicans.* Giving infants supplementary iron may interfere with the effectiveness of lactoferrin.

Immunoglobulins are present in highest amounts in colostrum but also present throughout lactation. Higher levels occur when the infant is born prematurely. Lymphocytes in the milk produce secretory IgA, which helps prevent viral or bacterial invasion of the intestinal mucosa, resulting in fewer intestinal infections in breastfed than in formula-fed infants. This protection is especially important because the infant does not produce adequate amounts of IgA in the intestinal tract until 6 to 12 weeks of age.

Infants who are breastfed may receive long-term protection against respiratory infections. Breastfeeding prevents absorption of foreign molecules that might precipitate development of allergies and is especially important for infants at high risk for allergic conditions such as eczema and asthma. During breastfeeding, the eustachian tubes remain closed, helping prevent ear infections. The eustachian tubes do not close during bottle feeding, and fluids may enter during feedings (Lawrence & Lawrence, 1999).

Effect of Maternal Diet

Although the fatty acid content of breast milk is influenced by the mother's diet, malnourished mothers have about the same proportions of protein, carbohydrates, and most minerals as those who are well nourished. Levels of vitamins in breast milk are affected by the mother's intake and stores, however. Breastfeeding women must eat a well-balanced diet to maintain their own health and energy levels (see Chapter 9, p. 207).

Formulas

Commercial formulas are produced to replace or supplement breast milk. Manufacturers adapt cow's milk to correspond with the components in breast milk as much as possible, although an exact match is not possible. A variety of formulas that differ in price and ingredients are available.

Cow's Milk

Unmodified cow's milk is not recommended for infants under 12 months of age. Modified cow's milk is the source of approximately 80% of commercial formulas. Manufacturers specifically formulate it for infants by reducing protein to decrease renal solute load. Saturated fat is removed and replaced with vegetable fats. Vitamins and other nutrients are added to simulate the contents of breast milk. Examples of formulas are Enfamil and Similac. Formulas with added iron are recommended by the American Academy of Pediatrics (AAP) for all formula-fed infants (AAP, 1999).

Soy and Protein Hydrolysate Formulas

Soy formulas may be given to infants with galactosemia or lactase deficiency or whose families are vegetarian. Soy milk is derived from the protein of soybeans and supplemented with amino acids. Examples of soy formulas are ProSobee and Isomil.

Because infants who are allergic to cow's milk also may be allergic to soy formulas, they are given casein-based protein hydrolysate formulas. The protein in these modified cow's milk formulas is treated to make them hypoallergenic. The formulas also are used for infants with fat malabsorption. Free amino acid–based formulas also are available for allergic infants.

Special Formulas

Some formulas are designed to meet the needs of infants with special problems. The preterm infant may require a more concentrated formula with more calories in less liquid, such as Enfamil Premature and Similac Special Care. Specific nutrients are added for the preterm infant's higher requirements in a more easily digestible form. Human milk fortifiers, such as Similac Natural Care, can be added to human milk to adapt it to the needs of preterm infants. Formulas such as Pregestimil are produced for infants with gastrointestinal problems. LactoFree formula is modified for infants who do not tolerate lactose. Lofenalac is low in the amino acid phenylalanine and given to infants with phenylketonuria (PKU), who are deficient in the enzyme to digest phenylalanine found in standard formulas.

CONSIDERATIONS IN CHOOSING A FEEDING METHOD

Many women decide on a feeding method well before birth. Some may not have questions about which method is best for them until late in their pregnancies. Nurses can help mothers decide on a method and gain confidence in feeding their infants. In fact, being advised during the prenatal period to breastfeed was the most important predictor of whether Mexican-American and non-Hispanic white women in one study breastfed their newborns (Balcazar, et al., 1995).

Although many woman who receive Women, Infants, and Children (WIC) assistance do not choose to breastfeed, those who receive breastfeeding advice and support from WIC staff are more likely to choose that method of feeding their infants. Breastfeeding rates for WIC participants have shown good increases in recent years because of increased WIC emphasis on breastfeeding education (Bocar & Riordan, 1999).

Nurses must be sensitive to mothers' feelings about feeding. Although nurses should encourage breastfeeding as the best method of feeding in most circumstances, they should be supportive of the mother's final decision. The early days of parenting are a very vulnerable time for new mothers, who may feel that their feeding abilities reflect their mothering abilities. The

Table 22-1
BENEFITS OF BREASTFEEDING

For the Infant	For the Mother
Breast milk does not cause allergic reactions or expose the infant to allergens. Immunologic properties help prevent infections. Infant may have fewer respiratory, ear, and gastrointestinal infections and less risk for hospitalization. Breast milk is species specific: its composition meets infant's specific nutritional needs. Nutritional and immunologic properties change according to infant's needs. Breast milk is easily digested, with nutrients that are well absorbed. Protein, fat, and carbohydrate occur in most suitable proportions. No possibility exists of improper (and potentially dangerous) dilution. Breast milk is unlikely to be contaminated, decreases growth of bacteria so that it can be unrefrigerated longer than formula, and is not affected by water supply. Breast milk is less likely to result in overfeeding. The infant is unlikely to have constipation.	Oxytocin release enhances involution of uterus. She is more likely to rest while feeding. She is likely to eat a balanced diet that improves healing. Breastfeeding may help with postpartum weight loss. Frequent, skin-to-skin contact may enhance bonding. Breastfeeding is convenient: it is always available, does not require preparation of bottles, does not require buying and heating of formula. Breastfeeding is economical: it eliminates cost of formula and bottles and time spent in preparation. It makes traveling easier: there are no bottles to prepare, carry, refrigerate, and warm. Breastfeeding reduces the risk for premenopausal breast cancer.

nurse's teaching and encouragement about the chosen feeding method are essential.

Breastfeeding

Breastfeeding offers many advantages (Table 22-1). Although breastfeeding was once the major method of feeding, the availability of refrigeration, commercial formulas, and the increased incidence of maternal employment have led many mothers to choose formula feeding.

It has been increasingly recognized, however, that formula feeding can never fully equal breastfeeding in terms of providing for the infant's optimal growth and development. Both the American Academy of Pediatrics (AAP) and the U.S. Surgeon General recommend breastfeeding. The AAP recommends that infants receive only breastmilk for the first 6 months after birth and that breastfeeding continue after the addition of solid foods until the infant is at least 12 months of age (AAP, 1997).

A goal set by the U.S. Department of Health and Human Services (USDHHS) for the year 2010 is for 75% of all new mothers to breastfeed at the time of birth facility discharge, at least 50% to be breastfeeding at 6 months, and 25% at 1 year. This is based on the 1998 figures of 64% of mothers breastfeeding at discharge from the birth facility, 29% still breastfeeding at 6 months, and 16% at 1 year (USDHHS, 2000).

Breastfeeding has increased in recent years. Between 1990 and 1998, the breastfeeding rate during the hospital stay increased 21%. The number of mothers breastfeeding at 3 and 6 months after birth also has increased. This increase has been greatest in mothers who are younger, African American, enrolled in the WIC program, and employed full time. These groups traditionally have had lower breastfeeding rates (Ross Products Division, 1999).

In an effort to promote breastfeeding, the United Nations Children's Fund (UNICEF) and the World Health Organization (WHO) advocate that birth facilities become certified as baby-friendly hospitals with policies to actively encourage breastfeeding. Guidelines to becoming certified as a baby-friendly hospital emphasize education of staff and parents about breastfeeding, early initiation of breastfeeding, demand feedings, avoidance of formula and pacifiers, and rooming in.

Formula Feeding

Mothers choose formula feeding for many reasons. Some mothers are embarrassed by breastfeeding, seeing the breast only in a sexual context. Many mothers have few relatives or friends who have had positive breastfeeding experiences. Some women feel a need to maintain a strict feeding schedule and are uneasy not knowing exactly how much milk the infant will take at each feeding. Occasionally, a woman must use formula because she must take medications that might harm the infant. A frequent reason that mothers choose formula feeding instead of breastfeeding may be a lack of adequate knowledge about the two methods.

Combination Feeding

Some parents prefer a combination of breastfeeding and bottle feeding. This combination is best delayed until lactation has been well established at 3 to 4 weeks of age, if possible. Either breast milk or formula may be given in the bottle. The mother may give a bottle each day or only occasionally, such as when a baby sitter is with the infant. This allows the mother to be away from the infant for longer periods of time, yet allows the closeness with the infant that many mothers enjoy and the physical advantages of breastfeeding to continue.

Factors Influencing Choice

Many factors influence a woman's choice of feeding method. These factors must be considered when educating women about their choices.

Culture

Cultural influences may dictate decisions about the way a mother feeds her infant. For example, many Mormon women believe that breastfeeding is an important part of motherhood. Muslim women often breastfeed for the first 2 years. Immigrants from countries where breastfeeding is the norm may breastfeed for shorter durations or not at all because they lack the support system they had in their own countries. In addition, formula feeding may be seen as a symbol of the new way of life and considered a way to help infants grow larger and be stronger. Nurses should be particularly watchful for ways to help mothers from other cultures who might wish to breastfeed but fail to do so because of lack of support.

In some Asian and Latino cultures, mothers give their infants formula while in the birth facility and do not begin to breastfeed until at home. This may be caused by modesty and embarrassment about nursing in front of others in the birth facility and lack of understanding about the value of colostrum. Some believe that breastfeeding before the milk comes in may drain heat and fluids from the mother (Mattson, 1995).

Women in some cultures believe that colostrum is "spoiled" because it has been in the breasts for a long time. Guatemalan women do not begin nursing until the third day because they believe the colostrum is bad for the baby (Callister, 1997). Women with these beliefs may manually express colostrum and discard it before they begin to breastfeed the infant. Some Indian mothers do not breastfeed the infant until the fifth or sixth day because they believe the milk may have "pus" in it. Instead, they give the infant special foods that include honey, sugar water, or *ghee,* made of clarified butter (Choudhry, 1997). This conflicts with beliefs in the United States, where honey is avoided in infants because it may cause botulism.

Some mothers may be amenable to nursing the infant with help while in the birth facility, especially if the antibody and laxative properties of colostrum are explained. Breastfeeding involves a learning process for both mother and infant, which is best started where assistance is available. Nurses can help women learn by offering to help them "practice" breastfeeding at least a few times before discharge. This helps build the woman's confidence and allows for early identification and correction of problems. If the mother is firm in her desire to wait until discharge to begin breastfeeding, nurses can support her by teaching her what she will need to know when she goes home. Cultural values about feeding, as in other areas of health care, must be respected.

The woman's culture also may influence the way she deals with common lactation problems. For example, the Sabbath-observing Jewish woman may follow special prohibitions to relieve engorgement that occurs on the Sabbath. Instead of using an electric breast pump, she may prefer to use hand expression or a manual breast pump. Less than 17 ml of breast milk will be removed at a time and then discarded. This quantity is considered equal to the volume of one third of an egg and less than the amount considered a violation of the Sabbath law. If heat or cold are used, a hot water bag or bag of ice or frozen vegetables may be used instead of hot or cold compresses. Cabbage leaves also are permitted to help her relieve breast engorgement (Chertok, 1999).

Employment

The need to return to employment soon after birth may cause concern about feeding methods. The mother may choose to use a combination of breastfeeding and bottle feeding with either stored breast milk or formula, plan a short period of breastfeeding before weaning the infant to formula, or use formula from the beginning. Nurses provide information about options, breastfeeding and working, use of breast pumps (see p. 597), and storage of breast milk. Pamphlets and books for the working breastfeeding mother are particularly helpful.

Support from Others

Family members and friends also may share in the decision-making process. The woman's own mother and the baby's father often are most important in helping her make a decision. The mother with little support or active discouragement from her family probably will have a difficult time nursing. Involvement of the father in feedings is important in some families and may be thought possible only if he can give a bottle regularly. Nurses can suggest other ways that fathers can participate in infant care, such as holding and rocking infants. Educating family members about the advantages of breastfeeding and ways to deal with problems may lead to their encouragement of the breastfeeding mother.

The support the mother receives from the nursing staff plays a significant part in whether she feels comfortable with her choice of feeding method. The woman who does not feel confident in her ability to breastfeed before she leaves the birth facility is less likely to continue breastfeeding if she encounters difficulties at home.

Other Factors

Other factors also may influence a woman's decision. Her knowledge and past experience with infant feeding are important. Very young mothers are less likely to breastfeed. Breastfeeding rates are highest in mothers over age 35 and those who have a college education. White mothers breastfeed more often than black and Latino women. Although African-American women still have the lowest rates of breastfeeding, they have shown a greater increase in breastfeeding than other groups in recent years (USDHHS, 2000).

The time when the decision is made is also important. Many mothers choose their feeding methods before pregnancy and the majority do so by the end of pregnancy. Those who have made the decision early are more likely to continue breastfeeding for a longer period (Biancuzzo, 1999).

Check Your Reading

4. What factors does breast milk contain that help prevent infection?
5. What types of commercial formulas are available?
6. What factors influence a woman's choice of feeding method?

NORMAL BREASTFEEDING

To be most helpful to lactating mothers, the nurse must have a good understanding of the physiology of lactation. The anatomy and physiology of the breast are discussed in Chapter 4 (p. 69), and breast changes occurring in pregnancy are discussed in full in Chapter 7 (p. 122) (see Figures 4-8 and 7-3).

Breast Changes during Pregnancy

Breast changes begin early in pregnancy with development of the ducts, lobules, and alveoli in response to the hormones estrogen, progesterone, placental lactogen, prolactin, and chorionic gonadotropin. The breasts begin to secrete colostrum by the second trimester, and women who give birth after the 16th week of gestation produce colostrum (Lawrence & Lawrence, 1999). During pregnancy, the anterior pituitary secretes high levels of prolactin, the hormone that causes the breasts to produce milk. However, milk production is prevented by estrogen, progesterone, and placental lactogen, which inhibit breast response to prolactin.

Milk Production

Milk is produced in the alveoli of the breasts through a complex process by which materials from the mother's blood stream are reformulated into breast milk. Thus amino acids, glucose, lipids, enzymes, leukocytes, and other materials are used to manufacture the nutrients needed by the infant. Most milk is synthesized when the infant is suckling (Lawrence & Lawrence, 1999).

The milk is ejected from the secretory cells of the alveoli into the alveolar lumen by contraction of the myoepithelial cells. From there, it travels into the lactiferous ducts, which lead from the alveoli to the nipple. The ducts widen in the area of the areola to become the lactiferous sinuses (ampullae), which the infant compresses during nursing to eject a stream of milk through pores in the nipple.

Hormonal Changes at Birth

Prolactin

At birth, loss of progesterone, estrogen, and placental lactogen from the placenta results in increasing levels and effectiveness of prolactin and brings about milk production. The tactile stimulation of suckling and the removal of colostrum or milk causes continued increased levels of prolactin.

Oxytocin

Oxytocin from the posterior pituitary increases in response to nipple stimulation. Oxytocin causes the milk-ejection reflex, commonly known as the *let-down reflex*. The resulting contraction of myoepithelial cells around the alveoli releases milk into the ducts, making it available to the infant.

When mothers see, hear, or think about their infants, they often have an increase in oxytocin level, bringing about a let-down of milk. Pain or lack of relaxation can inhibit oxytocin release. Oxytocin also is responsible for the uterine contractions mothers may feel at the beginning of nursing sessions. These contractions are beneficial because they hasten involution of the uterus (Figure 22-1).

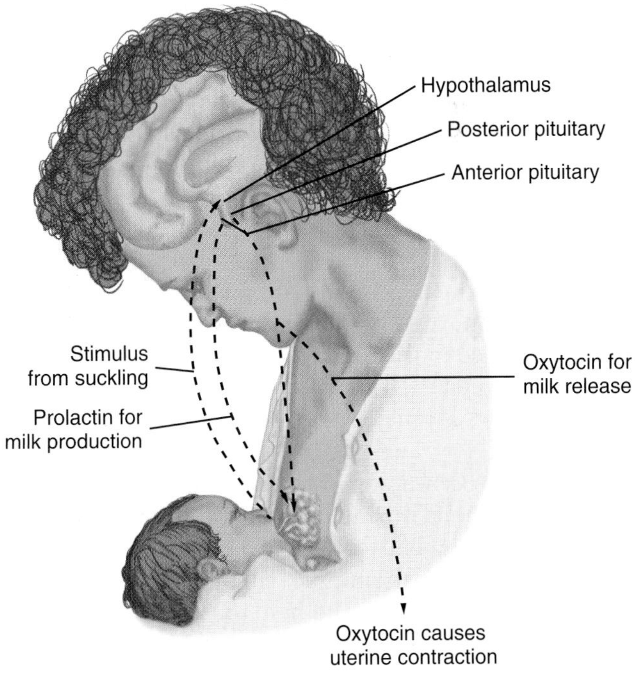

FIGURE 22-1 Effect of prolactin and oxytocin on milk production. When the infant begins to suckle at the breast, nerve impulses travel to the hypothalamus, which causes the anterior pituitary to secrete prolactin to increase milk production. Suckling also causes the posterior pituitary to secrete oxytocin, producing the let-down reflex, which releases milk from the breast. Oxytocin also causes the uterus to contract, which aids in involution.

Continued Milk Production

The amount of milk produced depends primarily on adequate stimulation of the breast and removal of the milk by suckling or a breast pump, which causes production of prolactin. This "supply and demand" effect continues throughout lactation. That is, increased demand with more frequent and longer nursing results in more milk available for the infant.

If milk (or colostrum) is not removed from the breasts, the alveoli become very distended. Pressure on the blood vessels reduces blood flow and prevents prolactin from reaching the secretory cells. Lack of nipple stimulation causes release of prolactin inhibiting factor by the hypothalamus, and milk production gradually ceases. The milk in the ducts is absorbed, the alveoli become smaller, and the cells return to a resting state.

Preparation of Breasts for Breastfeeding

Little preparation is needed during pregnancy for breastfeeding. The mother should avoid soap on her nipples to prevent removal of the natural protective oils from the Montgomery tubercles of the breasts. The use of creams, nipple rolling, pulling, and rubbing to "toughen" nipples does not necessarily decrease nipple pain after birth and may cause irritation or uterine contractions from release of oxytocin. In addition, some women feel that extensive nipple preparation is too much trouble or distasteful and may decide not to breastfeed if they believe that this preparation is necessary.

The breasts should be assessed during pregnancy to identify flat or inverted nipples (Figure 22-2). Normally, the nipples protrude. Flat nipples appear soft, like the areola, and do not stand erect unless stimulated by rolling them between the fingers. Nipples also may be inverted, or drawn into the breast tissue. Both conditions make drawing the nipples into the mouth difficult for infants. Some nipples appear normal but draw inward when the areola is compressed in the infant's mouth. Compressing the areola between the thumb and forefinger determines whether the nipple projects normally or becomes inverted.

Women with flat or inverted nipples sometimes use breast shells during the last weeks of pregnancy and after birth. The shells are worn in the bra with the opening over the nipple. They exert slight pressure against the areola and help the nipples protrude. Pumping the breasts for a few minutes before beginning nursing also helps bring the nipples out. Exercises for inverted nipples that involve stretching or manipulation of the nipple or areola (Hoffman technique) are not recommended during pregnancy because they are not effective and may cause uterine contractions.

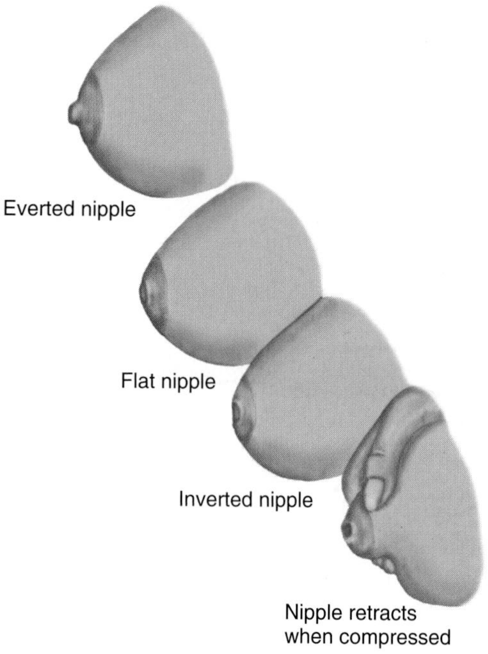

FIGURE 22-2 Normal everted nipple and other types of nipples that may cause the infant difficulty in latching-on. Nipples shown after stimulation.

Check Your Reading

7. What is the effect of suckling on the let-down reflex and milk production?
8. What preparation of the breasts is needed during pregnancy?

APPLICATION OF THE NURSING PROCESS: BREASTFEEDING

Assessment

Assess both the mother and the infant during the breastfeeding process. Various scoring tools have been developed to assess breastfeeding, but none is completely satisfactory. One method used is the LATCH breastfeeding assessment tool (Table 22-2).

Maternal Assessment

Assess the condition of the breasts and nipples and the mother's knowledge about breastfeeding to determine her needs for assistance.

Breasts and Nipples. Examine the breasts and nipples during pregnancy so that problems that might interfere with feeding can be corrected. If this assessment did not occur before birth, examine the breasts and nipples before the initial feeding. Assess the protrusion of the nipples to identify flat or inverted nipples.

Table 22-2
THE LATCH SCORING TOOL

	0	1	2
L Latch	Infant too sleepy or reluctant No sustained latch achieved	Repeated attempts and is able to sustain latch and suck Must hold nipple in infant's mouth Must stimulate infant to suck	Grasps breast Tongue down Lips flanged Rhythmic sucking
A Audible swallowing	None	A few with stimulation	Spontaneous and intermittent < 24 hr old Spontaneous and frequent > 24 hr old
T Type of nipple	Inverted	Flat	Everted (after stimulation)
C Comfort (breast/nipple)	Engorged Cracked, bleeding, large blisters, or bruises Severe discomfort	Filling Reddened or small blisters or bruises Mild to moderate discomfort	Soft Nontender
H Hold (positioning)	Full assist (staff holds infant at breast)	Minimal assist (e.g., elevate head of bed; place pillows for support) Teach one side; mother does other Staff holds and then mother takes over	No assist from staff Mother able to position or hold infant

The nurse can use the LATCH scoring system to assess and document need for assistance with breastfeeding. Each assessment area is scored 0 to 2. Modified from Jensen, D., Wallace, S., & Kelsay, P. (1994). LATCH: A breastfeeding charting system and documentation tool. *Journal of Obstetric, Gynecologic, and Neonatal Nursing,* 23(1), 27-32.

Ongoing assessments include identification of breast fullness and breast engorgement. Fullness is the swelling of the breasts that may occur early in lactation as a result of increased blood and lymph circulation. It may progress to engorgement if feedings are delayed, too short, or not frequent enough. Palpate the breasts to see if they are soft, filling, or engorged. Soft breasts feel like a cheek. If milk is beginning to come in, the breasts may be slightly firmer, which is charted as "filling." Engorged breasts are hard and tender, with taut, shiny skin. Note any redness, tenderness, and lumps within the breasts.

Assess the nipples, which may be red, bruised, blistered, fissured, or bleeding. Ask about nipple tenderness and when it occurs. Evaluate breastfeeding techniques of the mother having problems with her nipples.

Knowledge. The mother who is breastfeeding for the first time may have many questions and need substantial guidance during her first attempts. The mother who has nursed before may have more knowledge but have questions or be unaware of current information that was unavailable when she breastfed her last infant.

Infant Feeding Behaviors

Before initiating a breastfeeding session, assess an infant's readiness for feeding. The infant should be awake and hungry. Trying to feed an infant in a deep sleep period is frustrating to both mother and infant. Sucking on the hands, rooting when the cheek or side of the mouth is touched, smacking of the lips, and slight fussiness are signs that an infant is ready for feeding. Feeding should begin before crying, which is a late sign of hunger.

Analysis

Women with and without experience often need information to successfully breastfeed. Therefore a common nursing diagnosis for the breastfeeding mother is "Risk for Ineffective Breast-feeding related to lack of understanding of breastfeeding techniques."

Planning

Goals/expected outcomes for this nursing diagnosis are:

- The infant will breastfeed using nutritive suckling for a total average of 15 minutes/feeding before discharge.

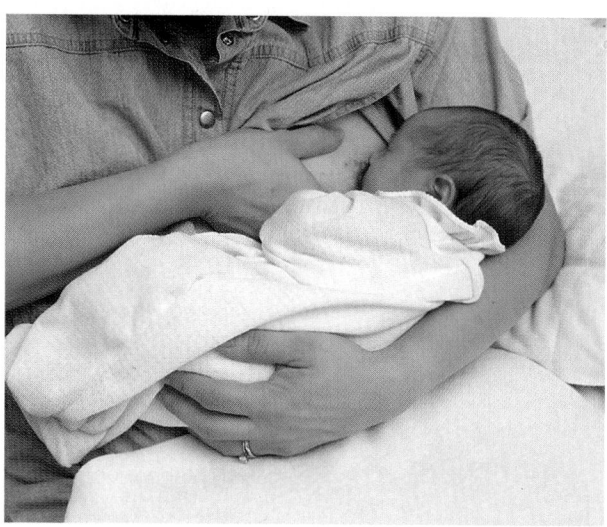

FIGURE 22-3 For the cradle hold, the mother positions the infant's head at or near the antecubital space and level with her nipple with her arm supporting the infant's body. Her other hand is free to hold the breast. Once the infant is positioned, pillows or blankets can be used to support the mother's arm, which may tire from holding the baby.

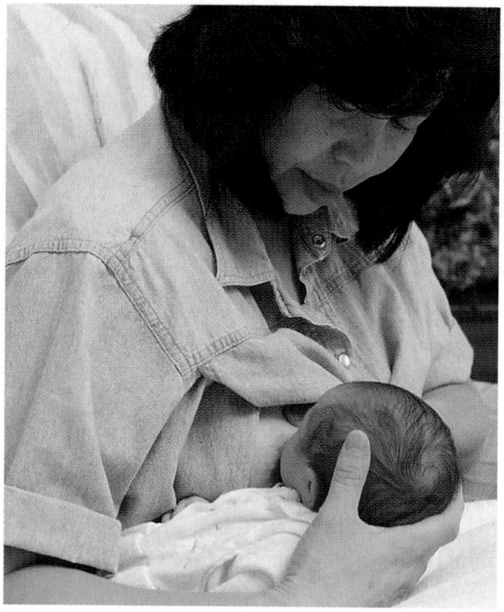

FIGURE 22-4 For the football hold, the mother supports the infant's head in her hand, with the infant's body resting on pillows alongside her hip. This method allows the mother to see the position of the infant's mouth on the breast, helps her control the infant's head, and is especially helpful for mothers with heavy breasts. This hold also avoids pressure against an abdominal incision.

- The mother will demonstrate breastfeeding techniques (such as positioning) as taught before discharge.
- The mother will verbalize satisfaction and confidence with the breastfeeding process before discharge.

Interventions

Inexperienced mothers may need detailed teaching. Experienced mothers often need only a review or clarification about techniques they have used previously. Interventions used for the first feeding session are summarized in "Keys to Clinical Practice: Assisting the Inexperienced Breastfeeding Mother" (see Appendix D, p. 985).

Assisting with the First Feeding

The first feeding should take place within the first hour after birth if both mother and infant are stable. At this time, infants are in an alert state and many begin to nurse at once. Others may nuzzle, lick, or suck intermittently at the breast, all of which stimulate production of prolactin necessary for lactation. Feeding at this time also helps establish early bonding. The mother may be very gratified to see her infant nurse right after birth.

Help the mother move to her side or into Fowler's position. Show her the way to hold the breast and explain proper positioning of the infant. This is a short session, and teaching should be repeated at the next feeding for reinforcement. Observe the infant's response to the feeding and watch for signs such as cyanosis or choking, which may indicate the presence of problems.

Teaching Feeding Techniques

Position of the Mother and Infant

Both the mother and the infant must be positioned properly for optimal breastfeeding. Make the mother as comfortable as possible before she begins to nurse. Pain or an awkward position may interfere with the let-down reflex and cause her to tire. Prevent interruptions and provide privacy so that she can concentrate on learning techniques.

The cradle and football holds and side-lying position are most commonly used (Figures 22-3 to 22-5). The cross-cradle hold is helpful for the very small infant. The infant's head is held in the hand opposite the breast used for feeding, with the mother's arm supporting the infant's body across her lap. The other hand holds the breast. This position provides more support for a small infant and allows the mother to see the infant's mouth on the breast.

Use pillows behind the mother's back to protect an abdominal incision or support her arms. Arrange folded blankets or pillows to elevate the infant to and prevent pulling and tension on the nipple, which would cause it to become sore. The infant's head and body should directly face the breast with the nose and chin lightly touching the breast. If the infant must turn the head to reach the breast, swallowing is difficult. The neck should be flexed because hyperextension also makes

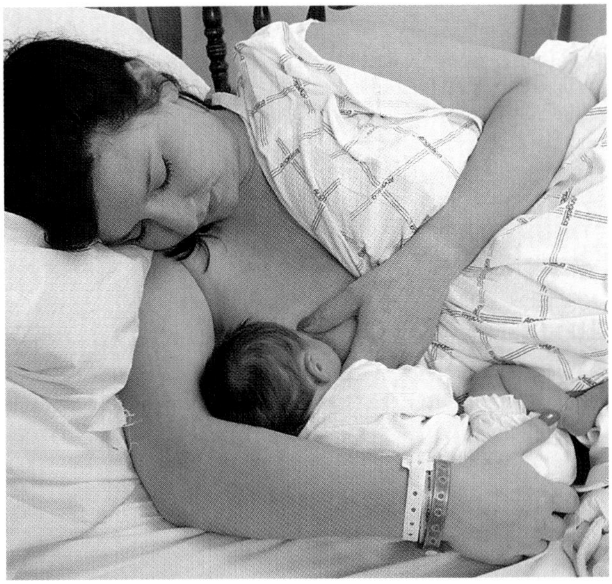

FIGURE 22-5 The side-lying position avoids pressure on episiotomy or abdominal incisions and allows the mother to rest while feeding. She lies on her side, with her lower arm supporting her head or placed around the infant. A pillow behind her back and between her legs provides comfort. Her upper hand and arm are used to position the infant on his or her side at nipple level and hold the breast. When the infant's mouth opens to nurse, the mother leans slightly forward or draws the infant to her to insert the nipple into the mouth.

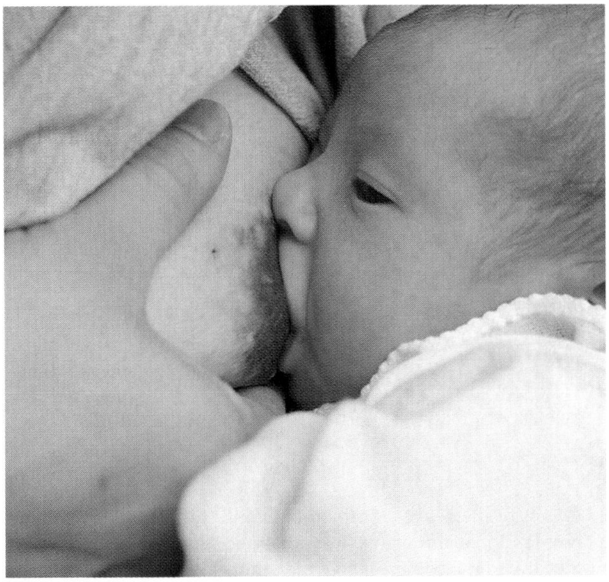

FIGURE 22-6 C position of hand on breast. The hand is positioned so that the thumb is on top of the breast while the fingers support the breast from below. Note the flaring of the infant's lips.

swallowing difficult. The infant's body should be aligned so that the ear, shoulder, and hips are on a straight line.

Position of the Mother's Hands

The mother may choose to use the palmar, or C hand position, or the "scissors," or V position. In the palmar position, the mother holds her breast with her thumb on top and the fingers against the chest wall and supporting the underside of the breast (Figure 22-6). This position often is preferred. Her fingers should be behind the areola and her thumb should not press on the breast enough to make the nipple tip upward, or the infant will suck improperly and the nipple may become sore.

In the "scissors hold" the woman uses her forefinger and middle finger to support the breast. She must be careful to place her fingers well back on the breast so that her fingers do not slip down the wet areola and interfere with the placement of the infant's mouth. The mother should support her breast in place if its weight makes it difficult for the infant to hold it in the mouth for the first few weeks. As the infant becomes more adept at breastfeeding, the mother will not need to hold the breast.

Although mothers worry about the infant's ability to breathe while nursing, indenting the breast tissue near the infant's nostrils is unnecessary. This might cause improper positioning of the nipple in the infant's mouth, interfere with the grasp of the nipple, or interfere with milk flow. Unless the mother's breasts are very heavy and the infant's nose is buried in the breast, breathing is not occluded. Lifting the infant's hips to a slightly more horizontal position or bringing them closer to the mother is usually sufficient if there appears to be a problem.

Latch-On Techniques

Teach the mother techniques to help the infant latch on to the breast. The infant should be awake and hungry. Talking and cuddling can help a sleepy infant awaken and calm an upset infant.

Eliciting Latch-On. After positioning the infant to face the breast, the mother holds her breast so that the nipple brushes against the center of the infant's lower lip. A hungry infant usually opens the mouth as soon as anything comes near it, but some need up to 1 minute of stroking the area around the mouth. The breast should not be inserted until the infant's mouth is opened wide, or the infant will compress the end of the nipple, causing pain and trauma and little milk flow. When the mouth opens wide with the tongue down and forward over the gum, the mother should quickly bring the infant close to her so that the infant can latch on to the areola. Suggesting to the mother that the infant's latch-on is like eating a very large sandwich may help her understand the need to wait until the infant's mouth is open wide (Wiessinger, 1999).

Position of the Mouth. Assess the position of the infant's mouth on the breast (Figure 22-7). As much of the areola as possible should be in the infant's mouth to allow the nipple to be drawn toward the back of the mouth. This prevents the infant from sucking on the

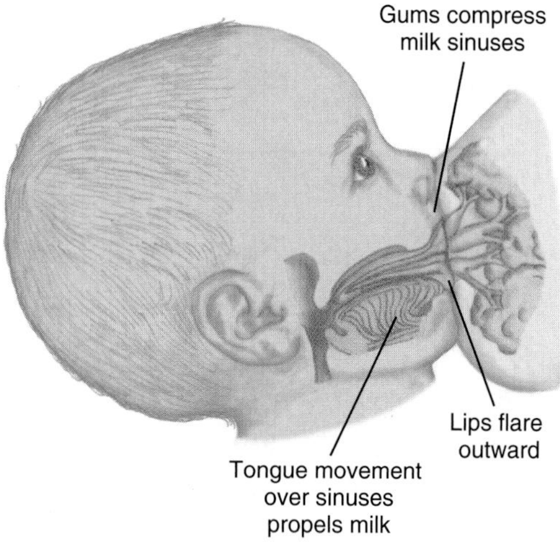
Gums compress milk sinuses
Lips flare outward
Tongue movement over sinuses propels milk

FIGURE 22-7 Position of infant's mouth while suckling. When the nipple and areola are properly positioned in the infant's mouth, the gums compress the milk sinuses behind the areola. The tongue is between the lower gum and breast. The tongue moves over the sinuses like a peristaltic wave to bring the milk forward into the infant's mouth. The infant's lips are flared outward.

nipple only, which leads to sore nipples and insufficient milk production. The infant's lips should be about 1 to 1.5 inches from the nipple base (Lawrence & Lawrence, 1999). This positions the gums over the milk sinuses behind the areola and causes milk to be released into the infant's mouth when the gums compress them.

Assess the position of the infant's tongue by gently pulling down on the lower lip. The tongue should be under the breast and over the top of the lower gums. The lips should be flared outward. Be sure that the lower lip is not turned in, which may result in a friction burn on the lower nipple.

Suckling Pattern

Observe the infant's suckling pattern. During nutritive suckling, the infant sucks with smooth, continuous movements with only occasional pauses to rest. Each suck may be followed by a swallow, or two or three sucks may occur before the swallow. Nonnutritive sucking often occurs when the infant is falling asleep. If a fluttery or choppy motion of the jaw not accompanied by the sound of swallowing occurs, the mother should remove the infant from the breast because her nipples may become sore. If she thinks that the infant should feed longer, she can try burping and waking the infant before resuming the feeding.

Explain the milk-ejection reflex to the mother. Many mothers learn to recognize a feeling of tingling in the nipples as the let-down occurs. The reflex occurs several times throughout the feeding. She sees the infant begin to swallow more rapidly each time a new let-down brings more rapid expulsion of milk.

> Mothers often wonder whether their infants are actually receiving milk from the breast. Call their attention to the sound of swallowing when it occurs. A soft "ka" or "ah" sound indicates the infant is swallowing colostrum or milk. The infant may suck several times before obtaining enough milk to swallow at first. Later, the infant swallows several times in succession when the milk-ejection reflex occurs and then does not swallow until another let-down of milk occurs.

Short pauses are normal during nursing. Caution mothers not to jiggle the breast in the infant's mouth in an effort to start the suckling again. This may cause the infant to lose the grasp on the nipple and areola, resulting in "chewing" on the nipple and soreness. If necessary, mothers should take their infants off the breast to awaken them, then start again.

Removal from the Breast

Teach the mother to remove the infant from the breast for burping midway in the feeding and whenever suckling becomes nonnutritive. Show her how to avoid trauma to the breast by inserting her finger into the corner of the infant's mouth between the gums to break suction. She then should remove the breast quickly before the infant begins to suck again. Another method is to indent the breast tissue with a finger near the infant's mouth and remove the infant when suction is released.

Frequency of Feedings

Because breast milk moves through the stomach within 1.5 to 2 hours, infants usually feed every 2 to 3 hours. Frequent feedings are especially important in the early days after birth, while lactation is being established and stomach capacity is small. Explaining that the hormone prolactin, which is responsible for milk production, is released in increased amounts while the infant is suckling helps the mother understand the relationship of frequent feeding to milk supply.

Infants who are fed frequently during the daytime often sleep longer during the night. During the early weeks of life, however, the infant usually should not be allowed to sleep beyond 4 to 5 hours at a time. Long periods between feedings increase the likelihood of breast engorgement. The resulting decreased stimulation of prolactin may reduce milk supply. Generally, the mother should nurse 8 to 12 times in each 24-hour period.

At times, some infants vary the length of feedings and time between each feeding. Several feedings close together (sometimes called "cluster feedings") may be followed by a longer interval between feedings. Strict scheduling of infant feedings is unnecessary and leads to frustration for both mother and infant. A mother should take her cues from her infant.

Length of Feedings

Although early feedings were once limited to only a few minutes per breast in an attempt to prevent sore nipples, improper positioning, rather than time at breast, is the usual cause of nipple trauma. When feedings are too short, the infant may receive little or no colostrum or milk. It may take as long as 5 minutes for the milk-ejection (let-down) reflex to occur during the early days after birth.

Generally, mothers can allow the infant to set the length of feedings. The infant should suckle vigorously for a period of time. When choppy, non-nutritive suckling without the sound of swallowing occurs, the mother should burp the infant and complete the feeding at the other breast. When the infant is satisfied, the suckling pattern changes and the infant may fall asleep.

Mothers who are uneasy without a specific length of time for feedings can be instructed to start with feedings lasting approximately 10 minutes on the first side, or longer if the infant continues to nurse vigorously. The feeding should continue on the second breast until the infant falls asleep or begins non-nutritive suckling, generally about 10 to 15 minutes.

Although variations in the length of feedings occur, feedings that last less than a total of 15 minutes may not be enough (Auerbach & Riordan, 1999). Feeding time increases as needed by the infant over the next few days. Teach the mother that longer feedings do not cause nipple tenderness.

Discuss the differences between foremilk, the watery first milk that quenches the infant's thirst, and hindmilk, which is richer in fat, more satisfying, and leads to weight gain. Feeding for too short a time prevents the infant from getting the hindmilk and decreases weight gain.

Switching back and forth between breasts several times during a feeding increases the amount of foremilk the infant receives but decreases the amount of hindmilk. Therefore the mother should continue feeding on the first side as long as the infant nurses vigorously before burping and continuing on the other breast.

Preventing Problems

Women who intend to breastfeed but encounter difficulties that cause them to switch to formula feeding may express guilt and disappointment for months after the experience (Mozingo, et al., 2000). Nurses can help prevent early problems in several ways.

Teaching. Once women leave the birth facility, they often have no one to advise them about breastfeeding. Help prevent problems by intensive teaching during the short birth facility stay. One study showed that mothers who received education about breastfeeding during the hospital stay were significantly more likely to still be breastfeeding at the end of the sixth month. Teaching both fathers and mothers was found to be very important (Susin, et al., 1999).

Include suggestions on how to improve positioning and techniques and common problems and solutions. Allow ample time to answer questions. Some facilities hold classes for groups of women during the birth facility stay. If the birth facility provides follow-up telephone calls or home visits, explain the service.

Give the mother breastfeeding pamphlets, and review them with her before discharge. Breastfeeding videos provide another means of providing education. Before using pamphlets or videos, review them to be sure that the information is correct and they contain no advertisements for formula.

Formula Gift Packs. Many nurses believe that breastfeeding women who receive formula gift packs at discharge are more likely to supplement with formula feedings because the gift packs may imply an expectation that nursing mothers will need formula. Using supplements may reduce milk supply and, for some women, lead to earlier weaning from the breast. Other nurses believe that gift packs have little effect on breastfeeding and attention should be focused on providing support and education to enhance lactation success (James, et al., 1999). In addition to formula samples, feeding formula in the hospital has been shown to be associated with shorter breastfeeding duration (Chezem, et al., 1998).

Insufficient Milk Supply. One of the major reasons mothers give for early weaning to formula is their perception of insufficient milk supply. Common causes of decreased milk supply include formula use, inadequate rest or diet, smoking by the mother or others in the home, and use of caffeine, alcohol, or some medications. Intervene appropriately if any common causes are found. Because the breasts are soft and the mother does not see large amounts of milk, she may believe that none is present. This may lead her to give the infant formula before or after the feeding, decreasing milk production.

To help her determine if the infant is receiving enough milk, assist her in assessing swallowing and nutritive suckling. Although mothers are not usually encouraged to weigh normal infants at home because it focuses too much attention on weight gain, the physician or nurse practitioner assesses weight gain at well-baby check-ups. After the initial weight loss after birth, infants generally gain approximately 15 to 30 g (0.5 to 1 oz) each day during the early months of life. Weight gain generally begins by the fifth day of life.

Mothers also can count the number of wet and soiled diapers to help them determine whether their infants are receiving enough milk. Generally an infant should have at least 6 to 10 wet diapers (after the first 2 days of life) and at least 4 stools a day.

The mother's general health may affect her continuation of breastfeeding. For example, one study shows that women who have hemoglobin levels below 10 g/dl are more likely to feel that they have insufficient milk (Henly, et al., 1995). Therefore advise the woman to take prescribed iron, eat foods high in iron content, and get adequate rest. If the mother needs to increase her

MOTHERS WANT TO KNOW *Is My Baby Getting Enough Milk?*

Your baby is probably getting enough milk if the following occur:

- You hear the baby swallow frequently during feedings. It sounds like a soft "ka" or "ah" sound.
- You see nutritive suckling, a smooth series of sucking and swallowing with occasional rest periods. This is different from short, choppy sucks that occur when the baby is falling asleep and not getting milk. After rest periods, you may feel a tingling of your nipples as a new let-down reflex occurs. This is followed by more nutritive suckling as the infant swallows the increased milk available.
- Your breast is getting softer during the feeding. (However, your breasts do not have to be hard [engorged] for you to have enough milk for the baby.)
- You can see milk in the baby's mouth or dripping from your breast occasionally.
- You feed your baby 8 to 12 times every 24 hours. You produce more milk when you nurse more often. (Keep track, at first, by writing down the time you start each feeding. Once breastfeeding is well established, keeping close track of the time is not necessary—your baby lets you know when it is time for feedings.)
- Your baby has at least 2 to 6 wet diapers a day for the first 2 days after birth and at least 6 to 10 wet diapers a day by the fifth day. Disposable diapers are very absorbent, and knowing whether they are wet is sometimes hard. If you are unsure, place a tissue or cotton ball inside the diaper to show even small amounts of urine. Urine should be light, not dark, yellow in color.
- Your baby passes at least 4 bowel movements daily during the first month and often more. The bowel movements are yellow in color by the end of the first week.
- Your baby seems satisfied after feedings. Babies remain quietly awake or go to sleep for at least an hour after most feedings. (An occasional fussy time is not unusual and does not mean that the baby is not getting enough to eat.)
- Your baby has gained weight at the first well-baby checkup.

milk supply, suggest that she feed more often and use a breast pump after feedings to increase milk production.

Women who continue to have difficulty with any aspect of breastfeeding should be referred to a lactation consultant. These professionals often are available in the birth facility and can help with the mechanics and psychosocial implications of breastfeeding.

Evaluation

Evaluation of interventions should be continued throughout the birth facility stay. Before discharge, the infant should be feeding well at each breast. The woman should demonstrate feeding techniques and voice satisfaction with breastfeeding and confidence in her ability. Satisfaction and confidence are major determinants of whether she continues breastfeeding at home.

Check Your Reading

9. How can the nurse help the mother establish breastfeeding during the initial feeding sessions?
10. What should the nurse teach the mother about frequency and length of feedings?

COMMON BREASTFEEDING CONCERNS

Because mothers may be discharged from the birth facility before problems arise, nurses should teach them ways to prevent and treat common difficulties. If the nurse is being consulted about problems that have developed after discharge, she should determine what the mother has done to solve the problem and ask about any complementary or alternative therapies the mother may have tried (Complementary/Alternative Therapy). The safety of any therapy should be determined.

Problems may be divided into those originating with the infant and those involving the mother.

Complementary/Alternative Therapy

To aid milk production—Acupuncture (especially in mothers under stress); tea from fennel, fenugreek, dill, or aniseed; reflexology; shiatsu

To relieve engorgement—Cabbage leaves, poultices of grated potato or carrot, hot compresses of parsley, reflexology

Sore nipples—Washing the nipples with infusions of marigolds or comfrey, ointments of yarrow, gel from fresh aloe vera leaf (washed off before nursing)

Cautions—Comfrey is recommended by some sources for engorgement and sore nipples but may cause hepatic toxicity and vascular problems (Lawrence & Lawrence, 1999).

(Data from Tiran & Mack, 2000, and Lawrence & Lawrence, 1999.)

Infant Problems

Infant problems generally involve a sleepy infant, suckling, and complications of the infant such as jaundice and prematurity. Crying and fussiness are common problems during the first weeks after birth for all infants (see Chapter 23).

MOTHERS WANT TO KNOW Solutions to Common Breastfeeding Problems

Problem: Infant is sleepy at feeding time or falls asleep shortly after beginning feeding.

Prevention
- Look for signs your baby is ready to wake up, such as movement of the eyes even though the eyelids are closed, small twitches of the face, sucking movements, stretching, and increased movements of the entire body.
- Gently awaken your baby. Talk, gently move the infant's arms and legs, and play with the infant for a short time before beginning the feeding.
- Unwrap the baby's blankets and change the diaper. Swaddling infants by wrapping them tightly with blankets is a calming technique that often helps them sleep. Leave the blanket off as you begin the feeding. Your body and a blanket draped over both of you after your baby begins to nurse will provide adequate warmth.

Solutions

If your baby goes to sleep during the feeding and has fed less than 5 minutes, try the following:

- Rub the baby's hair or cheeks gently, stroke around his or her mouth, or shift the baby's position slightly to see if he or she will wake up.
- Remove the baby from the breast and rub his or her back to bring up bubbles of air that may cause a sensation of stomach fullness. Rubbing the back also stimulates the central nervous system and awakens the baby.
- Express a few drops of colostrum onto the nipple. The baby tastes the colostrum as soon as the nipple is offered and often begins renewed suckling.
- Wash the baby's face with a lukewarm washcloth to help the infant wake up.

If your baby cannot be aroused with a few of the above gentle techniques, a longer sleep period may be needed. Let the infant sleep another half hour, then begin again. Watch for signs that indicate the baby is in a lighter phase of sleep and can be awakened more easily.

Problem: Infant who has taken bottles pushes the nipple out of the mouth and sucks poorly during breastfeeding. Infant has become confused about the way to suck from the breast.

Prevention
- Avoid all bottles and pacifiers unless absolutely necessary. If they are necessary, stop as soon as possible.
- Do not give the baby formula during the night. The extra sleep is not worth the possibility of later feeding difficulties.
- Avoid giving formula at the end of a breastfeeding session because it is unnecessary for healthy newborns. It may cause the infant's stomach to become distended, may result in more "spitting up," and may cause the infant to wait longer before nursing again. This decreases milk production.

Solution
- Stop all bottle feeding and pacifier use so that the baby gets used to suckling from the breast instead of the bottle. Nurse more often to stimulate milk and help the baby learn what to do.

Problem: Infant sucks on the end of the nipple or fails to open his or her mouth widely enough.

Prevention
- Do not insert the breast into the infant's mouth until the infant opens his or her mouth wide with the tongue down and forward.
- Pull down gently on the infant's chin to help the infant open the mouth if necessary.
- Be sure that the baby has the nipple at the back of the mouth and 1 to 1.5 inches of the areola in the mouth.

Solutions
- Stop the feeding and start again if you see dimples in the infant's cheeks or hear "smacking" or clicking sounds. Short, choppy movement of the jaw means that the infant is going to sleep or has finished feeding.
- If you believe that the infant should nurse longer, awaken the infant and begin again.

Problem: Breasts are hard and tender from engorgement.

Prevention
- Breastfeed the infant every 2 to 3 hours day and night. Do not give a bottle during the night, as this increases the risk of engorgement. Waiting even 4 hours between feedings may increase the risk of engorgement, but frequent breastfeeding often can prevent it.

Solutions
- Apply cold packs to the breasts after feedings to reduce edema and pain. Use commercial cold packs or make inexpensive cold packs by using a package of frozen vegetables, plastic bags filled with crushed ice, or frozen washcloths. Cover with a washcloth before applying to the skin.
- Just before feedings, apply heat with compresses or a shower to stimulate milk flow. Moisten disposable diapers with warm water and apply over each breast. Fasten the tabs to keep the diapers in place and prevent dripping.
- Massage the breasts before and during feedings to stimulate the let-down reflex so that the baby can nurse more easily. Massaging the breasts in the shower provides comfort and helps prepare for feeding.
- If the baby cannot latch on to a very hard areola, express a little milk by hand or with a breast pump. As soon as the areola is soft, begin to feed.
- Feed more often, such as every 1.5 to 2 hours.
- Wear a well-fitting bra for support, both day and night.
- Take prescribed pain medication to help you feel more comfortable.

Problem: Nipples are sore and may be cracked, blistered, or bleeding.

Prevention
- Position the baby at the breast with enough of the areola in the mouth that the nipple is not compressed between the baby's gums during nursing.
- Avoid engorgement by nursing frequently. Express enough milk to soften the areola if engorgement occurs.
- Do not use soap on the nipples because it removes the protective oils and causes drying.
- If you use breast pads for leaking milk, remove them when they become wet to prevent irritation of the skin. Avoid pads with plastic linings that retain moisture. Use a men's handkerchief or pieces of cotton cloth as inexpensive, washable substitutes for commercial breast pads.

Continued

Mothers Want to Know Solutions to Common Breastfeeding Problems—cont'd

- Breast creams may cause sensitivity and irritation. If you choose to use lanolin, use only purified lanolin to protect against allergens. Creams that have to be removed before each feeding may increase soreness.

Solutions

- Begin each feeding with the least sore side first. The hungry baby nurses more vigorously at first, which may be painful. The let-down reflex is started, causing milk to flow more quickly on the second breast.
- Vary the position of the infant during nursing. The area of the nipple directly in line with the infant's nose and chin is most stressed during the feeding.
- Massage the breasts during feedings to enhance milk flow.
- Apply colostrum or breast milk to the nipples after feedings because these have healing properties. Or try warm water or warm compresses to the nipples.
- Expose the nipples to air between feedings by lowering the flaps of your nursing bra. Use a hair dryer held 6 to 8 inches from the breast for 2 to 3 minutes to apply heat and dry the nipples.
- Do not use nipple shields (latex nipples that fit over your own nipples) without help from a lactation consultant. They decrease milk flow so that the baby does not get enough milk and milk production is decreased.
- If you have burning, itching, or stabbing pain throughout your breast, look in the baby's mouth for white patches of thrush, a yeast infection that can infect the nipples. Call the health care provider for medication to treat both you and your baby.

Problem: Flat or inverted nipples that the baby has difficulty drawing into his or her mouth.

Prevention

None. Can be treated during pregnancy or after birth with breast shells.

Solutions

- Wear breast shells in your bra for flat or inverted nipples to help make the nipples protrude.
- Just before beginning breastfeeding, roll the nipple between your thumb and forefinger to help it protrude.
- Use a breast pump just before feedings to draw out inverted nipples. Put the baby to your breast immediately after the pump causes the nipple to become erect. Once the infant gets the nipple in his or her mouth, the normal suckling process usually causes the nipple to stay erect.

NURSING CARE PLAN 22-1

Breastfeeding an Infant Who Has Complications

Assessment: Ruth James' son, David, is full term but develops respiratory complications at birth and is admitted to the neonatal intensive care unit. Ruth had looked forward to breastfeeding her infant, but David will probably not be able to feed at the breast for a few days. Although Ruth understands the situation, she sounds disappointed and discouraged. She states that she will probably have to use formula after David is better because "it will be too late to start breastfeeding."

Nursing Diagnosis: Interrupted Breastfeeding related to separation from infant secondary to illness.

Goals/Expected Outcomes:

Within 2 days Ruth will do the following:

1. Verbalize the importance of breastfeeding her infant and her desire to maintain lactation.
2. Pump her breasts as taught.
3. Breastfeed David successfully when it becomes possible.

Intervention	Rationale
1. Expore Ruth's perception of the problem and her understanding of the cause for separation and its effect on breastfeeding.	1. Discussion of the problem identifies misconceptions and determines what teaching and support are required.
2. Use therapeutic communication techniques to help Ruth express her feelings of disappointment with the unexpected change in plans.	2. Helping the mother express her feelings and accepting them helps her cope with the situation.
3. Explain to Ruth how valuable breast milk is for her infant and that she can use a breast pump to maintain lactation until David is able to breastfeed.	3. Reinforcing the value of breastfeeding and offering encouragement increase the chance of success.
4. Teach Ruth to use a breast pump and store her milk. Instruct her to pump her breasts for 15 to 20 minutes every 3 hours during the day and at least once at night.	4. Frequent use of a breast pump helps establish lactation by causing release of prolactin and oxytocin so that milk is produced and released from the breasts.

5. Feed David breast milk if possible, whether by bottle or gavage. Teach Ruth the way to store her milk and prepare it for use for her infant.	5. Breast milk has properties that are especially valuable for the sick infant.
6. Arrange for Ruth to spend as much time with David as possible. Stay with her during the early visits and when she begins to breastfeed to answer her questions and provide support.	6. Bonding occurs more easily if a mother is able to be with her baby. Being with a mother during visits with her infant allows the nurse an opportunity to offer support, encouragement, and teaching as needed.
7. When Ruth begins to breastfeed, offer the same teaching given to mothers of well infants. In addition, provide continued support if she has concerns.	7. Women who must delay breastfeeding may be more anxious about the process.
8. Offer praise and realistic encouragement frequently.	8. A mother needs reinforcement of her abilities to increase self-esteem as a mother. Encouragement must be suited to actual circumstances.
9. If Ruth must go home before David is ready for discharge, provide her with information about purchase or rental of a breast pump. Give her containers to bring her milk into the nursery.	9. The mother who must pump her breasts for a longer period of time may find that an electric pump is more efficient.

Critical Thinking: What other interventions might be necessary if Ruth had flat nipples?

Answer: Reassure Ruth that she can breastfeed even if her nipples are flat. Teach her to roll her nipples just before David latches on to begin feeding.

Evaluation: Ruth talks about her determination to provide breast milk for David. She maintains lactation and brings breast milk at each visit. At 5 days of age, David is ready to begin breastfeeding. Ruth is very patient in helping David learn to breastfeed with the nurses' help. David is able to nurse well at each feeding by discharge.

Sleepy Infant

During the first few days after birth, infants often sleep longer than expected or fall asleep at the breast after feeding for only a short time. They may be tired from the birth process and not recognize or respond appropriately to hunger.

The nurse should show mothers ways to arouse sleepy infants for breastfeeding. If infants start the feeding fully awake, they are more likely to stay awake to finish the feeding. Pointing out the various behavioral states to the mother helps her develop a greater understanding of her infant and recognize when attempts to feed will be most successful.

When the infant falls asleep during feedings, the nurse should evaluate whether the infant has fed adequately, should be awakened to feed longer, or should be fed again sooner than usual. Emphasizing that wake-up techniques should be gentle is important. Using excessively irritating techniques might cause the infant to associate them with feeding and be unwilling to breastfeed. Infants who continue to be excessively sleepy or nurse poorly need further evaluation. Poor feeding may be an early sign of a complication such as sepsis.

Nipple Confusion

Nipple confusion (or nipple preference) may occur when an infant who has been fed by bottle confuses the tongue movements necessary for bottle feeding and breastfeeding. Infants must push their tongue over the latex nipple of a bottle to slow the flow of milk and prevent choking (Figure 22-8). This can be demonstrated by noting the steady drip of milk when a bottle is held upside down. In bottle feeding, the infant's lips are relaxed because the infant does not need to hold the nipple in place. If the infant uses the same thrusting tongue motion and relaxed lips while nursing, the breast may be pushed out of the mouth.

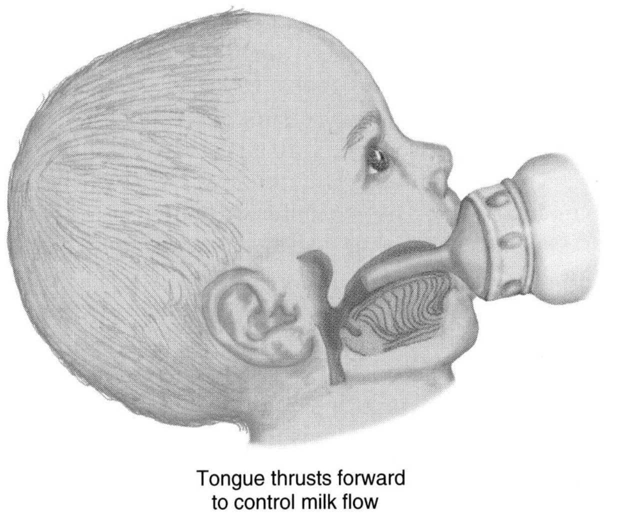
Tongue thrusts forward
to control milk flow

FIGURE 22-8 During bottle feeding, infants must thrust the tongue forward to slow the rapid flow of milk.

CRITICAL TO REMEMBER

Infant Signs of Breastfeeding Problems

Falling asleep after feeding less than 5 minutes
Refusal to breastfeed
Tongue thrusting
Smacking or clicking sounds
Dimpling of cheeks
Failure to open mouth wide at latch-on
Lower lip turned in
Short, choppy motions of jaw
No audible swallowing
Use of formula

During breastfeeding, suction holds the nipple in place near the soft palate. The tongue cups around the nipple and areola with the tip over the lower gum. With each compression of the lower jaw over the milk sinuses behind the areola, the tongue presses against the breast like a peristaltic wave, causing the milk to move forward from the sinuses and into the infant's mouth for swallowing.

Nurses should discourage use of formula in normal breastfeeding infants. It reduces breastfeeding time and decreases production of prolactin and thus milk supply. Formula takes longer to digest, and the infant is not hungry again for about 4 hours. This further limits breast stimulation and milk supply and may lead to engorgement. Women who avoid using bottles during the first month are more likely to continue breastfeeding over 6 months (Piper & Parks, 1996).

Pacifiers also may cause suckling problems. They also have been associated with an earlier weaning of infants from the breast (Biancuzzo, 1999). Although some infants can use a pacifier without ensuing problems with breastfeeding, use of pacifiers should be discouraged.

Suckling Problems

Suckling problems may occur when the nipple is poorly positioned in the mouth. Dimpling of the cheeks and smacking or clicking sounds may indicate that the infant needs more of the areola in the mouth and is sucking on the nipple only. Some infants do not open their mouth widely and suck on the end of the nipple. Short, choppy motions of the jaw signal non-nutritive suckling.

Inserting a gloved finger into the infant's mouth helps assess sucking. The peristaltic motion of the tongue should be felt as the infant sucks. The infant who is thrusting the tongue may have become confused by use of latex nipples, which should be avoided until the problem is resolved. If the infant tends to place the tongue on top of the nipple, placing a finger in the mouth and pressing the infant's tongue down just before latch-on may be effective. More complicated suckling problems may require assistance from a lactation educator or consultant.

Check Your Reading

11. What wake-up techniques should the nurse teach the mother of a sleepy infant?
12. How does sucking from a bottle differ from suckling from the breast?

Infant Complications

Infant complications may be minor and cause minimal interference with breastfeeding. However, the very preterm or ill infant may be unable to breastfeed for a long period.

Jaundice

Jaundice (hyperbilirubinemia) need not interfere with breastfeeding. Even when infants receive phototherapy, they usually can be removed from the lights for feedings. Concern with adequate intake may be more prevalent in caring for the infant with jaundice. Insensible water loss from the skin is increased as a result of the heat and lights used in treatment and could lead to dehydration.

Infants receiving phototherapy should not be given extra water, which may decrease the intake of breast milk. Decreased intestinal motility from insufficient milk intake allows reabsorption of bilirubin through the intestinal wall into the blood stream, increasing the work of the immature liver. Breastfeeding increases the number of stools and aids in excretion of bilirubin. Therefore frequent and adequate feedings are essential. (Jaundice is discussed in Chapters 19 [p. 492] and 30 [p. 846].)

Prematurity

If the preterm infant is unable to breastfeed immediately after birth, the mother needs encouragement and instruction on the way to use a breast pump to establish and maintain her milk supply. Breast milk offers immunologic and nutritional benefits and is adapted to preterm needs. It may help prevent necrotizing enterocolitis, a serious complication of preterm infants. It also helps the mother feel she is providing care for her infant even if she cannot take the infant home with her.

The woman can pump her milk and take it to the nursery for the infant's feedings. The nurse should provide sterile containers for the woman to take home and instruct her in special nursery requirements. In some cases, mothers are taught to separate the foremilk from the hindmilk to provide a higher caloric intake for their preterm infant. They may even learn to measure the fat content of the milk so that the milk with the highest fat levels is used (Griffin, et al., 2000). (Feeding the preterm infant is discussed in Chapter 29, p. 818.)

Some preterm infants or those with breastfeeding problems respond well to the use of supplementary feeding devices. These consist of a container of milk with a small plastic feeding tube attached to the breast. When the infant begins to breastfeed, milk flows from both the container and the breast, increasing the infant's intake and motivation to continue suckling. As the infant gains weight and feeding ability increases, use of the device is gradually decreased until it can be discontinued completely.

Women who provide breastmilk for their preterm infants may feel something is wrong with their milk when additions such as human milk fortifier are used. They should be reassured that their milk is very important in providing protection against infection and good nutrition but that the infant needs more of some nutrients during the period of very rapid growth (Meier, Brown, & Hurst, 1999).

Illness and Congenital Defects

Illness in the infant and congenital defects such as a cleft palate may cause breastfeeding problems. Parents of these infants need the same type of assistance as parents with preterm infants to maintain lactation until the mother is able to nurse the infant. Referral to support groups can be particularly helpful. Some groups focus on particular congenital defects, and others focus on breastfeeding infants with special problems.

Maternal Concerns

The most frequent breastfeeding problems of the mother involve problems of the breasts and nipples. The mother who is ill needs special help to continue breastfeeding. Other common concerns include feeding after multiple birth, working, and weaning.

Common Breast Problems

Engorgement, nipple trauma, flat or inverted nipples, plugged ducts, and mastitis are common problems involving the breasts.

CRITICAL TO REMEMBER

Maternal Signs of Breastfeeding Problems

Hard, tender breasts
Painful, red, cracked, blistered, or bleeding nipples
Flat or inverted nipples
Localized edema or pain in either breast
Fever, generalized aching, or malaise

Engorgement

Many women have a temporary swelling or fullness of the breasts in response to increased blood flow when the milk begins to "come in" or change from colostrum to transitional breast milk. This usually does not occur until the second or third day after birth but may begin earlier in women who have nursed previously. This normal, temporary engorgement should not interfere with breastfeeding.

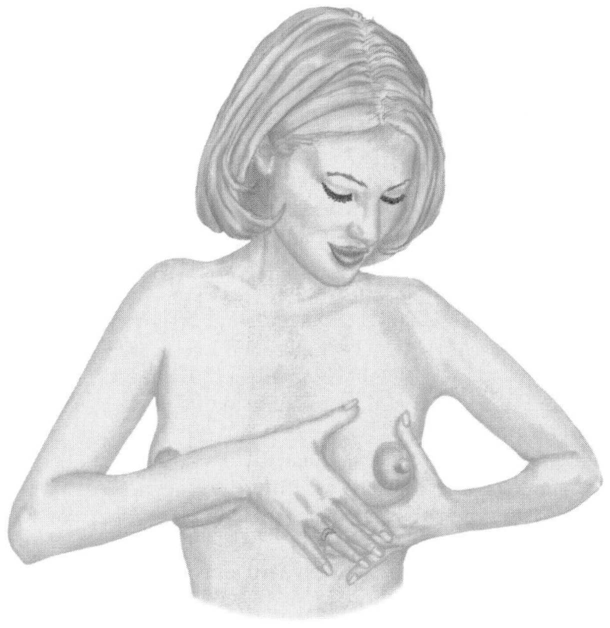

FIGURE 22-9 To massage the breasts, the mother places her hands against the chest wall with her fingers encircling the breasts. She gently slides her hands forward until the fingers overlap. The position of the hands is rotated to cover all breast tissue.

Engorgement becomes a problem if breastfeeding is delayed or infrequent. When this occurs, the breasts become edematous, hard, and tender, making feeding and even movement painful. The areola may become so hard that the infant cannot compress it for nursing. An engorged areola causes the nipple to become flat, making it more difficult for the infant to draw it into the back of the mouth. Engorgement may lead to nipple trauma, mastitis, and even the discontinuation of breastfeeding.

Nurses help prevent engorgement by assisting women to begin breastfeeding early and feed frequently. Encouraging mothers to breastfeed at night, unless extenuating circumstances are present, insures that the breasts are emptied regularly. The use of water and formula should be discouraged.

The nurse should teach women with engorgement about application of cold and heat, massage, and breastfeeding techniques. Cold is used after feedings to reduce edema and pain. Heat applied just before feedings increases vasodilation and milk flow. Prolonged heat may increase edema. Massage of the breasts causes release of oxytocin and increases the speed of milk release. This decreases the length of time the infant nurses on painful breasts (Figure 22-9). Cabbage leaves are sometimes applied to the breasts for short periods of time to provide relief from engorgement (Lawrence & Lawrence, 1999). A well-fitting bra should be worn both day and night to help support the breasts.

Therapeutic Communication

Anxiety about Breastfeeding

Jenny Lavelle gave birth to her second baby, Danny, by cesarean. She tells her nurse, Teresa Hernandez, that she breastfed her first infant for a week and then switched to bottle feeding because she didn't have enough milk. Danny is a sleepy baby but does nurse at times. Jenny's breasts are engorged, and her nipples are sore.

Jenny: I really wanted to nurse Danny, but I don't know if it's worth the effort. My breasts hurt, and I don't know if he's getting enough milk. I probably should just use the bottle again.

Teresa: You sound really discouraged! *(Reflecting the feelings expressed.)*

Jenny: When I couldn't nurse my daughter, I was so disappointed. I had this "Mother Earth" view of the kind of mother I was going to be. But the baby wouldn't stop crying, so I went to the bottle.

Teresa: That must have been hard for you! *(Reflecting the feelings expressed.)*

Jenny: It was awful, and now it looks like I'm going to fail again. Danny won't nurse half the time, and I'm going home this afternoon.

Teresa: And you're worried about what's going to happen at home. *(Seeking clarification of the mother's concerns.)*

Jenny: What if he won't nurse at home? I don't know what to do!

Teresa: Breastfeeding isn't always easy. Mothers and babies both have to learn the process, and that takes time and a lot of patience. Danny's hungry now—would you like to try again? I'll stay with you and answer your questions. *(Offering realistic encouragement and assistance in techniques.)*

Jenny: That would be great! Maybe I'll get the hang of this yet!

(By allowing Jenny to express her feelings of discouragement and disappointment before beginning to teach, the nurse learns how important breastfeeding is to Jenny and how best to go about teaching her. Jenny feels accepted even though she is discouraged.)

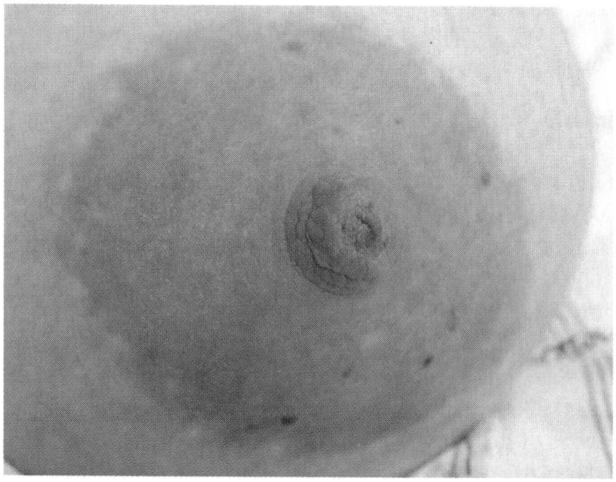

FIGURE 22-10 Note the cracked area on this nipple.

If the areola is too engorged for the infant to compress it, the nurse should help the mother express milk by hand or with a breast pump to soften the areola. Nurses should wear gloves if the possibility exists that they will come in contact with colostrum or breast milk, as for any other body fluid.

Mothers with engorgement may need medication for discomfort so that they can relax while breastfeeding. Medications safe for use during breastfeeding are ordered by the physician. Drugs such as ibuprofen, acetaminophen, and codeine given just before a feeding will not reach the milk for more than a half hour (Lawrence & Lawrence, 1999).

Nipple Trauma

Nipple pain is common during early breastfeeding. Pain for a minute or less may occur at the beginning of feedings because of tissue stretching and suction on the ductules before they fill with milk. Nipple trauma causes more sustained pain. Traumatized nipples appear red, cracked, blistered, or bleeding (Figure 22-10). Minor nipple trauma can be treated by independent nursing interventions. Redness of breast tissue, purulent drainage, and fever indicate mastitis or breast abscess and require antibiotic treatment (see Chapter 28, p. 792).

Improper positioning or latch-on techniques and exposure to soaps, prolonged moisture from wet breast pads, or irritating creams may cause sore nipples. Using a breast pump too long or with the suction set on high may be traumatic.

Care. Teaching includes correcting causes of nipple trauma. Helping the mother with proper positioning may be the most important solution. Increasing air flow to the nipples, feeding with the less inflamed side first, and varying positions for feeding to rotate strain on the nipples also may be helpful. Expressing a small amount of milk to begin the let-down reflex may decrease vigorous suckling on sore nipples.

Unfortunately, studies have not shown that any one comfort measure is significantly more effective than others in treating painful nipples. More research is needed in this area. Warm water compresses may have some effectiveness in reducing pain. Wet tea bags help some mothers but may cause dryness and cracking in others. Application of breast milk to the nipples after feedings is helpful for some women. Breast milk helps prevent infection and aids in healing because it contains lysozymes. Ointments are no more effective than other treatments. Women who plan to use lanolin should use only USP-modified lanolin that has no pesticides and is hypoallergenic. Many creams have to be removed before feeding and may further irritate sore nipples.

NURSING CARE PLAN 22-2

Engorged Breasts and Painful Nipples

Assessment: Sally Portner says during a feeding, "I'm going to give a bottle for the next few feedings. I'm too sore to nurse anymore today." Her breasts are engorged, warm, and tender. Her son, Grady, has difficulty grasping Sally's nipple and areola to feed. Her nipples are everted but red. There are no blisters, fissures, or bleeding. Sally says she has been breastfeeding for 3 minutes per side every 4 to 4½ hours. She holds Grady lying on his back with his hips and legs lower than the rest of his body during feedings. A few swallowing sounds are heard during nursing.

Critical Thinking: Evaluate the information above and assign a LATCH score that can be used in planning care for Sally and Grady. (See Table 22-2.)

Answer: The LATCH score is 6. One point is given for latch, audible swallowing, comfort, and hold. Two points are given for type of nipple. The focus of teaching will be on improving the areas where only one point is assigned.

Nursing Diagnosis: Impaired Skin Integrity related to incorrect positioning and engorgement.

Goals/Expected Outcomes:
Sally will do the following:
1. Demonstrate correct positioning within 1 day.
2. Describe prevention and treatment of engorgement and sore nipples within 1 day.
3. Have no engorgement or redness of the nipples within 2 days.

Intervention	Rationale
1. Apply warm compresses (such as clean wet disposable diapers) to Sally's breasts before feeding.	1. Heat dilates blood vessels and milk ducts, encourages the let-down reflex, and relieves pain.
2. Offer Sally ordered medication just before feedings. Be sure that the medication ordered is safe for the infant.	2. Medication relieves pain that could interfere with the let-down reflex, yet only minimal amounts reach breast milk within the feeding time.
3. Demonstrate gentle massage of the breasts before feedings.	3. Massage causes release of oxytocin, resulting in the let-down reflex. The infant gets milk more quickly, reducing nonproductive time on a painful breast.
4. Demonstrate hand expression or use of a breast pump if necessary to soften the areola enough so that Grady can grasp it to suckle.	4. If the areola is hard, the infant compresses the nipple rather than the milk sinuses because the nipple is not deep enough in the mouth. This causes nipple trauma, inadequate emptying, and decreased milk production.
5. Demonstrate correct positioning of the infant. Place Grady on his side so that he faces the nipple with his abdomen against Sally.	5. If the infant must turn his head to feed, it interferes with swallowing and causes traction on the nipple.
6. Have Sally begin the feeding on the less sore side.	6. The let-down reflex occurs in both breasts at once. Vigorous suckling on the sore side before let-down increases nipple trauma.
7. Assess Grady's mouth position by gently pulling down the lower lip to see that his tongue covers the lower gum. If the lower lip is turned in, gently pull it out so that the lips flare. Assess the position of the nipple.	7. The tongue cushions the lower gum compression of the areola. A turned-in lower lip causes a friction rub on the nipple and areola. If the lips are 1 to 1.5 inches from the base of the nipple, the nipple should be at the back of infant's mouth.
8. Instruct Sally to wear a well-fitting bra both day and night.	8. A bra provides support to painful breasts.
9. Prevent further engorgement by teaching Sally to feed Grady every 2 to 3 hours during the day and at least every 4 hours at night for a total of 8 to12 feedings/day. She should feed an average 15 minutes or more of effective suckling per feeding.	9. Frequent feedings empty the breasts, prevent stasis, stimulate milk production, and reduce the risk of mastitis. Adequate length allows time for the let-down reflex, which may be delayed at first, to occur.
10. Suggest that Sally use a variety of positions for feeding and demonstrate each.	10. Changing the area of stress on the nipple allows healing of the sore area.
11. Teach Sally to apply warm water compresses or colostrum to the sore nipples after feedings. Instruct her to leave the flaps of her nursing bra down between feedings. Ice packs can be used on the breasts after feeding for engorgement.	11. Warm water compresses are soothing. Colostrum has lysosomes and other healing properties. Increased air circulation promotes healing. Ice packs help reduce edema of the breast tissue.
12. Teach Sally to avoid creams that must be removed before nursing or to which she may have allergies. If she uses breast pads, suggest that she change them frequently. Tell her to avoid soap on her nipples.	12. Cream removal, allergies, and wet pads increase irritation. Prolonged exposure to wet pads can cause maceration and breakdown of skin. Soap removes protective oils from nipples.

Continued

Critical Thinking: Should Sally use a bottle for the next few feedings?

Answer: If Sally skips feedings, her engorgement will increase. Grady will not be ready to feed again for 3 to 4 hours after taking formula, increasing the time between breastfeedings. The lack of suckling and engorgement decrease milk production. Using the above interventions, Sally should be able to breastfeed with less discomfort and prevent further problems.

Evaluation: Sally breastfeeds Grady every 2 to 3 hours for approximately 10 minutes per side during the day and every 4 hours at night. She positions Grady correctly and discusses causes and care for sore nipples. When she is seen by the home visit nurse on the day after discharge, her engorgement, nipple redness, and tenderness have resolved. Sally verbalizes methods she will use to prevent further engorgement.

Mothers with vaginal candidiasis may transmit it to the infant during birth. If oral infection with *Candida albicans* (thrush) develops in the infant, the mother's nipples may become infected. The infant may have visible white patches in the mouth. The woman has burning, itching, or stabbing pain throughout the breast. The health care provider should be notified, and both mother and infant are usually treated with nystatin.

The use of nipple shields, nipples with wide bases that are placed over a mother's own nipple, is controversial. The shields are used by some mothers to decrease pain during feedings or help the baby latch on to inverted nipples but also interfere with adequate emptying of the breast and markedly reduce the amount of milk the infant receives. Although use of shields should be discouraged in general, they may be used temporarily in some situations to help an infant who cannot latch on to the breast. A lactation consultant should be involved in helping the mother avoid decreasing milk production and wean the baby away from the shield and back to the breast.

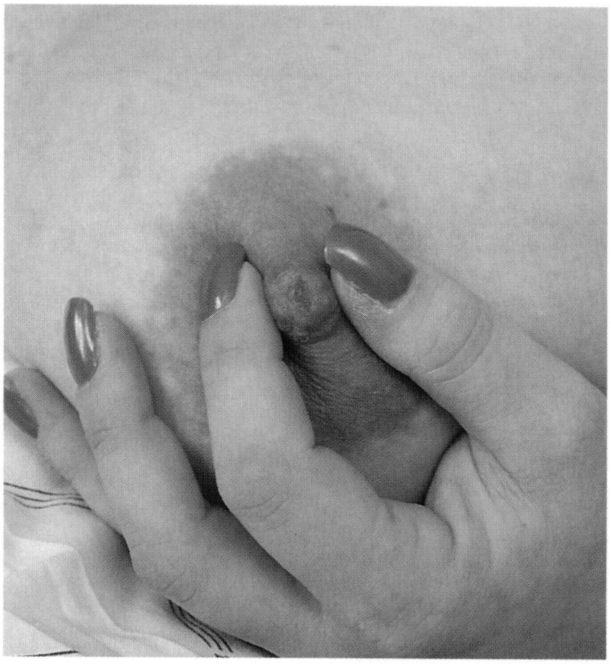

FIGURE 22-11 Rolling helps flat nipples become erect in preparation for latch-on.

Flat and Inverted Nipples

Nipple abnormalities should be treated during pregnancy if possible, but interventions can begin after birth if necessary. Use of breast shells can be taught at this time. Nipple rolling just before feeding helps flat nipples become more erect so that the infant can grasp them more readily (Figure 22-11). A breast pump may help draw out inverted nipples.

Check Your Reading

13. How can the nurse help the mother who has engorged breasts?
14. How should the nurse advise the mother with sore nipples?

Plugged Ducts

Although the exact cause of occlusion of a lactiferous duct is unknown, engorgement, missed feedings, or a constricting bra may be involved. Localized edema and tenderness are present, and a hard area may be palpated. A tiny, white area may be present on the nipple. Massage of the area followed by heat and continued breastfeeding using varied positions cause the duct to open. The infant should be allowed to nurse an adequate amount of time after let-down. A plugged duct may progress to mastitis if not treated promptly. Mastitis involves localized pain accompanied by fever, generalized aching, and malaise (Chapter 28, p. 792).

Drug Transfer to Breast Milk

Most medications taken by the mother cross into the breast milk to some degree, but many pass in very small amounts and are safe for the mother to take during lactation (Auerbach, 1999). Some interfere with milk production. Therefore both prescription drugs and over-the-counter drugs should be approved by a physician. Another drug often can be substituted for one that adversely affects the infant. Scheduling medication to be given after feedings decreases the amount that passes into the milk. If a mother must take a drug that will be harmful to her infant, she should pump her breasts while she is taking the medication. Once the drug clears her blood stream, she may resume breastfeeding (see Appendix C).

Illness in the Mother

When the mother is ill, breastfeeding may have to be postponed temporarily because of the mother's condition or the drugs she receives. When breastfeeding must be stopped, abrupt weaning may lead to mastitis and maternal depression from decreased prolactin, which has been associated with feelings of well-being (Lawrence, 1999). Another factor in depression may be the mother's emotional reaction to having to stop her chosen method of feeding. The nurse should help the mother use a breast pump, if she wishes, until she resumes breastfeeding.

Conditions in Which Breastfeeding Should Be Avoided

Some situations occur in which breastfeeding is contraindicated, such as a mother's serious illness that can be transmitted to the infant. Examples are active tuberculosis and human immunodeficiency virus (HIV) infection. Maternal drug abuse also is usually a contraindication.

Previous Breast Surgery

Women who have had previous surgery such as breast reduction or augmentation may have difficulty with lactation. The ability to produce and transfer the milk to the nipple depends on the surgical technique used and the amount of tissue involved. Disruption of neural pathways, ducts, and blood supply may occur. Some women can breastfeed without problems and others may be able to do so using a supplementation device to help build up milk supply when the breasts are able to produce only a small amount of milk.

Milk Expression

When milk expression is needed, the nurse helps the mother use hand expression (Figure 22-12) or a breast pump (Figure 22-13). Hand expression can be done without other equipment but is not as effective as a breast pump. Hand expression or manual pumps are useful for the mother who wants to save breast milk for another feeding or whose areola is so engorged that the infant cannot grasp it.

The mother who needs to pump her milk for a prolonged period may prefer using a battery-operated or electric breast pump. Battery-operated pumps are small, portable, and relatively inexpensive. Large electric pumps can be rented for home use. They are more efficient than hand or battery pumps and are indicated when the mother must pump to maintain her milk supply for a long period of time. Pumps that can be used on both breasts at once should be used to save time and increase production.

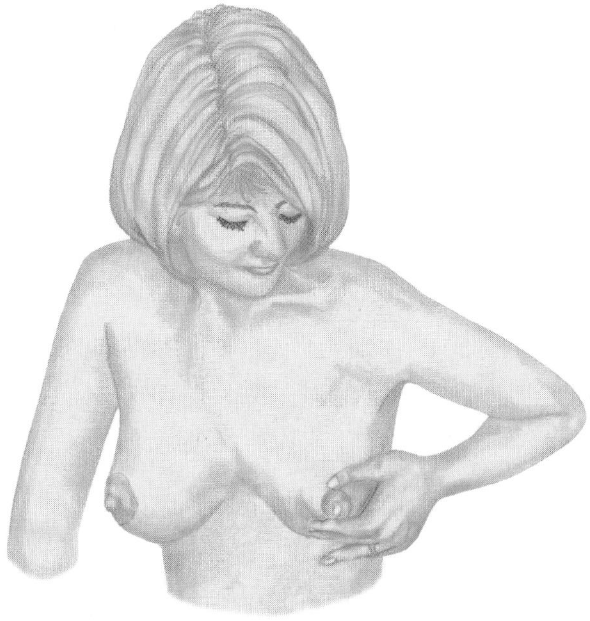

FIGURE 22-12 To express milk from the breast, the mother places her hand just behind the areola, with the thumb on top and the fingers supporting the breast. The tissue is pressed back against the chest wall, then the fingers and thumb are brought together and toward the nipple. This compresses the milk sinuses and causes milk to flow. The action is repeated to simulate the suckling of the infant. Moving the hands around the areola allows compression of all sinuses and complete removal of milk from the breast. Compression should be gentle to avoid trauma.

Use of the breast pump should begin within the first 24 hours after birth for the woman who cannot breastfeed her infant. She should pump her breasts approximately every 3 hours during the day and at least once at night when prolactin levels are elevated. Sessions last approximately 15 to 20 minutes. A total of eight or more sessions in each 24 hours is best to maintain milk supply.

Massage and application of heat before pumping helps initiate the flow of milk. Massage of each quadrant of the breast during pumping may increase the volume of milk obtained at each session. The amount of suction should be set at a low level in the beginning and gradually increased if necessary. Too much negative pressure traumatizes the breast. If the woman needs to increase her milk supply, pumping more often rather than for longer periods of time is more effective.

Breastfeeding after Multiple Births

Mothers who have more than one newborn have many questions about breastfeeding and need help and support from nurses and family members to be successful. Nursing every 2 to 3 hours to build up the milk supply is important. If the infants are unable to breastfeed, the woman will need help using a breast pump.

A

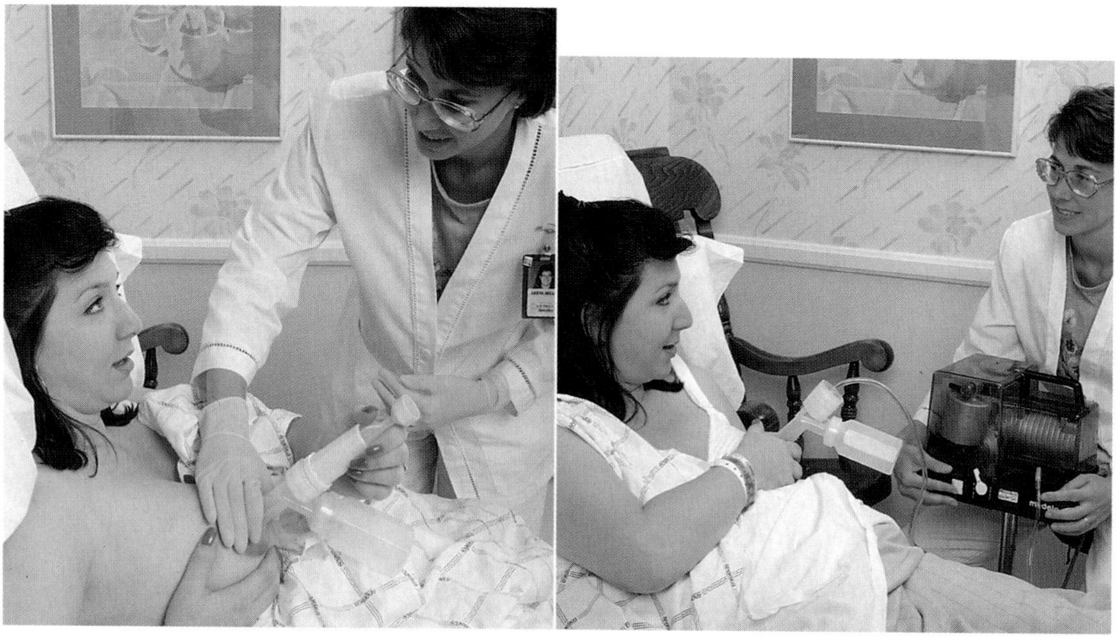

B

FIGURE 22-13 The nurse demonstrates methods of pumping breast milk. **A,** Manual breast pump. **B,** Electric breast pump.

MOTHERS WANT TO KNOW *Breastfeeding after the Birth of More than One Infant*

Ensuring Adequate Milk Production
Because the amount of milk produced depends on the amount of suckling the breasts receive, mothers can produce enough milk for more than one baby. Nursing frequently, every 2 to 3 hours, helps build up the milk supply. Production of milk may be more evenly stimulated if you alternate breasts for each infant, especially if one infant has a weaker suck.

Using a Breast Pump
If your infants are not ready for breastfeeding, use a breast pump to build up your milk supply and provide milk for them until they are ready to breastfeed. Use the pump every 2 to 3 hours while you are awake and at least once during the night. Pump for 15 to 20 minutes during at least 8 pumping sessions daily. Use a double pump on both breasts at the same time to decrease the time spent pumping and increase the production of milk. If one baby is ready to breastfeed before the other(s), nurse the baby and pump your breasts after each feeding to stimulate milk production. An alternative is to nurse the infant on one breast and use a breast pump on the other at the same time.

Feeding Simultaneously or Individually
You can feed each baby individually or feed two infants at once. Simultaneous nursing shortens feeding times, but both infants must be awake at once. You need help positioning the infants at first. Individual feeding can be done without help and on each infant's own schedule, but a larger portion of your day will be spent feeding.

Positioning Infants for Simultaneous Feeding
Use a variety of positions for breastfeeding two infants at once. Place pillows under both infants to bring them to the right height and keep them in place. Use pillows under your arms and behind your back so that you are comfortable.

Football Hold—Place each infant's head on your lap and support each infant's body with pillows alongside your body. Support each infant's head in your hand and bring the infants to the nipples.

Football and Cradle Hold—Place one infant in a cradle position on pillows across your lap. Place the other in a football position with the body supported on pillows alongside you. Once the infants are in position, help one and then the other latch on to the breast.

Criss-Cross Hold—Place pillows on your lap and hold each baby in the cradle position. The infants' legs criss-cross over each other.

Keeping Track
Keep track of when and for how long each baby eats, especially if you feed them individually. Record the number of wet diapers and bowel movements each infant has each day. Six to eight wet diapers and at least four bowel movements usually show adequate intake.

Care for Yourself
Eating well and getting enough rest is important. Ask for help from family and friends. Pamper yourself as much as possible, and leave care of the house and cooking to others if you can. Your major responsibility during this time should be to care for yourself and your new babies!

MOTHERS WANT TO KNOW *How to Wean from Breastfeeding*

Deciding When to Wean

Breastfeeding has many benefits, and you can continue to breastfeed as long as you are comfortable. Only you can make the decision about when to wean your baby. Before you decide to begin weaning, evaluate the reasons for continuing nursing or beginning weaning.

How to Proceed

Gradual weaning is best for both you and your baby. Abrupt weaning can lead to engorgement and mastitis for you and can upset your baby. You both need to get used to this change slowly.

- Eliminate one feeding at a time. Replace it with a bottle for the young infant who needs to continue sucking. Infants generally do not drink as much from a cup as they do from a bottle. They may need a bottle to get enough milk to meet their nutritional requirements. The older infant who has learned to use a cup may not need a bottle at all. Use formula instead of cow's milk until the infant is at least 1 year old because formula is more suited to an infant's needs.
- Wait several days before eliminating another feeding. This allows time for your milk production to adjust and the baby to accept the changes.
- Omit daytime feedings first. Begin with the feeding at which the baby seems least interested, then gradually eliminate others.
- Eliminate the baby's favorite feedings last. Many infants are particularly fond of morning and bedtime feedings.
- Expect your infant to want to nurse again when tired, ill, or hurt during the weaning process. This is sometimes called "comfort nursing." A few minutes of nursing may be all that are necessary to comfort the baby.

If the woman decides to feed two infants simultaneously, she will need help positioning them using the football hold, cradle hold, or a combination of both. She should be encouraged to eat well, get enough rest, and ask for help from family and friends. (See "Mothers Want to Know: Breastfeeding after the Birth of More than One Infant.")

Employment

Working and breastfeeding can be combined very well with some advance planning. Because breastfeeding infants have a lower incidence of some illnesses than those who are formula fed, nursing mothers are less likely to miss work because their baby is sick. Recent Federal legislation has been introduced to ensure that women are allowed to pump or breastfeed during their breaks and lunch time while working. The bills set up tax incentives for employers who promote a lactation-friendly environment by providing places for pumping and breast pumps or lactation consultants at the workplace (Hill, 2000).

Milk supply can be well established by frequent breastfeeding during the time before return to work. A week or two before she returns to work, the mother should use a breast pump once or twice a day to practice pumping her breasts and build up a small supply of frozen breast milk. This avoids the stress of having to learn the technique or worry about having enough milk while adjusting to the work situation.

Milk should be stored in rigid polypropylene plastic containers because antibodies in the milk adhere to glass. The rigid plastic containers maintain the stability of the milk components and are easier to use than plastic bottle liners, which spill easily. The milk can be kept in a refrigerator for 48 hours, a refrigerator freezer for 1 month, or a deep freeze at 0° F for 6 months (Lawrence & Lawrence, 1999). Leukocytes are destroyed by freezing, but most other immunologic properties are preserved. Containers should be labeled with the date so that the oldest is used first.

Breast milk can be thawed and warmed by holding the container under running water. It should not be refrozen or heated in a microwave. A microwave heats milk unevenly and may burn the infant because the container feels cooler than the milk inside. Refrigerated milk should be used as much as possible so that the leukocytes are available for the infant. Thawed breast milk should be gently inverted a few times to mix the foremilk and hindmilk.

Most working mothers use a battery-operated or an electric pump once or twice a day during lunch or coffee breaks. The woman needs to find a place at her work where she can pump her milk in privacy. The milk should be refrigerated or placed in an insulated container with ice and can be used for the next day's feeding. Breastfeeding just before leaving for work and again as soon as the mother returns home keeps the time between feedings at a minimum. The infant is breastfed frequently throughout the evening hours and on weekends to continue to build up the milk supply.

Some mothers choose to use formula during work hours but breastfeed when at home. They should prepare for this by gradually eliminating the feedings that occur during work hours and substituting a bottle. Although the total milk supply is diminished, breastfeeding can continue in the mornings and evenings.

Weaning

Mothers are sometimes subjected to pressure and opinions offered by family and friends about weaning. No one "right" time to wean the infant exists. Mothers choose to wean their infants for various reasons. The nurse should provide information so that women can

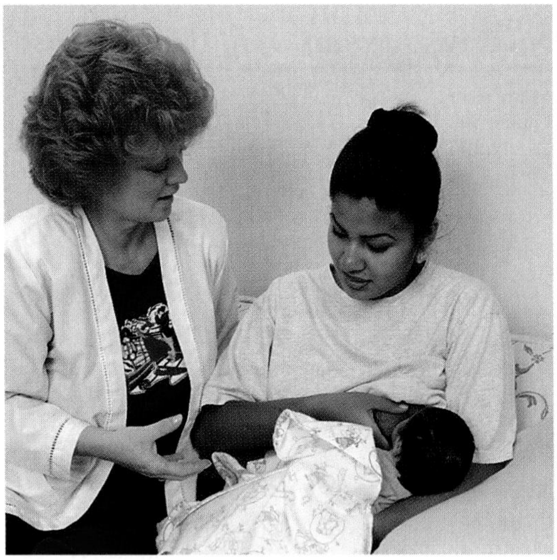

FIGURE 22-14 The nurse offers suggestions on hand position during the home visit.

make informed decisions about weaning and should support the woman once her decision is made. Explaining that even a short period of breastfeeding offers her infant many advantages is reassuring to the woman. Mothers may need help in planning a gradual weaning process, if possible. This allows them to avoid engorgement and infants can get used to a bottle or cup over a period of time.

Home Care

Many infants have not breastfed well by the time of discharge from the birth facility, placing them at risk for failure to gain weight, dehydration, and hyperbilirubinemia. Problems with engorgement and sore nipples are more likely to occur after discharge. These families need continued support after discharge.

Mothers can be referred to lactation specialists or organizations such as La Leche League, a support group that gives ongoing assistance to breastfeeding mothers. La Leche League chapters are available in most communities and are listed in the telephone book. Support groups also may be provided by the birth facility.

Some birth facilities provide one or two home visits for new mothers by a nurse who can assess both the mother's progress and the infant's progress and intervene appropriately. A home visit allows assessment of the breastfeeding process in the mother's own surroundings and intervention before serious problems develop. The nurse can observe a feeding session and offer suggestions. The mother can ask questions that were not answered during her birth facility stay (Figure 22-14).

Outpatient clinics are a less costly alternative to the home visit and provide care similar to that received during a home visit. "Warm lines" also may be available for mothers to call their birth facilities and talk to nurses about breastfeeding problems. Women with more serious breastfeeding problems need referral to a lactation consultant, a professional educated to deal with more complex situations. Assistance helps prevent infant readmission for dehydration and hyperbilirubinemia.

Check Your Reading

15. What types of care may be available after discharge for the breastfeeding mother?
16. What teaching should be included for the mother who plans to work and breastfeed?

FORMULA FEEDING

Although formula feeding may require less knowledge and skill than breastfeeding, the inexperienced mother often has many questions and may need assistance in learning to use formula correctly. Although breastfeeding is preferable, the nurse should support the woman who has decided to use formula.

APPLICATION OF THE NURSING PROCESS: FORMULA FEEDING

Assessment

Assess both the mother and the infant during the feeding process.

Mother's Knowledge

Assess the mother's knowledge of bottle feeding. Ask her whether she has fed an infant before and whether she has questions. Observe her technique during the initial and subsequent feedings. Note the way she holds the infant and the bottle, assess her burping technique, and identify areas in which she seems unsure. To determine her understanding of the correct method to prepare formula, ask her to describe the way she will do it at home.

Infant Feeding Behaviors

Hungry infants show the same behaviors whether breastfeeding or formula feeding (Table 22-3). They may fuss or cry, suck on their hands, and root for the nipple. Waiting until the infant is frantic may result in a feeding taken too fast, with excess swallowing of air or choking. Assess the way the infant sucks during the feeding to identify sucking problems.

Analysis

Because improper formula preparation and feeding techniques could harm the infant, an appropriate nursing diagnosis for the mother using formula feeding is "Risk for Altered Health Maintenance related to lack of understanding of formula preparation and feeding techniques."

Table 22-3
SIGNS OF HUNGER IN INFANTS
Licking movements
Lip smacking
Rooting
Hands to mouth
Sucking on the hands
Increased activity
Crying (a late sign)

Planning

The mother will demonstrate correct techniques in holding the infant and bottle during feedings and will describe the way to prepare formula and the frequency of feedings.

Interventions

Teaching about Formula

The mother must learn the type of formula to use and the way to prepare it. Improper preparation can cause problems for the infant. Infection may occur if the milk or water used for preparation is contaminated. Improper dilution of the formula may cause undernutrition or imbalances of sodium, which can be dangerous to the infant.

Types of Formula

Many types of formula are available, and the physician or nurse practitioner prescribes the type of formula the mother is to use. If milk allergies are prevalent in the family, a soy-based or protein hydrolysate formula may be chosen from the start. Formula may be purchased in three different forms.

Ready to Use. This formula is available in bottles to which a nipple is added or in cans to be poured directly into a bottle. Although expensive, it is practical when the formula is difficult to mix or the water supply is in question. An open can should be refrigerated and used within 24 hours.

Concentrated Liquid. This type must be diluted before use. Be sure that the mother understands the directions for dilution. Equal parts of concentrated liquid formula and water are mixed in a bottle to provide the amount desired for each feeding.

Powdered. Powdered formula is more economical and is particularly useful when a breastfeeding mother plans to give an occasional bottle of formula. Usually one scoop of powder is added to each 2 ounces of water in a bottle. Packets with enough powdered formula for one bottle are convenient when away from home. Formula should be well mixed to dissolve the powder and make the solution uniform.

Equipment

Many different types of bottles and nipples are available. Bottles may be glass or plastic, or a plastic liner that fits into a rigid container may be used. Some nipples are designed to simulate the human nipple to promote jaw development. Selection of type of bottles and nipples depends on individual preference.

Preparation

Discuss preparation of formula with the mother. She can prepare a single bottle or a 24-hour supply. If the water supply is safe, sterilization is not necessary. Bottles and nipples can be washed in hot, sudsy water, rinsed well, and allowed to air dry. Bottles may be washed in a dishwasher, but nipples tend to deteriorate quickly unless washed by hand. The top of the can and a can opener are washed just before opening the can. The formula and water are poured into the bottles, which then are capped. Be sure the mother understands to measure the exact the proportion of water and liquid or powdered formula to prevent illness in the infant.

When safety of the water supply is questionable, sterilization by aseptic or terminal method is required. In both methods, all equipment is washed and rinsed well before beginning. In the aseptic method, equipment needed for the procedure is boiled for 5 minutes in a sterilizer or deep pan. Water for diluting the formula is boiled separately. The bottles then are assembled using sterilized tongs to avoid contamination by the hands. The formula and boiled water are added, and the bottles are capped and refrigerated until needed.

In the terminal sterilization method, the formula is prepared in the bottles, which are loosely capped. The bottles then are placed in the sterilizer or pan of water, where they are boiled for 25 minutes. After the bottles cool, the caps are tightened and the bottles refrigerated.

Explaining Feeding Techniques

Positioning. Show the mother the way to position the infant in a semi-upright position such as the cradle hold. This allows the mother to hold the infant close in a face-to-face position. The bottle is held so that the nipple is kept full of formula to prevent excessive swallowing of air (Figure 22-15).

Burping. For the first few days, the infant should be burped or "bubbled" after every half ounce. Gradually, the infant is able to take more milk before burping. Demonstrate placing the infant over the shoulder or in a sitting position with the head supported while patting or rubbing the infant's back.

Frequency and Amount. Instruct the mother to feed the infant every 3 to 4 hours but to avoid rigid scheduling and take her cues from the infant. Explain that the bottle-fed infant takes only 0.5 to 1 ounce per feeding during the first day of life but gradually increases to 2 to 3 ounces per feeding within 3 to 7 days. An infant who is satisfied often goes to sleep.

Cautions. Caution the mother not to prop the bottle. Propping increases the likelihood of choking if re-

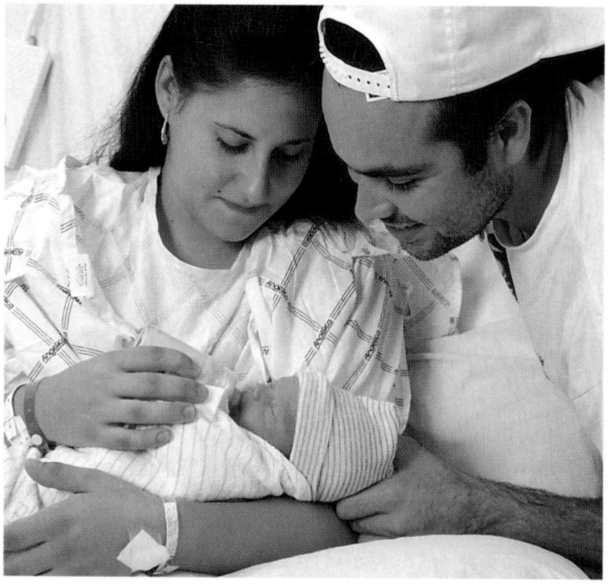

FIGURE 22-15 This mother holds her infant close during bottle feeding. The bottle is positioned so that the nipple is filled with milk at all times. The father offers encouragement.

gurgitation occurs and eliminates the holding and cuddling that should accompany feeding. Some mothers put an infant to bed with a bottle propped. This not only increases the danger of aspiration but allows milk to stay in the mouth for prolonged periods. The milk may pool in the mouth, promoting growth of bacteria and leading to cavities once the teeth are in. Ear infections also are more common in infants who sleep with a bottle.

The mother should not try to coax the infant to finish the bottle at each feeding. This could result in regurgitation and excessive weight gain. She should not save formula from one feeding to the next because of the danger of rapid growth of bacteria in warm milk. Any formula not used within an hour should be discarded.

Formula should not be heated in a microwave oven because the heating is uneven and may result in some parts of the liquid being very hot even when the outside of the bottle feels only warm. Formula can be heated by placing it in a container of hot water until it is warm. The mother should test the formula temperature by allowing a few drops from the bottle to fall on her inner arm.

Infant Variations. Infants vary in their feeding preferences. Some infants drink from the bottle reluctantly. Although formula usually is given at room temperature, some infants take heated formula better. The mother of a sleepy infant needs to use the same wake-up techniques discussed for the breastfeeding mother.

Soft nipples may be helpful for the infant with a weak suck or small mouth. Angling the tip of the nipple so that it rubs the palate triggers the suck reflex in most infants. Placing a finger under the chin for support may help some infants suck better. It often takes patience and persistence to find the most effective techniques.

Evaluation

The mother should hold the infant and bottle correctly during feedings. She should be able to describe formula preparation and the amount and frequency of feedings.

Check Your Reading

17. What questions might a mother have about formula feeding?
18. Why should mothers avoid propping bottles?

SUMMARY CONCEPTS

- The newborn may lose weight in the first few days after birth as a result of insufficient intake and normal loss of extracellular fluid.
- Colostrum is rich in protein, vitamins, minerals, and immunoglobulins. Transitional milk appears between colostrum and mature milk. Mature milk is present after the first 2 weeks of lactation.
- Breast milk has nutrients in proportions required by the newborn and in an easily digested form. The majority of commercial formulas are cow's milk adapted to simulate human milk.
- Breast milk contains factors that help establish the normal intestinal flora and prevent infection. These include bifidus factor, leukocytes, lysozymes, and immunoglobulins.
- A variety of commercial formulas are available. They include modified cow's milk formula, soy-based or protein hydrolysate formulas, and formulas for preterm infants or those with special problems.
- Factors that influence the mother's choice of feeding method include knowledge about each method, support from family and friends, cultural influences, and employment.
- Suckling at the breast causes the mother's posterior pituitary to release oxytocin, which triggers the let-down reflex. It also causes the anterior pituitary to release prolactin, which increases milk production.
- Milk production increases when the infant feeds frequently. When breastfeeding ceases, prolactin is decreased and eventually the alveoli of the breasts atrophy and stop producing milk. This is the principle of supply and demand.
- Flat and inverted nipples should be identified during pregnancy. Creams and methods to toughen the nipples are not necessary.
- The nurse can help the mother establish breastfeeding by initiating early feeding and assisting her with positioning and latch.
- Adequate intake in breastfeeding infants is shown by at least 6 to 10 voidings and 4 stools daily.
- The mother should feed the infant 8 to 12 times each day for an average of at least 15 minutes of effective suckling per feeding, nursing until the infant is satisfied at the second breast.

- When infants suck from a bottle, they must push the tongue against the nipple to slow the flow of milk. When they suckle at the breast, they position the nipple far into the mouth so that the gums compress the areola as the tongue moves over the milk sinuses in a wavelike motion.
- Nurses must intervene to prevent and treat engorged breasts and sore nipples and help with flat or inverted nipples.
- Teaching for the mother who plans to work and breastfeed includes expression of breast milk by hand or pump and proper storage of the milk.
- Mothers who use formula need information about the types of formula available, correct preparation, and feeding techniques.

REFERENCES & READINGS

American Academy of Pediatrics Committee on Nutrition. (2000). Hypoallergenic infant formulas. *Pediatrics,*106(2), 346-349.

American Academy of Pediatrics Committee on Nutrition. (1999). Iron fortification of infant formulas. *Pediatrics,*104(1), 119-123.

American Academy of Pediatrics Work Group on Breastfeeding. (1997). Breastfeeding and the use of human milk. *Pediatrics,* 100(6), 1035-1039.

American Academy of Pediatrics & American College of Obstetricians and Gynecologists. (1997). *Guidelines for perinatal care* (4th ed.). Elk Grove Village, IL: American Academy of Pediatrics.

Association of Women's Health, Obstetric and Neonatal Nurses. (1998). *Standards and guidelines for professional nursing practice in the care of women and newborns* (5th ed). Washington, D.C.: Author.

Auerbach, K.G. (1999). Breastfeeding and maternal medication use. *Journal of Obstetric, Gynecologic, and Neonatal Nursing,* 28(5), 554-563.

Auerbach, K.G. (1999). Maternal employment and breastfeeding. In J. Riordan & K.C. Auerbach (Eds.), *Breastfeeding and human lactation* (2nd ed., pp. 577-600). Boston: Jones & Bartlett.

Auerbach, K.G., Riordan, J., & Gross, A.G. (2000). The lactation consultant: An increasingly visible health care role. *Mother Baby Journal,* 5(1), 41-46.

Balcazar, H., Trier, C.M., & Cobas, J.A. (1995). What predicts breastfeeding intention in Mexican-American and non-Hispanic white women? Evidence from a national survey. *Birth,* 22(2), 74-80.

Barger, J. (1998). The ten steps to successful breastfeeding: Principles, practicalities, and practices, part I. *Mother Baby Journal,* 3(6), 41-44.

Biancuzzo, M. (1999). *Breastfeeding the newborn: clinical strategies for nurses.* St. Louis: Mosby.

Biancuzzo, M. (1999). Selecting pumps for breastfeeding mothers. *Journal of Obstetric, Gynecologic, and Neonatal Nursing,* 28(4), 417-426.

Bocar, D.L., & Riordan, J. (1999). Breastfeeding education. In J. Riordan & K.G. Auerbach (Eds.), *Breastfeeding and human lactation* (2nd ed., pp. 241-277). Sudbury, MA: Jones & Bartlett.

Brooks, S.L., Mitchell, A., & Steffenson, N. (2000). Mothers, infants, and DHA: Implications for nursing practice. *MCN: American Journal of Maternal/Child Nursing,* 25(2), 71-75.

Brown, S.G., & Johnson, B.T. (1998). Enhancing early discharge with home follow-up: A pilot project. *Journal of Obstetric, Gynecologic, and Neonatal Nursing,* 27(1), 33-38.

Chertok, H. (1999). Relief of breast engorgement for the Sabbath-observant Jewish woman. *Journal of Obstetric, Gynecologic, and Neonatal Nursing,* 28(4), 365-369.

Chezem, J., Friesen, C., Montgomery, P., Fortman, T., & Clark, H. (1998). Lactation duration: Influences of human milk replacements and formula samples on women planning postpartum employment. *Journal of Obstetric, Gynecologic, and Neonatal Nursing,* 27(6), 646-651.

Chapman, D.J., & Perez-Escamilla. (1999). Does delayed perception of the onset of lactation shorten breastfeeding duration? *Journal of Human Lactation,* 15(2), 107-111.

Callister, L.C., & Vega, R. (1998). Giving birth: Guatemalan women's voices. *Journal of Obstetric, Gynecologic, and Neonatal Nursing,* 27(3), 289-295.

Choudhry, U.K. (1997). Traditional practices of women from India: Pregnancy, childbirth, and newborn care. *Journal of Obstetric, Gynecologic, and Neonatal Nursing* 26(5), 533-539.

Coleman, C. (1999). Formula feeding: What new parents need to know. *International Journal of Childbirth Education,* 14(2), 15-17.

Fein, S.B., & Falci, C.D. (1999). Infant formula preparation, handling, and related practices in the United States. *Journal of the American Dietetic Association,* 99(10), 1234-1240.

Gomez, L.T. (2000). Breastfeeding: Increasing primary adjustment milk supply. *International Journal of Childbirth Education,* 15(1), 29-35.

Greenly, R.L., & Dunsworth, T. (1999). Drugs and the lactating woman. *Mother Baby Journal,* 4(6), 7-12.

Griffin, T.L., Meier, P.P., Bradford, L.P., Bigger, H.R., & Engstrom, J.L. (2000). Mothers' performing creamatocrit measures in the NICU: Accuracy, reactions, and cost. *Journal of Obstetric, Gynecologic, and Neonatal Nursing,* 29(3), 249-257.

Gromada, K.K., & Spangler, A.K. (1998). Breastfeeding twins and higher-order multiples. *Journal of Obstetric, Gynecologic, and Neonatal Nursing,* 27(4), 449-551.

Grover, G. (2000). Nutritional needs. In C.D. Berkowitz (Ed.), *Pediatrics: A primary care approach* (2nd ed., pp. 34-39). Philadelphia: W.B. Saunders.

Hamelin, K., & McLennan, J. (2000). Examination of the use of an in-hospital breastfeeding tool. *Mother Baby Journal,* 5(3), 29-37.

Hamosh, M., Peterson, J.A., Henderson, T.R., Scallan, C.D., Kiwan, R., Ceriani, R.L., Armand, M., Mehta, N.R., & Hamosh, P. (1999). Protective function of human milk: The milk fat globule. *Seminars in Perinatology,* 23(3), 242-249.

Hauck, C.L. (2000). Breastfeeding and the workplace: A review of the literature. *Mother Baby Journal,* 5(2), 45-51.

Henly, S.J., Anderson, C.M., Avery, M.D., Hills-Bonczyk, S.G., Potter, S., & Duckett, L.J. (1995). Anemia and insufficient milk in first-time mothers. *Birth,* 22(2), 87-92.

Hill, P.D. (2000). Update on breastfeeding: Health people 2010 objectives. *MCN: American Journal of Maternal/Child Nursing,* 25(5), 248-251.

Huggins, K. (1999). *The nursing mother's companion* (4th ed.). Boston: Harvard Common Press.

Humenick, S.S. (2000). Prenatal preparation for breastfeeding. In F.H. Nichols & S.S. Humenick. *Childbirth education: practice, research, and theory* (2nd ed., pp. 114-137). Philadelphia: W.B. Saunders.

Kopec, K. (1999). Herbal medications and breastfeeding. *Journal of Human Lactation,* 15(2), 157-161.
Jacobi, A.M., & Levin, M. (1997). Promotion and support of breastfeeding. In B. Worthington-Roberts & S.R. Williams (Eds.), *Nutrition in pregnancy and lactation* (6th ed.). St. Louis: Mosby.
James, D.C., Pimley, M., Curtis, C., & Griese, M. (1999). Second opinion: Should nurses offer discharge formula samples to women who plan to breastfeed. *MCN: American Journal of Maternal-Child Nursing,* 24(4), 166-175.
Johnson, T.S., Brennan, & R.A., & Flynn-Tymkow, C.D. (1999). A home visit program for breastfeeding education and support. *Journal of Obstetric, Gynecologic, and Neonatal Nursing,* 28(5), 480-485.
Kannan, S., Carruth, B.R., & Skinner, J. (1999). Cultural influences on infant feeding beliefs of mothers. *Journal of the American Dietetic Association,* 99(1), 88-90.
Lavergne, N.A. (1997). Does application of tea bags to sore nipples while breastfeeding provide effective relief? *Journal of Obstetric, Gynecologic, and Neonatal Nursing,* 26(1), 53-58.
Lawrence, R.A., & Lawrence, R.M. (1999). *Breastfeeding: A guide for the medical profession* (5th ed.). St. Louis: Mosby.
Locklin, M.P., & Jansson, M.J. (1999). Home visits: Strategies to protect the breastfeeding newborn at risk. *Journal of Obstetric, Gynecologic, and Neonatal Nursing,* 28(1), 33-40.
MacMullen, N.J., & Dulski, L.A. (2000). Factors related to sucking ability in healthy newborns. *Journal of Obstetric, Gynecologic, and Neonatal Nursing,* 29(4), 390-396.
Mattson, S. (1995). Culturally sensitive perinatal care for southeast Asians. *Journal of Obstetric, Gynecologic, and Neonatal Nursing,* 24(41), 335-341.
Meier, P., Brown, L.P., & Hurst. N.M. (1999). Breastfeeding the preterm infant. In J. Riordan & K.G. Auerbach (Eds.), *Breastfeeding and human lactation* (2nd ed., pp. 449-481). Sudbury, MA: Jones & Bartlett.
Mohrbacher, N., & Stock, J. (1997). *The breastfeeding answer book* (2nd ed.). Schaumburg, IL: La Leche League International.
Moore, K., Zale, M., & Moramarco, M.L. (1998). New guidelines for breastfeeding. *RN,* 61(8), 36-39.
Mozingo, J.N., Davis, M.W., Droppleman, P.G., & Merideth, A. (2000). "It wasn't working": Women's experiences with short-term breastfeeding. *MCN: American Journal of Maternal/Child Nursing,* 25(3), 120-126.
Novotny, R., Hla, M.M., Kieffer, E.C., Park, C., Mor, J., & Thiele, M. (2000). Breastfeeding duration in a multiethnic population in Hawaii. *Birth,* 27(2), 91-96.
Orr, S.S. (2000). Breastfeeding. In S. Mattson & J.E. Smith (Eds.), Core curriculum for maternal-newborn nursing (2nd ed., pp. 317-344). Philadelphia: W.B. Saunders.
Peeler, M.C. (1999). Teaching standards: Breastfeeding. *Mother Baby Journal,* 4(6), 25-33.
Piper, S., & Parks, P. (1996). Predicting the duration of lactation: Evidence from a national survey. *Birth,* 23(1), 7-12.
Righard, L. (1998). Are breastfeeding problems related to incorrect breastfeeding technique and the use of pacifiers and bottles? *Birth,* 25(1), 40-44 .
Riordan, J. (1998). Predicting breastfeeding problems. *AWHONN Lifelines,* 2(6), 31-33.
Riordan, J. (1999a). The biologic specificity of breastmilk. In J. Riordan & K.C. Auerbach (Eds.), *Breastfeeding and human lactation,* (2nd ed., pp. 121-161). Boston: Jones & Bartlett.
Riordan, J. (1999b). The cultural context of breastfeeding. In J. Riordan & K.C. Auerbach (Eds.), *Breastfeeding and human lactation* (2nd ed., pp. 29-52.) Sudbury, MA: Jones & Bartlett.
Riordan, J.M., & Koehn, M. (1997). Reliability and validity testing of three breastfeeding assessment tools. *Journal of Obstetric, Gynecologic, and Neonatal Nursing,* 26(2), 181-187.
Ross Products Division. (1999). *Updated breastfeeding trends through 1998: Mothers' survey.* Columbus, OH: Ross Products Division, Abbott Laboratories.
Saadeh, R., & Akre, J. (1996). Ten steps to successful breastfeeding: A summary of the rationale and scientific evidence. *Birth,* 23(3), 154-160.
Saarinen, U.M., & Kajosaari, M. (1995). Breastfeeding as prophylaxis against atopic disease: Prospective follow-up study until 17 years old. *Lancet,* 346, 1065-1069.
Smale, M. (1998). Working with breastfeeding mothers: The psychosocial context. In S. Clement. *Psychological perspectives on pregnancy and childbirth* (pp. 183-204). Edinburgh: Churchill Livingstone.
Susin, L.R.O., Giugliani, E.R.J., Kummer, S.C., Maciel, M., Simon, C., & daSilveira, L.C. (1999). Does parental breastfeeding knowledge increase breastfeeding rates? *Birth,* 26(3), 149-156.
Swett, W. (1999). Infant formulas in Canada. *International Journal of Childbirth Education,* 14(2), 14.
Timbo, B., Altekruse, S., Headrick, M., & Klontz, K. (1996). Breastfeeding among black mothers: Evidence supporting the need for prenatal intervention. *Journal of the Society of Pediatric Nurses,* 1(1), 35-40.
Tiran, D., & Mack, S. (Eds.). *Complementary therapies for pregnancy and childbirth.* Edinburgh: Balliere Tindall.
Tsang, R.C., DeMarini, S., & Rath, L.L. (1998). Fluids, electrolytes, vitamins, and trace minerals: Basis of ingestion, digestion, elimination, and metabolism. In C. Kenner, J.W. Lott, & A.A. Flandermeyer (Eds.), *Comprehensive neonatal nursing, a physiologic perspective* (2nd ed., pp. 336-353). Philadelphia: W.B. Saunders.
U.S. Department of Health and Human Services (USDHHS). (2000). *Healthy People 2010* (Conference edition, in 2 volumes). Washington, D.C.: Author.
Walker, M. (1997). Breastfeeding the sleepy baby. *Journal of Human Lactation,* 13(2), 151-153.
Wambach, K.A. (1998). Maternal fatigue in breastfeeding primiparae during the first nine weeks postpartum. *Journal of Human Lactation,* 14(3), 219-229.
Wiessinger, D. (1999). A breastfeeding teaching tool using a sandwich analogy for latch-on. *Journal of Human Lactation,* 14(1), 31-36.
Williamson, M.T., & Murti, P.K. (1996). Effects of storage, time, temperature, and composition of containers on biologic components of human milk. *Journal of Human Lactation,* 12(1), 31-35.
Worthington-Roberts, B. (1997a). Human milk composition and infant growth and development. In B. Worthington-Roberts & S.R. Williams (Eds.), *Nutrition in pregnancy and lactation* (6th ed.). St. Louis: Mosby.
Worthington-Roberts, B. (1997b). Lactation: Basic considerations. In B. Worthington-Roberts & S.R. Williams (Eds.), *Nutrition in pregnancy and lactation* (6th ed.). St. Louis: Mosby.

23 HOME CARE OF THE INFANT

OBJECTIVES

1. Explain why nurses need knowledge about care of the infant during the early weeks after birth.
2. Describe postdischarge nursing care included in home visits, clinic visits, and telephone follow-up.
3. Explain the safety features of infant equipment that parents must consider.
4. Explain methods of resolving common problems involving infant crying and sleep patterns during the early weeks of parenting.
5. Answer common questions that parents might have about care of the young infant.
6. Describe the normal changes in growth and development of the infant during the first 12 weeks of life.
7. Explain the purpose and importance of well-baby checkups and immunizations for infants.
8. List signs that indicate illness in the infant.
9. Discuss current knowledge about sudden infant death syndrome.

DEFINITIONS

EXTRUSION REFLEX Automatic nervous system response that causes an infant to push anything solid out of the mouth.

HYPERBILIRUBINEMIA Excessive amount of bilirubin in the blood.

JAUNDICE Yellow discoloration of the skin and sclera caused by excessive bilirubin in the blood.

MILIARIA (PRICKLY HEAT) Rash caused by heat.

OPHTHALMIA NEONATORUM Severe conjunctivitis in the newborn often caused by gonorrhea or chlamydia infection in the mother; may cause blindness.

PREPUCE Fold of skin covering the glans penis; foreskin; may be removed by circumcision.

REFLUX Condition in which stomach contents enter the esophagus and may be aspirated into the lungs.

SEBORRHEIC DERMATITIS (CRADLE CAP) Yellowish, crusty area of the scalp.

SUDDEN INFANT DEATH SYNDROME (SIDS) Sudden death of an infant that is unexplained by autopsy, examination of the scene of death, or history.

THERMOREGULATION Maintenance of body temperature.

Nurses often receive questions from parents about care of infants during the early weeks. This chapter provides information on caring for infants during the first 12 weeks of life. The focus is on teaching parents beyond the usual birth facility discharge teaching, which is included in Chapter 21. Detailed information about ill or older infants can be found in pediatric textbooks.

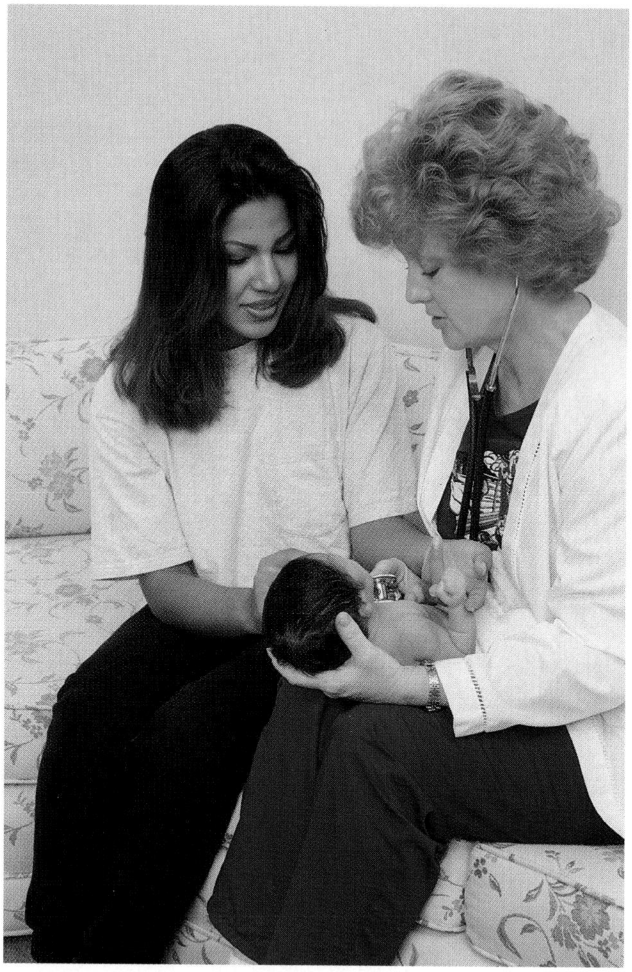

FIGURE 23-1 During the home visit, the nurse performs a complete assessment of the infant. Here she is checking the apical pulse and listening to breath sounds.

INFORMATION FOR NEW PARENTS

Needs

The early weeks after birth are often stressful for new parents. The mother is tired from the pregnancy and birth, both parents may be anxious about their new role, and the newborn may be awake much of the night or behave in unexpected ways. Parents have concerns about ongoing care of the infant and adjustment to parenthood.

Sources of Information

In the birth facility, parents often receive more information about care of the newborn than they can absorb in the short time available. New mothers' physical needs and anxieties often interfere with their ability to learn. This may leave parents inadequately prepared to deal with the multiple demands of early parenting.

Family members, once the primary source of support for new parents, frequently live far away, and parents must rely on friends, health care personnel, child care classes, television, books, and magazines. Many people get information from the Internet. Parents should determine the source of information obtained online because if from nonprofessional sources it may not be accurate. Friends can be important sources of support and information, but their knowledge may be incorrect or outdated. Nurses are ideal sources of assistance in these situations.

CARE AFTER DISCHARGE

The American Academy of Pediatrics and the American College of Obstetricians and Gynecologists recommend that women and their infants stay in the birth facility for 48 hours after vaginal birth and 96 hours after cesarean birth. The optimal time of discharge should be based on the individual needs of the woman and her infant. Although longer stays have been legislated, women may choose to go home before 48 hours after a vaginal birth. Early follow-up is essential for these families. The American Academy of Pediatrics recommends that infants discharged earlier than 48 hours after birth should have follow-up care within 48 hours after discharge (AAP & ACOG, 1997).

Various programs have been instituted to provide after-discharge care. They may include nursing contact with the family in the home, clinic, or by telephone. Follow-up may increase client satisfaction with care, result in longer breastfeeding, and decrease infant physician visits or hospital readmissions for conditions such as hyperbilirubinemia and dehydration (Johnson, Brennan, & Flynn-Tymkow, 1999; Williams & Cooper, 1996).

Home Visits

The home visit is scheduled during the first few days after discharge. This timing allows early assessment and intervention for problems in nutrition, jaundice, newborn adaptation, and maternal-infant interaction. During the first 3 to 5 days after birth, infections, feeding problems, excessive weight loss, jaundice, and other problems may become evident (Jacobson, Brock, & Keppler, 1999). Nurses may visit low-risk mothers and infants or may follow high-risk infants after discharge from the neonatal intensive care nursery (Figures 23-1 to 23-4).

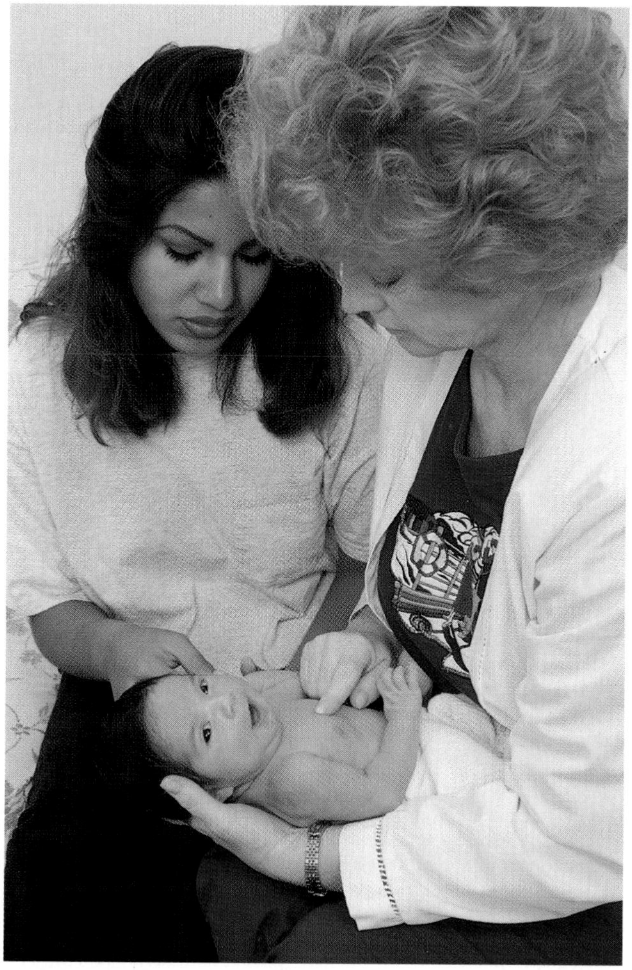

FIGURE 23-2 Jaundice is especially of concern when infants are discharged early after birth. The nurse shows the mother how to blanch the skin to check for jaundice and discusses what the mother should do if she sees it.

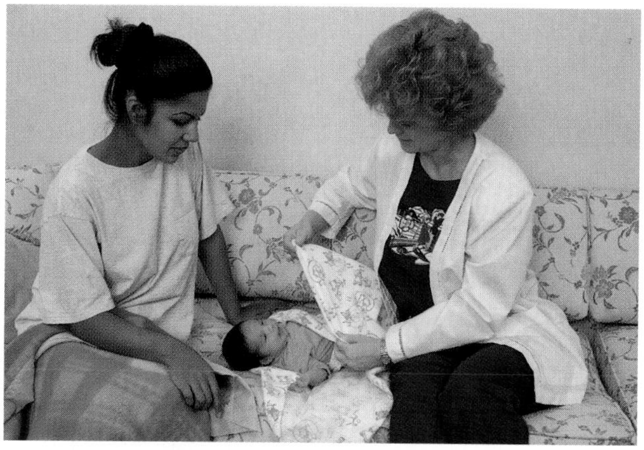

FIGURE 23-3 The nurse discusses thermoregulation with the mother and demonstrates swaddling.

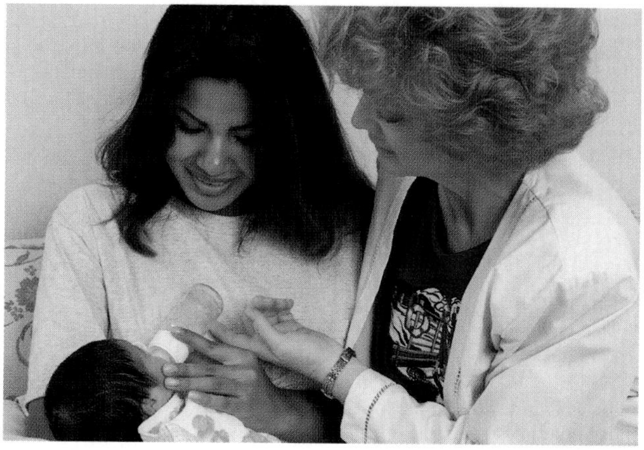

FIGURE 23-4 The nurse observes a feeding during the visit to assess feeding techniques and provide a chance for parents to ask questions about feeding concerns. This is a good time to assess parent-infant interaction. The infant is weighed to help determine adequacy of intake.

Visits to Low-Risk Families

During the home visit, the nurse performs a physical examination of the mother and infant. Family adaptation to the addition of a new member and the adequacy of the mother's support system are assessed. The nurse reinforces and continues the teaching that was begun at the birth facility. A feeding session should be assessed, especially if the mother is breastfeeding. Blood may be obtained for metabolic screening if the infant went home too early for reliable testing in the birth facility (Figure 23-5).

Home visits provide reassurance for parents and may increase a woman's confidence and competence in caring for herself and her infant. The visits are especially valuable in recognizing jaundice and intervening before bilirubin levels become dangerously high. When jaundice is found, the nurse can discuss the implications and draw blood for testing bilirubin levels. Appropriate care is discussed, as necessary, including hydration and phototherapy (see Parents Want to Know: Home Care for the Infant Receiving Phototherapy, Chapter 30, p. 848).

Feeding is an area of concern for many parents. Breastfeeding problems were found in one study in almost a third of infants (Williams & Cooper, 1996). When the nurse observes a feeding and helps a woman deal with problems, the infant's intake may increase. Increased intake helps to prevent dehydration and possible hospital readmission and leads to increased excretion of bilirubin, which may prevent a need for phototherapy at home or in the hospital.

Visits to Families with High-Risk Infants

High-risk infants (see Chapters 29 and 30) often need special care after discharge. Parents may be very anxious about assuming care of an infant who has had a prolonged hospitalization. Many hospitals have programs that enable parents to take over their infant's care gradually before discharge.

EXPECTED NEWBORN/FAMILY OUTCOMES	ASSESSMENTS	INTERVENTIONS	RESPONSE
Physical assessment: The newborn assessment is within normal limits.	Vital signs, weight Respiratory status (color, retractions, etc.) Skin (rash, jaundice, cord, circumcision) Fontanelles Activity, sleep, behavior, crying Elimination (number of voids and stools in 24 hours)	Complete systematic assessment.	Outcomes met. Outcome not met (requires further documentation).
Nutrition: Infant's intake is adequate. LATCH score is over 7 if infant breastfed. (See Chapter 22, p. 583.)	Infant's and mother's behaviors during a feeding	Discuss frequency, length of feedings, and amount (in oz. or time at breast). Discuss breastfeeding or other problems. Provide written educational materials.	Outcome met. Outcome not met (requires further documentation). Referral made
Caregiving: Parents correctly describe infant characteristics and needs and demonstrate care.	Parent's knowledge and performance of infant care	Teach and clarify as necessary. Provide written educational materials.	Outcome met. Outcome not met (requires further documentation).
Infant/family relationships: The family demonstrates attachment behaviors.	Interaction of parents and family members with infant	Discuss emotional adjustment of all family members, sibling rivalry, postpartum blues. Provide written educational materials.	Outcome met. Outcome not met (requires further documentation).
Support system: Parents have an adequate support system.	Interaction of family members, sources of support within and outside the immediate family	Discuss availability and need for support, resources. Provide written educational materials.	Outcome met. Outcome not met (requires further documentation). Referral made.
Environment: The home is safe and has adequate facilities and baby equipment and supplies are safe.	Safety and potential hazards in the home; availability of heat, electricity, telephone, sanitation, sleeping arrangements	Provide written educational materials.	Outcome met. Outcome not met (requires further documentation).
Need for care: The parents understand need for well baby care. They recognize signs of infant illness and how to get help.	Knowledge about well baby checkups and immunizations, signs of illness, how to take a temperature, where to get care	Discuss areas in which there is need; demonstrate temperature taking. Provide written educational materials.	Outcome met. Outcome not met (requires further documentation).

FIGURE 23-5 An example of a clinical pathway for a home visit by a nurse to the family of a normal newborn.

EXPECTED NEWBORN/FAMILY OUTCOMES	ASSESSMENTS	INTERVENTIONS	RESPONSE
Other care: Metabolic screening or other care is received, as ordered.	Need for specimen collection or other care	Collect blood specimens for newborn metabolic screening; give other care (phototherapy, etc.) as ordered. Provide written educational materials.	Outcome met. Outcome not met (requires further documentation).
Referrals: Parents receive necessary referrals.	Need for referrals	Refer to physician, lactation consultant, WIC, community resources, etc. Provide written educational materials.	Outcome met (document to whom referral made). Outcome not met (requires further documentation).

FIGURE 23-5, cont'd For legend see opposite page.

A nurse may visit the home before the infant's discharge to help the family plan for accommodating the equipment and the type of care the infant needs. The home is checked for the availability of electricity, heat, and a telephone. If the family has a technology-dependent infant, the nurse checks that they have notified the utility companies to ensure that no disruption of services occurs.

After the infant is discharged, nursing visits can help the family maintain the infant's health and decrease the need for rehospitalization. Components of each visit vary according to the infant's needs. The nurse provides assessment of the infant and the parents' caregiving ability in addition to necessary teaching and nursing care.

Medically fragile infants may require home treatment with mechanical ventilation, oxygen therapy, or apnea monitors. Parents may have to perform such nursing skills as tracheostomy care, tube feedings, suctioning, and care of intravenous sites. Mothers often have concerns about feeding the infant, which may differ from feeding a healthy full-term infant. Follow-up telephone calls from nurses between visits help families adapt to the needs of these infants and may also decrease the need for rehospitalization.

The home health nurse may be part of an interdisciplinary team of health care providers working with families in the home. The nurse may help coordinate care by different professionals. Some infants are eligible for home health aides who provide direct care in the home. The aide is supervised by a nurse.

Infants with complications often need more frequent visits to the pediatrician or nurse practitioner or are rehospitalized during the early months after birth. Common problems include respiratory illness, infections (gastroenteritis, sepsis, urinary tract infections, otitis media), and need for surgery. These parents need information on preventive measures and care of the infant with acute illness.

Although parents' greatest concerns involve the infant's health, other problems may exist. Finding a baby sitter who is qualified to care for an infant on oxygen or who might need resuscitation may be difficult. Siblings often have difficulty adjusting to the needs of the infant and may resent the diversion of the parents' attention. The nurse can make suggestions and put the parents in touch with parent groups that offer practical help in caring for a high-risk infant.

General Considerations in Home Visits

The nurse making a home visit is a guest of the family and must adapt nursing care usually given in the birth facility to the home setting. The needs of other family members may make care in the home quite different from care given in the hospital. For example, the examination of the infant may need to wait for a short time while the mother meets the needs of her other small children.

Careful planning before the visit is essential to make the most of the limited time available. Before visiting, the nurse calls to schedule the visit at a time convenient for the family and obtain directions to the home. Setting priorities carefully based on the needs identified by the nurse and the family is important, especially when only one visit is planned. After the home visit, the nurse may plan additional visits or provide the family with a telephone number where they may receive further help if needed.

Communication skills are particularly important when the setting is the home and the client is the family. The nurse must develop rapport with family members quickly and work with them to meet shared goals for the visit. A brief social interaction may be beneficial at the beginning of the visit to develop a trusting relationship. The purpose of the visit should be explained and the family's expectations and desires discussed. Open-ended questions and therapeutic communication techniques help the nurse identify and address the family's needs. Making suggestions in a positive manner is important.

The nurse should be aware of any cultural practices affecting the family's view of care. For example, many Asians are offended by direct eye contact, pointing a finger, or showing the bottom of the shoe. In patriarchal cultures, the father is the head of the family and teaching should be directed to him and the mother. The elder members of the family also may play a large role in determining essential health care. In some cultures, the mother-in-law is an important influence in the care of the mother and infant.

Documentation of the visit is essential. The results of the assessments, teaching, nursing care, referrals, and plans for follow-up should be recorded. Copies of the record usually are sent to the primary caregiver.

Outpatient Visits

Outpatient visits may be provided by the birth facility in clinics managed by nurses. The charge is often included in the maternity care package. Assessment and care are essentially the same as those provided for home visits. The advantage of outpatient visits is that the nurse does not have to travel to the home and can see more clients each day, thereby reducing the cost of the service. Assessment of the home setting and family interaction is not possible, however. Clinic visits usually last 30 to 45 minutes. Appointments may be made during the discharge procedure from the birth facility.

In some areas nurses take a van to various neighborhoods to provide nursing care. This allows clients with transportation problems easy access to care. Nurses in the van carry out the same assessment and care of the mother and infant that is provided during clinic visits. Care may begin in the prenatal period and extend through the postpartum period.

Telephone Counseling

Telephone counseling can occur during follow-up calls to discharged clients or when parents call "warm lines" for help with problems or questions. Telephone calls are much less expensive than home or clinic visits. The major disadvantage is that the nurse cannot perform an in-person assessment of the mother, baby, or home environment and must rely on the caller to present an accurate picture of the situation.

Follow-Up Calls

Follow-up calls are placed by nurses in the first few days after discharge. The nurse asks a series of questions to assess the physical condition of the mother and infant and to identify any needs or problems. All mothers may receive calls or only those considered at risk for problems. If problems are discovered, the nurse may schedule another call or a home visit, if available, or refer the woman to her primary care provider.

Warm Lines

Warm lines, also called *help lines,* provide parents with an opportunity to ask a nurse the questions arising from the daily challenges of parenting. They are used for troubling but not emergency situations. The service should be available 24 hours each day to best meet the needs of the callers. Parents often call about infant feeding, breastfeeding concerns, and basic care of the mother and infant. Calls last about 15 to 20 minutes. The nurse answers the caller's questions and assesses for other problems. The nurse may call back later to see if the situation has resolved.

Telephone Techniques

Nurses caring for clients by telephone must understand telephone counseling techniques. They need special education in telephone communication and triage.

Open-ended questions help the mother describe any problems in her own terms. Examples are as follows:

> "How have you been getting along since you left the hospital?"
> "What situations have occurred in which you weren't quite sure what to do?"

Telephone triage involves determining the existence of and solution to a serious problem. Callers may not describe the situation accurately. The nurse should help the mother (or caller) describe the major concerns, which may not be those discussed first. "What worries you most?" may help focus on the most important problems. Although most problems discussed are concerns about normal infants, the nurse must be alert for "red flags" that signal serious situations needing immediate referral.

CRITICAL TO REMEMBER

Red Flags of Telephone Triage

An emergency situation (such as respiratory difficulty, bleeding). Tell the parent to call 911 or take the infant to a hospital emergency department immediately. Call back in 5 minutes to ensure that parents did seek help.

Illness (fever, dehydration, change in feeding or behavior, unusual rashes).

Severe feeding problems (infant may become dehydrated or jaundiced, or fail to thrive).

Problem has been present for longer than usual or usual remedies are ineffective (such as prolonged crying or sleeping, rash is spreading).

Parent's affect seems inappropriate for situation (extremely emotional with apparently minor situation or unconcerned when situation could be serious).

Note: Callers should be referred to the primary health care provider or the hospital emergency room, if necessary, when a serious problem may be present. Being overcautious is preferable; refer parents to the primary care provider early rather than miss a serious situation.

Table 23-1
SAFETY CONSIDERATIONS FOR INFANT EQUIPMENT

CRIBS

Crib slats must be no more than 2⅜ inches apart so that the infant's head cannot become wedged between them. Remove corner posts that extend more than 1/16 inch above the end panel to prevent strangulation if clothing catches on them. Plastic teething guards should be firmly attached to side rails.

Bumper pads prevent the infant from hitting against the side rails. They should fit well around the entire crib and must be anchored to keep them in place so that infants cannot get caught between the side rail and the bumper.

The crib mattress should fit snugly, with less than an inch between the mattress and the sides of the crib so that the infant cannot become wedged in that space. The mattress should be firm. The crib should contain no loose bedding or pillows that would increase the risk of suffocation.

Crib toys or mobiles should be firmly attached, with no straps or strings in the infant's reach. Mobiles should be removed when the infant can reach them.

Cribs should be placed away from hanging cords of blinds or drapes, which could become wrapped around an active infant.

OTHER EQUIPMENT

Paint used to refurbish infant equipment should be marked lead-free and safe for children's equipment to prevent lead poisoning.

All parts should function properly: crib side rails must be secure, highchair trays must stay firmly in place, latches must remain fastened, etc. The frame and basic construction of all equipment should be sturdy.

All moving parts should be examined carefully to see whether little fingers could get caught or whether the infant could trigger a catch that would cause the equipment to become unsafe.

Safety straps for infant seats, swings, changing tables, high chairs, or other equipment must be in good condition. Straps should fit around the infant but not be long enough that the infant could become entangled.

Automatic swings should have legs that are stable, without a tendency to tip over. Note how difficult it is to put the infant into the swing and to remove the infant from the swing safely.

All toys should be examined carefully for parts that can be moved and swallowed.

Guidelines and Documentation

When nurses give care by telephone, they must have written protocols and policies that provide guidelines for care. This helps ensure that all who perform this service provide clients with similar information. A list of common questions can be compiled to help nurses obtain appropriate information when parents call about a problem.

Parents should always be told when and how to seek more care if problems are not resolved. If the infant seems ill, referral to the pediatrician or hospital emergency department is most appropriate. The nurse's judgment, based on education, expertise, and experience, determines how helpful the service is to clients.

All calls should be documented so that accurate, legal records are available for future reference. The nurse may use a checklist or a simple written description of the call. Documentation should include identifying information for the caller, including address and phone number. The reason for the call, problems described, advice given, and any referrals also should be recorded. In some agencies, all calls are audiotaped. A copy of the information is sent to the primary caregiver to provide continuity of care.

Check Your Reading

1. Where do parents obtain information about caring for their infant during the early weeks after birth?
2. What are some ways in which nurses offer follow-up services to new parents?

INFANT EQUIPMENT

Generally, parents obtain most of their infant equipment before the infant is born, but nurses may receive questions in the weeks after the birth. Although nurses should never recommend specific brand names of equipment, their guidance about features and safety is helpful.

Safety Considerations

Parents, especially those of limited means, need to understand that few, if any, pieces of equipment are absolutely essential for newborns. Infants sleep in padded dresser drawers and designer cribs with equal comfort. Safety is the most important consideration.

New equipment sold in the United States is generally safe because manufacturers are required to follow certain governmental standards for safety. However, hand-me-down equipment may have been produced before newer requirements were in effect. Older equipment should be checked carefully to ensure all parts are strong and working properly (Table 23-1).

Car Seats

An infant carried by an adult while riding in a car is never safe. A sudden stop or accident could cause the infant to be hurled against the dashboard or crushed by the adult, who would be thrown forward by the force of the impact. In the United States and Canada, laws require restraint of infants and young children in car seats when they are riding in automobiles.

Generally, laws require that special seats be used for children younger than 4 years or less than 40 pounds.

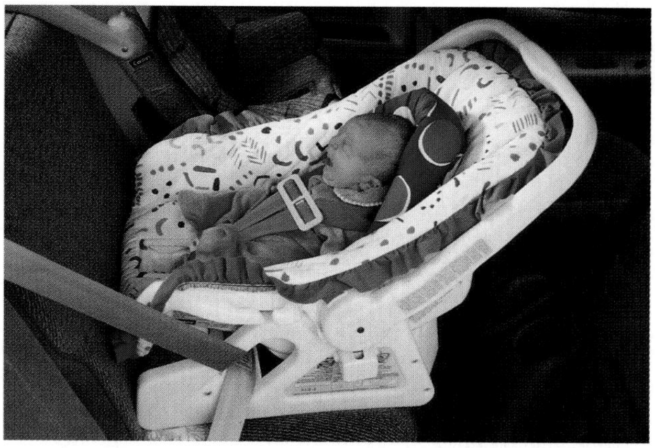

FIGURE 23-6 A car seat for an infant under 20 pounds should face the rear of the car. Note the clip that holds the straps together for a snug fit.

Table 23-2
SAFETY CONSIDERATIONS FOR INFANT CAR SEATS

Use only car seats that are approved for use in automobiles. Seats designed for use in the home do not provide adequate protection in a car.
Use car seats that are appropriate for the infant's age and size. Place the seat in the center of the back seat of the car, never where an air bag is installed.
Follow the manufacturer's directions for fastening the seat in the car and the infant in the car seat. Recheck the restraint straps each time the seat is used.
Be certain that the straps are tight enough to prevent the infant from getting out of the restraints or turning over in the seat. Infants who turn over can suffocate in the padding of the seat.
Check to see that the infant cannot become caught with the straps tightly around the neck.
Use car seats only in an automobile. Do not place them on a soft surface, such as a bed, where they might turn over and suffocate the infant.
Do not place them on surfaces from which they might fall, such as grocery carts.
Never leave infants alone in a car, even for a few minutes. They could be kidnapped or injured in an accident involving the car even though it is parked. Cars quickly become very warm, and the infant could become dangerously overheated.

Discharge teaching should include information about state car seat laws. In some birth facilities, car seat rentals or loans are available.

The many different car seats available may be confusing to parents. Some car seats are designed for infants younger than 1 year and weighing up to 20 pounds. Some of these are safe for infants up to 30 pounds. Seats for newborns face the rear of the car and recline at up to a 45-degree angle. Those for older children face forward and allow the child to sit up or recline. Convertible seats meet the needs of both newborns and young children. They are used in a rear-facing position for the infant and turned to face forward for the toddler.

The harness of the car seat should firmly restrain the infant yet be quick and easy to fasten. For the rear-facing infant, shoulder straps should be in the lowest position and at or slightly below the shoulder level (Figure 23-6). A restraint clip should be placed at mid-chest level to keep the straps in place on the infant's shoulders. Blankets should never be placed under the infant or behind the back or head.

All car seats should be secured by the automobile seat belt to prevent the infant from being thrown forward on impact. Car seats are safest when they are placed in the center back seat of the car. They never should be placed in the front passenger seat in a car with air bags, which can kill or injure the infant when they inflate. Some cars have switches to turn off air bags. If necessary to place a car seat in the front seat, the air bags should be disengaged. Even with the air bags turned off, however, the front seat of the car is not as safe as the back seat for infants and children.

Exceptionally small infants may need special adaptations. Blankets placed at the head, along the sides, and between the legs may improve the fit. They should not be placed under the infant. Special seats or beds designed specifically for preterm or low-birth-weight infants are also available.

According to the National Transportation Safety Board, four out of five parents make mistakes in using their car seat that could result in injury or death to their child. An incorrectly fastened harness may not restrain the infant in an accident and could cause damage, such as laceration of the liver. If the automobile seat belt is not routed through the correct area of the car seat, the seat may tip or become a flying missile during an accident. Car seats should be used only in cars and only according to manufacturer's directions (Table 23-2). Further information about proper use of car seats is available on the Internet from sources such as the National Transportation Safety Board, www.ntsb.gov/default.htm.

Check Your Reading

3. What advice can the nurse offer about safety features of equipment used for infants?
4. What should the nurse teach parents about buying and using a car seat?

EARLY PROBLEMS

Infant Crying

Crying is a major parental concern during the early weeks after birth. Crying is most frustrating to parents when they cannot find a cause for it. Infants cry for many reasons, including hunger, discomfort, fatigue, overstimulation, and boredom. Sometimes no specific cause can be determined.

When the cause for crying is not obvious, some parents are afraid that responding may spoil the infant. If the infant stops crying when picked up, their concern may increase. Changing the infant's position may help gas move in the intestines, relieve tired muscles, or distract the infant by changing the scenery, bringing about a temporary cessation of crying.

Infants cannot signal that they have unmet needs in any other way but crying and are not spoiled by parents meeting their needs. In fact, their needs must be met in a consistent, warm, prompt manner for the development of trust to occur. Infants of parents who intervene appropriately for crying are less likely to cry excessively as they get older.

Some families develop creative methods for dealing with crying infants. Others benefit from a nurse's suggestions about appropriate techniques to use.

When parents have searched for causes of crying and tried a variety of comfort measures with no success, the infant may need to spend some time alone. Some infants need to discharge excess tension by crying before going to sleep. Although this is difficult for parents, leaving the infant safely in the crib for 10 to 15 minutes may be enough to allow the infant to fall asleep.

Some parents find that setting a timer is helpful. At the end of the period allowed, they can quietly check to be sure that the infant is all right. Changing the diaper or holding the infant for a few minutes before putting the infant back to bed may be all that is necessary. Talking softly to provide reassurance and patting the infant's back without picking the infant up may be effective.

Colic

Description

Colic is characterized by irritable crying for no obvious reason, for 3 hours or more a day. It usually takes place during the late afternoon or early evening on at least 3 days a week. It occurs in 10% to 20% of all infants, beginning in the first 2 to 3 weeks of life (Grover, 2000a). Although it usually ends about 3 months after birth, some infants continue to have colic until 6 months of age. The infant is in good health, eats well, and gains weight appropriately, despite the daily crying episodes. Both breastfed and formula fed infants have colic.

Infants with colic cry as though in pain, draw their knees onto the abdomen or rigidly extend the legs, and may pass flatus. The crying is intense and may last until the infant falls asleep, exhausted. Persistent crying may interfere with the mother-infant relationship (Keefe, et al., 1996). Because crying causes so much parental distress and may be a factor in parenting disorders or child abuse, nurses should find ways to provide support to parents of colicky infants.

Although many theories have been investigated, the cause of colic remains unknown. Allergies, abnormal intestinal peristalsis, feeding techniques, parental tension, and exposure to smoking have all been considered. Colic may be due to immaturity of the gastrointestinal tract or nervous system or to a combination of factors.

Interventions

Nursing interventions include using therapeutic communication to help parents express their frustrations and teaching techniques for coping with the problem. Parents should be encouraged to talk about their feelings and should be reassured that colic does not indicate poor parenting. They often feel inadequate about their failure to manage the problem and guilty if their frustration develops into anger.

The nurse should explain that it is not abnormal to feel ambivalent or even angry with the infant. Taking time away from infant care to rest and recoup energy needed to deal with the demands of a crying infant is essential. Parents can leave the infant with a baby sitter for short periods or take turns consoling the infant to provide breaks from the crying.

The techniques listed in Parents Want to Know: Methods to Relieve Crying in Infants may alleviate crying from colic temporarily, but generally none gives prolonged relief. The colic holds may be particularly effective for some infants (Figure 23-7). Changing from a cow's milk formula to a protein hydrolysate formula may help the infant with allergies. Breastfeeding mothers whose diet includes cow's milk, orange juice, peanuts, the cabbage family, onions, or chocolate should try eliminating these foods for 5 to 7 days to see if improvement occurs.

A quiet environment, calm approach, and fairly regular schedule may help some infants with colic. Increasing the time spent carrying the infant often produces some improvement. Parents should be assured that spoiling does not result from responding to the infant's cries. In severe cases, the infant may be given an antiflatulent, sedative, antispasmodic, or antihistamine for a short time.

Shaken Baby Syndrome

One possible result of crying in infants is shaken baby syndrome. Shaken baby syndrome results from shaking an infant vigorously enough to cause the soft tissue of the brain to bounce against the skull. Subdural hemorrhage, retinal hemorrhage or detachment, skeletal fractures, and damage to the spinal cord may result.

PARENTS WANT TO KNOW *Methods to Relieve Crying in Infants*

Treating Common Causes

Hunger. Try feeding the infant if it has been more than ½ hour since the last feeding. A bubble of air may have caused a feeling of fullness too soon during the last feeding. The infant may be experiencing a "growth spurt" and need more frequent feedings for a day or two to provide necessary nutrients for rapid growth.

Air Bubbles. Fussy infants may need more frequent burping during and after feedings than other infants. Try burping during crying spells because the infant may swallow air.

Diapers. Although most infants do not mind wet or soiled diapers, they may become cold or their skin may be irritated when diapers are not changed frequently enough.

Clothing. Check the infant's clothing for anything that could cause discomfort. Be sure that pins are closed, no irritating seams or neck tags are irritating the infant, and that elastic on sleeves is not too tight.

Warmth. Be sure that the infant is warm enough, yet not too warm. The abdomen should feel warm even if the hands and feet are cool. Dress the infant as warm as an adult would want to be dressed, but add a receiving blanket. Infants who are overdressed rarely perspire but often cry because of their discomfort.

Overstimulation. Too many visitors handling the infant or too much noise and commotion in the household may be overstimulating. A quiet environment, rocking, or just being left to work off excess tension alone in the crib for a short time may be necessary.

Quieting Techniques

Rocking. The gentle motion of rocking, reminiscent of intrauterine life, is often soothing for infants.

Automatic Swings. Swings may be battery operated or wind-up. Check the noise level on wind-up swings to be sure that winding does not wake the infant going off to sleep. Small infants may need padding with blankets for safety and comfort.

Walking, Jiggling, Swaying. Sometimes newborns prefer a particular style of motion. Rocking sideways with the infant held in an upright position is helpful for some infants, whereas others prefer vertical rocking. Taking a walk outside with new sights and sounds may provide distraction.

Swaddling. Wrap the infant snugly. This is comforting because infants are used to restricted activity in the uterus. Swaddling is especially helpful during the first few weeks after birth.

Stroller or Buggy Rides. The motion of a stroller or buggy may be soothing to some infants. The ride can be in or outside the house. A parent can move a stroller back and forth with one foot while doing chores or eating meals. The stroller should allow the infant to lie down rather than sit. Padding may increase comfort.

Car Rides. Some infants go to sleep in a moving car. A short ride may put the infant to sleep. The infant may stay asleep when carried into the house.

Music. The sound of a parent singing may be reassuring to the infant. Some newborns respond well to a music box, radio, CD, or tape of music. Music with a steady beat or classical music may be particularly effective. Music should be played softly.

White Noise. Background noise sometimes puts infants to sleep by diffusing other noises. A radio set on low, a clock ticking, an indoor water fountain, or the sound of a dishwasher, dryer, or even a vacuum cleaner may be effective. Tapes of sounds heard in utero are available and work best if introduced in the first week of life.

Heat. A well-covered warm water bottle placed against the infant's abdomen may be soothing. (Take care not to burn the infant's skin.) A blanket warmed in the clothes dryer for a few minutes serves the same purpose. Do not use a heating pad. Placing the newborn in an infant seat on top of a dishwasher or clothes dryer provides heat and background noise. Be sure that the infant is well secured, of course.

Bathing. Although older infants love baths, young infants may not yet have reached that stage. However, giving a bath may be a distraction for both parent and infant, and the infant may sleep afterward.

Water. Infants who have been crying may be thirsty. Although extra water is not necessary, some mothers like to give it on occasion. It may help bring up bubbles of air that the infant has swallowed while crying. The breastfed infant's thirst can be alleviated by nursing.

Infant Carriers or Packs. Front carriers are designed for the young infant and may be especially helpful during crying episodes. A parent's warm body, soothing voice, and gentle swaying motion can often put an infant to sleep. At the same time, the parent can accomplish other tasks. Backpacks should be used only for older infants who are able to support the head alone.

Pacifiers. Parents may find pacifiers useful for an irritable infant. The infant may be comforted by sucking even though not hungry.

Position Changes. Try varying the infant's position. Laying the infant prone across a parent's lap (or over a warmed blanket) may help expel gas. Try the "colic holds" (Figure 23-7) to help the infant pass gas. Placing the infant in a supine position and flexing the knees on the abdomen may also help.

Mother's Diet. Breastfeeding mothers should review their diet. Some infants react when the mother's diet includes cow's milk, orange juice, foods in the cabbage family, onion, or chocolate. Others react to highly acidic or spicy foods. Caffeine passes into breast milk and can cause wakefulness and irritability. Omit the suspected food for 5 to 7 days; then try it again and watch for irritability after the next feedings to identify the cause of the crying.

Massage. Gentle massage may be soothing for some infants. Massage of the abdomen may help infants with colic.

Smoking. Ask anyone in the home who smokes to do so away from the infant, preferably outside.

A 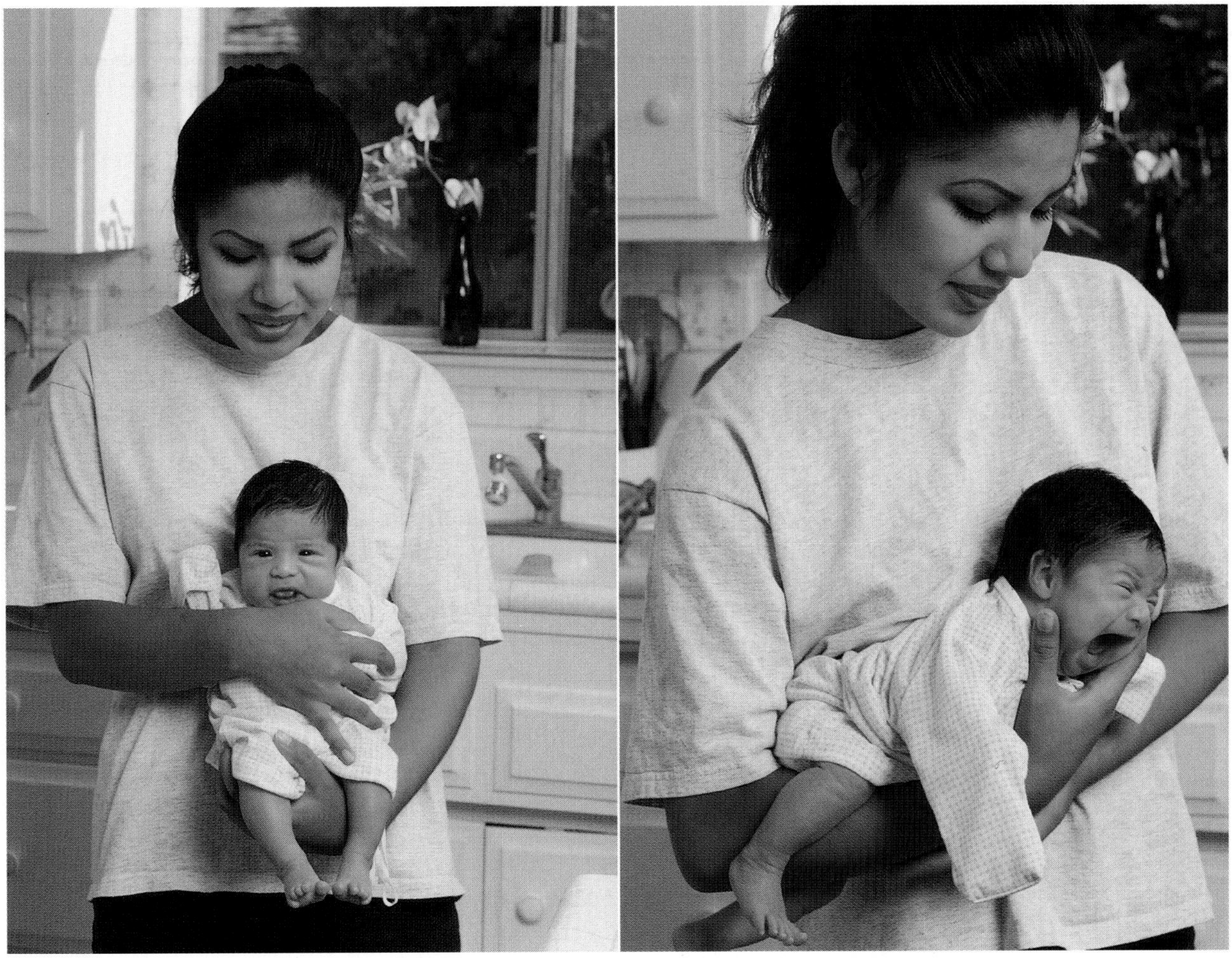 B

FIGURE 23-7 Positions for holding an infant with colic. **A,** The mother holds the infant facing forward. One hand creates slight pressure against the abdomen, while the other flexes the legs. This position may help the infant expel flatus. **B,** The prone hold is also effective for some infants. The mother holds the infant in a horizontal position along her arm.

Therapeutic Communication

Coping with Crying

Shannon Gray tells the nurse, Mark Winston, about her daughter, Marina, who has been having crying spells every day lasting 4 hours or longer. Shannon looks tired and worried. Marina, age 4 weeks, eats well, shows good weight gain, and is developing appropriately for her age.

Shannon: It seems like I can't do anything anymore, except try to stop Marina's crying.

Mark: You spend a lot of time trying to find ways to comfort her.

(Paraphrasing to encourage the mother to continue)

Shannon: I've tried everything! I rock her, walk with her, feed and change her. We go for car rides and put her in her swing, but nothing works for long. She just starts crying again.

Mark: It's so frustrating when nothing seems to work!

(Reflecting mother's feelings shows that the nurse is trying to understand them.)

Shannon: Sometimes I wonder if I was cut out to be a mother. I never thought it would be like this.

Mark: Being a mother is so much harder than you expected that sometimes you aren't sure you made the right choice.

(Reflecting the content of what the mother said helps her focus and shows acceptance.)

Shannon: But I really do love her. I just don't know how to help her. I must be a terrible mother (becomes teary).

Mark: Parents often feel guilty when they can't find a way to help an upset baby. And yet, we really don't know all the reasons why babies cry. You've tried very hard to help Marina. Maybe we can work together to think of some other techniques to use.

(Gives reassurance that what the mother is feeling is normal, then offers information and further help)

Shannon: I'd love that. It worries me to have Marina so unhappy. What else can I do for her?

PARENTS WANT TO KNOW ***How to Help Infants Sleep Through the Night***

Allow the infant to cry for a few minutes before responding. The infant may not be completely awake and often returns to sleep if undisturbed.

Keep night feedings for feeding only. Avoid unnecessary activity, or the infant may learn to think of this as a playtime.

Use a soft light that provides only the amount of light essential for care.

Give night feedings in the infant's room to further avoid stimulation.

Keep sounds subdued. Soft music or humming may help the infant return to sleep, but talking should be kept to a minimum.

Keep night feedings short, and put the infant back to bed immediately.

Change diapers in the middle of the feeding to avoid awakening the infant after feeding.

As the infants near 12 weeks, when sleeping through the night is more likely, try patting them on the back instead of feeding. Offer water instead of milk.

Allow infants to fall asleep at bedtime on their own instead of always rocking or feeding the infant. This may help infants go back to sleep alone after awakening in the night.

Nurses can help prevent shaken baby syndrome by making parents aware of the danger in shaking infants and by helping them learn methods to cope with infant crying. Birth facilities often include pamphlets and other information on shaken baby syndrome with discharge teaching. Further information on child abuse may be found in pediatrics textbooks.

Check Your Reading

5. Why should parents respond to crying without fear of spoiling the infant?
6. How can nurses help parents of crying infants?

Sleep

Parents

During the early months after birth, parents often wonder whether they will ever get a full night's sleep again. Because they are so often up during the night, they should try to make up lost sleep at other times. If the mother is not employed, she may be able to sleep during the day when the infant naps. If she is working, parents can alternate responsibility for night or early morning feedings. When mothers are breastfeeding, fathers can change the diaper, bring the infant to the mother for night feedings, and then settle the infant back in bed when the feeding is finished. This allows the mother more time to sleep and shares the middle-of-the-night care.

Infant Sleep Patterns

Infants spend less time than adults in deep sleep. They have a larger percentage of lighter rapid eye movement (REM) sleep. During this type of sleep, they make noises loud enough to wake parents in the same room, and they move about as if awakening. Going to them at this time is likely to wake them, but they may return to deep sleep if left alone.

Infants should be positioned on the back for sleep. The nurse should explain to parents that the prone position has been associated with sudden infant death syndrome (SIDS). No pillows or soft stuffed animals should be allowed in the crib, because they could cause suffocation. Some infants sleep better in an enclosed space and may scoot themselves into a corner of a large crib. The nurse should suggest to parents that they use rolled blankets around the infant to provide a "nest," which feels more like the circumscribed area of the uterus.

Sleeping Through the Night

Parents are often confused about when infants should sleep through the night. Newborns are neurologically unable to sleep through the night during the early weeks of life. By 12 weeks of age, many infants sleep at least 5 hours at night and most infants sleep that long by 4 months. By 12 months of age, infants take two naps during the day and sleep about 10 hours at night (Grover, 2000b).

Once infants establish longer sleep patterns, they often awaken at night again when they are teething or ill. Therefore parents can expect to be awakened frequently during the early years. Parents should be taught methods of helping infants achieve longer sleep periods at night.

Concerns of Working Mothers

Although it has been traditional for women who work to have at least 6 weeks of maternity leave, this is not always possible. Some women must return to work as early as 3 weeks after childbirth. The problems of working mothers are different from those of mothers who remain at home. They must find adequate child care, identify methods of managing the household, and try to find enough time and energy to meet the needs of the infant, other family members, and themselves (see Chapter 18, p. 463).

Working mothers should not become so involved in their many responsibilities that they have little time for their own needs. Some mothers regularly schedule time for themselves and for family activities. Many working mothers find that the time they can spend with their infant is particularly precious.

Concerns of Adoptive Parents

Although adoptive parents have not experienced pregnancy and childbirth, they must make adjustments similar to those of biologic parents. In some adoptive situations, the parents meet the biologic mother during pregnancy and may even be with her during birth. Other adoptive parents receive a call after months of waiting telling them that their new infant is ready for them. In either case, the lives of the parents abruptly change.

> **CRITICAL THINKING EXERCISE**
>
> Mary and Raymond Reynolds received their adopted daughter, Ashley, 3 days ago. They bring the 6-day-old infant to the pediatrician's office and discuss their concerns with the nurse. They received basic discharge teaching at the hospital where Ashley was born but have many questions about infant care. The last two nights Ashley slept very little, and both parents are exhausted, "We've waited so long to get Ashley," Mary says, "but I'm beginning to wonder if she's all right and if I'll be a good mother."
>
> QUESTIONS:
> 1. What are the priorities in this situation?
> 2. How should the nurse support Mary and Raymond?
> 3. What information should the nurse include in teaching these parents?
> 4. How should the nurse deal with Ashley's night wakefulness?

In some agencies, adoptive parents receive the same teaching given to other parents. However, their ability to absorb information may be impaired by the excitement of the situation. Although adoptive mothers have not been pregnant or undergone childbirth, they are still tired from the loss of sleep and sudden changes that they experience. This may be surprising and worrisome to some. They have many questions that nurses can answer.

Adoptive parents sometimes feel the need to be more perfect than biologic parents do and may feel guilt if they do not meet their own expectations. These parents need reassurance and emotional support as they go through this happy but exhausting change in their lives.

COMMON QUESTIONS AND CONCERNS

Dressing and Warmth

A room temperature of about 70° F is warm enough for the infant. The infant should be dressed as the parents would like to be dressed, with a receiving blanket added. The abdomen should be checked to see if the infant is warm enough. The hands and feet are slightly cooler than the rest of the body but should not be mottled or blue. The infant's head should be kept warm because many thermal skin sensors are located in the scalp. A hat is appropriate if the infant is outside when it is cold or windy.

Stool Patterns

Formula-fed infants generally pass at least one stool each day. Breastfed infants may pass a stool after every feeding or, occasionally in the older infant, only 1 every 2 to 3 days. Infants may get red in the face and appear to be straining when having a bowel movement, but this is normal behavior and does not indicate constipation. Stools that are dry, hard, and marble-like indicate constipation.

Watery stools indicate diarrhea. A watery stool is absorbed into the diaper with little or no solid material left at the surface. A "water ring" remains on the diaper, showing where the liquid was absorbed. Diarrhea stools occur more frequently than the infant's normal stools and are greenish from bile moving quickly through the intestines. Diarrhea can be serious because life-threatening dehydration develops quickly. Infants should be taken to the pediatrician or nurse practitioner for treatment.

Smoking

Many mothers quit smoking before or during pregnancy but may not realize that preventing infant exposure to smoke is just as important after birth as before. Infants exposed to smoke from parents' cigarettes are more likely to develop frequent respiratory problems. Smoking is a risk factor in SIDS. Smoke absorption by infants occurs even when smoking is done in another room. Parents who continue to smoke should do so outside the house and away from the infant.

Eyes

Parents can wipe away small amounts of mucus that accumulate in the corners of the eyes with a damp, clean washcloth. A large amount of mucus, redness, or excessive tearing indicates an infection or a blocked lacrimal duct. The infant should be seen by the pediatrician or nurse practitioner.

Transient strabismus, or crossing of the eyes, can be frightening to parents. The nurse should reassure them that this is normal for infants for the first few months, until they gain control of the small muscles of the eye. It does not indicate that the infant will have later problems.

Baths

Sponge and tub bathing are discussed in Chapter 21 (p. 568), as is care of the cord (p. 568) and the circumcision site (p. 565). If the infant is washed well at diaper changes and when milk is regurgitated, bathing the child every day is not necessary. Bathing should be a time for infant stimulation and parent-infant interaction. It can be done at any time of the day that is convenient for parents.

Nails

Nails should be cut straight across with either blunt-ended scissors or clippers. The edges can be carefully smoothed with an emery board. Mothers should not attempt to cut nails too short because this increases the danger of cutting the infant's fingertip. Some mothers prefer to cut nails while the infant is sleeping. Others have someone else hold the hand steady while the mother cuts the nails. Nails grow rapidly and may need trimming twice a week.

Sucking Needs

Parents often have questions about pacifiers and thumb or finger sucking. Nurses should explain that all infants have an urge to suck, although the amount of sucking needed varies with individual infants. Some seem satisfied by feedings, but others suck their hands or a pacifier even when not hungry.

Parents may be concerned that sucking a pacifier or thumb will cause the teeth to become maloccluded. The nurse should reassure them that sucking that ends before the secondary teeth begin to erupt is unlikely to cause malocclusion (Berkowitz, 2000b). Trying to stop an infant from sucking is difficult and may cause emotional problems if it becomes a major focus.

Some infants increase nonnutritive sucking because the time they spend sucking during feedings is too short. Using bottle nipples with small holes and replacing the nipples every couple of months before they get soft increase the amount of sucking that feedings provide. Breastfed infants should be allowed to continue sucking at the breast long enough to meet basic sucking needs. A short time of sucking after the infant is finished feeding generally satisfies sucking needs and increases production of milk.

When infants use a pacifier, parents should be instructed to examine it often to see if it is in good condition. Cracked, torn, or sticky nipples or nipples that can be pulled away from the shield should be discarded. Pacifiers should be replaced every month or two because they may come apart as they deteriorate and cause aspiration of parts.

Pacifiers should be kept clean by frequent washing, and parents should buy several so that one is always clean when needed. Pacifiers should never be placed on a string around the infant's neck. The string could become tangled tightly around the neck and cause strangulation. Clips with a short band to attach pacifiers to the infant's clothing without danger are available or several pacifiers can be placed in the bed for the infant to find.

Some parents find that an advantage to a pacifier is that the infant gives it up more quickly than a thumb or finger because it is not so easily accessible. Parents who resort to the pacifier as the first response when the infant is fussy are likely to reinforce its use and increase dependence on it. Pacifiers used only after other causes of distress are ruled out may be given up sooner. Because the need for nonnutritive sucking begins to diminish between 4 and 6 months of age, pacifier use may begin to decrease at that time with parents' help.

Teething

The timing of tooth eruption varies. The first tooth may appear as early as 3 months or as late as 13 months of age. Generally the two lower central incisors come through the gums at about 6 to 8 months. The average age for eruption of all deciduous teeth is 2½ years.

The actual time when teeth erupt has no relationship to the infant's development in other areas. Parents may think that teething has begun when the infant is about 3 months of age, when the normal increased production of saliva causes drooling. Infants must learn to swallow the extra saliva without drooling.

Some infants show signs of teething for weeks before the first tooth comes through the gums. These signs include excessive salivation, biting, irritability, slight fever, and decreased feedings. Many infants who were sleeping through the night begin to wake again as a result of teething discomfort. A rash around the mouth may result from drooling. The infant's gums may look red and swollen over the area where the tooth will erupt.

Instruct parents that high fevers or other signs of illness are not normal symptoms of teething. Infants may be more susceptible to illness at the time of teething because of poor eating and sleeping. In addition, teething begins at about the time many of the antibodies received in utero are disappearing.

Some teething infants like to bite on hard objects such as teething rings. Some rings can be frozen to soothe inflammation of the gums. Over-the-counter local anesthetics or analgesics, such as acetaminophen, are safe in small amounts for teething discomfort. Alcoholic beverages should never be rubbed on the gums because infants swallow the alcohol.

Common Rashes

Diaper Rash

Diaper rash occurs as a result of prolonged exposure of skin to wetness combined with a chemical reaction between the urine and fecal enzymes that increases skin sensitivity to irritation. A rash is more likely to develop when infants begin to sleep for longer periods and the time between diaper changes increases. Another cause may be sensitivity to commercial disposable washcloths or components of paper diapers.

Treatment of diaper rash is primarily keeping the diaper area clean and dry. The nurse should instruct the parents to change diapers as soon as they are wet or soiled. They should gently wash the perineum with mild soap and warm water, avoiding excessive washing. Removing the diapers and exposing the perineum to warm air helps healing.

Applying a thin layer of creams such as those with zinc oxide may speed healing and help prevent further outbreaks. The nurse should tell parents not to apply the ointments too thickly because they may be difficult to remove. Ointments contaminated with fecal matter may accumulate in the skin folds and hold bacteria. Low-potency corticosteroid preparations may be necessary for severe cases.

Severe rash or pustules or crusted areas signal infection. The infant should be taken to a pediatrician or nurse practitioner for treatment. *Staphylococcus* or *Candida albicans* are common causes of infections. Antifungal or antibiotic creams may be necessary for infections.

Miliaria (Prickly Heat)

Although most common during hot weather, miliaria or prickly heat develops in infants who are too warmly dressed in any weather. This rash is due to occlusion and inflammation of the sweat (eccrine) glands. It has a red base with papules or vesicles in the center.

Treatment is cooling the infant by removing excess clothing or by giving a soothing lukewarm bath. The condition clears quickly with removal of the cause, and ointments or other skin preparations should be avoided. The nurse should discuss the appropriate amount of clothing with parents when infants develop prickly heat.

Seborrheic Dermatitis (Cradle Cap)

Cradle cap is a chronic inflammation of the scalp or other areas of the skin characterized by yellow, scaly, oily lesions. It sometimes results when parents do not wash over the anterior fontanelle carefully for fear that they will hurt the infant.

Treatment is application of oil or shampoo to the area to help the lesions soften, then removal with a comb before shampooing the head. The nurse should teach parents how to shampoo the scalp and explain that they will not damage the fontanelle by normal gentle shampooing. The scalp should be rinsed well to remove all soap, which otherwise may cause irritation.

Check Your Reading

7. What are common signs of teething?
8. How can parents prevent or treat diaper rash?

NUTRITION DURING THE EARLY WEEKS

Infant feeding is discussed in detail in Chapter 22. This section addresses only the most frequent early concerns parents have about feeding.

Breastfeeding

Breastfeeding mothers should be taught not to set a strict timetable but to feed the infant when signs of hunger are present. This will be more often than if the infant were formula fed, about every 2 to 3 hours. Generally, feedings should last at least 15 minutes initially (see Chapter 22). As nursing becomes well established, mothers often feed approximately 15 minutes on the first side and then continue on the second side as long as the infant is interested. The feeding concludes when the infant falls asleep or after a short period of nonnutritive suckling.

The total time for each breastfeeding session varies with individual infants and from feeding to feeding. The time may be as short as 20 minutes or as long as 40 minutes. As infants become older, they become more efficient at nursing and obtain all the milk they need in a shorter period.

Mothers may be concerned when an infant suddenly seems fussy and wants to breastfeed much more often than previously. This is frequently a way of increasing milk production for an infant experiencing a growth spurt. Nurses can teach mothers to expect growth spurts at approximately 10 days, 2 weeks, 6 weeks, and 3 months after birth (Grodner, Anderson, & DeYoung, 2000).

Formula Feeding

Mothers using formula may be unsure about how much to feed the infant during the early weeks after birth. Although infants take about 1 ounce at a time during the first day or two of life, this rapidly increases to 2 or 3 ounces per feeding in the first 2 weeks. By 12 weeks they usually drink 5 to 6 ounces every 3 to 4 hours. Considerable variation is seen between infants, and mothers should be encouraged to adapt to their own infant's needs.

Formula-fed infants generally eat every 3 to 4 hours. Strict schedules are unnecessary and the mother should feed the infant when signs of hunger appear. Fussiness or crying, rooting, sucking on hands, and eagerly taking the bottle indicate that the infant is hungry.

Mothers should not urge infants to drink all of the formula if they do not seem interested. Infants vary, as adults do, in the amount taken at each meal. Encouraging the infant to complete all feedings places undue emphasis on the feeding and may lead to later feeding problems or obesity.

Water

Both formula and breast milk contain enough water for infants who are eating well. Additional water is not necessary. Some mothers give water to formula-fed infants who are fussy and do not respond to other interventions. Sips of water also can be given to infants with hiccups. Hiccups go away shortly, with or without water, however.

Infants should not be given water with sugar added. Sugar only adds empty calories and accustoms them to the sweet taste. Honey should never be used for young infants because of the risk of botulism.

Regurgitation

Infants often regurgitate ("spit up") because they may eat more than their stomach can easily hold and because their immature lower esophageal sphincter allows the stomach contents to flow into the esophagus easily. "Wet burps" result when air is trapped under stomach contents. As the air is expelled, a small amount of milk comes with it.

The nurse should teach parents to differentiate normal spitting up from vomiting, which is a sign of illness. Regurgitation may occur frequently, but usually only a small amount at a time. Vomiting may involve the entire feeding and it is expelled forcefully. Parents should always seek treatment for the infant with projectile vomiting, in which the vomitus is expelled with such force that it travels some distance. This is a sign of pyloric stenosis, which may require surgery.

If an infant has frequent regurgitation, parents can elevate the head of the bed or use an infant seat after feedings to help air rise and to decrease regurgitation. Turning the infant to the side promotes drainage of regurgitated fluids and prevents aspiration.

Some infants swallow excessive air because they eat very rapidly. Nurses can instruct parents to feed infants before they get too hungry and to stop often for burping. If the hole in a bottle nipple is too small, an infant may swallow air around the nipple. Enlarging the nipple hole slightly with a hot needle may prevent this.

Some infants experience reflux because of the flow of liquids across a dilated lower esophageal sphincter. Approximately 85% of these infants have vomiting within the first week of life. The condition improves in 60% of infants by age 2 years (Herbst, 2000). The infant who has excessive regurgitation or vomiting should be referred for follow-up with the pediatrician or nurse practitioner.

Introduction of Solid Foods

Infants do not need solid foods until 4 to 6 months of age. Some mothers introduce solids earlier in the hope that the infant will sleep longer at night. This is seldom successful because the infant receives no more calories from the small amounts of solids taken than from milk. In addition, early introduction of solids may precipitate allergies or cause intestinal upsets because they are incompletely digested. When infants start solids, they drink less milk, thus replacing a food that meets their nutrient needs well with a food that is poorly digested.

The extrusion reflex, in which infants push the tongue out against anything that touches it, continues until approximately 4 months of age. This makes feeding a younger infant difficult because the infant pushes almost all of every spoonful out of the mouth. The nurse should explain the problems involved with early introduction of solid foods and encourage parents to wait until the infant is physiologically ready, at 4 to 6 months of age. The concerns that made the parents consider changing the feeding routine should also be discussed.

Weaning

Some mothers decide to wean the infant from the breast to the bottle during the first 12 weeks after birth. Information about weaning is included in Chapter 22, p. 599.

Check Your Reading

9. How much should infants eat during the early weeks after birth?
10. Why should solid foods be avoided until the infant is 4 to 6 months old?

GROWTH AND DEVELOPMENT

Anticipatory Guidance

Parents often have questions about normal patterns of growth and stages of development. Nurses provide anticipatory guidance about these areas to help parents develop realistic expectations about infants' abilities at various ages. This also helps parents prepare for changes they must make to keep the infant's environment safe, especially during the second half of the first year of life, when the infant begins to explore the house alone.

Growth and Developmental Milestones

A brief summary of the changes that can be expected during the infant's first 12 weeks is included here. More in-depth information is included in pediatrics textbooks. The nurse should emphasize to parents that guidelines are only averages, the range of normal is often broad, and individual differences are expected.

During the first 6 months of life, growth proceeds at a predictable rate in normal infants. The weight lost after birth is usually regained by 10 days of age. Each month during the first 3 months, the average infant gains approximately 900 g (2 pounds), grows 3.5 cm

(1.4 inches), and has an increase in head circumference of 2 cm (0.8 inch). The posterior fontanelle closes by 2 to 3 months and the anterior fontanelle closes by 12 to 18 months of age. Tears appear 2 to 4 weeks after birth.

The Moro, grasp, tonic neck, and rooting reflexes especially are noticed by parents. The nurse should point out that their gradual disappearance helps prepare the infant to learn new skills, such as voluntary grasping or turning over, which are impossible if the reflexes continue. The infant gradually develops more control of the heavy head and has less bobbing or head lag by the end of the third month of life.

Infants are social beings. They stare at objects of interest within a range of 8 to 12 inches as newborns and learn to follow objects by turning the head a full 180 degrees during the first 12 weeks of life. A social smile begins as early as 3 to 5 weeks and is well developed by 6 to 8 weeks. Infants make vowel sounds (cooing) by 2 months and begin some consonant sounds (babbling) and may even squeal with delight at 3 months.

Accident Prevention

Knowing what infants can do helps prevent accidents. In the first 3 months after birth, they are totally helpless. Although they can communicate their needs through crying, someone must be available at all times to care for them. Parents must be taught the dangers of leaving the infant on any unprotected surface even for seconds. In a short time, an infant can wiggle from the middle to the edge of a large bed and fall. Crib sides should be raised whenever the infant is in bed. Cribs should be positioned away from hanging cords of blinds or drapes because these could become wrapped around an active infant and cause strangulation.

Parents should keep one hand on an infant lying on an unprotected surface if they must turn away. Infants should never be left for an instant in even an inch of water because of the danger of drowning. Parents should take the telephone off the hook and ignore the doorbell when bathing the infant, or take the infant out of the water and with them if they must leave the room.

As infants learn to grasp objects with increasing accuracy, parents must be certain that nothing is in the infant's reach that could be swallowed or otherwise cause harm. Help parents to think ahead to the time when the infant will be crawling and walking and make plans for how they will "child proof" their home.

WELL-BABY CARE

Well-Baby Checkups

Well-baby checkups are an opportunity for the pediatrician or nurse practitioner to assess the infant's growth and development, answer questions about feeding and infant care, observe for abnormalities, and give immunizations. These checkups may be provided by a private practitioner or in a well-baby clinic, where examinations and immunizations are free or at reduced cost. Infants are usually taken to their first well-baby checkup at 2 to 4 weeks of age. They generally receive well-baby checkups at 2, 4, 6, 9, and 12 months of age.

Well-baby checkups are a good time for mothers to learn about what is normal for their infants in terms of growth and behaviors. Anticipatory guidance is a major part of well-baby visits. Many mothers are reassured to find that such problems as wakefulness at night or changes in feeding habits are normal. Safety is discussed as the parents learn about skills infants will soon learn that might place them in danger.

Immunizations

Nurses often receive questions about the need for immunizations for uncommon diseases, such as diphtheria, that parents have never seen. Parents may consider a condition such as chickenpox to be a harmless childhood illness. When they do not understand the need for immunizations, parents may be reluctant to have their infants undergo painful procedures.

The nurse must explain to parents the importance of immunizations, briefly describing the serious illnesses immunizations prevent. Discuss the age at which each immunization is given and when boosters are needed (Table 23-3). A new vaccine that has recently been added to those recommended for infants prevents pneumococcal infections, which can cause serious illness in infants and young children (AAP, 2000a).

In the United States, national health objectives for the year 2010 include full immunization of at least 90% of children before the age of 3 years. In 1998 more than 90% of children under 3 years received Hib, MMR, and polio vaccines. Levels are much lower for varicella at 43% (USDHHS, 2000). Maintaining high levels of immunization rates is important to prevent the rise of communicable diseases, as happened in the late 1980s, when a resurgence of measles occurred in many U.S. communities.

Common reactions to immunizations should also be discussed with the parents. For example, infants may develop a fever and local tenderness after administration of vaccines. Many care providers suggest that infants receive acetaminophen at the time of the vaccine to decrease the reaction and increase comfort.

In addition to immunizations, infants also receive a tuberculin skin test at 12 to 15 months and every 1 to 2 years thereafter. This is to detect exposure to tuberculosis to allow early treatment when the disease is most treatable.

Because recommendations for immunizations change from time to time, parents should be referred to their pediatrician for the latest information. Another source is the American Academy of Pediatrics, which offers Internet information for parents as well as professionals. The Internet address is http://www.aap.org.

Table 23-3
RECOMMENDED IMMUNIZATION SCHEDULE FOR THE FIRST SIX YEARS

Immunization	Age for Original Immunization	Age for Booster
HBV (hepatitis B)	Birth-2 months, 1-4 months, 6-18 months*†	
DTaP (diphtheria, tetanus, and acellular pertussis)	2, 4, 6 months	15-18 months‡, 4-6 years
Hib (*Haemophilus influenzae* type b)	2, 4, 6 months or 2, 4 months§	12-15 months
Injectable polio vaccine‖	2, 4 months	6-18 months, 4-6 years
MMR (measles, mumps, rubella)	12-15 months	4-6 years¶
Varicella-zoster virus vaccine	12-18 months or at any time after 12 months	
Pneumococcal vaccine	2, 4, 6 months	12-15 months

From Advisory Committee on Immunization Practices of the Centers for Disease Control and Prevention, the American Academy of Pediatrics Committee on Infectious Diseases, and the American Academy of Family Physicians (2000) data.
*Infants of HBsAg negative mothers receive the first dose by age 2 months, the second dose at least 1 month following the first dose, and the third dose at least 4 months after the first dose and at least 2 months after the second dose, but not before the infant is 6 months of age.
†Newborns whose mothers are HBsAg positive should receive hepatitis B immune globulin and the first hepatitis B vaccine within 12 hours of birth and at different sites. The second dose of vaccine is at 1 to 2 months of age and third dose at 6 months. If the mother's HBsAg status is unknown, the infant is vaccinated within 12 hours of birth and hepatitis immune globulin is given as soon as possible (within 1 week) if testing shows the mother is positive.
‡The fourth dose may be given as early as 12 months of age if 6 months have passed since the third dose and if the child is unlikely to return at age 15 to 18 months.
§The number of doses of Hib depends on the vaccine used.
‖Injectable polio vaccine is now recommended for all routine polio vaccination of children.
¶The second dose of MMR may be given at any time at least 4 weeks after the first dose if necessary as long as both doses are after 12 months of age.

Check Your Reading

11. How can parents make use of knowledge about infant development to prevent accidents in the first 12 weeks of life?
12. What is the importance of well-baby checkups?
13. Why are immunizations important?

ILLNESS

Parents have many questions about illness in the infant. They have concerns about how to recognize an illness and when to call the pediatrician or nurse practitioner.

Recognizing Signs

Parents may need help in recognizing signs of illness in infants (Table 23-4). The nurse should explain that any time the infant appears sick or parents believe that something is wrong with the infant, they should call the pediatrician or nurse practitioner. Office staff are usually educated to help parents determine if the infant is sick enough to be seen.

Table 23-4
COMMON SIGNS OF ILLNESS IN INFANTS

Fever above 100° F axillary
Vomiting all of a feeding more than once or twice in a day
Watery stools or significant increase in number of stools over what is normal for the infant
Blisters, sores, or rashes that are unusual for the infant
Unusual changes in behavior: listlessness or sleeping much more than usual, irritability or crying much more than usual
Coughing, frequent sneezing, runny nose. (*Note:* Occasional sneezing may be due to lint from new clothes or blankets.)
Pulling or rubbing at the ear, drainage from the ear

Calling the Pediatrician or Nurse Practitioner

When calling the pediatrician or nurse practitioner about an illness, parents should prepare by writing down the information about the illness to avoid forgetting something. They should have the name and telephone number of a pharmacy available in case a prescription drug is needed, and they should be ready to write down instructions (Table 23-5).

Office staff are usually able to answer questions on the telephone about common concerns and simple illnesses. They can help determine if an infant should be brought into the office, but parents should be assertive in asking for an appointment if they believe that one is needed. They have a more complete picture of the infant's condition than can be given over the telephone. Parents should immediately identify emergencies so that the staff can act accordingly. Parents can expect the pediatrician or nurse practitioner to return calls about acute illness as soon as possible and those about other concerns near the end of the day.

Table 23-5

CALLING THE PEDIATRICIAN OR NURSE PRACTITIONER

Write down pertinent information before calling. Have your pharmacy name and telephone number handy and a pen and paper to write down instructions.

1. Give the infant's name and age first.
2. Describe the illness or problem.
   a. When did it start?
   b. How often does it occur (the number of times the infant vomits or passes a stool)?
   c. How does this compare with the infant's normal patterns?
   d. What does it look like? Describe the rash or the color and consistency of the stools.
3. Describe any fever.
   a. How high is it?
   b. Was it taken by axillary or rectal method?
   c. How long has the fever been present?
   d. Has it been higher than it is now?
4. Describe other signs of illness.
   a. Has eating behavior changed?
   b. Have sleep patterns changed?
5. Describe the infant's behavior.
   a. Does the infant seem sick?
   b. Is the infant irritable, lethargic, acting differently from normal?
6. Describe what has been done so far to treat the condition and the results.
7. Discuss other relevant information.
   a. Is there a similar illness in family members?
   b. Was the infant treated recently for a similar or different illness?
   c. Does the infant take any other medications?

Knowing When to Seek Immediate Help

Parents should take the infant to the pediatrician or to an emergency room if signs of dyspnea are present. An infant from birth to 3 months of age should not have a sustained respiratory rate above 60 breaths per minute. If retractions, cyanosis, or extreme pallor is present, parents should get immediate help. If respiratory difficulty occurs suddenly in an infant who is well, the infant may have aspirated a feeding or small object. Parents should call paramedics. Nurses should encourage all parents to take classes in cardiopulmonary resuscitation.

If an infant's respiratory rate is below 30, parents should stimulate the infant and see if the respirations increase and stay within the normal range of 30 to 60 breaths per minute. If the respiratory rate continues to be below normal, the infant should be seen by a pediatrician or nurse practitioner.

Parents should call the pediatrician if the infant is hard to arouse and keep awake. The infant could be semi-comatose and showing signs of central nervous system disease such as meningitis or encephalitis.

Learning About Sudden Infant Death Syndrome

Sudden infant death syndrome is the abrupt death of an infant that is unexplained by autopsy, examination of the scene of death, or history. In the United States, more than 2500 SIDS deaths occur each year. Although the incidence has decreased, SIDS is the third leading cause of death between birth and 1 year of age (Guyer, et al., 1999). It is the leading cause of infant deaths after the age of 1 month, accounting for 30% of infant deaths in this age range (USDHHS, 2000).

Sudden infant death syndrome occurs in apparently healthy infants during sleep, more often in males and during cold weather. It peaks between 2 to 4 months of age. In the United States, Native Americans and African-Americans have the highest rates of SIDS. The lowest rates occur in Asians and Latinos. The reasons for these differences are not known.

Although there have been many studies, the cause of SIDS remains unknown. Maternal smoking, young maternal age, late or no prenatal care, prematurity, low birth weight, low socioeconomic status, and maternal drug abuse are some of the factors that have been associated with SIDS. Associations have been found between SIDS and infants sleeping in the prone position, sleeping on a soft surface, overheating, and sleeping in the same bed with another person.

Current recommendations are that a healthy infant be placed in a supine position for sleep because the prone position may increase the risk of upper airway obstruction, rebreathing expired air, and hyperthermia. A 40% decrease in deaths from SIDS has occurred in the United States since 1992, when the change in position was recommended (AAP, 2000b). A national goal for the year 2010 is to reduce the number of SIDS death by increasing the number of infants put down to sleep on their backs to at least 70% (USDHHS, 2000).

Although the side position is also associated with a decreased incidence of SIDS, infants who sleep on their sides are more likely to have SIDS than those who sleep in the supine position. If infants are placed in the side position for sleep, the lower arm should be brought forward to lessen the chance the infant will roll into the prone position. The recommendation for supine positioning for sleep applies to all infants, regardless of their birth weight or gestational age, unless other circumstances necessitate an exception (AAP, 2000b).

Nurses should teach parents about proper positioning of their infants for sleep. Other modifiable factors that should receive increased parent education are not allowing infants to become overheated or to sleep on a soft surface and avoiding maternal smoking. Objects such as pillows, comforters, and loose bedding may be hazardous. Blankets should be tucked under the mattress so that they are not likely to cover the infant's face.

Because parents often have many concerns about SIDS, therapeutic communication techniques may assist them to talk about their fears. They may need reassurance that the chance that any one infant will experience SIDS is small.

Check Your Reading

14. When should immediate help be sought for an infant?
15. What should nurses teach parents about SIDS?

SUMMARY CONCEPTS

- Nurses assist parents after discharge by home or clinic visits and telephone calls.
- Careful planning, good communication skills, and knowledge of cultural practices are necessary during home visits.
- Clinic visits include the same assessment and teaching as home visits but do not allow the nurse to assess the home. They are more cost effective, however.
- Telephone calls after discharge from the birth facility are less expensive than home or clinic visits but do not allow the nurse to assess the client or home environment in person.
- All equipment, particularly older, used articles, should be checked by parents for safety.
- Infants under 1 year or 20 pounds should use a rear-facing car seat. Older infants need car seats that face forward. All should be placed in the back seat of the car.
- Crying is a major source of concern for parents. They should be reassured that infants are not spoiled by prompt attention to their needs.
- Colic, crying lasting 3 or more hours, usually occurs in the afternoon or evening and often disappears after 3 months. The cause is unknown, and infants with colic grow and develop appropriately.
- Infants may sleep 5 or more hours at night beginning about 12 weeks.
- Common signs of teething include drooling, irritability, decreased appetite and sleep, rash, and red and swollen gums. High fever or other signs of illness are not due to teething.
- Diaper rash may be caused by prolonged exposure to wet or soiled diapers or sensitivity to substances in diapers or disposable wash cloths. It can become infected.
- Both breastfed and formula-fed infants vary in amounts taken at each feeding but average about 1 ounce per feeding initially and 5 to 6 ounces per feeding at 12 weeks of age.
- Solid foods should be started at 4 to 6 months of age when the extrusion reflex is gone and solids can be digested by infants.
- Well-baby checkups are important for assessment of growth and development, guidance, and immunizations. Immunizations safeguard infants and communities from spread of communicable diseases.
- Parents should learn signs of illness in the infant and when immediate medical care is necessary. They should seek immediate medical attention if infants have respiratory difficulty or are difficult to arouse from sleep.
- The nurse should teach parents about current knowledge about SIDS and the fact that the cause remains unknown. Parents should be taught to place the infant in a supine position for sleep.

ANSWERS TO CRITICAL THINKING EXERCISE

1. The major priorities are to support the parents in their new role and to determine if Ashley is progressing normally.
2. Information should be based on the parent's concerns. Explain normal characteristics and behaviors of the newborn. Determine if Mary and Raymond need more information about basic infant care, such as feeding, sleeping, cord care, and signs of illness. Provide frequent opportunities for them to ask questions.
3. Obtain more information about Ashley's sleep patterns. Discuss normal sleep in newborns and methods of helping infants sleep. Offer suggestions for methods of dealing with crying. Help Mary and Raymond work out a plan for sharing the burdens and the joys of parenthood.
4. Use therapeutic communication techniques to allow Mary and Raymond to express their feelings adequately. If Ashley appears to be progressing normally, emphasize that she is doing well. Point out that the problems they are encountering are quite common for both biologic and adoptive parents.

REFERENCES & READINGS

American Academy of Pediatrics (AAP), Committee on Infectious Diseases. (2000a). Policy Statement: Recommendations for the prevention of pneumococcal infections, including the use of pneumococcal conjugate vaccine (Prevnar), pneumococcal polysaccharide vaccine, and antibiotic prophylaxis. *Pediatrics,* 106(2), 362-366.

American Academy of Pediatrics (AAP), Task Force on Infant Sleep Position and Sudden Infant Death Syndrome. (2000b). Changing concepts of Sudden Infant Death Syndrome: Implications for infant sleeping environment and sleep position. *Pediatrics,* 105(3), 650-656.

American Academy of Pediatrics (AAP). (1999). Safe transportation of newborns at hospital discharge. *Pediatrics,* 104(4), 986-987.

American Academy of Pediatrics (AAP) and American College of Obstetricians and Gynecologists (ACOG). (1997). *Guidelines for perinatal care* (4th ed.). Elk Grove, IL: American Academy of Pediatrics.

Association of Women's Health, Obstetric, and Neonatal Nurses. (2000). *Didactic content and clinical skills verification for professional nurse providers of perinatal home care* (2nd ed.). Washington, D.C.: Author.

Association of Women's Health, Obstetric, and Neonatal Nurses. (1998). *Standards & guidelines for professional nursing practice in the care of women and newborns* (5th ed.). Washington, D.C.: Author.

Berkowitz, C.D. (2000a). SIDS and ALTE. In C.D. Berkowitz, *Pediatrics: A primary care approach* (2nd ed., pp. 155-159). Philadelphia: W.B. Saunders.

Berkowitz, C.D. (2000b). Thumbsucking and other habits. In C.D. Berkowitz, *Pediatrics: A primary care approach* (2nd ed., pp. 127-131). Philadelphia: W.B. Saunders.

Brown, S.G. & Johnson, B.T. (1998). Enhancing early discharge with home follow-up: A pilot project. *Journal of Obstetric, Gynecologic, and Neonatal Nursing, 27*(1), 33-38.
Cady, R. (1999a). Pitfalls in telephone triage. *MCN: The American Journal of Maternal Child Nursing, 24*(3), 157.
Cady, R. (1999b). Telephone triage—Avoiding the pitfalls. *MCN: The American Journal of Maternal Child Nursing, 24*(4), 209.
Christian, A. (1996). Clinical nurse specialists: Creating new programs for neonatal home care. *Journal of Perinatal and Neonatal Nursing, 10*(1), 54-63.
Davis, L.J., Okuboye, S., & Ferguson, S.L. (2000). Healthy people 2010: Examining a decade of maternal & infant health. *AWHONN's Lifelines, 4*(3), 26-33.
Grodner, M., Anderson, S.L., & DeYoung, S. (2000). *Foundations and clinical applications of nutrition: A nursing approach* (2nd ed.). St. Louis: Mosby.
Grover, G. (2000a). Crying and colic. In C.D. Berkowitz (Ed.), *Pediatrics: A primary care approach* (2nd ed., pp. 111-114). Philadelphia: W.B. Saunders.
Grover, G. (2000b). Immunizations. In C.D. Berkowitz (Ed.), *Pediatrics: A primary care approach* (2nd ed., pp. 62-69). Philadelphia: W.B. Saunders.
Grover, G. (2000c). Sleep: Normal pattern and common disorders. In C.D. Berkowitz (Ed.), *Pediatrics: A primary care approach* (2nd ed., pp. 39-44). Philadelphia: W.B. Saunders.
Guyer, B., Hoyert, D.L., Martin, J.A., Ventura, S.J., MacDorman, M.F., & Strobino, D.M. (1999). Annual summary of vital statistics 1998, *Pediatrics, 104*(6), 1229-1245.
Herbst, J.J. (2000). Gastroesophageal reflux (chalasia). In R.E. Behrman, R.M. Kliegman, & A.M. Arvin (Eds.), *Nelson textbook of pediatrics* (16th ed., pp. 1125-1126). Philadelphia: W.B. Saunders.
Huffman, A.D., Smok-Pearsall, S.M., Silvestri, J.M., & Weese-Mayer, D.E. (1999). SIDS risk factor awareness: Assessment among nursing students. *Journal of Obstetric, Gynecologic, and Neonatal Nursing, 28*(1), 68-73.
Jacobson, B.B., Brock, K.A., & Keppler, A.B. (1999). The post birth partnership: Washington state's comprehensive approach to improve follow-up care. *Journal of Perinatal Neonatal Nursing, 13*(1), 43-52.
Johnson, T.S., Brennan, R.A., & Flynn-Tymkow, C.D. (1999). A home visit program for breastfeeding education and support. *Journal of Obstetric, Gynecologic, and Neonatal Nursing, 23*(5), 480-485.
Keefe, M.R., Kotzer, A.M., Froese-Fretz, A., & Curtin, M. (1996). A longitudinal comparison of irritable and nonirritable infants. *Nursing Research, 45*(1), 4-9.
Kemp, J.S., Unger, B., Wilkins, D., Psara, R. M., Ledbetter, T.L., Graham, M.A., Case, M., & Thach, B.T. (2000). Unsafe sleep practices and an analysis of bedsharing among infants dying suddenly and unexpectedly: Results of a four-year, population-based, death-scene investigation study of sudden infant death syndrome and related deaths. *Pediatrics, 106*(3), 41.
Kutner, L. (1999). The crying baby: Is it colic? *Mother Baby Journal, 4*(6), 35-38.
Lang, N.J. & Stewart, D.D. (1999). Child passenger safety: Clear reflections on gray areas. *Mother Baby Journal, 4*(4), 9-11.
Lang, N.J., & Stewart, D.D. (1999). Safe travel in the car: What parents need to know. *Mother Baby Journal, 4*(4), 13-18.
Lieu, T.A., Wikler, C., Capra, A.M., Martin, K.E., Escobar, G.J., & Bravemen, P.A. (1998). Clinical outcomes and maternal perceptions of an updated model of perinatal care. *Pediatrics, 102*(6), 1437-1444.
Lowe, M., Millea, D., & Simpson, K.R. (1996). Discharge planning. In K.R. Simpson & P.A. Creehan (Eds.), *AWHONN's perinatal nursing*. Philadelphia: Lippincott.
Lust, K.D., Brown, J.E., & Thomas, W. (1996). Maternal intake of cruciferous vegetables and other foods and colic symptoms in exclusively breastfed infants. *Journal of the American Dietetic Association, 96*(1), 46-48.
Mendler, V.M., Scallen, D.J., Kovtun, L.A., Balesky, J., & Lewis, C. (1996). The conception, birth, and infancy of an early discharge program. *MCN: American Journal of Maternal-Child Nursing, 21*(5), 241-246.
National Transportation Safety Board. (2000). NTSB addresses child transportation safety. Retrieved September 29, 2000 from http://www.ntsb.gov/surface/Highway/childseat.htm.
Pascale, J.A., Brittian, L., Lenfestey, C.C., & Jarrett-Pulliam, C. (1996). Breastfeeding, dehydration, and shorter maternity stays. *Neonatal Network, 15*(7), 37-43.
Peeke, K., Hershberger, M., Kuehn, D., & Levett, J. (1999). Infant sleep position: Nursing practice and knowledge. *MCN: The American Journal of Maternal/Child Nursing, 24*(6), 301-304.
Purdy, I.B. (2000). Shaken baby syndrome: The cry for universal prevention. *Mother Baby Journal, 5*(1), 21-25.
Rice, R., Birk, D., & Jenkins, R.L. (1999). Postpartum care. In R. Rice (Ed.), *Handbook of pediatric and postpartum home care procedures*. St. Louis: Mosby.
Simpson, K.R., Seibold, L., & Stremsterfer, K. (1996). Perinatal homecare services. In K.R. Simpson & P.A. Creehan (Eds.), *AWHONN's perinatal nursing*. Philadelphia: J.B. Lippincott.
Stevenson, A.M. (1999). Immunizations for women and infants. *Journal of Obstetric, Gynecologic, and Neonatal Nursing, 28*(5), 534-544.
U.S. Department of Health and Human Services (USDHHS), Public Health Service. (2000). *Healthy people 2010*. Washington, D.C.: Author.
Valaitis, R., Tuff, K., & Swanson, L. (1996). Meeting parents' postpartal needs with a telephone information line. *MCN: American Journal of Maternal-Child Nursing, 21*(2), 90-95.
Weekly, S.J., & Neumann, M.L. (1997). Speaking up for baby: The case for individualized neonatal discharge plans. *AWHONN's Lifelines, 1*(1), 24-29.
Williams, L.R., & Cooper, M.K. (1996). A new paradigm for postpartum care. *Journal of Obstetric, Gynecologic, and Neonatal Nursing, 25*(9), 745-749.

24

THE CHILDBEARING FAMILY WITH SPECIAL NEEDS

OBJECTIVES

1. Discuss the incidence and identify the factors that contribute to teenage pregnancy.
2. Identify the effects of pregnancy on the adolescent mother, her infant, and family.
3. Describe the role of the nurse in the prevention and management of teenage pregnancy.
4. Relate the major implications of delayed childbearing in terms of maternal and fetal health.
5. Describe the effects of substance abuse on both the mother and the infant.
6. Identify nursing interventions to reduce or minimize the effects of substance abuse in the antepartum, intrapartum, and postpartum periods.
7. Discuss parental responses when an infant is born with congenital anomalies, and identify nursing interventions to assist the parents.
8. Describe parental responses to pregnancy loss, and identify nursing interventions to assist parents through the grieving process.
9. Examine the role of the nurse when the mother relinquishes the infant for adoption.
10. Identify the factors that promote violence against women, and describe the role of the nurse in terms of assessment, prevention, and interventions.

DEFINITIONS

Abstinence Syndrome A group of symptoms that occur when a person who is addicted to a specific drug withdraws or abstains from taking that drug.

Addiction Physical or psychological dependence on a substance such as alcohol, tobacco, or drugs, either legal or illicit.

Alcohol-Related Neurodevelopmental Disorder (ARND) Neurologic conditions and delayed development resulting from prenatal exposure to alcohol.

Alcohol-Related Birth Defects (ARBD) Birth defects that are directly attributed to prenatal exposure to alcohol.

Alcoholism A chronic, progressive, and potentially fatal disease characterized by tolerance for and physical dependency on alcohol, pathologic organ changes resulting from alcohol abuse, or both.

Amphetamines Central nervous system stimulants that create a perception of pleasure unrelated to external stimuli.

Crack A highly addictive form of cocaine that has been processed to be smoked.

Egocentrism Interest centered on the self rather than the needs of others.

Fetal Alcohol Syndrome A group of physical and mental disorders of the offspring associated with maternal use of alcohol during pregnancy.

Methadone A synthetic compound with opiate properties; used as an oral substitute for heroin and morphine in the opiate-addicted person.

Neonatal Abstinence Syndrome A cluster of physical signs exhibited by the newborn who was exposed in utero to maternal use of substances such as cocaine or heroin. (See also *abstinence syndrome.*)

Opiate Any narcotic containing opium or a derivative of opium.

Prune-Belly Syndrome An absence of abdominal muscles resulting in a flabby, distended, and creased abdomen that may occur in the infant exposed to cocaine in utero.

Withdrawal Syndrome See *abstinence syndrome.*

All families must make major changes as they adapt to pregnancy and childbirth. For some families, however, the changes are particularly difficult. Such families have special needs related to parental age, substance abuse, birth of an infant with congenital abnormalities, loss of a pregnancy or neonate, or domestic violence. Perinatal nurses can make a difference in the lives of these families, particularly in the lives of infants born into them.

ADOLESCENT PREGNANCY

Incidence

Every year in the United States, more than 900,000 teenage girls become pregnant (USDHHS, 2000). A baby is born to an adolescent almost every minute of every day (James, 2000). For most of these young women, the pregnancy is unplanned and unwanted at conception. When compared to other developed countries, the pregnancy and birth rate for teenagers in the United States is one of the highest (Singh & Darroch, 2000).

The birth rate for adolescents in the United States has been declining, however. It has decreased each year since 1991, dropping 2% in 1998 to 51.1 births per 1000 women between the ages of 15 and 19 years (Ventura, et al., 2000) (Figure 24-1).

Factors Associated with Teenage Pregnancy

The high level of sexual activity among adolescents and the low incidence of contraceptive use are directly related to the incidence of teenage pregnancies in the United States. The recent declines in adolescent pregnancies are partially related to increased abstinence but mostly the result of more effective contraceptive practices. In spite of this, nearly half of sexually active teens report they did not use condoms during their most recent intercourse (Warren, et al., 1998).

Many adolescents fail to understand their vulnerability to pregnancy as a result of their sexual activity.

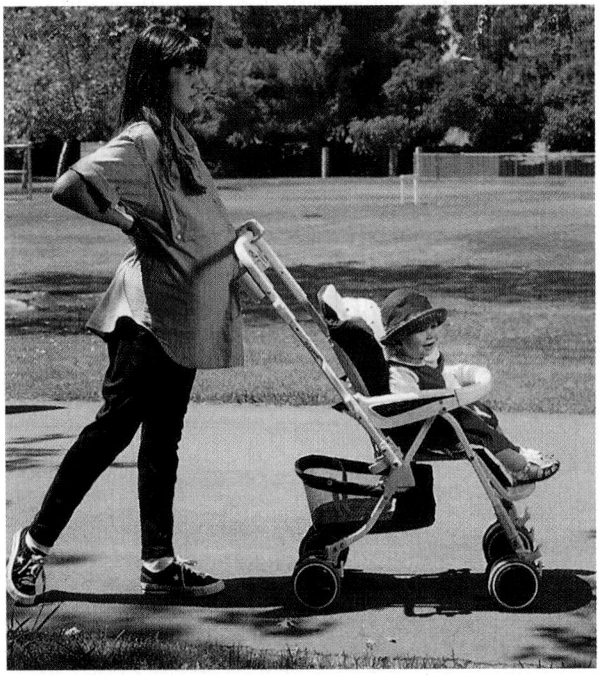

FIGURE 24-1 Pregnant adolescent. Approximately 20% of teenage girls who become pregnant have had one or more children previously.

Table 24-1
FACTORS CONTRIBUTING TO TEENAGE PREGNANCY

Lack of accurate information about ways to use contraceptives
Limited access to contraceptive devices
Fear of reporting sexual activity to parents
Ambivalence toward sexuality; intercourse not "planned"
Feelings of invulnerability
Peer pressure to begin sexual activity
Low self-esteem and consequent inability to set limits on sexual activity
Means to attain love or escape present situation
Lack of appropriate role models
Low level of education correlated with incorrect use of contraceptives

Some seem to believe that because they are unique, they are immune to pregnancy. Others risk pregnancy and parenthood as a means of gaining a love relationship. Still others see it as a means to gain independence. (Other factors that contribute to teenage pregnancy are listed in Table 24-1.)

National Health Goals

Teenage pregnancies result in numerous personal, social, and financial problems. A national goal for the year 2010 is to reduce the rate of pregnancies among female adolescents to not more than 46 per 1000 (U.S. Department of Health & Human Services, 2000).

Much controversy exists about the way to achieve the national health goals. The controversy centers on the debate over who should provide sex education. Some believe that information about sex and contraceptives should be provided only by the family. These people are convinced that providing sex education in schools gives tacit approval to sexual activity among teenagers.

Conversely, many families advocate early, continuing sex education in public schools. Within this context, ongoing information about prevention of pregnancy and sexually transmissible diseases (STDs) may be combined with other aspects of teenage sexuality, such as personal adjustments, interpersonal associations, and the establishment of values.

Sex Education

Most educators emphasize that two major strategies should be employed in education about sexuality. First, teenagers should be helped to understand ways to set limits on sexual activity. Second, they must be instructed in effective measures to prevent pregnancy and STDs. (Contraceptive methods are discussed in Chapter 31.)

Learning ways to set limits on sexual behavior is particularly important for younger teenagers, who may be pressured to become sexually active before they have developed the maturity to deal responsibly with intercourse, contraception, and unplanned pregnancy. They need advice about ways to handle pressure so that they can postpone sexual intercourse until they are emotionally and physically ready. Adolescent females often say they wish they had been taught how to say "not now," "not yet," and "not you."

When providing sex education, nurses must keep in mind that adolescent males and females mature at different rates, and forming segregated groups may be desirable until teenagers indicate they would feel comfortable in a combined group. Nurses should use simple but correct language such as "uterus," "testicles," "penis," and "vagina." Once the meanings of the terms are understood, most teenagers prefer to use them in their discussions.

Options When Pregnancy Occurs

An adolescent who becomes pregnant must choose one of three options: (1) terminate the pregnancy, (2) continue the pregnancy and place the infant for adoption, or (3) continue the pregnancy and keep the infant. Termination of pregnancy is not an acceptable alternative for some adolescents. Although they might consider termination, many teenagers do not acknowledge their pregnancies until late in the second trimester, when abortion is complicated.

The choice of abortion or adoption leaves the adolescent with no tangible evidence of her pregnancy and mixed messages from society regarding her decision. Unlike the teenager who decides to keep her infant, these adolescents receive less assistance about ways to deal with their experiences. They need recognition of the significance of the experience to them and assistance in dealing with their feelings. (See relinquishment by adoption, p. 650.)

Few teenagers choose to continue the pregnancy and place the infant for adoption. Those who do may have complicated feelings of grief, relief that a "bad" experience is over, and anger at parents who were unwilling to provide assistance and thus made adoption the only realistic option. For some young women, the autonomous decision to relinquish the child "for the child's good" may be an important step toward maturity.

The decision to keep the infant may result from the expectant mother's or her partner's desire for a baby or because of her belief that she could be a better parent than her own mother. Some choose to keep the baby because they are opposed to having an abortion or giving the baby up for adoption (Alan Guttmacher Institute, 2000).

Socioeconomic Implications

The financial cost of teenage pregnancy in the United States is estimated to be between $7 billion and $15 billion per year (USDHHS, 2000). Such figures may include funds for Temporary Assistance for Needy Families (TANF), Medicaid, food stamps, and direct payment to care providers. Teenage mothers are more likely than older mothers to be nonwhite, poor, less well educated, and unmarried.

In 1997, approximately 20% of teenagers giving birth had had one or more previous births (Ventura et al., 1999). Because they are more likely to have larger families at an earlier age, adolescent mothers have more children to feed and clothe on an already inadequate income.

Although the financial cost of teenage pregnancy is enormous, the cost in human terms is often tragic. The developmental tasks of adolescence, such as achieving independence from parents and establishing a lifestyle that is personally satisfying, are interrupted when a pregnancy increases the need for financial and emotional support from parents (Table 24-2). Educational goals often are curtailed, which limits employment opportunities and results in reliance on the welfare system. Research has found that in adolescent girls, having a child and not using contraceptives are associated with depression, low self-esteem, and little feeling of control over their lives (Kowaleski-Jones & Mott 1998).

Children born into this situation do not escape unscathed. They show a higher incidence of impaired intellectual functioning and poor school adjustment. The negative cycle often is repeated: A large percentage of teenage parents were children of teenage parents. As a result, children of adolescent parents often are among the poorest people in the United States.

Implications for Maternal Health

Pregnancy presents significant problems for the health of adolescent females. They are at increased risk for pregnancy-induced hypertension (PIH), but this may be related to the fact that PIH occurs more often in first pregnancies. Anemia and nutritional deficiencies are more common in pregnant teens (Cunningham, et al., 1997). In addition, the maternal mortality rate is higher for adolescents compared with older women. The high incidence of STDs among pregnant teenagers is another concern. Gonorrhea and chlamydial infection are particularly prevalent during these years.

The reason for the high incidence of complications among teenagers is unclear. It may be related to delayed prenatal care rather than age. Some pregnant adolescents do not start prenatal care until the third trimester, and others receive none at all. This is espe-

Table 24-2

IMPACT OF PREGNANCY ON THE DEVELOPMENTAL TASKS OF ADOLESCENCE

Developmental Task	Impact of Pregnancy	Nursing Considerations
Achievement of a Stable Identity: how the person sees himself or herself and perceives that others see and accept him or her; peer group approval provides confirmation and is a major component of identity development.	The ability to adapt and respond to stress is a good indicator of identity development, and adolescents who become pregnant before a stable identity is developed may not be able to accept the responsibilities of parenthood and plan for the future.	Explore the availability of a school-based mothers' program to provide the peer support that is so important. Emphasize the importance of prenatal classes and the effect of prenatal care on the pregnancy. Encourage both parents to attend parenting classes and describe the expected growth and development of infants. Focus on the infant's need to develop trust and parenting behaviors that promote this.
Achievement of Comfort with Body Image: requires internalization of mature body size, contour, and function.	The adolescent must learn to deal with body changes of pregnancy (increasing size, contour, increased pigmentation, and striae) before she has learned to accept the body changes associated with puberty. May deny pregnancy or severely restrict calories to avoid gaining weight. May be disgusted with the physical changes of pregnancy that make her look different from her peers.	Allow time for the teenager to verbalize her feelings about the body changes of pregnancy. Emphasize that dieting is harmful to the infant and will not stop the changes in body size and contour. Provide exercises that will help her regain her figure after the birth of the infant.
Acceptance of Sexual Role and Identity: requires internalization of strong sexual urges and achievement of intimacy with others.	The adolescent may need to achieve an intimate relationship with another and form an exclusive relationship before she is ready. The pregnant teenager also will need to cope with changes in relationships with friends. She often has difficulty seeing herself as a sexual being or as a mother.	Allow the teenager to express her feelings about sexuality and motherhood. Initiate groups designed specifically for adolescents (childbirth education or parenting classes, or special groups about nutrition). This will help her deal with the changing relationships with her peers and move toward a mothering role.

Modified from Mercer, R.T. (1990). *Parents at risk.* New York: Springer.

Continued

Table 24-2

IMPACT OF PREGNANCY ON THE DEVELOPMENTAL TASKS OF ADOLESCENCE—cont'd

Developmental Task	Impact of Pregnancy	Nursing Considerations
Development of a Personal Value System: able to consider the rights and feelings of others.	Pregnancy occurs before the adolescent is able to move from following rules to considering the rights and feelings of others and developing ethical standards. She may experience conflict when she must adjust to the responsibilities of premature motherhood.	Initiate a discussion of the teenager's feelings of conflict about her role as mother versus her role as student. Explore her views about motherhood: How does she expect it to change her life? What are her future plans? Present options and assist her to explore her goals.
Preparation for Vocation or Career: completing educational or vocational goals; youths living in poverty may not have the means or encouragement to accomplish this.	Pregnancy often interrupts school for both parents; this may be a major frustration and result in permanent withdrawal from school and limited access to jobs that pay more than the minimum wage.	Discuss the importance of continued education and elicit the teenager's feelings and plans to accomplish this. Determine the amount and availability of support from her parents. Refer her to social services for needed assistance.
Achievement of Independence from Parents: competent in the social environment and able to function without parental guidance.	Must adjust to the need for continued financial assistance and dependence on parents at a time when achieving independence is a major priority.	Assist the teenager to verbalize her feelings about continued dependence on parents. Discuss the reality of the situation and her need for financial support and help with the care of the infant. Determine whether she will continue to live at home and the reaction of her parents to the pregnancy. How much support will they provide? What are the conditions for her remaining at her parents' home with the infant?

Modified from Mercer, R.T. (1990). *Parents at risk.* New York: Springer.

cially true for the young adolescent: fewer than half of pregnant teenagers aged 15 years and under receive adequate care (USDHHS, 2000).

Delayed prenatal care may result from denial of the pregnancy, lack of knowledge of how to get care, or a negative view of health care providers. Early prenatal care that includes counseling about nutritional needs and close observation of the client for the onset of pregnancy-induced hypertension can reduce the high rate of fetal and maternal complications that occur when the expectant mother is very young.

Implications for Fetal-Neonatal Health

Infants of teenage mothers have an increased risk of long-term serious disabilites and death during the first year of life (Ventura, Curtin, & Matthews, 1998). An infant born to a teenage mother is at higher risk for two major complications: prematurity (birth before the end of the 37th week of gestation) and low birth weight (<2500 g).

The cause of low birth weight may be intrauterine growth restriction, which means that the fetus does not grow as expected. This may result from a variety of causes, such as poor placental perfusion or the underdeveloped vasculature of the uterus in young primigravidas. When placental perfusion is decreased, the newborn may have a low birth weight even if the pregnancy goes to term because transport of nutrients and oxygen to the fetus have been inadequate. Prematurity also is a major cause of low-birth-weight infants. An infant born before 38 weeks of gestation is likely to weigh less than 2500 g and has the added risks associated with immature organs.

The Teenage Expectant Father

Approximately 85% of adolescents are not married at the time of conception (Darroch, Landry, & Oslak, 1999). The partners of approximately 50% of pregnant adolescents are within 2 years of the adolescent's age, but approximately 29% are 3 to 5 years older, and 19% are 6 or more years older than the adolescent. These men may accept responsibility for the child, or they may become "phantom fathers," which means that they are absent and rarely involved in parenting the child.

Almost all adolescent expectant fathers indicate that they are not ready for fatherhood, and this attitude does not diminish as the pregnancy progresses. Many are depressed as they grapple with the conflicting roles of adolescence and fatherhood. Although some express interest in learning about childbirth and child care, those who do not want to be fathers are less likely to be supportive. Some do not wish to interact with the infant, leaving the pregnant girl to seek support elsewhere.

A disproportionate number of teenage expectant fathers are from environments of poverty and lack job skills or educational preparation. Many need job training before they are able to earn enough money to contribute to the support of their children.

Adolescent fathers often receive financial and emotional support from their own mothers. They may live in the parental home, and their own mothers (the paternal grandmothers) may encourage them to maintain contact with the baby and the mother (Dallas & Chen, 1999). Nurses should determine the involvement of both sets of grandparents when working with adolescent parents.

Impact on Parenting

Adolescent mothers are at risk of becoming nonnurturing parents and having negative parent-infant interactions (Kenner & Amlung, 1999). Having to focus on an infant at a time when most teenagers are absorbed in their own thoughts and activities may make parenting difficult. The ability to deal with stress plays an important part in mothering skills. Because of their immature coping mechanisms, young adolescents may be unable to separate the stress of other life events from that which occurs when the infant cries and cannot be consoled. They may respond with immature or punitive measures toward the infant when the source of stress is other factors such as social isolation or inadequate financial resources.

Teenage parents may have little understanding of the expected growth and development of infants. They may expect too much too soon from their children. For instance, they may expect that an infant will sleep through the night or be toilet trained before infants are able to do so. In addition, the infant may be in an neonatal intensive care unit for some time and the mother may have to learn to care for an infant with problems.

The mother's relationship with the father of the baby may affect her parenting abilities. A close and satisfying relationship with the baby's father may help increase attachment behaviors in the mother. Therefore it is important to include the father, when appropriate, in the care of the mother and baby (Bloom, 1998).

Check Your Reading

1. How does pregnancy affect the developmental tasks of adolescence?
2. What are the major problems associated with teenage pregnancy in terms of maternal and fetal health?

APPLICATION OF THE NURSING PROCESS: THE PREGNANT TEENAGER

Assessment

Physical Assessment

Assessment of pregnant teenagers is similar to that of older women in many respects. At the initial visit, obtain a thorough health and family history to determine the presence of conditions such as diabetes or infectious diseases that increase the risk for the mother and fetus. Monitor closely for signs of iron-deficiency anemia or pregnancy-induced hypertension. If STDs are diagnosed, elicit information about sexual partners so that therapeutic management can be initiated. Attempt to identify lifestyle behaviors, such as poor nutrition, smoking, and alcohol or drug use, that could harm the mother or fetus.

> Teenagers are sometimes defensive and inconsistent in their responses. Because they may not volunteer information about nutrition, exercise, and the use of alcohol or other drugs, the nurse needs to press for details. The teenager's statement "I eat okay, and I'm pretty active" requires follow-up questions worded to obtain specific information: "What did you eat yesterday? Begin with when you first got up." "What activities do you enjoy most?"

Structure the interview so that questions can be interspersed in a more general conversation that explores the teenager's likes and concerns. For example, a question such as "So, you are a member of the choir, will you be able to continue with that after the baby is born?" may establish rapport and help determine whether the teenager is making plans for the future.

Knowledge of Infant Needs

Assess knowledge of infant needs and parenting skills. How does the teenager plan to feed the infant? What will she do when the infant cries? How will she know when the infant is ill and should be taken to a pediatrician? Does she know how much the infant should sleep? What plans have been made to provide for the hygiene and safety needs of the infant?

Cognitive Development

Determine the teenager's cognitive development and ability to absorb health counseling. The three most important areas of cognitive development are the following:

1. *Egocentrism,* which involves the ability to defer personal satisfaction to respond to the needs of the infant: "What would you do if the baby were sick?" "How would you make the baby better?"

2. *Present-future orientation,* which involves the ability to make long-term plans: "What are your plans for finishing high school?" "What will you and the infant need in the first year of the infant's life?"
3. *Abstract thinking,* which involves identifying cause and effect: "Why is it important to keep clinic appointments?" "Why should condoms be used during sexual intercourse?"

Family Assessment

Begin assessment of the family unit by determining the degree of participation by the father of the infant. The father may deny responsibility for the pregnancy, be married to or plan to marry the expectant mother, or plan to participate in the pregnancy and rearing of the child without marriage.

Assessing the adolescent without the presence of her parents is important, yet determining the availability and amount of family support also is crucial. Will the pregnant teenager continue to live with her parents? How do her parents feel about the pregnancy? How will they incorporate the mother and her infant into the family?

Families generally respond in one of three ways:

1. A family member (often the adolescent's mother) assumes the mothering role, which the teenager may abdicate willingly.
2. All care and responsibilities are left to the adolescent mother, although shelter and food are provided.
3. The family shares care and responsibilities, which allows the teenager to grow in the mothering role while completing the developmental tasks of adolescence.

The pregnant teenager's mother is particularly important when assessing the family. How does she feel about becoming a grandmother? Many women feel embarrassed and disgraced. She may feel that she has "failed" as a mother, or she may resent the new cycle of child care in which the pregnancy involves her. Is communication with her daughter open? Is she aware of the difficult role conflict (as adolescent and mother) that her daughter will experience? If the family is unable or unwilling to provide care for an adolescent with an infant, what other social support can be located?

Analysis

Many adolescents wait until the second or third trimester to seek prenatal care because they either do not realize they are pregnant or continue to deny they are pregnant. In addition, many teenagers have little information about the physiologic demands that pregnancy imposes on their bodies, such as the increased need for nutrients. As a result, they may have a pattern of sporadic prenatal care and missed appointments (Nursing Care Plan 24-1). One of the most relevant nursing diagnoses is "Risk for Altered Health Maintenance related to lack of knowledge of measures to promote health during pregnancy and increased family stress."

Planning

For the nursing diagnosis "Risk for Altered Health Maintenance," the most appropriate goals or outcomes are the following:

- The expectant mother will keep scheduled prenatal appointments and actively participate in recommended group classes.
- She will communicate concerns and seek knowledge of measures that promote her health and the health of the fetus throughout the pregnancy.
- She will express knowledge of infant needs and the expected pattern of infant growth and development before the end of the third trimester.
- The family will verbalize emotions and concerns and maintain functional support of the expectant mother and her infant.

Interventions

Eliminating Barriers to Health Care

The two major barriers to health care are (1) scheduling conflicts and (2) negative attitudes of health care workers. Determine the most convenient location and time for appointments. Helping the adolescent locate the clinic closest to her and providing information about public transportation to that location may be necessary. In addition, appointments must be available when the girl (and her partner, if he wishes) are not in school. Some clinics are open in the evening or on Saturday. If this is not available, alternative plans may be necessary.

Pregnant women of all ages state that the attitude of health care workers can discourage attendance at prenatal clinics. Some health care workers, including nurses, physicians, and social workers, are described as rude, insensitive, patronizing, judgmental, hostile, and condescending. This attitude is particularly unfortunate because it discourages families that would benefit most from early, consistent prenatal care.

Nurses can be instrumental in finding ways to overcome these negative attitudes and thus encourage pregnant women, including teenagers, to return to prenatal clinics for needed follow-up care. Recommended strategies include the following:

- Identify pervasive attitudes of the health care team.
- Acknowledge that frustration, stress, and staff burnout are common when health care workers attempt to provide care for families with multiple problems.
- Recognize that health care workers who are parents of teenagers may feel vulnerable and fearful about their own children and project these feelings onto clients.

Text continued on p. 635

NURSING CARE PLAN 24-1
Adolescent's Responses to Pregnancy and Birth

Assessment: Ann Killian, a 16-year-old white female, presented at the neighborhood health clinic during the 20th week of her pregnancy. She lives with her mother and father, who both work long hours, and a younger sister. Ann remains in school but verbalizes concern about how she looks and feels: "How much bigger am I going to get?" "Why is my face so blotchy?" "My feet swell and it looks gross."

Nursing Diagnosis: Body Image Disturbance related to perceived negative effects of pregnancy as evidenced by verbalized concern about appearance

Goals/Expected Outcomes:
Ann will do the following:
1. Verbalize her feelings about pregnancy and her perception of herself during each antepartum visit.
2. Make two positive statements about herself during next antepartum visit.

Intervention	Rationale
1. Allow time at each prenatal visit for Ann to express concerns about weight gain and other physiologic changes of pregnancy, such as hyperpigmentation and stretch marks.	1. The adolescent often is ashamed and uncomfortable with her pregnant body. She feels more comfortable if she is allowed to share these feelings and be reassured that they are a normal part of pregnancy.
2. Initiate interaction about body changes by asking open-ended questions such as "How do you feel about wearing maternity clothes?"	2. Adolescents often are intimidated by health care professionals and may think that their own feelings are not important enough to discuss.
3. Provide anticipatory guidance about expected changes of pregnancy such as the pattern of weight gain during pregnancy and rate of weight loss after childbirth.	3. Most adolescents do not know what to expect during pregnancy, and their fears often are unexpressed. Anticipatory guidance reduces fear and provides information about expected changes.
4. Explain the reason for changes that are most troublesome at each prenatal visit (weight gain, hyperpigmentation, stretch marks, breast changes).	4. Knowing that some changes are temporary and that increasing weight indicates the fetus is growing and developing often is helpful for the adolescent. This often becomes a source of pride for the young teenager as well as for the older woman.
5. Involve Ann in scheduling follow-up prenatal appointments and other activities related to the birth of the infant (classes, plans for childbirth).	5. Participation in decision making promotes a positive sense of self.
6. Promote positive self-image by praising grooming, posture, and responsible behavior such as keeping prenatal appointments and following recommendations: "You have never missed an appointment, and your baby is growing so well."	6. Positive reinforcement is particularly important to help the adolescent meet the developmental tasks of developing a sense of identity and self-worth.

Evaluation: Ann discusses her concerns about how she looks and feels about herself and makes several positive statements about herself.

Assessment: Ann reveals that her father has said she has "shamed the family," and she is worried her friends will reject her when they learn that she is pregnant. Ann states that she will have to "drop out of everything." She confides, in a trembling voice, that she feels guilty for "putting her family through this."

Nursing Diagnosis: Situational Low Self-Esteem related to feelings of rejection by family and friends as manifested by statements indicating guilt and uncertainty about future support for herself and infant.

Goals/Expected Outcomes:
Ann will do the following:
1. Identify at least two new measures to cope with anxiety by the end of the current antepartum visit.
2. Demonstrate the ability to implement these measures during subsequent antepartum visits.
3. Make at least one positive statement about herself at each visit.

Continued

Intervention	Rationale
1. Use therapeutic communication techniques to help Ann express her feelings about her pregnancy and the reactions of significant others.	1. Listening to the adolescent helps her see her feelings as important to others and helps the nurse determine which areas have highest priority for nursing interventions.
2. Help Ann identify what she can do to overcome anxiety about rejection of her family and friends.	2. Planning how to approach the family and friends reduces anxiety.
a. Role play how Ann can initiate a conversation with friends to discuss activities that they can continue to share.	a. Acceptance by the peer group and participation in group activities are major concerns of the adolescent, and a change in status within the group is a threat to self-concept that precipitates acute anxiety.
b. Suggest that she request a family meeting and acknowledge her feelings of guilt for the unhappiness she is causing and her fear they will not assist her through the pregnancy and birth.	b. Although adolescents strive for independence, family values continue to be a significant influence. Rejection by the family at this time would leave her vulnerable to stress beyond her coping ability.
c. Recommend that she share her feelings with the father of the infant if she continues to see him.	c. Expectant fathers may be a source of emotional and financial support.
3. Assist Ann in locating and joining the school-aged mothers' program if available through her school district.	3. Teenagers who are either mothers or expectant mothers often replace the pregnant teenager's previous peer group. The shared concerns and activities provide an opportunity for growth.
4. Help Ann to discuss her economic needs and plans for continuing school when the infant is born.	4. Beginning to develop plans for the future provides some sense of control over the situation and increases feelings of competency.
5. Point out and praise any positive actions that Ann takes, such as keeping prenatal appointments or eating a balanced diet.	5. Sincere praise helps reinforce a positive self-image.

Evaluation: Ann talks with her family and reports relationships are somewhat improved. She enters a school-age mother's program and is very pleased. She often makes more positive statements about herself and her life in the future.

Assessment: Ann has given birth to a 6-lb, 3-oz girl at 38 weeks' gestation. She has decided not to breastfeed because she plans to go back to school as soon as possible. Ann will live at home, and her mother has agreed to work part time so that she can care for the infant while Ann is in school. Ann is very concerned about caring for the newborn. She seems unsure how to respond when the infant cries and handles her only during feedings.

Nursing Diagnosis: Risk for Altered Parenting related to knowledge deficit of infant needs and lack of confidence in ability to care for the infant, as evidenced by uncertain responses to infant.

Goals/Expected Outcomes:
Ann will do the following:
1. Demonstrate basic infant care (cord care, bathing, burping, feeding, swaddling) by discharge.
2. Verbalize infant needs for gentle, prompt response to crying.
3. Demonstrate attachment behaviors (eye contact, gazing, holding, verbal stimulation, and positive comments about infant) before discharge.

Intervention	Rationale
1. Demonstrate infant care on the first postpartum day, and obtain a return demonstration on the second postpartum day before discharge.	1. Confidence is increased by returning the demonstration of infant care and continued practice in caring for the infant.
2. Role play the way to respond when the infant cries, and emphasize the importance of promptness and gentleness.	2. Observing how nurses respond to the infant increases the likelihood that adolescents will respond in the same manner. Prompt, gentle responses help the infant develop trust.
3. Emphasize the importance of touch and verbal stimulation, and point out the reciprocal bonding behaviors that the infant exhibits (see p. 460).	3. Many teenage parents do not provide adequate tactile and verbal stimulation for their infants, which may decrease the infant's ability to learn. The infant has many behaviors that stimulate mutual attachment between parent and child.
4. Include the grandparents and father of the infant in as many demonstrations as possible.	4. When all primary caregivers are included, family cohesiveness and consistency of care are enhanced.
5. Instruct Ann in early growth and development of the infant (how often infants need to eat, how much they sleep, what to do when they cry).	5. Some teenage parents expect too much, too soon from infants and become frustrated when the infant does not respond as expected. Anticipatory guidance may help them have more realistic expectations.

Evaluation: Ann responds quickly and gently to infant crying. She cares for the infant as she was taught and discusses the infant's expected growth and development. She talks about her daughter in a positive manner.

- Allocate time for staff development, planning programs, and stress reduction.
- Find ways to obtain increased assistance from clerical and support personnel.
- Initiate a scheduling plan that allows health care workers to see the same families whenever possible so that a caring relationship can be established.

Applying Teaching/Learning Principles

Because peers are important to adolescents, they benefit from participating in small groups with common concerns. Specific needs that might be addressed are the benefits of prenatal care or education to eliminate unhealthful habits such as smoking, drug use, and alcohol consumption. Finding common goals, such as eliminating smoking, may be discussed in groups where the teens can assist each other to have more healthful pregnancies. As pregnancy progresses, needs and group focus change. For example, ways to prepare for labor and delivery and care for an infant become the priorities.

Repetition is an important method of teaching and clarifying misconceptions. Allow ample time for questions and discussions. Although teenagers do not read or benefit from printed materials to the same degree that older parents do, many learn well from audiovisual aids. Numerous well-made videos and slide presentations deal with all aspects of prenatal and infant care. Time spent waiting for clinic appointments can be used to view videos that reinforce information.

Maintain an open, friendly posture, and convey empathy by using attending behaviors such as eye contact, frequent nodding, and leaning toward the speaker. As with all expectant families, avoid closed posture (arms folded across the chest), finger pointing, and lack of attention to the person speaking. Avoiding sounding like a parent is particularly important. Refrain from using the words *should* and *ought,* offering unwanted advice, and making decisions for the teenagers. (Table 24-3 summarizes additional recommended methods for teaching adolescents.)

Table 24-3

RECOMMENDED METHODS FOR TEACHING PREGNANT ADOLESCENTS

Identify and correct barriers to prenatal care.
Communicate with kindness and respect.
Form small groups with like concerns.
Allow ample time for clarification and discussion.
Use audiovisual materials.
Provide information in appropriate language.
Convey empathetic concern by nonverbal communication skills.
Include other family members when appropriate.

Counseling

Allow time to counsel teenagers about their specific problems such as nutrition, stress reduction, and infant care.

Nutrition. Nutrition counseling can help reduce the incidence of low-birth-weight infants. Tailor information to the individual adolescent's likes and peer group habits. She often needs instruction in ways to make the most nutritious selection from fast-food menus and select and plan for healthy snacks when she is away from home (see Chapter 9).

Food preparation equipment and referrals to food stamp providers, the Special Supplemental Food Program for Women, Infants, and Children (WIC), surplus food distributors, and food banks may be necessary because many teenagers have limited access to food and lack the ability to store or prepare food. Nutrition education must be socially and culturally appropriate.

Stress Reduction. Stress is an important factor in perinatal outcome, and teenagers are vulnerable to many sources of stress. Stress may be related to basic needs such as food, shelter, and health care. Fear of labor and delivery and fear of being single, alone, and unsupported all create stress. Perhaps a major source of stress for teenagers occurs when they attempt to meet the developmental tasks of adolescence while working on the developmental tasks of pregnancy (overcoming ambivalence, attaining the role of parent).

A variety of measures may be used to reduce stress, depending on the teenager's age, situation, and available support. Adolescents with chronic life stress may require the concentrated efforts of a social worker to achieve stabilization.

The pregnant teenager often experiences stress because she has not told her parents or the father of the infant about the pregnancy. Exploring her reluctance to do this and role playing the encounter so that she can work out a plan for breaking the news may be helpful. If appropriate, encourage her to tell the prospective father so that he can work out his role. If the girl is very young or the pregnancy occurred as a result of rape or incest, social service and law enforcement agencies must become involved to provide protection and assistance.

Attachment to the Fetus. Because attachment begins during pregnancy, methods of helping the adolescent begin this process are important. Use of ultrasound may increase the expectant mother's awareness of the fetus and facilitate developing attachment. Seeing the fetus move often changes pregnant teenager's perceptions about the fetus (Colucciello, 1998). This may make her more likely to follow suggestions that will enhance fetal well-being. Discussion of the fetus as it changes month to month may lead to discussion of the capabilities and needs of the neonate.

Infant Care. The priorities for teaching gradually change from maternal to infant needs, with particular emphasis on normal growth and development. For example, to reduce the worry that many mothers feel when the newborn startles in response to loud noises, demonstrate reflexes and explain that the uncoordinated motor responses are normal. Explain that development proceeds from the head downward. This helps the young mother understand that the infant must learn to sit before walking and must walk before toilet training is possible.

Explain and demonstrate infant cues (using behaviors of the infants in videos or the group as examples) in terms of gaze, vocalization, facial expression, body position, and limb movement. Describe the way that infants use these behaviors to "talk" without words and ways in which parents can use the same behaviors to respond to their infants. Demonstrate ways that mothers (and fathers) can adjust their position, distance, face, voice, and touch to correspond to their infant's cues. Emphasize that eye contact, holding, cuddling, and verbal stimulation are important for the child's development.

Because adolescents tend to have a more rigid and punitive approach to child care, emphasize to them that infants develop a sense of *trust* when their needs are met promptly and gently. In addition, their future development depends on attaining a sense of trust during infancy. Emphasize that crying does not indicate the infant is spoiled but simply that the infant has a need. Perhaps the need is for food, warmth, or comfort and love.

Promoting Family Support

The pregnant teenager needs encouragement to include her family in her decision making and problem solving. The involvement of her mother, older sister, or other close relative is particularly important in terms of future plans. Adolescent mothers who have adequate emotional support, are enrolled in school, want to avoid pregnancy for at least 2 years, and believe pregnancy will occur without adequate contraception are more likely to use contraceptives reliably (Berenson & Wiemann, 1997).

Topics that should be discussed include who will care for the infant, whether the teenager will return to school, and what financial assistance is available from the family and the father of the infant. However, involving the family may be inappropriate if they have multiple problems such as substance abuse or domestic violence. In such situations the teenager should be encouraged to communicate instead with a family friend or other trusted adult.

Providing Referrals

Nurses who are knowledgeable about national and community resources for pregnant adolescents can make referrals to the closest and most convenient locations. These include well-baby clinics offered by the Public Health Service, programs for school-age mothers offered by many school districts, Temporary Assistance for Needy Families (TANF) offered by state social service agencies, and WIC. Church and community organizations also may provide needed assistance.

Evaluation

Nursing care has been effective if the pregnant adolescent keeps clinic appointments and participates actively in her plan of care, as demonstrated by asking questions, sharing concerns, and adhering to the recommended program of care. Demonstrating knowledge of the infant's needs and expected pattern of growth and development by the end of the pregnancy increases the teenager's confidence in her ability to provide a nurturing environment. Family support often is available, but if not, nurses often must make referrals to agencies that can provide assistance.

Check Your Reading

3. What methods are effective for teaching pregnant teenagers?
4. What should prospective teenage parents be taught about infant growth and development?

Delayed Pregnancy

An increasing number of women become pregnant relatively late in their reproductive lives. Pregnancies at advanced maternal age often are the result of contraceptive techniques that provide women with freedom to time the births of their first children. Furthermore, advances in reproductive medicine increase the chance for infertile women to have children. Some women may delay childbearing to pursue a career or establish financial security.

Maternal and Fetal Implications

When the mature woman decides to conceive, she may experience a delay in becoming pregnant. This is particularly true after the age of 35 years because of the normal aging of the ovaries and the increased incidence in reproductive tract disorders. For instance, pelvic inflammatory disease can cause pelvic and tubal adhesions that interfere with fertilization and implantation.

Once the mature woman conceives, she is at increased risk for complications associated with pregnancy. The risks may be considered in three categories: genetic, preexisting medical conditions, and obstetric complications. The increased risk of fetal chromosomal abnormalities with advancing maternal age is well documented. Trisomy 21 (Down syndrome) is the most common example. The likelihood of a 20-year-old woman having an affected child is approximately 1 in 1400, compared with a 1 in 100 risk for a 40-year-old woman (Cunningham, et al., 1997). The use of chorionic villus sampling or amniocentesis permits detection of some chromosomal abnormalities, and legalized abortion allows the woman to terminate the pregnancy if she wishes.

The most common examples of preexisting diseases that increase maternal or fetal jeopardy are hypertension and diabetes mellitus. Gestational diabetes and uterine myomas (fibroids) occur with greater frequency in women older than 35 years. Myomas may be associated with postpartum hemorrhage. The older primigravida also is at increased risk for obstetric complications such as pregnancy-induced hypertension, multiple gestation, preterm labor, dysfunctional labor, and cesarean birth. In addition, the risk of a small-for-gestational age infant increases with advanced maternal age.

Advantages of Delayed Childbirth

Unlike adolescents, for whom pregnancy may be unplanned and unwanted, women older than 35 years of age seldom make the decision to have a child without careful thought. They have a range of personal resources: psychosocial maturity, self-confidence, and a sense of control over their lives (Figure 24-2). They demonstrate high levels of empathy and flexibility in childrearing attitudes.

In addition, mature primigravidas are capable of solving complex problems and often are adept at maintaining interpersonal relationships. Because they are more likely to be financially secure, they can afford excellent care for their infants. They are experienced at setting priorities and developing plans. They usually are able to manage stress and will independently seek support and assistance.

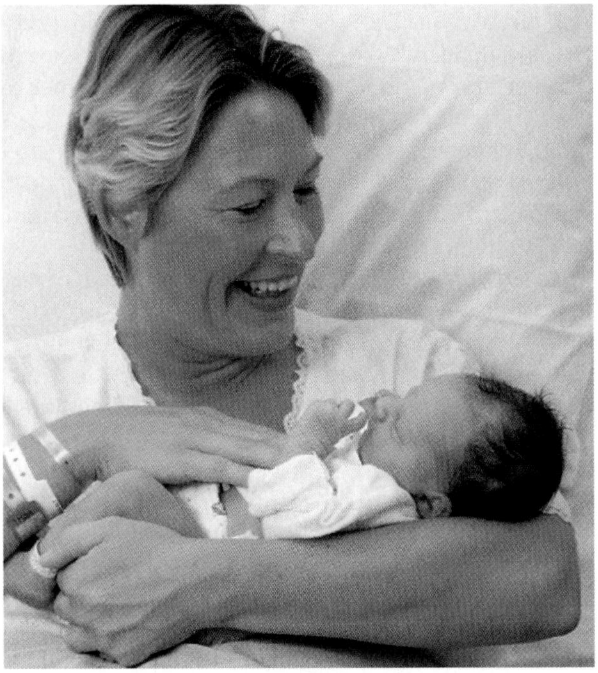

FIGURE 24-2 Older primigravidas bring maturity and problem-solving skills to the maternal role, but they are at somewhat increased risk for physiologic problems related to pregnancy and birth.

Disadvantages of Delayed Childbirth

Mature primiparas need more time to recover from childbirth, and they have less energy than their younger counterparts. They may find child care an exhausting experience for the first few weeks. This is particularly true if they had a cesarean birth or other complications of pregnancy, such as excessive bleeding.

Because their friends have teenage children instead of infants, mature primiparas may lack peer support. Many of their friends do not relate to the concerns of a new mother. Younger mothers have some of the same concerns, but they often do not share the perspective of older mothers. Family support also may be lacking for the older woman. Her parents are usually in their 60s or 70s and may not be able to assist with child care to the extent of younger grandparents.

Nursing Considerations

Reinforcing and Clarifying Information

Because the fetus of a mature gravida is at increased risk for chromosomal anomalies, the woman will be informed about available diagnostic tests. Professionals with special preparation in genetics provide genetic counseling, but all nurses must be prepared to reinforce and clarify the information that has been provided. The tests most often recommended are triple-marker screening (analysis of alpha-fetoprotein, human chorionic gonadotropin, and estriols), chorionic villus sampling, amniocentesis, and ultrasonography (see Chapter 10).

The family's beliefs and attitudes about abortion often determine whether to have the recommended tests. The woman who would not consider abortion regardless of the condition of the fetus may refuse diagnostic studies. Nurses must respect the decision and acknowledge that it may have been difficult to make.

Facilitating Expression of Emotions

Several days or weeks may pass between performance of diagnostic studies and when results of the tests are known. This is a particularly difficult time for many expectant parents, and nurses often assist the couple to express their concerns and emotions.

> A broad statement such as "Many couples find it difficult to wait for the results" often will elicit free expression of their feelings. Follow-up questions such as "What concerns you most?" may reveal anxiety about the procedure itself or the possible effects of the procedure on the fetus. Simply acknowledging that it is a stressful time helps the couple cope with their emotions.

Providing Parenting Information

Nurses often help the mature primipara prepare for effective parenting by pointing out her individual strengths and advantages. These often include financial security, a stable relationship, and personal maturity. The older mother may have unique needs, however. She often has less energy than younger mothers and must learn to conserve it, particularly during the early weeks after childbirth. Anticipatory guidance about measures that will help conserve energy after childbirth is very useful. Such measures may include meal planning and setting realistic housekeeping goals. In addition, many older mothers need to mobilize all available support so that they can reserve their energy for care of the infant.

During the first weeks after childbirth, the mother may experience feelings of social isolation, particularly if her friends have children who are a great deal older. If she is accustomed to a great deal of mental stimulation, she may miss it while staying at home. If she elects to return to work, she is likely to experience guilt and grief because she must leave her infant (see Chapter 18 for a discussion of this problem). Balancing the needs of the infant and those of what may be a demanding career or occupation may be difficult.

First-time mothers older than age 35 are especially receptive to prenatal classes. These include classes in childbirth education, preparation for cesarean birth, breastfeeding, and early parenting. When teaching infant care after childbirth, the nurse should allow time for demonstrations and return demonstrations so that the expectant parents feel comfortable with routine care. Older couples are particularly interested in learning the way the infant grows and develops and what they can do to provide nurturing care for the infant. They generally comprehend printed materials that can be used to reinforce teaching.

Check Your Reading

5. What special resources do mature primigravidas often have?
6. Why is it important to offer prenatal testing (triple-marker sceening, chorionic villus sampling, amniocentesis) to the mature primigravida?
7. What anticipatory guidance should the nurse provide the older mother for the first weeks at home after childbirth?

SUBSTANCE ABUSE

The use of legal substances such as alcohol and tobacco and illicit drugs such as cocaine, heroin, and marijuana increases the risk of medical complications in the mother and poor birth outcomes in the infant.

Incidence

More than 4.4 million women use illicit drugs (Lieberman, 1998). Approximately 1 in 10 infants is exposed to one or more mood-altering drugs during pregnancy (AAP & ACOG, 1997). Although tobacco, alcohol, and marijuana are the most commonly abused drugs, the use of cocaine and heroin have had a major impact on health care for pregnant women and their offspring.

Maternal and Fetal Effects

When the pregnant woman takes a substance by drinking, smoking, snorting, or injecting it, the fetus receives the same substance. The fetus experiences the same systemic effects as the expectant mother but often more severely. For instance, cocaine raises the blood pressure of the woman and fetus and puts both at risk for intracranial bleeding. A drug that causes intoxication in the woman causes it for prolonged periods of time in the fetus. This is because the fetus is unable to metabolize drugs as efficiently as the expectant mother and will experience the effects long after they have abated in the woman. Therefore substances taken by the woman can have great impact on the fetus and interfere with normal fetal development and health. (Maternal, fetal, and neonatal effects of commonly abused substances are summarized in Table 24-4.)

Tobacco

The active ingredients of cigarette smoke are nicotine, tar, and harmful gases such as carbon monoxide and cyanide. Nicotine, which causes vasoconstriction, transfers readily across the placenta and reduces placental blood circulation. This contributes to fetal hypoxia and increased incidence of fetal death. Carbon monoxide inactivates fetal and maternal hemoglobin and further reduces the amount of oxygen delivered to the fetus. Indirect effects of cigarette smoking include decreased maternal appetite, which results in inadequate intake of calories and added difficulties in absorbing nutrients such as calcium and vitamins A, B, and C.

Cigarette smoking is the most common form of substance abuse by pregnant women (Kearney, 1999). In 1998, 12.9% of pregnant women smoked during their pregnancies (Ventura, et al., 2000).

Neonatal consequences of smoking tobacco during pregnancy are low birth weight and prematurity. On average, neonates exposed to tobacco in utero weigh 200 g to 300 g less than those not exposed to tobacco (Kearney, 1999). In 1998, 12% of infants born to mothers who smoked weighed less than 2500 g (5 lb, 8 oz) while the rate for infants born to nonsmokers was 7.2% (Ventura, et al., 2000). Infants born to smokers are symmetrically smaller in all areas, including head circumference, weight, and length (Bauer, 1998).

Smoking during pregnancy also is associated with neurologic and intellectual development problems that affect later school achievement. Sudden infant death

Table 24-4

MATERNAL AND FETAL OR NEONATAL EFFECTS OF COMMONLY ABUSED SUBSTANCES

Substance	Maternal Effects	Fetal or Neonatal Effects
Caffeine (coffee, tea, cola, chocolate, cold remedies, analgesics)	CNS and cardiac function stimulation, vasoconstriction and mild diuresis results, half-life triples during pregnancy	Placental barrier is crossed, stimulating fetus; teratogenic effects are undocumented
Tobacco	Decreased placental perfusion, anemia, PROM, preterm labor, spontaneous abortion	Prematurity, LBW, fetal demise, developmental delays, increased incidence of SIDS, pneumonia
Alcohol (beer, wine, mixed drinks, after-dinner drinks)	Spontaneous abortion	Fetal demise, IUGR, FAS (facial and cranial anomalies, developmental delay, mental retardation, short attention span), fetal alcohol effects (milder form of FAS)
Narcotics (heroin, methadone, morphine)	Spontaneous abortion, PROM, preterm labor, increased incidence of STDs, HIV exposure, hepatitis, malnutrition	IUGR, perinatal asphyxia, intellectual impairment, neonatal abstinence syndrome, neonatal infections, neonatal death (SIDS, child abuse and neglect)
Sedatives (barbiturates, tranquilizers)	Lethargy, drowsiness, CNS depression	Neonatal abstinence syndrome, seizures, delayed lung maturity, possible teratogenic effects
Cocaine ("crack")	Hyperarousal state, generalized vasoconstriction, hypertension, increased spontaneous abortion, abruptio placentae, preterm labor, cardiovascular complications (stroke, heart attack), seizures, increased STDs	Stillbirth, prematurity, IUGR, irritability, decreased ability to interact with environmental stimuli, poor feeding reflexes, nausea, vomiting, diarrhea, decreased intellectual development; distended, flabby, creased abdomen (prune-belly syndrome) resulting from absence of abdominal muscles
Amphetamines ("speed" or "ice" when processed in crystals to smoke) Methamphetamines ("ecstasy")	Malnutrition, tachycardia, withdrawal symptoms (lethargy, depression)	Increased risk for cardiac anomalies and cleft palate, IUGR, withdrawal symptoms, fetal death
Marijuana ("pot" or "grass")	Often used with other drugs: alcohol, cocaine, tobacco; increased incidence of anemia and inadequate weight gain	Unclear, more study needed, believed related to prematurity, IUGR, neonatal tremors, sensitivity to light

CNS, Central nervous system; *FAS,* fetal alcohol syndrome; *HIV,* human immunodeficiency virus; *IUGR,* intrauterine growth restriction; *LBW,* low birth weight; *PROM,* premature rupture of membranes; *SIDS,* sudden infant death syndrome; *STDs,* sexually transmissible diseases.

syndrome is twice as frequent in children of smokers (Moran, 2000).

Alcohol

Fetal alcohol syndrome (FAS) is the leading cause of mental retardation and is the only cause that is preventable (Botham, 2000). Researchers are unsure in what way alcohol causes damage to the fetus. However, alcohol is known to pass easily through the placental barrier, and concentrations found in the fetus are believed to be at least as high as those found in the mother. During the first trimester, alcohol is believed to affect cell membranes and alter the organization of tissue. Throughout pregnancy, alcohol interferes with the metabolism of carbohydrates, lipids, and proteins and thus retards cell growth and division. The central nervous system (CNS) is probably most vulnerable during the third trimester, a time of rapid brain growth.

The teratogenic effects of alcohol are well known. FAS is the most serious condition related to drinking during pregnancy. This syndrome is characterized by three clinical features:

1. A recognizable combination of facial features—Common facial anomalies associated with FAS include short palpebral fissures (the openings between the eyelids), flat midface, indistinct philtrum (median groove on the external surface of the upper lip), and a thin upper lip (Figure 24-3).
2. Prenatal and postnatal growth restriction—Growth restriction in length, weight, and head circumference is present at birth and weight is low for height during childhood.
3. Central nervous system impairment—CNS developmental abnormalities include decreased head size, structural brain abnormalities and neurologic signs. Microcephaly, high activity level, short attention span, poor short-term memory, and lower intelligence quotient may occur.

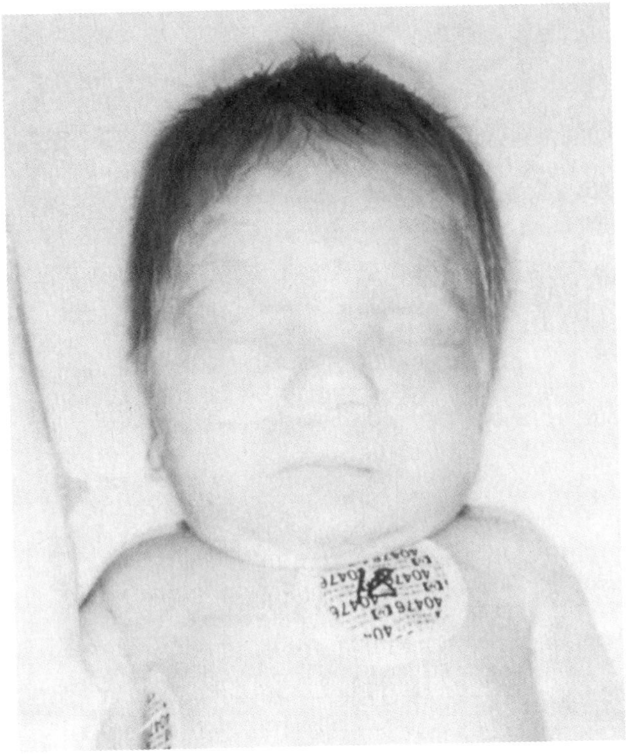

FIGURE 24-3 Infant with fetal alcohol syndrome. Subtle indicators present are flat midface, indistinct philtrum, and low-set ears. (Courtesy Trish Beachy, Perinatal Program Coordinator, University of Colorado Health Sciences, Denver.)

Fetal alcohol effects (FAE) describes infants who exhibit mild or partial manifestations of FAS, such as low birth weight, developmental delay that may not be obvious for 1 to 2 years, and hyperactivity. *Alcohol-related neurodevelopmental disorder (ARND)* and *alcohol-related birth defects (ARBD)* are other terms to describe problems caused by prenatal exposure to alcohol. ARND includes problems with judgment, problem solving, and memory, whereas ARBD includes cardiac, skeletal, renal, ocular, and auditory abnormalities. Because the amount of alcohol necessary to cause these problems is unknown, abstaining from drinking alcohol throughout pregnancy is recommended.

Cocaine

Actions of Cocaine. Cocaine is a powerful, short-acting stimulant of the CNS. Chemically, cocaine works by blocking the presynaptic reuptake of the neurotransmitters norepinephrine and dopamine, producing an excess of these substances at nerve terminals. The excess of neurotransmitters acts on the cerebral cortex to produce a hyperarousal state that results in euphoria, physical excitement, reduced fatigue, and a heightened sense of well-being and power. Anorexia, hyperglycemia, hyperthermia, and tachypnea are among the side effects of cocaine use.

When the initial euphoria wears off, a period of irritability, fatigue, lethargy, depression, and impatience occurs, which elicits a strong desire for additional cocaine so that the initial feelings can be recaptured. Physical effects of cocaine use are related to cardiovascular stimulation and vasoconstriction. The heart rate, systolic blood pressure, and demand for oxygen increase. Complications of generalized vasoconstriction include myocardial ischemia or infarction, cerebrovascular accidents, and pulmonary, renal, and gastrointestinal problems.

Maternal and Fetal Effects. Many women who use cocaine have a lifestyle that includes the use of additional drugs, such as alcohol, tranquilizers, or marijuana, to "come down" from the superarousal state that cocaine produces. In addition, women who abuse cocaine are less likely to seek prenatal care or eat a diet that contains adequate nutrition. In addition, sex is often exchanged for drugs, which places the woman at increased risk for STDs.

Cocaine directly stimulates uterine contractions, and one of the most common problems attributed to cocaine use in the pregnant woman is premature delivery. Increased incidence of spontaneous abortion and abruptio placentae also occur because of the cocaine-induced vasoconstriction of placental vessels. Additional complications include premature rupture of membranes, precipitous delivery, and stillbirths.

Cocaine crosses the placental barrier and causes the same physical stress on the fetus as on the expectant mother. In addition, clearance of the drug takes a prolonged period of time in the fetus. Fetal effects include tachycardia, decreased beat-to-beat variability of the fetal heart rate baseline, fetal overactivity, and intrauterine growth restriction.

Neonatal Effects. Clinical signs observed in neonates exposed to cocaine in utero include low birth weight, tremors, tachycardia, marked irritability, muscular rigidity, hypertension, and exaggerated startle reflex. These infants are difficult to console and exhibit an inability to respond to voices or environmental stimuli. They often are poor feeders and have frequent episodes of diarrhea.

The behavioral and developmental characteristics of cocaine-exposed infants may include learning problems, and delayed language and motor development. Infants may continue to be irritable and have limited interaction with people and objects in their environment. They are at increased risk for SIDS.

Marijuana

The active constituent of marijuana is delta-9-tetrahydrocannabinol (THC), which crosses the placenta and accumulates in the fetus. Marijuana is the most commonly used illicit drug and often is paired with other drugs such as cocaine and alcohol, making it difficult to determine the effects that are solely the result of marijuana use (Bauer, 1998).

An increased incidence in maternal anemia and inadequate maternal weight gain seems to occur with repeated use of marijuana. Clinically, the neonate may exhibit hyperirritability, tremors, sleep disruption, and unusual sensitivity to light. Long-term effects of marijuana on the development of the child are unclear.

Heroin

Heroin is an illegal opiate derived from morphine that produces severe physical addiction. Like all opiates, heroin is a CNS depressant that soothes and lulls. It produces a feeling of mental dullness, drowsiness, and finally stupor ("nodding out," or "on the nod"). Addiction may be said to exist when discontinuance causes withdrawal symptoms (abstinence syndrome) that are quickly relieved by a dose of the drug.

Women who abuse heroin have poor general health with multiple medical problems associated with their drug abuse and addicted lifestyle. Heroin is an appetite suppressant that also interferes with absorption of nutrients that are ingested, and many women are malnourished and anemic at the beginning of pregnancy. Additional problems include a high incidence of STDs and infections such as hepatitis and exposure to HIV from sharing unclean needles.

Fetal Effects. The fetus suffers both direct and indirect effects of heroin use by the expectant mother. The street supply of heroin usually is not steady, and direct effects on the fetus result from frequent episodes of maternal overdose alternating with periods of withdrawal from the drug. This exposes the fetus to intermittent episodes of hypoxia in utero, which increases the risk of prematurity, growth restriction, spontaneous abortion, and stillbirth. Indirect effects result from maternal malnutrition and fetal exposure to STDs.

Neonatal Effects. Infants born to mothers who are addicted to opiates including heroin, methadone, meperidine, and morphine exhibit a neonatal abstinence (withdrawal) syndrome. This syndrome affects all body systems with most signs involving the neurologic or gastrointestinal systems. Long-term developmental and learning problems may occur. In addition, the lifestyle of parents who are substance abusers is strongly associated with child neglect and abuse, which are major causes of infant death in this population. (Withdrawal signs and management of the neonate are discussed in Chapter 30, pp. 857.)

Diagnosis and Management of Substance Abuse

In addition to toxicology screening, the pregnant woman who uses illicit drugs must be tested throughout pregnancy for STDs, hepatitis, and exposure to HIV. Ultrasonography, nonstress tests, and biophysical profiles help pinpoint problems. Nurses monitor weight gain and provide guidance in nutrition at each opportunity to prevent maternal anemia and inadequate weight gain.

Therapeutic management depends on the type of drug used. In the case of opiates such as heroin, withdrawal during pregnancy has been associated with significant fetal stress and even fetal death. Pregnant women who use heroin often are placed on the alternative drug methadone. Methadone can be taken orally and is long acting, maintaining consistent blood levels, in contrast to the use of heroin, which is short acting and results in wide swings in blood level that can have severe adverse effects on the fetus. The woman receives a daily dose of methadone in a drug treatment program and is more likely to receive prenatal care. However, women using methadone often use other illicit drugs such as cocaine and marijuana (Brown, et al., 1998).

Treatment is aimed at establishing abstinence and preventing relapse. Combining education, individual and group therapy sessions, and peer support groups (such as Narcotics Anonymous, Alcoholics Anonymous, Cocaine Anonymous) often is helpful. All members of the health care team must understand that women have extremely positive memories associated with drug use, and thus relapse is common. Written contracts that focus on abstinence for 1 day at a time often are used to help the patient who has relapsed and experiences severe feelings of guilt and self-blame.

Various alternative therapies have been tried for treatment of addictions. Research about the various methods has been largely inconclusive. Acupuncture has shown positive effects in some studies, but further research is needed (Culliton, Boucher, & Bullock, 1999). Although no complementary or alternative therapy has been proven to be completely effective, some may be beneficial.

Complementary/Alternative Therapy

Acupuncture
Biofeedback
Hypnosis
Light therapy
Massage
Nutritional supplements such as zinc

Check Your Reading

8. How does smoking affect the neonate? What are the long-term effects on the child?
9. How does FAS compare with FAE?
10. What are the long-term effects of maternal cocaine use on the child?
11. Why are women who use heroin encouraged to use methadone during pregnancy?

APPLICATION OF THE NURSING PROCESS: MATERNAL SUBSTANCE ABUSE

ANTEPARTUM PERIOD

Assessment

Multiple drug abuse appears to be the most common substance abuse problem among women, and all women must be screened at the first prenatal visit for nicotine, alcohol, and other drugs. Because substance abuse occurs in all populations, the nurse must not make assumptions based on class, race, or economic status.

Certain behaviors are strongly associated with substance abuse: seeking prenatal care late in the pregnancy, failing to keep appointments, and following recommended regimens inconsistently. Physical appearance offers additional clues. Poor grooming, inadequate weight gain, or a pattern of weight gain that does not correspond to the stated gestational age may be signs of a lifestyle that includes substance abuse. Intravenous drug users may have fresh needle punctures, thrombosed veins, or signs of cellulitis.

Defensive and hostile behaviors may be overt signs of substance abuse. Women who use drugs have low self-esteem, and they are dealing with conflicting issues: the physical or psychological need for the substance, the need to deny that the substance is harming the fetus, guilt that they may be responsible for harming the fetus, and finally, fear that they will be prosecuted for use of illegal drugs. In addition, many women with substance abuse problems face the discrimination and resentment of health care professionals who direct their frustration at the woman rather than the problem.

CRITICAL TO REMEMBER

Behaviors Associated with Substance Abuse

- Prenatal care sought late in pregnancy
- Failure to keep prenatal appointments
- Inconsistent follow-through with recommended care
- Poor grooming, inadequate weight gain
- Needle punctures, thrombosed veins, cellulitis
- Defensive or hostile reactions
- Anger or apathy regarding pregnancy

Given the powerful deterrents to self-disclosure, extensive history taking provides the best opportunity to determine current and past substance use. The nurse taking the health history must exhibit patience, empathy, and tolerance and use a blend of approaches that reinforce concern for the woman and her infant.

Medical History

Determine whether the woman has medical conditions that are prevalent among women who use drugs, such as depression, seizures, hepatitis, pneumonia, cellulitis, STDs, hypertension, and suicide attempts. Current problems may include insomnia, panic attacks, exhaustion, and heart palpitations.

Obstetric History

Evaluate for past and current complications of pregnancy. Spontaneous abortions, premature deliveries, abruptio placentae, and stillbirths are associated with substance abuse, although they also occur in the population that has never used drugs. Current complications may include STDs, vaginal bleeding, and an inactive or hyperactive fetus. Fundal height may be inconsistent with gestational age, suggesting intrauterine growth restriction.

Investigate emotional responses regarding the pregnancy, such as anger or apathy. These feelings are particularly significant during the latter half of the pregnancy, when the normal feelings of ambivalence would be expected to be resolved. Negative feelings toward the pregnancy may interfere with prenatal compliance with follow-up care.

History of Substance Abuse

Obtaining an accurate history of substance abuse is difficult and depends in large part on the way the health care worker approaches the woman. A sincere, nonjudgmental, and empathetic approach promotes an open exchange of information.

Investigate all forms of drug use, including cigarettes, over-the-counter drugs, prescribed medications, and alcohol, as well as illicit drugs such as cocaine, marijuana, and heroin. Examine patterns of drug use, which can range from occasional recreational use to weekly binges to daily dependence on a particular drug or group of drugs. (Suggestions for interviewing are shown in Table 24-5.)

Analysis

Some women acknowledge the use of harmful substances but do not fully understand the effects. Other women acknowledge the use of drugs and are aware of their harmful effects but unable to stop using the substances. A nursing diagnosis that addresses both factors is "Risk for Altered Health Maintenance related to lack of knowledge of the effects of substance abuse on self and fetus and inability to manage stress without the use of drugs."

Planning

Goals and expected outcomes for this diagnosis are that the woman will do the following:

- Identify the harmful effects of substances on herself and the infant.
- Verbalize feelings related to continued use of harmful substances.
- Identify personal strengths and accept resources offered by the health care delivery system to stop using drugs.

Table 24-5

TECHNIQUES FOR INTERVIEWING A WOMAN ABOUT SUBSTANCE ABUSE

To determine whether the woman abuses substances:
- Express an accepting and nonjudgmental attitude.
- Explain why it is important to know about substance abuse: "We need to know about anything that might affect you or your baby during the pregnancy."
- Acknowledge that women may be reluctant to disclose information: "I know it's difficult to talk to us about this, but we need to know so that we can give you and your baby the best care possible."
- Begin with questions about over-the-counter or prescription drugs and lead up to use of tobacco, alcohol, and, finally, illicit drugs.
- Demonstrate knowledge of types and forms of drugs commonly used in the community: "Do you see much heroin in your area?" "Do you have friends who are using crack?"

When substance abuse is acknowledged, the important points in the drug history are the following:
- The type of drug used
- The amount of drug used
- The frequency of use
- The time of last dose

The nurse can ask specific questions:
- How often have you taken over-the-counter medications?
- What drugs did you take last month? Were they prescribed?
- How many cigarettes do you smoke on a daily basis? Are there times when you smoke more?
- How many times a week do you drink alcoholic beverages (beer, wine, mixed drinks)?
- How many in a day? Are there times when you have more drinks?
- How often did you use (drug used) before becoming pregnant? How often do you use it now? Do you snort? Smoke crack? Shoot cocaine? How many lines or rocks do you use? How long do you stay high?

Interventions

Effective interventions for substance abuse require the combined efforts of nurses, physicians, social workers, law enforcement, and numerous community and federal agencies. Nurses must be aware that progress is slow and frustrating. Keep in mind that the major priority is to protect the fetus and the expectant mother from the harmful effects of drugs.

Examining Attitudes

When working with substance-abusing pregnant women, nurses must identify and acknowledge their own feelings and prejudices. They may have limited knowledge about perinatal substance abuse and negative attitudes toward mothers who abuse substances (Selleck & Redding, 1998). Nurses commonly express anger at the woman who not only engages in self-destructive behavior but also may be inflicting harm on an innocent victim. Avoiding becoming judgmental or even unknowingly punitive to the pregnant woman may be difficult. Nurses also may feel helpless, incompetent, and discouraged when the pregnant woman continues to abuse drugs despite the best efforts of the health care team.

Inservice education, professional consultation, and peer support are helpful when working with pregnant women who abuse drugs. These processes can allow opportunities for discussion, sharing of feelings, problems, and particularly troublesome treatment issues.

Preventing Substance Abuse

The key to any preventive strategy is to provide accurate information in terms that the client can easily understand. Use posters, diagrams, pamphlets, and other visual aids to describe the effects of alcohol, tobacco, cocaine, and heroin on the fetus. Visual aids should be posted in high schools, colleges, supermarkets, shopping centers, and other areas where women of childbearing age will be exposed to them.

Focus on the benefits of remaining drug free. These benefits include a decrease in maternal and neonatal complications. For example, the effects of smoking tobacco are potentially dose related and cumulative, and nurses need to encourage and support cessation at any point during pregnancy.

Providing Follow-Up Care

At each antepartum visit, consider the current status of substance use, social service needs, education needs, and compliance with treatment referrals. In particular, address current drug use because women may change their pattern of drug use during pregnancy. For instance, they may stop using cocaine but increase their use of marijuana or alcohol.

Verify compliance with recommended treatment regimens such as antepartum clinics and chemical-dependence referral programs. Coordinate care among various service providers such as group therapy and prenatal classes. Establish communication with all agencies that provide care, and facilitate communication that helps the woman with a chaotic lifestyle meet treatment objectives.

Provide continuing prenatal education about the anatomy and physiology of pregnancy and consequences of prenatal substance abuse. Describe the way the newborn benefits when the mother abstains from using drugs including tobacco and alcohol. Praise any attempts at abstinence and encourage the expectant mother to try again if she relapses.

Communicating with the Woman

Ask the expectant mother about other stressors that may be contributing to the pattern of substance abuse. Additional stressors may include inadequate housing, economic predicaments, family discord, and emotional or physical illness.

Continue to exercise patience because a hurried or impatient nurse may lose the trust of the expectant mother. Be honest at all times while displaying a nonjudgmental attitude as well as genuine interest and concern. This is especially important when the woman relapses into substance-abusing patterns. Allow her to express guilt, and reassure her that abstinence is possible and she must simply begin again.

Helping the Woman Identify Strengths

Assist the substance-abusing pregnant woman in identifying personal strengths because she generally has a poor self-image. Acknowledge her actions when she abstains from the use of drugs or alcohol for even a short time. Praise for maintaining an adequate weight gain and attending prenatal classes may increase self-esteem and compliance with the recommended regimen of care.

Evaluation

Interventions have been successful if the expectant mother identifies the harmful effects of substance abuse on herself and on the fetus, discusses her strengths and her feelings about continued use of substances, and is receptive to assistance to stop using drugs.

INTRAPARTUM PERIOD

Assessment

Cocaine

Nurses who work in labor and delivery units must become skilled at identifying drug-induced signs and symptoms. Signs associated with frequent or recent use of crack cocaine include profuse sweating, high blood pressure, and irregular respirations combined with a lethargic response to labor and apparent lack of interest in the necessary interventions. Additional signs include dilated pupils, increased body temperature, and sudden onset of severely painful contractions. Fetal signs often include tachycardia and excessive fetal activity. Fetal bradycardia and late decelerations may occur.

CRITICAL TO REMEMBER

Signs of Recent Cocaine Use

Diaphoresis, high blood pressure, irregular respirations
Dilated pupils, increased body temperature
Sudden onset of severely painful contractions
Fetal tachycardia, excessive fetal activity
Angry, caustic, abusive reactions and paranoia

Emotional signs of recent cocaine use may include angry, caustic, or abusive reactions to those attempting to provide care. Emotional lability and paranoia are signs of cocaine intoxication.

Heroin

Typically, the pregnant woman addicted to heroin comes to the labor and delivery unit intoxicated from a recent drug administration. When the effects of the drug begin to wear off, withdrawal symptoms may be observed. These include yawning, diaphoresis, rhinorrhea, restlessness, and excessive tearing of the eyes.

Analysis

One of the most relevant nursing diagnoses during the intrapartal period is "Risk for Injury related to physiologic and psychological effects of recent drug use."

Planning

The major goal or expected outcome for this nursing diagnosis is that the woman and the fetus will remain free from injury during labor and childbirth.

Interventions

Preventing Injury

When a laboring woman has recently used a substance, the nurse must intervene to meet the needs of the woman and the fetus for safety, oxygen, and comfort.

Admitting Procedure. Two nurses may be needed to admit the woman into the labor unit and to persuade her to assume a safe position. One nurse helps the woman into the position, initiates electronic fetal monitoring, and begins administration of oxygen, as needed. The other nurse acts as communicator.

Because the woman who has recently used a drug such as cocaine often has difficulty following directions, she should hear only one voice telling her what to do. The second nurse states firmly what is happening and exactly what the woman must do: "Lie on your left side." "This helps us watch how the baby is doing." "This gives you more oxygen." This nurse maintains eye contact with the woman while giving her instructions.

Setting Limits. Realizing the importance of setting limits is critical to protect the safety of the mother and the fetus. For instance, the mother cannot smoke. The nurse may say, "It must be difficult not to smoke, but there is real danger to you and to all of us if you do smoke when oxygen is flowing." The mother who must remain in bed may become agitated. The nurse may say, "I know it is hard to stay in bed, but we can't take good care of the baby when you walk." If walking is safe for the woman, the nurse must set limits about where she can walk (in the labor room, not to the cafeteria).

Initiating Seizure Precautions. The laboring woman who recently used cocaine is at risk for hypertensive crisis and must be protected from injury in case of seizures. Seizure precautions are as follows:

- Keep the bed in a low, locked position.
- Pad side rails and keep them up at all times.
- Make sure suction equipment functions properly to prevent aspiration.
- Reduce environmental stimuli (lights, noise) as much as possible.

Maintaining Effective Communication

Establishing a therapeutic pattern of communication is one of the primary methods of providing care for the patient who has recently used cocaine. Avoid confrontation. Instead, acknowledge feelings: "I know you hurt, and I know how frightened you are. I will do everything I can to make you comfortable." When the woman is abusive, be careful not to take the abuse personally or react in a nontherapeutic manner.

Examine your own feelings when women are abusive and acknowledge when anger is getting in the way of providing care. Another nurse may need to assume care of the woman for a time to allow some relief from unrelenting abusive comments.

Providing Pain Control

Pain control for women who are substance abusers poses a difficult problem because determining the type or combination of drugs that were used before admission is often impossible. If the woman has used heroin, drugs such as morphine, hydromorphone, and meperidine must be used with caution. If medications can be administered safely, do not withhold them under the false assumption that their use will contribute to addiction. Comfort measures include sacral pressure, back rubs, a cool cloth on the head, and continual support and encouragement as for any other woman in labor.

Preventing Heroin Withdrawl

To prevent or stabilize heroin withdrawal during labor, administer methadone intramuscularly, as ordered, if the woman is nauseated or vomiting. Give methadone to the woman who usually receives methadone at chemical-dependence centers if she did not receive her daily dose. Avoid use of drugs such as butorphanol (Stadol) because they may cause acute withdrawal in the woman and fetus.

Evaluation

Both the expectant mother and the fetus may have experienced harmful effects of drugs throughout pregnancy. However, the interventions for this nursing diagnosis can be considered effective if neither the woman nor the fetus sustains additional injury during labor and childbirth.

POSTPARTUM PERIOD

In the postpartum unit, be aware of the signs of recent drug use and abstinence syndrome and continue to assess the vital signs and level of consciousness of the mother. Observe the mother-infant interaction so that bonding and attachment can be promoted. This is a major concern at this time (see Chapter 30, p. 861.) Encourage the woman to continue her efforts to stop taking substances. This is especially important because women who reduce or stop substance use in pregnancy often return to using it within 2 years (Kearney, 1999).

Check Your Reading

12. What prenatal behaviors indicate substance abuse?
13. What signs and symptoms indicate recent cocaine use?
14. How does nursing care differ during the intrapartum period when the woman has recently taken cocaine?

BIRTH OF AN INFANT WITH CONGENITAL ANOMALIES

Even when everything goes according to plan, childbirth is a time of stress for parents. Their anxiety about the condition of the infant is obvious as they carefully trace the features and count the fingers and toes of their newborn. When the infant is not perfect but is born with anomalies, the parents often are overwhelmed with feelings of shock and grief. Because nurses are with the parents more than other members of the perinatal team, they have an opportunity to help the family adjust and cope with their feelings.

Factors Influencing Emotional Responses of Parents

Timing and Manner of Being Told

At one time, common practice was to remove the infant born with congenital anomalies from the delivery area before parents could see the infant. Parents were told about the anomalies at a later time, often after the physician had prepared them for disturbing news. This practice changed, however, with the discovery that parents experienced less stress if they were told at once and permitted to hold their baby if the physical status of the infant allowed (Figure 24-4).

The manner of presenting information also changed. Physicians and nurses became aware of the importance of helping the parents accept and bond with the newborn. Many now present the infant to the parents in a very sensitive manner, as the following incident illustrates.

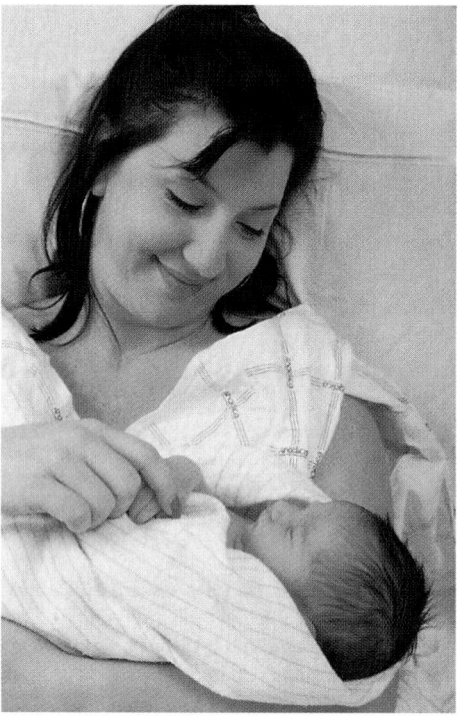

FIGURE 24-4 Touching and cuddling between parents and the infant with a congenital anomaly foster attachment and help resolve the grieving process.

A baby girl was delivered with a major irreparable anomaly: the right arm below the elbow was missing entirely. While the placenta was still intact and the cord attached, the physician placed the infant on the mother's abdomen and said, "Oh, we have a very special baby." As the mother and father stroked their baby, the physician pointed out how healthy and beautiful the child was and allowed time for the parents to hold their child.

Prior Knowledge of the Defect

In this age of sophisticated prenatal examinations, the parents may be aware of the existence of a congenital anomaly before the infant is born. These parents may not demonstrate the shock and disbelief at the birth that is seen in parents who are unprepared. This should not be interpreted to mean that they do not experience grief but rather that they have completed some of the early stages of grieving before the birth.

One young couple was aware from 18 weeks' gestation that the fetus had hydrocephalus and protrusion of brain tissue from the skull. The mother elected to carry the fetus to term so that the infant would have "every chance at life." When the infant died within minutes after birth, the parents calmly held their child and called the infant by the name they had selected several weeks previously. The only overt signs of grief were silent tears and a request to see their minister.

Type of Defect

Although any defect in a newborn produces feelings of extreme concern and anxiety, certain defects are associated with long-term parenting problems. Accepting an infant with facial or genital anomalies is particularly difficult for the family and community. The face is visible to everyone, and parents are fearful about whether the child will be accepted. If the defect is cleft lip and palate, the parents are extremely concerned about surgical repair. Common questions include "When can it be done?" "Will the child look normal?" "Will the child sound normal?" "Will the scars be obvious?" Parents often are anxious about the way grandparents and siblings will accept the child. With time and support, families often work out unique methods to help the family develop strong feelings of attachment.

One young father, profoundly disturbed about the birth of a daughter with a cleft lip and palate and extremely concerned about the way his 6-year-old daughter would respond to the infant, took control of the situation. He carefully presented the infant to her sister and pointed out that the baby was small and had special problems. She would need the love of her big sister to overcome them. The 6-year-old held the infant and promised to help care for her. After a long talk, the older child, with the help of a nurse, fashioned a sign that was placed in the infant's crib. The sign said, "Hello, my name is Rachel. As you can see, I have a problem, but I am going to be fine."

Gender is at the core of a person's identity, and any defect of the genitals, however slight or correctable, arouses deep concern in both parents. Some anomalies such as hypospadias (opening of the urethra on the underside of the penis) are repaired in early childhood. Other genital anomalies such as ambiguous genitalia (assignment of gender is in doubt) cause extreme concern in the family and affect such basic things as what to name the infant, ways to dress the infant, and ways to respond to questions about the infant's gender.

Irreparable Defect

Although the initial impact of any defect is profound disappointment and concern, when the defect is irreparable the parents have no time limit to their endeavors. Eventually, they must grapple with the knowledge that the infant will have a lifelong handicap. Examples of irreparable defects include Down syndrome, microcephaly, and amelia (absence of an entire extremity).

Grief and Mourning

Grief describes the emotional response to loss. *Mourning* is the process of going through the phases of grief until the loss can be accepted and resolved. Birth of an infant with an anomaly evokes a grief response, and the family must mourn the loss of the perfect infant they fantasized during pregnancy. Early emotions include denial, anger, and guilt.

Denial and disbelief are the initial reactions of most parents to the birth of an infant with a congenital defect. "This can't be true." "How could this happen?" Anger often is a pervasive response and may take the form of fault-finding or resentment. Anger may be directed toward the family, the medical personnel, or the self, but it is seldom directed toward the infant. Guilt may be expressed as a question of responsibility for the defect: "I shouldn't have taken that trip while I was pregnant."

Other emotions include fear, which may be expressed as concern about what must be done in the immediate or distant future (surgical procedures, complicated health care, the infant's potential for a normal life). Sadness and depression, manifested by crying, withdrawal from relationships, lack of energy, inability to sleep, and decreased appetite, may precede acceptance and resolution. Gradually—often after a prolonged time—the feelings of sadness abate and the family is able to accept and resolve its grief.

Check Your Reading

15. When should parents be told that the infant has anomalies?
16. What types of defects most affect parenting?
17. How can the reaction of parents to birth anomalies be described?

Nursing Considerations

Assisting with the Grieving Process

Parents must grieve the loss of the perfect infant that they expected before they can form an attachment with this newborn. Nurses can help by remaining with the parents through the initial phase of shock and disbelief and maintaining an atmosphere that encourages them to express their feelings. One way to do this is to listen carefully to what the parents say and respond by reflecting the content and feelings that they express.

For example, the mother of an infant girl with cleft palate says, "How could this happen? I should have gone to the doctor earlier." A helpful response might be, "Actually, we don't know what causes cleft palate, but let's talk about how you are feeling." This offers reassurance but keeps the interaction open to explore the underlying feelings of guilt that the mother may be expressing.

Grief responses vary with individuals, and cultural and religious beliefs affect the expression of grief. Some groups express grief openly by crying, becoming angry, or seeking comfort from a support group. Other cultures (such as Chinese, Japanese, and Native Americans) do not. They may appear stoic and not reveal the depths of their grief. In some cultures (such as Latino), public grieving is acceptable for women but not men.

Promoting Bonding and Attachment

A priority nursing intervention is to promote bonding and attachment, which may be disrupted when parents who expected a perfect infant give birth to an infant with an abnormality. The process often begins when the nurse communicates acceptance of the infant.

> To do this, the nurse handles the newborn gently and presents the infant as something precious. Parents are particularly sensitive to facial expressions of shock or distress. Many nurses emphasize the normal aspects of the infant's body: "She is so alert and she has the most beautiful eyes." Perhaps it is most important to help the parents hold their infant as soon as possible. Touching and cuddling are essential to caring.

Providing Accurate Information

Nurses who work in perinatal settings must become informed about follow-up treatment and timing of surgical procedures so that they can clarify and reinforce information provided by the physician. This involves discussing the plan of care with the physician and researching the nursing care that will be required. Parents develop trust in the health care team when consistent information is presented clearly and explained fully. Parents may need information repeated frequently because retaining it may be difficult.

Facilitating Communication

Nurses are sometimes fearful of being asked questions they are unable to answer, or they fear they will say the wrong thing.

> The most helpful course of action is to answer questions as honestly as possible. If unsure of information, say so: "I am not sure about that, but I will find out about that for you." In addition to answers, parents need kindness, support, and genuine concern.

It is crucial that family members communicate with one another as well as with the health professionals. Fathers should be included in all discussions, demonstrations, and care of the infant. Information and empathy should be offered consistently to both parents. Without this, the father cannot be expected to support his partner, explain the infant's condition to relatives and friends, or begin to deal with his own shock and sadness.

Planning for Discharge

Often the infant may require special feeding, holding, and positioning techniques. For example, parents may need to learn ways to feed an infant with cleft palate or ways to hold and position the infant with meningocele (protrusion of meninges through a defect in the vertebrae). Early participation in infant care fosters feelings of attachment and responsibility for the infant.

Anticipatory guidance may help prevent problems in the family when the infant is discharged to home care. Siblings' reaction and behavior depend on their ages and abilities to understand the needs of the infant. Young children, who often are jealous of the attention and care that the infant requires, may regress to infantile behaviors such as bed wetting and thumb sucking. Parents should be reminded that this indicates a need for attention rather than naughtiness.

Although grandparents can be a great source of strength and support, they also may have difficulty adjusting to the infant with an abnormality. When appropriate, or if the parents indicate their willingness, include grandparents when teaching special care that the infant will need.

Providing Referrals

Finally, nurses often initiate referrals to national and community resources. Besides a referral to the social worker in the hospital, parents also may benefit from information about the National Easter Seal Society for Crippled Children, the March of Dimes Birth Defects Foundation, or the handicapped children's services of the public health department. In addition, organizations such as the Shriners provide funds for the care of children. Support groups vary among communities, and perinatal nurses may wish to make a list of the names, addresses, and telephone numbers of these organizations.

Check Your Reading

18. How do nurses promote bonding and attachment in families with an infant with congenital anomalies?
19. What should be included in discharge planning for the family of an infant with congenital anomalies?

PREGNANCY LOSS

Perinatal death can occur at any time. Early spontaneous abortion, fetal demise during the latter half of pregnancy, stillbirth, or neonatal death when the infant survives for a few days or weeks can be equally devastating for the parents who experience profound sadness and grief.

Because many people do not consider perinatal loss to be on the same level as the loss of an older child or adult, parents experiencing perinatal death often feel alone in their grief. In addition, friends and family members often are hesitant to discuss the loss for fear of saying the wrong thing. They may be uncomfortable with the topic and change the subject when parents want to talk.

Early Pregnancy Loss

Early pregnancy loss from spontaneous abortion or ectopic pregnancy may precipitate intense grief by the parents. However, many people, even health professionals, minimize the grief that occurs at this time. Comments such as "You shouldn't have any problems getting pregnant again" discount the feelings of the mother and father.

When ectopic pregnancy is the reason for the loss, the woman has to deal with the loss of the pregnancy and the possible loss of one fallopian tube. Health care workers mean well when they say, "You still have one fallopian tube left; you'll get pregnant again," but this does not acknowledge to the mother that a child has been lost.

Concurrent Death and Survival in Multifetal Pregnancy

Parents experience conflicting and complex feelings of joy and grief when one or more infants in a multifetal pregnancy survive and one or more infants in the same gestation die. Contrary to common belief, parents do not grieve less for the dead infant because of the joy that they experience in the living child. They experience an acute sense of loss despite having an infant, and they grieve no less for the infant who did not survive.

For parents experiencing both survival and death of an infant, the grieving process may be more complicated. They may have fears about the health of the surviving infant, especially if the infant is preterm or ill. They may be unable to grieve for the dead child because of their concerns and responsibilities for the surviving child. They also may experience problems with attachment to the surviving infant because of grieving. In addition, they may receive less support from others than parents who lost the only child in a single gestation.

Parents who experience the death of one infant and the survival of another need the same interventions as those offered for parents who lose the only child in a single gestation. These interventions include allowing the parents to hold the dead infant and gathering mementos. In addition, nurses must be prepared to confirm the cause of death, if known, and the health status of the surviving infant.

APPLICATION OF THE NURSING PROCESS: PREGNANCY LOSS

Assessment

Nursing assessment of the family that has experienced the loss of a fetus or infant requires a great deal of sensitivity. In the case of infant death, collect as much information as possible before meeting with the woman and her family for the first time so that hurtful mistakes can be avoided. Knowing the child's sex, weight, length, and gestational age and whether any abnormalities were noted will help the nurse communicate effectively.

Many perinatal units design a sticker to place on the door, chart, and Kardex so that all staff who come into contact with the family, including auxiliary, housekeeping, laboratory, and radiology personnel, will be alerted the infant has not survived. Designs include a flower, teardrop, fallen leaf, or rainbow. This visual symbol diminishes the chance that an uninformed person will make inadvertent comments that cause the family pain.

> Nurses often are unsure about the way to interact with a family that has experienced the loss of an infant. Nurses can help by acknowledging the situation and clarifying their role at once: "I am Bette Turner. I will be your nurse for the next 8 hours. I am so sorry for your loss. Let me know if there is any way I can be of help." This is not an appropriate time for self-disclosure or for false reassurance. Keep the focus on the family's response and their ability to support one another.

Initial grief responses, such as crying and expressions of anger, often occur during the woman's stay in the birth facility. Nurses who provide home care or make follow-up telephone calls must be aware of subtle cues of grief, such as sighing, excessive sleeping, apathy, poor hygiene, and loss of appetite. This awareness is especially important when assessing members of cultural groups that do not display grief publicly.

Also evaluate the availability of a support system that includes family members or clergy. Asking whether a spiritual adviser would offer comfort may be necessary. Many religions emphasize the acceptance of God's will and the immortality of the soul, and hearing these beliefs affirmed may help the family cope with the grief that they are experiencing.

Fathers often feel a need to appear strong so that they can support their partners. As a result, they often hold back their own feelings of grief and pain and are sometimes perceived as needing less support than mothers.

Analysis

The most obvious nursing diagnosis for any woman who experiences perinatal death is "Grieving related to newborn (or fetal) death."

Planning

Grief reactions are unique to each person, and assigning a time frame in which parents will acknowledge or share their grief is inappropriate. Goals and expected outcomes for this diagnosis are that the parents will do the following:

- Acknowledge their grief and express the meaning of the loss.
- Share their grief with significant others.

Interventions

Acknowledging the Infant

For many years, the common belief was that when an infant was stillborn or died shortly after birth, the less parents knew of the infant, the less they would grieve. The infant often was whisked away so that the parents never saw their newborn. Relatives often disposed of the clothes and bassinet of the expected infant before the mother returned home, and the parents were left with very few memories of the birth or the infant.

The response to perinatal death changed as nurses discovered that the most helpful interventions for grieving parents were those that acknowledged the rights of the baby. These include the following rights:

- To be recognized as a person who was born and died
- To be named
- To be seen, touched, and held by the family
- To have life-ending acknowledged
- To be put to rest with dignity (Primeau & Lamb, 1995)

Presenting the Infant to the Parents. The way in which the infant is presented to the parents is extremely important because these are the memories that they will retain. If necessary, wash the infant and apply baby lotion or powder. Wrap the infant in a soft, warm blanket. If possible, bring the parents and infant together while the infant is still warm and soft. Keeping the infant in a warmed incubator may be necessary if some time elapses before the parents have contact with the infant. If this is not possible, tell the parents that the skin may feel cool. Allow parents to keep the infant as long as they wish, and make them feel free to unwrap the infant if they wish.

Many nurses are concerned about the way to present the stillborn infant with severe deformities. Explain the defect briefly and gently. Wrap the infant to expose the most normal aspect. Use diapers to cover genital defects, and use booties and mittens to cover abnormalities of the hands and feet. Trying to hide the defects completely is not advisable, however. Allow parents to progress at their own speed in inspecting the infant. Parents may look at the abnormality or choose to leave the infant wrapped. They may quietly discuss positive features of the infant: "He has my father's eyes." "Look at the long fingers."

In one case, a stillborn infant had a severely deformed head and face. The nurse wrapped the infant loosely and draped a corner of the blanket over the part of the face that was most affected before giving the infant to the father and mother to hold. Neither parent lifted the blanket, although they did reach under the blanket to hold the infant's hands and feet.

Allow as much privacy and time as the parents and other family members need to be together. Avoid prying, and remain sensitive to cues that members of the family want to or prefer not to talk. Keeping up a flow of conversation is not necessary. A sympathetic smile, a gentle touch of the hand, and a promise to return in a specific time and returning at that time are equally important. Asking "Do you want to talk?" and then listening quietly and reflecting the mother or father's feelings are all that are required.

Preparing a Memory Packet. The death of a newborn is a loss that must be mourned by the parents, and mourning requires memories. Nurses have explored measures that help the family create memories of the infant so that the existence of the child is confirmed and the parents can complete the grieving process.

Most parents treasure a memory packet that includes a photograph, handprints or footprints, a birth bracelet with the date and time of birth, the crib card with the infant's name, weight, and length, and if possible, a lock of hair. Some parents and grandparents want pictures taken of themselves with the infant. The memory packet should be kept on file if the parents do not wish to take it home because they may change their minds later.

Assisting with Other Needs. If the family includes other children, help the parents plan ways to tell them about the death of the expected infant. Provide reading material about perinatal loss, grieving, and children's responses to death. Parents can take it home for later reading when they are less overwhelmed with immediate concerns. Offer to call clergy for them and discuss plans for a funeral or memorial service, if they wish. Discuss common reactions that families and friends might have, and mention that some may minimize the loss or urge them to have another baby in a misguided attempt to offer comfort. Let them know that grandparents also go through grief because of the loss as well as the pain their children must endure.

Providing Referrals

Parents may find that friends and relatives expect them to recover quickly from perinatal loss and are unable to understand their continued grief. Because parents experience grief and go through the process in different ways, they may not understand each other's responses. Mothers who want to talk about the loss repeatedly may have partners who deal with their grief by being stoic or focusing their energy on work. Emphasize the individuality of grief and that no single method or duration of grieving is right for everyone.

The greatest help often comes from contact with persons who have experienced similar loss, and a variety of support groups have been formed. These include Resolve through Sharing, AMEND (Aiding a Mother Experiencing Neonatal Death), SHARE (Source of Help in Airing and Resolving Experiences), and HAND (Helping After Neonatal Death). Some birth agencies offer ongoing support groups. Telephone calls may be made by agency staff and cards may be sent to help parents with their grief.

Couples usually want to know the cause of death of their infant. An autopsy may be recommended even if the cause of death is obvious. This gives parents the most accurate diagnosis for risk of recurrence in a future pregnancy. In some cases, the cause may never be found. Referral for genetic counseling may be appropriate for some parents who are concerned about the risk of a repeated tragedy. Future pregnancies will be stressful, and the woman will need closer follow-up than usual to identify any possible problems as soon as possible. The anxiety may continue in the neonatal period, and parents may need education and emotional support during this time.

Evaluation

Nursing care has been successful if the parents acknowledge their feelings of loss and grief and communicate them to significant others.

Check Your Reading

20. How should the stillborn infant be presented to the parents? Why?
21. What is a memory packet, and what should it include?

RELINQUISHMENT BY ADOPTION

Some women carry the pregnancy to term and then relinquish the newborn to the care of another family by adoption. The decision to place the infant for adoption is a painful one that can produce long-lasting feelings of ambivalence and grief. On the one hand, the expectant mother may be satisfied that the infant is going into a stable home in which a child is wanted and will receive excellent care. On the other hand, the social pressures against giving up a child are often intense.

The process of adoption is relatively simple for the expectant mother. Each state and many organized churches have adoption agencies. In addition, private adoptions are available, although the legality of these adoptions may be questioned in some states. In private adoptions, an attorney acts as the intermediary between the expectant woman and the couple wanting to adopt the infant. The adoptive family usually agrees to pay the medical expenses of the woman, and sometimes a supportive relationship is established between the expectant mother and adoptive family. Some adoptive mothers want to experience as much of the birth as possible and elect to act as coach or support person during the birth.

Nurses are sometimes unsure of ways to communicate with the woman who is relinquishing her infant. First, the nursing staff who come into contact with the woman must be informed of her decision to place the infant for adoption. This prevents inadvertent comments that could cause distress. Second, nurses must remember that adoption is *an act of love, not one of abandonment* because the woman relinquishes the newborn to a family that is better able to provide financial and emotional support.

Nurses also must be prepared to respect any special wishes that the mother may have about the birth. For instance, most birth mothers want to know all about the infant—how big he or she is, how healthy, how beautiful. Encourage them to see and hold the newborn and give the baby a name. Prepare them for the appearance of the baby before they see the infant. Many parents take photographs or save mementos such as the birth bracelet or crib card. Such actions provide memories of the infant and help the mother through the grieving process that may accompany relinquishment of the child.

The nurse should try to establish rapport and a trusting relationship with the birth mother. The first step in this process is to acknowledge the situation at the initial contact with the woman: "Hello, my name is Denise, and I will be your nurse today. I understand the adoptive family is coming this morning. What can I do to help you get ready for that?" This is much more helpful than providing postpartum care without reference to an event that is of utmost concern to the mother. It also provides a broad opening for her to express feelings that may include strong attachment and love for the infant, ambivalence about her decision, and profound sadness.

Therapeutic communication techniques such as reflecting, paraphrasing, and summarizing are useful to help the mother explore her feelings. Although the mother has chosen to relinquish her baby, the grief she experiences may be similar to loss by death. Her grief may not be shared with family and friends, who may not understand her feelings. The nurse should acknowledge the feelings the mother may have, avoid offering advice, and remain nonjudgmental.

Nurses also teach adoptive families the way to care for the newborn and what to expect in terms of growth and development. This requires that adequate time and a private place be provided. This family benefits from all the teaching that is provided for new parents. They may be anxious, and demonstrations and return demonstrations are appropriate.

Check Your Reading

22. What is meant by the phrase "adoption is an act of love"?
23. What are the nurse's responsibilities to the adoptive parents?

VIOLENCE AGAINST WOMEN

Physical abuse may start or increase in frequency and severity during pregnancy and the postpartum period (Toohey, 2000). It has been recognized as a risk to the health of both mothers and infants (Figure 24-5). Estimates of the number of women affected by domestic violence vary from 1.9 million to 5 million women each year (Tjaden & Thoennes, 1998; American College of Obstetricians & Gynecologists, 1999). Approximately 31% of women report being physically or sexually abused by their husbands or boyfriends at some point in their lives (Commonwealth Fund, 1999). The incidence during pregnancy is reported to range from 4% to 16% (McFarlane, Parker, & Soeken, 1996a). It is higher among pregnant teenagers, with more than 37% reporting physical abuse within the past year in some studies (Curry, Doyle, & Gilhooley, 1998; Curry, 1998).

Physical abuse is recurrent, with 60% of abused women reporting two or more episodes of violence. Although all ethnic groups report similar rates of abuse, major ethnic differences exist, with white women experiencing more frequent and more severe abuse (McFarlane, Parker, & Soeken, 1996a). It is seen at all socioeconomic levels.

Physical abuse may involve threats, slapping, and pushing. It also may escalate to punching, kicking, and

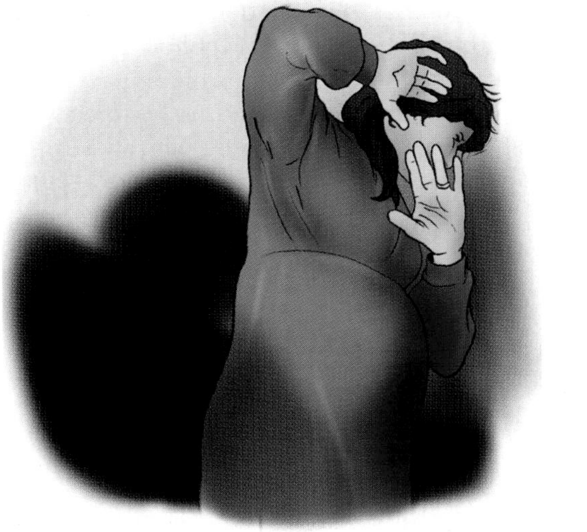

FIGURE 24-5 The woman who is abused by her partner lives with an ever-present risk of violence. Because they may not seek help, all women should be asked about abuse whenever they receive health care.

Table 24-6
MYTHS AND REALITIES OF VIOLENCE AGAINST WOMEN

Myths	Realities
The battered-woman syndrome affects only a small percentage of the population.	Battering is the single major cause of injury to women. 1.9 to 5 million women are battered each year by their partners.
Battering of women occurs only in lower socioeconomic classes and minority groups.	Violence occurs in families from all social, economic, educational, racial, and religious backgrounds.
The problem is really "spouse abuse," couples who assault each other.	Approximately 95% of serious assaults are male against female. Violence against women is about control and power.
Alcohol and drugs cause abusive behavior.	Substance abuse and violence against women are two separate problems. Substance abuse is a disease, but violence is a learned behavior that can be unlearned.
The abuser is "out of control."	He is not out of control. Instead, he is making a decision because he chooses who, when, and where he abuses.
The woman "got what she deserved."	No one deserves to be beaten. No one has the right to beat another person. Violent behavior is the responsibility of the violent person.
Women "like" it or they would leave.	Women are threatened with severe punishment or death if they attempt to leave. Many have no resources and are isolated, and they and their children are dependent on the abuser.
Couples counseling is a good recommendation for abusive relationships.	Couples counseling is not only ineffective for the couple, it can be dangerous for the abused woman.

beating that results in internal injury, wounds from weapons, or death. Sexual abuse, including rape, often is part of physical abuse, with almost half the abused women reporting being forced into sex by their male partners.

Physical violence occurs within the context of continuous mental abuse, threats, and coercion. As a result, the woman feels shame, lack of self-respect, and powerlessness. She often is isolated from sources of help and support.

In addition, physical abuse of the mother may be an indication of what life holds for the unborn child. In over 50% of homes in which domestic violence occurs, the children also are injured (Toohey, 2000). The majority of men who batter the woman also batter the children, and some women who are battered will physically abuse their children. Adults who abuse others often were abused as children.

Factors That Promote Violence

Family violence occurs in cultures in which the roles of males and females are gender based and little value is placed on the woman's role. Men hold power, and women are viewed as less worthy of respect than men. In these cultures, strength and aggression, the ability to "show her who is boss," are considered attractive and desirable in males.

In many cultures, women are seen as having less worth than men. Women earn less than men in the job market, and they often are victimized by marriage. For example, women who hold full-time jobs continue to carry the major responsibilities for housekeeping and child care. They often remain in unhealthy relationships because they are financially dependent on their partners. If they divorce, most women become single parents with a standard of living much lower than that of their former husbands.

Stereotyping males as powerful and females as weak and without value has a profound effect on the self-esteem of women. Many women internalize the messages and come to believe that they are less worthy than their partners and that they are the cause of their own punishment. They accept the message from society that women who are battered or raped "got what they deserved." Furthermore, American culture accepts and condones violence. Movies, television, and sports such as football, hockey, and boxing glorify aggression, physical strength, and the ability to hurt and dominate the opponent.

Although alcohol often is stated as a cause of violence against women, chemical dependence and domestic violence are two separate problems. Chemical dependence is a disease of addiction, but abuse is a learned behavior that can be unlearned. Violence may become more severe or bizarre when alcohol or drugs are involved, however. (See Table 24-6 for a summary of the myths and realities of violence against women.)

Characteristics of the Abuser

Physical abuse concerns power, and it is only one of many tactics that abusive men use to control their partners. Other tactics include isolation, intimidation, and threats. Extreme jealousy and possessiveness are typical of the abuser. An abusive male often attempts to control every aspect of the woman's life, including where she goes, to whom she speaks, and what she wears. He controls access to money and transportation

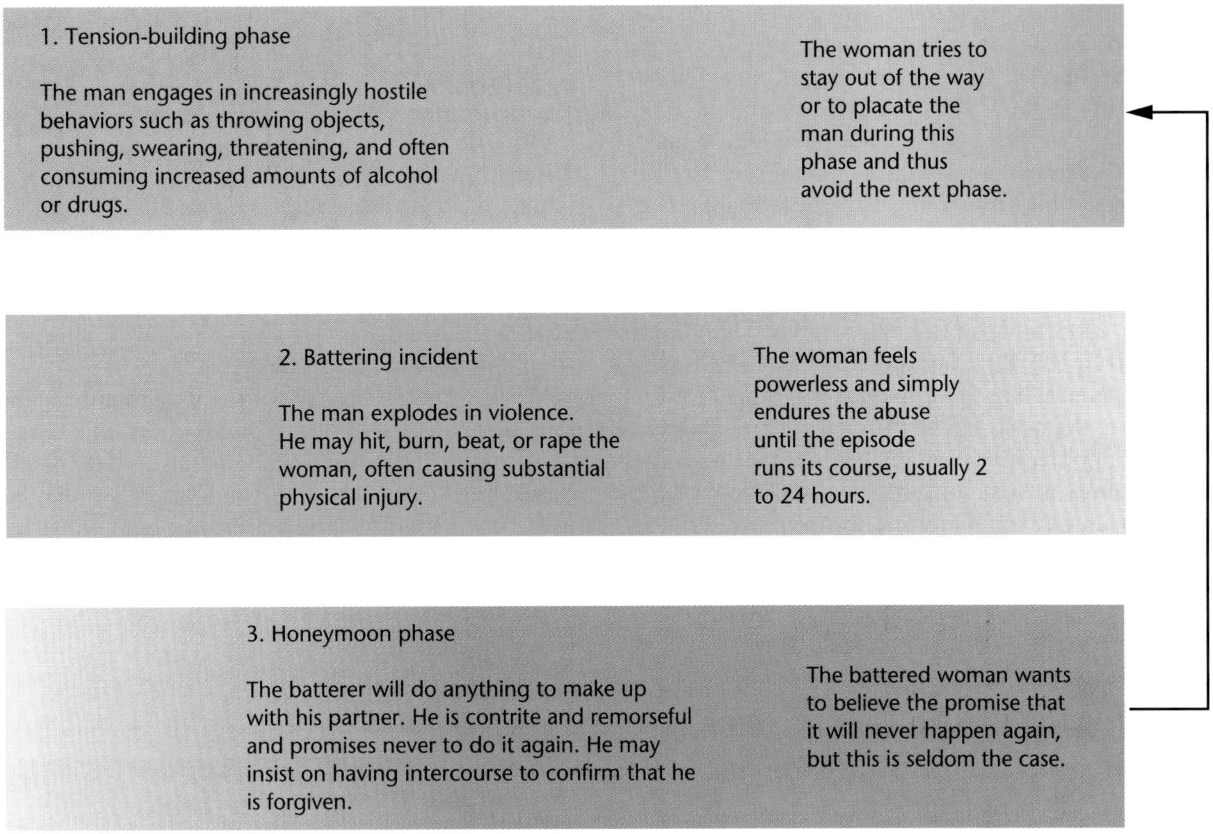

1. Tension-building phase
The man engages in increasingly hostile behaviors such as throwing objects, pushing, swearing, threatening, and often consuming increased amounts of alcohol or drugs.
The woman tries to stay out of the way or to placate the man during this phase and thus avoid the next phase.
2. Battering incident
The man explodes in violence. He may hit, burn, beat, or rape the woman, often causing substantial physical injury.
The woman feels powerless and simply endures the abuse until the episode runs its course, usually 2 to 24 hours.
3. Honeymoon phase
The batterer will do anything to make up with his partner. He is contrite and remorseful and promises never to do it again. He may insist on having intercourse to confirm that he is forgiven.
The battered woman wants to believe the promise that it will never happen again, but this is seldom the case.

FIGURE 24-6 Types of behaviors that are evident in each step of the cycle of violence.

and may force the woman to account for every moment spent away from him.

The abusive male often has a low tolerance for frustration and poor impulse control. He does not perceive his violent behavior as a problem and often denies responsibility for the violence by blaming the woman. Most abusive men come from homes in which they witnessed the abuse of their mothers or were abused as children. Men who inflict injury on their female partners are more likely to use alcohol and drugs, have problems with steady employment, and be estranged from the partner (Kyriacou, et al., 1999). Although many abusive men have alcohol problems, many also batter their partners when they are sober.

Cycle of Violence

Violence occurs in a cycle that consists of three phases: (1) a tension-building phase, (2) a battering incident, and (3) a "honeymoon phase." Being aware of behaviors that accompany each phase will enable the nurse to counsel the woman (Figure 24-6).

Effects of Battering

Abuse during pregnancy is correlated with health problems for the mother and infant. Women battered during pregnancy are more likely to have multiple injury sites, particularly of the abdomen, face, and breasts. Abused women tend to enter prenatal care late in the pregnancy, with up to 25% starting prenatal care in the third trimester. They are at increased risk for low weight gain and anemia, and a higher percentage report the use of tobacco, alcohol and illicit drugs (McFarlane, Parker, & Soeken, 1996b; Curry, 1998). Women may miss appointments because the batterer will not let them leave the house or because they wish to hide signs of recent injury. Pregnant women in battering relationships face an increased risk of prematurity and bearing low-birth-weight infants.

Abused women also have health problems unrelated to pregnancy. They are more likely to have conditions associated with stress, insomnia, chronic pain, and gynecologic problems. Severe pain during menstruation and intercourse and STDs are more often reported by women who have been abused (Letourneau, Holmes, & Chasedunn-Roark, 1999).

Nurse's Role in Prevention

Nurses can do a great deal to prevent physical abuse. First, they must examine their beliefs to determine whether they accept the prevailing attitude that blames the victim: "Why was she wearing that?" "She shouldn't have flirted with someone else." "Why does she stay with him?" Second, nurses can consciously practice in ways that empower women and make it clear that the woman owns her body. Once the woman is clear about ownership of her body, she has the right to decide the way it should be treated. Nurses must use language that indicates the woman is an active partner in her care: "You understand your body: what do you think?" "How did your body respond when you tried that?"

During examinations, nurses can introduce aspects of care that increase the woman's control over the situation. For example, make sure that the woman meets the physician or nurse practitioner who is to examine her while seated and clothed rather than while unclothed and in a lithotomy position. Nurses can place the examination table so that the woman's head, not her genitalia, meets the examiner's eye when he or she enters the room. When the woman is positioned for the examination, the table can be raised 45 degrees so that she has an opportunity to make eye contact with the examiner. Many nurses now provide the woman with a mirror so that she can view the examination and be fully informed about her body parts.

School nurses are in an excellent position to influence the way teenagers define gender roles: "Real men don't beat up women." "Girls don't have to put up with verbal or physical abuse from anyone." "Use a condom; it's not cool to give someone you care about sexually transmissible diseases or an unwanted pregnancy."

Nurses should be familiar with national resources that are designed to provide health care workers with technical assistance, training materials, posters, bibliographies, and relevant articles. The sources listed here provide information but are not crisis lines.

National Domestic Violence Health Resource Center
1-800-313-1310

National Clearinghouse for the Defense of Battered Women
1-215-351-0010

National Coalition Against Domestic Violence
1-303-839-1852
www.ncadv.org

National Domestic Violence Resource Center
1-800-537-2238

The National Domestic Violence Hotline (1-800-722-SAFE) offers information on crisis assistance throughout the United States. Their website, www.ndvh.org, is another source of information. Women who are being abused should be warned not to access Internet sources of information about abuse at home because their partners may be able to determine recently used Internet sites.

Check Your Reading

24. What is the effect of pregnancy on battering behavior?
25. How can nurses alter their practice to help prevent violence against women?

APPLICATION OF THE NURSING PROCESS: THE BATTERED WOMAN

Assessment

Stating that battered women can be found in every prenatal clinic and every obstetrician's or nurse-midwife's office is not an exaggeration. Unfortunately, few women identify themselves as such, and many remain unrecognized. Because of the prevalence of physical abuse during pregnancy, it is recommended that *every* woman be screened for physical abuse.

Nurses often are unsure of the way to approach the issue of suspected abuse. Women often seek care and are assessed in the "honeymoon phase" of the violence cycle. During this phase, the man often is overly solicitous (hovering husband syndrome) and eager to explain any injuries that the woman exhibits. Introducing the subject of violence in the presence of the man who may be responsible for it places the woman in danger. Separating the woman from the man for the interview is absolutely essential.

CRITICAL THINKING EXERCISE

Joan Piszarek, a 28-year-old primigravida, is admitted to the emergency room with contractions at 36 weeks' gestation. The right side of her face is swollen, evidence of old bruises that look like fingerprints are found on her upper arms, and a large bruised area is apparent on her abdomen. She is accompanied by her husband, who is very solicitous. He verbalizes concern about her labor status and remains close beside her at all times. Joan appears lethargic and avoids eye contact with the nurse who is admitting her. She states that she fainted at home and hurt herself when she fell against the bathtub. The nurse accepts the explanation and asks no further questions.

QUESTIONS:
1. What assumptions has the nurse made?
2. What should make the nurse examine the conclusion that the injuries resulted from falling?

Joan is transferred to the labor and delivery unit. Her new nurse waits for time alone with Joan and asks, "Did you get these injuries from being hit?" Joan appears extremely anxious and says, "Don't say anything to him! He got so mad when I was late getting home from shopping. It was my fault."

QUESTIONS:
3. Why did the nurse wait for time alone before asking questions?
4. How should the nurse respond? What bias must she guard against?
5. How can Joan be protected?

When a private, secure place has been found, the nurse can explain that many women experience abuse. For example, "Because abuse is very common and can affect the woman's health, it is the policy at this agency to ask all women about abusive situations." This lets the woman know that she is not being singled out for questioning. Screening questions often included are the following:

- Have you been hit, slapped, kicked, choked or otherwise hurt physically by someone within the last year?
- Has this happened since you have been pregnant?
- Within the last year, has anyone forced you to have sexual activities?
- Are you ever afraid of your partner?

A "yes" answer should prompt questions about who hurt the woman and the frequency and kinds of abuse. If a woman has old or new signs that might be from abuse, ask appropriate questions such as "Did someone hurt you?" "Did you receive these injuries from being hit?"

CRITICAL TO REMEMBER

Cues Indicating Violence against Women

Nonverbal—Facial grimacing, slow and unsteady gait, vomiting, abdominal tenderness, absence of facial response

Injuries—Welts, bruises, swelling, lacerations, burns, vaginal or rectal bleeding; evidence of old or new fractures of the nose, face, ribs, or arms

Vague somatic complaints—Anxiety, depression, panic attacks, sleeplessness, anorexia

Discrepancy between history and type of injuries—Wounds do not match woman's story, multiple bruises in various stages of healing, bruising on the arms (which she may have raised to protect herself), old, untreated wounds

The abused woman often appears hesitant, embarrassed, or evasive. She may be unable to look the nurse in the eye and appears guilty, ashamed, jumpy, or frightened. Reassure the woman that her privacy will be protected and confidentiality will be absolute. Document all information in the chart.

Because not all women are willing to acknowledge their situation when asked, provide written information about abuse in areas such as restrooms, where it will not be seen by the partner. Pamphlets or cards listing general community resources including a few devoted to domestic violence may be acceptable for her to take with her. The availability of such material signifies that health care professionals are interested and the woman can discuss her problems safely.

Asking women about abuse frequently during the pregnancy and when they come for other health care is essential. Women often deny the abuse when first approached. The woman who is not ready to seek help when she is first asked may be ready at a later time, however.

Evaluate and document all signs of injury, both past and present. This includes areas of welts, bruising, swelling, lacerations, burns, and scars. Injuries are most commonly noted on the face, breasts, abdomen, and genitalia. Many women have new or old fractures. These usually are fractures of the face, nose, ribs, or arms. If sexual abuse has occurred, a gynecologic examination is necessary because trauma to the labia, vagina, or cervix often is present. Types of forced sex may include vaginal intercourse, anal intercourse, and insertion of objects into the vagina and anus. Vaginal or rectal bleeding or trauma must be documented according to hospital protocol.

Be particularly alert for nonverbal cues that indicate that abuse has occurred. Facial grimacing or a slow, unsteady gait may indicate pain. Vomiting or abdominal tenderness may indicate internal injury. A flat affect (absence of facial response) is indicative of women who mentally withdraw from the situation to protect themselves from the horror and humiliation they experience during an abusive episode. Keep in mind that the woman may fear for her life because abusive episodes tend to escalate. Open-ended questions help prompt full disclosure and the expression of feelings.

Analysis

A variety of nursing diagnoses may be appropriate, but the most meaningful diagnosis for perinatal nurses to make may be "Fear related to possibility of severe injury to self and/or children during unpredictable cycles of violence (Table 24-7)."

Table 24-7

COMMON NURSING DIAGNOSES FOR FAMILIES WITH SPECIAL NEEDS

Altered Growth and Development
Anxiety
*Body Image Disturbance
Chronic Sorrow
Decisional Conflict
*Fear
*Grieving
Health Seeking Behaviors
Impaired Social Interaction
Ineffective Family Coping
Ineffective Individual Coping
Powerlessness
*Risk for Altered Health Maintenance
*Risk for Altered Parenting
*Risk for Injury
Risk for Spiritual Distress
Risk for Altered Family Processes
*Situational Low Self-Esteem

* Nursing diagnoses discussed in this chapter.

Planning

The abused woman may have difficulty developing a long-term plan of care without a great deal of specialized assistance. She often is unwilling to leave the abusive situation, and nurses often must focus on working with the woman to plan short-term goals that will protect her from future injury.

For realistic, short-term goals/expected outcomes, the woman will do the following:

- Acknowledge the physical assaults.
- Develop a specific plan of action to implement when the abusive cycle begins.
- Identify community resources that provide protection for her and her children.

Interventions

Developing a Personal Safety Plan

Help the woman make concrete plans to protect her safety and the safety of her children. For example, if the woman insists on returning to the shared home, describe the cycle of behavior that culminates in physical abuse and instruct her in factors that precipitate a violent episode. These include the use of alcohol or other drugs and behaviors that indicate an increasing level of frustration and anger. Additional plans will be needed to do the following:

- Locate the nearest shelter or safe house and make specific plans to go there once the cycle of violence begins.
- Identify the safest, quickest routes out of the home.
- Obtain extra keys to the car. Keep them and some necessities packed and hidden until needed.
- Devise a code word, and prearrange with someone to call the police when the word is used.
- Memorize the telephone number of the shelter or hotline because time often is a crucial element in the decision to leave. An easy number to remember is for the National Domestic Violence Hotline (1-800-799-SAFE) for immediate crisis intervention assistance in the caller's community.
- Review the safety plan frequently because leaving the batterer is one of the most dangerous times.

Affirming She Is Not to Blame

The abused woman often believes that she is responsible for the abuse. Let her know that no one deserves to be hit for any reason. The one who hit her is the person responsible. She did not provoke it, and she did not cause it. Nurses often are responsible for teaching basic family processes such as the following:

- Violence is not normal.
- Violence usually is repeated and escalates.
- Battering is against the law.
- Battered women have alternatives.

Providing Referrals

When contact with the battered woman is short term, acknowledge that many interventions are outside the scope of nursing practice. As a result, be prepared to refer the family to community agencies available to the victim. These include the local police department, legal services, community shelters, counseling services, and social service agencies.

Accepting the decisions of the battered woman and acknowledging that she is on her own timetable is essential. She may not contact the police, go to a shelter, or take any actions at the time they are recommended. Therefore listening to her, believing her, and providing information about resources may be the only help the nurse can provide.

Do not become negative or pass judgment on the partner of an abused woman. She often is tied to the man by economic and emotional bonds and may become defensive if her partner is criticized. Tell her that resources are available for her partner but he must admit abuse and seek assistance before help can be offered. To initiate referrals for the partner before he asks for help will increase the danger to the woman if her partner feels he has been betrayed.

Evaluation

The plan of care can be judged successful if the woman acknowledges the violent episodes in the home, makes concrete plans to protect herself and her children from future injury, and uses the community resources available to her.

Check Your Reading

26. What major cues indicate that a woman has been physically abused?
27. How can nurses intervene to help women protect their safety if they choose to remain in a home situation with a partner who physically abuses them?

SUMMARY CONCEPTS

- Teenage pregnancy is a major health problem in the United States that requires that adolescents receive accurate information about contraceptives and ways to set limits on sexual behavior.
- Adolescent pregnancy imposes serious physiologic risks that result in a higher incidence of complications for the mother and fetus.
- Teenage pregnancy interrupts the developmental tasks of adolescence and may result in childbirth before the parents are capable of providing a nurturing home for the infant without a great deal of assistance.

- The mature primigravida often has financial and emotional resources that younger women do not have. She may experience anxiety, however, about recommended antepartum testing and her ability to parent effectively.
- Multidrug substance abuse is a widespread problem that can have devastating fetal and neonatal effects, which may persist and become long-term developmental problems for the child.
- The lifestyle associated with illicit drug abuse includes inadequate nutrition, inadequate prenatal care, and increased incidence of STDs and necessitates interdisciplinary interventions to prevent injury to the expectant mother and fetus.
- The birth of an infant with congenital anomalies produces strong emotions of shock and grief in the family and calls for a sensitive response from the health care team to help the family grieve for the loss of the perfect or "fantasy" infant and form an attachment to the newborn.
- Pregnancy loss at any stage produces grief that must be acknowledged and expressed before it can be resolved. Nurses realize that mourning requires memories, and they intervene to arrange unlimited contact between the family and the stillborn infant and gather a memento packet for the family.
- Nursing care for the mother who is placing her infant for adoption is based on the knowledge that relinquishment (adoption) is an act of love, not abandonment.
- Multiple factors are associated with violence against women, which is deliberate, severe, and generally repeated in a predictable cycle that often causes severe physical harm (or death) to the woman.
- All perinatal nurses come into contact with abused women who require assistance to protect themselves and their children from serious injury.

ANSWERS TO CRITICAL THINKING EXERCISE

1. The nurse may have assumed that the husband's solicitous behavior indicated concern for his wife. Instead, it may have been a "hovering husband syndrome" that occurs in the honeymoon phase of the cycle of violence.
2. Facial injury, signs of previous bruising that resemble "grab marks," and abdominal bruising. Joan's story of falling and hurting herself is not congruent with the location of abdominal injury and injuries on her arms. Joan's lethargy and avoidance of eye contact also suggest that she is afraid.
3. The nurse should not question Joan's explanation of the injury in the presence of the husband because this can increase the danger of escalating violence when the mother and infant are discharged.
4. The nurse should respond, "No one deserves to be hurt; it's not your fault. How can I help you?" Nurses must examine their own thinking to be certain that they do not accept a common bias that physical abuse is deserved by the victim.
5. Joan needs information about ways to protect herself and the coming infant from future harm. However, this is not the appropriate time to give her this information. The nurse must inform the physician and the postpartum staff of the problem, and she must make the necessary referrals to the hospital's social service department for follow-up contact with the staff that intercedes for women who are admitted to the emergency department for injuries sustained during an episode of battering.

REFERENCES & READINGS

Allan Guttmacher Institute. (2000). *Occasional Report: Teenagers' pregnancy intentions and decisions.* Retrieved April 10, 2000 from http://www.agi-usa.org/pubs/or teen preg survey.html.

Allard-Hendren, R. (2000). Alcohol use and adolescent pregnancy. *MCN: American Journal of Maternal Child Nursing,* 25(3), 159-162.

American Academy of Pediatrics, Committee on Drugs. (1998). Neonatal drug withdrawal. *Pediatrics,* 101(6), 1079-1088.

American Academy of Pediatrics, Committee on Substance Abuse, & Committee on Children with Disabilities. (2000). Fetal alcohol syndrome and alcohol-related neurodevelopmental disorders. *Pediatrics,* 106(2), 358-361.

American Academy of Pediatrics (AAP) & American College of Obstetricians and Gynecologists (ACOG). (1997). *Guidelines for perinatal care* (4th ed.). Washington, D.C.: Author.

American College of Obstetricians and Gynecologists (ACOG). (1999). *Psychosocial risk factors: Perinatal screening and intervention.* ACOG Educational Bulletin 255. Washington, D.C.: Author.

ACOG. (1999). *Domestic violence: ACOG educational bulletin.* Washington, D.C.: Author.

ACOG. (1996). *Guidelines for women's health care.* Washington, D.C.: Author.

ACOG. (1999). *Psychosocial risk factors: Perinatal screening and intervention. ACOG educational bulletin.* Washington, D.C.: Author.

Askren, H.A., & Bloom, K.C. (1999). Postadoptive reactions of the relinquishing mother: A review. *Journal of Obstetric, Gynecologic, and Neonatal Nursing,* 28(4), 395-400.

Association of Women's Health, Obstetric and Neonatal Nurses. (1998). *Standards and guidelines for professional nursing practice in the care of women and newborns* (5th ed). Washington, D.C.

Austin, D.A., & Sheridan, M.E. (2000). Labor and delivery at risk. In *Core curriculum for maternal newborn nursing* (2nd ed., pp. 607-635). Philadelphia: W.B. Saunders.

Bauer, C.R. (1998). Perinatal effects of prenatal drug exposure. *Clinics in Perinatology,* 26(1), 87-106.

Bloom, K.C. (1998). Perceived relationship with the father of the baby and maternal attachment in adolescents. *Journal of Obstetric, Gynecologic, and Neonatal Nursing,* 27(4), 420-430.

Bloom, K.C., & Hall, D.S. (1999). Pregnancy wantedness in adolescents presenting for pregnancy testing. *MCN: American Journal of Maternal Child Nursing,* 24(6), 296-300.

Botham, S. (2000). Perinatal substance abuse. In J. Deacon & P. O'Neill, (Eds.), *Core curriculum for neonatal intensive care nursing* (2nd ed., pp. 618-634). Philadelphia: W.B. Saunders.

Brown, H.L., Britton, K.A., Mahaffey, D., Brizendine, E., Hiett, A.K., & Turnquest, M.A. (1998). Methadone maintenance in pregnancy: A reappraisal. *Obstetrics & Gynecology,* 179(2), 459-463.

Colucciello, M.L. (1998). Pregnant adolescents' perceptions of their babies before and after real-time ultrasound. *Journal of Psychosocial Nursing,* 36(11), 12-19.

Commonwealth Fund. (1999). *Health concerns across a woman's lifespan: The Commonwealth Fund 1998 survey of women's health.* New York: Author.

Cote-Arsenault, D., & Mahlangu, N. (1999). Impact of perinatal loss on the subsequent pregnancy and self: Women's experiences. *Journal of Obstetric, Gynecologic, and Neonatal Nursing,* 28(3), 274-282.

Culliton, P.D., Boucher, T.A., & Bullock, M.L. (1999). Complementary/alternative therapies in the treatment of alcohol and other additions. In J.W. Spencer & J.J. Jacobs. *Complementary/alternative medicine: An evidence-based approach,* (pp. 248-281). St. Louis, Mosby.

Cunningham, F.G., MacDonald, P.C., Gant, N.F., Leveno, K.J., Gilstrap, L.C., Hankins, G.D.U., et al. (1997). *Williams obstetrics* (20th ed.). Stamford, CT: Appleton & Lange.

Curry, M.A. (1998). The interrelationships between abuse, substance use, and psychosocial stress during pregnancy. *Journal of Obstetric, Gynecologic, and Neonatal Nursing,* 27(6), 693-699.

Curry, M.A., Doyle, B.A., & Gilhooley, J. (1998). Abuse among pregnant adolescents: Differences by developmental age. *MCN: American Journal of Maternal Child Nursing,* 23(3), 144-150.

Dallas, C.M., & Chen, S.C. (1999). Perspectives of women whose sons become adolescent fathers. *MCN: American Journal of Maternal Child Nursing,* 24(5), 247-251.

Darroch, J.E., Landry, D.J., & Oslak, S. (1999). Age differences between sexual partners in the United States. *Family Planning Perspectives,* 31(4), 160-167.

Deitch, K.V. (2000). Age-related concerns. In S. Mattson & J.E. Smith (Eds.), *Core curriculum for maternal-newborn nursing* (2nd ed., pp. 116-123). Philadelphia: W.B. Saunders.

DeMontigny, F., Beaudet, L., & Dumas, L. (1999). A baby has died: The impact of perinatal loss on family social networks. *Journal of Obstetric, Gynecology, and Neonatal Nursing,* 28(2), 151-156.

Dennison, C., & Coleman, J. (1998). Teenage motherhood: Experiences and relationships. In S. Clement. *Psychological perspectives on pregnancy and childbirth* (pp. 245-263). Edinburgh: Churchill Livingstone.

DeVille, K.A., & Kopelman, L.M. (1998). Moral and social issues regarding pregnant women who use and abuse drugs. *Obstetric and Gynecology Clinics of North America,* 25(1), 237-254.

Fishwick, N.J. (1998). Assessment of women for partner abuse. *Journal of Obstetric, Gynecologic, and Neonatal Nursing,* 27(6), 661-670.

Gantt, L., & Bickford, A. (1999). Screening for domestic violence. *Lifelines,* 3(2), 36-42.

Hartman, J.J. (2000). Battered woman in a small town. *AWHONN Lifelines,* 4(4), 35-39.

Heinonen, S., & Kirkinen, P. (2000). Pregnancy outcome after previous stillbirth resulting from causes other than maternal conditions and fetal abnormalities. *Birth,* 27(1), 33-37.

Hershberger, P. (1998). Smoking and pregnant teens. *Lifelines,* 2(4), 27-31.

Holmes, M., & Chasedunn-Roark, J. (1999). Gynecologic health consequences to victims of interpersonal violence. *Women's Health Issues,* 9(2), 115-120.

Hughes, P. (1998). Psychological effects of stillbirth and neonatal loss. In S. Clement. *Psychological perspectives on pregnancy and childbirth* (pp. 145-166). Edinburgh: Churchill Livingstone.

James, D.C. (2000). Managing teen pregnancy. *Mother Baby Journal,* 5(2), 53-55.

Kearney, M.H. (1999). *Perinatal impact of alcohol, tobacco and other drugs.* White Plains, NY: March of Dimes.

Kennell, J.H., & Klaus, M.H. (1998). Bonding: Recent observations that alter perinatal care. *Pediatrics in Review,* 19(1), 4-12.

Kenner, C., & Amlung, S. (1999). Families in crisis. In J. Deacon & P. O'Neill, *Core curriculum for neonatal intensive care nursing* (2nd ed., pp. 635-649). Philadelphia: W.B. Saunders.

Koniak-Griffin, D., Anderson, N.L.R., Verzemnieks, I., & Brecht, M. (2000). A public health nursing early intervention program for adolescent mothers: Outcomes from pregnancy through 6 weeks postpartum. *Nursing Research,* 49(3), 130-138.

Kowaleski-Jones, L., & Mott, F.L. (1998). Sex, contraception and childbearing among high-risk youth: Do different factors influence males and females? *Family Planning Perspectives,* 30(4), 163-169.

Kyriacou, D.N., Anglin, D., Taliaferro, E., Stone, S., Tubb, T., Linden, J.A., et al. (1999). Risk factors for injury to women from domestic violence. *New England Journal of Medicine,* 341(25), 1892-1898.

Leoni, L.C., Woods, J.R., & Woods, J.E. (1998) Caring for patients after pregnancy loss. *Lifelines,* 2(1), 56-58.

Lesser, J., & Escoto-Lloyd, S. (1999). Health-related problems in a vulnerable population: Pregnant teens and adolescent mothers. *Nursing Clinics of North America,* 34(2), 289-299.

Lieberman, L.D. (1998). Overview of substance abuse prevention and treatment approaches in urban, multicultural settings: The Center for Substance Abuse Prevention programs for pregnant and postpartum women and their infants. *Women's Health Issues,* 8(4), 208-217.

MacKay, A.P., Fingerhut, L.A., & Duran, C.R. (2000). *Adolescent health chartbook, Health, United States, 2000.* Hyattsville, MD: National Center for Health Statistics.

Mackey, M.C., & Tiller, C.M. (1998) Adolescents' description and management of pregnancy and preterm labor. *Journal of Obstetric, Gynecology, and Neonatal Nursing,* 27(4), 410-419.

McFarlane, J., Parker, B., & Soeken, K. (1996a). Abuse during pregnancy: Associations with maternal health and infant birth weight. *Nursing Research,* 45(1), 37-42.

McFarlane, J., Parker, B., & Soeken, K. (1996b). Physical abuse, smoking, and substance use during pregnancy: Prevalence, interrelationships, and effects on birth weight. *Journal of Obstetric, Gynecology, and Neonatal Nursing,* 25(4), 313-320.

Moore, M.L. (2000). Adolescent pregnancy rates in three European countries: Lessons to be learned? *Journal of Obstetric, Gynecology, and Neonatal Nursing,* 29(4), 355-362.

Moran, B.A. (2000). Substance abuse in pregnancy. In S. Mattson & J.E. Smith (Eds.), *Core curriculum for maternal-newborn nursing* (2nd ed., pp. 545-563). Philadelphia: W.B. Saunders.

Nichols, J.A. (1998). Bereavement: The state of having suffered a loss. In C. Kenner, J.W. Lott, & A.A. Flandermeyer (Eds.), *Comprehensive neonatal nursing: A physiologic perspective* (2nd ed., pp. 73-84). Philadelphia: W.B. Saunders.

Polaneczky, M., & O'Connor, K. (1999). Pregnancy in the adolescent patient. *Pediatric Clinics of North America,* 46(4), 649-670.

Primeau, M.R., & Lamb, J.M. (1995). When a baby dies: Rights of the baby and parents. *Journal of Obstetric, Gynecologic, and Neonatal Nursing,* 24(3), 206-208.

Renker, P.R. (1998). Physical abuse, social support, self-care, & pregnancy outcomes of older adolescents. *Journal of Obstetric, Gynecology, and Neonatal Nursing,* 28(4), 377-388.

Robertson, P.A., & Kavanaugh, K. (1998) Supporting parents during and after a pregnancy subsequent to a perinatal loss. *Journal of Perinatal & Neonatal Nursing,* 12(2), 63-71.

Ryan, J., & King, M.C. (1998). Scanning for violence: Educational strategies for helping abused women. *Lifelines,* 2(3), 36-41.

Selleck, C.S., & Redding, B.A. (1998) Knowledge and attitudes of registered nurses toward perinatal substance abuse. *Journal of Obstetric, Gynecologic, and Neonatal Nursing,* 27(1), 70-77.

Singh, S., & Darroch, J.E. (2000). Adolescent pregnancy and childbearing: Levels and trends in developed countries. *Family Planning Perspectives,* 32(1), 14-23.

Stark, M.A. (1997). Psychosocial adjustment during pregnancy: The experience of mature gravidas. *Journal of Obstetric, Gynecologic, and Neonatal Nursing,* 26(2), 206-211.

Tjaden, P., & Thoennes, N. (1998). *Prevalence, incidence, and consequences of violence against women: Findings from the National Violence Against Women Survey.* Washington, D.C.: National Institute of Justice & Centers for Disease Control and Prevention.

Toohey, J.S. (2000). Battered women. In E.J. Quilligan & F.P. Zuspan. *Current therapy in obstetrics and gynecology* (5th ed., pp. 453-456). Philadelphia: W.B. Saunders.

U.S. Department of Health and Human Services. (2000). *Healthy people 2010* (Conference edition). Washington, D.C.: Author.

Ventura, S.J., Curtin, S.C., & Mathews, T.J. (1998). *Teenage birth in the United States: National and state trends, 1990-1996.* National Vital Statistics System, Hyattsville, MD: National Center for Health Statistics.

Ventura, S.J., Martin, J.A., Curtin, S.C., & Mathews, T.J. (1999). Births: Final data for 1997. *National Vital Statistics Reports,* 47(18).

Ventura, S.J., Martin, J.A., Curtin, S.C., Mathews, T.J., & Park, M.M. (2000). Births: Final data for 1998. *National Vital Statistics Reports,* 48(3).

Walker, J.J. (1999). Drug addiction. In D.K. James, P.J. Steer, C.P. Weiner, & Gonic, B. *High-risk pregnancy: Management options* (2nd ed., pp. 599-616). Philadelphia: W.B. Saunders.

Warren, C.W., Santelli, J.S., Everett, S.A., Kann, L., Collins, J.L. Cassell, C., Morris, L., & Kolbe, L.J. (1998). Sexual behavior among US high school students, 1990-1995. *Family Planning Perspectives,* 30(4), 170-172, 200.

Wescott, C.S. (1997). The pain of grief. *Childbirth Instructor Magazine,* 7(5), 38-41.

Windridge, K.C., & Berryman, J.C. (1999). Women's experiences of giving birth after 35. *Birth,* 26(1), 16-23.

25 COMPLICATIONS OF PREGNANCY

OBJECTIVES

1. Describe the hemorrhagic conditions of early pregnancy, including spontaneous abortion, ectopic pregnancy, and gestational trophoblastic disease.
2. Explain how disorders of the placenta, such as placenta previa and abruptio placentae, result in hemorrhagic conditions of late pregnancy.
3. Discuss the effects and management of hyperemesis gravidarum.
4. Describe the development and management of hypertensive disorders of pregnancy.
5. Compare etiology, fetal and neonatal complications, and management of Rh and ABO incompatibility.
6. Explain nursing considerations for each complication of pregnancy.

DEFINITIONS

ABORTION Pregnancy that ends before 20 weeks' gestation, either spontaneously or electively. *Miscarriage* is a lay term for a spontaneous abortion.

ABRUPTIO PLACENTAE Premature separation of a normally implanted placenta.

ANTIPHOSPHOLIPID ANTIBODIES Autoimmune antibodies that are directed against phospholipids in cell membranes. It is associated with recurrent spontaneous abortion, fetal loss, and severe pregnancy-induced hypertension.

BICORNUATE (BICORNATE) UTERUS Malformed uterus having two horns.

CERCLAGE Encircling of the cervix with suture to prevent recurrent spontaneous abortion caused by early cervical dilation.

DILATION AND CURETTAGE (D&C) Stretching the cervical os to permit suctioning or scraping of the walls of the uterus. The procedure is performed in abortion, to obtain samples of uterine lining tissue for laboratory examination, and during the postpartum period to remove retained fragments of placenta.

DEFINITIONS—cont'd

Dilation and Evacuation (D&E) Wide cervical dilation followed by mechanical destruction and removal of fetal parts from the uterus. After complete removal of the fetus, a vacuum curet is used to remove the placenta and remaining products of conception.

Eclampsia Form of pregnancy-induced hypertension complicated by generalized (grand mal) seizures.

Ectopic Pregnancy Implantation of a fertilized ovum in any area other than the uterus; the most common site is the fallopian tube.

Erythroblastosis Fetalis Agglutination and hemolysis of fetal erythrocytes resulting from incompatibility between maternal and fetal blood. In most cases, the fetus is Rh-positive and the mother is Rh-negative.

Gestational Trophoblastic Disease Spectrum of diseases that includes both benign hydatidiform mole and gestational trophoblastic tumors, such as invasive moles and choriocarcinoma.

Hydatidiform Mole Abnormal pregnancy resulting from proliferation of chorionic villi that give rise to multiple cysts and rapid growth of the uterus.

Hypovolemic Shock Acute peripheral circulatory failure resulting from loss of circulating blood volume.

Kernicterus Staining of brain tissue caused by accumulation of unconjugated bilirubin in the brain. Bilirubin encephalopathy is the brain damage that results from these deposits.

Laparoscopy Insertion of an illuminated tube into the abdominal cavity to visualize contents, locate bleeding, and perform surgical procedures.

Linear Salpingostomy Incision along the length of a fallopian tube to remove an ectopic pregnancy and preserve the tube.

Maceration Discoloration and softening of tissues and eventual disintegration of a fetus that is retained in the uterus after its death.

Perinatologist Physician who specializes in the care of the mother, fetus, and infant during the perinatal period (from the twentieth week of pregnancy to 4 weeks after childbirth).

Preeclampsia A hypertensive disorder of pregnancy characterized by hypertension, edema, and proteinuria.

Salpingectomy Surgical removal of a fallopian tube.

Vacuum Curettage (Vacuum Aspiration) Removal of the uterine contents by application of a vacuum through a hollow curet or cannula introduced into the uterus.

Vasoconstriction Narrowing of the lumen of blood vessels.

Although childbearing is a normal process, numerous maternal and fetal adaptations must occur in an orderly sequence. If problems develop in these physiologic processes, complications may arise that threaten the well-being of the expectant mother, the fetus, or both. A nurse-midwife or family physician may co-manage some conditions, but women are often referred to an obstetrician or a perinatologist for management of severe complications.

Nurses who work at a primary care site or perinatal center frequently fill the role of case manager or coordinator of services provided for the woman. Often the nurse is the only consistent provider involved in the woman's care and therefore is the person on whom the woman relies to guide her through the system.

Conditions that complicate pregnancy are divided into two broad categories: (1) those that are related to pregnancy and are not seen at other times and (2) those that could occur at any time but when they occur concurrently with pregnancy may complicate its course. Concurrent conditions that affect pregnancy are covered in Chapter 26.

The most common pregnancy-related complications are hemorrhagic conditions that occur in early pregnancy, hemorrhagic complications of the placenta in late pregnancy, hyperemesis gravidarum, hypertensive disorders of pregnancy, and blood incompatibilities.

HEMORRHAGIC CONDITIONS OF EARLY PREGNANCY

The three most common causes of hemorrhage during the first half of pregnancy are abortion, ectopic pregnancy, and gestational trophoblastic disease.

Abortion

Abortion is the loss of pregnancy before the fetus is viable, or capable of living outside the uterus. The medical consensus today is that a fetus of less than 20 weeks' gestation or one weighing less than 500 g is not viable. Ending of pregnancy before this time is considered an abortion. Abortion may be either spontaneous or induced. Lay people often use the term *miscarriage* to denote an abortion that has occurred spontaneously. *Abortion* is the accepted medical term for either a spontaneous or induced ending of pregnancy, and this point should be clarified in discussions with women to avoid misinterpretation or confusion. Induced abortion is described in Chapter 33.

Spontaneous Abortion

Spontaneous abortion is a termination of pregnancy without action taken by the woman or another person.

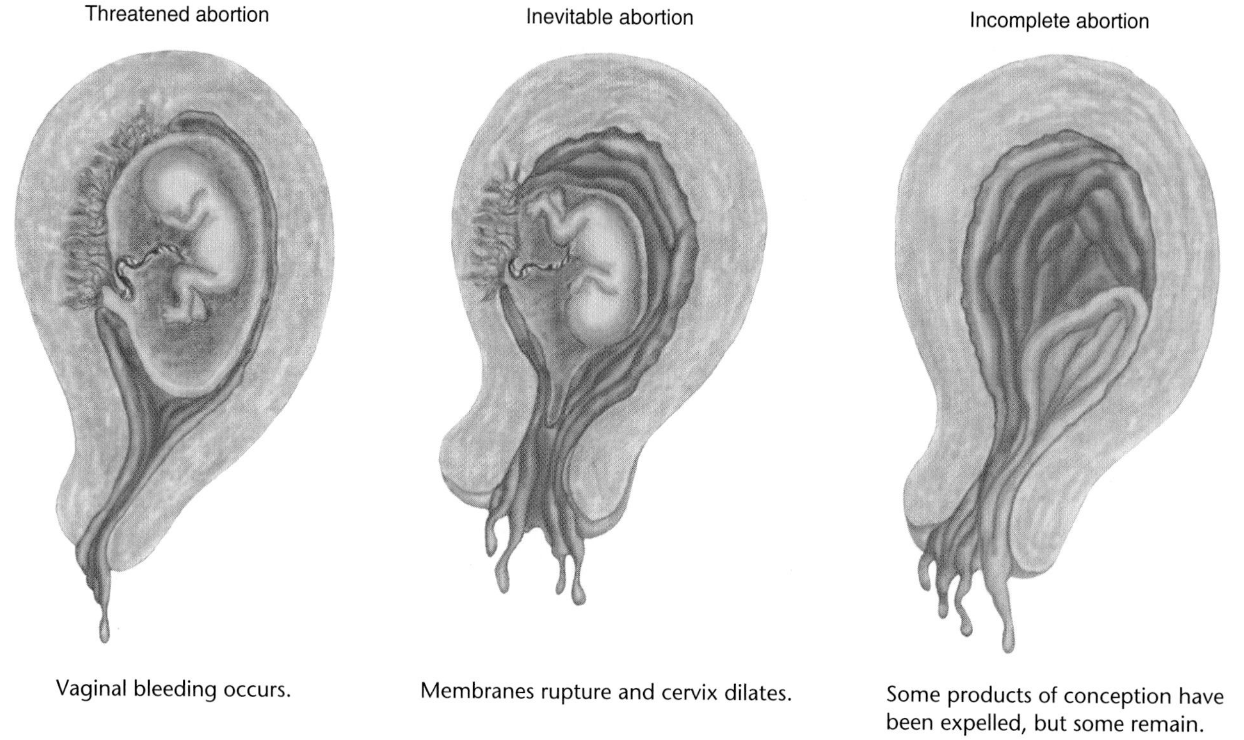
Threatened abortion
Inevitable abortion
Incomplete abortion
Vaginal bleeding occurs.
Membranes rupture and cervix dilates.
Some products of conception have been expelled, but some remain.

FIGURE 25-1 Three types of spontaneous abortion.

Incidence and Etiology

Determining the exact incidence of spontaneous abortion is difficult because many unrecognized losses occur in early pregnancy. However, 15% to 20% of pregnancies are lost spontaneously after pregnancy is recognized (Coulam, 2000). Most spontaneous abortions occur in the first trimester of pregnancy, with the rate declining thereafter.

The causes of spontaneous abortion are varied and often unknown. The most common cause is chromosomal abnormalities that are incompatible with life or that would result in gross deformity of the fetus. Additional causes may include maternal infections such as *Ureaplasma urealyticum,* bacterial vaginosis (BV), toxoplasmosis, and herpes simplex virus (HSV), although the role of infections is not always clear. (See Chapter 26 for more information about perinatal infections.) Endocrine disorders such as progesterone deficiency have been implicated in some spontaneous abortions. In addition, immunologic factors may be a cause of spontaneous abortion.

Spontaneous abortion is divided into six subgroups: threatened, inevitable, incomplete, complete, missed, and recurrent. Figure 25-1 illustrates threatened, inevitable, and incomplete abortion.

Threatened Abortion

Clinical Manifestations. The first sign of threatened abortion is vaginal bleeding, which is rather common during early pregnancy. Up to 25% of all women experience "spotting" or bleeding in early pregnancy. About half of these pregnancies end in spontaneous abortion. Pregnancies complicated by early bleeding that do not end with a spontaneous abortion are more likely to have further complications during late pregnancy such as prematurity, a small-for-gestational age infant, abnormal presentation, or perinatal asphyxia (Cunningham, et al., 1997; Rosevear, 1999).

Vaginal bleeding may be followed by rhythmic uterine cramping, persistent backache, or feelings of pelvic pressure. These symptoms increase the chance that the threatened abortion will progress to inevitable abortion.

Therapeutic Management. Bleeding in the first half of pregnancy should be considered a threatened abortion, and women must be advised to notify their physician or nurse-midwife if vaginal bleeding is noted. When a woman reports bleeding in early pregnancy, the nurse obtains a detailed history that includes length of gestation (or first day of her last menstrual period) and the onset, duration, and amount of vaginal bleeding. Any accompanying discomfort, such as cramping, backache, or abdominal pain also is noted.

Vaginal ultrasound examination is performed to determine whether a fetus is present and, if so, whether it is alive. Maternal serum chorionic gonadotropin and progesterone levels provide added information about the viability of the pregnancy.

Bedrest has been prescribed for threatened abortion but no evidence exists to support physical activity restrictions (Rosevear, 1999). The woman may be advised to curtail sexual activity until bleeding has ceased. The woman is instructed to count the number of perineal pads used and to note the quantity and color of blood on the pads. She should also look for evidence of tissue passage, which would indicate progression beyond a threatened abortion.

Bleeding episodes are frightening, and psychological support is important. The woman often wonders whether her actions may have contributed to the situation and is anxious about her own condition and that of the fetus. The nurse should offer accurate information and avoid false reassurance because the woman may lose her pregnancy despite every precaution.

Inevitable Abortion

Clinical Manifestations. Abortion is usually inevitable (that is, it cannot be stopped) when membranes rupture and the cervix dilates. Rupture of membranes generally is experienced as a loss of fluid from the vagina and subsequent uterine contractions and bleeding. If complete evacuation of the products of conception does not occur spontaneously, excessive bleeding or infection can occur.

Therapeutic Management. The usual treatment of inevitable abortion involves allowing a natural evacuation of the uterine contents. Vacuum curettage is used to clean out the uterus if the natural process is ineffective or incomplete. If the pregnancy is more advanced or if bleeding is excessive, a dilation and curettage (D&C) may be needed. Intravenous sedation or other anesthesia is used for either procedure.

Incomplete Abortion

Clinical Manifestations. Incomplete abortion occurs when some but not all products of conception are expelled from the uterus. The major symptoms are uterine bleeding and severe abdominal cramping. The cervix is open and fetal and placental tissues are passed.

Therapeutic Management. The retained tissue prevents the uterus from contracting firmly thus allowing profuse bleeding from uterine blood vessels. Initial treatment should focus on stabilizing the woman cardiovascularly. A blood specimen is drawn for crossmatching and blood typing, and an intravenous line is inserted for fluid replacement. When the woman's condition is stable, a D&C usually is performed to remove the remaining tissue. This procedure may be followed by intravenous administration of oxytocin (Pitocin) or intramuscular administration of methylergonovine (Methergine) to contract the uterus and control bleeding.

A D&C may not be performed if the pregnancy has advanced beyond 14 weeks because of the danger of excessive bleeding. In this case, oxytocin or prostaglandin is administered to stimulate uterine contractions until all products of conception (fetus, membranes, placenta, and amniotic fluid) are expelled.

Complete Abortion

Clinical Manifestations. Complete abortion occurs when all products of conception are expelled from the uterus. After passage of all products of conception, uterine contractions and bleeding subside and the cervix closes. The uterus feels smaller than the length of gestation would suggest. The symptoms of pregnancy are no longer present, and the pregnancy test becomes negative as hormone levels fall.

Therapeutic Management. Once complete abortion is confirmed, no additional intervention is required unless excessive bleeding or infection develops. The woman should be advised to rest and to watch for further bleeding, pain, or fever. She should schedule a follow-up visit with her health care provider.

Missed Abortion

Clinical Manifestations. Missed abortion occurs when the fetus dies during the first half of pregnancy but is retained in the uterus. When the fetus dies, the early symptoms of pregnancy (nausea, breast tenderness, urinary frequency) disappear. The uterus stops growing and decreases in size, reflecting the absorption of amniotic fluid and maceration of the fetus. Vaginal bleeding of a red or brownish color may or may not occur.

Therapeutic Management. Real-time ultrasound examination confirms fetal death by identifying a gestational sac or fetus that is too small for the presumed gestation. No fetal heart activity can be found. Serial pregnancy tests for chorionic gonadotropin should show a decline in placental hormone production.

In most cases, the woman would expel the contents of the uterus spontaneously, but this is emotionally difficult once she knows her fetus is not living. Therefore her uterus usually is emptied by the most appropriate method for the size when the diagnosis of missed abortion is made. For a first trimester missed abortion, a D&C can usually be done. If the missed abortion occurs during the second trimester, when the fetus is larger, a D&E may be done or vaginal prostaglandin E_2 (PGE_2) or misoprostol (Cytotec) may be needed to induce uterine contractions that expel the fetus.

Two major complications of missed abortion are infection and disseminated intravascular coagulation (DIC, see p. 664). If signs exist of uterine infection, such as elevation in temperature, vaginal discharge with a foul odor, or abdominal pain, evacuation of the uterus will be delayed until antibiotic therapy is initiated.

Recurrent Spontaneous Abortion

Clinical Manifestations. Recurrent spontaneous abortion usually is defined as three or more spontaneous abortions, although some authorities now use two or more pregnancy losses as the definition (Hill, 1999). The primary causes of recurrent abortion are believed to be genetic or chromosomal abnormalities and anomalies of the reproductive tract, such as bicornuate uterus or incompetent cervix. Other causes include inadequate progesterone secretion by the corpus luteum, systemic diseases such as lupus erythematosus and diabetes mellitus, and immunologic causes.

Therapeutic Management. The first step in management of recurrent spontaneous abortion is a thorough examination of the reproductive system to determine whether anatomic defects are the cause. If the cervix and uterus are normal, the woman and her partner are usually referred for genetic screening to identify chromosomal factors that would increase the possibility of recurrent abortions.

Additional therapeutic management of recurrent pregnancy loss depends on the cause. For instance, treatment may involve assisting the woman to develop a regimen to maintain normal blood glucose if diabetes mellitus is a factor. Supplemental hormones may be given if her progesterone or other hormone levels are lower than normal.

Recurrent spontaneous abortion may be due to cervical incompetence, an anatomic defect that results in painless dilation of the cervix in the second trimester. In this instance, the cervix may be sutured to keep it from opening in a cerclage procedure. The cerclage is most likely to be successful if done before much cervical dilation or bulging of the membranes through the cervix. Sutures may be removed near term in preparation for vaginal delivery or they may be left in place if a cesarean birth is planned. Prophylactic antibiotics are ordered if the woman is at increased risk for infection.

Rh immune globulin (RhoGAM) is given to the unsensitized Rh_0(D)-negative woman to prevent development of anti-Rh antibodies (see p. 695). A microdose (50 mcg) is given to the woman who is less than 13 weeks' gestational age at the time of the abortion.

Nursing Considerations

Nurses must consider the psychological needs of the woman experiencing spontaneous abortion. Vaginal bleeding is frightening, and waiting and watching is often difficult, although it may be the only treatment recommended. Many women and their families feel an acute sense of loss and grief with spontaneous abortion. Grief often includes feelings of guilt, wondering if the woman could have done something to prevent the loss. Nurses may help by emphasizing that abortions usually occur as the result of factors or abnormalities that could not be avoided.

Anger, disappointment, and sadness are commonly experienced emotions, although the intensity of the feelings may vary. For many people the fetus has not yet taken on specific physical characteristics, but they grieve for their fantasies of the unseen, unborn child. The couple may want to express their feelings of sadness but may feel that family, friends, and often health personnel are uncomfortable or unable to provide emotional support after early pregnancy loss.

Recognizing the meaning of the loss to each woman and her significant others is important. Nurses must listen carefully to what the woman says and observe how she behaves. Nurses must convey acceptance of the feelings expressed or demonstrated. A couple should be permitted to remain together as much as possible. Providing information and simple brief explanations of what has occurred and what will be done facilitates the family's ability to grieve.

The family should realize that grief may last from 6 months to a year, or even longer. Family support, knowledge of the grief process, spiritual counselors, and the support of other bereaved couples may provide needed assistance during this time. Chapter 24 provides additional information about pregnancy loss and grief.

Disseminated Intravascular Coagulation

Disseminated intravascular coagulation (DIC) is a life-threatening defect in coagulation that may occur with several complications of pregnancy. DIC is not limited to obstetric conditions. Complications of pregnancy that may have DIC as an added problem include the following:

- Missed abortion or retained dead fetus, more likely if the gestation reached the second trimester when fetal death occurred (Cunningham, et al., 1997)
- Abruptio placentae, or premature separation of the placenta (see p. 673)
- Severe pregnancy-induced hypertension (see p. 695)
- Amniotic fluid embolism (see p. 768)
- Sepsis

Something in one of these disease processes initiates clotting mechanisms inappropriately. The first result is a consumption of plasma factors including platelets, fibrinogen, prothrombin, factor V, and factor VIII. When these plasma factors are consumed, the circulating blood is then deficient in clotting factors and unable to clot. Fibrin degradation products accumulate and further interfere with coagulation.

While anticoagulation is occurring, inappropriate coagulation also is occurring in the microcirculation. The second result of DIC is that tiny clots form in the tiny blood vessels, blocking blood flow to the organs and causing ischemia.

Diseases that cause DIC fall into three major groups:

- Infusion of tissue thromboplastin into the circulation. Abruptio placentae and prolonged retention of the dead fetus cause this because the placenta is a rich source of thromboplastin.
- Conditions characterized by endothelial damage. Severe pregnancy-induced hypertension and the

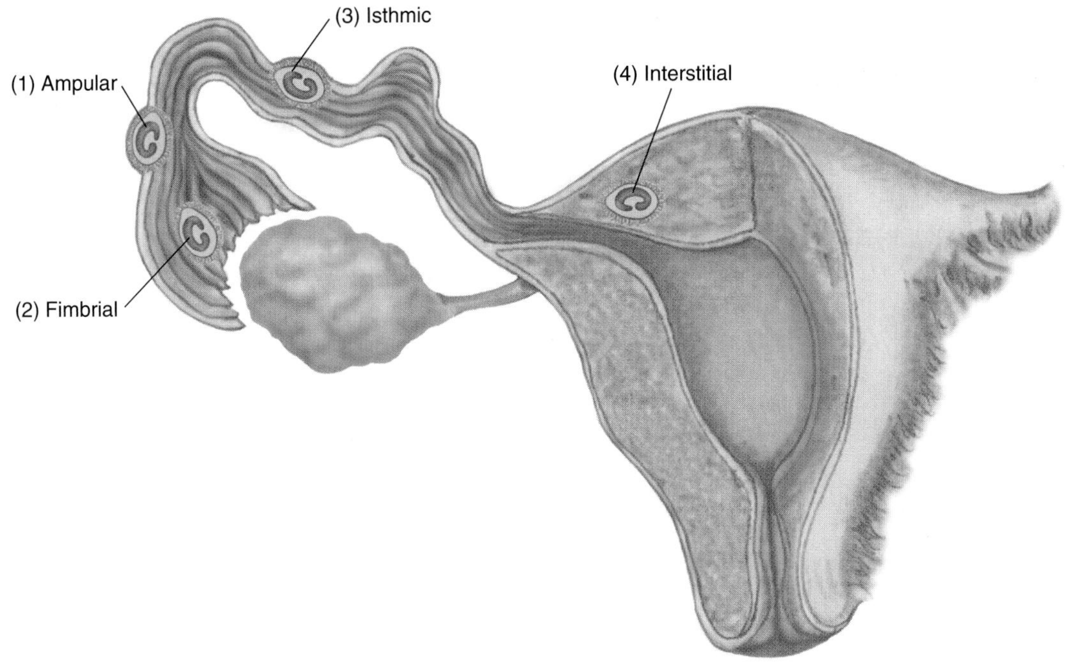

FIGURE 25-2 Sites of tubal ectopic pregnancy. Numbers indicate the order of prevalence.

HELLP syndrome (p. 691) are characterized by endothelial damage.

- Nonspecific effects of some diseases. Diseases such as maternal sepsis or the amniotic fluid embolism (see Chapter 30) are in this category.

DIC allows excess bleeding to occur from any vulnerable area, such as intravenous sites, incisions, or the gums or nose, and from expected sites such as the site of placental attachment during the postpartum period.

Laboratory studies help establish a diagnosis. Fibrinogen and platelets usually are decreased, prothrombin (PT) and activated partial thromboplastin (aPTT) times may be prolonged, fibrin degradation products, the most sensitive measurement, are increased. A newer test, the D-dimer study, confirms fibrin split products and is presumptive for DIC when positive.

The priority in treatment of DIC is to correct the cause. In the case of a missed abortion, delivery of the fetus and placenta ends production of thromboplastin, which is fueling the process. Blood replacement products, such as whole blood, packed red blood cells, and cryoprecipitate, are administered as needed to maintain the circulating volume and to transport oxygen to body cells.

Nursing Considerations

When caring for a woman who has any of the disorders that increase her risk for having DIC, the nurse should observe for bleeding from unexpected sites. Sites for intravenous insertion or lab work, nosebleeds, or spontaneous bruising may be early indicators of DIC and should be reported. Also, if her coagulation studies are severely abnormal, an epidural block may be contraindicated because of possible bleeding into the spinal canal, so other types of labor pain management should be anticipated.

Check Your Reading

1. What are the signs of threatened abortion, and how do they differ from those of inevitable abortion?
2. What are the major causes of recurrent spontaneous abortion?
3. How can nurses intervene for the grief families experience as a result of early pregnancy loss?
4. What is DIC?

Ectopic Pregnancy

Ectopic pregnancy is an implantation of a fertilized ovum in an area outside the uterine cavity. Although implantation can occur in the abdomen or cervix, more than 98% of ectopic pregnancies are in the fallopian tube (Pisarska & Carson, 1999). Figure 25-2 illustrates common sites of ectopic implantation.

Ectopic pregnancy has been called "a disaster of reproduction" for two reasons:

- It remains a significant cause of maternal death from hemorrhage.
- It reduces the woman's chance of subsequent pregnancies because of damage or destruction of a fallopian tube.

Table 25-1

RISK FACTORS FOR ECTOPIC PREGNANCY

History of sexually transmitted diseases (gonorrhea, chlamydial infection)
History of pelvic inflammatory disease
History of previous ectopic pregnancies
Failed tubal ligation
Intrauterine device
Multiple induced abortions
Maternal age older than 35 years
Assisted reproductive techniques such as gamete intrafallopian transfer (GIFT)

Incidence and Etiology

Ectopic pregnancies have increased in the United States since 1970 from a rate of 4.5 per 1000 pregnancies to 19.7 per 1000 pregnancies (Lipscomb & Ling, 2000). The increase in incidence is attributed to the growing number of women of childbearing age who experience scarring of the fallopian tubes because of pelvic infection, inflammation, or surgery. Additionally, sensitive tests that identify pregnancy earlier and transvaginal ultrasound allows diagnosis of some pregnancies within the fallopian tube that previously might have resolved spontaneously before diagnosis (Pisarska & Carson, 1999).

Pelvic infection often is due to *Chlamydia* or *Neisseria gonorrhoeae.* Failed tubal ligation and a history of previous ectopic pregnancy also increase the risk for an ectopic pregnancy that implants in the fallopian tube. Use of contraception that prevents intrauterine pregnancy, such as intrauterine contraceptive devices or low-dose progesterone agents, is associated with increased risk of extrauterine (ectopic) pregnancy (Cunningham, et al., 1997).

Additional causes of ectopic pregnancy are delayed or premature ovulation, with the tendency of the fertilized ovum to implant before arrival in the uterus, and altered tubal motility in response to changes in estrogen and progesterone levels. Multiple induced abortions increased the risk for tubal pregnancy, possibly because of salpingitis (infection of the fallopian tube) that has occurred after induced abortion (Table 25-1). Regardless of the cause of tubal pregnancy, the effect is that transport of the fertilized ovum through the fallopian tube is hampered.

Clinical Manifestations

The classic signs of ectopic pregnancy include the following:

- Missed menstrual period
- Abdominal pain
- Vaginal "spotting"

More subtle signs and symptoms depend on the site of implantation. If implantation occurs in the distal end of the fallopian tube, which can contain the growing embryo longer, the woman may at first exhibit the usual early signs of pregnancy and consider herself to be normally pregnant. Several weeks into the pregnancy, intermittent abdominal pain and small amounts of vaginal bleeding occur that initially could be mistaken for threatened abortion. Because routine ultrasound examination in early pregnancy is common, however, it is not unusual to diagnose an ectopic pregnancy before onset of symptoms.

If implantation has occurred in the proximal end of the fallopian tube, rupture of the tube may occur within 2 to 3 weeks of the missed period because the tube is narrow in this area. Symptoms include sudden, severe pain in one of the lower quadrants of the abdomen as the tube tears open and the embryo is expelled into the pelvic cavity, often with profuse hemorrhage. Radiating pain under the scapula may indicate bleeding into the abdomen caused by phrenic nerve irritation. Hypovolemic shock is a major concern because systemic signs of shock may be rapid and extensive without external bleeding.

Diagnosis

The combined use of transvaginal ultrasound examination (see Chapter 10) and determination of the beta subunit of human chorionic gonadotropin (β-hCG) are helpful in early detection of ectopic pregnancy. An abnormal pregnancy is suspected if β-hCG is present but at lower levels than expected. If a gestational sac cannot be visualized when β-hCG is present, a diagnosis of ectopic pregnancy may be made with great accuracy. Visualization of an intrauterine pregnancy, however, does not absolutely rule out an ectopic pregnancy. A woman may have an intrauterine pregnancy and concurrently have an ectopic pregnancy.

The use of sensitive pregnancy tests, maternal serum progesterone levels, and high-resolution transvaginal ultrasound has largely eliminated invasive tests for ectopic pregnancy. Laparoscopy (examination of the peritoneal cavity by means of a laparoscope) occasionally may be necessary to diagnose rupture of an ectopic pregnancy. A characteristic bluish swelling within the tube is the most common finding.

Therapeutic Management

Management of tubal pregnancy depends on whether the tube is intact or ruptured. Medical management may be possible if the tube is unruptured. The goal of medical management is to preserve the tube and improve the chance of future fertility. The chemotherapeutic agent methotrexate (a folic acid antagonist) is used to inhibit cell division in the developing embryo.

Surgical management of a tubal pregnancy that is unruptured may involve a linear salpingostomy to salvage

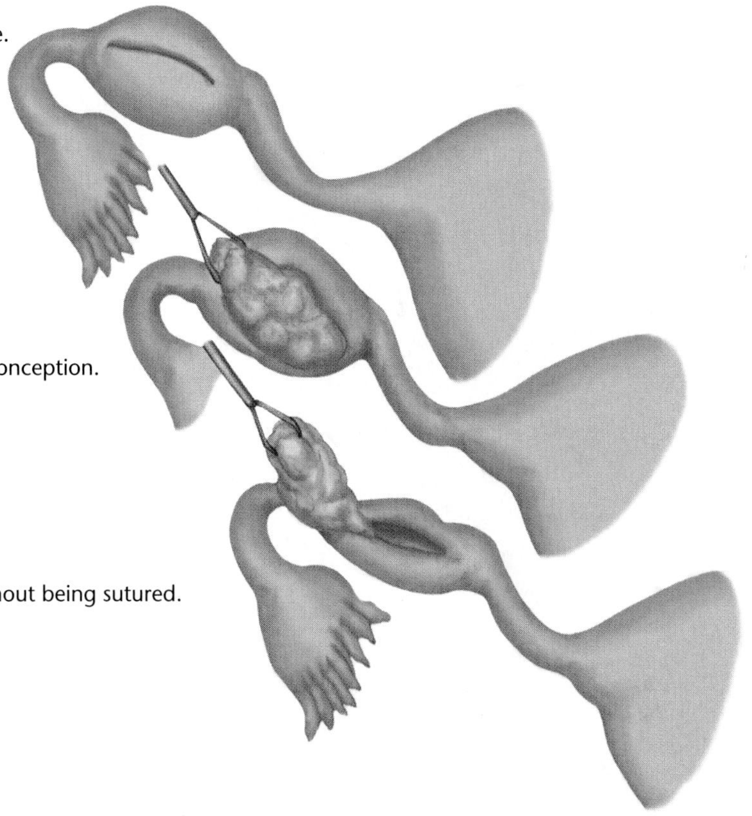
A linear incision is made in the intact tube.
Forceps are used to remove products of conception.
The incision is left to heal without being sutured.

FIGURE 25-3 Linear salpingostomy.

the tube (Figure 25-3). Linear salpingostomy also may be attempted if the tube is ruptured but damage to the tube is minimal. Salvaging the tube is particularly important to women concerned about future fertility.

When ectopic pregnancy results in rupture of the fallopian tube, the goal of therapeutic management is to control the bleeding and prevent hypovolemic shock. When the woman's cardiovascular status is stable, removal of the tube (salpingectomy) with ligation of bleeding vessels may be required. With early diagnosis and medical management, salpingectomy has become uncommon in the treatment of ectopic pregnancy.

Rh immune globulin is given to appropriate Rh_0(D)-negative women as it is after abortion.

Nursing Considerations

Nursing care focuses on prevention or early identification of hypovolemic shock, pain control, and psychological support for the woman who experiences an ectopic pregnancy. Nurses monitor the woman for decreasing hematocrit levels and pain that would indicate a ruptured ectopic pregnancy. Nurses administer analgesics and evaluate their effectiveness so that pain can be controlled.

If methotrexate is used, the nurse must explain adverse side effects, such as nausea and vomiting, and the importance of communicating any physical changes to the health care team. About 75% of the women will have an episode of increased pain during treatment, probably because of expulsion of the products of conception from the tube (Lipscomb & Ling, 2000). The woman must also be instructed to refrain from drinking alcohol, which decreases effectiveness, ingesting vitamins that contain folic acid, and having sexual intercourse until hCG is not detectable. If the treatment is successful, this hormone disappears from plasma within 2 to 4 weeks (Cunningham, et al., 1997). Keeping follow-up appointments is important.

The woman and her family will need psychological support to resolve intense emotions that may include anger, grief, guilt, and self-blame. The woman also may be anxious about her ability to become pregnant in the future. The nurses should clarify the physician's explanation and use therapeutic communication techniques that assist the woman to deal with her anxiety.

Gestational Trophoblastic Disease (Hydatidiform Mole)

Hydatidiform mole is one form of gestational trophoblastic disease that occurs when the trophoblasts (peripheral cells that attach the fertilized ovum to the uterine wall) develop abnormally. As a result of the abnormal growth, the placenta, but not the fetal part of the pregnancy, develops. The condition is characterized by proliferation and edema of the chorionic villi. The fluid-filled villi form grape-like clusters of tissue

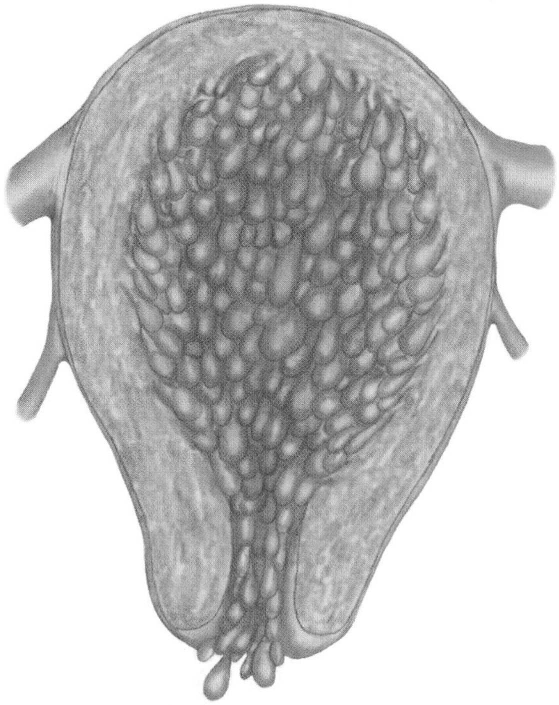

FIGURE 25-4 Hydatidiform mole.

that can rapidly grow large enough to fill the uterus to the size of an advanced pregnancy (Figure 25-4).

Incidence and Etiology

In the United States and Europe, the incidence of hydatidiform mole is 0.6 to 1.1 in every 1000 pregnancies. The rate is 3 to 10 times higher in Asian countries (Goldstein & Berkowitz, 2000b). Age is a factor, with the frequency of molar pregnancies highest at both ends of the reproductive life. Women who have had one molar pregnancy have 10 times the risk to have another in a subsequent pregnancy. Persistent gestational trophoblastic disease may undergo malignant change (choriocarcinoma) and may metastasize to distant sites such as the lung, vagina, liver, and brain.

Complete mole is thought to occur when the ovum is fertilized by a sperm that duplicates its own chromosomes while the maternal chromosomes in the ovum are inactivated. In a *partial mole,* the maternal contribution is usually present but the paternal contribution is double, and thus the karyotype is triploid (69,XXY or 69,XYY). If a fetus is identified with the partial mole, it is grossly abnormal because of the abnormal chromosome makeup.

Clinical Manifestations

Routine use of ultrasound allows earlier diagnosis of hydatidiform mole, usually before the more severe manifestations of the disorder develop. Possible signs and symptoms of molar pregnancy include the following:

- Elevated levels of hCG
- Characteristic ultrasonographic pattern that shows the vesicles and the absence of a fetal sac or fetal heart activity in a complete molar pregnancy
- A uterus that is larger than one would expect based on the duration of the pregnancy
- Vaginal bleeding, which varies from dark-brown spotting to profuse hemorrhage
- Excessive nausea and vomiting (hyperemesis gravidarum), which may be related to high levels of hCG from the proliferating trophoblasts
- Early development of pregnancy-induced hypertension, which is rarely diagnosed before 24 weeks in an otherwise normal pregnancy

Diagnosis

Measurement of the hCG levels detects the abnormally high levels of the hormone before treatment. Following treatment, hCG levels are measured to determine if they fall and then disappear.

In addition to the characteristic pattern showing the vesicles, ultrasound examination allows a differential diagnosis to be made between two types of molar pregnancies: (1) a partial mole that includes some fetal tissue and membranes and (2) a complete mole that is composed only of enlarged villi but contains no fetal tissue or membranes.

Therapeutic Management

Medical management includes two phases: (1) evacuation of the trophoblastic tissue of the mole and (2) continuous follow-up of the woman to detect malignant changes of any remaining trophoblastic tissue. At the same time, the woman is treated for any other problems such as pregnancy-induced hypertension or hyperemesis gravidarum.

Before evacuation, chest radiography, computed tomography (CT), or magnetic resonance imaging (MRI) may be performed to detect metastatic disease. A complete blood count, laboratory assessment of coagulation status, and blood typing and crossmatching are also necessary in case a transfusion is needed.

The mole usually is removed by vacuum aspiration. After tissue has been extracted, intravenous oxytocin is given to contract the uterus. Avoiding uterine stimulation with oxytocin before evacuation is important. Uterine contractions can cause trophoblastic tissue to be pulled into large venous sinusoids in the uterus, resulting in embolization of the tissue and respiratory distress (Berman, Di Saia, & Brewster, 1999). Curettage follows vacuum aspiration, and the tissue obtained is sent for laboratory evaluation. This is extremely important because, although a hydatidiform mole is usually a benign process, choriocarcinoma may occur.

Follow-up is critical to detect changes suggestive of trophoblastic malignancy. Follow-up protocol involves evaluation of serum hCG levels every 1 to 2 weeks until normal pre-pregnancy levels are attained. The test is then repeated every 1 to 2 months for a year. Pregnancy must be avoided during the 1 year follow-up because it would obscure the evidence of choriocarcinoma. Oral contraceptives are the preferred birth control method (Berman, Di Saia, & Brewster, 1999).

Nursing Considerations

Bleeding and infection are the early possible complications after a molar pregnancy. The nurse should observe the vital signs for an elevated temperature and pulse and observe vaginal bleeding for excessive amount or foul odor.

Women who have had a hydatidiform mole experience similar emotions as those who have had any other type of pregnancy loss. In addition, they may be anxious about follow-up evaluations, the possibility of malignant change, and the need to delay pregnancy for at least a year.

Check Your Reading

5. Why is ectopic pregnancy called a "disaster of reproduction"?
6. Why is the incidence of ectopic pregnancy increasing in the United States? How is it treated?
7. What is a hydatidiform mole, and why are two phases of treatment necessary?

APPLICATION OF THE NURSING PROCESS: HEMORRHAGIC CONDITIONS OF EARLY PREGNANCY

Regardless of the cause of early antepartum bleeding, nurses play a vital role in its management. Nurses are responsible for monitoring the condition of the pregnant woman and for collaborating with the physician to provide treatment.

Assessment

Confirmation of pregnancy and length of gestation are important initial data to obtain. Physical assessment focuses on determining the amount of bleeding and the description, location, and severity of pain. Estimate the amount of vaginal bleeding by examining linen and peripads. If necessary, make a more accurate estimation by weighing the linen and peripads (1 g weight equals 1 ml volume).

> When asking a woman how much blood she lost at home, ask her to compare the amount lost with a common measure such as a tablespoon or a cup. Ask also how long the bleeding episode lasted and what has been done to control the bleeding.

Bleeding may be accompanied by pain. Uterine cramping usually accompanies spontaneous abortion; deep, severe pelvic pain is associated with ruptured ectopic pregnancy. Remember that in ruptured ectopic pregnancy, bleeding may be concealed and pain could be the only symptom.

The woman's vital signs and urine output give a clue to her cardiovascular status. A rising pulse and respiratory rate and falling urine output are associated with hypovolemia. The blood pressure usually falls late in hypovolemic shock. Check laboratory values for hemoglobin and hematocrit and report abnormal values to the health care provider. Identify women who are Rh-negative so that they can receive Rh_0(D) immune globulin.

CRITICAL THINKING EXERCISE

All women who have experienced prenatal bleeding and invasive procedures are at increased risk for infection.

QUESTION:
What common assumptions do nurses make about those who are at risk for developing infections?

Because abortion or hydatidiform mole may be associated with infections, assess the woman for fever, elevated pulse, malaise, and prolonged or malodorous vaginal discharge. Determine the family's knowledge of needed follow-up care and how to prevent complications such as infection.

Analysis

A variety of complications and nursing diagnoses are possible. These include the possibility of "Hypovolemic Shock" (see p. 675) and "Risk for Infection." A more complete diagnosis might be "Knowledge Deficit of diagnostic and therapeutic procedures, signs and symptoms of infection, dietary measures to prevent infection, and recommended follow-up care."

Planning

Goals or expected outcomes for this nursing diagnosis are that the woman will do the following:

- Verbalize understanding of diagnostic and therapeutic procedures
- Verbalize signs of infection that should be reported to the health care provider
- Follow the designed plan for follow-up care

Interventions

Providing Information about Tests and Procedures

Women and their families experience less anxiety if they understand what is happening. Explain planned diagnostic procedures, such as transvaginal or transabdominal ultrasonography (see Chapter 10). Include the purpose of the tests, how long they will take, and whether the procedures cause discomfort. Briefly describe the reasons for blood tests such as hCG, hemoglobin, or hematocrit. Explain that diagnostic and therapeutic measures sometimes must be performed quickly to prevent excessive blood loss. If surgical intervention is necessary, reinforce explanations of the anesthesiologist or nurse-anesthetist about planned anesthesia. A signed informed consent is required before a surgical procedure such as a D&C or vacuum aspiration.

Teaching Measures to Prevent Infection

The risk for infection is greatest during the first 72 hours after spontaneous abortion or operative procedures. Personal hygiene should include careful hand washing before and after changing perineal pads and taking daily showers. Perineal pads, applied in a front-to-back direction, should be used instead of tampons until bleeding has subsided. The woman should consult with the health care provider about safe timing of resuming intercourse.

Providing Dietary Information

Nutrition and adequate fluid intake help maintain the body's defense against infection, and the nurse must promote adequate diet. The woman who has a hemorrhagic complication is also at risk for infection. She needs foods that are high in iron to increase hemoglobin and hematocrit values. These foods include liver, red meat, spinach, egg yolks, carrots, and raisins. In addition, she needs foods that are high in vitamin C, which increases the utilization of iron (Anderson, 2000; Fagen, 2000). These foods include citrus fruits, broccoli, strawberries, cantaloupe, cabbage, and green peppers. Adequate fluid intake (2500 ml per day) promotes hydration after bleeding episodes and maintains digestive processes.

Iron supplementation also frequently is prescribed, and the woman may require information on how to lessen the gastrointestinal upset that many people experience when iron is administered. Less gastric upset is experienced when iron is taken with meals. A diet high in fiber and fluid helps reduce the commonly associated constipation.

Teaching Signs of Infection to Report

Ensure the woman has a thermometer and knows how to use it. Tell her to take her temperature every 8 hours for the first 3 days at home. Teach the woman to seek medical help if her temperature rises above 37.8° C (100° F) or as her physician instructs. She also should report other signs of infection, even if she does not have a fever, such as vaginal discharge with foul odor, pelvic tenderness, or persistent general malaise.

Reinforcing Follow-Up Care

A variety of follow-up procedures such as repeat ultrasonic examinations or serum hCG levels may be necessary for women with gestational trophoblastic disease such as hydatidiform mole. Immunologic or genetic testing and counseling may be advised for couples having recurrent abortions. All couples who have had a pregnancy loss should be seen and counseled.

At this time, acknowledge their grief, which often manifests as anger. Many women have guilt feelings that must be recognized. They often need repeated reassurance that the loss was not due to anything they did or to anything they neglected.

Women who do not desire pregnancy right away will need contraception. Reliable contraception for at least 1 year also will be essential for women who have had a molar pregnancy. Teach the woman to use the contraceptive method appropriately so that it is effective (see Chapter 31).

CRITICAL THINKING EXERCISE

Alice Starkey, a 24-year-old primigravida, had an incomplete abortion at 12 weeks' gestation. When she was admitted to the hospital, intravenous fluids were administered and blood was taken for blood grouping and crossmatching. A vacuum curettage was performed to remove retained placental tissue. When bleeding subsided, Alice was discharged to go home. Helen Claude, the nurse providing discharge instructions, comments to Alice, "These things happen for the best, and you are so lucky it happened early." "You can have other children."

QUESTIONS:

1. What assumptions has Helen made? How might these affect Alice?
2. Is the comment that Alice can have other children comforting? Why or why not?
3. If the nurse's response was not helpful, what responses from the nurse would be most helpful for Alice?

Evaluation

Interventions are judged successful and the goals/expected outcomes are met if the woman does the following:

- Verbalizes understanding of diagnostic and therapeutic procedures
- Verbalizes signs of infection that should be reported to a health care professional
- Helps develop and participates in a follow-up plan of care

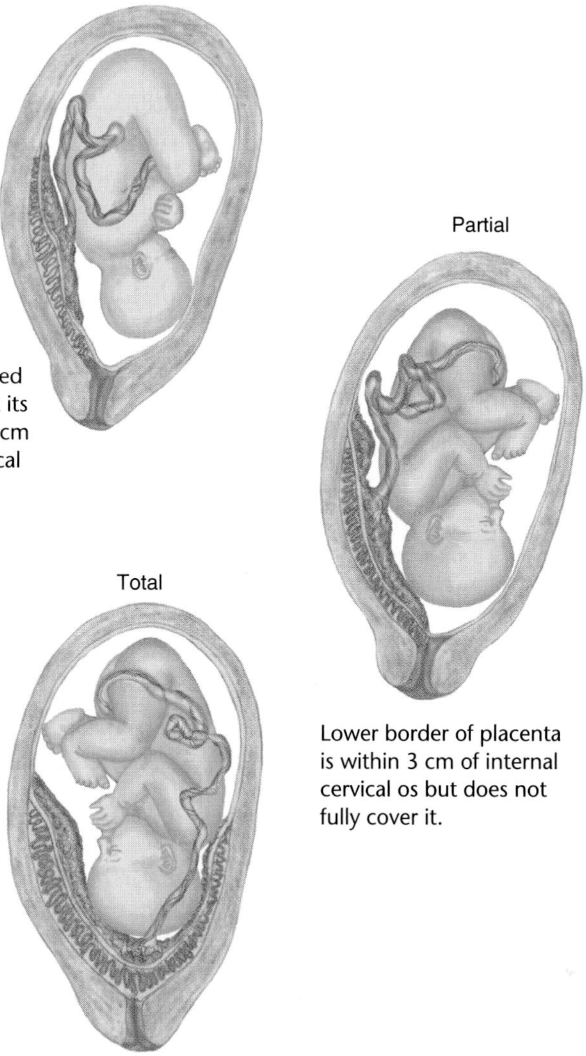
Marginal
Placenta is implanted in lower uterus but its lower border is >3 cm from internal cervical os.
Partial
Lower border of placenta is within 3 cm of internal cervical os but does not fully cover it.
Total
Placenta completely covers internal cervical os.

FIGURE 25-5 The three classifications of placenta previa.

HEMORRHAGIC CONDITIONS OF LATE PREGNANCY

After 20 weeks of pregnancy, the two major causes of hemorrhage are the disorders of the placenta called placenta previa and abruptio placentae. Abruptio placentae may be further complicated by DIC, which was discussed earlier.

Placenta Previa

Placenta previa is an implantation of the placenta in the lower uterus. As a result, it is closer to the internal cervical os than the presenting part (usually the head) of the fetus. The three classifications of placenta previa (total, partial, and marginal) depend on how much of the internal cervical os is covered by the placenta (Figure 25-5). High-resolution ultrasound allows measurement of the distance between the internal cervical os and the lower border of the placenta:

- Marginal (sometimes called *low-lying*): Placenta is implanted in the lower uterus but its lower border is more than 3 cm from the internal cervical os
- Partial: Lower border of the placenta is within 3 cm of the internal cervical os but does not completely cover the os
- Total: Placenta completely covers internal cervical os

Marginal placenta previa is common in early ultrasound examinations and often appears to move upward and away from the internal cervical os as the fetus grows and the upper uterus develops more than the lower uterus. Only about 10% of placenta previas diagnosed in the second trimester will remain a previa at term (Clark, 1999b).

Incidence and Etiology

In the United States, the incidence of placenta previa averages 1 in 200 births. It is more common in women who have had prior placenta previa, previous cesarean birth, previous pregnancy termination, and in older women. The multipara is more likely to have placenta previa than the nullipara. African or Asian ethnicity also increases the risk. Cigarette smoking and cocaine use are personal habits that add to a woman's risk for a previa.

Clinical Manifestations

The classic sign of placenta previa is the sudden onset of painless uterine bleeding in the last half of pregnancy. However, many cases of placenta previa are diagnosed by ultrasound examination before any bleeding occurs. Bleeding results from tearing of the placental villi from the uterine wall thus exposing uterine vessels. Bleeding is painless because it does not occur in a closed cavity and does not cause pressure on adjacent tissue. It may be scanty or profuse, and it may cease spontaneously, only to recur later.

Bleeding may not occur until labor starts, when cervical changes disrupt placental attachment. The admitting nurse may be unsure whether the bleeding is just heavy "bloody show" or a sign of a placenta previa.

If any doubt exists, the nurse never performs a vaginal examination or takes any action that would stimulate uterine activity. Digital examination of the cervical os when a placenta previa is present can cause additional placental separation or tear the placenta itself, causing severe hemorrhage and extreme risk to the fetus. Until the location and position of the placenta are verified by ultrasonography, no manual examinations should be performed, and administration of oxytocin should be postponed to prevent strong contractions that could result in sudden placental separation and rapid hemorrhage.

Therapeutic Management

When the diagnosis of placenta previa is confirmed, medical interventions are based on the condition of the expectant mother and fetus. The woman is evaluated to determine the amount of hemorrhage, and electronic fetal monitoring is initiated to evaluate the fetus.

Options for management include conservative management if the mother's cardiovascular status is stable and the fetus is immature and without signs of distress. Conservative management may take place at home or in the hospital. Antepartal units are often designed to consider the woman's needs for physical and occupational therapy and for diversion as well as care for her pregnancy complication.

Home Care. Criteria for home care include the following (Clark, 1999b):

- No evidence of active bleeding
- Ability to maintain bedrest at home
- Home is reasonable distance from the hospital
- Emergency systems available for immediate transport to the hospital 24 hours a day

Nurses are often responsible for helping the woman and family understand the physician's plan of care. Nurses help the woman and family develop a workable plan for home care that may include strict bedrest except for going to the bathroom, the presence of another adult to manage the home and be present if an emergency arises, and procedure if heavy bleeding begins. Teaching also includes emphasizing the importance of (1) assessing color and amount of vaginal discharge or bleeding, especially after each urination or bowel movement, (2) assessing fetal activity (kick counts) daily (see Chapter 10), (3) assessing uterine activity at prescribed intervals, (4) avoiding sexual intercourse to prevent disruption of the placenta, and (5) physician visits. Nurses may be responsible for making daily phone contact to assess the woman's perception of uterine activity (cramping, regular or sporadic contractions), bleeding, fetal activity, and adherence to the prescribed treatment plan. In addition, they may make home visits for comprehensive maternal-fetal assessments, including nonstress tests. The woman is instructed to report a decrease in fetal movement or if uterine contractions or vaginal bleeding occurs.

Nurses are also responsible for providing specific, accurate information about the condition of the fetus. For example, parents are reassured when they hear that the fetal heart rate is within the expected range and daily kick counts are reassuring. Nurses also may need to help the family understand the physician's plan of care. For instance, the nurse may explain why a cesarean birth is necessary when the placenta extends over the cervical os.

Inpatient Care. Women with placenta previa are admitted to the antepartum unit if they do not meet the criteria for home care or if they require constant assessment and care. When the expectant mother is confined to the hospital, nursing assessments focus on determining whether she experiences bleeding episodes or signs of preterm labor. Periodic electronic fetal monitoring is necessary to determine whether there are fetal heart activity changes in association with fetal compromise. A significant change in fetal heart activity, an episode of vaginal bleeding, or signs of preterm labor should be reported immediately to the physician.

At times conservative management is not an option. For instance, delivery is scheduled if the fetus is older than 36 weeks' gestation and the lungs are mature. Immediate delivery may be necessary regardless of fetal immaturity if bleeding is excessive, the woman demonstrates signs of hypovolemia, or signs of fetal compromise are present. If cesarean birth is necessary, nurses must prepare the expectant mother for surgery.

See Table 16-4 for a summary of care for the woman having cesarean birth.

The preoperative procedures are often performed quickly if the woman is hemorrhaging, and the family may be anxious about the condition of the fetus and the expectant mother. Nurses must use whatever time is available to keep the family informed.

> During the rapid preparations for surgery, the nurse can reassure both the woman and the family by briefly describing the necessary preparations: "I'm sorry we have to rush, but we need to start the IV in case she needs extra fluids." "Do you have questions I might answer as we prepare for the cesarean?"

Abruptio Placentae

Separation of a normally implanted placenta before the fetus is born (called *abruptio placentae, placental abruption,* or *premature separation of the placenta*) occurs in cases of bleeding and formation of a hematoma (clot) on the maternal side of the placenta. As the clot expands, further separation occurs. Hemorrhage may be apparent (vaginal bleeding) or concealed. The severity of the complication depends on the amount of bleeding and the size of the hematoma. If bleeding continues, the hematoma expands and obliterates intervillous spaces. Fetal vessels are disrupted as placental separation occurs, and fetal and maternal bleeding occur.

Abruptio placentae is a dangerous condition for both the pregnant woman and the fetus. The major danger for the woman is hemorrhage and consequent hypovolemic shock and clotting abnormalities (DIC, p. 664). The major dangers for the fetus are asphyxia, excessive blood loss, and prematurity.

Incidence and Etiology

Published incidence of abruptio placentae varies widely; however, it probably averages about 1 in 200 deliveries. Placental abruption extensive enough to cause the death of the fetus has declined to about 1 in 830 deliveries (Cunningham, et al., 1997).

The cause is unknown; however, several factors that increase the risk have been identified. Maternal use of cocaine, which causes vasoconstriction in the endometrial arteries, is a leading cause of abruptio placentae. Other risk factors include maternal hypertension, maternal cigarette smoking, multigravida status, short umbilical cord, abdominal trauma, and history of previous premature separation of the placenta.

Clinical Manifestations

The four classic signs and symptoms of abruptio placentae are the following:

- Bleeding, which may be evident vaginally or may be concealed behind the placenta
- Uterine tenderness

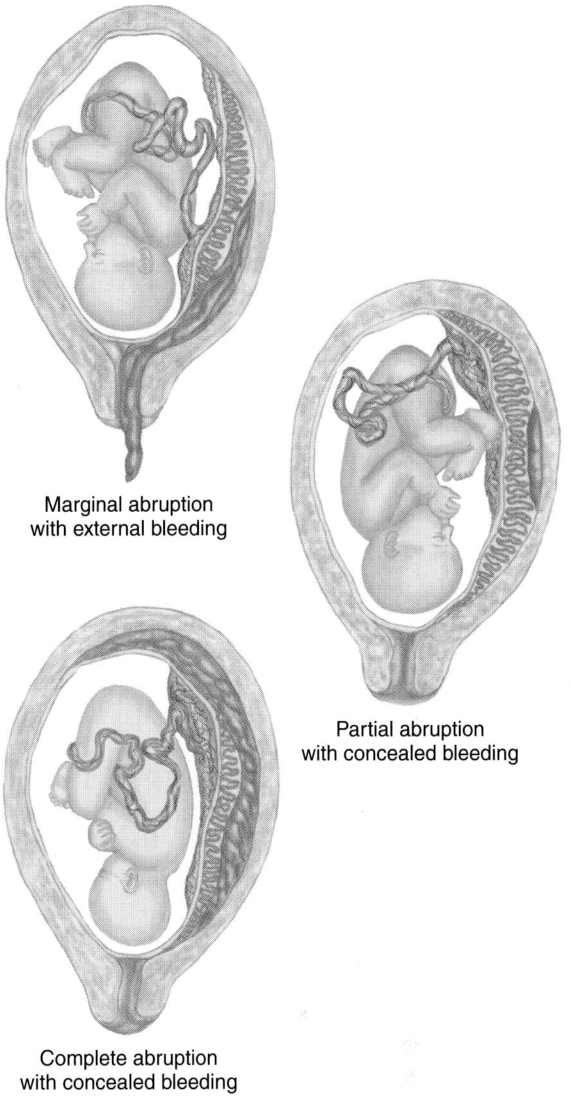

FIGURE 25-6 Types of abruptio placentae.

- Excess uterine activity with poor relaxation between contractions
- Abdominal pain

Additional signs include back pain, signs of hypovolemic shock, fetal distress, and fetal death. Many women have a normal blood pressure, however, because the blood loss masks an undiagnosed hypertensive disorder (Clark, 1999b).

Cases of abruptio placentae are divided into two main types: (1) those in which hemorrhage is concealed and (2) those in which hemorrhage is apparent. In either type, the placental abruption may be complete or partial. Concealed hemorrhage means bleeding occurs behind the placenta but the margins remain intact, causing formation of a hematoma. The hemorrhage is apparent when bleeding separates or dissects the membranes from the endometrium and blood flows out through the vagina. Figure 25-6 illustrates abruptio placentae with external and concealed bleeding. Apparent bleeding does not always correspond to the actual amount of blood lost, and signs of shock (tachycardia, hypotension, pale color, and cold, clammy skin) may be present when little or no external bleeding occurs.

Abdominal pain is also related to the type of separation. It may be sudden and severe when bleeding occurs into the myometrium (uterine muscle) or is intermittent and difficult to distinguish from labor contractions. The uterus may become exceedingly firm (board-like) and tender, making palpation of the fetus difficult. Ultrasound examination is helpful to rule out placenta previa as the cause of bleeding, but it cannot be used to diagnose abruptio placentae reliably because the separation and bleeding may not be obvious on ultrasonography.

Therapeutic Management

Any woman who exhibits signs of abruptio placentae should be hospitalized and evaluated at once. Evaluation focuses on the cardiovascular status of the expectant mother and the condition of the fetus. If the condition is mild and the fetus is immature and shows no signs of distress, conservative management may be initiated. This includes bedrest and may include administration of tocolytic medications to decrease uterine activity. Conservative management is rare, however, owing to the great risks of fetal death and maternal hemorrhage associated with abruptio placentae.

Immediate delivery of the fetus is necessary if signs of fetal compromise exist or if the expectant mother exhibits signs of excessive bleeding, either obvious or concealed. Intensive monitoring of both the woman and the fetus is essential because rapid deterioration of either can occur. Blood products for replacement should be available, and two large-bore intravenous lines should be started for replacement of fluid and blood.

Women who have experienced abdominal trauma are at increased risk for abruptio placentae. They may be monitored for 24 hours after significant trauma such as a motor vehicle accident, even if they are not having any signs of bleeding because it may take this long for an abruptio placentae to develop. If they are not having contractions after the trauma and the fetal heart rate pattern is reassuring, monitoring for 4 to 6 hours may be sufficient (Clark, 1999b).

Nursing Considerations

Abruptio placentae is frightening for a woman. She experiences severe pain and is aware of the danger to herself and to the fetus. She must be carefully assessed for signs of concealed hemorrhage.

If immediate cesarean delivery is necessary, the woman may feel powerless as the health care team hurriedly prepares her for surgery. If at all possible in the time available, nurses must explain anticipated procedures to the woman and her family to reduce their feelings of fear and anxiety.

Excessive bleeding and fetal hypoxia are always major concerns with abruptio placentae, and nurses are responsible for continuous monitoring of both the expectant mother and the fetus so that problems can be detected early before the condition of the woman or the fetus deteriorates.

CRITICAL TO REMEMBER

Signs of Concealed Hemorrhage

Abruptio Placentae

Increase in fundal height
Hard, board-like abdomen
High uterine baseline tone on electronic monitoring strip
Persistent abdominal pain
Systemic signs of early hemorrhage (tachycardia, falling blood pressure, falling urine output, restlessness)
Persistent late deceleration in fetal heart rate or decreasing baseline variability; absence of accelerations
Slight or absent vaginal bleeding

Check Your Reading

8. What are the signs and symptoms of placenta previa? How is it managed in the home?
9. What are the signs and symptoms of abruptio placentae?
10. What are the major dangers to the expectant mother and the fetus during the placental abruption?

APPLICATION OF THE NURSING PROCESS: HEMORRHAGIC CONDITIONS OF LATE PREGNANCY

Assessment

For hemorrhagic conditions of late pregnancy, some nursing assessments should be performed immediately and others can be deferred until initial interventions have been taken to stabilize the cardiovascular status of the woman. The priority nursing assessments are the following:

- *Amount and nature of bleeding* (time of onset, estimated blood loss before admission to hospital, and description of tissue or clots passed): The woman should be taught to save peripads and linen savers if she is at home so that blood loss can be determined accurately.
- *Pain* (type [constant, intermittent, sharp, dull, severe], onset [sudden, gradual], and location [generalized over abdomen, localized]): Is uterine tenderness apparent with gentle palpation?

- *Maternal vital signs:* Are these within normal limits or is hypotension, tachycardia, or both present? Hypertension may be present with early abruptio placentae.
- *Condition of the fetus:* An electronic fetal monitor determines fetal heart rate, presence of accelerations, and fetal response to uterine activity. Late decelerations or poor variability (if an internal spiral electrode is used) are of particular concern.
- *Uterine contractions:* Application of an external monitor determines frequency and duration of contractions. An intrauterine pressure catheter can identify hypertonic contractions and an increased resting tone associated with abruptio placentae. Palpation can identify that the uterus does not relax fully between contractions.
- *Obstetric history* (gravida, para, previous abortions, preterm infants, previous pregnancy outcomes)
- *Length of gestation* (date of last menstrual period, fundal height, correlation of fundal height with estimated gestation): If bleeding occurs into the myometrium, the fundus enlarges as bleeding progresses. A piece of tape can mark the top of the fundus at a given time and then the nurse can observe and report increasing fundal size, which indicates that bleeding into uterine muscles is occurring.
- *Laboratory data* (hemoglobin, hematocrit, blood type, coagulation studies): Laboratory data are obtained to prepare for transfusions should they become necessary and to determine whether signs of DIC are developing.

Despite the emphasis on physical assessment, the emotional response of the expectant mother and her partner must also be addressed. They will most likely be anxious, fearful, confused, and overwhelmed by the activity. They may have little knowledge of expected medical management and may not realize that the fetus will need to be delivered as quickly as possible and that a surgical procedure is necessary. They may fear for the life of the woman and the fetus.

Analysis

Nursing diagnoses vary, depending on the cause and severity of the bleeding. The most commonly used nursing diagnoses for antepartum bleeding appear in Nursing Care Plan 25-1. The most dangerous potential complication is *hypovolemic shock,* which jeopardizes the life of the mother as well as the fetus.

NURSING CARE PLAN 25-1

Antepartum Bleeding

Assessment: Beth Dixon, a 28-year-old gravida 2, para 1, is admitted to the antepartum unit at 34 weeks' gestation following an episode of vaginal bleeding resulting from total placenta previa. Vital signs are stable, and fetal heart rate is 140 beats per minute with a reassuring pattern. Beth and her husband, Bob, appear anxious about the condition of the fetus and the plan of care. Beth is particularly worried about her 5-year-old son who is at home with a neighbor.

Nursing Diagnosis: Anxiety related to unknown effects of bleeding and lack of knowledge of predicted course of management

Critical Thinking: Although this diagnosis is correct, what are priority nursing actions for Beth? Why?

Answer: To monitor the condition of the fetus and to observe Beth for vaginal bleeding or change in vital signs. These priorities are based on a hierarchy of needs; physiologic needs and the need for safety must be ensured before psychological needs are addressed.

Goals/Expected Outcomes:
1. The couple will verbalize expected routines and projected management by the end of the first day following admission.
2. The couple will relate less anxiety after learning.

Intervention	Rationale
1. Remain with the couple and acknowledge the emotions that they exhibit: "I know this is unexpected, and you must have many questions. Perhaps I can answer some of them."	1. The nurse's presence and empathetic understanding are potent therapeutic tools to prepare the family to cope with the unexpected situation.
2. Determine the couple's level of understanding of the situation and the projected management: "Tell me what you've been told to expect."	2. This allows the nurse to reinforce the physician's explanations and to notify the physician if additional explanations are necessary.
3. Provide the couple with factual information about projected management. a. Explain that Beth will need to remain in the hospital so that her condition and the condition of the fetus can be watched closely.	3. Patient education has proved to be an effective measure for preventing and reducing anxiety. Knowledge reduces fear of the unknown.

Continued

Intervention	Rationale
b. Explain why a cesarean birth is necessary this time even though she delivered vaginally before. c. Provide information about hospital routines (meals, visiting hours) and any fetal surveillance techniques (such as nonstress tests).	
4. Allow Beth and her family to participate in the routine as much as possible. This may mean scheduling nursing care around times when Bob and their son can visit.	4. Many women feel a sense of powerlessness when they are confined to bed and a course of treatment is prescribed without consultation.

Evaluation: The interventions are considered successful if the couple demonstrates knowledge of the projected management and why it is necessary and verbalizes reduced anxiety.

Assessment: Beth continues to have episodes of light vaginal bleeding, although none have been so heavy as to demand immediate delivery. Her doctor wants the fetus to mature at least 2 more weeks if possible. Beth cries frequently, telling the nurse, "I miss my son so much. He just started kindergarten and he is so shy. I feel useless and he really needs me now. It's hard on Bob, too; he has to do everything."

Nursing Diagnosis: Situational Low Self-Esteem related to temporary inability to provide care for family

Goals/Expected Outcomes:
Beth will do the following:
1. Identify positive aspects of self during hospitalization.
2. Identify ways of providing comfort and affection for her son during the hospital stay.

Intervention	Rationale
1. Encourage Beth to express her concerns about the need for hospitalization: "What bothers you most about being away from home?"	1. Major concerns may not be identified or may be misunderstood unless the woman clarifies them.
2. After acknowledging feelings, encourage examination of the need for hospitalization and its consequences: it provides time for the fetus to mature.	2. This identifies positive aspects of the situation and her important role.
3. Explore reality of Beth's self-appraisal ("I feel useless") by assisting her to investigate ways to provide nurturing care for her son while she is hospitalized: a. Keep in close touch by telephone (wake-up, goodnight, and after-school calls). b. Make small handmade items such as bookmarks. c. Explain in simple, nonfrightening terms why she must stay in the hospital. d. Offer reassurances of continued love.	3. Daily involvement in the life of the child helps reduce feelings of isolation and failure to meet obligations to her family.
4. Assist Beth to involve her son in plans for the newborn. He might benefit from sibling classes or playtime with the mother that involves caring for newborn-sized dolls.	4. This provides goals for combined family interaction that increase feeling of self-worth.

Evaluation: Beth is able to make positive comments about the importance of rest to the health of the new baby, and she initiates numerous activities that permit her to continue close, comforting contact with her child during the period of hospitalization.

Planning

The nurse cannot independently manage hypovolemic shock but must confer with physicians for medical orders for treatment. Planning should reflect the nurse's responsibility to do the following:

- Monitor for signs of hypovolemic shock
- Consult with the physician if signs of hypovolemic shock are observed
- Perform actions to minimize the effects of hypovolemic shock

Interventions

Monitoring for Signs of Hypovolemic Shock

Assess for any sign of developing hypovolemic shock. The body attempts to compensate for decreased blood volume and to maintain oxygenation of essential organs by increasing the rate and effort of the heart and lungs and by shunting blood from less essential organs, such as the skin and the extremities, to more essential organs, such as the brain and the kidneys. This compensatory mechanism results in the early signs and symptoms of hypovolemic shock:

- Tachycardia, diminished peripheral pulses
- Normal or slightly decreased blood pressure
- Increased respiratory rate
- Cool, pale skin and mucous membranes

The compensatory mechanism fails if hypovolemic shock progresses and insufficient blood exists to perfuse the brain, heart, and kidneys. Later signs of hypovolemic shock include the following:

- Falling blood pressure
- Pallor; skin becomes cold and clammy
- Urine output less than 30 ml per hour
- Restlessness, agitation, decreased mentation

CRITICAL TO REMEMBER

Signs and Symptoms of Hypovolemic Shock

Increased pulse rate, falling blood pressure, increased respiratory rate
Weak, diminished, or "thready" peripheral pulses
Cool, moist skin, pallor, or cyanosis (late sign)
Decreased (<30 ml/hr) or absent urinary output
Decreased hemoglobin, hematocrit levels
Change in mental status (restlessness, agitation, difficulty concentrating)

Monitoring the Fetus

Use continuous electronic fetal monitoring so that signs of fetal compromise, such as decreasing baseline variability or late decelerations, can be seen (see Chapter 14). If nonreassuring patterns are seen, contact the physician at once because the fetus often shows signs of compromise before maternal signs of hypovolemia are obvious.

Promoting Tissue Oxygenation

To promote oxygenation of tissues:

- Place the woman in a lateral position, with the head of the bed flat to increase cardiac return and thus to increase circulation and oxygenation of the placenta and other vital organs
- Limit maternal activity to decrease the tissue demand for oxygen
- Provide simple explanations, reassurance, and emotional support to the woman to reduce anxiety, which increases the metabolic demand for oxygen

Collaborating with the Physician for Fluid Replacement

To replace fluids:

- Obtain an order for blood typing and crossmatching so that blood is available for replacement if necessary.
- Insert IV lines according to hospital protocol; usually two lines that use large-gauge catheters (16- to 18-gauge) are recommended so that blood can be administered quickly if necessary.
- Administer fluids for replacement as directed by the physician to maintain a urinary output of at least 30 ml per hour.

Preparing the Woman for Surgery

Quick preparation of the woman for cesarean delivery may be necessary. The nurse is responsible for the following:

- Validating that preoperative permits have been correctly signed
- Validating that appropriate laboratory work has been done
- Surgical preparation and insertion of an indwelling urinary catheter
- Administering nonparticulate antacid or other medications as ordered by the anesthesiologist
- Providing information and reassurance to the family
- Assessing bleeding from the vagina as well as from any surgical sites or puncture wounds (epidural or intravenous sites) so that uncontrolled bleeding or bleeding from unexpected sites, which may indicate DIC, can be reported to the physician for prompt medical management

Providing Emotional Support

Once the safety of the woman and the fetus is ensured, nursing interventions promote comfort and provide emotional support. Explain what is causing the discomfort, and reassure the woman that pain relief measures will be initiated as soon as possible without causing harm to the fetus. Although offering false reassurance about the condition of the fetus is unwise, remain with the woman and provide accurate and timely information. Find time to explain what is going on to the woman and her family. They can feel overwhelmed by all the activity.

Evaluation

Although client-centered goals are not developed for collaborative problems, the nurse collects and compares data with established norms and judges whether the data are within normal limits. For hypovolemic shock, the maternal vital signs remain within normal limits and the fetal heart demonstrates no signs of compromise, such as abnormal rate, late decelerations, or decreasing baseline variability.

HYPEREMESIS GRAVIDARUM

Hyperemesis gravidarum (HEG) is persistent, uncontrollable vomiting that begins before the twentieth week of pregnancy. Hyperemesis gravidarum may continue throughout pregnancy, although its severity usually lessens. Unlike morning sickness, which is self-limited and causes no serious complications, hyperemesis gravidarum can have serious consequences. It can lead to loss of at least 5% of prepregnancy weight, dehydration, ketosis, acid-base imbalance, and electrolyte imbalance (both sodium and potassium are lost from gastric fluids). Metabolic alkalosis may develop because large amounts of hydrochloric acid are lost in the vomitus (Snell et al., 1999; Larson & Rayburn, 2000).

Etiology

The cause of hyperemesis gravidarum is not known but a number of factors seem to increase the risk for its occurrence. These include young age, first pregnancy, problems with nausea and vomiting in previous pregnancy, a history of intolerance to oral contraceptives, and previous gallbladder disease. Most research does not show an association between hyperemesis gravidarum and education, race, culture, or gender of the fetus (Snell, et al., 1998).

Four etiologic theories have been proposed (Snell, et al., 1998):

- *Endocrine theory:* The high levels of hCG and estrogen during pregnancy may be a causative factor. This theory is supported by the fact that in conditions such as gestational trophoblastic disease or multifetal pregnancy, in which these hormones are very high, hyperemesis gravidarum is more common. However, hyperemesis gravidarum occurs in women with low, normal, and elevated hormone levels. The woman's individual sensitivity to hormones of pregnancy may be the most important factor. Estrogen increases a woman's sensitivity to smell, which may trigger nausea in some women. Other hormones such as progesterone or thyroxine also may play a part.
- *Psychosomatic theory:* At one time, hyperemesis gravidarum was dismissed as totally psychosomatic, or "in the woman's mind." Although this is no longer an acceptable view, the role of psychological factors such as stress and lack of social support cannot be overlooked when caring for these women. At the very least, psychological stress adds to their physical problems.
- *Allergic theory:* This theory has been studied the least, but it hypothesizes that the introduction of a new antigen (the fetus and placenta) challenges the maternal immune system.
- *Metabolic theory:* Vitamin B_6 deficiency has been implicated as a cause for hyperemesis gravidarum, but research has been conflicting on this point. Another proposed premise is that some women have a lower liver function to metabolize the high hormones of pregnancy and therefore are more affected by the high blood levels.

Therapeutic Management

Treatment occurs primarily in the home, where the woman first attempts to control the nausea with methods that are used for morning sickness (see Chapter 7). In addition, some physicians prescribe vitamins, such as pyridoxine (vitamin B_6), that may provide some relief. A daily vitamin and mineral supplement may be recommended.

Drug therapy may be required if the vomiting becomes severe. Drugs prescribed may include the following:

- Promethazine (Phenergan)
- Diphenhydramine (Benadryl)
- Histamine-receptor antagonists such as famotidine (Pepcid) or ranitidine (Zantac)
- Metoclopramide (Reglan)
- Ondansetron (Zofran)
- Omeprazole (Prilosec)

Metoclopramide can be given with a subcutaneous infusion pump to provide continuous therapy at home (Buttino, Gambon, & Coleman, 1999). If drugs are required, a single drug is first prescribed in the lowest effective dose to minimize fetal effects. The benefit of the drug at controlling the adverse effects of the intractable vomiting is balanced against any fetal risk from the drug. The drugs listed are pregnancy category B or C.

If simpler methods are unsuccessful and weight loss or electrolyte imbalance persists, intravenous fluid and electrolyte replacement or total parenteral nutrition may be necessary. In some women, intravenous fluid replacement improves the nausea and vomiting quickly. The woman usually can be managed at home with periodic home nursing visits if she must have total parenteral nutrition.

Nursing Considerations

Because management frequently occurs in the home, nurses are often responsible for assessing and intervening for the woman with hyperemesis gravidarum. Physical assessment begins with determining the intake and output. Intake includes intravenous fluids and parenteral nutrition, as well as oral nutrition, which is allowed once vomiting is controlled. Output includes the amount and character of emesis and urinary output. As a rule of thumb, the normal urinary output is about 1 ml per kg (2.2 lb) per hour. A record of bowel elimination also provides significant information about oral nutrition.

Laboratory data may be evaluated to determine fluid and metabolic status. Elevated levels of hemoglobin and hematocrit may occur as a result of dehydration, which results in hemoconcentration. Concentrations of sodium, potassium, and chloride may be reduced, resulting in hypokalemia and alkalosis.

The woman weighs herself daily, first thing in the morning and in similar clothing. Her urine is tested for ketones. Weight loss and the presence of ketones in the urine suggest that fat stores and protein are being metabolized to meet energy needs.

Signs of dehydration include decreased fluid intake (less than 2000 ml/day), decreased urinary output, increased specific gravity of urine (more than 1.025), dry skin or dry mucous membranes, and nonelastic skin turgor.

Nursing interventions focus on reducing nausea and vomiting, maintaining nutrition and fluid balance, and providing emotional support.

Reducing Nausea and Vomiting

When food is offered to the woman, portions should be small so that the amount does not appear overwhelming. Food should be attractively presented, and foods with strong odors should be eliminated from the diet because food smells often incite nausea. Low-fat foods and easily digested carbohydrates, such as fruit, breads, cereals, rice, and pasta, provide important nutrients and help prevent low blood sugar, which can cause nausea. Soups and other liquids should be taken between meals, to avoid distending the stomach and triggering vomiting. Sitting upright after meals reduces gastric reflux.

Maintaining Nutrition and Fluid Balance

Women with nausea and vomiting should eat every 2 to 3 hours. Salting food helps replace chloride lost when hydrochloric acid is vomited. Potassium- and magnesium-rich foods should be encouraged because these nutrients are likely to be depleted and magnesium deficiency can exacerbate nausea. Potassium is found in fruits, vegetables, and meat. Sources of magnesium include seeds, nuts, legumes, and green vegetables.

Intravenous fluids and total parenteral nutrition are administered as directed by the physician. Small oral feedings of clear liquids are started when nausea and vomiting subside. When oral fluids are tolerated, parenteral nutrition is gradually discontinued. Any inability to tolerate oral feedings or continued episodes of vomiting should be reported to the physician so that continued parenteral fluids and nutrition can be prescribed.

Providing Emotional Support

The woman with hyperemesis gravidarum needs the opportunity to express how it feels to be pregnant and to live with constant nausea.

Often a curious lack of sympathy and support exists for these women, however. Nurses must use critical thinking to examine their own biases so that they can provide comfort and support. Case conferences or in-service educational programs may be necessary to overcome preset beliefs and to establish a level of care that meets the needs of the woman.

Check Your Reading

11. How do "morning sickness" and hyperemesis gravidarum compare in terms of onset, duration, and effect on the client?
12. What are the nursing goals in therapeutic management of hyperemesis gravidarum?
13. Why is critical thinking particularly important in the care of the woman with hyperemesis gravidarum?

HYPERTENSIVE DISORDERS OF PREGNANCY

Terminology used to describe hypertension in pregnancy is not always uniform. Several overlapping terms are commonly applied to different clinical manifestations of the same disease process. However, in clinical practice two distinct entities are commonly encountered: chronic hypertension and pregnancy-induced hypertension (PIH). Furthermore, these two conditions can coexist.

Pregnancy-Induced Hypertension

Pregnancy-induced hypertension is a multiorgan disease process that develops as a consequence of pregnancy and regresses in the postpartum period. Several clinical subsets have been given distinct labels, depending on end-organ effects (Table 25-2). In clinical

Table 25-2

CLASSIFICATION OF HYPERTENSIVE DISORDERS OF PREGNANCY

Pregnancy-induced hypertension	Development of hypertension (BP >140/90) during second half of pregnancy in previously normotensive woman
Preeclampsia	Renal involvement leads to proteinuria
Eclampsia	Central nervous system involvement leads to generalized seizures
HELLP	Clinical picture dominated by hematologic and hepatic signs and symptoms
Chronic hypertension	Elevation of blood pressure before 20 weeks' gestation

Adapted from American College of Obstetrics and Gynecology. (1996). Hypertension in pregnancy. *Technical Bulletin No. 219.* Washington, D.C.: ACOG.

Table 25-3

RISK FACTORS FOR PREGNANCY-INDUCED HYPERTENSION (PIH)

First pregnancy
Age <17 years
Family history of PIH
Chronic hypertension or preexisting vascular disease
Chronic renal disease
Obesity
Diabetes mellitus
Antiphospholipid syndrome
Multifetal pregnancy
Angiotensin gene T235
Mother or sister who had preeclampsia

From Leicht, T.G. & Harvey, C.J. (1999). Hypertensive disorders of pregnancy. In L.K. Mandeville & N.H. Troiano (Eds.), *AWHONN'S high-risk and critical care obstetrics* (2nd ed.). Philadelphia: Lippincott; Roberts, J.M. (1999). Pregnancy-related hypertension. In R.K. Creasy & R. Resnik (Eds.), *Maternal-fetal medicine* (4th ed.). Philadelphia: W.B. Saunders.

practice, the terms *PIH* and *preeclampsia* often are used interchangeably.

Preeclampsia

Preeclampsia is a condition in which hypertension develops during the last half of pregnancy in a woman who previously had normal blood pressure. In addition to hypertension, renal involvement may cause proteinuria. Many women also experience generalized edema. The only known cure is delivery of the fetus. Maternal and fetal morbidity can be minimized if preeclampsia is detected early and managed carefully.

Incidence and Risk Factors

Preeclampsia is relatively common, affecting 8% of all pregnancies (AAP & ACOG, 1997). It is a major cause of perinatal death, and it often is associated with intrauterine fetal growth restriction (IUGR).

Although the cause of preeclampsia is not understood, several factors are known to increase a woman's risk. Women with an increased risk for developing preeclampsia are those having their first baby, those under 17 years old, women who are obese, have diabetes mellitus, chronic hypertension, or preexisting vascular disease, and women with a multifetal gestation (Roberts, 1999; Leicht & Harvey, 1999). African Americans were once thought to have an increased risk, but newer studies have not supported this fact. Low socioeconomic status was once thought to be a risk factor, but the true contribution of socioeconomic status is not certain.

Less well-known risk factors include both genetic and immunologic factors. The presence of the angiotensinogen gene T235 greatly increases the woman's sensitivity to angiotensin, a powerful vasoconstrictor that could lead to hypertension. Also, a woman is more likely to have preeclampsia if her mother or sister also had the disorder. Antiphospholipid syndrome (APS) is also strongly associated with the development of PIH. This syndrome is due to the development of antiphospholipid antibodies (aPL). These antibodies are directed against phospholipids that are widely distributed in cell membranes. The clinical picture of APS includes thrombosis, recurrent fetal loss, intrauterine fetal growth restriction, and the presence of aPL. Not everyone with PIH has aPL, but women who have them and become pregnant are at increased risk to develop PIH (Silver & Branch, 1999). Table 25-3 summarizes major known risk factors for the development of PIH.

Pathophysiology

Preeclampsia is due to generalized vasospasm. The underlying cause of the vasospasm remains a mystery although some of the pathophysiologic processes are known. In normal pregnancy, vascular volume and cardiac output increase significantly. Despite these increases, blood pressure does not rise in normal pregnancy. This is probably because pregnant women develop resistance to the effects of vasoconstrictors, such as angiotensin II. Peripheral vascular resistance decreases because of the effects of certain vasodilators, such as prostacyclin (PGI_2), prostaglandin E (PGE), and endothelium-derived relaxing factor (EDRF).

In preeclampsia, however, peripheral vascular resistance increases because some women are sensitive to angiotensin II. They also may have a decrease in vasodilators. For instance, the ratio of thromboxane (TXA_2) to PGI_2 increases. Thromboxane, produced by

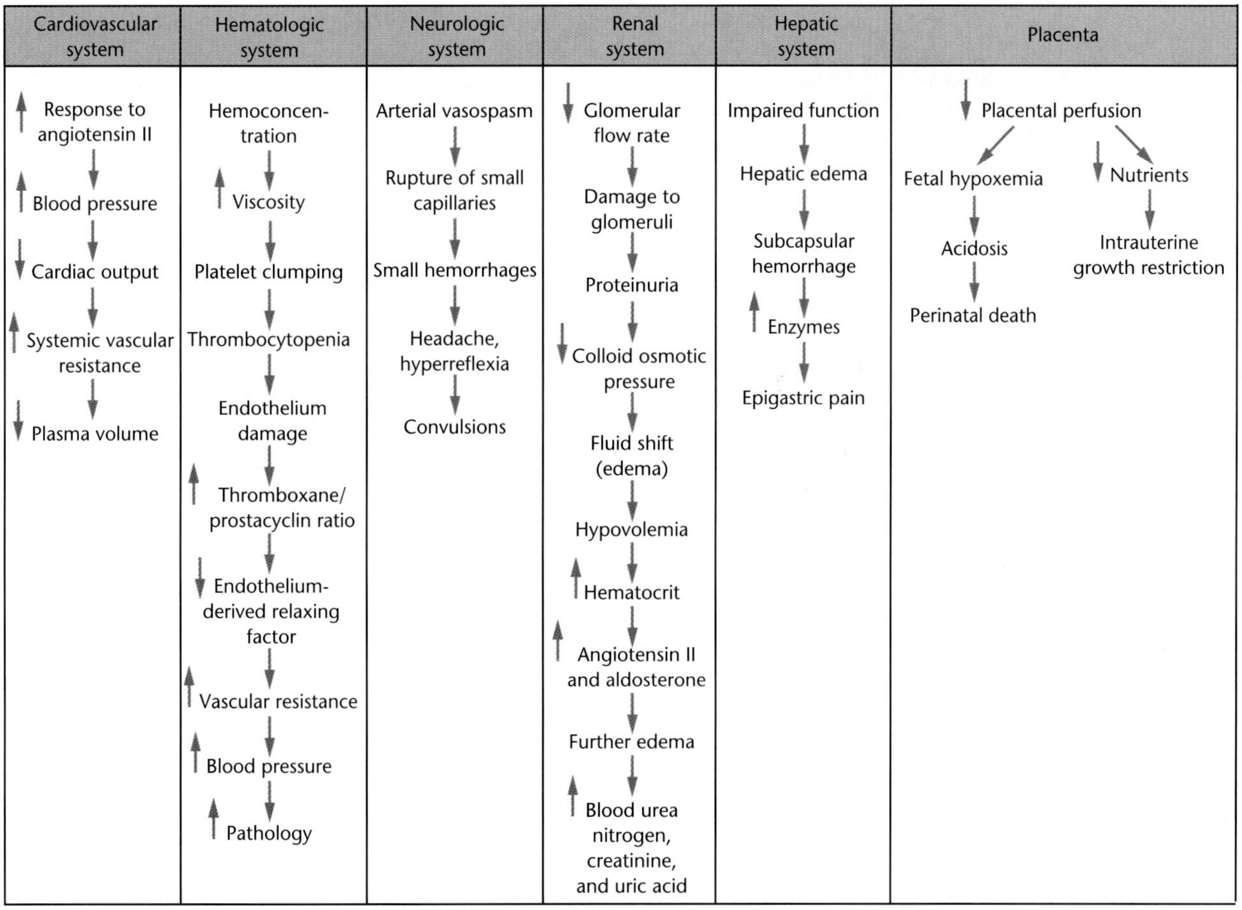

FIGURE 25-7 The pathologic processes of preeclampsia.

kidney and trophoblastic tissue, causes vasoconstriction and platelet aggregation (clumping). Prostacyclin, produced by placental tissue and endothelial cells, causes vasodilation and inhibits platelet aggregation.

Vasospasm decreases the diameter of blood vessels, which results in endothelial cell damage and decreased EDRF. Vasoconstriction also results in impeded blood flow and elevated blood pressure. As a result, circulation to all body organs, including the kidneys, liver, brain, and placenta, is decreased. The following changes are most significant:

- Decreased renal perfusion causes a decline in glomerular filtration rate; consequently, blood urea nitrogen, creatinine, and uric acid levels begin to rise.
- Reduced blood flow to the kidneys also results in glomerular damage. This allows protein to leak across the glomerular membrane, which is normally impermeable to large protein molecules. Loss of protein reduces colloid osmotic pressure and allows fluid to shift to interstitial spaces. This may result in edema and a reduction in intravascular volume, which causes increased viscosity of the blood and a rise in hematocrit. In response to reduced intravascular volume, additional angiotensin II and aldosterone are secreted to trigger the retention of both sodium and water. The pathologic processes spiral: additional angiotensin II results in further vasospasm and hypertension; aldosterone increases fluid retention, and edema is worsened.
- Decreased circulation to the liver leads to impaired liver function and to hepatic edema and subcapsular hemorrhage, which can result in hemorrhagic necrosis. This is manifested by elevation of liver enzymes in maternal serum.
- Vasoconstriction of cerebral vessels leads to pressure-induced rupture of thin-walled capillaries, resulting in small cerebral hemorrhages. Symptoms of arterial vasospasm include headache and visual disturbances, such as blurred vision, "spots" before the eyes, and hyperactive deep tendon reflexes.
- Decreased colloid oncotic pressure can lead to pulmonary capillary leak that results in pulmonary edema. Dyspnea is the primary symptom.
- Decreased placental circulation results in infarctions that increase the risk for abruptio placentae and DIC. In addition, when maternal blood flow through the placenta is decreased, the fetus is likely to experience intrauterine growth restriction and persistent fetal hypoxemia and acidosis. Figure 25-7 summarizes the pathologic processes of preeclampsia.

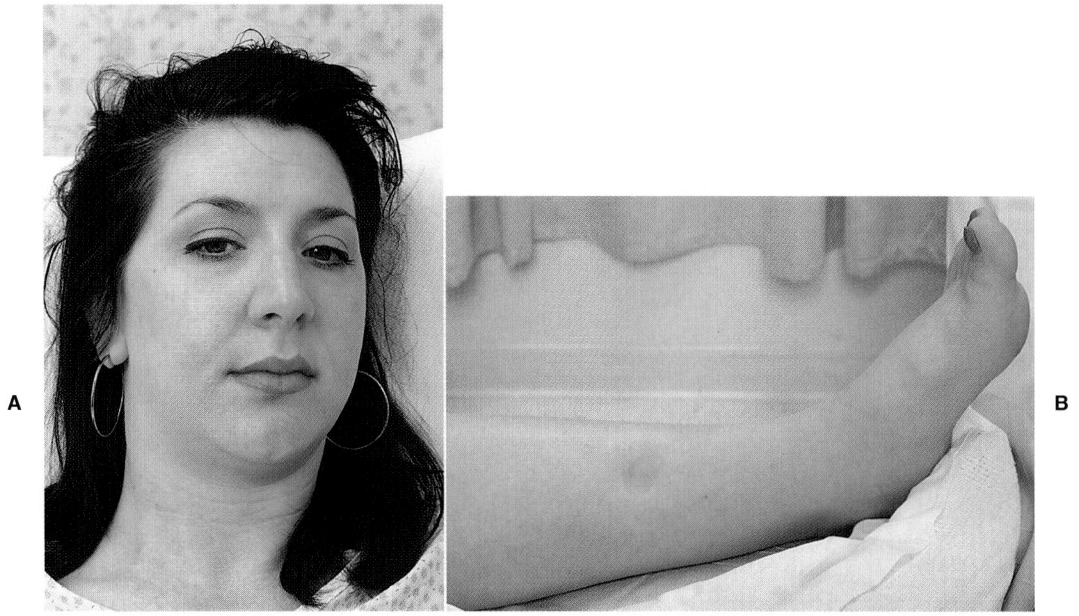

FIGURE 25-8 Generalized edema is a classic sign of preeclampsia. **A,** Facial edema may be subtle. **B,** Pitting edema of the lower leg.

Preventive Measures

Prenatal Care. Proper prenatal care with attention to pattern of weight gain and monitoring of blood pressure and urinary protein may minimize maternal and fetal morbidity and mortality by allowing early detection of the problem.

Low-Dose Aspirin. Low doses of aspirin (60 to 80 mg daily) have been prescribed for women at high risk for developing preeclampsia. Low-dose aspirin was thought to prevent injury to endothelial cells that line the blood vessels. This reduces the aggregation of platelets and allows increased production of EDRF. In addition, aspirin suppresses synthesis of TXA_2, the vasoconstrictor described earlier. The value of aspirin therapy for prevention of preeclampsia has yet to be proven, however. Additionally, a few reports exist of increased abruptio placentae with this form of therapy. Some feel that it might be useful in the woman who is at high risk for pregnancy-induced hypertension (Zuspan, 2000; Witlin & Sibai, 2000).

Calcium Supplementation. Calcium was hypothesized to lower maternal blood pressure, possibly through its effects on parathyroid hormone. However, larger trials did not support this theory and the value of calcium supplementation in prevention of preeclampsia remains unproven. Because calcium is a nutrient, it is considered safe for use, with the knowledge that its benefits in prevention of pregnancy-induced hypertension remain uncertain (Zuspan, 2000; Witlin & Sibai, 2000; Leicht & Harvey, 1999).

Clinical Manifestations of Preeclampsia

Classic Signs. Hypertension, generalized edema, and proteinuria are the three classic signs of preeclampsia. The first sign that the pregnant woman may notice is edema and a rapid weight gain, which are due to fluid retention. Edema is obvious in the lower legs, as is common in pregnancy, and above the waist, in the hands and face (Figure 25-8). She may notice that she cannot wear rings that she could wear just a few days ago. The edema in the legs is often more severe than normal pregnancy edema as well. However, edema may not be present in all women who develop preeclampsia.

Hypertension is defined as sustained blood pressure equal to or above 140/90. Earlier data suggested that an increase of 30 mm Hg systolic or 15 mm Hg diastolic from baseline was also of diagnostic value. However, this concept is no longer considered valid (ACOG, 1996). If a woman does not see her physician or nurse-midwife until the fifth or sixth month of pregnancy, a true baseline is not available for comparison.

Because of the potential errors associated with determination of blood pressure, blood pressure should be taken in the sitting position with the arm supported in a horizontal position at heart level. Outpatient and inpatient departments should use the same position. To reduce confusion among recorders, three sounds should be recorded: the systolic, the fourth Korotkoff's phase (muffling), and the fifth Korotkoff's phase (disappearance of sound) (Zuspan, 2000).

Proteinuria usually develops later than hypertension and edema, and the combination of proteinuria and hypertension indicates a worsening disease process. A clean-catch specimen is needed to prevent contamination of the specimen by vaginal secretions. Proteinuria is defined as the presence of 300 mg or more of protein in a 24-hour period or 100 mg/dL in two random urine samples 6 hours apart (Leicht & Harvey, 1999). The amount of protein lost in the urine varies over the course of a day, so a single urine sample is not sufficient to diagnose proteinuria.

Additional Signs. Careful assessment may reveal additional signs associated with preeclampsia. For instance, when the retina is examined, vascular constriction and narrowing of the small arteries are obvious in most women with preeclampsia. The vasoconstriction that can be seen in the retina is occurring throughout the body. Deep tendon reflexes may be very brisk (hyperreflexia) and clonus (see pp. 686-687) may be present. This suggests cerebral irritability secondary to decreased brain circulation and edema.

Signs and Symptoms. Preeclampsia is dangerous for the woman and fetus for two reasons: (1) it develops and progresses rapidly and (2) the earliest manifestations are not noticed by the woman. By the time she notices symptoms, the disease may have progressed to an advanced state and valuable treatment time has been lost.

Certain symptoms, such as continuous headache, drowsiness, or mental confusion, indicate poor cerebral perfusion and may be precursors of seizures. Visual disturbances, such as blurred or double vision or spots before the eyes, indicate arterial spasms and edema in the retina. Numbness or tingling of the hands or feet occurs when nerves are compressed by retained fluid. Some symptoms, such as epigastric pain or "upset stomach," are particularly ominous because they indicate distention of the hepatic capsule and often warn that a seizure is imminent. Decreased urinary output indicates poor perfusion of the kidneys and may precede acute renal failure.

Therapeutic Management of Mild Preeclampsia

The only cure for preeclampsia is delivery of the baby. However, the decision about delivery will be based on the severity of the hypertensive disorder and the degree of fetal maturity.

Preeclampsia is categorized as either mild or severe, depending on the presenting signs and symptoms. Yet because the disease may progress rapidly, an apparently mild condition can become severe in a very short time. Preeclampsia is considered mild when the diastolic blood pressure does not exceed 100 mm Hg; proteinuria is no more than 500 mg/day (trace to 1+), and symptoms, such as headache, visual disturbances, or abdominal pain, are absent. In addition, signs of kidney or liver involvement are absent, pulmonary edema is absent, and the fetus demonstrates normal growth (Cunningham, et al., 1997).

Home Care

Management in the home may be possible for selected women if the condition is mild and they are not good candidates to have their labor induced, usually because of fetal immaturity. In general the woman must be in stable condition with a reassuring fetal status. The woman must be willing to adhere to a prescribed treatment plan that may include bedrest or reduced activity; home blood pressure monitoring, although this increases cost with minimal proven benefit; and twice weekly visits to the physician (Branch & Porter, 1999). Fetal surveillance such as daily kick counts and weekly or twice-weekly nonstress tests or biophysical profiles (see Chapter 10) are usually prescribed when a woman has mild hypertension.

Activity Restrictions. The expectant mother should rest in the lateral position as much as possible. This position decreases pressure on the vena cava, thereby increasing cardiac return and circulatory volume and thus improving perfusion of vital organs and the placenta. Increased renal perfusion decreases angiotensin II levels, promotes diuresis, and lowers the blood pressure.

Blood Pressure. If prescribed, the family must be taught to use electronic blood pressure equipment. Blood pressure should be checked in the same arm and in the same position for the prescribed number of times each day. The blood pressures should be recorded for review on home visits and brought to antepartal visits.

Fetal Surveillance. Because the vasoconstriction can compromise placental flow, the woman will probably have increased fetal surveillance to observe for evidence of fetal compromise. Fetal compromise can be evidenced by reduced fetal movement, a nonreactive nonstress test, reduced amniotic fluid on ultrasound examination, or a biophysical profile score of 6 or lower.

The diet should have ample protein and calories. Sodium and fluid should not be limited (Cunningham, et al., 1997). The woman should be taught symptoms that indicate worsening of the preeclampsia and to report these at once. Indications of disease progression or fetal deterioration require admission to the hospital.

Therapeutic Management of Severe Preeclampsia

The disease is considered severe when blood pressure is higher than 160/110 mmHg, proteinuria is higher than 5 gm in 24 hours (3+ or more), and oliguria occurs (500 ml or less in 24 hours). If symptoms occur that were absent in the mild form of the disease, or if laboratory findings indicate liver involvement (elevated

DRUG GUIDE: HYDRALAZINE

Classification: Antihypertensive

Action: Relaxes arterial smooth muscle to reduce blood pressure.

Indications: Used in preeclampsia when blood pressure is elevated to a degree that might be associated with intracranial bleeding.

Dosage and Route: Obstetric uses in pregnancy-induced hypertension: Intravenous bolus infusion: 5 to 10 mg may be administered as often as every 20 minutes if necessary (ACOG, 1996). Continuous intravenous infusion: Add 100 mg hydralazine to 200 ml saline. Using an infusion pump, the dose is titrated to maintain the maternal diastolic blood pressure at approximately 80 to 90 mmHg (Zuspan, 2000).

Absorption: Widely distributed, crosses the placenta; enters breast milk in minimal concentrations

Excretion: Metabolized and excreted by the liver

Contraindications and Precautions: Contraindicated in coronary artery disease, cerebrovascular disease, and hypersensitivity to hydralazine. Used cautiously in pregnancy; pregnancy category C

Adverse Reactions: Headache, dizziness, drowsiness, hypotension that can interfere with uterine blood flow, epigastric pain, which may be confused with worsening preeclampsia

Nursing Implications: Obstetric clients are hospitalized before initiation of antihypertensive medications. Blood pressure and pulse must be monitored every 2 to 3 minutes for 30 minutes after initial dosage and periodically throughout the course of therapy. Therapy is repeated only when diastolic pressure exceeds limits set by physician or facility protocol (usually >110 mm Hg).

Table 25-4
MILD VERSUS SEVERE PREECLAMPSIA

	Mild	Severe
Systolic BP	<160	>160
Diastolic BP	<100	>110
Proteinuria	<500 mg/24 hr (Trace to 1+)	>500 mg/24 hr Elevated
Creatinine	Normal	
Thrombocytopenia	Absent	Present
Oliguria	Absent	<500 ml/24 hr
Liver enzyme elevation	Minimal	Marked
Fetal growth restriction	Absent	Present
Headache, visual disturbances, abdominal pain	Absent	Present

enzymes or hyperbilirubinemia) or kidney damage (elevated creatinine), the disease is judged to be severe (ACOG, 1996). Table 25-4 compares mild and severe preeclampsia.

Antepartum Management. The woman is hospitalized if preeclampsia becomes severe. If preeclampsia is severe, the fetus is usually delivered, regardless of gestation, because of compromised placental circulation. Goals of management are to maximize placental blood flow and fetal oxygenation and to prevent seizures and other maternal complications such as stroke as the woman is stabilized before delivery.

Bedrest. The woman is kept on bedrest in the lateral position and her environment is kept quiet. External stimuli (lights, noise) that might precipitate a seizure should be reduced.

Antihypertensive Medications. Blood pressure control is usually reserved for severe hypertension when the diastolic pressure exceeds 100 mm Hg to reduce the risk that the mother will have intracranial bleeding. When antihypertensive drugs are used, the fetal heart rate must be monitored closely because a sudden fall in the maternal blood pressure may precipitate fetal distress. Hydralazine (Apresoline), given by intravenous push or continuous infusion, is the primary antihypertensive given in preeclampsia. Other antihypertensive medications, such as nifedipine (Procardia, a calcium channel blocker) or labetalol (Normodyne, a β-adrenergic blocker), are alternate antihypertensives (Zuspan, 2000).

Anticonvulsant Medications. In the United States, magnesium sulfate ($MgSO_4$) is the drug of choice to prevent seizures because it has minimal adverse effects on the fetus. Phenytoin (Dilantin, Diphenylan) is sometimes used. Magnesium acts as a central nervous system depressant by blocking neuromuscular transmission and decreasing the amount of acetylcholine liberated. Magnesium is not an antihypertensive medication, but it relaxes smooth muscle and thus reduces vasoconstriction. Decreased vasoconstriction promotes circulation to the vital organs of the expectant mother and increases placental circulation. Increased circulation to the maternal kidneys leads to diuresis, as interstitial fluid is shifted into the vascular compartment and excreted.

Magnesium is generally administered by intravenous infusion, which allows for immediate onset of action and does not cause the discomfort associated with intramuscular administration. Intravenous magnesium is administered via a secondary ("piggyback") line so that the medication can be discontinued at any time while the primary line remains open and functional.

DRUG GUIDE: MAGNESIUM SULFATE

Classification: Miscellaneous anticonvulsant

Action: Decreases acetylcholine released by motor nerve impulses, thereby blocking neuromuscular transmission; depresses the central nervous system to act as an anticonvulsant; also decreases frequency and intensity of uterine contractions; produces flushing and sweating due to decreased peripheral blood pressure

Indications: Prevention and control of seizures in severe preeclampsia; prevention of uterine contractions in preterm labor

Dosage and Route: Magnesium sulfate generally is administered parenterally. An intravenous loading bolus (4 g over 20 minutes) is given and followed by continuous infusion (2 to 3 g/hour) via a controlled infusion device (ACOG, 1996). Therapeutic range for magnesium is generally considered to be 4 to 8 mg/dl (ACOG, 1996).

Absorption: Immediate onset after intravenous administration; duration of action is 3 to 4 hours

Excretion: Excreted by the kidneys

Contraindications and Precautions: Contraindicated in persons with myocardial damage, heart block, myasthenia gravis, or impaired renal function

Adverse Reactions: Result from magnesium overdose and include flushing, sweating, hypotension, depressed deep tendon reflexes, and central nervous system depression, including respiratory depression

Nursing Implications: Monitor blood pressure closely during administration. Assess client for respiratory rate above 12 per minute, presence of deep tendon reflexes, and urinary output greater than 25 ml per hour or 100 ml in 4 hours before administering magnesium or maintaining infusion. Place resuscitation equipment (suction, oxygen) in the room. Keep calcium gluconate, which acts as an antidote to magnesium, in the room along with syringes and needles.

Intrapartum Management. The fetus and the expectant mother must be monitored continuously to detect signs of decreased fetal oxygenation and imminent seizures. The woman should be kept in a lateral position to promote circulation through the placenta, and efforts should focus on controlling pain that may cause agitation and precipitate seizures.

Oxytocin to stimulate uterine contractions and magnesium sulfate to prevent seizures are often administered simultaneously during labor when a woman has preeclampsia. Infusion pumps should be used to ensure that the medications and fluids are administered at the prescribed rate, and equipment and intravenous lines should be checked carefully for correct placement and function.

Narcotic analgesics or epidural analgesia may be administered to provide comfort and to reduce painful stimuli that could precipitate a seizure. However, some women with severe preeclampsia have coagulation abnormalities and this may contraindicate use of epidural analgesia.

Continuous fetal electronic monitoring identifies changes in fetal heart rate patterns that suggest hypoxia. Interventions are tailored to the nonreassuring fetal heart pattern identified, such as maternal oxygen administration, stopping the oxytocin infusion, and increases in the intravenous fluid rates. See Chapter 14 for information about fetal monitoring.

A pediatrician, neonatologist, or neonatal nurse practitioner must be available to care for the newborn at birth.

Postpartum Management. Following birth, careful assessment of the mother's blood loss and signs of shock are essential because the hypovolemia caused by preeclampsia may be aggravated by blood loss during the delivery. Assessments for signs and symptoms of preeclampsia must be continued for at least 48 hours, and magnesium usually is continued to prevent seizures.

Signs that the woman is recovering from preeclampsia include the following:

- Urinary output of 4 to 6 liters per day, which causes a rapid reduction in edema and rapid weight loss
- Decreased protein in the urine
- Return of blood pressure to normal, usually within 2 weeks

Therapeutic Management of Eclampsia

Eclampsia is marked by generalized, or grand mal, seizures that typically begin with twitching about the mouth. The body then becomes rigid in a state of tonic muscular contractions that last 15 to 20 seconds. The facial muscles and then all body muscles alternatively contract and relax in rapid succession. This clonic phase of the seizure may last about 1 minute. Respiration is halted during the seizure because the diaphragm tends to remain fixed. Breathing usually resumes shortly after the seizure and is often rapid and deep (Usta & Sibai, 1995).

Magnesium may be given intravenously to control the seizures. Sedatives such as phenobarbital or diazepam are used only if magnesium fails to bring the seizures under control. Sedatives should not be given if birth is expected within an hour or two because of their depressant effects on the fetus.

Pulmonary edema, circulatory or renal failure, and intracranial hemorrhage are additional complications that may occur with eclampsia. The woman's lungs should be auscultated frequently, and furosemide (Lasix) may be administered if pulmonary edema develops. Digitalis may be needed to strengthen contraction of the heart if circulatory failure results. Urine output should be assessed hourly; if output drops below 25 ml per hour, renal failure should be suspected.

Disseminated intravascular coagulation is an added complication that may occur with severe preeclampsia or eclampsia, and the nurse must observe for unexpected bleeding. Coagulation studies listed in the discussion of DIC in Chapter 26 are often performed for these women.

The woman should be monitored for ruptured membranes, signs of labor, or abruptio placentae because eclampsia stimulates uterine irritability. While the woman is post-ictal (the unresponsive state after a seizure), she should be kept on her side to prevent aspiration and improve placental circulation. The side rails should be raised to prevent a fall and possible injury. After maternal and fetal conditions are stabilized, the fetus usually is delivered, either by induction of labor if the woman's cervix is favorable or by cesarean birth if she is farther from term.

Aspiration may cause maternal morbidity following an eclamptic seizure. After initial stabilization, the nurse should expect orders for chest radiographs and arterial blood gases to identify whether aspiration has occurred.

Check Your Reading

14. What are the effects of vasospasm on the fetus?
15. What are the signs and symptoms of preeclampsia? Why is reduced activity one part of management?
16. What is the effect of vasospasm on the brain?
17. What are the effects of magnesium sulfate, including the primary adverse effect?
18. What are the major complications of eclampsia?

APPLICATION OF THE NURSING PROCESS: PREECLAMPSIA

Assessment

Nursing assessment is one of the most important components of successful management of preeclampsia. Careful assessment is the only way to determine whether the condition is responding to medical management or whether the disease is worsening. A one-to-one nurse-patient ratio is needed for the woman with severe pregnancy-induced hypertension.

Weigh the woman on admission and daily. Check vital signs, and auscultate the chest for moist breath sounds that indicate pulmonary edema at least every 4 hours. Assess the location and severity of edema at least every 4 hours. Table 25-5 provides a useful method for describing edema. Insert an indwelling catheter to measure hourly urine output. Check the urine for protein every 4 hours. Apply an external electronic fetal monitor to identify nonreassuring patterns. Internal electronic fetal monitoring leads may be used for greater accuracy after the membranes are ruptured.

Table 25-5
ASSESSMENT OF EDEMA

Minimal edema of lower extremities	+1
Marked edema of lower extremities	+2
Edema of lower extremities, face, hands, and sacral area	+3
Generalized massive edema that includes ascites (accumulation of fluid in peritoneal cavity)	+4

Check brachial and patellar reflexes for hyperreflexia that indicates cerebral irritability. Determine if clonus is present by dorsiflexing the woman's foot sharply and then releasing it while her knee is held in a flexed position. Normally, no clonus is present. However, if oscillations or "jerking" motions occur as the foot drops, clonus is present and should be reported to the physician. Procedure 25-1 illustrates how to assess and rate deep tendon reflexes.

Question the woman carefully about symptoms she may be experiencing, such as headache, visual disturbances, epigastric pain, or increased edema.

> An open-ended question such as "How do you feel?" may not be adequate, and detailed questions are usually needed. Ask targeted questions, such as "Do you have a headache? Describe it for me." "Do you have any pain in the abdomen? Show me where it is and describe it." "Do you see spots before your eyes? Flashes of light? Double vision?" "Is your vision blurred?" "I see you have removed your rings. Did you do that because your hands were swollen? When did that happen?"

Assessments for Magnesium Toxicity

Adverse side effects of magnesium include central nervous system depression that includes depression of the respiratory center. As a result, nursing assessments should focus on these areas. Determine respiratory rate hourly. Assess the woman's level of consciousness (alert, drowsy, confused, oriented). Reflexes may be slightly hypotonic, but should not be absent, when magnesium levels are therapeutic (Table 25-6).

Psychosocial Assessment

The development of preeclampsia places a great deal of stress on the childbearing family. The woman may be on reduced activity at home or hospitalized. This creates anxiety about the condition of the fetus and that of

PROCEDURE 25-1
Assessing Deep Tendon Reflexes

Purpose: To determine whether there are exaggerated reflexes (hyperreflexia) or diminished reflexes (hyporeflexia)

Assess both the brachial and the patellar reflex, plus clonus. Equipment: reflex hammer.

1. To assess the brachial reflex, support the woman's arm and instruct her to let it go totally limp while it is being held. *This position partially relaxes and partially flexes the person's arm.*
2. Place your thumb over the woman's tendon, as illustrated, and strike the thumb with the small end of the reflex hammer. The normal response is slight flexion of the forearm. *The tendon response can be felt as well as seen when the tendon is tapped.*

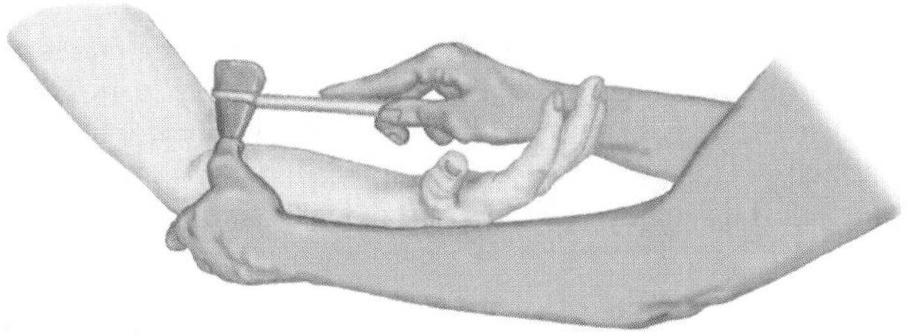

3. The patellar reflex can be assessed in two positions, sitting or lying. When the woman is sitting, allow her lower legs to dangle freely to flex the knee and stretch the tendons. Strike the tendon with the reflex hammer just below the patella. *This determines deep tendon reflexes in the lower extremities when the person is sitting.*

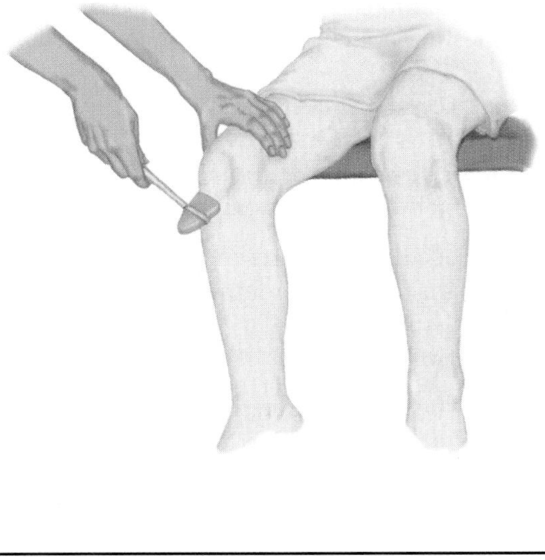

4. When the woman is in the supine position, the weight of her leg must be supported to flex the knee and stretch the tendons. Strike the partially stretched tendons just below the patella. Extension of the leg is the expected response. *It is necessary to support the leg because an adequate response requires that the limb be relaxed and the tendon partially stretched.*

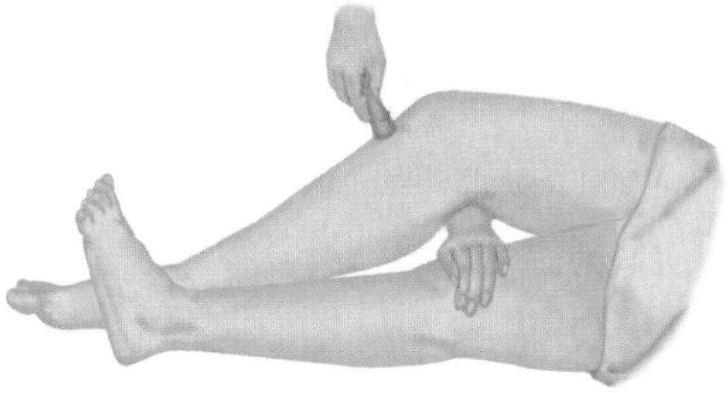

5. Clonus should be tested, particularly when the reflexes are hyperactive. The woman's lower leg should be supported, as illustrated, and the foot sharply dorsiflexed. Hold the stretch. With a normal response, no movement will be felt. When clonus is present, rapid rhythmic jerking motions of the foot are obvious. *Dorsiflexion stretches the tendon, and rapid rhythmic contractions indicate hyperreflexia.*

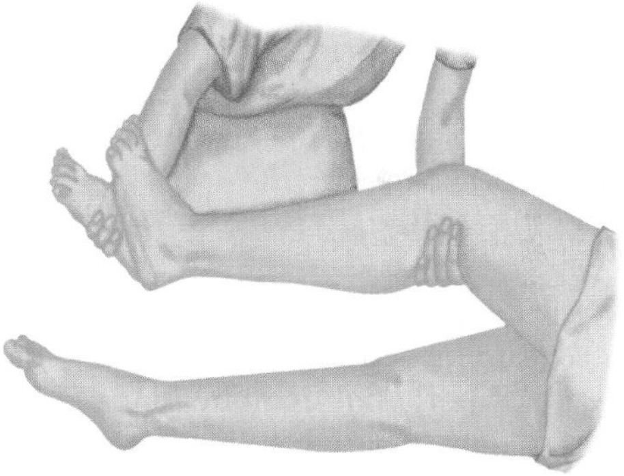

DEEP TENDON RATING SCALE

0 = Reflex absent
+1 = Reflex present, hypoactive
+2 = Normal reflex
+3 = Hyperactive reflex
+4 = Hyperactive reflex with clonus present

Table 25-6

NURSING ASSESSMENTS FOR PREECLAMPSIA AND MAGNESIUM TOXICITY

Assessment	Implications
Daily weight	Provides estimate of fluid retention
Blood pressure	To determine response to treatment
Respiratory rate	Drug therapy ($MgSO_4$) causes respiratory depression if the serum level becomes high, and drug should be held if respiratory rate is <12/min
Breath sounds	To detect onset of pulmonary edema
Deep tendon reflexes	Hyperreflexia indicates increased cerebral edema; absent reflexes indicates magnesium excess.
Edema	For estimation of interstitial fluid
Urinary output	More than 25 ml/hr indicates adequate perfusion of the kidneys and reduces the likelihood that magnesium, which is excreted by the kidneys, will reach excessively-high serum levels.
Level of consciousness	Drowsiness, dulled sensorium indicate therapeutic effects of magnesium; nonresponsive behavior or muscle weakness indicates magnesium excess
Headache, epigastric pain, visual problems	Indicate increasing severity of condition and development of eclampsia
Fetal heart rate and baseline variability	Rate should be between 110 and 160; decreasing or absent baseline variability may be due to magnesium or to fetal compromise. Late decelerations suggest poor uteroplacental perfusion.
Laboratory data	Elevated serum creatinine, elevated liver enzymes, or decreased platelets (thrombocytopenia) are significant signs of increasing severity of disease; serum magnesium levels should be in therapeutic range (4 to 8 mg/dL) or as designated by physician or facility protocol.

the expectant mother. Many families do not understand the seriousness of the disease. After all, the woman feels well for some time after its onset.

Explore how the family will function while the expectant mother is hospitalized. Determine how the woman is adapting to the "sick role" and the necessity of being dependent on others instead of functioning in her primary role. Ask how much support is available and who is willing to participate. Finally, determine the major concerns of the family.

Analysis

Analysis of the data collected can lead to both nursing diagnoses (see Nursing Care Plan 25-2) and collaborative problems or potential complications. Potential complications require that nurses monitor to detect onset or changes in status. Both physician-prescribed and nurse-prescribed interventions are used to minimize the complication. Potential complications for the woman with preeclampsia are eclamptic seizures and magnesium toxicity.

Planning

Client-centered goals are inappropriate for the potential complications of eclamptic seizures and magnesium toxicity because the nurse cannot independently manage these conditions but must confer with physicians for medical orders for treatment. For seizures, planning should reflect the nurse's responsibility to do the following:

- Monitor for signs of impending seizures
- Consult with the physician if signs of impending seizures are observed
- Perform actions that will minimize the risk of seizures occurring and prevent injury if seizures do occur

The following steps are necessary in cases of magnesium toxicity:

- Monitor for signs of magnesium toxicity
- Consult with the physician if signs of magnesium toxicity are observed
- Perform actions that will minimize the possibility of magnesium toxicity

Interventions

Interventions for Seizures

Monitoring for Signs of Impending Seizures

Signs of impending seizures include the following:

- Hyperreflexia or the presence of clonus, or both
- Increasing signs of cerebral irritability (headache, visual disturbances)
- Epigastric pain

None of these signs are an absolutely reliable predictor of imminent seizure. Nurses must be alert for subtle changes and prepared for seizures in all women with preeclampsia.

Initiating Preventive Measures

In the presence of cerebral irritability, generalized seizures may be precipitated by excessive visual or auditory stimuli. Nurses should reduce external stimuli by doing the following:

- Admitting the woman to a private room in the quietest section of the unit and keeping the door to the room closed
- Padding the door to reduce noise when the door must be opened and closed
- Keeping lights low and noise to a minimum; this may include blocking incoming telephone calls

NURSING CARE PLAN 25-2

Preeclampsia

Assessment: Julie Frost, a 16-year-old primigravida, is seen in the prenatal clinic at 30 weeks of gestation. She is experiencing blood pressure of 136/90, and some edema of the lower legs, and trace proteinuria. Because the signs are minimal at this time, she is given instructions about home care for pregnancy-induced hypertension. This includes rest at home, monitoring of blood pressure by her mother, and fetal "kick counts." She is told that she must return to the clinic in a week. Julie states that she feels fine and doesn't want to miss school. She says that she doesn't see the reason for rest.

Nursing Diagnosis: Impaired Adjustment related to lack of knowledge of health status and the need for a change in lifestyle

Goals/Expected Outcomes:
Julie will do the following:
1. Verbalize the benefits of the recommended regimen by the end of the first prenatal appointment.
2. Comply with the recommended care for the next week.
3. Keep prenatal appointments.

Intervention	Rationale
1. Allow Julie to verbalize her feelings about the recommended regimen: "What concerns you most about missing school?" Acknowledge her feelings as important: "It must be difficult to think of falling behind in your schoolwork." "It isn't any fun to miss all the after-school activities."	1. When feelings are identified and acknowledged as important, anxiety decreases and teaching and learning can begin.
2. Identify family support that will permit compliance with the recommended regimen of bedrest and home care.	2. Compliance with the regimen is unlikely without family assistance that includes assistance with activities of daily living and necessary assessments.
3. Describe in general terms the physiologic processes that are occurring and their effect on her and the fetus: "The small blood vessels in your body may be narrowed so they don't carry enough blood to your vital organs or to the baby." "Resting on your side helps the blood to move to all parts of your body and to carry oxygen to the baby."	3. Expectant mothers are more likely to comply with a therapeutic management that benefits the fetus, and knowledge of how the planned program provides the fetus with oxygen improves the possibility of compliance with bedrest and frequent assessments.
4. Explain that she may feel well even if the condition worsens and that she must be observed for painless symptoms daily at home and frequently at the clinic.	4. Hypertension and proteinuria are not noticed by the expectant mother. Edema is considered normal by many clients, and they may not identify edema above the waist as more significant than dependent edema.
5. Teach Julie to call the clinic if she notices headache, double vision, or spots before her eyes.	5. These signs indicate rapid progression of the disease and added medical management is needed.
6. Collaborate with Julie to arrange for contact with her boyfriend or selected friends and arrange for ongoing homebound classes.	6. Such an agreement will allow a schedule to be developed that provides peer support but that allows for prolonged periods of quiet. Homebound classes alleviate the concern that she is falling behind with schoolwork, and related anxiety will decrease.

Evaluation: Despite maintaining the recommended regimen of activity restrictions with the help of her mother and older sister, Julie experienced increasingly severe preeclampsia. She had a rise in blood pressure and a rapid gain in weight, indicating generalized edema.

Assessment: Julie is admitted to the hospital at 32 weeks of gestation with blood pressure 160/110, heart rate 92, and respirations 22. She has 2+ proteinuria and marked edema of her hands and face. External electronic fetal monitoring is started. The fetal heart rate is 136 and occasional accelerations with fetal movement are present. An intravenous infusion of magnesium sulfate ($MgSO_4$) is begun, seizure precautions are initiated, and environmental stimuli are reduced. Julie is agitated and verbalizes concern that the procedures are going to hurt her or the fetus. She frequently asks, "How sick am I?" "Is the baby going to be okay?" Her hands are perspiring, and they shake when she reaches for a tissue.

Nursing Diagnosis: Anxiety related to hospitalization and concern about her health and the health of the fetus

Goals/Expected Outcomes:
Julie will do the following:
1. Verbalize her concerns about the treatment.
2. Manifest less anxiety (agitation, physiologic signs such as tremors, tachycardia, and perspiration) after discussion of the treatment.

Continued

Intervention	Rationale
1. Initiate measures to reduce anxiety. a. Provide positive reassurance that a solution to anxiety can be found: "I can see you are really worried, and I will try to answer all your questions." b. Allow her to cry, get angry, or express any feeling that is present. c. Encourage a discussion of feelings: "Tell me more about how you feel." d. Reflect observations: "I see you wringing your hands; do you want to talk about it?" e. Convey empathy and positive regard; use nonverbal behavior, including touch, when appropriate.	1. Anxiety is an ominous feeling of tension resulting from a physical or emotional threat to the self. It is a global, often unnamed, sense of doom, a feeling of helplessness, isolation, and insecurity. Anxiety needs to be ventilated and then addressed by conveying that the person is not alone and that they will be protected.
2. Provide information about hospital procedures when anxiety is diminished enough for learning to take place. a. Be very specific about procedures, such as fetal monitoring, assessment of deep tendon reflexes, and vital signs. Explain what they are for, who will do them, and how long they will be maintained. b. Focus on Julie's present concerns; she is not able to be future-oriented at this time. c. Speak slowly and calmly, give short directions, and do not ask Julie to make decisions: "Turn on your side." "Breathe slowly." d. Allow a friend or family member to remain with Julie and instruct the person on the need for a low-stimulus environment.	2. Knowledge of the procedures that will be performed and the purpose of the procedures provides a sense of control that reduces anxiety. Perception is somewhat narrowed when anxiety is high; therefore, short, brief instructions are easier for the anxious person to understand than long explanations.

Evaluation: Julie discusses her feelings with the nurse and with her sister. She gradually shows a decrease in signs of agitation and physiologic signs (tachycardia, tachypnea) and by the ability to use relaxation techniques.

Critical Thinking:
1. What two potential complications cause the greatest concern for nurses who care for Julie?
2. Why do nurses not develop goals for these problems?
3. What are the nurses' responsibilities for these complications?

Answer:
1. The most common complications that cause the greatest concern are magnesium toxicity and generalized seizures.
2. These are collaborative problems that require collaboration with physicians for management. The nurse does not independently manage magnesium toxicity or seizures.
3. The nurse must monitor for signs of these conditions, administer prescribed medications, observe and report Julie's response to the medications, and collaborate with the physicians to lessen the chance that these complications will occur.

- Grouping nursing assessments and care to allow the woman long periods of undisturbed quiet
- Moving carefully and calmly around the room and avoiding bumping into the bed or startling the woman
- Collaborating with the woman and her family to restrict visitors

Preventing Seizure-Related Injury

The bed's side rails should be padded and the bed kept in the lowest position with the wheels locked to prevent trauma should the woman hit the side rails or fall from the bed during a seizure.

Oxygen and suction equipment should be assembled and ready to use to suction secretions and to provide oxygen after the seizure as necessary. Check equipment at the beginning of each shift because if seizures occur, sufficient time for setup will not exist.

A preeclampsia tray should be in the room. Typical contents include a medium plastic airway, an Ambu bag with mask, an ophthalmoscope, a tourniquet, a reflex hammer, syringes and needles. Medications that should be in the tray include magnesium sulfate, sodium bica bonate, heparin sodium, epinephrine, phenytoin, and calcium gluconate.

Protecting the Woman and Fetus during a Seizure

Nurses must protect the woman and the fetus during a seizure. The nurse's primary responsibilities are the following:

- Remain with the woman and press the emergency bell for assistance.
- If time is sufficient, attempt to turn the woman on her side when the tonic phase begins. A side-lying position permits greater circulation through the placenta and helps prevent aspiration.

- Note the time and sequence of the seizure. Eclampsia is marked by a tonic-clonic seizure that may be preceded by facial twitching that lasts for a few seconds. A tonic contraction of the entire body is followed by the clonic phase, which may last about a minute.
- Insert an airway following the seizure, and suction the woman's mouth and nose to prevent aspiration; administer oxygen by mask to increase oxygenation of the placenta and all maternal body organs.
- Notify the physician that a seizure has occurred. This is an obstetric emergency that is associated with cerebral hemorrhage, abruptio placentae, severe fetal hypoxia, and death.
- Administer medications and prepare for additional medical interventions as directed by the physician.

Providing Information and Support for the Family

Explain to the family what has happened, but do not minimize the seriousness of the situation. A generalized seizure is frightening for anyone who witnesses it, and the family often is reassured when the nurse explains that the seizure lasts for only a few minutes and that the woman will be unconscious, then drowsy for some time afterward. Acknowledge that the seizure indicates worsening of the condition and that it will be necessary for the physician to determine future management, which may include delivery of the infant as soon as possible.

Interventions for Magnesium Toxicity

Monitoring for Signs of Magnesium Toxicity

Magnesium excess depresses the entire central nervous system, including the brain stem, which controls respirations and cardiac function, and the cerebrum, which controls memory, mental processes, and speech. Carbon dioxide accumulates if the respiratory rate is reduced, leading to respiratory acidosis and further central nervous system depression, which could culminate in respiratory arrest.

Signs of magnesium toxicity include the following:

- Respiratory rate of less than 12 breaths per minute
- Absence of deep tendon reflexes
- Sweating, flushing
- Altered sensorium (confused, lethargic, slurring of speech, drowsiness, disorientation)
- Hypotension
- Serum magnesium above the therapeutic range of 4 to 8 mg/dL (ACOG, 1996)

Responding to Signs of Magnesium Toxicity

Discontinue magnesium if the respiratory rate is below 12 breaths per minute or if deep tendon reflexes are absent. These are signs of magnesium toxicity, and administration of additional magnesium will make the condition worse. Notify the physician of the woman's condition so that additional orders can be received. Magnesium is excreted by the kidneys, and if the urinary output falls below 25 ml per hour or less than 100 ml in the preceding 4 hours, the physician should be notified before additional magnesium is administered (Zuspan, 2000; Cunningham, et al.,1997; ACOG, 1996).

Calcium gluconate is the antidote for magnesium sulfate, because it antagonizes the effects of magnesium at the neuromuscular junction, and it should be readily available whenever magnesium is administered. Magnesium toxicity can be reversed by intravenous administration of 1 g (10 ml of 10% solution) calcium gluconate over 2 minutes (ACOG, 1996).

Evaluation

Collect and compare data with established norms and then judge whether the data are within normal limits. For seizures, interventions are judged to be successful if

- Reflexes are present, but hypoactive secondary to magnesium's therapeutic effect
- Clonus is absent
- The woman is free of visual disturbances, headache, and epigastric pain
- The woman remains free of seizures or free of injury if a seizure occurs

For magnesium toxicity, determine whether respiratory rates remain above 12 breaths per minute, deep tendon reflexes are present, and maternal plasma levels of magnesium do not exceed the therapeutic range of 4 to 8 mg/dL.

Check Your Reading

19. What nursing assessments should be made for the woman with preeclampsia? Why?
20. What measures may be initiated to prevent or manage seizures?
21. How can injury during seizure be prevented?
22. What are the signs of magnesium toxicity? How should it be managed?

HEMOLYSIS, ELEVATED LIVER ENZYMES, AND LOW PLATELETS (HELLP) SYNDROME

The hemolysis, elevated liver enzymes, and low platelets (HELLP) syndrome is a life-threatening variation of preeclampsia. HELLP often occurs at a preterm gestation of 26 to 34 weeks rather than late in pregnancy. *Hemolysis* is believed to occur as a result of the fragmentation and distortion of erythrocytes during passage through narrowed and damaged blood vessels. *Elevated liver* enzymes occur when hepatic blood flow is obstructed by fibrin deposits. Hyperbilirubinemia and jaundice also may be observed as a result of liver impairment. *Low platelets* are due to vascular damage resulting from vasospasm; platelets aggregate at sites of damage, resulting in thrombocytopenia elsewhere. A hepatic or subcapsular hematoma can cause massive bleeding.

The prominent symptom of HELLP syndrome is pain in the right upper quadrant, the lower chest, or epigastric area. Tenderness from liver distention also may occur. Additional signs and symptoms include nausea, vomiting, and severe edema.

Laboratory data is required to diagnose HELLP. A complete blood count may show a low hematocrit that cannot be accounted for by blood loss. Elevations in lactate dehydrogenase (LDH), bilirubin, aspartate aminotransferase (AST), and alanine aminotransferase (ALT) demonstrate liver impairment. Elevated uric acid and creatinine levels suggest reduced renal function. Coagulation studies may show the abnormalities discussed under DIC, particularly in the more severe forms of HELLP.

Avoid traumatizing the liver by abdominal palpation and use care in transporting the woman. A sudden increase in intraabdominal pressure could rupture the subcapsular hemotoma, which is most likely to occur during seizures (Usta & Sibai, 1995).

Management of women with HELLP syndrome should be in a setting with full intensive care facilities. The fetus is evaluated for gestational age and well-being through a nonstress test or biophysical profile. Steroids may be given to accelerate fetal lung maturity. High-dose corticosteroids are also being studied as a method to arrest maternal disease progression (Martin & Magann, 2000).

Treatment includes magnesium sulfate to control seizures and hydralazine to control the blood pressure. Fluid replacement is managed to avoid worsening the woman's reduced intravascular volume without giving her too much, which could cause pulmonary edema or ascites. Cervical ripening with labor induction usually is done if the gestation is at least 34 weeks. Delivery may be delayed up to 96 hours if the gestation is less than 34 weeks to give the steroids a chance to stimulate fetal lung maturation (Martin & Magann, 2000).

Most women improve within 48 to 72 hours postpartum. Their liver studies begin to normalize and urine output improves. Coagulation studies are not always repeated postpartum unless the coagulation deficiency was severe before birth. The woman's blood pressure begins to stay below 150 mm Hg systolic and 100 mm Hg diastolic. A 25% recurrence risk for HELLP syndrome, primarily in women who developed more severe disease at an earlier gestation, has been reported.

CHRONIC HYPERTENSION

A diagnosis of chronic hypertension is made whenever hypertension precedes pregnancy, or when a woman is hypertensive before 20 weeks' gestation. Chronic hypertension is seen most often in older women, in those who are obese, and in those with diabetes. Heredity, which includes racial factors such as being more common in African Americans, plays a role in the development of chronic hypertension (Cunningham, et al., 1997). Other factors may include renal or endocrine diseases or collagen vascular diseases such as systemic lupus erythematosus (Castro, 1998).

Pregnancy aggravates chronic hypertension. The most common hazard faced by women with chronic hypertension is the development of preeclampsia. The diagnosis is made when a sustained rise in blood pressure and proteinuria develop. Treatment of superimposed preeclampsia often requires hospitalization and measures to prevent the development of eclampsia.

Women with chronic hypertension have a higher risk for intrauterine fetal growth restriction and will be followed by fetal surveillance such as serial ultrasounds, nonstress tests, and biophysical profiles.

Because of the natural fall in blood pressure during early pregnancy, the woman's blood pressure may appear normal when she enters prenatal care. If she already is taking an antihypertensive drug, she usually continues this drug unless her blood pressure becomes unusually low. If she is not on an antihypertensive drug, she may be placed on one if her diastolic pressure is consistently above 90 mm Hg. Methyldopa (Aldomet) is the usual first antihypertensive drug because of its demonstrated safety for the fetus and infant. Diuretics may be used cautiously for women with chronic hypertension if antihypertensive drugs alone are insufficient.

In addition to drug therapy, reduced activity may be prescribed to increase placental blood flow. The diet should have adequate protein. Sodium may or may not be restricted.

Check Your Reading

23. What is the unabbreviated form of the term *HELLP?* What are the prominent signs and symptoms of this syndrome? Why should the liver not be palpated?
24. Compare preeclampsia with chronic hypertension in terms of onset and treatment.

INCOMPATIBILITY BETWEEN MATERNAL AND FETAL BLOOD

Rh Incompatibility

Rhesus (Rh) factor incompatibility during pregnancy is possible only when two specific circumstances coexist: (1) the expectant mother is Rh-negative and (2) the fetus is Rh-positive. For such a circumstance to occur, the father of the fetus must be Rh-positive. Rh incom-

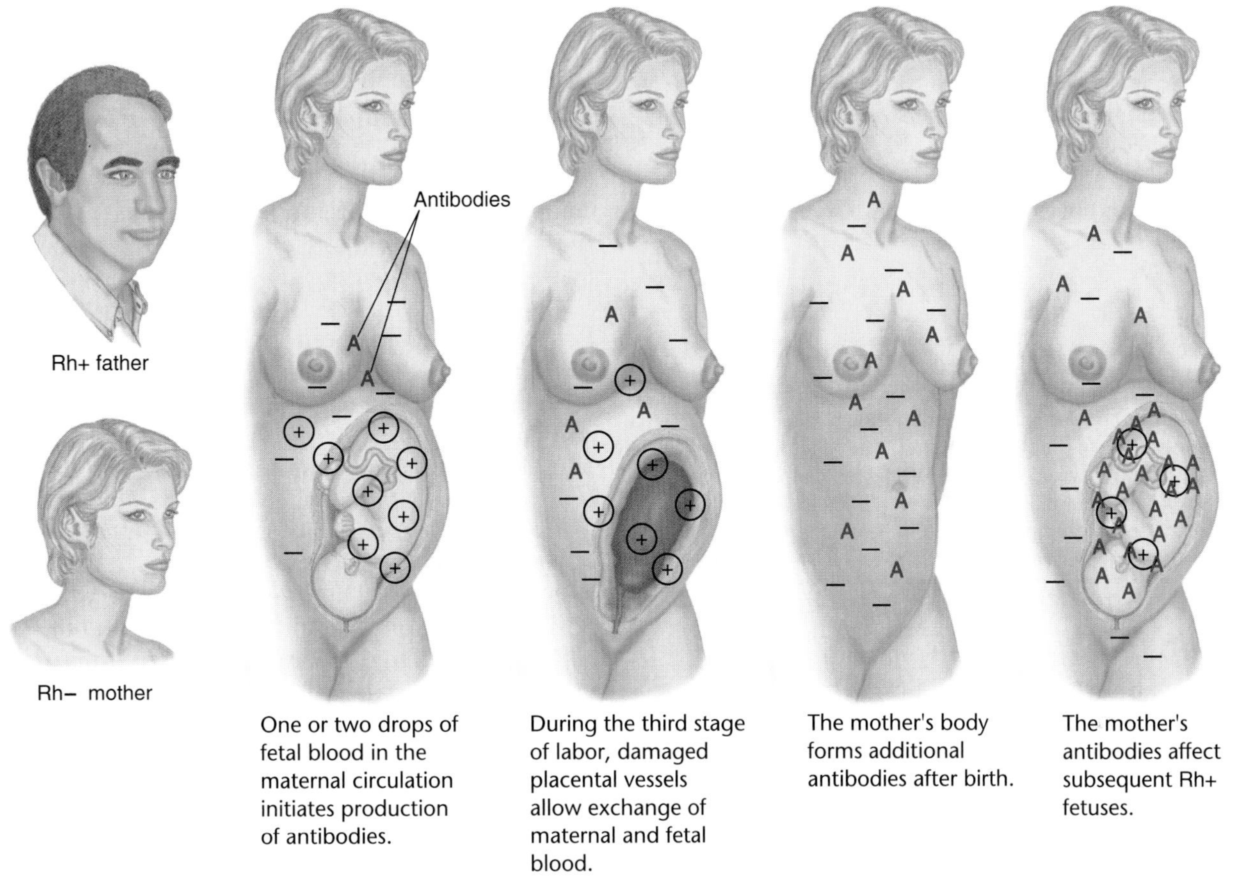

Rh+ father
Rh− mother
Antibodies
One or two drops of fetal blood in the maternal circulation initiates production of antibodies.
During the third stage of labor, damaged placental vessels allow exchange of maternal and fetal blood.
The mother's body forms additional antibodies after birth.
The mother's antibodies affect subsequent Rh+ fetuses.

FIGURE 25-9 The process of maternal sensitization to the Rh factor.

patibility is a problem that affects the fetus; it causes no harm to the expectant mother.

Rh-negative blood is a recessive trait and a person must inherit the same gene from both parents to be Rh-negative. Approximately 15% of the white population in the United States is Rh-negative. The incidence is lower in the African American and Asian populations.

Pathophysiology

People who are Rh-positive have the Rh antigen on their red blood cells, whereas people who are Rh-negative do not have the antigen. When blood from a person who is Rh-positive enters the bloodstream of a person who is Rh-negative, the body reacts as it would to any foreign substance: it develops antibodies to destroy the invading antigen. To destroy the Rh antigen, which exists as part of the red blood cell, the entire red blood cell must be destroyed.

Theoretically, fetal and maternal blood does not mix during pregnancy. In reality, small placental accidents occur that allow a drop or two of fetal blood to enter the maternal circulation and initiate the production of antibodies to destroy the Rh-positive blood. Sensitization also can occur during a spontaneous or elective abortion or during antepartal procedures such as amniocentesis and chorionic villus sampling (Figure 25-9). As little as 0.25 ml of Rh-positive blood can cause sensitization in an Rh-negative person (Queenan, 2000).

Most exposure of maternal blood to fetal blood occurs during the third stage of labor, when active exchange of fetal and maternal blood may occur from damaged placental vessels. In this case, the woman's first child is not affected because antibodies are formed after the birth of the infant. Subsequent Rh-positive fetuses may be affected, however, unless the mother receives Rh_0(D) immune globulin (RhoGAM) to prevent antibody formation after the birth of each Rh-positive infant.

Fetal and Neonatal Implications

If antibodies to the Rh factor are present in the expectant mother's blood, they cross the placental barrier and destroy fetal erythrocytes. The fetus becomes deficient in red blood cells, which are needed to transport oxygen to fetal tissue. As fetal red blood cells are destroyed, fetal bilirubin levels increase (icterus gravis), which can lead to neurologic disease (kernicterus, leading to bilirubin encephalopathy). This hemolytic process results in rapid production of erythroblasts (immature red blood cells), which cannot carry oxygen. The entire syndrome is termed *erythroblastosis fetalis*. The fetus may become so anemic that generalized fetal edema (hydrops fetalis) results and can end in fetal congestive heart failure.

Management of the infant born with erythroblastosis fetalis is discussed in Chapter 30.

CRITICAL TO REMEMBER

Treatment for Rh-Negative Women

All unsensitized Rh-negative women should receive Rh_0(D) immune globulin (RhoGAM) after abortion, ectopic pregnancy, chorionic villus sampling, amniocentesis, or birth of an Rh-positive infant. RhoGAM prevents the development of Rh antibodies that would result in destruction of fetal erythrocytes in subsequent pregnancies.

Prenatal Assessment and Management

All pregnant women should have a blood test to determine blood type and Rh factor at the initial prenatal visit. Rh-negative women should have an indirect Coombs' test to determine whether they are sensitized (have developed antibodies) as a result of previous exposure to Rh-positive blood. If the indirect Coombs' test is negative, it is repeated at 28 weeks of gestation to identify if they have developed subsequent sensitization.

Rh_0(D) immune globulin (such as RhoGAM) is administered to the unsensitized, Rh-negative woman at 28 weeks of gestation to prevent sensitization that may occur from small leaks of fetal blood across the placenta. Rh_0(D) immune globulin is a commercial preparation of passive antibodies against Rh factor. It effectively prevents the formation of active antibodies against Rh-positive erythrocytes.

If the indirect Coombs' test result is positive, indicating maternal sensitization and the presence of antibodies, it is repeated at frequent intervals throughout the pregnancy to determine whether the antibody titer is rising. An increase in titer indicates that the process is continuing and that the fetus will be in jeopardy.

Amniocentesis may be performed to determine the Rh factor of the fetus and to evaluate change in the optical density (ΔOD) of amniotic fluid. New techniques of DNA analysis allow determination of the Rh factor of the fetus from amniotic fluid cells with high accuracy. DNA testing eliminates uncertainty when other testing falls in the borderline zone. For example, if the optical density is slightly elevated, but DNA testing shows the fetus to be Rh-negative, it can eliminate the need to test further for Rh-related problems.

The optical density reflects the amount of bilirubin, the residue of red blood cell destruction, that is present in the amniotic fluid. If the fluid optical density remains low, it may indicate that the fetus is Rh-positive but in no jeopardy. An elevated optical density suggests fetal jeopardy.

Ultrasound examination also is used to evaluate the condition of the fetus. Generalized fetal edema, ascites, enlarged heart, or hydramnios indicates serious fetal compromise. A cordocentesis may be done to evaluate the fetal hematocrit, and an intrauterine transfusion may follow if the preterm fetus is anemic (Figure 25-10).

Postpartum Management

If the mother is Rh-negative, umbilical cord blood is taken at delivery to determine blood type, Rh factor, and antibody titer (direct Coombs' test) of the newborn. Rh-negative, unsensitized mothers who give birth to Rh-positive infants are given an intramuscular injection of Rh_0(D) immune globulin (RhoGAM) within 72 hours following delivery. If RhoGAM is given to the mother in the first 72 hours following delivery of an Rh-positive infant, any Rh antigens present in her blood are destroyed, and therefore the mother forms no natural antibodies. If the infant is Rh-negative, no possibility exists of Rh antibody formation and RhoGAM is not necessary.

Families often are concerned about the fetus, and nurses must be sensitive to cues that indicate that the family is anxious and must be able to offer honest reassurance. This is especially important if the expectant mother is sensitized and fetal testing is necessary throughout pregnancy (Table 25-7).

During labor, the nurse must carefully label the tube of cord blood obtained for analysis of the newborn's blood type and Rh factor. During the postpartum period, nurses are responsible for follow-up to determine whether RhoGAM is necessary and for administering the injection within the prescribed time.

ABO Incompatibility

ABO incompatibility occurs when the expectant mother is blood type O and the fetus is blood type A, B, or AB. Type A, B, and AB blood contains a protein component (antigen) that is not present in type O blood.

Table 25-7

NURSING DIAGNOSES FOR THE WOMAN WITH A COMPLICATION OF PREGNANCY
*Anxiety
Diversional Activity Deficit
Fear
*Impaired Adjustment
*Knowledge Deficit
Risk for Altered Family Processes
Risk for Infection
*Situational Low Self-Esteem

*Nursing diagnoses explored in this chapter.

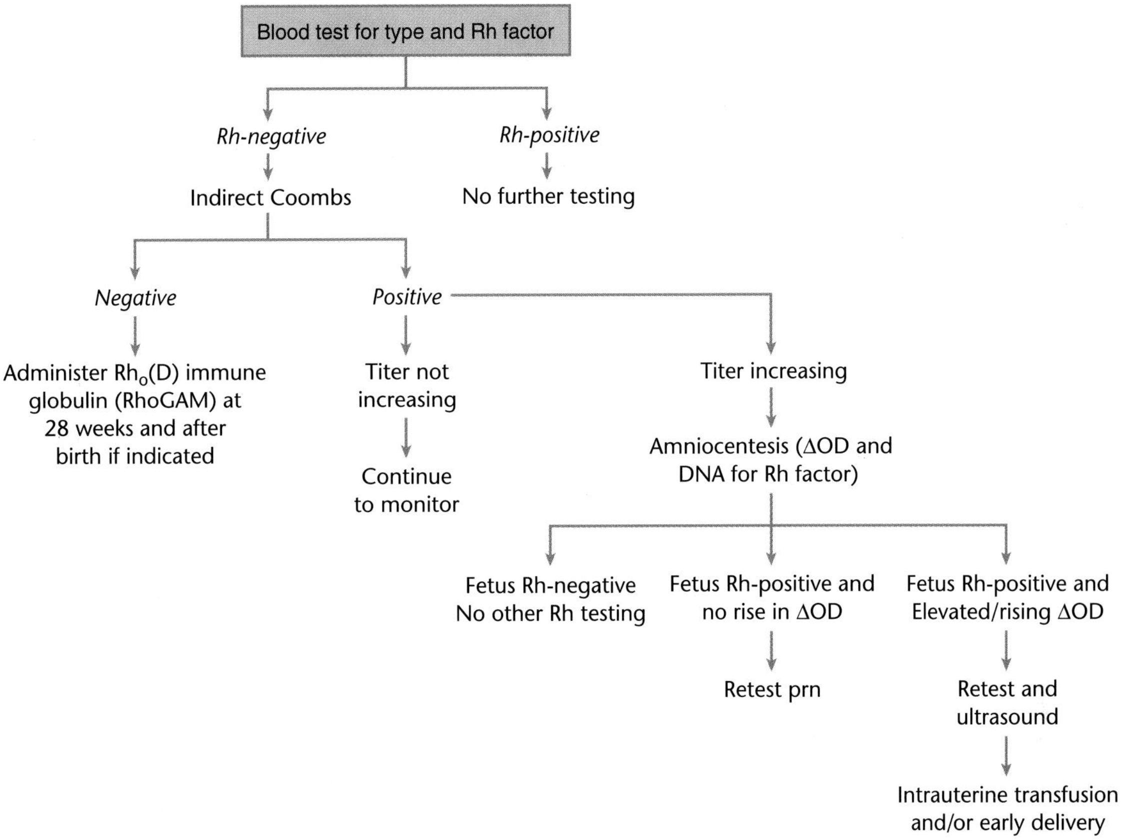

FIGURE 25-10 Sequence of assessments for Rh sensitization, as needed. *OD,* change in optical density of bilirubin.

DRUG GUIDE: $RH_o(D)$ IMMUNE GLOBULIN (RHOGAM, HYPRHOD, GAMULIN RH)

Classification: Concentrated immunoglobulins directed toward the red blood cell antigen $Rh_o(D)$

Action: Prevents production of anti-$Rh_o(D)$ antibodies in Rh-negative women who have been exposed to Rh-positive blood by suppressing the immune reaction of the Rh-negative woman to the antigen in Rh-positive blood; prevents antibody response and thus prevents hemolytic disease of the newborn in future Rh-positive pregnancies

Indications: Administered to Rh-negative women who have been exposed to Rh-positive blood by

1. Delivering an Rh-positive infant
2. Aborting an Rh-positive fetus
3. Having chorionic villus sampling, amniocentesis, or intraabdominal trauma while carrying an Rh-positive fetus
4. Receiving inadvertent transfusion of Rh-positive blood

Dosage and Route: One *standard* dose (300 mcg) administered intramuscularly:

1. At 28 weeks of pregnancy and within 72 hours of delivery
2. Within 72 hours following termination of a pregnancy of 13 weeks or more of gestation

One *microdose* (50 mcg) within 72 hours after the termination of a pregnancy of less than 13 weeks' gestation.

Dose is calculated based on the volume of blood erroneously administered in transfusion accidents. A standard dose will protect against 30 ml of Rh-positive blood (Queenan, 2000).

Absorption: Well absorbed from intramuscular sites

Excretion: Metabolism and excretion unknown

Contraindications and Precautions: Women who are Rh-positive or women previously sensitized to $Rh_o(D)$ should not receive $Rh_o(D)$ immune globulin. It is used cautiously for women with previous hypersensitivity reactions to immune globulins.

Adverse Reactions: Local pain at intramuscular site, fever, or both

Nursing Implications: Type and crossmatch of mother's blood and cord blood of the newborn must be performed to determine the need for the medication. The mother must be Rh-negative and negative for Rh antibodies. The newborn must be Rh-positive. If the fetal blood type after termination of pregnancy is uncertain, the medication should be administered. The drug is administered to the mother, not the infant. The deltoid muscle is recommended for intramuscular administration.

PARENTS WANT TO KNOW About Rh Incompatibility

What does it mean to be Rh-negative?

Those who are Rh-negative lack a substance that is present in the red blood cells of those who are Rh-positive.

How can the expectant mother be Rh-negative and the fetus be Rh-positive?

The fetus can inherit the Rh-positive factor from the father.

What does sensitization mean?

Sensitization means that the expectant mother has been exposed to Rh-positive blood and has developed antibodies against the Rh factor.

Do the antibodies harm the expectant mother?

No, because she does not have the Rh factor.

Do Rh-positive men always father Rh-positive children?

No. Rh-positive men who have an Rh-positive gene and an Rh-negative gene can father Rh-negative children.

Why is Rh_0(D) immune globulin (RhoGAM) necessary during pregnancy and following childbirth?

RhoGAM prevents the development of Rh antibodies in the mother, which might be harmful to subsequent fetuses who are Rh-positive.

Why will the next fetus be jeopardized if RhoGAM is not administered?

If RhoGAM is not administered when a baby is Rh-positive, the expectant mother may develop antibodies that cross the placental barrier and affect the next Rh-positive fetus.

People with type O blood develop anti-A or anti-B antibodies naturally as a result of exposure to antigens in the foods that they eat or to infection by gram-negative bacteria. As a result, some women with blood type O have developed high serum anti-A and anti-B antibody titers before pregnancy. The antibodies may be either IgG or IgM. When the woman becomes pregnant, the IgG antibodies cross the placental barrier and cause hemolysis of fetal red blood cells. Although the first fetus can be affected, ABO incompatibility is less severe than Rh incompatibility because the primary antibodies of the ABO system are IgM, which do not cross the placenta.

No specific prenatal care is needed; however, the nurse must be aware of the possibility of ABO incompatibility. During the delivery, cord blood is taken to determine the blood type of the newborn and the antibody titer (direct Coombs' test). The newborn is carefully screened for jaundice, which indicates hyperbilirubinemia. See Chapter 30 for medical and nursing management of hyperbilirubinemia in newborns.

Check Your Reading

25. Why do unsensitized Rh-negative expectant mothers receive Rh_0(D) immune globulin during pregnancy and after an abortion, amniocentesis, and childbirth?
26. What are the effects on the fetus of maternal Rh sensitization?
27. Why is the first fetus sometimes affected if ABO incompatibility occurs? Why are the effects of ABO incompatibility milder than Rh-sensitization?

SUMMARY CONCEPTS

- Spontaneous abortion is one of the leading causes of pregnancy loss. Treatment is aimed at preventing complications, such as hypovolemic shock and infection, and providing emotional support for grieving.
- The incidence of ectopic pregnancy is increasing in the United States as a result of pelvic inflammation associated with sexually transmissible diseases. The goals of therapeutic management are to prevent severe hemorrhage and to preserve the fallopian tube so that future fertility is retained.
- Management of hydatidiform mole involves two phases: (1) evacuation of the molar pregnancy and (2) continuous follow-up for 1 year to detect malignant changes in the remaining trophoblastic tissue.
- Disorders of the placenta (placenta previa and abruptio placentae) are responsible for hemorrhagic conditions of the last half of pregnancy. Either condition may result in maternal hemorrhage and fetal or maternal death.
- Disseminated intravascular coagulation is a life-threatening complication of missed abortion, abruptio placentae, and severe pregnancy-induced hypertension, in which procoagulation and anticoagulation factors are simultaneously activated.
- The cause of hyperemesis gravidarum remains unclear but the goals of management are to prevent dehydration, malnutrition, and electrolyte imbalance. Emotional support is an important responsibility of nurses in addition to physical care.
- Hypertensive disorders of pregnancy may include pregnancy-induced hypertension, preeclampsia, eclampsia, or preexisting (chronic) hypertension. The underlying process is generalized vasospasm, which decreases circulation to all organs of the body, including the placenta. Major maternal organs affected include the liver, kidneys, and brain.
- Treatment of preeclampsia includes reduced activity, reduction of environmental stimuli, and administration of medications to prevent generalized seizures.
- Magnesium sulfate, used to prevent preeclampsia from progressing to eclamptic seizures, is associated with adverse effects, the most serious being central nervous system depression, which includes depression of the respiratory center.
- Nurses monitor the woman with preeclampsia to determine the effectiveness of medical therapy and to identify signs that the condition is worsening, such as increasing hyperreflexia. Nurses also control external stimuli and initiate measures to protect her in case of eclamptic seizures.
- Nurses also monitor the woman with preeclampsia for signs of magnesium toxicity, which include decreased respiratory effort and absent deep tendon reflexes.

- Women who have chronic hypertension are at increased risk for preeclampsia and should be monitored for worsening hypertension, proteinuria, or generalized edema. Antihypertensive medication should be continued or initiated if diastolic blood pressure is consistently higher than 100 mmHg.
- Rh incompatibility can occur if an Rh-negative woman conceives a child who is Rh-positive. As a result of exposure to the Rh-positive antigen, maternal antibodies may develop that cause hemolysis of fetal Rh-positive red blood cells in subsequent pregnancies.
- Administration of Rh_0(D) immune globulin (RhoGAM) prevents production of anti-Rh antibodies thus preventing destruction of Rh-positive red blood cells in subsequent pregnancies.
- ABO incompatibility usually occurs when the mother has type O blood and naturally occurring anti-A and anti-B antibodies, which cause hemolysis if the fetus's blood is not type O. ABO incompatibility may result in hyperbilirubinemia of the infant, but it usually presents no serious threat to the health of the child.

ANSWERS TO CRITICAL THINKING EXERCISE, p. 669

Nurses often assume that patients know how to use a thermometer and that they know the signs of infection. Many nurses assume that patients realize the connection between blood loss and the tendency to develop infection. As a result, nurses may not emphasize the need for a diet that is high in nutrients that increase hemoglobin and hematocrit (iron and vitamin C). Nurses also may assume incorrectly that women know foods that contain these nutrients.

ANSWERS TO CRITICAL THINKING EXERCISE, p. 670

1. Many people wrongly assume that early pregnancy loss does not produce the grieving that accompanies loss at a later stage. Telling Alice that she is lucky ignores her feelings and invalidates any grief she feels.
2. The nurse also mistakenly assumes that little cause for grief exists over the loss of this one if later children are possible. However, a unique relationship exists between Alice and this fetus. Alice may experience an emotional upheaval when this special relationship comes to an abrupt end.
3. It would be beneficial if Helen examined her assumptions before having the interaction with Alice. She might then allow Alice to express her feelings and acknowledge the grief that she is feeling.

REFERENCES & READINGS

American Academy of Pediatrics (AAP) & American College of Obstetricians and Gynecologists (ACOG). (1997). *Guidelines for perinatal care.* (4th ed.). Elk Grove Village, IL: Author.

American College of Obstetricians and Gynecologists (ACOG). (1996). Hypertension in pregnancy. *Technical Bulletin No. 219.* Washington, D.C.: Author.

Anderson, J.J.B. (2000). Minerals. In L.K. Mahan & S. Escott-Stump (Eds.), *Krause's food, nutrition, and diet therapy* (10th ed., pp. 110-152). Philadelphia: W.B. Saunders.

Arias, F. (2000). Third-trimester bleeding. In E.J. Quilligan & F.P. Zuspan (Eds.), *Current therapy in obstetrics and gynecology* (5th ed., pp. 360-364). Philadelphia: W.B. Saunders.

Atterbury, J.L., Groome, L.J., Hoff, C., & Yarnell, J.A. (1998). Clinical presentation of women readmitted with postpartum severe preeclampsia or eclampsia. *Journal of Obstetric, Gynecologic, and Neonatal Nursing, 27*(2), 134-141.

August, P. (1999). Hypertensive disorders in pregnancy. In G.N. Burrow & T.P. Duffy (Eds.), *Medical complications during pregnancy* (5th ed., pp. 53-77). Philadelphia: W.B. Saunders.

Berman, M.L., Di Saia, P.J., & Brewster, W.R. (1999). Pelvic malignancies, gestational trophoblastic neoplasia, and nonpelvic malignancies. In R.K. Creasy & R. Resnik (Eds.), *Maternal-fetal medicine* (4th ed., pp. 1128-1150). Philadelphia: W.B. Saunders.

Bowman, J.M. (1999). Hemolytic disease (erythroblastosis fetalis). In R.K. Creasy & R. Resnik (Eds.), *Maternal-fetal medicine* (4th ed., pp. 736-767). Philadelphia: W.B. Saunders.

Branch, D.W., & Porter, T.F. (1999). Hypertensive disorders of pregnancy. In J.R. Scott, P.J. Di Saia, C.B. Hammond, & W.N. Spellacy (Eds.), *Danforth's Obstetrics and Gynecology* (8th ed., pp. 309-326). Philadelphia: Lippincott Williams & Wilkins.

Buttino, L., Gambon, C., & Coleman, S. (1999, June). *Home subcutaneous metoclopramide therapy for hyperemesis gravidarum.* Poster session presented at the annual convention of the Association of Women's Health, Obstetric, and Neonatal Nurses.

Carpenito, L.J. (1999). *Handbook of nursing diagnosis* (8th ed.). Philadelphia: Lippincott.

Carson, S.A. (2000). Spontaneous abortion. In S.B. Ransom, M.P. Dombrowski, S.G. McNeeley, K.S., Moghissi, & A.R. Munkarah (Eds.), *Practical Strategies in Obstetrics and Gynecology* (pp. 533-538). Philadelphia: W.B. Saunders.

Castro, L.C. (1998). Hypertensive disorders of pregnancy. In N.F. Hacker & J.G. Moore (Eds.), *Essentials of Obstetrics and Gynecology* (3rd ed., pp. 196-207). Philadelphia: W.B. Saunders.

Clark, S.L. (1999a). Critical care obstetrics. In J.R. Scott, P.J. Di Saia, C.B. Hammond, & W.N. Spellacy (Eds.), *Danforth's Obstetrics and Gynecology* (8th ed., pp. 471-484). Philadelphia: Lippincott Williams & Wilkins.

Clark, S.L. (1999b). Placenta previa and abruptio placentae. In R.K. Creasy & R. Resnik (Eds.), *Maternal-fetal medicine* (4th ed., pp. 616-631). Philadelphia: W.B. Saunders.

Coulam, C.B. (2000). Recurrent spontaneous abortion. In E.J. Quilligan & F.P. Zuspan (Eds.), *Current therapy in obstetrics and gynecology* (5th ed., pp. 349-354). Philadelphia: W.B. Saunders.

Crane, J.M., Van Den Hof, M.C., Dodds, L., Armson, A., & Liston, R. (1999). Neonatal outcomes with placenta previa. *Obstetrics and Gynecology, 93*(4), 541-544.

Cunningham, F.G., MacDonald, P.C., Gant, N.F., Leveno, K.J., Gilstrap, L.C., Hankins, G.D.V., et al. (1997). *Williams obstetrics* (20th ed.). Norwalk, CT: Appleton & Lange.

Emerson, R.J. (2000). Alterations in hemostasis and blood coagulation. In L.E.C. Copstead & J.L. Banasik (Eds.), *Pathophysiology: Biological and behavioral perspectives* (2nd ed., pp. 332-347). Philadelphia: W.B. Saunders.

Fagan, E.A. (1999). Diseases of liver, biliary system, and pancreas. In R.K. Creasy & R. Resnik (Eds.), *Maternal-fetal medicine* (4th ed, pp. 1054-1081). Philadelphia: W.B. Saunders.

Fagen, C. (2000). Nutrition during pregnancy and lactation. In L.K. Mahan & S. Escott-Stump (Eds.), *Krause's food, nutrition, and diet therapy* (10th ed., pp. 167-195). Philadelphia: W.B. Saunders.

Goldstein, D.P., & Berkowitz, R.S. (2000a). Gestational trophoblastic disease. In E.J. Quilligan & F.P. Zuspan (Eds.), *Current therapy in obstetrics and gynecology* (5th ed., pp. 210-212). Philadelphia: W.B. Saunders.

Goldstein, D.P., & Berkowitz, R.S. (2000b). Hydatidiform mole. In E.J. Quilligan & F.P. Zuspan (Eds.), *Current therapy in obstetrics and gynecology* (5th ed., pp. 213-217). Philadelphia: W.B. Saunders.

Hauth, J.C., Ewell, M.G., Levine, R.J., Esterlitz, J.R., Sibai, B., Curet, L.B., Catalano, P.M., & Morris, C.D. (2000). Pregnancy outcomes in healthy nulliparas who developed hypertension. *Obstetrics and Gynecology, 95*(1), 24-28.

Hewell, S.W., & Hammer, R.H. (1997). Antiphospholipid antibodies: A threat throughout pregnancy. *Journal of Obstetric, Gynecologic, and Neonatal Nursing, 26*(2), 162-168.

Hill, J.A. (1999). Recurrent pregnancy loss. In R.K. Creasy & R. Resnik (Eds.), *Maternal-fetal medicine* (4th ed., 423-443). Philadelphia: W.B. Saunders.

Huxley, R.R. (2000). Nausea and vomiting in early pregnancy: Its role in placental development. *Obstetrics and Gynecology, 95*(5), 779-782.

Iams, J.D. (1999). Cervical incompetence. In R.K. Creasy & R. Resnik (Eds.), *Maternal-fetal medicine* (4th ed., 445-464). Philadelphia: W.B. Saunders.

Kirkpatrick, S.J., & Laros, R.K. (1999). Maternal hematologic disorders. In R.K. Creasy & R. Resnik (Eds.), *Maternal-fetal medicine* (4th ed., 935-963). Philadelphia: W.B. Saunders.

Larry, C.D., & Yeo, S. (2000). The Circadian rhythm of blood pressure during pregnancy. *Journal of Obstetric, Gynecologic, and Neonatal Nursing, 29*(5), 500-508.

Larson, J.L., & Rayburn, W.F. (2000). Hyperemesis gravidarum. In E.J. Quilligan & F.P. Zuspan (Eds.), *Current therapy in obstetrics and gynecology* (5th ed., pp. 297-299). Philadelphia: W.B. Saunders.

Leicht, T.G., & Harvey, C.J. (1999). Hypertensive disorders in pregnancy. In L.K. Mandeville & N.H. Troiano (Eds.), *AWHONN'S High-Risk & Critical Care Intrapartum Nursing* (2nd ed., pp. 159-172). Philadelphia: Lippincott.

Lipscomb, G.H., Puckett, K.J., Bran, D., & Ling, F.W. (1999). Management of separation pain after single-dose methotrexate therapy for ectopic pregnancy. *Obstetrics and Gynecology, 93*(4), 590-593.

Lipscomb, G.H., & Ling, F.W. (2000). Ectopic pregnancy. In E.J. Quilligan & F.P. Zuspan (Eds.), *Current therapy in obstetrics and gynecology* (5th ed., pp. 273-277). Philadelphia: W.B. Saunders.

Lucas, L.S., & Jordan, E.T. (1997). Phenytoin as an alternative treatment for pre-eclampsia. *Journal of Obstetric, Gynecologic, and Neonatal Nursing, 26*(3), 263-269.

Maiolatesi, C.R., & Peddicord, K. (1996). Methotrexate for nonsurgical treatment of ectopic pregnancy: Nursing implications. *Journal of Obstetric, Gynecologic, and Neonatal Nursing, 25*(3), 205-208.

Maloni, J.A. (2000). Antepartum support group for women hospitalized on bedrest. *MCN: American Journal of Maternal/Child Nursing, 25*(4), 204-210.

Martin, J.N., & Magann, E.F. (2000). HELLP syndrome. In E.J. Quilligan & F.P. Zuspan (Eds.), *Current therapy in obstetrics and gynecology* (5th ed., pp. 288-293). Philadelphia: W.B. Saunders.

Pepper, G.A. (1999). Pharmacology of antihypertensive drugs. *Journal of Obstetric, Gynecologic, and Neonatal Nursing, 28*(6), 649-659.

Pisarska, M.D., & Carson, S.A. (1999). Ectopic pregnancy. In J.R. Scott, P.J. Di Saia, C.B. Hammond, & W.N. Spellacy (Eds.), *Danforth's Obstetrics and Gynecology* (8th ed., pp. 155-172). Philadelphia: Lippincott Williams & Wilkins.

Queenan, J.T. (2000). Rh and other blood group immunizations. In F.P. Zuspan & E.J. Quilligan (Eds.), *Current therapy in obstetrics and gynecology* (5th ed., pp. 429-432). Philadelphia: W.B. Saunders.

Riely, C.A., & Fallon, H.J. (1999). Liver diseases. In G.N. Burrow & T.P. Duffy (Eds.), *Medical complications during pregnancy* (5th ed., pp. 269-294). Philadelphia: W.B. Saunders.

Roberts, J.M. (1999). Pregnancy-related hypertension. In R.K. Creasy & R. Resnik (Eds.), *Maternal-fetal medicine* (4th ed., pp. 833-872). Philadelphia: W.B. Saunders.

Rosevear, S. (1999). Bleeding in early pregnancy. In D.K. James, P.J. Steer, C.P. Weiner, & B. Gonik (Eds.), *High-risk pregnancy: Management options* (2nd ed., p. 89). Philadelphia: W.B. Saunders.

Scott, J.R. (1999a). Early pregnancy loss. In J.R. Scott, P.J. Di Saia, C.B. Hammond, & W.N. Spellacy (Eds.), *Danforth's Obstetrics and Gynecology* (8th ed., pp. 143-153). Philadelphia: Lippincott Williams & Wilkins.

Scott, J.R. (1999b). Placenta previa and abruption. In J.R. Scott, P.J. Di Saia, C.B. Hammond, & W.N. Spellacy (Eds.), *Danforth's Obstetrics and Gynecology* (8th ed., pp. 407-418). Philadelphia: Lippincott Williams & Wilkins.

Sibai, B.M. (2000). Chronic hypertension in pregnancy. In F.P. Zuspan & E.J. Quilligan (Eds.), *Current therapy in obstetrics and gynecology* (5th ed., pp. 256-260). Philadelphia: W.B. Saunders.

Silver, R.M., & Branch, D.W. (1999). Immunologic disorders. In R.K. Creasy & R. Resnik (Eds.), *Maternal-fetal medicine* (4th ed., pp. 465-483). Philadelphia: W.B. Saunders.

Simon, E.P., & Schwartz, J. (1999). Medical hypnosis for hyperemesis gravidarum. *Birth, 26*(4), 248-254.

Sisson, M.C., & Ruth, D. (1999). Disseminated intravascular coagulation. In L.K. Mandeville & N.H. Troiano (Eds.), *AWHONN: High-Risk and Critical Care Nursing* (2nd ed., pp. 214-223). Philadelphia: Lippincott.

Snell, L.H., Haughey, B.P., Buck, G., & Marecki, G. (1998). Metabolic crisis: Hyperemesis gravidarum. *Journal of Perinatal and Neonatal Nursing, 12*(2), 26-37.

Thompson, W.B. (2000). Therapeutic abortion. In F.P. Zuspan & E.J. Quilligan (Eds.), *Current therapy in obstetrics and gynecology* (5th ed., pp. 358-360). Philadelphia: W.B. Saunders.

Tuncer, Z.S., Bernstein, M.R., Goldstein, D.P., Lu, K.H., & Berkowitz, R.S. (1999). Outcome of pregnancies occurring within 1 year of hydatidiform mole. *Obstetrics and Gynecology, 94*(4), 588-590.

Usta, I.M., & Sibai, B.M. (1995). Emergent management of puerperal eclampsia. *Obstetrics and Gynecology Clinics of North America, 22*(2), 315-335.

Witlin, A.G., & Sibai, B.M. (2000). Hypertensive diseases of pregnancy: Role of calcium and low-dose aspirin. In F.P. Zuspan & E.J. Quilligan (Eds.), *Current therapy in obstetrics and gynecology* (5th ed., pp. 299-303). Philadelphia: W.B. Saunders.

Zuspan, F.P. (2000). Preeclampsia. In F.P. Zuspan & E.J. Quilligan (Eds.), *Current therapy in obstetrics and gynecology* (5th ed., pp. 322-325). Philadelphia: W.B. Saunders.

26 Concurrent Disorders during Pregnancy

OBJECTIVES

1. Describe the effects of pregnancy on fuel metabolism.
2. Discuss the effects and management of preexisting diabetes mellitus during pregnancy.
3. Explain the effects and management of gestational diabetes mellitus.
4. Describe the major effects of pregnancy on the woman who has heart disease, and identify the goals of therapy.
5. Explain the maternal and fetal effects of specific anemias and the required management during pregnancy.
6. Identify the effects, management, and nursing considerations of specific preexisting conditions.
7. Identify the major causes of trauma during pregnancy and describe therapeutic management.
8. Discuss the maternal, fetal, and neonatal effects of the most common infections that may occur during pregnancy.

DEFINITIONS

Acquired Immunodeficiency Syndrome (AIDS) Syndrome caused by the human immunodeficiency virus (HIV), resulting in loss of defense against malignancies and opportunistic infections.

Cardiac Decompensation Failure of the heart to maintain adequate circulation to the tissues. See also *congestive heart failure.*

Caudal Regression Syndrome A malformation that results when the sacrum, lumbar spine, and lower extremities fail to develop.

Congenital Anomaly Abnormal intrauterine development of an organ or structure.

Congestive Heart Failure Condition resulting from failure of the heart to maintain adequate circulation; characterized by weakness, dyspnea, and edema in body parts that are lower than the heart.

Diabetes Mellitus A disorder of carbohydrate metabolism caused by a relative or complete lack of insulin secretion; characterized by glycosuria (glucose in the urine) and hyperglycemia.

DEFINITIONS—cont'd

Diabetogenic Condition such as pregnancy that produces the effects of diabetes mellitus.

Dystocia Difficult or prolonged labor; often associated with abnormal uterine activity and cephalopelvic disproportion.

Gestational Diabetes Impaired glucose tolerance that is induced by pregnancy and diagnosed during pregnancy; usually disappears after childbirth.

Gluconeogenesis Formation of glycogen by the liver from noncarbohydrate sources such as amino and fatty acids.

Human Immunodeficiency Virus (HIV) A retrovirus that results in the development of acquired immune deficiency syndrome (AIDS).

Hydramnios Excess volume of amniotic fluid (more than 2000 ml at term). Also called *polyhydramnios.*

Ketosis Accumulation of ketone bodies (metabolic products) in the blood; frequently associated with acidosis.

Lipogenic Substance such as insulin that stimulates the production of fat.

Macrosomia Unusually large fetal size; infant birth weight more than 4000 g.

Marfan's Syndrome A hereditary condition that involves weakness in connective tissue, bones, and muscles; the vascular system is affected, particularly the aorta.

Neonatologist A physician who specializes in the care of newborn infants (from birth until the 29th day of life).

Osmotic Diuresis Secretion and passage of large amounts of urine as a result of increased osmotic pressure that can result from hyperglycemia.

Perinatologist A physician who specializes in the care of the mother, fetus, and infant during the perinatal period (from the 20th week of pregnancy to 4 weeks after childbirth).

Polydipsia Excessive thirst.

Polyphagia Excessive ingestion of food.

Polyuria Excessive excretion of urine.

Seroconversion Change in a blood test result from negative to positive, indicating the development of antibodies in response to infection or immunization.

Pregnancy affects the care of women with a medical condition in two ways. First, pregnancy may alter the course of the disease. Second, the disease or its treatment may have unwanted effects on the pregnancy. As a result, the usual antepartum care must be adapted to include increased surveillance of the mother and fetus. Also, some disorders that are mild or even subclinical in the pregnant woman can produce massive damage to the fetus. This chapter describes some common disorders that can cause significant fetal jeopardy.

DIABETES MELLITUS

Pathophysiology

Etiology

Diabetes mellitus is a complex disorder of carbohydrate metabolism caused primarily by a partial or complete lack of insulin secretion by the beta cells of the pancreas. Some cells, such as those in skeletal and cardiac muscles and adipose tissue, rely on insulin to carry glucose across the cell membranes. Without insulin, glucose accumulates in the blood, resulting in hyperglycemia. The body attempts to dilute the glucose load by any means possible. The first strategy is to increase thirst (polydipsia), a classic symptom of diabetes mellitus. Next, fluid from the intracellular spaces is drawn into the vascular bed, resulting in dehydration at the cellular level but fluid volume excess in the vascular compartment. The kidneys attempt to excrete large volumes of this fluid and the heavy solute load of glucose (osmotic diuresis). This excretion produces the second hallmark of diabetes, polyuria, as well as glycosuria (glucose in the urine). Without glucose, the cells starve, so weight loss occurs even though the person ingests excessive amounts of food (polyphagia).

Because the body cannot metabolize glucose, it begins to metabolize protein and fat to meet energy needs. Metabolism of protein produces a negative nitrogen balance, and the metabolism of fat results in the buildup of ketone bodies (such as acetone, acetoacetic acid, or β-hydroxybutyric acid) or ketosis (accumulation of acids in the body).

If the disease is not well controlled, serious complications may occur. Hypoglycemia or hyperglycemia can result if the amount of insulin does not match the diet. In addition, fluctuating periods of hyperglycemia and hypoglycemia damage small blood vessels throughout the body. This damage can cause serious impairment, especially in the kidneys, eyes, and heart.

Effect of Pregnancy on Fuel Metabolism

To understand the relationship between diabetes mellitus and pregnancy, an understanding of the way pregnancy and diabetes alter the metabolism of food is necessary.

Early Pregnancy. Metabolic changes can be divided into those that occur early in pregnancy (from 1 to 20 weeks' gestation) and those that occur late in pregnancy (from 20 to 40 weeks' gestation). During early pregnancy, maternal metabolic rates and energy needs change little. During this time, however, insulin release in response to serum glucose levels accelerates. As a result, significant hypoglycemia may occur, particularly in women who experience the nausea, vomiting, and anorexia that often occur during the first weeks of pregnancy.

In an uncomplicated pregnancy, the availability of glucose and insulin, a lipogenic substance, favors the development and storage of fat during the first half of pregnancy. Accumulation of fat prepares the mother for the rise in energy use by the growing fetus during the second half of pregnancy.

Late Pregnancy. During the second half of pregnancy, when fetal growth accelerates, placental hormones rise sharply. These hormones, particularly estrogen, progesterone, and human placental lactogen, create *resistance to insulin* in maternal cells. This resistance allows an abundant supply of glucose to be available for the fetus. However, the hormones have a diabetogenic effect in that they may leave the woman with insufficient insulin and episodes of hyperglycemia.

For most women, insulin resistance is not a problem. The pancreas responds by simply increasing the production of insulin. If the pancreas is unable to respond, however, the woman will experience periods of hyperglycemia.

During late pregnancy, the fetus continually draws nutrients such as glucose and amino acids from maternal blood. The result is an earlier-than-normal switch from carbohydrate metabolism to gluconeogenesis (formation of glycogen from noncarbohydrate sources such as proteins and fat). Because the fetus uses many of the amino acids, the process becomes predominantly one of fat utilization. This process produces high levels of free fatty acids that further inhibit the uptake and oxidation of glucose, therefore preserving glucose for use by the central nervous system and fetus. These metabolic changes are similar to those occurring during "accelerated starvation," when fat is metabolized to meet many of the body's energy needs.

Classification

Diabetes that exists before pregnancy is classified as type 1 (insulin deficient) or type 2 (insulin resistant, with a relative deficiency of insulin to metabolize carbohydrate) according to whether the client requires the administration of insulin to prevent ketoacidosis. A third type is one in which any degree of glucose intolerance has its onset or first recognition during pregnancy. The onset of glucose intolerance during pregnancy is termed *gestational diabetes mellitus* (GDM) and accounts for 90% of cases of diabetes that occur during pregnancy (Expert Committee on the Diagnosis and Classification of Diabetes Mellitus, 1997). (See Table 26-1 for additional characteristics of the three types of diabetes.)

An additional classification of diabetes is sometimes used for descriptive purposes. The White classification describes the length of time the woman has had diabetes and any vascular complication, such as retinopathy, that is present. More recently, two categories were added to the White classification to describe whether the woman's gestational diabetes is controlled by diet alone (class A-1) or requires both diet and insulin (class A-2) for adequate control.

Table 26-1
CLASSIFICATION OF DIABETES MELLITUS

TYPE 1: INSULIN DEFICIENCY
Usual onset is in childhood or young adulthood
Usually dependent on insulin for survival
Prone to ketoacidosis
Associated with autoimmune destruction of beta cells
Not often obese at diagnosis, but obesity is not incompatible with this diagnosis
TYPE 2: INSULIN RESISTANT
Usual onset after 40 years
Hyperglycemia develops gradually
Associated with obesity, particularly with fat in abdominal area
Usually sufficient insulin produced to prevent ketosis
Occurs more often in women who had gestational diabetes in the past
GESTATIONAL DIABETES MELLITUS
Onset or first recognition of glucose intolerance during pregnancy
Exogenous insulin may or may not be needed
Glucose regulation returns to normal after birth in the majority of women
Is a risk factor for Type 2 diabetes later in life

From the Expert Committee on the Diagnosis and Classification of Diabetes Mellitus. (1997). *Diabetes Care,* 20(7), 1183-1197.

Incidence

The pregnant woman may have preexisting diabetes (type 1 or type 2), or she may develop gestational diabetes mellitus during the course of pregnancy. Diabetes mellitus is a common medical condition complicating pregnancy. One of every 100 pregnant women has preexisting diabetes. Between 2% and 5% of pregnant women will develop gestational diabetes (March of Dimes, 2000).

Preexisting Diabetes Mellitus

Maternal Effects

The course of pregnancy for women with diabetes mellitus has improved greatly as a result of new treatments and more effective methods of fetal surveillance. However, the incidence of complications affecting the mother and fetus remains higher than that experienced by nondiabetic women.

Diabetes can adversely affect a pregnant woman and her developing baby in several ways. During the first trimester, when major fetal organs are developing, the effects of the abnormal metabolic environment, such as hypoglycemia, hyperglycemia, and ketosis, may lead to increased incidence of spontaneous abortion or major fetal malformations. The risk of pregnancy-induced hypertension is four times greater than in the normal population even if no evidence of vascular or renal complications exists (Cunningham, et al., 1997). The development of ketoacidosis is a threat to women with type 1 diabetes and is most often precipitated by infection or missed insulin doses. In addition, ketoacidosis may develop in these women at lower thresholds of hyperglycemia than those seen in nonpregnant individuals. Untreated ketoacidosis can progress to fetal and maternal death. Urinary tract infections are more common, possibly because of glucose in the urine, which provides a nutrient-rich medium for bacterial growth.

Other effects include hydramnios, which may result from fetal hyperglycemia and consequent fetal diuresis, and premature rupture of membranes, which may be caused by overdistention of the uterus by hydramnios or a large fetus. Problems that arise during labor and childbirth if the fetus has macrosomia (more than 4000 g, or 8.8 lb) may include a difficult labor, shoulder dystocia (delayed or difficult birth of fetal shoulders after the head is born), and consequent injury to the birth canal or the infant. Large fetal size also increases the likelihood that a cesarean birth will be necessary and the risk of postpartum hemorrhage (Table 26-2).

Fetal Effects

Fetal and neonatal effects of preexisting diabetes depend on the timing and severity of maternal hyperglycemia and the degree of vascular impairment that has occurred.

Congenital Malformation. The most common major congenital malformations associated with preexisting diabetes are neural tube defects, caudal regression syndrome, and cardiac defects. The risk for a major congenital malformation is two to six times higher than that of the general population. The incidence correlates directly with the degree of maternal hyperglycemia during the first trimester. Fewer malformations occur if the woman is able to maintain a normal blood glucose level before conception and throughout early pregnancy (Fanaroff, Martin, & Miller, 1999).

Variations in Fetal Size. Fetal growth is related to maternal vascular integrity. In women without vascular impairment, glucose and oxygen are easily transported to the fetus; if the woman is hyperglycemic, so is the fetus. Although maternal insulin does not cross the placental barrier, the fetus produces insulin by the 10th week of gestation. Fetal macrosomia results when elevated levels of blood glucose stimulate excessive production of fetal insulin, which acts as a powerful growth hormone. This is a major neonatal effect with conse-

Table 26-2

MAJOR EFFECTS OF DIABETES MELLITUS ON PREGNANCY

Increased Maternal Risks	Probable Cause
Pregnancy-induced hypertension	Unknown but increased even with no renal or vascular impairment
Urinary tract infections	Increased bacterial growth in nutrient-rich urine Delayed bladder emptying because of diabetic neuropathy in some women
Hydramnios	Fetal diuresis caused by hyperglycemia
Ketoacidosis	Uncontrolled hyperglycemia
Difficult labor, injury to birth canal, cesarean birth, and postpartum hemorrhage	Fetal macrosomia and overdistention of uterus
Increased Fetal and Neonatal Risks	**Probable Cause**
Perinatal death	Poor placental perfusion because of maternal vascular impairment
Congenital anomalies	Maternal hyperglycemia in the first trimester
Macrosomia (>4000 g birth weight)	Fetal hyperglycemia stimulates production of insulin
Birth injury	Large fetal size
IUGR	Maternal vascular impairment
Preterm labor and premature rupture of membranes	Overdistention of uterus caused by hydramnios and fetal macrosomia
Preterm birth	Deterioration in fetal condition requiring delivery before maturity
Polycythemia; hyperbilirubinemia	Excess red blood cells manufactured in response to episodes of intrauterine hypoxia Breakdown of excessive red blood cells no longer needed after birth
Hypoglycemia	Neonatal hyperinsulinemia after birth when maternal glucose is no longer available
Hypocalcemia	Transfer of calcium abruptly stopped at birth
Respiratory distress syndrome	Delayed production of pulmonary surfactant

quent increase in cesarean birth or birth injury from shoulder dystocia.

Conversely, if vascular impairment occurs, placental perfusion may be decreased. Vascular impairment may be caused by complications of the diabetes, such as vasoconstriction that occurs in pregnancy-induced hypertension, a common added complication. When placental perfusion is impaired, the supplies of glucose and oxygen will be decreased. As a result, the infant is likely to be small for gestational age. This condition is called *intrauterine growth restriction (IUGR).*

Neonatal Effects

The four major neonatal complications of preexisting diabetes are hypoglycemia, hypocalcemia, hyperbilirubinemia, and respiratory distress syndrome.

Hypoglycemia. The neonate is at higher risk for hypoglycemia because fetal insulin production was accelerated during pregnancy to metabolize excessive glucose received from the expectant mother. The constant stimulation of hyperglycemia leads to hyperplasia and hypertrophy of the islets of Langerhans in the pancreas. At birth, when the maternal glucose supply is abruptly withdrawn, the level of neonatal insulin exceeds the available glucose and hypoglycemia develops rapidly. Poor maternal glycemic control during pregnancy and an elevated maternal glucose level during the intrapartum period increase the risk for neonatal hypoglycemia.

Hypocalcemia. During the last half of pregnancy, large amounts of calcium are transported across the placenta from the mother to the fetus. At the time of birth, this transfer is abruptly stopped, leading to a dramatic decrease in total and ionized calcium. Hypocalcemia, defined as 7 mg/dl or less, most often occurs between 24 and 36 hours after birth (Tyrala, 1996). It is associated with preterm birth, birth trauma, and perinatal asphyxia, all of which are common problems of the infant born to a mother with diabetes mellitus.

Hyperbilirubinemia. The fetus who experiences recurrent hypoxia compensates by production of additional erythrocytes to carry oxygen supplied by the mother. After birth, the excess erythrocytes are broken down, releasing large amounts of bilirubin into the neonate's circulation.

Respiratory Distress Syndrome. The infant of a diabetic mother is more likely to have delayed production of pulmonary surfactant, which is needed to keep the alveoli open after birth. A possible reason is that insulin administration disrupts the pulmonary maturation of the fetus, which is normally induced by glucocorticoids. This problem is most likely to occur if the mother's glycemic control is poor because of wide fluctuations in her insulin and glucose levels. Tests of fetal lung maturity, such as the lecithin/sphingomyelin (L/S) ratio and presence of phosphatidylglycerol (PG), will be done before elective delivery of the fetus by induction or cesarean if any questions about maturity exist. (See Chapter 10 for additional information on tests of fetal lung maturity.)

Maternal and fetal-neonatal complications can be greatly reduced by maintaining normal and stable blood glucose levels. The objective of the team providing treatment is to devise a plan that allows the woman to maintain a level as close to normal as possible (Nursing Care Plan 26-1).

Check Your Reading

1. What effects do the hormones of pregnancy have on maternal glucose metabolism?
2. What are the maternal effects of type 1 diabetes mellitus? What are possible fetal and neonatal effects?
3. How do insulin needs vary from the first trimester through the postpartum period?

Maternal Assessment

Whenever a pregnant woman with preexisting diabetes initiates prenatal care, a thorough evaluation of her health status must be completed. This evaluation includes history, physical examination, and laboratory tests.

History. A detailed history should include the onset and management of the diabetic condition. How long has she had the disease? How does she maintain normal blood glucose? Is she familiar with ways to monitor blood glucose and administer insulin? The degree of glycemic control before pregnancy is of particular interest. Effective management depends on her adherence to a plan of care. Therefore her knowledge of how diabetes affects pregnancy and pregnancy affects diabetes must be determined. The support person's knowledge also must be assessed, and specific learning needs should be identified. In addition, the woman's emotional status should be assessed to determine how she is coping with pregnancy superimposed on preexisting diabetes.

All women with diabetes should be seen by a qualified nurse-educator for an individualized assessment to ensure that they can monitor their blood glucose accurately. A variety of battery-powered, portable, blood glucose reflectance meters are currently available for home use. Accurate readings depend on performing the test correctly and at the times recommended. In addition to home monitoring of blood glucose, the nurse must observe the woman's skill in mixing and administering insulin.

Physical Examination. In addition to routine prenatal examination (see Chapter 7), specific efforts should be made to assess the effects of diabetes. A baseline electrocardiogram (ECG) should be obtained to determine cardiovascular status. Evaluation for retinopathy should be performed, with referral to an ophthalmologist if necessary. The woman's weight and blood pressure must be monitored because of the increased risk for pregnancy-induced hypertension. Fundal height should be measured, noting any abnormal increase in size that may indicate macrosomia or hydramnios, which may occur as a result of diuresis by the hyperglycemic fetus. Fundal height less than expected for the gestation may indicate fetal growth restriction or sometimes intrauterine death.

Laboratory Tests. In addition to routine prenatal laboratory examinations (see Chapter 7), baseline renal function should be assessed with a 24-hour urine collection for total protein excretion and creatinine clearance. The urine should be checked at each prenatal visit for possible urinary tract infections, which are common in women with diabetes. Urine also should be checked for the presence of glucose and ketones. Thyroid function tests should be performed because of the risk for coexisting thyroid disease.

Glycemic control should be evaluated on the basis of *glycosylated hemoglobin.* With prolonged hyperglycemia, a percentage of hemoglobin will remain saturated with glucose for the life of the red blood cell. The glycosylated hemoglobin assay (HbA1c) is an accurate measurement of the average glucose concentrations during the preceding 4 to 8 weeks (Homko & Khandelwal, 1996). Unlike other tests that reflect the amount of glucose in the plasma at that moment, the HbA1c is not affected by recent intake or restriction of food.

Fetal Surveillance

Because of the increased risk for congenital anomalies, growth abnormalities, and abnormal amniotic fluid accumulation, fetal surveillance should begin early for women with preexisting diabetes mellitus. Maternal serum alpha-fetoprotein should be offered at 16 weeks' gestation to screen for neural tube defects. A detailed ultrasonographic evaluation of the fetus should be recommended at 18 weeks' gestation, and an assessment of fetal cardiac structure by echocardiography should be done at 20 weeks' gestation (Gabbe & Landon, 2000).

During the third trimester, fetal surveillance may include maternal assessment of fetal movement ("kick counts"), nonstress tests, contraction stress tests, and biophysical profiles. Doppler velocimetry may be recommended if vascular complications exist or hypertension develops. (See Chapter 10 for a complete description of fetal diagnostic procedures.)

Therapeutic Management

The goals of therapeutic management for a pregnant woman with diabetes are to (1) maintain normal blood glucose levels, (2) give birth to a healthy baby, and (3) avoid accelerated impairment of blood vessels and other major organs. To achieve this outcome, an intensive, team approach to care is required.

Members of the team often include a diabetologist, who assists in regulation of maternal blood glucose; an obstetrician, who monitors the mother and fetus and determines the optimal time for birth; a dietitian, who provides a balanced meal plan; and a diabetes educator, often a nurse, who provides ongoing education and support. The team is completed by a neonatologist, who will care for the newborn, the family physician, and the pediatrician, who will provide ongoing care for the infant and mother. A maternal-fetal medicine specialist and support staff may be added if multiple fetal surveillance procedures are needed.

Preconception Care. Ideally, the team approach should begin before conception. Both prospective parents should participate in care sessions to learn more about the following issues (Moore, 1999):

- Establishing the optimal time for pregnancy based on maintenance of normal maternal blood glucose levels so that the risk of major fetal malformations can be reduced.
- Evaluating the degree of maternal cardiovascular, renal, and ophthalmologic complications.
- Determining the current degree of glucose control and providing information about the importance of maintaining normal blood glucose levels throughout the pregnancy. This is particularly important if excellent control has not been accomplished before conception.
- Providing instruction, if necessary, in the use of home glucose monitoring techniques and insulin administration for women who have previously taken oral hypoglycemic drugs.
- Taking a daily prenatal vitamin that includes 400 mcg (0.4 mg) of folic acid at least 3 months before conception to reduce the risk for neural tube defects in the fetus.
- Identifying support systems and financial resources that may be needed if extended hospitalization or reduced activity at home becomes necessary.

Diet. The average daily intake for the pregnant woman with diabetes ranges from 2200 to 2400 calories per day. Approximately 45% of the calories should be from carbohydrates, 20% from protein, and 35% from fat (Gabbe & Landon, 2000). Caloric intake should be distributed between three meals and two to four snacks. Women who are less active or gain excessive weight may require fewer calories.

Self-Monitoring of Blood Glucose. The schedule for self-monitoring of blood glucose is individualized but averages 4 to 6 times each day if the woman requires insulin. The woman usually tests her blood glucose on rising in the morning, 1 to 2 hours after breakfast, before and after lunch, before dinner, and at bedtime (Inzucchi, 1999; Moore, 1999). In addition to scheduled monitoring, women also should perform a glucose test whenever they have symptoms of hypoglycemia. They should record all test results on a log sheet for review by the health care provider at each visit.

Insulin Therapy. The need to maintain rigorous control of the maternal metabolism during pregnancy requires more frequent doses of insulin than usual. Most treatment regimens rely on three daily injections, with a combination of short-acting (regular) insulin and intermediate-acting (NPH) insulin given before breakfast, regular insulin before dinner, and NPH insulin at bedtime. Some regimens call for long-acting (Ultralente) insulin to be given once or twice daily, supplemented by regular insulin before meals. A new, short-acting insulin, lispro (Humalog), allows the woman to inject just before a meal. Lispro insulin has the advantage of limiting hypoglycemia later because it reaches its peak quickly and has a short duration of action (Moore, 2000). Because insulin needs change throughout pregnancy, insulin coverage will have to be adjusted as pregnancy progresses.

First Trimester. Insulin needs generally decline during the first trimester because the secretion of placental hormones antagonistic to insulin remains low. The woman also may experience nausea, vomiting, and anorexia, resulting in decreased intake of food, and thus require less insulin. In addition, the fetus receives its share of glucose, which reduces maternal plasma glucose levels and decreases the need for maternal insulin.

Second and Third Trimesters. Insulin needs increase markedly during the second and third trimesters when placental hormones, which initiate maternal resistance to the effects of insulin, reach their peak. In addition, the nausea of early pregnancy usually resolves and the diet includes 300 additional calories per day, which is needed to meet the increased metabolic demands of pregnancy.

During Labor. Insulin needs during labor are based on the blood glucose level. The muscular exertion and lack of oral intake should decrease the amount of insulin needed. Also, the woman may receive IV fluid containing dextrose. Capillary blood glucose monitoring every 1 to 2 hours guides the insulin administration to maintain the serum glucose level at approximately 100 mg/dL (Landon & Gabbe, 2000). If insulin is needed, regular insulin may be added to the IV solution and infused at a rate to maintain serum glucose levels. The woman also may receive insulin based on a sliding scale. Tight glucose control during labor reduces neonatal hypoglycemia in the hours immediately after birth.

Postpartum. Insulin needs should decline rapidly after the delivery of the placenta and abrupt cessation of placental hormones. However, blood glucose levels should be monitored at least four times daily so that the insulin dose can be adjusted to meet individual needs. Women with type 1 diabetes usually return to their prepregnancy dosages. Women with type 2 diabetes are monitored, and insulin is ordered only if needed

Timing of Delivery. If possible, the pregnancy should be allowed to progress to term so that the fetal lungs can mature and the risk of neonatal respiratory distress syndrome can be reduced. If evidence of fetal compromise exists, such as a low biophysical profile score, nonreactive nonstress test, or late decelerations on a contraction stress test, amniocentesis may be performed to evaluate the degree of fetal lung maturity (Moore, 1999). (See Chapter 10.) Delivery, often cesarean, will be carried out regardless of fetal lung maturity if the fetus is compromised.

Gestational Diabetes Mellitus

Risk Factors

Gestational diabetes is a carbohydrate intolerance of variable severity that develops or is first recognized during pregnancy. Diagnosis begins with a history to identify the woman at risk to develop gestational diabetes. Factors known to increase the risk include:

- Obesity (>90 kg, or 198 lb)
- Chronic hypertension
- Maternal age older than 25 years
- Family history of diabetes in close relatives
- Previous birth of a large infant (>4000 g)
- Previous birth of an infant with unexplained congenital anomalies
- Previous unexplained fetal death
- Gestational diabetes in previous pregnancy
- Fasting serum glucose >140 mg/dL or random serum glucose >200 mg/dL

Women with any of these factors should be screened for gestational diabetes at the first prenatal visit (Moore, 1999).

Screening

Glucose Challenge Test. The current recommendation is that pregnant women who have not been identified with glucose intolerance earlier in pregnancy be screened with a 50-g, 1-hour glucose challenge test (GCT) between 24 and 28 weeks of pregnancy unless they are in a low-risk group. Low-risk women include those younger than 25 years, of normal weight, with no known first-degree relatives having diabetes, and not a member of an ethnic group in which diabetes is prevalent. High-risk ethnic groups include African-Americans, Latinos, Pacific Islanders, and American

Indians (Centers for Disease Control and Prevention, 1998b).

The GCT can be done at a regular clinic visit, and the woman does not need to fast. The expectant mother drinks 50 g of oral glucose solution. Approximately 1 hour later, a blood sample is taken. If her blood glucose is equal to or above 140 mg/dl, a 3-hour oral glucose tolerance test (OGTT) should be recommended (Expert Committee on the Diagnosis and Classification of Diabetes Mellitus, 1997; ACOG, 1994). About one third of physicians prefer to use a lower cut-off of 130 mg/dL or 135 mg/dL on the GCT because the lower level improves the sensitivity of the screening test and avoids missing most women who will have gestational diabetes (Moore, 1999).

Oral Glucose Tolerance Test. The OGTT is diagnostic for diabetes mellitus. Although it is the gold standard for diagnosing diabetes, it is a more complicated test and requires the woman's participation. She must eat a high-carbohydrate diet for 3 days before the scheduled test and fast after midnight on the day of the test. After a fasting plasma glucose level is obtained, the woman ingests 100 g of oral glucose solution. Plasma glucose levels are obtained at 1, 2, and 3 hours. Gestational diabetes is the diagnosis if the fasting blood glucose is abnormal or two or more of the following values are found (Expert Committee on the Diagnosis and Classifi-cation of Diabetes Mellitus, 1997; ACOG, 1994):

- Fasting, greater than 105 mg/dl
- 1 hour, greater than 190 mg/dl
- 2 hours, greater than 165 mg/dl
- 3 hours, greater than 145 mg/dl

Maternal, Fetal, and Neonatal Effects

With a few important exceptions, the effects of gestational diabetes are similar to those associated with preexisting diabetes. The exceptions are that gestational diabetes is not associated with an increased risk for maternal ketoacidosis or spontaneous abortion. Because gestational diabetes develops after the first trimester, which is the critical period of major fetal organ development (organogenesis), it usually is not associated with an increase in major congenital malformations. Nevertheless, gestational diabetes, characterized by maternal hyperglycemia during the third trimester, is associated with increased neonatal morbidity and mortality. The major fetal complications are macrosomia, leading to birth injuries or necessitating cesarean birth, and neonatal hypoglycemia. Other problems such as hypocalcemia, hyperbilirubinemia, and respiratory distress also may occur. (See Table 26-2 for a summary of maternal, fetal, and neonatal effects of diabetes mellitus and their probable causes.)

Therapeutic Management

Diet. Nutritional counseling is the mainstay of therapy for women with gestational diabetes mellitus. The diet should provide the calories and nutrients needed for maternal and fetal health, result in euglycemia, and prevent ketosis caused by inadequate carbohydrate intake. Although the diet must be individualized and recommendations vary nationwide, in general an intake of 2200 to 2400 calories per day is recommended. Despite varied recommendations, one consistent recommendation is to limit carbohydrate intake at breakfast during pregnancy (Franz, 2000). One diet plan prescribes that complex carbohydrates from foods high in soluble fiber should provide 50% to 60% of total calories. Simple sugars found in concentrated sweets should be eliminated from the diet. Protein sources should supply 10% to 20%, with the remaining 25% to 30% coming from fat (Gabbe & Landon, 2000). Calories should be divided among three meals and at least two snacks.

Exercise. Exercise can play a significant role in normalizing blood glucose levels in women who develop gestational diabetes and women with type 2 diabetes who become pregnant. A contracting skeletal muscle increases its glucose uptake and helps regulate the capacity for glucose transport. Moderate exercise for active women and regular activity for sedentary women show promise for normalizing blood glucose levels (Artal, 1996; Inzucchi, 1999). The exercise program should be recommended by a physician who takes into account each woman's risk factors and risks to the fetus.

Blood Glucose Monitoring. Blood glucose levels should be evaluated to determine whether glucose levels are normal. The most common methods are *fasting blood sugar* (no food for the previous 4 hours) and *postprandial blood sugar* (2 hours after a meal). If fasting capillary blood glucose levels repeatedly exceed 95 mg/dL or postprandial values exceed 120 mg/dL, insulin is begun.

Fetal Surveillance. Testing to identify fetal compromise may begin as early as 28 weeks' gestation if the woman has poor glycemic control or by 34 weeks' gestation in lower-risk women with gestational diabetes. The surveillance testing often includes "kick counts," ultrasonography for fetal growth and amniotic fluid volume, biophysical profile, nonstress test, contraction stress test, or amniocentesis for fetal lung maturity (Moore, 1999).

Nursing Considerations

The care of a pregnant woman with diabetes mellitus focuses primarily on maintaining normal blood glucose. As stated earlier, this maintenance involves a rather rigid schedule of controlling the diet, blood glucose tests, administration of insulin, and fetal monitoring. Some women respond calmly to the intense medical supervision. Others respond with anxiety, fear, denial, or anger and feel inadequate or unable to control the diabetes to the degree expected by the health care team. These feelings may not be shared spontaneously, but they may affect the woman's ability to achieve the desired outcomes. Also, nurses should remember to provide for normal pregnancy care in addition to monitoring the pregnant woman's diabetes.

Increasing Effective Communication. A woman often does not volunteer information about her feelings and concerns, especially if she has negative feelings about her care. In addition, the woman and the nurse both may be unaware of misunderstandings or conflicts regarding the plan of care. Nurses must ask specifically about the feelings and concerns the woman and her family have about the pregnancy. Broad opening questions such as "What are your major concerns?" and "How do you feel about the plan of care?" are helpful. These should be followed with more specific questions such as "How do you feel about the fetal testing?" and "What would you like to change about the diet?" The woman's comments can provide valuable information about her emotional response to the care plan. One woman remarked, "I can tell you one thing, I don't feel like a person. I feel like an incubator, a faulty incubator." Another woman, who had a difficult time achieving the desired blood glucose level, said: "I feel as though my whole life has been taken over by diabetes. I'm tired of feeling like a sick person."

NURSING CARE PLAN 26-1

Pregnancy and Diabetes Mellitus

Assessment: Kathy Ringold is a 24-year-old primigravida of 9 weeks' gestation who was diagnosed with type 1 diabetes mellitus 6 years ago. She has been on a daily regimen of insulin and is comfortable with insulin administration and blood glucose monitoring. She is experiencing daily nausea and vomiting. Kathy states that she is concerned because she is not eating as much as before becoming pregnant. She also reveals that she had sometimes "binged" on food before becoming pregnant and didn't always monitor blood glucose as often as directed. She does not see why her blood glucose has to be watched so carefully now that she is pregnant.

Nursing Diagnosis: Risk for Altered Health Maintenance related to knowledge deficit of the effects of pregnancy on diabetes control.

Goals/Expected Outcomes:
Kathy will do the following:
1. Describe expected changes in insulin needs throughout pregnancy.
2. Follow prescribed schedule of blood glucose monitoring, insulin administration, diet, and exercise.
3. Describe the importance of frequent fetal surveillance and follow the prescribed schedule.

Intervention	Rationale
1. Reduce barriers to learning. a. Allow Kathy to express emotions and concerns before teaching. b. Examine her beliefs and past experiences related to diabetes. c. Assess her readiness to learn, based on interest, attention, and participation in scheduled learning sessions.	1. Motivation and readiness to learn are essential for permanent learning to occur. She will learn only if she sees the value of the information. Expressing her emotions and concerns are steps in her readiness to learn.
2. Teach Kathy about the predicted changes in insulin needs during pregnancy. Explain that she will need less insulin during the first trimester because of the nausea and vomiting that are common at this time. Insulin needs increase during the second and third trimesters as placental hormones increase and cause greater resistance to insulin. a. Explain the importance of blood glucose testing for control of glucose in the normal range. b. Teach Kathy that she will probably require more insulin during the second and third trimesters because of the effects of the placental hormones. c. Describe the importance of following the prescribed diet and exercise regimen to maintain normal blood glucose.	2. Behaviors change when learning occurs. Understanding why and how insulin needs change throughout pregnancy, labor, and the postpartum period increases the likelihood that a woman will follow the recommended regimen.

Continued

Intervention	Rationale
3. Inform Kathy about specific fetal surveillance techniques recommended during pregnancy (serial nonstress tests, contraction stress tests, biophysical profiles), and explain the importance of the tests.	3. Some frequently ordered tests are time consuming and expensive. The woman is more likely to accept the plan of care if she understands the importance of monitoring the fetal condition at frequent intervals.
4. Allow time for Kathy to focus on her feelings and concerns at each teaching session. Offer praise and encouragement for her adherence to the prescribed regimen.	4. Motivation to maintain the plan of care is strengthened by praise and the awareness that the woman's feelings are important.
5. Explain in simple, positive terms the advantages to the fetus of maintaining a normal maternal blood glucose level. These advantages include an optimal pattern of growth, the increased likelihood that the baby will be born near term, and fewer complications associated with prematurity.	5. Understanding how the fetus benefits when maternal glucose levels are normal and stable reduces anxiety and increases the likelihood that the mother will maintain the recommended treatment.
6. Review the recommended plan for diet and exercise during pregnancy, and determine whether Kathy knows the importance of these factors in her care. Identify any problems meeting diet or exercise recommendations.	6. Maintenance of normal blood glucose depends on coordinating the amount of food, insulin, and exercise. If any of these factors is altered, the others also must be altered to prevent hypoglycemia or hyperglycemia. Consulting the woman about possible problems allows them to be worked out, such as by having a dietician consult with her.

Evaluation: Kathy verbalizes her understanding of changing insulin needs and the importance of glucose monitoring. She states that she feels in better control of the diabetes and plans to keep the recommended schedule of fetal surveillance, diet, and exercise.

Assessment: At 32 weeks' gestation, Kathy's blood glucose is consistently above the desired level and daily nonstress tests are prescribed. The tests are reactive, indicating no present fetal compromise. Kathy verbalizes anxiety about the condition of the fetus and asks when it will be safe for the baby to be born.

Nursing Diagnosis: Anxiety related to perceived threat to the health of the fetus and lack of knowledge about the timing of the delivery.

Goals/Expected Outcomes:
Kathy will do the following:
1. Relate her perception of the condition of the fetus and the significance of the reactive nonstress test as the tests are performed.
2. Describe her concerns about timing of the delivery at the conclusion of the next nonstress test.

Intervention	Rationale
1. Ask Kathy to describe her concern about the fetus, and clarify her feelings.	1. Her concerns must be identified and clarified so that misconceptions do not occur. For example, Kathy may be anxious about labor and delivery or she may worry that the elevated blood glucose level poses an immediate threat to the baby.
2. Explain that a reactive nonstress test indicates the fetal heart rate accelerates whenever the fetus moves, a sign that the fetus is not in immediate jeopardy.	2. Reassurance that the fetus is not in jeopardy and the daily tests will detect early signs if a problem develops will reduce her anxiety about the fetal condition.
3. Ask Kathy how she feels about the labor and delivery. Determine whether she is taking childbirth education classes and has selected her labor partner.	3. Most women are concerned about the birth process and how they will cope with labor during the last few weeks of pregnancy. Health care professionals must remember that women with high-risk pregnancies also need routine care such as childbirth classes.
4. Assist her in locating a childbirth education class if she has not done so previously, and suggest that she and her labor partner begin classes.	4. Knowledge learned at childbirth classes may reduce the anxiety about the birth processes.

Evaluation: Kathy has been reassured by explanations about the reactive nonstress test but states she is concerned about how she will do in labor. She chooses a childbirth education class with her sister as her labor partner.

CRITICAL THINKING EXERCISE

Marcia Mahoney, a 28-year-old primigravida, is diagnosed with gestational diabetes in her 30th week of pregnancy. The health care team provides her with a diet and exercise regimen and tells her that she will need weekly tests to monitor her condition and that of the fetus. Although Marcia accepts the information without comment, she does not keep the next scheduled appointment.

QUESTIONS:

1. What assumptions has the health care team made?
2. What could the team have done to ensure that Marcia would keep the recommendations?

Marcia is located and agrees to return to the clinic for follow-up care. She states she does not "see what all the fuss is about." She understands she may have a large baby, but states that she was a 10-pound baby and did just fine. She wonders if the weekly tests are necessary and if they could harm the baby.

QUESTIONS:

3. How can the nurse respond to Marcia's comments about having a large baby without frightening her?
4. How can the nurse explain the need for weekly nonstress tests?

The nurse must be an active listener and allow time for the woman and her family to express concerns and feelings. The nurse must convey acceptance of both negative feelings and positive feelings that are expressed. Many women are reassured to hear that their feelings of stress or anger are normal and learn that the health care team understands those feelings. Sharing of emotions will help her avoid or diminish unnecessary guilt, anxiety, and frustration and thus promote positive feelings about her ability to participate successfully in her plan of care.

Most women benefit from praise when diabetic control is well maintained. They feel competent and trusted by the health care team and are motivated to continue their efforts.

Providing Opportunities for Control. Allowing the woman to make as many decisions as possible increases her sense of being in control. For instance, she can select foods from the exchange list that provide the necessary nutrients but still allow her some choice. A dietitian should be consulted if the list does not include food she likes or that suit her ethnic or cultural preferences. A regular schedule of exercise and sleep that helps keep the blood glucose level under control is important. The woman can develop the best schedule for rest and exercise that suits her lifestyle. Nurses should allow as much flexibility as possible when scheduling stressful events such as fetal monitoring tests and amniocentesis.

Some women resent being "treated as though ill" even though their diabetic control is excellent. These women may be capable of making more decisions regarding their care during pregnancy, but they need the support of an understanding team to do this.

Providing Normal Pregnancy Care. Some women express a need for more attention to the normal aspects of their pregnancies. This can be overlooked because of the intense focus on preventing complications that might occur as a result of diabetes. Women with diabetes also experience the discomforts that nondiabetic women experience during pregnancy, such as morning sickness, fatigue, backache, and difficulty sleeping. The nurse caring for women with diabetes should provide education and counseling regarding normal pregnancy.

Check Your Reading

4. What is the importance of glycosylated hemoglobin in monitoring diabetes mellitus?
5. How does gestational diabetes compare with type 1 diabetes mellitus in terms of onset and treatment?
6. What is the difference between a glucose challenge test and glucose tolerance test?
7. How do the maternal, fetal, and neonatal effects of gestational diabetes differ from those of preexisting diabetes?

APPLICATION OF THE NURSING PROCESS: THE PREGNANT WOMAN WITH DIABETES MELLITUS

Assessment

Determine how well the woman understands the prescribed management and how the family plans to carry out the recommended regimen. She may be newly diagnosed and have no experience in the necessary skills and procedures. On the other hand, she may be skilled in monitoring glucose and administering insulin but have no knowledge of the effects of diabetes on the pregnancy and the effects of pregnancy on diabetes. Or she may have been using premixed insulin exclusively and now must begin mixing insulin.

To determine whether her techniques are accurate, ask the expectant mother to demonstrate how she monitors blood glucose and observe as she mixes and injects insulins. Verify that she and her family are aware of the need to select appropriate sites and injection techniques that prevent insulin leakage.

Although diet is prescribed by a dietitian, assessing how well the family understands the diet is necessary. Determine whether special problems with food preferences or availability of recommended foods exist. Reviewing the exchange list and asking the woman how she plans to substitute and exchange foods may be necessary.

Identify the woman's knowledge of potential complications such as hypoglycemia and hyperglycemia so that she and her family can be provided with pertinent information.

Determine her knowledge of fetal surveillance techniques and her response to the need for frequent tests. Some women are highly motivated to continue the treatment regimen when test results indicate the fetus is thriving. Other women dread the tests and are puzzled by the need for such frequent testing.

Analysis

One of the most common nursing diagnoses is "Risk for Altered Health Maintenance related to knowledge deficit of specific measures to maintain normal blood glucose levels; signs, symptoms, and management of hypoglycemia and hyperglycemia; and recommended fetal surveillance procedures."

Planning

Goals and expected outcomes for this nursing diagnosis are that the woman (and her support person) will do the following:

- Demonstrate competence in home glucose monitoring and administration of insulin before home management is initiated.
- Describe a plan for meeting dietary recommendations.
- Identify signs and symptoms of hypoglycemia and hyperglycemia and the necessary management required for each.
- Verbalize knowledge of fetal surveillance procedures and keep scheduled appointments for testing.

Interventions

Although management of diabetes mellitus during pregnancy is a team effort, the nurse's major responsibility is to provide accurate information about the recommended therapeutic regimen and offer consistent support for the woman's efforts to comply with the recommendations. Demonstrating specific skills that the client and her support person must master and reviewing and reinforcing information from other members of the health care team may be necessary.

Teaching Self-Care Skills

Demonstrations and return demonstrations are the most effective ways to teach and evaluate psychomotor skills. The woman (and her support person) must learn to obtain a small sample of blood to test for glucose and to mix and inject insulin. Both procedures are invasive and cause mild discomfort, which may make the woman reluctant to start. Acknowledge these feelings before teaching begins.

Home Blood Glucose Monitoring. The blood glucose level is monitored several times a day, and the patient must be comfortable with the procedure. Spring devices available for sticking the finger make the procedure easier and less painful. Recommend that the expectant mother use the side of the finger, which is less sensitive than the tip. Teach her to cleanse the area with warm water before obtaining a sample to prevent infection. Each home monitoring kit contains specific instructions for use of the reagent strip, and these directions must be followed exactly to obtain an accurate reading.

Insulin Administration. Two types of insulin usually are prescribed: intermediate-acting and short-acting (regular) insulin. Teach the expectant mother the differences in onset, peak, and duration of each type of insulin. She also needs to learn the way to mix the two insulins in the same syringe.

Insulin is administered subcutaneously. Common sites include the upper thighs, abdomen, and upper arms. Aseptic technique is recommended to prevent infection. Because the pregnant woman is injecting insulin frequently, emphasize these precautions:

- To prevent hypoglycemia, a meal should be taken 30 minutes after insulin is injected, or within 15 minutes if lispro insulin is used.
- The angle of injection is usually 90 degrees unless the woman is very thin, in which case it is injected at a lesser angle.
- The needle should be inserted quickly to minimize discomfort.
- The tissue pinch, if used, is released after inserting the needle and before injecting insulin because pressure from the pinch can promote insulin leakage from the subcutaneous tissue.
- Aspirating when injecting into subcutaneous tissue is not necessary.
- Insulin is injected slowly (over 2 to 4 seconds) to allow tissue expansion and minimize pressure, which can cause insulin leakage.
- The needle is withdrawn quickly to minimize the formation of a track, which might permit insulin to leak out.

Emphasize the importance of administering the correct dose at the correct time. Teach the woman and her family the function of insulin and the importance of following the directions of her physician in regard to coordinating meals with the administration of insulin.

Continuous Subcutaneous Insulin Infusion. Many women use continuous subcutaneous insulin infusion and wish to continue with this method during pregnancy. The use of programmable insulin infusion pumps allows tailoring of insulin administration to the woman's individual lifestyle. Prompt, emergency counseling and assistance must be available 24 hours a day to deal with unexpected problems such as pump malfunction.

Teaching Dietary Management

Although a dietitian prescribes the recommended diet, the nurse must be aware of the general requirements and sensitive to the expectant mother's dietary habits and preferences. Often, reviewing and clarifying how the exchange lists are used to plan meals and snacks are necessary. Encourage the patient to avoid simple sugars (candy, cake, cookies), which raise the blood glucose levels quickly, and to include foods high in fiber, which are believed to help reduce glucose levels.

Finances often are a problem, and helping the woman select foods that are high in nutrients but low in cost may be necessary. Animal protein, such as meat or cheese, is especially expensive, and alternative sources of protein such as beans, peas, corn, and grains can be substituted to meet some protein needs.

Allow the expectant mother to verbalize her frustrations or problems with the diet, and collaborate with the dietitian if she has a particular problem.

Recognizing and Correcting Hypoglycemia and Hyperglycemia

Every woman and her family must be aware of the signs and symptoms that indicate abnormal blood glucose levels. Hypoglycemia and hyperglycemia pose a threat to the mother and fetus if they are not identified and corrected quickly.

Hypoglycemia. Treat hypoglycemia at once to prevent damage to the brain, which is dependent on glucose. The woman should take 15 g of carbohydrate if she can swallow. Examples of foods that supply this are 3 or 4 glucose tablets (depending on their carbohydrate quantity), ½ cup fruit juice or regular soft drink, or 6 saltine crackers (Franz, 2000). Large quantities of high-carbohydrate foods such as candy will increase the blood glucose excessively. The woman should retest 20 to 30 minutes after the carbohydrate intake. Depending on the time of her next scheduled meal, she also may eat a carbohydrate exchange after the hypoglycemic episode.

CRITICAL TO REMEMBER

Signs and Symptoms of Maternal Hypoglycemia

- Shakiness (tremors)
- Sweating
- Pallor; cold, clammy skin
- Disorientation; irritability
- Headache
- Hunger
- Blurred vision

CRITICAL TO REMEMBER

Signs and Symptoms of Maternal Hyperglycemia

- Fatigue
- Flushed, hot skin
- Dry mouth; excessive thirst
- Frequent urination
- Rapid, deep respirations; odor of acetone on the breath
- Drowsiness; headache
- Depressed reflexes

Teach family members how to inject glucagon in the event that the woman cannot swallow or retain food. Notify the physician at once. Intravenous glucose will be administered if she is hospitalized. If untreated, hypoglycemia can progress to convulsions and death.

To prevent hypoglycemia, instruct the woman to have meals at a fixed time each day and to plan snacks at 10 AM, 3 PM, and bedtime. Suggest that she carry glucose tablets or some crackers with her.

Hyperglycemia. Because infection is the most common cause of hyperglycemia, pregnant women must be instructed to notify the physician whenever they have an infection of any type.

If untreated, hyperglycemia can lead to ketoacidosis, coma, and maternal and fetal death. If signs and symptoms occur, notify the physician at once so that treatment can be initiated. Hospitalization often is necessary for monitoring blood glucose levels and IV administration of insulin and treatment of any underlying infection.

Explaining Procedures, Tests, and Plan of Care

Explain the schedule and the reasons for frequent checkups and necessary tests. Encourage the woman and her family to ask questions if any part of the schedule is confusing. This is particularly important for women who are aware that their prenatal care differs significantly from that of their nondiabetic friends. Knowing that the tests provide information about the condition of the mother and fetus reduces frustration and anxiety. Explain why more frequent antepartum surveillance testing is needed when diabetes complicates pregnancy. The woman needs to know that her diabetic care will require more time and effort than it did before pregnancy but that this care greatly improves her likelihood of having a healthy infant.

Evaluation

After procedures, tests, and plan of care have been explained, evaluation should ensure that:

- The expectant mother and one support person can demonstrate competence in blood glucose monitoring and administration of insulin.

- The woman can describe a plan for meeting dietary requirements.
- The woman and a support person can list the signs and symptoms of hypoglycemia and hyperglycemia and describe the initial management of these conditions.
- The woman can verbalize knowledge of the reason for fetal surveillance procedures and keeps appointments for tests.

HEART DISEASE

Alterations in cardiovascular function are necessary in pregnancy to meet additional maternal metabolic demands and the needs of the fetus. Plasma volume, venous return, and cardiac output all increase. Heart rate and stroke volume, the components of cardiac output, increase during pregnancy. The heart rate gradually rises above the baseline during the third trimester. However, increases in stroke volume are primarily responsible for the overall rise in cardiac output during early pregnancy.

A normal heart can adapt to the changes so that pregnancy and birth are tolerated without difficulty. For women with preexisting or underlying heart disease, however, the changes can impose an additional burden on an already compromised heart, which may result in cardiac decompensation and congestive heart failure.

Incidence and Classification

Heart disease complicates about 1% of pregnancies (Cunningham, et al., 1997). Pregnancy may unmask a previously asymptomatic heart condition, or it may aggravate known heart disease.

The two major categories of heart disease are rheumatic heart disease and congenital heart disease. Although rheumatic fever is uncommon in the United States, it is prevalent in less-developed countries, which may be the countries of origin for immigrant women seeking health care in the United States. The incidence of pregnancy complicated by congenital heart disease is increasing because women with congenital heart disease are more likely to survive to reproductive age. A third category, mitral valve prolapse, is a common but benign condition that usually does not cause problems during pregnancy.

Rheumatic Heart Disease

A remarkable decline in rheumatic heart disease has occurred in North America and western Europe as a result of early treatment of streptococcal pharyngitis (strep throat) in childhood, which often precedes the onset of rheumatic fever. Even one bout of rheumatic fever may cause scarring of the valves in the heart. This results in narrowing (stenosis) of the openings between the chambers of the heart.

The mitral valve is the most common site of stenosis. Mitral stenosis obstructs the free flow of blood from the left atrium to the left ventricle. The left atrium becomes dilated. As a result, pressure in the left atrium, pulmonary veins, and pulmonary capillaries is chronically elevated. This elevation may lead to pulmonary hypertension, pulmonary edema, or congestive heart failure. The first warnings of heart failure include persistent rales at the base of the lungs, dyspnea on exertion, cough, and hemoptysis. Progressive edema and tachycardia are additional signs of heart failure.

Congenital Heart Disease

Congenital heart defects can be grouped into those that cause a left-to-right shunt and those resulting in a right-to-left shunt. Those defects that produce left-to-right shunting include atrial and ventricular septal defects and patent ductus arteriosus. In contrast, right-to-left shunting occurs when a cyanotic heart defect such as tetralogy of Fallot is present. Right-to-left shunting also may occur through a septal defect or patent ductus arteriosus when pulmonary vascular resistance exceeds peripheral vascular resistance and pulmonary hypertension (Eisenmenger syndrome) occurs.

Left-to-Right Shunt

Atrial Septal Defect. Atrial septal defect often is first discovered in women of childbearing age because symptoms are absent or vague. This defect produces a left-to-right shunt because pressure in the left side of the heart is higher than in the right side. Pregnancy is well tolerated by patients with an uncomplicated atrial septal defect, and no specific treatment is recommended. Bacterial endocarditis is rare, and prophylactic antibiotics are not required (Caulin-Glaser & Setaro, 1999). Pulmonary hypertension occasionally develops because the additional blood that moves to the right side of the heart is transported to the lungs through the pulmonary artery.

Ventricular Septal Defect. Although ventricular septal defects are more common than atrial septal defects at birth, they usually are detected and corrected before childbearing age. Most women with ventricular septal defects who become pregnant are asymptomatic, but fatigue or symptoms of pulmonary congestion occur occasionally.

Pregnancy is well tolerated with small to moderate left-to-right shunts (Cunningham, et al., 1997). However, pregnancy occasionally precipitates heart failure or an arrhythmia, either of which is managed as in nonpregnant patients. Bacterial endocarditis is common with unrepaired defects, and antibacterial prophylaxis is recommended.

Patent Ductus Arteriosus. The communicating shunt between the pulmonary artery and aorta is usually discovered and treated in childhood. If untreated, the physiologic effects are related to size. If small, this lesion, like septal defects, may be well tolerated during pregnancy unless complicated by pulmonary hypertension. The patent ductus arteriosus tends to become infected, so antibiotic prophylaxis is recommended, particularly at the time of labor.

Right-to-Left Shunt

Tetralogy of Fallot. The primary cause of right-to-left shunting is tetralogy of Fallot, a combination of four defects (ventricular septal defect, pulmonary valve stenosis, right ventricular hypertrophy, and displacement of the aorta toward the right). Untreated patients with tetralogy of Fallot have obvious symptoms of heart disease that include (1) cyanosis, (2) clubbing of the fingers, indicating proliferation of capillaries to transport blood to the extremities, and (3) inability to tolerate activity.

Women who have undergone repair and in whom cyanosis did not reappear may do well during pregnancy. With uncorrected tetralogy of Fallot, maternal mortality approaches 10% (Cunningham, et al., 1997).

Eisenmenger Syndrome. Eisenmenger syndrome can develop in any cardiac lesion if right-to-left shunting occurs because of the development of pulmonary hypertension. The maternal and fetal mortality is high if this syndrome develops (Caulin-Glaser & Setaro, 1999).

Mitral Valve Prolapse

Mitral valve prolapse is one of the most common cardiac conditions among the general population. The incidence among otherwise normal young women is as high as 10% (Caulin-Glaser & Setaro, 1999; Cunningham, et al., 1997). Although the condition appears to be inherited, it is associated with a variety of other cardiac disorders such as atrial septal defects and Marfan's syndrome. In mitral valve prolapse, the leaflets of the mitral valve prolapse into the left atrium during ventricular contraction.

Mitral valve prolapse is considered a benign condition, and most women with mitral valve prolapse are asymptomatic. Some women experience arrhythmias or chest pain. However, most women with mitral valve prolapse tolerate pregnancy well. The condition is considered by some to be a significant risk factor for bacterial endocarditis, and some physicians administer prophylactic antibiotics before and during labor and delivery. If arrhythmia or chest pain occurs, β-blockers such as propranolol hydrochloride (Inderal) are administered to prevent stimulation of myocardial, vascular, and pulmonary receptor sites.

Peripartum and Postpartum Cardiomyopathy

Cardiomyopathy in the peripartum or postpartum period is a rare condition that is exclusively associated with pregnancy. Women with this condition have no underlying heart disease, but symptoms of cardiac decompensation appear during the last weeks of pregnancy or from 2 to 20 weeks postpartum. The symptoms are those of congestive heart failure: dyspnea, edema, weakness, chest pain, and heart palpitations. The condition is treated with digitalis, diuretics, sodium restriction, and prolonged bedrest. Peripartum cardiomyopathy tends to recur with subsequent pregnancies, and prognosis for future pregnancies is related to heart size. Because of its tendency to recur, future pregnancies are generally not advised (Drummond & Troiano, 1998).

Table 26-3

NEW YORK HEART ASSOCIATION FUNCTIONAL CLASSIFICATION OF HEART DISEASE

Class	Description
Class I	Uncompromised. No limitation of physical activity. Asymptomatic with ordinary activity.
Class II	Slightly compromised, requiring slight limitation of physical activity. Comfortable at rest, but ordinary physical activity causes fatigue, dyspnea, palpitations, or anginal pain.
Class III	Marked limitation of physical activity. Comfortable at rest, but less than ordinary activity causes excessive fatigue, palpitation, dyspnea, or anginal pain. Markedly compromised.
Class IV	Inability to perform any physical activity without discomfort. Symptoms of cardiac insufficiency even at rest.

In general, maternal and fetal risks for class I and II disease are small but are greatly increased with class III and IV.

Diagnosis and Classification

Early recognition of underlying heart disease is essential, and careful assessment for specific signs and symptoms of heart disease is part of every initial prenatal visit. Signs and symptoms include dyspnea, syncope (fainting) with exertion, hemoptysis, paroxysmal nocturnal dyspnea, and chest pain with exertion. Additional signs that confirm the diagnosis are (1) cyanosis; (2) clubbing; (3) diastolic, presystolic, or continuous heart murmur; (4) cardiac enlargement; (5) a loud, harsh systolic murmur associated with a thrill; and (6) serious arrhythmias (Shabetai, 1999).

Diagnosis of heart disease may be made from clinical signs and symptoms and physical examination. It often is confirmed by chest radiograph, electrocardiography, or echocardiography.

Once the diagnosis is made, the severity of the disease can be determined by the client's ability to endure physical activity. A clinical classification based on the effect of exercise on the heart has been developed by the New York Heart Association (Table 26-3).

Therapeutic Management

All pregnant women with heart disease should do the following:

- Limit physical activity so that demand does not exceed the functional capacity of the heart. In other words, the woman should remain free of symptoms of cardiac stress, such as dyspnea, chest pain, and tachycardia.
- Avoid excessive weight gain, which increases demands on the heart.
- Prevent anemia, which decreases the oxygen-carrying capacity of the blood and results in a compensatory increase in heart rate. Most anemia is prevented by administration of iron and folic acid.
- Prevent infection. This may include administration of prophylactic antibiotics in women at higher risk for bacterial endocarditis.
- Undergo careful assessment for the development of congestive heart failure, pulmonary edema, and cardiac arrhythmias.

For women with class III or IV heart disease, the primary goal of management is to prevent cardiac decompensation and development of congestive heart failure. Also, every effort is made to protect the fetus from hypoxia and IUGR, which can occur if placental perfusion is inadequate.

Drug Therapy

Anticoagulants. During pregnancy, clotting factors normally increase and thrombolytic activity decreases. These changes predispose the pregnant woman to thrombus formation. Superimposed cardiac problems such as mitral valve stenosis may require anticoagulant therapy during pregnancy. Warfarin is associated with fetal malformations and should be avoided during pregnancy. Heparin, which does not cross the placental barrier, is an effective alternative. Careful monitoring of partial thromboplastin time, activated partial thromboplastin time, and platelets is essential to achieve effective anticoagulation.

Antiarrhythmics. When medication to control arrhythmias is necessary during pregnancy, the effect on the fetus must be considered. Digoxin and quinidine are generally thought to be safe. β-blocker therapy has been successful in late pregnancy, although fetal growth restriction has been noted in early gestation (Caulin-Glaser & Setaro, 1999).

Anti-Infectives. Anti-infectives such as ampicillin and gentamicin may be administered as prophylaxis against bacterial endocarditis.

Diuretics. If possible, diuretics are avoided during pregnancy because they reduce the mother's blood volume and therefore reduce the perfusion of the placenta. Pregnant women who have been taking diuretics before pregnancy for hypertension may be changed to a different antihypertensive drug, or they may remain on the diuretic if their blood pressure control is optimal (Caulin-Glaser & Setaro, 1999).

Intrapartum Management

Every effort is made to minimize the effects of labor on the cardiovascular system. With every contraction, 300 to 500 ml of blood is shifted from the uterus and placenta into the central circulation. This extra fluid causes a sharp rise in cardiac workload. Therefore careful management of IV fluid administration is essential to prevent fluid overload. Central monitoring of her venous pressure and a transcutaneous oxygen saturation monitor provide added information about her cardiopulmonary status at this critical time.

The woman should be positioned on her side, with her head and shoulders elevated. Oxygen is administered to increase the amount of inhaled oxygen available. Sedation and epidural anesthesia are recommended early in labor to reduce discomfort. The environment is kept as quiet and calm as possible to decrease anxiety, which can cause tachycardia.

The fetus is electronically monitored, and nonreassuring fetal signs and maternal signs of cardiac decompensation (tachycardia, rapid respirations, moist rales, exhaustion) should be reported immediately to the physician.

A vaginal delivery produces less trauma and is recommended for a woman with heart disease unless indications for cesarean birth exist. A vacuum extractor or outlet forceps (see Chapter 16) often are used to shorten the second stage of labor and reduce pushing.

The fourth stage of labor is associated with special risks. After delivery of the placenta, about 500 ml of blood is added to the intravascular volume. To minimize the risks of overloading the circulation, the woman's legs are kept level with her body by avoiding the use of stirrups or lowering them during the third stage of labor. In addition, the uterus should not be massaged to expedite separation of the placenta. Careful assessment for signs of circulatory overload, such as a bounding pulse, distended neck and peripheral veins, and moist rales in the lungs, is performed during the third and fourth stages of labor.

Postpartum Management

Women who have shown no evidence of distress during pregnancy, labor, or childbirth may have cardiac decompensation during the postpartum period. The relief of vena caval compression and autotransfusion of blood from the uterus after placental delivery abruptly increases the blood returning to the right side of the heart.

The woman also must be observed closely for signs of infection, hemorrhage, and thromboembolism.

These conditions can act together to precipitate postpartum heart failure in women with underlying heart disease.

If no evidence of cardiac compromise during labor and the early postpartum period exists, breastfeeding usually is not contraindicated.

APPLICATION OF THE NURSING PROCESS: THE PREGNANT WOMAN WITH HEART DISEASE

Assessment

Begin with a review of the woman's medical record to determine the functional classification assigned (Table 26-3). Assess the woman at each prenatal appointment to determine how pregnancy affects the functional capacity of the heart.

CRITICAL TO REMEMBER

Signs and Symptoms of Congestive Heart Failure

- Cough (frequent, productive, hemoptysis)
- Progressive dyspnea with exertion
- Orthopnea
- Pitting edema of legs and feet or generalized edema of face, hands, or sacral area
- Palpitations of heart
- Progressive fatigue or syncope with exertion
- Moist rales in lower lobes, indicating pulmonary edema

- Take vital signs and compare them with preconception levels. Note any changes since the last prenatal appointment.

Table 26-4
OTHER CONDITIONS AND THEIR EFFECT ON PREGNANCY

Condition	Maternal-Fetal Effects	Nursing Considerations
APPENDICITIS		
Inflammation of the appendix. The most common nongynecologic surgical emergency during pregnancy.	Is difficult to diagnose during pregnancy. Early symptoms mimic common conditions of pregnancy. Ultrasonography may help rule out other diagnoses such as ectopic pregnancy.	When reasonable doubt exists that the patient has appendicitis, the appendix should be removed to prevent rupture and consequent complications. The location often is altered by the growing uterus.
ASTHMA		
An obstructive lung disease caused by airway inflammation. Characterized by dyspnea, cough, wheezing. Course in pregnancy is variable.	Effective therapy and avoidance of severe attacks are associated with a good pregnancy outcome. Medications used are well tolerated in pregnancy and appear to be safe for the fetus. Breastfeeding is safe for the newborn and may reduce the risk for allergies.	Early use of antiinflammatory agents such as inhaled corticosteroids may prevent severe attacks. Outpatient use of β-agonists often controls mild asthma.
GLUCOSE-6-PHOSPHATE DEHYDROGENASE DEFICIENCY		
Female-linked genetic disorder that predisposes to lysis of red blood cells when exposed to oxidizing drugs (salicylates, acetaminophen, phenacetin, and some sulfa drugs) and ingestion of fava beans in some people.	Is not affected by pregnancy unless complicated by anemia. Iron and folic acid supplementation is recommended. Newborn males have a higher incidence of severe jaundice.	Advise client of risks and suggest she consult with her health care provider for recommended list of drugs for minor discomforts.
HYPERTHYROIDISM		
An overactive, enlarged thyroid gland that is difficult to diagnose and manage during pregnancy because the normal changes of pregnancy increase the metabolic rate and mimic hyperthyroidism. Graves' disease is the most common cause during pregnancy.	Increased incidence of pregnancy-induced hypertension and postpartum hemorrhage if not well controlled during pregnancy. Treatment is complicated by the presence of the fetus, which may be jeopardized by surgery or antithyroid medications. Propylthiouracil has limited placental transfer and is widely used during pregnancy to control thyroid function.	Be aware of the major signs that should be reported. These include a resting pulse rate greater than 100/min, loss of weight or failure to gain weight in spite of normal intake of food, heat intolerance, and abnormal protrusion of the eyes (exophthalmos).

Continued

Table 26-4
OTHER CONDITIONS AND THEIR EFFECT ON PREGNANCY—cont'd

Condition	Maternal-Fetal Effects	Nursing Considerations
HYPOTHYROIDISM		
Characterized by inadequate thyroid secretion; confirmed by an elevated level of thyroid-stimulating hormone and low levels of triiodothyronine and thyroxine.	Women with hypothyroidism have a higher incidence of preeclampsia, abruptio placentae, and low-birth-weight or stillborn infants. If the expectant mother is untreated, there is an increased risk of neonatal goiter and congenital hypothyroidism; severity of symptoms depend on time of onset and severity of the deprivation but may include neurologic deficits. Treatment is with levothyroxine.	Suspect neonatal hypothyroidism when the infant is large for gestational age, with respiratory and feeding difficulties, rough and dry skin, and an umbilical hernia.
MATERNAL PHENYLKETONURIA (PKU)		
Inherited single-gene recessive defect leading to an inability to metabolize the essential amino acid phenylalanine, resulting in high serum levels of phenylalanine. Irreparable mental retardation occurs if the pregnant woman is not treated early with a diet that provides adequate protein but restricts phenylalanine.	The woman must be on a low-phenylalanine diet before conception and pregnancy. If not, the fetal risk for microcephaly, mental retardation, heart defects, and intraunterine growth restriction increases.	The child either will be a carrier of the gene or inherit the disease, depending on the presence of the gene in the father of the child. Special low-phenylalanine foods are expensive, but they may be obtained through the state's Supplemental Food Program for Women, Infants and Children (WIC), Medicaid, or may be covered by insurance.

- Assess the level of fatigue and any changes in fatigue since the last prenatal appointment. This is especially important when fluid volume peaks and the chance of cardiac decompensation is greatest (18 to 32 weeks' gestation).
- Observe for signs or symptoms of congestive heart failure.
- Note additional factors that may increase the workload of the heart (anemia, infections, anxiety, lack of adequate support to manage the activities of daily living).
- Weigh the client and compare the desired and actual patterns of weight gain to detect excessive weight gain or fluid retention.
- Assess the woman's knowledge of the prescribed regimen of care and her ability to comply with it.

Analysis

The pregnant woman with a cardiac defect may be unable to tolerate activity to the same degree as before pregnancy because of the stress imposed on the cardiovascular system. Arriving at the nursing diagnosis "Activity Intolerance related to insufficient knowledge of measures that reduce cardiac stress" is a priority.

Planning

Goals and outcomes are as follows:

- The woman (and her family) will identify factors that increase cardiac workload.
- They will describe measures that promote adaptation to activity restrictions.

Interventions

Prenatal nursing care focuses on teaching the woman and her family about the possible effects of the disease on their lives. This teaching may include specific instructions about factors increasing the workload of the heart and measures promoting adaptation to restrictions in activity.

Teaching about Increased Cardiac Workload

Excessive Weight Gain and Anemia. Excessive weight gain and anemia increase the workload of the heart just as they do in the nonpregnant state and should be avoided. A well-balanced diet that contains approximately 2200 calories is recommended, with adequate high-quality protein. Emphasize the importance of taking any prescribed iron supplements to prevent anemia and reduce the risk of tachycardia. Folic acid should be taken from before conception to avoid anemia and reduce the risk for neural tube defects in the fetus.

Exertion. Instruct the woman to modify approaches to activities to regulate energy expenditures and reduce cardiac workload. For example, she might take rest periods during the day and for an hour after meals. If possible, she should sit rather than stand when performing activities. She should rest every few minutes when performing an activity that increases the heart rate to allow the heart time to recover. Emphasize that she should stop an activity if she experiences dyspnea, chest pain, or tachycardia.

Exposure. Instruct the woman to avoid unnecessary exposure to environmental extremes. She should dress warmly during cold weather and create a barrier to cold temperatures by wearing layers of clothing. She must become aware that exertion in hot, humid weather or during extreme cold weather places additional demands on the heart and should be avoided.

Emotional Stress. Help the woman to identify areas of stress in her life, if applicable, and explain the effects of emotional stress on the cardiovascular system (increased blood pressure, heart rate, and respiratory rate). Discuss various methods for stress management, such as meditation, progressive relaxation of muscles, and biofeedback. Teach that cigarette smoking and use of illicit drugs such as cocaine and amphetamines greatly increase stress on the heart.

Helping the Family Accept Restrictions on Activity

Assist family members to accept the need for activity restriction. The amount of activity that can be tolerated depends on the severity of the disease. However, all women with heart disease require 8 to 10 hours of sleep each night, with a period of morning and afternoon rest. For some women, complete bedrest (with bathroom privileges only) is necessary during the last half of pregnancy, and this may create special problems for the family. Nurses often help family members plan ways to meet their needs while the expectant mother remains on bedrest. See the Nursing Care Plan for Preterm Labor (Chapter 27) for additional interventions when a prolonged period of bedrest is required.

Providing Postpartum Care

After childbirth, the mother may be unable to assume care of the newborn, especially after a prolonged period of bedrest. However, every effort should be made to promote contact between the mother and baby. Many nurses assess the baby and perform the necessary newborn care at the bedside, then allow the mother ample time to hold the infant. The father and other family members should be included in the care of the infant whenever possible.

The decision about breastfeeding will be individualized according to the mother's condition and its demands on her energy. She should be encouraged to feed the infant whenever possible to promote maternal-infant attachment, even if she feeds formula. Consult with physicians, and make referrals as necessary for follow-up care, which may include home care by a nurse or nursing assistant. Be certain that the family understands the signs and symptoms of cardiac complications and when to notify the physician that problems have developed.

Evaluation

The ability to identify the factors increasing cardiac workload offers reassurance that the woman and her family will initiate measures promoting adaptation to restricted activity.

Check Your Reading

8. How do the cardiovascular changes of pregnancy affect the condition of the woman who has a cardiac defect?
9. What are the two major categories of heart disease? What is the functional classification of heart disease?
10. What are the primary goals for management of heart disease in terms of diet, activity, and weight gain?
11. Why must the administration of fluids be monitored closely during labor?
12. Why is the fourth stage of labor particularly dangerous for the woman with heart disease?

ANEMIAS

Anemia is a condition in which a decline in circulating red blood cell mass occurs, which reduces the capacity to carry oxygen to the vital organs of the mother or fetus. During pregnancy and the puerperium, anemia is defined as a hemoglobin concentration of less than 10.5 to 11.0 g/dl (Kilpatrick & Laros, 1999).

Anemia is one of the most common problems of pregnancy. An estimated 20% to 60% of women will be anemic at some time during pregnancy (Kilpatrick & Laros, 1999). The incidence varies according to geographic location and socioeconomic group. Anemia may be caused by a variety of factors including nutrition, hemolysis, and blood loss. The most common types of anemia observed during pregnancy include iron-deficiency anemia, folic acid–deficiency anemia, sickle cell disease, and thalassemia.

Iron-Deficiency Anemia

The total iron requirement for a typical pregnancy with a single fetus is approximately 1000 mg (Cunningham, et al., 1997). Unfortunately, most women do not have iron stores that equal this amount. Furthermore, meeting pregnancy needs by diet alone is difficult, although iron is present in many foods. The primary sources are meat, fish, chicken, liver, and green leafy vegetables.

Maternal Effects

Signs and symptoms of iron-deficiency anemia include pallor, fatigue, lethargy, and headache. Clinical findings also may include inflammations of the lips and tongue. Pica (consuming nonfood substances such as clay, dirt, ice, and starch) also is a sign of iron-deficiency anemia (Kilpatrick & Laros, 1999). Laboratory findings for iron-deficiency anemia include red blood cells that are *microcytic* (small) and *hypochromic* (pale). The plasma iron and serum ferritin are low, whereas the total iron-binding capacity is higher than normal.

Fetal and Neonatal Effects

The effects of maternal iron-deficiency anemia on the fetus and neonate are unclear. In general, even with significant maternal iron deficiency, the fetus will receive adequate stores at a cost to the mother. If the mother is severely anemic, the fetus may have reduced red cell volume, hemoglobin, and iron stores. Profound maternal anemia can reduce fetal oxygen supply (Kilpatrick & Laros, 1999).

Therapeutic Management

Iron replacement is easily achieved in most patients with administration of ferrous sulfate tablets, 320 mg, 1 to 3 times per day. Giving the iron with a citrus drink or 500 mg ascorbic acid is believed to improve iron absorption from the gastrointestinal tract. Many women experience less gastrointestinal discomfort if iron is taken with meals, although doing so reduces absorption somewhat. Therapy often is continued for about 3 months after the anemia has been corrected. Parenteral therapy may be necessary if the woman cannot take oral preparations.

Folic Acid–Deficiency (Megaloblastic) Anemia

Folic acid, which functions as a coenzyme in the synthesis of deoxyribonucleic acid (DNA), is essential for cell duplication and fetal and placental growth. It also is an essential nutrient for the formation of red blood cells.

Maternal Effects

Maternal needs for folic acid double during pregnancy in response to the demand for greater production of erythrocytes and fetal and placental growth. A deficiency in folic acid results in a reduction in the rate of DNA synthesis and mitotic activity of individual cells, resulting in the presence of large, immature erythrocytes (megaloblasts). Folate deficiency is the primary cause of megaloblastic anemia during pregnancy.

Nonnutritional factors that contribute to folic acid deficiency include hemolytic anemias with increased red blood cell turnover, some medications such as phenytoin (Dilantin), and malabsorption entities. Folic acid deficiency often is present in association with iron-deficiency anemia.

Fetal and Neonatal Effects

Folate deficiency is associated with increased risk of spontaneous abortion, abruptio placentae, and fetal anomalies. A known association exists between folic acid–deficiency and an increase in neural tube defects.

Therapeutic Management

The recommended daily allowance for folic acid doubles during pregnancy, and some women have difficulty ingesting the amount needed even though it does occur widely in foods. The best sources of folic acid are liver, kidney beans, lima beans, and fresh, dark-green, leafy vegetables (see Table 9-5). Folic acid often is destroyed in cooking. As a result of the awareness of the association between folic acid deficiency and neural tube defects, it is now recommended that all women of childbearing age take 400 mcg (0.4 mg) of folic acid daily to reduce this risk. This supplementation should be increased to 600 mcg (0.6 mg) when pregnancy is confirmed. Most prenatal vitamins contain 1 mg folate to ensure sufficient intake. Higher doses of folate may be ordered according to individual needs.

Check Your Reading

13. Why is supplemental iron needed by most women who are pregnant?
14. What are the neonatal effects of iron-deficiency anemia?
15. What are the fetal and neonatal effects of folic acid deficiency?

Sickle Cell Disease

Sickle cell disease is an autosomal recessive genetic disorder. It occurs when the gene for the production of hemoglobin S is inherited from both parents. The defect in the hemoglobin causes erythrocytes to become shaped like a sickle, or crescent, under certain conditions. Low oxygen concentration usually causes the sickling, with acidosis and dehydration worsening the process. At first, the erythrocytes regain their normal shape, but eventually they remain permanently sickled. Because of their distorted shape, the erythrocytes cannot pass through small arteries and capillaries and tend to clump together and occlude the blood vessel.

The disease is characterized by chronic anemia, increased susceptibility to infection, and periodic episodes of obstruction of blood vessels by the abnormally shaped erythrocytes. Sickle cell disease occurs most often in people of African-American or Mediterranean ancestry. The incidence is 1 in 2000 persons in African-Americans (Nuwayhid, Nguyen, & Khalife, 1998).

Maternal Effects

Pregnancy may exacerbate sickle cell disease and bring on *sickle cell crisis.* This broad term includes several different conditions, particularly temporary cessation of bone marrow function, hemolytic crisis with massive erythrocyte destruction resulting in jaundice, and severe pain caused by infarctions located in the joints and the major organs. In addition, expectant mothers with sickle cell anemia are prone to pyelonephritis, bone infection, and heart disease.

Fetal and Neonatal Effects

The fetus is prone to serious complications including prematurity and IUGR. The incidence of fetal death is particularly high in the presence of maternal sickle cell crisis.

Therapeutic Management

Women with sickle cell disease should seek preconception or early prenatal care and be informed of the maternal and fetal risks associated with the pregnancy. Frequent evaluations of hemoglobin, complete blood count, serum iron, total iron-binding capacity, and serum folate are necessary to determine the degree of anemia and iron and folic acid stores.

Fetal surveillance studies (ultrasonography, nonstress tests, biophysical profiles) are necessary to assess fetal growth and development and placental function. A newer investigational treatment is to give the woman prophylactic transfusions during pregnancy. The objectives are to raise her hemoglobin level and reduce the total amount of abnormal hemoglobin S in her intravascular system. The risks of prophylactic transfusions are that the woman may have a transfusion reaction and she is likely to develop higher levels of antibodies to cells in the transfused blood. This means that it will become more difficult to find compatible blood for transfusion in the future.

The goal of nursing management is to help the pregnant woman maintain a healthy status and avoid hospitalization. Women must be encouraged to keep all prenatal care appointments, usually at least every other week. Topics in prenatal education include the need (1) to maintain adequate hydration to prevent sickling, (2) for adequate nutrition to meet metabolic needs, (3) for folic acid supplementation for erythrocyte production, (4) for rest periods throughout the day and good hygiene practices and the avoidance of persons with infectious illnesses, and (5) for prompt treatment for fever or other signs of infection.

Nurses must be alert for signs of sickle cell crisis. The most common indications are pain in the abdomen, chest, vertebrae, joints, or extremities; pallor; and signs of cardiac failure. Nurses also must provide comfort measures such as repositioning, good skin care, assisting with ambulation and movement in bed, and assisting the woman to splint the abdomen with a pillow when she must cough or breathe deeply.

Nurses must remember that pain is not always related to the sickling crisis but could be related to a complication of pregnancy. Women with sickle cell disease also can have ectopic pregnancy, abruptio placentae, appendicitis, and other painful complications not related to their blood disorder.

Intrapartum care focuses on preventing the development of sickle cell crisis. Oxygen is administered continuously, and fluids should be administered to prevent dehydration because hypoxemia, dehydration, exertion, infection, and acidosis stimulate the sickling process.

Thalassemia

Like sickle-cell anemia, thalassemia is a genetic disorder that involves the abnormal synthesis of α or β chains of hemoglobin. This abnormal synthesis leads to alterations in the red blood cell membrane and decreased life span of red blood cells. Thalassemia is named and classified by the type of chain that is abnormal. β-thalassemia is most frequently encountered in the United States. *β-thalassemia minor* refers to the heterozygous form that results from the inheritance of one abnormal gene from either parent. *β-thalassemia major* refers to inheritance of the gene from both parents (homozygous form). Females with *β-thalassemia major (Cooley's anemia)* usually die in childhood or adolescence. Those females who survive adolescence are often sterile (Cunningham, et al., 1997). β-thalassemia is most often found in those people of Mediterranean and Asian (particularly Chinese) origin.

Maternal Effects

Women with β-thalassemia minor often are mildly anemic but otherwise healthy. Laboratory values normally associated with β-thalassemia minor indicate a mild hypochromic and microcytic anemia. Large amounts of iron usually are not given despite the anemia because persons with β-thalassemia absorb and store iron in their bodies excessively and must take a chelating agent to rid the excess (Kotter & Osguthorpe, 2000; Honig, 2000).

Fetal and Neonatal Effects

Controversy exists regarding whether this disorder is associated with increased fetal or neonatal morbidity. There appears to be no increase in prematurity, low-birth-weight infants, or abnormal size for gestation. The fetus may inherit the serious problem of β-thalassemia major.

Therapeutic Management

No specific therapy for β-thalassemia minor during pregnancy exists. Generally, the outcomes for the mother and fetus are satisfactory (Cunningham, et al., 1997). Infections, which depress production of red blood cells and accelerate erythrocyte destruction, should be identified and treated promptly.

Check Your Reading

16. What are the maternal effects of sickle cell disease?
17. How is sickle cell disease treated during pregnancy?
18. Why is iron supplementation often not recommended for women with thalassemia?

MEDICAL CONDITIONS

Women with a preexisting medical condition should be aware of the effects that pregnancy will have on their conditions as well as the impact of their medical conditions on pregnancy outcome. Some conditions that complicate pregnancy are discussed in this section.

Immune-Complex Diseases

Systemic Lupus Erythematosus

Systemic lupus erythematosus (SLE) is a chronic, inflammatory, autoimmune disease that can affect any organ or system in the body. Although the cause is unknown, an imbalance appears to exist between immune response and tolerance of specific antigens in which the body produces antibodies to its own cells and tissue. Signs and symptoms result from inflammation of multiple organ systems, especially the joints, skin, kidneys, and nervous system. The most common signs and symptoms are joint pain, photosensitivity, and a characteristic "butterfly rash" on the face, which may be less apparent because of the pigmentation changes of pregnancy. The disease is marked by episodes of exacerbation (flares), when the symptoms become worse, and quiescence, when the symptoms recede.

The disease tends to affect young women but may occur in any age group. Females are affected more than 10 times as often as men. The incidence is approximately 1 per 1000 persons. SLE is more common in African-Americans.

The pregnant woman with SLE has an increased incidence of abortion and fetal death during the first trimester. After the first trimester, the prognosis for a live birth is as high as 90% if no active disease exists, but it may fall to 50% if hypertensive renal disease is present. The most serious potential complication for the neonate is a congenital heart block, which usually is permanent and will require a pacemaker (Shiffman & Josimovich, 2000).

Antiphospholipid Syndrome

Antiphospholipid syndrome is an autoimmune condition characterized by the production of antiphospholipid antibodies combined with certain clinical features. The most specific clinical features include arterial and venous thrombosis, decreased platelets, and pregnancy loss. Pregnancy complications that are more common with antiphospholipid syndrome include early-onset preeclampsia, intrauterine growth restriction, and preterm birth.

Although the syndrome occurs most often in women with other underlying autoimmune diseases such as SLE, it also is diagnosed in women with no other recognizable autoimmune disease.

Women with antiphospholipid syndrome should be informed of the potential maternal and obstetric problems, including a possible risk of stroke. They should be assessed for evidence of anemia, thrombocytopenia, and underlying renal disease. Some physicians believe that treatment with heparin may be warranted on the basis of increased risk for thrombosis, even in women with no previous clotting problems. Combinations of low-dose aspirin and subcutaneous heparin sometimes are recommended.

Rheumatoid Arthritis

Rheumatoid arthritis is a chronic inflammatory disease that usually affects the synovial (hinged) joints. Although the cause is unknown, an autoimmune mechanism is suspected. It is strongly associated with rheumatoid factor, an autoantibody present in 80% to 90% of patients with inflammatory rheumatoid arthritis (de Swiet, 1999). It occurs in 1% to 2% of the population and affects females two to three times more frequently than males (Gladman & Urowitz, 1999).

Marked improvement in symptoms of rheumatoid arthritis often occurs during pregnancy. The exact reason is unclear, but improvement is reported to parallel the rise in pregnancy-specific protein, which suppresses inflammatory reactions. Hormonal factors also have been suggested. For instance, increased levels of cortisol, estrogen, and progesterone may be beneficial in suppressing the immune response. Unfortunately, most women relapse within 6 weeks to 6 months postpartum.

In contrast to SLE, the risk of abortion does not increase in women with rheumatoid arthritis. Usually, obstetric problems do not occur at delivery unless the hips or cervical spine are significantly deteriorated (Gladman & Urowitz, 1999).

Neurologic Disorders

Seizure Disorders

Convulsive seizures are the most common form of epilepsy, which is a recurrent disorder of cerebral function. Epilepsy occurs in 0.3% to 0.6% of pregnant women (Aminoff, 1999).

The effect of pregnancy on the course of epilepsy is variable and unpredictable. The frequency of seizures may increase, decrease, or remain the same. In general, the longer the woman has been seizure free before pregnancy, the less likely she is to develop seizures during pregnancy. Women with epilepsy have a higher-than-normal incidence of stillbirth, and some studies have shown a higher incidence of preterm labor.

Maternal bleeding may occur due to a deficiency of clotting factors associated with anticonvulsant drugs such as diphenylhydantoin, or hydantonin, (Dilantin) and phenobarbital. Anticonvulsant drugs also compete with folate for absorption, which may result in folate deficiency.

A major concern is the teratogenic effects of anticonvulsant drugs. A specific syndrome known as *fetal hydantoin syndrome* has been described that includes craniofacial abnormalities, limb reduction defects, growth restriction, mental retardation, and cardiac anomalies. Other anticonvulsants such as trimethadione, paramethadione, and carbamazepine also are associated with malformation syndromes. The teratogenic effects of phenobarbital are difficult to assess because it often is combined with other drugs.

Health professionals should recommend that the woman consult a neurologist before conception. The goal of treatment is to prevent generalized (grand mal) seizures and also reduce the adverse effects of anticonvulsant medications. The family must be made aware of the risks involved when anticonvulsant drugs must be used. They also should realize that treatment cannot be stopped during pregnancy unless the woman has been seizure free for a prolonged time. Grand mal seizures result in fetal hypoxia and acidosis and thus pose a serious problem for the fetus.

Bell's Palsy

Bell's palsy is a sudden unilateral neuropathy of the seventh cranial (facial) nerve that causes facial paralysis with weakness of the forehead and lower face. It is thought to be caused by a virus. It is three times more common during pregnancy and generally occurs in the third trimester. Although the reason for the increase during pregnancy is unknown, one theory suggests that estrogen-induced edema puts pressure on the facial nerve, making the pregnant woman more vulnerable to the disease. Pregnancy does not affect recovery rate, and nearly 90% of women will recover function within a few weeks to months (Aminoff, 1999).

The face feels stiff and pulled to one side. Closing the eye on the affected side may be difficult or impossible. Difficulty with eating or fine facial movements may occur. The ability to taste also may be disturbed.

Treatment is controversial. However, many physicians prescribe steroids within the first few days. Supportive care may include patching the eye and applying ointment or eye drops to prevent dryness or injury to the exposed cornea. Facial massage may be helpful, and the woman should be cautioned to chew carefully. Psychological support is necessary to assist the woman and her family deal with anxiety they naturally feel when sudden paralysis of the face occurs. They must be reassured that the condition usually is temporary.

Check Your Reading

19. What are the maternal and fetal effects of SLE?
20. In what ways does pregnancy affect rheumatoid arthritis?
21. What is the major concern about administering anticonvulsant drugs for the woman with epilepsy?
22. What is the recommended supportive care for those with Bell's palsy?

TRAUMA IN PREGNANCY

Blunt Force Injuries

Automobile accidents cause most blunt force injuries to the pregnant woman. Maternal deaths are most often caused by head injury or intraabdominal hemorrhage. Fetal death may be secondary to maternal death or follow sudden premature separation of the placenta or rupture of the uterus. Fetal loss occurs in at least 40% of critically injured women, but the pregnancy outcome is poor in at least 4% of women even when maternal injuries are minor (Bobroski, 1999). Pelvic fracture also is a commonly reported nonfatal injury in automobile accidents, falls, and domestic violence.

During the first trimester, the fetus is protected from external forces by the bony pelvis, amniotic fluid, and soft tissue surrounding the pelvis. Later in pregnancy, the fetal compartment extends beyond the bony pelvis, and as a result the fetus is more vulnerable to blunt force injury. Fetal injury may include skull fracture and intracranial hemorrhage. In addition, disruption of uteroplacental blood flow because of premature separation of the placenta can result in fetal anoxia.

Use of seat belt restraints significantly improves maternal and fetal outcomes in automobile accidents. Current recommendations are that the pregnant woman wear three-point restraint seat belts during automobile travel, with the lap belt under her protruding abdomen.

Penetrating Injuries

Gunshot and knife wounds are the most common penetrating injuries and may be associated with assaults or suicide attempts. Mortality rates from penetrating wounds in the pregnant woman are less than those in nonpregnant women because the uterus acts as a shield for the abdominal structure (Daddario, 1998; Gonik, 1999). The fetus fares less well, with high injury and mortality rates.

Therapeutic Management

Initial management of trauma in pregnancy is similar to that in the nonpregnant state. Primary goals are evaluation and stabilization of maternal injuries. Basic rules are applied to resuscitation, including establishing ventilation and arrest of hemorrhage. During attempted resuscitation, however, prolonged supine positioning

Table 26-5

SEXUALLY TRANSMITTED DISEASES AND VAGINAL INFECTIONS: THEIR IMPACT ON PREGNANCY

Maternal, Fetal, and Neonatal Effects	Nursing Considerations
SEXUALLY TRANSMITTED DISEASES	
Syphilis (Causative Organism: Spirochete Treponema pallidum)	
If untreated, the infection may be passed across the placenta to the fetus and result in spontaneous abortion, a stillborn infant, premature labor and birth, or congenital syphilis. Major signs of congenital syphilis are enlarged liver and spleen, skin lesions, rashes, osteitis, pneumonia, and hepatitis.	Penicillin is the only treatment that will cure the disease without harming the fetus. Women who are allergic are desensitized to penicillin and then treated (CDC, 1998a).
Gonorrhea (Causative Organism: Bacterium Neisseria gonorrhoeae)	
Not transmitted via the placenta; vertical transmission from mother to newborn during birth may cause ophthalmia neonatorium. Endocervicitis and weakness of the fetal membranes increase the risk of premature rupture of membranes and preterm labor.	Dual treatment for chlamydia recommended because chlamydia infection also is present in 20% to 40% of those infected with gonococcus. A cephalosporin or spectinomycin is given for the gonococcal infection and either erythromycin or amoxicillin is recommended for the presumptive or diagnosed chlamydia infection (CDC, 1998a).
Chlamydial Infection (Causative Organism: Bacterium Chlamydia trachomatis)	
The fetus may be infected during birth and suffer neonatal conjunctivitis or pneumonitis, which manifests within 4 to 6 weeks. Conjunctivitis is prevented by erythromycin ophthalmic ointment. Chlamydia also may be responsible for premature rupture of membranes, chorioamnionitis, and premature labor.	Chlamydia is the most common sexually transmissible disease in the United States, and infection usually is asymptomatic. Both partners should be treated to prevent recurrent infection. As with all sexually transmitted diseases, the use of condoms decreases the risk of infection. Erythromycin or amoxicillin are recommended treatments (CDC, 1998a).
Trichomoniasis (Causative Organism: Protozoan Trichomonas vaginalis)	
Is not transmitted across the placental barrier; organism cannot survive in the infantile, nonestrogenized vagina. Associated with premature rupture of membranes and postpartum endometritis.	Metronidazole (Flagyl) 2 g in a single dose is recommended (CDC, 1998a). Some clinicians prefer to delay treatment until the second trimester because of concerns about fetal teratogenicity, although the drug has been used at this time without apparent problems (Pedler & Orr, 2000). Clotrimazole may provide relief of symptoms during first trimester.
Condyloma Acuminatum (Causative Organism: Human Papillomavirus)	
Transmission of condyloma acuminatum, also called venereal warts, may occur during vaginal birth and is associated with the development of epithelial tumors of the mucous membranes of the larynx in children. Pregnancy can cause proliferation of lesions, which are associated with cervical dysplasia and cancer. Large lesions can obstruct labor.	Podophyllin, imquimod, and podofilox should not be used during pregnancy because of the possible teratogenic effects. Applications of trichloracetic acid or removal by electrocoagulation, electrodessication, or laser is recommended instead (Peiris and Madeley, 2000).
VAGINAL INFECTIONS	
Candidiasis (Causative Organism: Yeast Candida albicans)	
Oral candidiasis (thrush) may develop in newborns if infection is present at birth. Thrush is treated with application of nystatin (Mycostatin) over the surfaces of the oral cavity four times a day for several days. Characteristic "cottage cheese" vaginal discharge with vulvar pruritus, burning, and dyspareunia. Vulva may be red, tender, and edematous.	Candidiasis is a persistent problem for many women during pregnancy. Effective treatment may be obtained with miconazole (Monistat), terconazole (Terazole), butoconazole (Femstat), and clotrimazole (Gyne-Lotrimin). Many experts recommend treating candidiasis for 7 days during pregnancy (CDC, 1998a).
Bacterial Vaginosis	
Has been associated with premature rupture of membranes, preterm birth, and low birth weight. May be associated with postpartum endometritis. Is marked by a shift in vaginal flora from the normal predominance of lactobacilli to a predominance of anerobic bacteria. Causes profuse, malodorous, "fishy" vaginal discharge, itching, and burning, although many are asymptomatic.	The causative organism is sensitive to metronidazole and clindamycin. Metronidazole may be delayed until the second trimester to avoid concerns about possible fetal teratogenicity.

Table 26-6
URINARY TRACT INFECTIONS AND THEIR EFFECTS ON PREGNANCY

Maternal, Fetal, and Neonatal Effects	Nursing Considerations
Asymptomatic Bacteriuria (Causative Organisms: Escherichia coli, Klebsiella, Proteus)	Treatment with sulfonamides, ampicillin, or nitrofurantoin is sufficient for most women. Follow-up urine cultures identify adequate treatment. Stress hygienic measures with the woman and the need to take all the medication as prescribed although symptoms are absent. Explain the importance of follow-up urine cultures.
Cystitis (Causative Organisms: E. coli, Klebsiella, Proteus) Signs and symptoms include dysuria, frequency, urgency, and suprapubic tenderness. Ascending infection may lead to pyelonephritis.	Treatment is the same as for asymptomatic bacteriuria. Provide information about hygiene measures. Stress the importance of taking all the medication prescribed even if the symptoms abate.
Acute Pyelonephritis (Causative Organisms: E. coli, Klebsiella, Proteus) Increased risk of preterm labor and premature delivery. Maternal complications include septic shock and adult respiratory distress syndrome.	Inform women with asymptomatic bacteriuria or cystitis of signs and symptoms, such as sudden onset of fever, chills, flank pain or tenderness, nausea, and vomiting, so that treatment can begin promptly. Usually hospitalized for intravenous administration of antibiotics.

should be avoided so that compression of the large blood vessels can be minimized. Lateral displacement of the uterus can be accomplished by placing a wedge along the right side of the woman. In addition, the need for large amounts of fluid replacement should be anticipated. After resuscitation, evaluation is continued for neurologic injuries, fractures, bleeding sites, and internal injuries. Exploratory abdominal surgery may be necessary to identify and control internal bleeding. The uterus and fetus must also be evaluated for injuries. Rh immune globulin (RhoGAM) will be given if a fetal-to-maternal hemorrhage is suspected in the $Rh_O(D)$-negative mother.

Electronic fetal monitoring may reflect the condition of the mother as well as that of the fetus. For example, although the mother is stable, electronic monitoring may detect signs of early maternal hypovolemia or premature separation of the placenta, such as uterine contractions, fetal tachycardia, and late decelerations. The duration of fetal monitoring varies according to the severity of the trauma.

The necessity for cesarean delivery of a live fetus depends on several factors, including the age of the fetus, fetal condition, and extent of uterine injury. Because placental abruption usually develops soon after trauma, electronic monitoring is begun as soon as the maternal condition is stabilized. It is continued as long as signs of uterine contractions, vaginal bleeding, uterine tenderness, and ruptured membranes exist.

INFECTIONS DURING PREGNANCY

A number of different infections can adversely affect the health of the fetus, mother, or both when acquired during pregnancy. Some infections are mild or even subclinical in the mother yet may cause severe birth defects or death of the fetus. Other infections may have adverse effects by increasing the risk for other pregnancy complications such as preterm labor. Some infections are transmitted primarily or exclusively by sexual means, whereas others may be transmitted in this way but also by other avenues.

The wide variety of infections affecting pregnancy care are divided into those caused by viruses and those caused by other organisms. Table 26-5 presents nursing considerations of major sexually transmissible diseases and vaginal infections. Table 26-6 summarizes urinary tract infections and their effect on pregnancy. (See also Chapter 33 for infection in the nonpregnant woman.)

Viral Infections

Pregnancy does not worsen the effects of most viral infections in the woman. However, although viral infections often are mild or even asymptomatic in adults, fetal and neonatal consequences can be catastrophic. Maternal infection with cytomegalovirus, rubella, varicella-zoster virus, herpes simplex, hepatitis B, and human immunodeficiency virus (HIV) have the greatest potential for harm to the fetus or newborn.

Cytomegalovirus

Cytomegalovirus (CMV), a member of the herpesvirus group, is widespread and eventually infects most humans. CMV has been isolated from urine, saliva, blood, cervical mucus, semen, breast milk, and stool. Transmission may occur from contamination with any of these fluids. The highest rate of infection occurs between the ages of 15 and 35 years, so the possibility of CMV infection occurring during pregnancy is high.

After primary infection, the virus becomes latent, but like other herpesvirus infections, periodic reactivation and shedding of the virus may occur. Seroconversion and a rise in the specific IgM antibody titer can detect a primary infection that has occurred within the past 4 to 8 months. Isolation of the virus in culture identifies infection but does not distinguish whether the infection is primary or recurrent (Gibbs & Sweet, 1999; Landry, 1999). However, most infections are asymptomatic, so they may not be suspected during pregnancy and no testing may be done. Diagnosis of neonatal infection is by urine culture.

Fetal and Neonatal Effects. Up to 2% of all live neonates may be infected with the virus at birth, and about 10% of these infected infants are affected at birth. The more severe effects include deafness, mental retardation, seizures, blindness, and dental abnormalities. Some effects of CMV infection may not be obvious for several months or even years. Infected infants shed the virus from the nasopharynx and urine for several years after birth and thus are a significant reservoir of infection for uninfected caregivers and family (Landry, 1999).

Therapeutic Management. No effective therapy is currently available for the treatment of congenital infection. Gancyclovir has been used in the treatment of congenitally infected infants, but little data are available to support its use during pregnancy. Prenatal diagnosis of cytomegalovirus infection of the fetus is not yet a reality for routine use (Peiris & Madeley, 2000).

Rubella

Rubella is caused by a virus transmitted from person to person by droplets or through direct contact with articles contaminated with nasopharyngeal secretions. Rubella is a mild disease. Major symptoms include fever, general malaise, and a characteristic maculopapular rash that begins on the face and migrates over the body. Although the overall incidence has declined since rubella vaccine became available, up to 10% of adults in the United States remain susceptible (Landry, 1999).

Fetal and Neonatal Effects. Rubella is a serious concern because the virus can cross the placental barrier and infect the fetus at any time during pregnancy. The greatest risk to the fetus occurs during the first trimester, when fetal organs are developing. If maternal infection occurs during this time, approximately one third of these cases will result in spontaneous abortions and the surviving fetuses may be seriously compromised. Deafness, mental retardation, cataracts, cardiac defects, IUGR, and microcephaly are the most common fetal complications. In addition, infants born to mothers who had rubella during pregnancy shed the virus for many months and thus pose a threat to other infants and susceptible adults who come in contact with them.

Therapeutic Management. Prevention is the only effective protection for the fetus. A Healthy People 2010 objective is to reduce the number of congenital rubella syndrome cases to zero through immunization of susceptible individuals. Women who are immune do not become infected, so determining the immune status of all women of childbearing age is critical. A serologic test, hemagglutination inhibition, determines rubella titers. A titer of 1:8 or greater provides evidence of immunity. Women who are not immune should be vaccinated before they become pregnant, and they should be advised not to become pregnant for 3 months after vaccination because of the possible risk to the fetus from the live-virus vaccine. Many women are vaccinated during the postpartum period so that they will be immune before becoming pregnant again. In most facilities, women of childbearing age must read and sign a document indicating they understand the risks to the fetus if they become pregnant before 3 months. (See Chapter 17 for the Drug Guide for rubella vaccine.)

Varicella-Zoster Virus

Varicella infection (chickenpox) is caused by varicella-zoster virus, a herpesvirus that is transmitted by direct contact or through the respiratory tract. The varicella virus can become latent in nerve ganglia. When the virus is reactivated, herpes zoster (shingles) results. Potential maternal complications of acute varicella infection may include preterm labor, encephalitis, and varicella pneumonia, which is the most serious complication associated with varicella-zoster virus. Between 5% and 15% of adults in the United States are susceptible to varicella (Cottrell, 1998).

Fetal and Neonatal Effects. Fetal and neonatal effects depend on the time of maternal infection. If the infection occurred during the first 20 weeks of pregnancy, the fetus may be at risk for congenital varicella syndrome. Clinical findings include limb hypoplasia, cutaneous scars, chorioretinitis, cataracts, microcephaly, and symmetric IUGR (Peiris & Madeley, 2000; Gibbs & Sweet, 1999). In later pregnancy, transplacental passage of maternal antibodies usually protects the fetus.

However, the infant who is infected during the perinatal period (4 days before or 2 days after birth) will not have the benefit of maternal antibodies. Just 4 days before birth is not sufficient time for the mother to develop antibodies to varicella and pass them to the fetus. A varicella infection occurring in the fetus or infant just before or after birth would not be inactivated by antibodies, leaving the infant at risk for life-threatening neonatal varicella infection (Peiris & Madeley, 2000).

Therapeutic Management. Immune testing may be recommended for pregnant women who are presumed to be susceptible. Varicella-zoster immune globulin should be administered to women who have been exposed and whose fetuses are at high risk for the congenital rubella syndrome (Peiris & Madeley, 2000; Landry, 1999). Those infected with chickenpox during pregnancy should be instructed to report pulmonary symptoms immediately. Hospitalization, fetal surveillance, full respiratory support, and hemodynamic monitoring should be available for women diagnosed with varicella pneumonia because it may become severe in a short time. Acyclovir is the primary drug used to treat varicella pneumonia.

For infants born to mothers infected with varicella during the perinatal period, immunization with varicella-zoster immune globulin as soon as possible but within 96 hours of birth provides passive immunity against varicella. Women and infants with varicella are highly contagious and should be placed in strict isolation. Only staff members known to be immune to varicella should come in contact with these clients.

A live attenuated vaccine is available for immunization of healthy children older than 12 months through adults. If the vaccine is given to a female of childbearing age, it is important to teach her to avoid pregnancy for 1 month after each of the two injections, which are given 4 to 8 weeks apart. Nonimmune healthcare workers should be immunized.

Herpesvirus Serotypes 1 and 2

Genital herpes is one of the most common sexually transmissible diseases. It may be caused by herpesvirus serotype 1 or 2. Most episodes of genital herpes are caused by type 2. Infection occurs as a result of direct contact of the skin or mucous membrane with an active lesion. Lesions form at the site of contact and begin as a group of painful papules that progress rapidly to become vesicles, shallow ulcers, pustules, and crusts. The woman sheds the virus until the lesions are completely healed. The virus then migrates along the sensory nerves to reside in the sensory ganglion, and the disease enters a latent phase. It can be reactivated later as a recurrent infection. A woman may not always have signs and symptoms of infection and may acquire and shed the virus without knowing she has it (Peiris & Madeley, 2000).

Vertical transmission (from mother to infant) generally occurs in one of two ways: (1) after rupture of membranes, when the virus ascends from active lesions; or (2) during birth, when the fetus comes into contact with infectious genital secretions or the fetal skin is punctured with a fetal scalp electrode.

Diagnosis usually is based on clinical signs and symptoms. Definitive diagnosis requires isolation of the virus from a lesion. (See Chapter 33 for implications of herpes genitalis in nonpregnant women.)

Fetal and Neonatal Effects. Complications of pregnancy from a recurrent infection are rare. However, if primary infection occurs during the first 20 weeks, the rates of spontaneous abortions, IUGR, and preterm labor increase (Peiris & Madeley, 2000). Neonatal herpes infection is uncommon but potentially devastating. The neonate may have infection that is limited to skin lesions or systemic (disseminated). Symptoms usually appear within the first week, and the disease progresses rapidly. The likelihood of death or serious sequelae for infants who have systemic herpes infection is about 50% (Gibbs & Sweet, 1999). The risk of neonatal infection is greatest if the mother has a primary (rather than recurrent) infection during the perinatal period. This is most likely because the amount of virus shed is higher during first infections than subsequent ones.

Therapeutic Communication

CONCERN ABOUT CONFIDENTIALITY

Mary Smith, who had a cesarean delivery because of an active herpes lesion, appears anxious and uncomfortable during the morning assessment by nurse Eileen Sinclair.

Mary: Why does everyone wear gloves whenever they come near me?

Eileen: You wonder why we wear gloves when we care for you? *(Reflecting content.)*

Mary: Well, it bothers me that you think I am so contagious.

Eileen: You seem to think we wear gloves because you have a herpes outbreak. *(Clarifying content and feeling.)*

Mary: Yes, why else would it be necessary?

Eileen: We wear gloves when we care for all patients, whenever there is a chance that we will come into contact with body fluids. I'm sorry you thought it was only because of your infection. *(Providing information and conveying empathy.)*

Mary: I'm just so touchy about having my family find out I have herpes.

Eileen: You don't want your family to know why you had a cesarean? *(Clarifying and reflecting feelings.)*

Mary: Yes, I'm so embarrassed. I wish they didn't have to know.

Eileen: They will know only if you tell them. We do everything possible to protect your privacy. I'd like to come back in a few minutes and we can talk more about how you feel. *(Offering reassurance about Mary's privacy and giving her the option to express her feelings more completely at a later time.)*

Therapeutic Management. No known cure for herpes infection exists, although antiviral chemotherapy (acyclovir) is prescribed in nonpregnant women to reduce symptoms and shorten the duration of the lesions. Acyclovir is sometimes administered in pregnancy; however, it is in pregnancy risk category C according to the U.S. Food and Drug Administration and should be used with caution. (See Appendix C: "Effects of Drug Use during Pregnancy and Breastfeeding.")

For women with a history of genital herpes, birth is managed normally if no genital lesions are present at the time of labor. Cesarean in these women is done only for obstetric indications. For women with active genital lesions (either recurrent or primary) at the time of labor or membrane rupture, cesarean birth usually is recommended. After delivery, isolation of the mother from her infant is not necessary as long as direct contact with lesions is avoided and mothers are instructed in careful hand-washing techniques. Mothers may breastfeed if no lesions are present on the breasts.

The infant is observed for signs of infection, including temperature instability, lethargy, poor sucking reflex, jaundice, seizures, and herpetic lesions.

Expectant mothers need information about effective ways to deal with the emotional and physical effects of herpes. Many women are concerned about privacy and do not want family members to know why cesarean birth is necessary. These women must be assured that their wishes will be respected. Many women need an opportunity to discuss their feelings of shame, anger, or anxiety about the disease.

After birth, the woman with active lesions, including the more common type 1 lesions, must be taught to avoid contact between the lesions and the infant.

Check Your Reading

23. What are the fetal and neonatal effects of cytomegalovirus infection?
24. Why is rubella infection most dangerous in the first trimester?
25. How can rubella be prevented?
26. How are infants born to mothers with varicella treated?
27. How does vertical transmission of the herpes virus occur?

Parvovirus B19

Erythema infectiosum (also called *fifth disease*), caused by human parvovirus B19, is an acute, communicable disease characterized by a highly distinctive rash. The rash starts on the face with a "slapped-cheeks" appearance, followed by a generalized maculopapular rash. Other symptoms include fever, malaise, and joint pain. Erythema infectiosum is more common among children and often occurs in community epidemics. The prognosis is usually excellent. However, if the disease occurs in pregnancy, potential fetal and neonatal effects exist. Parvovirus titers can be drawn if exposure during pregnancy is suspected.

Fetal and Neonatal Effects. In most instances of maternal infection, the fetus is not infected. About one fourth to one third of fetuses infected will have transient adverse effects, and the fetal death rate from parvovirus B19 infection is less than 5% (CDC, 1999). Fetal death usually results from failure of fetal red blood cell production, followed by severe fetal anemia, hydrops (generalized edema), and heart failure. Serial ultrasonography also can be performed to detect hydrops. Intrauterine transfusion may be done to correct fetal anemia and hydrops.

Therapeutic Management. No specific treatment exists. Starch baths may help reduce pruritus, and analgesics may be necessary to relieve mild joint pain.

Hepatitis B

Hepatitis B is one of five currently recognized serotypes of hepatitis. Hepatitis B is caused by a virus transmitted through blood, saliva, vaginal secretions, semen, and breast milk and across the placental barrier. The disease is prevalent in certain population groups such as Asians, Native Americans, Eskimos, Southeast Asian and sub-Saharan African immigrants, and intravenous drug users. It is more likely to occur if a person has a sexually transmitted disease. Symptoms may include vomiting, abdominal pain, jaundice, fever, rash, and painful joints. Fortunately, most infected adolescents and adults recover within 6 months and acquire long-lasting immunity.

Chronic hepatitis B develops in 1% to 6% of infected adults, who can continue to transmit the disease to others. Persons with chronic hepatitis B also are at greater risk for chronic liver disease, cirrhosis of the liver, and primary hepatocellular carcinoma.

Fetal and Neonatal Effects. The incidence of prematurity, low birth weight, and neonatal death increases when the mother has hepatitis B infection during pregnancy. Infants born to mothers who have hepatitis B during pregnancy or who are chronic carriers of hepatitis B surface antigen (HBsAg) are at risk for the development of acute infection at birth. Chronic hepatitis B infection develops in about 90% of infected newborns. The infected infant also is more likely to have chronic liver disease.

Therapeutic Management. Hepatitis B is preventable. Simple hygiene measures such as protected sex, avoidance of multiple sex partners, and standard precautions with body fluids are ways to begin. However, preexposure and postexposure prophylaxes are more effective. Highly effective hepatitis B vaccines also are available in the United States. A series of three intramuscular injections given during a 6- to 12-month period produces a protective antibody response for most infants, children, and adults. (See Chapter 21 for the drug guide for hepatitis B vaccine.)

All pregnant women should be screened for HBsAg. Women at high risk for hepatitis should be rescreened in the third trimester if the initial screen is negative. Household members and sexual contacts should be tested and offered vaccination if they are susceptible. No specific treatment exists for hepatitis. Recommended supportive treatment includes bedrest and a high-protein, low-fat diet.

Infection of the newborn whose mother is known to be HBsAg positive usually can be prevented by administration of hepatitis B immune globulin (H-BIG, Hep-B-Gammagee), followed by hepatitis B vaccine (Heptavax B) soon after birth. The newborn must be carefully bathed before any injections are given to prevent infections from skin surface contamination. The vaccine should be repeated at 1 and 6 months of age.

Infants born to mothers who were not screened for HBsAg should receive the vaccine soon after birth. If the mother is found to be HBsAg positive (infected), HBIG should be administered at birth and the second and third doses of vaccine should be given at regularly scheduled times. Some physicians give the first hepatitis B immunization to infants born to noninfected mothers while the infant is still in the birth facility rather than waiting until an early well-baby check to start the series. Infants of noninfected mothers will not receive HBIG.

Breastfeeding is considered safe as long as the newborn has been vaccinated. Vaccination is recommended for any population at risk, including healthcare workers who come in contact with potentially infectious secretions.

Human Immunodeficiency Virus

Acquired immunodeficiency syndrome (AIDS) is a breakdown in the immune function caused by a retrovirus known as *human immunodeficiency virus (HIV)*. The infected person develops opportunistic infections or malignancies that ultimately are fatal. The time from infection with HIV to development of AIDS has a median of 10 years with current antiretroviral therapy. Transmission of HIV infection is predominantly through three modes: (1) sexual exposure to genital secretions of an infected person, (2) parenteral exposure to infected blood or tissue, and (3) perinatal exposure of an infant to infected maternal secretions through birth or breastfeeding.

After rapid increases in cases during the early years of the epidemic, the incidence of the infection declined for the first time in 1996. Deaths from AIDS also have declined as a result of more effective combination antiretroviral therapies. However, many new cases are among women, African Americans, and Latinos. Heterosexual spread is now the major mode of transmission, although HIV was largely confined to gay men in the early years of the epidemic. The number of children with AIDS acquired during the perinatal period dropped 43% between 1992 and 1996 with the introduction of zidovudine prophylaxis during pregnancy (CDC, 1998c).

Pathophysiology. Like other retroviruses, HIV integrates its viral genetic makeup into the genetic makeup of the cell when infecting it. This results in an abnormal cell that cannot perform its functions properly. At the same time, this cell replicates and produces more viruses that invade more cells. The disease worsens as more cells cease to function, and at the same time a greater number of viruses are produced. The principal mechanism whereby HIV leads to immunodeficiency is through its effect on helper (CD4) lymphocytes. These cells play a key role in organizing the body's immune response.

As the number of CD4 cells declines, the immune response becomes inadequate and opportunistic infections are able to overwhelm the HIV-positive person. A CD4 count of less than 200 cells/mm^3 confirms the diagnosis of AIDS.

The clinical course of HIV infection follows fairly predictable stages:

- An early or acute stage occurs several weeks after HIV exposure. Flulike symptoms may develop and last a few weeks. Antibodies to HIV (seroconversion) generally appear within a few months, but delays of more than a year have been reported occasionally.
- A middle or asymptomatic period of minor or no clinical problems follows. This period is characterized by continuous low-level viral replication and CD4 cell loss.
- A transitional period of symptomatic disease follows.
- A late or crisis period of symptomatic disease follows, which consists of opportunistic infections lasting months or years.

During stages 1 and 2, the infected person is said to be HIV positive. During stages 3 and 4, the immune system no longer offers adequate protection, and opportunistic diseases occur. The person is then said to have AIDS, regardless of the CD4 count.

CRITICAL TO REMEMBER

Facts about HIV

- After initial exposure, there is a period of 3 to 12 months before seroconversion. The person is considered infectious during this time.
- There is a long period of time, averaging 10 years, from HIV infection to development of AIDS.
- As of now, AIDS will eventually develop in all those who are HIV positive.
- There is not yet a cure for the HIV infection or AIDS. Medications are available to slow replication of the virus and delay onset of opportunistic diseases.
- Zidovudine should be part of the medication regimen for a pregnant woman to reduce the transmission to her fetus. The newborn also should receive zidovudine after birth.
- HIV is transmitted by sexual contact with an infected person, by contact with infected body fluids, and through the placenta from mother to fetus.

Fetal and Neonatal Effects. An infant born to an HIV-positive mother has a 20% to 30% risk for developing the disease without prophylactic treatment during pregnancy (Duff, 2000). Typically, the newborn is asymptomatic at birth, but signs usually become obvious during the first year of life. The most common early signs are enlargement of the liver and spleen, lymphadenopathy, failure to thrive, persistent thrush, and extensive seborrheic dermatitis (cradle cap). Infants frequently experience chronic bacterial infections such as meningitis, pneumonia, osteomyelitis, septic arthritis, and septicemia.

Prevention. Prevention remains the only way to control HIV infection. Sexual transmission can be avoided by several methods. Abstinence would render a person safe from all sexually transmissible diseases including HIV. However, for many people, sexual expression adds to the quality of life, and many are not willing to practice abstinence. Transmission of HIV also can be prevented if infected persons do not have intercourse with susceptible persons. If intercourse does occur, barrier methods such as latex condoms reduce contact with infectious secretions. A condom offers protection from transmission through cunnilingus or fellatio (oral sex).

Intravenous drug users who refuse rehabilitative treatment must be taught to wash the equipment with water, soap, and bleach before each use to reduce transmission of the virus through a soiled needle.

Medical Management. No cure exists for HIV infection at this time, but several medications are beneficial in extending the lifespan after infection. Zidovudine (ZDV) is recommended for pregnant women who are HIV positive to reduce vertical transmission of the virus to about 8% (CDC, 1998a). Additional drugs are used for greatest treatment effectiveness for the woman, but zidovudine is included in multidrug regimens because so far it is the only one shown to inhibit HIV transmission to the fetus. Other drugs used for HIV therapy include neucleotide analogs, neucleoside analogs, reverse transcriptase inhibitors, and protease inhibitors. A medical-surgical nursing text should be consulted for greater detail about these drugs in the treatment of HIV infection.

The recommendations for zidovudine prophylaxis during pregnancy and for the newborn are:

- Oral zidovudine to the expectant mother during the antepartum period beginning after 14 weeks' gestation
- IV zidovudine during labor
- Zidovudine syrup to the newborn for 6 weeks

Zidovudine appears to be safe for the infant. A slight anemia appears to be the main adverse effect.

Additional steps to reduce the infant's exposure to the virus include formula feeding rather than breastfeeding because the virus is secreted in breast milk. The American College of Obstetricians and Gynecologists (1999b) recommends that HIV-positive women be offered elective cesarean delivery at 38 weeks' gestation, before labor or the rupture of membranes occurs. Elective cesarean delivery further reduces the risk for virus transmission to the infant to about 2% if the woman and newborn also take zidovudine therapy. However, if labor has begun or the membranes have ruptured, no added benefit is gained from a cesarean birth.

Nursing Considerations. Learning of HIV infection during pregnancy can have a devastating and immobilizing effect on the entire family. A nursing diagnosis of "Anticipatory Grieving related to multiple losses that include shortened life expectancy and possible death of the infant" should be considered. Initially, crisis intervention may be necessary to help the family cope.

Nurses frequently must determine what the family perceives as the most pressing needs and worries. Some of the most common fears are loss of control, loss of support and love, social isolation, and loss of privacy. The nurse's response may involve finding ways for the woman to retain control while she is physically able and assisting her to select those in her family who will provide continued love and emotional support. Above all, reassuring the woman that her right to privacy will not be violated is necessary.

Nurses can help the woman maintain the highest possible level of wellness. Adequate, high-quality nutrition decreases the risk of opportunistic infections and promotes vitality. A daily regimen should include sufficient rest and activity. Avoiding large crowds, travel to areas with poor sanitation, and exposure to infected individuals is important. Meticulous skin care is essential, especially during recurrent herpes infections.

The woman will need to know that breastfeeding is contraindicated but she can provide all other care for her infant. She almost certainly will experience a great deal of anxiety about whether the infant will be HIV positive. Nurses need to respond honestly that testing will be required but most infants do not get the virus if the medication regimen is followed carefully. In addition, nurses must reinforce information about medications that both slow the progression of the disease for the mother and decrease the incidence of vertical transmission.

Check Your Reading

28. What are the fetal and neonatal effects of parvovirus B19 infection?
29. How is hepatitis B virus transmitted? How are newborns treated?
30. How can HIV infection be prevented?
31. What is the medical management for HIV infection?

Nonviral Infections

Toxoplasmosis

Toxoplasmosis is a protozoan infection caused by *Toxoplasma gondii.* Infection is transmitted through organisms in raw and undercooked meat, through contact with infected cat feces, and across the placental barrier to the fetus if the expectant mother acquires the infection during pregnancy.

Toxoplasmosis often is subclinical. The woman may experience a few days of fatigue, muscle pains, and swollen glands but be unaware of the disease. If the infection is suspected, diagnosis can be confirmed by positive serologic test results, which include indirect fluorescent antibody tests for IgG and IgM.

Fetal and Neonatal Effects. Although toxoplasmosis may go unnoticed in the pregnant woman, it may cause abortion or result in the birth of a liveborn infant with the disease. About 50% of infants born to mothers who were infected during pregnancy acquire congenital toxoplasmosis. Affected infants may be asymptomatic at birth or have low birth weight, enlarged liver and spleen, jaundice, and anemia. Complications (usually chorioretinitis) or signs of neurologic damage may develop several years later.

Therapeutic Management. All pregnant women should be advised to do the following:

- Cook meat thoroughly, particularly pork, beef, and lamb.
- Avoid touching mucous membranes of the mouth and eyes while handling raw meat.
- Wash all kitchen surfaces that come into contact with uncooked meat.
- Wash the hands thoroughly after handling raw meat.
- Avoid uncooked eggs and unpasteurized milk.
- Wash fruits and vegetables before consumption.
- Avoid contact with materials that are possibly contaminated with cat feces (such as cat litter boxes, sandboxes, and garden soil).

The most serious consequences occur if the disease is contracted during the first 20 weeks of pregnancy, so abortion may be presented as an option for the woman to consider. One drug therapy regimen includes pyrimethamine-sulfadiazine plus folinic acid beginning after the 14th week of gestation to reduce the risk for causing birth defects. The neonate with congenital toxoplasmosis is given 6 months' treatment with the same drugs.

Group B Streptococcus Infection

Group B streptococcus (GBS) is a leading cause of life-threatening perinatal infections in the United States. The gram-positive bacterium colonizes the rectum, vagina, cervix, and urethra of pregnant and nonpregnant women. Approximately 10% to 30% of pregnant women are colonized with GBS in the vaginal or rectal area (CDC, 1996a). Often these women are asymptomatic, although symptomatic maternal infections can occur. These infections include urinary tract infection, chorioamnionitis, and metritis. Most women respond quickly to antimicrobial therapy. However, potentially fatal complications such as meningitis, fascitis, and intraabdominal abscess can occur.

Fetal and Neonatal Effects. Early-onset GBS disease occurs within 7 days of birth, usually within 48 hours. If the woman carries GBS, she has a 60% chance of transmitting the organism to the newborn, and about 1% to 2% of these infants will develop early-onset GBS disease (AAP & ACOG, 1997; Gibbs & Sweet, 1999; Savoia, 1999). Sepsis, pneumonia, and meningitis are the primary infections in early-onset GBS disease. Late-onset disease occurs after the first week of life, and meningitis is the most common clinical manifestation. Permanent neurologic consequences may be seen in up to 50% of those who survive meningeal infections (Savoia, 1999). (See Chapter 30 for additional information about manifestations and recommended management of neonatal sepsis.)

Therapeutic Management. Health care providers have difficulty identifying pregnant women who are asymptomatic GBS carriers because the duration of carrier status is unpredictable. Prenatal screening cultures may not identify the woman who will be a GBS carrier at the time of membrane rupture or onset of labor. Optimal identification of the GBS carrier depends on culture timing and technique.

Either of two approaches to preventing GBS disease is acceptable: (1) a risk-based approach or (2) a screening approach based on cultures (AAP & ACOG, 1997). The risk-based approach is somewhat simpler and likely to result in less overall use of antibiotics (Glantz & Kedley, 1998).

In the *risk-based approach,* the woman should receive antibiotics during the intrapartum period if she has any of the following risk factors:

- Previous infant with GBS disease
- The presence of GBS in urine during this pregnancy
- Birth before 37 weeks' gestation
- Maternal fever during labor (38° C [100.4° F])
- Membranes ruptured 18 or more hours before childbirth

If the care provider chooses the *screening approach,* cultures from the rectal and vaginal areas are collected at 35 to 37 weeks' gestation. If these are positive for GBS, the woman is offered intrapartum antibiotics because her infant is at higher risk for GBS infection. If they are negative, she is not given antibiotics unless risk factors develop during labor, such as a prolonged labor or fever.

The antibiotic options for intrapartum prophylaxis are as follows (AAP & ACOG, 1997):

- IV penicillin G, 5 million units initially and 2.5 million units every 4 hours until birth
- IV ampicillin, 2 g initially and 1 g every 4 hours until birth

Other antibiotics may be given for specific clinical indications.

Tuberculosis

Tuberculosis results from infection by *Mycobacterium tuberculosis.* It is transmitted by aerosolized droplets of liquid containing the bacterium, which are inhaled by a noninfected individual and taken into the lung. Initially, most individuals are asymptomatic. Women at risk should be screened for tuberculosis when obtaining prenatal care if they are not already known to be positive. This screening involves an intradermal injection of mycobacterial protein (purified protein derivative). If the reaction is positive or the woman is already known to have a positive reaction, her abdomen should be protected by a lead shield while a radiograph is taken of her chest, preferably after the first trimester. Diagnosis is confirmed by isolating and identifying the bacterium in the sputum.

Signs and symptoms include general malaise, fatigue, loss of appetite, weight loss, and fever. Symptoms occur in the late afternoon and evening and are accompanied by night sweats. As the disease progresses, a chronic cough develops and a mucopurulent sputum is produced.

Tuberculosis is associated with poverty, malnutrition, and HIV infection. It is more likely to occur in women from large urban areas and immigrants from third-world countries. The rate is rising overall and also is increasing among women of childbearing age. Additional problems include noncompliance with therapy and the emergence of strains resistant to multiple drugs.

Fetal and Neonatal Effects. Although perinatal infection is uncommon, it may be acquired as a result of the fetus aspirating infected amniotic fluid. Diagnosis is made by finding the bacilli in gastric aspirate of the neonate or placental tissue. Signs of congenital tuberculosis include failure to thrive, lethargy, respiratory distress, fever, and enlargement of the spleen, liver, and lymph nodes. If the mother remains untreated, the newborn is at high risk for acquiring tuberculosis by inhalation of infectious respiratory droplets from the mother.

Therapeutic Management. Treatment of tuberculosis is based on two principles. First, more than one drug must be used to prevent growth of resistant organisms. Second, treatment must continue for a prolonged period of time. The preferred treatment for pregnant women is isoniazid, pyrazinamide, and rifampin every day for 9 months. Ethambutol should be added if drug resistance is probable. Pyridoxine (vitamin B_6) should be given with isoniazid to prevent fetal neurotoxicity and because pregnancy itself increases the requirement for this vitamin. Short-course therapy is now preferred, meaning that after the first 1 to 2 months of therapy, an alternative to daily therapy is twice-weekly therapy. *Directly-observed therapy* is preferred, in which a responsible person observes the woman taking the medication at each dose to increase compliance and completion of the full regimen and reduce the emergence of drug-resistant organisms (Weinberger & Weiss, 1999).

Management of the infant born to a mother with tuberculosis involves preventing the disease and treating early infection (AAP & ACOG, 1997; de Sweit, 1999a). If the mother's sputum is free of organisms, the infant does not need to be isolated from the mother in the hospital. Prevention focuses on teaching family members how the disease is transmitted so that they can protect the infant from airborne organisms. The infant should be skin tested at birth and may be started on preventive isoniazid therapy. Skin testing should be repeated at 3 to 4 months, and isoniazid may be stopped if the skin test result remains negative. If the skin test result is positive, the infant should receive isoniazid for at least 6 months. Infants who also have HIV infection should receive therapy for 12 months. Breastfed infants of mothers who are taking isoniazid should receive pyridoxine (vitamin B_6) with a multivitamin supplement.

Check Your Reading

32. How can toxoplasmosis be prevented?
33. What are the risk factors for colonization of the newborn with GBS during the intrapartum period? How is colonization prevented?
34. How is tuberculosis treated in the mother? How is it diagnosed and treated in the newborn?

APPLICATION OF THE NURSING PROCESS: THE PREGNANT WOMAN WITH TUBERCULOSIS

Assessment

Question each pregnant woman about signs or symptoms of tuberculosis. These include fever, night sweats, fatigue, weight loss, and cough. Ask whether the cough is productive and the sputum is purulent. Administer and read a purified protein derivative (PPD) skin test as directed. Identify factors that increase the risk of tuberculosis, such as poverty, homelessness, recent immigration from an area that has a high incidence of tuberculosis, and HIV infection. Determine whether a family member or close friend has a history of tuberculosis.

If a woman has tuberculosis, determine the amount of knowledge she has about the disease. For example, does she know the ways in which the disease is transmitted, the importance of completing the lengthy course of prescribed medications, and the major side effects of medications? Does she know about drug resistance in tuberculosis, particularly if she does not adhere to the drug regimen? Ask about stressors in her life that increase the risk that she will not adhere to therapy, such as nonsupport of a significant other, substance abuse, unstable living conditions, and other factors.

Analysis

To achieve a cure, the woman with tuberculosis must adhere to a prolonged treatment regimen that has significant side effects. In addition, women with tuberculosis often have many other stressors in their lives, including poverty, uncertain housing, and other infections such as HIV. The most relevant nursing diagnosis for this woman might be "Ineffective Individual Management of Therapeutic Regimen related to lack of knowledge of disease process and expected course of treatment."

Planning

Goals and expected outcomes for this nursing diagnosis are that:

- The woman and at least one other responsible person will verbalize information about the mode of transmission of tuberculosis, the importance of medications, and possible side effects of antituberculosis medications.
- The woman will adhere to the prescribed treatment plan.

Interventions

Providing Information

1. Teach about the ways in which tuberculosis is transmitted to decrease the chance of transmission:
   - Isolating infants from persons who have infectious sputum is essential.
   - Covering the mouth when coughing, sneezing, and laughing helps prevent the organisms from entering the air.
   - Washing the hands carefully after any contact with body substances or soiled tissues decreases exposure to others.
2. Furnish reassuring information about pregnancy and tuberculosis:
   - Tuberculosis usually does not affect the course of pregnancy, type of delivery (vaginal, or cesarean), or birth weight of newborns.
   - Congenital tuberculosis of the newborn is rare.
   - Skin testing of the mother does not have adverse fetal effects.
   - Commonly used antituberculosis medications are in pregnancy risk category B or C (see Appendix C).
   - Tuberculosis may be cured or arrested if medication is taken as prescribed.
3. Instruct the woman and a responsible person about correct administration of medications:
   - Take medication at the same time each day.
   - Rifampin and isoniazid are best taken on an empty stomach (1 hour before or 2 hours after a meal). Isoniazid can be given with meals, but doing so will delay absorption. Ethambutol should be given with food.
   - Do not skip medications or double up on missed doses.
   - Avoid the use of alcohol, which increases the risk of liver toxicity.
   - Avoid antacids containing aluminum because they impair absorption of isoniazid.
4. Educate the woman and another responsible person about expected or potential side effects:
   - Oral contraceptives are less effective when a woman is taking rifampin.
   - Body fluids such as urine, saliva, and tears may become a characteristic red-orange when taking rifampin. Soft contact lenses may be stained.
   - Nausea, heartburn, diarrhea, and flatulence are fairly common side effects. Rifampin may cause drowsiness.
   - Symptoms of hepatitis (jaundice, anorexia, excessive fatigue) should be reported to the physician.
5. Teach the necessity of continuing medication after symptoms have disappeared to eradicate the organism and avoid development of drug-resistant organisms.
6. Emphasize the importance of keeping follow-up appointments.

Providing Support

Respiratory isolation may be necessary if the woman's sputum still contains organisms, and a new mother may be separated from her newborn. The nursing staff must provide emotional support and counseling so that the mother can deal with the anxiety and frustration she may feel because she is not allowed to care for the infant. Language barriers and cultural implications also should be addressed. A referral to social services may be necessary to arrange temporary care of the newborn outside the home until the infant and mother have received adequate treatment (Table 26-7).

Evaluation

Goals or outcomes are met if the following occur:

- The woman and another responsible person demonstrate knowledge of the mode of transmission, verbalize the importance of taking medications as prescribed, and can describe possible side effects of antituberculosis medications.

Table 26-7

COMMON NURSING DIAGNOSES FOR WOMEN WHO HAVE MEDICAL COMPLICATIONS OF PREGNANCY

** Activity Intolerance
** Anticipatory Grieving
** Anxiety
Fatigue
Fear
Health-Seeking Behaviors
** Ineffective Individual Management of Therapeutic Regimen
Risk for Altered Family Processes
Risk for Altered Parenting
** Risk for Altered Health Maintenance
Risk for Infection
Risk for Injury

** Nursing diagnoses explored in this chapter.

- The woman adheres to the treatment regimen as directed.

SUMMARY CONCEPTS

- The release of insulin accelerates during early pregnancy, which may result in episodes of maternal hypoglycemia. The availability of glucose and insulin favors the development and storage of fat that the mother will need later.
- Placental hormones, which reach their peak during the second and third trimesters, create resistance to insulin in maternal cells and precipitate increases in insulin needs throughout the rest of pregnancy.
- Diabetes is classified according to onset (before or during pregnancy) and whether the woman requires the administration of insulin to prevent ketoacidosis.
- Type 1 diabetes mellitus adversely affects the mother in a variety of ways, including increased risks of pregnancy-induced hypertension, urinary tract infections, and ketosis.
- Because maternal hyperglycemia during the first trimester increases the risk for congenital anomalies in the fetus, a major goal of management is to establish normal blood glucose levels before pregnancy occurs.
- Fetal growth depends on the condition of maternal blood vessels. If no vascular impairment occurs, placental perfusion is adequate and the infant is likely to be large (macrosomia). If vascular impairment does occur, placental perfusion may be reduced and the fetus may have IUGR.
- In addition to congenital anomalies, the infant of a diabetic mother is at increased risk for hypoglycemia, hypocalcemia, hyperbilirubinemia, and respiratory distress syndrome.
- Maternal adverse effects of gestational diabetes include increased urinary tract infections, hydramnios, premature rupture of membranes, and the development of pregnancy-induced hypertension.
- Gestational diabetes increases the risk for fetal macrosomia and neonatal hypoglycemia.
- Gestational diabetes usually can be treated by diet and exercise. However, insulin may be administered if blood glucose levels remain high.
- Cardiovascular changes occurring in normal pregnancy impose an additional burden that may result in cardiac decompensation if the expectant mother has preexisting heart disease.
- The primary goal of management of the pregnant woman with heart disease is to prevent the development of congestive heart failure. This may be done by restricting activity, limiting weight gain, and preventing anemia and infection so that cardiac demand does not exceed cardiac reserves.
- Intrapartum and postpartum management of heart disease focuses on preventing fluid overload, which can cause a sharp rise in cardiac effort.
- Iron supplementation often is needed during pregnancy because most women do not have sufficient iron stores to meet the demands of pregnancy with diet alone.
- Folic acid deficiency is associated with increased risk of spontaneous abortion, abruptio placentae, and fetal anomalies such as neural tube defects. Folic acid supplementation of 400 mcg (0.4 mg daily) is recommended for all women of childbearing age to reduce the risk for neural tube defects.
- Sickle cell disease often is worsened by pregnancy, and a primary goal is to prevent sickle cell crisis during pregnancy.
- Laboratory values for thalassemia are similar to those of iron deficiency. However, administration of iron is risky because increased iron absorption and storage makes the woman susceptible to iron overload.
- Although the woman with SLE can have a normal pregnancy and give birth to a normal newborn, the pregnancy must be treated as high risk because of the increased incidence of abortion, fetal death during the first trimester, and possible exacerbation of the disease.
- Antiphospholipid syndrome (an autoimmune disorder) is a cluster of clinical entities that includes increased risk for thrombosis, fetal loss, and the presence of antiphospholipid antibodies.
- Marked improvement in rheumatoid arthritis often occurs during pregnancy, possibly as a result of pregnancy-specific hormone and hormonal factors. However, most women relapse soon after childbirth.
- Management of epilepsy is complicated because of the teratogenic effects of anticonvulsant medications coupled with the importance of preventing seizures.
- Although Bell's palsy usually is temporary, the woman may be anxious. Supportive care and emotional support are essential.
- Motor vehicle accidents are a major cause of blunt force trauma that may result in premature separation of the placenta, hemorrhage, fractures, and internal injuries. Penetrating injuries caused by knife or gunshot wounds are particularly dangerous for the fetus.
- Treatment of trauma in the pregnant woman is similar to that in a nonpregnant woman. Cardiopulmonary resuscitation and controlling bleeding are the priorities. Careful evaluation of the uterus and fetus also are essential after even minor trauma.
- Viral infections that occur during pregnancy can be transmitted to the fetus in two ways: across the placental barrier or by exposure to organisms during birth. Although they may be mild or even subclinical in the mother, viral infections can have serious effects for the fetus.

- The health care team is responsible for teaching how infectious diseases can be prevented and that early treatment also may reduce fetal and neonatal exposure to infections.
- HIV is a retrovirus that invades the CD4 subset of lymphocytes and destroys them, producing AIDS, which allows opportunistic infections to overwhelm the immune system.
- Pregnant women who are HIV positive experience anxiety, fear, and grief as they contemplate potential losses resulting from the disease. Nurses must provide emotional support, information, and counseling, which will help the woman cope with her emotions and retain control of her care for as long as possible.
- Nonviral infections such as toxoplasmosis, GBS infection, and tuberculosis can be prevented or treated.

ANSWERS TO CRITICAL THINKING EXERCISE

1. The team may have assumed that Marcia knew the maternal and fetal effects of gestational diabetes and the importance of following the plan of care.
2. The team could have explained the reasons for the recommended plan and allowed adequate time to answer all questions. Emphasizing why it is necessary to monitor the condition of the fetus is particularly important because mothers usually are motivated to do whatever they can to ensure the health of the fetus.
3. The nurse should acknowledge Marcia's belief. "I realize that we haven't made our concerns clear to you. Let me explain why it is important for you and for your baby to be watched carefully during these last weeks." The nurse must then provide clear, simple explanations and allow time to answer questions.
4. The nurse must acknowledge that weekly tests are time consuming but that they provide valuable information about the well-being of the baby. Usually the information is reassuring, but additional tests can be performed if questions exist.

REFERENCES & READINGS

Abbott, J.T. (1999). Emergency management of the obstetric patient. Pregnancy and cardiovascular disease. In G.N. Burrow & T.P. Duffy (Eds.), *Medical complications during pregnancy* (5th ed., pp. 225-236). Philadelphia: W.B. Saunders.

American Academy of Pediatrics (AAP) & American College of Obstetricians and Gynecologists (ACOG). (1997). *Guidelines for perinatal care* (4th ed.). Elk Grove Village, IL: Author.

American College of Obstetricians and Gynecologists (ACOG). (1996). *Committee opinion: Prevention of early-onset group B streptococcal disease in newborns.* Washington, D.C.: Author.

American College of Obstetricians and Gynecologists (ACOG). (1999a). Management of herpes in pregnancy. *Practice bulletin no. 8.* Washington, D.C.: Author.

American College of Obstetricians and Gynecologists (ACOG). (1999b). *Scheduled cesarean delivery and the prevention of vertical transmission of HIV infection. Committee opinion no. 219.* Washington, D.C.: Author.

Aminoff, M.J. (1999). Neurologic disorders. In R.K. Creasy & R. Resnik (Eds.), *Maternal-fetal medicine: Principles and practice* (4th ed., pp. 1091-1119). Philadelphia: W.B. Saunders.

Anderson, G.D. (1997). Tuberculosis in pregnancy. *Seminars in Perinatology,* 21(4), 328-335.

Artal, P. (1996). Exercise: An alternative therapy for gestational diabetes. *The Physician and Sports Medicine,* 24(3), 54-66.

Atterbury, J.L., Munn, M.B., Groome, L.J., & Yarnell, J.A. (1997). The antiphospholipid antibody syndrome: An overview. *Journal of Obstetric, Gynecologic, and Neonatal Nursing,* 26(5), 522-530.

Bjorgen, S. (1998). Herpes zoster. *American Journal of Nursing,* 98(2), 46-47.

Bobroski, R. (1999). Trauma in pregnancy. In D.K. James, P.J. Steer, C.P. Weiner, & B. Gonik (Eds.) *High-risk pregnancy: Management options* (2nd ed., pp. 959-982). London: W.B. Saunders.

Brozanski, B.S., Jones, J.G., Krohn, J.A., & Sweet, R.L. (2000). Effect of a screening-based prevention policy on prevalence of early-onset group B streptococcal sepsis. *Obstetrics and Gynecology,* 95(4), 496-501.

Burpo, R.H. (2000). Common antiviral agents used in women's and children's care, part 1. *Journal of Obstetric, Gynecologic, and Neonatal Nursing,* 29(2), 181-190.

Burpo, R.H. (2000). Common antiviral agents used in women's and children's care, part 2. *Journal of Obstetric, Gynecologic, and Neonatal Nursing,* 29(2), 191-200.

Caulin-Glaser, T., & Setaro, J.F. (1999). Pregnancy and cardiovascular disease. In G.N. Burrow & T.P. Duffy (Eds.), *Medical complications during pregnancy* (5th ed., pp. 111-135). Philadelphia: W.B. Saunders.

Centers for Disease Control and Prevention (CDC). (1996a). Prevention of perinatal group B streptococcal disease: A public health prospective. *Morbidity and Mortality Weekly Report* 45(RR-7), 1-24.

CDC. (1996b). Recommendations of the U.S. Public Health Service Task Force on the use of zidovudine to reduce perinatal transmission of human immunodeficiency virus. *Morbidity and Mortality Weekly Report,* 43(RR-11), 81-84.

CDC. (1998a). Guidelines for the treatment of sexually transmitted diseases. *Morbidity and Mortality Weekly Report,* 47 (RR-1), 1-73.

CDC. (1998b). National Diabetes Fact Sheet. Retrieved September 17, 2000 from http://www.cdc.gov/diabetes/ubs/pdf/bw_eng.pdf.

CDC. (1998c). *Trends in the HIV and AIDS epidemic.* Retrieved September 21, 2000 from http://www.cdc.gov.hiv/stats/trends98.pdf.

CDC. (1999). Parvovirus B19 infection and pregnancy. Retrieved September 21, 2000 from http://www.cdc.gov/ncidod/diseases/parvob19preg.htm.

Classen, S.R., Paulson, P.R., & Zacharias, S.R. (1998). Systemic lupus erythematosus: Perinatal and neonatal implications. *Journal of Obstetric, Gynecologic, and Neonatal Nursing,* 27(5), 493-500.

Corrarino, J.E. (1998). Perinatal hepatitis B: Update and recommendations. *MCN: American Journal of Maternal/Child Nursing,* 23(5), 246-252.

Cottrell, B.H. (1998). Attention health care professionals: Have you had the chicken pox? *AWHONN Lifelines,* 2(4), 33-38.

Coustan, D.R. (1996). Screening and testing for gestational diabetes mellitus. *Obstetrics and Gynecology Clinics of North America,* 23(1), 125-136.

Cunningham, F.G., MacDonald, P.C., Gant, N.F., Leveno, K.J., Gilstrap, L.C., Hankins, G.D.V., et al. (1997). *Williams obstetrics* (20th ed.). Norwalk, CT: Appleton & Lange.

Daddario, J. (1998). Trauma in pregnancy. In L.K. Mandeville & N.H. Troiano (Eds.), *High-risk and critical care intrapartum nursing* (2nd ed., pp. 322-352). Philadelphia: Lippincott.

Davison, J.M., & Lindheimer, M.D. (1999). Renal disorders. In R.K. Creasy & R. Resnik (Eds.), *Maternal-newborn medicine: Principles and practice* (4th ed., pp. 873-894). Philadelphia: W.B. Saunders.

de Swiet, M. (1999a). Pulmonary disorders. In R.K. Creasy & R. Resnik (Eds.), *Maternal-newborn medicine: Principles and practice* (4th ed., pp. 921-934). Philadelphia: W.B. Saunders.

de Swiet, M. (1999b). Rheumatologic and connective tissue disorders. In R.K. Creasy & R. Resnik (Eds.), *Maternal-newborn medicine: Principles and practice* (4th ed., pp. 1082-1090). Philadelphia: W.B. Saunders.

Drummond, S.B., & Troiano, N.H. (1998). Cardiac disorders during pregnancy. In L.K. Mandeville & N.H. Troiano (Eds.), *High risk and critical care intrapartum nursing* (2nd ed., pp. 173-184). Philadelphia: Lippincott.

Duff, P. (2000). Human immunodeficiency virus in pregnancy. In F.P. Zuspan & E.J. Quilligan (Eds.), *Current therapies in obstetrics and gynecology* (5th ed., pp. 293-296). Philadelphia: W.B. Saunders.

Duffy, T.P. (1999). Hematologic aspects of pregnancy. In G.N. Burrow & T.F. Ferris (Eds.), *Medical complications during pregnancy* (5th ed., pp. 79-95). Philadelphia: W.B. Saunders.

Expert Committee on the Diagnosis and Classification of Diabetes Mellitus. (1997). Report of the expert committee on the diagnosis and classification of diabetes mellitus. *Diabetes Care, 20*(7), 1183-1197.

Fanaroff, A.A., Martin, R.J., & Miller, M.J. (1999). Identification and management of problems in the high-risk neonate. In R.K. Creasy & R. Resnik (Eds.), *Maternal-newborn medicine: Principles and practice* (4th ed., pp. 1151-1193). Philadelphia: W.B. Saunders.

Faro, S. (2000). Sexually transmitted diseases. In F.P. Zuspan & E.J. Quilligan (Eds.), *Current therapies in obstetrics and gynecology* (5th ed., pp. 161-168). Philadelphia: W.B. Saunders.

Fleming, D.R. (1999). Challenging traditional insulin injection practices. *American Journal of Nursing, 99*(2), 72-74.

Frank, S., Esch, J.F., & Margeson, N.E. (1998). Mandatory HIV testing of newborns: The impact on women. *American Journal of Nursing, 98*(10), 49-51.

Franz, M.J. (2000). Medical nutrition therapy for diabetes mellitus and hypoglycemia of nondiabetic origin. In L.K. Mahan & S. Escott-Stump (Eds.), *Krause's food, nutrition, & diet therapy* (10th ed., pp. 742-780). Philadelphia: W.B. Saunders.

Gabbe, S.G., & Landon, M.B. (2000). Diabetes mellitus in pregnancy. In F.P. Zuspan & E.J. Quilligan (Eds.), *Current therapies in obstetrics and gynecology* (5th ed., pp. 263-268). Philadelphia: W.B. Saunders.

Gibbs, R.S., & Sweet, R.L. (1999). Maternal and fetal infectious disorders. In R.K. Creasy & R. Resnik (Eds.), *Maternal-fetal medicine* (4th ed., pp. 659-724). Philadelphia: W.B. Saunders.

Gladman, D.D., & Urowitz, M.B. (1999). Rheumatic disease in pregnancy. In G.N. Burrow & T.P. Duffy (Eds.), *Medical complications during pregnancy* (5th ed., pp. 415-438). Philadelphia: W.B. Saunders.

Glantz, J.C., & Kedley, K.E. (1998). Concepts and controversies in the management of group B streptococcus during pregnancy. *Birth, 25*(1), 45-53.

Gonik, B. (1999). Intensive care monitoring of the critically ill pregnant patient. In R.K. Creasy & R. Resnik (Eds.), *Maternal-fetal medicine: Principles and practice* (4th ed., pp. 895-920). Philadelphia: W.B. Saunders.

Hewell, S.W. (1997). Antiphospholipid antibodies: A threat throughout pregnancy. *Journal of Obstetric, Gynecologic, and Neonatal Nursing, 26*(2), 162-178.

Homko, C.J., & Khandelwal, M. (1996). Glucose monitoring and insulin therapy during pregnancy. *Obstetrics and Gynecology Clinics of North America, 23*(1), 47-74.

Honig, G.R. (2000). Hemoglobin disorders. In R.E. Behrman, R.M. Kliegman, & H.B. Jenson (Eds.), *Nelson textbook of pediatrics* (16th ed., pp. 1478-1488). Philadelphia: W.B. Saunders.

Hutchinson, M.K. (1998). Something to talk about: Sexual risk communication between young women and their partners. *Journal of Obstetric, Gynecologic, and Neonatal Nursing, 27*(2), 127-133.

Inzucchi, S.E.. (1999). Diabetes mellitus. In G.N. Burrow & T.F. Ferris (Eds.), *Medical complications during pregnancy* (5th ed., pp. 25-51). Philadelphia: W.B. Saunders.

Kendrick, J.M. (1999). Diabetes mellitus in pregnancy. In L.K. Mandeville & N.H. Troiano (Eds.), *High risk and critical care intrapartum nursing* (2nd ed., pp. 224-255). Philadelphia: Lippincott.

Kilpatrick, S.J., & Laros, R.K. (1999). Maternal hematologic disorders. In R.K. Creasy & R. Resnik (Eds.), *Maternal-fetal medicine: Principles and practice* (4th ed., pp. 935-963). Philadelphia: W.B. Saunders.

Kirby, R.B. (1999). Maternal phenylketonuria: A new cause for concern. *Journal of Obstetric, Gynecologic, and Neonatal Nursing, 28*(3), 227-234.

Kotter, M., & Osguthorpe, S. (2000). Alterations in oxygen transport. In L.C. Copstead & J.L. Banasik (Eds.), *Pathophysiology: Biological and behavioral perspectives* (2nd ed., pp. 292-330). Philadelphia: W.B. Saunders.

Landon, M.B., & Gabbe, S.G. (2000). Diabetes mellitus. In W.M. Barron, M.D. Lindheimer, & J.M. Davison (Eds.). *Medical disorders during pregnancy* (3rd ed., pp. 337-362). St. Louis: Mosby.

Landry, M.L. (1999). Viral infections. In G.N. Burrow & T.F. Ferris (Eds.), *Medical complications during pregnancy* (5th ed., pp. 25-51). Philadelphia: W.B. Saunders.

Lee, K.A., Portillo, C.J., & Miramontes, H. (1999). The fatigue experience for women with human immunodeficiency virus. *Journal of Obstetric, Gynecologic, and Neonatal Nursing, 28*(2), 193-200.

Lilley, L.L., & Guanci, R. (1997). When 'look-alikes' and 'sound-alikes' don't act alike. *American Journal of Nursing, 97*(9), 12, 14.

Luppi, C.J. (1999). Cardiopulmonary resuscitation in pregnancy: What all nurses caring for childbearing women need to know. *AWHONN Lifelines, 3*(3), 41-45.

Mancuso, P. (2000). Dermatologic manifestations of infectious diseases in pregnancy. *Journal of Perinatal and Neonatal Nursing, 14*(1), 17-38.

March of Dimes. (2000). *Fact sheet: Diabetes in pregnancy.* Retrieved September 15, 2000 from http://www.modimes.org/HealthLibrary2/FactSheets/Diabetes_in_pregnancy.htm.

Minkoff, H.L. (1999). Human immunodeficiency virus. In R.K. Creasy & R. Resnik (Eds.), *Maternal-fetal medicine: Principles and practice* (4th ed., pp. 725-735). Philadelphia: W.B. Saunders.

Mitchell, A., Steffenson, N., Hogan, H., & Brooks, S. (1997). Group B streptococcus and pregnancy: Update and recommendations. *MCN: American Journal of Maternal/Child Nursing,* 22(5), 242-248.

Monga, M. (1999). Cardiovascular and renal adaptation to pregnancy. In R.K. Creasy & R. Resnik (Eds.), *Maternal-fetal medicine: Principles and practice.* (4th ed., pp. 783-792). Philadelphia: W.B. Saunders.

Montgomery, K.S. (1996). Caring for the pregnant woman with sickle cell disease. *MCN: American Journal of Maternal/Child Nursing,* 21(5), 224-228.

Moore, T.R. (1999). Diabetes in pregnancy. In R.K. Creasy & R. Resnik (Eds.), *Maternal-fetal medicine: Principles and practice* (4th ed., pp. 964-995). Philadelphia: W.B. Saunders.

Newshan, G. (1998). Use of combination antiretroviral therapy in pregnant women with HIV disease. *MCN: American Journal of Maternal/Child Nursing,* 23(6), 307-312.

Nuwayhid, B., Nguyen, T., & Khalife, S. (1998). Medical complications of pregnancy. In N.F. Hacker & J.G. Moore (Eds.), *Essentials of obstetrics and gynecology* (3rd ed., pp. 234-262). Philadelphia: W.B. Saunders.

Pedler, S.J., & Orr, K.E. (2000). Bacterial, fungal, & parasitic infections. In W.M. Barron, M.D. Lindheimer, & J.M. Davison (Eds.), *Medical disorders during pregnancy* (3rd ed., pp. 411-465). St. Louis: Mosby.

Peiris, J.S.M., & Madeley, C.R. (2000). Viral infections. In W.M. Barron, M.D. Lindheimer, & J.M. Davison (Eds.), *Medical disorders during pregnancy* (3rd ed., pp. 466-515). St. Louis: Mosby.

Savoia, M.C. (1999). Bacterial, fungal, and parasitic disease. In G.N. Burrow & T.F. Ferris (Eds.), *Medical complications during pregnancy* (5th ed., pp. 295-335). Philadelphia: W.B. Saunders.

Schmidt, G.A., & Hall, J.B. (2000). Pulmonary disease. In W.M. Barron, M.D. Lindheimer, & J.M. Davison (Eds.). *Medical disorders during pregnancy* (3rd ed., pp. 193-228). St. Louis: Mosby.

Scott, L.D. (1999). Gastrointestinal disease in pregnancy. In R.K. Creasy & R. Resnik (Eds.), *Maternal-fetal medicine: Principles and practice.* (4th ed., pp. 1038-1053). Philadelphia: W.B. Saunders.

Seely, B.L. (1999). Thyroid disease and pregnancy. In R.K. Creasy & R. Resnik (Eds.), *Maternal-fetal medicine: Principles and practice.* (4th ed., pp.996-1014). Philadelphia: W.B. Saunders.

Shabetai, R. (1999). Cardiac diseases. In R.K. Creasy & R. Resnik (Eds.), *Maternal-fetal medicine: Principles and practice.* (4th ed., pp. 793-819). Philadelphia: W.B. Saunders.

Shiffman, R., & Josimovich, J.B. (2000). Systemic lupus erythematosus in pregnancy. In F.P. Zuspan & E.J. Quilligan (Eds.), *Current therapies in obstetrics and gynecology* (5th ed., pp. 355-358). Philadelphia: W.B. Saunders.

Silver, R.M. (2000). Antiphospholipid antibodies in reproductive loss. In F.P. Zuspan & E.J. Quilligan (Eds.), *Current therapies in obstetrics and gynecology* (5th ed., pp. 8-12). Philadelphia: W.B. Saunders.

Silver, R.M., & Branch, D.M. (1999). Immunologic disorders. In R.K. Creasy & R. Resnik (Eds.), *Maternal-fetal medicine: Principles and practice* (4th ed., pp. 465-483). Philadelphia: W.B. Saunders.

Simpkins, S.M., Hench, C.P., & Bhatia, G. (1996). Management of the obstetric patient with tuberculosis. *Journal of Obstetric, Gynecologic, and Neonatal Nursing,* 25(4), 305-312.

Tyrala, E.E. (1996). The infant of the diabetic mother. *Obstetrics and Gynecology Clinics of North America,* 23(1), 221-241.

U.S. Department of Health and Human Services. (2000). Immunization and infectious diseases. Retrieved September 20, 2000 from www.health.gov.healthypeople/Document/pdf/volume1/14Immunizatioin.pdf.

Weinberger, S.E., & Weiss, S.T. (1999). Pulmonary diseases. In G.N. Burrow & T.P. Duffy (Eds.), *Medical complications during pregnancy* (5th ed., pp. 363-400). Philadelphia: W.B. Saunders.

Wendel, G.D., & Cunningham, F.G. (2000). Group B streptococcus in pregnancy. In F.P. Zuspan & E.J. Quilligan (Eds.), *Current therapies in obstetrics and gynecology* (5th ed., pp. 286-288). Philadelphia: W.B. Saunders.

Witlin, A.G. (1997). Asthma in pregnancy. *Seminars in Perinatology,* 21(4), 284-297.

27

INTRAPARTUM COMPLICATIONS

OBJECTIVES

1. Explain abnormalities that may result in dysfunctional labor.
2. Describe maternal and fetal risks associated with premature rupture of the membranes.
3. Analyze factors that increase a woman's risk for preterm labor.
4. Explain maternal and fetal problems that may occur if pregnancy persists beyond 42 weeks.
5. Describe the intrapartum emergencies discussed in this chapter.
6. Explain therapeutic management of each intrapartum complication.
7. Apply the nursing process to care of women with intrapartum complications and care of their families.

DEFINITIONS

ABRUPTIO PLACENTAE Premature separation of a normally implanted placenta.

AMNIOTIC FLUID EMBOLISM An embolism in which amniotic fluid with its particulate matter is drawn into the pregnant woman's circulation, lodging in her lungs.

AMNIOCENTESIS Transabdominal puncture of the amniotic sac to obtain a sample of amniotic fluid that contains fetal cells and biochemical substances for laboratory analysis.

CEPHALOPELVIC DISPROPORTION (CPD) Fetal head size that is too large to fit through the maternal pelvis at birth. Also called *fetopelvic disproportion.*

CERCLAGE Encircling of the cervix with suture to prevent recurrent spontaneous abortion caused by early cervical dilation.

CHORIOAMNIONITIS Inflammation of the amniotic sac (fetal membranes); usually caused by bacterial or viral infection. Also called *amnionitis.*

DYSTOCIA Difficult or prolonged labor; often associated with abnormal uterine activity and cephalopelvic disproportion.

HYDRAMNIOS Excessive volume of amniotic fluid (more than 2000 ml at term). Also called *polyhydramnios.*

HYPERTONIC LABOR DYSFUNCTION Ineffective labor characterized by erratic and poorly coordinated contractions. Uterine resting tone is higher than normal.

HYPOTONIC LABOR DYSFUNCTION Ineffective labor characterized by weak, infrequent, and brief but coordinated uterine contractions. Uterine resting tone is normal.

MACROSOMIA Unusually large fetal size; infant birth weight more than 4000 g.

MULTIFETAL PREGNANCY A pregnancy in which the woman is carrying two or more fetuses. Also called *multiple gestation.*

OCCULT PROLAPSE *See prolapsed cord.*

DEFINITIONS—cont'd

OLIGOHYDRAMNIOS Abnormally small volume of amniotic fluid (less than 500 ml at term).

PLACENTA ACCRETA A placenta that is abnormally adherent to the uterine muscle. If the condition is more advanced, it is called *placenta increta* (the placenta extends into the uterine muscle) or *placenta percreta* (the placenta extends through the uterine muscle).

PLACENTA PREVIA Abnormal implantation of the placenta in the lower uterus, at or very near the cervical os.

PRECIPITATE BIRTH A birth that occurs without a trained attendant present.

PRECIPITATE LABOR An intense, unusually short labor (less than 3 hours).

PRETERM LABOR Onset of labor after 20 weeks and before the beginning of the 38th week of gestation.

PROLAPSED CORD Displacement of the umbilical cord in front of or beside the fetal presenting part. An occult prolapse is one that is suspected on the basis of fetal heart rate patterns; the umbilical cord cannot be palpated or seen.

SHOULDER DYSTOCIA Delayed or difficult birth of the fetal shoulders after the head is born.

TOCOLYTIC A drug that inhibits uterine contractions.

UTERINE INVERSION Turning of the uterus inside out after birth of the fetus.

UTERINE RESTING TONE Degree of uterine muscle tension when the woman is not in labor or during the interval between labor contractions.

UTERINE RUPTURE A tear in the wall of the uterus.

For most women, birth is a normal process free of major complications. However, complications sometimes make childbearing hazardous for the woman or her baby. The nurse's challenge is to identify the complications promptly and provide effective care for these mothers while nurturing the entire family at this significant time in their life.

The complications addressed in this chapter are often interrelated. For example, a dysfunctional labor is likely to be prolonged, and the woman is more vulnerable to infection, psychological distress, and fetal compromise. Also, women who have complications are more likely to need interventions such as cesarean birth. The nurse should provide nursing care that relates to all problems experienced by the woman.

DYSFUNCTIONAL LABOR

Normal labor is characterized by progress. Dysfunctional labor is one that does not result in normal progress of cervical effacement, dilation, and fetal descent. *Dystocia* is a general term that describes any difficult labor or birth. A dysfunctional labor may result from problems with the powers of labor, the passenger, the passage, the psyche, or a combination of these. Dysfunctional labor often is prolonged but may be unusually short and intense.

An operative birth (assisted with a vacuum extractor or forceps, or cesarean birth) may be needed if dysfunctional labor does not resolve or fetal or maternal compromise occurs. Signs of possible compromise include persistent nonreassuring fetal heart rate (FHR) patterns (see Chapter 14), fetal acidosis, and meconium passage. Maternal exhaustion or infection may occur, especially with long labors. Nursing measures that enhance progress and maternal comfort and promote fetal well-being also are discussed in this chapter.

Problems of the Powers

The powers of labor may not be adequate to expel the fetus because of ineffective contractions or ineffective maternal pushing efforts.

Ineffective Contractions

Effective uterine activity is characterized by coordinated contractions that are strong and numerous enough to propel the fetus past the resistance of the woman's bony pelvis and soft tissues. It is not possible to say how frequent, long, or strong labor contractions must be. One woman's labor may progress with contractions that would be inadequate for another woman. Possible causes of ineffective contractions include the following:

- Maternal fatigue
- Maternal inactivity
- Fluid and electrolyte imbalance
- Hypoglycemia
- Excessive analgesia or anesthesia
- Maternal catecholamines secreted in response to stress or pain
- Disproportion between the maternal pelvis and fetal presenting part
- Uterine overdistention such as with multiple gestation or hydramnios

Two patterns of ineffective uterine contractions are hypotonic and hypertonic dysfunction. Hypotonic dysfunction is more common than hypertonic dysfunction. Characteristics and management of each are different, but either results in poor labor progress if it persists (Table 27-1).

Hypotonic Dysfunction. Hypotonic contractions are coordinated but too weak to be effective. They are infrequent and brief and can be indented easily with fingertip pressure at the peak.

Hypotonic dysfunction usually occurs during the active phase of labor, when progress normally quickens. Active phase usually begins at about 4 cm of cervical

Table 27-1

PATTERNS OF LABOR DYSFUNCTION

Hypotonic Dysfunction	Hypertonic Dysfunction
CONTRACTIONS	
Coordinated but weak Become less frequent and shorter in duration Easily indented at peak May cause minimal discomfort because the contractions are weak	Uncoordinated, irregular Short and poor intensity but painful and cramplike
UTERINE RESTING TONE	
Not elevated	Higher than normal. Important to distinguish from abruptio placentae, which has similar characteristics (p. 673).
PHASE OF LABOR	
Active. Typically occurs after 4 cm dilation. More common than hypertonic dysfunction.	Latent. Usually occurs before 4 cm dilation. Less common than hypotonic dysfunction.
THERAPEUTIC MANAGEMENT	
Amniotomy (may increase the risk of infection). Oxytocin augmentation. Cesarean birth if no progress.	Correct cause if it can be identified. Sedation; possible low-dose epidural block; possibly cautious low-rate oxytocin infusion to promote more coordinated contractions. Hydration. Tocolytics to reduce high uterine tone and promote placental perfusion.
NURSING CARE	
Interventions related to amniotomy and oxytocin augmentation. Encourage position changes. Ambulation if no contraindication and if acceptable to the woman. Emotional support: Allow her to ventilate feelings of discouragement. Explain measures taken to increase effectiveness of contractions. Include her partner and family in emotional support measures because they may have anxiety that will heighten the woman's anxiety.	Promote uterine blood flow: side-lying position. Promote rest, general comfort, and relaxation. Provide pain relief. Emotional support: Accept the reality of the woman's pain and frustration. Reassure her that she is not being childish. Explain reason for measures to break abnormal labor patterns and their expected results. Allow her to ventilate her feelings during and after labor. Include her partner and family (see hypotonic labor).

dilation. Uterine overdistention is associated with hypotonic dysfunction because the stretched uterine muscle contracts poorly.

The woman may be fairly comfortable because her contractions are weak. However, she often is frustrated because labor slows at a time when she expects to be making more rapid progress. Hypotonic dysfunction is tiring simply because it adds to labor's duration. Fetal hypoxia is not usually seen with hypotonic labor.

Management depends on the cause. Many women respond to simple measures. Providing IV or oral fluids corrects maternal fluid and electrolyte imbalances or hypoglycemia. Maternal position changes, particularly different upright positions, favor fetal descent and promote effective contractions. The woman who moves about actively typically has better labor progress and is more comfortable than the woman who remains in one position.

The nurse should use therapeutic communication to help the woman identify anxieties or beliefs about labor and its progress. Identifying her anxieties is the first step to managing them effectively so that the stress response does not slow her labor. For example, the nurse might ask, "What do you think is making your labor slow?" or "How do you feel that your labor is going?"

Many women need measures such as amniotomy and oxytocin infusion to promote labor progress. The birth attendant evaluates the woman's labor to confirm that she is having hypotonic active labor rather than a long latent phase of labor. The latent phase of labor occurs within the first 3 cm of cervical dilation. A prolonged latent phase may be annoying but is not associated with problems for the mother or fetus (Fraser & Boulvain, 2000). The maternal pelvis and fetal presentation and position are assessed to identify abnormalities.

Amniotomy or augmentation, usually with oxytocin, may be used to stimulate a labor that slows after it is established. The risks of amniotomy are umbilical cord prolapse, infection, and abruptio placentae. Reduced placental perfusion caused by excessive uterine contractions is the most common risk of oxytocin labor augmentation.

Hypertonic Dysfunction. Hypertonic dysfunction of labor is less common than hypotonic dysfunction. Contractions are uncoordinated and erratic in their frequency, duration, and intensity. The contractions are painful but ineffective. Hypertonic dysfunction usually occurs during the latent phase of labor.

Although each contraction varies in its intensity, the uterine resting tone between contractions is higher than normal, reducing uterine blood flow. This uterine ischemia decreases fetal oxygen supply and causes the woman to have almost constant cramping pain. Because high uterine resting tone and constant pain also are seen in abruptio placentae, this complication should be considered as well.

The mother becomes very tired because of nearly constant discomfort. She may lose confidence in her ability to give birth and cope with labor. She often thinks, "If it hurts this much so early, I must be a real baby about pain." Frustration and anxiety further reduce her pain tolerance and interfere with the normal processes of labor. The nurse should accept her frustration and discomfort. Cervical dilation should not be equated with the amount of pain a woman "should" experience.

Management of hypertonic labor depends on the cause. Relief of pain is the primary intervention to promote a normal labor pattern. Warm showers and baths promote relaxation and rest, often allowing a normal labor pattern to ensue. Systemic analgesics or occasionally low-dose epidural analgesia may be required to achieve this purpose.

Oxytocin is not usually given because it can intensify the already high uterine resting tone. However, very low doses of oxytocin sometimes are given to promote coordinated uterine contractions. Tocolytic drugs may be ordered to reduce uterine resting tone and improve placental blood flow. The decision to order uterine stimulant or relaxant drugs is very individualized, based on each woman's labor pattern.

Ineffective Maternal Pushing

A reflex urge to push with contractions usually occurs as the fetal presenting part reaches the pelvic floor during second-stage labor. However, ineffective pushing may result from the following:

- Use of incorrect pushing techniques and positions
- Fear of injury because of pain and tearing sensations felt by the mother when she pushes
- Decreased or absent urge to push
- Maternal exhaustion
- Analgesia or anesthesia that suppresses the woman's urge to push
- Psychological unreadiness to "let go" of her baby

Management focuses on correcting causes contributing to ineffective pushing. If maternal and fetal vital signs are normal, no maximum allowable duration for the second stage exists. Each woman is evaluated individually by her birth attendant to determine whether labor should be ended with an operative delivery or can continue safely. For most women, this occurs after about 2 to 3 hours of adequate pushing efforts that do not result in fetal descent to the pelvic floor.

Nursing care to promote effective pushing helps the mother make each effort more productive. Most women, even women who have had epidural analgesia, can detect the urge to push with today's techniques. The practice of *laboring down* or *delayed pushing*—encouraging the woman to wait until she feels the reflex urge to push—has been shown to have a lower incidence of adverse effects than pushing immediately upon full cervical dilation (Mayberry, et al., 2000). (See Chapter 13 for more information about the evidence-based nursing practice of laboring down.)

Upright positions such as squatting add gravity to the woman's pushing efforts. Semi-sitting, side-lying, and pushing while sitting on the toilet are other options. If she prefers to lie in bed on her side, she should pull her upper leg toward her chest with each push. Leaning forward while in a sitting or squatting position maintains the best alignment of the fetal head with the pelvis.

The woman who fears injury because of the sensations she feels when pushing may respond to accurate information about the process of fetal descent. If she understands that sensations of tearing often accompany fetal descent but her tissues can expand to accommodate the baby, she may be more willing to push with contractions.

A reduced urge to push may occur when epidural block analgesia is given. Today's epidural blocks for labor use a mixture of a local anesthetic agent (one of the *-caine* drugs) and an epidural opioid analgesic to provide pain control without the major loss of sensation that is likely if local anesthetic is used alone. However, if a woman cannot feel the urge to push at all or cannot feel it strongly after the fetus has descended, she can be coached to push with each contraction.

The woman who is exhausted may push more effectively if she is encouraged to rest and push only when she feels the urge, or she may push with every other contraction. Giving oral or IV fluids as ordered provides energy for the strenuous work of second-stage labor. Reassuring her about fetal well-being and the fact that she has no absolute deadline to meet helps her work with her body's efforts most effectively. This reassurance also helps the woman who may be emotionally readying herself to "let go" of her fetus in exchange for a newborn as she labors.

Problems with the Passenger

Fetal problems associated with dysfunctional labor are related to the following:

- Fetal size
- Fetal presentation or position

- Multifetal pregnancy
- Fetal anomalies

These variations may cause mechanical problems and contribute to ineffective contractions.

Fetal Size

Macrosomia. The macrosomic infant weighs more than 4000 g (8.8 lb) at birth. The head may be so large that it cannot mold enough to adapt to the pelvis. Even if the head makes it through the pelvis, the shoulders may be too large to pass. Uterine distention by the large fetus reduces contraction strength during and after birth.

Size is relative, however. The woman with a small or abnormally shaped pelvis may not be able to deliver an average-sized or small infant. The woman with a large pelvis may easily give birth to an infant heavier than 4000 g.

Shoulder Dystocia. Delayed or difficult birth of the shoulders may occur as they become impacted above the maternal symphysis pubis. After the head is born, it retracts against the perineum, much like a turtle's head drawing into its shell ("turtle sign"). Shoulder dystocia is more likely to occur when the fetus is large or the mother has diabetes, but many cases occur in pregnancies with no identifiable risk factors (Wright & Higgins, 1999; Simpson, 1999).

Shoulder dystocia is an urgent situation because the umbilical cord can be compressed between the fetal body and maternal pelvis. Although the infant's head is out of the vaginal canal, the chest is inside, preventing respirations. Any of several methods may be used to quickly relieve the impacted fetal shoulders (Figure 27-1). Fundal pressure should be avoided so that the shoulders are not pushed even harder against the symphysis. The infant's clavicles should be checked for crepitus, deformity, and bruising, each of which suggests fracture. Documentation of all care is essential, including a clear description if *suprapubic* pressure was used to avoid confusion with fundal pressure in any subsequent legal action (Simpson, 1999).

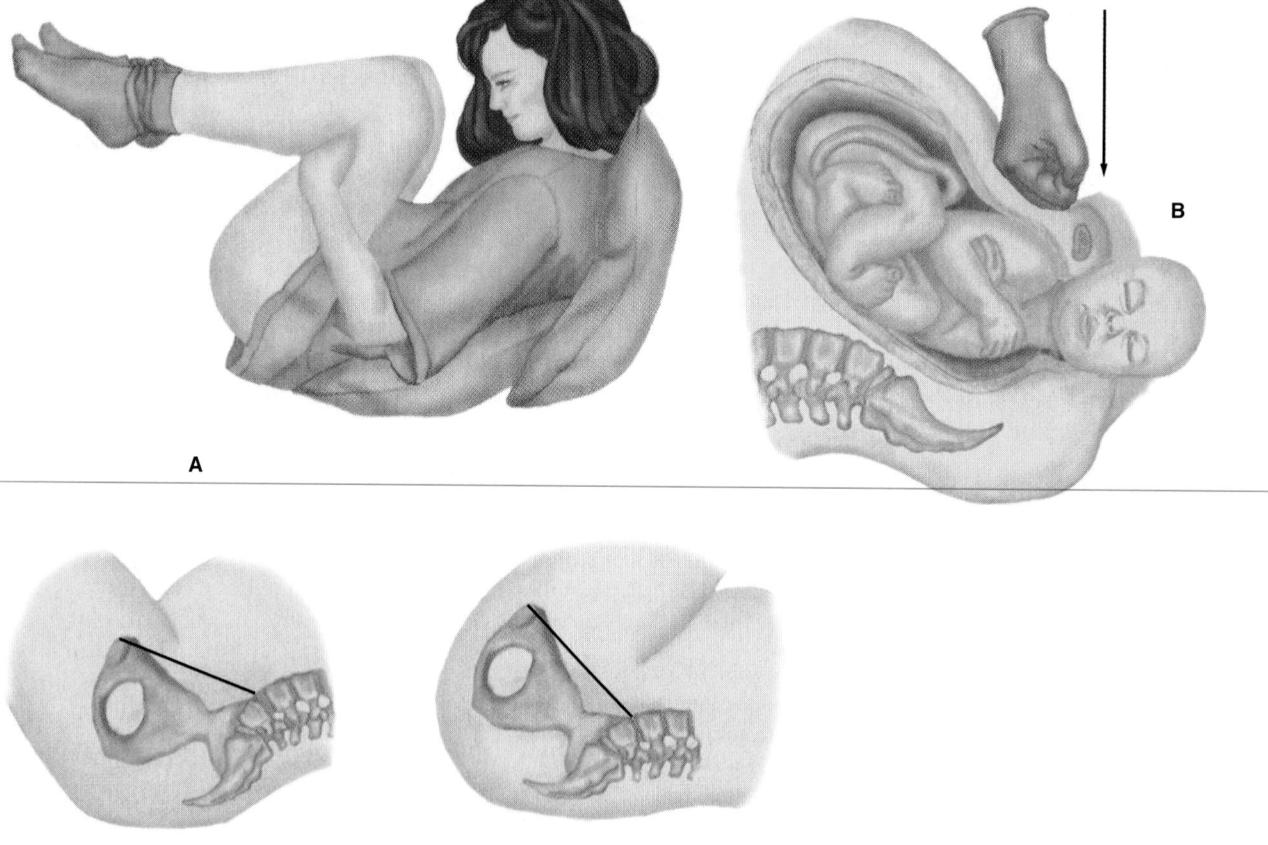

FIGURE 27-1 Methods that may be used to relieve shoulder dystocia. **A,** McRobert's maneuver. The woman flexes her thighs sharply against her abdomen, which straightens the pelvic curve somewhat. A supported squat has a similar effect and adds gravity to her pushing efforts. **B,** Suprapubic pressure by an assistant pushes the fetal anterior shoulder downward to displace it from above the mother's symphysis pubis. Fundal pressure should not be used because it will push the anterior shoulder even more firmly against the mother's symphysis.

Abnormal Fetal Presentation or Position

An unfavorable fetal presentation or position may interfere with cervical dilation or fetal descent.

Rotation Abnormalities. Persistence of the fetus in the occiput posterior or occiput transverse position can contribute to dysfunctional labor. These positions prevent the mechanisms of labor (cardinal movements) from occurring normally. Most fetuses that begin labor in an occiput posterior position rotate spontaneously to an occiput anterior position, promoting normal extension and expulsion of the head. The fetus may not rotate or may partly rotate and remain in an occiput transverse position. Although many women cannot readily deliver a fetus in the occiput posterior position, the woman with a large pelvis compared with the fetal size may be able to do so.

Labor usually is longer and more uncomfortable when the fetus remains in the occiput posterior or occiput transverse position. Intense back or leg pain that may be poorly relieved with analgesia makes coping with labor difficult for the woman. "Back labor" aptly describes the sensations a woman feels when her fetus is in an occiput posterior position. Some women who had a fetus in the occiput posterior position during labor continue to feel more back or coccyx pain during the postpartum period.

Maternal position changes promote fetal head rotation to an occiput anterior position and descent (see Figure 13-5). Examples are as follows:

- Hands and knees—Rocking the pelvis back and forth while on hands and knees encourages rotation. The woman's knees should be slightly behind her hips in this position.
- Side-lying (on the opposite side of the fetal occiput)
- Lunge—The mother places one foot on a chair with her foot and knee pointed to that side (Simkin, 1995). She lunges sideways repeatedly for 5 seconds at a time during a contraction. The lunge also can be done in a kneeling position. The nurse or her partner must secure the chair and help the woman balance.
- Squatting (for second-stage labor); sitting on a slightly underinflated birth ball gives a similar effect
- Sitting, kneeling, or standing while leaning forward

CRITICAL THINKING EXERCISE

A woman having her first baby has been in labor for several hours. Her nurse-midwife performs a vaginal examination and says that the cervix is 6 cm dilated and completely effaced, with the fetus in right occiput posterior position. The mother is having persistent back pain that worsens during contractions.

QUESTIONS:
How should the nurse interpret this information? Should the nurse take any specific action based on the nurse-midwife's examination?

Upright maternal positions promote descent, which usually is accompanied by fetal head rotation. The first two maternal positions promote rotation because the mother's abdomen is dependent in relation to her spine. In the hands-and-knees position, the convex surface of the fetal back tends to rotate toward the convex anterior uterus, similar to nesting two spoons (Figure 27-2). A side-lying position has a similar effect, although not quite as pronounced. These positions decrease the mother's discomfort by reducing fetal head pressure on her sacrum.

The lunge widens the side of the pelvis toward which the woman lunges. If the fetal position is known, she lunges toward the side where the occiput is located (Figure 27-3). If the fetal position is not known, the

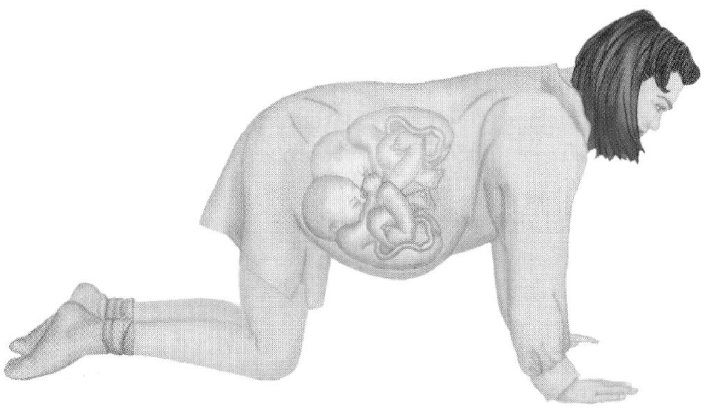

FIGURE 27-2 A "hands and knees" position helps the fetus rotate from a left occiput posterior (LOP) position to an occiput anterior position.

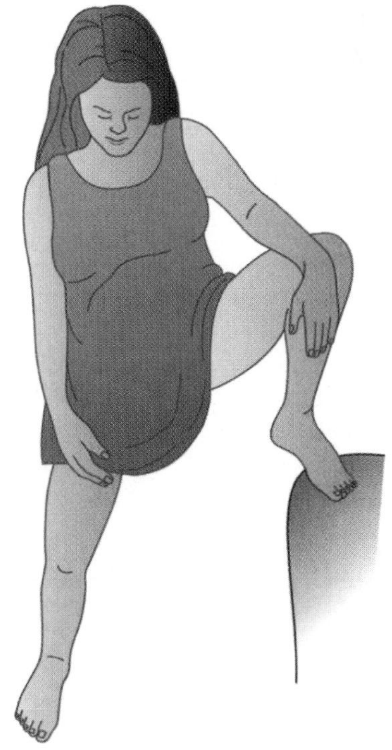

FIGURE 27-3 The "lunge" to one side promotes rotation of the fetal occiput from a posterior position to an anterior one.

woman can lunge toward the side that gives her greater comfort.

All variations of the squatting position aid rotation and fetal descent by straightening the pelvic curve and enlarging the pelvic outlet. They add gravity to the force of maternal pushing.

If spontaneous rotation does not occur, the physician may assist rotation and descent of the head with forceps. The vacuum extractor cannot always be applied to the fetal head when it remains in an occiput posterior position. However, some styles of vacuum extractors may be used for minor degrees of malrotation because the fetal head tends to rotate as it descends with downward traction. Cesarean birth may be needed if these methods are unsuccessful or cannot be used.

Deflexion Abnormalities. The poorly flexed fetal head presents a larger diameter to the pelvis than if flexed with the chin on the chest (see Figure 12-8). In the *vertex presentation,* the head diameter is smallest. In the *military* and *brow presentations,* the head diameter is larger. In the *face presentation,* the head diameter is similar to that of the vertex presentation but the maternal pelvis can be traversed only if the fetal chin (mentum) is anterior.

Breech Presentation. Cervical dilation and effacement often are slower when the fetus is in a breech presentation because the buttocks or feet do not form a smooth, round dilating wedge like the head. The greatest fetal risk is that the head—the largest fetal part—is last to be born. By the time the lower body is born, the umbilical cord is well into the pelvis and may be compressed. The shoulders, arms, and head must be delivered quickly so that the infant can breathe.

A breech presentation is common well before term, but only 3% to 4% of term fetuses remain in this presentation. Adverse outcomes for infants that remain in a breech presentation may relate to causes other than their mode of birth:

- Fetal injury with a difficult vaginal birth
- Prolapsed umbilical cord
- Low birth weight because of preterm gestation, multifetal pregnancy, or intrauterine growth restriction
- Fetal anomalies such as hydrocephalus
- Complications secondary to placenta previa or cesarean birth

External version may be attempted to change the fetus in a breech presentation or transverse lie to a cephalic presentation (see Chapter 16). If the fetus remains in the abnormal presentation, cesarean birth usually is performed to avoid complications of a difficult vaginal birth. Birth for the nulliparous woman with a fetus in a breech presentation is almost always cesarean. The fetus remaining in a transverse lie is delivered by cesarean.

However, a cesarean is not clearly beneficial for every woman with a fetus in a breech presentation. The physician may recommend that vaginal birth be attempted when the fetus is in a breech presentation in the following cases (Bowes, 1999):

- The maternal pelvis is of normal size and shape.
- The estimated fetal weight is 2000 to 3800 g (4.4 to 8.4 lb).
- The fetus is in either a frank or complete breech presentation (see Chapter 12).
- The fetal head is well flexed.

Some women are admitted in advanced labor with the fetus in a breech presentation, so birth attendants and intrapartum nurses must be prepared to care for the woman having either a planned or an unexpected vaginal breech birth. (Figure 27-4 illustrates the mechanisms of vaginal birth for an infant in a breech presentation.)

Multifetal Pregnancy

Multifetal pregnancy may result in dysfunctional labor because of uterine overdistention, which contributes to hypotonic dysfunction, and abnormal presentation of one or both fetuses (Figure 27-5). In addition, the potential for fetal hypoxia during labor is greater because the mother must supply oxygen and nutrients to more than one fetus. She also is at greater risk for postpartum hemorrhage resulting from uterine atony because of uterine overdistention.

Because of these problems, cesarean birth is more common for a woman with a multifetal pregnancy. If three or more fetuses are involved, the birth is almost always cesarean. The physician considers fetal presentations, maternal pelvic size, and presence of other complications such as pregnancy-induced hypertension.

Each twin's FHR is monitored separately during labor. When in bed, the woman should remain in a lateral position to promote adequate placental blood flow. After vaginal birth of the first twin, assessment of the second twin's FHR continues until birth, which usually occurs within about 30 minutes.

The delivery staff must be prepared for the care and possible resuscitation of multiple infants. Radiant warmers, resuscitation equipment, medications, blankets, hats, and identification materials must be prepared for each infant. One or more neonatal nurses, a neonatal nurse-practitioner, and a pediatrician or a neonatologist should be available to care for each infant. One nurse should be free to care for the mother.

Fetal Anomalies

Fetal anomalies such as hydrocephalus or a large fetal tumor may prevent normal descent of the fetus. Abnormal presentations such as breech or transverse lie also are associated with fetal anomalies. These abnormalities often are discovered by ultrasound exami-

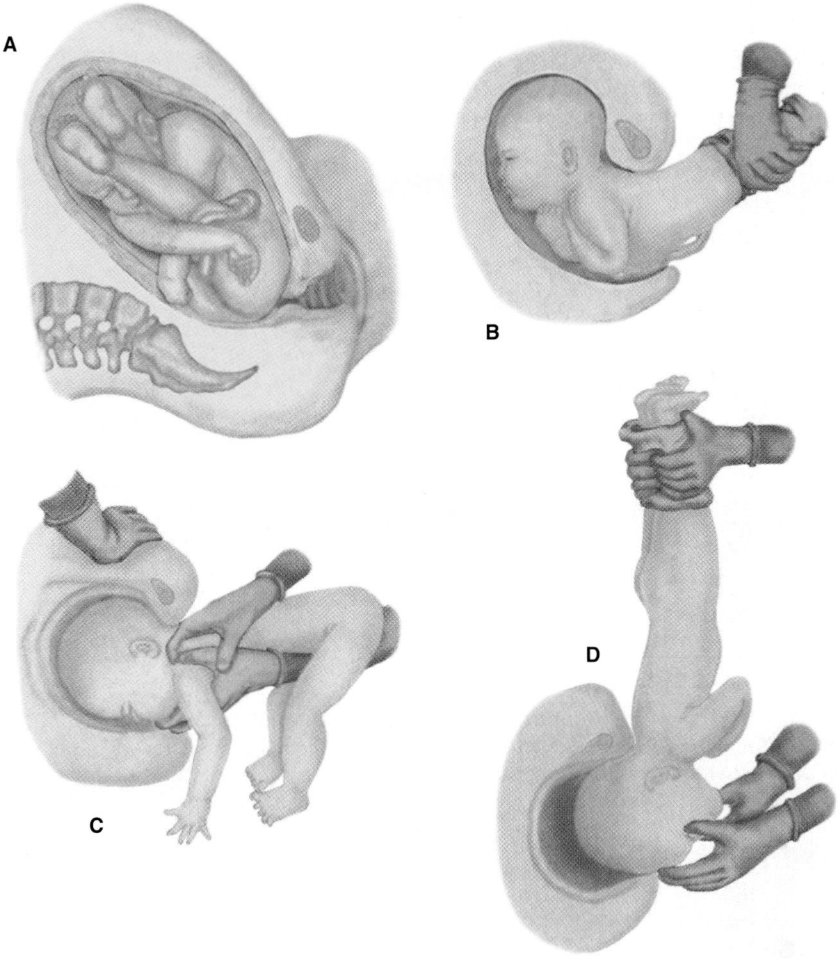

FIGURE 27-4 Sequence for vaginal birth in a frank breech presentation. **A,** Descent and internal rotation of the fetal body. **B,** Internal rotation complete; extension of the fetal back and neck as the trunk slips under the symphysis pubis. The birth attendant uses a towel for traction when grasping the fetal legs. **C,** After the birth of the shoulders, the attendant maintains flexion of the fetal head by using the fingers of the left hand to apply pressure to the lower face. The fetal body straddles the attendant's left arm. An assistant provides suprapubic pressure to help keep the fetal head well flexed. **D,** After the fetal head is brought under the symphysis pubis, an assistant grasps the fetal legs with a towel for traction while the attendant delivers the face and head over the mother's perineum.

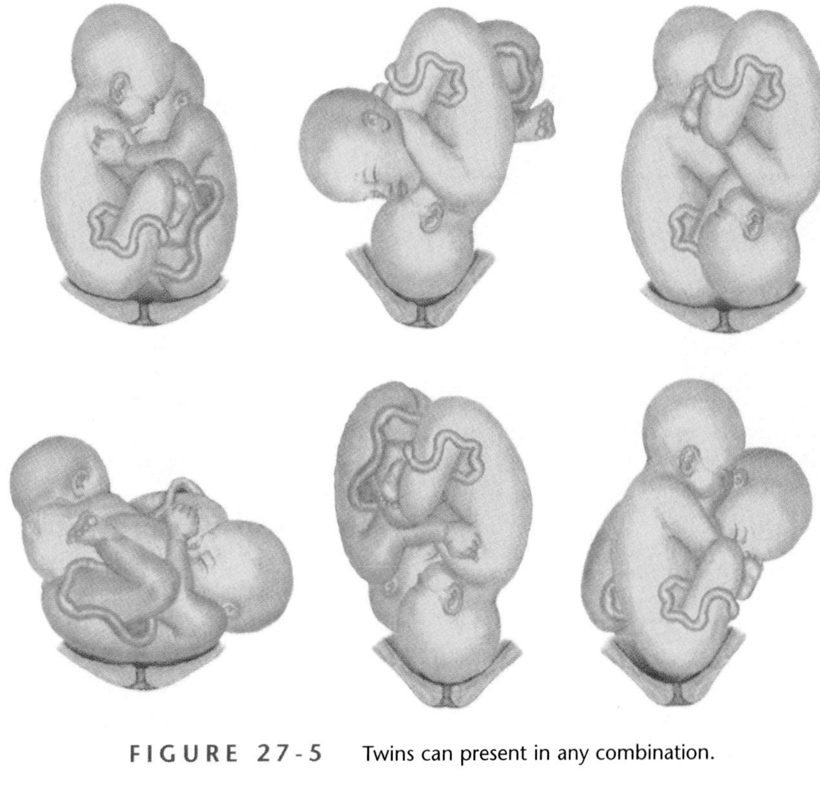

FIGURE 27-5 Twins can present in any combination.

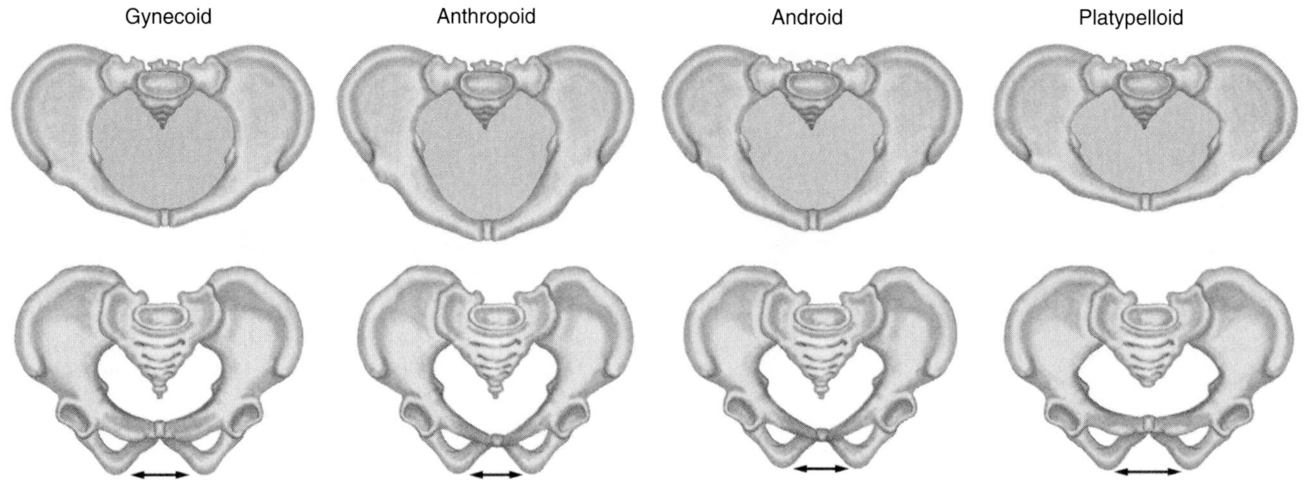

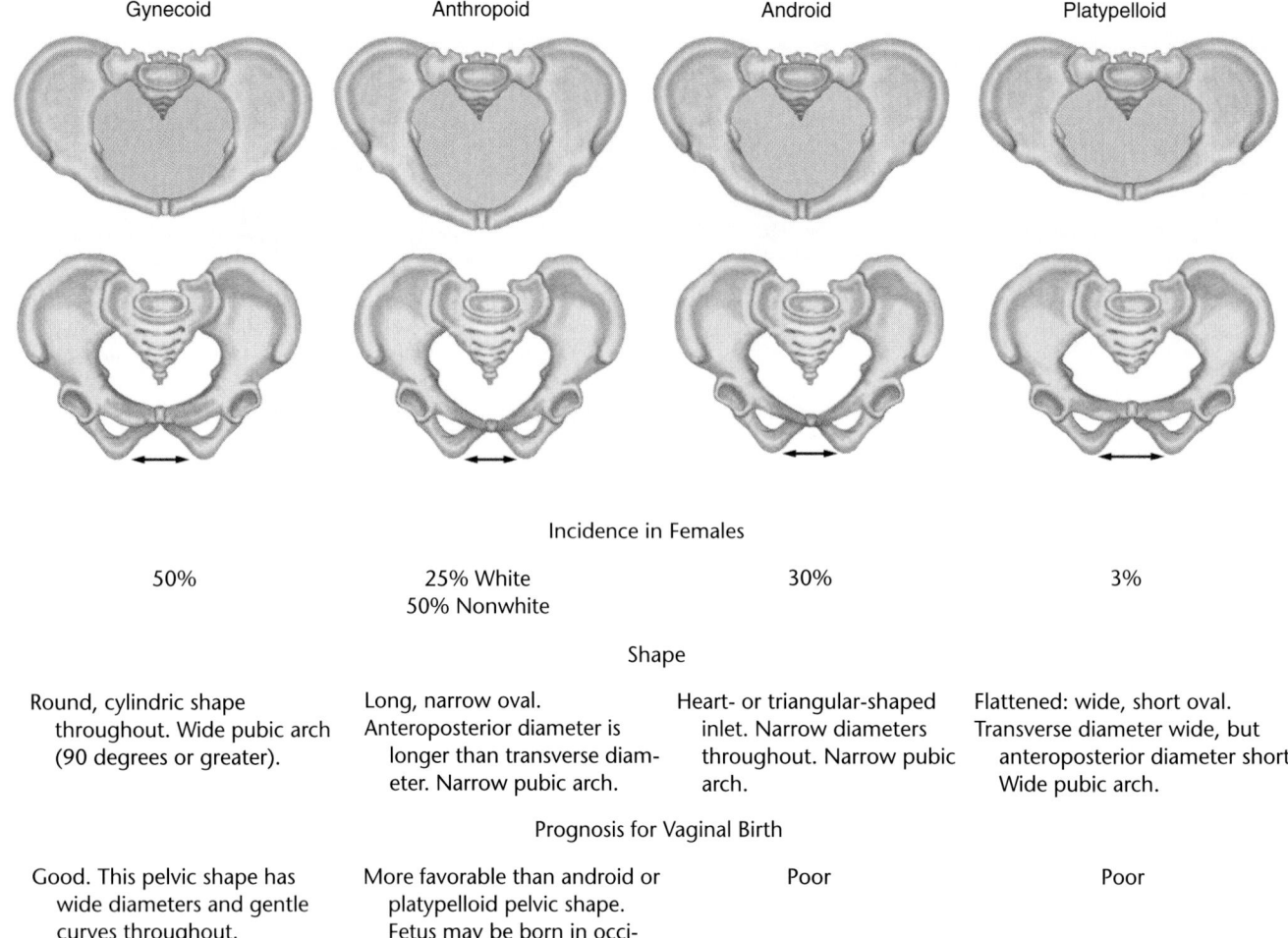

	Gynecoid	Anthropoid	Android	Platypelloid
Incidence in Females	50%	25% White 50% Nonwhite	30%	3%
Shape	Round, cylindric shape throughout. Wide pubic arch (90 degrees or greater).	Long, narrow oval. Anteroposterior diameter is longer than transverse diameter. Narrow pubic arch.	Heart- or triangular-shaped inlet. Narrow diameters throughout. Narrow pubic arch.	Flattened: wide, short oval. Transverse diameter wide, but anteroposterior diameter short. Wide pubic arch.
Prognosis for Vaginal Birth	Good. This pelvic shape has wide diameters and gentle curves throughout.	More favorable than android or platypelloid pelvic shape. Fetus may be born in occiput posterior position.	Poor	Poor

FIGURE 27-6 Pelvic shapes.

nation before labor. A cesarean birth is scheduled if vaginal birth is not possible or inadvisable.

Check Your Reading

1. How does hypotonic labor dysfunction differ from hypertonic labor in terms of the most common labor phase when it becomes evident? Uterine contractions? Presence of pain? Therapeutic management?
2. How can maternal position changes favor rotation of the fetus from an occiput transverse or occiput posterior position to an occiput anterior position?
3. Why does a cesarean birth not eliminate all adverse outcomes for infants in a breech presentation?
4. How does preparation for the birth of multiple infants (vaginal or cesarean) differ from preparation for a single infant's birth?

Problems of the Passage

Dysfunctional labor may occur because of variations in the maternal bony pelvis or soft tissue problems that inhibit fetal descent.

Pelvis

A small (contracted) or abnormally shaped pelvis may retard labor and obstruct fetal passage. The woman may experience poor contractions, slow dilation, slow fetal descent, and a long labor. The danger of uterine rupture is greater with thinning of the lower uterine segment, especially if contractions remain strong.

Four basic pelvic shapes exist, each with different implications for labor and birth (Figure 27-6). Most women do not have a pure pelvic shape but instead have mixed characteristics from two or more types.

Maternal Soft Tissue Obstructions

During labor, a full bladder is a common soft tissue obstruction. Bladder distention reduces available space in the pelvis and intensifies maternal discomfort. The woman should be assessed for bladder distention regularly and encouraged to void every 1 to 2 hours. Catheterization may be needed if she cannot urinate or an epidural depresses her urge to void.

Problems of the Psyche

Labor is a stressful event for most women. However, a perceived threat caused by pain, fear, nonsupport, or personal situation can result in excessive maternal stress and interfere with normal labor progress. The woman's perception of stress more than the actual existence of a threat is what is most important.

Responses to excessive or prolonged stress interfere with labor in several ways:

- Increased glucose consumption reduces the energy supply available to the contracting uterus.
- Secretion of catecholamines (epinephrine and norepinephrine) by the adrenal glands stimulates uterine beta-receptors, which inhibit uterine contractions (an action similar to that of tocolytic drugs such as terbutaline).
- Adrenal secretion of catecholamines diverts blood supply from the uterus and placenta to skeletal muscle.
- Labor contractions and maternal pushing efforts are less effective because these powers are working against the resistance of tense abdominal and pelvic muscles.
- Pain perception is increased and pain tolerance is decreased, which further increase maternal anxiety and stress.

Assisting the woman to relax helps her body work more effectively with the forces of labor. General nursing measures involve the following:

- Establishing a trusting relationship with the woman and her significant other
- Making the environment comfortable by adjusting temperature and light
- Promoting physical comfort such as cleanliness
- Providing accurate information
- Implementing nonpharmacologic and pharmacologic pain management

Chapters 13 and 15 describe specific methods to encourage relaxation and promote comfort.

Check Your Reading

5. Why should the nurse observe the laboring woman's bladder frequently?
6. Why is psychological support during labor important for effective physiologic function?

Abnormal Labor Duration

An unusually long or short labor may result in maternal, fetal, or neonatal problems.

Prolonged Labor

Prolonged labor results from problems with any of the factors in the birth process. After the woman reaches the active phase of labor, cervical dilation should proceed at a minimum rate of 1.2 cm per hour in the nullipara and 1.5 cm per hour in the parous woman. The fetal presenting part is expected to descend at a minimal rate of 1.0 cm per hour in the nullipara and 2.0 cm per hour in the parous woman (Bowes, 1999; Hayashi & Bashore, 1998; ACOG, 1995b). If all previous births were by cesarean before much cervical dilation occurred, the criteria that apply to a nullipara may be applied.

Possible maternal and fetal problems in prolonged labor include the following:

- Maternal infection, intrapartum or postpartum
- Neonatal infection, which may be severe or fatal
- Maternal exhaustion
- Higher levels of anxiety and fear during a subsequent labor

Maternal and neonatal infections are more likely if the membranes have been ruptured for a prolonged time because organisms ascend from the vagina. The mother is more likely to have an intrapartum infection, postpartum infection, or both.

Nursing measures for the woman who has prolonged labor include promotion of comfort, conservation of energy, emotional support, position changes that favor normal progress, and assessments for infection. Nursing care for the fetus includes observation for signs of intrauterine infection and compromised fetal oxygenation (see Chapter 14).

Precipitate Labor

Precipitate labor is one in which birth occurs within 3 hours of its onset. Intense contractions often begin abruptly rather than gradually increasing in frequency, duration, and intensity, as typical of most labors.

Precipitate labor is not the same as a precipitate birth. A precipitate birth occurs after a labor of any length, in or out of the hospital or birth center, when a trained attendant is not present to assist. However, a woman in precipitate labor also may have a precipitate birth. If the physician or nurse-midwife will not arrive in time for the baby's birth, the nurse should wear gloves and simply support the infant's body as it emerges. If the maternal pelvis is adequate and the soft tissues yield easily to fetal descent, little maternal injury is likely. However, if the soft tissues are firm and resist stretching, trauma (uterine rupture, cervical lacerations, hematoma) of the vagina or vulva may occur.

The fetus may suffer direct trauma such as intracranial hemorrhage or nerve damage during a precipitate labor. The fetus may become hypoxic because intense contractions with a short relaxation period reduce time available for gas exchange in the placenta. Nonreassuring electronic fetal monitoring patterns may include bradycardia and late decelerations.

Priority nursing care of the woman in precipitate labor includes promotion of fetal oxygenation and maternal comfort. A side-lying position enhances placental blood flow and reduces the effects of aortocaval compression. An added benefit of the side-lying position is to slow the rapid fetal descent and minimize perineal tears. Additional measures to enhance fetal oxygenation include administering oxygen to the mother and maintaining adequate blood volume with nonadditive IV fluids. If oxytocin is being used when rapid-fire contractions begin, it should be stopped. A tocolytic drug may be ordered.

Promoting comfort is difficult in a precipitate labor because intense contractions give the woman little time to prepare and use coping skills such as breathing techniques. Pharmacologic measures (opioid analgesia or regional block) may not be useful because quick labor progression does not allow time for them to become effective. Also, possible newborn respiratory depression must be considered when opioids are given near birth. The nurse helps the woman focus on techniques to cope with pain, one contraction at a time. The nurse must remain with her to provide support and assist with an emergency birth if it occurs.

Check Your Reading

7. During the active phase of labor, what is the minimal dilation and fetal descent rate expected for a nulliparous woman? For the parous woman?
8. What is the priority nursing care for a woman in prolonged labor?
9. What are the maternal and fetal risks when labor is unusually short?

APPLICATION OF THE NURSING PROCESS: DYSFUNCTIONAL LABOR

Several nursing diagnoses and collaborative problems may be appropriate when caring for a woman having dysfunctional labor. The potential complication of fetal compromise should be part of all intrapartum management (see Chapter 14). Pain management is especially important to women in dysfunctional labor because they may find that their coping skills are inadequate or difficult to use because of fatigue. Anxiety or fear often is higher with abnormal labor, which limits the woman's ability to cope with labor. Maternal or newborn injury may become apparent after the birth.

In addition to these problems, nursing care is directed toward two other nursing diagnoses: possible intrauterine infection and maternal exhaustion.

INTRAUTERINE INFECTION

Assessment

Infection can occur with both normal labors and dysfunctional labors. Assess the FHR and maternal vital signs for evidence of infection:

- Fetal tachycardia (>160 beats per minute [BPM] for a term fetus); a rising baseline fetal heart rate often is the first sign of intrauterine infection.
- Maternal temperature; assess every 2 to 4 hours in normal labor and every 2 hours after membranes rupture; assess hourly if elevated (38° C, or 100.4° F) or other signs of infection are present.
- Maternal pulse, respirations, and blood pressure; assess at least hourly to identify tachycardia or tachypnea, which often accompanies temperature elevation.

Assess amniotic fluid for normal clear color and mild odor. Yellow or cloudy fluid or fluid with a foul or strong odor suggests infection. The strong odor may be noted before birth or afterward on the infant's skin.

Analysis

For the woman without signs of infection but with risk factors, the nursing diagnosis selected is "Risk for Infection related to presence of favorable conditions for development."

Planning

Goals and expected outcomes relate to detecting the onset of infection:

- Maternal temperature will remain below 38° C (100.4° F).
- The FHR will remain near the baseline and below 160 BPM.
- The amniotic fluid will remain clear and without a foul or strong odor.

Interventions

Reducing the Risk for Infection

Nurses should wash their hands before and after each contact with the woman and her infant to reduce transmission of organisms. Limit vaginal examinations to reduce transmission of vaginal organisms into the uterine cavity, and maintain aseptic technique during essential vaginal examinations. The intrapartum nurse learns to estimate a woman's progress with few vaginal examinations. For example, increased bloody show and heightened anxiety may occur when the cervix is about 6 cm dilated. The woman may become irritable and lose control at about 8 cm dilation if she does not have epidural block analgesia.

Keep underpads as dry as possible to reduce the moist, warm environment that favors bacterial growth.

Periodically clean excess secretions from the vaginal area in a front-to-back motion to limit fecal contamination and promote the mother's comfort. Use personal protective equipment to avoid contact with body secretions.

Identifying Infection

Assess the woman and fetus for signs of infection. Increase the frequency of assessments if labor is prolonged, if other risk factors are present, or if any signs of infection are found. If signs of infection are noted, report them to the birth attendant for definitive treatment. Note the time at which the membranes ruptured to identify prolonged rupture, which adds to the risk for infection.

The birth attendant may collect specimens from the uterine cavity or placenta for culture to identify infectious organisms and determine antibiotic sensitivity. Aerobic and anaerobic culture specimens may be collected in containers specifically made for these two types of organisms. Follow directions on the container for proper handling and prevention of contamination with extraneous organisms, which would result in inaccurate results. Transport specimens to the laboratory promptly because living organisms are required for culture and sensitivity study.

Inform the newborn nursery staff if signs of infection are noted or increased maternal risk factors exist. Specimens of infant secretions also may be obtained for testing.

CRITICAL TO REMEMBER

Signs Associated with Intrapartum Infection

- Fetal tachycardia (rising baseline or >160 beats per minute)
- Maternal fever (38° C or 100.4° F)
- Foul or strong-smelling amniotic fluid
- Cloudy or yellow appearance to amniotic fluid

The infant often is given prophylactic antibiotics to prevent neonatal sepsis (see p. 851). If results of infant cultures indicate that no infection is present, the antibiotic usually is discontinued. Culture and sensitivity testing may reveal an infection and indicate that a different antibiotic would be more effective.

Evaluation

If the goals and expected outcomes are achieved,

- The woman's temperature will remain below 38° C (100.4° F).
- The amniotic fluid will have normal characteristics.
- Fetal tachycardia, either sudden or gradual in onset, will be absent.

Even if the woman has no signs of intrapartum infection, she remains at higher risk for postpartum infection and should be observed for signs and symptoms of infection.

MATERNAL EXHAUSTION

Assessment

Many women begin labor with a sleep deficit because of fetal movement, frequent urination, and shortness of breath associated with advanced pregnancy. As labor drags on, the mother's reserves are further depleted. Even with epidural block analgesia, a long labor drains the mother's energy. Also, some women do not choose or cannot take epidurals. Therefore the labor nurse must be prepared to deal with this problem.

Assess the mother for excessive fatigue:

- Verbal expression of tiredness, fatigue, or exhaustion
- Verbal expression of frustration with a prolonged, unproductive labor ("I can't go on any longer. Why doesn't the doctor just take the baby?")
- Ineffectiveness or inability to use coping techniques (such as patterned breathing) that she previously used effectively
- Changes in her pulse, respiration, and blood pressure (increased or decreased)

Analysis

The intense energy demands of a dysfunctional labor may exceed a woman's physical and psychological ability to meet them. For this reason, "Activity Intolerance related to depletion of maternal energy reserves" is an appropriate nursing diagnosis.

Planning

Contractions must continue for labor to progress. Two realistic goals or expected outcomes are that the woman will do the following:

- Rest between contractions with her muscles relaxed
- Use coping skills such as breathing and relaxation techniques

Interventions

Conserving Maternal Energy

Reduce factors that interfere with the woman's ability to relax. Lower the light level, and turn off overhead lights. Reduce noise by closing the door or using soft music, water sounds, or other comforting sounds. Maintain a comfortable maternal temperature with blankets or a fan. If not contraindicated, a warm shower or bath is soothing.

Position the woman to encourage comfort, promote fetal descent, and enhance fetal oxygenation. Support her with pillows to reduce muscle strain and added fatigue. Help her change positions regularly (about every 30 to 60 minutes) to reduce muscle tension from constant pressure.

A soothing back rub reduces muscle tension and thus decreases fatigue. Firm sacral pressure and use of some maternal positions discussed with fetal occiput posterior positions may reduce back pain. (See Chapters 13 and 15 for added comfort measures.)

Maintain IV fluids at the rate ordered to provide fluid, electrolytes, and occasionally glucose. Assess intake and output to identify dehydration, which may accompany prolonged labor. Dehydration also may cause maternal fever. If not contraindicated, provide juice, lollipops, frozen juice bars, or other clear liquids, as ordered by the physician or nurse-midwife, to moisten the woman's mouth and replenish her energy.

Promoting Coping Skills

When position changes or medical therapy is used to enhance labor, explain their purpose and expected benefits. Encourage the woman to visualize her baby passing downward smoothly through her pelvis as a result of her efforts. Provide her with mental images that allow her to "see" herself giving birth.

Generous praise and encouragement of the woman's use of skills such as breathing techniques motivate her to continue them even when she is discouraged. As with any laboring woman, tell her when she is making progress. Tell her that fetal heart rates and patterns are reassuring if this is true. Knowing that her efforts are having the desired results and her fetus is doing well gives the woman courage to continue.

Evaluation

Goals are met if the woman does the following:

- Rests and relaxes between contractions. If she is unable to relax, discuss analgesia options with her. Inability to relax between contractions is associated with pain beyond the woman's tolerance.
- Continues to demonstrate adequate use of learned skills to cope with labor.

In addition, solicit the woman's perceptions of her ability to relax and cope with labor.

PREMATURE RUPTURE OF THE MEMBRANES

Rupture of the amniotic sac before onset of true labor, regardless of length of gestation, is called *premature rupture of the membranes (PROM).* A related term, *preterm premature rupture of the membranes (PPROM),* describes ruptured membranes earlier than the end of the 37th week of gestation, with or without contractions. PPROM is associated with preterm labor and birth.

Etiology

Several conditions are associated with PROM, but the exact cause often remains unclear. Conditions associated with preterm ruptured membranes include the following:

- Infections of the vagina or cervix, such as group B streptococcal infection and bacterial vaginosis
- Chorioamnionitis, primarily a problem with PPROM
- Incompetent cervix or short cervical length ($\leq$25 mm by transvaginal ultrasonography)
- Fetal abnormalities or malpresentation
- Hydramnios
- Amniotic sac with a weak structure
- Recent procedures such as amniocentesis or cerclage
- Recent sexual intercourse
- Nutritional deficiencies
- Previous preterm birth related to PPROM
- Positive fetal fibronectin results (see p. 752)

Complications

Both mother and newborn are at risk for infection during the intrapartum and postpartum periods. Chorioamnionitis can be both a cause and a result of PROM. Organisms that cause chorioamnionitis weaken the amniotic membrane, leading to the rupture. The mother is at higher risk for postpartum infection, and the newborn is vulnerable to neonatal sepsis.

If chorioamnionitis does not precede PROM, it is more likely to occur if a long time elapses between membrane rupture and birth because vaginal organisms can readily enter the uterus. The exact time at which infection occurs cannot be predicted, but the risk is known to increase after 24 hours. However, infection may occur after just a few hours of ruptured membranes.

If preterm birth occurs, the infant is more likely to have respiratory distress syndrome (RDS) and complications related to prematurity. The hazards of prematurity are greatest before 34 weeks' gestation, especially if the woman did not receive steroids to accelerate fetal lung maturation before birth (see p. 757).

Other infant complications result from the loss of the amniotic fluid cushion (oligohydramnios). Umbilical cord compression, reduced lung volume, and deformities resulting from compression may occur.

Therapeutic Management

Management of PROM depends on the gestation and whether evidence of infection or other fetal or maternal compromise exists. For a woman at or near term (36 weeks' or more gestation), PROM may herald the imminent onset of true labor. Often, the cervix is soft with some dilation and effacement. If the fetus is immature or the woman's cervix is not soft and favorable for labor induction, therapeutic management is more complex. The risk of infection or prematurity for the fetus and newborn is weighed against the hazards of labor induction or cesarean birth.

Determining True Membrane Rupture

The first step is to determine whether the membranes are truly ruptured. Urinary incontinence, increased vaginal discharge, or loss of the mucus plug can make a woman think that her membranes have ruptured when they have not. A digital vaginal examination is avoided, particularly if the gestation is preterm and no evidence of labor exists. Instead, the physician or nurse-midwife performs a sterile speculum examination to look for a pool of fluid near the cervix and estimate cervical dilation and effacement. A Nitrazine or fern test may be done on the fluid to verify that the liquid is amniotic fluid. Tests to assess fetal lung maturity and identify infection are often done as well. A transvaginal ultrasound may be done to measure cervical length in higher-risk women (see Chapter 10).

Gestation Near Term

If the woman is at or near term and her cervix is soft, induction may be done if labor does not begin spontaneously. This will usually be done if the gestation is at least 36 weeks because the infant is unlikely to have severe problems associated with prematurity. Walking often helps stimulate the contractions of early labor as long as the woman takes adequate fluids and rests periodically. Labor is usually induced within 12 to 24 hours if contractions do not begin. Prostaglandin inserts such as Cervidil or Prepidil may assist cervical softening if needed before induction (see Chapter 16).

Preterm Gestation

If the gestation is preterm, the physician weighs the risks of maternal-fetal infection against the newborn's risk for complications of prematurity. The cervix usually is not favorable for induction far from term. Factors such as gestational age, amount of amniotic fluid remaining, fetal lung maturity, and any signs of fetal compromise are considered.

Between 32 and 35 weeks' gestation, the physician usually will test for fetal lung maturity from the amniotic fluid pooled in the vagina. The test, which measures the ratio of surfactant to albumin, may indicate that the fetal lungs are likely to be mature, immature, or borderline (transitional) when results are reported. Another test may indicate the presence (mature) or absence (immature) of phosphatidylglycerol (PG), but this test has limited usefulness because it remains negative in many women until late in pregnancy (Lenke & Ashwood, 2000). A lecithin/sphingomyelin (L:S) ratio may be done with an amniocentesis. At the time of amniocentesis, cultures for infecting organisms and glucose levels (which are low in infection) usually are done. If these tests show infection or the fetal lungs are mature, delivery usually is done by induction or cesarean. Antibiotics are given to the mother, including prophylactically if no infection exists. Prophylactic antibiotics have been shown to extend the interval to delivery and reduce neonatal morbidity (Hobel, 1998).

If no evidence of infection exists and the fetal lungs are immature, the woman usually is observed for infection or onset of labor in the hospital. Daily nonstress tests or biophysical profiles are done to watch for FHR nonreactivity, which often occurs with intraamniotic infection. Fetal lung maturity testing will be done periodically and the woman will be delivered when the fetal lungs are mature. Antibiotics are given during labor. An amnioinfusion (see Chapter 14) may be done prophylactically to reduce cord compression during labor (Garite, 2000b).

At very early gestations, management is more complex. Steroids given to the mother accelerate fetal lung maturity and antibiotics prolong gestation by about 1 week on average. Before 25 weeks' gestation, the likelihood of having a newborn who does well is low. The mother may elect to terminate the pregnancy or decide to be managed expectantly. For the women whose membranes rupture at these very early gestations, home care may be offered to spare them the extended hospitalization (Garite, 2000b).

Nursing Considerations

The woman usually remains hospitalized until birth unless a long stay is anticipated. The nurse observes for signs of infection along with the onset of labor and provides appropriate teaching. Care includes the following:

- Take her vital signs and the FHR every 4 hours, reporting any temperature above 38° C (100.4° F), or as her caregiver directs. A rise in the baseline of the FHR is a common indicator of infection.
- Note a foul or strong odor or cloudy or yellow appearance to the vaginal drainage.
- Teach her to avoid breast stimulation with preterm gestation because it causes release of oxytocin from the posterior pituitary and thus stimulates contractions. Breast stimulation can occur during a shower, from not wearing a bra, or during sexual activity.
- Avoid insertion of anything into the vagina to reduce the risk for carrying organisms into the area of the cervix. This includes vaginal examinations, vaginal suppositories, or, if she will be at home, vaginal intercourse. Additionally, seminal fluid contains prostaglandins, a potent stimulant of uterine contractions.
- Maintain any activity restrictions recommended.
- Note uterine contractions and report an increase in their frequency or intensity or a change in character.
- Teach the mother to observe fetal activity (kick counts) and report a decrease in the usual activity of the fetus.

Also see p. 758 for additional care of the woman with preterm labor.

Check Your Reading

10. How does PROM differ from PPROM?
11. What is the relationship of infection to PROM?
12. What is the usual therapeutic management of PROM if the woman is at or near term? What if the gestation is preterm?
13. What are the nursing considerations for a woman with PPROM?

PRETERM LABOR

Preterm labor begins after the 20th week but before the end of the 37th week of pregnancy. Preterm labor may result in the birth of an infant who is ill equipped for extrauterine life. The classification of preterm and low–birth weight (less than 2500 g) infants is second only to that of infants with birth defects in the top 10 causes for infant mortality in the United States (March of Dimes, 1999).

Associated Factors

Just as all causes of labor's onset at term are not known, the causes of preterm labor are not fully known. Several types of factors are associated with preterm labor:

- Medical conditions
- Present and past obstetric conditions
- Social and environmental factors
- Demographic factors such as race and age

See Table 27-2 for more detail about each of these factors. However, many women who have preterm labor and birth have no obvious risk factors.

Signs and Symptoms

Signs and symptoms of early preterm labor are more subtle than those of labor at term and often occur in normal pregnancies as well. The woman may be only vaguely aware that something seems different, or she may not detect that anything is amiss. Only when preterm labor reaches the active phase is it likely to have characteristics typical of term labor. Symptoms vary among women, but common ones are as follows:

- Uterine contractions that may or may not be painful (the woman may not feel contractions at all)
- A sensation that the baby is frequently "balling up"
- Cramps similar to menstrual cramps
- Constant low backache
- Sensation of pelvic pressure or a feeling that the baby is pushing down
- Pain, discomfort, or pressure in the vagina or thighs
- Change or increase in vaginal discharge (increased, watery, "spotting," bleeding)
- Abdominal cramps with or without diarrhea
- A sense of "just feeling bad" or "coming down with something"

Preventing Preterm Birth

Community Education

Preterm birth can impose substantial physical, emotional, and financial burdens on the child, family, and society. Nurses play an important role in preventing preterm birth. Ideally, strategies begin before conception, with community education. Programs often include teaching about the following:

- Duration of normal pregnancy
- Consequences of preterm birth

Table 27-2
MATERNAL RISK FACTORS FOR PRETERM LABOR

Medical History	Obstetric History	Present Pregnancy	Lifestyle and Demographics
Uterine or cervical anomalies Diethylstilbestrol (DES) exposure as a fetus History of cone biopsy History of pyelonephritis Low weight for height Chronic illness (such as cardiac, renal, hypertension)	Previous preterm birth Previous preterm labor with term birth First trimester abortions (>2) Second trimester abortions (≥2) Incompetent cervix Uterine anomaly	Uterine distention (such as multifetal pregnancy or hydramnios) Abdominal surgery during pregnancy Uterine irritability Uterine bleeding after 12 weeks Febrile illness Anemia Cervix dilated >1 cm at 32 weeks Cervical shortening <1 cm at 32 weeks Preeclampsia Preterm premature rupture of membranes (PPROM) Fetal or placental abnormalities	Little or no prenatal care Poor nutrition Age under 18 or over 40 Low education level Low socioeconomic status Smoking >10 cigarettes daily Cocaine abuse Nonwhite Chronic physical or psychological stress (such as stressful job or one requiring heavy work) Substance abuse (in addition to cocaine)

- Role of early and regular prenatal care in preventing preterm birth
- Conditions that increase risk for preterm birth

Women who are aware of the consequences of preterm birth may be more likely to take action to prevent it. If they recognize that they have risk factors, they may seek prenatal care earlier in gestation than they otherwise might.

During Pregnancy

During pregnancy, measures to prevent preterm birth include the following:

- Reducing barriers and improving access to early prenatal care for all women
- Assessing for risk factors to permit changes, if possible
- Promoting adequate nutrition
- Educating women and their partners about the subtle signs and symptoms of preterm labor and ways in which they differ from normal pregnancy changes
- Empowering women and their partners to take an active approach in seeking care if they have signs and symptoms of preterm labor

One group (Freston, et al., 1997) surveyed women about preterm labor and found that most could identify obvious symptoms such as having 4 to 5 contractions in an hour. For the more subtle symptoms that resembled common pregnancy discomforts, such as intermittent backache or vaginal heaviness, 35% of the women surveyed would have delayed care. This delay might mean the difference between preterm labor that could be stopped and preterm birth.

Improving Access to Care. Improving access to prenatal care must be customized for the community. What works in one area may be inappropriate for another. Difficult access is a serious problem for women who rely on public clinics for their care. Long waits, fragmented care, language barriers, and insensitivity of caregivers discourage women from obtaining care. Expanding the number of caregivers by using advanced-practice nurses, such as certified nurse-midwives and nurse practitioners, can reduce waits for care significantly. Nurses can help coordinate various aspects of care to limit the number of different appointments a woman needs to obtain complete care.

Identifying Risk Factors. Identification of risk factors may allow reduction or elimination of these factors. Women should be rescreened regularly to identify new risks that emerge as pregnancy progresses. Women with high-risk factors benefit from care such as more frequent prenatal care appointments, reinforcement of the symptoms of preterm labor, telephone contacts, and added assessments of fetal growth and health.

Some risk factors can be reduced or eliminated if the woman changes her lifestyle. Many women have stopped smoking or using drugs to benefit their babies, changes that may have been difficult for them. A woman may need to rest more or stop working, which may be difficult or impossible for many. Nurses can work with the woman to help reduce her risks as much as possible by helping her identify sources of support.

The role of subclinical infection in PPROM and preterm labor is becoming better known. Screening for pathogenic organisms in the urine, vagina, and cervix identifies women who may benefit from antibiotic therapy.

Promoting Adequate Nutrition. An adequate maternal diet contributes positively to the length of gestation and the infant's birth weight. In one study, low weight gain in pregnancy increased the risk for preterm birth in women who were underweight or of average weight before pregnancy (Schieve, et al., 2000). The mother's height should be measured at the first prenatal visit and her weight should be taken at each visit to evaluate adequacy of weight gain. Every pregnant woman should be offered culturally sensitive diet counseling. The Women, Infants, and Children (WIC) program is available to supplement the diet of some low-income women. Anemia can be corrected with appropriate supplements. (See Chapter 9 for added information about nutrition and pregnancy, including nutrition for cultural practices and vegetarianism.)

Educating Women and Their Partners about Preterm Labor. All pregnant women and their partners should be taught about symptoms of preterm labor because about half of preterm births occur in women with no identified risk factors. Interpreters and printed materials in the woman's primary language should be used if needed. Diagrams should supplement the words of any language for women of limited reading skills. Jones and Collins (1996) recommend that written materials have a reading level no higher than sixth grade.

The nurse should verify the woman's understanding by seeking feedback, such as having her restate the signs and symptoms of preterm labor and the appropriate responses to them.

Empowering Women and Their Partners. Delaying birth depends critically on early identification of preterm labor. Women should be encouraged to seek treatment promptly if they suspect preterm labor. The woman must communicate her concerns clearly when arriving at the clinic or hospital. She should tell the triage person that she should be checked for labor, regardless of the subtlety of the symptoms. Caregivers must not make the woman feel foolish if she reports signs and symptoms that could be preterm labor but turn out to be a false alarm. Otherwise, she may not seek care for recurrent episodes when she truly is in labor and the opportunity to delay preterm birth may be lost.

> The nurse might suggest that a woman who is seeking care for possible preterm labor say, "I'm not due for 8 more weeks but I think I may be in labor. I need to be seen right away or I might have a premature baby."

Therapeutic Management

Management focuses on predicting those at risk for preterm birth, identifying preterm labor early, delaying birth, and accelerating fetal lung maturity if preterm birth is likely.

Predicting Preterm Birth

Because treatment for preterm labor has been less than satisfactory at preventing preterm birth, research has focused on predicting those women who will deliver early. Better identification of these women would allow more intensive treatment, ideally before preterm labor or rupture of membranes occurs. Also, many signs and symptoms of preterm labor occur in women who deliver at term, possibly exposing them to unneeded treatment. The key is to identify which women with the symptoms are really at risk for preterm birth and treat those women intensively while continuing regular prenatal care for the women with these symptoms as a variant of normal pregnancy symptoms. A good screening test would be inexpensive, usable for all pregnant women, noninvasive, and highly specific for the condition. No screening test meeting these criteria is available to screen for preterm labor yet, but two tests, the fetal fibronectin and salivary estriol tests, help identify who is *unlikely* to deliver early.

The results of a major preterm prediction study looked at multiple factors and found that their relevance interrelated according to the mother's parity and obstetrical history. As might be expected, a woman's risk for preterm birth was substantially increased if she had several risk factors. In this study, factors most strongly associated with predicting preterm birth included (1) a short cervical length of ≤25 mm (1 cm), (2) a previous preterm birth caused by PPROM, and (3) a positive fetal fibronectin screening result (Mercer, et al., 2000). An additional test, the salivary estriol test, was not included in the study but has received FDA approval for preterm birth prediction.

Cervical Length. A short cervix (≤25 mm [≤1 cm]), measured by transvaginal ultrasound, may allow vaginal organisms easier access to the uterus, where they weaken the membranes and cause premature rupture. Alternately, the shortened cervix may reflect structural changes caused by an intrauterine infection or uterine contractions. Transvaginal ultrasound is expensive as a screening test in routine care but may have a place in pregnancies at higher risk for preterm birth, such as multifetal gestation (Mercer, et al., 2000; Creasy & Iams, 1999).

PPROM in a Previous Birth. Some women may have a predisposition to weak amniotic membrane structure that predates the actual leaking of fluid (Mercer, et al., 2000). This predisposition seems to repeat in subsequent pregnancies.

Fetal Fibronectin. Fetal fibronectin (fFN) is a protein present in fetal tissues. Fetal fibronectin is not normally found in the cervical and vaginal secretions between 22 weeks' gestation and term. It normally reappears in the cervical and vaginal secretions about 2 to 3 weeks before the onset of labor at term. If it appears too early, it suggests that labor may begin early, similar to the way elevated cardiac enzymes rise in the person with a myocardial infarction (Garite, 2000a; Creasy & Iams, 1999). The fetal fibronectin test may help the physician make a better judgment about whether the woman's symptoms are true preterm labor that should be treated aggressively or a variant of normal pregnancy symptoms that can be managed more conservatively. However, in a study of low-risk women (for whom the test is not designed), the fFN assay was not sensitive in predicting those who would deliver before 35 weeks (Iams, et al., 2001).

To reduce false positives from the fetal fibronectin test, the test must be collected before significant vaginal manipulation from examination. Cervical examination, sexual intercourse within 24 hours, and vaginal bleeding can cause a test to be positive when preterm labor is not truly present (Moore, 1999).

Salivary Estriol. Estriol rises in the saliva about 5 weeks before term or preterm birth. A negative test is reassuring that preterm birth is unlikely, but a positive test is less certain because false-positive tests are common. However, the test may prevent overtreatment of a woman with more Braxton-Hicks contractions than usual.

The woman can collect the specimen in her home. It is mailed to the lab at the company where it was developed. She must not smoke, eat, drink, chew gum, or care for her teeth for 1 hour before collecting the saliva, and the specimen must be collected between 9:00 AM and 8:00 PM because the estriol levels show a diurnal variation (different in the daytime than at night). Bleeding in her mouth will interfere with the accuracy of the test, and betamethasone, given to accelerate fetal lung maturity, suppresses estriol levels (Moore, 1999).

Identifying Preterm Labor

The reason to predict risk for preterm birth or identify preterm labor early is to delay birth, thus promoting further fetal maturation.

Frequent Prenatal Visits. Women at risk for preterm labor should have more frequent prenatal visits, at which time they are checked for evidence of preterm labor and their ability to follow preventive therapy, in addition to their regular prenatal checkup. They should be assessed for development of new risk factors with each visit. Gentle cervical examinations identify painless effacement or dilation. A transvaginal ultrasound may identify the shortened cervix that often precedes onset of labor. Infections can be identified and treated promptly before rupture of membranes or onset of labor occurs.

fFN testing can help the caregiver decide the best course of treatment. For example, if the woman in suspected preterm labor has a positive fFN test, she can be treated more aggressively with tocolytics or transported to a facility with available neonatal intensive care, rather than being treated conservatively. Salivary estriol testing serves a similar purpose.

Home Uterine Activity Monitoring. Home monitoring to detect early uterine contractions before they cause cervical change has not proven to be beneficial in reducing preterm birth (Creasy & Iams, 1999). It may be used occasionally to detect very early contractions that precede obvious labor. Data are transmitted through a modem to a central office, where nurses interpret the information and discuss it with the woman.

Stopping Preterm Labor

Once diagnosis of preterm labor is made, management focuses on stopping uterine activity before the point of no return, usually after about 3 cm dilation. If preterm delivery is inevitable, therapy is directed toward reducing the infant's risk for respiratory distress.

Initial Measures

The physician initially determines whether any maternal or fetal conditions contraindicate continuing the pregnancy. Examples of these conditions are severe preeclampsia, maternal hypovolemia, chorioamnionitis, and fetal compromise.

Initial measures to stop preterm labor include identifying and treating infections, identifying other causes of preterm labor that may be treatable, and reducing activity. Hydration with IV fluids has been used to reduce posterior pituitary secretion of oxytocin but has not been found beneficial (Creasy & Iams, 1999). Overhydration increases the risk for pulmonary edema if some drugs also are used to stop preterm labor.

Identifying and Treating Infections. Infection, both systemic and local, has a strong association with preterm birth, as it does with premature rupture of the membranes. Blood studies identify signs of infection and other conditions such as anemia that also are associated with preterm labor or affect its management. Common studies include a complete blood count with differential white blood cell analysis and vaginal or cervical cultures for group B streptococcus, chlamydia, and gonorrhea. Amniocentesis may be done to obtain amniotic fluid for culture if chorioamnionitis is suspected because this infection would contraindicate stopping preterm labor. Fetal lung maturity testing will likely be done on an amniotic fluid specimen as well. A catheterized urine specimen is usually obtained for analysis and culture and sensitivity testing (Iams, 2000; Creasy & Iams, 1999; Flynn, 1999).

If infection is suspected, it is treated with the anti-infective agent or agents expected to be effective against the organism before completion of cultures, which requires a minimum of 24 to 48 hours. If cultures show that a different drug would be best, the medication is changed.

Identifying Other Causes for Preterm Contractions. The woman with polyhydramnios, identified by ultrasonography, may have more contractions because her uterus is stretched more than normal. A therapeutic amniocentesis to remove some amniotic fluid can reduce uterine irritability. Multifetal gestations also can be identified by ultrasonography. These mothers may benefit from improved nutrition, stress reduction, assistance with household care, and other interventions.

Restricting Activity. Bed rest, usually on the left side, increases placental blood flow and reduces fetal pressure on the cervix. However, bedrest has not been shown to lengthen pregnancy significantly and is associated with serious maternal side effects. Studies have not found that bedrest is contraindicated as a therapy in preterm labor (Creasy & Iams, 1999; Maloni, 1998). Adverse physical effects include cardiovascular deconditioning, muscle and calcium loss, and weight loss (or failure to gain normally). Other adverse effects may include depression, anxiety, and sleep changes. Because of significant maternal problems with no clear benefit to the infant, lengthy bedrest is less often prescribed for women who are at risk for preterm labor. Activity restrictions may be modified, such as resting in a semi-Fowler's position or partial bedrest. Alternating sides from left to right reduces discomfort of constant side lying. Despite the lack of proven benefits and known drawbacks, bedrest or some degree of activity restriction continues to be prescribed for women who are diagnosed with preterm labor (Schroeder, 1998; Maloni, 1998).

The nurse in high-risk antepartum nursing is likely to encounter a variety of prescriptions for activity limitations when women have preterm labor or other complications of pregnancy. "Total" bedrest is fairly uncommon, and even then the woman often is allowed to go to the bathroom. Lesser amounts of activity restriction include stopping work with several hours of extra rest each day and simply increasing regular rest periods.

The woman and her family often are burdened by strict activity restriction. In addition to the physical effects mentioned, loss of the woman's income may make the critical difference in the family's economic survival, especially if the family includes other children. The family is at risk for domestic stress and violence because the woman cannot maintain her usual role. The woman who has other children may feel a great deal of ambivalence, wanting to do what is prescribed for the well-being of her fetus but also feeling the need to care for the older children (Schroeder, 1998).

Tocolytics

Tocolysis is most likely to be effective if the cervix is less than 3 cm dilated. However, tocolytic drugs have significant side effects, and physicians do not want to treat a nonexistent disorder. The decision about whether to treat for preterm labor is individualized, based on risk factors, cervical dilation, and other signs and symptoms. If the cervix is between 2 and 3 cm dilated, the physician will probably recheck the cervix for further dilation or effacement after 1 or 2 hours. A fetal fibronectin test also will be done to determine whether the woman is likely to be in preterm labor or is having stronger Braxton-Hicks activity.

Tocolysis is most likely ordered if preterm labor occurs before the 34th week of gestation because the infant's risk for respiratory and other complications of prematurity is high if born during this time. Tocolytic drugs do not typically *prevent* preterm birth but may delay it. This delay may provide time to allow use of corticosteroids to accelerate fetal lung maturity or transfer the woman to a facility with a neonatal intensive care unit.

Most tocolytic drugs are used primarily for conditions other than preterm labor and therefore have effects on body systems other than the reproductive system. The lowest possible dose that inhibits contractions is used. Four types of drugs are used for tocolysis: (1)

Table 27-3

DRUGS USED IN PRETERM LABOR

Drug/Purpose	Sample Dose Regimens*	Side or Adverse Effects
β-adrenergics (tocolysis) Ritodrine (Yutopar)	*IV:* Start at 0.05 mg/min (50 mcg/min). Increase by 0.05 mg/min increments every 20 min until labor stops, contraction frequency is 6 or fewer per hour, or significant side effects develop. Maximal dose is 0.35 mg/min (350 mcg/min). When contractions are 4 or fewer per hour, maintain the infusion for 1 hr and decrease dose to the lowest rate that maintains contractions at fewer than 4 per hour. Continue this dose for 12 hr. *Oral:* Give first oral dose 30 to 60 minutes before discontinuing IV ritodrine. 5 to 10 mg every 2 to 4 hr for 24 to 48 hr. Maximal daily oral dose: 120 mg/day.	Side effects are dose related and more prominent during increases in the infusion rate than during maintenance therapy. Cardiovascular: Maternal and fetal tachycardia. Wide pulse pressure. Pulmonary: Shortness of breath, chest pain; pulmonary edema (more likely if the woman receives corticosteroids at the same time and if IV drug is diluted in normal saline or Ringer's lactate). Gastrointestinal: Nausea, vomiting, diarrhea, ileus. Neurologic: Tremors, jitteriness, restlessness, feeling of apprehension. Metabolic alterations: Hyperglycemia; hypokalemia. Drug should be diluted in D_5W unless glucose solution is contraindicated (maternal diabetes) to reduce the risk for pulmonary edema.
Terbutaline (Brethine)	See "Drug Guide: Terbutaline" (p. 756). *IV:* Begin at 10 mcg/min. Increase by 5 mcg increments at 10- to 20-min intervals until contractions stop or maximum of 25 mcg/min is reached or significant side effects develop. Maintain dose for 30 to 60 min after contractions stop, then reduce rate at 30-min intervals to reach lowest effective dose. Continue maintenance dose for 8 hr after contractions stop before changing route of administration to subcutaneous or oral. *Subcutaneous (SC)* (most common parenteral route): 0.25 mg (250 mcg) every 3 to 4 hr (range, every 1 to 6 hr based on uterine activity and maternal pulse rate). Sometimes given by subcutaneous infusion pump. *Oral:* 5 to 10 mg every 2 to 4 hr for 48 hr. Maximal daily dose of 120 mg.	Cardiovascular: Maternal and fetal tachycardia, palpitations, cardiac arrhythmias, chest pain, wide pulse pressure. Respiratory: Dyspnea, chest discomfort; pulmonary edema. Central nervous system: Tremors, restlessness, weakness, dizziness, headache. Metabolic: Hyperglycemia, hypokalemia. Gastrointestinal: Nausea, vomiting, reduced bowel motility. Skin: Flushing, diaphoresis. Infection at injection site (subcutaneous infusion pump).

*Doses and frequency of administration are examples; actual protocols vary.

β-adrenergics, (2) magnesium sulfate, (3) prostaglandin synthesis inhibitors, and (4) calcium antagonists. (Table 27-3 summarizes doses and routes of administration for each of these drugs.)

A new drug, atosiban, which opposes the action of oxytocin, is being researched. Early trials on this drug suggest that it offers a delay until birth similar to that of other tocolytic drugs. Its side effects have been minimal. If further study confirms the beneficial effects of atosiban, it offers another drug to counteract preterm labor.

β-adrenergic Drugs. Although ritodrine (Yutopar) is the only β-adrenergic currently approved by the U.S. Food and Drug Administration (FDA) for tocolysis, terbutaline (Brethine) is the most widely used drug in this class.

The main side effects involve the cardiorespiratory system. Maternal and fetal tachycardia are common. Other side effects include decreased blood pressure, wide pulse pressure, arrhythmias, myocardial ischemia, and chest pain. Pulmonary edema is the most common serious side effect. Metabolic changes include hyperglycemia and hypokalemia. Tremors and restlessness are other side effects (Creasy & Iams, 1999).

The neonate may have hypoglycemia and myocardial hypertrophy. Some early evidence suggests that these drugs may increase the incidence of serious intraventricular hemorrhage in the newborn (Iams, 2000). (See the Drug Guide for nursing care related to terbutaline tocolysis.)

β-adrenergics may be given by the IV, intramuscular, subcutaneous, or oral route. Treatment usually is initiated by the intravenous route. When the preterm contractions are stopped, the dose is kept at that level for up to 24 hours or reduced to the lowest dose that inhibits contractions. If used, oral therapy begins 30 minutes before the IV dose is stopped to maintain consis-

Table 27-3
DRUGS USED IN PRETERM LABOR—cont'd

Drug/Purpose	Sample Dose Regimens*	Side or Adverse Effects
Magnesium sulfate (tocolysis)	*IV:* Loading dose: 6 g in 10% to 20% solution over 15 min. Maintenance dose is 2 g/hr; dose may be increased by 1 g/hr until woman has 1 contraction or fewer in 10 min or reaches a maximal dose of 4 g/hr. When contractions are fewer than 4 per hour, maintain magnesium infusion rate for 12 to 24 hr, then reduce magnesium by 1 g/hr. Discontinue magnesium infusion when rate reaches 2 g/hr. While woman is on magnesium, check vital signs and reflexes hourly; check intake and output every 2 to 4 hr.	Side and adverse effects are dose-related, occurring at higher serum levels. Depression of deep tendon reflexes. Respiratory depression. Cardiac arrest (usually at serum levels above 12/mg/dl). Less serious side effects: Lethargy, weakness, visual blurring, headache, sensation of heat, nausea, vomiting, constipation. Fetal-neonatal effects: Reduced FHR variability, hypotonia.
Indomethacin (Indocin) (nonsteroidal anti-inflammatory for tocolysis)	Loading dose of 100 mg rectally or 50 mg orally. May repeat in 1 hr if no decrease in contractions. Follow by 25 to 50 mg PO every 4 to 6 hr for 48 hr. Should be discontinued if birth appears imminent. Amniotic fluid volume should be checked before initiation of therapy and at 48 and 72 hr. Recommendation is to use only before 32 weeks' gestation (Iams, 2000).	Epigastric pain, nausea, gastrointestinal bleeding. Asthma in aspirin-sensitive women. Increased blood pressure in hypertensive women. May obscure a fever. Fetus: May have constriction of the ductus arteriosus and decreased urine output. Decreased urine output is associated with oligohydramnios, which may result in cord compression. Adverse fetal/neonatal effects are uncommon if treatment is 48 hr or less.
Nifedipine (Procardia) (calcium channel blocker for tocolysis)	*Oral:* 10 mg PO every 20 to 30 min up to 3 doses, then 10 to 20 mg PO every 4 to 6 hr.	Maternal flushing, headache, dizziness, nausea. Transient maternal tachycardia. Maternal hypotension.
Corticosteroids (accelerating fetal lung maturation) *Betamethasone (Celestone) *Dexamethasone (Decadron)	See "Drug Guide: Betamethasone and Dexamethasone" (p. 757). *Betamethasone:* 12 mg IM for two doses, 24 hr apart *Dexamethasone:* 6 mg IM q 12 hr for four doses Greatest fetal benefits if at least 24 hr elapse between first dose and birth	Concurrent administration with β-adrenergics and corticosteroids increases the risk for pulmonary edema. May worsen conditions such as diabetes and hypertension and may increase incidence of infections.

DRUG GUIDE: TERBUTALINE (BRETHINE)

Classification: β-adrenergic agent.

Action: Stimulates β-adrenergic receptors of the sympathetic nervous system. Action primarily results in bronchodilation and inhibition of uterine muscle activity. Increases pulse rate and widens pulse pressure.

Indications: Stop preterm labor. Reduce or stop hypertonic labor contractions, whether natural or stimulated.

Dosage and Route: Numerous protocols for terbutaline administration for tocolysis exist.

1. *IV infusion.* IV use is investigational. Begin at 10 mcg/minute. Increase by 5 mcg/minute increments at 10- to 20-minute intervals until contractions stop or a maximal dose of 25 mcg/minute is reached, or significant side effects develop. Maintain this dose for 30 to 60 minutes after contractions stop. Reduce infusion rate at 30-minute intervals to reach lowest effective maintenance dose. Continue maintenance dose for 8 hours after contractions stop before changing route of administration to subcutaneous or oral.
2. *Subcutaneous (SC)* (most common parenteral route). 0.25 mg (250 mcg) every 3 to 4 hours for up to 3 doses (range: every 1 to 6 hours, with frequency determined by uterine activity and maternal pulse rate).
3. *Oral.* 5 to 10 mg every 2 to 4 hours (maximal daily dose of 120 mg); oral therapy should be discontinued within 48 hours because of the likelihood of rapid pulse rate.

If changing from IV to oral therapy, give oral dose 30 minutes before discontinuing IV infusion.

Absorption:

1. *IV.* Prompt; duration about 2 hours.
2. *Subcutaneous.* 6 to 15 minutes; duration 1.5 to 4 hours.
3. *Oral.* 1 to 2 hours; duration 4 to 8 hours.

Excretion: Metabolized in the liver. Excreted in urine.

Contraindications: Hypersensitivity. Contraindicated before 20 weeks' gestation and if continuing the pregnancy is hazardous to the mother or fetus, as in fetal distress, hemorrhage, chorioamnionitis, and intrauterine fetal death. Contraindicated in conditions that may be adversely affected by β-adrenergic agents (uncontrolled diabetes, hyperthyroidism, bronchial asthma treated with other β-mimetic agents or steroids, cardiac dysrhythmias, hypovolemia, and uncontrolled hypertension).

Precautions: Terbutaline is not approved by the U.S. Food and Drug Administration for inhibiting uterine activity, although it is widely used for this purpose based on extensive clinical experience. All tocolytics are most effective if begun as soon as a diagnosis of preterm labor is made.

Adverse Reactions

1. *Cardiovascular:* Maternal and fetal tachycardia, palpitations, cardiac arrhythmias, chest pain, wide pulse pressure
2. *Respiratory:* Dyspnea, chest discomfort
3. *Central nervous system:* Tremors, restlessness, weakness, dizziness, headache
4. *Metabolic:* Hypokalemia, hyperglycemia
5. *Gastrointestinal:* Nausea, vomiting, reduced bowel motility
6. *Skin:* Flushing, diaphoresis

Nursing Considerations: Diagnostic studies that may be ordered related to terbutaline therapy include electrocardiogram, blood glucose, electrolytes, and urinalysis. Explain common side effects that are usually well tolerated, such as palpitations, tremors, restlessness, weakness, and headache. Assess FHR, usually with continuous electronic fetal monitoring, recording rate and patterns every 15 minutes during IV dose increases. Assess maternal pulse, respirations, and blood pressure by same schedule as for FHR. Assess lung sounds every 6 to 12 hours to identify pulmonary edema. Maintain adequate IV or oral hydration; intake should be about 1500 to 2500 ml per day (Creasy & Iams, 1999). Encourage the woman to empty her bladder every 2 hours. Output should be recorded to identify fluid retention. Notify the physician for significant or unacceptable side effects (maternal heart rate above 110/BPM, respirations above 24/minute, systolic blood pressure lower than 90 mmHg, FHR above 160/BPM, chest pain, dyspnea). Report continuing or recurrent uterine activity. Teach signs and symptoms of recurrent preterm labor and follow-up medical care after discharge.

tent blood levels of the drug. Oral therapy may continue until 36 to 37 weeks of gestation. After 24 hours on oral therapy, modified bedrest may be prescribed to the woman (Creasy & Iams, 1999).

Subcutaneous terbutaline may be given with a continuous, low-dose infusion pump at home or in the hospital. The pump is similar to an insulin pump in that it injects a continuous low dose of terbutaline with intermittent bolus doses at times of peak uterine activity. The benefits and risks for subcutaneous pump terbutaline have yet to be determined (Creasy & Iams, 1999).

Magnesium Sulfate. Magnesium sulfate is used in management of pregnancy-induced hypertension to prevent seizures (see the Drug Guide on p. 685). Because of its added effect of quieting uterine activity, it often is used to inhibit preterm labor. Magnesium sulfate therapy has a well-established record of safety during pregnancy. The woman who cannot tolerate other drugs or for whom other drugs are ineffective may benefit from magnesium sulfate tocolysis.

Magnesium sulfate for tocolysis is given intravenously using a similar protocol to that for pregnancy-induced hypertension. The criteria needed to continue magnesium sulfate therapy include the following:

- Urine output of at least 25 ml per hour
- Presence of deep tendon reflexes
- At least 12 respirations per minute

In addition, the nurse should check heart and lung sounds with hourly vital signs because fluid overload and electrolyte imbalances can lead to pulmonary edema or cardiac dysrhythmias. Bowel sounds are checked when therapy begins and every 4 to 8 hours because the smooth muscle in the intestinal tract may be relaxed just

DRUG GUIDE: BETAMETHASONE (CELESTONE) DEXAMETHASONE (DECADRON)

Classification: Corticosteroids.

Indications: Acceleration of fetal lung maturity to reduce the incidence and severity of respiratory distress syndrome and intraventricular hemorrhage in the preterm infant. Greatest benefits accrue if at least 24 hours elapse between the initial dose and birth of the preterm infant, but the drug is indicated if birth is not actually imminent.

Dosage and Route:
Betamethasone: 12 mg IM for two doses, 24 hours apart.
Dexamethasone: 6 mg IM every 12 hours for four doses.
The doses may be repeated if birth has not occurred within 7 days.

Absorption: Rapid and complete after IM administration.

Excretion: Metabolized in the liver. Excreted in urine.

Contraindications: Active infection such as chorioamnionitis is a relative contraindication, although further study is needed. The National Institutes of Health recommend use of corticosteroids for the woman who has preterm rupture of the membranes (24 to 32 weeks' gestation), and the American College of Obstetricians and Gynecologists (ACOG) and American Academy of Pediatrics (AAP) also recommend their use in *Guidelines for Perinatal Care* (4th ed.).

Precautions: Possible infection. Pregnancies complicated by diabetes.

Adverse Reactions: Few, in most cases owing to the short-term use of the drug. Pulmonary edema is possible secondary to sodium and fluid retention.

Nursing Considerations: Explain the potential benefits of corticosteroid administration to the preterm neonate. Explain that the drug cannot prevent or lessen the severity of all complications of prematurity. If the woman is diabetic, explain that more frequent blood glucose determinations are common because these levels often are slightly higher. Assess lung sounds at least every 6 to 12 hours or more frequently. Report chest pain or heaviness and dyspnea.

as the uterus is relaxed. Serum magnesium level measurements guide maintenance of therapeutic levels.

The magnesium sulfate infusion continues for 12 to 24 hours, when it is gradually reduced. Oral terbutaline may be given to maintain tocolysis when the magnesium sulfate is discontinued.

Calcium gluconate (10%) should be available to reverse magnesium toxicity and prevent respiratory arrest if serum levels become high. Excess serum levels of magnesium are less likely when the drug is given for preterm labor because the woman's renal function is usually normal. However, the nurse must remain alert for this complication of magnesium sulfate therapy.

Prostaglandin Synthesis Inhibitors. Because prostaglandins stimulate uterine contractions, drugs can be used to inhibit their synthesis. Indomethacin (Indocin) is the drug in this class that is most often used for tocolysis.

The main fetal and neonatal side effects are constriction of the ductus arteriosus, pulmonary hypertension, and oligohydramnios. These effects are unlikely if treatment is 48 hours or less. The drug's effect in reducing the amount of amniotic fluid makes indomethacin useful for normalizing the volume if hydramnios is present (Creasy & Iams, 1999; Iams, 2000).

The nurse should observe the woman for side effects such as nausea, heartburn, vomiting, and rash. Because indomethacin can prolong bleeding time, the nurse observes for abnormal bleeding such as prolonged bleeding from injections and bruising with no apparent cause. The antipyretic effect of indomethacin can mask infection because fever may not be present. Hypertensive women may have an increase in blood pressure. Checking the height of the fundus at the beginning of therapy and daily thereafter helps identify reduced amniotic fluid. Decreased fetal movements and absent fetal heart rate accelerations with fetal movement may occur if the fetal condition deteriorates.

Calcium Antagonists. Nifedipine (Procardia) is a calcium channel blocker usually given for problems such as hypertension. Calcium is essential for muscle contraction in smooth muscles such as the uterus, so blocking calcium reduces the muscular contraction. Flushing of the skin, headache, and a transient increase in the maternal and fetal heart rates are common side effects. Because nifedipine is a vasodilator, the woman may have postural hypotension.

The nurse should observe for side effects of nifedipine and report a maternal pulse greater than 110. The woman should be assisted when sitting or standing and should do so gradually to reduce the effects of postural hypotension.

Atosiban. Atosiban (Antocin) is an oxytocin-receptor antagonist that is undergoing clinical trials. Atosiban selectively antagonizes oxytocin-induced uterine contractions. In a major trial, atosiban prolonged pregnancy for up to 7 days (compared to an average of 48 hours for most β-adrenergics) in women who were at least 28 weeks pregnant and had fewer adverse maternal and fetal effects. The results in pregnancies under 28 weeks were less conclusive (Romero, et al., 2000).

Accelerating Fetal Lung Maturity

The physician may order corticosteroids to speed fetal lung maturation if birth before 34 weeks seems inevitable. Steroid therapy may reduce the incidence and severity of RDS and intraventricular hemorrhage in the preterm infant (Iams, 2000; ACOG, 1995c). Betamethasone (Celestone) or dexamethasone (Decadron) may be used for this purpose.

Corticosteroids are indicated if the woman is between 24 and 34 weeks' gestation because of the high incidence of RDS at this age. For greatest benefit in reducing RDS, the mother should have the drug at least 24 hours before birth, with effects lasting 7 days (Parsons & Spellacy, 1999). A dose of corticosteroid given to the mother less than 24 hours before birth appears to offer some benefits to the infant, so steroids are prescribed unless birth is imminent. The corticosteroid is repeated weekly until 34 weeks' gestation, when the risk for RDS is much lower.

Maternal adverse effects that can occur with corticosteroid administration include pulmonary edema, increased risk for infection, and more difficult glucose control in diabetic women. A significantly increased incidence of bacterial infections occurred when women received 3 or more doses of steroids during treatment for preterm labor in one study (Rotmensch, Vishne, Celentano, Dan, & Ben-Rafael, 1999).

Vital signs should be assessed to identify fever and elevated pulse that may indicate infection associated with steroid administration. Lung sounds should be assessed with vital signs because corticosteroids can cause sodium retention with accompanying fluid retention and pulmonary edema. The nurse should observe for and teach the woman about signs of pulmonary edema. The woman is taught to report any chest pain or heaviness or any difficulty breathing because these symptoms could indicate pulmonary edema or possibly pneumonia. Pain and burning with urination are symptoms of urinary tract infection that is common in pregnancy even when steroids are not given.

Check Your Reading

14. What symptoms of preterm labor should be taught to women at risk?
15. Why is it important to identify preterm labor early?
16. What four drugs may be used to stop preterm labor contractions?
17. What is the purpose of giving corticosteroids to a woman who is in preterm labor at 27 weeks' gestation? Why is it important that birth be delayed at least 24 hours?

APPLICATION OF THE NURSING PROCESS: PRETERM LABOR

Nursing care for the woman experiencing preterm labor often includes interventions related to tocolytic, corticosteroid, or antibiotic drug therapy. If labor cannot be halted, care is similar to that for other laboring women, with additional care to prepare for a preterm infant's needs at birth. Support for anticipatory grieving may be needed if the infant is very immature and expected to die.

Nursing care when an extremely preterm infant (20 to 23 weeks' gestation) is expected to be born can be heavily laden with ethical and legal issues. For example, if labor cannot be halted, should fetal monitoring be used if the infant's survival is unlikely? If no intervention is done for a nonreassuring pattern, it can distress parents and caregivers alike. Plus, less information is known about fetal monitor patterns at very early gestations compared with gestations nearer term. In addition, for women who are first entering care at this time, ultrasound estimates have greater uncertainty for dating gestation. A fetus who was presumed to be 23 weeks' gestation before birth may be assessed to be 26 weeks' gestation after birth and suited to more aggressive treatment than expected.

Much of the general nursing care for a woman having preterm labor also applies to women experiencing other types of high-risk pregnancies. Women may need multiple hospitalizations that occur in the middle of the night, disrupting sleep and family routines. Other women may have attended a routine prenatal visit and be shocked to discover that they may be in preterm labor. These women often have some activity restriction and may have to stop working. Therefore this section focuses on the family's psychosocial concerns, management of home care, and the woman's boredom.

PSYCHOSOCIAL CONCERNS

Assessment

The entire family is affected by stressors associated with a high-risk pregnancy. Assess how the woman and her family usually cope with crisis situations and how they are coping with this one. Identify their greatest concerns to prioritize care. For example, the nurse might say, "This development in your pregnancy must have been a shock." Other questions the nurse might ask include "How are you handling things?" "In what ways do you usually handle crisis situations in your family?" and "What concerns you the most right now?" Rather than asking questions in a rapid-fire manner, the nurse must give the woman time to answer assessment questions because stress has narrowed her focus.

The woman or her family may have physical, emotional, and cognitive impairments because of the unexpected problems. Physical signs of emotional distress, such as tremulousness, palpitations, and restlessness, also are side effects of β-adrenergic drugs. The woman may express fear, helplessness, or disbelief. She may be irritable and tearful. Her ability to concentrate may be impaired at a time when she needs to absorb new information.

Her partner often feels at loose ends. He struggles to keep the household running if she must be inactive. Young children pick up on their parents' anxiety and may misbehave or regress. They may feel abandoned if they must be temporarily placed with relatives or friends.

The woman often must curtail or stop working, straining family finances. If she does not have sick time or other benefits, the family sustains an abrupt drop in income at a time when medical expenses are mounting. The woman's career may not progress as expected if she must be off work for a prolonged time.

Overlaid on the sudden change in lifestyle is the family's concern for their baby's well-being. A woman may feel pulled in many directions by the needs of all her children—those already born and the fetus she is trying to mature. She may be concerned about the effects of drug therapy on the fetus and her own body.

Analysis

Unexpected development of complications during pregnancy can prevent a woman and her family from using their normal coping mechanisms. Therefore the nursing diagnosis selected for the woman and family is "Anxiety related to the inadequacy of their usual ways of coping with stress."

Planning

The outcome of any pregnancy is never certain, especially when the pregnancy is a high-risk one. Goals and expected outcomes should focus on the family's ability to cope with the crisis of preterm labor. Appropriate outcomes include the following:

- The family will identify one or more constructive methods to cope with this temporary disruption in their lives.

Interventions

Providing Information

Knowledge decreases anxiety and fear related to the unknown. Include appropriate family members so that they are more likely to be supportive. Appropriate family members may include the woman's partner, mother or mother-in-law, adult siblings, and others, which may vary with her culture. Determine the extent of the woman's knowledge about preterm birth and the specific therapy recommended. Determine what information the parents need about problems that a preterm infant may face. Use this opportunity to correct misinformation and reinforce accurate information.

Initially, the woman for whom activity restriction is prescribed may be highly motivated to maintain the restrictions. However, because she usually feels well, she may soon feel lazy and unproductive. Explain what is currently known about the benefits of activity restriction for her pregnancy complication because research continues in this area.

The Sidelines National Support Network is a growing network of local groups across the country for women experiencing high-risk pregnancy. Its website is www.sidelines.org. The site has information for women "sidelined" by pregnancy complications, including articles, information about reimbursement from insurance, and support contact via e-mail (Nursing Care Plan 27-1).

Promoting Expression of Concerns

Encourage the woman and her family to express their concerns. Begin by exploring common concerns of women with problem pregnancies. For example, say, "Most women are worried when they must stop work-

NURSING CARE PLAN 27-1

Preterm Labor

Assessment: Rhonda Ellis is a 28-year-old gravida IV, para III. Her first child was born at 40 weeks' gestation, the second at 28 weeks' gestation, and the third at 32 weeks' gestation. Her oldest child is a second grader, the second child is 4 years old, and the youngest is 18 months old. She is having her regular prenatal appointment today at 12 weeks' gestation. Her pregnancy has progressed normally with normal weight gain. Rhonda tells the nurse that she and her husband, Carl, are anxious to avoid having another premature baby.

Nursing Diagnosis: Health Seeking Behaviors related to Rhonda's expressed desire for a full-term pregnancy.

Goals/Expected Outcomes:
At the end of teaching, Rhonda will restate the following:
1. Actions that may prevent preterm labor
2. Signs and symptoms that suggest early preterm labor
3. What to do if she has symptoms of preterm labor

Intervention	Rationale
1. Ask Rhonda what she already knows about preterm labor related to her previous experience. For example, a. How long pregnancy should last for the baby to have minimal problems. b. How serious she believes preterm labor and birth are and her beliefs about the causes of preterm labor.	1. Knowledge is best retained if it is related to something the learner already knows and the learner is motivated to learn. Relating it to the woman's previous experience with preterm labor and birth helps identify her individual perceptions of and beliefs about her situation.

Continued

c. How likely preterm labor is to recur.
d. Whether preterm labor can be detected and stopped.
e. What measures she used to try to stop it previously and their effectiveness.

2. Discuss methods to prevent preterm labor that are appropriate for Rhonda's present situation.

2. Rhonda is in a high-risk group because she has already had two preterm infants. Prevention focuses on usual health-promoting activities, with preparation for other restrictions that may be needed.

a. Avoid physically or psychologically stressful activities.

a. Physical or psychological stress increases the risk for preterm labor. Rhonda has three young children, including two who are not yet in school.

b. Plan several rest periods during the day.

b. Rest promotes uterine blood flow and relieves some of the stress of everyday life.

c. Eat a well-balanced diet so that she gains about 1 lb per week.

c. A high-quality diet and adequate weight gain have a positive effect on pregnancy outcomes. Low prepregnancy weight and inadequate weight gain are associated with preterm labor and birth.

d. Drink eight glasses of fluid each day, excluding caffeine-containing beverages.

d. Adequate hydration reduces the risk for urinary tract infection, one type of infection associated with preterm labor.

e. Avoid excessive breast stimulation during sexual activity or bathing.

e. Breast stimulation may cause release of oxytocin from the posterior pituitary.

f. If preterm contractions do occur, sexual activity should stop.

f. Sexual activity can cause orgasm and semen contains prostaglandins, both of which may stimulate contractions.

3. Ask Rhonda how labor started in her other preterm births and how these differed from her term birth. Explain that she should promptly go to the hospital if she has any of these signs and symptoms of preterm labor:
a. Uterine contractions, painful or painless. These may feel like the baby is "balling up."
b. Cramping similar to menstrual cramps
c. A constant backache
d. A sensation of pelvic pressure or thigh pain
e. A change or increase in vaginal discharge
f. Abdominal or intestinal cramps, with or without diarrhea
g. A sense of "feeling bad" or that something is not quite right

3. Symptoms of early preterm labor are often vague and not as obvious as signs of early term labor. If preterm labor is considered as a possible cause for the symptoms, a woman is more likely to seek early therapy to halt it.

4. Teach Rhonda signs of a urinary tract infection:
a. Fever (either low or high)
b. Burning or pain on urination
c. Unusual urinary frequency
d. Flank pain
e. Strong-smelling or cloudy urine

4. Urinary tract infection is associated with preterm labor. Treatment of the infection improves effectiveness of other measures to halt preterm labor and birth.

Evaluation: Rhonda already knows about the need for rest but acknowledges that resting is difficult with small children. She tries to eat a well-balanced diet but often is rushed during meals because of the demands of her family. She dislikes water and prefers colas but says she will try to drink more water and fewer caffeinated drinks. Rhonda discusses several early symptoms of preterm labor, including those she had with her other pregnancies. She says she will come to the hospital right away if she suspects preterm labor.

Assessment: Rhonda has mild cramping and pelvic pressure at 28 weeks' gestation and comes to the hospital right away. The physician does a speculum examination of her cervix and finds that it is dilated 1 to 2 cm and is beginning to efface. She responds to IV magnesium sulfate to stop her contractions. The physician also orders betamethasone, 12 mg, IM for two doses, 24 hours apart. She will be discharged home in 48 hours if no recurrent symptoms develop.

Critical Thinking: What should you tell Rhonda about each of the prescribed drugs?

Answer: Explain that magnesium sulfate is eliminated by the kidneys, so you will be measuring her urine output to be sure it is adequate. Tell her that you will be checking her reflexes and vital signs to identify toxicity if it develops. Serum magnesium levels are often assessed as well.
Because Rhonda's fetus is likely to have significant respiratory and other problems if born at this early gestation, explain that the use of corticosteroids such as betamethasone help speed fetal lung maturity. Betamethasone will be repeated weekly.

Assessment: The physician recommends that she remain on modified bed rest in a semi-Fowler position for much of the day. She may be up for meals, showers, and use of the restroom. She says she is worried about how she will care for her three children. Her mother-in-law lives nearby but works part time.

Nursing Diagnosis: Impaired Home Maintenance Management related to activity restrictions and family demands.

Goal/Expected Outcome:
By hospital discharge, Rhonda will relate ways that she can maintain prescribed activity restrictions.

Intervention	Rationale
1. Assess what support systems are available and financially feasible to help Rhonda with child care and transportation, such as daycare, mother's day out programs at churches, family, and friends.	1. Responsibilities for other children may impede a woman's ability to maintain activity limits. Coordination among several resources helps provide all-day coverage for child care.
2. Encourage Rhonda to temporarily lower her standards for home management: a. Eat nourishing take-out or fast food. b. Prioritize household tasks that must be done. c. Let her children do tasks that are within their abilities. d. Make lists of tasks that need to be done for different people who will be available to help her.	2. Many usual roles must be reallocated during this time. Having alternative arrangements increases the chance that the woman can maintain therapy.
3. Encourage Rhonda to accept help from others. Remind her that this situation is temporary and that she may be able to help someone else at another time.	3. If a woman feels that she can help others at another time, she may be more willing to accept help when she needs it.

Evaluation: Rhonda identifies three friends in addition to her mother-in-law who may be able to help with child care. She says she cannot afford to continue sending her children to their daycare center if she is not working. She feels that if her children are cared for, her husband can handle her home management needs.

Assessment: At 31 weeks' gestation, Rhonda again experiences preterm labor and goes to the hospital. Her cervix is dilated 2 to 3 cm and is 75% effaced (about 0.5 cm long). Her contractions occur every 6 to 7 minutes, lasting about 20 to 30 seconds each. The physician again orders a magnesium sulfate infusion and betamethasone injections. The physician explains that preterm birth may be delayed but will probably occur within the next 24 hours. Rhonda begins crying, and says, "I did what I was supposed to do and now I'm still going to have another preemie! It will be weeks before I can be a real mother!"

Nursing Diagnosis: Rhonda will probably lose the experience of a term birth that she has been hoping for and working toward. The nursing diagnosis chosen is "Anticipatory Grieving related to loss of expected birth experience."

Goal/Expected Outcome:
Rhonda will express her feelings about the loss of her expected birth at term.

Intervention	Rationale
1. Sit down and spend time with Rhonda. Use therapeutic communication to encourage her to express her feelings.	1. Unhurried time allows expression of feelings, which is the first step in dealing with the anticipated loss.
2. When she has expressed her frustration about this development in her pregnancy, explain that much remains unknown about why labor begins, whether at term, preterm, or post-term.	2. If a woman knows that professionals do not have all the answers but must make recommendations based on what is known or appears to work for an individual woman, she may be more accepting of the inevitability of preterm birth.
3. Explain that Rhonda's efforts have paid off because she has gained 3 valuable weeks of gestation for her baby.	3. Knowing that her self-care has benefits, although not the hoped-for term birth, reduces the sense of failure that she may feel.

Evaluation: Rhonda cries and expresses her frustration about the developments in her pregnancy. She says that she knew she was more likely to have another preterm infant but hoped that this time would be different. As the day goes by, Rhonda gradually begins expressing feelings that she did do something positive for this baby because the baby is now 3 weeks more mature.

ing. How has this affected your family?" An open question gives the woman and her family a chance to ventilate their feelings so that they can take the next step: identifying constructive methods to cope with the situation. Collaboration with a social worker may identify financial or other community resources available.

Teaching What May Occur during a Preterm Birth

Because preterm birth often occurs despite all interventions, a pregnant woman and her partner should be prepared for this possibility. If the hospital has a neonatal intensive care unit, a nurse often visits the parents to explain what might occur if their baby is born early. One or both parents may tour the unit to see the equipment and care given to preterm infants. Often, just seeing the infants in the neonatal intensive care unit motivates a woman to maintain recommended therapy even though she is tired of doing so.

In hospitals with neonatal intensive care units, one or more neonatal nurses, a neonatal nurse-practitioner, a neonatologist, or a combination of these are present at birth to care for the infant. The woman who has planned to give birth in a hospital without a neonatal intensive care unit may be transferred to a facility with this type of unit before the birth to allow immediate care and stabilization of her newborn. The infant also may be transferred after birth if there is no time to transfer the woman before birth or the infant has more problems than were anticipated. Hospitalization of the mother, infant, or both at a distant location adds to the stress on the family and can impair the attachment process.

Evaluation

The goal or expected outcome for this nursing diagnosis is achieved if the woman and her family can identify constructive methods to deal with their anxiety. If a high-risk pregnancy situation is prolonged or the family has difficulty adapting constructively to the situation, a nursing diagnosis of "Altered Family Processes" may be more appropriate.

MANAGEMENT OF HOME CARE

Assessment

Despite their uncertain value in the treatment of preterm labor, activity restrictions continue to be widely prescribed. If the membranes are not ruptured, the woman may be managed at home rather than in the hospital, particularly if a longer course is anticipated. Therefore the nurse should expect that part of the care of women with high-risk pregnancies, including a risk for preterm birth, often occurs in the home. Many daily household activities are probably managed by the woman. When she is disabled, even briefly, the usual roles of family members are disrupted.

Determine the level of activity prescribed by the physician and identify the role of each family member. A good way to do this is to have the woman describe a usual day before any activity restrictions. Determine the number and ages of children in the home.

Evaluate the home itself, either by visual inspection or questions to the family. Does the home have more than one level? If it is an apartment, is it upstairs or downstairs? Determine whether a telephone is available for emergency contact.

Evaluate the family's resources and their willingness to use them. Ask whether family members and friends in the area are available to help. Explore local support groups such as churches and mother-to-mother networks that the family might contact for assistance. Determine whether insurance covers assistance such as homemaker services.

Analysis

The diagnosis chosen is "Impaired Home Maintenance Management related to change in usual roles and responsibilities."

Planning

Two goals or expected outcomes are appropriate for this nursing diagnosis:

- Short-term goal—The family will identify methods for management of daily household routines.
- Long-term goal—The woman will be able to maintain the prescribed levels of activity and drug therapy.

Interventions

The pregnancy threatened by preterm labor or other complications that require activity restriction is a self-limiting situation, making temporary adjustments somewhat easier. Needed changes in home routines may be brief but sometimes extend over several weeks. Even if the restriction consists only of added rest periods during the day, the woman still is unable to fulfill all her usual roles. For the woman who is prescribed more restricted activity, the disruptions are greater.

Caring for Children

The woman who has children has different concerns than the woman who does not. Toddlers and preschoolers rarely understand why their mother does not play with them as usual. If they already are in daycare, this can continue if the family can afford it. They may temporarily live with a relative or friend. Toddlers may feel that their parents have abandoned them if they are sent away, although this may be the only realistic solution if no one except the mother is available to supervise them.

School-aged children can understand the situation better and often are quite helpful. They may assist with care of other children, but they should not be put into the role of an adult. They may resent responsibility excessive for their age. The mother can visit with them after school and help them with homework while remaining in her rest position (usually sidelying).

Adolescents may welcome their parents' trust but also resent the intrusion on independent activities with their peers. Teenagers who drive can be very helpful in taking younger siblings to school and other activities. They may be enlisted for grocery shopping and meal preparation. If resentment flares, a reminder that the situation is temporary and they are valuable contributors to the health of the new baby may defuse the situation.

Maintaining the Household

The first step to home maintenance during this time may be for the woman to lower her standards of housekeeping. Things may not be as clean or organized as she would like. The partner may take over some household tasks, but these may compete with responsibilities outside the home. Talk to the woman about ignoring chores that are not performed exactly as she wants and tell her to remember that it is temporary.

Advise the woman to have a list of tasks ready when friends and family ask, "Can I do anything to help?" If they offer to bring a meal or do laundry, encourage her to accept. Remind her that people who offer to help mean it and she may be able to return the favor to someone else. Homemaker services may be an option to help the family deal with the woman's temporary disability.

Transportation of school-aged children may be a concern. If no family or friends are available, the school nurse or Parent-Teacher Association (PTA) may help find someone willing to take the children to school each day.

Evaluation

Goals and expected outcomes are met under the following conditions:

- The short-term goal is met if the family can identify ways to manage minimal household care.
- The long-term goal is met if she can maintain the prescribed therapy.

BOREDOM

Assessment

If activity is restricted, determine what skills the woman has for coping with boredom. At first, a prescription for rest may sound wonderful to a busy woman, but after a short time, it can become trying. One study described women on restricted activity for high-risk pregnancy as feeling like prisoners, whether they were at home or in the hospital. Most women in this study felt that they had fewer stresses when at home, however (Heaman & Gupton, 1998).

Ask about a usual day to identify activities that are still appropriate within the restrictions prescribed. Ask about hobbies, present and past. What type of leisure activities does the woman enjoy? Which activities are available or possible? Does she have good alternative places to maintain rest and still give her a change of scenery?

Assess her personality. Is she calm and composed, taking whatever comes with serenity? Or does she need to be busy most of the time? No matter how motivated, the woman who finds inactivity tiresome will find even limited activity restriction difficult to maintain.

Analysis

The nursing diagnosis is "Diversional Activity Deficit related to lack of knowledge about alternative activities."

Planning

Two goals are appropriate for this nursing diagnosis. The woman will do the following:

- Identify activities that are appropriate for her level of activity restriction.
- Pursue (with help of others) appropriate activities to relieve boredom.

Interventions

Identifying Appropriate Activities

Determine the woman's understanding about needed activity restrictions to identify misunderstandings and reinforce correct information. Help her identify which usual activities are permitted and which ones should not be done and why. If she understands the rationale, she may be more willing to maintain restrictions.

Computer connections allow some women to continue work activities. They may be able to do paperwork or other types of activities that can be done at home. Workplace deadlines can increase stress, even at home. However, the feeling of usefulness gained by such activities may be beneficial because it reduces some financial concerns.

Help the woman identify appropriate activities to stay busy and productive. These may include household activities that can be done at rest, volunteering for activities such as phone calls, and leisure activities such as puzzles, games, and hand needlework. Help her identify someone who can obtain the necessary supplies for her. This might be a good time to reactivate an old (quiet) hobby.

The woman can participate in some activities with her children while she is in bed. She can read to them and play board or card games. Encourage her to help the children with their homework and stimulate their development with thought-provoking discussions.

Changing the Physical Surroundings

Encourage the woman to identify at least two areas where she can maintain her prescribed rest. This gives her a change of scene and helps her feel more a part of the family activities. Each area should include pillows, blankets, and a clipboard with writing materials. An adjustable ironing board can provide a movable table for her things, and a shoe bag helps keep supplies organized and at hand. Ideally, the telephone is within reach or cordless and she has a television with a remote control unit.

Evaluation

The first goal is short term and may be met when activity restrictions are first instituted if the woman can accurately discriminate between appropriate and inappropriate activities. The second goal is met over time if she actually pursues only appropriate activities.

PROLONGED PREGNANCY

A prolonged pregnancy is one that lasts longer than 42 weeks. Most women who receive prenatal care today do not reach 42 weeks before their labor is induced if they have accurate due dates. Many apparent cases of prolonged pregnancy are actually miscalculations of the estimated date of delivery (EDD) because the woman has had irregular menstrual periods or forgotten the date of her last normal menstrual period.

Complications

The main physical risk in prolonged pregnancy is to the fetus or newborn. Insufficiency of the placental function secondary to aging and infarction reduces transfer of oxygen and nutrients to the fetus and removal of waste. Because the fetus with placental insufficiency has less reserve to tolerate uterine contractions, signs of fetal compromise, such as late decelerations and decreased variability, may develop during labor. In addition, reduced amniotic fluid volume (oligohydramnios) that often accompanies placental insufficiency can result in umbilical cord compression. Meconium in the amniotic fluid may cause respiratory distress in the newborn if it is aspirated before or during birth. The infant may have late growth retardation and appear to have lost weight, with a normal-sized head and thin body.

Many postterm fetuses do not suffer from placental insufficiency and may continue growing. If the fetus becomes large, the woman and fetus then may have complications related to dysfunctional labor, inadequate postpartum uterine contraction to control bleeding, and injury if the birth is traumatic.

Psychologically, the woman often feels as though her pregnancy will never end. The added fatigue imposed by a pregnancy that extends significantly beyond her due date diminishes her resources for tolerating the added stress and anxiety about labor and birth.

Therapeutic Management

If the woman has no prenatal care until late in pregnancy, therapeutic management begins by determining her gestation as accurately as possible. Several markers used to pinpoint gestation, such as ultrasonography, fundal height measurements, dates of quickening, and first auscultation of the fetal heart tones with a nonamplified fetoscope, may be lost if a woman presents late for prenatal care. Also, the woman may have forgotten her last menstrual period date.

Another factor in management decisions is whether the fetus is thriving in the uterus. If antepartum tests such as a biophysical profile indicate that the fetus is doing well, the birth attendant can take a more conservative approach than if the placental function is diminished and thus allow labor to begin naturally.

If the gestation appears to be truly postterm and no fetal urgency to deliver quickly exists, management depends on whether the cervix is favorable for induction of labor. If so, induction is usually begun. If the cervix is not favorable, the caregiver often uses a cervical ripening procedure (see Chapter 16) to soften the cervix. The cervical ripening also would be done if the fetal signs were nonreassuring and delivery was needed but the cervix was not favorable (unless the fetal situation was sufficiently nonreassuring that a cesarean was indicated).

Nursing Considerations

Nursing care for the woman with a prolonged pregnancy is tied to the medical management. The nurse's role may include the following:

- Teaching about procedures such as antepartum testing or induction of labor
- Support for her psychological and physical fatigue
- Nursing care related to specific procedures such as induction of labor

INTRAPARTUM EMERGENCIES

Placental Abnormalities

Women with placental abnormalities may experience hemorrhage during the antepartum or intrapartum period. Placenta previa is sometimes associated with an abnormally adherent placenta (placenta accreta). Placenta accreta may cause immediate or delayed hemorrhage immediately after birth because the placenta does not separate cleanly, often leaving small fragments that prevent full uterine contraction. More extreme degrees of abnormal adherence occur when the placenta penetrates the uterine muscle itself (placenta increta) or even all the way through the uterus (placenta percreta). All or only part of the placenta may be involved. A hysterectomy often is required if a large portion of the placenta is abnormally adherent.

Prolapsed Umbilical Cord

A prolapsed umbilical cord slips downward after the membranes rupture, subjecting it to compression between the fetus and pelvis (Figure 27-7). It may slip down immediately with the fluid gush or long after the membranes rupture. Interruption in blood flow through the cord interferes with fetal oxygenation and is potentially fatal.

Causes

Prolapse of the umbilical cord is more likely when the fit is poor between the fetal presenting part and the maternal pelvis. When the fit is good, the fetus fills up the pelvis, leaving little room for the cord to slip down.

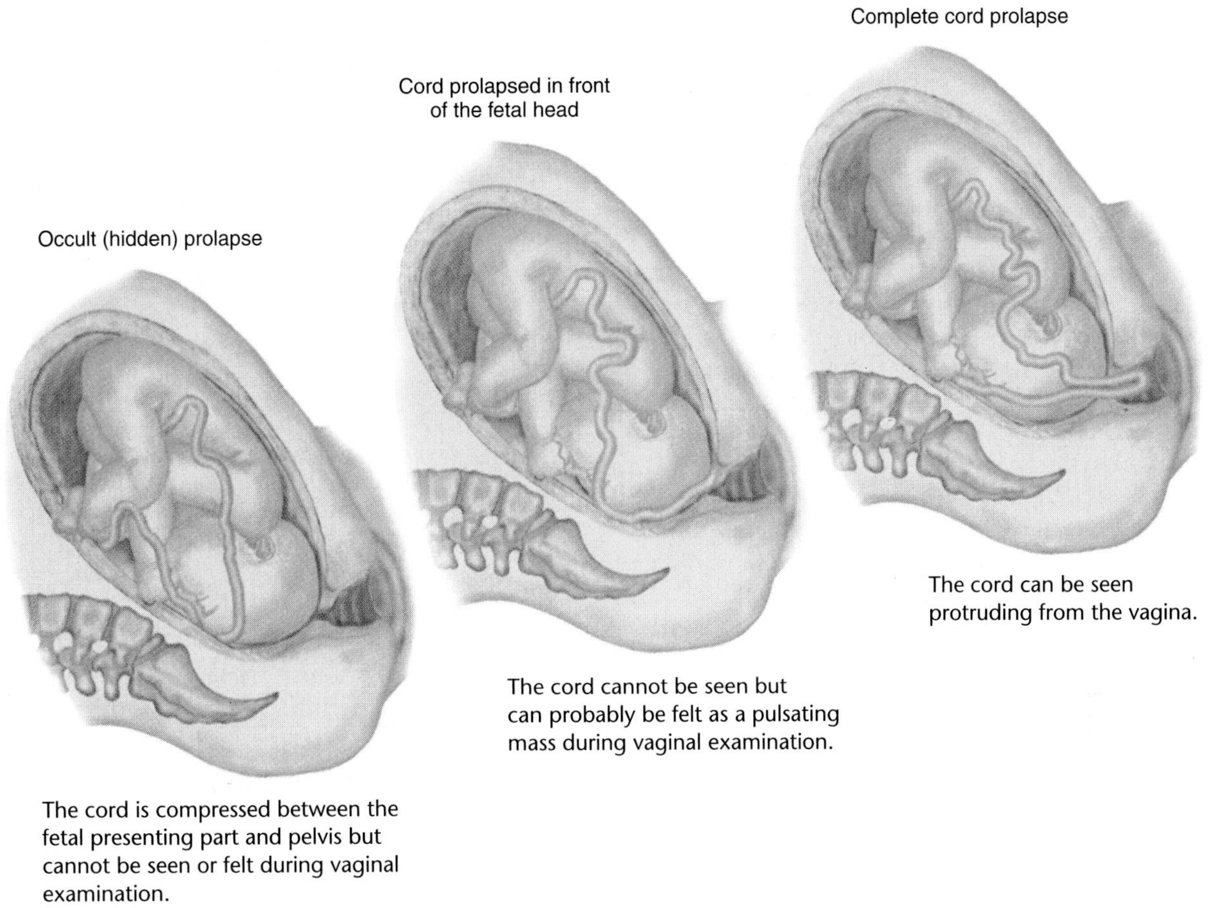

Occult (hidden) prolapse
The cord is compressed between the fetal presenting part and pelvis but cannot be seen or felt during vaginal examination.
Cord prolapsed in front of the fetal head
The cord cannot be seen but can probably be felt as a pulsating mass during vaginal examination.
Complete cord prolapse
The cord can be seen protruding from the vagina.

FIGURE 27-7 Variations of prolapsed umbilical cord.

Although prolapse of the cord is possible during any labor, it is more likely if these conditions are present:

- A fetus that remains at a high station
- A very small fetus
- Breech presentations (the footling breech is more likely to be complicated by a prolapsed cord because the feet and legs are small and do not fill the pelvis well)
- Transverse lie
- Hydramnios (often associated with abnormal presentations; also, the unusually large amount of fluid exerts more pressure to push the cord out)

Signs of Prolapse

Prolapse may be complete, with the cord visible at the vaginal opening. A prolapsed cord may not be visible but may be palpated on vaginal examination as it pulsates synchronously with the fetal heart. An occult prolapse of the cord is one in which the cord slips alongside the fetal head or shoulders. The prolapse cannot be palpated or seen but is suspected because of changes in the FHR, such as sustained bradycardia or variable decelerations.

CRITICAL TO REMEMBER

Factors That Increase a Woman's Risk for a Prolapsed Umbilical Cord

Ruptured membranes *and*

- The fetal presenting part at a high station
- A fetus that poorly fits the pelvic inlet because of small size or abnormal presentation
- Excessive volume of amniotic fluid (hydramnios)

Therapeutic Management

Medical and nursing management often overlap, as they do in many emergency situations. Either the nurse or the birth attendant may be the first to discover umbilical cord prolapse. Birth is almost always cesarean unless vaginal delivery can be accomplished more quickly and less traumatically.

When cord prolapse occurs, the priority is to relieve pressure on the cord to improve blood flow through it until delivery. None of these interventions should delay the promptest possible delivery. Push the call light to summon help. Others should call the physician and prepare for birth while the nurse caring for the woman relieves pressure on the cord, if the physician or nurse-

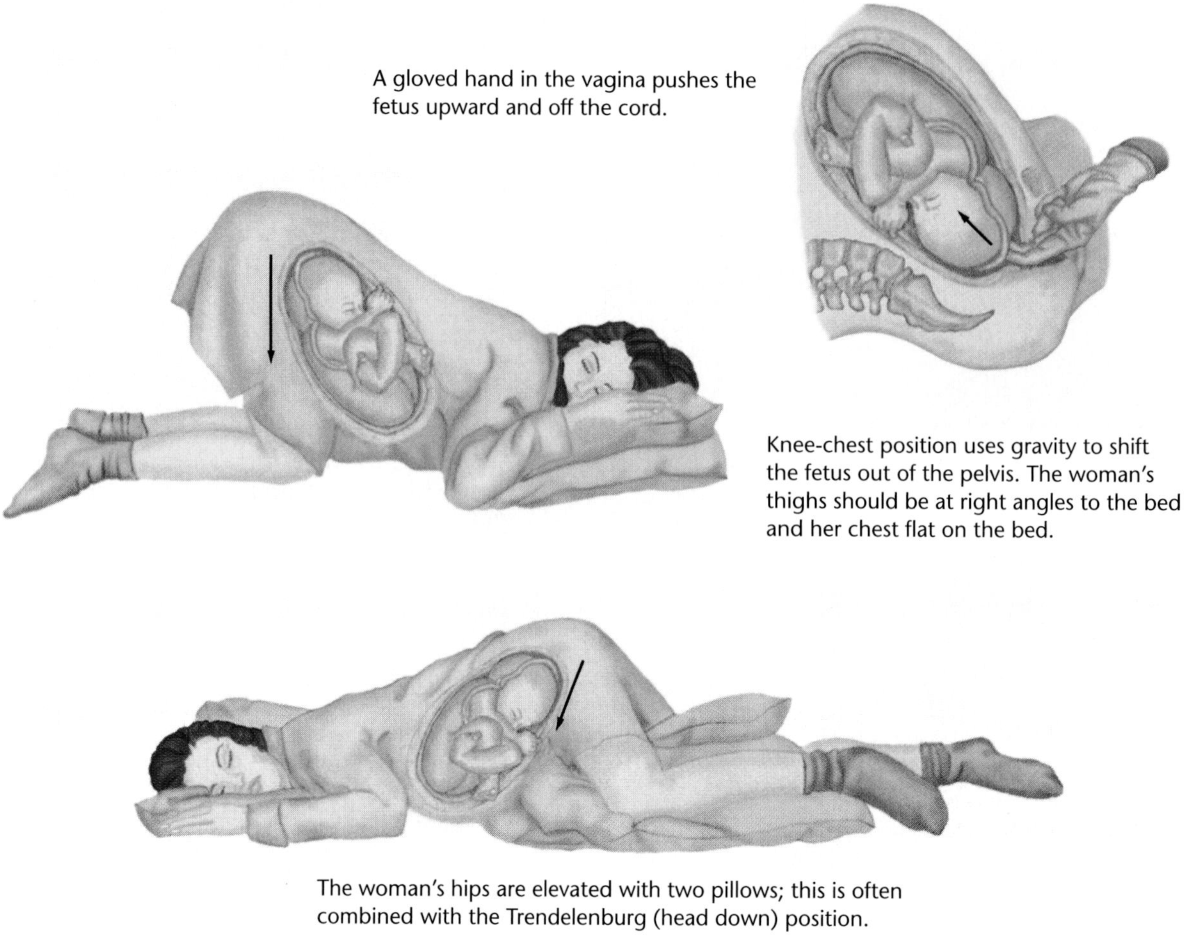

A gloved hand in the vagina pushes the fetus upward and off the cord.
Knee-chest position uses gravity to shift the fetus out of the pelvis. The woman's thighs should be at right angles to the bed and her chest flat on the bed.
The woman's hips are elevated with two pillows; this is often combined with the Trendelenburg (head down) position.

FIGURE 27-8 Measures that may be used to relieve pressure on a prolapsed umbilical cord until delivery can take place.

midwife is not doing so. Neonatal nurses and a pediatrician or neonatologist should be notified, and the staff should prepare for neonatal resuscitation.

Prompt actions reduce cord compression and increase fetal oxygenation:

1. Position the woman's hips higher than her head to shift the fetal presenting part toward her diaphragm. Any of these methods (Figure 27-8) may be used:
   a. Knee-chest position
   b. Trendelenburg position
   c. Hips elevated with pillows, with side-lying position maintained
2. With a gloved hand, push the fetal presenting part upward. Maintain this position until the physician orders it stopped, which may not be until a cesarean incision is made.

Give oxygen at 8 to 10 liters per minute by face mask while preparing for surgery to increase maternal blood oxygen saturation, making more available for the fetus.

Other actions may be used to enhance fetal oxygenation, but prompt delivery is the priority. A tocolytic drug such as terbutaline inhibits contractions, increasing placental blood flow and reducing intermittent pressure of the fetus against the pelvis and cord. Warm, saline-moistened towels retard cooling and drying of the cord. If the cord is protruding from the vagina, no attempt should be made to replace it because doing so could traumatize and further reduce blood flow through the cord. Manipulating the cord can induce umbilical artery spasm, which would reduce blood flow between the fetus and placenta.

Prognosis for the woman is good because the only additional risks are those associated with cesarean birth. Prognosis for the infant depends on how long and how severely blood flow through the cord has been impaired. With prompt recognition and corrective actions, the infant usually does well.

Nursing Considerations

In addition to prompt corrective actions, the nurse must consider the woman's anxiety. The nurse must remain calm while working quickly during this time and acknowledge the woman's anxiety. Explanations must be simple because anxiety interferes with the woman's

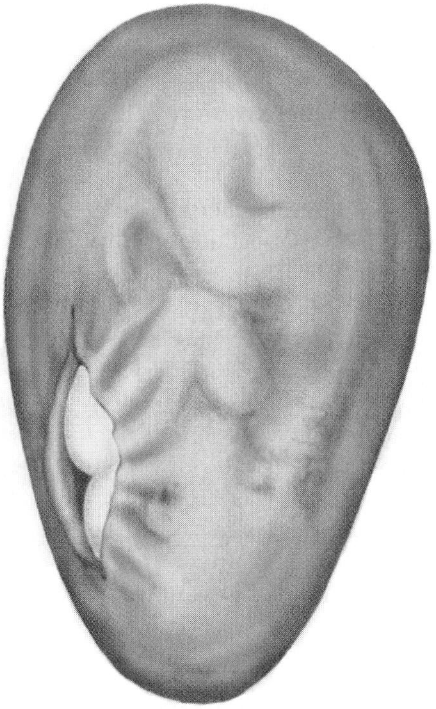

FIGURE 27-9 Uterine rupture in the lower uterine segment.

ability to comprehend them. Her partner and family should be included as much as possible.

Uterine Rupture

Sometimes a tear in the wall of the uterus occurs because the uterus cannot withstand the pressure against it (Figure 27-9). Three variations of uterine rupture exist.

- Complete rupture—A direct communication between the uterine and peritoneal cavities
- Incomplete rupture—A rupture into the peritoneum covering the uterus or into the broad ligament but not the peritoneal cavity
- Dehiscence—A partial separation of an old uterine scar. Little or no bleeding may occur. No signs or symptoms may exist, and the rupture ("window") may be found incidentally during a subsequent cesarean birth or other abdominal surgery.

Causes

Although uterine rupture is rare, dehiscence is not unusual. Uterine rupture is associated with previous uterine surgery such as cesarean birth or surgery to remove fibroids. The risk for rupture in a woman who has had a prior cesarean birth depends on the type of uterine incision. The risk for rupture is greater in the woman with a classic incision (vertical into the upper uterine segment) than the woman with a low transverse incision. For this reason, vaginal birth after cesarean is not recommended for women who have had a previous classic cesarean birth.

Rupture of the unscarred uterus is more likely for women of high parity with a thin uterine wall, women sustaining blunt abdominal trauma, and women having intense contractions, especially if fetopelvic disproportion is present. Excessively strong contractions (hypertonic) may cause the intrauterine pressure to exceed the tensile strength of the uterine wall. If the fetus cannot be expelled downward through the pelvis, contractions may push it through the lower uterine segment. Intense contractions are more likely to occur when uterine stimulants such as oxytocin and misoprostol are administered for induction or augmentation of labor, but they also may occur spontaneously.

Signs and Symptoms

Dehiscence does not have symptoms initially and may not interfere with labor or vaginal delivery if the area is small. However, labor progress may stop because the open area prevents efficient expulsion of the fetus. Intrauterine pressures may have little change during contractions. A larger area of dehiscence may cause abdominal pain that persists despite analgesia.

Manifestations of uterine rupture vary with the degree of rupture and may mimic other complications. Possible signs and symptoms of uterine rupture are as follows:

- Abdominal pain and tenderness—The pain may not be severe; it may occur suddenly at the peak of a contraction. The woman may describe a feeling that something "gave way" or "ripped."
- Chest pain, pain between the scapulae, or pain on inspiration—Pain occurs because of the irritation of blood below the woman's diaphragm.
- Hypovolemic shock caused by hemorrhage—Falling blood pressure, tachycardia, tachypnea, pallor, cool and clammy skin, and anxiety. Signs of shock may not occur until after birth.
- Signs associated with impaired fetal oxygenation, such as late decelerations, reduced variability, tachycardia, and bradycardia
- Absent fetal heart tones with a large disruption of the placenta
- Cessation of uterine contractions
- Palpation of the fetus outside the uterus (usually occurs only with a large, complete rupture). The fetus is likely to be dead.

If the rupture is incomplete, blood loss is slower and signs of shock, chest pain, or intrascapular pain may be delayed. Complete rupture results in massive blood loss. Signs of shock and pain develop quickly. External bleeding may not be impressive, however, because most blood is lost into the peritoneal cavity. The fetus often dies in complete rupture because the placental blood supply is disrupted.

Therapeutic Management

Initial management is to stabilize the woman and fetus and perform cesarean delivery. If the rupture is small and the woman wants other children, it may be repaired. A woman with a large uterine rupture requires hysterectomy. Blood is replaced if needed.

Nursing Considerations

The nurse must be aware of women who are at increased risk for uterine rupture and stay alert for the signs and symptoms. Administer uterine stimulant drugs cautiously to reduce the likelihood of excessive contractions. The nurse must keep in mind that hypertonic contractions also can occur spontaneously. Notify the birth attendant if hypertonic contractions occur. A tocolytic drug may be needed to reduce excessive contractions.

Uterine rupture may not be detected before birth. If postpartum bleeding is excessive and the fundus is firm, injury to the birth canal, including uterine rupture, is possible. Bleeding may be concealed if the ruptured area bleeds into the broad ligament. In this case, signs of hypovolemic shock are likely to develop quickly.

Check Your Reading

18. What are three risks to the fetus or neonate when pregnancy lasts longer than 42 weeks?
19. What is the immediate management if prolapse of the umbilical cord occurs?
20. How can contractions stimulated with drugs such as oxytocin or misoprostol increase the risk for uterine rupture?

Uterine Inversion

An inversion occurs when the uterus completely or partly turns inside out, usually during the third stage of labor. Such an event is uncommon but potentially fatal.

Causes

Often, no single cause is identified. Predisposing factors are as follows:

- Pulling on the umbilical cord before the placenta detaches from the uterine wall
- Fundal pressure during birth
- Fundal pressure on an incompletely contracted uterus after birth
- Increased intraabdominal pressure
- An abnormally adherent placenta
- Congenital weakness of the uterine wall
- Fundal placenta implantation

Signs and Symptoms

The birth attendant notes that either the uterus is absent from the abdomen or a depression in the fundal area is present. The interior of the uterus may be seen through the cervix or protruding into the vagina. Massive hemorrhage, shock, and pain quickly become evident. The woman has severe pelvic pain.

Management

Quick action by nursing and medical personnel is required to reduce maternal morbidity and mortality. The birth attendant tries to replace the uterus through the vagina into a normal position. If that is not possible, laparotomy with replacement is done. Hysterectomy may be required.

Two IV lines are established to allow rapid fluid and blood replacement. A tocolytic drug or general anesthesia usually is needed to relax the uterus enough to replace it. After the uterus is replaced and the placenta removed, oxytocin is given to contract the uterus and control blood loss. Oxytocin is not given until the uterus is repositioned to avoid trapping the inverted fundus in the cervix.

Nursing Considerations

Nursing care during the emergency supplements that of other staff members. Postpartum nursing care is directed toward observing and maintaining maternal blood volume and correcting shock. The woman may be transferred to the intensive care unit.

Assess the uterine fundus for firmness, height, and deviation from the midline. Assess vital signs every 15 minutes or more frequently until stable, then according to recovery room routine. Observe for tachycardia and a falling blood pressure, which are associated with shock. A cardiac monitor identifies dysrhythmias, which may occur with shock, and a pulse oximeter provides information about oxygenation. Invasive hemodynamic monitoring is common.

An indwelling catheter often is inserted to observe fluid balance and keep the bladder empty so that the uterus can contract well. Assess the catheter for patency, and record intake and output. Urine output should be at least 25 to 30 ml per hour. A fall in urine output may indicate hypovolemia or an obstructed catheter.

The woman is allowed nothing by mouth until her condition is stable. She usually can receive fluids and progress to solid foods quickly because uterine inversion does not usually recur in the current postpartum period. It may recur in a future pregnancy if conditions favor its development.

Amniotic Fluid Embolism

Amniotic fluid embolism (AFE) occurs when amniotic fluid is drawn into the maternal circulation and carried to the woman's lungs. Fetal particulate matter (skin cells, vernix, hair, meconium) in the fluid obstructs pulmonary vessels. The fetal cells are foreign antigens in the maternal circulation, causing an anaphalactoid response. The woman has abrupt onset of respiratory distress, seizures, heart failure, and circulatory collapse. Coagulation abnormalities such as disseminated intravascular coagulopathy (DIC) (see p. 664) may occur because thromboplastin-rich amniotic fluid interferes with blood clotting. Fetal bradycardia quickly becomes evident if delivery has not occurred at the time of the embolism. This uncommon disorder often is fatal to mothers, with a mortality rate of 60% to 70% and often permanent neurologic impairment occurs in survivors (Clark, 2000).

Earlier data seemed to indicate that intense labor increased the risk for amniotic fluid embolism, but the current belief is that labor intensity itself does not increase the risk for the complication. Instead, the intense contractions often seen with AFE may occur as the uterus reacts to large amounts of norepinephrine released in response to the massive insult of the embolism on the body (Clark, 2000).

Therapeutic management of amniotic fluid embolism is supportive and includes the following:

- Cardiopulmonary resuscitation
- Oxygen with mechanical ventilation
- Fluid volume expansion; blood transfusion as indicated
- Inotropic agents such as dopamine (Intropin)
- Hemodynamic monitoring
- Correction of coagulation deficits with platelets or fibrinogen

The mother's well-being takes precedence in most cases of AFE. However, if she is in full cardiac arrest, her survival is unlikely and the fetus may be delivered to improve survival odds for the baby (Luppi, 1999; Clark, 2000).

Check Your Reading

21. What are the primary complications of a uterine inversion? How are they managed?
22. What are the specific factors about amniotic fluid embolism that make this type different from other embolisms?
23. What are important nursing considerations for each kind of intrapartum emergency: Prolapsed umbilical cord? Uterine rupture? Uterine inversion? Amniotic fluid embolism?

APPLICATION OF THE NURSING PROCESS: INTRAPARTUM EMERGENCIES

Nursing care of the woman with an intrapartum emergency overlaps with care in other situations discussed elsewhere. Much of the nursing care is collaborative and supports medical management. Parents may suffer loss if the fetus dies or the mother loses her ability to bear future children, as may occur with uterine rupture. One problem expected in any emergency situation is the emotional distress of the woman and her family.

Assessment

When an emergency occurs, the woman and her family have little time to absorb what has happened, simply because of its suddenness. In umbilical cord prolapse, for example, labor often has been uneventful up to that point. Suddenly, nurses place the woman in a strange position, apply oxygen, and pull her toward the operating room. The staff is clearly excited as well.

Under such circumstances, the woman and her family have a very narrow focus. They are obviously apprehensive and feel out of control. The woman or her partner may be immobilized by fear.

Analysis

The nursing diagnosis is "Anxiety related to unexpected occurrences because of the sudden development of complications." This diagnosis is expected to differ from the anxiety associated with preterm labor because the onset is acute. The anxiety also may lessen more quickly because the emergency is sometimes resolved quickly.

Planning

The focus of a goal is very narrow in an emergency situation. Two appropriate goals, during and after the emergency, are that the woman and her family will do the following:

- Indicate an understanding of emergency procedures.
- Express their feelings about the complication.

Interventions

Although little time for discussion exists, explain honestly and simply what is occurring. To reduce fear and anxiety of the unknown, tell the woman what is happening and why. Include her partner and family if appropriate. Provide continued reassurance and support to the woman because her partner often must be excluded from the emergency or operating room when an emergency occurs.

The infant born in an emergency situation may need resuscitation or other supportive measures. Nurses and a neonatal nurse-practitioner or pediatrician from the neonatal intensive care unit, if available, usually are present at the birth to attend the infant. A neonatologist also may be present. Explain to the family who the other professionals are and their roles. If possible, explain what is being done to care for the baby.

After the emergency, give the woman and her family a chance to ask questions. The ability to absorb new knowledge during periods of severe anxiety is very limited. Adequate explanations afterward help them understand and assimilate the experience (Table 27-4).

Table 27-4

NURSING DIAGNOSES TO CONSIDER WHEN CARING FOR WOMEN WITH INTRAPARTUM COMPLICATIONS

*Activity intolerance
Altered Family Processes
Altered Health Maintenance
*Anticipatory Grieving
*Anxiety
*Diversional Activity Deficit
*Health-Seeking Behaviors
*Impaired Home Maintenance Management
Ineffective Individual or Family Coping
Powerlessness
*Risk for infection

*Nursing diagnoses explored in this chapter.

> Although the nurse is usually anxious in an emergency situation too, keeping a calm attitude is important. The woman and her family quickly pick up on the staff's anxiety, and consequently their anxiety escalates. Remain with the woman to reduce fears of abandonment. If possible, hold her hand. Speak in a low, calm voice. The nurses involved should take time to talk out anxieties with colleagues after the emergency situation is over as well.

Evaluation

Evaluation of the goals is probably impossible until the emergency is over and the woman's physical condition stabilizes. Goals for this nursing diagnosis are achieved if the woman and her family do the following:

- Indicate that they understand the problem and the rationale for emergency procedures.
- Express, over several days, their feelings about what has occurred.

SUMMARY CONCEPTS

- Dysfunctional labor may occur because of abnormalities in the powers, the passenger, the passage, or the psyche. Combinations of abnormalities are common.
- Nursing care in dysfunctional labor focuses on prevention or prompt identification and action to correct additional complications such as fetal hypoxia, infection, injury to the mother or fetus, and postpartum hemorrhage.
- Premature rupture of the membranes is associated with infection as both a cause and a complication.
- The early indications of preterm labor are often vague. Prompt identification of preterm labor enables the most effective therapy to delay preterm birth.
- Nursing care for the woman at risk for a preterm birth before 34 weeks' gestation focuses on helping her delay birth long enough to provide time for fetal lung maturation with corticosteroids, allow transfer to a facility that has neonatal intensive care, or reach a gestation at which the infant's problems with immaturity are minimal.
- The main risk in prolonged pregnancy is reduced placental function. This may compromise the fetus during labor and result in meconium aspiration in the neonate. Dysfunctional labor may occur if a fetus continues growing during the prolonged pregnancy.
- The key intervention for umbilical cord prolapse is to relieve pressure on it and to expedite delivery.
- Be aware of women at risk for uterine rupture, and observe for signs and symptoms such as signs of shock, abdominal pain, a sense of tearing, chest pain, pain between the scapulae, abnormal FHR patterns, cessation of contractions, and palpation of the fetus outside the uterus.
- Uterine inversion often is accompanied by massive blood loss and shock. Recovery care promotes uterine contraction and maintenance of adequate circulating volume.
- Amniotic fluid embolism is more likely to occur when labor is intense and the membranes have ruptured.

ANSWERS TO CRITICAL THINKING EXERCISE

When the fetus is in one of the occiput posterior positions, back pain is usually persistent because the fetal head presses on the mother's sacrum with each contraction, often called "back labor." Additionally, the fetal head has to rotate internally through a wider arc to ultimately reach an occiput anterior position for birth. This process prolongs labor in most women.

The nurse should take actions to make the woman more comfortable and promote rotation of the fetal head to an occiput anterior position. The nurse should encourage the woman to change positions regularly. Positions that cause her uterus to fall forward reduce pressure on her sacrum and straighten the pelvic curve somewhat to encourage fetal rotation. Examples of these are leaning forward while sitting, kneeling, standing, or a hands-and-knees position. Lunging toward her right side provides slightly more room on that side of her pelvis. If she wants to lie in bed, a left side-lying position favors fetal rotation toward an occiput anterior position. Consult with the nurse-midwife if the woman wants analgesia or anesthesia.

REFERENCES & READINGS

Abbott, J.T. (1999). Emergency management of the obstetric patient. In G.N. Burrow & T.F. Ferris (Eds.), *Medical complications during pregnancy* (5th ed., pp. 228-236). Philadelphia: W.B. Saunders.

Alexander, J.M., McIntire, D.D., & Leveno, K.J. (2000). Forty weeks and beyond: Pregnancy outcomes by week of gestation. *Obstetrics & Gynecology, 96*(2), 291-294.

American College of Obstetricians and Gynecologists (ACOG). (1995a). *Technical bulletin no. 196: Operative vaginal delivery.* Washington, D.C.: Author.

ACOG. (1995b). *Technical bulletin no. 218: Dystocia and the augmentation of labor.* Washington, D.C.: Author.

ACOG. (1995c). *Technical bulletin no. 206: Preterm labor.* Washington, D.C.: Author.

Asrat, T., & Quilligan, E.J. (2000). Postterm pregnancy. In E.J. Quilligan & F.P. Zuspan (Eds.), *Current therapy in obstetrics and gynecology* (5th ed., pp. 321-322). Philadelphia: W.B. Saunders.

Bachman, J., & Kendrick, J.M. (1996). Childbirth. In K.R. Simpson and P.A. Creehan (Eds.), *AWHONN's perinatal nursing* (pp. 151-186). Philadelphia: Lippincott.

Bowes, W.A. (1999). Clinical aspects of normal and abnormal labor. In R.K. Creasy & R. Resnick (Eds.), *Maternal-fetal medicine: Principles and practice* (4th ed., pp. 541-568). Philadelphia: W.B. Saunders.

Boyle, J.G. (1995). Beta-adrenergic agonists. *Clinical Obstetrics and Gynecology,* 38(4), 688-696.

Burke, M.E., & Poole, J. (1996). Common perinatal complications. In K.R. Simpson & P.A. Creehan (Eds.), *AWHONN's perinatal nursing* (pp. 109-148). Philadelphia: Lippincott.

Clark, S.L. (2000). Amniotic fluid embolism. In E.J. Quilligan & F.P. Zuspan (Eds.), *Current therapy in obstetrics and gynecology* (5th ed., pp. 232-236). Philadelphia: W.B. Saunders.

Colombo, D.F., & Iams, J.D. (2000). Preterm birth. In S.B. Ranson, M.P. Dombrowski, S.G. McNeeley, K.S. Moghissi, & A.R. Munkarah (Eds.), *Practical strategies in obstetrics and gynecology* (pp. 344-352). Philadelphia: W.B. Saunders.

Creasy, R.K., & Iams, J.D. (1999). Preterm labor and delivery. In R.K. Creasy & R. Resnick (Eds.), *Maternal-fetal medicine: Principles and practice* (4th ed., pp. 498-531). Philadelphia: W.B. Saunders.

Crowther, C.A. (1995). Commentary: Bed rest for women with pregnancy problems: Evidence for efficacy is lacking. *Birth,* 22(1), 13-14.

Cruikshank, D.P. (1999). Malpresentations and umbilical cord complications. In J.R. Scott, P.J. Di Saia, C.B. Hammond, & W.N. Spellacy (Eds.), *Danforth's obstetrics & gynecology* (8th ed., pp. 419-436). Philadelphia: Lippincott Williams & Wilkins.

Cunningham, F.G., MacDonald, P.C., Gant, N.F., Leveno, K.J., Gilstrap, L.C., Hankins, G.D.V., et al. (1997). *Williams obstetrics* (20th ed.). Norwalk, CT: Appleton & Lange.

de Veciana, M., Porto, M., Major, C.A., & Barke, J.I. (1995). Tocolysis in advanced preterm labor: Impact on neonatal outcome. *American Journal of Perinatology,* 12(4), 294-298.

Dorman, K. (1999). Pulmonary disorders in pregnancy. In L.K. Mandeville and N.H. Troiano (Eds.), *High-risk & critical care intrapartum nursing* (2nd ed., pp. 185-199). Philadelphia: Lippincott.

Dudley, D.J. (1999). Complications of labor. In J.R. Scott, P.J. Di Saia, C.B. Hammond, & W.N. Spellacy (Eds.), *Danforth's obstetrics & gynecology* (8th ed., pp. 437-455). Philadelphia: Lippincott Williams & Wilkins.

Edwards, R.K., Duff, P., & Ross, K.C. (2000). Amniotic fluid indices of fetal pulmonary maturity with preterm premature rupture of membranes. *Obstetrics & Gynecology,* 96(1), 102-105.

Ellings, J.M., & Bowers, N.A. (1998). Intrapartum care for women with multiple pregnancy. *Journal of Obstetric, Gynecologic, and Neonatal Nursing,* 27(4), 466-472.

Flynn, K. (1999). Preterm labor and premature rupture of membranes. In L.K. Mandeville and N.H. Troiano (Eds.), *High-risk & critical care intrapartum nursing* (2nd ed., pp. 102-122). Philadelphia: Lippincott.

Fraser, W.D., & Boulvain, M. (2000). Dysfunctional labor. In E.J. Quilligan & F.P. Zuspan (Eds.), *Current therapy in obstetrics and gynecology* (5th ed., pp. 271-273). Philadelphia: W.B. Saunders.

Fraser, W.D., Marcoux, S., Krauss, I., Douglas, J., Goulet, C., & Boulvain, M. (2000). Multicenter, randomized, controlled trial of delayed pushing for nulliparous women with second stage of labor with continuous epidural analgesia. *Obstetrics & Gynecology,* 182(5), 1165-1172.

Freda, M.C. (1995). Arrest, trial, and failure. *Journal of Obstetric, Gynecologic, and Neonatal Nursing,* 24(5), 393-394.

Freston, M.S., Young, S., Calhoun, S., Fredericksen, T., Salinger, L., Malchodi, & Egan, J.F.X. (1997). Responses of pregnant women to potential preterm labor symptoms. *Journal of Obstetric, Gynecologic, and Neonatal Nursing,* 26(1), 35-41.

Gahart, B.L., & Nazareno, A.R. (2000). *2000 intravenous medications.* St. Louis: Mosby.

Garite, T.J. (1999). Premature rupture of the membranes. In R.K. Creasy & R. Resnick (Eds.), *Maternal-fetal medicine: Principles and practice* (4th ed., pp. 644-658). Philadelphia: W.B. Saunders.

Garite, T.J. (2000). Fetal fibronectin: Its role in obstetrics. In E.J. Quilligan & F.P. Zuspan (Eds.), *Current therapy in obstetrics and gynecology* (5th ed., pp. 277-279). Philadelphia: W.B. Saunders.

Garite. T.J. (2000a). Fetal fibronectin: Its role in obstetrics. In E.J. Quilligan & F.P. Zuspan (Eds.), *Current therapy in obstetrics and gynecology* (5th ed., pp. 277-279). Philadelphia: W.B. Saunders.

Garite, T.J. (2000b). Premature rupture of the membranes. In E.J. Quilligan & F.P. Zuspan (Eds.), *Current therapy in obstetrics and gynecology* (5th ed., pp. 644-658). Philadelphia: W.B. Saunders.

Gupton, A., Heaman, M., & Ashcroft, T. (1997). Bed rest from the perspective of the high-risk pregnant woman. *Journal of Obstetric, Gynecologic, and Neonatal Nursing,* 26(4), 423-430.

Hall, S.P. (1997). The nurse's role in the identification of risks and treatment of shoulder dystocia. *Journal of Obstetric, Gynecologic, and Neonatal Nursing, 26* (1), 25-32.

Hayashi, R.H., & Bashore, R.A. (1998). Gap junctions, uterine contractility, and dystocia. In N.F. Hacker & J.G. Moore (Eds.), *Essentials of obstetrics and gynecology* (3rd ed., pp. 301-311). Philadelphia: W.B. Saunders.

Heaman, M., & Gupton, A. (1998). Perceptions of bed rest by women with high-risk pregnancies: A comparison between home and hospital. *Birth,* 25(4), 252-258.

Helal, K.J., Gordon, M.C., Lightner, C.R., & Barth, W.H. (2000). Adrenal suppression induced by betamethasone in women at risk for premature delivery. *Obstetrics & Gynecology,* 96(2), 287-290.

Hobel, C.J. (1998). Preterm labor and premature rupture of the membranes. In N.F. Hacker & J.G. Moore (Eds.), *Essentials of obstetrics and gynecology* (3rd ed., pp. 312-323). Philadelphia: W.B. Saunders.

Hodnett, E. (1996). Nursing support of the laboring woman. *Journal of Obstetric, Gynecologic, and Neonatal Nursing,* 22(4), 311-315.

Iams, J.D. (2000). Preterm birth. In E.J. Quilligan & F.P. Zuspan (Eds.), *Current therapy in obstetrics and gynecology* (5th ed., pp. 329-334). Philadelphia: W.B. Saunders.

Iams, J.D., Goldenberg, R.L., Mercer, B.M., et al. (2001). The preterm prediction study: Can low-risk women destined for spontaneous birth be identified? *American Journal of Obstetrics and Gynecology,* 184(4),652-655.

Janke, J. (1999). The effect of relaxation therapy on preterm labor outcomes. *Journal of Obstetric, Gynecologic, and Neonatal Nursing,* 28(3), 255-263.

Joffe, G.M., Symonds, R., Alverson, D., & Childton, L. (1995). The effect of a comprehensive prematurity prevention program on the number of admissions to the neonatal intensive care unit. *Journal of Perinatology,* 15(4), 305-309.

Jones, D.P., & Collins, B.A. (1996). The nursing management of women experiencing preterm labor: Clinical guidelines and why they are needed. *Journal of Obstetric, Gynecologic, and Neonatal Nursing,* 25(7), 569-592.

Lenke, R., & Ashwood, E. (2000). Lung maturity testing. In E.J. Quilligan & F.P. Zuspan (Eds.), *Current therapy in obstetrics and gynecology* (5th ed., pp. 418-420). Philadelphia: W.B. Saunders.

Luppi, C.J. (1999). Cardiopulmonary resuscitation in pregnancy. In L.K. Mandeville and N.H. Troiano (Eds.), *High-risk & critical care intrapartum nursing* (2nd ed., pp. 353-379). Philadelphia: Lippincott.

Malone, F.D., & D'Alton, M.E. (1999). Multiple gestation: Clinical characteristics and management. In R.K. Creasy & R. Resnick (Eds.), *Maternal-fetal medicine: Principles and practice* (4th ed., pp. 598-615). Philadelphia: W.B. Saunders.

Maloni, J.A. (1996). Bed rest and high-risk pregnancy: Differentiating the effects of diagnosis, setting, and treatment. *Nursing Clinics of North America,* 31(2), 313-325.

Maloni, J.A. (1998). *Antepartum bed rest: Case studies, research, & nursing care.* Washington, D.C.: Association of Women's Health, Obstetric and Neonatal Nurses.

Maloni, J.A. (2000a). Antepartum support group for women hospitalized on bed rest. *MCN: American Journal of Maternal/Child Nursing,* 25(4), 204-210.

Maloni, J.A. (2000b). Preventing preterm birth: Evidence-based interventions shift toward prevention. *AWHONN Lifelines,* 4(4), 26-33.

March of Dimes. (1999). Ten leading causes of infant mortality, United States, 1997. Retrieved September 30, 2000 from modimes.org/HealthLibrary2/InfantHealthStatistics/ten_new.htm.

Mark, S.P., Croughan-Minihane, M.S., & Kilpatrick, S.J. (2000). Chorioamnionitis and uterine function. *Obstetrics & Gynecology,* 95(6), 909-912.

Martin-Arafeh, J.M., Watson, C.L., & Baird, S.M. (1999). Promoting family-centered care in high-risk pregnancy. *Journal of Perinatal and Neonatal Nursing,* 13(1), 27-42.

Mayberry, L.J., Wood, S.H., Strange, L.B., Lee, L., Heisler, D.R., & Nielsen-Smith, K. (2000). *AWHONN symposium: Second stage labor management: Promotion of evidence-based practice and a collaborative approach to patient care.* Washington, D.C.: Association of Women's Health, Obstetric, and Neonatal Nurses.

Mercer, B.M., Goldenberg, R.L., Meis, P.J., Moawad, A.H., Shellhaas, C., Das, A., Menard, M.K., Caritis, S.N., Thurnau, G.R., Dombrowski, M.P., Miodovnik, M., Roberts, J.M., & McNellis, D. (2000). The Preterm Prediction Study: Prediction of preterm premature rupture of membranes through clinical findings and ancillary testing. *Obstetrics & Gynecology,* 183(3), 738-745.

Miltner, R.S. (2000). Identifying labor support actions of intrapartum nurses. *Journal of Obstetric, Gynecologic, and Neonatal Nursing,* 29(5), 491-499.

Moore, M.L. (1999). Biochemical markers for preterm labor and birth: What is their role in the care of pregnant women? *MCN: American Journal of Maternal/Child Nursing,* 24(2), 80-86.

Mozurkewich, E.L., Luke, B., Avni, M., & Wolf, F.M. (2000). Working conditions and adverse pregnancy outcome: A meta-analysis. *Obstetrics & Gynecology,* 95(4), 623-635.

Nicholson, W.K., Frick, K.D., & Powe, N.R. (2000). Economic burden of hospitalizations for preterm labor in the United States. *Obstetrics & Gynecology,* 96(1), 95-101.

Papatsonis, D.N.M., Kok, J.H., Van Geijn, H.P., Bleker, O.P., Adèr, H.J., & Dekker, G.A. (2000). Neonatal effects of nifedipine and ritodrine for preterm labor. *Obstetrics & Gynecology,* 95(4), 477-481.

Parsons, M.T., & Spellacy, W.N. (1999). Preterm labor. In J.R. Scott, P.J. Di Saia, C.B. Hammond, & W.N. Spellacy (Eds.), *Danforth's obstetrics & gynecology* (8th ed., pp. 257-267). Philadelphia: Lippincott Williams & Wilkins.

Ray, D., & Dyson, D. (1995). Calcium channel blockers. *Clinical Obstetrics and Gynecology,* 38(4), 713-721.

Resnik, R., & Calder, A. (1999). Post-term pregnancy. In R.K. Creasy & R. Resnick (Eds.), *Maternal-fetal medicine: Principles and practice* (4th ed., pp. 532-539). Philadelphia: W.B. Saunders.

Rippin, C.S. (1996). The experience of precipitate labor. *Birth,* 23(4), 224-228.

Romero, R., Sibai, B.M., Sanchez-Ramos, L., Valenzuela, G.J., Veille, J.C., Tabor, B., Perry, K.G., Varner, M., Goodwin, T.M., Lane, R., Smith, J., Shangold, G., & Creasy, G.W. (2000). An oxytocin receptor antagonist (atosiban) in the treatment of preterm labor: A randomized, double-blind, placebo-controlled trial with tocolytic rescue. *American Journal of Obstetrics & Gynecology,* 182(5), 1173-1183.

Ross, M.G., & Hobel, C.J. (1998). Normal labor, delivery, and the puerperium. In N.F. Hacker & J.G. Moore (Eds.), *Essentials of obstetrics and gynecology* (3rd ed., pp. 150-167). Philadelphia: W.B. Saunders.

Rotmensch, S., Vishne, T.H., Celentano, C., Dan, M., & Ben-Rafael, Z. (1999). Maternal infectious morbidity following multiple courses of betamethasone. *Journal of Infection,* 39, 49-54.

Rouse, D.J., Owen, J., & Hauth, J.C. (1999). Active phase labor arrest: Oxytocin augmentation for at least 4 hours. *Obstetrics & Gynecology,* 93(3), 323-328.

Ruiz, R.J. (1998). Mechanisms of full-term and preterm labor: Factors influencing uterine activity. *Journal of Obstetric, Gynecologic, and Neonatal Nursing,* 27(6), 652-660.

Ruiz, R.J., & Pearson, A.J. (1999). Psychoneuroimmunology and preterm birth: A holistic model for obstetrical nursing practice and research. *MCN: American Journal of Maternal/Child Nursing,* 24(S):230-235.

Schieve, L.A., Cogswell, M.E., Scanlon, K.S., Perry, G., Ferre, C., Blackmore-Prince, C., Yu, S.M., & Rosenberg, D. (2000). Prepregnancy body mass index and pregnancy weight gain: Associations with preterm delivery. *Obstetrics & Gynecology, 96*(2), 194-200.

Schroeder, C.A. (1996). Women's experience of bed rest in high-risk pregnancy. *Image: Journal of Nursing Scholarship, 28*(3), 253–258.

Schroeder, C.A. (1998). Bedrest in complicated pregnancy: A critical analysis. *MCN: American Journal of Maternal/Child Nursing, 23*(1), 45-49.

Simkin, P. (1995). Reducing pain and enhancing progress in labor: A guide to nonpharmacologic methods for maternity caregivers. *Birth, 22*(3), 161-171.

Simpson, K.R. (1999). Shoulder dystocia: Nursing interventions and risk-management strategies. *MCN: American Journal of Maternal/Child Nursing, 24*(6), 305-310.

Wright, M., & Higgins, P.G. (1999). How competent are you (or your staff) with shoulder dystocia? *AWHONN Lifelines, 3*(1), 35-38.

28 POST-PARTUM MATERNAL COMPLICATIONS

OBJECTIVES

1. Describe postpartum hemorrhage in terms of predisposing factors, causes, clinical signs, and therapeutic management.
2. Explain major causes, clinical signs, and therapeutic management of subinvolution.
3. Describe three major thromboembolic disorders (superficial venous thrombosis, deep vein thrombosis, pulmonary embolism) in terms of predisposing factors, causes, clinical signs, and therapeutic management.
4. Discuss puerperal infection in terms of location, predisposing factors, causes, signs and symptoms, and therapeutic management.
5. Describe two major affective disorders (postpartum depression and psychosis).
6. Describe the role of the nurse in the management of women who have a postpartum complication.

DEFINITIONS

ATONY Absence or lack of usual muscle tone.

DILATION AND CURETTAGE (D&C) Stretching of the cervical os to permit suctioning or scraping of the walls of the uterus. The procedure is performed in abortion, to obtain samples of uterine lining tissue for laboratory examination, and during the postpartum period to remove retained fragments of placental tissue.

EMBOLUS A clot, usually part or all of a thrombus, or amniotic fluid brought by the blood from another vessel and forced into a smaller one thus obstructing circulation.

HEMATOMA Localized collection of blood in a space or tissue.

HYDRAMNIOS Excess volume of amniotic fluid (more than 2000 ml at term). Also called *polyhydramnios.*

HYPOVOLEMIA Abnormally decreased volume of circulating fluid in the body.

HYPOVOLEMIC SHOCK Acute peripheral circulatory failure resulting from loss of circulating blood volume.

PLACENTA ACCRETA A placenta that is abnormally adherent to the uterine muscle. If the condition is more advanced, it is called *placenta increta* (the placenta extends into the uterine muscle) or *placenta percreta* (the placenta extends through the uterine muscle).

DEFINITIONS—cont'd

PSYCHOSIS Mental state in which a person's ability to recognize reality, communicate, and relate to others is impaired.

SUBINVOLUTION A slower-than-expected return of the uterus to its nonpregnancy size after childbirth.

THROMBUS Collection of blood factors, primarily platelets and fibrin, that may cause vascular obstruction at the point of formation.

Pregnancy and childbirth are natural functions that most women recover from without complication. However, nurses must be aware of problems that may occur and their effect on the family. The most common physiologic complications are hemorrhage, thromboembolic disorders, and infection. Complications that are psychogenic in origin include postpartum depression and postpartum psychosis.

POSTPARTUM HEMORRHAGE

Postpartum hemorrhage is defined as blood loss that exceeds 500 ml after vaginal childbirth or 1000 ml after cesarean birth. Blood loss to this extent in the first 24 hours after childbirth is termed *early postpartum hemorrhage.* When it occurs after 24 hours, it is called *late postpartum hemorrhage.*

Estimating blood loss is difficult, especially when bleeding is brisk or when hemorrhage is concealed. Furthermore, blood loss during childbirth is frequently underestimated and constitutes only about half the actual loss (Cunningham, et al., 1997). This information is important to remember when excessive bleeding occurs later.

Postpartum hemorrhage complicates approximately 4% of deliveries (Hayashi, 1998). Hemorrhage, along with pulmonary embolism, infection and hypertensive disorders, are leading causes of maternal morbidity and mortality.

Early Postpartum Hemorrhage

The two major causes of early postpartum hemorrhage are uterine atony and trauma to the birth canal during labor and delivery. Abnormalities of the third stage of labor, such as placenta accreta (abnormal adherence of the placenta to the uterine wall), and inversion of the uterus are described in Chapter 27.

Uterine Atony

Uterine atony causes 75% to 80% of cases of early hemorrhage (Hayashi, 1998). Atony is lack of muscle tone that results in failure of the uterine muscle fibers to contract firmly around blood vessels when the placenta separates. The relaxed muscles allow rapid bleeding from the endometrial arteries at the placental site. Bleeding continues until the uterine muscle fibers contract to stop the flow of blood. Figure 28-1 illustrates the effect of uterine contraction on the size of the placental site and the amount of bleeding that occurs.

Predisposing Factors. Knowledge of factors that increase the risk of uterine atony can be used to anticipate and thus reduce excessive bleeding. Overdistention of the uterus from any cause (multiple gestation, a large infant, hydramnios) makes it more difficult for the uterus to contract with enough firmness to prevent excessive bleeding. Multiparity results in muscle fibers that have been stretched repeatedly, and these flaccid muscle fibers may not remain contracted after birth.

Intrapartum factors include contractions that were barely effective, resulting in prolonged labor, or contractions that were excessively vigorous, which may have resulted in precipitate labor. Labor that was induced or that was augmented with oxytocin is more likely to be followed by postdelivery uterine atony and hemorrhage. Retention of a large segment of the placenta does not allow the uterus to contract firmly and thus can result in uterine atony. Disseminated intravascular coagulation (DIC) also may be the cause of postpartum hemorrhage. Table 28-1 summarizes predisposing factors.

Clinical Signs. Major signs of uterine atony are as follows:

- A uterine fundus that is difficult to locate
- A soft or "boggy" feel when the fundus is located
- A uterus that becomes firm as it is massaged, but loses its tone when massage is stopped

Table 28-1
COMMON PREDISPOSING FACTORS FOR POSTPARTUM HEMORRHAGE

Overdistention of the uterus (multiple gestation, large infant, hydramnios)
Multiparity (more than 5)
Use of tocolytic drugs
Precipitate labor or delivery
Prolonged labor
Use of forceps or vacuum extractor
Cesarean birth
Manual removal of the placenta
Previous postpartum hemorrhage
General anesthesia
Placenta previa or accreta
Administration of magnesium sulfate
Clotting disorders
Previous uterine surgery
Disseminated intravascular coagulation

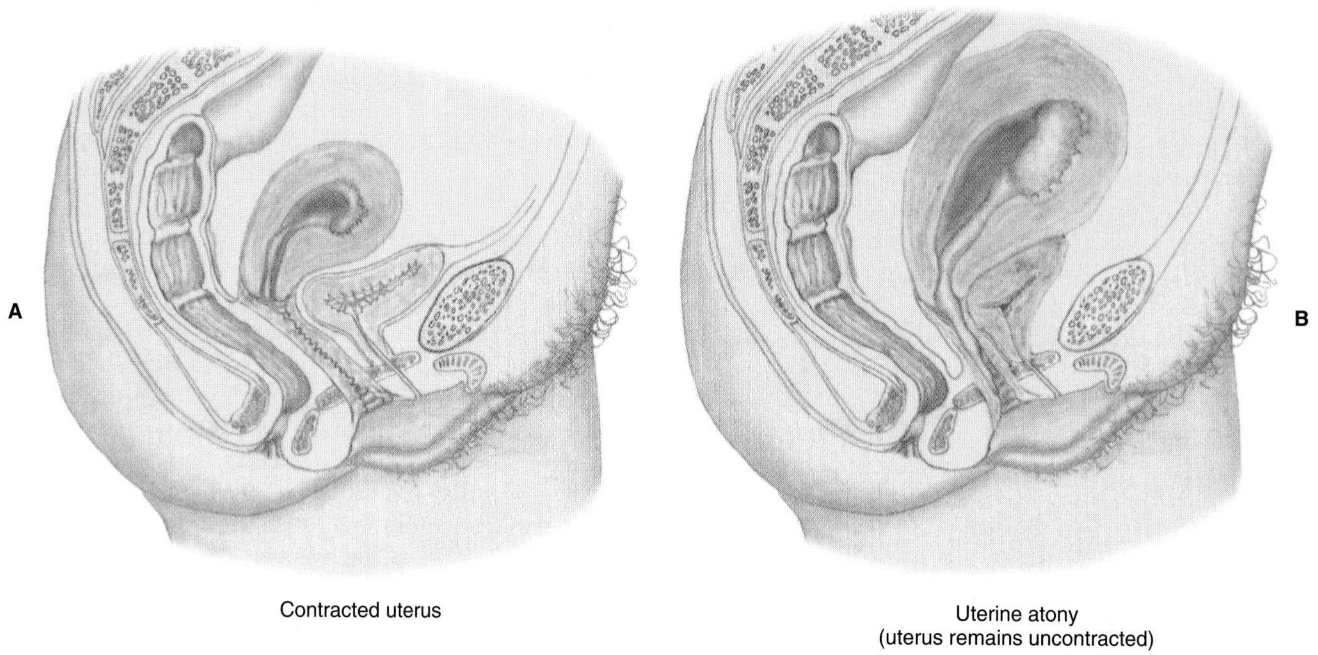

FIGURE 28-1 **A,** When the uterus remains contracted, the placental site is smaller, so bleeding is minimal. **B,** If uterine muscles fail to contract around the endometrial arteries at the placental site, hemorrhage occurs.

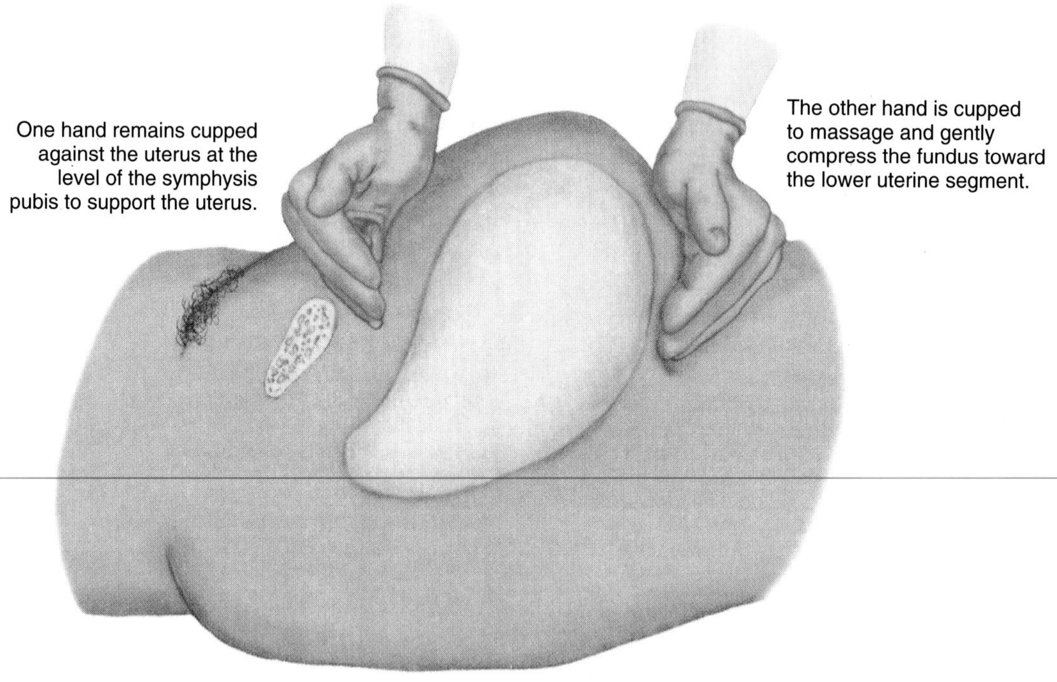

One hand remains cupped against the uterus at the level of the symphysis pubis to support the uterus.
The other hand is cupped to massage and gently compress the fundus toward the lower uterine segment.

FIGURE 28-2 Technique for fundal massage.

- Uterine fundus located above the expected level, which is at or near the umbilicus
- Excessive lochia, especially if it is bright red
- Excessive clots expelled

For the first 24 hours after birth, the uterus should feel like a firmly contracted ball roughly the size of a large grapefruit. It should be located easily at about the level of the umbilicus. Lochia should be dark red and moderate in amount. Saturation of more than one peripad per hour is considered excessive, even in the early postpartum period. The nurse must realize that although bleeding may be profuse and dramatic, a constant steady trickle is just as danger-

DRUG GUIDE: METHYLERGONOVINE (METHERGINE)

Classification: Oxytocic

Action: Stimulates contraction of the uterus and causes arterial vasoconstriction

Indications: Used for the prevention and treatment of postpartum or postabortion hemorrhage caused by uterine atony or subinvolution

Dosage and Route: Usual dosage is 0.2 mg intramuscularly (IM) every 2 to 4 hours for a maximum of five doses. Change to oral route 0.2 mg every 6 to 8 hours for a maximum of 7 days.

Absorption: Well absorbed after oral or IM route

Excretion: Metabolized by the liver, excreted in the urine

Contraindications and Precautions: It should never be used during pregnancy or to induce labor. Do not use IM if the mother is hypersensitive to ergot. Contraindicated for women with hypertension, severe hepatic or renal disease, coronary artery disease, peripheral vascular disease, hypocalcemia, sepsis and before the fourth stage of labor.

Adverse Reactions: Nausea, uterine cramping, vomiting, hypertension, dizziness, headache, dyspnea, chest pain, palpitations, peripheral ischemia, and uterine and gastrointestinal cramping

Nursing Considerations: Before administering medication, assess blood pressure. Follow facility protocol if medication must be withheld (usually a reading of 136/90). Caution the mother to avoid smoking because nicotine constricts blood vessels. Remind her to report any adverse reactions.

ous. (See Chapter 17 for assessment of the uterus and lochia.)

Therapeutic Management. Nurses are with the mother during the hours after childbirth and are responsible for assessments and initial management of uterine atony. If the uterus is not firmly contracted, the first intervention is to massage the fundus until it is firm and to express clots that may have accumulated in the uterus. One hand is placed just above the symphysis pubis to support the lower uterine segment while the fundus is gently but firmly massaged in a circular motion. Figure 28-2 illustrates correct hand placement for fundal massage.

Clots that may have accumulated in the uterine cavity are expressed by applying firm but gentle pressure on the fundus in the direction of the vagina. The uterus must be contracted firmly before clots are expressed. *Pushing on an uncontracted uterus could invert the uterus and cause massive hemorrhage and rapid shock.*

If the uterus does not remain contracted as a result of uterine massage, the problem may be a distended bladder. A full bladder lifts and displaces the uterus and prevents effective contraction of the uterine muscles. Nurses should assist the mother to urinate or catheterize her, if necessary, to correct uterine atony caused by bladder distention.

Pharmacologic measures also may be necessary to maintain firm contraction of the uterus. A rapid IV infusion of dilute oxytocin (Pitocin) often increases uterine tone and controls bleeding. Approximately 20 units in 1000 ml of lactated Ringer's or normal saline at a rate of 600 ml per hour may be recommended (Cunningham, et al., 1997).

If the uterus remains atonic and bleeding continues, methylergonovine (Methergine) may be given by intramuscular or, rarely, IV injection. Methylergonovine has the side effect of elevating blood pressure and should not be given to a woman who is hypertensive. Analogues of prostaglandin F_{2a} (carboprost tromethamine, Hemabate, Prostin/15M) may be given intramuscularly. Misoprostol (Cytotec) given rectally or orally is being studied as another method of controlling bleeding. It has fewer side effects and is less expensive. Table 28-2 summarizes management for early postpartum hemorrhage.

Table 28-2
THERAPEUTIC MANAGEMENT FOR EARLY POSTPARTUM HEMORRHAGE

Cause	Treatment
Uterine atony	Massage of the fundus, express clots from uterus, assist to empty bladder Rapid IV infusion of dilute oxytocin Parenteral administration of methylergonovine or analogues of prostaglandin carboprost tromethamine (Hemabate, Prostin/15M) Misoprostol (Cytotec) IV replacement of intravascular fluids and blood Bimanual compression of the uterus Abdominal hysterectomy if other interventions fail to control bleeding
Trauma	Locate and repair lacerations and hematomas in the genital tract
Retained placental fragments	Oxytocin, methylergonovine, prostaglandins, or evacuation or curettage if hemorrhage continues; antibiotics if infection suspected

If uterine massage and pharmacologic measures are ineffective in stopping uterine bleeding, the physician or nurse-midwife may use bimanual compression of the uterus to stop the bleeding. In this procedure, one hand is inserted into the vagina and the other compresses

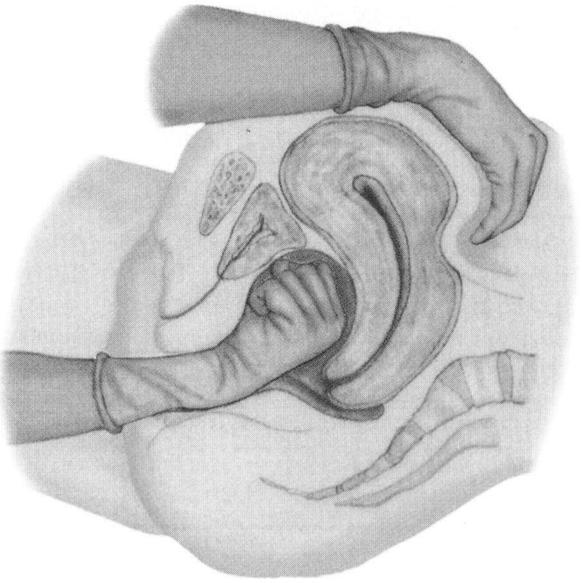

FIGURE 28-3 Bimanual compression. One hand is inserted in the vagina, and the other compresses the uterus through the abdominal wall.

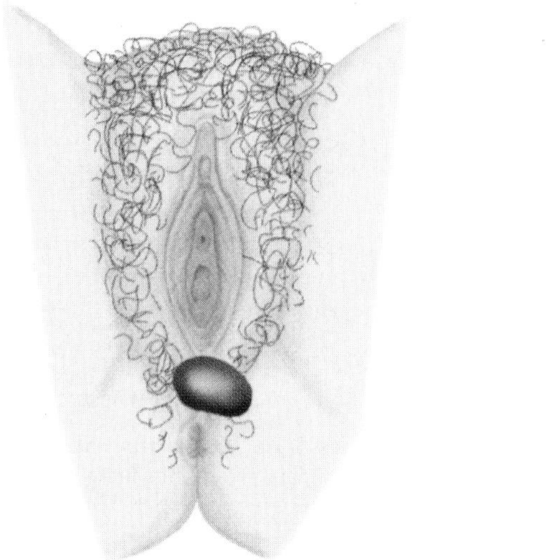

FIGURE 28-4 A vulvar hematoma is caused by rapid bleeding into soft tissue, and it causes severe pain and feelings of pressure.

the uterus through the abdominal wall (Figure 28-3). The woman may need to return to the delivery area to explore the uterine cavity and remove placental fragments that interfere with uterine contraction.

Hemorrhage requires prompt replacement of intravascular fluid volume. Lactated Ringer's solution or other plasma extenders, whole blood, or packed cells may be used. Enough fluid should be given to maintain urine flow of at least 30 ml per hour (Cunningham, et al., 1997). The nurse often is responsible for obtaining properly typed and crossmatched blood and, if they are not already present, inserting large-bore IV lines that are capable of carrying whole blood.

Operative procedures are the last resort. A hysterectomy may be necessary to save the life of a woman with uncontrollable postpartum hemorrhage.

Trauma

Trauma to the birth canal is the second most common cause of early postpartum hemorrhage. Trauma can include vaginal, cervical, or perineal lacerations as well as hematomas.

Predisposing Factors. Many of the same factors that increase the risk of uterine atony increase the risk of soft tissue trauma during childbirth. For example, trauma to the birth canal is more likely to occur if the infant is large or if labor and delivery occur rapidly. Induction and augmentation of labor and use of assistive devices increase the risk of tissue trauma.

Lacerations. The perineum, vagina, cervix, and the area around the urethral meatus are the most common sites for lacerations. Cervical lacerations occur frequently when the cervix dilates rapidly during the first stage of labor. Lacerations of the vagina, perineum, and periurethral area usually occur during the second stage of labor, when the fetal head descends rapidly or when assistive devices such as forceps or a vacuum extractor are used to assist in delivery of the fetal head.

Lacerations of the birth canal should always be suspected if excessive uterine bleeding continues when the fundus is contracted firmly and is at the expected location. Bleeding from lacerations of the genital tract often is bright red, in contrast to the darker red color of lochia.

Hematomas. Hematomas occur when bleeding occurs into loose connective tissue while overlying tissue remains intact. Hematomas develop as a result of blood vessel injury in spontaneous deliveries and deliveries in which forceps or vacuum extractors are used. Hematomas may be found in vulvar areas, on the wall of the vagina, or in retroperitoneal areas.

Visible vulvar hematomas appear as a discolored bulging mass caused by rapid bleeding into soft tissue. Hematomas produce deep, severe, unrelieved pain and feelings of pressure. Formation of a hematoma also should be suspected if the mother demonstrates systemic signs of concealed blood loss, such as falling blood pressure or tachycardia, when the fundus is firm and lochia is within normal limits. Figure 28-4 illustrates a vulvar hematoma.

Therapeutic Management. When postpartum hemorrhage is caused by trauma of the birth canal, surgical repair often is necessary. Visualizing lacerations of the vagina or cervix is difficult, and it is necessary to return the mother to the delivery area, where surgical lights are available. She is placed in a lithotomy position and carefully draped. Surgical asepsis is required while the laceration is being visualized and repaired. Small hematomas usually reabsorb naturally, but large hematomas may require incision, evacuation of the clots, and location of the bleeding vessel so that it can be ligated.

Late Postpartum Hemorrhage

The most common causes of late postpartum hemorrhage are subinvolution (delayed return of the uterus to its nonpregnant size and consistency) and fragments of placenta that remain attached to the myometrium when the placenta is delivered. Clots form around the retained fragments, and excessive bleeding can occur when the clots slough several days after delivery.

Late postpartum hemorrhage caused by retained placental fragments is generally preventable. The placenta should be inspected carefully by the nurse-midwife or physician to determine whether it is intact. If a portion of the placenta is missing, the health care provider can explore the uterus, locate the missing fragments, and remove them soon after delivery of the placenta.

Late postpartum hemorrhage, which typically occurs without warning usually at 7 to 14 days after delivery, can be dangerous for the unsuspecting mother. Families must be taught how to assess the fundus and the normal duration of lochia. They must be instructed to notify their health care provider if bleeding persists or becomes unusually heavy.

Predisposing Factors

Attempts to deliver the placenta before it separates from the uterine wall, manual removal of the placenta, and placenta accreta are the primary predisposing factors for retention of placental fragments.

Therapeutic Management

Initial treatment for late postpartum hemorrhage is directed toward control of the excessive bleeding. Oxytocin, methylergonovine, and prostaglandins are the most commonly used pharmacologic measures. Placental fragments often are dislodged and swept out of the uterus by the bleeding, and if the bleeding subsides when oxytocin is administered, no other treatment is necessary. Sonography can exclude placental fragments as the cause of delayed postpartum hemorrhage (Cunningham, et al., 1997). If bleeding continues or recurs, suction evacuation of the fragments or curettage may be carried out. Curettage should be performed only when other treatment has failed, because it may cause trauma and additional bleeding. Broad-spectrum antibiotics also may be given if postpartum infection is suspected because of uterine tenderness, foul-smelling lochia, or fever.

APPLICATION OF THE NURSING PROCESS: EXCESSIVE BLEEDING

Assessment

The initial postpartum assessment includes a chart review to determine whether any factors such as prolonged labor or birth of a large infant increase the risk for the woman to bleed excessively.

Check Your Reading

1. Why does the nurse examine the mother's prenatal record and her labor and delivery record?
2. Why is a mother who has given birth to twins at increased risk for postpartum hemorrhage?
3. Can the nurse be positive that bleeding is controlled when the fundus is firm and the lochia is moderate? Why or why not?
4. How is uterine atony treated?
5. How are hematomas treated?

Uterine Atony

Priority assessments for uterine atony include the fundus, bladder, lochia, vital signs, and skin temperature and color. Assess the consistency and the location of the uterine fundus. The fundus should be firmly contracted, at or near the level of the umbilicus, and midline. If the uterus is not firmly contracted, the fundus feels soft (boggy) and bleeding from the placental site is rapid and continuous. If the fundus is above the level of the umbilicus and displaced, a full bladder may be the cause of excessive bleeding. A full bladder lifts the uterus and impedes contraction, which allows excessive bleeding. The accumulation of clots also expands the uterus, making contraction difficult and resulting in continued bleeding. See Procedure 17-1 (p. 441) for complete information about assessing the fundus.

Estimating the volume of lochia is difficult by visual examination of peripads. More accurate information is obtained by weighing peripads and bed liners before and after use and subtracting the difference. Approximately 1 gram (weight) equals 1 ml (volume). When inspecting for blood loss, always ask the woman to turn on her side because blood that pools under her is not visible when checking pads from the front. Large amounts of blood could be pooling undetected underneath her. Although bleeding may be profuse and dramatic, a continuing steady trickle may lead to significant blood loss that becomes increasingly life threatening.

Measure vital signs at least every 15 minutes to detect trends, such as tachycardia or a decrease in pulse pressure (difference between systolic and diastolic blood pressure), that may reveal a deteriorating status

Table 28-3
NURSING ASSESSMENTS FOR POSTPARTUM HEMORRHAGE

Assessments	Abnormal Signs/Symptoms	Nursing Implications
Chart review	Presence of predisposing factors	Perform more frequent evaluations.
Fundus	Soft, boggy, displaced	Massage, express clots, assist to void or catheterize, notify primary health care provider if measures are ineffective.
Lochia	Excessive bleeding (saturation of more than 1 pad/hr, steady trickle or profuse flow)	Assess for trauma, save and weigh pads and bed liners so that estimation of blood loss will be more accurate. Notify physician or nurse-midwife.
Vital signs	Tachycardia, decreasing pulse pressure, falling blood pressure	Report signs of hypovolemia.
Comfort level	Severe pelvic or rectal pain	Signs of hematoma, usually perineal or vaginal; examine vulva for masses or discoloration.
Skin	Cool, damp, pale	Signs of hypovolemia, vigilant assessment and management by entire health care team is necessary.

in a woman with significant blood loss. Initially the body compensates for excessive bleeding by constricting the blood vessels and shunting blood to vital organs. As a result, vital signs may remain normal although the woman is becoming hypovolemic. (See p. 782 for a discussion of hypovolemic shock.)

The skin should be warm and dry, mucous membranes of the lips and mouth should be pink, and capillary return should occur within 3 seconds when the nails are blanched. These signs confirm adequate circulating volume to perfuse the peripheral tissue.

Trauma

If the fundus is firm but bleeding is excessive, the cause may be lacerations of the cervix or birth canal. Inspect the perineum to determine whether a laceration is visible in that area. Lacerations of the cervix or vagina are not visible, but bleeding in the presence of a contracted uterus is suggestive of a laceration. This sign warrants examination of the vaginal walls and the cervix by the health care provider.

Assess comfort level. If the mother complains of deep, severe pelvic or rectal pain or if vital signs or skin changes suggest hemorrhage but excessive bleeding is not obvious, the cause may be concealed bleeding and the formation of a hematoma. Examine the vulva for bulging masses or discoloration of the skin. However, a hematoma may be developing in the vagina or in the retroperitoneal area and will not be obvious when the vulva is examined. Table 28-3 summarizes assessments, abnormal signs and symptoms, and nursing implications.

Analysis

Certain signs and symptoms, such as uterine atony that does not respond to massage, excessive lochia, pelvic or rectal pain, or changes in vital signs, may be the earliest signs of postpartum hemorrhage. Postpartum hemorrhage is a potential complication that requires the efforts of the health care team to control the hemorrhage and prevent further complications such as hypovolemic shock.

Planning

Client-centered goals are inappropriate for this potential complication because the nurse cannot manage postpartum hemorrhage independently but must confer with the physician or nurse-midwife for medical orders to treat the condition. Planning should reflect the nurse's responsibility to do the following:

- Monitor for signs of postpartum hemorrhage
- Perform actions that will minimize postpartum hemorrhage and prevent hypovolemic shock
- Consult with the health care provider if signs of postpartum hemorrhage are observed

Interventions

Preventing Hemorrhage

Every nurse should be aware of factors that put the new mother at risk for postpartum hemorrhage. This knowledge alerts the nurse to be particularly vigilant in monitoring these women so that excessive bleeding can be anticipated and minimized.

When predisposing factors are present, initiate frequent assessments. Many hospitals and birth centers have a standard of care that calls for assessments every 15 minutes during the first hour after delivery, every 30 minutes for the next 2 hours, and hourly for the next 4 hours. This may not be adequate for the woman at known risk for postpartum hemorrhage, however, because bleeding occurs rapidly. A delay in assessment may result in a great deal of blood loss.

CRITICAL TO REMEMBER

Signs of Postpartum Hemorrhage

An uncontracted uterus
Large gush or slow, steady trickle of blood from the vagina
Saturation of more than one peripad per hour
Severe, unrelieved perineal or rectal pain
Tachycardia

Collaborating with the Health Care Provider

Notify the physician or nurse-midwife when excessive bleeding is suspected. In addition, initiate actions such as uterine massage to control bleeding. In some hospitals or birth centers, protocols permit nurses to initiate specific laboratory studies, such as hemoglobin and hematocrit levels and typing and crossmatching of blood, so that blood is available should transfusions be necessary. Other laboratory studies that may be ordered include platelets, prothrombin time, activated partial thromboplastin time, fibrinogen, fibrin degradation products, and fibrin split products. Many protocols also allow the nurse to start IV fluids while the health care provider is being informed of the mother's condition. These actions do not substitute for notifying the health care provider, but they do allow nurses to make initial interventions quickly.

CRITICAL THINKING EXERCISE

Dolores Stanton, a 26-year-old multipara, is admitted to the postpartum unit after rapid labor and the birth of her fourth infant 2 hours ago. The baby weighed 4000 g (8 pounds, 12 ounces). At the initial assessment, Dolores' fundus is firm, at the level of the umbilicus. Lochia is heavy, with occasional small clots expressed. Vital signs are unchanged from prenatal norms.

QUESTIONS:

1. Do any "red flags" suggest a potential problem or complication? What actions should the nurse take?
2. The nurse observes that the fundus is soft and that lochia is excessive. What are the priority interventions? Why?
3. Within an hour, the fundus becomes "boggy" again and is located 3 cm above the umbilicus and displaced to the right. What is the priority nursing action? Why?
4. Dolores voids 500 ml. The fundus is difficult to locate, however, and lochia is excessive. What is the next nursing action? Why?

Maintain the woman on bedrest to increase venous return and maintain cardiac output. The Trendelenburg position may interfere with cardiac function and is not advised. Continue the assessments described earlier, call for assistance, and save all pads, linen savers, and linen for an accurate estimation of blood loss. Assistance is necessary because one nurse must continue to massage the uncontracted uterus and perform and record assessments while the other notifies the health care provider of the mother's condition.

When notifying the health care provider, document the time and the content of each communication. For example, "1300: Dr. X notified of difficulty maintaining uterine contraction and continued excessive bleeding. Requested Dr. X to see client. Orders received."

Administer medications and fluids ordered by the health care provider and evaluate their effect. For example, add the prescribed amount of oxytocin to the IV solution and infuse the solution at the prescribed rate. Evaluate the effect of the medication on the uterus, and relay this information to the health care provider. Physicians and nurse-midwives depend on the nurse for accurate information, and they base medical management on information relayed by the nurse.

If measures fail to control bleeding, notify the health care provider so that additional procedures can be initiated. These may include preparation for operative intervention (surgical prep, consent signed for operative procedure, or confirmation that blood replacement is available).

Providing Support for the Family

The unusual activity of the hospital staff may make the mother and her family anxious. Be alert to their nonverbal cues, and when they appear frightened, acknowledge their feelings. Keeping them informed is one of the most effective ways of reducing anxiety.

Acknowledge the anxiety and provide simple appropriate explanations of the activity. "I know all this activity must be frightening. She is bleeding a little more than we would like and we are doing several things at once."

Posthemorrhage Care

After the hemorrhage is controlled, continue to assess the woman frequently for a resumption of bleeding. The woman may be anemic and fatigued. Allow rest periods and organize work to help her conserve energy. Because the woman may experience orthostatic hypotension, assist her in getting out of bed after dangling her legs and assessing for dizziness and low blood pressure. Encourage intake of foods high in iron.

Evaluation

Although client-centered goals are not developed for potential complications (collaborative problems), the nurse collects and compares data with established norms and judges whether the data are within normal limits. If problems arise, the nurse acts to minimize hemorrhage and notifies the health care provider.

HYPOVOLEMIC SHOCK

During and after giving birth, the woman can tolerate blood loss that approaches the volume of blood added during pregnancy with little or no drop in hematocrit (Cunningham, et al., 1997). When more than this reserve is lost, hypovolemic shock can ensue. A woman who was anemic before birth has less reserve than a mother with normal blood values.

Hypovolemia endangers vital organs by depriving them of oxygen. The brain, heart, and kidneys are especially vulnerable to hypoxia and may suffer damage in a brief period. When blood loss is high enough, hypovolemic shock can ensue. Hypovolemia endangers vital organs by depriving them of oxygen. The brain, heart, and kidneys are especially vulnerable to hypoxia and may suffer damage in a brief period.

How the Body Compensates for Hypovolemia

Recognition of hypovolemic shock may be delayed because the body activates compensatory mechanisms that mask the severity of the problem. For example, carotid and aortic baroreceptors are stimulated to constrict peripheral blood vessels. This shunts blood to the central circulation and away from less essential organs, such as the skin and extremities. This causes the skin to become pale and cold but maintains cardiac output and perfusion of vital organs.

In addition, the adrenal glands release catecholamines, which compensate for decreased blood volume by promoting vasoconstriction in nonessential organs, increasing the heart rate, and raising the blood pressure. As a result, blood pressure remains normal initially, although a decrease in pulse pressure may be noted. The tachycardia that develops is an early sign of compensation for excessive blood loss.

Pathophysiology of Hypovolemic Shock

As shock worsens, the compensatory mechanisms fail and physiologic insults spiral. Inadequate organ perfusion and decreased cellular oxygen for metabolism result in a buildup of lactic acid and the development of metabolic acidosis. Decreased serum pH (acidosis) results in vasodilation, which further increases bleeding. In this instance, the effects of hemorrhage now become additional causes of further blood loss.

Eventually, circulating volume becomes insufficient to perfuse cardiac and brain tissue. Cellular death occurs as a result of anoxia, and the mother dies.

Clinical Signs and Symptoms

Tachycardia is one of the earliest signs of hypovolemic shock, and even gradual increases in the pulse rate should be noted. A decrease in blood pressure and narrowing of pulse pressure (see p. 780) occurs when the circulating volume of blood is sufficiently decreased. The respiratory rate increases as the woman becomes more anxious and as she attempts to take in more oxygen to overcome the need that is created when hemoglobin is inadequate to transport oxygen to all of her organs.

Skin changes also provide early cues. Increased catecholamine levels initiate vasoconstriction in the skin, and the skin becomes pale and cool to the touch. As hemorrhage worsens, the skin changes become more obvious; pallor increases, and the skin temperature changes from warm and dry to cold and clammy.

As shock progresses, changes also occur in the central nervous system. The mother becomes anxious, then confused, and finally lethargic when blood loss totals 30% to 40% of the total blood volume. Urine output also progressively decreases from more than 30 ml per hour in early shock to less than 5 ml per hour when more than 40% of the blood is lost. Eventually, urine output stops.

Therapeutic Management

The goals of therapy are to control bleeding and prevent hypovolemic shock from becoming irreversible. Assessment and intervention goals include those described for postpartum hemorrhage. In addition, a second IV line should be inserted with a large-bore (16- to 18-gauge) catheter that is capable of carrying whole blood. Sufficient fluid volume is infused to produce a urinary output of at least 30 ml per hour. At the same time, every effort is made by the health care team to locate the source of bleeding and to stop the loss of blood. Interventions may include uterine packing; ligation of the uterine, ovarian, or hypogastric artery; or hysterectomy.

Nursing Considerations

An automatic blood pressure device should be used to monitor the blood pressure and pulse every 3 to 5 minutes. The location and consistency of the fundus, amount of lochia, skin temperature and color, and capillary return also are assessed. Nurses collaborate with the physician or nurse-midwife to provide initial care. Many facilities also have protocols that allow nurses to initiate specific procedures. Blood should be drawn for hemoglobin, hematocrit, clotting studies, and type and crossmatch. In addition, a pulse oximeter should be applied to determine oxygen saturation of the blood.

A urinary catheter should be inserted so that hourly urinary output can be measured. The indwelling catheter is also necessary if a surgical procedure to control the hemorrhage is required. Oxygen may be needed to increase the saturation of fewer red blood cells. It should be administered by tight face mask at 8 to 10 liters per minute or as directed by the health care provider.

Nurses are also responsible for administering fluids, whole blood, and medications as directed and for reporting on their effectiveness. Nurses must make every effort to provide information and emotional support for the woman and her family.

Home Care

Nurses involved in home care or who work in nurse-managed postpartum clinics must be aware that women who have postpartum hemorrhage are subject to a variety of complications. In general, they are exhausted, and it may take weeks for them to feel well again. Anemia often results, and a course of iron therapy may be prescribed to restore hemoglobin level. Activity may be restricted until strength returns. Some women need extra assistance with housework and care of the new infant. Exhaustion may interfere with bonding and attachment. Because extensive blood loss increases the risk of postpartum infection, the woman and her family must be taught to observe for specific signs and symptoms.

SUBINVOLUTION OF THE UTERUS

Subinvolution refers to a slower-than-expected return of the uterus to its nonpregnancy size after childbirth. Normally, the uterus descends at the rate of about 1 cm or one fingerbreadth per day. By 2 weeks, it is no longer palpable above the symphysis pubis. The endometrial lining has sloughed off as part of lochia, and the site of placental attachment is well healed by 6 weeks after childbirth if involution progresses as expected.

The most common causes of subinvolution are retained placental fragments and pelvic infection. Signs of subinvolution include prolonged lochial discharge, irregular or excessive uterine bleeding, and sometimes profuse hemorrhage (Cunningham, et al., 1997). Pelvic pain or feelings of pelvic heaviness, backache, fatigue, and persistent malaise are reported by many women. On bimanual examination, the uterus feels larger and softer than normal for the particular period of the puerperium.

Therapeutic Management

Treatment is tailored to correct the cause of subinvolution. Oral methylergonovine maleate (Methergine), 0.2 mg every 3 to 4 hours for 24 to 48 hours, provides long, sustained contraction of the uterus. Infection responds to antimicrobial therapy.

Nursing Considerations

In most cases, subinvolution is not obvious until the mother has returned home after childbirth. For this reason, nurses must teach the mother and her family how to assess for the condition and how to recognize its occurrence.

The nurse should demonstrate how to locate and palpate the fundus and how to estimate fundal height in relation to the umbilicus. The nurse should request return demonstrations until the mother is confident of her skill. The uterus should become smaller each day (by approximately one fingerbreadth). The nurse also explains the progressive changes from lochia rubra, to lochia serosa, and then to lochia alba (see Chapter 17).

The mother is instructed to report any deviation from the expected pattern or duration of lochia. A foul odor often indicates uterine infection, for which treatment must be sought. Additional signs must be reported to the physician or midwife, such as pelvic or fundal pain, backache, or feelings of pelvic pressure or fullness.

Check Your Reading

6. Why is it sometimes difficult to recognize that the woman is becoming hypovolemic?
7. What are the major signs of subinvolution?
8. What is the nurse's primary responsibility in the management of subinvolution?

THROMBOEMBOLIC DISORDERS

Thromboembolic disorders encountered during pregnancy and the postpartum period include superficial venous thrombosis, deep venous thrombosis, and occasionally, pulmonary embolism. Superficial venous thrombosis generally involves the saphenous venous system and is confined to the lower leg. Deep venous thrombosis can involve veins from the foot to the iliofemoral region. It is a major concern because it predisposes to pulmonary embolism. Pulmonary embolism is a potentially fatal complication that occurs when the pulmonary artery is obstructed by a blood clot that was swept into circulation from a vein. Figure 28-5 illustrates the venous system of the leg.

Incidence and Etiology

The incidence of thromboembolic disease in pregnancy and the puerperium is five times higher than that in non-pregnant women of a similar age. Thromboembolic disease remains a major cause of maternal death in the United States. Deep venous thrombosis occurs in 1 in 2000 women during pregnancy and 1 in 700 women after birth (Nuwayhid, Nguyen, & Khalife, 1998).

A *thrombus* is a collection of blood factors, primarily platelets and fibrin, on a vessel wall. Thrombi can form whenever the flow of blood is impeded. Once started, the thrombus can enlarge with successive layering of platelets, fibrin, and blood cells as the blood flows past the clot. Thrombus formation is often associated with an inflammatory process in the vessel wall, which is termed *thrombophlebitis*.

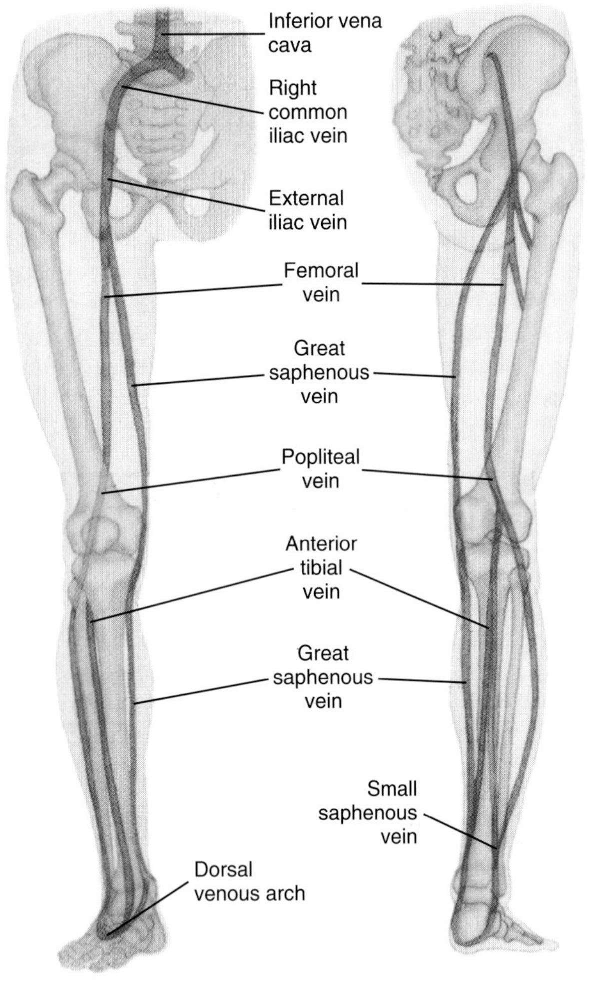

FIGURE 28-5 The venous system of the leg is affected when deep venous thrombosis occurs.

The three major causes of thrombosis are venous stasis, hypercoagulable blood, and injury to the intima (the innermost layer) of the blood vessel. At least two of these conditions, venous stasis and hypercoagulable blood, are present in all pregnancies.

Venous Stasis

Pregnancy is characterized by an increase in venous stasis in the lower extremities and pelvis as a result of compression of the large vessels by the enlarging uterus. Stasis is most pronounced when the pregnant woman stands for prolonged periods of time. Stasis results in dilated vessels and the potential for continued pooling of blood postpartum. Relative inactivity during pregnancy also leads to venous pooling and stasis of blood in the lower extremities.

Prolonged time in stirrups for delivery and repair of the episiotomy also may promote venous stasis and increase the risk of thrombus formation.

Hypercoagulation

Pregnancy also is characterized by changes in the coagulation and fibrinolytic systems that persist in the postpartum period. During pregnancy, the levels of most coagulation factors (particularly fibrinogen and factors VII, VIII, IX, and X) are elevated. In addition, the fibrinolytic system (plasminogen activator and antithrombin III), which causes clots to disintegrate (lyse) is suppressed. The net result is that factors that promote clot formation are increased to prevent maternal hemorrhage and factors that prevent clot formation are decreased, resulting in a higher risk for thrombus formation during pregnancy and the postpartum period.

Table 28-4 FACTORS THAT INCREASE THE RISK OF THROMBOSIS
Inactivity
Obesity
Cesarean birth
Smoking
History of previous thrombosis
Varicose veins
Diabetes mellitus
Prolonged time in stirrups in second stage of labor
Maternal age older than 35 years
Parity greater than 3

Blood Vessel Injury

Injury to the intima of the blood vessel generally does not occur, except possibly during cesarean births, which could trigger a pelvic vein thrombosis. Thrombosis is nine times more likely to occur if the birth was cesarean (Laros, 1999).

Additional Predisposing Factors

Certain factors create additional risk for some women. These factors include varicose veins, obesity, a history of thrombophlebitis, and smoking. Women older than 35 years or who have had more than three pregnancies are also at increased risk (Table 28-4).

Superficial Venous Thrombosis

Clinical Signs and Symptoms

Thrombosis of superficial veins usually is accompanied by signs and symptoms of inflammation. Superficial thrombophlebitis usually is associated with varicose veins and limited to the calf area. Signs and symptoms include swelling of the involved extremity as well as redness, tenderness, and warmth. Palpating the enlarged, hardened vein may be possible. The woman may experience pain when she walks. Some women have no signs at all.

Therapeutic Management

Superficial venous thrombosis often is seen in association with varicose veins. Thrombosis that is limited to the superficial veins of the saphenous system is

WOMEN WANT TO KNOW How Do I Prevent Thrombosis (Blood Clots)?

Methods to improve peripheral circulation will help prevent the occurrence of thrombophlebitis:

- Improve your circulation with a regular schedule of activity, preferably walking.
- Avoid prolonged standing or sitting in one position.
- When sitting, elevate your legs and avoid crossing them. This will increase the return of venous blood from the legs.
- Maintain a daily fluid intake of 12 or more 8-oz glasses to prevent dehydration and consequent sluggish circulation.
- Stop smoking. Smoking is a risk factor for thrombosis and can cause respiratory problems in you and your newborn.

treated with analgesics, rest, and elastic support. Elevation of the lower extremity to improve venous return also may be recommended. Warm packs may be applied to the affected area to promote healing. Anticoagulants or antiinflammatory agents are not needed unless the condition persists. After a period of bedrest and when symptoms have disappeared, the woman may ambulate gradually. She should avoid standing for long periods of time and continue to wear support hose to help prevent venous stasis and a subsequent episode of superficial thrombosis. Little chance exists of pulmonary embolism if thrombosis occurs and remains in the superficial veins of the lower leg.

Deep Venous Thrombosis

Deep venous thrombosis is much more difficult to diagnose on the basis of clinical manifestations because signs and symptoms are often absent or diffuse. If they are present, they are caused by an inflammatory process and obstruction of venous return; calf swelling, erythema, heat and tenderness, and pedal edema are the most common signs.

Many believe that a positive Homans' sign (presence of pain behind the knee when the foot is dorsiflexed) is an indicator of deep venous thrombosis in postpartum women. Homans' sign has proved to be of little value in the diagnosis, however, because pain may also be caused by a strained muscle or contusion and the sign may not be present in many women who have a venous thrombosis.

Reflex arterial spasms may cause the leg to become pale and cool to the touch with decreased peripheral pulses. At one time, this condition was called *milk-leg.* Additional symptoms may include pain on ambulation, chills, general malaise, and stiffness of the affected leg.

Diagnosis

Noninvasive tests to diagnose deep venous thrombosis include duplex Doppler scanning of the deep veins of the upper legs to detect alterations in blood flow. Impedance plethysmography measures changes in venous blood volume and flow. Magnetic resonance imaging (MRI) may also be used, especially for pelvic veins. Venography is an accurate method for diagnosing deep venous thrombosis, but significant risks are associated with the radiographic dye that is used. These include pain, anaphylaxis, and radiation exposure (Clarke-Pearson, 2000).

Therapeutic Management

Preventing Thrombus Formation. During pregnancy it is important to identify women at increased risk. Those with high risk (such as previous deep vein thrombosis or pulmonary embolism) may be placed on prophylactic heparin throughout pregnancy. Heparin may be discontinued during labor and birth, and resumed 6 to 24 hours after birth. Long-term use of heparin is associated with a form of osteoporosis, but bone mineralization improves when heparin is discontinued (DeSwiet, 1999).

After birth, all new mothers are encouraged to ambulate frequently and as early as possible. Ambulation prevents stasis of blood in the legs and decreases the likelihood of thrombus formation.

If the woman is unable to ambulate, range of motion and gentle leg exercises, such as flexing and straightening the knee and raising one leg at a time, should begin within 8 hours after childbirth. In addition, the mother should avoid using pillows or the knee gatch to prevent sharp flexion at the knees, pressure on the popliteal space, and consequent pooling of blood in the lower extremities.

Antiemboli stockings are used for mothers with varicose veins, a history of thrombosis, or a cesarean birth. The stockings should be applied before the mother rises in the morning to prevent venous congestion, which begins as soon as she gets up. She must understand the correct way to put on the antiemboli stockings. Improperly applied stockings can roll or bunch and may cause slower venous return from the legs.

Stirrups should be padded during childbirth to prevent prolonged pressure against the popliteal angle during the second stage of labor. Another option is decreasing the time in stirrups to no more than 1 hour.

Before discharge from the birth facility, the mother should be taught about lifestyle changes that can improve peripheral circulation.

Initial Treatment. Initial treatment of deep venous thrombosis consists of the following:

- Bedrest, with the affected leg elevated to decrease interstitial swelling and to promote venous return from that leg
- Gradual ambulation, which is allowed when symptoms have disappeared; sitting with the legs dependent should be avoided
- Anticoagulant therapy, which usually begins with continuous infusion of IV heparin to prevent extension of the thrombus by delaying the clotting time of the blood; activated partial thromboplastin time should be monitored and the heparin dose should be adjusted to maintain a therapeutic level of 1.5 to 2.5 times control (Laros, 1999)
- Analgesics, as necessary, to control pain
- Antibiotic therapy, if necessary, to prevent or control infection
- Continuous, moist heat for possible relief of pain and increased circulation

Subsequent Treatment. The long-term management of deep venous thrombosis depends on whether the woman is pregnant or in the postpartum period. After several days of treatment with heparin, the postpartum woman is started on warfarin (Coumadin). Anticoagulants are continued for 6 weeks to as long as 6 months (DeSwiet, 1999; Laros, 1999). The usual anticoagulating dose of warfarin is 10 to 15 mg daily until a therapeutic level is reached. Prothrombin time and the international normalized ratio (INR) are used to monitor coagulation time when warfarin is used. The INR corrects for variations in the potency of the thromboplastins used by different laboratories. An appropriate ratio for treatment of deep venous thrombosis is 2.0 to 3.0 (Laros, 1999).

Warfarin is contraindicated during pregnancy because of teratogenic effects and the increased risk of fetal hemorrhage. Therefore pregnant women are given heparin, which is administered subcutaneously. Heparin does not cross the placenta. Postpartum women may breastfeed without fear of harm to the infant from either drug.

APPLICATION OF THE NURSING PROCESS: THE MOTHER WITH DEEP VENOUS THROMBOSIS

Assessment

Assessment focuses on determining the status of the venous thrombosis. Palpate pedal pulses to determine whether they are absent, diminished, or easily palpable and equally strong on both sides. Inspect the affected leg for unusual warmth or redness, which indicates inflammation, or for unusual coolness or cyanosis, which indicates venous obstruction. Compare the affected and unaffected leg for size and color. Sometimes the nurse measures the legs and compares the circumference to obtain an accurate estimation of the edema that may be present in the affected leg.

Determine the degree of discomfort present. Pain is caused by tissue hypoxia, and increasing pain indicates progressive obstruction.

Evaluate the laboratory reports of clotting studies to monitor circulating heparin levels. In addition to activated partial thromboplastin time, whole-blood partial thromboplastin time and platelets may be evaluated when heparin is used. Thrombocytopenia is a concern when heparin is administered for a prolonged time (Laros, 1999). Prothrombin time and international normalized ratio are evaluated when the anticoagulant for the postpartum woman is changed to warfarin.

Analysis

The treatment of deep venous thrombosis includes the administration of anticoagulants for a prolonged time. As a result, "Hemorrhage secondary to anticoagulation therapy" is one of the most troubling potential complications.

Planning

Client-centered goals are inappropriate for potential complications because the nurse cannot independently manage them. The nurse must confer with physicians for medical orders to treat the condition. Planning should reflect the nurse's responsibility to complete the following tasks:

- Monitor for signs of hemorrhage
- Consult with the physician if signs of hemorrhage are observed
- Perform actions that will minimize the risk of hemorrhage

Interventions

Monitoring for Signs of Bleeding

At least twice a day, visually inspect the mother for the appearance of bruising or petechiae. Instruct her to report the appearance of any bleeding: bloody nose, blood in urine, bleeding gums, or increased vaginal bleeding. Be alert to signs of hemorrhage, such as tachycardia, falling blood pressure, or other signs of shock that may indicate internal bleeding.

Observe for excessive or bright red lochia. If the uterus is boggy, the cause is uterine atony. Massage the uterus and express clots. If the fundus is firm, bleeding may be from trauma or anticoagulant therapy. In either case the physician should be notified.

Unless frank hemorrhage is present, the usual treatment for excessive anticoagulation is temporary discontinuance of the anticogulant. However, keep protamine sulfate, the antidote for heparin, available. The antidote for warfarin is vitamin K.

Explaining Continued Therapy

Instruct the woman in measures to prevent excessive anticoagulation. Carefully explain the treatment regimen, including the schedule of medication and possible side effects, such as unexplained fever, unusual fatigue, or sore throat (signs of agranulocytosis or diminished number of neutrophils). Assist her to devise a method for remembering to take the medication as directed, for example, marking a calendar each time the drug is taken. Caution her not to "double up" if a dose is missed. If necessary, teach her and another family member how to inject heparin.

Because oral anticoagulants are associated with many clinically significant drug interactions, emphasize the importance of keeping the health care provider informed about any medications the mother takes. Caution the woman that common over-the-counter medications, such as aspirin and nonsteroidal antiinflammatory drugs, increase the risk of hemorrhage.

Complementary/Alternative Therapy

The woman should avoid herbs such as ginko biloba, garlic, and feverfew, which increase the anticoagulant effect of warfarin, and ginseng that may decrease the effectiveness of warfarin (Miller, 1998).

Suggest that the mother use a soft toothbrush and floss her teeth gently to prevent bleeding from the gums. She should postpone dental appointments until the therapy is completed. A depilatory to remove unwanted hair is safer than a razor during anticoagulant therapy.

Caution the new mother against going barefoot, about the importance of avoiding activities that may cause injury, and against the use of alcohol, which inhibits the metabolism of oral anticoagulants. Also emphasize the importance of reporting unusual bleeding.

Helping the Family Adapt to Home Care

In addition to the assessments, physical care, and teaching described above, nurses often must help the family adapt to home care. The first step may be to assess family structure and function to determine how prepared the family is to cope with the mother's illness. How many children are in the family? What are their ages? Who is usually the primary caregiver? Are family members available to provide care while the mother is confined to bed or on limited activity? Who helps the family in times of need?

Note interactions between the mother and the newborn and between the father and the newborn. If the father is not present, determine who else will be available to support the mother during the subsequent weeks.

The nurse may need to help the family develop a plan of care that includes temporary assistance by members of the extended family. Although the health of the mother is of primary importance, care must be taken that the attachment process between her and the infant progresses normally.

Evaluation

Although client-centered goals are not developed for potential complications, the nurse collects and compares data with established norms and judges whether the data are within normal limits. Abnormal data are reported to the physician.

- The mother demonstrates no signs of unusual bleeding or other side effects of the medication.

Pulmonary Embolism

Pathophysiology

Pulmonary embolism is a serious complication of deep venous thrombosis and a leading cause of maternal mortality. It occurs when fragments of a blood clot dislodge and are carried to the pulmonary artery or one of its branches. The embolus occludes the vessel and obstructs the flow of blood into the lungs, either entirely or partially. If pulmonary circulation is compromised severely, death may occur within a few minutes. If the embolus is small, adequate pulmonary circulation may be maintained until treatment can be initiated.

Clinical Signs and Symptoms

Clinical signs and symptoms depend on how much the flow of blood is obstructed. Dyspnea, sudden, sharp chest pain; tachycardia; syncope; tachypnea; pulmonary rales; cough; and hemoptysis are the most common. Arterial blood gas determinations show decreased partial pressure of oxygen, and chest radiography reveals areas of atelectasis and pleural effusion.

Therapeutic Management

Treatment of pulmonary embolism is aimed at dissolving the clot and maintaining pulmonary circulation. Heparin therapy is initiated and may be continued for many months to prevent further emboli. Oxygen is used to decrease hypoxia, and narcotic analgesics are used to reduce pain and apprehension. The woman is kept at bedrest, with the head of the bed slightly elevated to reduce dyspnea. Intensive care, support of ventilation, and other measures depend on her pulmonary status. Pulse oximetry should be initiated and arterial blood gases should be evaluated. Emergency medications, such as dopamine, may be used to support falling blood pressure. Thrombolytic drugs, such as streptokinase or urokinase, may be used for life-threatening pulmonary emboli but are associated with high fever and bleeding. Embolectomy (surgical removal of the embolus) may be attempted if no time exists to allow the clot to dissolve.

Nursing Considerations

Monitor for Signs. When caring for a woman with deep venous thrombosis, nurses must be aware of the danger of pulmonary embolism and focus the assessment for early signs and symptoms. This includes frequent assessment of respiratory rate and auscultation of breath sounds. Abnormalities, such as diminished or unequal breath sounds, or coughing should be reported immediately to the health care provider. Additional signs that require immediate attention include air hunger, dyspnea, tachycardia, pallor, and cyanosis.

Facilitate Oxygenation. Oxygen should be administered at 8 to 10 liters by tight face mask (Simpson & Creehan, 1996). The nurse should remain with the mother to allay fear and apprehension. The head of the bed should be raised to facilitate breathing, and the woman should be kept warm. Narcotic analgesics, such as morphine, may be used to relieve pain.

Seek Assistance. The woman's condition is precarious until the clot is lysed or until it adheres to the pulmonary artery wall and is reabsorbed. The primary nurse should call for assistance to initiate interventions. These include IV administration of heparin, continuous assessment of vital signs, and administration of emergency drugs that may be needed. The woman who has pulmonary embolism requires critical-care nursing skills and is transferred to an intensive care unit.

Check Your Reading

9. Why is the risk of thrombus formation increased in pregnancy and in the postpartum period?
10. What are the signs and symptoms of superficial venous thrombosis?
11. How does the long-term treatment for deep venous thrombosis differ for the pregnant woman from that of the woman who is in the postpartum period?
12. Why is strict bedrest prescribed for the woman with deep venous thrombosis?
13. What additional nursing assessments are necessary when the mother is receiving anticoagulation medication?
14. In addition to assessment, physical care, and teaching, what are the home care nurse's responsibilities?

PUERPERAL INFECTION

Puerperal infection is a term used to describe bacterial infections after childbirth. It occurs in 2% to 5% of women who have vaginal births and in 15% to 20% of those who have cesarean births (Savoia, 1999). Until the advent of antibiotics, puerperal infection resulting in death was not uncommon. Even today, it is one of the leading causes of maternal deaths.

The most common postpartum infections are metritis, wound infections, urinary tract infections, mastitis, and septic pelvic thrombophlebitis.

Definition

The definition of puerperal infection, according to the Joint Committee on Maternal Welfare, is a fever of 38° C (100.4° F) or higher after the first 24 hours and occurring on at least 2 days during the first 10 days following childbirth. Although a slight elevation of temperature may occur during the first 24 hours because of dehydration or the exertion of labor, any mother with fever should be assessed for other signs of infection.

Effect of Normal Anatomy and Physiology on Infection

To understand the seriousness of infection of the reproductive tract, consider the anatomy of the region. Every part of the reproductive tract is connected to every other part, and organisms can move from the vagina, through the cervix, into the uterus, up the fallopian tubes, and out the tubes to infect the ovaries and the peritoneal cavity. The entire reproductive tract is particularly well supplied with blood vessels during pregnancy and after childbirth. Bacteria that invade or are picked up by the blood vessels or lymphatics can carry the infection to the rest of the body, which can result in life-threatening septicemia.

The normal physiologic changes of childbirth increase the risk of infection. During labor, the acidity of the vagina is reduced by the amniotic fluid, blood, and lochia, which are alkaline. An alkaline environment encourages growth of bacteria.

Necrosis of the endometrial lining and the presence of lochia provide a favorable environment for the growth of anaerobic bacteria. Many small lacerations, some microscopic in size, occur in the endometrium, cervix, and vagina during birth and allow bacteria to enter the tissue. Although the uterine interior is not sterile until 3 to 4 weeks after delivery, infection does not develop in most women. This is partly because of the presence of granulocytes in the lochia and endometrium that prevent infection. Scrupulous aseptic technique during labor and birth and careful hand washing during the postpartum period are also major preventive factors.

Other Risk Factors

In addition to the normal physiologic changes of the puerperium, other factors may predispose a woman to infection (Table 28-5). Cesarean birth, a major predisposing factor, increases the risk 5 to 30 times above that for vaginal delivery (Gibbs & Sweet, 1999). This is because of the trauma to the tissue that occurs in surgery,

Table 28-5
RISK FACTORS FOR PUERPERAL INFECTION

Risk Factor	Reason
History of previous infections (urinary tract infection, mastitis, thrombophlebitis)	May be more vulnerable to infectious process
Colonization of lower genital tract with pathogenic organisms such as group B streptococcus, *Chlamydia trachomatis, Staphylococcus aureus, Escherichia coli,* and *Gardnerella vaginalis*	Infections usually caused by several microbes that have ascended to the uterus from the lower genital tract
Cesarean birth	Increased portals of infection
Trauma	Provides entrance for bacteria and makes tissues more susceptible
Prolonged rupture of membranes	Removes barrier of amniotic fluid and allows access for organisms to interior of uterus
Prolonged labor	Increases number of vaginal examinations; allows time for bacteria to multiply
Catheterization	Could introduce organisms into bladder
Excessive number of vaginal examinations	Increases chance that organisms from vagina or outside source are carried into the uterus
Retained placental fragments	Provide growth medium for bacteria and may interfere with flow of lochia
Hemorrhage	Loss of infection-fighting components of blood
Poor general health (excessive fatigue, anemia, frequent minor illnesses)	Increases vulnerability to infections and complications of labor
Poor nutrition (decreased protein, vitamin C)	Less able to repair tissue and defend against infection
Poor hygiene	Excessive exposure to pathogens
Medical conditions, such as diabetes mellitus	Decreases ability to defend against infections of any kind. Diabetes increases glucose in urine
Low socioeconomic status	More likely to have poor nutrition and inadequate prenatal care

the incision, which provides an entrance for bacteria, the possibility of contamination during surgery, and the presence of foreign bodies such as sutures. In addition, women who must have a surgical delivery because of a problem that develops during labor may have other risk factors, such as prolonged labor, that raise the chances of infection. Colonization of the vagina with virulent organisms, such as group B streptococcus, *Chlamydia trachomatis, Mycoplasma hominis,* and *Gardnerella vaginalis,* also predisposes to the development of infection after childbirth.

Any trauma to maternal tissues increases the hazard of infection. Trauma may occur with rapid delivery, birth of a large infant, use of forceps or a vacuum extractor, or the need for manual delivery of the placenta as well as lacerations and episiotomies. Catheterization during labor increases the chance of introduction of organisms into the bladder and adds to the trauma of the urinary tract that occurs during normal childbirth.

When prolonged rupture of membranes occurs during labor, organisms from the vagina are more likely to ascend into the uterine cavity. This is especially true if more than 24 hours pass before delivery. A long labor or many vaginal examinations during labor increase the danger of infection. Each vaginal examination increases the possibility of contamination from gloves or from organisms in the vagina being pushed through the open cervix. If part of the placenta remains inside the uterus after delivery, the tissue becomes necrotic and provides a good place for bacteria to grow.

Additional factors include postpartum hemorrhage, which causes loss of some of the infection-fighting components of the blood, such as leukocytes, and leaves the mother in a weakened condition. Prenatal conditions (poor nutrition, anemia) interfere with the mother's ability to resist infection. Lack of knowledge of hygiene or lack of access to facilities that permit adequate hygiene increases the risk of postpartum infection.

Check Your Reading

15. Why is the woman who had an assisted birth or cesarean birth at increased risk for postpartum infection?
16. Why do the normal physiologic changes of childbearing make a mother especially susceptible to infection of the reproductive system?
17. Why is infection more likely to develop in a mother who had prolonged labor?

Specific Infections

Metritis

Infections of the uterus have been called endometritis, endomyometritis, and endoparametritis. The preferred term is *metritis with pelvic cellulitis* because infection involves the decidua, myometrium, and parametrial tissues (Cunningham, et al., 1997).

Etiology. Metritis is usually caused by organisms that are normal inhabitants of the vagina and cervix. More than one organism is responsible for most infections. Organisms most often involved include gram-negative coliform bacteria, such as *Escherichia coli, Klebsiella, Gardnerella vaginalis, Bacteroides, Staphylococcus,* and anaerobic nonhemolytic *Streptococcus.* Although group A hemolytic streptococcal infections were once the source of epidemics of puerperal infections (then known as "childbed fever"), improved routine care has made it uncommon today. Group B streptococcus often is involved and is a major cause of neonatal sepsis in the newborn.

Clinical Signs and Symptoms. The mother with severe metritis looks sick. She presents a different picture from the typical happy new mother. The major signs and symptoms of metritis are fever, chills, malaise, lethargy, anorexia, abdominal pain and cramping, uterine tenderness, and purulent, foul-smelling lochia. Additional signs include tachycardia and subinvolution. In most cases, the signs and symptoms occur within the first 2 to 7 days (Gibbs & Sweet, 1999). When the causative organisms are group A or group B streptococci, the woman may exhibit no signs except fever.

Laboratory data may confirm the diagnosis. The results of a complete blood count may show an elevation of leukocytes. Leukocytes are normally elevated to 20,000 or as high as 30,000 during labor and for a short time afterward, however. Leukocytosis above 30,000 after the first day should lead to further evaluation.

Specimens may be taken from the blood, endocervix, and uterine cavity for cultures. A catheterized urine specimen should also be obtained. The antibiotic sensitivity from these cultures may be used to determine the appropriate second-line antibiotic therapy in case the broad-spectrum therapy is unsuccessful in halting the infection.

Therapeutic Management. IV administration of antibiotics is the initial treatment for metritis. The goal of this therapy is to confine the infectious process to the uterus and to prevent spread of the infection throughout the body. Broad-spectrum antibiotics, such as ampicillin and cephalosporins, are rapidly effective for mild to moderate infection after vaginal birth. Response to antibiotics after cesarean birth is less dramatic, and a combination of clindamycin plus gentamicin or cephalosporins may be necessary (Gibbs & Sweet, 1999; Savoia, 1999).

Improvement in clinical signs usually follows within 48 to 72 hours. If the symptoms persist, additional investigation is needed to determine the cause and precise location. Oral antibiotics may be used after completion of an IV course of treatment. Some physicians give prophylactic antibiotics intravenously, orally, or both for any woman who is having a cesarean birth or who is particularly at risk for infection. Other drugs include antipyretics for fever and oxytocics, such as methylergonovine, to increase drainage of lochia and promote involution.

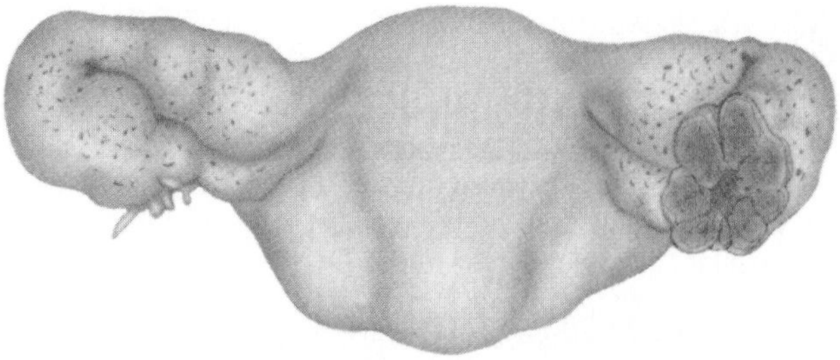

Salpingitis: Infection in fallopian tubes causes them to become enlarged, hyperemic, and tender.

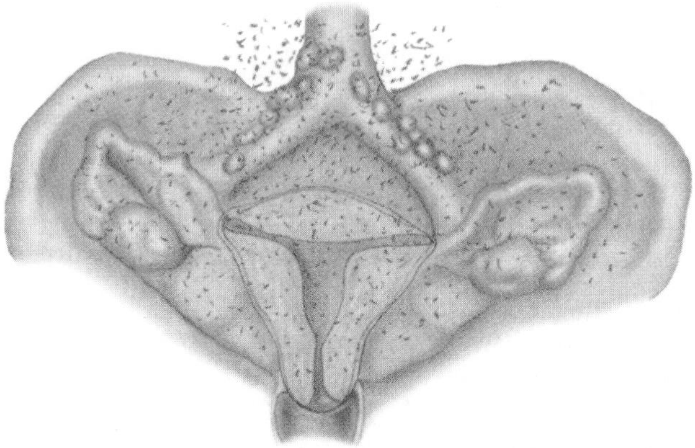

Peritonitis: Infection spreads through the lymphatics to the peritoneum; a pelvic abscess may form.

FIGURE 28-6 Areas of spread of uterine infection.

Complications. If the infection spreads outside the uterine cavity, the fallopian tubes *(salpingitis)* or the ovaries *(oophoritis)* may be infected, which could result in sterility. *Peritonitis* (inflammation of the membrane lining the walls of the abdominal and pelvic cavities) may occur and lead to formation of a pelvic abscess. In addition, the risk of pelvic thrombophlebitis is increased when pathogenic bacteria enter the blood stream during episodes of metritis. Figure 28-6 illustrates complications of metritis.

Signs and symptoms that the infection is spreading may be similar to those of metritis, but more severe. Fever and abdominal pain will be particularly pronounced. Peritonitis may result in paralytic ileus and a distended, board-like abdomen with absent bowel sounds.

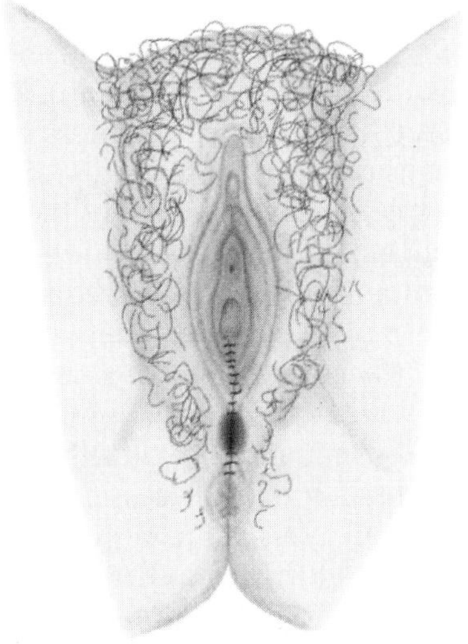

FIGURE 28-7 Any break in the skin, such as the episiotomy site, provides a portal of entry for bacteria and can result in localized infection.

Nursing Considerations. The mother with metritis should be placed in a Fowler's position to promote drainage of lochia. She may be medicated as needed for abdominal pain or cramping, which may be severe. The nurse should give the medications as directed and observe the mother for signs of improvement or new symptoms, such as nausea and vomiting, abdominal distention, absent bowel sounds, and severe abdominal pain. Comfort measures include warm blankets, cool compresses, sponge baths, perineal care, cold or warm drinks, or use of a heating pad.

Teaching incorporates signs and symptoms of worsening condition, side effects of therapy, and the importance of adhering to the treatment plan and follow-up care. If the woman must be isolated from her infant, a nursing diagnosis of "Risk for Altered Parenting related to separation from infant" should be considered. If the mother is breastfeeding, she will need help to pump her breasts to establish and maintain lactation. If she is not isolated from the infant, a nursing diagnosis "Risk for Infection related to knowledge deficit of preventive measures" is appropriate. In that instance, she can be instructed in methods to prevent the spread of infection to her infant.

Wound Infection

Wound infections are common types of puerperal infection because any break in the skin or mucous membrane provides a portal of entry for bacteria. The most common sites are the perineum, where episiotomies and lacerations are common (Figure 28-7); the vagina; and cesarean surgical incisions.

Clinical Signs and Symptoms. Signs of wound infection are edema, warmth, redness, tenderness, and pain. The edges of the wound may pull apart, and seropurulent drainage may come from the wound. If the wound remains untreated, generalized signs of infection, such as fever and malaise, may develop as well.

As with other puerperal infections, cultures may reveal mixed aerobic and anaerobic bacteria. The most common pathogens of early abdominal wounds are group A streptococcus or *Clostridium* (Gibbs & Sweet, 1999). Lower genital tract wounds usually are colonized with organisms typically found in that area and include *E. coli, Proteus,* and *Bacteroides* species.

Therapeutic Management. If healing has begun, an incision and drainage of the affected area may be necessary. Broad-spectrum antibiotics may be ordered until a report of the antibiotic-sensitive organism is returned. Analgesics are often necessary, and warm compresses or sitz baths may be used to provide comfort and to promote healing by increasing circulation to the area.

Nursing Considerations. Wound infections are painful and annoying to the mother, out of proportion to their size. Perineal infections cause discomfort during many activities, such as walking, sitting, or defecating, and are particularly troublesome because they are not expected by the new mother.

Wound infections may require readmittance to the hospital or home health care visits. The woman requires reassurance and supportive care. Comfort measures might include sitz baths, warm compresses, and frequent perineal care. The woman is taught to wipe from front to back and to change perineal pads frequently. Good hand washing techniques are emphasized. Adequate fluid intake and diet are important. Activity may be modified depending on the site, severity, and treatment of the wound infection.

The infant is not routinely isolated from the mother with a wound infection, but she must be advised how to protect her infant from contact with contaminated articles. Anticipatory guidance should include teaching side effects of medication, signs of worsening condition, and any necessary self-care measures.

Check Your Reading

18. What are the signs and symptoms of metritis? How is it usually treated?
19. What are the most common sites for wound infections?
20. How does the nurse assess for wound infection?

Urinary Tract Infections

Etiology. During childbirth, the bladder and urethra are traumatized by pressure from the descending fetus. Insertion of a catheter, with its risk of infection, occurs at least once during many labors. After birth, the bladder and urethra are hypotonic, with stasis of urine and urinary retention common problems. Residual urine and reflux of urine may occur during voiding.

Women who had bacteria in the urine during pregnancy are at increased risk. These women may have asymptomatic bacteruria, which may be discovered during urine screens at prenatal visits. Urinary tract infections are usually caused by coliform bacteria, such as *E. coli.*

Clinical Signs and Symptoms. Symptoms typically begin on the first or second postpartum day. They include dysuria (a burning pain on urination), urgency, and frequency of urination. A low-grade fever is sometimes the only symptom. In some women, an upper urinary tract infection, such as pyelonephritis, may develop the third or fourth day, with chills, spiking fever, costovertebral angle tenderness, flank pain, and nausea and vomiting. This infection of the kidney pelvis may result in permanent damage to the kidney if not promptly treated.

Therapeutic Management. With the exception of pyelonephritis, most urinary tract infections can be treated on an outpatient basis. If the mother is breastfeeding, medications such as ampicillin or other antibiotics safe during lactation are used.

Pyelonephritis warrants IV hydration and IV administration of broad-spectrum antibiotics until the causative organism and its sensitivity are known. The antibiotic therapy can then be adjusted, if necessary, to a drug that is effective against organisms identified on the culture.

Nursing Considerations. The woman with a urinary tract infection must be instructed to take the medication for the entire time it is prescribed and not to stop when symptoms abate. In addition, she must drink at least 3000 ml of fluid each day to help dilute the bacterial count and flush the infection from the bladder. Acidification of the urine inhibits multiplication of bacteria, and drinks that acidify urine, such as apricot, plum, prune, or cranberry juices, are frequently recommended. Carbonated drinks should be avoided because they increase urine alkalinity.

Teaching should also include measures to prevent urinary tract infections, such as proper perineal care, increasing fluid intake, and urinating frequently.

Mastitis

Mastitis, an infection of the lactating breast, occurs most often during the second and third weeks after birth, although it may develop at any time during breastfeeding. It is more common in mothers nursing for the first time and usually affects only one breast.

Etiology. Mastitis is generally caused by *S. aureus*, although *E. coli* may also be involved. The bacteria are most often carried on the hands of the mother or staff or in the mouth of the newborn. The organism may enter through an injured area of the nipple, such as a crack or blister, although only redness is present or no obvious signs of injury are apparent. Soreness of a nipple may result in insufficient emptying of the breast resulting from pain during breastfeeding.

Engorgement and stasis of milk frequently precede mastitis. This may occur when a feeding is skipped, when the infant begins to sleep through the night, or when breastfeeding is suddenly stopped. Constriction of the breasts from a bra that is too tight may interfere with emptying of all the ducts and may lead to infection. A blocked duct is a significant predictor of mastitis (Featherston, 1998). The mother who is fatigued or stressed or who has other health problems that might lower her immune system is also at increased risk for mastitis.

Clinical Signs and Symptoms. At first, the mother may think that she has the flu because of fatigue and aching muscles. Symptoms progress to include fever of 38.4° C (101.1° F) or higher, chills, malaise, and headache. Mastitis is characterized by a localized area of redness and inflammation (Figure 28-8). Although rare, purulent drainage may be present. Untreated mastitis may progress to breast abscess.

Therapeutic Management. Antibiotic therapy and continued decompression of the breast by breastfeeding or breast pump constitute the first line of treatment. With early antibiotic treatment, mastitis usually resolves within 24 to 48 hours and abscess formation is unusual. Supportive measures include moist heat or ice packs, breast support, bedrest, and analgesics (Lawrence & Lawrence, 1999).

In most cases, the mother can continue to breastfeed from both breasts. An infant may temporarily reject the affected breast because of changes in milk composition such as increased sodium in that breast (Hager, 1998). If the affected breast is too sore, she can pump the breast gently. Regular emptying of the breast is important in preventing abscess formation. If an abscess forms and ruptures into the ducts of the breasts, breastfeeding should be discontinued and a mechanical pump used to empty the breast. Milk obtained should be discarded.

Nursing Considerations. Because mastitis rarely occurs before discharge from the birth facility, the nurse must concentrate on providing adequate information for the family. Measures to prevent the development of mastitis include correct positioning of the infant and avoiding trauma to the nipples and milk stasis. The mother should breastfeed every 2 to 3 hours. She should avoid formula supplements and nipple shields,

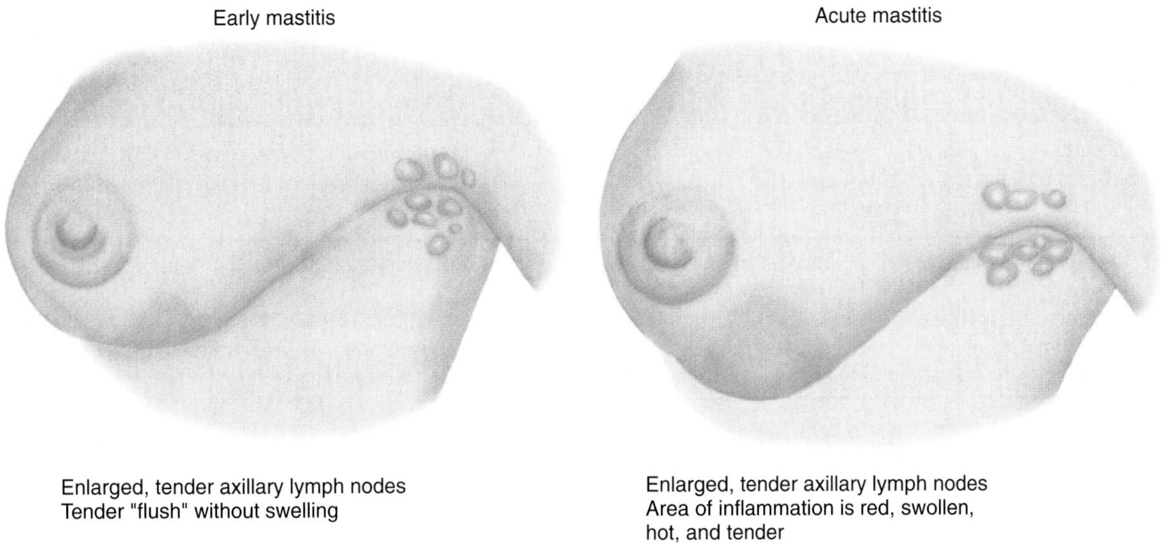

FIGURE 28-8 Mastitis typically occurs 2 to 3 weeks after birth in the breast of a woman who breastfeeds.

and she should change nursing pads when they are wet. She should also avoid continuous pressure on the breasts from tight bras or infant carriers.

Once mastitis occurs, nursing measures are aimed at increasing comfort and helping the mother maintain lactation. Moist heat promotes comfort and increases circulation. A shower or hot packs should be used before feeding or emptying the breasts. One way to apply heat to the breast is to use a disposable diaper moistened with warm water. The thickness helps to retain heat, and the plastic cover prevents dripping. Some mothers find ice packs more comfortable for short periods.

The breast should be completely emptied at each feeding to prevent stasis of milk, which can result in an abscess. If the mother is too sore to breastfeed on the affected side or if she must take antibiotics that are contraindicated during lactation, she should be instructed in how to empty the breasts by expressing the milk or using a mechanical pump. Breastfeeding or pumping every 1½ to 2 hours makes the mother more comfortable and prevents stasis. Starting the feeding on the unaffected side causes the milk-ejection reflex to occur in the painful breast and makes the process more efficient. Massage over the affected area before and during the feeding helps to ensure complete emptying.

The mother should stay in bed during the acute phase of her illness. Her fluid intake should be at least 3000 ml per day. Analgesics may be required to relieve discomfort.

The mother with mastitis is likely to be very discouraged. Some mothers decide to stop breastfeeding because of the discomfort involved. The nursing diagnosis "Interrupted Breast Feeding related to discomfort, infectious process, or effects of therapy" may be appropriate. Weaning during an episode of mastitis may increase engorgement and stasis, leading to abscess formation or recurrent infection. The mother may need much encouragement, and she will need help in arranging care for other children or with other responsibilities so that she can remain in bed.

Septic Pelvic Thrombophlebitis

Septic pelvic thrombophlebitis is the least common of the puerperal infections. It usually is not seen until 2 to 4 days after childbirth. It occurs when infection spreads along the venous system and thrombophlebitis develops. It occurs more often in women with wound infection and usually involves the ovarian, uterine, or hypogastric veins.

Clinical Signs and Symptoms. The primary symptom is pain in the groin, abdomen, or flank. Also present may be fever, tachycardia, gastrointestinal distress, and decreased bowel sounds. Fever that does not respond to antibiotics may be the only sign. Laboratory data may be used to exclude other diagnoses and usually include complete blood count with differential, blood chemistries, coagulation studies, and cultures.

Therapeutic Management. Readmittance to the hospital is usually necessary. Primary treatment includes IV antibiotics and anticoagulation therapy with IV heparin. The use of heparin, however, has been questioned (Brown, et al., 1999). Supportive care is similar to that for deep venous thrombosis and includes monitoring for safe levels of anticoagulation therapy and for signs and symptoms of pulmonary embolism.

NURSING CARE PLAN 28-1

Postpartum Infection

Assessment: Lisa Pyle, a thin, pale, 16-year-old primipara, is admitted to the postpartum unit after a cesarean birth because of fetal distress. Her membranes were ruptured for 14 hours, and she was in labor for 16 hours before the birth. She was catheterized twice during labor, with insertion of an indwelling catheter shortly before her surgery.

Critical Thinking: What data indicate that Lisa is at increased risk for infection? What additional data should be obtained?

Answer: Factors that increase the risk for metritis include a cesarean birth and rupture of membranes several hours before the surgery was performed. Catheterization increases the risk for urinary tract infection. Additional necessary data to better evaluate the risks for infection include estimated blood loss and prenatal conditions such as anemia or other infections.

Nursing Diagnosis: Risk for Infection related to presence of favorable conditions for infections

Goals/Expected Outcomes:
Before discharge Lisa will:
1. Demonstrate no signs of infection
2. Discuss methods she will use to prevent infections
3. List signs of infection she will report to her health care provider

Intervention	Rationale
1. Assess vital signs every 4 hours.	1. Temperature above 38° C (100.4° F) or tachycardia suggests an infectious process and should be reported.
2. Observe the surgical incision for redness, tenderness, edema, drainage, approximation and note the odor of lochia every 4 hours. Determine character of urine and whether Lisa experiences frequency urgency or pain with urination after the catheter is removed.	2. Redness, pain, or edema of the incision suggests wound infection. Drainage could be bleeding or a sign of infection. Separation also can indicate infection. Foul odor of lochia suggests endometrial infection. Frequency, urgency, or painful urination may indicate urinary tract infection.
3. Instruct Lisa in hygienic practices to prevent infection:	3. Good hygiene helps prevent infection.
a. Careful hand washing before and after perineal care	a. Hand washing is the most important defense against infection and its spread.
b. Perineal cleansing after elimination	b. Perineal cleansing helps prevent growth of bacteria.
c. Changing peripads frequently	c. Frequent pad changes remove accumulated lochia, an excellent culture medium for bacteria.
d. Wiping the perineum from front to back	d. Wiping from front to back prevents fecal contamination of the vagina.
4. Initiate measures to reduce the risk of urinary tract infection. a. Provide fluids of Lisa's choice when she is able to take them, and emphasize the importance of drinking at least 12 glasses per day. b. Monitor bladder distention to prevent overfilling. Teach Lisa the importance of emptying her bladder every 2 to 3 hours during the first days after childbirth. c. Use methods to promote bladder emptying, such as running water in the shower or sink, running warm water over the perineum, and providing pain medication as needed.	4. Adequate hydration and frequent emptying of the bladder help prevent stasis of urine, which increases the risk of urinary tract infection. Relief of pain may allow the mother to relax enough to void.
5. Offer and encourage Lisa to eat well-balanced meals when she progresses to a regular diet. Emphasize the importance of a diet high in protein and vitamin C.	5. Adequate protein and vitamin C are necessary for healing damaged tissues.

Evaluation: Lisa is free of signs and symptoms of infection throughout her hospital stay and at her postpartum check-up. She verbalizes measures she will take to reduce her risk of infection when she is discharged from the hospital. She is able to list signs of infection that would require treatment.

APPLICATION OF THE NURSING PROCESS: INFECTION

Assessment

Although all women are observed for indications of infection as part of routine nursing assessments, the nurse must practice increased vigilance for mothers who are at increased risk of infection.

Pay particular attention to signs that may be expected in infection, such as fever; tachycardia; pain; or unusual amount, color, or odor of lochia. Generalized symptoms of malaise and muscle aching may also be significant. Examine all wounds each shift for the presence of signs of localized infection, such as redness, edema, tenderness, discharge, or pulling apart of incisions or sutured lacerations. Particularly note whether the mother experiences difficulty emptying her bladder or discomfort related to urination.

Assess the mother's knowledge of hygiene practices that prevent infections, such as proper hand washing, perineal care, and handling of perineal pads. Evaluate her knowledge of breastfeeding and any problems that might result in breast engorgement and stasis of milk in the ducts. Assess the nipples for signs of injury that might provide a portal of entry for organisms.

Analysis

Because all women are at risk for infection after childbirth, most facilities have developed standards of practice that protect postpartum women from infection and individual nursing care plans are usually not necessary. When predisposing factors increase the likelihood of infection, however, routine assessments and care must be modified and preventive measures intensified. In this case, the most relevant nursing diagnosis is "Risk for Infection related to the presence of significant risk factors."

Planning

The goals/expected outcomes for this nursing diagnosis are that the mother will:

- Remain free of signs of infection during the postpartum period
- Describe methods to prevent infection
- List signs of infection that should be reported immediately

Interventions

Preventing Infection

Promoting Hygiene. Nursing responsibilities for the woman at risk for puerperal infection focus on prevention of initial infection. Preventive measures include aseptic technique for all invasive procedures and meticulous attention to hand washing. Hand washing is important for the nursing staff and the mother. She should wash her hands before and after changing pads or touching the perineum. Instruct her on care of the perineum and episiotomy site (see Chapter 17), making sure that she can demonstrate cleansing methods before she is discharged.

Preventing Urinary Stasis. An adequate intake of fluids (at least 2500 to 3000 ml/day) is important for preventing stasis of urine. Encourage the woman to empty her bladder at least every 2 to 3 hours during the day. Measure the first two voidings after delivery or removal of an indwelling catheter, and assess the bladder and fundus to be certain the bladder is empty. Instruct her to report any signs of urinary tract infection immediately so that early treatment can be obtained.

Use appropriate measures to promote bladder emptying if she has difficulty. Drinking hot fluids, such as tea, helps some mothers to void. Running water or having the mother blow bubbles in a glass of water uses the sound of water to stimulate the urge to urinate. Pouring warm water over the perineum or having the mother void in a sitz bath or shower may help relax the urinary sphincter. Administration of analgesics may help her relax enough to urinate.

Teaching Breastfeeding Techniques. Mothers often need assistance in establishing an effective pattern of breastfeeding that results in complete emptying of the breasts at each feeding and that reduces the risk of nipple trauma (see Chapter 22).

Providing Information. Advise mothers to obtain adequate rest and sufficient food of high nutritive value to replenish their energy and prevent infection. If necessary, identify foods high in protein, necessary for repair of damaged tissue. Whole-grain breads, cereals, or pasta; cheese; eggs; chicken; fish; and meat are some of the best sources of protein. This is particularly important if the mother is breastfeeding.

CRITICAL TO REMEMBER

Signs and Symptoms of Postpartum Infection

Fever, chills
Pain or redness of wounds
Purulent wound drainage or wound edges not approximated
Tachycardia
Uterine subinvolution
Abnormal duration of lochia, foul odor
Elevated white blood cell count
Frequency or urgency of urination, dysuria, or hematuria
Suprapubic pain
Localized area of warmth, redness, or tenderness in the breasts
Body aches, general malaise

Obtaining adequate rest is a problem for many mothers. Nursing interventions focus on helping them plan a schedule that allows them to rest while the infant sleeps and to identify family members or friends who are available to provide support and assistance.

Teaching Signs and Symptoms That Should Be Reported

Because many women are discharged 24 to 48 hours after childbirth, they must be taught signs and symptoms of infection that should be reported to their health care provider. These include fever, chills, dysuria, and redness and tenderness of a wound. Malodorous lochia or discharge from a wound as well as prolonged lochial discharge also should be reported.

Evaluation

The interventions can be judged to be successful if the mother does the following:

- Remains free of signs of infection during the puerperium
- Explains methods she will use to prevent infection
- Lists signs and symptoms that she should report to her health care provider

If infection occurs, the problem is no longer amenable to independent nursing actions but becomes a collaborative problem requiring medical and nursing interventions.

Check Your Reading

21. What measures can the woman take to decrease the risk of urinary tract infection? How does the treatment for cystitis differ from that of pyelonephritis?
22. How may mastitis be prevented?

AFFECTIVE DISORDERS

Affective (mood) disorders are disturbances in function, affect, or thought processes that can impact the family after childbirth as severely as physiologic problems. They include postpartum blues, postpartum depression, and postpartum psychosis. Postpartum blues is discussed on p. 468. Postpartum depression and postpartum psychosis are more serious disorders that disrupt the family and require intervention to resolve.

Postpartum Depression

Incidence

Postpartum depression (PPD) is the most common affective disorder of the postpartum period. It occurs in 15% to 20% of women (Hayashi & Zettelmaier, 2000). The incidence may be as high as 25% in women after multifetal pregnancy (Leonard, 1998). All ethnic groups are affected. Many investigators believe that PPD is underdiagnosed and underreported.

Predictors of Postpartum Depression

The cause of PPD is unknown, but is probably due to a combination of biologic, psychosocial, and situational life-stresses (Beck, 1999). It is associated with a personal or family history of depression, poor social support, and problems during the pregnancy and birth (Stewart & Robinson, 1998). Factors that are believed to increase the risk include the following:

- Hormonal fluctuations that follow childbirth
- Medical problems during pregnancy or after birth, such as pregnancy-induced hypertension, preexisting diabetes mellitus, anemia, or postpartum thyroid dysfunction
- History of depression, mental illness, or alcoholism, either in the woman or in her family
- Personality characteristics, such as immaturity and low self-esteem
- Marital dysfunction or difficult relationship with significant other, resulting in lack of support
- Anger about the pregnancy
- Feelings of isolation, lack of social support, or support that does not meet the mother's needs
- Fatigue, sleep deprivation, financial worries, and birth of an ill infant or an infant with anomalies
- Multifetal pregnancy
- Chronic stressors

Clinical Signs and Symptoms

Postpartum depression usually starts in the first 4 weeks after childbirth and may last for several months or more, especially if untreated. The woman shows less interest in her surroundings and a loss of her usual emotional response toward her family. Even though she cares for the infant in a loving manner, she is unable to feel pleasure or love. She may have intense feelings of unworthiness, guilt, and shame, and she often expresses a sense of loss of self. Generalized fatigue, complaints of ill health, and difficulty in concentrating are also present. She often has little interest in food and experiences sleep disturbances. She often describes panic attacks and relentless obsessive thinking. Thoughts of suicide may occur.

PPD is differentiated from the normal labile emotions of pregnancy and the postpartum period by the number, intensity, and persistence of symptoms. A majority of the symptoms are intensely and consistently present for at least a 2-week period. These are not mood swings but a persistent depressed state.

Women with PPD may go through a 4-stage process. This includes the following:

1. Encountering terror—The beginning of severe anxiety, obsessive thinking, and loss of concentration
2. Dying of self—A feeling of unreality, isolating oneself, and contemplating and sometimes attempting self-destruction
3. Struggling to survive—Efforts to battle the system to find help, praying for relief, and seeking solace in support groups
4. Regaining control—Unpredictable transitioning with good and bad days, mourning lost time with their infants, and guarded recovery where mothers feel fragile and vulnerable, though recovered (Beck, 1999)

Impact on the Family

Postpartum depression has an impact on the entire family. It creates strain on each member's usual methods of coping and often causes difficulties in relationships. Stressors tend to be magnified, and, as a result, family members may decrease their interactions with the depressed mother when she needs support the most. Communication is impaired because she gradually withdraws from contact with others. The decreased libido commonly associated with depression may also affect the relationship with the significant other.

Partners of depressed women report many changes in their lives after the birth. These include a sense of loss of the partner and the relationship they had known previously, feelings of loss of control, anger, and frustration. Fathers may take on household chores and child care that the depressed mother is unable to manage. They may be suffering from depression along with their partners (Meighan, et al., 2000).

Depressed mothers interact differently with their infants than do women who are not depressed. They appear tense, are more irritable, and feel less competent as mothers. They may not pick up on their infants' cues or smiles, thus failing to meet the infants needs and to enjoy their positive feedback (Beck, 1995). Infants of depressed mothers tend to be fussier, more discontented, and make fewer positive facial expressions. Possible long-term effects on the infant include behavioral and cognitive problems (Beck, 1999).

Therapeutic Management

Depression responds best to a combination of psychotherapy, social support, and medication. Some women need electroconvulsive therapy. Psychotherapy may be helpful to assist the woman to cope with changes in her life. The partner and immediate family must be included in counseling sessions so that they can develop an understanding of what the woman feels and needs.

Antidepressants are often used for PPD and may be continued for 6 months or more. If the woman wants to continue breastfeeding, medications safe for use during lactation should be used because this may enhance the bonding process (Riordan & Auerbach, 1999b). Abrupt weaning may increase the severity of depression (Lawrence & Lawrence, 1999).

APPLICATION OF THE NURSING PROCESS: POSTPARTUM DEPRESSION

Assessment

All women should be assessed for PPD during pregnancy, at the birth facility, and during follow-up visits. Observe for subjective symptoms, such as apathy, lack of interest or energy, anorexia, or sleeplessness. Ask the mother about her feelings. The mother's verbalizations of failure, sadness, loneliness, anxiety, or vague confusion are important cues. Assess for objective data, such as crying, poor personal hygiene, or inability to follow directions or to concentrate. Screening tools are available for assessment or risk factors or actual depression.

Determine whether family support is available. Single mothers or mothers with an absent or unavailable support system may feel increasingly isolated, leading to stress that they are unable to manage. Inappropriate expressions of blame or anger toward the partner and unmet expectations of the baby or the parenting role are sometimes present.

Analysis

A likely nursing diagnosis, particularly if predisposing factors are present, is "Risk for Ineffective Individual Coping related to depression in response to stressors associated with childbirth and parenting."

Planning

To achieve the goals and expected outcomes for this nursing diagnosis, the new mother will do the following:

- Verbalize feelings with the health care provider and significant other throughout the postpartum period
- Discuss her own strengths
- Identify resources that are available during the postpartum period

Interventions

Demonstrating Care

Conveying a caring attitude is one nursing strategy to help mothers decrease their emotional distress and to guide them in regaining their well-being during the postpartum period. Acknowledge that something is wrong and that the woman seems depressed. Spend time with the woman and explain that the condition is

CRITICAL THINKING EXERCISE

Aricella Nunez, a 23-year-old multipara, gave birth several days ago to her second baby. It is obvious to the nurse making a telephone follow-up call after discharge that Aricella is crying. She says, "I feel so stupid. I can barely get out of bed in the morning and I am worn out just trying to take care of the kids." The nurse, Sharon Greenspan, responds, "Oh, that is just the 'baby blues.' Just look at those beautiful babies and you will feel better."

QUESTIONS:

1. Has the nurse made any assumptions?
2. Is the nurse's response helpful for Aricella? Why or why not?
3. What would be a more therapeutic response?
4. What additional action should the nurse take?

not her fault. It is an illness that can be treated and it will end.

Providing Anticipatory Guidance

Some mothers, particularly young mothers, are unprepared for the rapid change in lifestyle that follows the birth of an infant. During the prenatal period, initiate a discussion of the changes to present anticipatory guidance about the early weeks at home. Discuss the need for frequent contact with other adults so that the new mother does not become isolated. Emphasize the need for continued communication with the partner or with a close friend who is available to provide support when loneliness or anxiety becomes a problem. Explain the importance of adequate rest and nutrition for maintaining energy and a feeling of health and well-being.

Helping the Mother Verbalize Feelings

Many women and their families minimize depression because they cannot find the exact cause. Many in the health care delivery system also trivialize the problem by making comments such as, "You'll get over it. After all, you have a beautiful baby."

Recommend that although some of her feelings may seem "unreasonable" (anger, guilt, shame), the woman should acknowledge negative feelings to herself and insist that others acknowledge them too. It may be helpful to rehearse some of the situations that may occur, such as a fussy baby or being home alone and feeling lonely, as a means to develop perspective and to find solutions before the situation occurs.

Enhancing Sensitivity to Infant Cues

The nurse can model behavior to show the mother how to respond to the infant's cues. Measures to help the mother relax may help improve her mood and her response to her infant. Some that may be helpful are listed here.

Complementary/Alternative Therapy

Music
Relaxation therapy
Massage and aromatherapy using jasmine, sandalwood, or rose oil
Reflexology (Tiran, 2000)
CAUTION: St. John's Wort is often used to treat depression. It has not been proven to be safe for use by lactating women, however.

Helping Family Members

Include the father in discussions about depression, before and after the birth. Acknowledge his feelings as well as those of the mother. Stress his role in helping his partner and other family members. Give practical suggestions of ways he can help manage the changes in their lives.

Discussing Options and Resources

Encourage the new mother to determine if stressors in her life may be contributing to her feelings of depression. Help her plan ways to reduce common areas of stress.

Assist the mother and her partner in identifying those persons who are available to provide support. Suggest that she explain her anticipated needs to those persons before the development of symptoms. In addition, provide them with telephone numbers of support groups in the area.

Additional information and support are supplied by national and international programs:

Depression After Delivery (DAD)
Morrisville, PA 19067
1-800-994-4773
Provides the telephone numbers and address of the nearest DAD support group.
Website: http://www.behavenet.com/dadinc/

Postpartum Support International
927 North Kellogg Avenue
Santa Barbara, CA 93111
1-805-967-7636
Provides information and has a website: http://www.postpartum.net

Evaluation

The interventions have been successful if the mother does the following:

- Verbalizes her feelings to staff and family members
- Discusses her personal strengths
- Identifies community and family resources she can access

Postpartum Psychosis

Postpartum psychosis is a rare condition that causes psychiatric admission in 2 in 1000 postpartum women (Hayashi & Zettelmaier, 2000). It generally surfaces within 3 weeks of delivery. Women who have one episode of postpartum psychosis have a 50% chance of having another episode (Pearlstein, et al., 1998). A history of bipolar disorder is an important risk factor. The condition usually fits one of two categories:

1. *Bipolar disorder* is characterized by the occurrence of manic and depressive episodes.
2. *Major depression* is characterized by depression without manic episodes.

Women with bipolar disorder suffer from irritability, hyperactivity, euphoria, and grandiosity. They exhibit little need for sleep and are seldom aware they have a problem. The delusions, poor judgment, and confusion they experience make self-care and infant care impossible. They can create a dangerous, even life-threatening set of conditions for mother and infant because the mother may harm herself or her infant.

The depressions of the bipolar disorder and major depression are similar and are characterized by tearfulness, preoccupations of guilt, feelings of worthlessness, sleep and appetite disturbances, and an inordinate concern with the baby's health. Delusions about the infant being dead or defective are common and hallucinations may be present.

Assessment and management of postpartum psychosis are beyond the scope of maternity nurses, and mothers who experience these conditions must be referred to specialists for comprehensive therapy.

Hospitalization is usually necessary to treat women with postpartum psychosis. Women who have manic symptoms are usually treated with the standard medications (lithium, antidepressants, antipsychotics). Lithium is not recommended during pregnancy, but it may be resumed in the postpartum period if the mother is not breastfeeding. Women who have depressive symptoms must be assessed for suicidal potential and treated according to the severity of the threat. Antipsychotics and antidepressants are used for treatment, and careful monitoring is required because of the effect of hormonal imbalances on the mother's reaction to the prescribed medication.

Check Your Reading

23. What are the symptoms of postpartum depression and how does it differ from postpartum "blues"?
24. How can nurses intervene for postpartum depression?
25. What is the therapeutic management for postpartum psychosis?

Table 28-6

COMMON NURSING DIAGNOSES FOR THE WOMAN WITH A POSTPARTUM COMPLICATION
Activity Intolerance
Fatigue
*Interrupted Breast Feeding
Pain
*Risk for Altered Parenting
*Risk for Ineffective Individual Coping
*Risk for Infection

*Nursing diagnoses discussed in this chapter.

SUMMARY CONCEPTS

- Postpartum hemorrhage sometimes can be anticipated and prevented by careful examination of antepartum and intrapartum factors that predispose to excessive bleeding.
- Overstretching of the muscle fibers during pregnancy or repeated stretching during past pregnancies predispose to uterine atony and excessive uterine bleeding.
- Uterine atony is not the only cause of hemorrhage; soft tissue trauma (lacerations, hematomas) also can cause rapid loss of blood even when the uterus is firmly contracted.
- Initial management of uterine atony focuses on measures to contract the uterus and provide fluid replacement.
- Management of trauma of the reproductive tract involves locating the trauma and repairing it before excessive blood loss occurs.
- Compensatory mechanisms maintain the blood pressure so that vital organs, such as the brain, heart, and kidneys, receive adequate oxygen. When compensatory mechanisms fail, hypovolemic shock follows.
- The process of uterine involution is delayed (subinvolution) when placental fragments are retained or when the inner lining of the uterus is infected (metritis).
- Subinvolution of the uterus develops after the mother has been discharged from the hospital. The nurse teaches the family the process of normal involution and the signs and symptoms that should be reported to the health care provider.
- Venous stasis that occurs during pregnancy, increased levels of coagulation factors, and decreased thrombolytic factors that persist into the postpartum period increase the risk of thrombus formation during the puerperium.
- Treatment for deep venous thrombosis includes anticoagulants, analgesics, and bedrest, with the affected leg elevated.
- Nurses who administer anticoagulant therapy are responsible for assessing the mother to determine whether her clotting time is within the recommended therapeutic level so that overmedication with anticoagulants does not result in bleeding from unusual sites.
- Pulmonary embolism is a complication of deep venous thrombosis that occurs when a clot is partially or completely dislodged from the vein and carried by the blood to a pulmonary vessel, which may be completely or partially occluded by the clot.

- The risk of infection is increased with childbearing because the anatomy of the reproductive tract provides open access to bacteria from the vagina through the fallopian tubes and into the peritoneal cavity. Increased blood supply to the pelvis and the alkalinization of the vagina by the amniotic fluid further increase the risk of metritis.
- Any break in the skin or mucous membranes during childbirth provides a portal of entry for pathogenic organisms and increases the risk of puerperal infection. Nurses must assess women with an incision or laceration for signs of localized wound infections.
- Urinary stasis and trauma to the urinary tract increase the risk of postpartum urinary tract infection. Nurses must initiate measures to prevent urinary stasis.
- Nurses must provide information about the importance of completely emptying the breasts at each feeding and about measures to prevent nipple trauma to prevent mastitis.
- Postpartum depression is a disabling affective disorder that affects the entire family. It is often underdiagnosed and underreported. Nurses must help the woman to acknowledge her feelings and assist her in identifying measures that will help her cope with the condition.

ANSWERS TO CRITICAL THINKING EXERCISE, p. 781

1. Some data (multiparity, birth of large infant, rapid labor and delivery) in her history indicate that she is at risk for postpartal hemorrhage. The nurse will increase the frequency of her assessments of the fundus, lochia, vital signs, and skin temperature and color.
2. Massage the fundus, express clots that may have accumulated in the uterus. Massage often stimulates uterine contractions that compress torn myometrial blood vessels and stop excessive bleeding. Continued assessment of the fundus and lochia are imperative to determine whether the uterus relaxes again leading to resumption of bleeding.
3. Assist Dolores to void, because a distended bladder lifts the uterus, making contraction more difficult and resulting in excessive bleeding.
4. Continue to massage the fundus and turn on the call light to ask a colleague for help. Ask that another nurse notify the physician, the nurse-midwife, or both because excessive bleeding requires the combined efforts of primary health care providers and nurses to prevent postpartum hemorrhage.

ANSWERS TO CRITICAL THINKING EXERCISE, p. 798

1. The nurse assumes that the feelings Aricella has are transient, self-limiting moods of depression that come and go in the majority of women who give birth. The nurse fails to obtain additional data that may indicate whether Aricella is experiencing postpartum depression that requires additional therapy.
2. The nurse's response is not helpful because it minimizes the feelings Aricella has expressed and it offers no measures for dealing with the feelings.
3. It would be more therapeutic for the nurse to acknowledge the feelings and ask follow-up questions that allow Aricella to express those feelings fully.
4. The nurse must convey genuine interest and caring. She can do this best by
   a. Indicating awareness that something may be wrong
   b. Sharing as much time as Aricella needs to express her feelings
   c. Providing hope by reassuring Aricella that this is not her fault and that it can be cured
   d. Making appropriate referrals that try to provide as much continuity of care as possible

REFERENCES & READINGS

American Academy of Pediatrics & American College of Obstetricians and Gynecologists. (1997). *Guidelines for perinatal care* (4th ed.). Elk Grove Village, IL: Author.

Beck, C.T. (1995). The effects of postpartum depression on maternal-infant interaction: A meta-analysis. *Nursing Research, 44*(5), 298-304.

Beck, C.T. (1998). A checklist to identify women at risk for developing postpartum depression. *Journal of Obstetric, Gynecologic, and Neonatal Nursing, 27*(1), 39-46.

Beck, C.T. (1999). *Postpartum depression: Case studies, research, and nursing care.* Washington, D.C.: Association of Women's Health, Obstetric, & Neonatal Nurses (AWHONN).

Brown, C.E., Stettler, R.W., Twickler, D., & Cunningham, F.G. (1999). Puerperal septic pelvic thrombophlebitis: Incidence and response to heparin therapy. *American Journal of Obstetrics & Gynecology, 181*(1), 143-148.

Brumfield, C.G., Hauth, J.C., & Andrews, W.W. (2000). Puerperal infection after cesarean delivery: Evaluation of a standardized protocol. *American Journal of Obstetrics & Gynecology* 182(5), 1147-1151.

Clarke-Pearson, D.L. (2000). Venous thromboembolic disease in pregnancy. In E.J. Quilligan & F.P. Zuspan (Eds.), *Current therapy in obstetrics and gynecology* (5th ed., pp. 368-371). Philadelphia: W.B. Saunders.

Cunningham, F.G., MacDonald, P.C., Gant, N.F., Leveno, K.J., Gilstrap, L.C., Hankins, G.D.V., et al. (1997). *Williams obstetrics* (20th ed.). Norwalk, CT: Appleton & Lange.

DeSwiet, M. (1999). Thromboembolic disease. In D.K. James, P.J. Steer, C.P. Weiner, & B. Gonik (Eds.). *High-risk pregnancy: Management options* (2nd ed., pp. 901-909). London: W.B. Saunders.

Featherston, C. (1998). Risk factors for lactation mastitis. *Journal of Human Lactation,* 14(2), 101-109.

Gibbs, R.S., & Sweet, R.L. (1999). Maternal and fetal infectious disorders. In R.K. Creasy & R. Resnik (Eds.), *Maternal-fetal medicine: Principles and practice* (4th ed., pp. 659-724). Philadelphia: W.B. Saunders.

Hager, W.D. (1998). Puerperal mastitis. *Contemporary Obstetrics and Gynecology,* 43(4), 27-33.

Hauth, J.C. (2000). Postpartum hemorrhage. In E.J. Quilligan, & F.P. Zuspan (Eds.). *Current therapy in obstetrics and gynecology,* (5th ed., pp. 317-320). Philadelphia: W.B. Saunders.

Hayashi, R.H. (1998). Postpartum hemorrhage and puerperal sepsis. In N.F. Hacker, & J.G. Moore (Eds.). *Essentials of obstetrics and gynecology* (3rd ed., pp. 333-342). Philadelphia: W.B. Saunders.

Hayashi, R.H., & Zettelmaier, M.A. (2000). Postpartum management. In S.B. Ransom, M.P. Dombrowski, S.G. McNeeley, K.S. Moghissi, & A.R. Munkarah, (Eds.), *Practical strategies in obstetrics and gynecology* (pp. 321-325). Philadelphia: W.B. Saunders.

Higgins, P.G. (2000). Postpartum complications. In S. Mattson & J.E. Smith (Eds.), *Core curriculum for maternal-newborn nursing* (2nd ed.), pp. 637-655.

Hodgson, B.B., & Kizior, R.J. (2000). *Saunders nursing drug handbook 2000.* Philadelphia: W.B. Saunders.

Klock, S.C. (1999). Psychological aspects of women's reproductive health. In K.J. Ryan, R.S. Berkowitz, R.L. Barbieri, & A. Dunaif (Eds.). *Kistner's gynecology and women's health* (7th ed., pp. 519-539.). St. Louis: Mosby.

Laros, R.K. (1999). Thromboembolic disease. In R.K. Creasy & R. Resnik (Eds.), *Maternal-fetal medicine: Principles and practice* (4th ed., pp. 821-831). Philadelphia: W.B. Saunders.

Lawrence, R.A., & Lawrence, R.M. (1999). *Breastfeeding: A guide for the medical profession* (5th ed.). St. Louis: Mosby.

Leonard, L.G. (1998). Depression and anxiety disorders during multiple pregnancy and parenthood. *Journal of Obstetric, Gynecologic, and Neonatal Nursing, 27*(3), 329-337.

Logsdon, M.C., Birkimer, J.C., & Usui, W.M. (2000). The link of social support and postpartum depressive symptoms in African-American women with low incomes. *MCN: The American Journal of Maternal/Child Nursing, 25*(5), 262-266.

Luegenbiehl, D.L. (1997). Improving visual estimation of blood volume on peripads. *MCN: The American Journal of Maternal/Child Nursing, 22*(6), 294-298.

Meighan, M., Davis, M.W., Thomas, S.P., & Droppleman, P.G. (2000). Living with postpartum depression: The father's experience. *MCN: The American Journal of Maternal/Child Nursing, 24*(4), 202-208.

Miller, L.G. (1998). Herbal medicinals. *Archives of Internal Medicine, 158*, 220-221.

National Institute of Mental Health. (1999). Depression: What every woman should know. (Online). Available at http://www.nimh.gov/depression/women/wom_pr.htm.

Nuwayhid, B., Nguyen, T., & Khalife, S. (1998). Medical complications of pregnancy. In Hacker, N.F. & Moore, J.G. (Eds.), *Essentials of obstetrics and gynecology* (3rd ed., pp. 234-262). Philadelphia: W.B. Saunders.

O'Brien, P., El-Refaey, H., Gordon, A., Geary, M., & Rodeck, C.H. (1998). Rectally administered misoprostol for the treatment of postpartum hemorrhage unresponsive to oxytocin and ergometrine: A descriptive study. *Obstetrics & Gynecology, 92*(2), 212-214.

Park, E.H., & Sachs, B.P. (1999). Postpartum hemorrhage and other problems of the third stage. In D.K. James, P.J. Steer, C.P. Weiner, & B. Gonik (Eds.). *High risk pregnancy: management options* (2nd ed., pp. 1231-1246). London: W.B. Saunders.

Park, E.H., & Sachs, B.P. (1999). Puerperal problems. In D.K. James, P.J. Steer, C.P. Weiner, & B. Gonik (Eds.). *High risk pregnancy: Management options* (2nd ed., pp. 1269-1280). London: W.B. Saunders.

Pearlstein, T., Diaz, S., Howard, M., Zlotnick, C., & Jain, N. (1998). Dysphoric disorders in women: A case of perinatal depression. *Medscape Women's Health,* 3(4). From http://www.Medscape.com.

Rickert, V.I., Wiemann, C.M., & Berenson, A.B. (2000). Ethnic differences in depressive symptomatology amoung young women. *Obstetrics & Gynecology, 95*(1), 55-60.

Riordan, J., & Auerbach, K.G. (1999a). Breast-related problems. In *Breastfeeding and human lactation* (2nd ed., pp. 483-511). Boston: Jones & Bartlett.

Riordan, J., & Auerbach, K.G. (1999b). Women's health and breastfeeding. In *Breastfeeding and human lactation* (2nd ed., pp. 541-576). Boston: Jones & Bartlett.

Savoia, M.C. (1999). Bacterial, fungal, and parasitic disease during pregnancy. In G.N. Burrow & T.F. Ferris (Eds.), *Medical complications during pregnancy* (5th ed., pp. 295-335). Philadelphia: W.B. Saunders.

Scott-Conner, C.E.H. (1997). Diagnosing and managing breast disease during pregnancy and lactation. *Medscape women's health, 2*(5). From www.medscape.com.

Seguin, L., Potvin, L., St-Denis, M., & Loiselle, J. (1999). Depressive symptoms in the late postpartum among low socioeconomic status women. *Birth, 26*(3), 157-163.

Selig, C. (1996, June). *Clinical guidelines for detection of depression in women's health.* Paper presented at the national AWHONN Conference, Anaheim, CA.

Simpson, K.R., & Creehan, P.A. (1996). *AWHONN perinatal nursing.* Philadelphia: Lippincott-Raven.

Sorokin, Y. (2000). Obstetric hemorrhage. A Postpartum management. In S.B. Ransom, M.P. Dombrowski, S.G. McNeeley, K.S. Moghissi, & A.R. Munkarah, (Eds.). *Practical strategies in obstetrics and gynecology* (pp. 311-320). Philadelphia: W.B. Saunders.

Stewart, D.E., & Robinson, G.E. (1998). Postpartum depression. In L.A. Wallis, A.S. Kasper, G.G. Reader, D.M. Barbo, W. Brown, O.R. Etingin, C.C. Nadelson, & V.W. Pinn (Eds.). *Textbook of Womens Health* (pp. 675-677). Philadelphia: Lippincott.

Straub, H., Cross, J., Curtis, S., Iverson, S., Jacobsmeyer, M., Anderson, C., & Sorenson, M. (1998). Proactive nursing: The evolution of a task force to help women with postpartum depression. *MCN: The American Journal of Maternal/Child Nursing, 23*(5), 262-265.

Tiran, D. (2000). Massage and aromatherapy. In D. Tiran & S. Mack (Eds.), *Complementary therapies for pregnancy and childbirth* (2nd ed., pp. 129-168). London: Bailliere Tindall.

Tiran, D. (2000). Reflexology in midwifery practice. In D. Tiran & S. Mack (Eds.), *Complementary therapies for pregnancy and childbirth* (2nd ed., pp. 169-188). London: Bailliere Tindall.

Williams-Judge, S. (1998). Managing postpartum hemorrhage. *Mother Baby Journal,* 3(6), 5-12.

Wood, A.F., Thomas, S.P., Droppleman, P.G., & Meighan, M. (1997). The downward spiral of postpartum depression. *MCN: The American Journal of Maternal/Child Nursing, 22*(6), 308-316.

29

High-Risk Newborn: Complications Associated with Gestational Age and Development

OBJECTIVES

1. List risk factors that may lead to complications of gestational age and development in the newborn.
2. Explain the special problems of the preterm infant.
3. Identify common nursing diagnoses for preterm infants, and explain the nursing care for each.
4. Describe the complications that may result from premature birth.
5. Describe the characteristics and problems of the infant with postmaturity syndrome.
6. Explain the effects of intrauterine growth restriction.
7. Compare the problems of the large-for-gestational age infant with those of the small-for-gestational age infant.

DEFINITIONS

Apneic Spells Cessation of breathing for more than 15 seconds, accompanied by cyanosis or bradycardia.

Bronchopulmonary Dysplasia Chronic pulmonary condition in which damage to the infant's lungs requires prolonged dependence on supplemental oxygen.

Compliance Stretchability or elasticity of the lungs and thorax that allows distention without resistance during respirations.

Containment A method of increasing comfort in infants by using swaddling or other methods to keep the extremities in a flexed position near the body.

Corrected Age Gestational age that a preterm infant would be if still in utero. Also may be called *developmental age;* the chronologic age minus the number of weeks the infant was born prematurely.

Enteral Feeding Nutrients supplied to the gastrointestinal tract orally or by feeding tube.

Intrauterine Growth Restriction Failure of a fetus to grow as expected for gestational age. Also may be called *intrauterine growth retardation.*

Large-for-Gestational-Age Infant An infant whose size is above the 90th percentile for gestational age.

Low-Birth-Weight Infant An infant weighing less than 2500 g at birth.

Macrosomia Unusually large fetal size; infant birth weight more than 4000 g.

Necrotizing Enterocolitis A condition of injury, invasion by bacteria, and possible necrosis of the intestines.

Noncompliance Resistance of the lungs and thorax to distention with air during respirations.

Parenteral Nutrition Intravenous infusion of all nutrients needed for metabolism and growth.

Periventricular-Intraventricular Hemorrhage Bleeding around and into the ventricles of the brain.

Postmaturity Syndrome Condition in which a postterm infant shows characteristics indicative of poor placental functioning before birth.

Postterm Infant An infant born after 42 weeks of gestation.

Preterm Infant An infant born before the beginning of the 38th week of gestation. Also called *premature infant.*

Pulse Oximetry Method of determining the level of blood oxygen saturation by sensors attached to the skin.

Respiratory Distress Syndrome Condition caused by insufficient production of surfactant in the lungs; results in atelectasis (collapse of the lung alveoli), hypoxemia, and hypercapnia.

Retinopathy of Prematurity Condition in which interference with blood supply to the retina may cause decreased vision or blindness.

Small-for-Gestational-Age Infant An infant whose size is below the 10th percentile assigned for gestational age.

Transcutaneous Oxygen/Carbon Dioxide Monitoring Method of continuous noninvasive measurement of oxygen and carbon dioxide levels in the blood by transducers attached to the skin.

Very-Low-Birth-Weight Infant An infant weighing 1500 g or less at birth.

Maternity nurses identify and care for the immediate needs of infants who are transferred to the neonatal intensive care unit (NICU) and provide information and emotional care for parents. Neonatal intensive care is a nursing specialty. Nurses who work in an NICU (also called *special care nursery* or *special care unit*) need additional education and experience to prepare them for this role.

CARE OF HIGH-RISK NEWBORNS

Nurses care for minor illness in the normal newborn nursery, but more serious problems in newborns require care in specialized nurseries, which are designed for that purpose.

Levels of Care

Not every hospital is equipped to provide an NICU with staff members who are specialized clinical experts able to provide complex treatment with expensive technical equipment. Hospitals are categorized according to the level of care they provide. Facilities at each level also provide care for infants with less acute needs.

Basic care facilities treat normal, low-risk mothers and newborns and identify and stabilize mothers and newborns with complications before transfer to another facility. They perform resuscitations of infants when necessary and care for minor problem that do not require specialized care.

Specialty care facilities provide care for high-risk mothers and fetuses where delivery is expected at 32 weeks' gestation or more. They also care for stable or moderately ill newborns with conditions that will resolve rapidly and preterm infants with a birth weight of 1500 g or more.

Subspecialty care facilities (previously called "tertiary care centers") offer comprehensive perinatal care for mothers and neonates belonging to all risk categories (Figure 29-1). Any fetus that will require immediate, complex care should be delivered at a subspecialty care facility (American Academy of Pediatrics & American College of Obstetricians and Gynecologists, 1997).

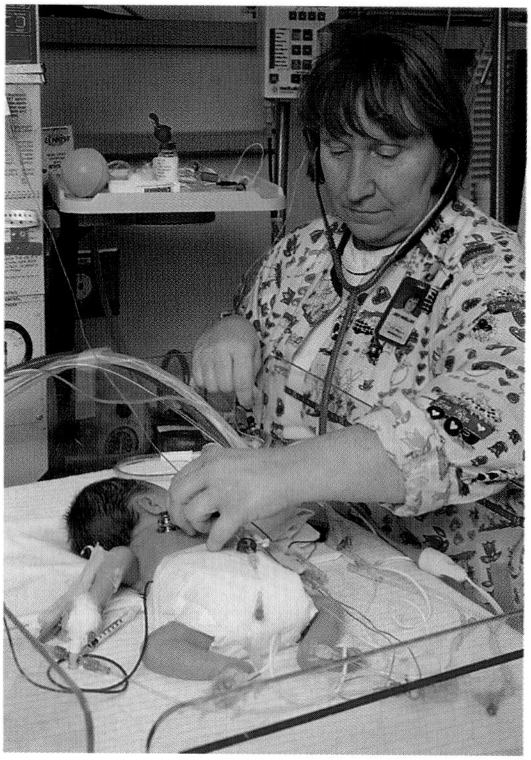

FIGURE 29-1 The infant in an NICU is cared for by nurses with highly specialized skills.

Multidisciplinary Approach

The care of infants with problems at birth often necessitates collaboration between many different professionals. In the hospital setting, this care may include nurses, nurse practitioners, physicians with different specialties, respiratory therapists, laboratory personnel, and pharmacists. Care from social workers, physical therapists, feeding specialists, occupational therapists, and infant development experts may begin during the hospital stay and continue after the infant is discharged. Nurses often must coordinate this care and explain or clarify it to parents.

Case Management and Clinical Pathways

Neonates with complications may remain in the NICU for many days at a cost of thousands of dollars. Methods to reduce the length of stay and cost of hospitalization include case management and clinical pathways.

The case manager is a nurse who follows infants from admission to discharge to identify or prevent situations that would interfere with progression toward discharge. Clinical pathways are guidelines developed collaboratively by staff members from all disciplines. They list the care infants will need along a time line and the expected outcomes of that care. This allows staff members and parents to know when to expect changes in care. (Figure 29-2 is an example of a clinical pathway used for infants in the NICU.)

PRETERM INFANTS

Preterm infants (also called *premature infants*) are born before the beginning of the 38th week of gestation. A gestational age assessment of preterm infants' size and development may show that they are small, appropriate, or large for the amount of time they have spent in the uterus. Most preterm infants are appropriate for their gestational age.

The word *preterm* is sometimes confused with the term *low birth weight (LBW),* which refers to infants weighing 2500 g (5 lb, 8 oz) or less at birth and of any gestational age. *Very-low-birth-weight (VLBW)* infants weigh 1500 g (3 lb, 5 oz) or less at birth. *Extremely-low-birth-weight (ELBW)* infants weigh 1000 g (2 lb, 3 oz) or less at birth. Although most of these infants are preterm, others are full-term and have failed to grow normally while in the uterus, a condition called *intrauterine growth restriction (IUGR).*

Incidence and Etiology

Scope of Problem

Advances in technology have resulted in survival at much lower birth weights than ever before. Approximately 85% to 90% of infants weighing 1250 g to 1500 g at birth and 20% of infants weighing 500 to 600 g at birth now survive (Stoll & Kliegman, 2000).

Although advances in technology have allowed very small infants to survive, the rate of preterm births is not decreasing. In 1996, 11% of all births were preterm and 7.4% were to low-birth-weight infants (March of Dimes, 1999). In terms of medical expense, lost potential, and suffering of infants and their parents, preterm birth is extremely costly.

Disorders related to short gestation and low birth weight are the second leading cause of infant mortality. Only congenital anomalies cause more infant deaths. Infant mortality increases as gestational age decreases. The risk of infant death in 1997 was 5 times higher for infants weighing 1500 to 2499 g and 92 times higher for infants born under 1500 g than for those over 2500 g (Guyer, et al., 1999).

Care of very preterm infants raises ethical questions concerning the benefit of saving them at great expense versus the risk that they may have permanent, serious disabilities and little chance to live normal lives. The incidence of problems such as blindness, hearing loss, developmental retardation, and cerebral palsy increases as the gestational age decreases.

Causes

The exact causes of preterm birth are not known, but all risk factors in pregnancy are potential causes of complications for the newborn. Problems during pregnancy may lead to preterm birth, and complications may occur during labor or delivery that result in decreased oxygenation of the fetus or trauma during delivery. Multifetal pregnancy is an increasing cause of early birth because of infertility treatment to achieve pregnancy.

One major factor associated with prematurity is low socioeconomic status of the pregnant woman because many risk factors often are present in low-income women. They are more likely to be malnourished, young, unmarried, and have frequent, closely spaced pregnancies. With little money and inadequate transportation, these women may begin pregnancy in poor health and receive little or no prenatal care. Complications may not be discovered until late in the pregnancy or labor, when they are more difficult to treat. Substance abuse may occur more often among (but is not limited to) the poor. Together, these factors increase the risk of complications for women and infants who live in poverty.

Prevention

Prevention of preterm birth is best accomplished by provision of adequate prenatal care for every pregnant woman to identify and treat risk factors as early as possible. Teaching women signs of preterm labor will help them seek care when halting labor is still a possibility (see Chapter 27, p. 750).

Characteristics of Preterm Infants

Characteristics of preterm infants vary by gestational age. For example, the appearance and problems of infants born at 34 weeks' gestation are different from those of infants born at 26 weeks' gestation. However, some characteristics are common to all preterm infants.

Appearance

Preterm infants often appear frail and weak, and they have underdeveloped flexor muscles and muscle tone. Their extremities are limp and offer little or no resistance when moved. Premature newborns typically lie in an extended position (see Figure 20-20). The head of the normal preterm infant is large in comparison with the rest of the body.

Preterm infants lack subcutaneous fat, which makes their thin skin appear red and translucent, with blood vessels clearly visible. The nipples and areola may be barely perceptible, but vernix caseosa and lanugo may be abundant. Plantar creases are absent in infants of less than 32 weeks' gestation (see Figure 20-26).

The pinna of the ear are flat and soft and contain little cartilage (see Figure 20-28). In the female infant, the clitoris and labia minora appear large and are not covered by the small, separated labia majora. The male infant may have undescended testes, with a small, smooth scrotal sac (see Figures 20-29 and 20-30).

Behavior

The behavior of preterm infants varies according to gestational age. It often differs from that of full-term infants because of the stress of having to adjust to extrauterine life before they are ready. They may have little excess energy for maintaining muscle tone and poor development of flexion. Premature newborns are easily exhausted from noise and routine activities. Their responses are varied, including lowered oxygenation levels and behavior changes. Their cries may be feeble.

Assessment and Care of Common Problems

Because preterm infants are "unfinished" in their growth and development, they are prone to problems affecting all systems and body processes. Some of the most common problems are discussed here. Problems with environmental stress, nutrition, and parenting are discussed in the section on application of the nursing process.

Problems with Respiration

Problems of the respiratory system are a major concern because preterm newborns must go through the same processes as the full-term infant to begin breathing but with less mature lungs. The presence of surfactant in adequate amounts is of primary importance. Surfactant reduces surface tension in the alveoli and prevents their collapse with expiration. Infants born before surfactant production is adequate develop respiratory distress syndrome (p. 831).

Assessment. The infant's respiratory status must be observed constantly. The lungs are assessed for adventitious breath sounds or areas of absent breath sounds. The Silverman-Andersen index is a useful tool for evaluating the degree of respiratory distress (Figure 29-3).

The nurse differentiates periodic breathing from apneic spells. Periodic breathing is the cessation of breathing for 5 to 10 seconds without other changes, interspersed with 10- to 15-second periods of rapid respirations. Changes in color or heart rate do not occur. Although periodic breathing sometimes occurs in term infants, preterm infants experience it more often.

Apneic spells generally last more than 15 seconds and are accompanied by cyanosis and bradycardia. Apnea lasting a shorter time with heart rate or color changes also are a concern. Apneic spells are common in preterm infants, increasing in incidence with lower gestational age. Apnea without an identified cause in a preterm infant is called *apnea of prematurity* and generally improves as the infant matures. Spells may occur along with periodic breathing, and the infant may require gentle stimulation or bag and mask ventilation. Apnea from any cause should be investigated because it may be related to other causes.

The nurse observes the effort required for breathing and the location and severity of retractions. Retractions are particularly noticeable in preterm infants, whose weak chest wall is drawn in with each inspiration. The

Text continued on p. 811

YORK HEALTH SYSTEM
YORK, PENNSYLVANIA

NICU CLINICAL PATHWAY

Page 1

Gest. age ________ wks. Birthweight __________ gms. DOB ________

Admitting diagnosis ______________________________

Family Care Team Members ______________________________

____

Mother's/Father's names ______________________________

Phone No. (home) ______________ alternative ______________

CODES:

Initials = Completed
N = Not applicable
D = Deferred
* = See progress notes

PROBLEM LIST:

1. Altered Pulmonary Status
2. Altered Nutritional Status
3. Altered Skin Integrity
4. Parental Knowledge Deficit
5. Thermoregulation
6. Immunological Impairment
7. Altered Parenting
8. Altered Cardiovascular Status
9. Altered Neuro Status
10. Altered Metabolic Status

	PHASE 1: ADMISSION/CRITICAL	PHASE 2: CONVALESCENT	PHASE 3: DISCHARGE
PSYCHOSOCIAL/ DISCHARGE PLANNING	☐ Orient parents to NICU environment, visitation & handwashing policies, provide phone numbers ☐ Provide NICU booklet ☐ Review equipment in use ☐ Discuss disease process and plan of care ☐ Review Family Care Team ☐ Assess family learning needs, family structure and support systems ☐ Social Services consult completed ☐ Encourage verbalization of fears/ concerns ☐ Document parental interaction/ teaching ☐ Provide Support Group information ☐ Informed of Lactation Consultant Support **EXPECTED OUTCOME:** Prob #4: Parents verbalize understanding of disease process and plan of care OUTCOME MET __________	☐ Provide Support Group information ☐ Parents introduced to Developmental F/U Services (i.e., Growth & Development, Early Intervention) ☐ Discharge Booklet given ☐ Discuss/demonstrate infant care techniques Parents safely perform/verbalize understanding of: ☐ axillary temp & normal range ☐ eye/oral care ☐ diapering/elimination patterns ☐ nail care ☐ cord care ☐ bath (sponge/tub) & skin care ☐ umbilicus care ☐ bulb syringe ☐ feeding techniques ☐ duration/amount ☐ scheduled/demand ☐ positioning ☐ burping ☐ formula preparation ☐ vitamin administration ☐ appropriate clothing/weather ☐ visitors/outings ☐ sleep/wake cycles ☐ temperament/disposition ☐ stress management ☐ "Back to Sleep" positioning ☐ s/s of illness/when to call the M.D. ☐ safety ☐ Assess home readiness ☐ has car seat/provide loaner information ☐ car seat safety reviewed ☐ has adequate supplies (i.e., diapers, clothing, formula) ☐ discuss rooming in ☐ circ consent signed ☐ CPR class scheduled ☐ CPR class completed /reviewed ☐ Begin teaching specialized care ☐ gastrostomy feeds ☐ home O_2 ☐ ostomy care ☐ trachea care ☐ other: __________ **EXPECTED OUTCOME:** Prob #4: Parents safely perform/verbalize understanding of infant care techniques. OUTCOME MET __________	☐ Review Discharge Booklet ☐ Age appropriate vaccinations given ☐ Vitamins relabeled ☐ prescriptions filled prior to D/C ☐ Circ completed ☐ Circ care reviewed ☐ Car seat check passed ☐ Rooming-in scheduled _____ ☐ Review s/s of illness ☐ Specialized instruction completed ☐ monitor training completed ☐ home O_2 training completed ☐ F/U home care arranged ☐ Other: _____ ☐ Ongoing Social Service intervention ☐ Home visits scheduled ☐ Lactation consultant ☐ Nursing ☐ Pediatrician/follow-up physician identified **EXPECTED OUTCOME:** Prob #4: discharged to home OUTCOME MET __________

	PHASE 1: ADMISSION/CRITICAL	PHASE 2: CONVALESCENT	PHASE 3: DISCHARGE
CARDIOVASCULAR Indocin / Lasix 1. ______ 2. ______ 3. ______ 4. ______	☐ Assess CV status, auscultate for murmur/PDA ☐ VS q 1°, H.O. q 8° ☐ VS q 2°, H.O. q 4° when stable ☐ Continuous B/P monitoring via UAC or PAL ☐ Cuff B/P when stable ☐ Echocardiogram as ordered **EXPECTED OUTCOME:** Prob #8: Hemodynamically stable without evidence of PDA OUTCOME MET ______	☐ Assess CV status ☐ VS as ordered ☐ Cuff B/P q shift ☐ F/U echo as ordered **EXPECTED OUTCOME:** Prob #8: Hemodynamically stable with B/P in normal range OUTCOME MET ______	☐ Assess CV status ☐ VS $\overline{ac}$ ☐ Cuff B/P daily **EXPECTED OUTCOME:** Prob #8: Discharged with VS WNL OUTCOME MET ______
RESPIRATORY surfactant administered 1. ______ 2. ______ 3. ______ 4. ______	☐ Assess respiratory status ☐ Pulse oximetry within prescribed range ☐ Noted @ bedside ☐ Mechanical ventilation ☐ Suction to pre-measured depth ☐ ETT placement depth @ bedside ☐ CXR as ordered ☐ G + 3 as ordered ☐ CPT as ordered ☐ Aerosol therapy as ordered ☐ TCOM as ordered ☐ Meds started ☐ Caffeine ☐ Aminophylline ☐ Albuterol ☐ Vancenase ☐ Decadron ☐ Other: ______ **EXPECTED OUTCOME:** Prob #1: Extubated OUTCOME MET ______	☐ Assess respiratory status ☐ Pulse oximetry within prescribed range ☐ Noted @ bedside ☐ NCPAP ☐ TCOM as ordered ☐ CXR as ordered ☐ CPT as ordered ☐ Aerosol therapy as ordered ☐ G + 3 as ordered ☐ Wean to NC as tolerated ☐ Meds continued ☐ Caffeine ☐ Aminophylline ☐ Albuterol ☐ Decadron ☐ Vancenase ☐ Monitor training scheduled ☐ Completed ☐ Pneumogram done **EXPECTED OUTCOME:** Prob #1: CPAP D/C'd OUTCOME MET ______	☐ Assess respiratory status ☐ Maintain oximetry while on O_2 ☐ Discharge Meds ______ ______ ______ ______ **EXPECTED OUTCOME:** Prob #1: Nasal Cannula D/C'd OUTCOME MET ______
THERMOREGULATION INTEG.	☐ Minimize insensible H_2O loss ☐ Initiate skin care guidelines **EXPECTED OUTCOME:** Prob #5: Transferred to isolette OUTCOME MET ______	☐ Wean isolette as tolerated ☐ Maintain skin care guidelines **EXPECTED OUTCOME:** Prob #5: Temp stable out of heat OUTCOME MET ______	☐ Maintain skin care guidelines **EXPECTED OUTCOME:** Prob #5: Maintains temp in open crib OUTCOME MET ______

Note: Each patient requires an individual assessment & treatment plan. This clinical path is a recommendation for the average patient which requires modification when necessary by the professional staff.

FIGURE 29-2 An example of a clinical pathway for infants in an NICU. The pathway is adapted to meet the needs of each individual infant. *CPT,* Chest physiotherapy; *CXR,* chest x-ray; *ETT,* endotracheal tube; *HAL/lipids,* hyperalimentation; *H.O.,* hands-on; *NCPAP,* nasal continuous positive airway pressure; *NGT,* nasogastric tube; *OGT,* orogastric tube; *PDA,* patent ductus arteriosus; *TCB,* transcutaneous bilirubinometer; *TCOM,* transcutaneous oxygen monitor; *TPN,* total parenteral nutrition. (Courtesy Women and Children Services of the York Health System, York, Penn. Modified with permission.)

Continued

YORK HEALTH SYSTEM
YORK, PENNSYLVANIA

NICU CLINICAL PATHWAY

Page 2

	PHASE 1: ADMISSION/CRITICAL	PHASE 2: CONVALESCENT	PHASE 3: DISCHARGE

FLUIDS, ELECTROLYTES, NUTRITION
Extended metabolic screen drawn
Date ______
Repeated ______
	☐ Assess abdomen for bowel sounds, distention, tenderness
	☐ Assess fluid/hydration status
	  ☐ IV fluids as ordered
	  ☐ Blood glucose as ordered
	  ☐ TPN, lipids as ordered
	☐ NPO ☐ OGT/NGT change q 72°
	☐ Trophic feeds initiated
	☐ Advance to full OG feeds as tolerated
	☐ Lactation consultation
	  ☐ Breastfeeding Care Plan initiated
	  ☐ Pumping started within 24 hrs
	  ☐ Breast milk storage reviewed
	  ☐ Received NICU Breastfeeding Information Folder
	
	EXPECTED OUTCOME:
	Prob #2: HAL/lipids D/C'd
	OUTCOME MET ______
	Prob #2: Returned to birthweight
	OUTCOME MET ______
	Prob #4: Mother verbalized/demonstrated understanding of pumping frequency, storage & cleaning
	OUTCOME MET ______
		☐ Assess abdomen for bowel sounds, distention, tenderness
		☐ Assess fluid/hydration status
		  ☐ IV fluids as ordered
		  ☐ C/S as ordered
		☐ Advance to breast/nipple feeds as tolerated
		☐ Lactation consultation assessment
		  ☐ Reports maintaining milk supply
		
		EXPECTED OUTCOME:
		Prob #2: Weight gain pattern achieved
		OUTCOME MET ______
		Prob #2: Nippling/breastfeeding all feeds
		OUTCOME MET ______
		Prob #4: Breastfeeding support/education continued
		OUTCOME MET ______
			☐ Assess abdomen for bowel sounds, distention, tenderness
			☐ Lactation consultation assessment
			  ☐ Discharge Breastfeeding Care Plan reviewed
			
			EXPECTED OUTCOME:
			Prob #2: Ad lib feeds with overall weight
			OUTCOME MET ______
			Prob #4: Verbalizes understanding of Discharge Breastfeeding Care Plan
			OUTCOME MET ______

HEME/BILI
Vitamin K given ______
Type & cross as ordered
______
Transfusion Dates:
______
______
______
	☐ Assess for S/S jaundice
	  ☐ TCB as ordered
	  ☐ Phototherapy as ordered
	  ☐ Serum bili as ordered
	☐ Assess for S/S of anemia
	☐ CBC, IT, retic as ordered
	
	EXPECTED OUTCOME:
	Prob #10: Phototherapy discontinued
	OUTCOME MET ______
		☐ Assess for S/S jaundice
		  ☐ TCB as ordered
		  ☐ Serum bili as ordered ______
		☐ Assess for S/S anemia
		  ☐ CBC, IT, retic as ordered
		
		EXPECTED OUTCOME:
		Prob #10: Jaundice resolved
		OUTCOME MET ______
			☐ Assess for S/S anemia
			
			EXPECTED OUTCOME:
			Prob #4: Discharged with stable HCT
			OUTCOME MET ______

	PHASE 1: ADMISSION/CRITICAL	PHASE 2: CONVALESCENT	PHASE 3: DISCHARGE
NEURO	☐ Assess neuro status ☐ Assess for & document seizure activity ☐ Head sono as ordered **EXPECTED OUTCOME:** Prob #9: Free of seizure activity OUTCOME MET ________	☐ Assess neuro status ☐ Assess for & document seizure activity ☐ Algo as ordered ☐ Eye exam as ordered ☐ F/U head sono as ordered **EXPECTED OUTCOME:** Prob #9: Hearing & eyes evaluated OUTCOME MET ________	☐ Late sono as ordered ☐ F/U referrals made ________ ________ ________ **EXPECTED OUTCOME:** Prob #9: Appropriate referrals for F/U will be made OUTCOME MET ________
INFECTIOUS DISEASE	☐ Assess for S/S of infection ☐ Blood culture as ordered ☐ Antibiotics as ordered ☐ Warmer changed after swamping D/C'd **EXPECTED OUTCOME:** Prob #6: D/C Amp/Gent if blood cultures negative OUTCOME MET ________	☐ Assess for S/S nosocomial infection ☐ Blood cx as ordered ☐ Antibiotics as ordered **EXPECTED OUTCOME:** Prob #6: Free of signs and symptoms of infection OUTCOME MET ________	☐ Med assessment for Synargis ☐ Synargis given ☐ RSV education reviewed **EXPECTED OUTCOME:** Prob #6: Age appropriate vaccination administered OUTCOME MET ________ Prob #4: Parents verbalize understanding of RSV prophylaxis OUTCOME MET ________
DEVELOPMENTALLY SENSITIVE CARE	☐ Maintain minimal stimulation, ↑ noise & light, cluster care ☐ Position flexed using H_2O beds, rolls, nesting, etc. ☐ Offer non-nutritive sucking ☐ Provide comfort measures such as swaddling, music, position changes ☐ Provide opportunities for touching, holding as tolerated ☐ Kangaroo care as tolerated ☐ Pain scale reviewed q shift **EXPECTED OUTCOME:** Prob #4: Developmentally sensitive care techniques implemented OUTCOME MET ________ Prob #9: Infant's comfort maximized as demonstrated by minimal pain scores OUTCOME MET ________	☐ Provide as appropriate: ☐ Visual stimulation ☐ HSS ☐ Soft music ☐ Swaddling ☐ Holding, rocking ☐ Social interaction ☐ Kangaroo care ☐ Cluster care, enforce undisturbed time-out periods ☐ Position flexed ☐ OT/PT as ordered ☐ Infant massage as tolerated ☐ Pain scale reviewed prn **EXPECTED OUTCOME:** Prob #4: Parents verbalize understanding and demonstrate developmentally sensitive care techniques OUTCOME MET ________ Prob #9: Infant cues indicative of comfort OUTCOME MET ________	☐ Referral to Growth & Development Clinic ☐ Referral to Early Intervention ☐ Pain assessment prn **EXPECTED OUTCOME:** Prob #4: Appropriate discharge referrals and appointments made OUTCOME MET ________ Prob #9: Pain assessment zero OUTCOME MET ________

Note: Each patient requires an individual assessment & treatment plan. This clinical path is a recommendation for the average patient which requires modification when necessary by the professional staff.

FIGURE 29-2, cont'd For legend see p. 807.

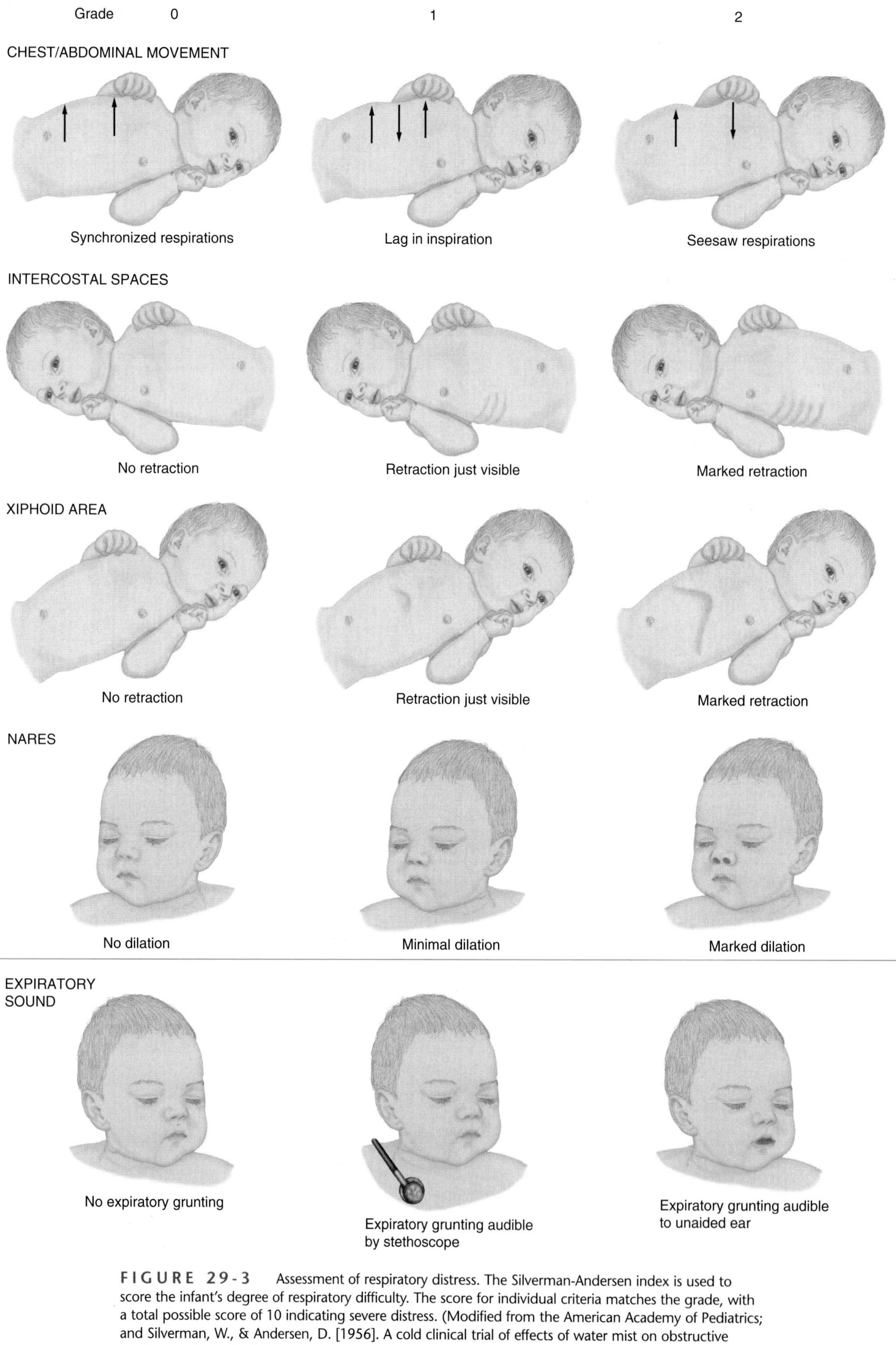

FIGURE 29-3 Assessment of respiratory distress. The Silverman-Andersen index is used to score the infant's degree of respiratory difficulty. The score for individual criteria matches the grade, with a total possible score of 10 indicating severe distress. (Modified from the American Academy of Pediatrics; and Silverman, W., & Andersen, D. [1956]. A cold clinical trial of effects of water mist on obstructive respiratory signs, death rate and necropsy findings among premature infants. *Pediatrics,* 17, 4.)

excessive compliance (elasticity) of the chest cage during retractions occurs because the bones of the chest wall are very pliable. This may interfere with full expansion of the lungs.

Grunting may be an early sign of respiratory distress syndrome. It closes the glottis and increases the pressure within the alveoli. This keeps the alveoli partially open during expiration and increases the amount of oxygen absorbed.

Nursing Interventions. Interventions focus on collaborating with other team members such as the respiratory therapist to manage technical equipment and facilitate removal of secretions.

Working with Respiratory Equipment. An oxygen hood often is used for infants who are able to breathe alone but need extra oxygen. The hood is a plastic, box-like device that fits over the infant's head. The infant breathes the higher levels of oxygen surrounding the head, and the hood does not interfere with access to the rest of the infant's body for care (Figure 29-4).

Oxygen also may be given by nasal cannula to the infant who breathes well alone. After discharge, many preterm infants continue to receive oxygen delivered via nasal cannula at home. Oxygen must be humidified to prevent insensible water loss and drying of the delicate mucous membranes. It is warmed to maintain body temperature. The infant also may need an endotracheal tube and mechanical ventilation.

Continuous positive airway pressure may be necessary to keep the alveoli open and improve expansion of the lungs. It can be delivered with nasal prongs or an endotracheal tube. High-frequency ventilation may be used to provide very fast, frequent respirations with less pressure and volume. This prevents injury to the tissue from pressure (barotrauma) and volume (volutrauma) than other methods.

Inhaled nitric oxide and liquid ventilation are newer methods that have been used for infants who have not responded well to other treatments. Nitric oxide is a gas that causes pulmonary vasodilation and improves oxygenation. Liquid ventilation is the use of a perfluorochemical fluid for ventilation of the infant. This fluid has a low surface tension and is a solvent for oxygen and carbon dioxide, so gas exchange can take place through the fluid introduced into the lungs.

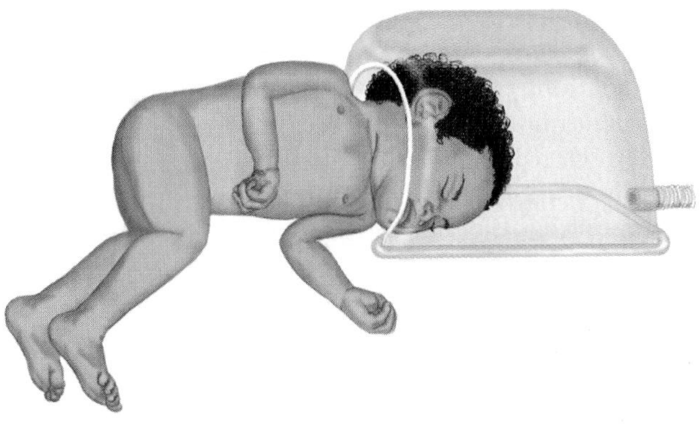

FIGURE 29-4 The oxygen hood is one way of delivering oxygen to an infant who can breathe unassisted.

When oxygen is administered, the level of oxygen in the infant's blood must be monitored. Arterial blood may be drawn for testing arterial oxygen levels. Pulse oximetry or transcutaneous monitoring also may be used. These methods are less invasive and provide continuous information about oxygen partial pressure (PO_2) levels through sensors attached to the skin.

The nurse must observe the infant's increasing or decreasing dependence on breathing assistance and need for oxygen. The infant's response to activity that may increase oxygen need, such as handling, feeding, and linen changes, may require changes in settings on equipment to meet the infant's needs. Oxygen flow should be increased when suctioning is necessary.

Positioning the Infant. Frequent position changes help drain air passages and prevent stasis of secretions. The side-lying and prone positions facilitate drainage of respiratory secretions and regurgitated feedings. The prone position is not recommended for normal newborn infants because it is associated with increased incidence of sudden infant death syndrome (SIDS). In the preterm infant, however, the prone position allows more efficient use of the respiratory muscles. It improves oxygenation and lung mechanics, decreases energy expenditure, and reduces gastric reflux if the head of the bed is elevated 30 degrees. (Gardner & Lubchenco, 1998). This should be explained to parents. The supine position should be used for sleep when infants have recovered enough to tolerate it. By changing to the supine position as soon as possible before discharge, infants will become used to sleeping on the back whenever possible.

If the infant must be in a supine position, the nurse can elevate the head of the bed and turn the infant's head to the side. Placing rolled blankets by the head can prevent movement, if necessary. A small roll under the shoulders straightens the airway.

Suctioning Secretions. The weak or absent cough reflex and very small air passages make the preterm infant susceptible to obstruction by mucus. Suction equipment must be available at all times. The nurse checks equipment at the beginning of each shift to ensure proper functioning. A bulb syringe is less likely to be traumatic than wall suction, but it may not reach mucus deep in the respiratory tract.

The infant is suctioned as mucus becomes apparent. The mouth is always suctioned before the nose to prevent aspiration of fluids if the infant gasps when the nose is suctioned. Suction always should be gentle to avoid traumatizing the delicate mucous membranes. Trauma could cause edema, which could further decrease the size of the air passages and lead to more respiratory difficulty.

Performing Chest Physiotherapy. Chest physiotherapy (postural drainage, percussion, and vibration) and suctioning are used in some hospitals to help keep the airway clear. Postural drainage helps the affected areas of the lung drain into the major bronchi.

Percussion helps loosen secretions and bring them into the bronchi, where they can be removed by suction. The procedure may not be used on small infants, however, because the stimulation causes stress and may increase intracranial pressure.

Maintaining Hydration. Adequate hydration is essential to keep secretions thin so that they can be removed by drainage or suction. If infants become dehydrated, secretions will become thick and viscous and could obstruct tiny air passages. Fluid intake should be increased (within the limits of the overall treatment plan ordered by the physician) if secretions seem to indicate even minimal dehydration. Small amounts of saline may be administered through endotracheal tubes just before suctioning to thin secretions.

Check Your Reading

1. Why are low-income women at increased risk of having preterm infants?
2. How does the appearance of a preterm infant differ from that of a full-term infant?
3. What factors contribute to respiratory problems in preterm infants?
4. What nursing responsibilities relate to care of preterm respiratory problems?

Problems with Thermoregulation

Although heat loss can be a problem for full-term infants, it is even more significant in preterm infants. Because the skin is thin, with blood vessels near the surface, and little subcutaneous fat is present to serve as insulation, rapid heat loss results. The shorter time in the uterus allows less brown fat to accumulate before birth, impairing the preterm infant's ability to produce heat by nonshivering thermogenesis.

Preterm infants have a larger head and more body surface area in proportion to size than full-term infants. Although full-term infants maintain heat by flexion of the extremities, the limp, extended body of preterm newborns exposes a greater surface area to the air for heat loss. The temperature control center of the brain of preterm infants is less mature and may be further impaired by asphyxia.

Complications from heat loss, such as hypoglycemia and respiratory problems, are more likely to develop in preterm infants. This limits the glucose and oxygen available to increase metabolism as a method of heat production. Vasoconstriction, which occurs when body temperature drops, may lead to metabolic acidosis, pulmonary vasoconstriction, interference with production of surfactant, and more respiratory difficulty.

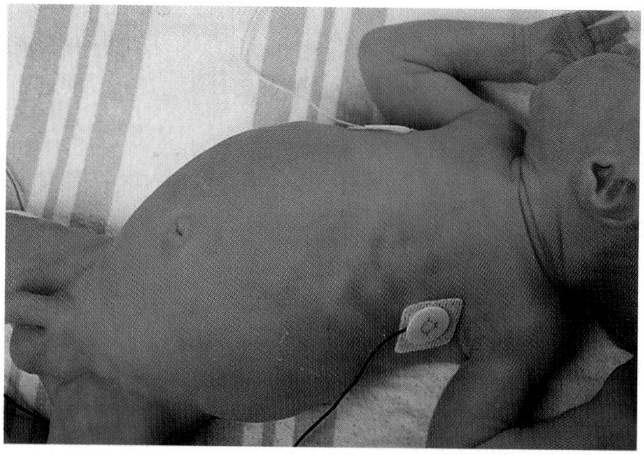

FIGURE 29-5 This preterm infant has mildly mottled skin and slight abdominal distention and retractions.

Assessment. The infant's temperature is monitored continuously by a skin probe on the infant's abdomen, which is attached to the heat control mechanism of the radiant warmer or incubator. The infant's temperature as shown on the monitor should be recorded at least every 30 to 60 minutes initially and every 4 hours when the infant is stable. The nurse should assess the axillary temperature every 4 to 8 hours and compare it with the heat control reading to ensure that the machinery is functioning properly.

The normal axillary temperature for preterm infants is between 36.3° and 36.9° C (97.3° and 98.6° F), slightly lower than the temperature for full-term infants, which is 36.5° and 37.5° C (97.7° and 99.5° F) (Blake & Murray, 1998). The abdominal skin temperature is usually maintained at 36° to 36.5° C (96.8° and 97.7° F). If the infant has accumulated brown fat, a normal axillary temperature when the monitor shows a decreased skin temperature may indicate that brown fat in the axillary space is being used to maintain the infant's core temperature.

Indications of inadequate thermoregulation include poor feeding or intolerance to feedings in an infant who previously had little difficulty, lethargy, irritability, poor muscle tone, cool skin temperature, and mottled skin (Figure 29-5). Hypoglycemia and respiratory distress may be the first signs that the infant's temperature is low. Because temperature instability may be an early sign of infection, the nurse should assess for other evidence that infection may be present. A decrease in weight gain or weight loss may occur over time.

CRITICAL TO REMEMBER

Signs of Inadequate Thermoregulation

Axillary temperature < 36.5° C or > 37.5° C (full term), <36.3° C and >36.9° C (preterm)
Abdominal skin temperature < 36° C or > 36.5° C
Change in feeding behavior
Lethargy
Irritability
Decreased muscle tone
Cool skin temperature
Mottled skin
Signs of hypoglycemia
Signs of respiratory difficulty

Nursing Interventions. Maintenance of heat in preterm infants involves the same basic nursing care principles as for the full-term infant (see Chapter 21). These principles must be adapted to meet the needs of the preterm infant, however.

Maintaining a Neutral Thermal Environment. A neutral thermal environment is especially important to help the infant maintain body temperature. Radiant warmers or incubators are used until infants can maintain normal body temperature alone. Charts are available that indicate the appropriate temperature setting to maintain a neutral thermal environment according to the infant's size and maturity. Because they lose more heat and produce heat less effectively, smaller, less mature infants will need more warmth to maintain body heat than larger or older preterm infants.

Infants needing many procedures are usually placed under the open radiant warmer to make it easier to see them and work with equipment. However, air currents around an unclothed infant can cause heat loss by convection despite the heat generated by the warmer. Doors near the warmer should be closed and traffic kept to a minimum to further decrease convective heat loss. The infant should receive only warmed oxygen because thermal receptors in the face are very sensitive to cold. Cold oxygen could quickly lead to cold stress.

Equipment and caregivers should not come between the infant and the heat source, preventing heat from reaching the infant. A transparent plastic blanket over the infant allows heat from the warmer to pass across to the infant and decreases insensible water loss and heat loss from evaporation while maintaining visibility of the infant's body parts.

When infants are in incubators, the nurse should keep portholes and doors closed as much as possible. Temperature in the incubator can drop several degrees in just a few minutes and much more if a longer time is involved. It may take 10 to 20 minutes for the temperature to reach the original level (Amlung, 1998). On removal from the incubator for procedures or holding, the infant should be placed in heated blankets and head coverings should be used. Incubator doors should be closed while the infant is outside to retain heat inside.

Infants should be placed under a radiant warmer or on a surface padded with warm blankets for procedures that cannot be performed inside the incubator. A heat lamp provides an alternative source of heat.

Although temperature loss is the most common concern, overheating also is a problem for preterm infants. This may occur when heating devices such as radiant warmers are set too high or the skin probe is inadvertently removed. Overheating leads to an increase in the metabolic rate, with increased oxygen and glucose needs, and insensible water losses.

Weaning to an Open Crib. Preparation of infants for moving to an open crib should begin early. When they are stable, they can be dressed in a shirt, diaper, and hat while in the incubator. This conserves heat and helps them adjust to a different temperature on the face than the rest of the body. Infants who weigh about 1500 g and have a consistent weight gain for approximately 5 days can begin gradual weaning from external heat (Medoff-Cooper, 1994).

Each NICU has its own protocol for the weaning process. The incubator temperature usually is decreased 1° to 1.5° C each day. It is raised if the infant's temperature falls below 36° C. If the temperature remains stable, the process can continue the next day.

When infants can tolerate the incubator setting at 28° C, they are ready for transfer to an open crib. They should be double wrapped with warm blankets at first to help insulate body heat. The temperature is assessed at gradually increasing intervals until the infant is on a routine schedule. A blanket is added for a low temperature, but if the temperature does not rise to normal, infants are returned to the incubator.

Nurses should observe infants carefully during the first few days after transfer to an open crib. Signs that may indicate inadequate thermoregulation include decreased weight gain, poor feeding, and increased oxygen need.

Problems with Fluid and Electrolyte Balance

Preterm infants lose fluid very easily. Their thin skin has little protective subcutaneous fat and a greater water content, and it is more permeable than the skin of term infants. The large surface area in proportion to body weight and lack of flexion further increase transepidermal water losses. Radiant warmers and the heat from phototherapy lights cause even more fluid loss through the skin. Radiant warmers heighten insensible water losses enough to result in a 40% to 50% increase in fluid needs (Blake & Murray, 1998). Water loss also occurs through the respiratory and gastrointestinal tracts. The rapid respiratory rate and use of oxygen can increase fluid loss from the lungs. Loose stools will lead to rapid dehydration.

Development of the kidneys is not complete until approximately 35 weeks of gestation. The ability of the kidneys to concentrate or dilute urine is poor before that time, causing a fragile balance between dehydration and overhydration. Monitoring intake and output of fluids is important in determining fluid balance. Normal urinary output is 1 to 3 ml/kg per hour for full-term infants. Although some variation occurs according to gestational age, values are similar for preterm infants. For ELBW infants, urine output should be 1 to 3 ml/kg per hour after the second day but may be less in the first two days of life (Gomella, et al, 1999).

Great variation in fluid needs occurs depending on many variables such as the infant's size, gestational age, insensible water loss from radiant warmers or phototherapy, and medical needs. During the first few days, 60 to 100 ml/kg/day may be given, with more given to extremely preterm infants as needed. Fluids are increased to 150 to 175 ml/kg daily gradually over the next few days unless restriction of fluids is needed (Stokowski, 1999).

Regulation of electrolytes by the kidneys also is a problem. Preterm infants need higher intakes of sodium because the kidneys do not reabsorb it well. If they receive too much sodium, however, they may be unable to increase sodium excretion adequately and are susceptible to sodium and water overload.

Assessment. The nurse must be alert for fluid overload or deficit. The infant's intake and output by all routes is carefully calculated. Parenteral, feeding tube, or oral fluids are included when measuring intake. Output from drainage tubes and urine should be measured. A urine output of less than 1 ml/kg per hour may indicate inadequate fluid intake or decreased kidney function, whereas more than 3 ml/kg per hour is a sign of overhydration (Gomella, et al., 1999). The nurse also must keep track of the amount of blood taken for laboratory tests, which can be substantial.

Urinary Output. Several methods of measuring urinary output are available. Plastic bags that adhere to the perineum are not suitable for the preterm infant because they may damage the fragile skin. Weighing diapers is less harmful. The weight of dry diapers is subtracted from the weight of wet diapers to determine the amount of urine excreted. Approximately 1 gram is equivalent to 1 ml of urine. However, humidification may add moisture to the diaper and a radiant warmer may cause evaporation of urine on the diaper. When precise measurement is essential, diapers can be fastened instead of placed open under the infant.

Specific gravity should be checked to determine if urine is more concentrated or dilute than expected. Urine is collected by placing cotton balls at the perineum. The specific gravity should range approximately between 1.005 and 1.015. For ELBW infants, the range should be between 1.008 and 1.015 (Gomella, et al., 1999).

Weight. Changes in the infant's weight can give an indication of fluid gain or loss, especially if they are sudden and greater than would be expected from feeding changes. The undressed infant should be weighed daily at the same time each day with the same scale. Very small infants often are placed in a bed with a scale so that they do not have to be disturbed for daily weighing. They may be weighed twice a day to monitor their fluid status more closely.

Signs of Dehydration or Overhydration. The nurse should observe for signs that indicate the infant has received too little or too much fluid. Early signs of dehydration include decreased urine output and increased specific gravity. Weight loss may exceed that expected for the infant's age and general condition. Dry skin or mucous membranes, sunken anterior fontanelle, and poor tissue turgor are late signs. Changes in the blood include increased sodium, protein, and hematocrit levels resulting from decreased plasma volume.

Signs of overhydration include increased output of urine with a below-normal specific gravity. Edema and weight gain occur from retention of fluids. Bulging fontanelles and decreased blood sodium, protein, and hematocrit levels also are present. Complications of excess fluid may include patent ductus arteriosus and congestive heart failure.

CRITICAL TO REMEMBER

Signs of Fluid Imbalance in the Newborn

Dehydration

Urine output < 1 ml/kg per hr
Urine specific gravity > 1.015
Weight loss greater than expected
Dry skin and mucous membranes
Sunken anterior fontanelle
Poor tissue turgor
Blood: elevated sodium, protein, and hematocrit levels
Tachycardia
Hypotension

Overhydration

Urine output > 3 ml/kg per hr
Urine specific gravity < 1.005
Edema
Weight gain greater than expected
Bulging fontanelles
Blood: decreased sodium, protein, and hematocrit levels
Moist breath sounds
Difficulty breathing

Nursing Interventions. The nurse must carefully regulate IV fluids with infusion control devices to help prevent fluid volume overload. IV medications should be diluted in as little fluid as is consistent with safe administration of the drug and be included when measuring intake. Starting IV lines on infants with poor veins is a lengthy, difficult procedure. Infants must be restrained as necessary to prevent infiltration. Some fluids will cause extensive damage as a result of tissue sloughing with infiltration.

Problems with the Skin

Preterm infants have fragile, permeable, easily damaged skin. They often have endotracheal tubes, IV lines, electrodes, and other equipment that must be maintained in place, but adhesive tape can be very damaging to the skin. Removal of adhesive tape may strip the epidermal layer of the skin, causing pain and increasing transepidermal water loss and the risk of infection. Alcohol, povidone-iodine, and other preparations used to disinfect the skin before invasive procedures can be damaging to fragile skin and may be absorbed.

Assessment. The nurse should frequently assess the condition of the infant's skin and note any changes. The infant's response to products used for cleansing and disinfection should be noted.

Nursing Interventions. Care of the skin is a subject of much research. Evidence-based practice guidelines for care of the neonate's skin have been developed and endorsed by the Association of Women's Health, Obstetric and Neonatal Nurses (AWHONN) and the National Association of Neonatal Nurses (NANN) (Lund, et al., 1999). A research-based practice project was being conducted in 58 sites in the United States using guidelines from this research in various settings across the country.

Tape should be used as little as possible. Backing tape with cotton, waiting more than 24 hours to remove it, and using gauze wraps decrease skin damage. Products that use pectin, hydrogel, and hydrocolloid adhesive are less disruptive to the skin surface.

The nurse should avoid the use of chemicals that can injure the skin or may be absorbed through it. If these solutions are used, sterile saline or water can be used to remove them and minimize damage. In some agencies, sterile saline or water is used to clean the skin before invasive procedures. Sterile water may be safest for bathing infants less than 26 weeks' gestational age.

Humidity in incubators should be regulated to reduce the drying effects of heat. Petrolatum, Aquaphor ointment, and similar products may be used as emollients to reduce transepidermal water loss and for healing. Transparent adhesive dressings may be placed on uninfected wounds and excoriations but should not be removed daily because the adhesive can further injure the skin (Lund, et al., 1999).

Infants and their equipment should be positioned to avoid undue pressure on the skin. Frequent position changes are important but should be based on the infant's ability to tolerate changes.

Problems with Infection

The incidence of infection in preterm infants is 3 to 10 times greater than that in full-term newborns (Gotoff, 2000). Many preterm infants have one or more episodes of sepsis during their hospital stay. They have several risk factors for infections. A maternal infection may have caused labor to begin prematurely and exposed the infant to the same infection. The infant may not have received adequate passive immunity from the transfer of immunoglobulin G from the mother that takes place during the third trimester. In addition, the immune response of a preterm infant is less mature than that of the full-term newborn.

Preterm infants often are exposed to situations that may cause infection. In addition to their fragile skin, they are subject to invasive procedures such as insertion of IV lines and drawing of blood specimens.

Assessment. The nurse should be on the alert for signs of infection at all times (see Chapter 30, p. 853).

Nursing Interventions. Handwashing is one of the most important aspects of preventing infections. Nursing care involves scrupulous cleanliness and maintenance of the infant's skin integrity. Even normal flora on the hands of caretakers may cause sepsis. Therefore parents and staff members should thoroughly wash their hands and arms before handling infants. Exposure to family members and staff members with contagious diseases should be prevented.

Problems with Pain

Infants in the NICU undergo many painful procedures each day. Caregivers once thought that newborns, particularly preterm infants, were too neurologically immature to feel pain. Pain stimuli are now recognized to cause physiologic and behavioral changes in infants. Preterm infants may be even more sensitive to pain than older infants (Evans, et al., 1997). The long-term effects of pain in the neonate are not yet fully understood. The American Academy of Pediatrics and the Canadian Paediatric Society recommend that environmental, nonpharmacologic, and pharmacologic interventions be used to prevent, reduce, or eliminate pain in neonates (2000).

Assessment. The nurse must assess the infant for pain level and response to potentially painful stimuli. Physiologic changes include changes in heart rate and respirations, increased blood pressure and intracranial pressure, and decreased oxygen saturation. Hormonal and metabolic changes also occur. Physiologic changes may be unpredictable and cannot be used alone to assess pain.

Behavioral changes include high-pitched, intense, harsh crying. In infants who are intubated or too weak to cry, a "cry face" is seen, with a crying facial expression without the sound of a cry.

CRITICAL TO REMEMBER

Common Signs of Pain in Infants

High-pitched, intense, harsh cry
"Cry face"
Eyes squeezed shut
Mouth open
Grimacing
Rigidity or flailing of extremities
Color changes: red, dusky, pale
Increased or decreased heart rate
Increased respirations
Increased blood pressure
Decreased oxygen saturation
Increased intracranial pressure

Nursing Interventions. Nurses should prepare infants for potentially painful procedures by waking them slowly and gently and using containment. Containment simulates the enclosed space of the uterus and is comforting to infants. It involves keeping the extremities in a flexed position near the body by swaddling, rolled blankets, commercial nesting or positioning devices, or the nurse's hands. At least one hand should be near the mouth for sucking.

Comfort measures help the infant cope with short-term, mild pain and reduce agitation. Nonnutritive sucking, sometimes with a pacifier that has been dipped in a sucrose solution, has been shown to be effective in reducing pain response for short-term procedures such as heel sticks (Stevens, et al., 1999). Soft talking, restraining the extremities to prevent flailing, and holding and rocking are other common methods of pain relief. Measures should be adapted according to the infant's response.

The nurse should discuss the infant's pain with the primary care provider to ensure that medications are available for long-term and more severe pain. Narcotics such as morphine and general anesthesia are tolerated by preterm infants. The nurse should give ordered medications before painful procedures and when the infant demonstrates pain signs. The nurse should carefully note the infant's response to allow increasing or decreasing dosage as necessary.

Check Your Reading

5. How do nurses help infants adjust to the cooler environment of an open crib?
6. How does the nurse keep track of an infant's intake and output?
7. What special problems related to fluid balance, infections, and pain occur in preterm infants?

APPLICATION OF THE NURSING PROCESS: THE PRETERM INFANT

Preterm infants commonly have difficulty with stress from the NICU environment and inability to obtain adequate nutrition. Their parents may have difficulty with bonding.

Environmentally Caused Stress

Preterm infants are constantly exposed to a bright, loud environment. Sounds of alarms, ventilators, incubators, doors, and people create a noise level that may increase the risk for hearing loss and other complications. In addition, stimulation of any kind can cause increased energy expenditure by the preterm infant. Noise and routine nursing interventions often are accompanied by changes in heart rate and respirations, oxygen saturation levels, and behavior states.

Although touch is generally thought to be comforting to infants, it often is associated with painful events for preterm infants. This can cause infants to develop touch aversion, a negative response to touch of any kind. During uterine life, the fetus sleeps as much as 80% to 90% of the time. Preterm infants undergo multiple assessments and treatments that may cause frequent interruptions of sleep and interfere with the development of normal sleep-wake cycles. Energy that must be directed toward coping with an overstimulating and stressful environment may be unavailable for normal growth and development.

Assessment

Assess the amount of noise to which the infant is exposed. Determine how often interruptions occur and how the infant responds to different types of care.

Assess the infant's ability to tolerate activity and noise. Overstimulation results in changes in oxygenation and behavior. Signs of alteration in oxygenation include pulse and respiratory rate variations from baseline, apnea, rapid color changes and cyanosis, nasal flaring, and drop in oxygen saturation levels.

Behavioral indications of stress (sometimes called *avoidance cues* or *behavior*) include stiffening and extension of the extremities with fisting or splaying (spreading) of the fingers. The infant may appear hyperalert with a worried facial expression or may turn away from eye contact. Coughing, yawning, hiccuping, and regurgitation also are signals that infants are receiving more stimulation than they can tolerate. All signs may be accompanied by increased fatigue.

Analysis

A nursing diagnosis appropriate for preterm infants having difficulty enduring the multiple stimuli in their environment is "Risk for Altered Growth and Development related to stress from an overstimulating environment." Use of this nursing diagnosis can help the nurse plan ways to increase the infant's ability to tolerate interventions.

CRITICAL TO REMEMBER

Signs of Overstimulation in Preterm Infants

Oxygenation Changes
Increase or decrease in pulse and respiratory rate
Cyanosis, pallor, or mottling
Flaring nares
Decreased oxygen saturation levels

Behavior Changes
Stiff, extended arms and legs
Fisting of the hands or splaying of the fingers
Alert, worried expression
Turning away from eye contact
Hiccuping
Regurgitation
Fatigue
Coughing
Yawning

Planning

The goals or expected outcomes for this nursing diagnosis are that the infant will do the following:

- Conserve energy for growth and development by showing decreased signs of overstimulation during routine activity.
- Gradually show an ability to withstand more activity before signs of overstimulation occur.

Interventions

Interventions are focused on providing developmentally supportive nursing care that meets the preterm infant's ability to tolerate stimulation. Developmental care keeps stressors in the environment to a minimum based on the infant's physiologic and behavioral responses.

Scheduling Care

Schedule periods of undisturbed rest throughout the day to allow the infant to recover from treatments. Avoid disturbing rest by arranging routine care to correspond with the infant's awake periods. If the infant must be awakened for care, try to do it during an active period of sleep and use quiet talking and gentle touch. Group care activities so that several tasks are performed at one time to allow for more rest between interruptions. However, be alert to the infant's signs of stress. Too many activities may be more than the infant can tolerate without rest.

Provide short rest periods within grouped activities or during long or painful procedures if the infant shows signs of overstimulation. Decrease the frequency of taking vital signs and providing other routine care as soon as possible. Even routine sponge bathing may cause changes in heart rate and oxygenation saturation levels in small infants (Peters, 1996a). If this procedure causes stress responses in an infant, it should be limited to necessary cleaning to conserve energy.

An important nursing responsibility is managing the infant's care by coordinating activities of different health care workers. For example, many different tests often are needed, and the nurse must see that they are done properly while protecting the infant from overstimulation.

Reducing Stimuli

Keep noise around the infant as low as possible. Place incubators away from traffic and congestion of people. Avoid talking near the incubator. Set volume on alarms on low and respond quickly when they sound. Open and close portholes and doors on incubators and cupboards gently. Do not place objects on top of the incubator or use it as a writing surface, which increases the noise inside. Teach parents and others to avoid tapping on the incubator.

Lights that are on 24 hours a day in the nursery may interfere with the development of sleep cycles. Position the incubator so that the infant is not facing bright lights, and drape a blanket or commercial incubator cover over it to decrease light and noise further. Use a dimmer switch to vary the intensity of lights as needed. Place infants in a prone position to help them avoid looking at ceiling lights.

Promoting Rest

When possible, schedule "quiet periods," when lights and noise in the unit are kept to a minimum, to promote rest. Scheduled naps when infants are disturbed as little as possible help increase sleep, decrease waking, and lead to longer uninterrupted sleep (Gardner & Lubchenco, 1998). They may be associated with decreased periods of apnea and increased weight gain for some infants. A daytime and evening nap and two naps during the night will help the infant begin to differentiate between day and night sleeping patterns.

Contain the infant's arms and legs to promote flexion and reduce energy loss from flailing extremities. Containment also promotes quieting and improves physiologic stability. Provide a "nest" with rolled blankets or commercial nesting or positioning devices placed around the infant for boundaries. Use the prone position to increase flexion and quiet sleep periods. In the side or supine position, arrange the infant's arms and legs in a flexed position, with the hands near midline.

Promoting Motor Development

Preterm infants may have musculoskeletal and developmental problems from prolonged immobilization and the effects of gravity on their immature neuromuscular system. Because the extensor muscles mature before the flexor muscles, the infant tends to remain in an extended, "frog-leg" position. Shoulder retraction, abduction of the lower extremities, and lateral flexion of the arms may result. When possible, position the infant in a side-lying or prone position with the extremities flexed and the hands placed near the mouth to allow the infant to suck the hands for comfort. The prone position also facilitates development of head control. Swaddling, when appropriate, may help keep the infant in a contained position. Turn the infant every 2 hours and use blankets, rolls, and positioning devices to maintain flexion.

Individualizing Care

The ability to tolerate stress varies with each infant. Adapt general care according to the infant's ability to tolerate it. When possible, the same nurse should care for the infant each day. This allows the nurse to learn the infant's unique behavior and response to stress. Even positive stimuli such as playing soft music and talking quietly to the infant can cause overstimulation. Use stimuli judiciously and according to the infant's tolerance level.

Infants often require extra energy to adjust to changes in care. Observe how well infants tolerate changes such as moving from assisted to more independent breathing or introduction of new feeding methods. Increase rest periods during these times.

Communicating Infants' Needs

Use the nursing care plan, Kardex, and shift reports to inform other caregivers of techniques that are especially effective for certain infants. Tape notes at the bedside as reminders of needs unique to each infant. Doing so also alerts parents to the methods nurses use to help their infant. Explain all techniques to parents.

Evaluation

As a result of interventions, the infant displays signs of overstimulation less often and shows an increasing tolerance before signs appear.

NUTRITION

The need for adequate nutrition in the preterm newborn is especially acute because the infant is born before full accumulation of nutrient stores and digestive capacity is achieved. The problem increases with decreasing gestational age.

Full-term newborns have reservoirs of calcium, iron, and other substances, but these are lacking in preterm infants. Between 30% and 90% of preterm infants develop hypocalcemia (Putman, 1999). Fat stores are minimal or absent, and glucose reserves are used soon after birth. Nutrients are needed not only to promote growth but to prevent injury to the brain. Hypoglycemia is a major concern because of the lack of glucose and fat reserves. Low blood glucose develops very quickly and must be prevented or treated quickly because the brain needs a steady supply of glucose.

Preterm infants need an average of 110 kcal/kg per day, although much variation exists among infants, especially when they have conditions that increase caloric need (Georgieff, 1999). They need more protein, iron, calcium, and phosphorus.

The gastrointestinal tract of preterm infants does not absorb nutrients as well as that of full-term infants. Although they digest protein well, preterm infants have insufficient bile acids and pancreatic lipase to absorb fat adequately. Lactase activity is low until the end of pregnancy, interfering with digestion and absorption of lactose. Glucose and sucrose are used adequately. Although their smaller stomach capacity limits the volume that they can tolerate at each feeding, preterm infants need more of many nutrients per kilogram than do full-term infants and require supplementation.

Although much variation exists among infants, coordination of sucking and swallowing generally occurs at about 34 weeks' gestation. The infant's respiratory status, other problems, and distractions in the environment can greatly affect this. Infants of less than 34 weeks' gestation or those weighing less than 1500 g generally have difficulty coordinating sucking, swallowing, and breathing. The gag reflex, which helps prevent aspiration, may function poorly. Oral feeding may cause an increased need for oxygen and glucose in very weak infants. When sucking is uncoordinated or requires too much energy, the infant must receive IV or gavage feedings.

Preterm infants do not have the well-developed buccal sucking pads in the cheeks that term infants use to form a seal around the nipple for efficient sucking. The jaw is less stable and the infant tires easily during oral feedings.

Assessment

Feedings often are changed according to the nurse's assessment of an infant's adjustment to feedings and signs indicating complications or readiness for change.

Readiness for Nipple Feeding

Preterm infants often are fed parenterally or by gavage (feeding tube) initially to conserve energy for growth and basic functioning. During feedings, watch for signs that nipple feeding may soon be possible, such as rooting and an increasing ability to tolerate holding and handling. Although sucking on the gavage tube, a finger, or a pacifier may be a sign of readiness, it alone is not enough. Infants also must have an intact gag reflex. Note whether the infant gags on the tube or a gloved finger inserted into the mouth. Infants who do not have a gag reflex are more likely to aspirate feedings. Infants born at more than 34 weeks' gestation usually can begin with oral feeding if they are healthy (Bakewell-Sachs, 1999).

CRITICAL TO REMEMBER

Signs of Readiness to Nipple

Signs of Readiness for Nipple Feedings
Rooting
Sucking on gavage tube, finger, or pacifier
Able to tolerate holding
Respiratory rate < 60 breaths per minute
Presence of gag reflex

Signs of Nonreadiness for Nipple Feedings
Respiratory rate > 60 breaths per minute
No rooting or sucking
Absence of gag reflex
Excessive gastric residuals

Adverse Signs during Nipple Feedings
Tachycardia
Bradycardia
Increased respiratory rate
Markedly decreased oxygen saturation level
Apnea
Coughing
Gagging
Falling asleep early in feeding
Feeding time beyond 25 to 30 minutes

Feeding Tolerance

Assess how well the infant tolerates feedings, whether by feeding tube or nipple. Before beginning a gavage feeding, withdraw the gastric contents to measure the amount left from the previous feeding. This helps determine whether the stomach is emptying and prevents overdistention. An excessive residual indicates that the amount or type of formula may need changing. It also may be an early sign of a complication such as obstruction, ileus, necrotizing enterocolitis, or sepsis, and it should be reported to the physician.

Practice varies on whether to replace gastric residuals (Bakewell-Sachs, 1999). If they are not replaced, observe carefully for signs of electrolyte imbalance.

When the infant begins to feed by nipple, assess coordination of suck, swallow, and breathing and observe for aspiration. Frequent choking, gagging, or cyanosis during feedings may indicate that the infant is unable to coordinate sucking, swallowing, and breathing well enough for nipple feeding. Some infants are so weak that the usual signs of aspiration are minimal or absent.

Assess the respiratory rate before and during feedings. When the respiratory rate is more than 60 to 70 breaths per minute before feedings, gavage feed to prevent aspiration. An increased respiratory rate, tachycardia, bradycardia, color changes, decreased oxygen saturation levels, or excessive fatigue demonstrate that the effort of nipple feeding requires too much energy for the infant. Gulps or shallow "catch" breaths during nippling may indicate the infant is having difficulty coordinating breathing with sucking and swallowing. Swallowing several times in succession without breathing may be caused by a bolus of fluid that is too big for the infant to swallow at once. A brief rest period allows time for the infant to clear the mouth, take some deep breaths, and reorganize the breathing (Shaker, 1999).

Observe for signs of intestinal complications. Obtain objective data about abdominal distention by using a tape to measure abdominal girth. Place the tape at the level of the umbilicus, and record the placement on the nursing care plan to ensure consistency. Stool may be sent to the lab for tests for reducing substance, which indicates malabsorption of carbohydrates. It also may be tested for occult blood.

Vomiting or frequent regurgitation may indicate that the feedings are too large. Vomitus containing bile may be a sign of intestinal obstruction and may require surgery. Diarrhea may be caused by rapid advancement of the feeding or intolerance to the type of formula. Report signs of feeding intolerance to the physician or nurse practitioner because they may be early indications of complications such as ileus, sepsis, obstruction of the gastrointestinal tract, and necrotizing enterocolitis.

Analysis

When the infant's nutritional needs are met by parenteral methods, the nursing care is mainly collaborative. However, once the infant is able to take formula or breastfeed, many nursing interventions are involved. They address the nursing diagnosis "Risk for Altered Nutrition: Less Than Body Requirements related to uncoordinated suck and swallow and fatigue during feedings."

Planning

Goals or expected outcomes written for an individual infant with this nursing diagnosis take into consideration the specific needs of that infant. The infant will:

- Consume adequate amounts of breast milk or formula to meet nutrient needs for age and weight.
- Gain weight as appropriate for age.

The actual amount of feedings and weight gain will vary according to the infant's gestational age and other conditions. Discuss what is appropriate for a particular infant with the physician or nurse practitioner.

Interventions

Administering Parenteral Nutrition

The nurse manages the administration of parenteral nutrition, which may be necessary for very immature infants. Parenteral nutrition is the IV infusion of solutions containing the major nutrients needed for metabolism and growth. It provides calories, amino acids, fatty acids, vitamins, and minerals in amounts adapted to the specific needs of infants.

Administering Gavage Feedings

Enteral feedings (feeding into the gastrointestinal tract, either orally or by feeding tube) are started as soon as possible because they may improve intestinal hormone production and help promote intestinal growth and maturity (Townsend, Johnson, & Hay, 1998). Infants of less than 34 weeks' gestation or those weighing less than 1800 g (4 lb) may need special formulas or fortified breast milk. Special formulas are adapted to meet the need for easily digestible, concentrated nutrients in a smaller volume of fluid. Preterm infants may need 22 or 24 kcal per ounce (instead of 20 kcal/oz used for the full-term infant) to meet their needs. Preterm formulas contain added calcium, phosphorus, and vitamins needed by the preterm infant. The addition of long-chain polyunsaturated fatty acids may be especially important for brain growth and the blood vessels (Brooks, Mitchell, & Steffenson, 2000). Breast milk fortifiers add needed nutrients to breast milk to make it more concentrated. Very small infants begin with half-strength breast milk or formula, and the amount and strength are gradually increased.

Gavage feedings usually are started before oral feedings for preterm infants (Procedure 29-1). A small, soft catheter may be inserted through the mouth or nose at each feeding for intermittent (bolus) feedings. Or the catheter may be left in place for a period to provide for intermittent or continuous feedings. Indwelling catheters decrease the vagal stimulation with apnea and bradycardia and are less traumatic than frequent, multiple insertions. Continuous feedings may be better for very small infants who cannot tolerate the larger quantities of bolus feedings. However, continuous feedings have a higher risk of aspiration because the infant is not attended at all times during the feeding.

An orogastric or nasogastric catheter may be used. The orogastric catheter often is used because a naso-

PROCEDURE 29-1
Administering Gavage Feeding

Purpose: Gavage feeding is used for infants who are unable to take the full feeding by nipple. It may be used alone or along with nipple feedings.

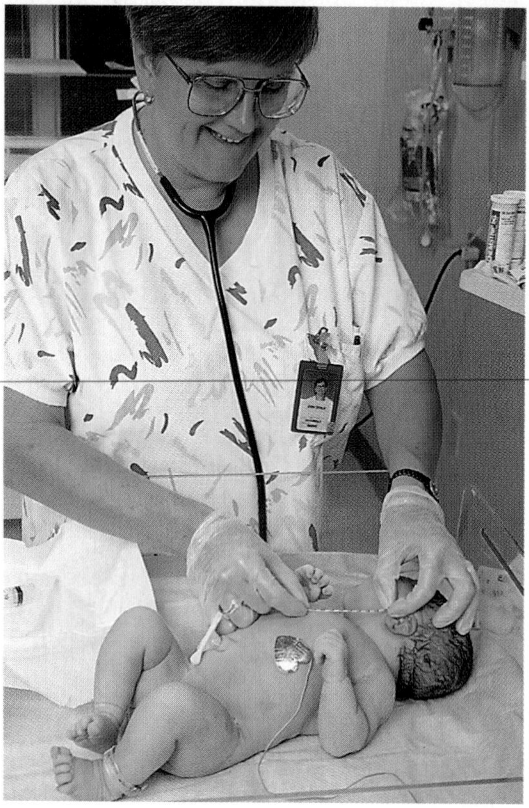

1. Wash hands and gather equipment, including gavage tube of proper size (3.5, 5, or 8 French, depending on size of the infant), medicine cup or other measured container, and 20-ml syringe. Warm breast milk or formula to room temperature. Check the chart to determine how previous feedings were tolerated. Add fortifier to breast milk if necessary. *Having all equipment ready helps the procedure go smoothly and avoids disturbing the infant or delaying feedings. Cold milk could interfere with thermoregulation. Information about previous feedings will help meet the infant's needs.*
2. If the infant has a tendency to regurgitate when moved after feedings, position him or her on the right side or prone. If parents are present, they may hold the infant in their arms once the tube is inserted or hold the hands if the infant cannot be held. *Positioning uses gravity to help avoid reflux of milk into the trachea and promotes emptying of the stomach. Feeding is important to parents, and helping increases their sense of involvement.*
3. Determine the length of catheter to insert. For orogastric insertion, measure from the mouth to the ear to the xiphoid process. For nasogastric feedings, measure from the infant's nose to the earlobe and then to the xiphoid process and add 1 cm. Mark the tube at the proper point with a piece of tape. *The measured distance is equal to the distance from the mouth to the stomach.*
4. While holding the infant's head steady, gently insert the tube through the mouth or nose to the point marked. Remove the tube immediately if persistent coughing, choking, cyanosis, apnea, or bradycardia occurs. *Moistening the tip provides lubrication. Signs may indicate that the tube is entering the trachea instead of the esophagus. Stimulation of the vagus nerve may cause bradycardia or apnea.*

5. Check for placement when the tube is first placed, before beginning bolus feedings, and at least once a shift for continuous feedings. Attach a syringe to the tube and gently aspirate stomach contents. Move or rotate the tube slightly if the plunger does not withdraw easily. *Aspirating stomach contents provides further proof that the feeding tube is in the proper place. Some NICUs check the pH of the aspirate. Use of force could traumatize the stomach lining if the end of the tube is resting against it. Moving the tube may draw it away from the stomach lining.*
6. Insert 2 to 3 cc (depending on tube size) of air through the tube while listening over the stomach with a stethoscope. Gently draw back on the plunger to withdraw the inserted air. *Hearing air enter the stomach ensures that the catheter is in place. Withdrawing the inserted air provides more room for feeding and helps prevent regurgitation.*
7. Tape the tube in place. *Taping ensures the tube will remain inserted to the proper length during the procedure.*
8. Withdraw stomach contents. Observe amount, color, and consistency of the aspirate. During continuous feedings, check the gastric residual every 2 to 4 hours. Do not feed the infant if the aspirate is abnormal. Report abnormal appearance or amount of stomach contents. *Stomach contents that are red or dark brown may indicate blood. If the aspirate is green with bile or brown with feces, intestinal obstruction may have occurred. An excessive amount may mean that the infant is receiving too much or that stomach emptying is delayed. For continuous feedings, residual equal to 2 to 3 hours of volume may be normal if no other signs of feeding intolerance exist.*

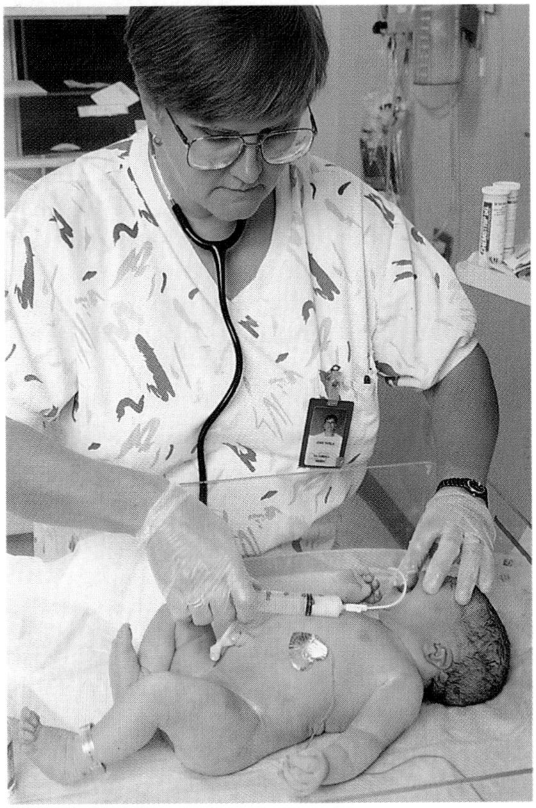

9. Replace the aspirate before beginning feeding or discard according to agency policy. If it is replaced, subtract the amount of gastric residual from the amount of milk to be given. *Replacement of aspirate prevents loss of electrolytes. Overdistention of the stomach is avoided by subtracting the residual from the feeding to be given.*
10. Remove the plunger and attach the syringe to the feeding tube. Pour the correct amount of solution into the syringe. Attach to a feeding pump that will regulate the amount of flow. *A gravity flow or regulation of the flow by pump causes less trauma and prevents filling the stomach too fast.*
11. If using gravity flow, raise or lower the syringe to increase or decrease the rate of flow so that the feeding moves slowly into stomach over 15 to 30 minutes. *The higher the syringe, the faster the flow of solution and the greater the pressure. Feedings should be given slowly to prevent sudden distention or trauma from pressure.*

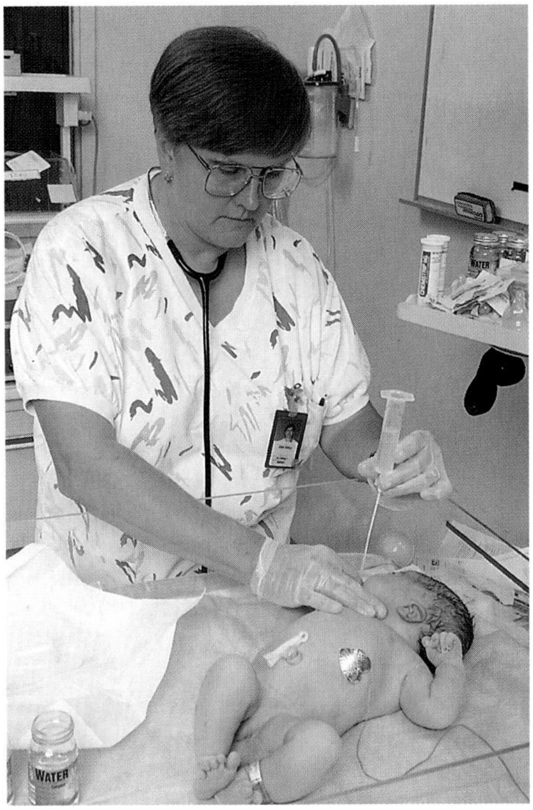

12. For continuous feedings, place no more than a 2- to 4-hour supply of milk in a feeding bag or syringe. Set the pump to deliver the correct rate of flow. Change the equipment every 4 hours or according to hospital policy. *Limiting the amount and changing equipment prevents excessive growth of bacteria in the milk or tubing. Infusion pumps deliver the feeding at a constant, measured rate.*
13. Give the infant a pacifier during the feeding. *The pacifier stimulates the sucking reflex, helps prepare the infant for nippling, is comforting, and helps the infant associate sucking with feeding.*
14. For intermittent feedings with a tube that remains in place, clear the tube with air or sterile water and close off the end when the feeding is completed. *This prevents air from entering the tube or formula from coming back through it.*
15. When the catheter is to be withdrawn, pinch the tube and remove quickly. *Pinching prevents drops of milk from entering the trachea as the tube is removed, and quick removal decreases irritation.*
16. Burp the infant, and position on the right side or prone, with the head of the bed elevated 35 to 45 degrees. If movement tends to cause regurgitation, omit burping. Allow the infant to remain on the right side or prone. *Air is swallowed around the tube and can cause the infant to regurgitate and aspirate. Position helps prevent reflux of feeding into the esophagus and promotes emptying of the stomach by gravity. If regurgitation occurs, the milk will flow out of the mouth.*
17. Record time, amount, and characteristics of gastric residual, type and amount of feeding given, and how the infant tolerated it. *Documentation allows monitoring of infant's ability to tolerate feedings and meet nutritional needs.*

gastric catheter may interfere with airflow through the infant's small nasal passages. Nasogastric tubes may be used in some situations. In addition, bacteria counts in the milk or formula may become too high, and fats tend to adhere to the tubing during continuous feeding.

Gavage feedings are begun with "minimal enteral nutrition," where a few milliliters of feeding are given at a time to promote maturation and hormone production, and help increase later feeding tolerance and weight gain. Feedings are gradually increased according to the infant's tolerance. Carefully observe the infant's tolerance at each feeding to determine when the feeding type or amount can be changed. Parenteral nutrition continues until the infant is able to take adequate enteral feedings.

Preterm infants have been exposed to aversive stimulation around the mouth, such as intubation and suctioning. As a result, they may react negatively to any additional oral stimulation, thus interfering with feedings. Using a pacifier for an infant who is able to suck during gavage feedings provides positive oral stimulation and helps associate the comfortable feeling of fullness with sucking. Nonnutritive sucking also increases later success in oral feedings, decreases behavior changes during feedings, and helps bring the infant to an alert state, which improves feeding success (Koch, 1999).

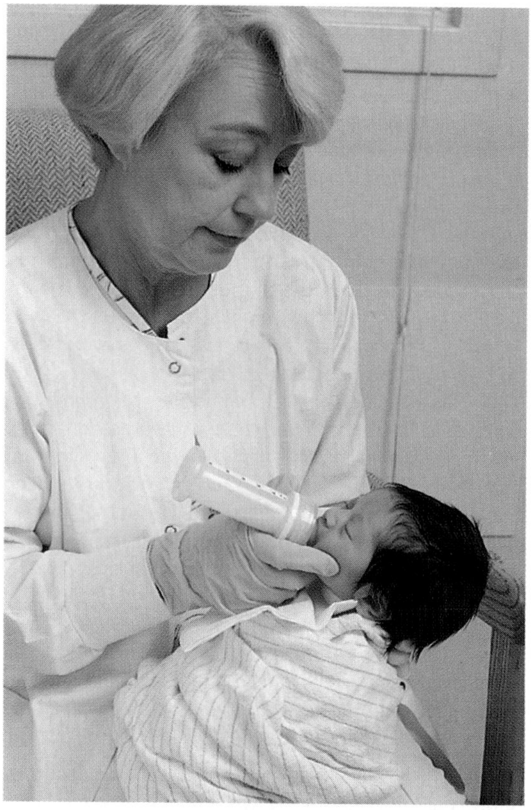

FIGURE 29-6 The nurse positions her hands to provide cheek and jaw support for feeding this preterm infant.

Administering Oral Feedings

Oral feedings often are begun when the infant reaches 34 weeks' corrected gestational age and weighs at least 1500 g, although some infants are able to begin earlier. At this time, most healthy preterm infants are able to coordinate sucking with swallowing and breathing, have a functional gag reflex, and have enough energy to feed orally without compromising oxygenation (Figure 29-6). The first nipple feedings may be only a few milliliters once a day and completed by gavage. Placing the gavage tube before beginning oral feedings helps prevent regurgitation stimulated by passing the catheter. Gradually increase the amount and frequency of oral feedings until the infant feeds by breast or bottle once a shift, then every second or third feeding, and eventually every feeding.

Critical Thinking Exercise

QUESTION:
What are the major differences between formula feeding a preterm infant and a full-term infant?

Preparing for Feedings. Provide for maintenance of heat during feeding times. When infants have stable temperature maintenance, wrap them in warm blankets and hold them for feedings. If thermoregulation is a problem, use a heat lamp over the infant or feed the infant in the radiant warmer or incubator.

Nipple feedings involve a greater expenditure of energy by the infant than gavage feedings. Allow for a period of rest before and after feedings. Use of a pacifier before feedings helps bring preterm infants to an inactive awake state that enhances oral feeding success. Infants may be fed according to a feeding schedule or at times when they demonstrate cues that they are ready.

Giving Bottle Feedings. Nursing interventions for bottle feeding the preterm infant are presented in Nursing Care Plan 29-1.

Facilitating Breastfeeding

Encourage mothers who would like to breastfeed. Contributing her milk helps the mother realize she has something important to offer at a time when she may feel that she can do little to help her baby. The immunologic benefits of breast milk are particularly important to the preterm infant who did not receive passive immunity during fetal life. Nutrients in breast milk are more easily digested, and enzymes, hormones, and growth factors important for the preterm infant are provided. Although milk from mothers of preterm infants is higher in protein, fat, and electrolytes during the early weeks, adding special fortifiers may be necessary to meet total nutrient needs.

NURSING CARE PLAN 29-1

The Preterm Infant

Assessment: Giovanni was born at 33 weeks' gestation and weighs 1800 g (4 lb). He breathes on his own with oxygen by hood. Giovanni needs many treatments throughout the day. He demonstrates pallor and increased respiratory rate when tired. Noises often cause a drop in oxygen saturation. When held or disturbed for care, Giovanni may stiffen and extend his arms with the fingers splayed. He sleeps most of the time when he is undisturbed.

Nursing Diagnosis: Activity Intolerance related to weakness, fatigue, and possible overstimulation.

Goals/Expected Outcomes

1. Giovanni will not show signs of overstimulation (increased respirations, pallor, decreased oxygen saturation level, stiffening of arms and legs, and splaying of fingers) as a result of normal activity.
2. Giovanni will increase tolerance to activity gradually as demonstrated by fewer signs of fatigue or stress.

Intervention	Rationale
1. Arrange to provide routine care to correspond with Giovanni's natural awake periods, whenever possible.	1. Preterm infants need undisturbed sleep to promote growth.
2. Schedule periods of uninterrupted rest, especially before and after energy-draining activities.	2. Infants tolerate activities best when they begin in a rested state and are allowed to recover from them before other activities are necessary.
3. Experiment with grouping care to determine the number and combination of care activities that Giovanni tolerates best.	3. Flexible nursing care allows individualization to meet the infant's needs. Grouping accomplishes more tasks at once so that longer rest periods are possible between tasks. However, too many activities are too fatiguing.
4. Assess carefully to determine what activities bring about signs of overstimulation and fatigue: changes in color, respirations, or pulse; stiff, extended extremities; worried, hyperalert expression. Stop and allow a short rest period.	4. Careful observation allows the nurse to be sensitive to the infant's ability to tolerate care.
5. Reduce the noise level around Giovanni. Avoid unnecessary talking, open and close doors softly, and keep alarm volumes low.	5. Noise may be overstimulating and result in increased oxygen need.
6. Reduce nonessential lighting. Place Giovanni's bed facing away from bright lights. Partially cover the incubator over Giovanni's head to keep out light but allow visualization of the infant.	6. Continuous lighting interferes with infant's sleep. Reducing light in the infant's face will increase rest.
7. Use blanket rolls or positioning devices to form "boundaries" around Giovanni and keep the extremities flexed.	7. Enclosed space promotes rest and comfort because it is similar to the small space of the uterus. Positioning devices also prevent the infant from hitting the hard walls of the bed.

Critical Thinking: Who else besides the primary nurse needs to know about methods to maintain appropriate stimuli in Giovanni's environment? How can this information be made available to other people?

Answer: Everyone involved in caring for Giovanni—other nurses, members from other disciplines, and parents—need to know about the plan for appropriate stimuli so that everyone will follow the same methods for developmental care. See interventions below.

Intervention	Rationale
8. Inform everyone working with Giovanni about what works best in decreasing fatigue and stimulation for him. Use shift report, the nursing care plan and Kardex, and arrange an interdisciplinary team conference. Ask for suggestions. Tape signs on the bed to provide this information to parents and others.	8. All caregivers should have information available to help meet the infant's needs consistently.
9. Explain Giovanni's needs for rest and low stimulation to his parents. Suggest ways that they can interact appropriately to meet Giovanni's needs, and point out signs that he is receiving too much stimulation. Ask for their input.	9. Parents who are informed can care for the infant appropriately and feel that they are members of the team and parenting their child by learning his needs.

Evaluation: Giovanni gradually shows increased ability to tolerate progressive activity with fewer episodes of overstimulation. His respirations and oxygen saturation levels remain stable, and he rarely stiffens his arms and legs during activity.

Continued

Assessment: Giovanni begins to take feedings by nipple supplemented by gavage when he becomes too tired. He has occasional episodes of increased respirations or short cyanotic spells when fed. He sometimes takes only half the feeding before falling asleep and must receive the rest by gavage. Giovanni's mother has decided to formula feed.

Nursing Diagnosis: Risk for Altered Nutrition: Less Than Body Requirements related to fatigue during feedings.

Goals/Expected Outcomes:
Giovanni will do the following:
1. Take approximately 198 kcal per day to meet his needs at a weight of 1800 g.
2. Gain approximately 30 g daily.
3. Complete nipple feedings without signs of excessive fatigue (such as increased respiratory rate or falling asleep during feeding).

Intervention	Rationale
1. Schedule nursing care to provide rest periods before and after nipple feedings.	1. Nippling consumes a great deal of energy. Rest helps prevent excessive fatigue that might prevent the infant from completing the feeding.
2. Gather equipment. Use a feeding container (such as a Volutrol) on which each milliliter is marked. Place the container in warm water to warm the milk to room temperature or slightly warmer. Do not use a microwave oven to warm.	2. Having all equipment ready prevents wasted motion and ensures that infant is fed without interruption. Exact measurement of the amount taken is important to ensure that infants receive required nutrients. Some infants will take slightly warmed milk better. Microwaving provides uneven heating of formula and may cause the infant to be burned.
3. Determine the type of nipple that works best for Giovanni. Choose between various sizes and consistencies.	3. A "preemie" nipple is more pliable than regular nipples and requires less energy for sucking. Some infants need firmer nipples because soft nipples allow milk to flow too fast, cause choking, and interfere with breathing between sucking bursts. Infants with a very small mouth require a smaller nipple.
4. Wrap Giovanni in warmed blankets and place a hat on his head. Feed him in the incubator or under the warmer if needed.	4. A hat and blankets help maintain temperature when infants are out of the incubator. If infants have difficulty with temperature maintenance, an incubator or warmer provides warmth during feedings.
5. Position Giovanni at a 45- to 60-degree angle facing the nurse. Position the head slightly forward and the chin slightly down. Place a finger on each cheek and one under the jaw at the base of the tongue midway between the chin and the throat. Provide gentle pressure.	5. This position allows the nurse to observe the infant's suck, response to feeding, and any regurgitation. The finger position increases sucking efficiency and jaw stability.
6. Feed slowly, with frequent stops to burp and allow the infant to stop for rest.	6. Slow feeding is necessary because of the infant's decreased energy. Preterm infants may swallow more air than full-term infants because sucking is less efficient. They need rest periods during feedings because they have difficulty regulating their breathing while feeding.
7. Observe for coughing, gagging, cyanosis, changes in heart rate or respirations, and apnea. Evaluate the infant's ability to continue.	7. These signs show difficulty coordinating sucking, swallowing, and breathing, and possible aspiration.
8. Assess for signs of overfatigue: falling asleep during feedings, feedings lasting more than 25 to 30 minutes, increased respirations.	8. Feedings may require more energy than the infant has available. Infants who are overfatigued are more likely to aspirate.
9. Finish the feeding by gavage if necessary.	9. Completing the feeding by gavage conserves energy and prevents aspiration.
10. Position Giovanni on the right side or prone with his head elevated approximately 30 degrees after feeding.	10. The right-side position and elevation of the head allow gravity to help empty the stomach and fluids to drain if the infant regurgitates.
11. Include parents in the feedings. Teach them how to assess the infant's response to feedings.	11. Feeding allows parents to participate in the infant's care. Their comfort with feedings and learning about the infant's responses will help them prepare for discharge.

Evaluation: Giovanni consumes an average of 196 calories a day and gains an average of 31 g daily. He gradually takes more of his feeding by nipple and rarely needs gavage feeding to finish it. His respiratory rate remains under 60 breaths/minute, and he stays awake for the entire feeding.

Breast milk may increase feeding tolerance, reduce later allergies, improve retinal function, enhance neurologic development, and help prevent necrotizing enterocolitis (Meier & Brown, 1996). Breastfeeding may be less stressful than bottle feeding for preterm infants, and some infants can tolerate breastfeeding earlier and better than bottle feeding. Oxygenation levels often are higher during breastfeeding because the infant can regulate breathing and suckling better than with bottle feeding. In addition, the mother's body temperature helps keep the infant warm.

When the mother plans to breastfeed, she will need help with maintaining lactation until the infant is mature enough for nipple feedings. Teach her how to use a breast pump and give her sterile containers to store her milk. Tell her to place her milk in a refrigerator or freezer until she brings it to the NICU for the infant. If fortifiers will be added to the milk, explain the higher needs of the preterm infant so that the mother does not believe that her milk is inadequate.

Support the mother in her efforts in feeding, which may be difficult at first. Remind her that even full-term infants must learn how to breastfeed. Relaxation needed for feeding is difficult in the busy NICU. Provide as much privacy as possible, using a separate room or screens. Help the mother feel comfortable holding the tiny infant and any attached equipment such as monitor leads.

Adapt breastfeeding teaching to the needs of a very small infant. Show the mother how to use the cross cradle hold, which is very effective for small infants. The mother holds her breast with the hand on the same side, pressing slightly back and downward behind the areola to make the nipple prominent. She holds the infant's head in the other hand with the infant across her body and supported by her arm. This allows the mother to see the infant well during latching on and throughout the feeding.

A supplemental nursing system, a device that holds expressed breastmilk in a bag with a small tube attached to the mother's nipple, may be used to help infants receive more milk with less effort during early feedings. Other methods to increase the amount of milk received include supplementation with gavage or cup feedings. These methods avoid bottle feeding and may increase the length and success of breastfeeding.

Make the same observations of the infant during breastfeeding as during bottle feeding. Signs of fatigue, bradycardia, tachypnea, and apnea may show lack of readiness for breastfeeding. Be sure that the infant stays warm. The mother's body heat will help maintain the infant's temperature during feedings. Kangaroo care (p. 828) often can be combined with breastfeeding.

Making Ongoing Assessments

Continuously assess the infant's responses to all feeding methods. Watch for signs of distress, especially when feedings are first initiated. These may include changes in pulse or respiratory rate, decreased oxygen saturation, color changes, gagging, choking, and fatigue. Record the amount of breast milk or formula that the infant takes by gavage or bottle feeding and compare it with the amount needed to meet nutrient needs for the infant's age and weight. Because accurate estimation of milk intake is difficult, infants may be weighed on an electronic scale before and after breastfeedings. This allows supplementary gavage feeding amounts to be calculated based on the infant's oral intake.

Note the infant's response to other stimuli during feeding. Some infants respond well to being talked to and rocked during feedings. Others become distracted by any noise, motion, or nearby activities.

Weigh the infant daily at the same time of day with the same scale. Record the length and head circumference each week. Plot measurements on a growth chart for preterm infants to see whether changes are within expected ranges. Weight increase not accompanied by increased length may be caused by edema and may be a sign of a complication such as congestive heart failure.

Observe changes in the infant's ability to take feedings. The suck and swallow coordination should gradually improve with maturity and practice. As the infant becomes more mature, less energy should be expended during the feeding sessions. The infant will take the feedings more quickly and show fewer signs of fatigue, such as falling asleep during feedings.

Evaluation

If the goals have been met, the infant will consume adequate amounts of formula or breast milk to meet nutrient needs for age and weight and will gain weight as appropriate for age.

Check Your Reading

8. What can the nurse do for the infant at risk for overstimulation?
9. How does the nurse assess feeding tolerance?
10. How can the nurse help the mother who wants to breastfeed her preterm infant?

PARENTING

The birth of a preterm infant is generally unexpected and always emotionally traumatic to parents. Infants often are hurried to the NICU shortly after birth. Later, when parents see the infant attached to an array of machines, they may have difficulty developing feelings of attachment to a tiny baby who looks so different from what they expected. At first, parents cannot hold, feed, or offer any of the usual care that parents give their infants who do not have problems. The infant may not be capable of usual expected newborn behaviors such as making eye contact and grasping the parent's finger. When the infant's appearance and behavior are different from the parents' expectations, attachment may be delayed (Bialoskurski, Cox, & Hayes, 2000). Interference in the attachment process increases vulnerability for parents in establishing a nurturing relationship with the infant (Kenner & Amlung, 1999).

The extended hospitalization of the preterm infant results in separation of the parents from their newborn and disrupts family life. Parents must relinquish the role of primary caregiver during their infant's hospitalization. Loss of the parental role is a major stressor for parents of infants needing prolonged hospitalization. Some parents later say that they didn't feel like parents until they were able to hold or take the baby home (Miles, Wilson, & Docherty, 1999). Other stressors include worry about the infant's condition and potential outcome (Holditch-Davis & Miles, 2000).

Parents need help in understanding the infant's condition and what is expected to occur throughout the hospital stay. Parents perceive nurses as being among the most helpful in aiding them to cope with these stresses (Miles, Carlson, & Funk, 1996; Miles, Wilson, & Docherty, 1999). Nurses must evaluate the progress of attachment and assist parents to feel important in caring for their infant.

Assessment

Assess for signs of parental attachment on the first and subsequent visits to the NICU. Expect parents to be fearful at first but more able to focus on the infant as they get over the initial shock of preterm birth. Assess for common behaviors that show normal progression of attachment. These include talking about the infant in positive terms, pointing out physical characteristics, naming the infant, making eye contact, and calling the infant by name. Parents should ask questions about the infant. When they are able to hold and participate in the care of the infant, observe for gradual increase in comfort and skill. The parents should smile and talk to the infant and verbalize increasing confidence in their caretaking abilities.

Watch for signs that bonding is not occurring as expected. These include failure to perform usual attachment behaviors or a decrease in behaviors that were previously present. Parents who seem as interested in other infants in the NICU as in their own infant or talk about the infant in an impersonal way may be having difficulty. Note how often the parents make visits or calls to the NICU and changes that may indicate a need for support. Determine whether other stressors exist in the parents' lives that may interfere with their ability to visit and attach to the infant.

After the critical period in the early days after birth, healthy preterm infants become more stable. They still require specialized nursing care and hospitalization but gradually need fewer technologic interventions. They are sometimes called "growers" at this time. This is a time when parent participation in the infant's care should increase in preparation for discharge.

Analysis

Whenever parents and infants must be separated because of hospitalization during the newborn period, a risk for disruption of the attachment process exists. The nursing diagnosis that fits this concern is "Risk for Altered Parent/Infant Attachment related to separation of parents from infant and lack of understanding about the preterm infant's condition and characteristics."

CRITICAL TO REMEMBER

Signs That Bonding May Be Delayed

- Using negative terms to describe the infant
- Discussing the infant in impersonal or technical terms
- Failing to give the infant a name or to use the name
- Visiting or calling infrequently or not at all
- Decreasing the number and length of visits
- Showing interest in other infants equal to that in their own infant
- Refusing offers to hold and learn to care for the infant
- Showing a decrease in or lack of eye contact
- Spending less time talking to or smiling at the infant

Planning

The goals or expected outcomes for this nursing diagnosis are that the parents will:

- Demonstrate bonding behaviors, including visiting frequently and interacting as appropriate for the infant's condition throughout the hospital stay.
- Verbalize understanding of the preterm infant's condition and characteristics within 2 days.
- Express increasing comfort in caring for the infant within 1 week.

Interventions

Making Advance Preparations

Preparing for threatening situations such as preterm birth helps parents cope with the actual event. Parents at higher risk for a preterm birth should visit the NICU before delivery. If the mother is confined to bed, arrange for a nurse from the NICU to visit her so that she feels a link with the nursery and can ask questions. The father or another support person should have a tour of the nursery so that he will know where to go and can discuss the nursery environment with the mother.

Parents have many questions before the birth, which should be answered truthfully but in an encouraging manner. A major question is whether the infant is likely to survive, especially for infants born very early. One way physicians use to help parents understand is to inform them that at 24 weeks' gestation, approximately

40% of infants survive. The percent that survive increases approximately 10% for each additional week of gestation at birth and will be approximately 80% at 28 weeks (Koh, Harrison, & Morley, 1999). The nurse can help the parents get the information they desire and clarify it as necessary.

Assisting Parents at Birth

After the birth, allow the parents to see and touch the newborn in the delivery room, even if only for a few moments, so that they have a realistic idea of the infant's appearance and condition. If possible, allow the father or primary support person to watch the initial care in the NICU. Explain what is happening and why. This allows him to see the intensive efforts made on behalf of his infant, increases his confidence in the staff, and enables him to give the mother a full description later. Support the father and mother by using therapeutic communication techniques during this difficult time.

If the infant must be transported to another facility, having the transport team visit the parents just before they leave, if possible, is important. This helps the parents feel connected to their infant and the staff providing care. Leaving photographs with the parents is one way of helping them bond even though the infant is not with them.

Supporting Parents during Early Visits

Take the mother to the NICU as soon as she is able. If she is too ill to be with her infant, bring her photographs. Before parents first visit the infant, prepare them for what they will see by describing the equipment and its purposes, the various attachments to the infant, and the sounds of alarms (Figure 29-7). Explain how the infant will look and behave. (Table 29-1 provides specific steps that the nurse can follow to help parents become familiar with the NICU setting.)

At first, stay with the parents during visits. When they are comfortable, allow them time alone with the infant so that they can interact in private. Answer questions

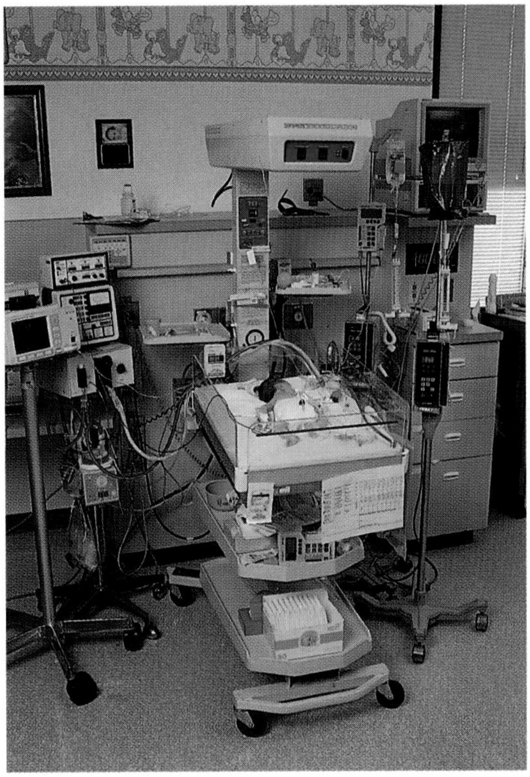

FIGURE 29-7 An infant in the NICU is surrounded by highly technologic equipment. This can be very frightening to parents at first. Preparation of parents before they visit is an important nursing responsibility.

Table 29-1

INTRODUCING PARENTS TO THE NICU SETTING

BEFORE PARENTS VISIT THE NICU

Describe the NICU environment. Include the noise of alarms, the busyness of the staff, and the number of people and sick infants.

Show parents photographs of the infant. This helps prepare them, but it is not as overwhelming as seeing the infant in person.

Describe the infant. Include the size, lack of fat, breathing, and weak cry.

Explain that no sound of crying can be heard if the infant is intubated. Include some human aspects: "He's a real fighter" or "She makes the funniest faces during her feedings."

Describe the equipment. Include ventilators, IV lines, and monitors. Explain how they look and how they are attached to the infant. Keep the explanations simple, without technical details.

WHEN PARENTS VISIT THE NICU

Help parents perform thorough handwashing or scrubbing with a brush and explain its purpose.

Stay with the parents during their visit. Having a familiar person nearby will help them feel more comfortable while they adjust to this unfamiliar environment.

Introduce them to their infant's nurse. Ask the NICU nurse to explain some of the things being done for the infant.

Provide parents with written information about the NICU so that they can take it home with them to read later. This usually includes visiting hours, telephone updates about the infant, availability of classes on infant care, and support groups.

Tell the parents that they will receive instruction on how to care for their infant in time. Encourage them to visit the infant as much as possible. Emphasize how important they are to their infant.

Offer realistic encouragement based on the infant's condition.

Provide an opportunity for the parents to express their concerns and feelings and ask questions.

Therapeutic Communication

Reassuring Parents during Visits to the NICU

Ann Gibson gave birth to a preterm infant, Molly, at 30 weeks' gestation. Ann is visiting the NICU for the first time the day after the birth. The nurse, Lee Wills, has talked to her about what to expect and stays with her during the visit.

Ann: Oh, she looks so tiny! I saw her for only a minute after she was born, and I didn't really get a good look. How can she ever survive when she's so small and covered with tubes?

Lee: So far, Molly is doing very well. Her vital signs are stable, and she's holding her own. But it is frightening when she looks so small and vulnerable, isn't it? *(Offering realistic reassurance and reflecting Ann's fearful feelings. Using infant's name to promote bonding.)*

Ann: I stayed in bed like they told me to do. I thought she wouldn't be born so soon if I stayed in bed.

Lee: It must have been a shock, especially when you tried so hard to prevent it. *(Reflecting feelings and acknowledging that Ann did what she could to prevent early birth.)*

Ann: Now she's so tiny and so sick! She looks so different from what I expected.

Lee: Molly's small, but babies her size grow very quickly. Would you like to touch her? *(Offering realistic reassurance and attempting to bring Ann closer to her infant.)*

Ann: Oh, I might hurt her. Maybe I should wait until she's bigger.

Lee: Even tiny babies like to have their mothers stroke their skin and talk to them. She listened to your voice all through your pregnancy, so it is familiar to her. Why don't you hold her hand while I work with her? And I can tell you about all this equipment and what we are doing for Molly. *(Emphasizing the mother's importance, involving her in care being given, and offering information about the infant's equipment and care.)*

and explain changes in the infant's condition and treatment. Use therapeutic communication as the parents cope with feelings of grief, guilt, and emotional turmoil.

Parents should touch the infant as soon as possible because this helps promote the development of attachment. They may be hesitant initially because of fear that they will interfere with equipment. The smaller the infant, the more reluctant parents may be. Some parents may hesitate to touch because they are afraid of becoming attached to an infant whom they may lose. They will need sensitive support from the nurse until they are ready to progress in their relationship with the infant.

Show parents how to touch in ways appropriate for the infant, such as holding the infant's hand through the portholes of the incubator or stroking the small areas of skin not encumbered by equipment. Explain to parents that handling is kept to a minimum for physiologically unstable infants because it is too stressful to them. As the infant becomes more stable and mature, help parents learn various kinds of touch and determine which ones work best with their infant. This helps parents feel more a part of the infant's plan of care. Gentle massage and structured tactile stimulation may be used with stable infants and may improve the infant's ability to respond positively to touch.

Holding the baby is particularly important to parents who may interpret it as a very positive sign of the infant's condition. Yet it also may be frightening, especially if the infant is attached to various kinds of equipment. Help the parents find a comfortable position for themselves and the infant and point out signs of a positive response from the infant.

Providing Information

Explain all nursing care, its purpose, and the expected response. Point out ways in which preterm infants are similar to and different from full-term infants to help parents develop a realistic understanding of the infant's capabilities.

Offer realistic reassurance about the infant's condition. This means emphasizing positive aspects yet being truthful in all communication with the parents. If they have misconceptions or did not understand a physician's explanations, clarify or ask the physician to go over specific information again. Translate medical terms into words that the parents can understand. Use an interpreter if the parents do not understand English.

Repeat explanations, especially at first. Because of their emotional distress, parents often are unable to fully comprehend or remember what is said to them.

Offer written information in the language of the parents about NICU policies and procedures. Explanations about visiting hours, regulation of visitors, routines for handwashing or scrubbing with a brush, and the role of parents can be reinforced in writing so they are available for later reading by overwhelmed parents.

Instituting Kangaroo Care

Begin kangaroo care (KC) as soon as possible. KC is a method of providing skin-to-skin contact between preterm infants and their parents. The infant, wearing only a diaper and hat, is placed under the mother's clothes between her breasts (Figure 29-8). Mothers may breastfeed if they wish and if the infant is able. Fathers also are encouraged to participate in KC (Figure 29-9).

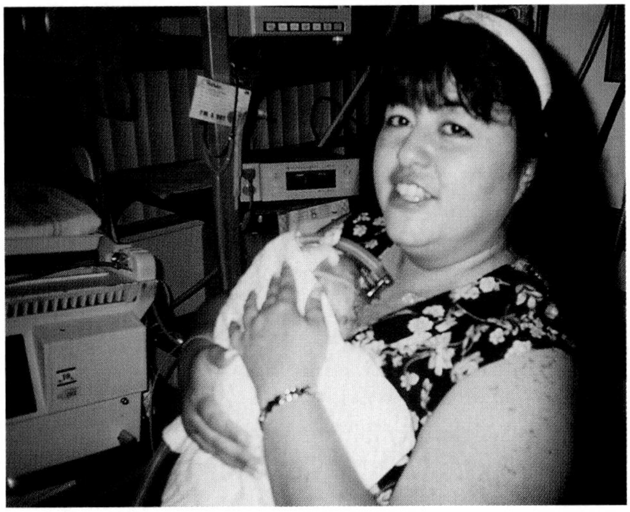

FIGURE 29-8 This mother has her 27-week-gestation preterm infant tucked under clothes against her skin as she gives kangaroo care. Such care enhances bonding and has many other benefits for infants and parents.

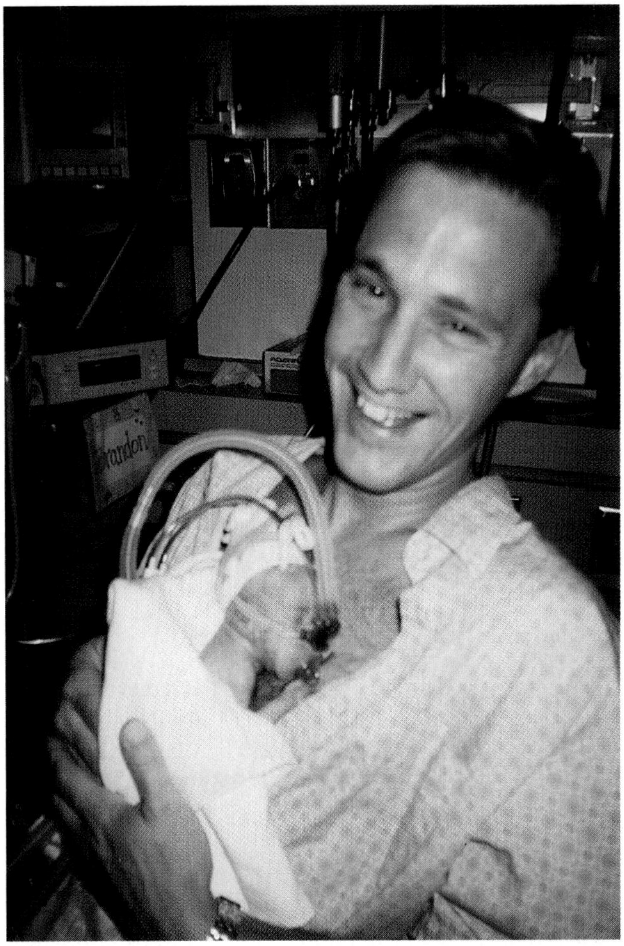

FIGURE 29-9 Even though he is intubated, this 1-lb, 8-oz preterm infant goes to sleep against his father's chest.

Explain the advantages of KC to parents and elicit their participation. This method of care has been found safe for stable infants, even if intubated; provides an opportunity for parents to participate in the infant's care; and increases parental attachment. KC provides developmental care that is so important for the preterm infant. The upright position of the infant against the parent's chest improves oxygen saturation and improves pulmonary function (Koch, 1999). The containment of the extremities decreases purposeless movements that use valuable oxygen and calories. Direct contact with the parent's skin helps the infant to maintain body temperature, and quiet sleep is doubled during KC (Luddington-Hoe & Engler, 1999). Parents often are gratified to see how they are able to cause this positive response in their infants.

Facilitating Interaction

Parents may feel rejected by the infant's lack of the expected response during interactions. Explain to them that infants born at less than 34 weeks of gestation may not be able to cope with socialization. The talking, smiling, and eye contact so effective with full-term infants may be too stimulating for very young or ill preterm infants. Encourage forms of touch and interaction based on the individual infant's capacity. Quiet holding or gentle stroking may be better until the infant is able to tolerate more.

Teach parents signs of overstimulation so that they can adapt their interaction to meet the infant's needs. Let them know that stress signs like gaze aversion help protect the infant from overstimulation and the infant should be allowed a short rest period without added stimuli. Discuss methods to avoid too much stimulation and ways to calm the infant. If several types of stimulation (such as rocking, eye contact, and talking) cause signs of distress, suggest they stop one or more activities until the infant has had a period of rest. Show them ways to position the infant with the hands near the mouth so that the infant can suck on them as a self-comforting measure.

As the infant matures, show parents signs that the infant is ready for more interaction and suggest appropriate types of stimulation. Point out small signs of improvement and even minor strengths. Talk about individual characteristics that make this infant different from all others. The way the infant eats, reacts to sounds, or even how the infant seems to get tangled in the monitor leads may help parents feel closer to their newborn and understand the infant's special characteristics.

Involve the parents in care of the infant as soon as possible (Figure 29-10). As they become familiar with the NICU setting and equipment, more involvement will help them feel a sense of control. At first, plan to change

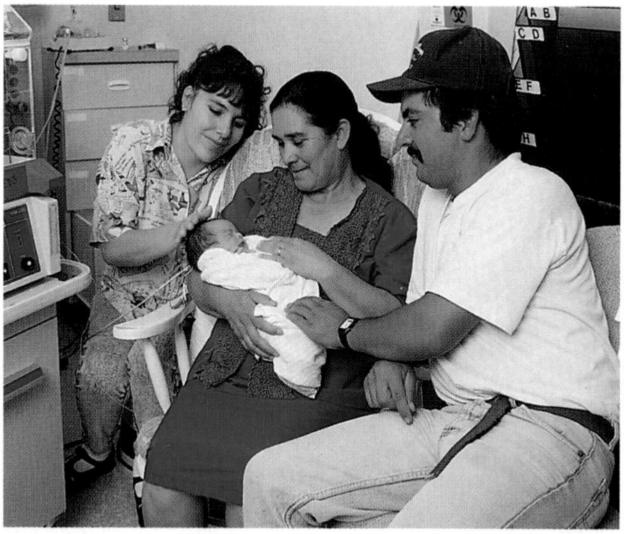

FIGURE 29-10 The parents look on while the grandmother holds the infant in the NICU.

the linens in the incubator or radiant warmer when the parents are there so that they can hold their infant, even if for only a few moments. As the infant's condition improves, parents can develop skill in caring for a tiny infant by changing diapers, feeding, and bathing.

Increasing Parental Decision Making

Encourage parents to help make large and small decisions about care of the infant. Give them the information they need to take an active part in decisions made about the infant's treatment plan. This will increase their feelings of control over a situation in which many parents feel they have little power.

Alleviating Concerns

Encourage parents to call the NICU at any time for information about their infant. This helps allay worry when parents wake up at night and wonder how the infant is doing. It is especially beneficial for parents not able to visit the infant because of distance or other reasons.

Parents also need support from others besides nursing staff. Put them in touch with other parents who have had a preterm infant. Talking with those who have faced the same problems can be very comforting. They can compare notes and get down-to-earth suggestions from an experienced parent's point of view.

Helping with Ongoing Problems

Parents often are unprepared for the inconsistent progress that infants often make after surviving the risks of the early days. They expect steady progress once the infant can eat and breathe alone. However, complications such as necrotizing enterocolitis can cause major setbacks at this time. Parents need extensive support from the nurse to cope with a new crisis. Use therapeutic communication techniques to help them express and cope with their extreme disappointment. Give information about the infant's changing condition and what to expect in the days ahead.

Preparing for Discharge

Because infants go home very early, the parents need to understand the expected hospital course. If a clinical pathway is being used for the infant, give them a copy. They can chart the infant's achievement of major milestones in development and changes in care as the infant moves toward discharge. This helps them prepare themselves and their home to provide the special care that their infant may need after discharge.

Teach parents any special procedures that the infant will need after discharge. Begin early to show them ways to manage treatments and medications. Observe the parents as they perform care until they are comfortable and can do it safely. Help them learn what is normal for their infant and ways to recognize and respond to abnormal signs. Some hospitals have parents spend a night in a special "parent room," where they take over full 24-hour care of the infant. This provides an opportunity to practice complete care of the infant in an environment where help is available if needed.

Help the parents determine what adaptations they will need to make at home before discharge. Utility companies should be notified if the infant is considered medically fragile. This ensures the family receives priority service in cases of power failure. Ordering special equipment and supplies may be necessary before the infant can go home. Home nursing services arrangements should be completed.

Discuss what to expect in care of the infant after discharge. Infants may require oxygen, suctioning, or tube feedings, which parents will have to learn to perform. Some infants have such complex treatments as apnea monitors or even home mechanical ventilation (Vargo & Trotter, 1998). Many infants need feedings every 3 hours, day and night, to help them gain the 20 to 40 g a day expected when the infant is at home (Sifuentes, 2000). Feedings may be time consuming, and parental fatigue resulting from interruptions to their sleep may be more than they expected. Infants are used to the noises of a nursery 24 hours a day and may not sleep well at first in a quiet home environment. Suggest parents play soft music and use a night light for the first week. They should gradually eliminate these aids to avoid conditioning the infant to their use. Visitors and noise or activity may be too much for the infant at first and should be limited.

Explore with parents what kind of help they might need to meet the everyday requirements of the infant and the rest of the family. Help them identify where they might find assistance from family and friends. Refer the parents to a family support group, if available, so that they can learn from the experiences of other parents and receive encouragement and emotional support for the problems they will encounter. Many hospitals offer these groups, which often are facilitated by nurses and social workers.

Help parents form realistic expectations of the infant. For example, they should know that the infant will accomplish developmental tasks, such as crawling and walking, later than full-term infants. Parents should base expectations on the infant's developmental or corrected age rather than chronologic age.

Assist the parents in planning for integrating the new infant into the family. Meeting the needs of their other children, in addition to the new responsibilities of caring for the preterm infant, is a major source of worry. Listen to their concerns about other children, and encourage siblings to visit, if possible. Caution parents that siblings with infections should not visit the infant who cannot fight off infections well. Help parents explain to the other children what they will see when they visit the infant. Siblings should touch or hold the infant, if possible, to help them bond. Taking photographs of the siblings with the infant will help them remember the visit.

Evaluation

Goals are met if parents visit often and interact appropriately with the infant, express their understanding of and comfort with the infant's needs, and take an increasingly active role in the care of the infant.

Check Your Reading

11. How can the nurse help parents be comfortable with their preterm infant?
12. How should the nurse prepare parents for the discharge of their preterm infant?

COMMON COMPLICATIONS OF PRETERM INFANTS

The preterm infant is at risk for a number of complications that increase as the infant's gestational age and birth weight decrease. Some complications that occur in full-term and preterm infants, such as hyperbilirubinemia and patent ductus arteriosus, are discussed in Chapter 30. Complications most often associated with preterm birth are discussed in this section.

Respiratory Distress Syndrome

Although more than 90% of affected infants now survive respiratory distress syndrome (RDS), also called "hyaline membrane disease," it causes 20% of all neonatal deaths in the United States (Gomella, et al., 1999). The syndrome occurs most often in preterm infants. Approximately 50% of infants born at 26 to 28 weeks' gestation, but fewer than 20% to 30% of those born at 30 to 31 weeks' gestation, develop the condition (Whitsett, et al., 1999). RDS also occurs in birth asphyxia, birth by cesarean, and infants of diabetic mothers because these conditions interfere with surfactant production. It is less frequent, however, when chronic fetal stress such as heroin addiction, pregnancy-induced hypertension, and smoking causes the lungs to mature more quickly (Casey, 1999).

Pathophysiology

RDS is caused by insufficient production of surfactant, a phospholipid that lines the alveoli. Surfactant is first produced in the alveoli at 22 weeks of gestation. By 34 to 36 weeks, production of surfactant is usually mature enough to enable the infant to breathe normally outside the uterus (Hagedorn, Gardner, & Abman, 1998).

Surfactant decreases surface tension to allow the alveoli to remain open when air is exhaled. It must be continuously produced as it is being used. When too little surfactant exists, the alveoli collapse each time the infant exhales. The lungs become noncompliant, or "stiff," and resist expansion. Noncompliant lungs require a much higher negative pressure for the alveoli to open each time the infant inhales. Severe retractions occur with each breath, drawing the weak muscles of the chest wall inward. The resulting pressure on the lungs further interferes with expansion.

As fewer alveoli expand, atelectasis (collapse) and hypoxia occur. This causes pulmonary vasoconstriction and decreased blood flow to the lungs because of the high resistance within the vessels of the lungs. Persistent pulmonary hypertension can result in a return to fetal circulation patterns, with opening of the ductus arteriosus. Respiratory and metabolic acidosis and alveolar necrosis further complicate the condition by interfering with surfactant synthesis. Hyaline membranes consisting of debris from necrotic cells in a proteinaceous material are an added problem.

Tests of amniotic fluid can detect lecithin, sphingomyelin, phosphatidylglycerol, and phosphatidylinositol, which are components of surfactant. These tests can predict whether the fetal lungs are mature enough so that survival outside of the uterus is possible (see Chapter 10, p. 227). The incidence and severity of RDS may be reduced by giving the mother corticosteroids at least 24 hours before birth (Chapter 27, p. 757).

Manifestations

Signs of RDS begin during the first hours after birth, often become worse on the next day, and may begin to improve within 72 hours after birth. They include tachypnea, nasal flaring, retractions, and cyanosis. Audible grunting on expiration is characteristic and signifies physiologic efforts to maintain lung expansion. Breath sounds may be decreased or wet. Acidosis develops as a result of hypoxemia. Chest radiographs show the "ground glass" appearance of the lungs that is characteristic of RDS. Areas of atelectasis are present.

Therapeutic Management

Surfactant replacement therapy is used prophylactically to prevent RDS or as "rescue" treatment once RDS has occurred. It is instilled into the infant's trachea during stabilization after birth or as soon as signs of RDS become apparent. Improvement in breathing occurs in minutes. Doses are repeated if necessary. Infants treated with surfactant have higher survival rates and decreased severity and fewer complications of RDS, although they may have other complications resulting from their prematurity.

Other treatment is supportive, including mechanical ventilation, correction of the acidosis, IV fluids, and care of additional complications.

Nursing Considerations

The nurse observes for signs of developing RDS at birth and during the early hours after the delivery. Changes in the infant's condition are constantly assessed. For example, diuresis may occur with improvement in the disease. Changes in ventilator settings may be necessary as the infant's ability to oxygenate increases. Observation for complications such as patent ductus arteriosus and bronchopulmonary dysplasia is important. Other care is similar to general care for the preterm infant.

Bronchopulmonary Dysplasia

Bronchopulmonary dysplasia (BPD), also known as "chronic lung disease," is a chronic condition occurring most often in infants weighing less than 1500 g at birth. The condition is said to be present when an infant remains dependent on oxygen at 36 weeks' postconceptional age (Stoll & Kliegman, 2000). Mortality rate increases with decreasing gestational age. The rate is 85% in infants born at 700 g but only 5% in infants who weigh more than 1500 g at birth (Casey, 1999).

Pathophysiology

BPD results from a combination of factors. High levels of oxygen, damage from oxygen-free radicals, and high positive-pressure ventilation that causes lung injury are major factors in the condition. The result is inflammation, atelectasis, edema, and airway hyperreactivity with loss of cilia, thickening of the walls of the alveoli, and fibrotic changes.

Manifestations

The major sign of BPD is an increased need for ventilation or an inability to be weaned from the ventilation and oxygen. Other signs include retractions, rales, respiratory acidosis, increased secretions, bronchospasm, and characteristic changes in the lungs on chest radiographs. Pulmonary edema may occur.

Therapeutic Management

Prevention includes use of maternal steroids to reduce prematurity and RDS, minimal exposure to oxygen and pressure with ventilation, and avoidance of fluid overload and nutrition management. High-frequency ventilation or other newer modalities also may help prevent BPD. Treatment is supportive, with gradual decreases in the amount of oxygen, bronchodilators, diuretics, and antibiotics as necessary. Corticosteroids are controversial because they improve lung function in a short time, but complications of use may occur and long-term outcomes may not be improved. The infant may go home on long-term oxygen therapy, and some need frequent rehospitalization for respiratory infections.

Alveoli normally increase in number from 20 to 70 million at birth to as many as 300 to 400 million at 2 to 8 years of age (Whitsett, et al., 1999). Many infants who survive the first year have gradual improvement of lung function, but some pulmonary problems may remain.

Periventricular-Intraventricular Hemorrhage

Periventricular-intraventricular hemorrhage (PIVH) occurs in 20% to 30% of infants of less than 32 weeks' gestation or weighing less than 1500 g (Moe & Paige, 1998).

Pathophysiology

PIVH results from rupture of the fragile blood vessels in the germinal matrix, located around the ventricles of the brain. It is most often associated with hypoxic injury to the vessels, increased or decreased blood pressure and increased or fluctuating cerebral blood flow, and rupture of blood vessels. Rapid volume expansion, hypercarbia, anemia, and hypoglycemia are other causes.

Hemorrhage is graded 1 through 4, according to the amount of bleeding. Grade 1 is a very small bleed outside ventricle walls, producing few, if any, clinical changes. Grade 2 hemorrhage extends into the lateral ventricles, and grade 3 distends at least one ventricle. Grade 4 hemorrhage extends into cerebral tissue.

Although fewer complications and less mortality occurs with grade 1 or 2 hemorrhages, infants with grade 3 and 4 hemorrhages may have neurologic abnormalities and developmental delays. The degree of neurologic deficits may not always correlate with the amount of hemorrhage, however. The mortality rate for all infants with PIVH ranges from 5% to 20% for infants with moderate bleeding and 50% for those with severe hemorrhage (Blackburn, 1998).

Manifestations

Signs of PIVH are determined by the severity of the hemorrhage. They may include lethargy, poor muscle tone, deterioration of respiratory status with cyanosis or apnea, drop in hematocrit level, decreased reflexes, full or bulging fontanelle, and seizures.

Therapeutic Management

Screening by ultrasound is performed at 1 week and repeated in 2 weeks if bleeding is present. Treatment is supportive and focuses on maintaining respiratory function and dealing with other complications. Hydrocephalus may develop from blockage of cerebrospinal fluid flow. Lumbar taps or a ventriculoperitoneal shunt may be necessary to drain the fluid.

Nursing Considerations

Many aspects of care may increase cerebral blood flow. These include mechanical ventilation, suctioning, exchange transfusions, and others. Therefore the nurse must be alert for early signs of PIVH. Nursing care includes measurement of the head circumference daily and observation for changes in neurologic status, which may be subtle. Increases in blood pressure from excessive handling or crying and suctioning should be avoided. Developmental care has been found helpful in preventing or minimizing the problem.

Parents will need assistance to cope with the diagnosis and their concerns regarding long-term implications. They should learn ways to assess for signs of hydrocephalus and understand that follow-up care may include periodic ultrasound examinations.

Retinopathy of Prematurity

Retinopathy of prematurity (ROP), previously known as "retrolental fibroplasia," may result in visual impairment or blindness in preterm infants. It occurs more often in infants weighing less than 1000 g.

Pathophysiology

ROP is caused by damage to immature blood vessels in the retina of the eye. Once thought to be caused only by too much oxygen, ROP can result from too much or not enough oxygen, acidosis, prolonged mechanical ventilation, sepsis, and shock (Lee, 1999). Oxygen concentration and mechanical ventilation are important variables. The condition has become more common with the increase in survival of VLBW infants. These infants need higher levels of oxygen to survive, and their immature retinas are more prone to the condition.

In ROP, immature blood vessels in the retina of the eye constrict and become permanently occluded. New vessels proliferate, extending throughout the retina and into the vitreous of the eye. Hemorrhages from the fragile vessels may cause scarring, traction on the retina, and retinal detachment.

Therapeutic Management

Infants delivered at less than 28 weeks' gestation or those weighing less than 1500 g should be screened 4 to 6 weeks after birth or at 31 to 33 weeks' corrected age to detect changes of the eye (AAP/ACOG, 1997). Many NICUs screen infants at younger ages to obtain baseline data with a series of follow-up examinations for early identification of changes. Laser surgery and cryotherapy have been used to destroy the proliferating blood vessels. Reattachment of the retina also may be necessary. Studies of use of vitamin E supplements and decreased exposure to lights have been conducted; however, results are inconclusive. Many infants have a spontaneous regression with little or no impairment of vision.

Nursing Considerations

The nurse should check the pulse oximeter equipment and readings frequently for any infant receiving oxygen. Parents should be informed about ophthalmology tests and receive explanation of results. Mydriatic eye drops, given to dilate the eyes, may cause feeding intolerance. If surgery is performed, the eye is assessed for drainage. Ice packs may be used for edema over the eye and pain medication should be given.

Necrotizing Enterocolitis

Necrotizing enterocolitis (NEC) is a serious condition of the intestinal tract, with necrotic lesions of the mucosa of the intestines. The mortality rate is 25% to 30% (Berseth & Abrums, 1998).

Pathophysiology

Although the exact causes are unknown, NEC may be caused by interference with blood supply to the intestinal mucosa. During asphyxia, blood is diverted from the gastrointestinal tract to the brain, heart, and kidneys. Sepsis, polycythemia, and maternal cocaine use are other causes of decrease in intestinal blood flow. The resulting ischemia may make the mucosa more susceptible to invasion with bacteria. When infants are fed, bacteria proliferate and gas-forming organisms may invade the intestinal wall. Eventually, necrosis, perforation, and peritonitis may occur. Other factors may be feeding the infant too early or too late, or advancing feedings too quickly. Breast milk may have a preventive effect on the development of NEC.

Manifestations

Signs include increased abdominal girth caused by distention, increased gastric residuals, decreased or absent bowel sounds, loops of bowel seen through the abdominal wall, vomiting, bile-stained residuals, signs of infection, and blood in the stools. Apnea, bradycardia, temperature instability, and lethargy also may be present. On radiographs, loops of bowel dilated with air and layers of gas within the intestinal wall are present. The presence of free air in the peritoneum indicates that perforation has occurred.

Therapeutic Management

Treatment includes antibiotics, discontinuation of oral feedings, continuous or intermittent gastric suction, and use of parenteral nutrition to rest the intestines.

Surgery may be necessary if perforation or continued lack of improvement occurs. The necrotic area is removed, and an ostomy may be performed.

Nursing Considerations

Early recognition of signs of NEC is essential to decrease mortality. Because nurses are constantly observing the infant, they often are able to detect the early, subtle signs that lead to prompt diagnosis. Noting one or more signs will prompt the nurse to withhold the next feeding and notify the physician. The infant should be positioned on the side to minimize the effects of pressure on the diaphragm from the distended intestines. During recovery, the nurse must observe for signs of feeding intolerance when feedings are resumed. Scar tissue may cause partial or complete bowel obstruction.

POSTTERM INFANTS

Postterm infants are those born after the 42nd week of gestation. Their longer-than-normal gestation places them at risk for a number of complications.

Scope of the Problem

Approximately 6% to 12% of all pregnancies are considered postterm. Postterm infants have a two to three times higher perinatal mortality rate than infants born at term. The major concern is with placenta functioning during the last weeks of pregnancy. In 20% to 30% of postterm pregnancies, placental insufficiency occurs because placental function deteriorates, causing interference with oxygen and nutrient supply. This results in hypoxia and malnourishment in the fetus and is called *postmaturity syndrome* or *dysmaturity syndrome* (Ogundipe & Hamilton, 1998).

Generally, however, the fetus continues to be well supported by the placenta. Some may grow to more than 4000 g (8 lb, 13 oz) and are at risk for birth injuries or cesarean birth because of their size.

Assessment

If placental insufficiency occurs, prenatal asphyxia and decreased amniotic fluid volume may be present. Fetal distress may occur during labor and the fetus may pass meconium as a result of hypoxia, increasing the risk of meconium aspiration at delivery. Meconium passage may occur shortly before birth or the cord, skin, and nails may be stained at birth, indicating that meconium was present for some time.

Postterm infants should be assessed for hypoglycemia because of rapid use of glycogen stores. If loss of subcutaneous fat has occurred, the infant is at risk for low temperature. Skin changes also may occur with peeling, sloughing, and even maceration (Putman, 1999). Vernix and lanugo are sparse or absent, and fingernails are long.

Therapeutic Management

Therapeutic management focuses on prevention and symptomatic treatment. Expectant mothers who are "overdue" are scheduled for tests of placental functioning, and labor is induced if signs of placental deterioration exist. If the fetus cannot tolerate labor, a cesarean birth is necessary. Apgar scores less than 7 are more likely in postterm infants. In cases of asphyxia or meconium aspiration, respiratory support is needed at birth (Chapter 30, pp. 841 and 844).

Nursing Considerations

The nurse's role is primarily one of prevention of complications, where possible, and monitoring of changes in status. During labor and delivery, the nurse responds appropriately to fetal heart rate decelerations, prepares for and assists in emergency delivery, and cares for respiratory problems at birth. Initial assessments should include a thorough assessment for injuries if the infant is large.

Signs of postmaturity syndrome in infants are noted during the initial assessment. If the mother's due date was calculated incorrectly, the condition will be unexpected. Attention to thermoregulation and early feeding will be important if the infant was poorly nourished by a poorly functioning placenta.

SMALL-FOR-GESTATIONAL AGE INFANTS

Small-for-gestational age (SGA) infants are those who fall below the 10th percentile in size on growth charts. They have had IUGR. Some infants who do not meet the definition for SGA may have IUGR and fail to grow to full potential in utero for a variety of reasons. However, the terms *SGA* and *IUGR* often are used interchangeably.

Infants who are SGA may be preterm, full-term, or postterm but have failed to grow at the rate expected for the time spent in utero. Approximately one third of all infants who have a low birth weight are full term but IUGR (Stoll & Kliegman, 2000).

Causes

Many risk factors may cause an infant to be SGA. Congenital malformations, chromosomal anomalies, and fetal infections from rubella or cytomegalovirus may cause IUGR. Poor placental function resulting from aging, small size, separation, or malformation may interfere with fetal growth. Illness in the expectant mother, including pregnancy-induced hypertension and severe diabetes, restricts uteroplacental blood flow and decreases fetal growth. Smoking, drug or alcohol abuse, and severe maternal malnutrition also impair fetal growth.

Scope of Problem

Intrauterine growth restriction occurs in 3% to 10% of all pregnancies, and affected infants have a four to eight times higher perinatal mortality rate than infants who are not growth restricted. Approximately half of infants who survive have serious problems (Gomella, et al, 1999).

Full-term infants who are SGA are subject to many of the same complications as those who are preterm or postterm. Specific complications and their severity depend on the cause and degree of growth restriction. Infants with congenital defects also have problems at birth associated with the anomaly. Drug-exposed infants may have the added complication of drug withdrawal. SGA infants are more likely to experience fetal distress and asphyxia. Problems tend to be greatest in infants who are preterm in addition to being SGA.

Low Apgar scores, meconium aspiration, and polycythemia are increased in the SGA infant. Hypoglycemia is common because little storage of glycogen exists in the liver. Although muscle tone enables the SGA infant to maintain better flexion than the preterm infant, SGA infants are prone to inadequate thermoregulation because subcutaneous and brown fat stores have been used to survive in utero. If hypoglycemia develops, inadequate glucose is available for increased metabolism to produce heat, increasing the problem.

Characteristics

The appearance of the SGA infant varies according to whether the cause of growth restriction began early or late in the pregnancy. This is because growth restriction affects the weight first. If it continues, the length and then the head size eventually will be affected.

Symmetric growth restriction involves the entire body. It may be caused by congenital anomalies or exposure to infections or drugs early in pregnancy. Although the infant's weight, length, and head circumference are all below the 10th percentile, the body is proportionate and appears normally developed for size. The total number of cells decreases, and the infant may have long-term complications. These infants often are small throughout their lives.

Asymmetric restriction is caused by complications that begin after 28 weeks of gestation, such as pregnancy-induced hypertension. In asymmetric restriction, the head is normal in size but seems large for the rest of the body. Brain growth and heart size are normal, but other organs may be small in size. The length is normal, but the weight is below the 10th percentile for gestational age. The infant appears long and thin. The loose skin has longitudinal thigh creases from loss of subcutaneous fat. The infant has sparse hair, a thin cord, dry skin, and the wide-eyed look associated with intrauterine hypoxia. These infants generally "catch up" in growth if they are adequately nourished after birth (Putman, 1999).

Therapeutic Management

Therapeutic management is focused on prevention with good prenatal care to identify and treat problems early. When growth restriction cannot be prevented, ultrasound examination may permit early discovery of the condition so that the infant can be delivered early, if necessary, and preparation can be made for the expected complications at birth. Problems after birth are treated as they occur.

Nursing Considerations

Because the causes of growth restriction are so varied, care of the SGA infant must be adapted to meet the specific problems that the infant demonstrates. When signs of growth restriction are present, the nurse must observe for complications that commonly accompany it. The general appearance and measurements will give an indication of the type of growth restriction that has occurred. Measurements of the head, chest, length, and weight will be below normal in the infant with symmetric growth restriction. If the restriction is asymmetric, the head circumference and length will be normal and the chest circumference and weight will be low.

The nurse should assess for hypoglycemia, especially in asymmetric, growth-restricted infants. The brain of the infant is normal and needs large amounts of glucose, but the liver is small and has inadequate stores of glycogen. Calorie needs will be higher than for a normal infant, making early and more frequent feedings important. Temperature regulation and respiratory support are added nursing concerns.

LARGE-FOR-GESTATIONAL AGE INFANTS

Large-for-gestational age (LGA) infants are those who are above the 90th percentile on intrauterine growth charts. They may weigh more than 4000 g (8 lb, 13 oz) and are usually born at term, although they may be preterm or postterm. The preterm LGA infant may be mistaken for full-term but has the same problems as other preterm infants.

Causes

Infants who are LGA may be born to multiparas, large parents, and certain ethnic groups known to have large infants. Diabetes in the mother may also cause increased size (Chapter 30, p. 855), as may erythroblastosis fetalis (Chapter 30, p. 847).

Scope of the Problem

The LGA infant is more likely to go through a longer labor, have injury during birth, or need a cesarean birth. Shoulder dystocia may occur because the

Table 29-2
COMMON NURSING DIAGNOSES FOR PRETERM INFANTS

*Activity Intolerance
Altered Family Processes
Ineffective Airway Clearance
Ineffective Thermoregulation
Pain
*Risk for Altered Growth and Development
*Risk for Altered Nutrition: Less Than Body Requirements
*Risk for Altered Parent/Infant Attachment
Risk for Altered Parenting
Risk for Caregiver Role Strain
Risk for Fluid Volume Deficit or Fluid Volume Excess
Risk for Impaired Skin Integrity
Risk for Infection

*Nursing diagnoses explored in this chapter.

shoulders are too large to fit through the pelvis. Fractures of the clavicle or skull, damage to the brachial plexus or facial or phrenic nerves, cephalhematoma, and bruising occur more often in these infants than those of normal size. Congenital heart defects and a higher mortality rate also are more common (Stoll & Kliegman, 1999).

Therapeutic Management

Therapeutic management is based on identification of macrosomia (large size) during pregnancy by measurements of fundal height and ultrasound examination. Delivery problems may lead to use of forceps, vacuum extraction, or cesarean birth. Specific treatment involves identification and treatment of birth injuries and complications as they arise.

Nursing Considerations

The nurse assists in a difficult delivery or cesarean birth resulting from dystocias when the infant is LGA. After birth, the infant is carefully assessed for injuries or other complications such as hypoglycemia or polycythemia (pp. 516 and 856). Nursing care is geared to problems presented. (See Table 29-2.)

Check Your Reading

13. What is the typical appearance of the infant with postmaturity syndrome?
14. What special problems might a postmature infant have?
15. How are symmetric and asymmetric IUGR different?
16. What problems may occur in infants who are LGA?

SUMMARY CONCEPTS

- Low socioeconomic status increases risk of preterm birth because of possible decreased general health, nutrition, and medical care and lack of economic, social, and emotional support.
- Preterm infants differ in appearance from full-term infants. Some differences include small size, limp posture, red skin, abundant vernix and lanugo, and immature ears and genitals.
- The lungs of preterm infants may lack adequate surfactant, which may cause the lungs to be noncompliant, increasing the amount of energy necessary for breathing and leading to atelectasis.
- Other factors that may increase respiratory problems are poor cough reflex, narrow respiratory passages, and weak muscles.
- Preterm infants should be positioned on the side or prone to increase drainage of respiratory secretions. The prone position decreases breathing effort because respiratory muscles are used efficiently. In the supine position, a small roll should be placed under the shoulders to straighten the airway.
- Preterm infants are prone to cold stress because they have thin skin with blood vessels near the surface, little subcutaneous or brown fat, a large surface area, a limp position, and an immature temperature control center.
- Maintaining a neutral thermal environment at all times for infants is important. The nurse should prevent air drafts, use warmed oxygen, and keep incubator doors and portholes closed. After being taken out of heating devices, the infant should be wrapped in warmed blankets and wear a hat.
- Preterm infants are subject to increased insensible water losses and have difficulty maintaining fluid balance. Their kidneys do not concentrate or dilute urine as well as those of full-term infants. Intake and output must be carefully measured.
- Preterm infants are subject to infections because they lack passive antibodies from the mother, have an immature immune system, have fragile skin, and are subjected to many invasive procedures.
- The nurse must watch carefully for signs of pain and use comfort measures and medications to alleviate it.
- Infants demonstrate that they are receiving too much stimulation by changes in oxygenation and behavior. The nurse should schedule care to allow rest periods, keep noise to a minimum, and teach parents ways to interact with the infant appropriately.
- Preterm infants lack nutrient stores and need more nutrients but do not absorb them well. They lack coordination in sucking and swallowing and fatigue easily.
- Signs indicating that an infant may be ready for nipple feeding include rooting, sucking on a gavage tube or pacifier, presence of gag reflex, and respiratory rate below 60 breaths per minute. Some infants, however, suck vigorously on a pacifier but are not yet ready for all the steps involved in nipple feeding.
- The nurse should teach mothers who wish to breastfeed their preterm infants ways to use a breast pump and store breast milk. Nurses provide privacy, give support and encouragement, explain the infant's behavior, and answer general questions about breastfeeding.

- Nurses can increase parents' comfort with their preterm infant by providing information, spending time with parents during visits, offering therapeutic communication and realistic encouragement, and involving parents in care of the infant.
- Preparation for discharge should be started early in the infant's hospital stay. This allows parents to gradually learn about and take on increasing responsibility in the care of the infant until they are comfortable with complete care.
- Common complications of preterm birth are respiratory distress syndrome, bronchopulmonary dysplasia, periventricular-intraventricular hemorrhage, retinopathy of prematurity, and necrotizing enterocolitis.
- Infants with postmaturity syndrome may appear thin with loose skin folds, cracked peeling skin, and meconium staining. They appear hyperalert and worried. They may have respiratory difficulties at birth and suffer hypoglycemia and inadequate temperature regulation.
- Infants with IUGR may be SGA at birth. In symmetric growth restriction, the infant is proportionately small; in asymmetric growth restriction, the head and length are normal and the body is thin.
- LGA infants may have birth injuries such as fractures, nerve damage, or bruising as a result of their size. They may have hypoglycemia or polycythemia.

ANSWERS TO CRITICAL THINKING EXERCISE

The preterm infant may need a special formula and smaller amounts. The preterm infant will take longer to feed, might need gavage feedings before introduction of a bottle, and would be more prone to complications in feeding. See Nursing Care Plan 29-1 for interventions appropriate for bottle feeding the preterm infant.

REFERENCES & READINGS

Adcock, E.W., & Consolvo, C.A. (1998). Fluid and electrolyte management. In G.B. Merenstein & S.L. Gardner (Eds.), *Handbook of neonatal intensive care* (4th ed., pp. 243-258). St. Louis: Mosby.

Als, H. & Gilkerson, L. (1997). The role of relationship-based developmentally supportive newborn intensive care in strengthening outcome of preterm infants. *Seminars in Perinatology,* 21(3), 178-189.

American Academy of Pediatrics. (1999). Hospital discharge of the high-risk neonate: Proposed guidelines. *Pediatrics,* 102(2), 411-417.

American Academy of Pediatrics & American College of Obstetricians and Gynecologists. (1997). *Guidelines for perinatal care* (4th ed.). Elk Grove Village, IL: American Academy of Pediatrics.

American Academy of Pediatrics & Canadian Paedriatric Society. (2000). Prevention and management of pain and stress in the neonate. *Pediatrics,* 105(2), 454-461.

American College of Obstetricians and Gynecologists. (2000). *Intrauterine growth restriction.* ACOG Practice Bulletin Number 12. Washington, D.C.: Author.

Amlung, S.R. (1998). Neonatal thermoregulation. In C. Kenner, J.W. Lott, & A.A. Flandermeyer (Eds.), *Comprehensive neonatal nursing, a physiologic perspective* (2nd ed., pp. 207-219). Philadelphia: W.B. Saunders.

Association of Women's Health, Obstetric, and Neonatal Nurses. (1995). *Clinical commentary: Pain in neonates.* Washington, D.C.: Author.

Bakewell-Sachs, S. (1999). Neonatal nutrition. In J. Deacon & P. O'Neill, *Core curriculum for neonatal intensive care nursing* (2nd ed., pp. 294-325). Philadelphia: W.B. Saunders.

Bell, R.P., & McGrath, J.M. (1996). Implementing a research-based kangaroo care program in the NICU. *Nursing Clinics of North America,* 31(2), 387-403.

Berseth, C.L., & Abrums, S.A. (1998). Special gastrointestinal concerns. In H.W. Taeusch & R.A. Ballard (Eds.), *Avery's diseases of the newborn* (7th ed., pp. 965-978). Philadelphia: W.B. Saunders.

Bialoskurski, M., Cox, C.L., & Hayes, J. (2000). The nature of attachment in a neonatal intensive care unit. *Journal of Perinatal Neonatal Nursing,* 13(1), 66-77.

Blackburn, S.T. (1998). Assessment and management of neurologic dysfunction. In C. Kenner, J.W. Lott, & A.A. Flandermeyer (Eds.), *Comprehensive neonatal nursing: A physiologic perspective,* (2nd ed., pp. 564-607). Philadelphia: W.B. Saunders.

Blake, W.W., & Murray, J.A. (1998). Heat balance. In G.B. Merenstein & S.L. Gardner (Eds.), *Handbook of neonatal intensive care* (4th ed., pp. 100-175). St. Louis: Mosby.

Bracht, M., Ardal, F., Bot, A., & Cheng, C.M. (1998). Initiation and maintenance of a hospital-based parent group for parents of premature infants: Key factors for success. *Neonatal Network,* 17(3), 33-37.

Brooks, S.L. , Mitchell, A., & Steffenson, N. (2000). Mothers, Infants, & DHA: Implications for nursing practice. *MCN: American Journal of Maternal Child Nursing,* 25(2), 71-75.

Buschbach, D. (1999). Physical assessment of the newborn infant. In J. Deacon & P. O'Neill, *Core curriculum for neonatal intensive care nursing* (2nd ed., pp. 74-100). Philadelphia: W.B. Saunders.

Casey, P.M. (1999). Respiratory distress. In J. Deacon & P. O'Neill, *Core curriculum for neonatal intensive care nursing* (2nd ed., pp. 118-150). Philadelphia: W.B. Saunders.

Cox, C.A., Wolfson, M.R., & Shaffer, T.H. (1996). Liquid ventilation: A comprehensive overview. *Neonatal Network,* 15(3), 31-43.

De Roo-Merritt, L. (2000). Lasers in medicine: Treatment of retinopathy of prematurity. *Neonatal Network,* 19(1), 21-26.

Dodd, V. (1996). Gestational age assessment. *Neonatal Network,* 15(1), 27-36.

Evans, J.C., Vogelpohl, D.G., Bourguignon, C.M., & Morcott, C.S. (1997). Pain behaviors in LBW infants accompany some "nonpainful" caregiving procedures. *Neonatal Network,* 16(3), 33-40.

Fanaroff, A.A., & Martin, R.J. (1997). *Neonatal-perinatal medicine* (6th ed.). St. Louis: Mosby.

Forsythe, P.L. (1999). Transition of the high-risk neonate to home care. In J. Deacon & P. O'Neill, *Core curriculum for neonatal intensive care nursing* (2nd ed., pp. 772-780). Philadelphia: W.B. Saunders.

Gardner, S.L., & Lubchenco, L.O. (1998). The neonate and the environment: Impact on development. In G.B. Merenstein & S.L. Gardner (Eds.), *Handbook of neonatal intensive care* (4th ed., pp. 197-242). St. Louis: Mosby.

Georgieff, M.K. (1999). Nutrition. In G.B. Avery, M.A. Fletcher, & M.G. MacDonald (Eds.), *Neonatology, pathophysiology and management of the newborn* (5th ed., pp. 363-394). Philadelphia: Lippincott.

Gomella, T.L., Cunningham, M.D., Eyal, F.G. & Zenk, K.E. (Eds.) (1999). *Neonatology* (4th ed.). Norwalk, CT: Appleton & Lange.

Gordon, M., & Montgomery, L.A. (1996). Minimizing epidermal stripping in the very low birth weight infant: Integrating research and practice to affect infant outcome. *Neonatal Network,* 15(1), 37-44.

Gotoff, S.P. (2000). Infections of the neonate. In R.E. Behrman, R.M. Kliegman, & A.M. Arvin (Eds.), *Nelson textbook of pediatrics* (15th ed., pp. 538-552). Philadelphia: W.B. Saunders.

Gray, K., Dostal, S., Ternullo-Retta, C., & Armstrong, M.A. (1998). Developmentally supportive care in a neonatal intensive care unit: A research utilization project. *Neonatal Network,* 17(2), 33-38.

Griffin, T. (1999). Visitation patterns: Parents who visit "too little." *Neonatal Network,* 18(6), 75-76.

Guyer, B., Hoyert, D.L., Martin, J.A., Ventura, S.J., MacDorman, M.F., & Strobino, D.M. (1999). Annual summary of vital statistics: 1998. *Pediatrics,* 104(6), 1229-1245.

Hagedorn, M.I., Gardner, S.L., & Abman, S.H. (1998). Respiratory diseases. In G.B. Merenstein & S.L. Gardner (Eds.), *Handbook of neonatal intensive care* (4th ed., pp. 437-499). St. Louis: Mosby.

Hansen, T., & Corbet, A. (1998) Disorders of the transition. In H.W. Taeusch & R.A. Ballard (Eds.), *Avery's diseases of the newborn* (7th ed., pp. 602-629). Philadelphia: W.B. Saunders.

Higley, A.M., & Miller, M.A. (1996). The development of parenting: Nursing resources. *Journal of Obstetric, Gynecologic, and Neonatal Nursing,* 25(9), 707-713.

Hill, A.S., Kurkowski, T.B., & Garcia, J. (2000). Oral support measures used in feeding the preterm infant. *Nursing Research,* 49(1), 2-10.

Holditch-Davis, D., & Miles, M.S. (2000). Mothers' stories about their experiences in the neonatal intensive care unit. *Neonatal Network,* 19(3), 13-21.

Kelly, D.D., & Bullock, L.F.C. (2000). A student nurse intervenes to foster grandfather/grandchild bonding. *Journal of Obstetric, Gynecologic, and Neonatal Nursing,* 25(4), 211-213.

Kenner, C., & Amlung, S. (1999). Families in crisis. In J. Deacon & P. O'Neill, *Core curriculum for neonatal intensive care nursing* (2nd ed., pp. 635-649). Philadelphia: W.B. Saunders.

Kirkpatrick, J.M., Alesander, J., & Cain, R.M. (1997). Recovering urine from diapers: Are test results accurate? *MCN: American Journal of Maternal Child Nursing,* 22(2), 96-102.

Kliethermes, P.A., Cross, M.L., Lanese, M.G., Johnson, K.M., & Simon, S.D. (1999). Transitioning preterm infants with nasogastric tube supplementation: Increased likelihood of breastfeeding. *Journal of Obstetric, Gynecologic, and Neonatal Nursing,* 28(3), 264-273.

Koch, S. (1999). Developmental support in the neonatal intensive care unit. In J. Deacon & P. O'Neill (Eds.), *Core curriculum for neonatal intensive care nursing,* (2nd ed., pp. 522-539). Philadelphia: W.B. Saunders.

Koh, T.H.H.G., Harrison, C., & Morley, C. (1999). Gestation versus outcome table for parents of extremely premature infants. *Journal of Perinatology,* 19(6), 452-453.

Lee, S. (1999). Retinopathy of prematurity in the 1990s. *Neonatal Network,* 18(2), 31-38.

Lefrak, L., & Dowling, D.A. (1998). Nutrition: Physiologic basis of metabolism and management of enteral and parenteral nutrition. In C. Kenner, J.W. Lott, & A.A. Flandermeyer (Eds.), *Comprehensive neonatal nursing: A physiologic perspective,* (2nd ed., pp. 354-370). Philadelphia: W.B. Saunders.

Liaw, J. (2000). Tactile stimulation and preterm infants. *Journal of Perinatal Neonatal Nursing,* 14(1), 84-103.

Logsdon, M.C., & Davis, D.W. (1998). Guiding mothers of high-risk infants in obtaining social support. *MCN: American Journal of Maternal Child Nursing,* 23(4), 195-199.

Lockridge, T. (1999). Following the learning curve: The evolution of kinder, gentler neonatal respiratory technology. *Journal of Obstetric, Gynecologic, and Neonatal Nursing,* 28(4), 443-455.

Lockridge, T., Taquino, L.T., & Knight, A. (1999). Back to sleep: Is there room in that crib for both AAP recommendations and developmentally supportive care? *Neonatal Network,* 18(5), 29-33.

Ludington-Hoe, S.M., & Swinth, J.Y. (1996). Developmental aspects of kangaroo care. *Journal of Obstetric, Gynecologic, and Neonatal Nursing,* 25(8), 691-703.

Ludington-Hoe, S.M., Anderson, G.C., Simpson, S., Hollingsead, A., Argote, L.A., & Rey, H. (1999). Birth-related fatigue in 34 to 36 week preterm neonates: Rapid recovery with very early kangaroo (skin-to-skin) care. *Journal of Obstetric, Gynecologic, and Neonatal Nursing,* 28(1), 94-103.

Ludington, S.M., & Engler, A. (1999). Kangaroo Care Congress report. *Neonatal Network,* 18(4), 55-56.

Lund, C., Kuller, J., Lane, A., Lott, J.W., & Raines, D.A. (1999). *Journal of Obstetric, Gynecologic, and Neonatal Nursing,* 28(3), 241-254.

March of Dimes. (1999). *Live births by gestational age and birthweight, United States, 1996.* Retrieved November 11, 1999 from http://www.modimes.org/HealthLibrary2/facts-figures/livebirthsxage.htm.

McGrath, J.M., & Conliffe-Torres, S. (1996). Integrating family-centered developmental assessment and intervention into routine care in the neonatal intensive care unit. *Nursing Clinics of North America,* 31(2), 367-386.

Medoff-Cooper, B. (1994). Transition of the preterm infant to an open crib. *Journal of Obstetric, Gynecologic, and Neonatal Nursing,* 23(4), 329-335.

Medoff-Cooper, B., McGrath, J.M., & Bilker, W. (2000). Nutritive sucking and neurobehavioral development in preterm infants from 34 weeks PCA to term. *MCN: American Journal of Maternal Child Nursing,* 25(2), 64-70.

Meier, P., & Brown, L.P. (1996). State of the science: Breastfeeding for mothers and low birth weight infants. *Nursing Clinics of North America,* 31(2), 351-365.

Meier, P., Engstrom, J.L., Fleming, B.A., Streeter, P.L., & Lawrence, P.B. (1996). Estimating milk intake of hospitalized preterm infants who breastfeed. *Journal of Human Lactation,* 12(1), 21-26.

Meier, P., Brown, L.P., & Hurst. N.M. (1999). Breastfeeding the preterm infant. In J. Riordan & K.G. Auerbach (Eds.), *Breastfeeding and human lactation* (2nd ed., pp. 449-481). Sudbury, MA: Jones & Bartlett.

Miles, M.S., Carlson, J., & Funk, S.G. (1996). Sources of support reported by mothers and fathers of infants hospitalized in a neonatal intensive care unit. *Neonatal Network,* 15(3), 45-51.

Miles, M.S., Shandor, M., & Holditch-Davis, D. (1997). Parenting the prematurely born child: Pathways of influence. *Seminars in Perinatology,* 21(3), 254-266.

Miles, M.S., Wilson, S.M., & Docherty, S.L. (1999). African American mothers' responses to hospitalization of an infant with serious health problems. *Neonatal Network,* 18(8), 17-25.

Militello, L., & Lim, L. (1995). Patient assessment skills: Assessing early cues of necrotizing enterocolitis. *Journal of Perinatal Neonatal Nursing,* 9(2), 42-52.

Moe, P., & Paige, P.L. (1998). *Neurologic disorders.* In G.B. Merenstein & S.L. Gardner (Eds.), *Handbook of neonatal intensive care* (4th ed., pp. 571-603). St. Louis: Mosby.

Ogundipe, O.A., & Hamilton, L.A. (1998). Intrauterine growth restriction, postterm pregnancy, and intrauterine fetal demise. In N.F. Hacker & J.G. Moore (Eds.), *Essentials of obstetrics and gynecology* (3rd ed., pp. 324-332). Philadelphia: W.B. Saunders.

Palmer, M.M., & VandenBerg, K.A. (1998). A closer look at neonatal sucking. *Neonatal Network,* 17(2), 77-79.

Peters, K.L. (1996a). Research update: Dinosaurs in the bath. *Neonatal Network,* 15(1), 71-73.

Peters, K.L. (1996b). Selected physiologic and behavioral responses of the critically ill premature neonate to a routine nursing intervention. *Neonatal Network,* 15(1), 74.

Philip, A. (1996). *Neonatology: A practical guide* (4th ed.). Philadelphia: W.B. Saunders.

Pickler, R.H., Mauck, A.G., & Geldmaker, B. (1997). Bottle-feeding histories of preterm infants. *Journal of Obstetric, Gynecologic, and Neonatal Nursing,* 26(4), 414-420.

Premji, S.S. (1998) Ontogeny of the gastrointestinal system and its impact on feeding the preterm infant. *Neonatal Network,* 17(2), 17-24.

Putman, M. (1999). Risks associated with gestational age and birth weight. In S. Mattson & J.E. Smith, *Core curriculum for maternal-newborn nursing* (2nd ed., pp. 658-686). Philadelphia: W.B. Saunders.

Raines, D.A. (1998). Values of mothers of low birth weight infants in the NICU. *Neonatal Network,* 17(4), 41-46.

Roberts, K.L., Paynter, C., & McEwan, B. (2000). A comparison of kangaroo mother care and conventional cuddling care. *Neonatal Network,* 19(4), 31-35.

Robison, M., Pirak, C., & Morrell, C. (2000). Multidisciplinary discharge assessment of the medically and socially high-risk infant. *Journal of Perinatal Neonatal Nursing,* 13(4), 67-86.

Schwoebel, A., & Jones, M.L.H. (1999). A clinical pathway system for the neonatal intensive care nursery. *Journal of Perinatal Neonatal Nursing,* 13(3), 60-69.

Shaker, C.S. (1999). Nipple feeding preterm infants: An individualized, developmentally supportive approach. *Neonatal Network,* 18(3), 15-22.

Short, M.A., Brooks-Brunn, J.A., Reeves, D.S., Yeager, J., & Thorpe, J.A. (1996). The effects of swaddling versus standard positioning on neuromuscular development in very low birth weight infants. *Neonatal Network,* 15(4), 25-31.

Sifuentes, M. (2000). Well child care for preterm infants. In C.D. Berkowitz (Ed.), *Pediatrics: A primary care approach* (2nd ed, pp. 84-88). Philadelphia: W.B. Saunders.

Simpson, K.R., & Creehan, P.A. (Eds.), (1996). *AWHONN's perinatal nursing.* Philadelphia: Lippincott-Raven.

Stevens, B., Johnston, C., Franck, L., Petryshen, P., Jack, A., & Foster, G. (1999). The efficacy of developmentally sensitive interventions and sucrose for relieving procedural pain in very low birth weight neonates. *Nursing Research,* 48(1), 35-43.

Stoll, B.J., & Kliegman, R.M. (2000). Respiratory tract disorders. In R.E. Behrman, R.M. Kliegman, & H.B. Jenson (Eds.), *Nelson textbook of pediatrics* (16th ed., pp. 496-510). Philadelphia: W.B. Saunders.

Stokowski, L.C. (1999). Metabolic disorders. In J. Deacon & P. O'Neill, *Core curriculum for neonatal intensive care nursing* (2nd ed., pp. 326-356.). Philadelphia: W.B. Saunders.

Sullivan, J.R. (1999). Development of father-infant attachment in fathers of preterm infants. *Neonatal Network,* 18(7), 33-39.

Townsend, S.F., Johnson, C.B., & Hay Jr., W.W. (1998). Enteral nutrition. In G.B. Merenstein & S.L. Gardner (Eds.), *Handbook of neonatal intensive care* (4th ed., pp. 275-299). St. Louis: Mosby.

Tsang, R.C., DeMarini, S., & Rath, L.L. (1998). Fluids, electrolytes, vitamins, and trace minerals: Basis of ingestion, digestion, elimination, and metabolism. In C. Kenner, J.W. Lott, & A.A. Flandermeyer (Eds.), *Comprehensive neonatal nursing, a physiologic perspective* (2nd ed.). Philadelphia: W.B. Saunders.

VandenBerg, K.A. (1999). What to tell parents about the developmental needs of their baby at discharge. *Neonatal Network,* 18(1), 57-59.

Vanderhoof, J.A., Zach, T.L., & Adrian, T.E. (1999). Gastrointestinal disease. In G.B. Avery, M.A. Fletcher, & M.G. MacDonald (Eds.), *Neonatology: pathophysiology and management of the newborn* (5th ed., pp. 739-763). Philadelphia: Lippincott.

Vargo, L.E., & Trotter, C.W. (1998). *The premature infant: Nursing assessment and management.* White Plains, NY: March of Dimes.

Vecchi, C.J., Vasquez, L., Tadin, T., & Giovannison, P. (1996). Neonatal individualized predictive pathway (NIPP): A discharge planning tool for parents. *Neonatal Network,* 15(4), 7-13.

Wereszczak, J., Miles, M.S., & Holditch-Davis, D. (1997). Maternal recall of the neonatal intensive care unit. *Neonatal Network,* 16(4), 33-40.

Whitsett, J.A., Pryhuber, G.S., Rice, W.R., Warner, B.B., & Wert, S.E. (1999). Acute respiratory disorders. In G.B. Avery, M.A. Fletcher, & M.G. MacDonald (Eds.), *Neonatology: pathophysiology and management of the newborn* (5th ed., pp. 485-508). Philadelphia: Lippincott.

Wilson, S.K. (1998) Incubator to open crib: a three-phase process. *Mother Baby Journal,* 3(3), 7-13.

30

High-Risk Newborn: Acquired and Congenital Conditions

OBJECTIVES

1. Describe the steps involved in neonatal resuscitation.
2. Explain the common respiratory problems in the newborn.
3. Explain the causes and significance of pathologic jaundice.
4. Describe the nursing care of the infant with pathologic jaundice.
5. Describe causes of neonatal infections and nursing care for infants with infections.
6. Explain the effect of maternal diabetes on the newborn and the implications for nursing care.
7. Describe the effect of maternal substance abuse on the newborn and the nursing care.
8. Describe common congenital anomalies.

DEFINITIONS

Asphyxia Insufficient oxygen and excess carbon dioxide in the blood and tissues.

Bilirubin Encephalopathy Brain damage resulting from deposits of unconjugated bilirubin in the brain tissue.

Erythroblastosis Fetalis Agglutination and hemolysis of fetal erythrocytes caused by incompatibility between the maternal and fetal blood types, such as when the fetus is Rh-positive and the mother is Rh-negative.

DEFINITIONS—cont'd

ESOPHAGEAL ATRESIA Condition in which the esophagus is separated from the stomach and ends in a blind pouch.

GASTROSCHISIS Protrusion of the intestines through a defect in the abdominal wall. Intestines are not covered by a peritoneal sac or skin.

HYDROPS FETALIS Heart failure and generalized edema in the fetus secondary to severe anemia resulting from destruction of erythrocytes.

KERNICTERUS Staining of brain tissue caused by accumulation of unconjugated bilirubin in the brain.

MECONIUM ASPIRATION SYNDROME Obstruction and air trapping caused by meconium in the infant's lungs, which may lead to severe respiratory distress.

MENINGOCELE Protrusion of the meninges through a defect in the vertebrae; a form of neural tube defect.

MYELOMENINGOCELE Protrusion of the meninges and spinal cord through a defect in the vertebrae; a form of neural tube defect.

NEONATAL ABSTINENCE SYNDROME A cluster of physical signs exhibited by the newborn who was exposed in utero to maternal use of substances such as heroin.

OMPHALOCELE Protrusion of the intestines into the base of the umbilical cord. Intestines are covered by a peritoneal sac.

PERSISTENT PULMONARY HYPERTENSION Vasoconstriction of the infant's pulmonary vessels after birth; may result in right-to-left shunting of blood flow through the ductus arteriosus, the foramen ovale, or both.

SPINA BIFIDA Defective closure of the bony spine that encloses the spinal cord; a type of neural tube defect.

TRACHEOESOPHAGEAL FISTULA Abnormal connection between the esophagus and trachea.

TRANSIENT TACHYPNEA OF THE NEWBORN Condition of rapid respirations caused by inadequate absorption of fetal lung fluid.

In addition to the high-risk conditions related to gestational age discussed in Chapter 29, the newborn at risk may have acquired or congenital complications. Acquired conditions may be associated with prenatal complications or may occur at birth or shortly thereafter.

RESPIRATORY COMPLICATIONS

Respiratory distress is one of the most common problems of the neonate. It may be caused by asphyxia before or during birth, disease of the respiratory system, and other conditions that affect the infant's ability to breathe. The nurse is responsible for identification and evaluation of respiratory status at birth and throughout the hospital stay. The degree of respiratory distress must be monitored for change, the need for intervention, and the effectiveness of treatment. Charts like the Silverman-Andersen index help evaluate the degree of respiratory distress (see Figure 29-2, p. 810).

Asphyxia

Asphyxia is a lack of oxygen and increase of carbon dioxide in the blood. It may occur in utero, at birth, or later. Asphyxia may cause the fetus to pass meconium (see meconium aspiration syndrome, p. 844). When asphyxia occurs at birth, it may be a continuation of asphyxia that began in utero or the result of other factors such as preterm lungs with insufficient surfactant to function adequately.

Infants may have primary apnea, in which a few gasping breaths at birth are followed by cessation of respirations and a rapid fall in heart rate. Stimulation, alone or with oxygen, may restart respirations. If asphyxia continues without intervention, gasping respirations may resume weakly until the infant enters a period of secondary apnea. In secondary apnea, the oxygen levels in the blood continue to decrease, the infant loses consciousness, and stimulation is ineffective. Resuscitative measures must be initiated immediately to prevent permanent damage to the brain or death.

Lack of oxygen to the cells leads to anaerobic metabolism and the production of lactic acid. Metabolic acidosis develops when available bicarbonate is no longer able to buffer the accumulating acids. A high partial pressure of carbon dioxide occurs in arterial blood ($PaCO_2$) as well as a low partial pressure of oxygen (PO_2), pH, and bicarbonate. Vasoconstriction decreases blood flow to all organs except the brain, myocardium, and adrenal glands. The ductus arteriosus and foramen ovale may remain open because of the low oxygen in the blood, high resistance to blood flow through constricted pulmonary vessels, and elevated pressure on the right side of the heart. Thus even circulating blood remains low in oxygen. Progress toward brain damage and death is rapid unless intervention is prompt.

Infants at Risk

Whenever complications occur during pregnancy, labor, or birth, the infant may be at risk for asphyxia. In addition, if the expectant mother receives narcotics for analgesia shortly before delivery, the infant may be too depressed at birth to breathe spontaneously. Naloxone (Narcan) may be given to these infants (Table 30-1).

Neonatal Resuscitation

Although 90% of newborns have no difficulty with breathing at birth, approximately 10% require some help to begin respirations and 1% require extensive resuscitative measures (AAP & AHA, 2000). Therefore, all personnel involved in deliveries should know the way to perform resuscitative measures. Courses in neonatal resuscitation are usually required of all staff

Table 30-1

COMMON DOSAGES OF NALOXONE HYDROCHLORIDE (NARCAN)

Dosage must be calculated based on weight (0.1 mg/kg). The amount for various weights is given below for *two different drug concentrations.*

Infant's Weight	Total Dose	Drug Concentration 0.4 mg/ml	Drug Concentration 1.0 mg/ml
1 kg (2 lb, 3 oz)	0.1 mg	0.25 ml	0.1 ml
2 kg (4 lb, 7 oz)	0.2 mg	0.50 ml	0.2 ml
3 kg (6 lb, 10 oz)	0.3 mg	0.75 ml	0.3 ml
4 kg (8 lb, 13 oz)	0.4 mg	1.00 ml	0.4 ml

DRUG GUIDE: Naloxone Hydrochloride (Narcan)

Classification: Opioid antagonist.

Action: Reverses central nervous system and respiratory depression caused by narcotics (opiates). Competes with narcotics at receptor sites.

Indications: Severe respiratory depression when the mother has received narcotics within 4 hours of delivery.

Dosage and Route: Available in 0.4 mg/ml and 1 mg/ml. Dosage is 0.1 mg/kg. Given intravenously, intramuscularly, subcutaneously, or into an endotracheal tube. Intravenous and endotracheal routes are preferred during resuscitation.

Absorption: Well absorbed by all routes. Onset of action is 1 to 2 minutes if given intravenously.

Excretion: Metabolized by the liver and excreted by kidneys.

Contraindications and Precautions: Duration of effect is 1 to 4 hours. The dose may need to be repeated because the opioid may have a longer half life than naloxone. If given to an infant of a mother addicted to drugs, it will cause withdrawal and may cause seizures. Resuscitative measures should be used as necessary.

Nursing Considerations: Note the strength of the medication available when calculating the dose. Prepare the syringe before birth by drawing up more than is needed. After birth, the excess is removed from the syringe, and the amount is given according to the estimate of the infant's weight. Inject rapidly. Monitor for response, and be prepared to give repeated doses if necessary. See Table 30-1 for correct dose for various weights.

members working with newborns, and many agencies expect these skills to be updated annually. (Neonatal resuscitation is presented in Procedure 30-1.)

Nurses must be prepared for situations in which asphyxia may develop. Equipment should be readily available and functioning properly at all times so that no delay occurs when starting resuscitation. Nurses begin resuscitation measures as necessary and assist the physician with intubation, insertion of umbilical vein catheters, and administration of medications. Some nurses and neonatal nurse practitioners are taught to intubate infants in emergency situations.

Once the infant is stabilized, the nurse continues to assess for changes. Infants with asphyxia often have other complications. Communication with the parents is a vital nursing function. They will be confused and frightened and will need explanation and realistic reassurance. Parents often need continued support after the crisis to talk about their fears and concerns.

Transient Tachypnea of the Newborn (Retained Lung Fluid)

Infants who experience transient tachypnea of the newborn (TTN) develop rapid respirations soon after birth. The condition, which resolves within a few days, is also called *retained lung fluid and respiratory distress syndrome, type II.* It occurs in approximately 11 of 1000 live births (Whitsett, et al., 1999). Risk factors include cesarean birth without labor, asphyxia, and maternal analgesia, bleeding, or diabetes. Mild immaturity of surfactant production also may be a factor. Infants may be term or preterm.

Cause

Although the exact cause of TTN is unknown, it is thought to be caused by a delay in absorption of fetal lung fluid by the pulmonary capillaries and lymph vessels. This causes decreased lung compliance and air trapping and brings about signs similar to respiratory distress syndrome.

Manifestations

In TTN, respirations as high as 120 per minute develop within hours of birth. Grunting, retractions, nasal flaring, and mild cyanosis also are present. Chest radiography shows streaking from engorgement of pulmonary vessels and lymphatics, hyperinflation, and presence of fluid in the fissures between the lobes and in the pleural space. The condition is self-limiting and usually lasts 24 to 48 hours, although it may continue longer.

Therapeutic Management

Treatment is supportive. Usually, moderate amounts of oxygen are sufficient to prevent cyanosis. Intravenous (IV) or gavage feeding may be necessary while the respiratory rate is high to prevent aspiration and conserve

PROCEDURE 30-1

Performing Resuscitation in the Newly Born

Purpose: To ensure adequate oxygenation of the neonate with asphyxia.

NOTE: Although the procedure is listed by steps, several steps may be performed at the same time. Resuscitation is performed as an integrated process rather than individual steps. Because two people often are working together, more than one step can be performed at one time.

1. Place the infant under a preheated radiant warmer immediately. *Prevention of cold stress is important to prevent increased oxygen need.*
2. Position the infant with the neck in a neutral or slightly extended ("sniffing") position. Avoid hyperextension or flexion of the neck. Place a small, folded blanket under the shoulders. *Proper positioning will help maintain an open airway. Hyperextension or flexion may obstruct the airway.*

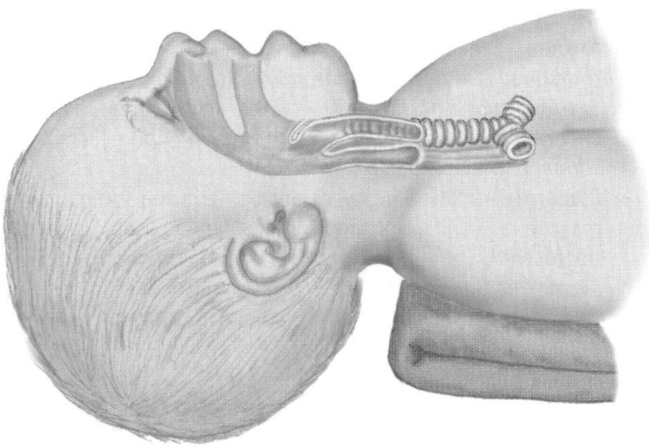

3. Suction the mouth and then the nose. Endotracheal intubation may be necessary to clear the airway if meconium is present. *Suctioning removes mucus from the airways. Infants often gasp when the nose is suctioned and may aspirate secretions from the mouth into the lungs. An endotracheal tube may be inserted at this time or later, if necessary, to provide an open airway.*
4. Dry and stimulate the infant if necessary. Gently rub the infant's back or body, or flick or slap the soles of the feet. *Drying helps prevent cold stress and increased oxygen need. If two people are present, one can be drying the infant while the other positions and suctions. The tactile stimulation of drying the infant and suctioning the mouth and nose may cause spontaneous respirations. If the baby does not respond adequately, additional stimulation may be needed. Stimulation should be gentle to avoid injury.*
5. Remove wet linens and reposition the head as necessary. *Removal of wet linens prevents heat loss. Repositioning may be necessary because the infant has been moved.*
6. If no response occurs after stimulating once or twice, stop and initiate immediate resuscitation. Do not delay resuscitation to continue stimulating or until the Apgar scores are given. *Resuscitation becomes more difficult the longer it is delayed.*
7. Give 100% oxygen if the infant is breathing but cyanotic. Hold the oxygen mask or tubing close to the infant's nose. *Oxygen will help relieve cyanosis and prevent damage to vital tissues. Holding the source close to the nose helps provide 100% oxygen rather than diluting it by combining with room air.*
8. Evaluate the respirations, heart rate, and color. Use a stethoscope or feel the pulsations at the base of the cord. Count the heart rate for 6 seconds and multiply by 10 to obtain the heart rate per minute. Positioning, clearing the airway, drying, stimulating, and providing oxygen should take no more than 30 seconds. *Evaluation determines whether further resuscitation is necessary. Immediate resuscitation is necessary to prevent hypoxic brain damage.*
9. Begin positive-pressure ventilation with a bag and mask if the infant fails to breathe spontaneously with initial stimulation, has gasping respirations, or the heart rate is less than 100 beats per minute when respirations have begun. *Positive-pressure ventilation ensures oxygen entry into the lungs.*
10. Attach the bag to an oxygen source with 100% oxygen. Place the mask snugly over the infant's nose and mouth. Squeeze the bag gently to force air into the infant's lungs. Use a bag with a manometer to show the amount of pressure being used and a flow-control valve that can be adjusted to control the pressure delivered to the infant. Or use a bag with a pressure release valve that releases if the pressure is high enough to cause lung damage. The initial breaths require pressures of 30 to 40 cm H_2O to inflate the lungs. Less pressure is used for subsequent breaths but varies with the infant's condition. *Great care must be taken to use a pressure that will deliver enough pressure to inflate the lungs without causing damage from overinflation. More pressure is needed for the first breaths and diseased lungs.*
11. Observe the rise and fall of the chest during ventilation. If the chest does not move, suction secretions and reposition the head and the mask. Ventilate the infant at a rate of 40 to 60 breaths per minute until the infant is breathing spontaneously and the heart rate is above 100 beats per minute. *The airway must not be occluded by positioning or secretions.*
12. If the heart rate is less than 60 beats per minute after 30 seconds of effective assisted ventilation, a second person should begin chest compressions while the first continues to ventilate the infant. *Adequate ventilation causes improvement of bradycardia in most infants. Evaluation of the infant's status determines whether ventilation can be discontinued or chest compressions must be added for the infant to survive.*
13. Compress the chest by placing the hands around the infant's chest with the fingers under the back to provide support and the thumbs over the lower third of the sternum (just above the xiphoid process). An alternate method is to use two fingers of one hand to compress the chest with the other hand under the back to provide support. *Correct hand position compresses the heart but avoids or minimizes injury to the liver or spleen, fractures of the ribs, and pneumothorax. The alternative method may be necessary to allow access to umbilical vessels or for people with small hands.*

Data from Kattwinkel, J., American Academy of Pediatrics, & American Heart Association. (2000). *Textbook of neonatal resuscitation* (4th ed.) Elk Grove, IL: American Academy of Pediatrics and American Heart Association.

Continued

PROCEDURE 30-1

Performing Resuscitation in the Newly Born—cont'd

Purpose: To ensure adequate oxygenation of the neonate with asphyxia.

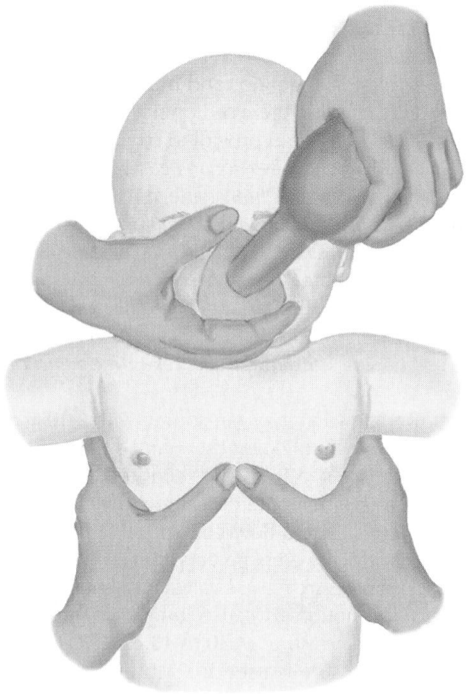

14. Compress the sternum to a depth of approximately one third of the anterior posterior diameter of the chest and sufficient to cause a palpable pulse. Use three compressions followed by one ventilation for a combined rate of compressions and ventilations of 120 each minute. This is 90 compressions and 30 ventilations each minute. Pause for ½ second after every third compression for ventilation. *The size of the infant determines the depth of compressions to avoid injury. Simultaneous compression and ventilation may interfere with adequate ventilation. The short pause allows air to enter the lungs.*
15. Check the heart rate after approximately 30 seconds. If it is 60 beats per minute or more, discontinue compressions but continue ventilation until spontaneous breathing begins. If the heart rate is less than 60 beats per minute, medications will be necessary. Endotracheal intubation may be performed at this point if not performed previously. *Periodic evaluation is necessary to ensure that treatment is appropriate to the infant's status. Endotracheal intubation may be used to ensure adequate airway. Medications may be necessary to stimulate the heart.*
16. Prepare medications, if necessary. Epinephrine and naloxone may be given through an umbilical vein catheter or endotracheal tube. Volume expanders may include normal saline, Ringers lactate, or O-negative red blood cells. Sodium bicarbonate is given intravenously only after prolonged arrest and with effective ventilation. *Epinephrine stimulates the heart. Naloxone counteracts the effects of opioids given to the mother in labor. Volume expanders may be used for fluid or blood loss. Sodium bicarbonate corrects acidosis after prolonged asphyxia that does not respond to other treatment.*

energy. Because the signs are similar to respiratory distress syndrome and sepsis, the infant is observed for those complications. Antibiotics may be given and later discontinued if cultures show that sepsis is not present.

Nursing Considerations

The nurse may be the first person to see signs of TTN, especially if they are not apparent at birth. After identifying signs, the nurse notifies the appropriate caregiver and carries out treatment. General nursing care is similar to that of the respiratory care of the preterm infant (see p. 805).

Check Your Reading

1. What is the result of asphyxia before or during birth?
2. What is the role of the nurse in care of the infant with asphyxia?
3. How is TTN different from respiratory distress syndrome?

Meconium Aspiration Syndrome

Meconium aspiration syndrome (MAS) occurs most often in postterm infants who have decreased amniotic fluid and are prone to cord compression. It also occurs in term infants who have suffered intrauterine asphyxia. It is rare before 36 to 38 weeks' gestation. MAS results in obstruction of the airways, pneumonitis, and air trapping. It may lead to persistent pulmonary hypertension of the newborn (Figure 30-1).

Causes

Although the normal fetus may pass meconium, it is most often seen when hypoxia causes increased peristalsis of the intestine and relaxation of the anal sphincter previous to or during labor. MAS develops when meconium in the amniotic fluid enters the lungs during fetal life or at birth. Meconium may be drawn into the lungs if gasping movements occur in utero as a result of asphyxia and acidosis, or the meconium in the upper airways may be pulled deep into the respiratory passages when the infant takes the first breaths after birth.

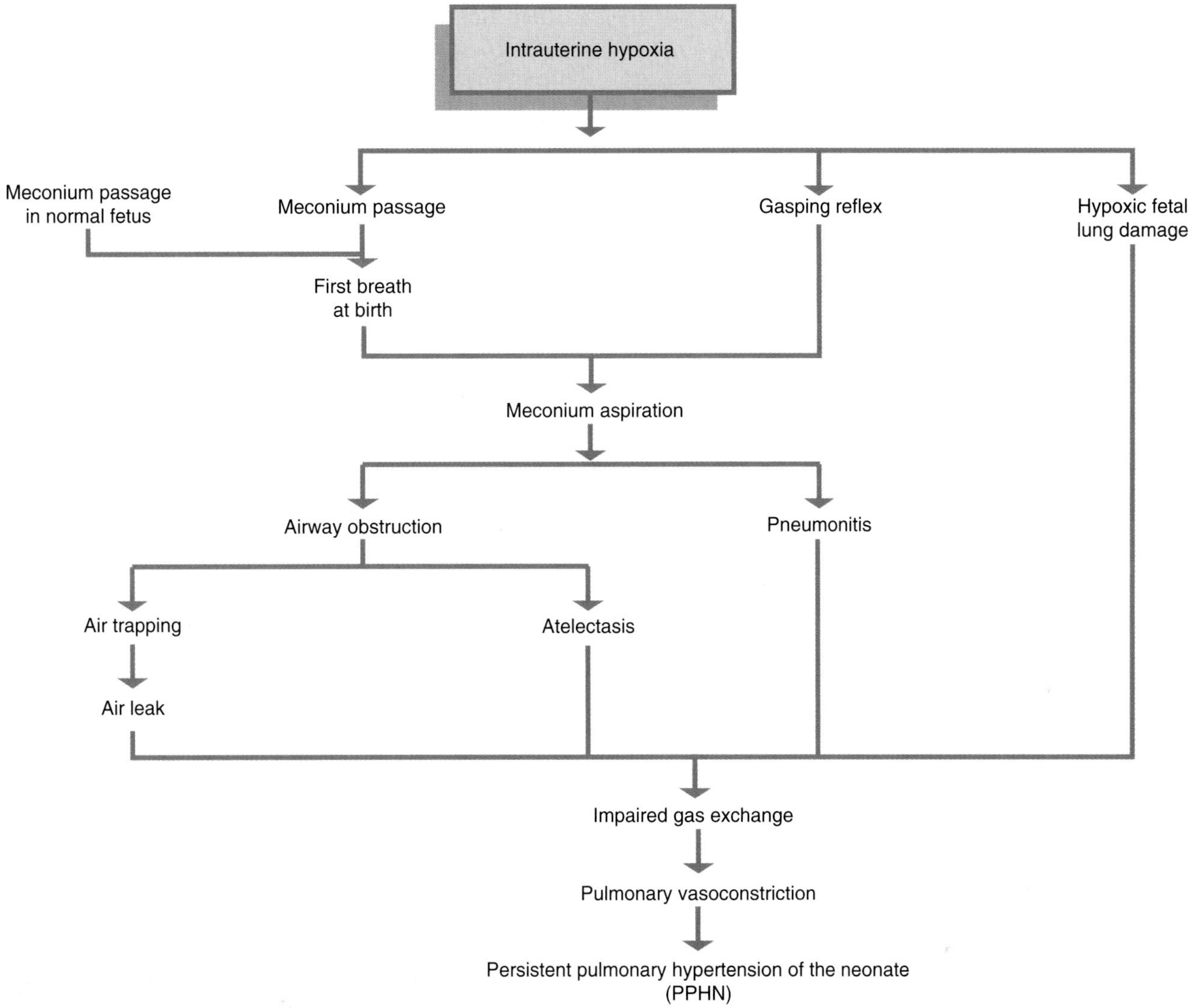

FIGURE 30-1 Flow chart showing the effects of meconium aspiration syndrome.

Obstruction of the airways may be complete or partial. In partial obstruction, air can enter but not escape from the alveoli. During inhalation, the bronchioles expand slightly as air flows into them past the meconium. During exhalation, the passages constrict and meconium blocks the passage of air out of the lungs.

This ball-valve mechanism results in air trapping. The overdistended alveoli may develop an air leak, with escape of air into the pleural cavity (pneumothorax) or mediastinum (pneumomediastinum). In addition, meconium is irritating to lung tissue and causes an inflammatory reaction and chemical pneumonitis. Persistent pulmonary hypertension may result.

Severe MAS develops in only a small number of the approximately 4% of newborns with meconium below the vocal cords. It most often occurs when the fetal heart rate during labor and delivery indicated asphyxia (Whitsett, et al., 1999). The addition of meconium to a lung damaged by asphyxia may increase the severity of the condition. Damage from asphyxia interferes with clearing of lung fluid and surfactant production and causes pulmonary vasoconstriction that can result in return to fetal circulation. (See p. 846.)

Manifestations

If meconium in the amniotic fluid is light, respiratory problems usually do not develop. However, thick meconium may cause serious respiratory pathology. Signs of mild to severe respiratory distress are present at birth, with tachypnea, cyanosis, retractions, nasal flaring, grunting, coarse breath sounds, and a barrel-shaped chest from hyperinflation. Radiography shows atelectasis, consolidation, and hyperexpansion from air trapping.

Therapeutic Management

At birth, the airway must be cleared, especially if meconium is thick. The infant's mouth and pharynx are suctioned as soon as the head is delivered and before delivery of the rest of the body. This helps prevent drawing the meconium from the upper air passages deep into the lungs during the infant's first breath.

Immediately after birth and before the infant is stimulated to breathe, a laryngoscope is inserted and the trachea suctioned. An endotracheal tube is inserted to allow deep suction of meconium and ventilation, if necessary. If the infant is vigorous and shows no respiratory difficulty, intubation and suction may not be necessary.

Infants may only need warmed, humidified oxygen, or extensive respiratory support with a ventilator may be required. High-frequency ventilation may be used. Ongoing management consists of supportive care to meet the problems presented.

Infants with severe MAS who do not respond to conventional treatment may benefit from extracorporeal membrane oxygenation (ECMO). ECMO, which is available in some larger hospitals, oxygenates the blood while bypassing the lungs, much like heart-lung machines used during heart surgery. It allows the infant's lungs to rest temporarily and recover. Surfactant therapy is a new treatment that may decrease the need for ECMO (Whitsett, et al., 1999).

Nursing Considerations

When meconium is noted in the amniotic fluid during labor, the nurse notifies the primary caregiver of the amount of meconium present so that delivery care can be adapted as necessary. The nurse ensures that equipment is available and functioning and assists with care at delivery. After the infant's birth, nursing care is adapted to the problems presented. Although meconium is sterile, lung damage promotes the growth of bacteria. Infants should be closely observed for infection, which may further complicate the condition.

Persistent Pulmonary Hypertension of the Newborn

Persistent pulmonary hypertension of the newborn (PPHN) is a condition in which the vascular resistance of the lungs does not decrease after birth and normal changes to neonatal circulation are impaired. For this reason, the condition also is called *persistent fetal circulation.*

Causes

The cause of PPHN may be abnormal lung development, maternal use of nonsteroidal antiinflammatory agents or aspirin, or hypoxia, or it may develop for unknown reasons. It often is associated with hypoxemia and acidosis from conditions such as asphyxia, meconium aspiration, sepsis, and respiratory distress syndrome.

Inadequate oxygenation results in vasoconstriction, instead of the normal dilation, of the pulmonary artery and small pulmonary vessels and produces increased resistance in the lungs. It also causes relaxation, instead of constriction, of the ductus arteriosus. The elevated pulmonary vascular resistance causes a rise in pressure on the right side of the heart. This results in a right-to-left shunt of blood through the foramen ovale and patent ductus arteriosus, as occurs during fetal circulation.

Manifestations

Infants with PPHN are usually term or postterm and develop signs of PPHN within the first 24 hours after birth. Tachypnea, respiratory distress, and progressive cyanosis often become worse with handling. Oxygen saturation and partial pressure of oxygen in arterial blood (PaO_2) are decreased. Other signs may result from associated conditions.

Therapeutic Management

Management involves treating the underlying cause of poor oxygenation and relieving pulmonary vasoconstriction. Arterial pH may be increased with respiratory and drug therapy to cause pulmonary vasodilation. High-frequency ventilation, surfactant therapy, and ECMO therapy may be necessary. Inhalation of nitric oxide, which dilates pulmonary vessels, also is used and may reduce the need for ECMO. Nursing care is similar to care of other infants with severe respiratory disease. Because infants become hypoxic with activity and other stimuli, handling and noise are kept to a minimum.

Check Your Reading

4. How does meconium get into an infant's respiratory tract? Why is it a problem?
5. What is the role of the nurse when meconium is discovered in amniotic fluid?

HYPERBILIRUBINEMIA (PATHOLOGIC JAUNDICE)

Conjugation of bilirubin and physiologic jaundice are discussed in Chapters 19 and 20, pp. 495 and 522, respectively. This discussion focuses on pathologic jaundice. When the bilirubin level reaches 5 to 7 mg/dl, jaundice is visible in the skin (Stoll & Kliegman, 2000). Jaundice is considered pathologic when it appears in the first 24 hours after birth; total bilirubin rises above 12 mg/dl in a full-term infant or 10 to 14 mg/dl in a preterm infant, or more than 5 mg/dl in 24 hours; direct bilirubin is above 2 mg/dl or continues beyond 10 to 17 days of life (Stoll & Kliegman, 2000).

Pathologic jaundice is a concern because it may lead to kernicterus. In kernicterus, bilirubin deposits cause yellowish staining of the brain, especially the basal ganglia, cerebellum, and hippocampus. It is more likely to occur in infants who have suffered sepsis, hypoxia, or respiratory acidosis, which impairs the blood-brain barrier and allows unconjugated bilirubin to enter the brain. Kernicterus causes bilirubin encephalopathy.

Although bilirubin encephalopathy is rare today because of improved treatment measures, the mortality rate of affected infants is high. Those who survive may suffer from cerebral palsy, mental retardation, hearing loss, or more subtle long-term neurologic and developmental problems. The exact level at which bilirubin encephalopathy begins to develop is not known. It may occur when total bilirubin levels are more than 20 mg/dl in full-term infants and at lower levels in preterms or neonates with other complications, but higher levels may not be a problem in healthy term infants. Causes and other factors must be considered in each case.

Causes

The most common cause of pathologic jaundice is hemolytic disease of the newborn caused by incompatibility between the blood of the mother and that of the fetus. The best known cause is Rh incompatibility, in which the Rh-negative mother forms antibodies when Rh-positive blood from the fetus enters her circulation. Antibodies may have developed during a previous pregnancy or after injury, abortion, amniocentesis, or a transfusion of Rh-positive blood. The antibodies cross the placenta and attach to fetal red blood cells and destroy them. Excessive hemolysis causes erythroblastosis fetalis.

Infants with erythroblastosis fetalis are anemic from destruction of red blood cells. However, jaundice usually does not develop until soon after birth because bilirubin crosses the placenta and is excreted by the mother. Severely affected infants may experience hydrops fetalis, a severe anemia that results in heart failure and generalized edema. Use of $Rh_O(D)$ immune globulin (RhIG) such as RhoGAM to prevent the mother from forming antibodies against Rh-positive blood has greatly decreased the incidence of erythroblastosis fetalis. (See Rh incompatibility, p. 692.)

ABO incompatibility also causes pathologic jaundice. Mothers with type O blood have natural antibodies to type A or B blood. The antibodies cross the placenta and cause hemolysis of fetal red blood cells. However, the destruction is much less severe than with Rh incompatibility and causes milder signs.

Other causes of pathologic jaundice include infection, hypothyroidism, glucuronyl transferase deficiency, polycythemia, glucose-6-phosphate dehydrogenase deficiency, and biliary atresia. Any condition that causes destruction of erythrocytes or impairment of the liver may result in pathologic bilirubin levels.

Therapeutic Management

Therapeutic management is focused on preventing the development of kernicterus. The cause is determined by history and diagnostic tests to identify infections or blood abnormalities. During pregnancy, an Rh-negative expectant mother will have an indirect Coombs test to determine the presence of antibodies against fetal blood. If the test is positive, amniocentesis may be performed to determine the fetal Rh factor and degree of hyperbilirubinemia.

When infants are jaundiced, the infant's blood type and a direct Coombs' test are performed on the cord blood. A positive Coombs' test indicates that antibodies from the mother have attached to the infant's red blood cells. Bilirubin levels are followed closely for changes that indicate that treatment should be initiated or changed.

Phototherapy

The most common treatment of jaundice is phototherapy, the use of special fluorescent lights. During phototherapy, bilirubin in the skin absorbs the light and changes into water-soluble products, the most important of which is lumirubin. These products do not require conjugation by the liver and can be excreted in the bile and urine. Because bilirubin encephalopathy develops in preterm infants at lower bilirubin levels than in full-term infants, phototherapy is begun at lower levels for them.

Phototherapy can be delivered in several ways. The most common is a bank of phototherapy or "bili" lights. The infant, wearing only a diaper to provide maximal exposure of the skin to the lights, often is placed inside an incubator for warmth. The lights are placed above the incubator at a distance determined by the type of bulb used (usually 12 to 30 inches) (Figure 30-2).

A fiberoptic phototherapy blanket that is placed against the infant's skin is another option. The infant can be swaddled and does not require patches over the eyes when the blanket is used. Double phototherapy lights or a combination of blanket and lights may be used if the bilirubin level is high. Another option is a phototherapy bed, a device containing phototherapy lights that fits into a crib and on which the infant lies. Although the infant must remain in the bed during therapy, the bed can be moved into the mother's room and eye shields are not necessary.

Side effects of phototherapy include frequent, loose, green stools that result from increased bile flow and peristalsis. This causes more rapid excretion of the bilirubin but may be damaging to the skin and result in fluid loss. African-American infants may experience a tanning effect from the light. Bronze baby syndrome, a grayish-brown discoloration of the skin, occurs in infants with cholestatic jaundice in whom liver function and production or flow of bile are impaired. A skin rash similar to erythema toxicum also may occur. The color changes

PARENTS WANT TO KNOW Home Care for the Infant Receiving Phototherapy

Fiberoptic Blankets

If you are using a fiberoptic blanket, keep it next to the baby's skin at all times. Be sure the baby does not roll off the blanket. You may wrap the baby with a receiving blanket over the "bili" blanket and hold the baby for feedings and other activities. It is not necessary to cover the infant's eyes if the blanket alone is used.

Phototherapy Bed

Keep the infant positioned correctly in the bed. It is not necessary to use eye covering.

Phototherapy Lights

Position the phototherapy or "bili" light at the proper distance from your baby according to the manufacturer's directions. Placing it too close to the infant could result in fever or burns. Placing it too far away will make the treatment ineffective.

Close the baby's eyes, and place patches over the eyes before placing the infant under the lights. Check at least every hour to see that the patches remain in place. They must cover the eyes but not press on the nose because they can interfere with breathing. There should be no pressure on the eyes from the patches.

Change your baby's position about every 2 hours so that the light reaches all areas of the body. Keep diapers on your infant but no other clothing that would prevent exposure of the skin to the light. You may have to keep the room temperature higher than usual to keep the baby warm.

When the baby is under the lights, you can talk to her or him. The sound of your voice will be comforting.

All Types of Phototherapy

The infant may be removed from phototherapy for feedings, diaper changes, and other general care but should receive phototherapy for 18 hours every day (or number of hours ordered by the physician). Hold and cuddle your infant during that time, especially if he or she must remain in the "bilibed" or under lights.

Check your baby's temperature under the arm before every feeding. The temperature should remain between 97.7 and 99.5° F. If it is abnormal, verify whether the heat in the room is too low or high or the phototherapy light source is positioned correctly. Use warm blankets when you remove the baby from the warmth of phototherapy. Call your physician if the baby has a temperature less than 97.7° F or above 100° F.

Feed your baby every 2 to 3 hours. It is important for the infant to eat well while receiving phototherapy, which causes the baby to lose fluid from the skin and have loose stools. This could cause dehydration. The infant needs protein, which helps eliminate the bilirubin that causes the jaundice.

Keep a list of your baby's wet diapers and stools. If there are less than 6 wet diapers a day or the urine appears dark, increase the feedings. Call the physician or home care nurse if you have questions about care, if the baby has a fever or appears sick to you, if the mouth seems dry, or if the urine is dark or less than normal.

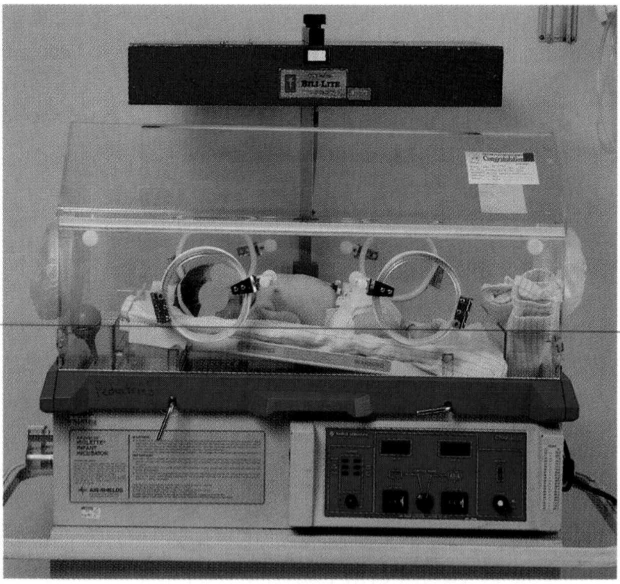

FIGURE 30-2 The infant receiving phototherapy is wearing eye patches to protect the eyes.

and rash disappear when phototherapy is ended. Some infants experience a temporary lactose intolerance during therapy and need formula without lactose.

Home phototherapy is a way to avoid prolonged hospitalization, separation from parents, and interference with breastfeeding. Parents using phototherapy at home need extensive teaching on ways to manage the equipment and the infant's requirements. Home visits by nurses are important to help ensure that the infant is making adequate progress and the parents understand how to provide care.

Exchange Transfusions

Exchange transfusions are necessary when phototherapy cannot reduce dangerously high bilirubin levels quickly enough. This treatment removes antibodies, unconjugated bilirubin, and sensitized red blood cells before they break down, and it corrects severe anemia. When an immediate transfusion is needed for Rh incompatibility, type O, Rh-negative blood is used so that circulating antibodies will not destroy the erythrocytes.

Procedure. During the exchange transfusion, blood is removed from the infant and replaced with an equal amount of donor blood in small portions or simultaneously. Because the donor blood mixes with the infant's blood, approximately twice the infant's blood volume is usually administered. Normal blood volume is 80 to 85 ml/kg in a full-term infant and 100 ml/kg in a preterm infant. At the end of the transfusion, approximately 85% of the infant's red blood cells have been replaced.

The bilirubin level after transfusion is about 45% of the pre-exchange level. When the level in the blood decreases, bilirubin from the tissues moves into the plasma. This may increase the blood level to 60% or more of the original level (Frank, Cooper, & Merenstein, 1998). This rebound elevation of bilirubin may necessitate repeat transfusions, but phototherapy is generally adequate to resolve it.

Complications. Many complications may occur during exchange transfusion, including electrolyte imbalances, infection, hypervolemia or hypovolemia, cardiac arrhythmias, increased or decreased blood glucose, decreased perfusion to the intestines, bleeding, thrombosis, and embolism. Samples of blood are analyzed before and after the exchange, including a complete blood count, bilirubin and calcium levels, and other tests as needed.

Role of the Nurse. The nurse's role during exchange transfusion is to prepare equipment, assess the infant during and after the procedure, and keep accurate records. A cardiac monitor is attached to the infant, and warmth is provided by a radiant heater. The nurse also must clarify any misunderstandings that the parents may have about the treatment and help allay their anxiety.

APPLICATION OF THE NURSING PROCESS: HYPERBILIRUBINEMIA

Although collaborative care of the infant with jaundice is an important part of the nurse's role, several nursing diagnoses are appropriate. "Risk for Injury associated with bilirubin increases and phototherapy" is discussed in this section. The diagnoses "Risk for Fluid Volume Deficit and Impaired Skin Integrity" are discussed in Nursing Care Plan 30-1.

Assessment

Assess the level of jaundice at the initial assessment each shift. Press the skin over a bony prominence, and note the color in the area before the blood returns. Determine the areas of the body affected by the jaundice, and document carefully to use for comparison

NURSING CARE PLAN 30-1

The Infant with Jaundice

Assessment: Holly, a 2-day-old, full-term infant born by cesarean, is jaundiced secondary to ABO incompatibility and is receiving phototherapy. She weighs 3.2 kg (7 lb, 1 oz) and her mucous membranes appear slightly dry. Skin turgor is good with quick recoil, and the anterior fontanelle is flat. Urine appears slightly dark in color. Holly had three loose green stools with no water ring on this shift. She is being formula fed but only takes ½ to 1 oz. when her mother, Valerie, feeds her. Valerie states that the infant keeps falling asleep during feedings.

Nursing Diagnosis: Risk for Fluid Volume Deficit related to inadequate oral intake to meet needs of increased insensible water loss and frequent loose stools.

Goals/Expected Outcomes:

Holly will do the following:

- Take at least 320 to 480 ml of fluid per day (100 to 150 ml/kg/day) to meet normal needs
- Show adequate hydration (moist mucous membranes, elastic skin turgor, flat fontanelles, pale yellow urine)

Intervention	Rationale
1. Instruct Valerie to feed Holly every 2 to 3 hours. Feed Holly in the nursery at night or when Valerie needs rest, if she prefers.	1. Adequate intake of formula is necessary to meet the infant's nutrient and fluid needs and ensure excretion of bilirubin in the stools. The mother's need for rest must be met without interfering with the infant's needs.
2. Explain to Valerie why Holly needs frequent feedings.	2. The mother's understanding of the reasons will increase her willingness to work with the infant.
3. Observe Valerie feeding Holly and offer suggestions as needed. Show her how to waken the infant by unwrapping and gentle stimulation. Try warming the formula slightly. Stroke around Holly's mouth, and insert a finger to elicit the suck reflex before feedings.	3. Observation of feedings may identify problems and interventions that work for this situation. A wide-awake infant is more likely to feed well. Some infants prefer warm milk. Oral exercise may help infant suck effectively.
4. Tell the parents about the need for frequent feeding to provide added fluid, protein, and other nutrients.	4. Infants under phototherapy have a greater than normal insensible water loss. Albumin (protein) is necessary to carry bilirubin to the liver for conjugation. Heightened intestinal motility decreases absorption of nutrients.

Continued

Intervention	Rationale
5. Avoid offering water or dextrose water. Use formula instead.	5. Water supplements may decrease the intake of formula and its necessary nutrients. Formula increases motility of intestines and expedites excretion of bilirubin in stools, but water does not have the same effect.
6. If water loss appears excessive, weigh all diapers. Urine output should be 1 to 3 ml/kg/hr.	6. Weighing the diapers will identify inadequate output and dehydration early. The diaper weight in grams minus the weight of the dry diaper equals the amount of urine.
7. Use therapeutic communication techniques to help Valerie vent her frustrations. Offer praise for her attempts to feed Holly.	7. Helping the mother deal with her feelings helps her meet the infant's needs. Feeding difficulties often interfere with the mother's view of herself as a "good" mother. Praise increases her sense of adequacy.

Evaluation: Holly drinks a total of 450 ml (15 oz) of formula during 24 hours. Valerie is able to wake Holly, who begins to suck more vigorously. Holly's mucous membranes are moist and she has 10 diapers with pale yellow urine during the 24 hours.

Assessment: Holly's diaper area is slightly red and irritated from her frequent loose stools.

Nursing Diagnosis: Impaired Skin Integrity related to frequent loose stools.

Goals/Expected Outcomes:
Skin will return to normal within 2 days without further signs of irritation or breakdown.

Intervention	Rationale
1. Check diapers at least every hour. Cleanse the diaper area with soap and water after each stool.	1. Extended exposure of the skin to stool and urine may cause skin breakdown. Thorough cleansing removes irritating substances from the skin.
2. Expose the entire diaper area to air for short periods when the phototherapy light is off. Place a diaper under Holly to catch urine and stools.	2. Exposure to air dries the area and aids healing.
3. Avoid lotions, powders, ointments, or wipes containing alcohol.	3. Skin preparations may irritate the skin and increase the risk of burns from the phototherapy lights.
4. Explain the reason for loose stools and methods of treatment of skin irritation to Valerie.	4. The mother may need help to understand that the condition is not the result of poor care. She should learn how to care for diaper rash at home.

Evaluation: Holly's diaper area returns to normal within 1 day.

during future assessment. Jaundice begins at the head and moves down the body as the bilirubin levels rise. Monitor laboratory bilirubin levels for change, especially because visibility of jaundice in the skin may be affected by phototherapy.

Assess for risk factors that might further increase bilirubin levels. Note temperature fluctuations, hypoglycemia, and infection. Determine the infant's oral intake and number of stools.

Analysis

Nurses can do many things to prevent situations that might cause further rises in bilirubin. They also must protect the infant from injury from the light during phototherapy. Therefore an appropriate nursing diagnosis is "Risk for Injury related to preventable causes of further elevation of bilirubin and damage to the eyes secondary to phototherapy."

Planning

The goal or expected outcome for this nursing diagnosis is that the infant will avoid injury from increased bilirubin or exposure of the eyes to phototherapy lights.

Interventions

Interventions are designed to prevent situations that might cause injury to the infant from rising bilirubin levels or effects of treatment.

Maintaining a Neutral Thermal Environment

Prevent situations, such as cold stress and hypoglycemia, that could result in increased fatty acids in the blood caused by acidosis, thereby decreasing the availability of albumin-binding sites for unconjugated bilirubin. Prevent cold stress at birth and during all care by maintaining the infant in a neutral thermal environment. Check the infant's axillary temperature every 2 to 4 hours to identify an early decrease before it becomes a problem. Dress the infant in warmed clothes and blankets upon removal from phototherapy lights.

Prevent elevation of the infant's temperature from exposure to the heat of the "bili" lights. Use a skin probe when the infant is in an incubator to maintain the appropriate environmental temperature. Position the lights according to the manufacturer's guidelines to prevent overheating or burning the skin.

Providing Optimal Nutrition

Ensure that the infant receives feedings every 2 to 3 hours, whether by breast or bottle. This prevents hypoglycemia, provides protein to maintain the albumin level in the blood, and promotes gastrointestinal motility and prompt emptying of bilirubin from the bowel. Avoid offering water because the infant may take less milk, which is more effective in removing bilirubin from the intestines. If breastfeeding must be supplemented, use formula instead of water.

Protecting the Eyes

Provide patches to protect the eyes from possible retinal damage from the phototherapy lights. Close the infant's eyes before placing the patches to avoid abrasions to the cornea. Check the position of the patches at least every hour. Infants often wiggle enough to push the patches above or below the eyes, leaving them exposed. The edges of the patches can dig into the eyes or compress the nose and interfere with breathing. If adhesive is used to fasten patches, check for skin irritation.

CRITICAL THINKING EXERCISE

QUESTION:
Why is it important to remove the patches from the eyes each time the infant is taken from the phototherapy for feeding?

Enhancing Response to Therapy

Expose as much skin as possible to the light. Remove all clothing except a diaper. Turn the infant frequently to prevent irritation of the skin from lack of position change and to expose the areas evenly.

If a fiberoptic blanket is used, check the position of the blanket frequently. Infants sometimes need to be repositioned so that the blanket remains in contact with the skin.

Controversy exists regarding the amount of time that the infant can be removed from phototherapy lights without decreasing the effectiveness. Generally, short periods out of the lights do not decrease effectiveness. The policy in most nurseries is to keep infants under the lights except during feedings. When bilirubin levels are high, some feedings may be given while the infant remains under the lights.

Use a light meter to check the level of irradiance to be sure the apparatus is functioning appropriately.

Observe for other complications. Although bilirubin encephalopathy is rare today, monitor for signs that indicate its presence. These include lethargy, poor muscle tone, decreased or absent Moro reflex, high-pitched cry, opisthotonos, and seizures.

Note the presence of rashes or changes in the color of the skin. Inform parents that they are not harmful and will disappear when phototherapy is discontinued.

Evaluation

No signs of injury should exist. The eyes will not have been exposed to the phototherapy lights.

Check Your Reading

6. When is jaundice considered pathologic?
7. What is the role of the nurse in caring for the infant receiving phototherapy?

INFECTION

Neonatal infection affects 1 to 4 in every 1000 live births (Gotoff, 2000). It is responsible for more than 30% of all neonatal deaths (Lott, et al., 1998). The nurse must be constantly alert for this condition.

Transmission of Infection

Newborns acquire infections in two ways:

1. Vertical infection:
   - In utero by passage of organisms across the placenta. These infections may cause long-term consequences. Examples are rubella, cytomegalovirus, syphilis, and toxoplasmosis.
   - During labor and birth as bacteria ascend the vagina. Examples are group B streptococci, hepatitis B, and herpes.
2. Horizontal infection:
   - After birth from hospital staff members, contaminated equipment (nosocomial infections), or family members.

Some common infections and their effects on the neonate are listed in Table 30-2. Some infections also are discussed in Chapter 26, p. 723.

Sepsis Neonatorum

Infection that occurs during or after birth may result in sepsis neonatorum, systemic infection with bacteria in the blood stream. Newborns are particularly susceptible to sepsis because their immune system is immature and they react more slowly to invasion by organisms. They fail to localize infection as well as older children, and this allows infection to spread easily from one organ to another. The blood-brain barrier is less effective in keeping out organisms, and central nervous system infection may occur. In addition, they have fewer antibodies. Preterm and low-birth-weight infants are especially susceptible to infection.

Table 30-2
COMMON VERTICAL INFECTIONS IN THE NEWBORN*

Infection	Transmission	Effect on Newborn	Nursing Considerations
VIRAL INFECTIONS			
Cytomegalovirus	Transplacental.	Most infants asymptomatic at birth. LBW, IUGR, enlarged liver and spleen, jaundice, mental retardation, hearing loss, blindness, seizures. May have no signs for months or years.	Most common perinatal infection. A major cause of mental retardation. Diagnosed by urine culture. May shed virus in saliva and urine for months or years. Antiviral drug therapy.
Hepatitis B	Usually during birth through contact with maternal blood. Also transplacental and in breast milk.	Asymptomatic at birth. LBW, prematurity. Most become chronic carriers. Risk of later liver cancer.	Wash well to remove all blood before skin is punctured for any reason. After cleaning, administer hepatitis B immune globulin and hepatitis B vaccine to prevent infection.
Herpes	Usually during birth through infected vagina or ascending infection after rupture of membranes. Transplacental rarely. Transmission highest with primary infection.	Clusters of vesicles, temperature instability, lethargy; poor suck, seizures, encephalitis, jaundice, purpura. Death or severe neurologic impairment is very high with disseminated infection.	Contact precautions. Obtain lesion specimens for culture. If untreated, approximately half die or have severe morbidity. Antiviral drug therapy improves outcome.
Human Immunodeficiency Virus/ Acquired Immunodeficiency Syndrome	Transplacental, during birth from infected blood and secretions or from breast milk. Transmission rate is greatly decreased if mother takes antiretroviral drugs during pregnancy.	Asymptomatic at birth, signs usually apparent at 4 to 12 months. Enlarged liver and spleen, lymphadenopathy, failure to thrive, pneumonia, persistent candida and bacterial infections.	Diagnosis may be delayed due to maternal antibodies. Some early tests available. Wash early and before skin is punctured to remove blood. Treat with antiretroviral drugs and prophylaxis against other infections.
Rubella	Transplacental.	Asymptomatic or IUGR, cataracts, cardiac defects, deafness, mental retardation. Damage greatest if infected in first trimester.	Contact precautions. Virus may be shed by infant as long as 1 year after birth. Diagnosed by presence of antibody. No treatment.
Varicella Zoster Virus (Chickenpox)	Transplacental.	Congenital varicella syndrome (skin scarring, IUGR, limb hypoplasia, CNS involvement), rash, eye damage, death. Damage greatest before the 20th weeks of gestation.	Immune globulin for pregnant woman exposed in pregnancy or for mothers and infants of mothers infected just before delivery. Acyclovir. Airborne isolation precautions for infants with lesions.
OTHER INFECTIONS			
Group B Streptococcal Infection	During birth or ascending after rupture of membranes.	Sudden onset of respiratory distress in infant usually well at birth, pneumonia, shock, meningitis. May have early or late onset.	Early identification essential to prevent death. Treated with IV antibiotics to mother in labor or to infant after birth.
Gonorrhea	Usually during birth.	Conjunctivitis (ophthalmia neonatorum), with red, edematous lids and purulent eye drainage. May result in blindness if untreated.	All infants receive erythromycin or tetracycline eye ointment for prevention. Silver nitrate previously used. Antibiotics if infection occurs.
Chlamydial Infection	During birth.	Conjunctivitis, pneumonia, otitis media.	Erythromycin eye ointment for prevention of conjunctivitis. Infection treated with erythromycin.

*Standard precautions for infection control apply to all patients and are not listed above. They include precautions for contact with blood; all body fluids, secretions, and excretions except sweat; nonintact skin; and mucous membranes. Contact precautions are used when transmission of the disease may occur from direct contact with patient's dry skin or articles in the patient's environment. See Appendix A for more information about infection control.

LBW, Low birth weight; *IUGR,* intrauterine growth restriction; *IV,* intravenous; *CNS,* central nervous system.

Table 30-2
COMMON VERTICAL INFECTIONS IN THE NEWBORN*—cont'd

Infection	Transmission	Effect on Newborn	Nursing Considerations
OTHER INFECTIONS—CONT'D			
Candidiasis	During birth	White patches in mouth (thrush) that bleed if removed. Rash on perineum. May be systemic.	Administer nystatin drops or cream and teach parents how to administer them. Assess mother for vaginal or breast infection.
Toxoplasmosis	Transplacental	Asymptomatic, or LBW, thrombocytopenia, enlarged liver and spleen, jaundice, anemia, seizures, microcephaly, hydrocephalus, chorioretinitis. Signs may not develop for years.	Consider in infants with IUGR. Confirmed by serum tests. Treatment: pyrimethamine, sulfadiazine, leucovorin calcium, and folinic acid.
Syphilis	Transplacental	Asymptomatic or enlarged liver and spleen, jaundice, lymphadenopathy anemia, rhinitis, pink or copper-colored peeling rash, pneumonitis, osteochondritis, CNS involvement.	Diagnosed by blood and cerebrospinal fluid testing. Administer penicillin as ordered.

LBW, Low birth weight; *IUGR,* intrauterine growth restriction; *IV,* intravenous; *CNS,* central nervous system.

CRITICAL TO REMEMBER

Signs of Sepsis in the Newborn

General Signs
Temperature instability (usually low)
Nurse's feeling that infant is not doing well
Rash

Respiratory Signs
Tachypnea
Respiratory distress (nasal flaring, retractions, grunting)
Apnea

Cardiovascular Signs
Color changes (cyanosis, pallor, mottling)
Tachycardia
Hypotension
Decreased peripheral perfusion

Gastrointestinal Signs
Decreased oral intake
Vomiting
Excessive gastric residuals

Gastrointestinal Signs—cont'd
Diarrhea
Abdominal distention
Hypoglycemia or hyperglycemia

Central Nervous System Signs
Decreased muscle tone
Lethargy
Irritability
Bulging fontanelle

Signs That May Indicate Advanced Infection
Jaundice
Evidence of hemorrhage (petechiae, purpura, pulmonary bleeding)
Anemia
Enlarged liver and spleen
Respiratory failure
Shock
Seizures

Causes

Common causative agents of neonatal sepsis include group B streptococci, *Escherichia coli, Haemophilus influenzae,* and coagulase negative staphylococci. Sepsis may be divided into early onset and late onset according to when signs of disease begin.

Early-onset sepsis often is caused by complications of labor such as prolonged rupture of membranes, prolonged labor, and chorioamnionitis. It usually begins within the first 3 days after birth. The mortality rate is 15% to 50% (Klein & Marcy, 1995). It often involves pneumonia or meningitis.

Late-onset sepsis generally develops 3 days to 2 months after birth. It usually involves the central nervous system with meningitis common. Mortality rate is 10% to 20% (Klein & Marcy, 1995), and serious long-term effects frequently occur.

Therapeutic Management

Testing. Neonatal sepsis may be confused with other illnesses. For example, group B streptococcal pneumonia has the same initial symptoms as respiratory distress syndrome. Therefore a variety of tests are ordered. Cultures of the blood, urine, gastric aspirate, and cerebral spinal fluid are obtained.

A complete blood count may show decreased neutrophils, increased bands (a form of immature neutrophils), an increased ratio of immature neutrophils to total neutrophils, and decreased platelets. Presence of elevated immunoglobulin M levels in cord blood or shortly after birth indicates that infection was acquired in utero because this immunoglobulin does not cross the placenta. It often indicates transplacental infection.

A C-reactive protein, a sign of an inflammatory process, may be elevated after the first day of infection. Chest radiography will help differentiate between respiratory distress syndrome and sepsis. Blood glucose levels should be checked because they may be unstable (high or low) in sepsis.

Treatment. Broad-spectrum antibiotics are given intravenously until culture and sensitivity results are available. Continued antibiotic therapy is based on culture results. Commonly used antibiotics include ampicillin, cefotaxime, gentamicin, and penicillin G. IV immunoglobulins also may be used in prevention and treatment of sepsis in some preterm infants. Other care is supportive to meet the infant's specific needs. The infant may require oxygen or intubation and mechanical ventilation. Fluid balance maintenance, monitoring of the blood pressure, and hourly urine output are important.

Nursing Considerations

Assessment

Risk Factors. The nurse should identify infants at risk for infection. The mother who had a prolonged or precipitous labor, prolonged rupture of membranes, signs of infection, or foul smelling or meconium-stained amniotic fluid may have an infant with sepsis. Women who are colonized in the vagina or rectum during pregnancy are treated with antibiotics during labor to reduce risk to the infant. Preterm or low-birth-weight infants and those with other complications also are at risk. Invasive procedures such as the use of IV catheters and endotracheal tubes are other sources of infection.

Signs of Infection. In the newborn, signs of infection are not as specific or obvious as those in the older infant or child. Instead, they tend to be subtle and could indicate other conditions. Temperature instability may occur, usually with low temperatures (Muchmore, 1999). Respiratory problems are common, and changes may occur in feeding habits or behavior. Often, the nurse is the person who notices the early, subtle changes that indicate sepsis. Experienced nurses may have a feeling that the infant is not doing well even before specific signs of infection are present. When this occurs, the nurse expands the assessment and watches carefully for the development of other signs. Early identification and treatment are important because infants can develop septic shock with little warning.

Nursing Interventions

The nurse is responsible for obtaining or helping obtain specimens for laboratory analysis and checking that other tests ordered by the physician are completed.

Providing Antibiotics. Because the signs of sepsis are nonspecific and the disease can be fatal, physicians may order antibiotics before an actual diagnosis is made for infants who are at high risk or show early signs. Broad-spectrum antibiotics are given intravenously until culture and sensitivity results are available. Continued antibiotic therapy is based on the organisms that are positive on culture. The nurse must be knowledgeable about the specific antibiotics used and possible side effects.

The nurse starts IV fluids and ensures that medications are administered on time. If more than one antibiotic is ordered, the timing of administration must be coordinated to increase effectiveness. Laboratory analysis of peak and trough levels may be ordered to measure blood levels of the medications at times when they are expected to be at the highest and lowest points. This requires planning with the laboratory so that blood is drawn at the correct time in relation to medication administration. Changes in dosage will be based on results of the laboratory tests. Antibiotics usually are continued for 10 days or longer.

Providing Other Supportive Care. Oxygen or other respiratory support is used if needed. The infant may need treatment for shock, hypoglycemia or hyperglycemia, electrolyte imbalances, and problems in temperature regulation. Gavage feeding may be necessary if the infant is unable to take oral feedings.

Infants with sepsis may have additional problems. They may be premature or have other transplacentally acquired infections. These may require other intensive nursing care.

Preventing Spread of Infection. Transmission of infection to other infants in the nursery must be prevented. This is accomplished with the same techniques used to prevent cross-contamination between normal infants (such as hand washing, separation of supplies, and standard precautions for infection control). They must be conscientiously performed by all who come in contact with the infant. Placing the infant in an incubator provides a physical separation between infected and well infants, similar to placing adults in isolation in private rooms. The nurse can observe the infant in an incubator more easily.

Supporting Parents. Nurses should support parents of newborns with sepsis and help them understand their infant's illness and treatment. The infant with sepsis often appears healthy at birth but suddenly becomes critically ill. Parents have feelings of shock, fear, and disappointment when their apparently healthy newborn is suddenly moved to the intensive care nursery. They will benefit from a chance to talk about their feelings with an understanding nurse who can explain the infant's treatment and care. Keeping the parents informed of the infant's changes in condition and involving them in care are essential.

INFANT OF A DIABETIC MOTHER

Scope of Problem

The infant of a diabetic mother (IDM) faces many risks that depend on the type of diabetes the mother has and how well it is controlled. Infants of mothers with long-term diabetes and vascular changes may be small-for-gestational age (SGA) because decreased placental blood flow causes intrauterine growth restriction. Hypertension occurs more often in diabetic women and further compromises uteroplacental blood flow.

Macrosomia (Figure 30-3) occurs in approximately one third of IDMs, even with good control of maternal glucose (Fanaroff, Martin, & Miller, 1999). When the mother is hyperglycemic, large amounts of amino acids, free fatty acids, and glucose are transferred to the fetus, but maternal insulin is not. This causes hypertrophy of the islet cells of the fetal pancreas. The islet cells produce large amounts of insulin, which acts as a growth hormone. The accelerated protein synthesis and the deposit of fat and glycogen in fetal tissues result in macrosomia. Macrosomic infants are at risk for trauma during birth, including fractures, facial nerve and brachial plexus damage, cephalhematoma, and skull fractures.

Congenital anomalies are two to six times more likely to occur in all IDMs (Fanaroff, Martin, & Miller, 1999). Anomalies of the neural tube, heart, and kidney and caudal regression syndrome are most common. The incidence of anomalies is less if blood glucose levels remain within normal limits, especially before conception and in the early weeks of gestation, when organs are forming.

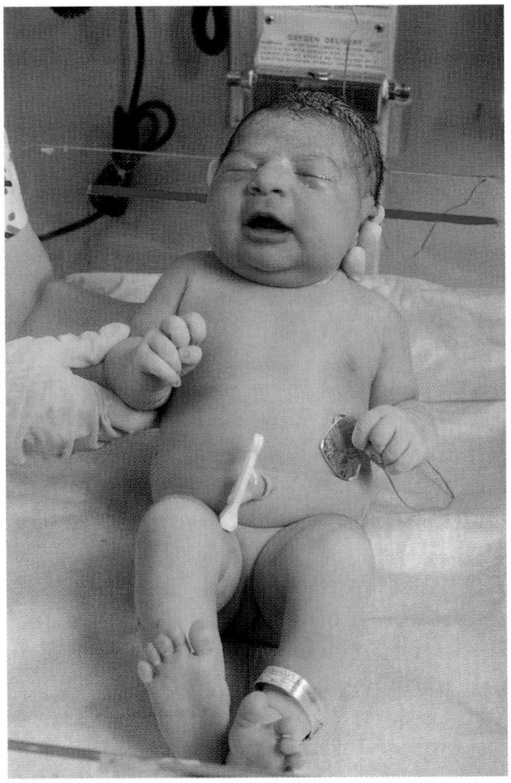

FIGURE 30-3 Macrosomia is common in infants of diabetic mothers.

IDMs have a higher risk of asphyxia and respiratory distress syndrome (RDS) than normal infants. RDS occurs because high levels of insulin interfere with the production of surfactant. Maintaining strict control of the diabetes and allowing the pregnancy to progress to full term reduces the incidence of RDS.

Other complications for which the IDM is at risk include hypoglycemia after birth, when the maternal supply of glucose ends but the infant's high level of insulin production continues. Hypocalcemia (p. 856) may occur as a result of decreased parathyroid hormone production, especially when the mother's diabetes was poorly controlled. Polycythemia also may be a problem (p. 856) and could lead to high bilirubin levels.

Characteristics of Infants of Diabetic Mothers

The SGA IDM is similar to other SGA infants but is more likely to have congenital anomalies. The macrosomic IDM is different from other large-for-gestational age (LGA) infants. The infant's size results from fat deposits and hypertrophy of the liver, adrenals, and heart. All organs except the brain are larger than normal. The length and head size are generally within the normal range for gestational age. Other LGA infants do not have enlargement of the organs and tend to be long, with large heads to match the rest of their bodies. Infants of diabetic mothers have a characteristic appearance. The face is round and red, and the body is obese. Poor muscle tone exists at rest, but the infant becomes irritable and may have tremors when disturbed.

Therapeutic Management

Therapeutic management includes controlling the mother's diabetes throughout the pregnancy to decrease complications of the fetus and newborn (see Chapter 26). If the infant is large, delivery may be difficult and a cesarean birth may be required. Immediate care of respiratory problems and continued observation for complications determine treatment.

Nursing Considerations

Assessment

The IDM is assessed for signs of complications, trauma, and congenital anomalies at delivery and during the early hours after birth. Hypoglycemia occurs in 25% to 50% of infants of mothers with pregestational diabetes and 15% to 25% of those with gestational diabetes (Stoll & Kliegman, 2000). It may be present without observable signs. The blood glucose is screened according to hospital protocol. An example is testing shortly after birth, every 2 hours for the first 8 hours, and every 4 hours for 24 hours or until stable (Johnson, 2000).

Glucose levels of less than 40 to 45 mg/dl measured with beside glucose screening should be reported and verified by laboratory analysis.

The most frequent sign of low glucose is jitteriness or tremors. Diaphoresis is uncommon in newborns but may occur with hypoglycemia. Rapid respirations, low temperature, and poor muscle tone also are common (Chapter 20, p. 520). Because these signs are not specific for hypoglycemia, the nurse must be alert for other complications, particularly if signs continue after feeding.

Nursing Interventions

If hypoglycemia develops, infants must be fed immediately to prevent further decreases in glucose. Gavage feeding may be used if the infant does not suck well or the respirations are high. Some infants need IV glucose to maintain balance and prevent damage to the brain.

> **CRITICAL THINKING EXERCISE**
>
> QUESTION:
> Although 5% or 10% dextrose water was often used for the first feeding for infants with low blood glucose in the past, using breast milk or formula is now more common. What is the rationale for this?

The nurse must be alert for signs of other complications that occur in IDMs. Signs of respiratory distress syndrome or other respiratory complications may exist. Cold stress, which increases the need for oxygen and glucose, could increase respiratory problems and exacerbate hypoglycemia.

Infants with polycythemia need adequate hydration and should be observed for jaundice. Infants also are at increased risk for low calcium levels. If jitteriness occurs and the glucose levels are normal, the infant may have hypocalcemia.

Providing support to parents is important. They may not understand why their infant, who appears fat and healthy to them, needs close observation and frequent blood tests. The mother may have had a difficult pregnancy and may feel guilty, even if she followed a program of good diabetic control. Ample opportunity for discussion of feelings and information about the care of the infant is important.

> **Check Your Reading**
>
> 8. What is the difference between vertical and horizontal transmission of infection?
> 9. What is the role of the nurse in caring for the infant with sepsis?
> 10. What problems occur in infants of diabetic mothers?
> 11. What are the major nursing responsibilities in caring for infants of diabetic mothers?

POLYCYTHEMIA

In polycythemia, infants have a hemoglobin above 22 g/dL and a hematocrit higher than 65% during the first week of life. The increased viscosity of the blood interferes with circulation and may result in organ damage, renal vein thrombosis, and necrotizing enterocolitis. Polycythemia also may result in hyperbilirubinemia as the excessive red blood cells break down after birth.

Causes

Polycythemia may occur when poor intrauterine oxygenation causes the fetus to produce more erythrocytes than normal to compensate. Maternal hypertension or diabetes, SGA infants, and delayed clamping of the cord may cause the condition.

Therapeutic Management

Treatment is primarily supportive but may include partial exchange transfusion. Blood is replaced with albumin or plasma to decrease the total number of red blood cells.

Nursing Considerations

Infants may be plethoric (red) but have no other signs, or they may have lethargy, jitteriness, cyanosis, respiratory problems, and hypoglycemia. Monitoring of bilirubin levels is important if jaundice occurs as blood cells break down. Infants must be hydrated adequately to prevent dehydration and watched for complications of an exchange transfusion.

HYPOCALCEMIA

Hypocalcemia is a total serum calcium concentration of less than 7.0 mg/dl. It is divided into early onset (<48 hours of age) and late onset (at about 1 week of age).

Causes

Early-onset hypocalcemia occurs most often in IDMs, asphyxia, prematurity, and low-birth-weight infants. Late hypocalcemia is caused by maternal hyperparathyroidism or vitamin D deficiency, high phosphate formula, low magnesium levels, and congenital hypoparathyroidism. Other causes of hypocalcemia include alkalosis, administration of bicarbonate or citrate-preserved blood, furosemide therapy, and renal disease.

Therapeutic Management

Laboratory testing of serum calcium determines the presence of the problem. Oral or IV calcium gluconate is given if feeding alone does not raise the calcium level. A cardiac monitor is necessary when IV calcium is given because bradycardia can occur.

Nursing Considerations

The nurse must be alert for signs of hypocalcemia, including irritability, tremors, poor feeding, high-pitched cry, tachycardia, apnea, muscle twitching, seizures, and electrocardiogram changes. Hypocalcemia often is asymptomatic.

Oral calcium should be given with feedings because it may cause gastric irritation. IV calcium should be administered slowly and stopped immediately if bradycardia or arrhythmia develops. The IV site should be assessed frequently because infiltration can cause necrosis and ulceration.

PRENATAL DRUG EXPOSURE

Substance abuse affects the fetus at any time during pregnancy. Most drugs readily cross the placenta and cause a variety of problems. Abuse during the first 2 months of pregnancy may cause congenital anomalies. Later abuse may interfere with development or functioning of organs already formed. Abuse of more than one substance is common, making it difficult to determine which substance led to individual effects.

The effects of substance abuse on pregnancy, the fetus, and the neonate are discussed in Chapter 24. This section includes nursing care for infants with neonatal abstinence syndrome, the disorder in which neonates demonstrate signs of drug withdrawal.

Identification of Drug-Exposed Infants

Maternal substance abuse may be identified before an infant is born, but many infants are born to women whose substance use is not known to the health professionals caring for them during labor and delivery. Lack of prenatal care or the mother's behavior during labor may cause nurses to suspect substance abuse. Placental abruption may occur after cocaine use. When any cause exists to suspect drug use, the infant is observed closely for signs of prenatal drug exposure.

CRITICAL TO REMEMBER

Signs of Intrauterine Drug Exposure

Behavioral Signs
- Irritability
- Jitteriness, tremors
- Muscular rigidity, increased muscle tone
- Restless, excessive activity
- Exaggerated Moro reflex
- Prolonged high-pitched cry
- Difficult to console

Signs Relating to Feeding
- Uncoordinated sucking and swallowing
- Frequent regurgitation or vomiting
- Diarrhea

Other Signs
- Poor sleeping patterns
- Yawning
- Nasal stuffiness, sneezing
- Fever
- Tachypnea
- Apnea
- Seizures
- Diaphoresis
- Excoriation

NOTE: Some infants with prenatal drug exposure will have no abnormal signs at all, or signs may be delayed.

Neonatal abstinence syndrome occurs in infants who have suffered prenatal opiate exposure sufficient to cause withdrawal signs after birth. Infants with prenatal cocaine exposure do not experience an abstinence syndrome or withdrawal, unlike opiate-exposed infants. Instead, problems in these infants are related to neurotoxicity from the drug (Kandall, 1998).

Signs of drug exposure usually begin during the first 48 to 72 hours after birth for opiates, 2 to 3 days for cocaine, and within 3 to 12 hours for alcohol, depending on the time of the mother's last use. Polydrug use is common, and signs vary according to the drug or combination of drugs and time of last use. Signs often include neurologic and gastrointestinal abnormalities, but some infants with prenatal drug exposure show no abnormal signs or do not show signs until after the first week.

Infants with neonatal abstinence syndrome may be irritable and have hyperactive muscle tone and a high-pitched cry. Although they have tremors, the blood glucose level is normal. They appear hungry and suck vigorously on their fists but have poor coordination of suck and swallow. Frequent regurgitation, vomiting, and diarrhea are common. Infants are restless, and their excessive activity coupled with poor feeding ability result in failure to gain weight. Seizures may occur.

Various scoring systems are available to determine the number, frequency, and severity of behaviors that may indicate neonatal abstinence syndrome. The score is used when considering whether drug therapy to alleviate withdrawal signs is needed and to determine dosage.

Congenital anomalies and other effects of prenatal drug exposure may be apparent at birth. Many of these infants are SGA. They also may be preterm and suffer from related complications. Infants are more likely to have respiratory problems at birth, jaundice, or sudden infant death syndrome. Infants with fetal alcohol syndrome have a characteristic appearance (see Figure 24-3).

When exposure is suspected, a urine specimen is collected from the infant for analysis. Drugs or their metabolites are present in the newborn's urine for various lengths of time after the mother has used them. Some drugs last several days because of the infant's difficulty in excreting them, whereas others disappear very soon. Therefore obtaining a urine specimen as early as possible is important, preferably during the first 24 hours after birth (Procedure 30-2). Meconium also may be tested because it shows drug use for a longer period before birth.

Therapeutic Management

Because many signs of drug exposure are similar to those for other conditions, testing may be performed to rule out other causes. Sepsis, hypoglycemia, hypocalcemia, and neurologic disorders are possible causes for the infant's problems. In addition, the infant may have been exposed to infections from the mother, such as hepatitis or sexually transmissible infections.

PROCEDURE 30-2

Applying a Pediatric Urine Collection Bag

Purpose: To collect a nonsterile urine specimen from an infant.

1. Wash and dry the genitalia. Apply tincture of benzoin according to hospital policy. Allow to dry until "tacky." *Removal of gross contaminants prevents contamination of the specimen. The bag adheres to a clean, dry surface best. Tincture of benzoin increases adherence of the bag to the skin.*
2. Remove the paper covering the posterior adhesive tabs of the bag first. To apply to female infants, stretch the perineum (skin between the rectum and the vagina). Fold the bag in half and apply smoothly over the perineum, extending the tabs to the side. For male infants, place the penis and scrotum (if small) inside the bag and apply the posterior adhesive tabs to the perineum. If the scrotum will not fit in the bag easily, apply the tabs smoothly over the scrotum. *Covering the perineum with the posterior tabs first helps ensure smooth fit at this area, where leakage of urine may occur in the female infant especially, and prevents contamination with feces. Care in application prevents losing the specimen.*
3. Remove the paper covering the anterior adhesive tabs, and apply to cover genitalia. Be sure that there are no wrinkles in the tabs. *Wrinkles allow openings for urine to leak out of the bag.*

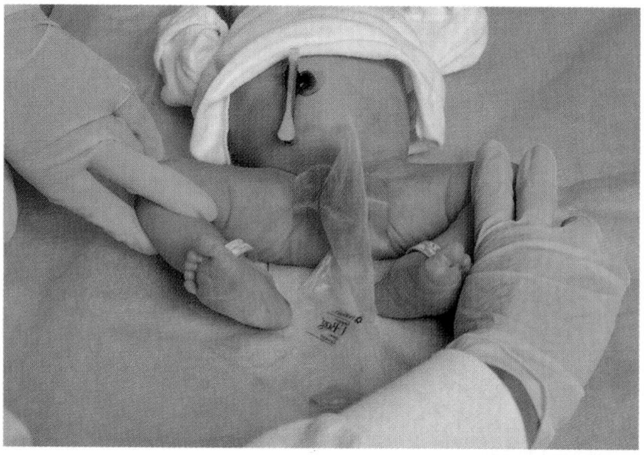

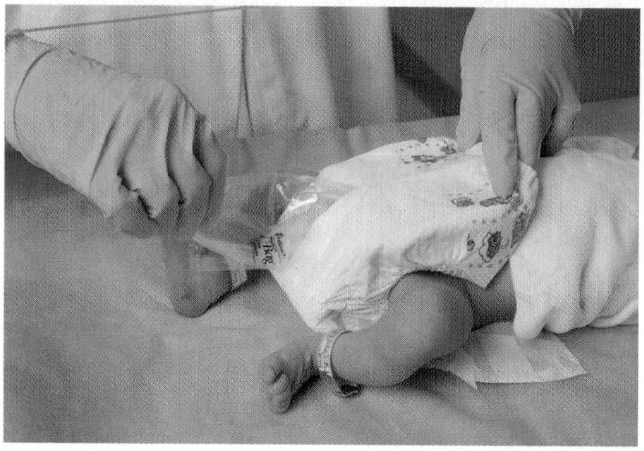

4. Place the diaper loosely over the bag or cut a slit in the diaper and gently pull the bag through the slit. *Cutting a slit in the diaper allows visualization of the bag. Placing the diaper too tightly over the bag might pull against the adhesive, causing trauma to the skin and providing an opening through which the specimen is lost.*
5. Check the bag for urine frequently and remove as soon as urine is present. Transfer the urine to a specimen cup by removing the tab over the hole in the bottom or cutting the lower corner and pouring. The specimen also can be aspirated with a syringe after cleaning the puncture site with alcohol. *Ensures removal of the bag before urine loosens the adhesive. Prepares the specimen to be sent to the laboratory for analysis.*
6. Clean the genitalia, and observe for irritation. *Removes urine and adhesive from the skin.*
7. Label the specimen and transport to the lab or refrigerate if necessary. Record in the infant's chart. *Ensures proper disposition of the specimen.*

Therapeutic management includes dealing with the complications common to drug-exposed infants during and after birth. Respiratory problems and those related to prematurity are treated as for other infants. Drug therapy may be necessary for approximately 50% to 60% of these infants, who may have vomiting, diarrhea, marked irritability, and high scores on abstinence scales (Weiner & Finnegan, 1998). Drugs used include phenobarbital, oral morphine, tincture of opium, paregoric, methadone, diazepam, and chlorpromazine. Drug dosage is gradually tapered over time. Although these drugs help relieve the signs of withdrawal, all have side effects that may be undesirable.

Because the infant's suck and swallow are uncoordinated, gavage or IV feeding may be required. Some infants may need more than the normal caloric requirements because of their excessive activity. Involvement by social services in and out of the hospital is important to deal with the long-term effects of the drugs, placement of the infant after hospitalization, and follow-up of the mother or other caretaker to help provide for the infant's needs.

Nursing Considerations

The infant who has been exposed to drugs prenatally will need special care to cope with drug withdrawal. Care is focused on feeding, rest, and enhancing parental attachment, if possible (Nursing Care Plan 30-2).

Feeding

Feeding can be difficult and time consuming. The poor suck and swallow coordination of drug-exposed infants interferes with caloric intake, yet their excessive activity increases their caloric needs.

NURSING CARE PLAN 30-2

The Drug-Exposed Infant

Tracy was born at 38 weeks' gestation to Gloria, who was on a methadone maintenance program. However, Tracy tested positive not only for methadone but also for heroin, which Gloria admitted using several times in the days just before she began labor.

Assessment: Tracy weighs 2240 g (4 lb, 15 oz) and is small for gestational age. She is jittery, becomes agitated easily, and has a poor suck and swallow. Tracy regurgitates her feedings frequently. She has been fed by gavage but is now taking formula feedings orally.

Nursing Diagnosis: Altered Nutrition: Less Than Body Requirements related to abnormal coordination of suck and swallow and excessive activity.

Goals/Expected Outcomes:
Tracy will do the following:
- Take and retain 246 to 269 kcal daily (110 to 120 kcal/kg/day)
- Gain at least ½ ounce each day

Intervention	Rationale
1. Feed Tracy as soon as she begins to wake at feeding times.	1. Drug-exposed infants often move from sleeping to an agitated state very quickly. This makes feeding more difficult.
2. Swaddle Tracy with her extremities in a flexed position during feeding.	2. Infants become more agitated if they are allowed to startle. Swaddling provides a sense of security and prevents excessive movement.
3. Try warming the formula slightly before feeding.	3. Some infants take warmed formula more readily.
4. Use chin and cheek support during the feedings as needed.	4. Chin and cheek support increases sucking strength and increases intake.
5. Feed slowly with frequent stops for burping Tracy. If frantic sucking continues when the feeding is stopped, use a pacifier to soothe her.	5. Frequent burping while keeping the infant calm helps prevent regurgitation.
6. Place Tracy on her right side with her head elevated 30 to 45 degrees after feedings. Keep the environment as nonstimulating as possible after feedings.	6. Positioning uses gravity to promote gastric emptying and helps prevent aspiration during regurgitation. Quiet surroundings promote sleep and weight gain and decrease agitation.

Evaluation: Tracy's intake averages 250 calories each day. She gains slightly more than ½ ounce daily.

Assessment: Tracy sleeps less than an hour after feedings. When she awakens, her high-pitched cry and agitation begin immediately. She wiggles out of her blankets, and her activity elicits the Moro reflex, which leads to more agitation. She is irritable and does not respond to care taking activities as quickly as other infants.

Nursing Diagnosis: Sleep Pattern Disturbance related to agitation from own activity and irritability.

Goals/Expected Outcomes:
Tracy will do the following:
- Sleep for periods of 2 hours or more after feedings within 3 days.
- Decrease crying by at least 1 hour a day within the first week.

Intervention	Rationale
1. Place Tracy's crib in the quietest corner of the nursery. Place a sign nearby to remind others of the need for quiet in that area. For example, "Quiet, please! Tracy is resting!"	1. Drug-exposed infants are easily overstimulated by noise and activity.
2. Keep lights turned down as much as possible. Place a blanket over the head end of the crib to decrease light.	2. Lowered lighting provides a more restful environment.
3. Keep Tracy tightly swaddled in a flexed position during sleep and feedings.	3. The drug-exposed infant's own movements can cause startling, awakening, and agitation.
4. Use a pacifier, and position her hands near her mouth.	4. Nonnutritive sucking may have a calming effect on the infant. Positioning the hands near the mouth allows the infant to self-comfort by sucking.
5. Use a slow vertical rocking motion or a vibrating infant seat when Tracy is upset.	5. Vertical rocking or a vibrating infant seat may increase rest, decrease agitation, and help infants move more smoothly from one behavior state to another.

Continued

Intervention	Rationale
6. Use a front infant carrier during Tracy's awake periods.	6. An infant carrier provides the same effect as swaddling. In addition, it provides warmth and a rocking motion from the caretaker's body that may be soothing.
7. Organize nursing care so that Tracy is not disturbed unnecessarily especially when sleeping.	7. Drug-exposed infants may have difficulty going back to sleep if awakened.

Evaluation: Tracy gradually lengthens her sleep periods to 2 hours and decreases crying episodes within the first week.

Assessment: Gloria visits Tracy sporadically. She seems hesitant when she comes into the nursery and afraid to touch or care for Tracy. She asks, "Why does she cry so much?" When the nurse helps her hold Tracy, Gloria states, "I don't think she likes me."

Nursing Diagnosis: Altered Parenting related to lack of understanding of the infant's characteristics and how to relate to an irritable infant.

Goals/Expected Outcomes:
Gloria will do the following:
- Visit at least every other day
- Participate in Tracy's care by holding and feeding her
- Make positive statements about her daughter

Intervention	Rationale
1. Show acceptance of Gloria when she comes to visit Tracy. Greet her and provide her with an update on Tracy's progress.	1. A mother is more likely to visit her infant if she feels accepted by staff. The more she visits, the more she is likely to learn to parent her infant.
2. Assist Gloria to hold and feed Tracy. Explain nursing actions such as placing the crib in a secluded corner and covering the top.	2. Encouraging the mother to participate in care of the infant helps her get to know her infant and how to care for the infant more quickly.
3. Show Gloria how to make Tracy more comfortable. Demonstrate and explain swaddling and rocking. Show her how to place a rolled blanket around the infant to provide a feeling of security and help promote sleep.	3. When the mother learns ways to comfort her infant, the positive response from the infant may increase bonding.
4. Explain the behavioral characteristics of infants who are drug exposed. Explain that Tracy's stiff body posture and failure to "mold" to the mother's body are normal for her. Point out signs that Tracy is overstimulated such as gaze aversion and increase in irritability. Explain that the high pitched cry is common.	4. The mother needs to learn that the infant's behavior is part of the infant's problem and is not caused by the mother's handling of her.
5. Model ways of interacting with Tracy and calming her when she becomes agitated. Demonstrate holding quietly and point out signs that Tracy is ready to interact. Suggest only one stimulus at a time, such as talking softly without rocking.	5. The mother learns appropriate interaction when she sees it performed by the nurse. Infants may need short time-outs before they are ready for more stimulation. Decreasing the number of stimuli may be more effective.
6. Point out positive points about Tracy, such as her long eyelashes or delicate fingers. Point out signs that show that Tracy is making progress.	6. The mother needs help to focus on positive aspects of the infant as well as the problems.
7. Explain the routine care of a newborn. Spread teaching out over Gloria's visits.	7. The mother needs to learn the usual care of any newborn as well as the infant's special needs.
8. Give praise and encouragement frequently as Gloria works with Tracy.	8. The mother needs positive reinforcement and help to feel that she is capable of mothering her infant.
9. Use therapeutic communication techniques to help Gloria discuss her feelings as she cares for Tracy.	9. Mothers often find it frustrating to care for the drug-exposed infant. Helping them vent their feelings may increase their ability to cope with the infant's special needs.
10. Discuss sources of support from family members or friends. Refer her to social services or support groups in the community.	10. Ongoing support is necessary for the woman with addiction problems. Support for the mother will help her care more effectively for her infant.
11. If Gloria will have custody of Tracy, help her begin to make plans for discharge. Discuss ongoing problems and concerns such as continued withdrawal signs and sudden infant death syndrome (SIDS).	11. Preparation for discharge must be made well in advance. Infants will have ongoing problems that will continue in the home setting. Infants exposed to heroin have an increased incidence of SIDS.

Evaluation: Gloria begins to visit more often, coming four to five times a week. She participates in care, begins to talk about her "pretty little girl," and discusses her plans for when she can regain custody and take Tracy home with her.

Assessment. The nurse should assess the infant's ability to coordinate sucking and swallowing. Infants often suck frantically on their fists or a nipple but are unable to coordinate feeding behaviors well. Changes in the frequency and amount of regurgitation, vomiting, or the time it takes infants to finish feedings should be noted.

Nursing Interventions. Gavage feedings may be necessary to save the infant's energy and prevent aspiration if the infant is excessively agitated, unable to suck and swallow adequately, or has rapid respirations. When oral feedings begin, infants may need chin and cheek support similar to that used for preterm infants to help them suck more efficiently. Formula with 24 calories per ounce instead of the usual 20 calories per ounce may be used because the infant's excessive activity, poor sleeping, vomiting, and diarrhea increase the caloric need.

Distractions during feedings can be prevented by choosing a quiet, low-activity area of the nursery for feedings. Infants should be swaddled to prevent the startling that occurs when drug-exposed infants are handled. Stimuli such as rocking and talking should be kept to a minimum during feedings. After feedings, infants should be positioned on the right side with the head of the bed elevated 30 to 45 degrees.

Rest

The excessive activity and poor sleep patterns of drug-exposed neonates interfere with their ability to rest.

Assessment. The infant's muscle tone, tremors, and tendency for excessive activity with and without being disturbed should be assessed. The degree of tremors and stimuli that increase or decrease irritability are important. The nurse also keeps track of the number of hours that the infant sleeps after each feeding.

Nursing Interventions. Stimulation of the drug-exposed infant should be kept to a minimum, especially at first when the infant is excessively irritable. The number of different types of stimulation should be kept to a minimum and adapted to each infant's needs. Noise and bright lights are reduced as much as possible. If the infant shows signs of overstimulation, all activity should be stopped briefly to allow a rest. Swaddling or placing the excessively agitated infant in a dark, quiet room may be necessary. As the infant shows the ability to withstand stimulation, new types can be gradually added, one at a time.

The nurse should organize nursing care to reduce handling and disturbances. A calm approach and slow, smooth movements during care help avoid startling the infant. Swaddling the infant in a flexed position helps prevent startling and agitation. Nonnutritive sucking also helps quiet the infant. Some infants benefit from being placed in special rocking beds or infant seats that gently vibrate. This must be evaluated on an individual basis, however. One small study found that rocking beds caused an increase in withdrawal behaviors in infants during the acute phase (D'Apolito, 1999). Skin abrasions from excessive activity and rubbing of the face, elbows, and knees may increase discomfort and agitation. Diaper rash from frequent diarrhea also may occur. Skin breakdown should be prevented if possible and treated promptly if it occurs.

Bonding

Infants who test positive for drugs may not be released to the mother until her ability to care for her infant safely has been assessed by social services or a court. She may be required to enter a drug rehabilitation program before she can obtain custody of the infant. After hospital discharge, some infants must be cared for in a foster home or by family members approved by the court. The mother will most likely gain custody of the infant eventually if she complies with court-ordered treatment, and attachment to the infant should be encouraged.

Assessment. The frequency of her visits and her response to the infant may give an indication of the mother's apparent interest in the infant. Although some substance-abusing mothers are uninterested in their infants, for others the infant provides a reason to attempt to overcome their addiction. Bonding behaviors such as calling the infant by name and smiling at the infant should be noted.

Nursing Interventions. Child neglect, child abuse, and failure to respond to infant signals and cues are associated with alcohol and drug abuse. Because the mother may become the infant's primary caretaker, nurses must do whatever they can to enhance mother-infant bonding. Helping the mother feel welcome when she visits the infant provides a challenge. It is sometimes easy to be judgmental and difficult to be accepting when the mother's behavior has been harmful to her infant. Yet a friendly approach will make the mother more likely to visit the infant and accept teaching from the nurse.

The nurse can promote bonding by encouraging mothers to participate actively in infant care during visits. Including the mother will help her feel that the nurses trust her to care for the infant. This may help increase her determination to go through recovery to regain her newborn.

The mother's participation also provides a chance to assess the mother's infant care skills and areas in which further discussion of the newborn's needs will be helpful. In addition, it gives the nurse an opportunity to demonstrate parenting skills. Many mothers who use drugs have not had good parenting role models and do not know what to do. Frequent positive feedback about the mother's participation also is important.

PARENTS WANT TO KNOW: *Measures to Prevent Frantic Crying in a Drug-Exposed Infant*

Swaddle the infant with the hands brought to the midline and secured (see Figure 30-4).

Provide a pacifier.

Keep the infant's back toward you and support the head while flexing the knees. Slowly and smoothly rock in a vertical motion.

Coo softly and gently.

Place the infant over your shoulder and gently stroke the back.

Keep the room fairly dark because some infants are particularly sensitive to light.

Avoid simultaneous auditory and visual stimuli.

Curtail stimulation if infant shows signs of stress (yawning, sneezing, jerky movements, or spitting up).

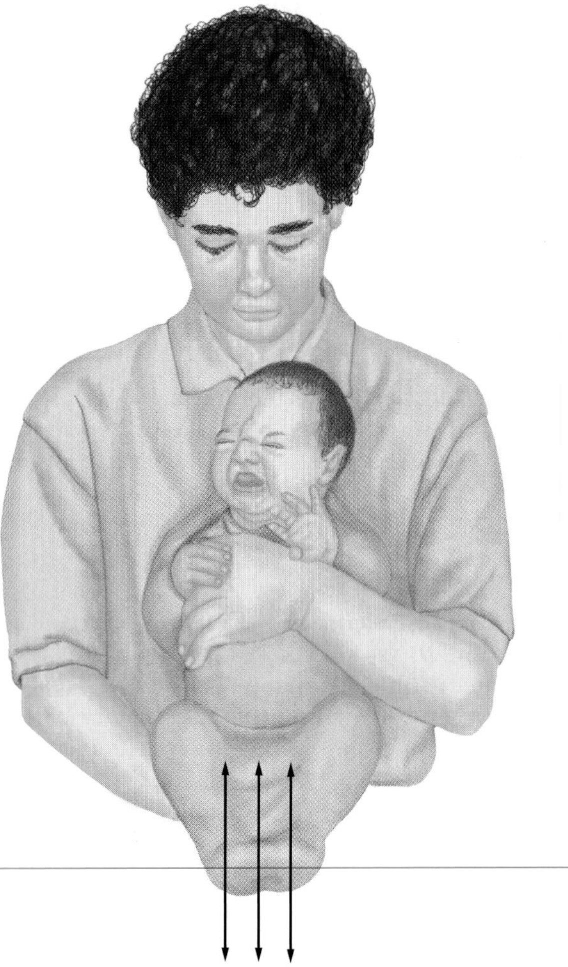

FIGURE 30-4 Consoling behaviors for a drug-exposed infant. Note that the infant is swaddled with the hands positioned in the midline, facing away from the caregiver to reduce simultaneous stimuli, and that the caregiver uses vertical rocking.

The mother needs the same teaching given to all new parents, as well as special techniques necessary to meet the needs of drug-exposed infants. The nurse should teach her about her newborn's special characteristics and help her take on more of the infant's care as she demonstrates readiness. For example, she will need to learn the way to swaddle the infant in a flexed position to prevent excessive startles and tremors (see Figure 30-4, opposite, and Parents Want to Know, above).

Parents of a drug-exposed infant need to know that they may experience feelings of rejection, frustration, and even hostility. These feelings are likely to occur when the infant stiffens while being held, cries after being fed, or looks away. Parents also must know that drug-exposed infants are easily stressed because of the decreased stability of their central nervous systems. Emphasize that the infant needs gentle handling. Also explain that crying indicates a need, not a spoiled infant.

Some infants are comforted when they are snugly swaddled with their hands brought to midline. These infants cannot tolerate simultaneous visual and tactile stimulation. Some infants are consoled more easily if positioned with their faces away from the caregiver and if vertical, rather than horizontal, rocking movements are used (see Figure 30-4).

Signs of overstimulation in drug-exposed infants have some similarities with those for the preterm infant. In addition, some infants cannot tolerate more than brief periods of interaction. They may not make eye contact, or they may avert their eyes after 30 to 60 seconds of social interaction. Cuddling and soothing to console the infant may not elicit the same response in these infants as in other infants. The nurse should teach the mother that the infant responds poorly to everyone so that she does not think she is being rejected.

Many drugs pass into breast milk. Trying to breastfeed an infant with poorly developed feeding skills may be too much stress for the mother who is trying to recover from addiction. Therefore mothers who are likely to continue drug use after delivery should be discouraged from breastfeeding. However, breastfeeding may be acceptable in some situations. If the woman has a strong desire to breastfeed, the nurse should consult the health care provider.

The nurse can provide information and referral to any special programs available to help parents learn special stimulation techniques appropriate for drug-exposed infants. Some withdrawal signs may continue for as long as 6 months, and the mother needs to know how to deal with them (Weiner & Finnegan, 1998). If the mother is unable to care for the newborn, the same

Check Your Reading

12. What common problems occur in infants with prenatal exposure to drugs?
13. What special nursing care measures are needed for drug-exposed infants?

interventions can be used to help the person who will take over care of the infant on hospital discharge.

PHENYLKETONURIA

Phenylketonuria (PKU) is a genetic disorder that causes central nervous system damage from toxic levels of the amino acid phenylalanine in the blood. All newborns are screened for this condition before or shortly after discharge from the birth facility. Mental retardation occurs in untreated infants and children.

Causes

PKU is caused by a deficiency of the enzyme phenylalanine hydroxylase, which is necessary to convert phenylalanine to tyrosine for use. It is an autosomal recessive disorder.

Therapeutic Management

Positive screening tests are followed with other testing. Treatment is a low phenylalanine diet. Small amounts of phenylalanine are allowed because it is a necessary amino acid. Early and continued treatment are necessary to prevent mental retardation.

Nursing Considerations

The nurse should determine whether the newborn received screening for PKU. Screening performed before 24 to 48 hours of age should be repeated because the infant must have consumed enough protein for the test to be accurate.

Signs of the disease include digestive problems, vomiting, seizures, musty or mousy odor of the urine, and mental retardation. Older children have eczema, hypertonia, hyperactive behavior, and hypopigmentation of the hair, skin, and irises.

The nurse assists parents in regulating the diet to meet the infant's changing phenylalanine needs. Parents can be reassured that good control should allow normal infant growth and development.

CONGENITAL ANOMALIES AND CONGENITAL CARDIAC DEFECTS

Approximately 2% to 3% of newborns have major congenital anomalies at birth. These defects are responsible for approximately 20% of all neonatal deaths (Lott, 1998). Some infants have more than one anomaly, which may be part of a syndrome or result from unrelated causes. Although congenital anomalies generally are treated in the pediatric setting, they usually are identified soon after birth. Common congenital anomalies are noted in Table 30-3. (See a pediatric nursing textbook for more detailed information.) Congenital cardiac conditions are discussed in this section.

Approximately 1% of newborns have congenital heart defects (Daberkow & Washington, 1998). Congenital heart defects are a major cause of death in the first year. Genetics, teratogens, maternal diabetes, and rubella are known to be possible factors. The heart forms by the sixth week of gestation, and problems in development during this period may be associated with anomalies of other structures as well.

Classification of Cardiac Defects

Cardiac defects are generally categorized according to the pattern of blood flow and whether cyanosis results from the defect. Some of the most common defects are illustrated in Figure 30-5.

Acyanotic Defects

In acyanotic conditions, an obstruction of blood flow from the left side of the heart or a defect that causes increased flow of blood to the lungs occurs. Both increase the work of the heart. In addition, congestion in the lungs may eventually cause increased resistance of the pulmonary vessels and pulmonary hypertension. Infants are prone to respiratory infections because of the pulmonary congestion and increased work of the heart and lungs. Growth is slowed, and the infant fatigues easily. The heart may fail from overwork. Patent ductus arteriosus is an example of this group.

Cyanotic Defects

In cyanotic defects, a decrease in blood flow to the lungs, mixing of venous and oxygenated blood into the general systemic circulation, or both occurs, decreasing the oxygen carried to the tissues and resulting in cyanosis. This results in a right-to-left shunt where venous blood from the right side of the heart flows through an abnormal opening to the left side of the heart and into the systemic circulation. Although the heart and lungs work harder, adequate oxygenation may be impossible, resulting in hypoxia of the major organs. Infants usually have serious problems from birth. The infant grows poorly, has frequent infections, and is easily fatigued. Heart failure may be an early complication. Transposition of the great vessels is an example of a cyanotic heart defect.

The presence of cyanosis depends on the severity and combination of defects and the child's ability to compensate. Some infants with cyanotic heart disease may be pink, and some with acyanotic heart defects may develop cyanosis. Because of this potential change in classification, further classification by blood flow is helpful.

Text continues on p. 869

Table 30-3
COMMON CONGENITAL ANOMALIES
Gastrointestinal Tract

Cleft Lip and Palate

These are among the most common congenital anomalies, and they occur together or separately, on one or both sides. *Lip:* minor notching of the lip or completely through the lip and into floor of nose. *Palate:* only the soft palate or division of entire hard and soft palate. Both genetic and environmental factors are included in cause.

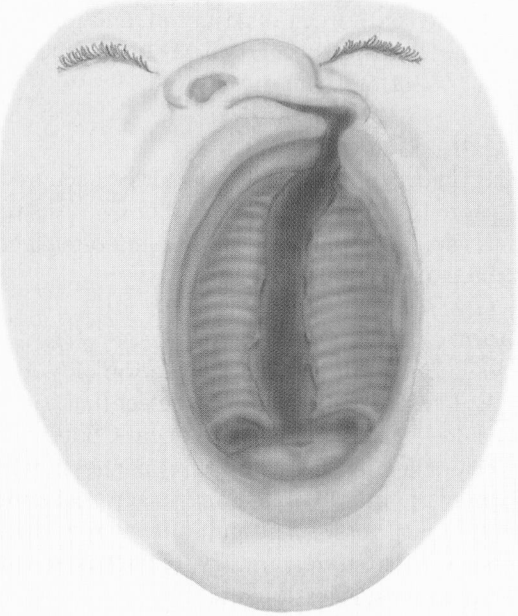

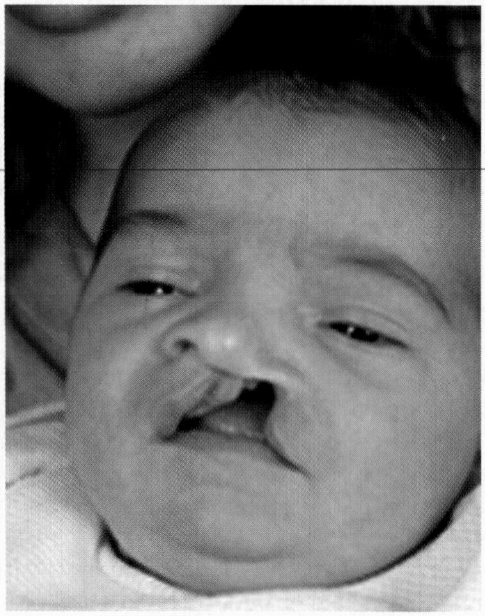

Assessment

Severe clefts are obvious at birth.

Palpate hard and soft palate of all neonates during initial assessment.

Therapeutic Management

Lip surgery should be done as soon as possible within the first few days or weeks after birth to enhance appearance and parental bonding.

Palate repair surgery is done in stages, depending on the degree, beginning at about 1 year to minimize speech problems.

Long-term follow-up should be done for orthodontia, speech therapy, and possible hearing problems.

Nursing Considerations

Degree of cleft determines approach to feeding.

Experiment to find method that works best for individual infant. Try:

1. Breastfeeding (soft breast tissue fills in the cleft)
2. Soft preemie nipple directed away from a cleft palate
3. Nipple with enlarged hole
4. Compressible bottles
5. Special long nipples that extend beyond cleft
6. Nipples with extensions to cover cleft
7. Medicine dropper
8. Asepto syringe with soft tubing attached

Feed infant in upright position because milk enters nasal passages through palate, causing increased tendency to aspirate.

Feed slowly with frequent stops to burp because infant tends to swallow excessive air.

Wash away milk curds with water after feeding.

Help parents deal with disappointment over infant with obvious anomaly. Show before and after pictures of plastic surgery.

Reinforce physician's explanation of plans for surgery.

Teach parents feeding techniques. Have parents observe at first, then take over gradually. Discuss positioning infant upright during feedings and on side after feedings to prevent aspiration.

Prevent infections. Infants are especially susceptible to respiratory and ear infections, which can delay surgery. Ear infections may lead to hearing loss.

Emphasize the need for long-term follow-up. Refer to agencies that help with expense of long-term care and to support groups for help and emotional support from other parents.

Esophageal Atresia and Tracheoesophageal Fistula

The esophagus is most commonly divided into two unconnected segments (atresia) with a blind pouch at the proximal end. The distal end is connected to the trachea, resulting in tracheoesophageal fistula (TEF). Cause is failure of normal development during the fourth week of pregnancy.

Table 30-3
COMMON CONGENITAL ANOMALIES—cont'd

Gastrointestinal Tract—cont'd

Common variations of the condition are shown in the figure.

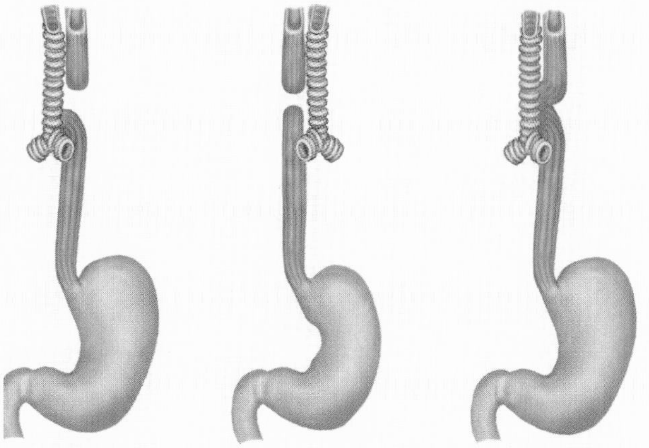

Assessment

Watch for TEF when polyhydramnios occurs because the excessive fluid may be caused by fetal inability to swallow amniotic fluid.

Other defects (cardiovascular and gastrointestinal most common) occur in 30% to 50% of infants with TEF.

Signs vary by type of defect.

Suspect TEF in infant with excessive frothy drooling and more suction needed than usual, when regurgitation occurs from secretions that pool in blind pouch, and when catheter will not pass into stomach.

If upper esophagus connects with trachea, feedings enter lungs and cause immediate coughing, choking, and cyanosis.

If fistula is between distal esophagus and trachea, stomach becomes distended with air from trachea. Gastric secretions are aspirated into the lungs, causing severe inflammatory reaction.

Therapeutic Management

Diagnosis is confirmed by symptoms and radiography.

Continuous suction should be used for upper pouch and gastrostomy if infant is too unstable for surgery.

Long-term follow-up should be done for esophageal reflux and dilation of strictures that form at surgical site.

Nursing Considerations

Observe all infants carefully during first feeding for respiratory difficulty or other signs.

Prevent aspiration by maintaining in a semi-upright position to prevent reflux of gastric fluids.

Maintain suction equipment.

Care after surgery involves ventilator, chest tubes, IV lines, and gastrostomy feedings.

Omphalocele and Gastroschisis

Both are caused by congenital defects in the abdominal wall. In omphalocele, the intestines protrude into the base of the umbilical cord. Other anomalies often occur with omphalocele.

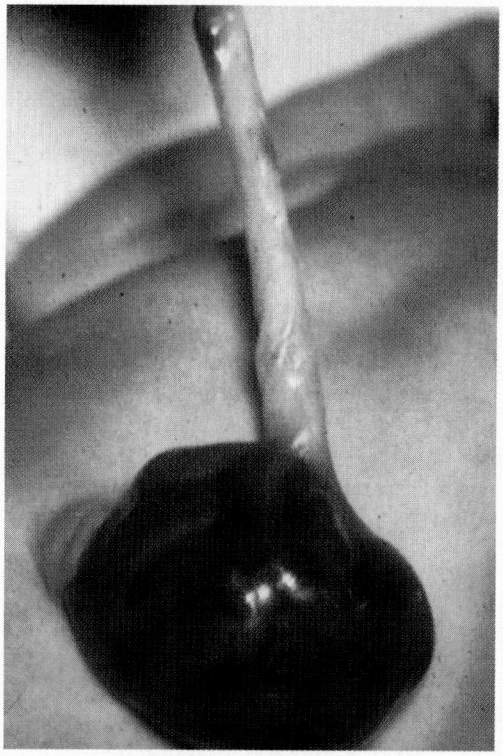

Gastroschisis is a defect to the side of the abdomen, next to and not involving the cord. The intestines protrude through the defect and float freely in the amniotic fluid.

Assessment

Diagnosis is made by prenatal ultrasound or is obvious at birth.

Therapeutic Management

Infant should be intubated at delivery, with gastric tube placed to decrease air in stomach. Gastric suction, parenteral nutrition, and antibiotics should be given.

Surgery should be performed as soon as infant is stable. A Silastic silo (pouch) may be used to replace the intestine gradually over a week.

Nursing Considerations

Cover intestines with sterile saline dressings and plastic to prevent drying.

Prevent infection and trauma.

Continued

Table 30-3

COMMON CONGENITAL ANOMALIES—cont'd

Gastrointestinal Tract—cont'd

Diaphragmatic Hernia

The diaphragm fails to fuse during the eighth to tenth weeks of gestation. A large or small part of the abdominal contents moves into the chest cavity, usually on the left side.

If herniation is large enough, the lungs may fail to develop (hypoplastic lungs). When gas fills bowel, further pressure on heart and lungs results.

Assessment

Mild to severe respiratory distress may occur at birth, with breath sounds diminished over the affected area, and barrel chest. The heart beat may be displaced to the right.

The abdomen may be scaphoid (concave).

The condition may be diagnosed prenatally by ultrasound.

Therapeutic Management

An endotracheal tube is placed for ventilation and a gastric tube for decompression of stomach.

Surgery to replace intestines and repair defect in diaphragm should be done as soon as possible.

Extracorporeal membrane oxygenation (ECMO) may be used.

Fetal surgery has been performed.

Nursing Considerations

Position the infant on the affected side to allow unaffected lung to expand. Elevate the head to decrease pressure on the heart and lungs. Assist with ventilation, and monitor respiratory status. Expect surgery as soon as infant is stable.

Continue to monitor respiratory status after surgery to determine whether lung function will be adequate.

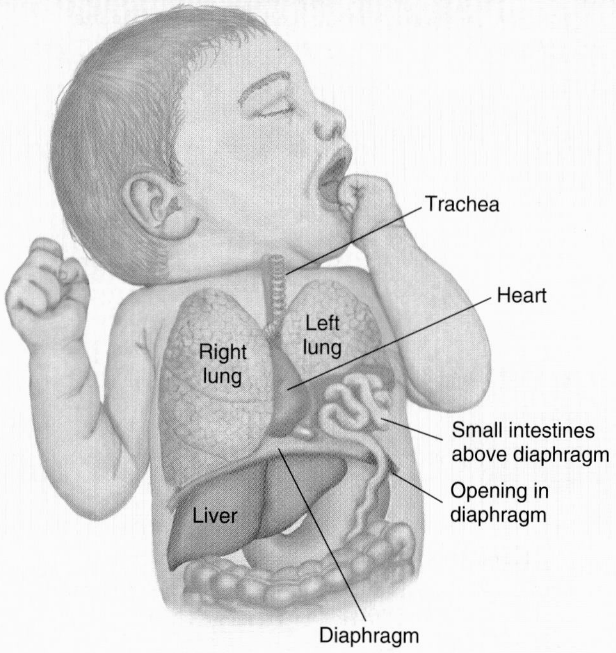

Central Nervous System

Neural Tube Defects

Forms of spina bifida are the most common central nervous system defects.

Folic acid supplements in pregnancy may help prevent neural tube defects.

Spina bifida occulta is failure of the vertebral arch to close, usually without other anomalies. It is seen by a dimple on the back, which may have a tuft of hair over it.

Meningocele is protrusion of meninges through the spina bifida, covered by skin or thin membrane. Because the spinal cord is not involved, paralysis does not occur.

Myelomeningocele is protrusion of meninges and spinal cord covered with membrane through spina bifida. The degree of paralysis depends on the location of defect. The infant may also have hydrocephalus, or it may develop after surgery.

Assessment

Note the position and covering of defect at birth.

Observe movement below the defect to determine degree of paralysis.

Examine for relaxed anus and dribbling of stool and urine.

Check for other anomalies.

Therapeutic Management

Surgery is performed for meningocele and myelomeningocele.

A shunt is placed to divert cerebrospinal fluid if hydrocephalus develops.

Antibiotics are given to prevent infection.

Long-term follow-up should be done, with physical therapy and other care as needed.

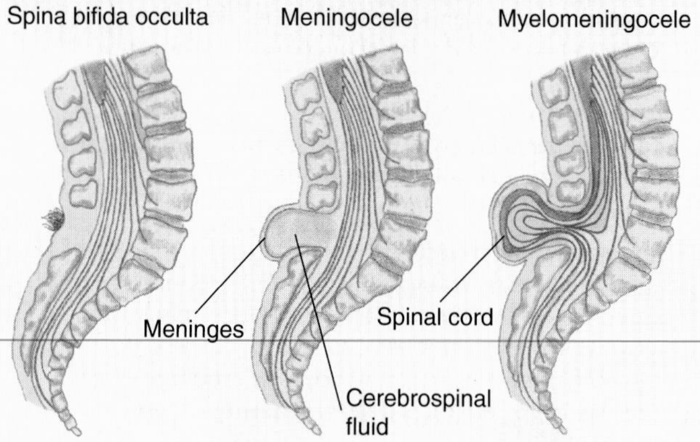

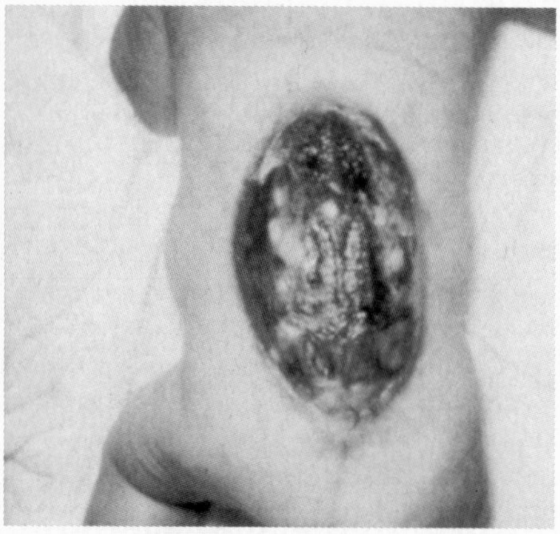

Table 30-3
COMMON CONGENITAL ANOMALIES—cont'd

Central Nervous System—cont'd

Nursing Considerations
Apply sterile saline dressing and plastic over a defect covered by membrane to prevent drying.
Handle the infant carefully, and position prone or to the side to prevent trauma to sac.
Prevent infection. Keep free of contamination from urine and feces.
Inspect sac for intactness before surgery. Monitor for signs of infection.
Every shift, check for increasing head circumference, bulging fontanelles, separation of sutures, intermittent apnea, and other signs of increased intracranial pressure to identify early hydrocephalus.

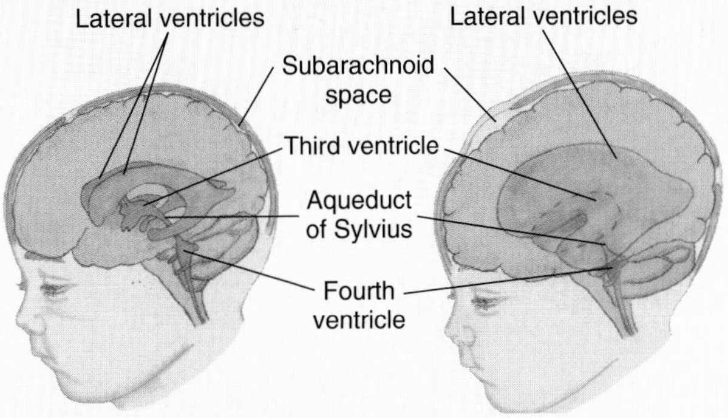

CONGENITAL HYDROCEPHALUS
This is a problem with absorption or obstruction to flow of cerebral spinal fluid in the ventricles of the brain, causing compression of the brain and enlargement of the head.

Assessment
A full or bulging fontanelle or separation of sutures exists.
The head is enlarged, especially in the frontal area.
The setting-sun sign is apparent (sclera visible above the pupils of the eyes).

Therapeutic Management
This disorder is corrected surgically, and a shunt is inserted to drain fluid. A ventriculoperitoneal shunt is used most often to drain fluid into the peritoneal cavity.

Nursing Considerations
Measure head circumference daily.
Prevent pressure areas.
Observe for signs of infection.
Teach parents how to care for shunt and observe signs of increased intracranial pressure.

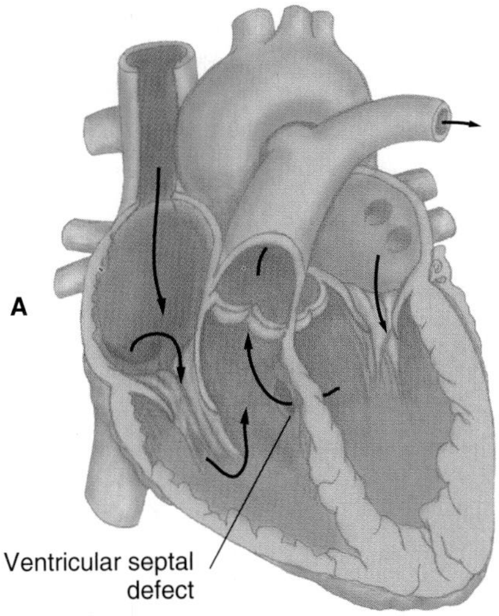

This is the most common type of congenital heart defect. It occurs alone or with other defects. The opening in the septum ranges from the size of a pin to very large. Many small defects close spontaneously. When the pressure in the left ventricle increases after birth, oxygenated blood is shunted through a large ventricular septal defect into the right ventricle and then recirculated to the lungs (a left-to-right shunt). Increased pulmonary resistance may cause pulmonary hypertension, hypertrophy of the right ventricle, heart failure, or a combination of these. Surgery is necessary for a large ventricular septal defect and increasing symptoms.

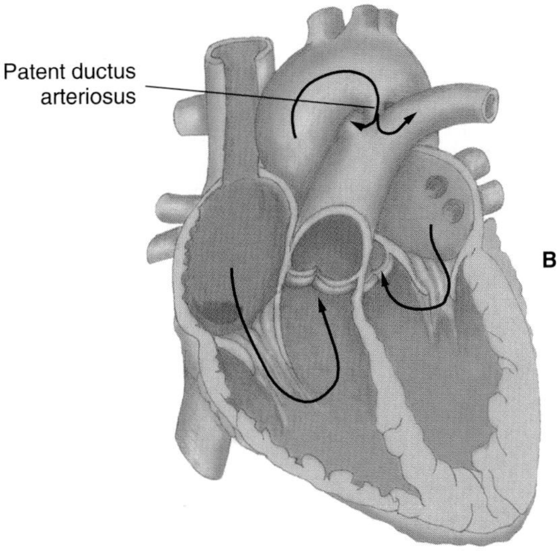

This condition is a failure of the ductus arteriosus to close after birth. Blood flows from the higher pressure of the aorta to the pulmonary artery and the lungs (left-to-right shunt). It is most common in the preterm infant. Symptoms vary from none to early congestive heart failure. Prostaglandins cause vasodilation and may interfere with closure of the ductus arteriosus. Indomethacin, a prostaglandin inhibitor, may be effective in causing closure. Surgical ligation is used when necessary. Devices to close the defect nonsurgically are also used.

FIGURE 30-5 Common congenital heart defects. **A,** Ventricular septal defect; **B,** patent ductus arteriosus;

Continued

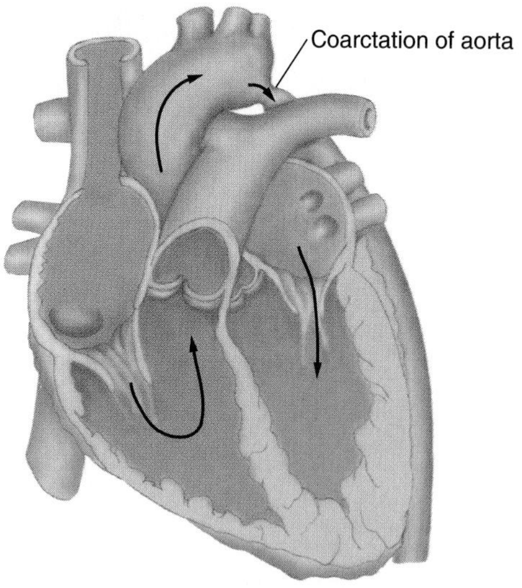

In this condition, blood flow is impeded through a constricted area of the aorta, increasing pressure behind the defect. The constriction is near the ductus arteriosus. The blood pressure is higher in the upper extremities than in the lower extremities. Carotid, brachial, and radial pulses are bounding, but pulses in the legs are weak or absent. The increased pressure in the left ventricle causes hypertrophy from the added workload. Congestive heart failure may result.

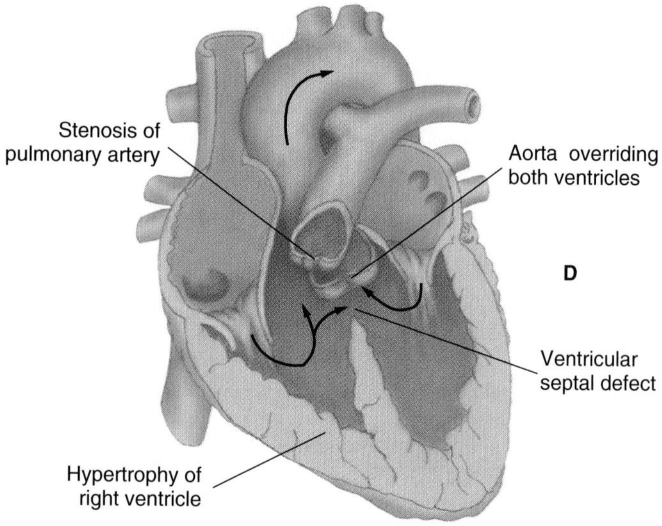

Tetralogy of Fallot has four characteristics: a ventricular septal defect, aorta positioned over the ventricular defect, pulmonary stenosis, and hypertrophy of the right ventricle. Cyanosis occurs if venous blood from the right ventricle flows through the septal defect and into the overriding aorta and blood flow to the lungs is diminished because of the narrowed pulmonary valve. The amount of right-to-left shunting and cyanosis varies according to the degree and position of each defect.

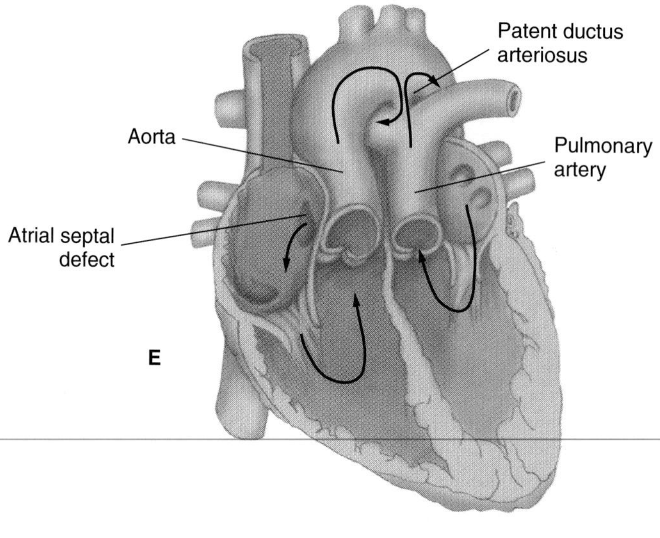

In this condition, the positions of the aorta and the pulmonary artery are reversed. The aorta carries venous blood from the right ventricle back to the general circulation. The pulmonary artery returns oxygenated blood from the left ventricle to the lungs. Unless there is another source for mixing oxygenated and venous blood, the infant cannot survive. A septal defect, open foramen ovale, or patent ductus arteriosus may be present. Prostaglandins may be given to keep the ductus open, and surgical correction is performed.

FIGURE 30-5, cont'd **C,** coarctation of the aorta; **D,** tetralogy of Fallot; **E,** transposition of the great arteries.

Defects with Increased Pulmonary Blood Flow

These heart defects allow blood to flow from the higher pressure of the left side of the heart to the right side or from the aorta to the pulmonary artery. This increases blood flow to the lungs and is called a *left-to-right shunt.* It causes some oxygenated blood to be sent to the lungs instead of to the rest of the body, increasing the work of the right side of the heart. Examples are ventricular septal defects and patent ductus arteriosus.

Defects with Obstruction of Blood Flow

In defects with obstruction of blood flow, a decrease in the blood flow through a narrowed vessel or valve occurs. This adds to the work of the heart, causes hypertrophy of the heart or major blood vessels, and may cause heart failure. Coarctation of the aorta fits into this classification.

Defects with Decreased Pulmonary Blood Flow

An impairment in the flow of blood from the right side of the heart to the lungs, combined with abnormal openings between pulmonary and systemic circulations, occurs in defects with decreased pulmonary blood flow. An example is tetralogy of Fallot.

Mixed Defects

Mixed defects allow survival only if a mixing of venous and oxygenated blood in the heart occurs. There is increased blood flow to the lungs and a mixture of venous and oxygenated blood in the systemic circulation. Transposition of the great vessels is a mixed defect.

Manifestations

Congenital heart defects may present obvious signs at birth or may not become apparent until later, when changes from fetal to neonatal circulation are completed. Some infants have no difficulty for months or years, but others experience early heart failure. The most common indications of cardiac problems are cyanosis, heart murmurs, tachycardia, and tachypnea.

Cyanosis

Cyanosis is a major sign of cardiac anomaly when respiratory disease does not exist. If the cyanosis is caused by a right-to-left shunt, giving oxygen will not improve the infant's color. Cyanosis increases with crying, feeding, or other activity. Pallor, mottling, or gray color may be present in infants who do not have cyanosis.

Heart Murmurs

Murmurs may sound like clicks, machinery, rumbling, swishing, or other muffled noises. It takes much practice to detect heart murmurs accurately. Although many infants have a temporary murmur until the fetal structures are closed, all abnormal sounds must be referred to the physician.

CRITICAL TO REMEMBER

Common Signs of Cardiac Anomalies

Cyanosis increasing with crying
Pallor
Murmurs
Tachycardia
Tachypnea
Dyspnea
Choking spells
Falling asleep during feedings
Diaphoresis

Tachycardia and Tachypnea

Tachycardia and tachypnea may occur anytime the heart and lungs must work harder to provide sufficient oxygen to the body. Thus they are present in both respiratory conditions and cardiac conditions. They increase in congestive heart failure.

Feeding Difficulties

Fatigue may interfere with the infant's ability to eat. The infant may feed slowly or fall asleep before the feeding is finished. Although diaphoresis is uncommon in the newborn, it may appear during feedings in the infant with a heart defect.

Therapeutic Management

Therapeutic management involves diagnosis of the specific defect and supportive and surgical treatment as indicated. Various tests such as echocardiograms and cardiac catheterizations confirm the diagnosis. The decision for surgery depends on the status of the infant and whether surgery can be delayed safely. Palliative surgery may be performed to partially correct a defect or make another defect to allow greater amounts of oxygenated blood to get to the systemic circulation.

Oxygen and drugs such as digitalis, diuretics, potassium supplements, and sedatives may be prescribed for the infant. Prostaglandins may be given to prevent the ductus arteriosus from closing in those cases in which keeping it open will increase the flow of oxygenated blood to the infant's body.

Nursing Considerations

Nursing care is focused on assessing for changes in condition and reducing the infant's need for oxygen. The need for rest is especially important. Infants with rapid respirations are at risk for aspiration and may need feeding by gavage. Oxygen may be increased during feedings or other exertion, but only enough oxygen to maintain saturation levels adequately should be used.

Support of the parents and education about the infant's condition and expected treatment are important.

Table 30-4
COMMON NURSING DIAGNOSES FOR FAMILIES OF NEWBORNS WITH COMPLICATIONS

Altered Family Processes
*Altered Nutrition: Less Than Body Requirements
*Altered Parenting
Anxiety
Disorganized Infant Behavior
*Risk for Fluid Volume Deficit
Ineffective Individual Coping
Ineffective Thermoregulation
*Impaired Skin Integrity
Risk for Injury
*Sleep Pattern Disturbance

*Nursing diagnoses discussed in this chapter.

The nurse uses drawings to help parents understand the defect. The parents are taught techniques for accurate administration of medications because the range between the therapeutic and toxic dosage of the drugs is narrow.

Check Your Reading

14. How are heart defects classified?

SUMMARY CONCEPTS

- Asphyxia before or during birth may cause apnea, acidosis, pulmonary hypertension, and possible death. Neonatal resuscitation must be initiated immediately.
- Nurses must identify conditions that increase the risk of asphyxia, begin resuscitation promptly, and assist other members of the team during treatment. Continued follow-up of the infant and parental support are important.
- In transient tachypnea of the newborn, respiratory difficulty in full-term or preterm infants is caused by failure of fetal lung fluid to be absorbed completely. It usually resolves spontaneously with supportive care.
- In meconium aspiration syndrome, meconium enters the lungs before birth or during the first breaths after birth. It causes inflammation and blocks air flow.
- The nurse's role in meconium aspiration syndrome is to prepare for care at birth, assist with care, and continue aftercare.
- Pathologic jaundice appears in the first 24 hours of life, and bilirubin levels rise faster and to higher levels than physiologic jaundice, or they may last longer. Pathologic jaundice may result in damage to the brain from kernicterus.
- The nurse's role in phototherapy is to decrease situations such as cold stress or hypoglycemia that might further elevate bilirubin levels, see that lights are used properly, observe for excessive fluid loss or skin impairment, ensure adequate oral intake, and teach parents.
- Infection in neonates is a problem because their immune system is immature, infection spreads easily, and the blood-brain barrier is less effective.
- The infant of a diabetic mother may have congenital anomalies, may be large or small for gestational age, and may suffer from respiratory distress syndrome, hypoglycemia, hypocalcemia, and polycythemia.
- Nursing responsibilities in caring for infants of diabetic mothers include early identification and follow-up of complications, monitoring of blood glucose levels, attention to early and adequate feedings, and support of parents.
- Infants with prenatal exposure to drugs may have congenital defects and behavioral and feeding abnormalities. They may have difficulty relating to others and may fail to gain weight.
- Nursing care for infants with neonatal abstinence syndrome includes decreasing stimuli from lights, noise, or handling; increasing feeding abilities; and fostering the mother's attachment to and ability to care for her infant.
- In cyanotic heart defects, unoxygenated blood flows into the systemic circulation, producing cyanosis. In acyanotic heart defects, impairment of blood flow or flow of oxygenated blood into the pulmonary system occurs. Defects may increase or decrease blood to the lungs.

ANSWERS TO CRITICAL THINKING EXERCISE, p. 847

Patches hide the eye area and an infection might not be noticed immediately. Removal of the patches at feedings allows inspection for signs of infection such as redness, edema, and drainage. Removal also allows a time for visual stimulation for the infant. If parents give the feeding, being able to see the infant's eyes enhances attachment.

ANSWERS TO CRITICAL THINKING EXERCISE, p. 856

Giving infants fluids with high levels of glucose will correct the immediate problem of hypoglycemia but also will stimulate the production of additional insulin. This causes a rebound hypoglycemia. Giving glucose in a form that will be metabolized more slowly provides longer normal glucose levels. If dextrose water is given, it should be followed within an hour by colostrum or formula.

REFERENCES & READINGS

American Academy of Pediatrics & American College of Obstetricians and Gynecologists. (1997). *Guidelines for perinatal care* (4th ed.). Elk Grove, IL: American Academy of Pediatrics.

American Academy of Pediatrics, Committee on Drugs. (1998). Neonatal drug withdrawal. *Pediatrics,* 101(6), 1079-1088.

American Academy of Pediatrics, Provisional Committee for Quality Improvement and Subcommittee on Hyperbilirubinemia. (1994). Practice parameter: Management of hyperbilirubinemia in the healthy term newborn. *Pediatrics,* 94(4), 558-565.

Berkowitz, C.D. (2000). Infants of substance abusing mothers. In C.D. Berkowitz, *Pediatrics: A primary care approach* (2nd ed., pp. 486-489). Philadelphia: W.B. Saunders.

Botham, S. (2000). Perinatal substance abuse. In J. Deacon & P. O'Neill, (Eds.), *Core curriculum for neonatal intensive care nursing* (2nd ed., pp. 618-634). Philadelphia: W.B. Saunders.

Carey, B.E., & Trotter, C. (2000). Radiology basics, Part III: TTN, meconium aspiration, and neonatal pneumonia. *Neonatal Network,* 19(4), 37-50.

Casey, P.M. (1999). Respiratory distress. In J. Deacon & P. O'Neill, *Core curriculum for neonatal intensive care nursing* (2nd ed., pp. 118-150). Philadelphia: W.B. Saunders.

Contributors and Reviewers for the Neonatal Resuscitation Guidelines. (2000). International guidelines for neonatal resuscitation: An excerpt from the guidelines 2000 for cardiopulmonary resuscitation and emergency cardiovascular care: International consensus on science. *Pediatrics,* 106(3), e29.

Cordero, L., Treuer, S.H., Landon, M.B., & Gabbe, S.G. (1998). Management of infants of diabetic mothers. *Archives of Pediatric Adolescent Medicine,* 152, 249-253.

Corrarino, J.E. (1998). Perinatal hepatitis B: Update and recommendations. *MCN: American Journal of Maternal/Child Nursing,* 23(5), 246-252.

Cottrell, B.H., & Carter, C.C. (1998). Attention health care professionals: Have you had chickenpox? *AWHONN Lifelines,* 2(4), 33-38.

Crockett, M. (2000). Cardiovascular conditions. In J. Deacon & P. O'Neill, (Eds.), *Core curriculum for neonatal intensive care nursing* (2nd ed., pp. 206-253). Philadelphia: W.B. Saunders.

Daberkow, E., & Washington, R.L. (1998). Cardiovascular diseases and surgical interventions. In G.B. Merenstein & S.L. Gardner (Eds.), *Handbook of neonatal intensive care* (4th ed., pp. 500-534). St. Louis: Mosby.

D'Apolito, K. (1999). Comparison of a rocking bed and standard bed for decreasing withdrawal symptoms in drug-exposed infants. *MCN: American Journal of Maternal/Child Nursing,* 24(3), 138-144.

D'Apolito, K., & McRorie, T.I. (1996). Pharmacologic management of neonatal abstinence syndrome. *Journal of Perinatal and Neonatal Nursing,* 9(4), 70-80.

Doshier, S. (1995). What happens to the offspring of diabetic pregnancies? *MCN: American Journal of Maternal/Child Nursing,* 20(1), 25-29.

Fanaroff, A.A., Martin, R.J., & Miller, M.J. (1999). Identification and management of problems in the high-risk neonate. In R.K. Creasy & R. Resnik, *Maternal-Fetal Medicine,* (4th ed, pp. 1151-1193). Philadelphia: W.B. Saunders.

Flandermeyer, A.A. (1998). The drug-exposed neonate. In C. Kenner, J.W. Lott, & A.A. Flandermeyer (Eds.), *Comprehensive neonatal nursing: A physiologic perspective* (2nd ed., pp. 864-892). Philadelphia: W.B. Saunders.

Frank, D.G., Cooper, S.C., & Merenstein, G.B. (1998). Jaundice. In G.B. Merenstein & S.L. Gardner (Eds.), *Handbook of neonatal intensive care* (4th ed., pp. 393-412). St. Louis: Mosby.

French, E.D., Pituch, M., Brandt, J., & Pohorecki, S. (1998). Improving interactions between substance-abusing mothers and their substance-exposed newborns. *Journal of Obstetric, Gynecologic, & Neonatal Nursing,* 27(3), 262-269.

Gotoff, S.F. (2000). Infections of the neonatal Infant. In R.E. Behrman, R.M. Kliegman, & H.B. Jenson (Eds.), *Nelson textbook of pediatrics* (16th ed., pp. 538-543). Philadelphia: W.B. Saunders.

Hagedorn, M.I., & Gardner, S.L. (1999). Hypoglycemia in the newborn, part I: Pathophysiology and nursing management. *Mother Baby Journal,* 4(1), 15-21.

Hagedorn, M.I., Gardner, S.L., & Abman, S.H. (1998). Respiratory diseases. In G.B. Merenstein & S.L. Gardner (Eds.), *Handbook of neonatal intensive care* (4th ed., pp. 437-499). St. Louis: Mosby.

Halamek, L.P., & Stevenson, D.K. (1997). Neonatal jaundice and liver disease. In A.A. Fanaroff & R.J. Martin (Eds.), *Neonatal-perinatal medicine* (Vol. 2, 6th ed., pp. 1345-1389). St. Louis: Mosby.

Harvey, D., Holt, D.E., & Bedford, H. (1999). Bacterial meningitis in the newborn: A prospective study of mortality and morbidity. *Seminars in Perinatology,* 23(3), 218-225.

Healy, K., Jovanovic-Peterson, L., & Peterson, C.M. (1995). Pancreatic disorders of pregnancy: Pregestational diabetes. *Endocrinology and Metabolism Clinics of North America,* 24(1), 73-101.

Johnson, W.L. (2000). Infant of a diabetic mother. In S. Mattson & J.E. Smith (Eds.), *Core curriculum for maternal-newborn nursing* (2nd ed., pp. 730-743). Philadelphia: W.B. Saunders.

Kaftan, H., & Kinney, J.S. (1998). Early onset neonatal bacterial infections. *Seminars in Perinatology,* 22(1), 15-24.

Kandall, S.R. (1998). Treatment strategies for drug-exposed neonates. *Clinics in perinatology: Prenatal drug exposure and child outcome,* 26(1), 231-243.

Kattwinkel, J., American Academy of Pediatrics, & American Heart Association. (2000). *Textbook of neonatal resuscitation* (4th ed.). Elk Grove, IL: American Academy of Pediatrics & American Heart Association.

Kearney, M.H. (1999). *Perinatal impact of alcohol, tobacco and other drugs.* White Plains, NY: March of Dimes.

Klein, J.O., & Macy, S.M. (1995). Bacterial sepsis and meningitis. In J.S. Remington & J.O. Klein (Eds.), *Infectious diseases of the fetus & newborn infant* (4th ed.). Philadelphia: W.B. Saunders.

Klein, J.O., & Remington, J.S. (1995). Current concepts of infections of the fetus and newborn infant. In J.S. Remington & J.O. Klein (Eds.), *Infectious diseases of the fetus & newborn infant* (4th ed.). Philadelphia: W.B. Saunders.

Lott, J.W. (1998). Fetal development: Environmental influences and critical periods. In C. Kenner, J.W. Lott, & A.A. Flandermeyer (Eds.), *Comprehensive neonatal nursing: A physiologic perspective.* (2nd ed., pp. 112-132). Philadelphia: W.B. Saunders.

Lott, J.W., & Kenner, C. (1998). Assessment and management of immunologic dysfunction. In C. Kenner, J.W. Lott, & A.A. Flandermeyer (Eds.), *Comprehensive neonatal nursing: A physiologic perspective* (2nd ed., pp. 496-519). Philadelphia: W.B. Saunders.

Ludwig, M.A., Marecki, M., Wooldridge, P.J., & Sheman, L.M. (1996). Neonatal nurses' knowledge of and attitudes toward caring for cocaine-exposed infants and their mothers. *Journal of Perinatal Neonatal Nursing,* 9(4), 81-85.

MacMahon, J.R., Stevenson, D.K., & Oski, F.A. (1998). Management of neonatal hyperbilirubinemia. In H.W. Taeusch & R.A. Ballard (Eds.), *Avery's diseases of the newborn* (7th ed., pp. 1033-1043). Philadelphia: W.B. Saunders.

MacMahon, J.R., Stevenson, D.K., & Oski, F.A. (1998). Physiologic jaundice. In H.W. Taeusch & R.A. Ballard (Eds.), *Avery's diseases of the newborn* (7th ed., pp. 1003-1007). Philadelphia: W.B. Saunders.

Maisels, M.J. (1999). Jaundice. In G.B. Avery, M.A. Fletcher, & M.G. MacDonald (Eds.), *Neonatology: Pathophysiology and management of the newborn* (5th ed., pp. 765-819). Philadelphia: Lippincott.

Meaux, J.B. (1996). Intravenous immunoglobulin: What nurses need to know. *Journal of Perinatal and Neonatal Nursing, 9*(4), 63-69.

Merenstein, G.B., Adams, K., & Weisman, L.E. (1998). Infection in the neonate. In G.B. Merenstein & S.L. Gardner (Eds.), *Handbook of neonatal intensive care* (4th ed., pp. 413-436). St. Louis: Mosby.

Mitchell, A., Steffenson, N., Hogan, H., & Brooks, S. (1997). Neonatal group B streptococcal disease. *MCN: American Journal of Maternal/Child Nursing, 22*(5), 249-253.

Muchmore, P. (2000). Respiratory distress. In J. Deacon & P. O'Neill, (Eds.), *Core curriculum for neonatal intensive care nursing* (2nd ed., pp. 687-703). Philadelphia: W.B. Saunders.

Muchmore, P. (2000). Sepsis in the newborn. In J. Deacon & P. O'Neill, (Eds.), *Core curriculum for neonatal intensive care nursing* (2nd ed., pp. 717-729). Philadelphia: W.B. Saunders.

Nash, P. (1996). Common neonatal complications. In K.R. Simpson & P.A. Creehan (Eds.), *AWHONN's perinatal nursing.* Philadelphia: Lippincott-Raven.

Paxton, J.M. (1999). Neonatal infections. In J. Deacon & P. O'Neill, (Eds.), *Core curriculum for neonatal intensive care nursing* (2nd ed. pp. 413-441). Philadelphia: W.B. Saunders.

Putnam, M., & Smith, J.E. (2000). The drug-dependent neonate. In S. Mattson & J.E. Smith (Eds.), *Core curriculum for maternal-newborn nursing* (2nd ed., pp. 730-743). Philadelphia: W.B. Saunders.

Reinarz, S.E., & Ecord, J.S. (1999). Drug-of-abuse testing in the neonate. *Neonatal Network,* 18(8), 55-61.

Robinson, T.M.S. (1999). Perinatal substance abuse: Working with neonates and families. *Neonatal Network,* 18(2), 68-70.

Ruchala, P., Seibold, L., & Stremsterfer, K. (1996). Validating assessment of neonatal jaundice with transcutaneous bilirubin measurement. *Neonatal Network,* 15(4), 33-37.

Sampson, J.E., & Gravett, M.G. (1999). Other infectious conditions in pregnancy. In D.K. James, P.J. Steer, C.P. Weiner, & B. Gonic. *High risk pregnancy: Management options,* (2nd ed., pp. 559-598). Philadelphia: W.B. Saunders.

Schwartz, R., & Teramo, K.A. (2000). Effects of diabetic pregnancy on the fetus and newborn. *Seminars in Perinatology,* 24(2), 120-135.

Shaw, N. (1998). Assessment and Management of hematologic dysfunction. In C. Kenner, J.W. Lott, & A.A. Flandermeyer (Eds.), *Comprehensive neonatal nursing: A physiologic perspective* (2nd ed., pp. 520-563). Philadelphia: W.B. Saunders.

Smith, J. (2000). Hyperbilirubinemia. In J. Deacon & P. O'Neill, (Eds.), *Core curriculum for neonatal intensive care nursing* (2nd ed., pp. 705-715). Philadelphia: W.B. Saunders.

Smith, J.B., Baker, A.L., Moynihan, P.J., Lincoln, P., & Kane, P.L. (1996). Cardiovascular critical care problems. In M.A.Q. Curley, J.B. Smith, & P.A. Moloney-Harmon (Eds.), *Critical care nursing of infants and children.* Philadelphia: W.B. Saunders.

Stoll, B.J., & Kliegman, R.M. (2000). Digestive system disorders. In R.E. Behrman, R.M. Kliegman, & H.B. Jenson (Eds.), *Nelson textbook of pediatrics* (16th ed., pp. 510-519). Philadelphia: W.B. Saunders.

Stoll, B.J., & Kliegman, R.M. (2000). The endocrine system. In R.E. Behrman, R.M. Kliegman, & H.B. Jenson (Eds.), *Nelson textbook of pediatrics* (16th ed., pp. 531-535). Philadelphia: W.B. Saunders.

Suevo, D.M. (1997). The infant of the diabetic mother. *Neonatal Network,* 16(5), 25-33.

Tyrala, E.E. (1996). The infant of the diabetic mother. *Obstetric Clinics of North America,* 23(1), 221-241.

Wang, E.C. (1999). Methadone treatment during pregnancy. *Journal of Obstetric, Gynecologic, & Neonatal Nursing,* 28(6), 615-622.

Watson, R.L. (1999). Gastrointestinal disorders. In J. Deacon & P. O'Neill (Eds.), *Core curriculum for neonatal intensive care nursing* (2nd ed., pp. 254-293). Philadelphia: W.B. Saunders.

Weiner, S.M., & Finnegan, L.P. (1998). Drug withdrawal in the neonate. In G.B. Merenstein & S.L. Gardner (Eds.), *Handbook of neonatal intensive care* (4th ed., pp. 129-145). St. Louis: Mosby.

Wheeler, B.J. (2000). Kernicterus: Ancient history or ongoing threat? *Mother Baby Journal,* 5(2), 21-30.

Whitsett, J.A., Pryhuber, G.S., Rice, W.R., Warner, B.B., & Wert, S.E. (1999). Acute respiratory disorders. In G.B. Avery, M.A. Fletcher, & M.G. MacDonald (Eds.), *Neonatology: Pathophysiology and management of the newborn* (5th ed., pp. 485-508). Philadelphia: Lippincott.

Wolach, B. (1997). Neonatal sepsis: Pathogenesis and supportive therapy. *Seminars in Perinatology,* 21(1), 28-38.

Wolkoff, L.I., & Davis, J.M. (1999). Delivery room resuscitation of the newborn. *Clinics in Perinatology,* 26(3), 641-658.

Wyckoff, M.M. (2000). Neonatal herpes simplex virus. *MCN: American Journal of Maternal/Child Nursing,* 25(2), 100-103.

Zahka, K.G., & Patel, C.R. (1997). Cardiovascular problems of the neonate. In A.A. Fanaroff & R.J. Martin. *Neonatal-perinatal medicine* (6th ed., pp. 1158-1167). St. Louis: Mosby.

31 FAMILY PLANNING

OBJECTIVES

1. Describe the role of the nurse in helping couples choose contraceptive methods.
2. Compare and contrast contraceptive methods in terms of safety, effectiveness, convenience, education needed to use, interference with spontaneity, availability, expense, and preference.
3. Explain why informed consent is important for contraception.
4. Compare and contrast contraceptive needs of adolescent and perimenopausal women.
5. Explain the mechanism of action of each method of family planning available: sterilization, hormonal contraceptives, intrauterine devices, barrier, and natural family planning.

DEFINITIONS

BASAL BODY TEMPERATURE Body temperature at rest.

CERVICAL CAP A small cuplike device placed over the cervix to prevent sperm from entering, thus preventing pregnancy.

COITUS Sexual union between a male and female.

COITUS INTERRUPTUS Withdrawal of the penis from the vagina before ejaculation.

CONDOM Latex, polyurethane, or natural membrane shield covering the penis or lining the vagina to prevent sperm from entering the cervix and prevent infection.

CONTRACEPTION Prevention of pregnancy.

DIAPHRAGM A contraceptive device consisting of a latex dome that covers the cervix and prevents entrance of sperm; must be used with a spermicide to be effective.

HORMONE IMPLANT Small capsules of progestin inserted subcutaneously to provide contraception.

INTRAUTERINE DEVICE (IUD) A mechanical device inserted into the uterus to prevent pregnancy.

LIBIDO Sexual desire.

MITTELSCHMERZ Low abdominal pain that occurs at ovulation.

NATURAL FAMILY PLANNING Method of predicting ovulation based on normal changes in a woman's body.

ORAL CONTRACEPTIVE Drug that inhibits ovulation; contains progestins alone or in combination with estrogen.

PROGESTIN Any natural or synthetic form of progesterone.

SEXUALLY TRANSMISSIBLE (OR TRANSMITTED) DISEASE (STD) A disease that is passed to others primarily through sexual contact. Also called *sexually transmissible (or transmitted) infection (STI).*

SPERMICIDE A chemical that kills sperm.

DEFINITIONS—cont'd

Spinnbarkeit Clear, slippery, stretchy quality of cervical mucus during ovulation.

Tubal Ligation Occluding the fallopian tubes to prevent passage of ova or sperm, thus preventing pregnancy.

Vasectomy Occluding the vas deferens to prevent passage of sperm, thus preventing pregnancy.

Family planning involves choosing when to have children. It includes contraception—the prevention of pregnancy—as well as methods to achieve pregnancy. Chapter 32 describes methods used by couples having difficulty attaining pregnancy. This chapter focuses on techniques used to avoid pregnancy.

If both partners are fertile, approximately 90% of women will conceive within 1 year if they do not use contraception (Cunningham, et al., 1997). Therefore those who wish to control the timing of pregnancies cannot leave contraception to chance. Unplanned pregnancies may cause a major disruption of the woman's life. In addition, they may have an impact on the health of the woman or neonate. For example, infants conceived less than 6 months after a previous birth are at increased risk for low birth weight, preterm birth, and small size for gestational age (Zhu, et al., 1999).

Because the majority of contraceptive methods available must be practiced by women, women often choose the type of contraception used. In the United States, more than 90% of all women at risk for pregnancy use some method of contraception (Alan Guttmacher Institute, 2000). During a woman's reproductive lifetime, her needs for contraception change. Most women use a variety of methods before they reach menopause. Because the average woman in the United States bears only two children, she may make contraceptive decisions for more than 30 years.

INFORMATION ABOUT CONTRACEPTION

Common Sources

Women often obtain information about contraception from friends, relatives, newspapers, magazines, and the Internet. They seek answers to practical questions about comfort, partners' responses, and problems encountered. They may receive incomplete facts or misinformation when their source is not a qualified health care professional, however.

Women frequently turn to nurses in clinics, physicians' offices, birth settings, and even social settings for accurate information about family planning. Some women are more comfortable asking a nurse about contraception than a physician, particularly when they are unsure of what technique they desire.

Role of the Nurse

The nurse's role in family planning is that of counselor and educator. To fulfill this role, nurses need current, correct information about contraceptive methods. Approximately half of all pregnancies are unintended. This has led to a national goal in the United States to increase intended pregnancies from the 1995 baseline of 51% to 70% (US Department of Health and Human Services, 2000).

Almost half of unintended pregnancies occur in women who are using a contraceptive method but use it incorrectly or inconsistently or have a contraceptive failure (Alan Guttmacher Institute, 1998). This would occur much less frequently if women had adequate education about their chosen method. The initial teaching that accompanies selection of the contraceptive technique may be insufficient to meet the woman's needs. Reinforcing teaching and providing an opportunity to ask questions after initial use can help ensure the woman is using her method correctly.

Nurses must feel comfortable discussing contraception and be sensitive to the woman's concerns and feelings. In discussing family planning, the woman's preferences take precedence. Nurses must be careful not to introduce their own biases toward or against specific methods. The nurse's personal experiences and choices regarding contraception are not pertinent. The focus of counseling must be the needs and feelings of the woman and her partner (Figure 31-1).

Nurses working in maternity settings should discuss family planning with every woman after birth to provide an opportunity to clarify misinformation and answer questions. Then the woman will be ready to discuss contraception further with her primary caregiver, if necessary.

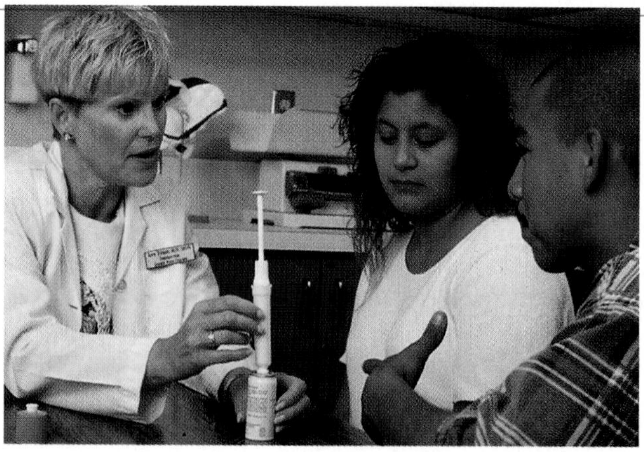

FIGURE 31-1 Success of contraception is more likely when both the woman and her partner are involved in discussions. The nurse demonstrates filling a foam applicator.

CONSIDERATIONS WHEN CHOOSING A CONTRACEPTIVE METHOD

The perfect contraceptive method does not exist. Each has advantages and disadvantages (Table 31-1). Women change contraceptive methods as circumstances in their lives change and may try several before finding one that is satisfactory. (The rate at which women discontinue the use of various contraceptive methods is shown in Table 31-2.) The nurse can help women weigh factors involved in choosing a family planning method. Careful consideration of all factors can help women choose methods that best meet their needs.

Safety

The safety of the method is a primary consideration. Medical conditions may make some methods unsafe for

Table 31-1
ADVANTAGES AND DISADVANTAGES OF THE MOST COMMON CONTRACEPTIVE METHODS

Method	Advantages	Disadvantages
Sterilization (tubal ligation and vasectomy)	Ends concern about contraception. Tubal ligation can be performed right after childbirth while still in the hospital or as an outpatient at another time. Vasectomy may be performed in the physician's office under local anesthesia. Although expensive initially, long-term cost is low.	Does not protect against STDs. Reversal is difficult, expensive, and may be unsuccessful. Requires surgery with potential complications of all surgeries. Vasectomy requires another contraceptive method until semen is free of sperm.
Implant (Norplant) (Presently not available)	In place at all times. Unrelated to coitus. Low long-term cost.	Does not protect against STDs. Expensive initially (although lower overall cost). Requires minor surgery to place and remove. Slightly visible. Side effects may lead to early removal.
Progestin injections (DepoProvera)	Unrelated to coitus.	Must be repeated every 4 to 12 weeks. Side effects similar to other progestin contraceptives. Does not protect against STDs.
Oral contraceptives	Taken at time unrelated to coitus. See Table 31-4 (Potential Benefits and Risks of Oral Contraceptives).	Must be taken at same time each day. May cause side effects and complications. Does not protect against STDs. See Table 31-4.
Intrauterine devices	In place at all times. Low long-term cost.	Does not protect against STDs. High initial cost. Can be expelled without woman's knowledge; woman must check for strings. Potential side effects or complications: menorrhagia, infection, ectopic pregnancy, abortion, perforation.
Barrier		
All methods	Avoid use of systemic hormones. Offer some protection against STDs.	Most coitus related (must be used just before coitus). May interfere with sensation. Some people are sensitive to components of spermicide or latex.
Chemical (spermicides)	Quick and easy. No prescription needed. Inexpensive per single use.	Films and suppositories must melt to be effective. Usually effective for only 1 hr. May be messy. New application needed for subsequent intercourse.
Condoms	Quick and easy. No prescription needed. Best protection available for STDs, especially if combined with spermicide. Inexpensive per single use. Can be carried discreetly. Vaginal condoms increase women's control over contraceptive use and protection from STDs.	Must be checked for expiration date and holes. Can break or slip off. Can be used only once. Vaginal condom may seem unattractive.

STD, Sexually transmissible disease.

Continued

Table 31-1

ADVANTAGES AND DISADVANTAGES OF THE MOST COMMON CONTRACEPTIVE METHODS—cont'd

Method	Advantages	Disadvantages
Barrier—cont'd		
Diaphragm	Can be inserted several hours before coitus.	Initially expensive. Requires nurse practitioner, certified nurse-midwife, or physician to fit. Requires education on proper use. Some women have difficulty with correct insertion or removal. Added spermicide necessary for repeat coitus. Possibility of toxic shock syndrome. Should be checked for fit annually and after birth, abortion, or weight change of 10 lb or more. Pressure against bladder may cause infections.
Cervical cap	Smaller than diaphragm and may fit women who cannot wear a diaphragm. Requires less spermicide and no additional spermicide for repeated intercourse. No pressure against bladder. Less noticeable than diaphragm. Can remain in place 48 hr.	Sizes are limited. Initially expensive. Requires nurse practitioner or physician to fit. Requires education on proper use. Somewhat more difficult to insert than diaphragm. Can be dislodged during intercourse. Possibility of toxic shock syndrome. Must be refitted each year and after birth, abortion, or surgery.
Natural family planning		
All methods	Inexpensive. No drugs or hormones. Help woman learn about her body. Can be combined with barrier methods to increase effectiveness. Acceptable to most religions. May be used to achieve pregnancy.	Requires high level of motivation and extensive education. Requires abstinence for large part of each cycle. High risk of pregnancy from error. Many factors may change ovulation time.

Table 31-2

DISCONTINUATION OF VARIOUS TYPES OF CONTRACEPTION

Method	Women Who Discontinue Use at 1 Year (%)
Norplant	12
DepoProvera	30
Oral contraceptives	29
Intrauterine devices	
Progestasert	19
Paragard (Copper T 380A)	22
Condoms	
Male	39
Female	44
Diaphragm	44
Cervical cap	
Nulliparous women	44
Parous women	58
Spermicides, gel, foam, films, suppositories (used alone)	60
Natural family planning (all types)	37

Data from Hatcher, R.A., Trussell, J., Stewart, J., Cates, W., Stewart, G.K., Guest, F., & Kowal, D. (1998). *Contraceptive technology* (17th ed.). New York: Ardent Media.

certain women. For example, oral contraceptives (OCs) should not be used by women who have had thrombophlebitis or strokes because the hormones used may increase the risk that these conditions will recur. The diaphragm and cervical cap are unsafe for women with a history of toxic shock syndrome, a possible complication of these methods.

Protection from Sexually Transmissible Diseases

No contraceptive (other than abstinence) is 100% effective in preventing sexually transmissible diseases (STDs). The risk of exposure to STDs should be considered in counseling women about contraceptive choices. The male condom offers the best protection available. It should be used whenever a risk exists that one partner may have an STD, even when another form of contraception is practiced. Although women are aware of the protection offered by condoms, the number of women reporting use at last intercourse is often low.

Effectiveness

The importance of avoiding pregnancy must be considered when choosing a contraceptive method. A

Table 31-3
COMPARISON OF EFFECTIVENESS OF COMMON TYPES OF COMMON TYPES OF CONTRACEPTION

Method	Effectiveness Rate: Actual or Typical Use (%)
Sterilization	
Vasectomy	99.85
Tubal ligation	99.50
Norplant	99.95
DepoProvera	99.70
Oral contraceptives	95.00
Intrauterine devices	
Progestasert	98.00
Paragard (Copper T 380A)	99.20
Mirena (LNG)	99.90
Condoms	
Male	86.00
Female	79.00
Diaphragm	80.00
Cervical cap	
Nulliparous women	80.00
Parous women	60.00
Spermicides, gel, foam, films, suppositories (used alone)	74.00
Natural family planning (all types)	75.00
Coitus interruptus (withdrawal)	81.00
No contraceptive use	15.00

Effectiveness rate of contraceptives shown as percent of women remaining free of unintended pregnancy during first year of use. Data from Hatcher, R.A., Trussell, J., Stewart, J., et al. (1998). *Contraceptive technology* (17th ed.). New York: Ardent Media.

woman may wish to put off pregnancy for a time but may not care if pregnancy occurs earlier. Other women may be extremely upset about an accidental pregnancy because it would affect their health or have a major impact on their financial stability.

Effectiveness is determined by how often the method prevents pregnancy or fails to prevent pregnancy (see Table 31-3). It involves two different types of failure rates:

1. The ideal, perfect, or theoretic failure rate refers to perfect use of the method with every act of intercourse. Failures are caused by a problem with the method itself rather than with the use of the method.
2. The typical, actual, or user failure rate is taken from studies of occurrence of pregnancy in real people using the method. Failure is presumably the result of incorrect or inconsistent use of the technique. Failures are most often caused by not using the method for every act of intercourse.

The difference between the two rates of failure shows how forgiving a method is; that is, how likely pregnancy is to occur if use is occasionally imperfect. The typical failure rate is more meaningful when counseling women and their partners. When comparing different methods, the same method of analysis must be used.

Failure rates are listed as the number of pregnancies in 100 women per year. Although a typical failure rate of 12% for a method might seem fairly good, it means that 12 of every 100 women using that method experience unintended pregnancies each year. For women who feel that a one-in-eight yearly risk of pregnancy is too great, a more effective method should be chosen.

Effectiveness varies according to accuracy of use. It drops greatly when the user does not understand the way to use the method. The failure rate commonly decreases after the first year of use because experience with the method leads to more accurate use. Methods that are less reliable can sometimes be combined to increase effectiveness, such as using a condom with a spermicide.

The effectiveness of the method must be balanced against the acceptability to the couple. Surgical sterilization is the most effective method but is unacceptable to couples planning to have children at a later time. OCs or intrauterine devices (IUDs) also are highly effective, but some women may dislike the side effects or have religious objections.

Convenience

Convenience is another important factor in choosing a contraceptive method. If the woman perceives her contraceptive as difficult to use, time consuming, or too much "bother," she is unlikely to use it consistently unless her level of motivation is very high. The education she receives about the method may affect her perception of its difficulty. Women who are knowledgeable about their family planning method are less likely to feel that the contraceptive is difficult to use.

Contraceptives that are "messy" may seem inconvenient and unattractive. Spermicide may drip from the vagina and decrease satisfaction for both the woman and the man. Less spermicide may decrease dripping but increase the risk of pregnancy.

Education Needed

Some methods of contraception, such as condoms, involve very little education, whereas others depend on one or more teaching sessions to ensure adequate knowledge. Natural family planning methods rely on extensive education about body changes that denote ovulation. Women using these methods need rather sophisticated information to practice them successfully.

Side Effects

Many methods of contraception have side effects that women may dislike. Side effects must be explained clearly when discussing the advantages and disadvantages of each method. When women know what to expect, they often are more willing to tolerate side effects, especially if they know they do not indicate a health risk. This may help them to continue an effective contraceptive method instead of discontinuing it and using no method or a less-effective one.

Interference with Spontaneity

Coitus-related contraceptive methods, such as spermicides and barrier methods, must be used just before sexual intercourse. They interrupt lovemaking, increasing the chance that the method will not be used. Some couples remedy this by including placement of the contraceptive device, such as a condom or diaphragm, as a part of foreplay. Others prefer methods such as OCs, IUDs, or hormone injections that do not interrupt sexual activity.

Availability

Condoms and spermicides are readily available without prescriptions. They can be purchased anonymously at any time without a trip to a health care provider. This may be important to an adolescent who wants to hide her sexual activity or to any woman who is embarrassed to discuss contraception with a health care provider.

Expense

The cost of family planning methods per use can be compared with long-term expense. The price of condoms and spermicides is relatively low, but frequent use makes them expensive over a period of years. Couples may find them economical for occasional sexual intercourse or until they can afford a more expensive method. However, they have a higher chance of failure and pregnancy than other, more expensive, methods. The yearly cost of any contraceptive method is less than the cost of a pregnancy.

Methods that depend on periodic visits to a nurse practitioner or physician are more costly than over-the-counter methods. However, the professional counseling given may enhance contraceptive effectiveness. Visits also provide opportunities for health teaching and screening for health problems. In spite of the fact that they require a health practitioner visit, the copper T IUD, implants, and injectable contraceptives are the most cost-effective reversible contraceptives available over a 5-year period because they prevent pregnancy so well.

Low-income women, especially those without insurance or Medicaid, may not be able to afford contraception on an ongoing basis. Contraceptive information and services often are available at publicly funded family planning clinics at little or no cost. A major purpose of these clinics is to prevent unintended pregnancies, thus reducing the cost incurred during pregnancy in a woman with Medicaid. These clinics provide professional counseling about all contraceptive methods and follow-up services. However, women may object to a long wait and the fact that they may see a different health care provider at each visit.

Women who have insurance may find that pregnancy is covered but contraceptives are only partially covered or not reimbursed at all. Health maintenance organizations (HMOs) provide the best coverage for contraception, but approximately half of fee-for-service (indemnity) insurance plans do not cover contraceptive costs. However, sterilization is covered in most plans (Alan Guttmacher Institute, 2000).

Organizations such as the Association of Women's Health, Obstetric, and Neonatal Nurses support legislation to increase contraceptive insurance coverage for women. State and federal legislation is in process to require full insurance coverage for contraceptives. More than one fourth of states now require insurance companies to cover contraception services.

Preference

The woman makes the final decision about her contraceptive method, and her satisfaction with her choice is crucial. Consistent use of any method depends on whether it meets the needs of the woman and her partner. If the woman feels pressured into choosing a method or the chosen method fails to live up to her expectations, use is likely to be inconsistent. The opinions of the woman's partner and friends also may influence what method she chooses.

Some women are uncomfortable with their bodies and embarrassed by methods that involve touching the vagina. Inserting a diaphragm or cervical cap or performing a daily assessment of cervical mucus may be unacceptable to them.

Religious and Personal Beliefs

Religious or other personal beliefs also affect the choice of contraceptives. Roman Catholics may not believe in the use of any contraceptives other than natural family planning methods.

Culture

Culture also may influence the method chosen. In the African-American culture, OCs and female sterilization are most often chosen and male sterilization is rare (Lethbridge, 1995). For some Latinas, condoms may not be acceptable because they suggest infidelity (Edwards, 1994). Traditional Latinas place a high cultural value on motherhood and often desire large families. Desire for a son may cause the woman to continue to become pregnant until she has a son (Unger & Molina, 1998). Hmong women may report that their husbands do not believe in contraception (Jambunathan & Stewart, 1995).

Informed Consent

Because some methods have potentially dangerous side effects, signing an informed consent form is important to show that the woman received and understands information about risks and benefits. For example, written consent may be obtained from women choosing surgical sterilization, OCs, hormone implants or injections, and IUDs. Of course, regardless of whether a consent form is used, every woman should receive information about the chosen contraceptive method and its proper use, risks and benefits, and alternative methods available.

Check Your Reading

1. Why do women usually choose the method of contraception that a couple uses?
2. What is the role of the nurse in helping women with contraceptive choices and use?
3. What are some important considerations in choosing a contraceptive technique?
4. Which contraceptive methods may involve an informed consent form?

ADOLESCENTS

Adolescent pregnancy is a major problem. In 1999, half of all high school students reported they had been sexually active. This included 66% of 12th-grade females and 64% of 12th-grade males who had ever had intercourse. At the 9th-grade level, 33% of females and 45% of males reported they were sexually active (MacKay, Fingerhut, & Duran, 2000).

As a result of such figures, the United States has set the following goals for the year 2010:

- Increase the number of sexually active, unmarried adolescents aged 15 to 17 who use contraceptives that are effective against pregnancy and STDs
- Increase condom use at first intercourse to 75% of adolescent females from a baseline of 68% and for males to 83% from a baseline of 72%
- Reduce pregnancies in women aged 15 to 17 to no more than 46 per 1000 adolescents from the 1995 baseline of 72 per 1000 in this age group (US Department of Health and Human Services, 2000)

The major impact of pregnancy on the lives of teenagers makes finding methods to enhance adolescent contraception use of major importance. (See Chapter 24 for information about adolescent pregnancy.)

Adolescent Knowledge

Many adolescents have little knowledge about their own anatomy and physiology, including how and when conception occurs. They are likely to learn about contraception from other teenagers, who often pass on incorrect information. Even adolescents who have been pregnant often are misinformed about contraceptive techniques, and they may become pregnant again because of lack of information about family planning.

Misinformation

Misinformation and erroneous beliefs cause adolescents to use ineffective methods of contraception or no method at all. Some teenagers think they cannot become pregnant the first time they have intercourse, unless they have an orgasm, or have been menstruating a certain length of time. However, pregnancy can result from any intercourse near ovulation. Although many adolescents have anovulatory menstrual cycles during the early months after menarche, they cannot depend on it to prevent pregnancy.

Teenagers may douche (insert a solution into the vagina) after intercourse to prevent pregnancy. Douching is ineffective, however, because sperm may enter the cervix soon after ejaculation. Coitus interruptus (withdrawal) is another unreliable method used by teenagers. It requires more control than most adolescent boys have over timing of ejaculation. Semen spilled near the vagina can enter and cause pregnancy, even without penetration by the penis. In addition, preejaculatory fluid may contain sperm.

Risk-Taking Behavior

Adolescents are more likely to take risks in sexual activity because they believe that their chances of becoming pregnant are small. They often do not plan intercourse and therefore are not prepared with contraceptives. Their risk-taking behavior may lead to STDs and pregnancy.

Counseling Adolescents

Nurses who counsel adolescents about sexuality must be sensitive to the feelings, concerns, and needs of the teenager. They must be prepared to be accepting of the teenager regardless of personal feelings about adolescent sexuality. For an adolescent to seek information about contraception, she must admit that she is and plans to continue to be sexually active. The teenager may be afraid to ask about contraception because she does not want anyone to know she is sexually active or she fears she will be lectured about her behavior. Her need for secrecy may cause her to miss appointments for family planning. The nurse must be adept at determining the adolescent's needs and reassure her about confidentiality.

Opportunities to provide counseling must not be missed. Adolescent visits to a health care provider for well checks or minor illnesses provide such opportunities. Another is when a young woman seeks a pregnancy test. If the test is negative, she can be asked about her desire to become pregnant. The nurse can assess the adolescent's use of contraception and adequacy of knowledge and provide information as appropriate.

Although nurses should encourage adolescents to discuss contraception with their parents, many teenagers will forgo contraception rather than talk to their parents about it. Therefore they need other sources of information. Schools have helped increase birth control use among adolescents by offering information about family planning and prevention of STDs. Contraceptive services also are available on some school campuses.

Family planning clinics in most states may provide information and supplies to minors without parental permission. Some family planning clinics are designed to meet the special needs of teenagers. They may be open after school, evenings, and on weekends and have staff who are especially skilled in working with adolescents.

Because adolescent girls frequently fear the pelvic examination, clinic staff may wait to perform it until the second visit. During the first visit, the teenager receives information about contraceptive techniques. Taking this extra time to explain different methods helps allay the common concern of adolescents about potential adverse health effects of contraceptives. It also helps the teenager to feel comfortable in the clinic setting.

Because of her youth and possible lack of knowledge about anatomy and physiology, the adolescent often needs more extensive teaching than the older woman. Liberal use of audiovisual materials such as pictures, anatomic models, and samples of various methods helps the teenager understand the information more easily. Using a banana and condom or showing her the packet of pills she will be using are important aids.

Using understandable terminology is especially important when teaching adolescents. The nurse must know street terms for body parts and sexual intercourse because they may be the only words with which the teenager is familiar.

Adolescents are most successful when they choose contraceptive methods that are easy to use and seem unrelated to coitus. Many teenagers choose oral or injectable contraceptives. These methods are safe, seem unrelated to sex, and are not difficult or messy. Long-term OC use has not been found to cause problems in healthy women.

Adolescent girls may be inconsistent in taking pills every day, however. They are more likely to discontinue any method for minor side effects such as nausea or spotting. Their concerns should be taken seriously, and attempts should be made to alleviate side effects. Otherwise, adolescents will stop using the method, with pregnancy as a possible result. They should understand all aspects of management of their contraceptive method and when a backup method is necessary.

Condom use should be encouraged to help prevent STDs, even when using another contraceptive method (Figure 31-2). A national goal is to increase the use of contraceptives at last intercourse by adolescent girls to 41% from a baseline of 38% (US Department of Health and Human Services, 2000).

Discussing perceived barriers to using condoms will help dispel misconceptions about them. Many young women are uneasy about asking a partner to use a condom. They benefit from learning ways to negotiate condom use with a partner. Adolescent males often are more concerned about avoiding pregnancy than STDs. They may not want to use a condom if they know their partner is using another contraceptive method.

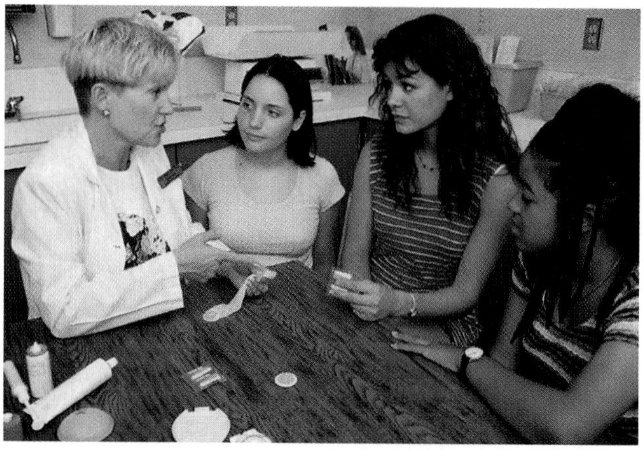

FIGURE 31-2 Although many adolescents choose oral contraceptives, the nurse emphasizes the need to use condoms for protection against sexually transmissible diseases. Demonstrating with actual contraceptives increases understanding.

CRITICAL THINKING EXERCISE

A 15-year-old girl approaches the nurse with questions about contraception. She says she does not want to become pregnant, but her boyfriend does not want to use condoms and she is too embarrassed to go to see a physician for other contraceptive methods.

QUESTION:

1. How should the nurse handle the situation?

PERIMENOPAUSAL WOMEN

Perimenopausal women may continue to ovulate as long as they have regular menstrual periods, and some ovulate even when indications of menopause are present. Pregnancy is rare after age 50, and contraception can be discontinued sooner if menstruation has ceased for at least 2 years (Cunningham, et al., 1997). The mature woman who does not smoke and has no other contraindications can use any method of contraception. She should have regular physical examinations to identify any conditions that would necessitate a change in contraceptive method. Many couples who do not plan to have more children choose sterilization. This ends their concerns about contraception permanently.

Check Your Reading

5. What are some erroneous beliefs about contraception commonly held by adolescents?
6. Why might teenagers be hesitant to seek contraceptive information?
7. How can the nurse increase effectiveness in teaching adolescents about contraception?
8. What considerations are necessary in contraception for perimenopausal women?

METHODS OF CONTRACEPTION

Sterilization

Sterilization is an extremely popular method of contraception for couples who have completed their families. In the United States, approximately 1 million sterilizations are performed annually (Stewart & Carignan, 1998). Although sterilization is expensive at the time of surgery, it ends all further contraceptive costs. It always should be considered a permanent end to fertility because reversal surgery is difficult, expensive, and usually not covered by insurance. Reversal surgery is not always successful and increases the risk of ectopic pregnancy.

Couples considering sterilization need counseling to ensure that they understand all aspects of the procedure. When surgery is planned for immediately after childbirth, the decision should be made well before labor begins. Future marriage, divorce, or death of a child may cause couples to regret their decision. In one study, 18% of women who had a tubal ligation during the postpartum period or within 1 year of the birth of their last child and 20% of women who were less than 30 years of age when the procedure was done expressed regret over their decision (Hillis, et al., 1999).

Complications of sterilization are those of any surgery, including hemorrhage, infection, and anesthesia complications. Although pregnancy is rare, the risk of failure should be discussed. Pregnancies occurring after tubal ligation are more likely to be ectopic.

Tubal Ligation

Female sterilization is the method of contraception used by more than 10 million women in the United States (Stewart & Carignan, 1998). It is the most widely used contraceptive method in the world (Grimes, 2000). The effectiveness rate is 99.5%. The surgery can be performed at any time. It is easiest during the immediate postpartum period, when the fundus is located near the umbilicus and the fallopian tubes are directly below the abdominal wall. Interval sterilization, performed when the woman is 4 or more weeks postpartum, often is performed as outpatient surgery. General anesthesia is most common, but regional or local anesthesia may be used.

The procedure is usually performed in one of three ways. In the first method, a minilaparotomy incision is made near the umbilicus in the postpartum period or just above the symphysis pubis for interval sterilization. The surgeon brings the tubes through the incision, where a piece is removed and the ends are tied. Rings or clips also can be used to occlude the tubes.

In the second method, surgery is performed through a laparoscope inserted through a small incision. The surgeon visualizes the fallopian tubes and blocks them with clips or rings or destroys a portion of the tubes with electrocoagulation.

The third method is performed during other surgery, generally along with cesarean birth, when a woman is sure that she wants the procedure regardless of the outcome of the birth.

Vasectomy

Vasectomy, the male sterilization procedure, is 99.85% effective. It involves making a small incision in the scrotum and cutting the vas deferens, which carries sperm from the testes to the penis. Cautery also may be used. After vasectomy, semen no longer contains sperm.

Although performed less frequently than tubal ligation, vasectomy is a very popular method of contraception. It involves lower morbidity rates than tubal ligation, and because it can be performed in a physician's office under local anesthesia, it is less expensive as well. After surgery, the man applies ice to the area and watches for excessive swelling or bleeding.

The couple should understand that complete sterilization does not occur until all sperm have left the system, which may be 1 month or longer. The man should submit semen specimens for analysis until two specimens show no sperm present.

Hormonal Contraceptives

Hormonal contraceptives alter the normal hormone fluctuations of the menstrual cycle. They may be given by implant, by injection, or orally.

Hormone Implant

The progestin implant (Norplant system) consists of six soft, flexible capsules about 1.5 inches long (the size of a match) that are inserted subcutaneously into the upper inner arm under local anesthetic. The capsules, which contain levonorgestrel, release a very low dose of progestin continuously at gradually decreasing levels over 5 years, after which they should be removed.

At the time of publication, the Norplant system is not available for use until completion of an investigation into the long-term effectiveness of certain implant lots inserted after October 1999. A back-up method of contraception is recommended for women who have implants from the affected lots until further information is available.

Other implant systems are being studied and may be available in the United States in the future. Systems with fewer capsules that are easier to insert and remove are used in other countries and may be available in the future.

Hormone Injections

DepoProvera (medroxyprogesterone acetate or DMPA) is an injectable progestin that prevents ovulation for 12 weeks. It is 99.7% effective, is convenient, and does not contain estrogen. Action and side effects are similar to those of other progestin contraceptives. Menstrual irregularities are the major reason for discontinuation. Although spotting and breakthrough bleeding are common, amenorrhea occurs in 50% of women at 1 year. Weight gain may approximate 4 lb per year. Other side effects include headaches and hair loss. Women who should not use other hormone contraceptives generally should avoid DepoProvera as well.

DepoProvera is given by deep intramuscular injection. The site should not be massaged after injection because this accelerates absorption and decreases the period of effectiveness. The injection is best given within 5 days of the menstrual period. If given later in the cycle, an additional form of contraception should be used for the first week. If the woman is more than 1 week late returning for a subsequent injection, she will need to use a back-up method for 1 week after receiving the injection.

Women can use DepoProvera at any age and for any length of time if they are in good health. For breastfeeding women, it often is started 6 weeks after delivery, when lactation is well established. Fertility returns in approximately 6 to 12 months (Hatcher, 1998).

Lunelle, a monthly injectable contraceptive, is a new contraceptive choice for women. Lunelle contains medroxyprogesterone acetate like DepoProvera but also includes estradiol cypionate. It provides immediate, very effective contraception if given within 5 days of the last normal menstrual period. Action is similar to combined oral contraceptives but has the advantage of monthly rather than daily doses and a faster return to fertility (average 2 to 4 months). In addition, women have regular menses that are less painful and have less blood loss than with DepoProvera. Bleeding occurs 2 to 3 weeks after the first injection and 22 days after subsequent injections. Bleeding lasts 5 to 6 days.

Oral Contraceptives

OCs are the most widely used reversible contraceptive method in the United States (Trussel & Kowal, 1998). Combination OCs contain both estrogen and progestin, whereas "minipills" contain only progestin. Both types have much lower hormone levels than the original OCs, thus decreasing the risk of long-term side effects. Oral contraceptives have a 95% typical effectiveness rate.

Combination. Estrogen and progestin combinations are the most common OCs and have an action similar to pregnancy in preventing ovulation. The high level of estrogen and progestin prevents the discharge of follicle-stimulating and luteinizing hormones from the pituitary. This inhibits maturation of the follicle and ovulation. (See Chapter 4 for information about the menstrual cycle.) In addition, the cervical mucus becomes too thick for sperm to penetrate, and the endometrium becomes less hospitable to implantation.

Combination OCs are available in packets of 21 or 28 tablets. With 21-tablet packets, the woman takes one pill daily for 3 weeks, then stops for a week, during which time menses occurs. Packets of 28 tablets include 7 tablets made of an inert substance that the woman takes during the fourth week. The extra pills avoid disrupting the everyday routine of taking pills.

Monophasic or multiphasic dosages are available. Monophasic pills have an estrogen and progestin content that remains constant throughout the cycle. With multiphasic pills, the estrogen dose may be constant or increased in the later part of the cycle. The progestin dose is low at the beginning and is increased later. This helps reduce side effects. Because two or three phases of dose changes may occur, women must take the pills in the proper order.

A low-dose combined OC is available that contains less estrogen than commonly used. The lower dose of estrogen is advantageous for some women with risk factors, such as smokers. This formulation may be slightly less effective, especially if women miss doses. Breakthrough bleeding is more likely to occur with low-dose pills.

Progestin Only. OCs that contain progestin but no estrogen are called *minipills.* They are useful for women who cannot take estrogen. They are less effective at inhibiting ovulation but cause thickening of the cervical mucus to prevent penetration by sperm and make the endometrial lining unfavorable for implantation. These pills have a lower dose of hormones and may avoid some side effects and risk factors associated with estrogen. Another method of contraception should be used during the first cycle. If the woman misses any pills or does not take them at the same time each day, however, chances of pregnancy increase. The woman who misses any minipills should continue to use the pills but use an additional method of contraception for the rest of the cycle. Breakthrough bleeding and higher risk of pregnancy have made these OCs less popular than the combination OCs.

Benefits, Risks, and Cautions. When choosing OCs, the balance between the benefits and the risks

Table 31-4
POTENTIAL BENEFITS AND DISADVANTAGES OR RISKS OF ORAL CONTRACEPTIVES

Benefits	Disadvantages or Risks*
Highly effective contraception. Reduces ovarian and endometrial cancer by as much as 50%. Protection continues for years after use. Regulates menstrual cycles and reduces cramping, menstrual blood loss, and associated anemia. Decreased incidence of the following: • Benign breast disease • Ovarian cysts • Pelvic inflammatory disease • Ectopic pregnancy • Rheumatoid arthritis Improves the following: • Acne • Endometriosis • Premenstrual syndrome (for some) • Dysmenorrhea • Fibroids (leiomyomas)	No protection against sexually transmissible diseases. May change insulin need in diabetics. Slightly increased risk of breast and cervical cancer. Increased incidence of the following: • Deep and superficial vein thrombosis • Pulmonary embolism • Myocardial infarction • Stroke • Hypertension • Migraines • Chlamydial infection • Benign liver tumors • Gallbladder disease • Depression (may increase or decrease)

*Incidence of many risks is significantly reduced with low-dose oral contraceptives presently used. Avoiding oral contraceptive use in women who smoke or have other risk factors significantly lowers risk for cardiovascular disease.

must be weighed for each individual (Table 31-4). The method has many benefits in addition to safe, reliable contraception. Women often exaggerate the health risks and underestimate the health benefits of OCs, however (Tessler & Peipert, 1997). Although risks in using OCs exist, women should know that the chances of complications and death during pregnancy and childbirth are greater (Hatcher & Guillebaud, 1998).

Although OCs were once thought unsafe for older women, studies show that women in good health who do not smoke can continue to take OCs until age 50 (Hatcher & Guillebaud, 1998). Some women using OCs go directly to hormone replacement therapy. Smoking increases the incidence of complications for women of all ages. Other risk factors include hypertension, high cholesterol levels, obesity, and diabetes.

Many risks were associated with the higher doses of hormones used in the original OCs but are less of a problem with current OCs. Hazards are decreased by careful screening for risk factors in each woman. OCs provide no protection against STDs and may increase susceptibility to some. Therefore women should be advised to use condoms and spermicide if their partners may be infected.

Side Effects. Approximately 29% of women who do not wish to become pregnant discontinue OCs within a year. Side effects are a major reason. Most side effects are minor and include signs and symptoms often seen in pregnancy. Decreasing the amount of estrogen helps relieve nausea, headaches, and breast tenderness, whereas increasing the estrogen content prevents breakthrough bleeding. Other side effects include weight gain or loss, fluid retention, amenorrhea, and chloasma. Side effects often decrease after the first few months of use and are less frequent in low-dose OCs.

CRITICAL TO REMEMBER

Cautions in Using Oral Contraceptives

Oral contraceptives should not be used by women with a history of any of the following:
- Thrombophlebitis and thromboembolic disorders
- Cerebrovascular or cardiovascular diseases
- Any estrogen-dependent cancer or breast cancer
- Benign or malignant liver tumors

Oral contraceptives should not be used by women who currently have any of the following:
- Any of the above conditions
- Impaired liver function
- Suspected or known pregnancy
- Undiagnosed vaginal bleeding
- Heavy cigarette smoking (more than 15 per day in women older than 35; any use of cigarettes is discouraged and should be evaluated individually)

Teaching. Education about proper use of OCs greatly increases their effectiveness. Teaching should be extensive when the woman begins to use the hormones. Follow-up is necessary to ensure that her questions and unanticipated problems are resolved. Because the instructions can be complicated, they should be written clearly and simply in her own language, if she can read.

Side effects are the most common reason for discontinuing OCs. The nurse should listen carefully to women's concerns about side effects and help them find

WOMEN WANT TO KNOW *What to Do if an Oral Contraceptive Dose Is Missed*

The following provides one example of information given to women who miss contraceptive pills. Talk with your nurse practitioner, nurse-midwife, or physician for specific information suited to your needs.

COMBINED ORAL CONTRACEPTIVES

One Hormonal Pill Missed

- Take the pill as soon as you remember it.
- Take the next pill at the normal time.
- Use another contraceptive method for 7 days or consider using emergency contraception if unprotected sexual intercourse occurred.

Two Hormonal Pills Missed

- Take one pill as soon as you remember and the next pill at the usual time.
- If the missed pills were from the first week of a new pack, use an additional method of contraception for the next 7 days and consider emergency contraception if unprotected intercourse occurred.
- If the missed pills were later than the first week, a backup method of contraception may not be necessary but can be used if you are very concerned about pregnancy. Also consider emergency contraception.
- NOTE: Some health care providers suggest taking 2 missed pills when you realize you missed them and taking 2 more pills the next day. Check with your provider for more information.

Inactive Pills Missed between Days 21 and 28

- Throw away pills missed, and continue to take the rest as scheduled. Contraception will not be affected.
- Begin a new packet of pills on the same day as usual.

Progestin-Only Oral Contraceptives (Minipills)

- Minipills missed or taken as much as 12 hours late: continue to take the pills for the rest of the cycle as usual.
- Use another method of contraception for the entire cycle.

(Information from Hatcher & Guillebaud [1998], & Hatcher, et al. [1999] [see "References" on p. 893]).

methods to relieve them. Accidental pregnancies may occur in many women who discontinue OCs owing to side effects. In one study of women who discontinued using OCs, 69% used a less effective contraceptive method and 19% used no contraception at all, yet these women did not wish to become pregnant (Rosenberg & Waugh, 1998). Women should be instructed that they need a back-up contraceptive method readily available should they decide to stop taking their OCs.

Blood Hormone Levels. Because maintaining a constant blood hormone level is important for effectiveness, the woman must take the pills at the same time each day. Many women make them a part of their bedtime routine, whereas others take them with a meal to avoid nausea. Breakthrough bleeding is more likely when a significant time variation occurs between doses. Unless they begin the pills during the first 7 days of the menstrual cycle, women should use another contraceptive method during the first week of the first cycle until the blood hormone levels are established (Cunningham, et al., 1997). Women also should understand that some pills must be taken in a certain order and that changing the order will decrease the effectiveness of the method.

Missed Doses. Instructions for the woman who misses one or more doses should be provided. Women who frequently miss OCs should be counseled about other contraceptive methods that might be more effective for them.

If a woman misses a period and thinks she may be pregnant because she missed one or more doses, she should stop taking the pills and get a sensitive pregnancy test immediately. Using another contraceptive method during this time is essential. Although association with fetal anomalies has not been established, continued use of OCs during pregnancy is not advisable.

Nutrition. Low-estrogen OCs currently used do not interfere with nutritional status as those in the past did. Women in good health do not need to take vitamin supplements just because they are taking OCs (Haken, 2000).

Postpartum and Lactation. Because of their increased risk for thrombosis, postpartum women who are not breastfeeding should wait 3 weeks to begin OCs (Kennedy & Trussell, 1998). Combination OCs reduce milk production in lactating women, and very small amounts may be transferred to the milk. Many experts recommend that OCs not be used during lactation (Kennedy & Trussell, 1998; Adams, 2000). Progestin-only contraceptives may be a better choice if a woman wishes to use a hormonal contraceptive because they do not affect milk production. They can be started 6 weeks after birth.

Other Medications. OCs may interact with other medications, and the effectiveness of each may be changed. Antibiotics and anticonvulsants such as phenobarbital, phenytoin, topirimate, carbamazepine, and primidone decrease the effectiveness of OCs. Therefore the woman should always tell any health care provider prescribing medications for her about other drugs she is taking.

Follow-up. The woman who takes OCs should have a yearly pelvic examination and a Papanicolaou (Pap) smear, breast examination, and blood pressure measurement. She should report any signs of adverse reaction immediately. Use of the acronym *ACHES* may help

Table 31-5
"ACHES"* WARNING SIGNS OF ORAL CONTRACEPTIVE COMPLICATIONS

	Warning Sign	Possible Complication
A	Abdominal pain (severe)	Benign liver tumor, gallbladder disease
C	Chest pain, dyspnea, hemoptysis	Pulmonary emboli or myocardial infarction
H	Severe headache, weakness or numbness of extremities	Stroke
E	Eye problems (visual changes such as blurred or double vision or visual loss, speech disturbance)	Stroke
S	Severe leg pain or swelling (calf or thigh)	Deep vein thrombosis

*The acronym *ACHES* can be used to help women remember warning signs that may indicate complications when using oral contraceptives. Other signs include jaundice, a breast lump, and depression. The woman should contact her health care provider if any of these signs develop. (Data from Hatcher, R.A., Trussell, J., Stewart, J., Cates, W., Stewart, G.K., Guest, F., & Kowal. D. [1998]. *Contraceptive technology* [17th ed.]. New York: Ardent Media.)

the woman remember signs that may indicate complications (Table 31-5). Return of fertility usually occurs within 2 to 3 months after the pills are discontinued. A woman should wait until her menstrual cycle is reestablished before conceiving so that she can date the beginning of her pregnancy more accurately.

Postcoital Emergency Contraception

Postcoital contraception (often called *emergency contraceptive pills [ECP]* or the "morning-after pill") is a method to prevent pregnancy after unprotected intercourse. It may be used after contraceptive failure, such as a condom breaking or diaphragm dislodging during intercourse. It also may be used after rape or in other situations when contraceptives were used incorrectly or not at all.

The most common method involves taking a larger-than-usual dose of a combined OC as soon as possible and no later than 72 hours after unprotected intercourse. A second dose is taken 12 hours after the first. A kit is available (Preven) that contains the proper ECP dose. Because of the short time frame during which ECP is effective, some health care providers give women prescriptions to use if necessary at a later date. Treatment reduces the risk of pregnancy by 75%.

The high hormone levels prevent or delay ovulation to prevent fertilization and may have some effect on endometrial development. The treatment is ineffective if pregnancy has already occurred and does not harm a developing fetus (Van Look & Stewart, 1998). Antiemetics may be prescribed to treat the side effects of nausea and vomiting. They may be started an hour before the woman takes the first dose of ECP.

Combined OC treatment should not be used in women who have contraindications for their use. High doses of progestin-only contraceptives may be preferable for these women. A progestin-only emergency contraceptive (Plan B) is available. A tablet of levonorgestrel is taken as soon as possible and within 72 hours of intercourse, and a second tablet is taken 12 hours later. Because it contains no estrogen, nausea and vomiting are less with this method.

Insertion of the copper T 380A IUD within 5 days of intercourse also may be used and provides 99% effectiveness. It has the added advantage of providing long-term (10 years') protection from pregnancy for those who choose this method.

Check Your Reading

9. What factors should a couple consider in deciding which method of sterilization to use?
10. What is the mechanism of action of hormonal contraceptives?
11. What side effect is most likely to cause some women to discontinue use of DepoProvera?
12. What do women taking OCs need to know about this contraceptive method?
13. How soon after unprotected intercourse should ECP be used?

Intrauterine Devices

Intrauterine devices (IUDs) are inserted into the uterus to provide continuous pregnancy prevention. The copper T 380A (ParaGard), the progestin IUD (Progestasert), and the levonorgestrel IUD (LNG or Mirena) are shaped like the letter T (Figure 31-3). They are 98% to 99.2% effective. Although safety was a concern with early models, IUDs are considered very safe at this time. They often are inserted at the 6 weeks' postpartum checkup and are safe during lactation. Although they are expensive at the time of insertion, IUDs have a relatively low long-term cost.

Action

The exact mechanism of action is unknown, but IUDs appear to affect sperm, ova, and the endometrium to prevent fertilization. Sperm are immobilized, and ova move through the fallopian tubes more quickly. The endometrium undergoes a sterile inflammatory response

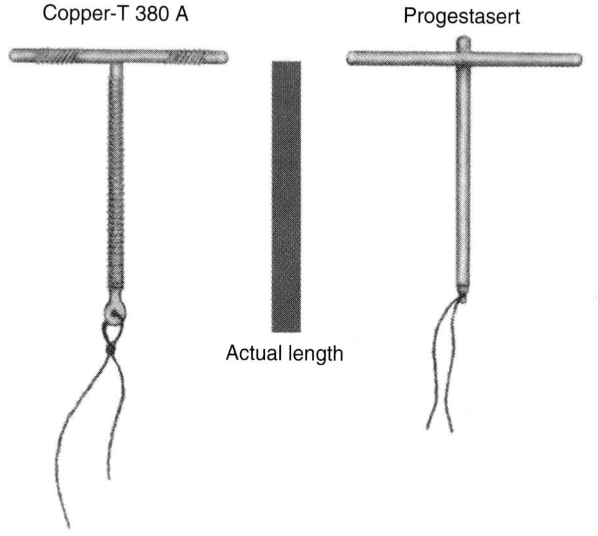

FIGURE 31-3 The Copper T 380A (ParaGard) and progestin (Progestasert) intrauterine devices (IUDs). Currently, IUDs are considered a very safe method for preventing pregnancy.

that is toxic to sperm and may prevent implantation. The ParaGard IUD has copper wire wound around it and remains effective for 10 years. Progestin is continuously released from the Progestasert and Mirena IUDs. Progestasert is replaced yearly, but Mirena is effective for 5 years.

Side Effects

Side effects include cramping and bleeding with insertion. Menorrhagia (increased bleeding during menstruation) and dysmenorrhea (painful menstruation) are common reasons for removal. They may be more frequent with the copper device. Spotting may occur during the early months with Mirena but may be followed by amenorrhea. Ibuprofen may relieve cramping, and some women need iron for anemia. Pelvic infections are less common than with the original models. They occur most often in the first few weeks after insertion or are caused by STDs. Therefore only women in mutually monogamous relationships and at low risk for STDs should use IUDs.

Complications include expulsion and perforation of the uterus. Women who become pregnant using the IUD are more likely to have ectopic pregnancies, spontaneous abortions, and preterm deliveries. Nulliparous women and those with recent or recurrent pelvic infections, a history of ectopic pregnancy, bleeding disorders, and abnormalities of the uterus should choose another contraceptive method.

Teaching

Teaching the woman about side effects and ways to check for the presence of the plastic strings or "tail" extending from the IUD into the vagina is important. The woman should feel for the strings once a week during the first 4 weeks, then monthly after menses, and if she has signs of expulsion (cramping or unexpected bleeding). If the strings are longer or shorter than previously, she should see her health care provider. Signs of infection such as unusual vaginal discharge, pain or itching, low pelvic pain, and fever should prompt a call to the health care provider. Any signs of pregnancy should be reported to rule out ectopic pregnancy and remove the device if pregnancy has occurred. The woman should return yearly for a Pap smear and to check for anemia if menses are heavy.

Barrier Methods

Barrier methods of contraception involve chemicals or devices that prevent sperm from entering the cervix. The method may kill the sperm or place a temporary partition between the penis and cervix. All barrier methods are coitus-related and may interfere with spontaneity. However, they avoid use of systemic hormones and provide some protection from STDs. Infection with human papillomavirus, an STD, may increase the risk of cervical cancer. Therefore use of barrier contraceptives may lower the incidence of cervical cancer.

Chemical Barriers

Chemicals that kill sperm are called *spermicides* and come in many forms. Creams and gels are generally used with mechanical barriers such as the diaphragm or cervical cap. Foams, suppositories, and vaginal film may be used alone. They are inserted into the vagina just before sexual intercourse and are effective for about 1 hour. Vaginal films and suppositories must melt before they become effective, which takes approximately 15 minutes.

Spermicides are readily available without a prescription, inexpensive per use, and easy to use. Spermicides may provide some protection against some STDs. Using spermicides with condoms increases lubrication, which decreases the risk of condom breakage. This may be an advantage, especially during lactation when vaginal secretions are decreased.

Women should avoid douching for at least 6 to 8 hours after intercourse and should add more spermicide if coitus is repeated. Sensitivity to the products may cause genital irritation, which could increase susceptibility to infection. Some women and their partners feel that spermicides are messy and interfere with sensation during intercourse. When used alone, spermicides are about 74% effective. Effectiveness is increased when spermicides are used with a mechanical barrier method.

Mechanical Barriers

Mechanical barriers are devices placed over the penis or cervix to prevent passage of sperm into the uterus. They include the condom, diaphragm, and cervical cap.

COUPLES WANT TO KNOW *What Is the Proper Way to Use Condoms?*

Although condoms are easy to use, proper use increases their effectiveness.

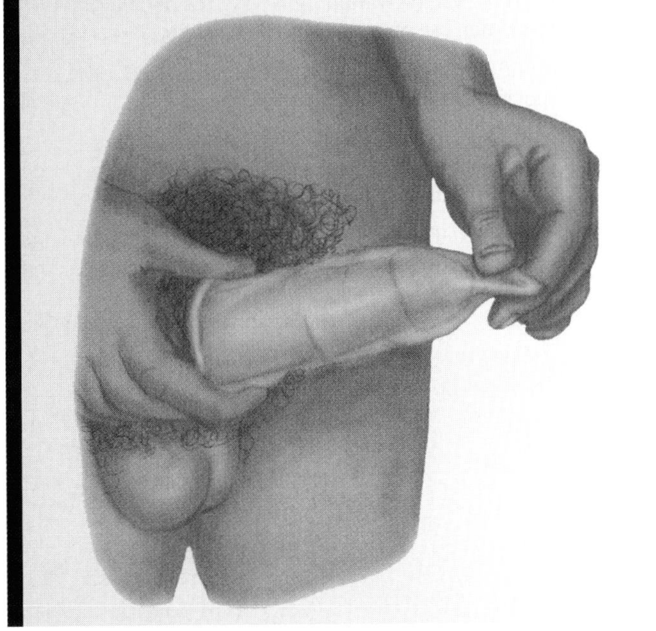

- Condoms are available in a variety of colors, textures, and materials, but those made of latex are most effective. Others may help protect against pregnancy but not protect against sexually transmissible diseases.
- Check the expiration dates on packages because condoms may deteriorate after 5 years.
- Lubrication may increase comfort for the woman and reduce the risk of breakage. Use a water-soluble lubricant or a spermicide because oil-based products (such as petroleum jelly or baby oil) cause deterioration of the latex.
- Always apply the condom before any contact of the penis with the vagina occurs because sperm may be present in preejaculatory fluid.
- Squeeze the air out of the tip of the condom, and leave one-half inch of space at the tip as the condom is rolled onto the erect penis. This allows a place for sperm to collect and helps prevent breakage.
- Withdraw the penis from the vagina before it becomes soft and hold the condom in place so that it does not slip off and no semen spills into the vagina.
- Use a new condom each time intercourse is repeated.

Male Condom. Condoms, the only male contraceptive device currently available, are one of the most popular contraceptive methods in the United States. They cover the penis to prevent sperm from entering the vagina. Condoms are most often made of latex and may be coated with spermicide. Some condoms are made from polyurethane or natural membrane. Polyurethane condoms are thinner than latex and can be used by people who are allergic to latex. They may require lubrication to avoid breakage. Natural-membrane condoms do not prevent passage of viruses and do not provide protection from STDs caused by viruses. Latex condoms provide the best protection available (other than abstinence) against many STDs. For this reason, they should be used during any possible exposure to an STD, even if another contraceptive technique is practiced or if the woman is pregnant.

Condoms are readily available, are inexpensive, and can be carried inconspicuously by the man or woman. The typical failure rate of 14% can be decreased greatly by combining condom use with another method such as a vaginal spermicide. Reservoir tips and water-based lubricants help prevent breakage. Because condoms must be applied just before intercourse, some couples object to the interference with spontaneity. Others feel that condoms interfere with sensation. People who are allergic to latex should avoid the use of latex condoms because severe reactions are possible. Condoms may be affected by vaginal medications and should not be used concurrently.

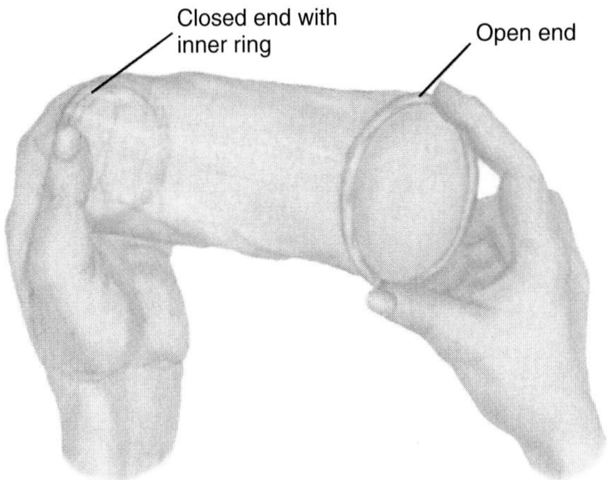

FIGURE 31-4 The female condom. A woman can protect herself from sexually transmissible diseases without relying on use of the male condom.

Female Condom. The female condom is a polyurethane pouch inserted into the vagina. A flexible ring fits over the cervix like a diaphragm, and another ring extends outside the vagina to partially cover the perineum (Figure 31-4). The female condom is the first contraceptive device to allow a woman some protection from STDs without relying on the male condom. It is less effective, however, and many women object to it on esthetic grounds. It has a typical failure rate of approximately 21%. Some women use the female condom some of the time and the male condom at other times (Macaluso, et al., 2000).

WOMEN WANT TO KNOW *How to Use a Diaphragm*

Follow instructions carefully when using your diaphragm. Skill at insertion and removal increases with practice.

- Plan to insert the diaphragm during intercourse or several hours before. Empty your bladder before insertion.
- Spread about a teaspoon of spermicidal cream or gel inside the dome and around the rim.

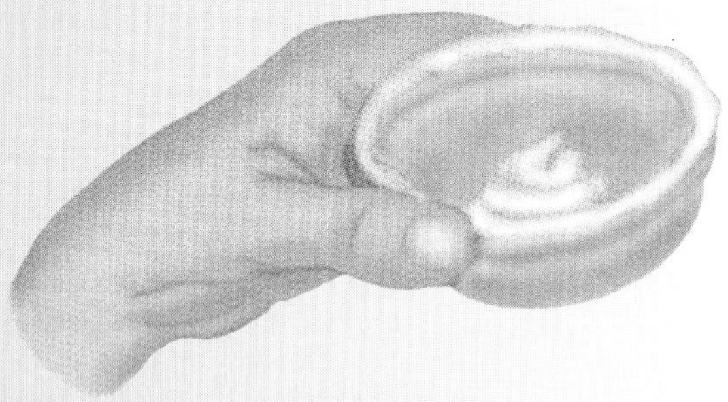

- Fold the diaphragm, and insert it into the vagina with the spermicide toward the cervix. A squatting position or placing one foot on a chair makes insertion and removal easier.

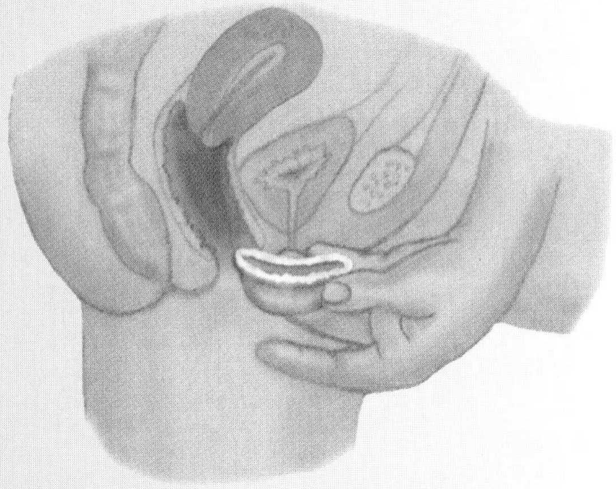

- Be sure that the front rim fits behind your pubic bone and that you can feel the cervix through the center of the diaphragm.

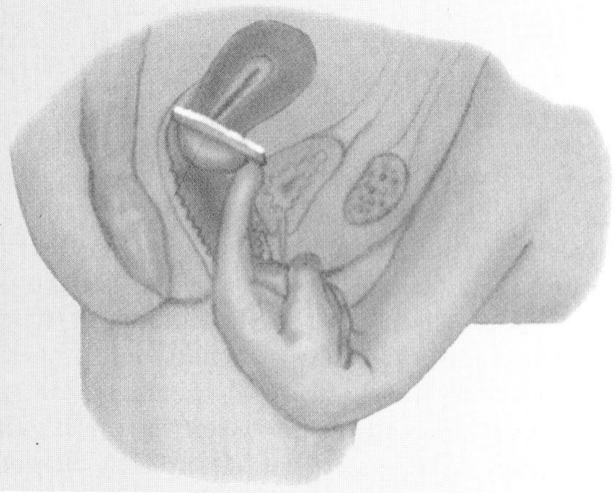

- If more than 6 hours pass between the insertion and intercourse or if you have intercourse again, insert more spermicide into the vagina without removing the diaphragm. Some women use more spermicide after 2 to 3 hours.
- Leave the diaphragm in place at least 6 hours after the last intercourse, but leave it in place for no more than a total of 24 hours to reduce risk of infection.
- Douching with the diaphragm in place is unnecessary and will lessen the effectiveness.
- To remove the diaphragm, assume a squatting position and bear down. Hook a finger around the front rim to break the suction, and pull down.

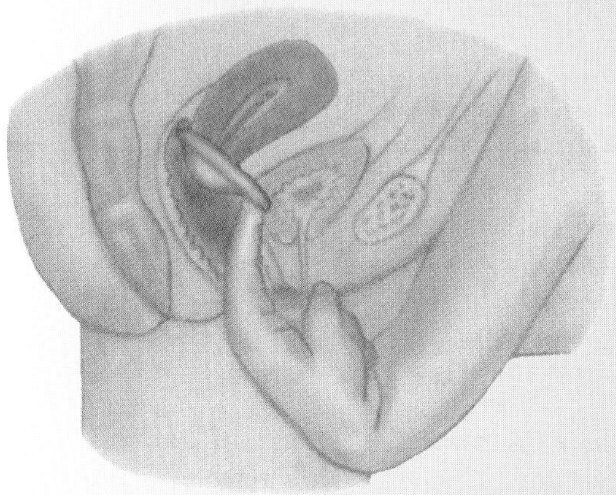

- Wash the diaphragm with mild soap, and dry well after each use. Inspect it occasionally for small holes by holding it up to a light. If you find one, use another contraceptive method and go to your physician, nurse-midwife, or nurse practitioner for a new diaphragm.

Diaphragm. The diaphragm is a latex dome surrounded by a spring or coil. The woman places spermicidal cream or gel into the dome and around the rim, then inserts it over the cervix by hand or with a plastic introducer. When folded, some models arch to form a half-moon shape, which assists in proper placement.

Because it covers the cervix, the diaphragm prevents passage of sperm while holding spermicide in place for additional protection. The failure rate is 20%. Diaphragms must be fitted by a nurse practitioner, nurse-midwife, or physician. The woman should be checked for size changes yearly, after a weight gain or loss of more than 10 lb, and after each pregnancy or abortion. The diaphragm should be replaced every 2 years. The correct size may not be available for all women.

To eliminate interference with spontaneity, some women insert the diaphragm hours in advance when intercourse is possible, although not necessarily planned. Although some women cannot feel the diaphragm once it is in place, others find it noticeable or uncomfortable. Pressure on the urethra may cause irritation and urinary tract infections. Allergies to latex or history of toxic shock syndrome preclude use. The diaphragm may be damaged by some medications used for vaginal candida infections and should not be used during treatment.

Cervical Cap. The cervical cap is similar to the diaphragm but smaller. The flexible latex cup fits over the cervix and remains in place by suction (Figure 31-5). Women who are difficult to fit with a diaphragm may be able to use the cervical cap. However, cap sizes are limited, and women with cervical abnormalities may not be able to use it. It is 80% effective for nulliparous women but only 60% effective for women who have already given birth.

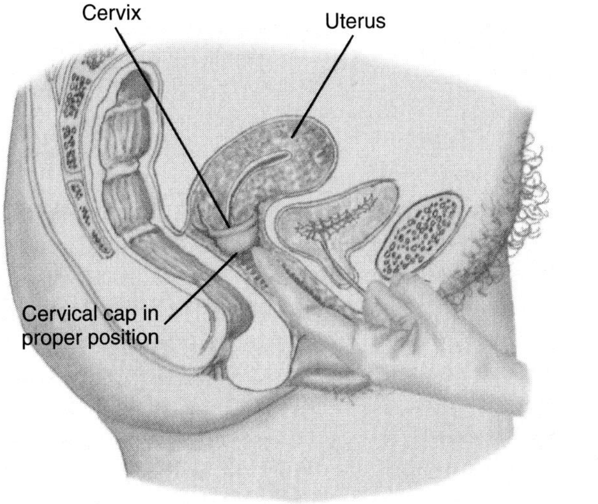

FIGURE 31-5 The cervical cap is inserted much like the diaphragm. The woman should check to be certain that it is placed over the cervix.

Because it is smaller than the diaphragm, the cervical cap is less noticeable and causes no pressure on the bladder. It can remain in place for 48 hours, and more spermicide is not needed if intercourse is repeated. It should not be removed for 6 hours after the last intercourse. Insertion and removal are similar to those for the diaphragm but may be more difficult because the cap is smaller. The nurse should teach the woman to feel her cervix to check placement before and after intercourse because the cap can be dislodged. It should not be used during menses or in women with a history of toxic shock syndrome.

The cap fitting should be checked yearly; after abortion, childbirth, or surgery; or if it dislodges frequently. A Pap smear is required 3 months after the original fitting because some users have had changes indicating cervical neoplasia. If the Pap smear is normal at 3 months, only yearly examinations are necessary.

Natural Family Planning Methods

Natural family planning methods, also called *fertility awareness* or *periodic abstinence methods,* use physiologic cues to predict ovulation and avoid coitus when conditions are favorable for fertilization. They also can help women who wish to become pregnant (see Chapter 32).

Natural family planning helps women learn about the ways in which their bodies change throughout the menstrual cycle. It is acceptable to most religious groups and avoids the use of drugs, chemicals, and devices. However, couples must be highly motivated because they must abstain from intercourse for as much as half the menstrual cycle. Natural family planning methods may be very effective if used perfectly. The method is very unforgiving, however, and errors in predicting ovulation or intercourse during the forbidden times carry a high risk of pregnancy. Some women use the method to determine when they are fertile and use a barrier contraceptive at that time.

Calendar

The calendar method is based on the fact that ovulation occurs approximately 14 days before the onset of menses. The woman keeps track of the length of her cycles for 6 months to determine the range in cycle length and uses it to estimate when ovulation will occur (Table 31-6). The calendar method is unreliable because many factors such as illness or stress can affect the time of ovulation.

Basal Body Temperature

In the basal body temperature method, the woman charts her temperature each morning before getting out of bed or increasing her activity, which would cause her temperature to rise (see Procedure 32-1, p. 902). Her basal body temperature may drop slightly before

Table 31-6
NATURAL FAMILY PLANNING METHODS

Method and Failure Rate (Perfect Use)	Application	Comments
Calendar: 9%	Subtract 18 to 21 days from shortest cycle and 9 to 11 days from longest cycle to determine fertile period.	Example: 28 to 32 day cycle—fertile between days 7 and 23 (28 − 21 = 7, 32 − 9 = 23).
Basal body temperature	See Procedure 32-1, p. 902.	Avoid intercourse until third day after temperature rise. Unreliable if used alone. Affected by illness, lack of sleep, stress.
Cervical mucus (ovulation or Billings): 3%	Assess mucus at vaginal orifice daily. Avoid intercourse during menses and from the time of thick, sticky mucus until 4 days after peak of clear, slippery, stretchy mucus.	Intercourse allowed only every other day because semen interferes with assessment of mucus. See Procedure 32-1.
Symptothermal: 2%	Combine all above methods and assess weight gain, libido, bloating, and mittelschmerz.	Requires much education and motivation.

ovulation and then rise approximately 0.2° to 0.45° C (0.4° to 0.8° F) with ovulation. The temperature remains higher throughout the second half of the cycle because of progesterone. Used alone, this method is not reliable because errors are frequent. It often is used along with other methods.

Cervical Mucus

Also called the *ovulation* or *Billings method,* the cervical mucus technique is based on changes in cervical mucus caused by rising estrogen levels during the follicular phase of the menstrual cycle. The woman assesses the cervical mucus by wiping it from the vaginal orifice with tissue each day (see Procedure 32-1, p. 902). The couple avoids intercourse during the time when the mucus indicates ovulation is near.

Symptothermal Method

The symptothermal method combines the calendar, basal body temperature, and cervical mucus methods. In addition, other symptoms that occur near ovulation, such as weight gain, abdominal bloating, mittelschmerz (pain on ovulation), and increased libido, are noted. This increases awareness of when ovulation occurs and increases effectiveness.

Check Your Reading

14. What education is important for women choosing an IUD?
15. How do barrier methods of contraception work?
16. What are the advantages and disadvantages of natural family planning methods?

Abstinence

Abstinence can be defined as the avoidance of sexual intercourse or the avoidance of all forms of sexual activity. Some people choose abstinence throughout their lives and others practice abstinence at various times. Abstinence is encouraged for adolescents and endorsed by many religious groups. If practiced perfectly, it is the only totally effective method of preventing pregnancy. If all sexual activity is avoided, abstinence also prevents STDs.

Nurses should support women who choose to be abstinent. Sexual education programs in schools often include information on ways to maintain abstinence. Adolescents especially need assistance to define their values and in practical methods of reaching their goal of abstinence. Role playing often is used to help them work through situations in which they might have difficulty maintaining abstinence.

Abstinence has no cost, avoids the use of hormones, and has no side effects or medical risks. It must be practiced perfectly to avoid risking pregnancy or STDs, however. Therefore women should know where to get information about other contraceptive methods should they decide to become sexually active at a later time.

Least Reliable Methods of Contraception

The following methods of contraception are not considered reliable. However, they are used by women who lack information about their risks and other options or who will not use other methods for medical or personal reasons. The nurse needs to be familiar with these methods to help women understand the risks involved.

Breastfeeding

Breastfeeding inhibits ovulation because suckling and prolactin interfere with secretion of gonadotropin-releasing hormone and luteinizing hormone. During lactation, the ovarian response to follicle-stimulating hormone and luteinizing hormone may be altered. The frequency, intensity, and duration of suckling are very important in inhibiting ovulation.

Women who breastfeed completely (at least 10 times in 24 hours with no supplementary feedings) may avoid ovulation and resumption of menstrual cycles. However, use of formula or solid foods decreases the frequency and duration of breastfeeding, increases the length of time between feedings, and reduces night feedings. This may cause ovulation and a return of menses. After the first 3 to 6 months, prolactin levels decrease and the menstrual cycle generally resumes by 6 months. Another method of contraception should be used before or at this time.

Coitus Interruptus

Also called *withdrawal,* coitus interruptus is the removal of the penis from the vagina before ejaculation. Although it has an effectiveness rate of 81%, it requires great control by the man and may be unsatisfying for both partners. Even a man who wishes to use the method may misjudge the timing and withdraw too late. Fluid that escapes from the penis before ejaculation is not felt by the man or woman and may contain sperm. Sperm spilled on the vulva may enter the vagina and cause pregnancy.

APPLICATION OF THE NURSING PROCESS: CHOOSING A CONTRACEPTIVE METHOD

Contraceptive failure often occurs because women lack knowledge of ways to use their contraceptive methods correctly or choose methods unsuited to their needs. When contraception fails, the woman is exposed to the physical, psychological, and social consequences of unplanned pregnancy. Lack of understanding also may expose her to unnecessary side effects, possible complications, or STDs.

Assessment

Because contraception is a very private matter, approach it in a sensitive manner. Perform the assessment in a quiet area where interruptions are unlikely, and keep voices low to increase the woman's comfort. Assure the woman that her confidentiality will be maintained.

Introducing the Subject

In the postpartum setting, introduce the subject by asking the woman whether she plans to have more children. Most women indicate a desire to wait some time before the next pregnancy. Ask, "What method of family planning are you thinking about using now?" or "How did you feel about the method you used before pregnancy?" These kinds of questions may identify problems that the woman has had with contraception. In other settings, a woman may make some reference to her contraceptive method. The nurse can respond by asking, "How do you like using (name method)?" This shows the nurse is interested if the woman wishes to pursue the topic.

Determining the Woman's Understanding

Determine the woman's understanding of her contraceptive technique. For example, ask how she inserts her diaphragm, when and where she adds spermicide, or what time of day she takes her OC. The woman should know how to use her technique effectively and what to do in special circumstances, such as when she misses an OC pill or has difficulty removing her diaphragm. Explore any misinformation, concerns, or problems that she may have in regard to effectiveness, technique, or common side effects of the method.

Assessing the Woman's Satisfaction

Assess the woman's satisfaction with her contraceptive. The length of time that she has used the method is important. Women may be unsure about their method in the early months until they gain comfort from repetitive use. Satisfaction and effectiveness increase with greater familiarity with the method. Side effects also affect satisfaction. They may be severe enough to cause the woman to consider another method, or they may be relieved by simple techniques. Determine whether what the woman considers simple side effects are indications of complications that necessitate referral for treatment.

Discussing Available Choices

If the woman is considering a change in contraceptive method, discuss available choices with her. Assess for factors that would help determine the best method for her. Include past history of medical conditions that might eliminate certain methods, childbearing history, cultural and religious beliefs, and intensity of desire to prevent pregnancy. The woman's ability to understand and follow complicated directions is important as well.

The type of relationship that a couple has is important in terms of contraceptive choice and protection against STDs. If the relationship is mutually monogamous, STDs are not a risk if neither partner is infected. If either of the couple has more than one partner, protection against STDs with a barrier method is essential, even if the woman uses another type of contraceptive.

Frequency of coitus may help determine the best choice of contraception. For occasional sexual intercourse, a barrier method may be most satisfactory. If intercourse is frequent, the woman may desire a method that is always in place, such as an IUD or a hormone implant. Explore her past experience with other methods, what she considers important, and her individual preferences. The woman who wants to avoid hormones that have a systemic effect is not a candidate for OCs or implants. Ask about beliefs and values that might eliminate certain choices.

Analysis

Lack of knowledge about family planning is common and can lead to physical, psychological, and social complications in a woman's life. A nursing diagnosis that addresses this problem is "Risk for Altered Health Maintenance related to lack of understanding about contraceptive methods chosen and available."

Planning

Goals and expected outcomes for this diagnosis are that the woman will:

- Correctly describe the way to use her contraceptive method, including solving common problems.
- Describe common side effects, indications of complications, and correct follow-up.
- Report that she and her partner are satisfied with their contraceptive method.
- Describe other methods available, and choose one if she desires a different form of contraception.

Interventions

Interventions involve follow-up of problems that may interfere with the woman's ability to maintain health. Increasing her understanding of contraceptive techniques will be the basis of the teaching plan.

Increasing Understanding of the Chosen Method

Fill in gaps in the woman's knowledge about the way her contraceptive method works, its effectiveness, advantages and disadvantages, common side effects and complications, and when to seek help. Use demonstrations and return demonstrations of the way to use the method (such as inserting a cervical cap or checking for IUD strings). Give suggestions for managing side effects and common problems.

Teaching about Other Methods

Provide information about other forms of contraceptives, if the woman wishes. Compare other methods with the one the woman is using. Discuss aspects most important to the individual woman and her lifestyle. If the woman expresses interest in one or two other methods, provide her with detailed information about them so that she can make an informed choice. She may wish to have written information to take home to discuss with her partner before making a final decision. If a fitting will be needed for a new method, discuss what may happen during the visit.

Protecting against Sexually Transmissible Diseases

Address defense against STDs, particularly if the woman is using a method that does not provide protection. This is a delicate subject. A way to approach it might be to say, "The method you are using is very effective against pregnancy but does not protect you against diseases like HIV. If there is any chance that you or your partner might have sex with more than one person or that your partner might have an infection, you should protect yourself by using one of the barrier types of contraception along with the one you are using. Let me explain about those further."

Including the Woman's Partner

Invite the woman to include her partner in discussions, if possible. He may influence the woman's choice of contraception and whether she actually uses it and uses it correctly. If the partner understands the proper method of use, he may be more cooperative, which will help ensure contraceptive success.

Evaluation

The woman should accurately describe all aspects of her contraceptive method, including ways to solve common problems and when to seek help for side effects or complications. At later visits, evaluate continued understanding, compliance with proper use, and satisfaction with the method. The woman who wishes to change her contraceptive method should describe other contraceptives available and ways to use them. She should choose a new method and, if necessary, visit a nurse practitioner, nurse-midwife, or physician for further discussion, examination, fitting, or prescription.

SUMMARY CONCEPTS

- The average woman must consider use of contraception for as many as 30 years of her life.
- The nurse helps women with family planning by providing current, accurate information about contraception and assisting them to find methods that best meet their needs.
- Because some methods have potential for serious complications, an informed consent form may be necessary.
- Adolescents may lack knowledge about their own bodies, conception, and methods of contraception. Risk-taking behaviors are common.
- Because teenagers often do not wish to talk to their parents about contraception, they need alternative sources of information and counseling.
- The most successful methods of contraception for adolescents are often those unrelated to coitus. They need information about methods from a nurse with an accepting attitude.
- Contraception is necessary until menstruation has ceased for 2 years. The healthy perimenopausal woman with no risk factors such as smoking can use any method of contraception safely.
- Sterilization offers permanent contraception. A tubal ligation can be performed soon after birth or at any time. Vasectomy is less expensive and can be performed in an office under local anesthesia. Although surgery to reverse sterilization is possible, it is expensive and not always successful.
- Hormonal contraceptives include the progestin implant, hormone injections, and OCs. They inhibit ovulation and make the cervical mucus unreceptive to sperm. Side effects and complications make these unsuitable for some women.

- Intrauterine devices are very effective and safe in women with no risk of STDs. Women must check for the device's strings each month.
- Barrier methods may be chemical or mechanical. They kill or prevent sperm from entering the cervix and provide some protection against STDs.
- Natural family planning methods involve avoidance of coitus when physiologic cues suggest that ovulation is likely. Women need high motivation and extensive education about their bodies to be successful with these methods.

ANSWERS TO CRITICAL THINKING EXERCISE

1. Find a private place to talk without interruption. Use therapeutic communication techniques to explore her feelings further. Help her think through the ways in which a pregnancy might change her life and the way she would feel about those changes. Discuss what happens when a woman is examined during a visit for contraceptive counseling. Explore what she feels would be most embarrassing about seeing a physician. Would a female nurse practitioner, midwife, or physician be more acceptable? Discuss common contraceptive methods and determine her understanding and feelings about them. Also discuss negotiation skills for condom use because condoms are important for prevention of STDs as well as pregnancy. Try role playing, with the adolescent acting the role of her partner and the nurse taking the role of the adolescent.

REFERENCES & READINGS

Ackerman, J.A., & Gray, M.J. (2000). Oral contraceptives. In E.J. Quilligan & F.P. Zuspan (Eds.), *Current therapy in obstetrics and gynecology* (5th ed, pp. 119-122). Philadelphia: W.B. Saunders.

Adams, D.M. (2000). Breastfeeding and oral contraceptives: Exploring opinions on the options. *AWHONN Lifelines,* 4(3), 45-46.

Alan Guttmacher Institute (AGI). (2000). *Facts in brief: Contraceptive use.* Internet: http://www.agi-usa.org/pubs/fb_contr_use.html.

AGI. (1998). *Issues in brief: Contraception counts: State-by-state information.* Internet: http://www.agi-usa.org/pubs/ib22.html.

AGI. (2000). *Issues in brief: US policy can reduce cost barriers to contraception.* Internet: http://www.agi-usa.org/pubs/ib_0799.html.

American Academy of Pediatrics. (1999). Policy statement: Contraception & adolescents. *Pediatrics,* 104(5), 1161-1166.

American College of Obstetricians and Gynecologists. (1996). Emergency oral contraception. *ACOG Practice Patterns, Number 2.* Washington, D.C.: Author.

Archer, D.F., Maheux, R., DelConte, A., & O'Brien, F.B. (1999). Efficacy and safety of a low-dose monophasic combination oral contraceptive containing 100 mcg levonorgestrel and 20 mcg ethinyl estradiol (Alesse). *American Journal of Obstetrics & Gynecology,* 181(5), S39-44.

Association of Women's Health, Obstetric, & Neonatal Nurses. (1999). *Position statement: Issue: Insurance coverage for contraceptives.* Washington, D.C.: Author.

Auerbach, K.D. (1999). Breastfeeding and maternal medication use. *Journal of Obstetric, Gynecologic, and Neonatal Nursing,* 28(5), 554-563.

Burns, V.E. (1999). Factors influencing teenage mothers' participation in unprotected sex. *Journal of Obstetric, Gynecologic, and Neonatal Nursing,* 28(5), 493-500.

Chez, R.A., & Strathman, I. (1999). Contraception and sterilization. In J.R. Scott, P.J. DiSaia, C.B. Hammond., & W.N. Spellacy. *Danforth's obstetrics and gynecology* (8th ed., pp. 553-565). Philadelphia: Lippincott.

Cunningham, F.G., MacDonald, P.C., Gant, N.F., Leveno, K.J., Gilstrap, L.C., Hankins, G.D.V., & Clark, S.L. (1997). *Williams obstetrics.* (20th ed.). Norwalk, CT: Appleton & Lange.

Deitch, K.V. (2000). Family planning. In S. Mattson & J.E. Smith (Eds.), *Core curriculum for maternal-newborn nursing* (2nd ed., pp. 338-344). Philadelphia: W.B. Saunders.

Edwards, S.R. (1994). The role of men in contraceptive decision making: Current knowledge and future implications. *Family Planning Perspectives,* 26(2), 77-82.

Glasier, A., & Baird, D. (1998). The effects of self-administering emergency contraception. *New England Journal of Medicine,* 339(1), 1-4.

Grimes, D.A. (2000). Updates in contraception from the XVI World Congress of the International Federation of Gynecology and Obstetrics, Washington, D.C. *Medscape Women's Health,* 5(5).

Haken, V. (2000). Interactions between drugs and nutrients. In L.K. Mahan & S. Escott-Stump. *Krause's food, nutrition, and diet therapy* (10th ed., pp. 399-414). Philadelphia: W.B. Saunders.

Hatcher, R.A. (1998). Depo-Provera, Norplant, and progestin-only pills (minipills). In R.A. Hatcher, J. Trussell, F. Stewart, W. Cates, G.K. Stewart, F. Guest, & D. Kowal. *Contraceptive technology* (17th ed., pp. 467-509). New York: Ardent Media.

Hatcher, R.A., & Guillebaud, J. (1998). The pill: Combined oral contraceptives. In R.A. Hatcher, J. Trussell, F. Stewart, et al. *Contraceptive technology* (17th ed, pp. 405-466). New York: Ardent Media.

Hatcher, R.A. (2001). Suspect Norplant lots still undergoing tests. *Contraceptive Technology Update,* 22(4), 48.

Hatcher, R.A., Zieman, M., Watt, A.P., Nelson, A., Darney, P.D., & Pluhar, E. (1999). *A pocket guide to managing contraception* (2nd ed.). Tiger, GA: Bridging the Gap Foundation.

Hillis, S.D., Marchbanks, P.A., Tylor, L.R., & Peterson, H.B. (1999). Poststerilization regret: Findings from the United States collaborative review of sterilization. *Obstetrics & Gynecology,* 93(6), 889-895.

Jambunathan, J., & Stewart, S. (1995). Hmong women in Wisconsin: What are their concerns in pregnancy and childbirth? *Birth,* 22(4), 204-210.

Kennedy, K.I. (1999). Fertility, sexuality, and contraception during lactation. In J. Riordan & K.G. Auerbach, *Breastfeeding and human lactation* (2nd ed., pp. 675-705). Boston: Jones & Bartlett.

Kennedy, K.I., & Trussell, J. (1998). Postpartum contraception and lactation. In R.A. Hatcher, J. Trussell, F. Stewart, W. Cates, G.K. Stewart, F. Guest, & D. Kowal. *Contraceptive technology* (17th ed., pp. 589-614). New York: Ardent Media.

Kowal, D. (1998). Abstinence and the range of sexual expression. In R.A. Hatcher, J. Trussell, F. Stewart, W. Cates, G.K. Stewart, F. Guest, & D. Kowal. *Contraceptive technology* (17th ed., pp. 297-302). New York: Ardent Media.

LaRose, K. (1999). Championing contraceptive coverage. *AWHONN Lifelines,* 3(2), 17-18.

Lawrence, R.A. & Lawrence, R.M. (1999). *Breastfeeding: A guide for the medical profession* (5th ed.). St. Louis: Mosby.

Lethbridge, D.J. (1995). Fertility management in Taiwanese and African-American women. *Journal of Obstetric, Gynecologic, and Neonatal Nursing,* 24(5), 459-463.

Lindberg, C.E. (1997). Emergency contraception: The nurse's role in providing postcoital options. *Journal of Obstetric, Gynecologic, and Neonatal Nursing,* 26(2), 144-152.

Macaluso, M., Demand, M., Artz, L., Fleenor, M., Robey, L., Kelaghan, J., Cabral, R., & Hook, E.W. (2000). Female condom use among women at high risk of sexually transmitted disease. *Family Planning Perspectives,* 32(3),138-144.

MacKay, A.P., Fingerhut, L.A., & Duran, C.R. (2000). *Adolescent health chartbook, Health, United States, 2000.* Hyattsville, MD: National Center for Health Statistics.

Martin, K., & Wu, Z. (2000). Contraceptive use in Canada: 1984-1995. *Family Planning Perspectives,* 32(2), 65-73.

McClanahan, P., & Edwards, M.R. (2000). Characteristics of Norplant users. *Journal of Obstetric, Gynecologic, and Neonatal Nursing,* 29(3), 275-281.

Osathanondh, R. (1999). Conception control. In K.J. Ryan, R.S. Berkowitz, R.L. Barbieri, & A. Dunaif. *Kistner's gynecology and women's health* (7th ed., pp. 285-324.) St. Louis: Mosby.

Rawlins, S., Burkman, R.T., & Schwarz, B.E. (2000). The power of the pill: Making evidence-based decisions. *American Journal for Nurse Practitioners,* 4(1), 25-40.

Rosenberg, M.J., & Waugh, M.S. (1998). Oral contraceptive discontinuation: A prospective evaluation of frequency and reasons. *American Journal of Obstetrics & Gynecology,* 179(3), 577-582.

Soler, H., Quadagno, D., Sly, D.F., Reihman, K.S., Eberstein, I.W., & Harrison, D.F. (2000). Relationship dynamics, ethnicity and condom use among low-income women. *Family Planning Perspectives,* 32(2), 82-88, 101.

Stewart, G.K., & Carignan, C.S. (1998). Female and male sterilization. In R.A. Hatcher, J. Trussell, F. Stewart, W. Cates, G.K. Stewart, F. Guest, & D. Kowal. *Contraceptive technology* (17th ed., pp. 545-588). New York: Ardent Media.

Stubblefield, P.G. (2000). Contraception. In L.J. Copeland & J.F. Jarrel (Eds.), *Textbook of gynecology* (2nd ed., pp. 287-333). Philadelphia: W.B. Saunders.

Stubblefield, P.G. (2000). Intrauterine devices. In E.J. Quilligan & F.P. Zuspan (Eds.), *Current therapy in obstetrics and gynecology* (5th ed., pp. 92-97). Philadelphia: W.B. Saunders.

Tessler, S.L., & Peipert, J.F. (1997). Perceptions of contraceptive effectiveness and health effects of oral contraception. *Women's Health Issues,* 7(6), 400-406.

Trussell, J., & Kowal, D. (1998). The essentials of contraception. In R.A. Hatcher, J. Trussell, F. Stewart, W. Cates, G.K. Stewart, F. Guest, & D. Kowal. *Contraceptive technology* (17th ed., pp. 211-247). New York: Ardent Media.

Unger, J.B., & Molina, G.B. (1998). Contraceptive use among Latina women: Social, cultural, and demographic correlates. *Women's Health Issues,* 8(6), 359-369.

U.S. Department of Health and Human Services. (2000). *Healthy people 2010: Healthy People 2010 (Conference edition, in two volumes).* Washington, D.C.

Van Look, P.F.A., & Stewart, F. (1998). Emergency contraception. In R.A. Hatcher, J. Trussell, F. Stewart, W. Cates, G.K. Stewart, F. Guest, & D. Kowal. *Contraceptive technology* (17th ed., pp. 277-295). New York: Ardent Media.

Zhu, B., Rolfs, R.T., Nangle, B.E., & Horan, J.M. (1999). Effect of the interval between pregnancies on perinatal outcomes. *New England Journal of Medicine,* 340(8), 589-594.

INFERTILITY 32

OBJECTIVES

1. Describe settings in which the nurse may encounter couples with infertility problems.
2. Explain factors that can impair a couple's ability to conceive.
3. Explain factors that may cause repeated pregnancy losses.
4. Specify evaluations that may be performed when a couple seeks help for infertility.
5. Explain the use of procedures and treatments that may aid a couple's ability to conceive and carry the fetus to viability.
6. Analyze ways in which infertility can affect a couple and other family members.
7. Summarize the nurse's role when caring for couples experiencing problems with fertility.

DEFINITIONS

ANOVULATORY (OR ANOVULAR) Menstrual cycles occurring without ovulation.

AZOOSPERMIA Absence of sperm in semen.

CLIMACTERIC Endocrine, body, and psychic changes occurring at the end of a woman's reproductive period. Also informally called *menopause.*

ENDOMETRIOSIS Presence of endometrial tissue (uterine lining) outside the uterine cavity.

ERECTILE DYSFUNCTION Consistent inability of a man to achieve or maintain an erection of the penis that is sufficiently rigid to permit successful sexual intercourse. Also called *impotence.*

FERNING (OR FERN TEST) The microscopic, fernlike appearance of dried cervical mucus that is most apparent at the time of ovulation.

GAMETE Reproductive cell; in the female, an ovum; in the male, a sperm.

GAMETOGENESIS Development and maturation of the sperm and ova.

GESTATIONAL SURROGATE A woman who carries the embryo of an infertile couple and relinquishes the child to the couple after birth.

IMPOTENCE See *erectile dysfunction.*

INCOMPETENT CERVIX Inability of the cervix to remain closed long enough during pregnancy for the fetus to reach a maturity sufficient to survive.

INFERTILITY Inability of a couple to conceive after 1 year of regular intercourse (two to three times weekly) without using contraception; also, the involuntary inability to conceive and produce viable offspring when the couple chooses. Primary infertility occurs in a couple who has never conceived; secondary infertility occurs in a couple who has conceived at least once before.

OLIGOSPERMIA A decreased number of sperm in semen, usually considered to be under 20 million per milliliter.

RETROGRADE EJACULATION Discharge of semen into the bladder rather than from the end of the penis.

SEMEN Spermatozoa with their nourishing and protective fluid; discharged at ejaculation.

SPINNBARKHEIT Clear, slippery, stretchy quality of cervical mucus during ovulation.

STERILITY Total inability to conceive.

DEFINITIONS—cont'd

SURROGATE MOTHER A fertile woman who is inseminated with the purpose of conceiving and relinquishing a child to an infertile couple.

VARICOCELE Abnormal dilation or varicosity of veins in the spermatic cord.

Infertility nursing is a specialty, but general practice nurses also meet couples who are seeking help or have had treatment for infertility in varied settings. The nurse's own friends and family members often turn to the nurse as a source of information when they have problems conceiving. Nurses working in the perioperative area may care for these couples during diagnostic or therapeutic surgery. Nurses in urology settings often see men who are being evaluated or treated for infertility. In the emergency department, nurses may care for women who are having a spontaneous abortion of a hard-won pregnancy.

Nurses in antepartum, intrapartum, and postpartum settings often encounter women with high-risk pregnancies or couples who have a new baby after infertility therapy. In addition, parenthood after infertility is not always easy, and nurses in pediatric and psychosocial settings may counsel families about parenting and changes in their personal relationships.

EXTENT OF INFERTILITY

The extent of infertility depends on its definition. Infertility is not an absolute condition but is a reduced ability to conceive. *Infertility* is strictly defined as the inability to conceive after 1 year of unprotected, regular sexual intercourse. A more workable definition does not specify a time limit but recognizes that infertility is any involuntary inability to conceive when desired. The definition is commonly expanded to include couples who conceive but repeatedly lose a pregnancy (pregnancy wastage) before the fetus is old enough to survive. Couples with primary infertility have never conceived. Couples with secondary infertility may have conceived before but are unable to conceive again.

In 1995, about 15% of U.S. couples sought infertility services because they could not have a baby when desired (Abma, Chandra, Mosher, Peterson, & Piccinino, 1997). Couples who delay childbearing until their mid- to late-30s or later feel pressured by the approaching end of the woman's reproductive years. To older couples, delay in achieving pregnancy or having a living baby is more significant than for young couples, who have more time to pursue pregnancy and make treatment decisions. As new methods of diagnosis and treatment emerge, couples who once accepted childlessness may enter infertility therapy or resume therapy they abandoned. Also, some women want to have a child without a male partner and may be served by infertility services.

FACTORS CONTRIBUTING TO INFERTILITY

Conception depends not only on normal reproductive function in each partner but also on a sensitive interaction between the partners. For some couples, identification and treatment of infertility are simple, but others require complex evaluation and treatment.

Because some factors contributing to infertility remain unknown, treatment of an identified problem does not always lead to a successful pregnancy. For example, it may be likely that a couple will be infertile because of problems in either or both partners, yet the couple nevertheless has several children. About 20% of infertile couples have no identified problem, yet some never conceive despite having undergone all available treatments.

Factors in the Man

The test of a man's fertility is his ability to initiate pregnancy in a fertile woman. Few absolute criteria exist to distinguish normal from abnormal male fertility, although an adequate number of sperm having normal structure and function must be deposited near the woman's cervix. Problems may exist with the sperm, erection or ejaculation, or the seminal fluid that carries the sperm into the woman's reproductive tract.

Abnormalities of the Sperm

Many factors can impair the number, structure, or function of sperm. Some conditions are temporary, such as an acute illness. Other conditions are permanent, such as a genetic disorder. A single or several findings may be abnormal. Further complicating evaluation of a man's fertility are the normal daily variations in semen.

Evaluation of the semen may reveal that the man has azoospermia or oligospermia. The average number of sperm released at ejaculation is 400 million. Approximately 20 million sperm with normal motility per milliliter of semen is probably the minimum number adequate for unassisted fertilization (Guyton & Hall, 2000).

A sufficient number of normal sperm must move in a purposeful direction to reach the ovum in the fallopian tube. Abnormal sperm structure or movement may reduce fertility, regardless of the actual number of sperm (Figure 32-1). Inflammatory processes in the man's reproductive organs may cause the sperm to clump, inhibiting their motility and fertilizing ability. Other sperm may look normal yet be unable to penetrate the ovum. No standard definition exists, but the impairment in sperm function may be classified according to sperm count and motility to promote the best choice of treatment when male factors contribute to infertility (Chantilis & Carr, 2000):

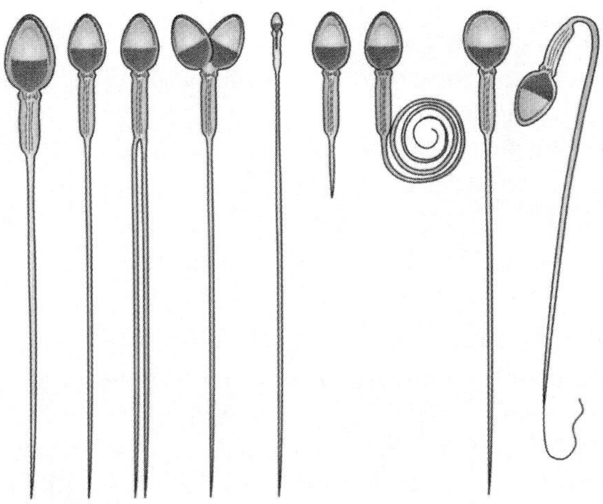

FIGURE 32-1 Abnormal infertile sperm compared with a normal sperm on the left. (From Guyton, A.C., & Hall, J.E. [2000]. *Textbook of medical physiology* [10th ed., p. 920]. Philadelphia: W.B. Saunders.)

- Mild—15 to 20 million sperm/mL, 35% to 50% motility
- Moderate—5 to 15 million sperm/mL, 20% to 35% motility
- Severe— <5% sperm/mL, or <20% motility

Factors that can impair the number and function of the sperm include the following:

- Abnormal hormonal stimulation of sperm production
- Acute or chronic illness such as mumps, cirrhosis, or renal failure
- Infections of the genital tract
- Anatomic abnormalities such as a varicocele or obstruction of the ducts that carry sperm to the penis
- Exposure to toxins such as lead, pesticides, or other chemicals
- Therapeutic treatments such as antineoplastic drugs or radiation for cancer
- Excessive alcohol intake
- Use of illicit drugs such as marijuana or cocaine
- An elevated scrotal temperature resulting from febrile illness or repeated use of saunas or hot tubs
- Immunologic factors, produced by the man against his own sperm (autoantibodies) or by the woman, causing the sperm to clump or be unable to penetrate the ovum

Abnormal Erections

Abnormal erections reduce the man's ability to deposit sperm-bearing seminal fluid in the woman's upper vagina. Erections are influenced by physical and psychological factors. Central nervous system dysfunction, which may be caused by drugs, psychiatric disturbance, or chronic illness, can interfere with erections. Surgery and disorders affecting the spinal cord or autonomic nervous system also may disrupt normal erections. Peripheral vascular disease reduces the amount of blood entering the penis and thus reduces the ability to maintain an erection. Drugs such as antihypertensives may reduce the erection or shorten its duration.

Abnormal Ejaculation

Abnormal ejaculation prevents deposition of the sperm in the ideal place to achieve pregnancy. Retrograde ejaculation is the release of semen backward into the bladder rather than forward through the tip of the penis. Conditions that may cause retrograde ejaculation are diabetes, neurologic disorders, surgery that impairs function of the sympathetic nerves, and drugs such as antihypertensives and psychotropics. Men who have suffered spinal cord injury may retain the ability to ejaculate, depending on the level of cord damage.

Anatomic abnormalities such as hypospadias (urethral opening on the underside of the penis) may cause deposition of semen near the vaginal outlet rather than near the cervix.

Excessive alcohol intake or use of illicit drugs can adversely affect ejaculation as well as sperm number and function. Ejaculation may be slow, absent, or retrograde when a man takes drugs that affect neurologic coordination of this event. Premature ejaculation is usually related to psychological disorders such as performance anxiety or unresolved conflicts.

Abnormalities of Seminal Fluid

The seminal fluid nourishes, protects, and carries sperm into the vagina until they enter the cervix. Only sperm enter the cervix; the seminal fluid remains in the vagina. Semen coagulates immediately after ejaculation but liquefies within 30 minutes, permitting forward movement of sperm. Seminal fluid that remains thick traps the sperm, impeding their movement into the cervix. The pH of seminal fluid is slightly alkaline to protect the sperm from the acidic secretions of the vagina. Adequate fructose must be present to provide energy for the sperm.

The specific abnormality found in the seminal fluid suggests the cause of the abnormality, such as obstruction or infection in a specific area of the genital tract. Seminal fluid that is abnormal in amount, consistency, or chemical composition suggests obstruction, inflammation, or infection. The presence of large numbers of leukocytes suggests infection.

Check Your Reading

1. How is infertility defined? What is the difference between primary and secondary infertility?
2. What are normal characteristics of sperm and the seminal fluid that carries sperm into the woman's vagina?
3. What problems in the man can occur with erection? With ejaculation of semen?
4. What can cause abnormalities in the sperm, ejaculation, and seminal fluid?

Factors in the Woman

A woman's fertility depends on the following:

- Regular production of normal ova
- An open path from her cervix to the fallopian tube to permit fertilization and movement of the embryo into the uterus for implantation
- A uterine endometrium that supports the pregnancy after implantation

See Chapter 4 for a complete discussion of the interrelated factors that contribute to normal female fertility.

Disorders of Ovulation

Normal ovulation depends on delicately timed and balanced secretions from the hypothalamus and pituitary and an ovarian response to mature and release an ovum. The hypothalamus secretes gonadotropin-releasing hormone (GnRH) beginning even before the obvious changes of puberty. GnRH stimulates the pituitary to release follicle-stimulating hormone (FSH) and luteinizing hormone (LH). FSH stimulates maturation of several follicles in the ovary. As the follicles mature, the ovary secretes estrogen to thicken the endometrium. About 24 to 36 hours before ovulation, a marked increase of LH occurs, which stimulates final maturation and release of one ovum from its follicle. The other follicles regress permanently. The collapsed follicle from which the ovum was released, now called a corpus *luteum,* produces progesterone and estrogen, which further prepare the endometrium for implantation and nourishment of the fertilized ovum.

Ovulation can be disrupted by many factors, including the following:

- A dysfunction in the hypothalamus or pituitary gland that alters the secretion of GnRH, FSH, and LH
- Failure of the ovaries to respond to FSH and LH stimulation, preventing maturation and release of the ovum

Disruption of hormone secretion or the ovarian response to hormone secretion can be caused by many factors such as cranial tumors, stress, obesity, anorexia, systemic disease, and abnormalities in the ovaries or other endocrine glands.

A woman does not produce new oocytes after her birth. Her existing oocytes therefore are vulnerable to cumulative toxic effects from therapeutic drugs, social or abused drugs, and environmental agents until the end of her reproductive life. Examples of factors that may impair normal ovulation include cancer chemotherapeutic agents, excessive alcohol intake, and cigarette smoking.

Women with ovulation disorders often have abnormal menses because hormone levels do not permit normal development and shedding of the endometrium. The woman may have absent, scant, or heavy menstrual periods. However, other women may have no menstrual disorders and the inability to conceive may be their only complaint.

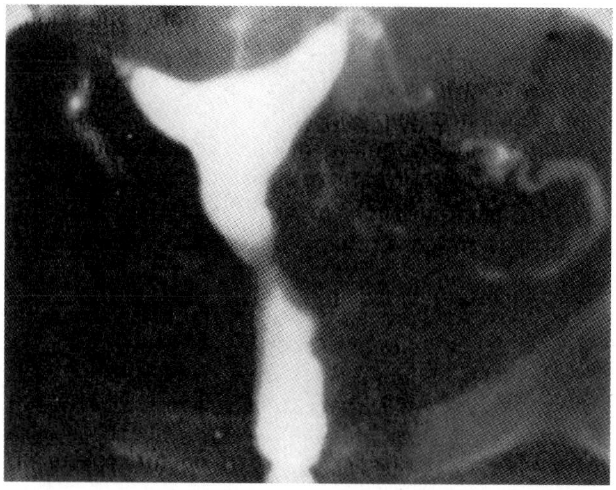

FIGURE 32-2 A hysterosalpingogram can determine whether fallopian tubes are patent. When tubes are open, as in this photograph, contrast medium that was injected through the cervix spills out of the fallopian tubes into the peritoneal cavity. (From Hacker, N.F., & Moore, J.G. [1998]. *Essentials of obstetrics and gynecology* [3rd ed., p. 617]. Philadelphia: W.B. Saunders.)

As a woman approaches the end of her reproductive life, she ovulates and menstruates more erratically. Thus her fertility naturally declines with age, falling dramatically after age 40. An occasional woman may be infertile at a younger age because of premature ovarian failure, causing her to have premature menopause.

Abnormalities of the Fallopian Tubes

At least one open fallopian tube is needed for natural conception and implantation to occur (Figure 32-2). Tubal obstruction may occur because of scarring and adhesions following reproductive tract infections. Infections such as chlamydia and gonorrhea are responsible for many cases of infertility from tubal obstruction. Prevention or prompt treatment and eradication of pelvic infections can reduce the incidence of fallopian tube damage.

Endometriosis may cause tubal adhesions, painful menstrual periods, and painful intercourse. Small lesions are unlikely to affect tubal function, but large lesions can distort tubal anatomy and lead to infertility.

Tubal obstruction also may occur if adhesions develop after pelvic surgery, ruptured appendix, peritonitis, or ovarian cysts. In addition, the fallopian tubes and other reproductive organs may have congenital anomalies that disrupt normal function.

The conditions that cause obstruction also may interfere with normal motility within the fallopian tube. Poor movement of the fimbriated (distal) end of the tube may prevent the pickup of the ovum from the ovarian surface after ovulation. Abnormal action of the cilia within the tube prevents normal transport of the ovum toward the uterine cavity.

Depending on the extent and location of the blockage, fallopian tube obstructions can prevent fertilization of the ovum or lead to an ectopic pregnancy. Complete tubal occlusion prevents fertilizing sperm from reaching the ovum, and the woman will be sterile without the use of advanced techniques such as in vitro fertilization. Partial obstruction may result in a tubal ectopic pregnancy because sperm can reach the ovum to fertilize it but the embryo cannot reach the uterine cavity to implant.

Abnormalities of the Cervix

Estrogen levels from the ovary peak twice during the menstrual cycle, once before ovulation and again about 1 week after ovulation. The first peak occurs about 2 days before ovulation and causes the woman's cervix to dilate slightly and produce a clear, thin, slippery mucus that is similar to egg white in consistency. This mucus facilitates passage of sperm into the uterus and capacitation to prepare one sperm for fertilization. Low estrogen levels prevent development of this mucus and are usually associated with anovulation.

Polyps or scarring from past surgical procedures such as cauterization or conization may obstruct the woman's cervix. Abnormal cervical mucus caused by estrogen deficiency, surgical destruction of the mucus-secreting glands, and cervical damage secondary to infection or other factors prevent normal capacitation and movement of the sperm into the uterus and fallopian tubes for fertilization.

Check Your Reading

5. What factors can result in abnormal ovulation?
6. Why does a woman with ovulation problems often have abnormal menstrual periods?
7. What are some causes of fallopian tube obstruction?
8. How do abnormalities of cervical mucus contribute to infertility?

Repeated Pregnancy Loss

Couples who repeatedly lose pregnancies have the same result as those unable to conceive: no living child. Repeated losses may result from abnormalities in the fetus or placenta or from maternal factors.

Abnormalities of the Fetal Chromosomes

Errors in the fetal chromosomes may result in spontaneous abortion, usually in the first trimester. Chromosome abnormalities often severely disrupt development, and the embryo or fetus cannot survive to live birth.

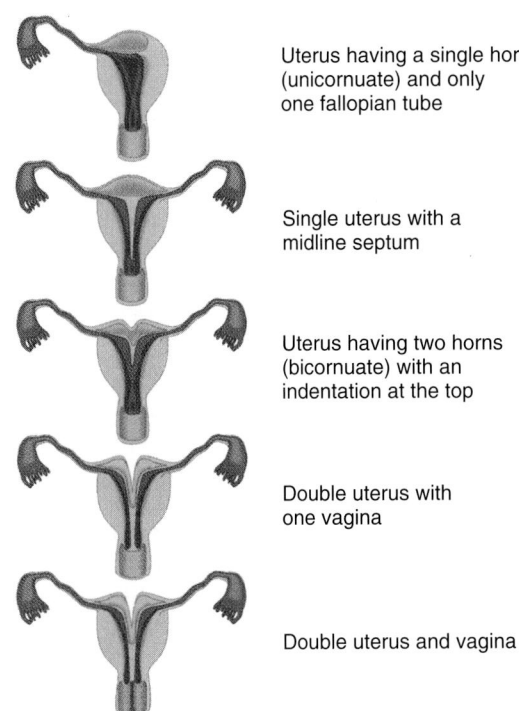

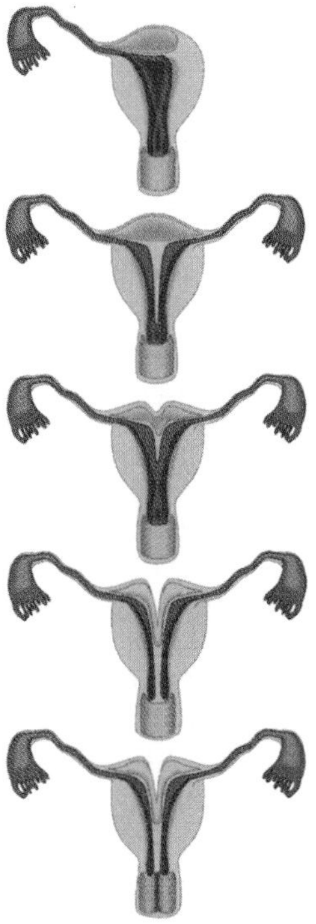

FIGURE 32-3 Types of uterine malformations that may cause infertility or repeated pregnancy loss.

Most chromosome abnormalities are sporadic, occurring randomly. Others occur because one parent has a balanced chromosome translocation that is passed on to the offspring. The parent with the balanced translocation has a normal total amount of chromosome material, but the chromosome material is rearranged. When the chromosomes are divided during gametogenesis, the resulting sperm or ovum may receive too much or too little chromosome material, or it may receive a balanced translocation like the parent. The sperm or ovum also may receive a normal chromosome complement with no translocation.

Abnormalities of the Cervix or Uterus

Stenosis or congenital malformations of the cervix or uterine cavity may cause repeated loss of a normal embryo or fetus (Figure 32-3). These malformations may prevent normal implantation of the fertilized ovum or normal prenatal growth of the placenta or fetus.

Women who were exposed prenatally to diethylstilbestrol (DES) are more likely to have uterine malformations or an incompetent cervix. Cervical or uterine abnormalities also may occur after surgery or trauma from a previous birth. Painless and premature cervical dilation, often early in the second trimester, is characteristic in the woman with an incompetent cervix. Uterine malformations occur in many forms and may result in early spontaneous abortion or preterm labor.

Uterine myomas (benign tumors of the uterine muscle) and adhesions inside the uterine cavity may cause repeated fetal losses. These problems can alter the blood supply to the developing fetus or cause uterine irritability that results in preterm labor and birth.

Endocrine Abnormalities

Inadequate progesterone secretion by the corpus luteum (luteal phase defect) prevents normal implantation and establishment of the placenta. The embryo may not implant, or it may implant poorly. In other cases, the corpus luteum may develop and function properly but the woman's endometrium may not respond to its progesterone secretion.

Hypothyroidism and hyperthyroidism may be associated with the inability to conceive and with recurrent pregnancy loss. Poorly controlled diabetes can result in repeated pregnancy loss and many other complications of pregnancy because of its effects on maternal blood glucose levels and the vascular system (see Chapter 26).

Immunologic Factors

Immunologic factors are implicated in some cases of recurrent pregnancy loss, although not all are established conclusively. The embryo has antigens different from those of the mother and ordinarily would be rejected like any other foreign tissue. However, the mother's body normally blocks this rejection response and tolerates the developing baby. Some women's bodies respond inappropriately to the embryo, rejecting it as any other foreign tissue. These women often have recurrent spontaneous abortions.

Women with autoimmune disease such as lupus erythematosus are more likely to experience fetal loss. Pregnancy loss in these women appears related to thrombosis or other damage in placental blood vessels. Women with lupus often have other complications during pregnancy, such as exacerbation of their symptoms, fetal heart block, and fetal death.

Environmental Agents

Some environmental agents have a well-established relationship to impairment of fertility and pregnancy loss. Others are believed to be damaging but do not show a conclusive link to pregnancy loss. In addition, the amount of exposure (dose) relates to the pregnancy outcome in most cases. For example, radiation exposure in the form of a chest radiograph is unlikely to have an adverse effect on pregnancy, whereas the larger doses used for cancer therapy might be toxic.

Examples of established toxins are ionizing radiation, alcohol, and isotretinoin (Accutane). Suspected toxins are numerous; for example, cigarette smoke, anesthetic gas, chemicals such as organic solvents or pesticides, and lead and mercury in occupational settings. These agents may be directly toxic to the embryo or fetus, causing its death, or they may interfere with the normal placental function necessary to sustain the pregnancy.

Infections

Infections of the reproductive tract are associated with poor pregnancy outcomes in general, and they also may be related to early pregnancy losses. These infections often are asymptomatic, making their link to pregnancy loss difficult to establish. Chapter 26 provides greater details about significant infections affecting pregnancy.

Check Your Reading

9. How can anatomic abnormalities of a woman's uterus or cervix cause her to lose a normal pregnancy?
10. What endocrine factors can cause repeated pregnancy loss?
11. What immunologic factors may cause loss of a normal fetus?

EVALUATION OF INFERTILITY

When a couple seeks help to conceive, both partners are evaluated in a systematic, timely, and cost-effective manner. Some tests such as semen evaluation must be repeated sequentially for an accurate picture. Infertility specialists use the history, physical examinations, and diagnostic testing to identify the best course of treatment. The treatment proposed will consider their ages, especially the woman's, and the results of their histories, physical examinations, and diagnostic testing. Therapy may require a series of steps rather than a single treatment.

The prolonged evaluation and treatment process is frustrating to many couples, especially older ones who are anxious for a child before the end of the woman's reproductive years. Another frustration for couples undergoing an infertility workup is that some diagnostic tests are investigational and their usefulness and normal values are not well established. Other tests are commonly used, but well-accepted, normal values have not always been established.

Numerous professionals may be involved in evaluation and care of infertile couples: nurses, physicians specializing in reproductive medicine, gynecologists, urologists, microsurgeons, embryologists, and ultrasonographers. In addition, general and specialized laboratory facilities may provide diagnostic services. Nurses working in infertility clinics often coordinate communication among the many providers and help the couple negotiate the maze of evaluation and treatment.

History and Physical Examination

A thorough history and physical examination of each partner can help identify the appropriate diagnostic tests and therapy.

History

The partners' general health history is reviewed to determine problems that affect their general health and

INFERTILE COUPLES WANT TO KNOW *What Is Infertility Treatment Like?*

General Information

- Both members of the couple are evaluated.
- Usually, simpler evaluations and therapies are done before more complex ones are undertaken.
- A complete medical and reproductive history and physical examination are taken for each partner.
- The ages of the partners, particularly the woman's, are considered. Evaluations and therapy may be instituted more quickly if the woman is in her mid-30s or older.
- Costs for some tests and therapy may be partially covered by insurance. Check to see what your insurance covers.
- Difficult decisions may be required at different times during evaluation and treatment; for example, whether to proceed to more complex and expensive tests and therapies, whether to take a break from treatment, or whether to abandon treatment altogether. Evaluating the likelihood of success is sometimes difficult when making a decision about whether to proceed with or abandon treatment.
- Infertility treatment often is stressful, can occupy many hours per week, and requires a substantial commitment to self-care.
- Infertility remains unexplained in about 20% of couples.

Men

- Semen analysis is usually the first test. Several semen specimens are obtained over a period of several weeks to obtain the best evaluation.
- Depending on your medical and reproductive history, physical examination, and semen analysis, other diagnostic tests may be done (hormone assay, an ultrasonogram of your reproductive organs, a biopsy of your testicles, and tests of sperm function).
- Corrective measures may include medications, surgery, and methods to reduce the scrotal temperature.

Women

- The first evaluation is usually to determine whether you are ovulating each month. You may be taught to take your basal body temperature each morning and assess your cervical mucus as the first step. These assessments are often done at the same time as other tests.
- Other evaluations may include an ultrasound examination, a hysteroscopy or laparoscopy, and a hysterosalpingogram (x-ray of your uterus and tubes). A postcoital test to determine how your partner's sperm react in your body is sometimes done.
- For some tests and therapies, an operative procedure is required (hysteroscopy, laparoscopy, laser surgery, or microsurgery) on an outpatient or inpatient basis.
- Typically, infertility evaluations and treatments require more of the woman in terms of time, energy, physical discomfort, and risk, compared with the man. Corrective measures depend on the problem that is identified; for example, medications, surgery, and advanced reproductive techniques such as in vitro fertilization.

fertility. A reproductive history also is taken, including the following:

- The woman's menstrual pattern, including age at onset, length of cycle, and characteristics of menstrual periods
- Any pregnancies, complications, and their outcomes
- Contraception methods, past and present
- Previous fertility of the man or woman with other partners
- Pattern of intercourse in relation to the woman's menstrual cycles
- Length of time the couple has had intercourse without using contraception
- Home tests the couple has used, such as basal body temperature or over-the-counter ovulation predictor kits
- Past surgeries, pelvic inflammatory disease, sexually transmitted disease, abnormal Pap tests and treatment

The past medical history, including childhood illnesses and surgery, and a history of exposure to toxins may give clues about the cause of infertility. The couple's past and present occupations may identify toxin exposure, stresses, or other adverse influences on reproduction. Investigation of their usual frequency and timing of intercourse may identify the need for a change to promote conception. Identifying a family history of birth defects, mental retardation, or problems with reproduction may provide a clue about chromosome abnormalities or other inherited problems that affect reproduction.

Physical Examination

Couples who seek help for infertility are usually healthy. However, a thorough physical examination of each partner may identify endocrine disturbances, cranial tumors, or undiagnosed chronic disease. Examination of the reproductive organs may reveal structural defects, infection, cysts, or other abnormalities. Chromosomal analysis may be performed for couples experiencing repeated pregnancy loss that is not explained by other factors.

Diagnostic Tests

Each couple's evaluation is individualized, but testing generally proceeds from the tests that are simple, least invasive, and less expensive to the more complex and expensive diagnostics expected to pinpoint the problem based on their history and physical examinations. Simple evaluations are done simultaneously, but more complex tests are delayed until their need is established. Two methods of identifying ovulation—basal body temperature and assessment of cervical mucus—can be used as contraceptive measures in addition to their use in infertility care (Procedure 32-1). Table 32-1 describes diagnostic tests that may be offered to an infertile couple and the nursing care associated with each.

Text continued on p. 906

PROCEDURE 32-1

Teaching Women about Fertility Awareness

Purpose: To identify whether ovulation occurs and the probable time of ovulation. These techniques can be used in infertility care or as a contraceptive method. When used as a contraceptive method, fertility awareness has a failure rate of about 25% in typical use (Planned Parenthood, 1999).

Basal Body Temperature

The basal body temperature (BBT) is designed to detect the slight elevation in temperature that accompanies increased progesterone secretion in response to the luteinizing hormone (LH) surge and ovulation.

1. Teach the woman the relationship between her BBT and ovulation:
   a. Explain that the BBT is the lowest, or resting, temperature of the body.
   b. During the first half of the woman's menstrual cycle, her temperature is lower than during the second half.
   c. The basal temperature often drops slightly just before ovulation. Not all women experience this preovulatory fall in basal temperature.
   d. Progesterone is secreted during the second half of the cycle, rising just after ovulation. The BBT rises after the slight drop near ovulation and remains higher during the second half of the cycle.
   e. The BBT remains high if conception occurs and falls about 2 to 4 days before menstruation if conception does not occur.

   This method of fertility awareness requires careful assessment and record keeping by the woman. She is more likely to have an accurate record if she understands the relationship between her basal temperature and ovulation.
2. Explain the occurrences that can interfere with the accuracy of her BBT; for example, illness, restless or inadequate sleep (fewer than 6 hours), waking later than usual, traveling across time zones (jet lag), alcohol intake the evening before, sleeping under an electric blanket or on a heated water bed, or any activity before taking the temperature. *Temperature changes are very slight at ovulation. These factors can cause the temperature to rise even if ovulation has not occurred.*
3. Show the woman a glass fever thermometer and a glass basal thermometer. Explain that the range of temperatures on the glass basal thermometer is smaller (96° to 100° F) and each degree is divided into tenths of a degree. Explain how to read the marks on the thermometer. Electronic basal thermometers digitally display the temperature in tenths of a degree. These require less time for accurate assessment than glass ones. The woman should read the instructions that come with her specific thermometer. Both types come with charts for recording the basal temperatures each day. The kits cost between $5 and $12, depending on the model chosen. *Allows the woman to see the differences between a fever thermometer, which may be familiar to her, and a basal thermometer. The temperature rise is very slight (about 0.4° to 0.8° F higher than during the first half of the cycle). A special glass thermometer is needed to detect the change more accurately, although electronic thermometers always register temperature in tenths of a degree. Glass thermometer kits are less expensive*

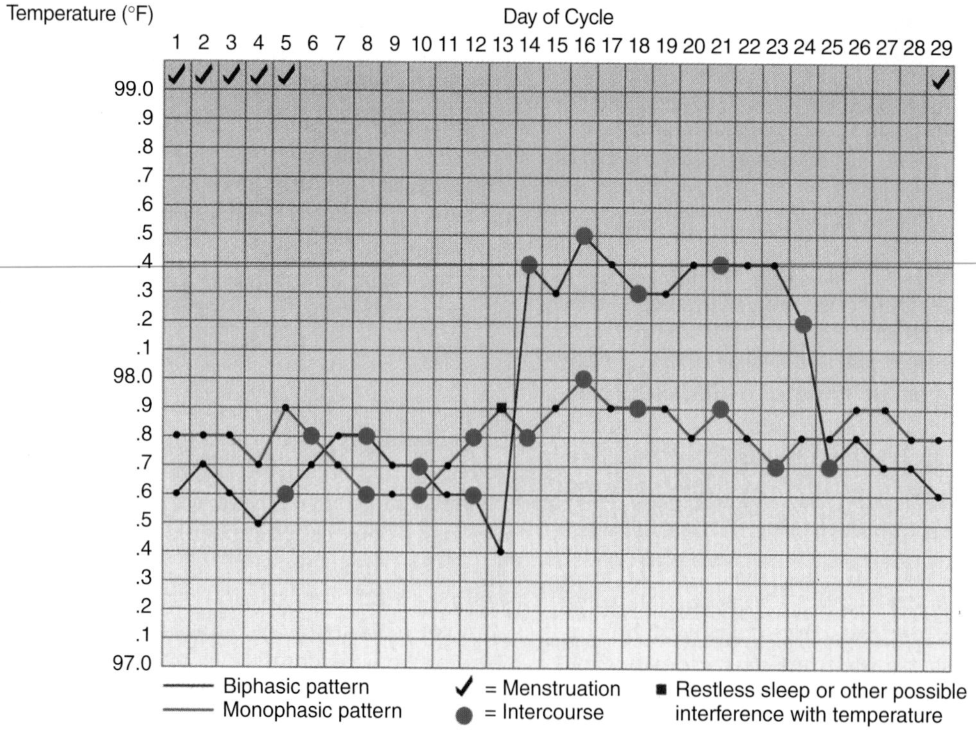

than digital thermometer kits. Some women may not know how to read a glass thermometer and should be taught if they will not be using the digital one. Reading and following instructions specific for the thermometer increases the accuracy of the assessment.

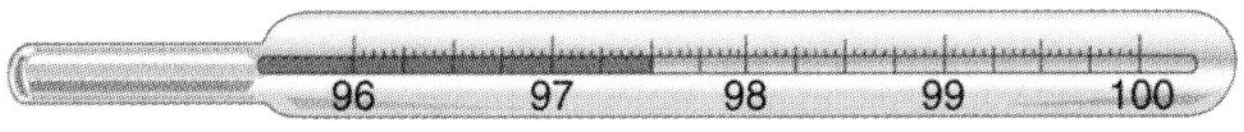

4. Basal temperatures with glass thermometers can be taken orally, rectally, or vaginally. The woman should use the same site for all readings. *Body temperatures vary from one site to another. The basal temperature identifies very small fluctuations, and varying sites may show changes unrelated to ovulation.*
5. Show the woman how to mark the chart for her BBT and the symbols for marking relevant events, such as menstrual periods, intercourse, illness, or other occurrences, which may alter her BBT. *Allows a consistent, more accurate interpretation of temperature fluctuations.*

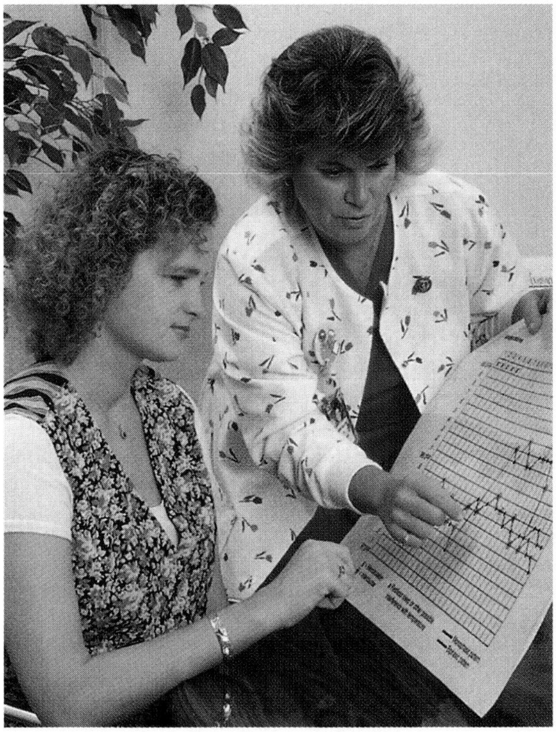

6. Teach the woman how to take her basal temperature:
   a. Shake down a glass thermometer the night before.
   b. As soon as she awakens but before any activity, the basal thermometer should be placed under her tongue until the electronic thermometer beeps. A glass thermometer requires up to 10 minutes for an accurate reading if the oral site is used. The thermometer should remain still while it is registering the temperature.
   c. Record the reading on the chart provided.

   Any activity before taking the basal temperature, including shaking the thermometer down, can alter the reading enough to cause inaccurate interpretation.
7. Encourage the woman to demonstrate taking her temperature and recording the result. Ask her to list events other than ovulation that can alter the BBT. *Verifies that she understands what has been taught and allows correction of misunderstandings.*
8. As a method to avoid pregnancy: Explain that for the greatest effectiveness, a woman should avoid intercourse from the onset of the menstrual period through the second day of elevated temperature. *The most conservative approach requires a long period of abstinence while a viable ovum could be present because the BBT primarily identifies that ovulation has already occurred. Not all women have a temperature drop at the time of ovulation, and the rise in BBT occurs after ovulation. Also, most sperm die within 24 hours, but some may live much longer. To reduce the time of abstinence, couples using fertility awareness as a method of contraception usually combine methods, such as BBT and the cervical mucus assessment.*
9. As used in infertility therapy: Emphasize that the BBT primarily identifies that ovulation has already occurred and whether progesterone is being secreted to prepare her endometrium during the second half of her menstrual cycle. The BBT is less effective for timing intercourse to coincide with ovulation because of the short life span (about 1 to 3 days) of the ovum after ovulation. *The woman receiving infertility therapy should understand the limitations of the BBT in terms of enhancing conception but know that it is useful to identify whether ovulation is occurring.*

Cervical Mucus Assessment

The cervical mucus normally changes just before ovulation to facilitate survival of the sperm and promote their passage into the woman's uterus.

1. Teach the woman how her cervical mucus changes throughout the menstrual cycle. Spinnbarkheit describes how much the mucus can be stretched between her fingers or between a microscope slide and coverslip. Before and after ovulation, the cervical mucus is scant, thick, sticky, and opaque. It stretches less than 6 cm (2.4 inches). Just before and for 2 to 3 days after ovulation, the cervical mucus is thin, slippery, and clear and is similar to raw egg white. It stretches 6 cm or more. When this ovulatory mucus is present, the woman probably has ovulated and could become pregnant. *As with the BBT, this method requires careful assessment and record keeping by the woman. She is more likely to perform the assessment and record changes in her cervical mucus accurately if she understands how the changes relate to fertility.*

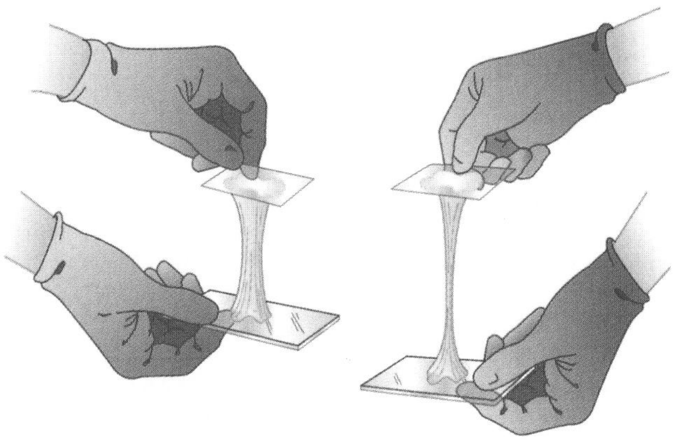

2. Explain the factors that can interfere with the accuracy of her assessment. The mucus may be thicker if she takes antihistamines or clomiphene citrate (Clomid, Serophene). Vaginal infections, contraceptive foams or jellies, sexual arousal, and semen can make the mucus thinner even if ovulation has not occurred. Tell her to record these factors.

Continued

PROCEDURE 32-1

Teaching Women about Fertility Awareness—cont'd

3. Demonstrate how to stretch mucus between the thumb and forefinger using raw egg white. Have the woman return demonstrate the process. *Provides visual and tactile experiences to enhance learning. Return demonstration allows the nurse to determine whether the woman has misunderstood the teaching.*
4. Teach the woman to wash her hands before and after assessing her mucus. *Reduces the chance of introducing infection into the reproductive tract and of transferring infectious organisms from the vagina to other areas.*
5. Teach the woman to obtain a small mucus sample several times a day from just inside her vagina and to note the following:
   a. The general sensation of wetness (around ovulation) or dryness (not near ovulation) on her labia.
   b. The appearance and consistency of the mucus: thick, sticky, and whitish or thin, slippery, and clear or watery.
   c. The distance the mucus will stretch between her fingers, usually at least 6 cm at the time of ovulation.
   Allows the woman to identify cyclic changes in her mucus over the entire duration of her menstrual cycle.
6. Have the woman record the day's typical mucus characteristics (often combined with the BBT recording). *Provides a means of evaluating signs and symptoms associated with ovulation during the entire cycle.*
7. As a method of contraception, the woman should avoid intercourse from the time the thin, stretchy ovulatory mucus appears until 48 to 72 hours after the mucus returns to its preovulatory characteristics. *Reduces the chance that sperm are available for fertilization while the ovum is viable.*
8. As a method to enhance conception, the couple should have intercourse every 2 days during the period of ovulatory mucus (approximately days 12 to 16 if the woman has a 28-day cycle). *Makes sperm available to fertilize the ovum while it is viable.*

Table 32-1
SELECTED DIAGNOSTIC TESTS IN INFERTILITY

Test/Purpose	Nursing Implications
Male	
SEMEN ANALYSIS	
Evaluates structure and function of sperm and composition of seminal fluid. Analysis may be done by manual and/or computer-assisted means. Semen volume: 2.0 to 6.0 ml pH: 7.2 to 7.8 Sperm concentration: >20 million/mL Motility: >50% with forward progression; ≥25% with rapid progression Normal forms: >30% Viability: 50% or more live Liquefaction: within 10 to 30 min Leukocytes (white blood cells): Fewer than 1 million/mL Fructose: 150 to 600 mg/dl	Explain purpose of semen analysis: three or more specimens are usually collected over several weeks' time for more accurate analysis. Explain to the man that he should collect the specimen by masturbation after at least a 2-day abstinence, but no more than 7 days. Semen may be collected in a condom during intercourse if masturbation is unacceptable. The man should note the time the specimen was obtained so the laboratory can evaluate liquefaction of the semen. The specimen should be transported near the body to maintain warmth and should arrive in the laboratory within 1 hr if not obtained at the lab.
ENDOCRINE TESTS	
Evaluate function of hypothalamus, pituitary gland, and the response of the testicles if an endocrine cause for the infertility is suspected. Assays are made to determine levels of hormones such as testosterone, luteinizing hormone (LH), and follicle-stimulating hormone (FSH). Additional tests may be made on the basis of history, physical findings, or diagnostic studies, but endocrine disorders are not a frequent cause for male factor infertility.	Teach the man about the relationship between hypothalamic and pituitary endocrine secretions and sperm formation: LH stimulates testosterone production by Leydig cells of the testes (needed for normal sperm production and development of secondary sex characteristics); FSH stimulates Sertoli cells of the testes to produce sperm.
ULTRASONOGRAPHY	
Evaluates structure of prostate gland, seminal vesicles, and ejaculatory ducts by use of a transrectal probe.	Teach the man that ultrasonography uses sound waves to evaluate these structures. No radiation is involved.
TESTICULAR BIOPSY	
An invasive test for obtaining a sample of testicular tissue. Identifies pathology and obstructions.	Explain the purpose of the test; a local anesthetic is used, and little discomfort should occur.

Table 32-1

SELECTED DIAGNOSTIC TESTS IN INFERTILITY—cont'd

Test/Purpose	Nursing Implications
Male—cont'd	
SPERM PENETRATION ASSAY	
Evaluates fertilizing ability of sperm; assesses ability of sperm to undergo changes that allow penetration of a hamster ovum from which the zona pellucida has been removed.	Explain the purpose of the test. Abnormal penetration does not necessarily mean that the sperm cannot fertilize a human ovum.
HEMIZONA ASSAY	
Measures ability of sperm to bind to the zona pellucida and penetrate the ovum.	Explain that the purpose of the test is to evaluate the ability of the sperm to fertilize an ovum. General usefulness of test is uncertain.
Female	
OVULATION PREDICTION	
Uses any of several methods to identify the surge of LH, which precedes ovulation by 24 to 36 hr. Enables the timing of intercourse to coincide with ovulation and identifies the absence of ovulation. Other tests that can identify ovulation are listed in this table: ultrasonography, endometrial biopsy.	Explain the purpose of the tests (commercial ovulation predictor kits, serum progesterone levels, basal body temperature, and cervical mucus assessment). Teach the woman to follow the instructions on the commercial products. Teach her how to do the basal body temperature and cervical mucus assessment (see Procedure 32-1).
ULTRASONOGRAPHY	
Evaluates structure of pelvic organs. Identifies number and maturation of ovarian follicles to determine best time for intrauterine insemination or ova retrieval and also to reduce the risk for high multifetal gestations. Identifies release of ova at ovulation. Evaluates for presence of ectopic or multifetal pregnancy or other abnormalities.	Teach the woman that ultrasonography uses sound waves to evaluate these structures; no radiation is involved. Ultrasonography may be performed transvaginally, with a covered probe inserted into the vagina, or transabdominally. Explain preparations needed for specific evaluations.
POSTCOITAL TEST	
Evaluates characteristics of cervical mucus and sperm function within it shortly before ovulation. Ovulation predictor kit or ultrasonography ensures proper timing for test. Used only if test results are expected to influence treatment because interpretation of results is subjective.	Explain that the test is performed 4 to 12 hr after intercourse and is similar to other pelvic examinations. The woman may have to rearrange her personal or work commitments each time this test is done.
ENDOCRINE TESTS	
Evaluates functions of hypothalamus, pituitary gland, and ovary. Assays are made to determine LH, FSH, estrogen, and progesterone levels. Other hormone evaluations that influence reproduction, such as thyroid or adrenal hormones, also are done if indicated.	Explain the purpose of each test: FSH and LH stimulate ovulation; estrogen and progesterone prepare endometrium for implantation of a fertilized ovum. Explain the importance of timing within the cycle to provide best information.
HYSTEROSALPINGOGRAPHY (HSG)	
X-ray that uses contrast medium to evaluate the structure and patency of the uterus and fallopian tubes.	The test is performed after the menstrual period during the first half of the cycle to avoid flushing menstrual debris through the tubes into the pelvic cavity and disrupting a pregnancy that might be in place. Explain the purpose of the test. Contrast medium is injected through the cervix, and x-ray films are made at the same time. A nonsteroidal anti-inflammatory drug (NSAID) taken before the test can reduce uterine cramping.
ENDOMETRIAL BIOPSY	
An invasive test for obtaining a small sample of endometrial tissue. Determines whether endometrium is responding properly to estrogen and progesterone stimulation from ovary.	Explain the purpose of the test. The test is done 2 to 3 days before the woman expects her menstrual period. Some cramping may occur that should be relieved with mild analgesics such as ibuprofen.
HYSTEROSCOPY AND LAPAROSCOPY	
Examines uterine interior and/or pelvic organs with a flexible endoscope. General anesthesia or conscious sedation is needed. Identifies congenital or acquired abnormalities (malformations, polyps, endometrial adhesions). Some corrective procedures can be done via the endoscope.	Explain the purpose of the test and any procedures that will be done at the same time. The woman takes nothing by mouth and should urinate before the procedure. Carbon dioxide gas, used to separate pelvic organs for better visualization, may cause temporary shoulder pain.

Therapies to Facilitate Pregnancy

Evaluation of the couple identifies whether therapy might improve their chances to conceive and complete a pregnancy. A variety of procedures may be used, depending on the couple's initial and ongoing evaluations and their personal choices. Some therapy is simple, such as timing intercourse to better coincide with ovulation. Other procedures may involve considerable expense, discomfort, or unpleasant side effects. Many infertile couples need a combination of treatments to improve their chances of conception.

Identification of appropriate infertility therapy is not always straightforward. Many factors must be considered, including the couple's history, medical evaluations, financial resources, ages and other time constraints, and religious and cultural values. Simple treatments are indicated before more complex ones, but the needs of each couple are considered individually. More aggressive diagnostic testing and therapy may be appropriate if the woman is approaching the end of her reproductive years.

Statistical success rates for various procedures often are difficult for couples to evaluate and vary widely among facilities. Factors that affect a center's success rate for a procedure are numerous. For example, a referral center that is willing to help couples with long-standing infertility may have lower success rates than one that accepts only couples with less severe problems.

Medications

Hormones and other medications may be given to either the man or the woman. A medication may be given to improve semen quality, induce ovulation, prepare the uterine endometrium, or support the pregnancy once it is established. Medications may be given to correct infections. Sildenafil (Viagra) may help men for whom erectile dysfunction is the primary problem. Table 32-2 summarizes many of the medications used in infertility therapy.

Ovulation Induction

Medications to induce ovulation may be prescribed for the woman who does not ovulate or who ovulates erratically. Medications also may be given to induce multiple ova if a woman plans to have advanced reproductive techniques such as gamete intrafallopian transfer (GIFT). Clomiphene citrate is a drug often used to stimulate ovulation in specific types of ovulatory dysfunction.

Ovulation induction increases the risk of multiple births because several ova may be released and fertil-

Table 32-2
MEDICATIONS USED IN INFERTILITY THERAPY

Drug	Primary Use
Bromocriptine (Parlodel)	Corrects excess prolactin secretion by anterior pituitary, improving GnRH secretion, in turn normalizing follicle-stimulating hormone (FSH) and luteinizing hormone (LH) release. These drug actions increase ovulation and support early pregnancy by stimulating progesterone secretion by the corpus luteum.
Clomiphene citrate (Clomid)	Induction of ovulation in women who have specific types of ovulatory dysfunction. The drug increases frequency of GnRH secretion from the hypothalamus, thus increasing FSH and LH release and maturing the ovarian follicle and release of the ovum.
Chorionic gonadotropin, human (hCG; Pregnyl)	Used in conjunction with menopausal gonadotropins to stimulate ovulation in the female or sperm formation in the male. Stimulates progesterone production by corpus luteum.
FSH (Metrodin)	Stimulation of ovarian follicle growth; ovulation induction
FSH, Recombinant DNA origin gonadotropin (Follitropin [Gonal-F])	Stimulation of ovarian follicle growth; ovulation induction
Gonadotropin-releasing hormone (GnRH; Lutrepulse)	Stimulates release of FSH and LH from the pituitary gland in men and women who have deficient GnRH secretion by their hypothalamus. FSH and LH, in turn, stimulate ovulation in the female and stimulate testosterone production and spermatogenesis in the male. The drug is given with an automated pump at 75- to 90-minute intervals (Daly, 2000).
Leuprolide (Lupron)	Reduces endometriosis; adjunct to drug given to stimulate ovulation
Mentropins (Humegon, Pergonal, Repronex)	Induction of ovulation; each ampule contains equal amounts of FSH and LH
Nafarelin (Synarel)	Reduces endometriosis
Progesterone (suspension; Crinone gel)	Prepares uterine lining and promotes implantation of embryo
Sildenafil (Viagra)	Increases blood flow to the penis, improving erectile function.
Urofollitropin (uFSH [Fertinex])	Induction of ovulation; contains primarily FSH and a small amount of LH

ized. Another serious complication is *ovarian hyperstimulation syndrome,* in which marked ovarian enlargement occurs, with exudation of fluid into the woman's peritoneal and pleural cavities. Careful adjustment of medication dose and serial ultrasound examinations prevent most cases of high multifetal pregnancy (triplets or more) and ovarian hyperstimulation syndrome. Twins remain a risk, however.

Surgical Procedures

In some men, correction of a varicocele improves sperm quality and quantity. Endoscopic procedures may be used to correct obstructions with minimal invasiveness in either the man or the woman. The woman may need a laparotomy to release pelvic adhesions and obstructions caused by endometriosis, infection, or previous surgical procedures if these cannot be corrected with laparoscopic surgery. Medications also may reduce endometriosis. Laser surgical techniques may be used to reduce adhesions because they are minimally invasive, precise, and less likely to cause formation of new adhesions. Microsurgical techniques are needed for surgical correction of obstructions in the fallopian tubes or tubal structures in the male genital tract because these structures are very narrow.

Transcervical balloon tuboplasty may be used to open a woman's fallopian tubes without more invasive procedures such as laparoscopy or laparotomy. A thin catheter is threaded through the uterus into the fallopian tube, and the balloon is inflated to clear the blockage.

Therapeutic Insemination

Therapeutic insemination may use either the partner's semen or that of a donor to overcome a low sperm count. Donor insemination also may be used if the woman's partner carries a genetic defect or if a woman wants a biologic child without having a relationship with a male partner. Intrauterine insemination (IUI) is a variation of therapeutic insemination that allows the sperm to be placed directly into the uterus, thus bypassing the cervical mucus and reducing some immunologic incompatibilities.

The man collects the semen by masturbation after a 3- to 5-day abstinence. Sperm that are to be placed directly in the uterus or fallopian tube are prepared by washing and spinning the semen in a centrifuge to remove seminal fluid. A technique called *sperm swim-up* may be used to concentrate sperm having the best motility. Although the total number of sperm is lower, the remaining ones (those with normal structure and highest motility) are more likely to fertilize the ovum and result in a normal embryo.

If retrograde ejaculation is the man's problem, he takes sodium bicarbonate 2 hours before obtaining the semen to render the urine alkaline. After collecting the semen in a sterile container with a special medium, the sperm are quickly separated from the urine. The sperm are then further prepared for intrauterine insemination.

Men who donate semen for intrauterine insemination are screened to reduce the risk of transmitting diseases or genetic defects. They are questioned about their per-

DRUG GUIDE: CLOMIPHENE CITRATE (CLOMID, SEROPHENE)

Classification: Ovarian stimulant.

Action: Stimulates pituitary gland to increase secretion of luteinizing hormone (LH) and follicle-stimulating hormone (FSH). LH and FSH stimulate maturation of the ovarian follicle, ovulation, and development of the corpus luteum.

Indications: Female infertility in which estrogen levels are normal.

Dosage and Route

Female sterility: *First course:* 25 to 50 mg p.o. daily for 5 days. *Second course:* Same dose if ovulation occurred with first course. If ovulation did not occur, increase dose to 100 mg daily for 5 days. Some women require up to 250 mg daily. An increased dose is not beneficial if ovulation is triggered.

Absorption: Readily absorbed from the gastrointestinal tract. Time to peak effect is 4 to 10 days after last day of treatment.

Excretion: Excreted in the feces.

Contraindication and Precautions: Pregnancy, liver disease, abnormal bleeding of undetermined origin, ovarian cysts, neoplastic disease. Therapy is ineffective in women with ovarian or pituitary failure.

Adverse Reactions: Ovarian enlargement; symptoms similar to premenstrual syndrome. Ovarian hyperstimulation syndrome. Multiple gestation, if more than one ovum is released. Visual disturbances. Abdominal distention, discomfort, nausea, vomiting. Abnormal uterine bleeding. Breast tenderness. Insomnia, nervousness, headache, depression, fatigue, lightheadedness, dizziness. Hot flashes, increased urination, allergic symptoms, weight gain, reversible alopecia. Dry cervical mucus.

Nursing Considerations: Take the history to determine whether the woman has a history of liver dysfunction or abnormal uterine bleeding. Rule out the possibility of pregnancy. Teach the woman to report abdominal distention, pain in the pelvis or abdomen, and visual disturbances. Teach her to avoid tasks requiring mental alertness or coordination because the drug can cause lightheadedness, dizziness, and visual disturbances. Instruct her to stop taking clomiphene and report to the physician if she suspects she might be pregnant. Teach the woman and her partner that she may notice irritability, mood swings, and other symptoms similar to those in premenstrual syndrome but that these are temporary.

sonal and family health history, including genetic disorders and birth defects. Questions about their social habits and personality can disclose high-risk behaviors and also give recipient parents information about traits their child might have. Physical and laboratory examinations are performed to evaluate the man's general health, determine his blood type and Rh factor, and screen for infections such as sexually transmissible diseases, hepatitis B and C, and human immunodeficiency virus (HIV). Carrier testing for some genetic defects such as sickle cell and Tay-Sachs diseases reduces the risk of passing on these disorders. Donor semen is frozen and held for 6 months before use to reduce the risk of transmitting diseases that may not be apparent at the initial screening.

The American Society for Reproductive Medicine (1997b) publishes *Guidelines for Gamete and Embryo Donation* that specify stringent safeguards for donation of sperm, ova, and embryos. These safeguards reduce but do not eliminate the risk for transmitting infections and genetic disorders. The full text of the guidelines can be viewed at the Society's website at www.asrm.org.

Surrogate Parenting

A surrogate mother may enter the picture if the woman is infertile or cannot carry a fetus to live birth. The surrogate mother may supply her uterus only (gestational surrogate), with the infertile couple supplying the sperm and ovum. Or she may be inseminated with the male partner's sperm and carry the fetus to birth, thus supplying both the genetic component and the gestational component. Surrogacy is different from therapeutic insemination with donor sperm because it is not anonymous. In addition, the woman who carries the child inevitably forms bonds with the fetus during the months of pregnancy.

Money paid to the surrogate mother can raise ethical issues. Could a poor but fertile woman feel compelled to provide her body for a more well-to-do couple? However, not compensating a woman for the real physical and emotional risks of this undertaking can be construed as coercive as well.

Custody of the resulting child has been the issue in several court cases involving surrogate mothers. In the *Baby M* case, a woman who was inseminated with the man's sperm refused to relinquish the baby as stated in the contract between the birth mother and the infertile couple. Ultimately, custody was awarded to the man providing the sperm and his spouse, but visitation rights were granted to the surrogate mother.

Custody issues when the birth mother is a gestational surrogate are clearer than when she also donates her ovum to the child. Courts have more often recognized the genetic parents as the legal parents and upheld the contracts between them and the gestational surrogate. Laws vary among states, however.

Advanced Reproductive Techniques

Advanced reproductive techniques bypass many natural obstacles to conception by placing intact gametes together to allow fertilization. These techniques include in vitro fertilization (IVF), gamete intrafallopian transfer (GIFT), and tubal embryo transfer (TET). Each procedure begins with ovulation induction to permit retrieval of several ova, thus improving the likelihood of a successful pregnancy. Sperm are prepared and concentrated as they are for therapeutic insemination.

Another class of advanced reproductive techniques involves assisting fertilization with microsurgical techniques. These techniques bypass obstacles to fertilization by penetrating the ovum with tiny needles to allow placement of the sperm within the ovum. The sperm also may be obtained by advanced techniques.

In Vitro Fertilization

The technique of IVF involves bypassing blocked or absent fallopian tubes. The physician removes the ova by laparoscope or ultrasound-guided transvaginal retrieval and mixes them with prepared sperm from the woman's partner or a donor. About 2 days later, two to five embryos, depending on the woman's prognosis for a successful pregnancy, are returned to the uterus to increase the likelihood of a successful pregnancy. The woman may receive supplemental progesterone to enhance the receptivity of her endometrium to implantation. Excess embryos may be frozen for future attempts at embryo transfer to the uterus.

IVF success rates vary among infertility centers. Bypassing the obstructions does not necessarily result in pregnancy. Not every ovum is successfully fertilized when this technique is used. Embryos transferred to the woman's uterus may not always implant, which is why several are transferred. However, multiple embryos also may implant.

Gamete Intrafallopian Transfer

For GIFT to take place, the woman must have at least one open fallopian tube. The procedure begins in a manner similar to that of IVF, with retrieval of multiple ova and washed sperm. Ova may be retrieved either laparoscopically or transvaginally with ultrasound guidance.

The retrieved ova are drawn into a catheter that also carries prepared sperm. Sperm and up to two ova per tube are injected into each fallopian tube through a laparoscope, in which fertilization may occur (Figure 32-4). Occasionally, as many as four ova are used. Additional prepared sperm may be injected into the uterus through the cervix to improve the chance of successful fertilization. Progesterone is often given to enhance implantation of any fertilized ova.

Tubal Embryo Transferr

Tubal embryo transfer, also called *zygote intrafallopian transfer (ZIFT),* is a hybrid of IVF and GIFT. The

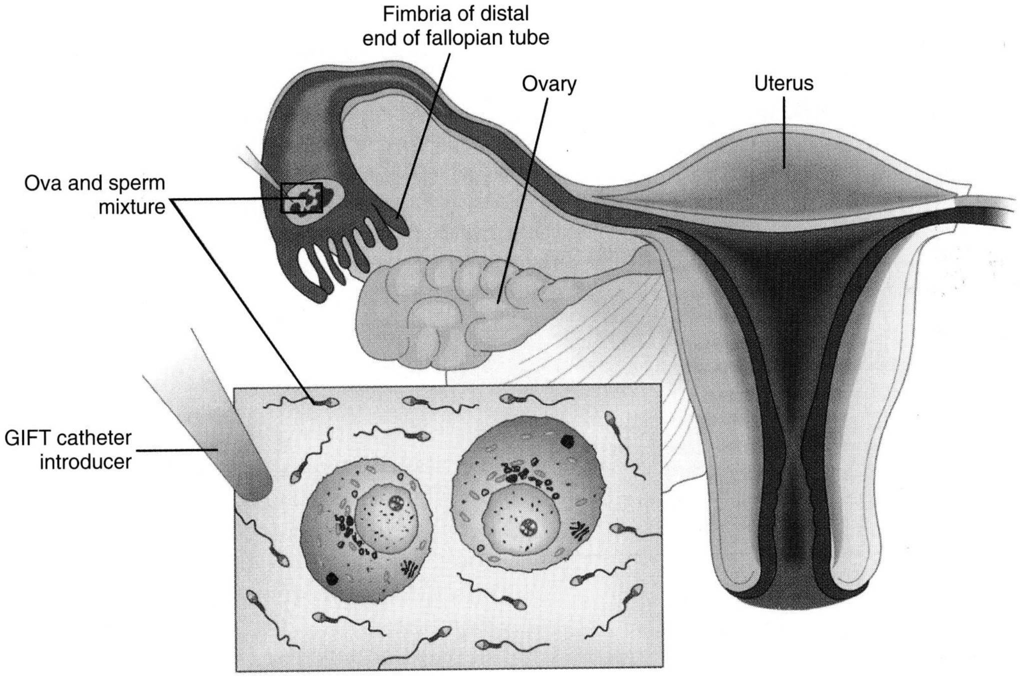

FIGURE 32-4 Gamete intrafallopian transfer (GIFT). Multiple ova and washed sperm are injected into the fallopian tube, where fertilization may occur.

woman's ova are fertilized outside her body, but the resulting fertilized ova are placed in the fallopian tubes and enter the uterus naturally for implantation. The woman must have at least one patent fallopian tube.

Comparison of In Vitro Fertilization, Gamete Intrafallopian Transfer, and Tubal Embryo Transfer

The primary advantage of GIFT and TET over IVF is a higher pregnancy rate. With IVF and TET, evidence of fertilization exists before placement in the uterus or tubes. The disadvantage of these procedures is that the woman may need to have a laparoscopy to retrieve gametes (IVF) or place the gametes (GIFT) or fertilized ova (TET) into the fallopian tube. Either GIFT or TET may result in a tubal pregnancy if the embryo cannot reach the uterine cavity to implant.

These reproductive techniques can result in multifetal pregnancy, sometimes higher than triplets. Pregnancies of more than twins carry a substantially higher risk to both mother and infants because of preterm labor and birth, placental insufficiency, and a high demand on maternal body systems. Selective reduction in the number of fetuses may be done to give the remaining ones a better chance to progress to a live birth. Also, selective reduction of some fetuses may inadvertently cause the loss of all fetuses. Such a procedure is, of course, heavily laden with emotional and ethical overtones.

Microsurgically Assisted Fertilization

Microsurgical techniques are related to IVF but considerably more complex. These techniques now help couples conceive despite severe male factor infertility when standard IVF, GIFT, and TET are unlikely to be successful.

Intracytoplasmic sperm injection (ICSI) is the direct injection of a spermatozoon into the cytoplasm of the ovum and can help men with very low sperm counts have biological children. If the low or absent sperm count is related to an obstruction such as an irreversible vasectomy, microsurgical techniques or aspiration of the sperm from the epididymis may permit retrieval of sperm to perform ICSI. For these techniques, the retrieval of oocytes and placement of the resulting embryo into the uterus are similar to IVF.

Preimplantation Genetic Testing

Preimplantation genetic testing may be offered to couples with higher risks for conceiving an embryo with a diagnosable genetic abnormality. A few cells are withdrawn for analysis before the embryo is implanted. The DNA from the cells is amplified to allow genetic analysis. Because cells are undifferentiated into specialized organ cells at this early stage, their loss is quickly made up. If a genetic defect is identified, the couple has the option of not implanting the embryo.

A recent situation had a different twist on preimplantation genetic testing. A 6-year-old girl had Fanconi anemia, failure of the bone marrow which would shorten her life. Her parents conceived several embryos through advanced reproductive techniques. They selected an embryo for implantation to both avoid the Fanconi anemia and supply umbilical cord blood for a bone marrow graft to their ill child. This situation raised many ethical questions about having a "made-to-order" child.

Check Your Reading

12. What elements are included in the history and physical examination for an infertility workup?
13. What medications may be used to induce ovulation?
14. What screening tests are performed if donor sperm is used for therapeutic insemination or GIFT?
15. What are the differences in technique among IVF, GIFT, and TET?

RESPONSES TO INFERTILITY

The desire for children is strong in many people. Even if they delay childbearing, most couples expect to have one or more children before the end of the woman's reproductive years. Those who chose childlessness earlier may reevaluate their decision when they are older. If a couple does not achieve pregnancy or produce a living child as expected, the man and woman often experience psychological distress and a threat to their self-images. Either or both partners may feel like failures. Their marital and family relationships may be stressed, and they may withdraw from relationships with others that they previously found satisfying. Every couple is unique, and many reactions depend on the importance attached to having biologic children. The following discussion describes the ways infertility can alter the lives of those affected.

Assumption of Fertility

Many couples practice contraception for a number of years before they decide to have a baby. They may want to establish a career and financial security, acquire a comfortable home and lifestyle, or perhaps travel and live freely without the responsibility of a child. They usually assume that they are fertile and must take steps to avoid pregnancy until they are ready.

When they do want a child, they discontinue contraception and assume that pregnancy will occur within a few months at most. They may plan conception so that the baby will be born at a certain time of year (such as not during the hottest weather) or to avoid major holidays.

Either or both partners may experiment with the role of parent as they anticipate pregnancy. They develop a heightened awareness of children and parenting. Being with others who are expecting or already have children is exciting because they plan to join their ranks shortly. They may discuss issues like full-time parenting by one partner, child care, and imminent lifestyle changes. The woman often finds that she enjoys shopping in the maternity and children's departments. They may begin acquiring toys and furnishings a child will need. Both partners may develop a fantasy child or a concept of what their baby will be like.

Growing Awareness of a Problem

As the months pass, the couple gradually becomes concerned about the inability to conceive. If the woman is older, they feel the urgency of the limited time before her reproductive years end. The plan to have a baby at a certain time of year is replaced by the desire for a baby any time—and soon.

The couple begins to feel uneasy with child-related activities. Now they are not so sure when they will be parents. They begin to feel hurt when other family members or friends have babies. Events such as baby showers and christenings become melancholy rather than joyful occasions to them. They bypass toy stores and children's departments because of the uncertainty. Family members and friends who are having children may feel guilty when they are around the couple who cannot conceive.

The potential grandparents may feel that their children are waiting too long to start a family or even that they are selfish. If they are aware the couple is trying to conceive, they become even more worried as the months pass without the longed-for announcement of a pregnancy. They are twice saddened by the lack of a grandchild and the hurt their adult children are enduring.

Seeking Help for Infertility

Eventually, couples must decide whether to seek help to conceive. They may reach this point after only a few menstrual cycles or, at the opposite extreme, may never seek help. Many factors enter into their decision, such as their age (especially the woman's), how long they have been unable to conceive, how much they want a biologic child, how they regard adoption, and how they feel about a life without children.

Identifying the Importance of Having a Baby

Each partner may place a different priority on having a baby. Conflicts may arise when one partner wants help to conceive sooner than the other. In addition, cultural or religious beliefs influence the way each feels about procreation and whether options such as assisted reproductive procedures or adoption are acceptable. The way in which the couple resolves these differences is crucial to the stability of the relationship.

Men and women often differ in their reactions to infertility. Women may want to talk about their feelings and frustrations, but men often internalize their feelings or feel that they must be strong for their partners.

The woman may interpret her partner's stoicism and reluctance to express his feelings as disinterest or lack of concern and care for her.

Sharing Intimate Information

Although the infertility specialist will limit questions to the necessary ones, evaluation and treatment for infertility require that both partners reveal information about their sexual relationship, such as the frequency and timing of intercourse. This is difficult for those who regard this information as intimate. In addition, infertile couples may feel that the evaluation calls their sexual adequacy into question. They may feel defensive if they perceive a threat to their self-image.

Considering Financial Resources

Financial concerns enter into the couple's decision about whether to seek treatment and how far to carry it. Techniques such as basal body temperature assessment and over-the-counter ovulation predictor kits are inexpensive but have limited usefulness in achieving successful pregnancy. Advanced techniques such as IVF are expensive and may have a low likelihood of success. Health insurance may not cover infertility treatment at all or may not cover all procedures because the problem is not always seen as an illness. Treatments that are investigational are usually not covered. Expense and restricted coverage limit treatment choices for many low- or middle-income couples. Those who seek and pursue infertility treatment usually have greater financial resources than those who do not.

Committing to Involvement in Care

Infertility evaluation and treatment require a great commitment from the couple in terms of time, energy, and money. Couples can be involved in this process for several years. They participate on a day-to-day basis as they do home assessments, take medications, and keep detailed records. For infertility diagnosis and therapy to be most effective, couples must consider their ability and desire to be directly involved in the process over a long time.

Reactions during Evaluation and Treatment

Couples undergoing infertility evaluation and treatment have different reactions to the process. Their reactions may change as care progresses.

Influences on Decision Making

If their evaluation shows that a treatment or procedure may enable them to conceive, the couple must then decide whether to proceed. The decision-making process begins early and must be repeated during therapy if pregnancy does not occur. A complex array of factors enters into their decisions about beginning and continuing treatment or whether to end their pursuit of pregnancy. Although discussed separately, these factors interact dynamically as the couple makes each decision. The nurse helps them examine each factor and arrive at a decision that is best for them.

Social, Cultural, and Religious Values. Some medically appropriate options are not acceptable to every couple within their personal social, cultural, and religious framework. Surrogate parenting, IVF, and therapeutic insemination (especially with donor sperm) are not consistent with the personal or religious beliefs of many people. If a procedure offers the partners hope for a child but is incompatible with their beliefs, their choices are two: use the technology despite their beliefs or be willing to accept childlessness. Adoption may be a third alternative for some couples if the desire for a biologic child is not absolute. As in other decisions, couples must work out conflicting personal values about what therapy is acceptable.

Difficulty of Treatment. The couple must consider how difficult, risky, and uncomfortable therapy will be. The level of difficulty involves physical, psychological, geographic, and time factors. Employment constraints also may affect treatment decisions.

Several infertility treatments involve invasive procedures or surgery. The person who undergoes the procedure must be the one who ultimately decides whether to do it. That person alone can decide whether the hope of a child is worth the risks and discomfort of the procedure.

Infertility treatment is stressful. Often partners feel or are willing to tolerate different levels of stress. To reduce the stress, they may abandon treatment completely or take a vacation for a few months from the constant preoccupation with conceiving. Women nearing or in their 40s often do not feel they have the luxury of skipping a treatment cycle.

Some couples encounter geographic difficulties if they must travel a long distance for therapy. Time stresses are substantial. The partners, particularly the woman, feel that achieving pregnancy is their new career. One or both partners may spend many hours every week in pursuit of pregnancy.

Employment constraints may be a barrier to infertility therapy because of the time required for treatment. The impact of time is usually greatest on the woman. Time away from work may burden the employer or coworkers. Stopping work may not be an option because the family needs the money and often needs the insurance coverage that comes with employment.

Probability of Success. Couples often have a biased interpretation of their statistical probability of success, especially when they begin treatment with a new procedure. For example, if a procedure has a 15% likelihood of success with each cycle, they tend to expect that they will be in the successful group rather than in the 85% who do not meet with success. As time goes by, however, they must weigh the likelihood of success of any therapy against financial concerns and their own willingness to accept the discomfort and difficulty associated with it. Again, the woman's age imposes an inescapable factor.

Financial Concerns. Some couples, particularly those with ample resources and a strong desire for a biologic child, pursue expensive treatments and do so longer than others of more limited means, despite a low probability of success. Couples with financial limitations find that they must abandon treatment sooner than they want. Other couples go heavily into debt, adding financial strain to the other stresses of treatment in their quest for a biologic child.

Psychological Reactions

A couple's initial reaction to infertility often is one of shock because the partners are usually healthy and did not expect to have problems conceiving. Their reactions vary according to how easily their infertility is alleviated, their personality and self-image, and the strength of their relationship.

Guilt. A partner having the only identified problem might feel that he or she is depriving the other of children. This feeling may be compounded if the "normal" partner has children from another relationship. It may be difficult for this person to understand that not all factors affecting fertility are known and what seems like the problem of only one partner may actually be a couple problem.

Either partner may feel guilty about past choices that now affect fertility. A woman with adhesions resulting from a sexually transmitted infection may regret her past sexual choices. The man who wanted to delay pregnancy longer than the woman may feel guilty if her age is now reducing her fertility.

Isolation. Infertile couples may withdraw from friends and relatives who have children to insulate themselves from painful reminders of their infertility. Some couples develop supportive relationships with others who also are infertile, which somewhat diminishes their sense of isolation.

Depression. One or both partners may experience depression as their sense of competence and control over their bodies is challenged, especially if therapy is not successful quickly. They often feel as though they are on a roller coaster of hope alternating with despair when the woman has her menstrual period each month. In an attempt to reduce their disappointment, couples with long-term infertility try not to expect too much with each cycle.

The couple may feel envy toward those who conceive easily. They may become judgmental and angry when they see those who seem to "have no business having a baby," such as an adolescent or a poor woman who has several children.

Stress on the Relationship. Because infertility can challenge a person's identity and self-esteem, partners may find less satisfaction in their relationship. They may feel unlovable or unappealing to their mate.

The man may have difficulty performing on demand for semen specimens or postcoital tests, feeling that others will judge his sexual function. The fact that semen samples are best obtained by masturbation is unacceptable to some men. Both partners are stressed when intercourse must be scheduled to coincide with specific evaluations or ovulation. Intercourse can become a chore more than an expression of love. It may come to be associated with failure rather than fulfillment if a child is not forthcoming.

If sperm from an anonymous donor is used for therapeutic insemination or other techniques, the man may feel that his masculinity is further threatened. He does not want to deprive his wife of a child, but he may be ambivalent about use of sperm from a third party. He may have difficulty distinguishing between fatherhood as a biologic achievement and fatherhood as a relationship.

The partners find their relationship strained if they disagree on which treatments are appropriate and how long they should be pursued. One partner may want to keep trying "one more month," and the other may want to abandon treatment. If they are considering adoption, their relationship may be strained if they differ on whether to adopt and what kind of child they are willing to accept.

Check Your Reading

16. What factors do couples consider when they are deciding whether to seek help for their infertility?
17. What factors must couples consider when they reach decision points during infertility evaluation and treatment?
18. What are possible psychological reactions to infertility?

OUTCOMES AFTER INFERTILITY THERAPY

After infertility therapy, three outcomes are possible: 1) the pregnancy may be lost, resulting in mixed emotions of grief and pain; 2) the couple may become parents, either biologically or through adoption; or 3) infertility therapy may be unsuccessful and the couple must decide whether to pursue adoption.

Pregnancy Loss after Infertility Therapy

Couples who suffer pregnancy loss after infertility therapy may interpret the experience with mixed feelings of loss and gain. Couples undergoing infertility evaluation and treatment often are aware of a pregnancy much earlier than fertile couples. They want to hope yet expect to be disappointed again. If a spontaneous abortion occurs, they may grieve profoundly for what they achieved and then lost.

Yet despite their grief about the pregnancy loss, the partners may be encouraged because they have proved that they can achieve a pregnancy. They may feel that if they succeeded once, they can do it again. A spontaneous abortion may give them the courage to continue treatment.

When pregnancy loss has occurred because of an ectopic pregnancy, the woman may lose a fallopian tube (see p. 898). These couples may have an added threat to their fertility because of the uncertainty of getting pregnant again in addition to the possible loss or blockage of one or even both fallopian tubes.

Parenthood after Infertility Therapy

Couples who conceive experience varied emotions. If they have been disappointed before, they may hardly believe the good news. They are thrilled but worry about whether they can complete the pregnancy and take home a baby. Pregnancy after infertility therapy is emotionally tentative for many infertile couples, especially those who have been trying to conceive for a long time or lost a pregnancy. They may distance themselves from the reality of the pregnancy until much later in gestation than normally fertile couples. The woman has learned to sense and report every symptom and may interpret normal changes of pregnancy as a threat.

The previously infertile couple may find little sympathy from those who do not understand their fear of investing in the pregnancy. Others are annoyed because they expect the couple to be overjoyed at a successful and apparently normal pregnancy. Outsiders may feel that the partners are self-centered and cannot decide what they want. Other infertile couples, who have been a source of mutual support, may either withdraw from the couple who achieves a pregnancy or rejoice in their success.

The parents' anxiety may be heightened during labor. They are afraid that something will go wrong at the last moment. Even after the birth of a healthy infant, some parents need time to relax and grasp the fact that their baby is really here.

These new parents often need much support as they gain experience with their child. Infertile couples who eventually have biologic or adopted children may have unrealistic expectations about parenting. After investing so many financial, physical, and emotional resources in having a child, they may be reluctant to express any unhappiness or frustration over the difficulties of childrearing.

Choosing to Adopt

Not every couple who seeks treatment for infertility achieves a "take-home" baby. Some couples discontinue treatment sooner than others, depending on their age and tolerance for the fatigue, stress, and expense. Some couples investigate adoption early in infertility treatment because advanced age may make them ineligible to adopt through many agencies or because a nonbiologic child is acceptable to them.

Couples who consider adoption must confront their personal preferences, limitations, and prejudices. As much as they want a child, many couples are not willing to adopt any child. Most couples prefer to adopt a newborn or an infant of their race. Some prefer an infant but also are willing to adopt an older child, one with special needs, one of a mixed or different race, or a group of siblings. Other couples will not consider adopting these children for a variety of reasons.

Some couples fear adopting a child because the woman might become pregnant. Although pregnancy has been their goal for a long time, they may worry that they would love their adopted child differently from their biologic child. If the couple plans to continue trying for a biologic child, they also must come to grips with this issue.

Couples who decide to adopt face further scrutiny of their personal lives. Agencies investigate their home, financial means (which may have been seriously drained), and fitness as parents. Once again, they may feel that their personal competence is questioned.

The couple who decides on adoption may have emotions similar to those who achieve a pregnancy. They may be slow to invest in the process emotionally because they expect disappointment again. In addition, the adopted child often arrives suddenly and unexpectedly. Although they may have been waiting months for this happy event, they may have little time to adjust to the reality of becoming parents.

Check Your Reading

19. If the partners become parents, either through birth or adoption, how may they react to parenthood?
20. What are the issues couples must face if they consider adoption?
21. What emotions do couples often experience if they lose a pregnancy after infertility treatment?

APPLICATION OF THE NURSING PROCESS: CARE OF THE INFERTILE COUPLE

Nurses may encounter couples facing infertility in many different settings and identify numerous nursing care needs. Regardless of the setting, the nurse often addresses the couple's emotional needs associated with infertility evaluation, treatment, and outcomes of therapy.

Assessment

In many instances, infertile couples previously have had a positive self-image and feelings of competence about themselves. The diagnosis of infertility shakes their positive view. The nurse should be aware that these feelings may be present, regardless of the practice setting in which the couple is encountered.

Determine at what point the couple is in their infertility treatment. Couples who have just discovered that they may have difficulty conceiving may be shocked yet optimistic that therapy will result in a baby. Other couples for whom simple treatments were unsuccessful may face shock again if the more high-tech treatments such as IVF or ICSI are recommended, particularly if these treatments require them to go into debt. Couples with long-standing infertility may have a deeper sense of failure and a pessimistic outlook. Listen for remarks that are negative, expressing guilt or helplessness.

Evaluate the way infertility has affected the partners' relationship with each other. Are there conflicts or differences in values between the two? Observing their body language, such as eye contact, may provide clues about similarities and differences in their commitment to diagnosis and treatment. Ask them how their relationship has changed. Are they more or less satisfied with their marital relationship than they were before they had problems conceiving? How is each member of the couple adjusting to the situation?

Ask about support systems. Couples suffering from infertility often withdraw from old relationships yet do not form new supportive ones. Do others who are significant in the partners' lives know that they are trying to conceive? Are family members and friends nearby, and are they supportive? Ask whether they have encountered assumptions by others that infertility is the "fault" of one partner or the other. Are they subjected to questions that invade their privacy, such as "When are you two going to have a baby of your own?"

Determine how the couple's culture or religion views infertility and the impact of these values on therapy. Are some therapies unacceptable to one or both partners? The partners may have differing views that can cause conflict during treatment, and they will need help to work these out.

Determine how the couple is coping with the stresses of treatment. How much has infertility cost them in terms of time, money, and discomfort? Identify the successes and failures they have experienced. Their age, especially the woman's, adds another unavoidable stressor.

If the woman is pregnant or has given birth recently or the couple has adopted a child recently, observe for high levels of anxiety in either or both parents. Assess them for negative behaviors and comments, such as reluctance to feel joy or a sense that they will "fail" again.

Analysis

A nursing diagnosis commonly encountered is "Situational Low Self-esteem related to loss of control secondary to the couple's infertility diagnosis and treatment."

Planning

Three goals are appropriate for this nursing diagnosis, and they may apply to the man, the woman, or both partners. The person(s) will do the following:

- Express feelings about infertility and its evaluation and treatment.
- Explore ways to increase control within the situation of infertility.
- Identify aspects of self that are positive.

Interventions

Assisting Communication

Therapeutic communication is the primary technique for assessment and intervention related to this nursing diagnosis. Use a variety of communication techniques such as active listening and exploration to encourage the partners to express their feelings honestly. Provide privacy and acceptance of their feelings. Nurses must recognize the validity of the couple's views and emotions, even if they differ from the nurse's own feelings.

Encourage the partners to accept their feelings, both positive and negative. For example, the couple who has finally achieved pregnancy may be living a lie to some extent. The partners may act elated because they believe they should feel happy, yet inside they are cautious and hesitant to become attached to their baby. Explain that feelings are not right or wrong but simply exist. Opening the subject of negative feelings (fear of attachment) within a successful situation (pregnancy or birth) may be helpful to reinforce the normality of their emotions. This technique gives them the opportunity to talk about emotional reactions that they or others feel are inappropriate and might otherwise be reluctant to discuss.

Discuss possible differences in ways the man and the woman communicate. For example, explain that the woman may feel more comfortable than the man in talking about their problem and concerns about treatment. Explain that these differences in communication style can cause misunderstandings because one partner believes that the other does not care as much about their problem. Encourage them to be open with each other for the best mutual support. Support groups provide another means for communication and ventilation of feelings among those who are most likely to understand what an infertile couple is going through.

Increasing the Couple's Sense of Control

Explore how the couple has dealt with stressors in the past and how these techniques might be used to cope with the present crisis. A couple's pattern of dealing with stress in other parts of life is likely to carry over into infertility diagnosis and treatment and throughout pregnancy and parenthood. Reinforce positive coping skills such as learning more about infertility and the proposed therapy for it.

Couples who experience undue stress may benefit from relaxation techniques such as visualization and moderate exercise. Frequent strenuous exercise may reduce the woman's ability to ovulate. Although a hot tub is relaxing for many people, it should be avoided because the high temperatures may inhibit spermatogenesis. In addition, the woman could become pregnant with any cycle, and high body temperatures may be associated with fetal anomalies.

Discuss behaviors that enhance the ability to handle stress and provide a good environment for a pregnancy that might occur. Reinforce healthy choices such as good nutrition and a balance between exercise and rest. Teach the couple ways to enhance general health if deficiencies are identified.

Explain any procedures and their purpose in language that the couple can understand. Reinforce any medical explanations that may have been given. Encourage questions so that the couple is fully informed. Have the partners restate what was explained to reduce misunderstandings.

Help the couple explore options at each decision point. The couple must decide the best course of action, but the nurse can help identify pros and cons of each choice so that the partners can arrive at a decision appropriate for them. Be nondirective so that the choices are theirs and do not reflect the biases of the nurse or other caregivers.

Reducing Isolation

Because couples often distance themselves from friends and family relationships that they find painful, they may have few social supports. Refer them to available support groups to provide emotional outlets, a sense of belonging, and a source of information.

Couples who achieve pregnancy or adopt a child may again find themselves isolated if infertile couples in their circle of support are no longer comfortable with them. Encourage them to take the initiative to reestablish ties with relatives and friends, who can be an important source of aid during pregnancy and childrearing. Help them identify ways they can improve communication with these significant others. Remind them that they have undergone significant shifts in self-image, which also have affected those around them.

Promoting a Positive Self-Image

Because infertility work often is such a dominant factor in their lives, a continuing inability to conceive erodes the partners' perception of themselves. Explore with them other areas of competence and activities that make them feel good about themselves. Reinforce positive attitudes and self-evaluations. Encourage them to maintain activities such as hobbies, sports, or volunteer work. The career of either partner may be a source of stress that needs relief, or it may be an avenue that fosters a positive self-perception.

Encourage them to avoid activities such as baby showers if these events make them sad. Help them identify the best way to cope with these activities if they cannot be avoided.

Some people benefit from self-improvement activities such as continuing education courses or enhancement of appearance. Encourage these activities if they help the individuals feel better about themselves. If the activity might impair fertility treatments, such as strict dieting, also inform the person of this fact.

Evaluation

The goals established are achieved if the individual or both partners do the following:

- Can express their feelings about their situation, usually over a period of time.
- Can explore ways to increase personal control over their lives, as evidenced by expressing feelings of reduced helplessness and dependence.
- Can identify one or more aspects of self perceived as positive, identifying areas of competence.

SUMMARY CONCEPTS

- Nurses may encounter persons having infertility problems in a variety of settings other than infertility clinics, such as maternity and gynecology services, urology services, the perioperative area, and the emergency department. Friends and family members also see the nurse as an information resource about infertility care.
- About 20% of infertile couples have no identified problem that is explained by current evaluation techniques.
- Because many unknown factors in reproduction exist, identification and correction of problems in one or both partners does not necessarily resolve their infertility.
- A variety of structural and functional abnormalities may contribute to a couple's infertility. The man may have abnormalities of the sperm or the seminal fluid or with ejaculation. The woman may have ovulation disorders, anatomic problems such as fallopian tube occlusion, or physiologic disorders such as hormone imbalances.

- A systematic evaluation of both partners, proceeding from simple to more complex, identifies therapy that is most likely to be successful and cost effective.
- Infertility is a crisis for the couple and often for the extended family. Either or both partners may feel that the inability to conceive represents a personal failure. They may have a variety of psychological reactions.
- Infertile couples must make choices at many points before and during evaluation and therapy. Some major factors that enter into their decisions involve social, cultural, and religious values; difficulty of treatment; probability of success; financial resources; and age, particularly the woman's.
- The possible outcomes after infertility therapy may present new challenges to the couple and their families: unsuccessful therapy and the choice of whether to pursue adoption, pregnancy loss after infertility, and parenthood after infertility.
- Many nursing care needs may be identified as the couple negotiates infertility evaluation and treatment.

REFERENCES & READINGS

Abma, J., Chandra, A., Mosher, W., Peterson, L., & Piccinino, L. (1997). Fertility, family planning, and women's health: New data from the 1995 national survey of family growth. *Vital & Health Statistics* 23(19).

American Society for Reproductive Medicine. (2000a). *Committee opinion: Effectiveness and treatment for unexplained infertility.* Birmingham, AL: Author.

American Society for Reproductive Medicine. (1999a). *Committee opinion: Guidelines on number of embryos transferred.* Birmingham, AL: Author.

American Society for Reproductive Medicine. (1999b). *Committee opinion: New techniques for sperm acquisition in obstructive azoospermia.* Birmingham, AL: Author.

American Society for Reproductive Medicine. (2000b). *Committee opinion: Optimal evaluation of the infertile woman.* Birmingham, AL: Author.

American Society for Reproductive Medicine. (1997a). *Fact sheet: Diagnostic testing for male factor infertility.* Birmingham, AL: Author.

American Society for Reproductive Medicine. (1997b). *Guidelines and minimum standards: Guidelines for gamete and embryo donation.* Birmingham, AL: Author.

American Society for Reproductive Medicine. (1998). *Technical Bulletin: Induction of ovarian follicle development and ovulation with exogenous gonadotropins.* Birmingham: AL: Author.

Andreyko, J. (2000). Hypopituitarism. In E.J. Quilligan & F.A. Zuspan (Eds.), *Current therapy in obstetrics and gynecology* (5th ed., pp. 73-76). Philadelphia: W.B. Saunders.

Angard, N.T. (1999). Diagnosis infertility: These treatments can help couples achieve pregnancy. *AWHONN Lifelines,* 3(3), 22-29.

Angard, N.T. (2000). Seeking coverage for infertility: Insurers should offer reasonable services to help couples achieve pregnancy. *AWHONN Lifelines* 4(3), 22-24.

Bowers, N.A. (2000). The multiple birth explosion: Implications for nursing practice. *Journal of Obstetric, Gynecologic, and Neonatal Nursing,* 27(3), 302-310.

Boxer, A.S. (1996). Images of infertility. *Nurse Practitioner Forum,* 7(2), 60-63.

Cady, R. (1999). Legal issues in the treatment of infertility. *MCN: American Journal of Maternal/Child Nursing,* 24(5), 264.

Carcio, H.A. (1998a). Causes of infertility. In H.A. Carcio (Ed.), *Management of the infertile woman* (2nd ed., pp. 25-48). Philadelphia: W.B. Saunders.

Carcio, H.A. (1998b). Intrauterine insemination. In H.A. Carcio (Ed.), *Management of the infertile woman* (2nd ed., pp. 25-48). Philadelphia: W.B. Saunders.

Carcio, H.A. (1998c). The investigation. In H.A. Carcio (Ed.), *Management of the infertile woman* (2nd ed., pp. 195-216). Philadelphia: W.B. Saunders.

Chantilis, S.J., & Carr, B.R. (2000). Infertility. In E.J. Quilligan & F.A. Zuspan (Eds.), *Current therapy in obstetrics and gynecology* (5th ed., pp. 83-90). Philadelphia: W.B. Saunders.

Daly, D.C. (2000). Induction of ovulation. In E.J. Quilligan & F.A. Zuspan (Eds.), *Current therapy in obstetrics and gynecology* (5th ed., pp. 80-83). Philadelphia: W.B. Saunders.

Doctors call blood transplant a success. (2000, October 19). *The Dallas Morning News,* p. 8A.

Edwards, R.G., & Brody, S.A. (1995). *Principles and practices of assisted human reproduction.* Philadelphia: W.B. Saunders.

Engstrom, J.L., Giglio, N.N., Takacs, S.M., Ellis, M.C., & Cherwenka, D.I. (2000). Procedures used to prepare and administer intramuscular injections: A study of infertility nurses. *Journal of Obstetric, Gynecologic, and Neonatal Nursing,* 29(2), 159-168.

Grow, D.R. (1998). The art of assisted reproductive technologies (ART). (1998). In H.A. Carcio (Ed.), *Management of the infertile woman* (2nd ed., pp. 243-257). Philadelphia: W.B. Saunders.

Guyton, A.C., & Hall, J.E. (2000). *Textbook of medical physiology* (10th ed.). Philadelphia: W.B. Saunders.

Habecker-Green, J., & Cohn, G.M. (1998). Preconception counseling. In H.A. Carcio (Ed.), *Management of the infertile woman* (2nd ed., pp. 51-73). Philadelphia: W.B. Saunders.

Handyside, A.H. (1995). In vitro fertilization and preimplantation genetic diagnosis for prevention of inherited disease. In W.R. Keye, R.J. Chang, R.W. Rebar, & M.R. Soules (Eds.), *Infertility: Evaluation and treatment* (pp. 859-867). Philadelphia: W.B. Saunders.

Hardy, R.I. (1998). Induction of ovulation. In H.A. Carcio (Ed.), *Management of the infertile woman* (2nd ed., pp. 169-193). Philadelphia: W.B. Saunders.

Hirsch, A.M., & Hirsch, S.M. (1995). The long-term psychosocial effects of infertility. *Journal of Obstetric, Gynecologic, and Neonatal Nursing,* 24(6), 517-522.

Israel, R. (2000). Intrauterine adhesions. In E.J. Quilligan & F.A. Zuspan (Eds.), *Current therapy in obstetrics and gynecology* (5th ed., pp. 90-92). Philadelphia: W.B. Saunders.

Jirka, J., Schuett, S., & Foxall, M.J. (1996). Loneliness and social support in infertile couples. *Journal of Obstetric, Gynecologic, and Neonatal Nursing,* 25(1), 55-60.

Johnson, C.L. (1996). Regaining self-esteem: Strategies and interventions for the infertile woman. *Journal of Obstetric, Gynecologic, and Neonatal Nursing,* 25(4), 291-295.

Jones, G.S. (2000). Luteal phase defect. In E.J. Quilligan & F.A. Zuspan (Eds.), *Current therapy in obstetrics and gynecology* (5th ed., pp. 80-83). Philadelphia: W.B. Saunders.

Leibowitz, D., & Hoffman, J. (2000). Fertility drug therapies: Past, present, and future. *Journal of Obstetric, Gynecologic, and Neonatal Nursing,* 29(2), 201-210.

Mastroianni, L. (1996). Forty years of infertility management exponential progress and a demanding future. *Nurse Practitioner Forum, 7*(2), 87-91.

Meldrum, D.R. (1998). Infertility. In N.F. Hacker & J.G. Moore (Eds.), *Essentials of obstetrics and gynecology* (3rd ed., pp. 610-620). Philadelphia: W.B. Saunders.

National Kidney and Urologic Diseases Clearinghouse, National Institutes of Health. (2000). *Impotence.* Retrieved October 14, 2000 from http://www.niddk.nih.gov/health/urolog/pubs/impotnc/impotnc.htm.

O'Connell, E., & Domar, A. (1998). The emotional cost of infertility: Helping patients cope. In H.A. Carcio (Ed.), *Management of the infertile woman* (2nd ed., pp. 297-312). Philadelphia: W.B. Saunders.

Patrizio, P. (2000). Male infertility: Intrauterine insemination. In E.J. Quilligan & F.A. Zuspan (Eds.), *Current therapy in obstetrics and gynecology* (5th ed., pp. 104-107). Philadelphia: W.B. Saunders.

Patrizio, P., & Asch, R.H. (2000). Microsurgical and percutaneous epididymal sperm aspiration (MESA/PESA). In E.J. Quilligan & F.A. Zuspan (Eds.), *Current therapy in obstetrics and gynecology* (5th ed., pp. 113-115). Philadelphia: W.B. Saunders.

Patrizio, P., & Khorram, O. (2000). GIFT procedure. In E.J. Quilligan & F.A. Zuspan (Eds.), *Current therapy in obstetrics and gynecology* (5th ed., pp. 64-66). Philadelphia: W.B. Saunders.

Planned Parenthood Federations of America, Inc. (1999). Facts about birth control: Periodic abstinence and fertility awareness methods. Retrieved November 4, 2000 from http://www.plannedparenthood.org.bc/bcfacts13.html.

Reshef, E., & Sanfilippo, J.S. (2000). Hysteroscopic evaluation and therapy of mullërian anomalies. In E.J. Quilligan & F.A. Zuspan (Eds.), *Current therapy in obstetrics and gynecology* (5th ed., pp. 77-80). Philadelphia: W.B. Saunders.

Schaper, A.M., Hellwig, M.S., Murphy, P., & Gensch, B.K. (1996). Ectopic pregnancy loss during fertility management. *Western Journal of Nursing Research,* 18(5), 503-518.

Schoener, C.J., & Krysa, L.W. (1996). The comfort and discomfort of infertility. *Journal of Obstetric, Gynecologic, and Neonatal Nursing,* 25(2), 167-172.

Sherrod, R.A. (1995). A male perspective on infertility. *MCN: American Journal of Maternal-Child Nursing,* 20(5), 269-275.

Soules, M.R. (1995). Luteal phase deficiency: A subtle abnormality of ovulation. In W.R. Keye, R.J. Chang, R.W. Rebar, & M.R. Soules (Eds.), *Infertility: Evaluation and treatment* (pp. 178-194). Philadelphia: W.B. Saunders.

Stansberry, J. (1996). The infertile couple: An overview of pathophysiology and diagnostic evaluation for the primary care clinician. *Nurse Practitioner Forum, 7*(2), 70-86.

Surrey, E.S. (1995). Hyperstimulation syndrome. In W.R. Keye, R.J. Chang, R.W. Rebar, & M.R. Soules (Eds.), *Infertility: Evaluation and treatment* (pp. 145-153). Philadelphia: W.B. Saunders.

Surrey, E.S. (2000). Endometriosis and adenomyosis. In E.J. Quilligan & F.A. Zuspan (Eds.), *Current therapy in obstetrics and gynecology* (5th ed., pp. 77-80). Philadelphia: W.B. Saunders.

Tietz, N.W. (1995). *Clinical guide to laboratory tests* (3rd ed.). Philadelphia: W.B. Saunders.

Timbers, K.A., & Feinberg, R.F. (1996). Recurrent pregnancy loss: A review. *Nurse Practitioner Forum, 7*(2), 64-75.

Trantham, P. (1996). The infertile couple. *American Family Physician,* 54(3), 1001-1011.

Urry, R.L. (1995). Tests of sperm function. In W.R. Keye, R.J. Chang, R.W. Rebar, & M.R. Soules (Eds.), *Infertility: Evaluation and treatment* (pp. 592-608). Philadelphia: W.B. Saunders.

Wang, C., & Swerdloff, R.S. (1995). In W.R. Keye, R.J. Chang, R.W. Rebar, & M.R. Soules (Eds.), *Infertility: Evaluation and treatment* (pp. 609-620). Philadelphia: W.B. Saunders.

33

WOMEN'S HEALTH CARE

OBJECTIVES

1. Explain examinations and screening procedures recommended to maintain the health of women.
2. Explain benign disorders of the breast, relate them to usual age of onset, and describe the diagnostic procedures used to rule out cancer of the breast.
3. Describe the incidence, risks, pathophysiology, management, and nursing considerations related to malignant breast tumors.
4. Discuss cardiovascular disease in women, including risk factors, signs and symptoms, and prevention measures.
5. Discuss four common menstrual cycle disorders.
6. Explain premenstrual syndrome, management options, and nursing considerations.
7. Discuss induced abortion in terms of procedures, possible complications, and follow-up care.
8. Describe the physical and psychological changes associated with menopause and the risks versus benefits of hormone replacement therapy.
9. Discuss preventive measures for osteoporosis.
10. Describe the major disorders associated with pelvic relaxation in terms of cause, treatment, and nursing considerations.
11. Discuss the most common benign and malignant disorders of the reproductive tract in terms of signs and symptoms, management, and nursing considerations.
12. Describe care of the woman with an infectious disorder of the reproductive tract, including sexually transmitted diseases, pelvic inflammatory disease, and toxic shock syndrome.
13. Explain use of selected complementary and alternative therapies in the management of women's health.

DEFINITIONS

Adjuvant Therapy Additional treatment that increases or enhances the action of the primary treatment.

Adnexa Accessory parts or organs, such as the fallopian tubes and ovaries, associated with the uterus.

Amenorrhea Absence of menstruation. Primary amenorrhea is a delay of the first menstruation. Secondary amenorrhea is cessation of menstruation after its initiation.

Angina Pectoris Myocardial pain usually brought on by physical activity or stress; usually called simply *angina.*

Atrophic Vaginitis Inflammation that occurs when the vagina becomes dry and fragile, usually as a result of estrogen deficit after menopause.

Autogenous Graft Tissue that is moved from one part of the body to another part of the same person's body.

Axillary Tail Wedge of tissue extending from the breast into the axilla (also called the *tail of Spence*).

Body Mass Index (BMI) A formula that defines the degree of adiposity according to the relationship of weight to height. Calculated by the following equation:

$$BMI = \frac{\text{weight (lb)}}{\text{height (in)}^2} \times 705$$

Carcinoma in Situ Malignant neoplasm in surface tissue that has not extended into deeper tissue.

Climacteric Endocrine, body, and psychic changes occurring at the end of a woman's reproductive cycle. Also informally called *menopause.*

Colposcopy Examination of the vaginal and cervical tissue with a colposcope for magnification of cells.

Condyloma A wart-like growth of the skin seen on the external genitalia, in the vagina, on the cervix, or near the anus; may be caused by human papillomavirus (condyloma acuminatum) or by syphilis (condyloma latum).

Cryotherapy Destruction of tissue using extreme cold.

Cystocele Prolapse of the urinary bladder through the anterior vaginal wall.

Dysmenorrhea Painful menstruation.

Dyspareunia Difficult or painful coitus in women.

Dysplasia Abnormal development of tissue.

Dysuria Painful urination, often associated with urinary tract infection.

Endometrial Hyperplasia Excessive proliferation of normal cells of the uterine lining; may be due to administration of estrogen during the postmenopausal period.

Endometriosis Presence of tissue resembling the endometrium outside the uterine cavity.

Laparoscopy Insertion of an illuminated tube into the abdominal cavity to visualize contents, locate bleeding, and perform surgical procedures.

Laparotomy Incision through the abdominal wall to examine the abdominal or pelvic organs or perform other surgical procedures.

Mammogram Study of breast tissue using very-low-dose x-ray; primary tool in the diagnosis of breast tumors.

Menarche Onset of menstruation; average age is 12.8 years.

Menometrorrhagia Uterine bleeding irregular in frequency and excessive in amount.

Menopause Permanent cessation of menstruation during the climacteric.

Menorrhagia Excessive bleeding at the time of menstruation in number of days' duration, amount of blood lost, or both.

Metrorrhagia Bleeding from the uterus at any time other than during the menstrual period.

Osteoporosis Increased spaces (porosity) in bone; process greatly accelerates after menopause.

Paroxysmal Nocturnal Dyspnea Respiratory distress occurring when lying down, often associated with congestive heart failure.

Peau d'Orange Dimpled skin condition that resembles an orange peel; associated with lymphatic edema and often seen over the area of breast cancer.

Phytoestrogen Estrogen of plant origin.

Rectocele Herniation (protrusion) of the rectum through the posterior vaginal wall.

Toxic Shock Syndrome Rare, potentially fatal disorder caused by toxin produced by *Staphylococcus aureus;* has been associated with improper use of tampons.

This chapter focuses on primary and preventive care of women: routine assessments, screening procedures, and management of specific health concerns. Nurses provide many of the services most valued by women. Some, such as nurse practitioners, provide primary care. Others act as educators and advocates for women. They are responsible for explaining screening and diagnostic procedures and for clarifying options so that women can make informed decisions about care. Finally, nurses traditionally have offered support and comfort to women when they experience disruptions in their health.

NATIONAL EMPHASIS ON WOMEN'S HEALTH

Two national programs have a potential to influence women's health positively. They are the Women's Health Initiative of the National Institutes of Health and the Healthy People 2010 health promotion and disease prevention agenda coordinated by the U.S. Department of Health and Human Services.

Women's Health Initiative

The Women's Health Initiative is a 15-year health study sponsored by the Heart, Lung, and Blood Institute within the National Institutes of Health (NIH), targeting the top causes of death and disability in older women of every race:

- Heart disease
- Breast cancer
- Colorectal cancer
- Osteoporosis

Three long-term studies of these diseases will be done in multiple centers across the United States: (1) a randomized, controlled trial, (2) an observational study, and (3) a community prevention study. For detailed information about the initiative and to determine the status of each study, see the Initiative's web site at www.nhlbi.nih.gov/whi/index.html.

The randomized, controlled trial will address how hormone replacement therapy, dietary patterns, and calcium plus vitamin D intake affect these four devastating diseases. This clinical trial has enrolled more than 68,000 women, 50 to 79 years old in 40 nationwide centers.

The observational study will examine the relationship between lifestyle, health, and risk factors and specific disease outcomes. This study will correlate the medical history and health habits of about 100,000 women over an 8- to 12-year period.

The community prevention study is a collaborative venture between the Centers for Disease Control and Prevention and the National Institutes of Health. Eight community centers will conduct and critically evaluate health programs that encourage women of all races and socioeconomic backgrounds to adopt healthful behaviors. These programs may consist of diet improvement, smoking cessation, exercise, and early detection of treatable health problems.

Healthy People 2010 Goals

The Healthy People 2010 national health promotion and disease prevention initiative has been discussed in other chapters in this text. The Healthy People 2010 home page may be found at http://www.health.gov/healthypeople/default.htm. Several Healthy People 2010 goals also relate to women's health and many address the goals in the Women's Health Initiative.

- Reverse the rise in breast cancer deaths from 27.7 per 100,000 women in 1998 to no more than 22.2
- Increase the number of women age 40 or older who have received a mammogram within the preceding 2 years from 68% in 1998 to 70%
- Reduce deaths from cancer of the cervix from 3 per 100,000 women in 1998 to no more than 2.0
- Increase from 79% in 1998 to 90% the number of women (18 years or older) who received a Pap test for cervical cancer within the last 3 years
- Increase from 34% in 1998 to 50% the number of adults 50 years and older who receive a fecal occult blood test within the preceding 2 years
- Reduce the proportion of adults who are hospitalized for vertebral fractures associated with osteoporosis from 14.5 per 10,000 in 1997 to 11.6 per 10,000
- Reduce the incidence of gonorrhea in women between the ages of 15 and 44 from 123 per 100,000 in 1997 to 19
- Reduce the prevalence of *Chlamydia trachomatis* infections among women under the age of 25 years to no more than 3%
- Reduce congenital syphilis from an incidence of 91.0 per 100,000 live births to no more than 1
- Increase the proportion of adolescents in grades 9 through 12 who abstain from sexual intercourse or use condoms if they are sexually active to at least 95%

HEALTH MAINTENANCE

Health maintenance includes all measures taken to prevent or detect specific diseases early, when they are most treatable. The most common health maintenance measures include periodic health examinations, immunizations, and screening procedures. Unfortunately, many women do not take advantage of recommended health maintenance measures. Some seek care only when they have a problem. The only regular health care other women receive comes from a gynecologist or nurse practitioner who conducts a gynecologic examination. Therefore those who provide health care for women must be familiar with principles of screening and counseling in areas that are not traditionally associated with gynecology, such as assessing for colon cancer and heart disease.

Health History

The health history identifies risk factors for a variety of conditions and may be obtained from sources such as questionnaires, interviews, and previous records. The focus of a health history depends on the woman's age, but some topics should be discussed with all women. Table 33-1 provides a summary of information to obtain. These topics include dietary intake, physical activity, habits, and sexual practices. Discussions of drugs must include long-term use of prescription and over-the-counter medications. Illicit drugs must also be discussed to provide the safest care for the woman.

Table 33-1
HEALTH HISTORY

PERSONAL HISTORY

Demographic data (name, age, marital status or whether living with a partner)
Reason for seeking health care (also termed chief complaint)
Current and past state of health, previous surgeries
Allergies
Regular medications (prescribed, over-the-counter, and illicit)
Use of complementary or alternative therapies, including herbal or botanical preparations
Habits (smoking, use of alcohol, drugs)
Appetite, usual dietary intake
Exercise pattern (type, frequency)
Sleep and rest patterns
Patterns of elimination (current or chronic problems)
Degree of stress and stress management techniques

MENSTRUAL HISTORY

Age of menarche
Regularity, duration of menstrual cycle
Menstrual discomfort (time during cycle, intensity, relief measures)
Age at menopause, if applicable

OBSTETRIC HISTORY

Gravida, para, duration of gestation, weight of infant(s) at birth
Labor experience and method of delivery

SEXUAL HISTORY

Sexually active? (number of partners, sexual activity patterns of partner(s), age when first sexually active)
Method of contraception (satisfaction with method, adverse reactions, accuracy of use)
Knowledge/practice of measures to protect self from sexually transmitted diseases

FAMILY HISTORY

Cardiovascular problems (anemia, hypertension, clotting disorders, stroke, heart disease)
Cancer (breast, uterine, ovarian, bowel, lung)
Osteoporosis

PSYCHOSOCIAL HISTORY

Primary language, additional languages spoken or understood
Marital status, employment, occupation, education (relevant to determine financial, social, and emotional support)

Complementary/Alternative Therapy

Many people take herbal or other botanical preparations but do not mention them because they do not consider them drugs. The nurse must specifically ask about use of these preparations or any therapies the woman may use in addition to medically prescribed interventions to obtain the most complete information for the medical history.

Check Your Reading

1. How is the Women's Health Initiative expected to affect the health of women?
2. Why is a family history an important part of a health history?
3. What questions should be asked when taking a sexual history?

Family history identifies many risk factors that cannot be modified. History of hyperlipidemia, heart disease, osteoporosis, and thyroid disease suggests the best choice of screening tests. A list of family members who had cancer, the type of cancer they had, and their ages when it was discovered provides important information about the woman's risk of cancer, particularly breast and colon cancer.

A family history of heart disease is especially important when the woman is postmenopausal because estrogen, which provides some protection against coronary artery disease, decreases after menopause. Therefore a family history that includes myocardial infarctions increases the risk of coronary artery disease in a postmenopausal woman who does not take estrogen replacement. In this case, a baseline electrocardiogram, stress test, and analysis of cholesterol and lipid profiles may identify additional risk factors that can be modified.

Physical Assessment

A complete physical examination is essential to detect general health problems. (See a physical assessment text for full explanation of the process of physical examination.) Blood pressure, temperature, pulse, respirations, and weight are measured at each visit. Height is taken at the initial examination and yearly after that. Loss of height, abnormal curvature of the vertebral column (dorsal kyphosis or scoliosis), and a thickening waistline in the absence of weight gain are important observations in evaluating osteoporosis in the postmenopausal woman.

The heart is auscultated to determine rate and rhythm and to detect heart murmurs. Auscultation of the lungs identifies abnormal sounds that may suggest the presence of fluid secondary to heart dysfunction. The extremities are observed for varicosities or edema, and pedal pulses are palpated for strength and equality. The abdomen is palpated for tenderness, masses, or disten-

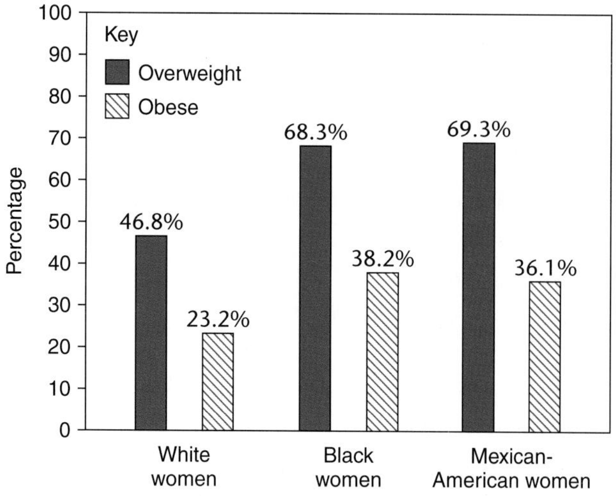

FIGURE 33-1 The extent of the problem of excess weight in the U.S. Overweight is defined as a body mass index (BMI) of 25 to 29.9; obese is defined as 30 to 39.9.

tion that may indicate presence of benign or malignant tumors.

Additional assessments are necessary if the woman is in a high-risk group. For instance, if she has a family history of diabetes mellitus, tests such as fasting glucose or a glucose tolerance test may be indicated. If she has a history of multiple sexual partners or a sexual partner with multiple contacts, she may require testing for sexually transmitted diseases.

Preventive Counseling

Physical examination provides an excellent opportunity to counsel women about preventive care. Major preventable problems are overweight and obesity, inactivity, and smoking. Overweight and obesity are associated with numerous health problems such as diabetes, hypertension, and coronary artery disease. The incidence of overweight, defined as a body mass index (BMI) of 25 to 29.9, is 46.8% in white women, 68.3% in black women, and 69.3% in Mexican-American women ages 20 to 74. The incidence of obesity in these groups, defined as a BMI of 30 to 39.9, is 23.2% in white women, 38.2% in black women, and 36.1% in Mexican-American women (American Heart Association, 2000f) (Figure 33-1).

Physical inactivity is associated with overweight and obesity, osteoporosis, high cholesterol levels, and coronary artery disease. Women, older adults, and the less affluent are more likely to be inactive. Blacks and Hispanics are less active when compared with whites (American Heart Association, 2000g). Smoking is increasing in females younger than 18, increasing the risk for cardiovascular problems and several types of cancer (American Heart Association, 2000d; American Cancer Society, 2000a).

Counseling about diet should be offered and positive health behaviors, such as adequate physical activity or smoking cessation, should be reinforced. Use of latex condoms should be emphasized for high-risk women with multiple sexual partners or those whose partner has multiple sexual partners. Latex condoms provide some protection against transmission of viruses, such as human immunodeficiency virus (HIV) and human papillomavirus (HPV), which is strongly implicated as a risk factor for cervical cancer.

The history or physical examination may identify other areas for client counseling. These include the dangers of malignant melanoma with repeated exposure to ultraviolet rays of the sun. In addition, counseling and referral for alcohol and other substance abuse may be needed for some women.

Screening Procedures

The value of screening procedures is based on two assumptions: (1) prevention is better than cure, and (2) early diagnosis allows early treatment while the pathologic process is most curable.

Some screening procedures are recommended for all women of reproductive age, including some screening procedures for early detection of breast cancer as well as vulvar self-examination and screening for cervical cancer. Other screening procedures are recommended for older women or those with higher risk.

Breast Self-Examination

Breast self-examination (BSE) supplements rather than replaces screening by professional examination and mammography. In many parts of the world, however, BSE is the only realistic means of early cancer detection.

Breast self-examination should be performed monthly by all women after the age of 20 years. Women should perform a BSE about 1 week following the onset of menses, when hormonal influences on the breasts are at a low level. If the woman no longer menstruates, she may choose a day that is easy to remember and perform the examination on that day every month. An example is the first day of the month.

Professional Breast Examination

Professional breast examination is similar to BSE but professional examiners are more experienced and may identify questionable areas that the woman misses. The examination includes both inspection and palpation. It should be part of every gynecologic examination.

Inspection

1. While the woman is in an upright position, the examiner inspects the breasts for size, symmetry, color, and skin changes. The nipples and areola are inspected for differences in size and color, unilateral retraction of a nipple, and asymmetric nipple direction, which may indicate an underlying tumor.

WOMEN WANT TO KNOW *How to Perform Breast Self-Examination*

- Lie down. Flatten your right breast by placing a pillow under your right shoulder. If your breasts are large, use your right hand to hold your right breast while you do the examination with your left hand.
- Use the sensitive pads of the middle three fingers on your left hand and a massaging motion to feel for lumps or changes in the breast tissue.
- Press firmly enough to distinguish different breast textures.
- Completely palpate or feel all parts of the breast and chest area. Be sure to examine the breast tissue that extends toward the shoulder. The amount of time required to completely palpate all the breast tissue depends on the size of the breast. Women with small breasts need at least 2 minutes to examine each breast. Larger breasts take longer.

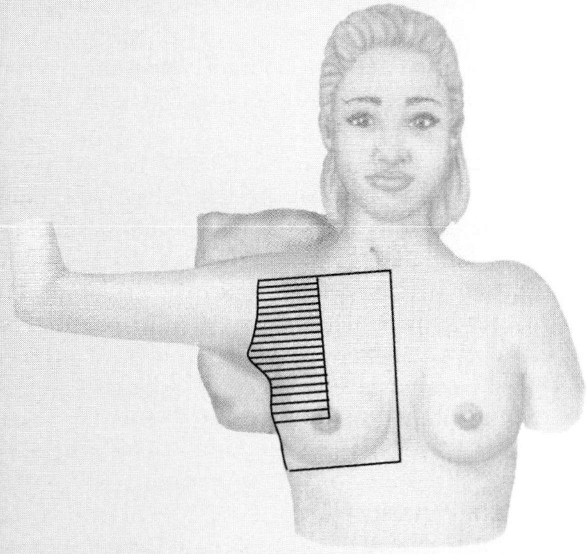

- Use the same routine or pattern to feel every part of the breast tissue. Any of three patterns can help you to make sure you have covered your entire breast: the circular pattern, the vertical strip, and the wedge. Choose the method you find easiest.

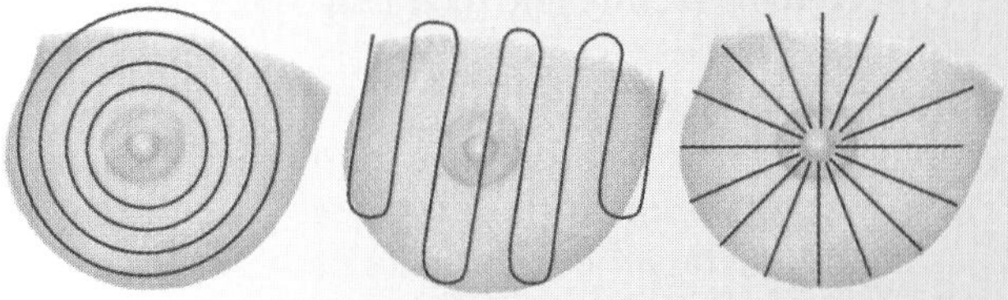

- When you have completely examined your right breast, the left breast should be examined using the same method. Compare what you feel in one breast with the other.
- You may also want to examine your breasts while bathing, when the skin is wet and lumps may be easily palpated.
- You can check your breasts in a mirror by raising your arms and looking for an unusual shape, dimpling of the skin, and any changes in the nipple.

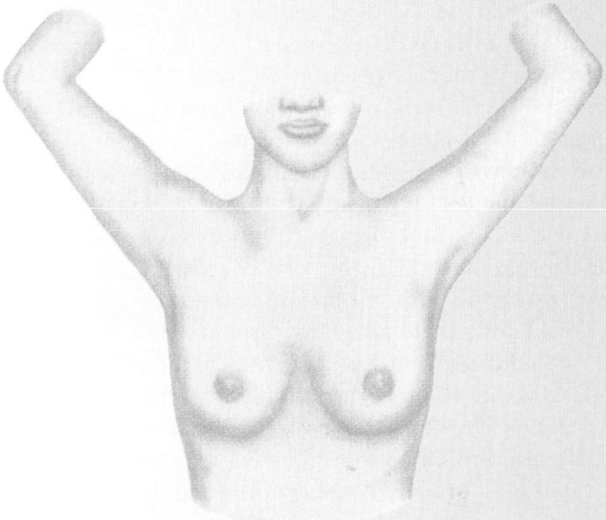

Adapted from the American Cancer Society (ACS) (2000). *How to perform a breast self-exam.* Available at the ACS website, http://www.cancer.org.

2. The woman raises her hands above her head, and the examiner inspects the sides and underneath portions of the breast for asymmetry and differences in color.
3. The woman places her hands on her hips and presses down; this action reveals skin dimpling or masses.

Palpation

1. The axillary, supraclavicular, and suprasternal lymph nodes are palpated for tenderness or enlargement.
2. The woman lies in a supine position for palpation of the breasts. A small pillow or folded towel is placed under the shoulder to stretch the tissue and flatten the breast. The examiner uses the flat part of the first three fingers to palpate the breast, rotating the fingers against the chest wall. Tissue that extends into the axilla, the axillary tail (or tail of Spence) also should be palpated. The procedure is repeated on the opposite side. Normal breast tissue is described as firm, lumpy, nodular, tender, and thickened. Abnormal breast tissue is often likened to a raisin, watermelon seed, or grape. In other words, a discrete mass can be felt and measured. If a suspicious area is found, follow-up by diagnostic mammography and/or ultrasonography is recommended.

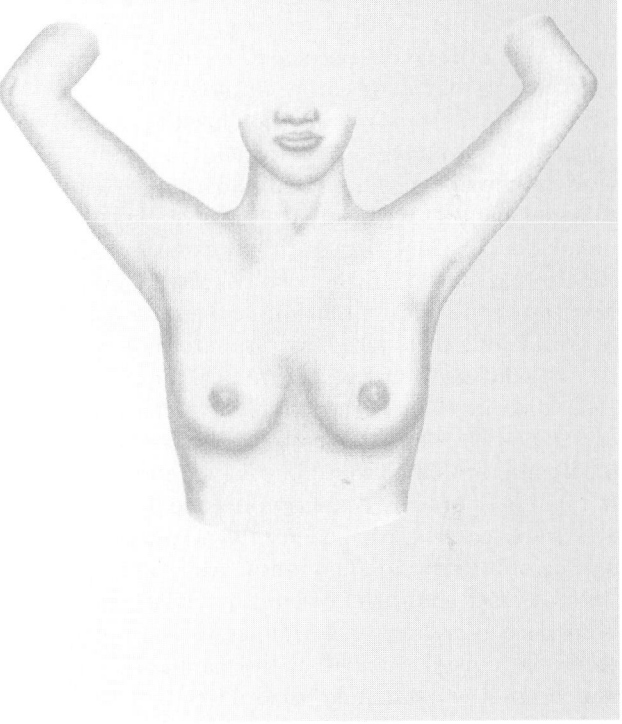

3. The nipples are compressed to detect the presence of discharge. A sample of any discharge should be collected for culture and examination of cells.

Mammography

Mammography may be used either to screen for cancer or to assist in the diagnosis of a palpable mass in the breast. Mammography is a screening tool that can detect breast lumps well before they are large enough to be palpated. This allows early diagnosis and treatment and thus increases the chance of long-term survival.

No consensus exists on the frequency of mammography for women in their forties. The American Cancer Society (2000a) recommends screening mammography each year for women age 40 and older. The American College of Obstetricians and Gynecologists recommends that women age 40 to 49 have a mammogram every 1 to 2 years, and yearly after age 50. Women at high risk for breast cancer (see p. 930 for a summary of risk factors) may need earlier or more frequent mammography and should consult their health care provider.

Despite the known value of mammography, many women have never had a mammogram. Reasons for this include lack of a health care professional's recommendation, expense, fear that x-ray exposure will cause cancer, fear of pain, and reluctance to hear "bad news." Nurses provide information and reassurance whenever possible and, in this way, help the woman overcome her objections to the use of this valuable screening tool. Mammography is relatively expensive but part of its cost is often covered by health insurance, Medicaid, or Medicare. Screening mammograms are frequently offered by community agencies at low cost. The American Cancer Society (www.cancer.org) is a source of information about low-cost mammograms. Acknowledge that brief discomfort occurs when the breast is compressed between two plates while the radiograph is taken. Scheduling the mammography after a menstrual period, when the breasts are less tender, reduces the discomfort. Knowledge that the risk of mammography is minimal to nonexistent, because very low-dose exposure to x-rays is used, may help women to overcome some of their fear.

Specific groups of women need to be particularly encouraged to have screening mammography (National Cancer Institute, 1999):

- Older women, who often are less likely to have annual mammograms, but an increasing risk for breast cancer as they age
- African-American women, who have a higher mortality rate for breast cancer
- Hispanic women because breast cancer is increasing more rapidly in this group
- American Indian or Alaskan Native women because of a higher incidence of breast cancer and lower survival rate
- Asian or Pacific Islander women because some studies suggest that their rates of breast cancer increase as they become acculturated to the United States

The Mammography Quality Standards Act of 1992 requires all mammography facilities to be certified by the Food and Drug Administration (FDA). The facilities are responsible for meeting quality standards for film processing, interpretation, and record keeping. Furthermore, mammography units must be monitored to ensure appropriate radiation levels and overall operation. Quality assurance programs ensure that positive results are followed up quickly and properly.

Vulvar Self-Examination

Vulvar self-examination should be performed monthly by all women older than 18 and by those younger than 18 who are sexually active. Vulvar self-examination is visual inspection and palpation of the female external genitalia to detect signs of precancerous conditions or infections.

The woman should sit in a well-lighted area and use a hand mirror to see her external genitalia. She is taught to examine the vulva in a systematic manner, starting at the mons pubis and progressing to the clitoris, labia minora, labia majora, perineum, and anus. Palpation of the vulvar area should accompany visual inspection. She should report new moles, warts or growths of any kind, ulcers, sores, changes in skin color, or areas of inflammation or itching to her health care provider as soon as possible.

Pelvic Examination

The complete gynecologic assessment includes a pelvic examination. The woman should schedule the examination between menstrual periods and not douche or have sexual intercourse for at least 48 hours before the examination. She also is advised not to use vaginal medications, sprays, or deodorants that might interfere with interpretation of cytology specimens that are collected.

The procedure is carefully explained before the examination and the woman empties her bladder. Although pelvic examinations are relatively painless, most women dislike them and welcome sensitive, considerate support. Women who have undergone female genital mutilation (Table 33-2) need extra consideration. The nurse must avoid displaying shock, despite the fact that most nurses in Western countries have an aversion to this often-unfamiliar practice. A pediatric vaginal speculum may be needed for these or other women with a very small vaginal opening. Routine preventive pelvic examinations may be impossible for women who have only a tiny opening left for drainage of urine and menstrual blood.

The adolescent having her first examination also benefits from an understanding nurse who takes the time to explain the equipment and steps of the examination

Table 33-2

FEMALE GENITAL MUTILATION

Female genital mutilation, sometimes called *female circumcision,* refers to the ritual disfigurement and the partial or total removal of a girl's external genitalia or other injury to her external genitalia for cultural, religious, or other nontherapeutic reasons.

The practice exists in Africa and in some areas of the Middle East and Asia. It may be found in immigrant groups in Europe, Australia, New Zealand, Canada, and the United States. More than 130 million girls and women are estimated to have undergone female genital mutilation and another 2 million are at risk annually (WHO, 1998).

The age when the procedure is performed varies from a few days old to adult. Most are performed when the girl is between 4 and 10 years, an age when she cannot give informed consent for a procedure with lifetime consequences for her health.

Female genital mutilation may be done by a village practitioner using crude tools, such as knives, razor blades, broken glass, thorns, or scissors, and without anesthesia. Parents in more developed countries may seek the procedure from a physician to assure pain relief and sterility.

Female genital mutilation is considered a part of the coming-of-age ceremonies in some societies, and a girl may not be considered marriageable unless she has undergone the procedure. Some societies believe that the practice enhances female chastity and increases male sexual pleasure. Other societies consider the external female genitalia to be unsightly and dirty. Thus they are removed to promote hygiene and the woman's attractiveness.

Female genital mutilation is illegal and subject to criminal prosecution in several countries, including the United States.

Four major types of female genital mutilation exist:

- Type I: Excision of the skin surrounding the clitoris, with or without excision of all or part of the clitoris
- Type II: Removal of all of the clitoris and part or all of the labia minora. The vaginal opening is visible.
- Type III (infibulation): In this, the most severe form, the entire clitoris is removed, some or all of the labia minora are removed, and raw surfaces are created on the labia majora. The raw surfaces on the labia majora are stitched together, leaving only a small posterior opening for urine and menstrual flow. A firm band of tissue replaces the labia and the urethral and vaginal openings cannot be seen.
- Type IV: Various practices of pricking, piercing, cutting of the clitoris and labia; stretching of the clitoris or labia; cauterization of the clitoris; and scraping or introducing corrosive substances or herbs to narrow the vagina.

Health consequences may include the immediate results of severe pain, shock, hemorrhage, ulceration, urinary retention, and infection. Transmission of HIV is a concern if unsterile materials are used, or if the vaginal opening is so small that anal intercourse is used as an alternative to vaginal intercourse. Infibulation may result in scar formation that causes dyspareunia, difficulty urinating, difficulty with menstruation, recurrent urinary tract infections, and infertility. Painful intercourse and reduced sexual sensitivity may have consequences on psychological health.

Several groups worldwide are working together to target societies and parents where the practice prevails about its harm to girls and women. The intent is to eradicate the harmful practice through education and legislation.

carefully before having her undress. If she is anxious and fidgeting, she will appreciate a hand to hold and an explanation before each step. Some of the breathing techniques used for birth, such as slow, paced breathing, or use of a focal point (see Chapter 15), may be helpful.

The pelvic examination is done usually with the woman in a lithotomy position, with a pillow under her head. If she wishes, she may be placed in a semi-sitting position and offered a hand mirror so that she can observe the external genitalia and the examination, and learn more about her body. She is draped so that only the parts being examined are exposed.

Women who cannot tolerate a lithotomy position, such as a frail elderly woman, may benefit from a side-lying pelvic examination. The pelvic can also be done with the woman in a semi-Fowler's position, with her knees bent and feet on the exam table, rather than using the stirrups and having her hips at the edge of the table. The paraplegic woman, with no control over her lower extremities, usually can be examined with her legs separated in a V shape without her knees being bent.

Necessary equipment to be assembled before the examination begins includes gloves, speculum (several sizes, including pediatric, should be available), slides, cotton swabs, a fixative agent, and a cytobrush and spatula for obtaining material for the cytology specimen, or Papanicolaou (Pap) test (see later in this chapter). A stool specimen may be obtained by the examiner during the rectal examination, and a slide for this specimen also should be available.

External Organs. The pelvic examination is conducted systematically and gently. The external organs are inspected for the degree of development or atrophy of the labia, the distribution of hair, and the character of the hymen. Any cysts, tumors, or inflammation of Bartholin's glands is noted. The urinary meatus and Skene's glands are inspected for purulent discharge. Perineal scarring resulting from childbirth is noted.

Speculum Examination. A bivalve speculum of the appropriate size is used to inspect the vagina and cervix. The speculum is warmed with tap water and gently inserted into the vagina. No other lubrication is used because it interferes with accurate cytology results. The size, shape, and color of the cervix are noted. A sample is taken for the Pap test. In addition, a sample of any unusual discharge is obtained for microscopic examination or culture.

Bimanual Examination. The bimanual examination provides information about the uterus, fallopian tubes, and ovaries. The labia are separated, and the gloved, lubricated index finger and middle finger of one hand are inserted into the vaginal introitus.

The cervix is palpated for consistency, size, and tenderness to motion. The uterus is evaluated by placing the other hand on the abdomen with the fingers pressing gently just above the symphysis pubis so that the uterus can be felt between the examining fingers of both hands. The size, configuration, consistency, and mobility of the uterus are evaluated (Figure 33-2).

Feeling the fallopian tubes is usually impossible, although the ovaries may be palpated between the fingers of both hands. Because ovaries atrophy following menopause, palpating the ovaries of a postmenopausal woman is usually not possible.

The Papanicolaou Test

Purpose. It is known that, in virtually all cases, changes occur in cells of the cervix before cervical cancer develops. These changes have variously been called *cervical intraepithelial neoplasia, dysplasia, squamous intraepithelial lesions (SIL),* and *carcinoma in situ.* Cervical cytology, or the Pap test, is the most useful procedure for detecting precancerous and cancerous cells that may be shed by the cervix. Regular Pap tests can increase the survival for those women who develop cervical cancer by identifying it when it is most treatable.

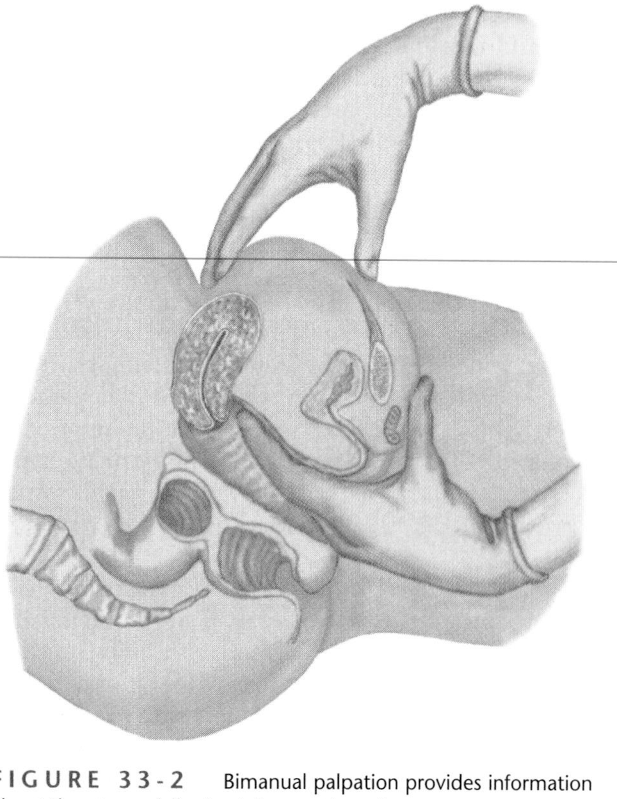

FIGURE 33-2 Bimanual palpation provides information about the uterus, fallopian tubes, and ovaries.

Procedure. With the speculum blades open and the cervix in view, samples of the superficial layers of the cervix and endocervix are obtained. Samples are best obtained with a spatula or a cytobrush at the squamocolumnar junction (the border where developing squamous tissue meets the immature columnar epithelium).

The material is placed on slides that are then either sprayed with or immersed in a fixative solution before being sent to the laboratory for analysis. Newer methods of computer analysis can improve the accuracy of the Pap cervical screenings and reduce false-negative results. The computer analysis costs more, but detects and displays abnormal cells on a high-resolution color video screen for interpretation and diagnosis.

Classification of Cervical Cytology. A great deal of variation existed in how cervical cytology findings were reported until recently. The Bethesda system was devised to offer standard terminology and give a narrative, descriptive diagnosis. It consists of three elements: (1) a statement of specimen adequacy, (2) a general categorization (normal or abnormal), and (3) a descriptive diagnosis regarding abnormal cytology.

Categories for epithelial cell abnormalities include the following:

1. Atypical squamous cells of undetermined significance (ASCUS)
2. Squamous intraepithelial lesion, which is subdivided into (a) low-grade SIL (including cellular changes of HPV) and (b) high-grade SIL (previously categorized as carcinoma in situ). The high-grade SIL is more likely to become cancerous without definitive treatment.
3. Squamous cell cancer

Glandular cell abnormalities are categorized as follows:

1. Atypical glandular cells of uncertain significance (AGCUS)
2. Adenocarcinoma

The woman's follow-up depends on the nature of the abnormality and whether it is persistent. Pap tests that have persistent ASCUS findings after a 3- to 6-month interval also usually are evaluated colposcopically. Suspicious lesions are examined with colposcopy and biopsy.

Rectal Examination

The anus is inspected for hemorrhoids, inflammation, and lesions. The examiner's lubricated index finger is gently inserted, and sphincter tone is noted. A slide may be prepared to test for the presence of occult blood in stool.

Fecal occult blood testing (FOBT) is a useful yearly screening measure for colorectal cancer beginning at age 50. Special instructions are necessary to prevent false test results when the woman is given materials for FOBT. She should be instructed to do the following:

- Avoid vitamin C, acetylsalicylic acid, and nonsteroidal antiinflammatory drugs (NSAIDs) such as ibuprofen or naproxen for at least 48 hours before collecting the specimen.
- Avoid red meat, turnips, beets, and horseradish for 48 hours before testing.
- Collect a specimen from three consecutive stools.
- Return slides as directed within 4 to 6 days after the specimens are collected.

Laboratory Screening Tests

Additional laboratory tests depend on the age, history, and risk assessment of the woman and might include the following:

- Testing for sexually transmitted diseases, such as chlamydial infection, gonorrhea, syphilis, and HIV
- Testing for rubella immunity, which is particularly important in the childbearing years
- Tuberculosis skin testing or chest x-ray
- Cholesterol and other lipid profile testing of women at risk for coronary artery disease (particularly important after menopause for women who do not take estrogen hormone replacement therapy)
- Fasting glucose testing or other tests to identify development of diabetes, recommended every 3 years after age 45 or earlier if the woman has high-risk factors
- A urinalysis to detect signs of urinary tract infection
- A thyroid function test, which may be indicated if the woman exhibits signs of thyroid dysfunction, such as heart palpitations and heat intolerance
- Serum testing for genes associated with specific cancers, such as the BRCA1, BRCA2, or p53 genes associated with breast and some other cancers
- Serum testing for CA 125, a tumor marker that may be elevated with ovarian cancer
- Transvaginal ultrasonography, which may be recommended for women who are at increased risk for malignant disorders of the reproductive tract (see p. 219)
- A sigmoidoscopy (every 3 to 5 years after age 50). A yearly colonoscopy may be recommended if the woman has a family history of colon cancer because the sigmoidoscopy only examines about half the length of the colon.

See Table 33-3 for a summary of recommended procedures.

Table 33-3

SUMMARY OF SCREENING PROCEDURES

Procedure and Frequency as Indicated	Purpose
Breast self-examination *Monthly 1 week after the menses begin or on a day that is easy to remember*	To inspect and palpate the breasts monthly for changes or masses that might indicate breast tumors
Professional breast examination *Every 3 years between age 20 and 39; yearly beginning at age 40 (American Cancer Society, 2000a)*	To allow experienced health care provider to detect masses that the woman might miss
Mammography *Every 1-2 yr from 40-49 yr; yearly after 50 yr (ACOG, 1999) [American Cancer Society recommends yearly beginning at age 40]*	To detect breast lumps before they become palpable. Early diagnosis of breast cancer promotes long-term survival
Vulvar self-examination *Monthly after age 18; monthly before 18 if sexually active*	To detect signs of precancerous conditions or infections
Pelvic examination *Yearly when sexually active, or by age 18*	To inspect and palpate the organs of reproduction for confirmation that no disease exists, or for early detection if disease does exist
Papanicolaou (Pap) test *Yearly when sexually active, or by age 18; may decrease to every 3 years if low risk at patient and physician discretion (ACOG, 1999)*	To detect abnormal cervical cell cytology early, thus preventing cervical cancer or identifying it at its most treatable stage
Cholesterol and/or lipid profile *Cholesterol every 5 years beginning at age 45*	To identify risk factors for coronary artery disease
Fasting glucose test *Every 3 years after age 45*	To identify development of diabetes
Urinalysis *Yearly*	To screen postmenopausal women; those with diabetes mellitus; history of urinary infections. Almost always performed.
Rectal examination *With pelvic examination*	To check for hemorrhoids and lesions and to evaluate sphincter control

STD, Sexually transmitted disease; *HIV,* human immunodeficiency virus; *IV,* intravenous.

Continued

Table 33-3
SUMMARY OF SCREENING PROCEDURES—cont'd

Procedure and Frequency as Indicated	Purpose
Fecal occult blood test *Yearly beginning at age 50*	To determine if blood is in stool, often an early sign of colon cancer
Sigmoidoscopy *Every 3-5 years after age 50*	To identify precancerous growths such as polyps in their most treatable stage.
Procedure and Frequency as Indicated	**Risk Factors**
ADDITIONAL PROCEDURES BASED ON RISK FACTORS	
STD testing	History of multiple sexual partners or a partner with multiple contacts, history of STDs
HIV testing	Identification of STDs; IV drug use; sexual partner who is HIV positive, bisexual, or injects drugs; recurrent or persistent episodes of STDs such as candidiasis and herpes
Thyroid-stimulating hormone (TSH)	Strong family history of thyroid disease
Rubella antibody testing	Questionable immunity to rubella
Tuberculosis skin testing *Yearly in areas where prevalent or with occupational exposure*	Identify possible development of new infection that requires treatment
Genetic studies for breast cancer genes (BRCA1 & BRCA2; p53) *Women thought to be at high risk for familial breast cancer*	Strong family history of breast cancer in multiple close relatives; may allow prophylactic treatment to reduce risk
Transvaginal ultrasound examination and/or blood test for CA 125	Family history of ovarian cancer
Colonoscopy *May be preferred to sigmoidoscopy at 3- to 5-year intervals after age 50 if visualization of entire colon is very important*	Family history of bowel cancer

Check Your Reading

4. What are the three screening procedures to identify cancer of the breast?
5. Why is vulvar self-examination recommended?
6. What is a Pap test, and why is it performed?
7. Why is fecal occult blood testing important?

BENIGN DISORDERS OF THE BREAST

Four relatively common benign disorders of the breast tend to occur at different ages.

Fibroadenoma

Fibroadenomas are the most common benign tumors of the breast, and although they may occur at any age, they are most common during the teenage years and the twenties. Fibroadenomas are composed of both fibrous and glandular tissue. They are firm, freely mobile nodules that may or may not be tender when palpated. Fibroadenomas do not change during the menstrual cycle. They are generally located in the upper, outer quadrant of the breast, and more than one is often present.

Treatment may involve careful observation for a few months, or the tumor may be excised and the specimen analyzed to rule out malignancy.

Fibrocystic Breast Changes

Fibrocystic breast changes, also called *benign breast disease,* often occur before menopause. The early stage is characterized by fibrosis, or thickening of the normal breast tissue, whereas cysts form in the latter stages and are felt as multiple, smooth, well-delineated nodules, which are usually present bilaterally.

The most common symptom of fibrocystic breast changes is pain and tenderness. The pain is often bilateral and most noticeable during the premenstrual phase of the normal cycle. This is believed to be the result of an imbalance in the estrogen-progesterone production. Women with fibrocystic breast changes improve dramatically during pregnancy and lactation because of the large amounts of progesterone produced.

The initial therapy is to rule out malignancy. The bilateral nature of the changes and pain suggest that the condition is benign, but definitive studies such as mammogram, fine needle aspiration of the cysts, or biopsy may be needed to identify malignancy. Fibrocystic breast changes may fall into three categories (Hacker, 1998):

- Nonproliferative lesions
- Hyperplasia without atypical cells
- Atypical hyperplasia

Hyperplastic lesions with atypical cellular changes have an increased risk to become malignant, but most women with fibrocystic breast changes do not have an increased risk for breast cancer.

Medical treatment is not standardized but the following drugs may be useful (Hacker, 1998). Medroxyprogesterone acetate (MPA, or Provera) may be prescribed for 5 to 10 days at the end of each cycle to balance an absolute or relative excess of estrogen. Tamoxifen (Nolvadex), an antiestrogen, may be prescribed to reduce the estrogen effects and restore the balance with progesterone. Danazol (Danocrine) is a pituitary gonadotropin inhibitory drug that has been successful in about 80% of women if taken over a period of several months, although the pain often returns after therapy ends.

Complementary/Alternative Therapy

Evening primrose oil, 250 to 500 mg/day, is a botanical preparation that has been beneficial in reducing cyclic breast pain (Fontaine, 2000; Johnston, 2000).

Although controversy exists about whether caffeine contributes to the development of fibrocystic breast changes, some physicians and nurse practitioners recommend limiting consumption of tea, coffee, colas, and chocolate. Some women benefit from a diuretic and restricting sodium intake to reduce fluid retention the week before menstruation starts, when symptoms are often most acute.

Ductal Ectasia

Ductal ectasia generally occurs as the woman approaches menopause. It is characterized by dilation of the collecting ducts that become distended and filled with cellular debris. This initiates an inflammatory process resulting in

- A mass that feels firm and irregular
- Enlarged axillary nodes
- Nipple retraction and discharge

These signs are similar to those of breast cancer, and accurate diagnosis is vital. Once a surgical biopsy confirms that the condition is benign mammary duct ectasia, no further treatment is necessary.

Intraductal Papilloma

Intraductal papilloma develops most often just before or during menopause. It occurs when papillomas (small elevations or protuberances) develop in the epithelium of the ducts of the breasts. Most lesions are located under the areola. As the papilloma grows, it causes trauma and erosion within the ducts that result in serous or bloody discharge from the nipple. Ultrasonography and diagnostic mammography aid in the diagnosis of the intraductal papilloma. Treatment consists of excision of the mass and ductal area, plus analysis of nipple discharge to rule out a malignant tumor. Long-term follow-up is essential to identify any malignancy early.

Diagnosis of Disorders of the Breast

When a lesion or lump is discovered in the breast, the physician must determine if it is benign or malignant. *Ultrasound* examination can be used to differentiate fluid-filled cysts from solid tissue that is more likely to be malignant. *Fine needle aspiration biopsy* can be performed to remove fluid or small tissue fragments for analysis of the cells. *Core needle biopsy* uses a larger needle to obtain a cylinder of tissue from an area of abnormal breast tissue. *Open, or surgical, biopsy* is performed under these conditions to remove all or part of the lump of breast tissue:

- Suspicious mass that persists through a menstrual cycle
- Bloody fluid aspirated from a cyst
- Failure of the mass to disappear completely after fluid aspiration
- Recurrence of the cyst after one or two aspirations
- Solid dominant mass not diagnosed as fibroadenoma
- Serous or serosanguineous nipple discharge
- Nipple ulceration or persistent crusting
- Skin edema and erythema suspicious for inflammatory breast carcinoma
- Suspicious mammography findings

Nursing Considerations

The nurse must acknowledge the anxiety that all women feel when a breast disorder is discovered. Furthermore, the apprehension continues for most women while they await a final diagnosis. Some women may find it helpful to learn that most breast disorders are benign. However, as discussed, some benign disorders do increase the risk for later occurrence of cancer. For others, the most helpful intervention is to encourage them to express their concerns.

The nurse should explain the diagnostic procedures that are planned, such as ultrasound examination, mammography, needle biopsy, or surgical biopsy. Explanations should include what the procedures entail and how long the woman will have to wait for results to be known. The woman's anxiety may be high and she will likely need reinforcement of explanations that she has forgotten.

Check Your Reading

8. How are fibrocystic breast changes treated?
9. What four diagnostic procedures are used to determine whether a breast disorder is benign or malignant?

MALIGNANT TUMORS OF THE BREAST

Incidence

A woman's risk of developing breast cancer anytime in her lifetime in the United States is one in eight, or about 12.6%. The risk is not equal at all ages, however, but rises significantly after age 50. Conditional age-specific probabilities are more useful than lifetime probabilities. For example, a 50-year-old black woman without breast cancer has a 2.4% chance of developing the disease by age 60 (National Cancer Institute, 2000). The estimated number of new cases of invasive breast cancer was 175,000 in 1999, with 43,000 deaths in women from breast cancer. Although the disease is much less common in men, 1300 cases of male breast cancer and 400 deaths were estimated during the same period. Cancer of the breast is second only to lung cancer as a cause of death from cancer among women (American Cancer Society, 2000a).

Risk Factors

Although the actual cause of breast cancer remains unknown, several factors are known to increase the risk for the development of breast cancer (Table 33-4). Two genes (BRCA1 and BRCA2), thought to be responsible for the majority of cases of familial breast cancer, have been identified.

Although risk factors are important, many women who do not fit into any high-risk category develop breast cancer. Therefore all women, not only those at high risk, should use the available screening procedures.

Table 33-4

RISK FACTORS FOR BREAST CANCER

Female
Age older than 50 yr
Mutations in the BRCA1 and BRCA2 genes; mutations in the p53 tumor suppressor gene
Personal history of breast cancer
Family history in first-degree relatives (mother, sister, daughter)
White race (African Americans are more likely to die of breast cancer because they are often diagnosed later)
Previous irradiation of the chest area as a child or young woman as treatment for another cancer (such as Hodgkin's disease or non-Hodgkin's lymphoma)
Breast biopsy results:

- Atypical hyperplasia increases the risk 4 to 5 times
- Proliferative breast disease without atypical cells or usual hyperplasia increases the risk 1.5 to 2 times
- Fibrocystic changes without proliferative changes does not change breast cancer risk

Nulliparity or first pregnancy after 30 yr
Early menarche (<12 yr), late menopause (>50 yr)
Possibly hormone replacement therapy when progesterone is prescribed as part of the replacement
Lifestyle factors: high intake of dietary fat, excessive consumption of alcohol, possibly physical inactivity

Data from American Cancer Society. (2000). *Breast cancer resource center.* See www.cancer.org.

Pathophysiology

About 80% of breast cancer is infiltrating ductal carcinoma, which originates in the epithelial lining of the mammary ducts. The cancer becomes invasive when it is no longer confined to the duct and spreads to surrounding breast tissue. Growth occurs in irregular patterns and invades the lymphatic channels, eventually causing lymphatic edema and the dimpling of the skin that resembles an orange peel (peau d'orange).

Cancer cells are carried by the lymph channels to the lymph nodes, and 40% to 50% of patients have involvement of axillary lymph nodes at the time of diagnosis. By the time a patient consults a physician, breast cancer is often already a systemic disease rather than being confined to the local tissue (Hacker, 1998). Metastasis occurs when the malignant cells are spread by both blood and lymph systems to distant organs. The most common sites of metastasis are the lungs, liver, and bones.

Staging

Although confirmation of malignancy is the first step in evaluating the woman with cancer, staging is necessary to understand the severity of the cancer. Staging is generally based on the TNM (tumor, node, metastasis) system used to describe the cancer's anatomic extent. Stages of breast cancer progress from stage 1, indicating a small tumor without lymphatic involvement or metastases, to stage 4, which indicates spread to lymph nodes and metastases to other organs. The stages are used to guide treatment and help provide a prognosis. The type of cancer cell, the presence of hormone receptors, and the proliferative rate of the breast cancer cells are also important factors in the rate of recurrence and determination of most appropriate treatment.

Management

Many new treatments have emerged over the last decade. Radical procedures now receive less emphasis, and a combination of surgical excision of the tumor and adjuvant therapy is often recommended.

Surgical Treatment

The surgical procedure depends on the type, stage, and location of the disease. The most common surgeries are the following:

- *Breast conservation treatment,* which involves wide local excision (sometimes called *lumpectomy* or *quadrantectomy*) of the tumor to microscopically clean margins for tumors that are small relative to the breast size. Some axillary lymph nodes are removed to determine spread of the disease. Radiation or other adjuvant therapy is indicated to complete the treatment.

- *Simple mastectomy,* which is removal of the entire breast. Axillary dissection is omitted, although some lymph nodes may be removed for staging purposes. It may be recommended for selected cases in which prophylactic removal of the breast is considered when a woman is at high risk for development of breast cancer. Simple mastectomy does not eradicate the risk for breast cancer, however, because a small amount of breast tissue remains. The woman will need regular mammography follow-up for the residual breast tissue (Johnston, 2000).
- *Modified radical mastectomy,* which involves removal of breast tissue, axillary nodes, and some chest muscles; however, the pectoralis major muscle is preserved. This surgical procedure may be recommended when a large primary lesion is found in a relatively small breast, other cosmetic limitations of a conservative procedure, if radiation therapy is contraindicated, to avoid local recurrence of the cancer, or as prophylaxis for patients at high risk (Smith, 1999).

Sentinel lymph node biopsy is a technique to remove only one or two key lymph nodes to evaluate cancer spread rather than removing most of the nodes in the area (axillary dissection). A radioactive suspension or a special dye is injected near the tumor site, where it is transported by the lymphatics toward the axillary nodes and trapped by the first one or two lymph nodes, or the "sentinel" nodes. The surgeon uses a modified Geiger counter or sees the dye while still in the operating room to identify the sentinel node or nodes, which are then excised for examination. If cancer has not spread to this sentinel node, the surgeon does not have to remove a large number of lymph nodes for staging of the cancer. Reducing the number of lymph nodes removed helps avoid some of the problems caused by lymphedema (see discussion later in chapter). Studies are underway to establish the most appropriate patients for the sentinel lymph node biopsy and the amount of surgical experience necessary for this technique to be accurate (American Cancer Society, 2000a).

Adjuvant Therapy

Adjuvant therapy is supportive or additional therapy that may be recommended after the surgical procedure. Radiation, chemotherapy, hormone therapy, and immunotherapy are adjuvant therapies that are often recommended. The decision about whether to use adjuvant therapy is based on the woman's age, the stage of the disease, the woman's preference, and the hormone receptor status of the lesion. Radiation and chemotherapy are known to improve the chance of long-term survival, and one or the both are usually recommended after surgical excision of the tumor. For a more in-depth discussion of cancer treatment, see a medical-surgical nursing text.

Radiation Therapy

Radiation uses high-energy rays to destroy cancer cells that remain in the breast, the chest wall, and the underarm area after surgery. It may be used occasionally to reduce the size of a large tumor before surgery. The lymph nodes above the clavicle and the internal mammary lymph nodes are also irradiated as well. The skin in the treated area may have a reaction similar to sunburn. Lymphedema (see p. 933) is more likely to occur if the axillary lymph nodes are treated.

Chemotherapy

Chemotherapy is considered standard for premenopausal patients and for those with lymph node involvement of their cancer. A combination of drugs such as cyclophosphamide, methotrexate, and 5-fluorouracil is given. Chemotherapy drugs are designed to kill the proliferating cancer cells. However, these medications also kill normal cells, especially rapidly dividing cells such those in the mucosa, the blood cells, and the platelets. For this reason, the woman may have sore, bleeding gums or other bleeding tendencies and be more susceptible to infection during treatment. Many chemotherapeutic drugs cause hair loss (head and body hair) or menstrual irregularities during treatment. Anemia, with resulting fatigue, is common because erythrocyte production is impaired.

Hormonal Therapy

Estrogen-blocking medications are prescribed because some tumors are estrogen receptor–positive, meaning that their growth is stimulated by estrogen. Tamoxifen (Nolvadex) is currently the hormone therapy most recommended. Tamoxifen blocks estrogen by binding to estrogen receptors, thereby suppressing tumor growth by reducing the effects of estrogen. It is taken daily for 5 years.

Side effects of tamoxifen vary from woman to woman. The most commonly mentioned side effects are hot flashes, vaginal dryness or increased vaginal discharge, nausea, and anorexia. A recent finding indicates that the risk of endometrial cancer is increased for women taking tamoxifen (Kiebeck & Beller, 2000). Laboratory values for cholesterol and triglycerides may also increase. All side effects should be discussed with the woman before tamoxifen is administered so that she can weigh the risks and benefits.

Raloxifene (Evista) is an estrogen modifier prescribed to reduce osteoporosis. Because its action is to block the effect of estrogen in the breast, it is being tested to determine if it can reduce a woman's chance of developing breast cancer. Raloxifene has cardiovascular benefits: it lowers low-density lipoproteins and cholesterol. It has not had sufficient testing to determine if it is therapeutic for women who have been diagnosed with breast cancer (American Cancer Society, 2000a; Johnston, 2000).

Other hormonal therapies may be used in advanced breast cancer that has metastasized, such as toremifene (Fareston), an antiestrogen drug, and anastrozole (Arimidex), a drug that inhibits an enzyme in estrogen production, or letrozole (Femara), a drug that inhibits conversion of androgens to estrogens.

Immunotherapy

Trastuzumab (Herceptin), is the first monoclonal antibody therapy approved for breast cancer. Some tumors produce excessive amounts of the HER-2 protein, which is important in regulation of cancer cell growth. Trastuzumab blocks the effect of this protein to inhibit growth of the cancer cells. Research is ongoing into other immunotherapy for breast and other cancers.

Breast Reconstruction

Timing. Breast reconstruction is a standard option in the treatment of breast cancer, and the timing of reconstruction should be discussed with the woman before surgical treatment. Immediate reconstruction has a psychological appeal. The prospect of having a life-threatening breast cancer and simultaneously facing the loss of a breast may be overwhelming for many women. Conversely, delayed reconstruction may give a woman time to learn about the procedure, to heal from the mastectomy, and to consider the extent of the disease and the side effects associated with adjuvant therapy.

Method. Several methods of breast reconstruction are available. The *tissue expansion method* uses an empty silicone prosthesis fitted with a valve that can be accessed by percutaneous needle puncture. The bag is filled with saline in small increments to slowly expand the tissue. When the desired volume is attained, the incision is reopened, the device is removed, and the expander is exchanged for the appropriate implant. In some models, only the valve must be removed, and the expander serves as the permanent implant (American Cancer Society, 2000a).

Muscle flap grafts move autogenous tissue from the back, abdomen, or buttocks to create a breast mound. Although these procedures do not involve implants of a foreign substance as the tissue expansion method does, they involve at least two incisions: one at the breast and one at the site of the donor tissue. All women are not suitable for muscle flap grafts, particularly those with diabetes, connective tissue disorders, or smokers because these procedures involve altering the blood supply to the transplanted tissue with the possibility of poor wound healing for these women (American Cancer Society, 2000a; Wagner & Ruth-Sahd, 2000).

Nipple-Areola Reconstruction. The nipple can be reconstructed in a variety of ways. Tissue may be taken from the opposite nipple, from skin that covers the prosthesis mound, or from other body tissue. After the nipple has been reconstructed, the plastic surgeon may inject pigment into the area to create an areola.

Psychosocial Consequences of Breast Cancer

The time from discovery to treatment of breast cancer is the most stressful time for many women. Factors that contribute to presurgery distress include a sense of uncertainty, incomplete information, the need to make difficult treatment decisions, and scheduling problems. Treatment usually involves consultations with several specialists, including a surgeon, a radiotherapist, a plastic surgeon, and a medical oncologist. Scheduling difficulties arise when women must travel significant distances for treatment. Members of the health care team may express conflicting opinions. This results in frustration and confusion for the woman and often leads to additional consultations.

Concerns frequently expressed during treatment for breast cancer include fear of death, uncertainty about the quality of life, changes in body image, the effect on sexuality, and side effects of recommended therapy. For most women, the knowledge that they will lose their hair as a result of chemotherapy creates one of the most difficult situations in therapy, adding yet another assault on their body image.

Breast cancer has psychological consequences for women and their husbands, significant others, and other family members. Difficulties reported include sleep disturbances, eating disorders, and problems with work responsibilities. Breast cancer can create strain on the marital relationship, primarily in the areas of sexual relations and communication about matters related to the illness. Women and their partners sometimes differ in regard to how much they want to discuss the illness. Some women have a great need to discuss their diagnosis, treatment, and fears of recurrence. Other women and many men view discussion of such fears as negative thinking that delays adjustment.

Nursing Considerations

The woman who is diagnosed with breast cancer depends on the nurse for emotional support and accurate information. The woman needs time to express her feelings and the nurse must convey a sense of empathetic understanding by quiet presence, touch, and close attention to the woman's concerns. Many women feel that they have lost control and that their lives have been taken over by cancer and the recommended treatment. Some women are concerned about family relationships, and, as indicated earlier, how their sexual partner will respond. Each woman should be allowed to express her fears and worries. In addition to providing time and demonstrating genuine interest in the woman's concerns, use communication techniques, such as clarifying, paraphrasing, and reflecting feelings, so that the woman can participate in decisions about her care.

Most women experience a reduction in anxiety with a clear understanding of procedures and care. Preoperative teaching is often part of the nurse's responsibility, and husbands and significant others should be included as much as possible in the teaching. Many women are relieved to learn that the hospital stay is short after mastectomy, and they may be relieved by knowing exactly what to expect. For instance, a pressure dressing may be applied over the wound to prevent further bleeding after surgery. Drainage tubes may be attached to portable suction apparatus (Hemovac or Jackson-Pratt drains) to prevent accumulation of fluid under the skin flaps. The incision may appear red and raised for the first few weeks. Lymphedema of the arm on the same side as the mastectomy is possible as a result of lymphedema. Specific exercises such as armlifts and pulley exercises may be necessary. Compression armsleeves, similar to TED hose, can be ordered if needed.

Discharge teaching focuses on the need for follow-up care and treatment. Some areas of concern include how to reduce the risk of wound infection, care of the arm on the affected side, side effects of adjuvant therapy, and signs and symptoms that should be reported to the physician. If she will be discharged with the drains in place, she should be taught how to empty them.

Most women also benefit from information about such groups as Reach to Recovery and Encore, which provide support, information, and guidance following mastectomy. Many surgeons ask for a Reach to Recovery volunteer to visit the woman before she leaves the hospital.

Relevant nursing diagnoses may include the following:

- Fear of death or pain
- Body image disturbance related to loss of breast and temporary loss of hair during chemotherapy
- Altered family processes related to illness of primary caregiver or lack of information about the course of the disease
- Altered sexuality patterns related to concern about changed body structure or discomfort with intercourse secondary to chemotherapy effects

Check Your Reading

10. What are the major risk factors for breast cancer?
11. Why is staging for breast cancer important?
12. What is meant by adjuvant therapy, and why is it used?
13. How and when may breasts be reconstructed following mastectomy?
14. What should preoperative teaching include?
15. What should discharge planning emphasize?

Cardiovascular Disease

Cardiovascular diseases include disorders of the heart and blood vessels, such as myocardial infarction, congenital abnormalities, and stroke. Those discussed here primarily relate to diseases of the blood vessels, particularly coronary artery disease (CAD). The topic is extensive and only an overview will be presented in this text. A medical-surgical text should be consulted for more extensive information.

Although most women fear dying from cancer, often breast cancer, cardiovascular disease is the leading cause of death in women after age 50. Almost twice as many U.S. women die of heart disease and stroke as from all forms of cancer, including breast cancer. Most people tend to think of heart and other blood vessel diseases as a male problem. Yet in 1997, 43.7% of the deaths of white women were from cardiovascular diseases while only 22.3% of their deaths were from any type of cancer. Women have heart attacks, or myocardial infarctions (MIs), when they are older than men, and they are more likely to die from them: 42% of women die from heart attacks compared to 24% of men. Women have less favorable outcomes after therapeutic procedures. Black women are affected more frequently than white women by all types of cardiovascular disease (American Heart Association, 2000h & 2000i; AWHONN, 1999c).

Recognition of Coronary Artery Disease

Women are more likely to die from a myocardial infarction than men. In part, this is because they are older and may have other complicating diseases, but it also happens because the MI tends to present with atypical, vague symptoms that can delay recognition and treatment. The classic crushing or stabbing chest pain or pressure in the chest is not the usual presentation in women as it is with men. Some of the symptoms of CAD in women include the following (Mosca, et al., 1997; Halm & Penque, 1999; AWHONN, 1999c):

- Fatigue, weakness
- Angina (chest pain with exertion) or pain at rest
- Dyspnea, sometimes paroxysmal nocturnal dyspnea
- Dizziness, faintness
- Upper abdominal pain, heartburn, loss of appetite
- Nausea, vomiting, sweating
- Pain in the upper body, but other than the chest (arm, neck, back, jaw, throat, teeth)

Because the pain is often atypical, the woman may not consider heart attack as a possibility. Caregivers must be aware that the woman's symptoms could be cardiac-related. For example, a dentist must consider that a woman with a toothache but no apparent tooth disease could have a cardiac ischemia and an MI.

Risk Factors

Several risk factors increase the woman's chances for developing cardiovascular disease. Risk factors may be fixed, or unmodifiable, or may be factors that can be changed. Aging is a major risk factor because the woman loses the protection that estrogen, secreted before menopause, exerts on the blood vessels unless she takes estrogen replacement. Estrogen's protective effect delays onset of cardiovascular disease, making most women older at the onset of the disease than men. Other risk factors are listed in Table 33-5 and are similar to those for men (Mosca, et al., 1997). Several risk factors deserve added discussion.

The leading preventable cause of CAD and other diseases in women is smoking. Cigarette smoking is increasing among young women and is expected to exceed that of men in 2000, adding to the burden of heart, blood vessel, respiratory, cancers, and many other diseases in females (Mosca, et al., 1997).

Table 33-5

RISK FACTORS FOR CORONARY ARTERY DISEASE IN WOMEN

Cigarette smoking
Hypertension (including isolated systolic hypertension)
Dyslipidemia:
- Elevated total cholesterol (normal: <200 mg/dL; borderline: 200-239 mg/dL; elevated: >240 mg/dL)
- Low level of high-density lipoprotein (HDL) cholesterol: <35 mg/dL
- Cholesterol ratio: The ratio of cholesterol to HDL cholesterol may be used instead of total blood cholesterol. The goal is to keep the ratio lower than 5 (total cholesterol): 1 (HDL cholesterol), with an optimum ratio of 3.5 to 1.
- Elevated triglyceride levels may be a risk factor, although the role of this plasma lipid in contributing to cardiovascular disease has not been fully determined

Possibly elevated homocysteine levels
Diabetes mellitus
Obesity
Sedentary lifestyle
Poor nutrition
Post-menopause status, without estrogen replacement
Family history of coronary artery disease

Data from Mosca, et al. (2000). Cardiovascular disease in women, *Circulation,* 96(7), 2468-2482; AWHONN. (1999). *Monograph I: Postmenopausal health risks and the importance of prevention.*

WOMEN WANT TO KNOW *Reducing the Risk for Coronary Artery Disease*

- Stop smoking. Your risk begins to decrease within a few months of stopping and reaches the level of a person who has never smoked within 3 to 5 years. Stopping also reduces your risk for lung cancer and many other respiratory diseases.
- Maintain a normal weight. Your risk is much higher if your weight is 30% or more than your ideal weight. See your health care provider about an ideal weight management plan, which usually includes a balanced diet and moderate exercise to lose weight gradually.
- Eat right. A variety of fruits, vegetables, grains, low-fat or nonfat dairy products, fish, legumes, poultry, and lean meats provides a basic healthy eating pattern. Substitute unsaturated fat from vegetables, fish, legumes, and nuts for foods high in saturated fats and cholesterol. Limit salt to less than 6 grams per day.
- Limit alcohol to 1 drink per day if you are a woman. Do not drink when pregnant or trying to become pregnant to avoid fetal alcohol syndrome and do not drink when breastfeeding.
- Control high blood pressure. Even modest blood pressure elevations can be deadly, causing heart attack and stroke. Measures to reduce your blood pressure include weight reduction, exercise, diet improvement, and stress management. If your physician prescribes drugs to control your blood pressure, take them faithfully, even if you feel fine. Let the doctor know if you are having problems with your drugs for high blood pressure–a change in the drug may be possible.
- Exercise. Aerobic exercise helps reduce your blood pressure, control your weight, and keep your blood glucose levels normal. Resistance and weight-bearing exercise also helps slow osteoporosis. You need at least 30 minutes of moderate-intensity exercise 3 to 4 days each week (American Heart Association, 2000).
- Control diabetes. Diabetes in a woman cancels many of estrogen's protective benefits, so you must work harder to control your diabetes as well as your cardiovascular risks.
- Consider taking hormone replacement therapy (HRT, or estrogen) after menopause. Taking estrogen after menopause continues its protective benefits on the cardiovascular system. Not every woman can take estrogen, however.
- To learn more about cardiovascular disease and its prevention, visit these web sites: American Heart Association: www.americanheart.org, and American Dietetic Association: www.eatright.org.

Both systolic and diastolic blood pressure elevations are associated with coronary artery disease. Older women (more than 65 years) have an increased risk from isolated systolic hypertension, not only sustained hypertension (Mosca, et al., 1997). Adequate control of hypertension reduces death and disability from myocardial infarction, stroke, and other blood vessel disorders.

Diabetes increases the risk for CAD in women as it does in men, but the increase in risk is greater. Diabetes is such a strong risk factor for coronary artery disease that its presence nearly eliminates the protective effects of estrogen for the premenopausal woman (AWHONN, 1999c; Mosca, et al., 1997).

Inadequate exercise contributes to many of the risk factors listed. Overweight and obesity are more likely when a person is sedentary, and these weight problems increase the likelihood that diabetes and hypertension will occur. Dyslipidemia is more likely in both women and men who do not get adequate exercise, adding further to the risk.

Prevention

Prevention is the key to reducing the death and illness from all cardiovascular diseases among women. Much of prevention includes modification of risk factors that can be changed. In addition to these factors, hormone replacement therapy (p. 945) is another important preventive measure for CAD and other diseases.

Hypertension. Lowering hypertension, including isolated systolic hypertension in older women, to levels lower than 140 mmHg systolic and lower than 90 mmHg diastolic reduces the risk of CAD and stroke. Even borderline hypertension is now known to be dangerous. Medication should be considered if regular aerobic exercise, weight reduction, improved nutrition, and stress management do not lower the blood pressure adequately (Halm & Penque, 1999).

Smoking Cessation. Stopping smoking may cause women to gain weight, but smoking cessation has a positive effect on reducing angina and stopping the progression of CAD. Stopping smoking also reduces the risk for lung cancer, the number one cancer in women. Improvement in other respiratory conditions is likely as well.

Diet and Glucose Control. Women with diabetes have a relatively greater risk for CAD than men, so maintaining weight and glucose within normal limits is especially important. Diet is the primary means to control the lipid profile. Diet recommendations should be individualized, but general guidelines are that fat intake should be a maximum of 30% of daily calories, and saturated fat (found in foods like meat, butter, cream, and cheese) make up no more than 10% of daily calories. Cholesterol intake should be maintained lower than 300 mg/day. Increased evidence shows that fish, especially fatty fish, confers cardiovascular benefits, and at least 2 servings per week are recommended. A diet high in vegetables, fruits, and low-fat dairy products and limiting salt intake to under 6 g per day and alcohol to a maximum of 1 drink per day for women has shown to be beneficial at reducing blood pressure (Krauss, et al., 2000).

Increased Activity. Aerobic exercise helps control weight, blood pressure, and glucose. It reduces body fat while increasing muscle mass and improving muscle tone. At least one-half hour of aerobic exercise, such as a brisk walk, 3 to 4 times per week can reduce serum cholesterol and improve the lipid profile (American Heart Association, 2000e; AWHONN, 1999a & 1999c). Exercise also helps manage stress, another contributor to CAD.

Aspirin. The American Heart Association recommends that women who have had an MI, unstable angina, stroke, or a transient ischemic attack (TIA, often called "little stroke") take aspirin, 80 to 325 mg per day, after consultation with her physician. Aspirin reduces the risk of recurrence for some cardiovascular disorders because it inhibits platelet aggregation. However, aspirin's pharmacologic action also increases vulnerability to bleeding problems such as gastrointestinal bleeding or hemorrhagic stroke. Therefore each woman should consult her physician about whether aspirin therapy is right for her. It has not yet been established whether aspirin is desirable for primary prevention of MI (before the first occurrence) in women as it has been in men, but this may soon be determined (American Heart Association, 2000a).

Check Your Reading

16. What are the symptoms of coronary artery disease, such as a myocardial infarction, in a woman?
17. List appropriate measures to reduce the risk for coronary artery disease.

MENSTRUAL CYCLE DISORDERS

The four most common menstrual cycle disorders are absence of menses (amenorrhea), abnormal uterine bleeding, pain associated with the menstrual cycle, and cyclic mood changes, including premenstrual syndrome. Although most of the disorders are benign, all require comprehensive gynecologic assessment. Nurses must be knowledgeable about underlying processes, diagnostic procedures, and expected treatment in order to fulfill the basic core of nursing activities, which include client advocacy, education, and supportive counseling.

Amenorrhea

Amenorrhea is a symptom that can indicate either normal physiologic processes or pathology in the reproductive system. Amenorrhea before menarche, during pregnancy, during the puerperium and lactation, and following menopause is normal. Amenorrhea at other times is abnormal, and it is called either *primary* or *secondary amenorrhea,* depending on when it occurs.

Primary Amenorrhea

Menstrual periods should begin within 2 years of breast development, usually between ages 10 and 16 (Riddick, 2000). Lack of breast development or other secondary sexual development or a shortened growth spurt in addition to the absence of menstruation provides additional diagnostic clues. The causes for primary amenorrhea may be genetic (ovarian failure), systemic, or may involve anomalies of the reproductive tract.

Ovarian failure may occur in girls who have Turner's syndrome, in which only one of the normal two X chromosomes is present. They have a total of 45 chromosomes, with a single X chromosome. Chemotherapy or radiation therapy may cause premature ovarian failure, which may or may not be permanent.

A common systemic cause of primary amenorrhea is low body weight for height. This may occur in competitive athletes and dancers but also occurs in girls with eating disorders, such as anorexia nervosa, who have a very low body weight. If the girl began sexual development and then restricted calories (or began an intense exercise program), her sexual development may be arrested at the point of the calorie restriction (Riddick, 2000). Other systemic causes of primary amenorrhea include chronic stress, hypothyroidism, Cushing's disease, central nervous system diseases, and drug use (Blackwell & Farah, 2000).

Abnormalities in the uterus, vagina, or hymen can obstruct the outflow of the menstrual flow. Congenital enzyme abnormalities may disable different aspects of the reproductive cycle.

The condition causes a great deal of concern for the young woman and her family. Amenorrhea is a symptom, not a diagnosis, and they may worry that it indicates a serious disease. Menstruation is a unique function of women, and absence of menstruation may provoke concerns about femininity and the ability to have children. Concern increases if medical treatment is not successful.

Medical management depends on the cause. Counseling for eating disorders, such as anorexia nervosa, and reducing excessive exercise to allow adequate weight gain may prove helpful. Hormone therapy may establish normal menses if the cause is hormone imbalance. However, some conditions cannot be successfully treated. For example, if the cause is reproductive tract or congenital anomalies, normal menses and fertility may not be possible, and psychological support becomes the most important therapy.

Secondary Amenorrhea

Secondary amenorrhea is the cessation of menstruation for a period of at least three cycles or 6 months in a woman who has established a pattern of menstruation (Kim, 2000). The most common cause is pregnancy. Other causes include systemic diseases such as diabetes mellitus, tuberculosis, and hypothyroidism. Hormonal imbalances, low weight for height, stress, systemic illness, poor nutrition, use of oral contraceptives or antidepressants, and tumors of the ovary, pituitary, or adrenal gland also may be the cause.

Assessment includes a thorough medical and obstetric history and questions about eating habits, history of dieting, and current exercise pattern. Women are also questioned about their uses of drugs, such as oral contraceptives, phenothiazines, and antihypertensives, which can cause secondary amenorrhea.

Medical treatment aims at identifying and correcting the underlying cause after ruling out pregnancy and determining if the woman wants children. Clomiphene citrate (Clomid, see Drug Guide, p. 907) may be given to induce ovulation if the woman's estrogen levels are normal and she wants to conceive. Progestin or oral contraceptives prevent hyperplasia of her endometrium if she does not want children (Kim, 2000).

She will need treatment of the underlying problem (such as anorexia) if her estrogen levels are low and she wants children. If she does not want children, estrogen-progestin replacement helps delay some of the estrogen deficiency effects on bone density, blood vessels, and vaginal mucosa.

Bromocriptine (Parlodel) may be prescribed if elevated prolactin levels are the problem.

Abnormal Uterine Bleeding

The normal menstrual cycle was described in Chapter 4. Abnormal bleeding is bleeding that occurs with abnormal frequency, lasts an abnormal length of time, occurs irregularly, or is excessive in amount. Most abnormal bleeding occurs in cycles without ovulation, often near puberty and perimenopause (McGovern & Little, 2000). Complications of an unrecognized pregnancy, such as spontaneous abortion, must be considered when making the diagnosis.

Etiology

The most common causes of abnormal bleeding fall into five basic categories:

1. Pregnancy complications, such as spontaneous abortion
2. Anatomic lesions, either benign or malignant, of the vagina, cervix, or uterus
3. Drug-induced bleeding, such as "breakthrough" bleeding that may occur in women who are on some oral contraceptives, or who have progestin implants, such as Norplant
4. Systemic disorders, such as diabetes mellitus, uterine myomas (fibroids), and hypothyroidism
5. Failure to ovulate (dysfunctional uterine bleeding)

Management

Evaluation of abnormal uterine bleeding may include a sensitive pregnancy test, coagulation studies, and tests to determine whether ovulation is occurring (see Procedure 32-1). Hormone and liver function tests, plus tests to determine if the woman is anemic will often be done. Ultrasonography or hysteroscopy may be used to look for polyps and check the condition of the uterine lining.

A common hormone treatment is progestin-estrogen combination oral contraceptives that suppress ovulation and allow a more stable endometrial lining to form. Surgical therapy may include dilation and curettage (D&C) to remove polyps or to diagnose endometrial hyperplasia, which may be treated with progesterone that will suppress the excess uterine lining. Hysterectomy may be performed if the uterus is enlarged as a result of fibroids or adenomyosis (benign invasive growth of the endometrium into the muscular layer of the uterus) and if the woman does not want more children. Laser ablation may be used to permanently remove the endometrial lining without hysterectomy.

Prolonged menorrhagia may result in decreased hemoglobin, and the woman may need treatment for iron-deficiency anemia.

Nursing Considerations

Nurses are often responsible for encouraging women to seek medical attention promptly when irregular or prolonged bleeding occurs. Nurses also help the woman keep a record of the bleeding episodes and the amount of blood lost. This involves keeping a calendar and noting any vaginal bleeding (spotting, menses) that occurs in addition to the number of pads and tampons saturated each day.

The nurse teaches the importance of adequate nutrition and discourages rigorous dieting. For women who are concerned about amenorrhea, the nurse should explain that, although exercise is beneficial, excess workouts or aerobic training can cause amenorrhea. In addition, the nurse teaches methods to reduce stress and promote relaxation. Finally, nurses must provide support for women who fear that irregular bleeding indicates a serious disease, such as cancer. Offering false reassurance is unwise, but information about diagnostic procedures, such as pelvic examinations, Pap test, and other tests is helpful.

Check Your Reading

18. How does primary amenorrhea differ from secondary amenorrhea in terms of onset, cause, and treatment?
19. What are possible causes of abnormal uterine bleeding, and why should it not be ignored?

Cyclic Pelvic Pain

Cyclic pelvic pain must be distinguished from acute pelvic pain. Acute pelvic pain is sudden in onset and is not experienced with each menstrual cycle. It may indicate a serious disorder, such as ectopic pregnancy or appendicitis. On the other hand, cyclic pelvic pain occurs repetitively and predictably in a specific phase of the menstrual cycle. The most common causes of cyclic pelvic pain are mittelschmerz, primary dysmenorrhea, and endometriosis.

Mittelschmerz

Mittelschmerz ("middle" pain) refers to pelvic pain that occurs midway between menstrual periods, or at the time of ovulation. The pain is due to growth of the dominant follicle within the ovary or rupture of the follicle and subsequent spillage of follicular fluid and blood into the peritoneal space. The pain is fairly sharp and is felt on the right or left side of the pelvis. It generally lasts from a few hours to 2 days, and slight vaginal bleeding may accompany the discomfort. Generally, women do not need medical treatment beyond simple explanation of the discomfort or mild analgesics.

Primary Dysmenorrhea

Primary dysmenorrhea refers to menstrual pain without identified pathology. Commonly called "cramps," primary dysmenorrhea affects as many as half of all young women and causes 10% to miss work or school (Dawood, 2000). The pain begins within hours of the onset of menses, and it is spasmodic or colicky in nature. It is felt in the lower abdomen but often radiates to the lower back or down the legs. Primary dysmenorrhea occurs in ovulatory cycles, and it is most common in young nulliparous women. The duration of the pain is usually 48 to 72 hours.

Current evidence suggests that some women produce excessive endometrial prostaglandin during menstruation. Prostaglandins (particularly E2) diffuse into endometrial tissue and cause abnormal uterine muscle contractions, uterine ischemia, hypoxia, and greater sensitivity of the pain fibers from the pelvis. This process accounts for the cramp-like uterine pain and symptoms that often accompany it, such as low back pain, fatigue, diarrhea, nausea, and vomiting. Some women also may have increased vasopressin release, which could cause abnormal uterine activity (Dawood, 2000).

Two recommended treatments of primary dysmenorrhea provide marked relief: oral contraceptives and prostaglandin inhibitors. Oral contraceptives decrease the amount of endometrial growth that occurs during the menstrual cycle and thus reduce the production of endometrial prostaglandin. For women who do not wish to take oral contraceptives, prostaglandin inhibitors offer relief. The most effective prostaglandin inhibitors are NSAIDs such as ibuprofen (Motrin, Advil) and naproxen (Naprosyn, Anaprox). To be effective, the NSAID should be taken around the clock for at least 48 to 72 hours beginning when menstrual flow starts. Nifedipine, a calcium channel blocker, is an investigational therapy that may help women who are not relieved by oral contraceptives and NSAIDs (Dawood, 2000).

Complementary/Alternative Therapy

For women who want to try nonmedical therapy or to reduce the medication dose, TENS (transcutaneous nerve stimulation) may be beneficial (Dawood, 2000). Herbal remedies such as black cohosh or blue cohosh, black haw, or valerian may help some women (Chavez & Chavez, 2000; Fontaine, 2000). Either type of cohosh should not be taken during pregnancy, however, and unrecognized pregnancy with an early bleeding complication is always a possibility. Cohosh should therefore be taken with medical supervision. Valerian should not be used with alcohol and it also has a bad odor. Herbal therapy typically requires a prolonged time to be effective and this must be considered when using it for a short-term, recurrent problem such as primary dysmenorrhea. Other alternative therapy that may be used for menstrual discomfort includes aromatherapy, yoga, and hydrotherapy.

Endometriosis

Pathophysiology. Endometriosis is defined as the presence outside the uterus of tissue that resembles the endometrium in both structure and function. The response of this tissue to the stimulation of estrogen and progesterone during the menstrual cycle is identical to that of the endometrial tissue. That is, it grows and proliferates during the follicular and luteal phases of the cycle and then sloughs during menstruation. The menstruation from endometriosis lesions, however, occurs in a closed cavity, which causes pressure and pain on adjacent tissue. In addition, prostaglandins secreted by the endometriosis lesions irritate nerve endings and stimulate uterine contractions that further increase pain. Cyclic bleeding into the pelvic cavity causes chronic inflammatory changes that may make conception and implantation difficult. The most common sites of endometriosis lesions are illustrated in Figure 33-3.

Although endometriosis occurs in 5% to 15% of all women, the cause remains unknown (Surrey, 2000). One theory is that menstrual discharge contains viable endometrial cells that can attach to sites outside the uterus, where they grow and produce patches of endometrial tissue. It is possible that the endometrial cells are disseminated primarily by retrograde menstruation, that is, reflux of menstrual flow through the fallopian tubes. The cells attach to nearby structures and proliferate, creating spots of endometrial tissue. Also endometriosis may represent an autoimmune process that has a genetic basis.

Signs and Symptoms. The two major problems associated with endometriosis are pain and infertility. The pain of endometriosis differs from that of primary dysmenorrhea. Endometriosis pain is deep, unilateral or bilateral, and either sharp or dull. It is constant, as opposed to the spasmodic or colicky pain of primary dysmenorrhea. Dyspareunia (painful intercourse) is common, particularly with deep penetration. Rectal pain is common, especially during defecation. Diarrhea, constipation, and sensations of rectal pressure or urgency are other symptoms of endometriosis. Although the cause of infertility is not completely understood, pelvic adhesions and tubal pathology because of chronic inflammatory changes are certainly contributing factors.

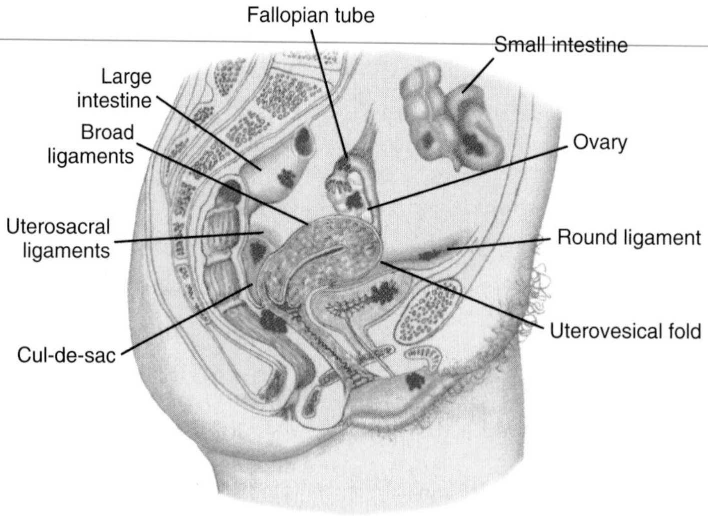

FIGURE 33-3 Common sites of endometriosis.

Management. Treatment may be either medical or surgical, and the therapy chosen must weigh the need for relief of pain and the desire to maintain fertility against the side effects that accompany many treatment regimens. Because growth of endometriosis depends on the production of ovarian hormones during the menstrual cycle, medical therapy is aimed at interrupting the menstrual cycle, thus leaving the woman in a state of "pseudomenopause." As a result, she experiences symptoms associated with estrogen deficit, such as hot flashes and vaginal dryness. In addition, she is at increased risk for postmenopausal conditions, such as adverse serum lipid changes and osteoporosis (see p. 948).

Oral contraceptives, medroxyprogesterone, and danazol are current therapies. Oral contraceptives are taken continuously rather than in the usual cyclic fashion, to induce a hormone state similar to pregnancy, which suppresses the endometrial tissue. The medroxyprogesterone has a similar effect. Danazol (Danocrine) causes atrophy of both the normal and ectopic endometrial tissue and also inhibits pituitary gonadotropic hormones. Side effects of danazol include headache, dizziness, irritability, and decreased libido. In addition, danazol often produces masculinizing effects, such as deepening of the voice, increased facial and body hair, and weight gain. These side effects limit danazol's acceptance for many women.

The GnRH agonists, such as leuprolide acetate (Lupron) and goserelin acetate (Zoladex), and nafarelin (Synarel), which may be administered by nasal spray, are newer alternatives that may be better accepted than danazol. Both danazol and GnRH agonists interfere with production of gonadotropins (follicle-stimulating hormone and luteinizing hormone) and thus stop the menstrual cycle, creating a "pseudomenopause." The most common side effects of GnRH agonists are hot flashes, vaginal dryness, decreased libido, and reversible loss of bone mineral density. New research has shown that it may be possible to give the GnRH agonists with low-dose estrogens without compromising the effectiveness of the GnRH agonists in the treatment of endometriosis (Surrey, 2000).

Pregnancy also interrupts menstruation, and if the woman wishes to conceive, she may be advised not to delay conception. If pregnancy is not an immediate option, continuous noncyclic oral contraceptives are sometimes recommended, although the effectiveness in treating symptoms of endometriosis is not well documented.

Surgical treatment can take many forms. For the older woman with severe pain who no longer wishes to have children, a hysterectomy with bilateral salpingo-oophorectomy (removal of the uterus, both fallopian tubes, and both ovaries) and excision of all lesions offers the greatest chance for cure. This surgery results in early menopause with permanent estrogen deficit. Postoperative hormone replacement therapy may be recommended if all lesions are removed. More conservative surgery includes laparoscopy for lysis of adhesions and laser vaporization of the lesions of endometriosis.

Nursing Considerations

Dysmenorrhea varies from mild "menstrual awareness" to incapacitating pain that affects the quality of life for several days out of each month. Too often the pain is belittled ("It's just cramps"). One of the most important nursing actions is to acknowledge the pain: "I understand this is really uncomfortable, and you are concerned that you have this much pain every month."

Complementary/Alternative Therapy

Women should be instructed in nonpharmacologic measures to relieve pain, such as frequent rest periods, application of heat to the lower abdomen, moderate exercise, and a well-balanced diet. If they want to try a herbal remedy, they should be advised to consult their healthcare provider for safety and effectiveness, particularly because the possibility of unrecognized pregnancy is always present.

The nurse should advise the woman to schedule stress-provoking situations so that they will not coincide with the menstrual period if possible. If nonsteroidal antiinflammatory drugs are recommended, these should be taken with meals to reduce gastrointestinal irritation. The woman should be counseled to report unusual side effects, such as headache, dizziness, or unusual fluid retention, to the physician or nurse practitioner.

The nurse must allow time for the woman to express her concerns about the therapy. She should be instructed to use a form of contraception other than oral contraceptives when medical therapy, such as GnRH or danazol, is used. Some women benefit from information about measures that promote sleep and relaxation, and, most importantly, from the knowledge that someone is available to provide support and guidance when needed.

Check Your Reading

20. What causes primary dysmenorrhea, and how may it be treated?
21. How does endometriosis cause dysmenorrhea, and how can it be treated?
22. What are the major side effects of danazol? Of the GnRH agonists?

Premenstrual Syndrome

Many women notice some minor physical and emotional changes related to their menstrual cycles. However, a few women have severe problems associated with these cyclic changes. Premenstrual syndrome (PMS), also called *premenstrual dysphoric disorder (PDD)* or *luteal phase dysphoric disorder (LPDD)*, may affect as many as 10% of women severely enough to cause significant disruption with their daily lives (Eden, 1998). The following criteria must be met for the condition to be diagnosed as premenstrual syndrome:

- The signs and symptoms must be cyclic and recur in the luteal phase (after ovulation) of the menstrual cycle.
- The woman should be symptom-free during the follicular phase (before ovulation) of the menstrual cycle, and the cycle must include 7 symptom-free days.
- Symptoms must be severe enough to have an impact on work, lifestyle, and relationships.
- Diagnosis should be based on *prospective* symptom charting by the woman, or charting of symptoms as they occur, rather than recall of symptoms that occurred in the past (Baram, 2000; ACOG, 2000).

Women who are on oral contraceptives, have chronic amenorrhea, or have undergone oophorectomy (removal of the ovaries) or who are menopausal do not have PMS because ovulation is a critical part of the syndrome (Baram, 2000). Some women who have medical or psychiatric disorders have an increased intensity of symptoms during the last half of their cycles, often leading them to assume that they have PMS.

Numerous symptoms have been ascribed to PMS but a relatively small number make up the majority of complaints. They can be divided in behavioral and physical symptoms. Table 33-6 lists those that are most common. Several PMS diaries are available for the woman to record her symptoms and their severity (Figure 33-4).

Table 33-6

SYMPTOMS OF PREMENSTRUAL SYNDROME

Physical Symptoms
Headaches
Bloating
Breast tenderness
Hot flashes
Muscle and joint pain
Fatigue
Appetite changes: binge eating, cravings
Sleep changes: excessive or insomnia
Behavioral Symptoms
Depressed mood
Feelings of hopelessness
Marked anxiety
Emotional lability
Irritability and anger
Feelings of being out of control
Reduced interest in activities of living
Difficulty concentrating
Lethargy

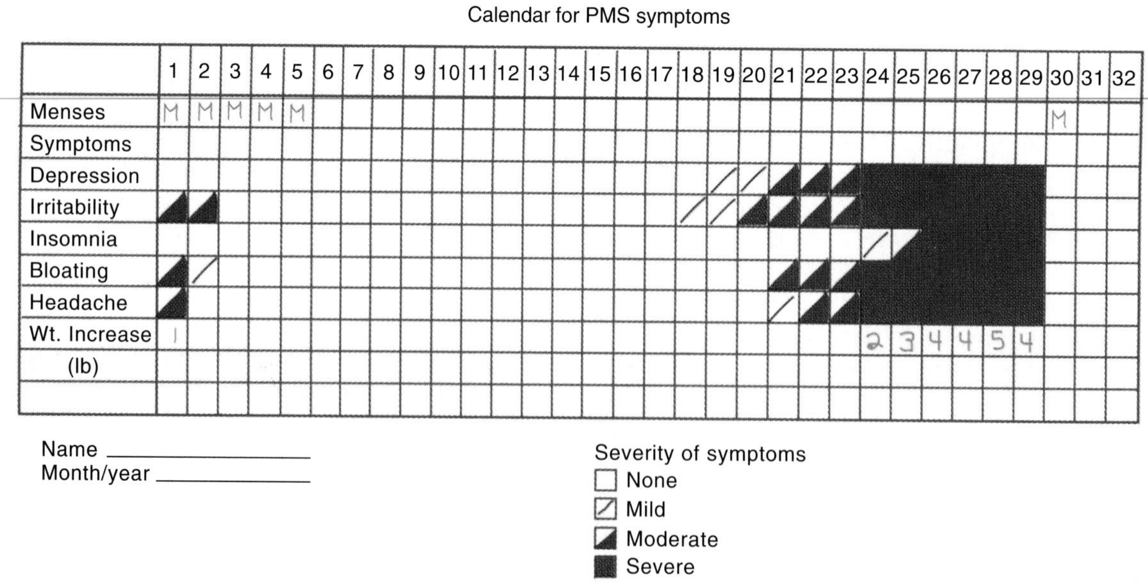

FIGURE 33-4 One type of diary to record occurrence and severity of premenstrual symptoms.

Etiology

Although the cause of PMS is unknown, several theories or predisposing factors have been suggested. These include the following:

- Prior affective disorder such as major depression or postpartum depression is often associated with PMS
- Identical twins have a high concordance for PMS
- Abnormal levels of estrogen or progesterone
- Greater sensitivity to the effect of ovarian hormones on the central nervous system neurotransmitters that affect mood, behavior, and cognition
- Possibly altered prolactin and thyroid secretion
- Low levels of beta-endorphins
- Abnormal production of prostaglandins
- Increased adrenal activity
- Fluid imbalance
- Nutritional deficiency: hypoglycemia; vitamin deficiencies
- Possibly a conditioned response in our society; may be expected if a mother or sibling was symptomatic, and males may reinforce stereotypes of how women are expected to behave premenstrually (Baram, 2000)

Impact on Family

Premenstrual syndrome puts a consistent strain on family relationships because symptoms recur monthly. The episodes of PMS affect the functioning of the entire family. Clinical descriptions of severe family disruptions include increased family conflict, disrupted communication, and decreased family cohesion. Of particular concern is the group of women who report symptoms of loss of control, child battering, self-injury, and increased accidents. Work and social relationships may likewise suffer.

Management

Treatment of PMS is based on the symptom profile of each woman after ruling out other problems, especially psychiatric diagnoses such as depression (Baram, 2000). Vitamin B_6 (pyridoxine), which is an important cofactor in the synthesis of neurotransmitters that influence mood, has often been prescribed, but has not been proved effective and excessive doses can cause peripheral neuropathy. Other trials have shown that supplements of calcium (1200 mg/day) have some effectiveness and magnesium (200 to 400 mg/day) is minimally effective. Carbohydrate-rich food and beverages may improve the mood and reduce food cravings in some women (ACOG, 2000). Also, reducing caffeine and taking vitamin E (400 IU/day) during the luteal phase of the cycle may help with mastalgia (breast pain).

A mild potassium-sparing diuretic such as spironolactone (Aldactone) 50 to 100 mg/day, may be prescribed for women with fluid retention and weight gain. Migraines related to the menstrual cycle are treated first with NSAIDs and prophylactically with a beta-blocker drug like propanolol (Inderal) (Baram, 2000).

Women with physical, emotional, and cognitive symptoms may be prescribed antidepressant medications, oral contraceptives to suppress ovulation, or both. Preferred antidepressants are selective serotonin reuptake inhibitors (SSRIs) such as fluoxetine (Prozac), sertraline (Zoloft), or paroxetine (Paxil), although tricyclic antidepressants may also be useful. Antianxiety medications help reduce the irritability and anxiety of severe PMS. Progesterone has often been prescribed, but has not been proven effective. Oral contraceptives have not been effective in relief of the psychological symptoms of PMS. Danazol in small doses has given women some symptomatic relief (Baram, 2000; ACOG, 2000).

Complementary/Alternative Therapy

Alternative therapy may help some women. Measures include acupuncture, biofeedback, hypnosis, psychotherapy, and stress management. A recent randomized controlled trial has found that reflexology is helpful in relief of some PMS symptoms (Baram, 2000). Evening primrose oil may be useful in treating breast tenderness but not other symptoms of PMS (ACOG, 2000).

Nursing Considerations

Many women experience some of the symptoms and diagnose themselves as having PMS. Nurses must discourage this practice because serious systemic disease can be missed if the criteria for diagnosis are ignored. Instead of self-diagnosis, nurses should recommend that the woman consult with her health care provider so that a complete history and physical examination can be performed to rule out other causes or a problem that may coexist with PMS.

Once the diagnosis of PMS is confirmed, nurses can teach the family about lifestyle changes that are known to relieve some symptoms of PMS and reduce the severity of others. Regular aerobic exercise helps relieve some symptoms of PMS. After the woman has received clearance from the physician or nurse-practitioner, the nurse can help her determine how to work an exercise program into her schedule. Regular exercise also has weight control, heart, and bone-strengthening benefits as well.

One study (Morse, 1999) showed that a health promotion program helped women diminish the impairment caused by PMS. In the program, women received education about the menstrual cycle and psychological help reframing their negative perceptions. For example, rather than viewing the menstrual cycle as a disease requiring treatment, the women in this study identified positive aspects of the menstrual cycle.

WOMEN WANT TO KNOW *How to Relieve Symptoms of Premenstrual Syndrome*

DIET
- Decrease consumption of caffeine (coffee, tea, colas, chocolate), which increases irritability, insomnia, anxiety, and nervousness.
- Avoid simple sugars (cookies, cake, candy) to prevent high blood glucose followed by a rapid decline and a period of low blood glucose (hypoglycemia).
- Decrease intake of salty foods (chips, pickles) to reduce fluid retention.
- Drink at least 2000 ml (2 quarts) of *water* per day, and do not include other beverages in this total.
- Eat six small meals a day to prevent hypoglycemia. Meals should be well balanced, with emphasis on fresh fruits and vegetables, complex carbohydrates, and nonfat milk products.
- Avoid alcohol, which aggravates depression.

EXERCISE
- Increase physical exercise to relieve tension and to decrease depression. Aerobic activity, such as jogging or walking, several times a week is recommended.

STRESS MANAGEMENT
- During the time when there are no symptoms of PMS, acknowledge the effect of PMS on daily life and make plans to avoid stressful situations during the premenstrual period when symptoms are acute.
- Use guided imagery, conscious relaxation techniques, warm baths, and massage to reduce stress.

SLEEP AND REST
To reduce fatigue and combat insomnia:
- Adhere to a regular schedule for sleep.
- Drink a glass of milk, which is high in tryptophan and is known to promote sleep, before bedtime.
- Schedule exercise in the morning or early afternoon rather than late afternoon.
- Engage in relaxing activities, such as reading, before bedtime, and avoid excitement at this time.

Acknowledge that dietary changes are particularly difficult because many women crave salty or sweet foods, which should be restricted. As they learn to predict the pattern of symptoms and gain a sense of control over them, the symptoms often diminish.

Education and support must be expanded to include the family. When the woman exhibits symptoms of PMS, family members often respond by withdrawing or confronting the woman. This increases the woman's feelings of anxiety and vulnerability.

It is more helpful if the family acknowledges feelings they believe the woman is experiencing. For instance saying "It must be disturbing to feel so irritable. What can I do to help?" provokes a different emotional response than confronting or blaming comments.

The family also should be encouraged to express their feelings so that anger and resentment within the family can be diminished.

Nurses must help the woman make concrete arrangements to obtain relief if she feels she is losing control or if she fears that she may harm herself or a child. A neighbor, friend, or family member should be identified to provide immediate relief, without questions or explanations, when the woman feels she is losing control. The telephone number of this important support person should be posted so that it is easily accessible, and the designated person should be called before symptoms are severe.

INDUCED ABORTION

Induced abortion is a voluntary method of terminating a pregnancy. It may be performed to preserve the health of the mother, to prevent the birth of an infant with severe birth defects, or to end a pregnancy caused by rape or incest. A woman may also choose to terminate a pregnancy for economic or social reasons. Termination of pregnancy for the purpose of safeguarding the health of the mother is termed "therapeutic" abortion. Interruption of the pregnancy at the request of the woman but not for reasons of impaired maternal health or fetal disease is often called "elective" abortion. Therapeutic and elective abortions involve many social and ethical issues (see Chapter 3). In 1996, the induced abortion rate was 22.9 per 1000 women, a decline from the peak of 29.4 per 1000 in 1980 (Ventura, et al., 1999).

Methods of Abortion

The technique used to induce abortion depends on the length of gestation and may be medical, if only drugs are used to end the pregnancy, or surgical, if a surgical procedure is required. A surgical procedure may sometimes be required to completely evacuate the uterine contents when a medical abortion is done.

Drugs that may be used in medical abortion regimens include the following:

- Mifepristone (Mifeprex), also known as RU 486, a drug that inhibits progesterone, which is necessary for maintenance of the embryo, can be used through the seventh week.

- Methotrexate (Folex, Mexate), a drug that interferes with DNA synthesis in rapidly-dividing cells such as embryonic or cancer cells.
- Prostaglandin analogs, which cause uterine contractions and expulsion of the uterine contents.
- Misoprostol (Cytotec), a prostaglandin drug normally given to prevent gastric ulcers. Its use for this purpose is investigational.

Although newly approved in the United States, mifepristone has been used for a number of years in Europe. The FDA-approved regimen for use for mifepristone is as a single 600-mg oral dose followed two days later by 400 mg of misoprostol to complete uterine evacuation. Expulsion may occur 1 to 2 hours after the misoprostol. The woman should receive Rh_O(D) immune globulin (RhoGAM) if she is Rh-negative, usually at the time of mifepristone administration, because some women expel the products of conception prior to the misoprostol. The woman should return to the office or clinic 14 days after taking the mifepristone to determine if the abortion is complete (Newhall & Winikoff, 2000; U.S. Department of Health and Human Services, 2000b). Regimens other than the one approved by the FDA have been used in other countries.

Methotrexate, an antineoplastic agent, has been used prior to the release of mifepristone in the United States to end pregnancies of 7 weeks or less. Misoprostol must be used to fully evacuate the products of conception as in the mifepristone abortion. Abortion with methotrexate takes longer than mifepristone, 1 to 5 weeks to complete (Pymar and Creinin, 2000).

Prostaglandin drugs alone can be used to effect abortion by causing uterine contractions but have a high rate of nausea, vomiting, fever, and diarrhea. These side effects make the drug unacceptable if there are better alternatives. However, prostaglandin can induce abortion in second-trimester pregnancy, when other methods are not effective.

Surgical methods or often a combination of medical and surgical methods of abortion are used in later pregnancy. Up to 13 weeks' gestation, *vacuum aspiration* or *curettage* is the method of choice. The cervix is dilated gently by inserting a series of tapered metal rods that increase progressively in size. When the cervical canal is open, a plastic cannula is inserted into the uterine cavity. The contents are aspirated with negative pressure within approximately 5 minutes. Many health care providers then gently scrape the uterine cavity with a curet to ensure that the uterus is empty. Cramping may last 20 to 30 minutes after the procedure is completed. Complications include uterine perforation, hemorrhage, cervical lacerations, and adverse reactions to the anesthetic agent.

For second-trimester abortions, *dilation with removal of the fetus and placenta* is generally performed. The procedure is similar to vacuum curettage but requires greater cervical dilation and a larger aspirator because the products of conception are larger and must be removed gradually. The cervix is dilated with laminaria that have been placed 24 hours before the procedure. Laminaria are short, rounded pieces of material that are hygroscopic (absorb water). When laminaria are inserted into the cervix, they draw fluid from the cervical canal and expand, causing the cervix to dilate. Cervical dilation occurs slowly and is less traumatic to the cervix.

Medical methods exist for abortion in the second trimester, but these involve hours of labor. Retention of the placenta often occurs, requiring a dilation and curettage to fully clean the uterus. *Labor induction* can be carried out with several agents that produce uterine contractions or cause fetal death. Laminaria are usually inserted about 12 hours before the procedure to start cervical dilation. Prostaglandin E_2, which stimulates contractions, may be given via vaginal suppository or intraamniotic infusion. Prostaglandin may also be combined with either hypertonic saline or hypertonic urea. Either may be injected into the amniotic sac. Hypertonic saline carries significant maternal risk for electrolyte imbalance if it accidentally moves into the maternal circulation. These solutions are feticidal, and labor usually starts within 24 hours. Giving oxytocin shortens labor, but second trimester abortion requires overnight hospitalization. Because of the emotional distress caused by the longer procedure and the increased risks involved, medical termination of pregnancy is not often chosen in the second trimester.

Nursing Considerations

The nurse's role in caring for women seeking induced abortion is one of providing physical and emotional support and information. History taking and collection of laboratory data depend on the routine of the health care setting in which the nurse is functioning. Counseling and lending emotional support are nursing responsibilities although a designated counselor may also perform these services.

Nurses are also responsible for providing information for self-care following an abortion. Self-care is similar to that following spontaneous abortion: observation for excessive bleeding or signs of infection (fever, foul-smelling vaginal drainage) and information about follow-up visits and contraception.

Check Your Reading

23. What are the criteria for diagnosing PMS?
24. What lifestyle changes can be made to reduce the symptoms of PMS?
25. What drugs can be used in a medical abortion?
26. What discharge teaching is appropriate after an induced abortion?

WOMEN WANT TO KNOW ***Guidelines for Self-Care after Early Induced Abortion***

- Resume normal activities, but avoid strenuous work or exercise for a few days.
- Bleeding or cramping may occur for a week or two. If either becomes severe, seek medical advice. Light "spotting" may occur for about a month.
- Use sanitary pads rather than tampons after the abortion to avoid infection.
- Avoid douching, to prevent infection.
- Curtail intercourse for 1 week after the abortion because of the possibility of infection until the uterine lining heals.
- Use birth control measures if sex is resumed before menstruation begins because it is possible to become pregnant during this time. Menstruation usually resumes in 4 to 6 weeks.
- Take temperature twice a day to detect possible infection; a temperature above 37.8° C (100° F) should be reported to the health care provider.
- Keep the follow-up appointment in 2 weeks.

MENOPAUSE

Menopause means the end of menstruation. However, most people use the term to include the array of endocrine, somatic, and psychic changes that occur at the end of the reproductive period. The entire process, frequently called the "change of life," is correctly termed the *climacteric*. Premenopause refers to the early part of the climacteric, before menstruation ceases but after the woman experiences some of the climacteric symptoms, such as irregular menses. Perimenopause includes premenopause, menopause, and at least 1 year after menopause. Postmenopause refers to the phase following menopause, when menstrual periods have ceased.

Unexpected postmenopausal bleeding should be investigated as soon as possible because it suggests endometrial cancer. Conversely, planned or scheduled postmenopausal bleeding is generally not a cause for concern. It occurs when the woman who takes estrogen and progesterone sequentially stops taking the drugs, usually once a month. This allows the uterine lining to be sloughed and prevents endometrial hyperplasia.

Age of Menopause

The average age for natural menopause is 51 years (Wren, 1998). The natural climacteric takes place over 3 to 5 years. Menopause can be induced or created artificially, however, at any age. Surgical removal of the ovaries or destruction of the ovaries by radiation causes abrupt, permanent cessation of ovarian function, including the production of estrogen. The most common reason for performing these procedures is treatment of gynecologic cancer or endometriosis. Young women who experience artificial menopause often have more symptoms associated with menopause than do women who go through the process naturally because theirs is not a gradual process.

Women can now expect to live another 30 years following menopause. During this period they must deal with physical, psychological, and social changes that often require a reevaluation of their primary roles and restructuring of personal goals.

Physiologic Changes

During the normal reproductive cycle, the ovaries respond to gonadotropins (follicle-stimulating hormone and luteinizing hormone) in a predictable pattern: (1) a follicle matures, (2) the ovary secretes estrogen, (3) ovulation occurs, and (4) the corpus luteum produces progesterone. During the premenopausal period, however, the ovaries are less responsive to gonadotropins, and, although increased amounts of follicle-stimulating hormone are secreted, ovulation is sporadic and menstrual periods are irregular. With progressive aging, the ovaries become unresponsive, even to high levels of gonadotropins, and ovulation, menstruation, and the secretion of ovarian hormones (estrogen and progesterone) cease.

Estrogen is responsible for the secondary sex characteristics of women; when estrogen levels decline, the organs of reproduction undergo regression. The labia become thin and pale. The vaginal mucosa atrophies, and vaginal tissue loses its lubrication and thus is easily traumatized. Dyspareunia is not uncommon, and bacterial invasion of the epithelium may occur and lead to frequent vaginal infections. This entire process is referred to as atrophic vaginitis. Breasts become smaller, and atrophy of the uterus occurs. However, a concurrent benefit is that uterine myomas (fibroids) and endometriosis lesions also atrophy. Estrogen deficit can also result in atrophic changes in the bladder and urethra that may cause loss of urethral tone and frequent atrophic cystitis.

In addition, absence of estrogen is associated with an adverse change in serum lipids. Serum levels of low-density lipoproteins, which carry cholesterol to blood vessels, increase. At the same time, levels of high-density lipoproteins, which are known to carry cholesterol to the liver and to protect against the development of coronary artery disease, decrease.

Most menopausal women experience hot flashes or flushes, which are the result of vasomotor instability.

The cause of vasomotor instability is not known, but it is closely associated with increased secretion of gonadotropins. Hot flashes are characterized by a sudden feeling of heat or burning of the skin, followed by perspiration. They occur more frequently during the night, and fatigue as a result of interrupted sleep is a major problem for some women.

Evidence is persuasive that estrogen may lower the risk and delay the onset of Alzheimer's disease in elderly women. Alzheimer's disease is a chronic, progressive, irreversible brain dysfunction that causes loss of memory. Eventually the person will be unable to function independently. Research is ongoing to determine the exact nature of the link between estrogen depletion and memory loss.

Psychological Responses

It is easy to understand why menopause is called the "change of life." It is accompanied by physical, psychological, and social changes, and individual responses vary widely. Many women are relieved that their childbearing and childrearing tasks are ending. They see this as an exciting time, when they can pursue personal development. Other women grieve that the possibility of childbearing is past. This may be particularly true for women who have never had a child. However, artificial reproductive techniques have blurred the line between the age when it is and is not possible to bear a child (see Chapter 32).

Menopause requires a woman to come to terms with aging. It may be difficult to accept aging in a society that reveres youth, and many women become extremely concerned with measures that slow the signs of aging. Many women become grandmothers at this time, which also confirms aging and requires a major adjustment in how the woman views herself. A large population of "baby boomers"—those born from 1946 to 1964—are entering menopause. These women are likely to change many of society's ideas about menopause by the sheer size of their group and because they have changed the social fabric of the United States dramatically as they have grown up and matured.

Some symptoms do not have a physiologic explanation, but they are no less real to women who experience them. Depression, mood swings, irritability, and agitation are common climacteric complaints. Insomnia and fatigue are often mentioned as major problems.

One of the most puzzling aspects of menopause is the wide variation in both physical and psychological symptoms that women experience. For some women, the only changes are mild, infrequent hot flashes and amenorrhea. Other women experience severe, debilitating hot flashes, atrophic vaginitis, and multiple psychological symptoms, such as irritability and prolonged depression.

Hormone Replacement Therapy

Hormone replacement therapy is the treatment of choice for many of the common discomforts of menopause. The type of hormone replacement, either estrogen only or estrogen in combination with progestin, depends on whether or not the woman has had a hysterectomy (removal of the uterus). Estrogen alone is prescribed for women who have had a hysterectomy. Estrogen and progestin are prescribed for women who still have a uterus and are at risk for endometrial hyperplasia if estrogen unopposed by progestin is administered.

Benefits

Although hormone replacement therapy is the primary medical treatment for the symptoms of menopause, the risks and the benefits of estrogen must be evaluated for each woman. Ample evidence exists that estrogen controls hot flashes and alleviates genital atrophy, which is associated with atrophic vaginitis, atrophic cystitis, and urinary incontinence. Either oral or topical estrogen may be administered for atrophic vaginitis.

Estrogen also offers protection from cardiovascular disease, which increases dramatically in postmenopausal women. The cardiovascular benefits of estrogen are believed to be due to its ability to increase high-density lipoprotein and to decrease total cholesterol and low-density lipoprotein. Progestin reverses some of estrogen's beneficial effects on serum lipids. However, this action of progestin may not be clinically relevant because myocardial infarction rates are lower in women who take estrogen replacement therapy. Endogenous estrogen's other protective effects on the heart include a lower blood pressure, lower fibrinogen levels, reduced platelet aggregation, vasodilation, increased cardiac stroke volume, and slowed deposits of fatty materials (atheromas) in the coronary arteries (Evans & Dumesic, 2000). Estrogen may promote normal memory function. Estrogen also slows bone loss and reduces osteoporosis, which is described later.

Many women expect more from estrogen than it can deliver. Estrogen does not prevent aging of the skin, and evidence is inconclusive about whether it relieves depression or other psychological symptoms. However, clinical experience suggests that estrogen replacement relieves insomnia, promotes increased energy, and improves the overall quality of life.

Risks

Hormone replacement at menopause is not for every woman. Some women have had breast cancers that were dependent on estrogen and/or progesterone and should not take the exogenous hormones. Likewise, a woman who has a close family history of breast cancer might not want to take it. Other significant risks associated with hormone replacement include stroke; uterine cancer; gallbladder disease, pancreatic disease, and acute liver disease; recent blood clot; any undiagnosed vaginal bleeding. Other possible contraindications include cigarette smoking, hypertension, a history of

DRUG GUIDE: ESTROGENS (PREMARIN, ESTRACE, OGEN, CLIMARA [PATCH])

Classification: Hormone, estrogen

Action: Increases synthesis of DNA, RNA, and various proteins in responsive tissues. Reduces release of gonadotropin-releasing hormone, thus reducing follicle-stimulating hormone and luteinizing hormone. Promotes normal growth and maintenance of female genital organs, maintaining genitourinary function and vasomotor stability. Restores hormone balance in deficiency states, reduces blood cholesterol, and retards bone resorption. Decreases serum concentration of testosterone.

Indications: Treatment of vasomotor symptoms of menopause, such as hot flashes; prevention of postmenopausal osteoporosis; management of atrophic vaginitis

Dosage and Route: Dosage varies with the drug. For relief of menopausal symptoms and prevention of osteoporosis:

- Conjugated estrogens (Premarin): 0.3 to 1.25 mg daily
- Estradiol (Estrace): 0.5 to 2 mg daily
- Estropipate (Ogen): 0.625 to 5 mg daily
- Estradiol transdermal (Climara): 0.025 to 0.1 mg daily

Schedule of administration depends on whether the woman has had a hysterectomy. If she has no uterus, estrogen alone may be administered daily or in a repeating cycle. If the woman has a uterus, both estrogen and progesterone are administered. Estrogen may be given for 21 days, with progesterone added for the final 10 days. Both medications are then stopped for 7 days. When medication is stopped, predictable bleeding occurs. An alternative schedule involves the administration of estrogen, 0.625 mg, and progesterone, 2.5 to 5 mg daily. This schedule eliminates episodes of planned bleeding. Vaginal cream applied daily for 21 days, off for 7 days, and then repeated, may be useful for atrophic vaginitis. Transdermal patch (Climara) reapplied weekly.

Absorption: Well absorbed following oral administration; readily absorbed through skin and mucous membranes

Excretion: Metabolized largely by the liver; as hepatic recirculation occurs, more absorption occurs from the gastrointestinal tract

Contraindications and Precautions: Contraindicated in thromboembolic diseases, undiagnosed vaginal bleeding, pregnancy, and lactation. Used cautiously in underlying cardiovascular disease and severe hepatic or renal disease; use of estrogen unopposed by progesterone may result in endometrial carcinoma.

Adverse Reactions: Headache, dizziness, intolerance to contact lenses, nausea, jaundice

Nursing Considerations: Assess blood pressure, pulse, and weight gain periodically throughout therapy; assess frequency and severity of hot flashes. Instruct the woman to report skin changes and to protect skin from excessive exposure to sunlight to prevent hyperpigmentation. Assess for vaginal bleeding, amenorrhea, or changes in menstrual flow, and instruct the woman to report these signs to her health care provider. Caution the woman to avoid use of any medication not approved by her health care provider.

DRUG GUIDE: MEDROXYPROGESTERONE (AMEN, DEPO-PROVERA, PROVERA)

Classification: Hormone progestin

Action: A synthetic form of progesterone that transforms the endometrium from a proliferative to a secretory phase and promotes withdrawal bleeding when estrogen is also present. Promotes relaxation of uterine smooth muscle and growth of mammary alveolar tissue.

Indications: Used to reduce the risk of endometrial carcinoma when estrogen is administered to control postmenopausal symptoms or to prevent osteoporosis. Prevention of pregnancy.

Dosage and Route: For induction of secretory endometrium after estrogen priming, 5 to 10 mg orally for 10 days. To prevent endometrial hyperplasia, 2 to 10 mg daily with exogenous estrogen. Also used for secondary amenorrhea and abnormal uterine bleeding. For pregnancy prevention: 150 mg IM every 3 months.

Absorption: Unknown; metabolized by the liver

Excretion: Unknown

Contraindications and Precautions: Contraindicated in pregnancy, thromboembolic disease, carcinoma of the breast, and liver disease. Use with caution with cardiovascular disease, seizure disorders, and mental depression. Distributed in breast milk.

Adverse Reactions: Depression, thrombophlebitis, edema, weight gain, dizziness, fatigue, headache, insomnia. Fluid retention may complicate other conditions such as asthma, heart disease, and renal disorders.

Nursing Considerations: Assess blood pressure throughout therapy. Monitor weight gain, and emphasize that steady weight gain should be reported to health care provider. Advise women to anticipate withdrawal bleeding 3 to 7 days after discontinuing medication. Emphasize the importance of reporting the following signs and symptoms: visual changes, sudden weakness, headache, leg or calf pain, shortness of breath, jaundice, depression, and skin rash. When used as contraceptive, teach women that their menstrual periods may be temporarily changed (spotting, change in flow, amenorrhea). Unsubstantiated reports of decreased volume of breast milk following contraceptive dose (Hale, 2000).

endometriosis, seizure disorder, migraines, and benign breast or uterine disease (DeMasters, 2000).

Dosage Forms

Estrogen replacement is available in three dosage forms: oral, dermal patch, and vaginal cream. The oral and dermal patch forms allow estrogen in the serum to reach levels high enough to exert the protective effects on the heart and bone as well as relieve other menopausal symptoms. Estrogen given by vaginal cream has serum levels no higher than 50% of the oral or dermal forms and does not offer significant protection from heart disease or bone loss, but is useful for atrophic vaginitis. Both dermal patch and cream forms of estrogen avoid the hepatic first-pass metabolism because they are not taken internally and thus have little effect on serum lipids. Dermal patch estrogen can treat symptoms of menopause, such as hot flashes, while providing protection against osteoporosis.

Table 33-7

CONTRAINDICATIONS AND CAUTIONS RELATED TO ESTROGEN REPLACEMENT THERAPY

Previous episode of breast cancer or other estrogen-dependent tumor
Close family history of breast cancer (first-degree relative)
Uterine cancer
Active thromboembolic disease or prior thromboembolic disorder when on estrogen
Stroke
Acute or chronic liver disease
Undiagnosed abnormal vaginal bleeding
Gallbladder or pancreatic disease
Diabetes mellitus
Conditions that may be aggravated by fluid retention, such as migraine, epilepsy, cardiac, renal dysfunction, depression

Treatment Regimens

Three treatment regimens are currently used for hormone replacement therapy. (1) *Cyclic regimen,* in which estrogen is given at specific intervals (such as 25 days per month) with the addition of progestin for the last 10 to 14 days. Many women dislike the monthly "period" that occurs when the hormones are stopped for several days before restarting. (2) *Combined regimen,* in which estrogen and a low dose of progestin are given daily, and planned bleeding is avoided. (3) *Estrogen only,* in which estrogen is given for 25 days per month or daily, without treatment-free intervals or the addition of progestin. This regimen is used for women who have had a hysterectomy. Estrogen cream is usually used as an adjuvant treatment to oral estrogen therapy and does not have serum levels to achieve the benefits of oral estrogen.

Risks

Administration of estrogen unopposed by a progesterone drug has been associated with an increased risk of endometrial cancer. To overcome this risk, small doses of progestin are given with estrogen. This eliminates the constant stimulation of the endometrium that occurs when estrogen alone is used. Some data suggest a minimally increased risk of breast cancer for women who used estrogen for more than 10 to 20 years, but the risk is unclear (Evans & Dumesic, 2000).

Some women should not take estrogen. Growth of existing breast cancer may be stimulated by estrogen, and women who have had estrogen receptor–positive breast cancer usually do not take estrogen. Oral contraceptives have been associated with venous thrombosis, and women who have developed a thrombosis should cease estrogen replacement therapy. Because estrogen is metabolized by the liver, it should not be taken by women who have hepatitis or liver disease. Not being able to take estrogen presents a dilemma for some women. Not only is osteoporosis an increased risk, but the atrophic changes of menopause and vasomotor instability remain major problems. When estrogen is contraindicated, women also have increased risk of coronary artery disease because they do not receive the protective effects of increased high-density lipoproteins that estrogen provides. Table 33-7 summarizes contraindications to estrogen replacement therapy.

When estrogen replacement therapy is contraindicated, alternative therapy may be prescribed. Clonidine hydrochloride (Catapres), an antihypertensive, is sometimes prescribed to decrease the severity and frequency of hot flashes. Other drugs include medroxyprogesterone acetate, bromocriptine, and naloxone (Narcan) and (Evans & Dumesic, 2000).

Complementary/Alternative Therapy

Products made from soybeans such as tofu, soy cheese, soy milk, and soy flour are high in phytoestrogens. Evidence exists that increased soy intake may reduce many of the discomforts of menopause. In addition, soy protein causes less calcium to be excreted in the urine and may reduce the risk for osteoporosis. Soy may also be beneficial in reducing the risk for heart disease, hypertension, and breast and other cancers (Lindsay, 1999; Lindsay & Claywell, 1998). It is not yet clear whether phytoestrogens are potent enough to stimulate growth of estrogen-dependent tumors such as breast cancers (Hendrix, 2000).

Continued

Complementary/Alternative Therapy—cont'd

Black cohosh, sold as an extract under the name Remifemin, is a botanical preparation containing phytoestrogen. Black cohosh causes uterine contractions and should not be used if pregnancy is a possibility. Chaste berry may reduce hot flashes but must be taken for a prolonged time to be effective, like most botanical preparations. Ginseng has estrogenic effects in women and may also help relieve some of the discomforts of menopause. However, it may cause breast tenderness and overstimulation, and some women are allergic to it. Ginseng has potential interactions with warfarin (Coumadin), MAO inhibitors, and digitalis, and it may reduce the amount of insulin the diabetic woman needs.

Nursing Considerations

Nursing care focuses on helping women understand the physical changes that occur and the psychological responses that may occur during menopause. Nurses must clarify the individual regimen of hormone replacement therapy as well as the risks and benefits of the therapy. For instance, women should be told that although hormone replacement therapy effectively treats atrophic vaginitis and reduces dyspareunia, it may not overcome the loss of libido that some women experience.

If hormone replacement therapy is contraindicated, nurses are often the primary source of information about alternative measures that mitigate symptoms:

- Using water-soluble lubricants, such as K-Y Liquid, Lubrin, Replens, or K-Y Silk-e to relieve vaginal dryness and dyspareunia. Oil-based lubricants should not be used because they adhere to the mucous membrane for long periods of time and provide a medium for bacterial growth.
- Discussing alternatives to estrogen, such as botanical preparations, if the woman does not want estrogen replacement therapy. The woman should discuss these with her health care provider because some have side or adverse effects or interactions with other drugs.
- Doing Kegel exercises to increase muscle tone around the vagina and urinary meatus and counteract the effects of genital atrophy.
- Drinking at least eight glasses of water a day decreases the concentration of urine, flushes urine from the bladder, and reduces bacterial growth, thereby preventing atrophic cystitis.
- Wiping from front to back following urination and defecation reduces the transfer of bacteria from the anus to the urinary meatus and helps prevent cystitis.

Check Your Reading

27. What are the effects of estrogen depletion at menopause (either natural or artificial) on the body?
28. What are the major psychological symptoms associated with menopause?
29. How does hormone replacement affect menopausal and postmenopausal women?

Osteoporosis

Osteoporosis is one of the greatest hazards of the postmenopausal years. It is characterized by decreased bone density, leaving the bones porous, fragile, and susceptible to fractures. The vertebrae, wrists, and hips are the most common sites of fractures.

Osteoporosis is a major public health problem which will likely increase as baby boomers age. More than 28 million people in the United States presently have either low bone mass or osteoporosis, and 80% of them are women. Approximately 8 million American women have osteoporosis. One in two women over age 50 will have a fracture related to osteoporosis in their lifetime. Osteoporosis causes as many as 300,000 hip fractures, 700,000 vertebral fractures, and 250,000 wrist fractures in addition to other fractures. About 24% of those

Women Want to Know *About Hormone Replacement Therapy*

- Take the medication with meals to reduce nausea.
- If you miss a dose, take the medication as soon as you remember, but not immediately before the next scheduled dose. *Do not take double doses.*
- Expect withdrawal bleeding (if your uterus is present) when estrogen and progestin are temporarily discontinued.
- Report unexpected bleeding to your health care provider.
- Stop smoking to reduce the risk of thromboembolism.
- Use sunscreen and protective clothing to prevent increased pigmentation.
- Continue follow-up physical examinations, including blood pressure measurements, Pap tests, and examinations of breasts, abdomen, and pelvis.

who have a hip fracture die within a year. Long-term care is needed for 25% of those who were ambulatory before their hip fracture (National Institutes of Health, Osteoporosis and Related Bone Diseases, National Resource Center, 2000).

Risk Factors

Small-boned, fair-skinned, white and Asian women are at greatest risk for osteoporosis. Other risk factors include a family history of the disease, early menopause, and a sedentary lifestyle. Women who smoke, drink alcohol, or take corticosteroids or anticonvulsants, as well as those who consume excessive amounts of caffeine, also have an increased risk for osteoporosis (National Institutes of Health, Osteoporosis and Related Bone Diseases, National Resource Center, 2000). Inadequate intake of calcium is a major risk factor because it results in failure to achieve peak bone mass during youth.

Signs and Symptoms

Osteoporosis has been called the "silent thief" because bone mass is lost over many years with no signs or symptoms. The first noticeable evidence is loss of height and back pain that occurs when the vertebrae collapse. Later signs include the "dowager's hump," which occurs when the vertebrae can no longer support the upper body in an upright position. Secondary to this, the waistline disappears and the abdomen protrudes as the rib cage moves closer to the pelvis. Depending on the number of fractures, several inches of height may be lost. Figure 33-5 illustrates progressive changes in posture associated with osteoporosis.

Diagnosis of osteoporosis requires a thorough history, physical examination, and bone mineral analysis. Conventional x-ray is of little help because more than 30% of the bone mass must be lost before changes are apparent. Dual-energy x-ray absorptiometry is highly accurate, fast, and relatively inexpensive. In addition, it involves low exposure to radiation. However, single-energy x-ray absorptiometry is becoming more popular for assessment of bone mass because it is cost effective and easier to use (Bailey, Combs, Rogers, & Stanley, 2000). Ultrasound can be used to measure the density of the shin (Hendrix, 2000).

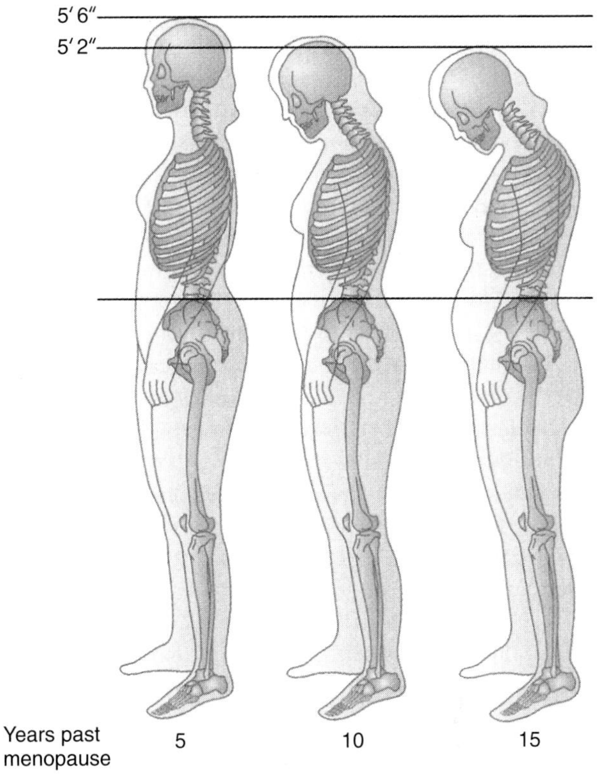

FIGURE 33-5 With progression of osteoporosis, the vertebral column collapses, causing loss of height and back pain. "Dowager's hump" is the term used for this curvature of the upper back.

Prevention and Medical Management

The main goal of treatment is to prevent the development of osteoporosis and to stabilize remaining bone mass. The most effective measures are estrogen replacement, supplemental calcium plus vitamin D, and exercise.

Estrogen Replacement. Estrogen halts bone loss and reduces the incidence of fractures. It is best to start estrogen before menopause because a great deal of bone calcium can be lost before the final menstrual period. Minimum effective doses of estrogen to prevent bone loss depend on the route:

- Conjugated equine estrogens 0.625 mg
- Transdermal estrogen 50 to 100 mcg
- Oral ethinyl estradiol 20 mcg

Starting therapy within 5 years of menopause and continuing it for 10 years can reduce fractures by as much as 50%. Starting therapy after bone loss has occurred does not offer the same benefits (Evans & Dumesic, 2000). Many women continue hormone therapy throughout their lives because of its added benefits to the cardiovascular system and memory.

Calcium and Vitamin D. Calcium does not prevent bone loss, but other therapies cannot be effective if it is deficient. Calcium intake between ages 25 and 50 should be 1000 mg per day. A postmenopausal woman should ingest 1200 to 1500 mg per day of elemental calcium (Association of Women's Health, Obstetric, and Neonatal Nurses, 1999b). Because it is difficult to take this amount daily from food alone, supplements may be needed. Vitamin D is necessary for calcium to be absorbed from the intestine. Supplemental vitamin D, 400 IU daily, is recommended for healthy women. Elderly women should receive 800 to 1000 IU daily (AWHONN, 1999b; National Institutes of Health, 2000b). Vitamin D is a fat-soluble vitamin that can accumulate to dangerous levels, and intakes higher than 1200 IU/day should be avoided without regular monitoring.

Exercise. Muscle-strengthening and high-impact exercise has been shown to be beneficial in slowing loss of bone mass, if there is adequate calcium and vitamin D intake. Most of the bone mass is acquired by age 18, but muscle-strengthening exercise may continue to build bone into the thirties. The premenopausal woman gains the greatest benefit from muscle loading and high-impact activities. The postmenopausal woman who does not take estrogen replacement will gain some protective effect if she exercises, but she cannot fully offset the loss of estrogen on bone health. Exercise in the ninth decade of life has been shown to increase both muscle mass and strength twofold or more in frail individuals (National Institutes of Health, Osteoporosis and Related Bone Diseases, National Resource Center, 2000a; National Institutes of Health, 2000b).

High-impact exercise improves bone mineral density but should be avoided in a woman who already has fragile vertebrae from osteoporosis. Lower-impact exercise, such as walking, benefits bone health less but improves cardiovascular health. Regular activities such as walking, weight training, and low-impact aerobics can help stabilize the bone loss and reduce the risk of fractures (National Institutes of Health, Osteoporosis and Related Bone Diseases, National Resource Center, 2000a).

Alternative Medications. Calcitonin is recommended for those women who already have low bone densities and for those with high rates of bone turnover. Formerly available only in injection form, calcitonin is now available in a nasal spray (Miacalcin). Side effects include nausea, flushing, rhinitis or epistaxis (with nasal administration), and arthralgias.

Biophosphonates such as alendronate (Fosamax) are potent inhibitors of bone resorption. The most common side effects are nausea, stomach irritation, and abdominal pain due to esophageal irritation. Alendronate should be taken exactly as directed to avoid side effects and to maximize absorption. Directions include (1) taking first thing on arising in the morning with 6 to 8 ounces of water, (2) remaining upright for at least 30 minutes, and (3) waiting at least 30 minutes before taking food, other fluids, or any other medications (including antacids, calcium supplements, and vitamins). Etidronate (Didronel) is another drug in this class, and research continues into other biophosphonate medications.

Newer drugs include selective estrogen receptor modifiers (SERMs) such as raloxifene (Evista). Raloxifene has the dual benefits of increasing bone mineral density while lowering blood cholesterol and LDL levels, thus also reducing the chance of cardiovascular disease. However, raloxifene may be contraindicated in women who have a history of blood clots because of its estrogen-like effects on coagulation. The woman should be taught to avoid one position for a prolonged time and to report any pain, swelling, or redness in her calves, all possible manifestations of thrombophlebitis.

Nursing Considerations

Nurses often counsel women about lifestyle factors that contribute to bone loss, such as cigarette smoking, excessive alcohol or caffeine intake, and the importance of following the recommended medical regimen. Nurses are also concerned about how to prevent falls and thus reduce the risk of fractures. A major responsibility is to help the woman make her environment as safe as possible. Lighting should be ample, with switches easily accessible. Loose electrical cords should be kept out of the way, and area rugs should have nonskid backing. The bathtub should have nonskid devices, and grab bars should be installed near toilets and tubs. Stairways should have handrails, and loose items should be kept out of the walking pathways. Consultation with an occupational or physical therapist may be needed if the woman has serious mobility problems.

Nursing Diagnoses

A variety of nursing diagnoses may be relevant for the woman with osteoporosis, depending on the severity of the condition. Examples that may apply include the following:

- Pain related to pressure and inflammation of nerves that exit the vertebral column
- Activity Intolerance related to discomfort and fear of falling
- Body Image Disturbance related to altered posture and functional limitations
- Self-Care Deficit (specify deficit) related to physical limitations and depression

Check Your Reading

30. Why is osteoporosis called the "silent thief"?
31. How can osteoporosis be prevented?
32. What can nurses do to prevent fractures in women with osteoporosis?

PELVIC FLOOR DYSFUNCTION

Pelvic floor dysfunction occurs when muscles, ligaments, and fascia that support the pelvic organs are damaged or weakened. This relaxation of pelvic support allows the pelvic organs to prolapse into, and sometimes out of, the vagina. Pelvic disorders generally occur in the perimenopausal period and may be the delayed result of traumatic childbirth or the effects of aging.

Vaginal Wall Prolapse

The vagina may prolapse at either the anterior or posterior wall. Anterior wall prolapse involves the bladder and urethra and is called cystocele. Prolapse of the posterior wall produces enterocele or rectocele.

Cystocele

When the weakened upper anterior wall of the vagina is no longer able to support the weight of urine in the bladder, cystocele develops. The bladder protrudes downward into the vagina, resulting in incomplete emptying of the bladder. Cystitis is likely to occur because of the stagnant urine. Urethral displacement, formerly termed *urethrocele,* may occur when the urethra bulges into the lower anterior vaginal wall, producing stress urinary incontinence (Figure 33-6, *A*).

Stress incontinence is the loss of urine that occurs with a sudden increase in intraabdominal pressure, such as that generated by sneezing, coughing, laughing, lifting, or sudden jarring motions. The two most common causes of stress incontinence are damage to the normal supports of the bladder neck and urethra that occurs during pregnancy and childbirth, and tissue atrophy that occurs following menopause.

Enterocele

Enterocele refers to prolapse of the upper posterior vaginal wall between the vagina and rectum. This is almost always associated with herniation of the pouch of Douglas (a fold of peritoneum that dips down between the rectum and the uterus) and may contain loops of bowel. Enterocele often accompanies uterine prolapse (Figure 33-6, *B*).

Rectocele

Rectocele occurs when the posterior wall of the vagina becomes weakened and thin. Each time the woman strains at defecation, feces are pushed against the thinned wall, causing further stretching, until finally the rectum protrudes into the vagina. Many rectoceles are small and produce few symptoms. If the rectocele is large, the patient may have difficulty emptying the rectum. Some women facilitate bowel elimination by applying digital pressure along the posterior vaginal wall to keep the rectocele from protruding during a bowel movement (Figure 33-6, *C*).

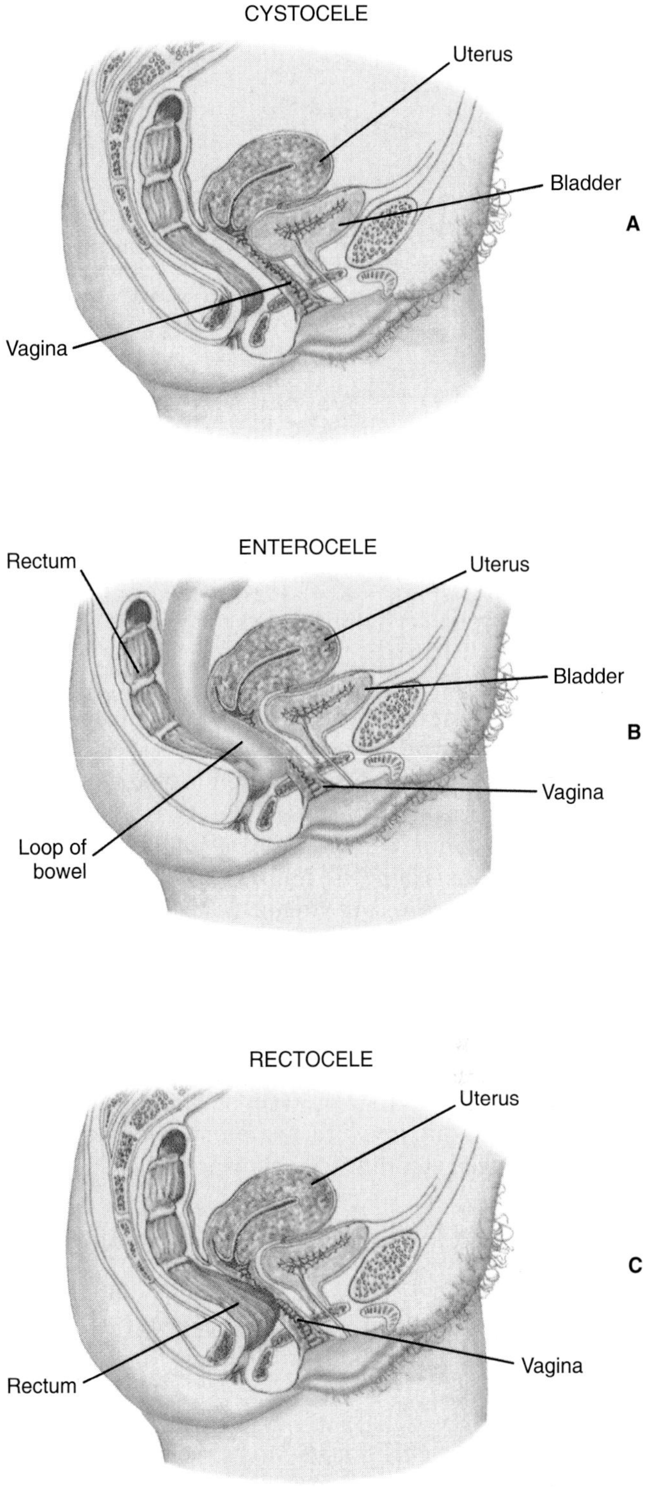

FIGURE 33-6 Three types of vaginal wall prolapse. **A,** Note bulging of bladder into the vagina. **B,** Note loop of bowel between rectum and uterus. **C,** Note bulging of rectum into vagina.

Uterine Prolapse

Uterine prolapse occurs when the cardinal ligaments, which support the uterus and vagina, are unduly stretched during pregnancy and do not return to normal following childbirth. This allows the uterus to sag backward and downward into the vagina. Uterine prolapse is less common than in the past, largely because of a decrease in traumatic vaginal deliveries. The condition continues to exist, however, particularly when the woman has had many vaginal deliveries or when

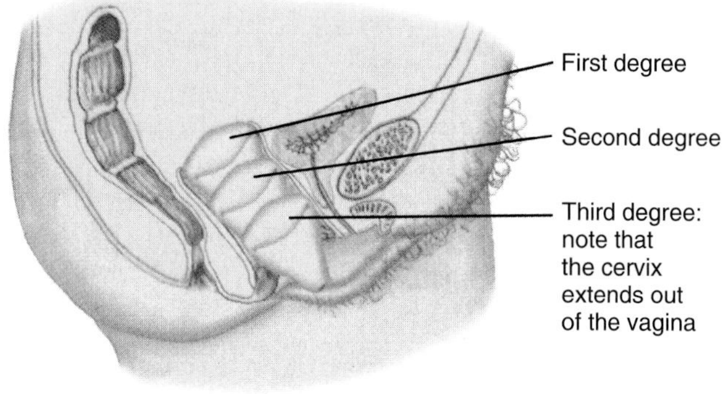

FIGURE 33-7 Three degrees of uterine prolapse.

the infants were large. Figure 33-7 illustrates three degrees of uterine prolapse from first degree, in which the uterus remains in the vagina, to third degree, in which the cervix protrudes through from the vagina.

Symptoms

Symptoms generally become obvious during the menopausal period. This is because estrogen diminishes at this time, resulting in atrophic changes in the supporting structures.

The most common symptoms of vaginal wall prolapse are feelings of pelvic fullness, a dragging sensation, pelvic pressure, and fatigue. Low backache and a feeling that "everything is falling out" are sometimes described. Symptoms also relate to the structures involved. For instance, urinary frequency, urgency, and urinary incontinence are seen in patients with cystocele. Constipation, flatulence, and difficulty defecating are major symptoms of rectocele. Regardless of the location or structure involved, symptoms become worse after prolonged standing, and they are relieved by lying down.

Symptoms of uterine prolapse are produced by the weight of the descending structures and may include sensations of pelvic pressure, backache, and fatigue. Cervical ulceration and bleeding occur if the cervix protrudes from the vaginal introitus.

Management

Treatment of disorders related to pelvic floor dysfunction depends on the woman's age, physical condition, sexual activity, and degree of prolapse. Surgical procedures provide the most satisfactory therapy for women who have significant discomfort. In general, all defects, even if they are currently asymptomatic, will be repaired at once (Nichols, 2000). The most common procedures are the anterior and posterior colporrhaphy. The anterior colporrhaphy involves suturing the pubocervical fascia to support the bladder and urethra when a cystocele exists. If a rectocele exists, a posterior colporrhaphy (suturing the fascia and perineal muscles that support the perineum and rectum) is performed. The two colporrhaphy surgeries are often described as an *A and P (anterior and posterior) repair.*

Vaginal hysterectomy, in which the uterus is removed through the vaginal canal rather than through an abdominal incision, is the most common surgery to correct vaginal prolapse. Vaginal hysterectomy often is combined with anterior and posterior repair.

If surgery is contraindicated, a pessary (a device to support pelvic structures) may be inserted into the vagina. The pessary must be inspected and changed frequently by a physician or nurse practitioner to prevent vaginal ulceration, fistula formation, stool impaction, or infection. Vaginal estrogen cream may improve the woman's tolerance of the pessary (Bhatia, 1998).

Medical therapy may include hormone replacement, which helps reduce the genital atrophy that contributes to pelvic relaxation. Some women have fears about hormone therapy and are reluctant to take it. See p. 945 for information about the benefits and risks of hormone replacement therapy.

Nursing Considerations

Pelvic Exercises. Kegel exercises are known to strengthen the pubococcygeal muscle, which surrounds the urethra, vagina, and rectum and is the main support of the pelvic floor. Before teaching Kegel exercise, determine if the woman can contract the pubococcygeal muscle by asking her to sit with her legs apart while she urinates and to squeeze the muscles to stop the stream of urine. If she can accomplish this, the muscle is contracted and it is possible for her to perform the exercise.

Some women mistakenly believe that the Kegel exercise should be performed while urinating, and this idea should be corrected. The stream of urine is stopped only to determine if it is possible for the woman to contract the muscles and to show the woman which muscles she should contract. Kegel exercises involve conscious contracting and relaxing of the pelvic muscles. Only the pelvic muscles should be used; the abdomen, thighs, and buttocks should NOT tighten. The woman should be taught to exhale and keep the mouth open to avoid bearing down when contracting the pelvic muscles. Each contraction should be held for at least 3 seconds, building to a hold of 10 seconds, and the contraction should be gradually relaxed. For greatest benefit, the woman should repeat the contractions at least 30 times per day, with a relaxation period of 10 seconds between each contraction. The woman must understand that for muscle tone to be maintained, the exercise must be continued for the rest of her life (Sampselle, et al., 1997).

Graduated weight cones may be used as an adjunct to pelvic muscle exercise. Incrementally weighted cones are inserted into the vagina and the woman attempts to hold the weights in place. As the weight of the cones increases, the resistance against which the pelvic muscles contract increases, thereby strengthening the pelvic muscles.

Measures that help reduce the symptoms of pelvic relaxation may also prove helpful. These include lying down with the legs elevated for a few minutes several times a day. Some women are relieved by assuming a knee-chest position for a few minutes. In addition, teaching may include measures to prevent constipation.

Urinary Incontinence. Nurses must acknowledge the reluctance many women feel about discussing incontinence and help them overcome these feelings and seek medical intervention. The types of incontinence most often experienced by women are stress urinary incontinence, discussed previously, and urge incontinence. *Urge incontinence* is involuntary loss of urine associated with a strong urge to urinate, often associated with contraction of the detrusor muscle (Sampselle, et al., 1997). Some women have mixed stress and urge incontinence.

> Direct questions, such as "Do you have trouble with your bladder?" or "Do you ever unintentionally lose urine?" may encourage women to discuss urine control problems. After the subject is introduced, follow up questions are asked to determine urinary frequency. For instance, can she sit through a 2 hour movie without emptying her bladder? How many times does she get up to urinate each night? Does she often feel that she must hurry to empty her bladder and that she will lose urine while going to the restroom?

Nursing research has shown that continence can be improved by teaching specific health promotion activities, such as Kegel exercises and bladder training, which involves adhering to a prescribed schedule for emptying the bladder (Sampselle, et al., 1997; Sampselle, et al., 2000a). Women who cannot execute even a weak pelvic muscle contraction or are unable to implement bladder training may benefit from biofeedback or electrical stimulation provided by a skilled practitioner. Women often benefit from knowing about some of the commercial products that protect the skin and prevent odor. These products are made of material that traps urine and prevents constant contact with the skin.

Women often restrict fluids, believing that this will decrease urinary incontinence. Restricting fluids may actually make the condition worse because the bladder does not fill to its normal capacity. Furthermore, decreased fluid intake can lead to concentrated urine that can irritate bladder mucous membranes and increase the urge to void. Alcohol and caffeine can also irritate the bladder and worsen incontinence.

Check Your Reading

33. How does cystocele differ from rectocele in terms of location? Symptoms?
34. What causes uterine prolapse, and how is it treated?
35. What are nursing actions to alleviate problems associated with pelvic floor relaxation? Urinary incontinence?

DISORDERS OF THE REPRODUCTIVE TRACT

Benign Disorders

The most common benign conditions of the reproductive tract include cervical polyps, uterine leiomyomas (fibroids), and ovarian cysts.

Cervical Polyps

Polyps are small tumors, usually only a few millimeters in diameter, that are generally on a pedicle (a stalk, or stemlike structure). They are caused by proliferation of cervical mucosa, and often cause intermittent vaginal bleeding.

Cervical polyps are surgically removed in an outpatient setting, and the specimen is sent for pathologic examination to rule out malignancy.

Uterine Leiomyomas

Leiomyomas, also called *fibroids,* are one of the most common gynecologic conditions encountered. About 25% of women have fibroids that are clinically detectable (Friedman, 2000). Although the cause is unknown, they develop from uterine smooth muscle cells and are estrogen dependent. As a result, they grow rapidly during the childbearing years when estrogen is abundant but shrink during menopause, unless growth is maintained by estrogen replacement therapy. Fibroids may occur throughout the muscular layer of the uterus (Figure 33-8).

Uterine fibroids often produce no symptoms. However, uterine size is sometimes increased and excessive menstrual bleeding may occur. Excessive bleeding may result in anemia, weakness, and fatigue. Additional symptoms include feelings of pelvic pressure, bloating, and urinary frequency that occurs when the tumor applies pressure on the bladder. Pressure on the ureter may cause hydroureter (dilation of the ureter).

Treatment depends on the size of the fibroids and the symptoms experienced. In the absence of symptoms, treatment may consist of observation only. If abnormal bleeding is a problem, surgical intervention may be necessary. The two most common surgeries are myomectomy or removal of the tumor only, and hysterectomy, which is removal of the uterus. Medical treat-

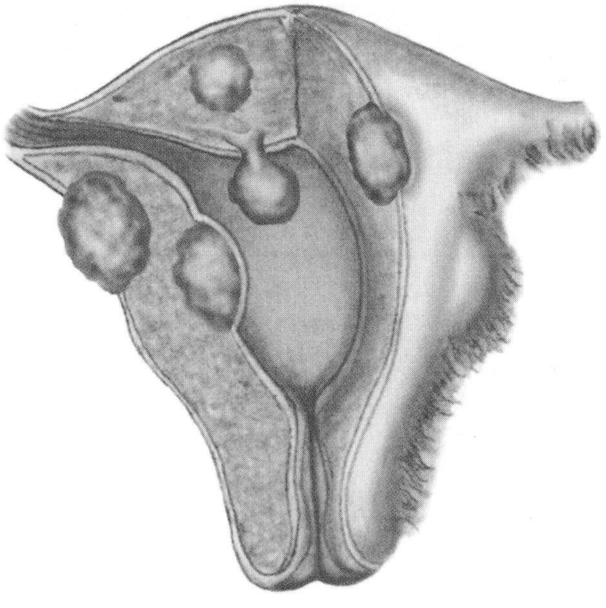

FIGURE 33-8 Sites within the uterus where fibroids commonly occur.

ment with GnRH agonists may be effective in reducing the size of myomas and lessen the need for surgical removal of the tumor. GnRH agonists cause hot flashes, vaginal dryness, and other discomforts similar to menopause, and thus are not tolerated well by some women. Loss of bone mineral density is an adverse effect of long-term therapy as well.

Ovarian Cysts

An ovarian cyst may be either follicular or luteal. If the ovarian follicle fails to rupture during ovulation, a follicular cyst may develop. These cysts are usually asymptomatic and may be an incidental finding on an ultrasound. They generally regress during the subsequent menstrual cycle. A lutein cyst may develop if the corpus luteum becomes cystic and fails to regress. A lutein cyst is more likely to cause pain and delay in the next menstrual cycle. Occasionally, an ovarian cyst can rupture or twist on its pedicle and become infarcted, causing pelvic pain and tenderness.

Treatment depends on differentiating a cyst from a solid ovarian tumor that is more likely to indicate cancer. If the woman is in her childbearing years, when the risk of ovarian cancer is less, the physician may wait until after the next menstrual cycle and examine the woman again. Transvaginal ultrasound examination is useful to determine if it is a fluid-filled cyst or a solid tumor. Laparoscopy may be helpful in ruling out endometriosis. Laparotomy may be necessary to remove the cyst from the ovary for examination by a pathologist.

Malignant Disorders

The primary sites for cancer in the female reproductive organs are the uterus, ovaries, and cervix. Cancer of the vagina, vulva, and fallopian tubes is relatively uncommon. Although cancer can occur at any age, the incidence increases with age.

Table 33-8 RISK FACTORS FOR CANCER OF THE REPRODUCTIVE ORGANS

UTERUS
Obesity
Nulliparity
Late menopause
Diabetes mellitus
Hypertension
Gallbladder disease
Breast, colon, or ovarian cancer
Chronic unopposed estrogen stimulation
CERVIX
First coitus before 20 yr
History of sexually transmitted diseases (strong link with human papillomavirus)
Multiple sexual partners
Lower socioeconomic status (may be related to infrequent gynecologic examinations)
Race (incidence higher in African-Americans)
OVARIES
Race (increased in white women)
Menopause >52 yr
Family history of ovarian or uterine cancer
Nulliparity

Signs and Symptoms

Cancer of the reproductive organs may not be diagnosed until it is advanced because few symptoms are experienced in the early stages. When symptoms occur, they are often nonspecific and could be caused by infection or other benign conditions. Cancer of the ovaries is particularly difficult to diagnose because it may remain "silent" until far advanced, when the chance of long-term survival is greatly reduced.

Risk Factors

Risk factors vary according to the site of the cancer. Risk factors for cervical cancer include a history of sexually transmitted diseases, particularly condyloma acuminatum, or genital warts, caused by HPV. Prolonged use of unopposed estrogen replacement therapy predisposes to overgrowth (hyperplasia) of endometrial tissue and is a significant risk factor for uterine cancer.

Family history is an important risk factor for ovarian cancer. Other factors such as the use of talcum powder and feminine hygiene products that contain talc have also been implicated but their role is inconclusive (Furniss, 2000). See Table 33-8 for a summary of risk factors for cancer of the reproductive organs.

Diagnosis

Early diagnosis is strongly associated with long-term survival. Many screening and diagnostic tests are useful. Screening tests include periodic pelvic examinations, Pap tests, ultrasonography, and serum tests for tumor markers such as CA 125, which may be increased with ovarian or other cancers. Diagnostic procedures such as endometrial biopsy for endometrial cancer and colposcopy can identify patterns of abnormality near the cervical os, where most cancers of the cervix develop.

CRITICAL TO REMEMBER

Symptoms That Must Always Be Investigated

- Irregular vaginal bleeding
- Unexplained postmenopausal bleeding
- Unusual vaginal discharge
- Dyspareunia
- Persistent vulvar or vaginal itching
- Elevated or discolored lesions of the vulva
- Persistent abdominal bloating or constipation
- Persistent anorexia or vomiting
- Blood in stools

Management

Cervical Cancer. Treatment of cancer of the reproductive organs is based on location and extent of the disease and the age and desire of the woman to have children. Early treatment of cervical cancer may consist of cryosurgery, destruction of abnormal tissue by laser, loop electrosurgical excision procedure, or surgical conization of the cervix. After treatment, a surveillance schedule should be established because of the risk of recurrent cervical squamous intraepithelial lesion (SIL).

Treatment for advanced cervical cancer usually consists of a total abdominal hysterectomy and bilateral salpingooophorectomy and may include adjuvant therapy with radiation or chemotherapy. Invasive cervical cancer may be treated with radical hysterectomy or radiation therapy. Survival results are similar, but the woman retains ovarian function with the hysterectomy (Kohler & DiSaia, 2000).

About 15% of male sexual contacts of women with candidiasis will have symptomatic inflammation of the glans penis (balanitis). Symptomatic males should be treated to prevent recurrent infection of the woman (Eschenbach, 1999).

Endometrial Cancer. Treatment for endometrial cancer is often complicated by the fact that women with the disease are often elderly, obese, and diabetic (Berchuck and Cirisano, 2000). The highest cure rate is with surgery (hysterectomy and salpingo-oophorectomy), but poor surgical candidates may be treated with radiation therapy alone, and radiation therapy may be given as adjuvant therapy to women at risk for metastatic disease or in the upper vagina (vaginal cuff).

Ovarian Cancer. A diagnostic workup identifies the effects of the tumor on adjacent organs in the abdomen and identifies metastases to distant sites. Chemotherapy may be given to reduce the tumor's size, followed by oophorectomy to remove it. Added chemotherapy is given after surgery. Many patients with advanced tumors relapse or have disease progression despite treatment.

Check Your Reading

36. What are the signs and symptoms of leiomyomas (uterine fibroids), and how are they treated?
37. Why is ultrasonography used to evaluate ovarian cysts?
38. What signs and symptoms are suggestive of cancer of the reproductive organs and should always be investigated?
39. How may cancer of the following reproductive organs be treated? Cervix? Endometrium? Ovary?

INFECTIOUS DISORDERS OF THE REPRODUCTIVE TRACT

Sexually Transmitted Diseases

Many diseases can be transmitted through sexual activity. For some diseases, such as syphilis, gonorrhea, and chlamydial infection, sexual activity is almost the only method of transmission. For other diseases, such as candidiasis and trichomoniasis, sexual activity may or may not be the mode of transmission.

Incidence

Sexually transmitted diseases are epidemic today, with the highest incidence among adolescents and young adults. Furthermore, the number of untreated infected individuals with no symptoms is most likely immense. For many reasons these diseases remain a major health problem despite advancements in the development of antibiotics. The age of the first sexual experience has been declining steadily, and sexual activity is high among adolescents and young adults. Multiple sexual partners, inadequate knowledge of transmission and prevention, and feelings of invincibility, are common among this age group.

Methods of contraception have a significant impact on the risk of sexually transmitted diseases. Barrier methods, such as condoms and female condoms, offer the best protection from infection. Diaphragms, cervical caps, and spermicidal foams and jellies do not offer the same protection as condoms, although they can decrease the risk of cervical and upper genital tract infections. When counseling teenagers, nurses must emphasize that oral contraceptives prevent pregnancy, but they do nothing to prevent exposure to sexually transmitted diseases.

Major concerns include the following:

- The vulnerability of women to sexually transmitted diseases
- The resistance of some organisms to antibiotics
- The relationship between HIV infection and other sexually transmitted diseases
- Failure of asymptomatic persons to seek treatment when their sexual partner is infected

See Chapter 26 for the impact of sexually transmitted diseases on pregnancy and the fetus.

Types of Sexually Transmitted Diseases

Candidiasis. Candidiasis, also known as *moniliasis* and *yeast infection,* is the most common form of vaginitis. Some conditions, such as pregnancy, diabetes mellitus, oral contraceptive use, and systemic antibiotic therapy, result in changes in vaginal flora that favor accelerated growth of *Candida albicans.* The vaginal pH is often in the normal range of 3.8 to 4.2 (Faro, 2000).

The hallmark presenting symptom for candidiasis is itching. Vulvar and vaginal tissues are inflamed, so burning on urination is also present. Vaginal discharge is white with a typical "cottage cheese" appearance; vaginal and perineal itching is common. Diagnosis is made by identifying the spores of *C. albicans.*

Treatment consists of vaginal application of miconazole (Monistat), clotrimazole (Gyne-Lotrimin), or nystatin (Mycostatin). These medications are available without prescription. However, women should be advised to seek medical attention with the first infection or if the infection persists or recurs frequently. Additional prescription drugs include oral fluconazole (Diflucan), or vaginal terconazole (Terazol) and ticonazole) (Vagistat-1). Many women prefer the oral fluconazole over vaginal preparations. Recurrent yeast infections that resist treatment are associated with diabetes mellitus or HIV infection.

Trichomoniasis. Trichomoniasis is caused by *Trichomonas vaginalis,* an anerobic protozoon that thrives in an alkaline environment. Most infections are believed to be transmitted by sexual contact. The presenting symptoms include a purulent vaginal discharge that is thin or frothy, malodorous, and yellow green or brownish-gray in color. The pH of the discharge is usually greater than 4.5. Vulvar itching, edema, and redness may also be present. The diagnosis is made by identifying the organism in a wet mount preparation.

If the woman is not pregnant, the treatment of choice is metronidazole (Flagyl, Protostat). Some clinicians prefer to avoid use of metronidazole in the first trimester of pregnancy. Clotrimazole (Gyne-Lotrimin) may provide symptom relief at this time. Metronidazole may be used during the second and third trimesters. Alcohol ingestion when taking metronidazole may result in a disulfiram-like (Antabuse) reaction. Women should be advised to avoid using alcohol during treatment with metronidazole and for 24 hours thereafter.

Sexual partners should refrain from intercourse until a cure is established. Reinfection may result when the woman's partner is not treated. In particular, emphasize that all sexual partners should be treated and that condoms should be used with a new partner.

Bacterial Vaginosis. This infection, previously referred to as nonspecific vaginitis or *Gardnerella* vaginitis, is most often caused by the bacillus *Gardnerella vaginalis,* which inhabits the vagina of healthy women. At times, the organism proliferates or "overgrows" and produces an extremely contagious vaginitis. Cause of the proliferation is not known, although tissue trauma and vaginal intercourse have been identified as contributing factors. The infection appears to be related to the frequency of intercourse and the number of sexual partners (Faro, 2000).

Chief signs and symptoms are a thin grayish white vaginal discharge that typically exudes a fishy odor. The diagnosis is made by preparing a saline wet mount and identifying characteristic clue cells (epithelial cells with numerous bacilli clinging to their surface).

Treatment for bacterial vaginosis is directed toward reestablishing the balance of flora in the vagina. Metronidazole has been shown to relieve symptoms and to improve vaginal flora. Clindamycin cream and metronidazole gel are alternative treatments. The woman should refrain from sexual intercourse until cured or her partner should use a condom. The partner also may be treated.

Chlamydial Infection. The most common sexually transmitted disease in Western countries is caused by the gram-negative bacterium *Chlamydia trachomatis.* The incidence is particularly high in the teenage population. Chlamydial infection is often asymptomatic in women, which makes diagnosis and control of the disease difficult. It should be suspected when the male sexual partner is treated for nongonococcal urethritis and when the culture results for gonorrhea are negative, yet the woman exhibits symptoms similar to those of gonorrhea, such as a yellowish vaginal discharge and painful urination. Gonorrhea and chlamydial infections often coexist.

Diagnosis of chlamydial infection can be made by isolating the bacterium in tissue culture, by enzyme-linked immunosorbent assay (ELISA), or by direct fluorescent monoclonal antibody.

Untreated, chlamydial infection ascends from the cervix to involve the fallopian tubes, and it is one of the chief causes of tubal scarring that results in pelvic inflammatory disease (PID), infertility, or ectopic pregnancy. Treatment is usually directed to eradicate both chlamydia and gonorrhea since the two often coexist. Treatment options include ceftriaxone (Rocephin) for the gonorrhea, plus azithromycin (Zithromax), doxycycline (Vibramycin), clindamycin (Cleocin), ofloxacin (Floxin), trovofloxacin (Trovan), ampicillin, or ampicillin/clavulanate. Treatment of all sexual partners is essential to prevent recurrence. Use of condoms until a cure is established is essential as well.

Gonorrhea. Gonorrhea is an infection of the genitourinary tract that is caused by the gonococcus *Neisseria gonorrhoeae.* Gonorrhea may be asymptomatic in women but when symptoms do occur, they usually include purulent discharge, dysuria, and dyspareunia. Diagnosis is based on a positive culture for the gonococcus. Gonorrhea is associated with PID, which increases the risk of tubal scarring and can result in infertility or ectopic pregnancy, as is chlamydial infection.

Currently, two factors influence the treatment of gonorrhea: the high numbers of organisms that have become resistant to previously used antibiotics, such as penicillin and tetracycline, and the high frequency of chlamydial infections in persons with gonorrhea. Ceftriaxone (Rocephin), in combination with one of the antibiotics listed above, appears to be effective for treatment of all gonococcal infections. Spectinomycin (Trobicin) is an option for those allergic to ceftriaxone. Doxycycline, oflaxacin, trovofloxacin, and azithromycin are often effective against both *C. trachomatis* and *N. gonorrhoeae.* All sexual partners should be treated simultaneously and intercourse should be avoided or the man should use a condom until a cure is confirmed.

Syphilis. Syphilis is caused by the spirochete *Treponema pallidum,* and it is divided into primary, secondary, and tertiary stages. The first sign of primary syphilis is a painless chancre that develops on the genitalia, anus, or lips or in the oral cavity. At this time, diagnosis is made by identifying the spirochete on darkfield microscopy in material scraped from the base of the chancre. A serologic test is generally negative in the primary stage. If untreated, the chancre heals in about 6 weeks. The disease is highly infectious at the primary stage.

Although the chancre disappears, the spirochete lives and is carried by the blood to all parts of the body. About 2 months after the initial infection, infected people exhibit symptoms of secondary syphilis, including enlargement of the spleen and liver, headache, anorexia, and a generalized maculopapular skin rash. Skin eruptions, called *condylomata lata,* may develop on the vulva during this time. Condylomata lata resemble warts; they contain numerous spirochetes and are highly contagious. Serologic tests are generally positive at this time.

If untreated, the disease enters a latent phase that may last for several years. Tertiary syphilis, which follows the latent phase, may involve the heart, blood vessels, and central nervous system. General paralysis and psychosis may result.

In addition to identification of the spirochete in material scraped from a chancre, diagnosis is also made by serology. The usual screening test is the Venereal Disease Research Laboratory (VDRL) serum test, which is based on the presence of antibodies produced in response to the infection. The rapid plasma reagin (RPR) and fluorescent treponemal antibody absorption (FTA-ABS) tests are more specific and are commonly performed to confirm a positive VDRL.

Best treatment of all stages of syphilis is with penicillin. Ceftriaxone can also be useful. Tetracycline is an alternative if the woman is not pregnant. A woman who is allergic to penicillin can be admitted to the hospital for desensitization to penicillin and followed by administration of the drug.

Herpes Genitalis. Herpes genitalis is a sexually transmitted disease caused by the herpes simplex virus (HSV). Two types of HSV have been identified: type 1 and type 2. HSV 2 usually causes genital lesions and HSV 1 usually causes oral-pharyngeal infection. However, either organism may infect the less-frequent location. Transmission occurs through direct contact with an infected person. A person infected with HSV 1 develops antibodies that may reduce the severity of the first HSV 2 infection. A *primary* HSV 2 infection is one in which the person had no preceding HSV 1 infection, and thus has no antibodies.

Within 2 to 12 days after the primary infection, vesicles (blisters) appear in a characteristic cluster on the vulva, perineum, or perianal area. The initial lesions may cause severe vulvar pain and tenderness as well as dyspareunia. Lesions may also occur on the cervix or in the vagina. With primary infection, the woman may also experience flu-like symptoms, including fever, general malaise, and enlarged lymph nodes. The vesicles rupture within 1 to 7 days and form ulcers that take an average of 7 to 10 days to heal.

When symptoms abate, the virus remains dormant in the nerve ganglia and periodically reactivates, particularly in times of stress, fever, and menses. Recurrent episodes are seldom as extensive or painful as the initial episode but they are just as contagious. Diagnosis is often based on clinical signs and symptoms and confirmed by viral culture of fluid from the vesicle.

No cure exists, but acyclovir, an antiviral drug, helps reduce or suppress symptoms, shedding, and recurrent episodes. The safe use of acyclovir in pregnancy has not been established. Women should be advised to abstain from sexual contact while the lesions are present. If it is an initial infection, they should continue to abstain until they become culture-negative, because prolonged viral shedding may occur in such cases.

Condylomata Acuminata. Condylomata acuminata, also known as *venereal* or *genital warts,* are caused

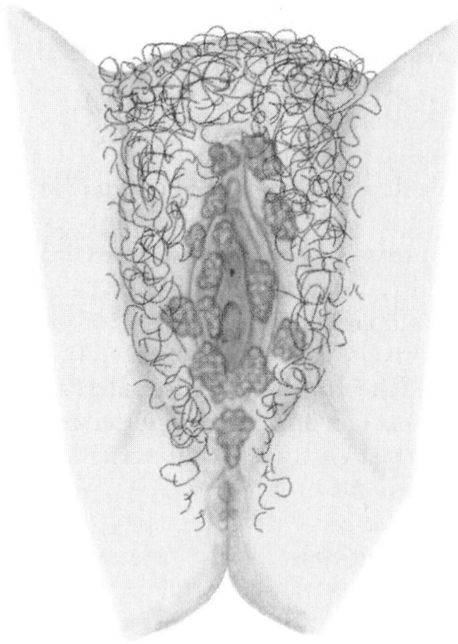

FIGURE 33-9 Condylomata acuminata, also called *venereal warts,* are caused by the human papillomavirus (HPV).

by human papilloma virus, or HPV. The dry, wart-like growths may be small and discrete, or they may cluster and resemble cauliflower (Figure 33-9). Common sites include the vagina, labia, cervix, and perineal area.

Condylomata acuminata are of particular concern because of the association of HPV with cervical cancer. Colposcopy, examination by a magnifying instrument called the colposcope, is generally recommended to evaluate abnormal cervical tissue and to identify HPV. Women with condylomata acuminata should be advised to have semiannual or annual Pap tests to detect cervical dysplasia.

The goal of treatment is to remove the warts, which easily transmit the virus back and forth between sexual partners. Treatment is determined by the site and extent of the warts and the woman's preference. Topical treatment options include podophyllin, trichloroacetic acid (TCA), bichloroacetic acid (BCA), and imiquimod cream. More extensive warts or those that do not respond to topical therapy may require removal by cryotherapy, electrodessication, electrocautery, or laser. Interferon, an antineoplastic drug, is sometimes used to treat condylomata acuminata in women older than 18 years of age who have not responded to conventional therapy.

The woman must understand that none of these treatments eradicate the virus and that she may have recurrences. Furthermore, all sexual partners must be treated. Sexual contact should be avoided until all lesions are healed, and the use of condoms is recommended to reduce transmission.

Acquired Immunodeficiency Syndrome. Acquired immunodeficiency syndrome (AIDS), caused by HIV, remains the most devastating sexually transmitted disease in the world today, although new treatments have improved the outlook considerably. Human immunodeficiency virus has been isolated from blood, semen, vaginal secretions, urine, saliva, tears, cerebrospinal fluid, amniotic fluid, and breast milk. The primary modes of transmission are intimate contact with infected bodily secretions, exposure to infected blood and blood products, and perinatal transmission from mother to infant.

HIV testing usually is offered to high-risk groups such as users of injectable drugs. It is also offered during pregnancy because use of zidovudine can substantially reduce transmission of the virus to the fetus. Diagnosis of another sexually-transmitted disease is an indication to offer HIV testing, as is the patient who has manifestations of HIV infection (recurrent candidiasis infection, profound weight loss, prolonged fever, recurrent herpes, and generalized lymphadenopathy) with no other explanation for the signs and symptoms (Wininger, 2000).

Although no cure exists, new medications show a great deal of promise. In addition to zidovudine and didanosine (a reverse transcriptase inhibitor), which have been used for some time, a newer category of drug has been introduced. These drugs, known as protease inhibitors, block the working of protease, an enzyme crucial to one step in the reproductive cycle of HIV. Recent studies are focusing on combination therapies and new reverse transcriptase inhibitors. See Chapters 26 and 30 for a discussion of HIV and AIDS management in pregnant women and neonates.

Nursing Considerations

As teachers and counselors, nurses can play a major part in preventing the spread of STDs. To fulfill this role, nurses must be prepared to do the following:

- Teach the signs and symptoms that require medical attention
- Explain diagnostic or screening tests
- Teach preventive measures and follow-up to assure a cure

Check Your Reading

40. What four conditions may change the normal flora of the vagina and result in *Candida albicans* vaginitis?
41. How does the vaginal discharge of candidiasis differ from that of trichomoniasis?
42. Why are barrier-type contraceptives recommended to prevent STDs?
43. How do primary and secondary syphilis differ in terms of signs and symptoms and potential for transmitting the disease?
44. How are condylomata acuminata associated with cervical cancer?

WOMEN WANT TO KNOW About Sexually Transmitted Diseases

What are the most common signs and symptoms of sexually transmitted diseases (STDs)?

- Unexpected nonbloody vaginal discharge (increased amount, unusual color, or odor) or vaginal bleeding
- Vulvar itching or swelling
- Pelvic pain, including painful intercourse, painful urination, and abdominal tenderness
- Skin eruptions or changes (rashes, chancres, warts, painful papules, or vesicles)
- Flu-like symptoms (fever, swollen or painful lymph glands, loss of appetite, nausea or vomiting)
- Presence of symptoms in a sexual partner, even if symptoms are absent in the woman

What are the common methods of diagnosis?

- Culture (vaginal discharge, cervix, lesions) to identify organism
- Blood test (serology) to determine if antibodies for specific diseases are present
- VDRL, RPR, or FTA-ABS test for syphilis, HIV test for human immunodeficiency virus)

How can STDs be prevented?

- Establish monogamous relationship with uninfected partner.
- Limit number of sexual partners.
- Use mechanical and chemical barriers such as a latex condom with every act of intercourse
- Remember that one episode of an STD offers no protection from future infection.
- Make sure partner is simultaneously treated to prevent reinfection.

What are the most important things to know about the treatment?

- The entire course of medication must be completed even if symptoms subside.
- Comply with follow-up evaluation as recommended by health care provider.
- Curtail sexual intercourse until free of infection.
- The partner must be examined, treated, and a follow-up evaluation done before resuming sexual intercourse.
- Side effects of medications, such as skin rashes, difficulty breathing, or headaches must be reported.
- Not all STDs can be cured (herpes, AIDS, venereal warts), and treatment is aimed at slowing the disease and preventing complications.

Are there measures that provide comfort and prevent secondary infections?

- Keep the vulva clean but avoid strong soaps, creams, and ointments unless prescribed by health care provider.
- Keep the vulva dry; using a hair dryer on low heat is helpful.
- Wear absorbent cotton underwear and avoid pantyhose and tight pants as much as possible.
- Take analgesics (aspirin or acetaminophen) as directed by health care provider.
- Cool or tepid sitz baths may provide relief from itching.
- Wipe vulva from front to back following urination or defecation and then carefully wash hands.

Pelvic Inflammatory Disease

Pelvic inflammatory disease (PID), infection of the upper genital tract, is a serious health problem in the United States. Pelvic inflammatory disease causes 200,000 hospitalizations and 100,000 surgical procedures annually, with another 2.5 outpatient visits each year. The estimated costs for PID in the United States are estimated to be approximately $10 billion (Culver & Martens, 2000). Numerous other women with "silent" sexually transmitted diseases face the risk of chronic pelvic pain, infertility, and ectopic pregnancy, which are common sequelae.

Etiology

About 12% of PID cases are caused by *C. trachomatis* and 30% by *N. gonorrhoeae.* The remainder are caused by a mixture of organisms such as *E. coli, Gardnerella vaginalis, Streptococcus, Peptostreptococcus, bacteroides, Prevotella, Mycoplasma,* and *Ureaplasma.* Bacterial vaginosis has also been associated with PID (Culver & Martens, 2000). These organisms invade the endocervical canal, where they cause cervicitis. Bacteria ascend and infect the endometrium, fallopian tubes, and pelvic cavity. The chronic inflammatory response results in tubal scarring and peritubal adhesions, which interfere with conception or with transport of the fertilized ovum through the obstructed fallopian tubes.

Symptoms

Signs and symptoms of PID vary widely. Some women are asymptomatic, whereas others experience pelvic pain, fever, purulent vaginal discharge, nausea, anorexia, and irregular vaginal bleeding. Findings during physical examination may include abdominal or adnexal tenderness, and tenderness of the uterus and cervix when they are moved during bimanual examination (cervical motion tenderness). Laboratory evaluation may reveal a marked leukocytosis and increased sedimentation rate. A urinalysis is needed to rule out urinary tract infection, and cervical cultures for suspected organisms help diagnose the disease.

Management

Women with serious infection, as manifested by fever, abdominal pain, and leukocytosis, may be admitted to a hospital. They are most often treated with intravenous administration of broad-spectrum antibiotics such as cefoxitin (Mefoxin), cefotetan (Cefotan), doxycycline, clindamycin, or gentamicin (Garamycin). Laparoscopy may be required to rule out surgical emergencies such as appendicitis or ectopic pregnancy, which present with similar signs and symptoms, and to obtain specimens for culture. Ambulatory treatment is appropriate for some women who are not as ill and are able to comply with the recommended regimen.

Nursing Considerations

Nurses can play an important role in preventing PID by teaching women how to prevent sexually transmitted diseases in themselves and in their partners. Prevention can be thought of as occurring on two levels: primary and secondary. Primary prevention involves avoiding exposure to these diseases or preventing acquisition of infection during exposure. Primary preventive measures include limiting the number of sexual partners and avoiding intercourse with those who have had multiple partners or other high-risk behaviors such as injectable drug use, which is associated with HIV infection. Barrier methods (latex condoms) used consistently and correctly during all sexual activity help prevent sexually transmitted diseases.

Secondary prevention involves keeping a lower genital tract infection from ascending to the upper genital tract or from being further transmitted within the community. This involves seeking medical attention promptly after having unprotected sex with someone who is suspected of having a sexually transmitted disease and when vaginal discharge or genital lesions are apparent. Periodic medical assessment is necessary if the woman is not in a mutually monogamous relationship, even if she is asymptomatic. Additional measures include taking medication as prescribed and returning for follow-up evaluation.

Toxic Shock Syndrome

Although toxic shock syndrome is rare, it is a potentially fatal condition caused by toxin-producing strains of *S. aureus.* The toxin that is produced alters capillary permeability, which allows intravascular fluid to leak from the blood vessels, leading to hypovolemia, hypotension, and shock. The toxin also causes direct tissue damage to organs and precipitates serious defects in coagulation.

If toxin-producing strains of *S. aureus* inhabit the vagina, certain factors increase the risk that the toxin will gain entry into the bloodstream. These include the use of high-absorbency tampons during menstruation and barrier methods of contraception (cervical cap or diaphragm), both of which may trap and hold bacteria if left in place for a prolonged time.

Symptoms of toxic shock syndrome include a sudden spiking fever and flulike symptoms (headache, sore throat, vomiting, diarrhea), hypotension, a generalized rash resembling sunburn, and skin peeling from the palms of the hands and the soles of the feet 1 and 2 weeks after the onset of the illness.

Treatment consists of fluid replacement, administration of vasopressor drugs, and antimicrobial therapy. Corticosteroids may be used to treat skin changes.

Nurses are often responsible for providing information that may help to prevent toxic shock syndrome.

Tampon Use

Nurses should instruct women to do the following:

- Wash the hands thoroughly to remove bacteria before inserting tampons.
- Change tampons at least every 4 hours to prevent excessive bacterial growth on a tampon that is left in place for a longer time.
- Do not use superabsorbent tampons at any time because they may be left in the vagina for a prolonged period, allowing bacteria to proliferate.
- Use pads rather than tampons during hours of sleep, which usually exceeds 6 to 8 hours.

Diaphragm Use

Nurses should tell women to do the following:

- Wash hands thoroughly before inserting diaphragm.
- Do not use diaphragm during menstrual periods.
- Remove diaphragm within time recommended by health care provider.

Check Your Reading

45. What organisms cause pelvic inflammatory disease?
46. How can the risk of toxic shock syndrome be reduced?

SUMMARY CONCEPTS

- Health maintenance refers to examinations and screening procedures that provide early detection of specific conditions, such as breast or cervical cancer, and allow for early treatment that increases the chance of long-term survival.
- A major role of nurses is to explain screening procedures and to encourage women to have them on a regular basis. The most common screening procedures include BSE, professional breast examination, and mammography for breast cancer; vulvar self-examination to detect precancerous conditions or infections; pelvic examination to detect abnormalities of the uterus or ovaries; Pap test for cervical cancer; and screening for fecal occult blood. Additional tests may include transvaginal ultrasonography and CA 125 if the woman is at risk for ovarian cancer.
- Disorders of the breast may be benign, such as fibrocystic changes that occur in relation to the menstrual cycle, or malignant. The discovery of any breast disorder creates anxiety in women, and nurses must be prepared to explain diagnostic procedures, such as ultrasonography, fine needle aspiration, core needle biopsy, and surgical biopsy.

- One in eight women in the United States develops breast cancer. Besides gender, the greatest risk factors are advancing age, a prior history of breast cancer, and genetic mutations in the BRCA 1 and BRCA 2 and p53 genes. Additional factors include family history (grandmother, mother, sister) of breast cancer and previous uterine, ovarian, or colon cancer. Lifestyle factors such as a high intake of dietary fat, smoking, and consumption of alcohol are also suspected to increase risk.
- Management of breast cancer includes surgical removal of the tumor plus varying amounts of surrounding tissue and lymph glands. Adjuvant therapy includes radiation, chemotherapy, hormone therapy, and immunotherapy.
- Breast reconstruction is an integral part of the surgical management of breast cancer. Methods include tissue expansion and autogenous grafts.
- Nursing care for women with cancer of the breast focuses on providing emotional support and accurate information.
- Cardiovascular disease kills more women than breast cancer. Preventive measures include modifying all risk factors that can be modified, such as maintaining a normal weight and stopping smoking. Added preventive measures include controlling hypertension, diet and glucose control, increasing activity, and, for certain women, use of aspirin on a daily basis.
- Menstrual cycle disorders include amenorrhea, abnormal uterine bleeding, cyclic pelvic pain, and premenstrual syndrome. Some of the disorders, such as premenstrual syndrome, respond to lifestyle alterations such as changes in diet, exercise habits, and stress management.
- Induced abortion may be performed by medical or surgical methods, and each method is associated with social and ethical conflicts.
- The climacteric, is a combination of endocrine, somatic, and psychic changes that occur at the end of the reproductive cycle. Menopause is the final menstrual period, although most people use the term interchangeably with climacteric. Women's responses to menopause vary widely, but all women are in a permanent state of estrogen deficit after menopause that can result in bone loss (osteoporosis), increased risk for coronary artery disease, atrophic vaginitis, and Alzheimer's disease.
- Hormone replacement therapy is commonly prescribed to manage the symptoms of estrogen deficit, such as hot flashes and atrophic vaginitis, and to decrease bone mineral loss that results in osteoporosis. Hormone replacement therapy also reduces a woman's risk for cardiovascular disease after menopause.
- Estrogen replacement has risks and benefits and is contraindicated for women who have thromboembolic disease, undiagnosed vaginal bleeding, previous episodes of breast cancer or untreated uterine cancer, or chronic liver disease. For these women, alternative measures are needed to control the symptoms of menopause.
- Relaxation of pelvic support structures occurs as a delayed result of traumatic childbirth and becomes troublesome when a deficiency in estrogen hastens genital atrophy.
- Many infections of the reproductive tract are transmitted by sexual contact. The incidence of sexually transmitted diseases is reduced by barrier methods of contraception, particularly the condom, which prevents contact between infected skin or mucosal surfaces and prevents potentially infected ejaculate from entering the woman's lower genital tract.
- Pelvic inflammatory disease is often a complication of untreated sexually transmitted diseases, and a large number are caused by chlamydial or gonorrheal infections. PID can cause infertility or ectopic pregnancy because of scarring of fallopian tubes resulting from inflammatory processes in the pelvic cavity.
- Toxic shock syndrome is a life-threatening condition resulting from infection with toxin-producing strains of *Staphylococcus aureus.* The infection may be related to use of high-absorbency tampons that trap and hold bacteria in nutrient-rich menstrual blood for an extended time. Tampons should be removed every 4 hours, and other items that trap bacteria, such as cervical caps and diaphragms, should be removed as directed by the health care provider.

REFERENCES & READINGS

Affara, F.A. (2000). Correspondence from abroad: When tradition maims. *American Journal of Nursing,* 100(8), 52-60.

American Academy of Pediatrics, Committee on Bioethics. (1998). Female genital mutilation. *Pediatrics,* 102(1), 153-156.

American Cancer Society. (2000a). *Cancer resource center.* Retrieved November 8, 2000 from http://www.cancer.org.

American Cancer Society. (2000b). *How to perform a breast self-exam.* Retrieved November 8, 2000 from http://www.cancer.org/NBCAM_breast_self_exam.html.

American College of Obstetricians and Gynecologists (ACOG). (1999a). *Medical management of endometriosis: ACOG Practice Bulletin.* Washington, D.C.: Author.

American College of Obstetricians and Gynecologists (ACOG). (2000). *Premenstrual syndrome: ACOG Practice Bulletin.* Washington, D.C.: Author.

American College of Obstetricians and Gynecologists (ACOG). (1999b). *Primary and preventive care: Periodic assessments: ACOG Committee Opinion.* Washington, D.C.: Author.

American Heart Association. (2000a). Aspirin in heart attack and stroke prevention. Retrieved November 18, 2000 from http://www.americanheart.org/Heart_and_Stroke_A_Z_Guide/aspirin.html.

American Heart Association. (2000b). Cholesterol levels. Retrieved November 18, 2000 from http://www.americanheart.org/Heart_and_Stroke_A_Z_Guidechollev.html.

American Heart Association. (2000c). Cholesterol ratio. Retrieved November 18, 2000 from http://www.americanheart.org/Heart_and_Stroke_A_Z_Guidecholr.html.

American Heart Association. (2000d). Cigarette and tobacco smoke: Biostatistical fact sheet. Retrieved November 8, 2000 from http://www.americanheart.org/statistics/biostats/bioci.htm.

American Heart Association. (2000e). Exercise (physical activity). Retrieved November 20, 2000 from http://www.americanheart.org/Heart_and_Stroke_A_Z_Guide/exercise.html.

American Heart Association. (2000f). Overweight and obesity: Biostatistical fact sheet. Retrieved November 6, 2000 from http://www.americanheart.org/statistics/biostats/bioow.htm.

American Heart Association. (2000g). Physical inactivity: Biostatistical fact sheet. Retrieved November 8, 2000 from http://www.americanheart.org/statistics/biostats/biopi.htm.
American Heart Association. (2000h). Women and cardiovascular diseases: Biostatistical fact sheet. Retrieved November 9, 2000 from http://www.americanheart.org/statistics/biostats/biowo.htm.
American Heart Association. (2000i). Women, heart disease and stroke. Retrieved November 20, 2000 from http://www.americanheart.org/Heart_and_Stroke_A_Z_Guide/women.html.
Association of Women's Health, Obstetric, and Neonatal Nurses (AWHONN). (1999a). *Monograph I: Postmenopausal health risks and the importance of prevention.* Washington, D.C.: Author.
Association of Women's Health, Obstetric, and Neonatal Nurses (AWHONN). (1999b). *Monograph II: Disease prevention strategies among postmenopausal women.* Washington, D.C.: Author.
Association of Women's Health, Obstetric, and Neonatal Nurses (AWHONN). (1999c). *Monograph III: Enhancing women's health through partnership.* Washington, D.C.: Author.
Bailey, K., Combs, M.C., Rogers, L.J., & Stanley, K.L. (2000). Measuring up: Could this simple nursing intervention help prevent osteoporosis? *AWHONN Lifelines,* 4(2), 41-44.
Baram, D.A. (2000). Premenstrual syndrome. In E.J. Quilligan and F.P. Zuspan (Eds.), *Current therapy in obstetrics and gynecology* (5th ed., pp. 139-143). Philadelphia: W.B. Saunders.
Bennet, M.J. (1998). Abortion. In N.F. Hacker & J.G. Moore (Eds.), *Essentials of obstetrics and gynecology* (3rd ed., pp. 477-486). Philadelphia: W.B. Saunders.
Berchuck, A., & Cirisano, F.D. (2000). Endometrial carcinoma. In E.J. Quilligan and F.P. Zuspan (Eds.), *Current therapy in obstetrics and gynecology* (5th ed., pp. 207-210). Philadelphia: Saunders.
Bhatia, N.N. (1998). Genitourinary dysfunction: Pelvic organ prolapse, urinary incontinence, and infections. In N.F. Hacker & J.G. Moore (Eds.), *Essentials of obstetrics and gynecology* (3rd ed., pp. 455-476). Philadelphia: W.B. Saunders.
Blackwell, R.E., & Farah, L.A. (2000). Amenorrhea. In S.B. Ransom, M.P. Dombrowski, S.G. McNeeley, K.S. Moghissi, & A.R. Munkarah (Eds.), *Practical strategies in obstetrics and gynecology* (pp. 551-559). Philadelphia: W.B. Saunders.
Chavez, M.L., & Chavez, P.I. (2000). Herbal medicine. In D.W. Novey (Ed.), *Clinician's complete reference to complementary & alternative medicine* (pp. 545-563). St. Louis: Mosby.
Christin-Maitre, S., Bouchard, P., & Spitz, I.M. (2000). Medical termination of pregnancy. *New England Journal of Medicine,* 342(13), 946-956.
Cotter, V.T. (1997). Harmonic convergence: Finding balance through hormone replacement therapy. *AWHONN Lifelines,* 1(1), 37-42.
Creehan, P.A. (1995). Toxic shock syndrome: An opportunity for nursing intervention. *Journal of Obstetric, Gynecologic, and Neonatal Nursing,* 24(6), 557-561.
Culver, S.M., & Martens, M.G. (2000). Pelvic inflammatory disease. In E.J. Quilligan and F.P. Zuspan (Eds.), *Current therapy in obstetrics and gynecology* (5th ed., pp. 122-131). Philadelphia: W.B. Saunders.
Czerwinski, B.S. (2000). Variation in feminine hygiene practices as a function of age. *Journal of Obstetric, Gynecologic, and Neonatal Nursing,* 29(6), 625-633.
Darrow, V.C. (2000). Annual examination. In E.J. Quilligan & F.P. Zuspan (Eds.), *Current therapy in obstetrics and gynecology* (5th ed., pp. 444-451). Philadelphia: W.B. Saunders.
Dawood, M.Y. (2000). Dysmenorrhea. In E.J. Quilligan & F.P. Zuspan (Eds.), *Current therapy in obstetrics and gynecology* (5th ed., pp. 31-36). Philadelphia: W.B. Saunders.
DeLancey, J.O.L. (2000). Genital prolapse. In E.J. Quilligan and F.P. Zuspan (Eds.), *Current therapy in obstetrics and gynecology* (5th ed., pp. 61-64). Philadelphia: W.B. Saunders.
DeMasters, J. (2000). HRT & menopause: A clinician's guide to understanding the dilemma. *AWHONN Lifelines,* 4(2), 26-35.
De Remer, P. (2001). Improving adherence to abnormal Pap smear follow-up. *Journal of Obstetric, Gynecologic, and Neonatal Nursing,* 30(1), 80-88.
Dowd, R. (1999). Help your patient live with osteoporosis: Identifying risk, managing pain, overseeing treatment. *American Journal of Nursing,* 99(4), 55-60.
Eden, J.A. (1998). Dysmenorrhea and premenstrual syndrome. In N.F. Hacker & J.G. Moore (Eds.), *Essentials of Obstetrics and Gynecology* (3rd ed., pp. 386-392). Philadelphia: W.B. Saunders.
Eschenbach, D.A. (1999). Pelvic infections and sexually transmitted diseases. In J.R. Scott, P.J. Di Saia, C.B. Hammond, et al. (Eds.), *Danforth's obstetrics and gynecology,* (8th ed., pp. 579-600). Philadelphia: Lippincott.
Eschenbach, D.A. (2000). Vaginosis (Bacterial). In E.J. Quilligan and F.P. Zuspan (Eds.), *Current therapy in obstetrics and gynecology* (5th ed., pp. 183-187). Philadelphia: W.B. Saunders.
Evans, M., & Dumesic, D.A. (2000). Menopause. In E.J. Quilligan & F.P. Zuspan (Eds.), *Current therapy in obstetrics and gynecology* (5th ed., pp. 108-113). Philadelphia: W.B. Saunders.
Faro, S. (2000). Sexually transmitted diseases. In E.J. Quilligan & F.P. Zuspan (Eds.), *Current therapy in obstetrics and gynecology* (5th ed., pp. 161-169). Philadelphia: W.B. Saunders.
Ferreira, N. (1996). Sexually transmitted *Chlamydia trachomatis. Nurse Practitioner Forum,* 7(1), 40-46.
Fleschler, R. (1998). Heart-healthy eating: Good nutrition can help prevent CAD in women. *AWHONN Lifelines* 2(2), 32-37.
Fontaine, K.L. (2000). *Healing practices: Alternative therapies for nursing.* Upper Saddle River, NJ: Prentice Hall.
Foulks, M.J. (1998). The Papanicolaou smear: Its impact on the promotion of women's health. *Journal of Obstetric, Gynecologic, and Neonatal Nursing,* 27(4), 367-373.
Friedman, A.J. (2000). Leiomyomata uteri. In E.J. Quilligan and F.P. Zuspan (Eds.), *Current therapy in obstetrics and gynecology* (5th ed., pp. 97-101).
Freund, K.M. (1995). Osteoporosis. In P.L. Carr, K.M. Freund, & S. Somani (Eds.), *The medical care of women* (pp. 643-651). Philadelphia: W.B. Saunders.
Furniss, K. (2000). Tomatoes, Pap smears, and tea? Adopting behaviors that may prevent reproductive cancers and improve health. *Journal of Obstetric, Gynecologic, and Neonatal Nursing* 29(6), 642-652.
Galsworthy, T.D. (1996). It steals more than bone. *American Journal of Nursing,* 96(6), 27-33.
Ginsburg, K.A., & Dinsay, R. (2000). Premenstrual syndrome. In S.B. Ransom, M.P. Dombrowski, S.G. McNeeley, K.S. Moghissi, & A.R. Munkarah (Eds.), *Practical strategies in obstetrics and gynecology* (pp. 684-694). Philadelphia: W.B. Saunders.

Grabo, T.N., Fahs, P.S., Nataupsky, L.G., & Reich, H. (1999). Uterine myomas: Treatment options. *Journal of Obstetric, Gynecologic, and Neonatal Nursing,* 28(1), 23-31.

Hacker, N.F. (1998). Breast disease: A gynecologic perspective. In N.F. Hacker & J.G. Moore (Eds.), *Essentials of obstetrics and gynecology* (3rd ed., pp. 507-515). Philadelphia: W.B. Saunders.

Hale, T. (2000). *Medications and mother's milk,* 9th ed. Amarillo, TX: Pharmasoft Publishing.

Halm, M.A., & Penque, S. (1999). Heart disease in women. *American Journal of Nursing,* 99(4), 26-31.

Heaney, R.P. (1998). Pathophysiology of osteoporosis. *Endocrinology & Metabolism Clinics of North America* 27(2), 255-265.

Hendrix, S.L. (2000). Menopause. In S.B. Ransom, M.P. Dombrowski, S.G. McNeeley, K.S. Moghissi, & A.R. Munkarah (Eds.), *Practical strategies in obstetrics and gynecology* (pp. 593-608). Philadelphia: W.B. Saunders.

Higgins, P.G., & Smith, P.E. (1997). Assessing cervical cancer risk. *AWHONN Lifelines* 1(6), 43-47.

Hindle, W.H. (2000). Mastalgia and fibrocystic changes of the breast. In E.J. Quilligan and F.P. Zuspan (Eds.), *Current therapy in obstetrics and gynecology* (5th ed., pp. 494-495). Philadelphia: W.B. Saunders.

Huff, B.C. (2000). Screening for cervical cancer: It's time to check your Pap technique. *AWHONN Lifelines* 4(3), 53-55.

Jenkins, P., Bernier, F., Davila, G.W., & Harris, L. (1996). *Nonsurgical treatment of urinary stress incontinence with the bladder neck support prosthesis; Extended experience.* Clinical Research Paper, AWHONN Conference, June 2-6.

Johnson, S.T. (2000). From incontinence to confidence. *American Journal of Nursing,* 100(2), 69-76.

Johnston, C. (2000). Diseases of the breast. In S.B. Ransom, M.P. Dombrowski, S.G. McNeeley, K.S. Moghissi, & A.R. Munkarah (Eds.). *Practical strategies in obstetrics and gynecology* (pp. 170-186). Philadelphia: W.B. Saunders.

Kiebeck, D., & Beller, F.K. (2000). Breast cancer: Principles of therapy. In E.J. Quilligan and F.P. Zuspan (Eds.), *Current therapy in obstetrics and gynecology* (5th ed., pp. 456-461). Philadelphia: W.B. Saunders.

Kim, M. (2000). Secondary amenorrhea. In E.J. Quilligan and F.P. Zuspan (Eds.), *Current therapy in obstetrics and gynecology* (5th ed., pp. 146-150). Philadelphia: W.B. Saunders.

Klingman, L. (1999). Assessing the female reproductive system. *American Journal of Nursing,* 99(8), 37-43.

Kohler, M.F., and DiSaia, P.J. (2000). Cervical carcinoma. In E.J. Quilligan and F.P. Zuspan (Eds.), *Current therapy in obstetrics and gynecology* (5th ed., pp. 204-207). Philadelphia: W.B. Saunders.

Krauss, R.M., Eckel, R.H., Howard, B., Appel, L.J., Daniels, S.R., Deckelbaum, R.J., et al. (2000). AHA Dietary guidelines: Revision 2000: A statement for healthcare professionals from the Nutrition Committee of the American Heart Association. *Circulation,* 102(10), 2296-2311.

Kuehn, J., McMahon, P., & Creekmore, S. (1999). Stopping a silent killer: Preventing heart disease in women. *AWHONN Lifelines,* 3(2), 31-35.

Lammers, S.E., Schaefer, K.M., Ladd, E.C., & Echenberg, R. (2000). Caring for women living with ovarian cancer: Recommendations for advanced practice nurses. *Journal of Obstetric, Gynecologic, and Neonatal Nursing,* 29(6), 567-573.

La Quatra, I. (2000). Nutrition for weight management. In L.K. Mahan and S. Escott-Stump (Eds.), Krause's food, nutrition, and diet therapy (10th ed., pp. 485-515). Philadelphia: W.B. Saunders.

Learn, C.D., & Higgins, P.G. (1999). Harmonizing herbs: Managing menopause with help from Mother Earth. *AWHONN Lifelines,* 3(5), 39-43.

Lebherz, T.B. (1998). Infectious and benign diseases of the vagina, cervix, and vulva. In N.F. Hacker & J.G. Moore (Eds.), *Essentials of obstetrics and gynecology* (3rd ed., pp. 393-411). Philadelphia: W.B. Saunders.

Lindsay, S.H., & Claywell, L.G. (1998). Considering soy: Its estrogenic effects may protect women. *AWHONN Lifelines,* 2(1), 41-44.

Lindsay, S.H. (1999). Menopause, naturally: Exploring alternatives to traditional hormone replacement therapy. *AWHONN Lifelines,* 3(5), 32-38.

Marchant, D.J. (2000). Breast mass and nipple discharge. In E.J. Quilligan & F.P. Zuspan (Eds.), *Current therapy in obstetrics and gynecology* (5th ed., pp. 462-465). Philadelphia: W.B. Saunders.

McGovern, P.G., & Little, A.B. (2000). Dysfunctional uterine bleeding. In E.J. Quilligan & F.P. Zuspan (Eds.), *Current therapy in obstetrics and gynecology* (5th ed., pp. 27-31). Philadelphia: W.B. Saunders.

McNeeley, S.G. (2000). Lower genital tract infection. In S.B. Ransom, M.P. Dombrowski, S.G. McNeeley, K.S. Moghissi, & A.R. Munkarah (Eds.), *Practical strategies in obstetrics and gynecology* (pp. 57-64). Philadelphia: W.B. Saunders.

Moore, J.G. (1998). Dysfunctional uterine bleeding. In N.F. Hacker & J.G. Moore (Eds.), *Essentials of obstetrics and gynecology* (3rd ed., pp. 441-445). Philadelphia: W.B. Saunders.

Moore, J.G. (1998). Obstetric and gynecologic evaluation. In N.F. Hacker & J.G. Moore (Eds.), *Essentials of obstetrics and gynecology* (3rd ed., pp. 12-26). Philadelphia: W.B. Saunders.

Morse, G. (1999). Positively reframing perceptions of the menstrual cycle among women with premenstrual syndrome. *Journal of Obstetric, Gynecologic, and Neonatal Nursing,* 28(2), 165-174.

Mosca, L., Manson, J.E., Sutherland, S.E., Langer, R.D., Manolio, & Barrett-Connor, E. (1997). Cardiovascular disease in women. *Circulation,* 96(7), 2468-2482.

Muscari, M.E. (1999). Adolescent health: The first gynecologic exam. *American Journal of Nursing,* 99(1), 66-67.

National Cancer Institute. (2000). *CancerNet: Cancer facts: Lifetime probability of breast cancer in American women.* Retrieved November 12, 2000 from http://www.cancernet.nci.nih.gov/index.html.

National Cancer Institute. (1999). *CancerNet: Cancer facts: Screening mammogram.* Retrieved November 8, 2000 from http://www.cancernet.nci.hih.gov/index.html.

National Institutes of Health. (2000a). *National Institutes of Health Consensus Development Conference Statement: Adjuvant therapy for breast cancer, November 1-3, 2000.* Retrieved November 17, 2000 from http://odp.od.nih.gov/consensus/cons/114/114_intro.htm.

National Institutes of Health. (2000b). *National Institutes of Health Consensus Development Conference Statement: Osteoporosis prevention, diagnosis, and therapy, March 27-29, 2000.* Retrieved November 17, 2000 from http://odp.od.nih.gov/consensus/cons/111/111_intro.htm.

National Institutes of Health. (2000c). *National Institutes of Health (NIH), National Heart, Lung, & Blood Institute (NHLBI): Women's Health Initiative.* Retrieved November 6, 2000 from http://www.nhlbi.nih.gov/whi/index.html.

National Institutes of Health, Osteoporosis and Related Bone Diseases, National Resource Center. (2000a). *Exercise & bone health,* 1(1). Washington, D.C.: Author.

National Institutes of Health, Osteoporosis and Related Bone Diseases, National Resource Center. (2000b). *Fast facts on osteoporosis.* Washington, D.C.: Author.

Newhall, E.P., and Winikoff, B. (2000). Abortion with mifepristone and misoprostol: Regimens, efficacy, acceptability and future directions. *American Journal of Obstetrics and Gynecology,* 183(2), S44-S53.

Nichols, D.H. (2000). Disorders of pelvic support. In E.J. Quilligan & F.P. Zuspan (Eds.), *Current therapy in obstetrics and gynecology* (5th ed., pp. 22-27). Philadelphia: W.B. Saunders.

Pymar, H.C., & Creinin, M.D. (2000). Alternatives to mifepristone regimens for medical abortion. *American Journal of Obstetrics and Gynecology,* 183(2), S54-S64.

Riddick, D.H. (2000). Primary amenorrhea. National Institutes of Health, Osteoporosis and Related Bone Diseases, National Resource Center, 2000a.

Rogers, R.E. (2000). Cancer screening. In E.J. Quilligan and F.P. Zuspan (Eds.), *Current therapy in obstetrics and gynecology* (5th ed., pp. 201-203). Philadelphia: W.B. Saunders.

Rousseau, M.E. (1999). Selected hormonal agents in gynecology. *Journal of Obstetric, Gynecologic, and Neonatal Nursing,* 28(5), 545-553.

Sampselle, C.M., Burns, P.A., Dougherty, M.C., Newman, D.W., Thomas, K.S., & Wyman, J.F. (1997). Continence for women. *Journal of Obstetric, Gynecologic, and Neonatal Nursing,* 26(4), 375-385.

Sampselle, C.M., Wyman, J.F., Thomas, K.S., Newman, D.W., Gray, M., Dougherty, M., & Burns, P.A. (2000a). Continence for women: A test of AWHONN's evidence-based protocol in clinical practice. *Journal of Obstetric, Gynecologic, and Neonatal Nursing,* 29(1), 18-26.

Sampselle, C.M., Wyman, J.F., Thomas, K.S., Newman, D.W., Gray, M., Dougherty, M., & Burns, P.A. (2000b). Continence for women: Evaluation of AWHONN's third research utilization project. *Journal of Obstetric, Gynecologic, and Neonatal Nursing,* 29(1), 9-17.

Schlaff, W.D., & Kletzkyt, O.A. (1998). Amenorrhea, hyperprolactinemia, and chronic anovulation. In N.F. Hacker & J.G. Moore (Eds.), *Essentials of obstetrics and gynecology* (3rd ed., pp. 580-593). Philadelphia: W.B. Saunders.

Smith, A. (1998). The estrogen dilemma. *American Journal of Nursing,* 98(4), 17-20.

Smith, B.L. (1999). The breast. In K.J. Ryan, R.S. Berkowitz, R.L. Barbieri, & A. Dunaif (Eds.), *Kistner's gynecology and women's health* (7th ed., pp. 191-217). St. Louis: Mosby.

Speroff, L. (2000). Dysfunctional uterine bleeding. In S.B. Ransom, M.P. Dombrowski, S.G. McNeeley, K.S. Moghissi, & A.R. Munkarah (Eds.), *Practical strategies in obstetrics and gynecology* (pp. 560-569). Philadelphia: W.B. Saunders.

Spiegel, K.S. (1997). On your markers: Research advances in breast cancer in women. *AWHONN Lifelines,* 1(5), 33-38.

Surrey, E.S. (2000). Endometriosis and adenomyosis. In E.J. Quilligan & F.P. Zuspan (Eds.), *Current therapies in obstetrics and gynecology* (5th ed., pp. 44-47). Philadelphia: W.B. Saunders.

Taylor, R.R., & Birrer, M.J. (2000). Ovarian cancer. In E.J. Quilligan and F.P. Zuspan (Eds.), *Current therapy in obstetrics and gynecology* (5th ed., pp. 217-220). Philadelphia: W.B. Saunders.

United States Department of Health and Human Services. (2000a). *Healthy People 2010* (Conference Edition, in Two Volumes). Washington D.C.: Author.

United States Department of Health and Human Services. (2000b). *HHS News: FDA Approves mifepristone for the termination of early pregnancy.* Retrieved from https://www.fda.gov/bbs/topics/news/NEW00737.html.

Ventura, S.L., Mosher, W.D., Curtin, S.C., Abma, J.C., & Henshaw, S. (1999). *Highlights of trends in pregnancies and pregnancy rates by outcome: Estimates for the United States, 1976-1996.* Hyattsville, MD: National Center for Health Statistics, Centers for Disease Control.

Wagner, L.H., & Ruth-Sahd, L.A. (2000). Pregnancy after a TRAM flap procedure: Principles of nursing care. *Journal of Obstetric, Gynecologic, and Neonatal Nursing,* 29(4), 363-368.

Walsh, B.W., & Ginsburg, E.S. (1999). Menopause. In K.J. Ryan, R.S. Berkowitz, R.L. Barbieri, & A. Dunaif (Eds.), *Kistner's gynecology and women's health* (7th ed., pp. 540-569). St. Louis: Mosby.

Wilbur, J., Miller, A.M., Montgomery, A., & Chandler, P. (1998). Women's physical activity patterns: Nursing implications. *Journal of Obstetric, Gynecologic, and Neonatal Nursing,* 27(4), 383-392.

Wilmoth, M.C., & Spinelli, A. (2000). Sexual implications of gynecologic cancer treatments. *Journal of Obstetric, Gynecologic, and Neonatal Nursing,* 29(6), 413-421.

Wininger, D.A. (2000). AIDS and HIV infection. In E.J. Quilligan and F.P. Zuspan (Eds.), *Current therapy in obstetrics and gynecology* (5th ed., pp. 440-444). Philadelphia: W.B. Saunders.

World Health Organization (WHO). (1998). *Female genital mutilation: Fact sheet N 153.* Retrieved November 30, 2000, from http://www.who.int/inf-fs/en/fact153.html.

Wren, B.G. (1998). Menopause. In N.F. Hacker & J.G. Moore (Eds.), *Essentials of obstetrics and gynecology* (3rd ed., pp. 602-609). Philadelphia: W.B. Saunders.

APPENDIX A

Infection Control in Maternity and Women's Health Care

Pathogens such as human immunodeficiency virus (HIV) and hepatitis B virus (HBV) have resulted in significant changes in infection control. Early infection control practices were based on segregation of infected persons or disease-specific categories of isolation, such as respiratory, wound and skin, or blood precautions. The major shortcoming of these systems was that they were applied after the infection status of the person was known. They also involved use of warning signs on the doors to the person's room, which compromised privacy.

Increases in HIV and HBV infections required a new approach because these pathogens could be transmitted long before the signs and symptoms became evident. To prevent transmission of blood-borne pathogens to caregivers, the infection control practice of *universal precautions* was established. Universal precautions stressed that all clients are presumed infectious for HIV and other blood-borne pathogens. Universal precautions required use of protective equipment if contact with certain fluids, or articles contaminated with these fluids, was likely. A major advantage of universal precautions was that they could protect the worker from blood-borne pathogens even if the client's infection status was unknown. A shortcoming of universal precautions was that the guidelines did not address sources of infection other than blood-borne. However, universal precautions did specify use of general infection control practices such as hand washing.

Because *all* body substances may contain pathogens, the more comprehensive guidelines of body substance isolation were adopted by many hospitals in the late 1980s. These guidelines specified use of barriers, primarily gloves, for contact with all moist body substances, mucous membranes, and nonintact skin. They also included placing signs on the doors to check with the nurse before entering the rooms of clients who might have infections transmitted by the airborne route. The advantages of using body substance isolation guidelines were that they protected the client's privacy better and protected workers from more pathogens than did universal precautions.

CURRENT INFECTION CONTROL GUIDELINES

Current guidelines for infection control have two levels of protection. The first level, *standard precautions,* combines features from universal precautions and body substance isolation and applies to all clients. Standard precautions specify the use of personal protective equipment for potential contact with the following:

- Blood
- All body fluids, secretions, and excretions except sweat
- Nonintact skin
- Mucous membranes

Hand washing before and after care is essential. Immediate, thorough hand washing should follow unexpected contact with body substances.

The second level of protection, *transmission-based precautions,* is used for care of specific clients. Transmission-based precautions are designed to limit spread of pathogens that may not be confined by use of standard precautions. These pathogens can be spread by air, droplet, or contact with dry skin or contaminated surfaces. Transmission-based precautions are used in addition to standard precautions.

Gloves are a major component of personal protective equipment, but gloves do not prevent injuries from needles or sharp instruments. Caregivers should never recap needles, purposely bend or break them by hand, remove them from disposable syringes, or otherwise manipulate used needles and other sharp instruments by hand. Use of equipment with safety features designed to prevent recapping and injury are widely available and should be used correctly. Use of such devices is mandated by legislation in some states. When possible, needleless or protected needle systems should be used for procedures such as the administration of IV medications. After use, disposable syringes and needles, scalpel blades, and other sharp items are placed in puncture-resistant containers for disposal.

SOURCES OF INFECTION IN MATERNAL, NEWBORN, AND WOMEN'S HEALTH CARE

Maternal, newborn, and women's health care nursing includes many situations in which the nurse must expect exposure to pathogens, both blood-borne and other infectious agents:

- Handling tissue specimens or specimens of body secretions
- Surgical procedures, including circumcision of the neonate (scrub personnel near the operative site need more protective equipment than circulating personnel)
- Contact with nonintact skin, including surgical incisions
- Contact with mucous membranes, such as vaginal examinations or assessment of the infant's mouth
- Parenteral procedures, such as venipunctures, injections, finger sticks, and heel sticks
- Application of medication to nonintact skin or mucous membranes, such as placement of rectal or vaginal suppositories, application of topical preparations, infant eye prophylaxis, and care of the umbilical cord
- Preoperative shaving
- Perineal care, enemas
- Handling linens, gowns, underpads, perineal pads, and dressings, especially during the intrapartum and postpartum periods, when these items are likely to be contaminated with amniotic fluid, blood, or both
- Handling the infant before the first bath
- Changing diapers and cleaning the infant's diaper area
- Assessing breasts or contact with colostrum or breast milk
- Suture or staple removal

APPENDIX B

Laboratory Values in Pregnant and Nonpregnant Women and the Newborn

LABORATORY VALUES IN PREGNANT AND NONPREGNANT WOMEN

Value	Nonpregnancy	Pregnancy
Blood volume, total (ml/kg)	60 to 80	Increases 45%
Plasma volume (ml/kg)	40 to 50	Increases 45% by 32 weeks (average 4700 to 5200 ml)
Red blood cell mass (ml/kg)	20 to 30	Increases 20% to 30% (average increase of 250 to 450 ml)
Red blood cell count (million/mm^3)	3.8 to 5.1	Increases 20-30%, 4.5-6.5
Hemoglobin (g/dl)	12 to 16	11 to 12 (<10.5 g/dl during late pregnancy suggests anemia)
Hematocrit, packed cell volume (%)	36 to 48	33 to 46
White blood cell count	5000 to 10,000/mm^3	9000 to 15,000/mm.^{3} Rises during labor and postpartum up to 25,000/mm^3 to 30,000/mm^3. Returns to normal by 6 days postpartum.
Platelets	150,000 to 400,000/mm^3	Slight decrease (values <100,000/mm^3 are considered abnormal)
Prothrombin time (sec)	11 to 15	Slight decrease
Activated partial thromboplastin time (sec)	21 to 35	Slight decrease
Glucose, serum		
Fasting (mg/dl)	65 to 110	Decreases approximately 11 mg/dl
Postprandial (mg/dl)	<140	<140
Creatine, serum (mg/dl)	0.5 to 1.1	Decreased
Creatinine clearance, urine (ml/min)	85 to 120	110 to 150
Fibrinogen (mg/dl)	200 to 400	300 to 600

Data from Creasy, R.K., & Resnik, R. (1999). *Maternal-fetal medicine: Principles and practice* (4th ed.). Philadelphia: W.B. Saunders; Cunningham, F.G., MacDonald, P.C., Gant, N.F., Leveno, K.J., Gilstrap, L.C., Hankins, G.D.V., et al. (1997). *Williams obstetrics* (20th ed.). Norwalk, CT: Appleton & Lange; Fischbach, F. (1996). *A manual of laboratory and diagnostic tests* (5th ed.). Philadelphia: Lippincott; Harvey, M.G. (1999). Physiologic changes during pregnancy. In L.K. Mandeville & N.H. Troiano (Eds.), *High-risk and critical care intrapartum nursing* (2nd ed., pp. 2-31). Philadelphia: Lippincott; and Pagana, K.D., & Pagana, T.J. (2001). *Mosby's diagnostic and laboratory test reference* (5th ed.) Philadelphia: Mosby.

LABORATORY VALUES IN THE NEWBORN

Test, Specimen, and Unit of Measurement	Age	Normal Ranges (Conventional Units)
Erythrocyte (RBC or red blood cell) count, whole blood (million/mm^3)	Cord	3.9 to 5.5
	1 to 3 days	4.0 to 6.6
	1 week	3.9 to 6.3
	1 month	3.0 to 5.4
Hemoglobin, whole blood (g/dl)	1 to 3 days (capillary)	14.5 to 22.5
	2 months	9.0 to 14.0
Hematocrit, whole blood (%)	1 day (capillary)	48 to 69
	2 days	48 to 75
	3 days	44 to 72
	2 months	28 to 42
White blood cell count, whole blood (thousand/mm^3)	Birth	9.0 to 30.0
	1 day	9.4 to 34.0
	1 month	5.0 to 19.5
White blood cell differential count, whole blood		
Myelocytes (%)		0
Neutrophils ("bands") (%)		3 to 5
Neutrophils ("segs") (%)		54 to 62
Lymphocytes (%)		25 to 33
Monocytes (%)		3 to 7
Eosinophils (%)		1 to 3
Basophils (%)		0 to 0.75
Platelet count, whole blood (thousand/mm^3)	Newborn	84 to 478
	>1 week	150 to 400
Glucose, serum (mg/dl)	Cord	45 to 96
	Newborn at 1 day	40 to 60
	Newborn, >1 day	50 to 90
Calcium, serum (mg/dl)	Cord	9.0 to 11.5
	Newborn 3 to 24 hours	9.0 to 10.6
	24 to 48 hours	7.0 to 12.0
Magnesium, plasma(mg/dl)	Newborn 0 to 6 days	1.2 to 2.6

		Preterm	Full-Term
Bilirubin, total serum (mg/dl)	Cord	<2.0	2.0
	0 to 1 day	<8.0	<6.0
	1 to 2 days	<12.0	<8.0
	2 to 5 days	<16.0	<12.0
	>5 days	<2.0	0.2 to 1.0
Bilirubin, direct (conjugated) serum (mg/dl)			0 to 0.2

Adapted from Nicholson, J.F., & Pesce, M.A. (2000). Reference ranges for laboratory tests and procedures. In R.E. Behrman, R.M. Kliegman, & H.B. Jenson (Eds.). *Nelson textbook of pediatrics* (16th ed., pp. 2181-2229). Philadelphia: W.B. Saunders.

APPENDIX C

Use of Drugs and Botanical Preparations during Pregnancy and Breastfeeding

FDA PREGNANCY RISK CATEGORIES

The U.S. Food and Drug Administration (FDA) has assigned pregnancy risk categories to many drugs on the basis of their known relative safety or danger to the fetus and whether safer alternative drugs exist. For many drugs, little is known about the fetal risk. The categories are as follows:

A: No evidence of risk to the fetus exists.

B: Animal reproduction studies have not demonstrated a risk to the fetus. No adequate and well-controlled studies have been done in pregnant women.

C: Animal reproduction studies have shown an adverse effect on the fetus but no adequate, well-controlled studies have been done in humans. Potential benefits may warrant use of the drug in pregnant women despite fetal risks. Or, animal studies show adverse effect on fetus but human studies with pregnant women have not demonstrated a risk to the fetus in any trimester of pregnancy.

D: There is positive evidence of human fetal risk based on adverse reaction data, but potential benefits may warrant use of the drug in pregnant women despite fetal risks. Essentially, no safer alternatives to the drug are available.

X: There is positive evidence of human fetal risk based on animal or human studies and/or adverse reaction data. The risks of using the drug in pregnant women clearly outweigh potential benefits. Safer alternatives to these drugs may be available.

DRUG USE DURING LACTATION

The effects of many drugs, when used during lactation, have not been studied. In general, if a drug is safe for use in infants, it is probably safe for the lactating woman to take. Other drugs are known not to be excreted in breast milk or excreted in an inactive form or very low concentrations. Modifying the time of maternal ingestion may reduce transfer of the drug to the infant. Some drugs are undesirable because they suppress lactation, which is a problem primarily in the earliest stages of breastfeeding.

The American Academy of Pediatrics (AAP) has established classifications for safety of some drugs during lactation. The categories are as follows:

AAP compatible: Usually compatible with breastfeeding

AAP contraindicated: Contraindicated for use in breastfeeding mothers

AAP reason for concern: Reports of infant side effects cause concern about use in breastfeeding mothers

Social and illicit drugs, such as alcohol and cocaine, are discussed in Chapters 22 and 24.

Complementary/Alternative Therapy

Herbal preparations should be used cautiously after consulting a lactation consultant or herbalist who is familiar with their use in the breastfeeding mother. Pure herbs should be used, in minimal amounts, and mixtures of unknown herbs should be avoided (Hale, 2000).

Drug	Use during Pregnancy	Use during Breastfeeding
AMEBICIDES		
Metronidazole (Flagyl)	Risk category B. Some practitioners remain concerned about use during pregnancy because of animal studies that suggest teratogenicity when high and prolonged doses were used. However, this teratogenicity has not been substantiated in humans in a recent analysis (CDC, 1998).	AAP reason for concern (primarily for oral form). Breastfeeding may be discontinued during treatment and for 12 to 24 hr after last dose to allow mother to excrete last dose, then restarted.
ANALGESICS		
Aspirin	Risk category C (D in 3rd trimester). Antiprostaglandin effects may prolong pregnancy. May cause bleeding disorders in mother or newborn if used during late pregnancy.	AAP reason for concern. Toxicity unlikely in normal doses, but higher doses could cause bleeding in infant.
Acetaminophen (Tylenol, Datril, Tempra)	Risk category B. Problems have not been documented, but drug crosses placenta in low concentrations. High doses may result in fetal liver toxicity.	AAP compatible. Very small amounts secreted into breast milk.
Opiate analgesics (butorphanol [Stadol], hydrocodone [Lortab, Vicodin], hydromorphone [Dilaudid], meperidine [Demerol], morphine, nalbuphine [Nubain], oxycodone [Percocet, Tylox, percodan])	Most are risk category B or C. Neonatal respiratory depression is the most significant adverse effect when large amounts of opiates are used during labor, making them a category D at this time. Neonatal withdrawal may occur if the woman is addicted to an opiate drug.	Most narcotics given briefly and in therapeutic doses are compatible with breastfeeding. Sedation, poor suckling reflex, and neurobehavioral delay make these drugs hazardous for the nursing mother during the *neonatal* period. Prolonged use may result in infant drug dependence and subsequent withdrawal when the mother no longer takes the drug or stops nursing.
Nonsteroidal antiinflammatory drugs (NSAIDs) (fenoprofen [Nalfon], flurbiprofen [Ansaid], ibuprofen [Advil, Motrin, Nuprin], indomethacin [Indocin], ketoprofen [Actron, Orudis], naproxen [Aleve, Anaprox])	Risk category B. Category D after 34 weeks (not recommended). May prolong pregnancy or labor because of antiprostaglandin effects. Associated with premature closure of ductus arteriosus in newborn.	Ibuprofen, indomethacin, and naproxen are AAP compatible. All should be used cautiously owing to potential for infant bleeding. Naproxen has a long half-life and may remain in mother's blood for a long time.
COX-2 inhibitors: celecoxib (Celebrex), rofecoxib (Vioxx)	Risk category C.	No problems reported, but observe for gastrointestinal (GI) cramping, diarrhea.
Migraine agent: Sumatriptan (Imitrex)	Risk category C.	Milk concentrations low.
ANTIALLERGIC AND ANTIASTHMATIC DRUGS (SEE ALSO *BRONCHODILATORS, DECONGESTANTS, HORMONES, CORTICOSTEROIDS*)		
Antihistamines	Risk category B: chlorpheniramine (Chlor-Trimeton), clemastine (Contac, Tavist), diphenhydramine (Benadryl), loratadine (Claritin), meclizine (Antivert, Dramamine). Risk category C: astemizole (Hismanal), brompheniramine (Dimetane), phenylephrine (Neo-Synephrine), terfenadine (Seldane), triprolidine (Alleract).	All should be used with caution. Most are safe but may cause infant drowsiness. If these adverse effects occur, a different drug may be tried. Clemastine is rated as AAP reason for concern and should be given with caution.
Cromolyn (Intal, Nasalcrom, Opticrom)	Risk category B.	Minimal oral absorption, so it is unlikely to adversely affect infant.
Epinephrine (Primatene)	Risk category C.	Unlikely to be absorbed in infant's gastrointestinal tract unless in the early newborn period, or if preterm.
Metaproterenol (Alupent)	Risk category C. May inhibit uterine contractions.	Unknown if secreted in milk; use cautiously.

Drug	Use during Pregnancy	Use during Breastfeeding
ANTICOAGULANTS		
Enoxaparin (Lovenox)	Risk category B.	Not reviewed by AAP, but molecular weight is too large to produce clinically relevant levels in breast milk.
Heparin	Risk category C.	AAP compatible. Not excreted in breast milk
Warfarin (Coumadin)	Risk category D. Associated with facial abnormalities and neurologic deficit. Traumatic intracranial hemorrhage may occur in neonate if ingested near term. If used, it is typically avoided between 6 and 12 weeks' gestation and for 2 to 3 weeks before term.	AAP compatible, but should be used with caution. Very small amounts secreted in milk. No reported bleeding abnormalities in infant, but observe for bruising or petechiae.
ANTICONVULSANTS		
Carbamazepine (Tegretol)	Risk category C. Associated with craniofacial abnormalities, underdeveloped fingernails, neural tube defects, and developmental delay.	AAP compatible. Small amounts secreted in breast milk; accumulation does not seem to occur. Observe infant for sedation.
Magnesium sulfate	Risk category A during early pregnancy. Infants exposed to magnesium sulfate shortly before birth may exhibit respiratory depression, hypotonic muscle tone, depressed reflexes, hypocalcemia, or cardiac dysrhythmias.	AAP compatible. Moderate amounts secreted in milk, but most remains in infant's gastrointestinal tract. Milk levels return to normal about 24 hr after drug is stopped.
Phenobarbital	Risk category D. Fetal addiction with subsequent withdrawal is possible but rare at dose levels used for seizure control. Abnormalities similar to those seen in infants exposed to carbamazepine, phenytoin, and valproic acid have been reported.	AAP reason for concern. Should be given with caution. Significant amounts accumulate in infant's plasma. Psychomotor delay and sedation possible.
Phenytoin (Dilantin)	Risk category D. Prenatal-onset growth deficiency, small head, developmental delay, craniofacial and other anomalies, underdeveloped nails or distal phalanges.	AAP compatible. Minimal effects if maternal dose is low. Observe for sedation and decreased sucking.
Topiramate (Topamax)	Risk category C.	No studies available. Use with caution.
Trimethadione (Tridione)	Risk category D. Associated with growth and developmental delay, craniofacial abnormalities, cardiovascular abnormalities.	Enters breast milk. Use cautiously.
Valproic acid (Depakene)	Risk category D. Associated with neural tube defects, craniofacial, cardiac, and hand abnormalities.	AAP compatible. Secreted in small amounts. May cause drowsiness. Used for infant seizures.
ANTIDIABETIC AGENTS		
Insulin	Risk category B. Insulin is only appropriate drug to control diabetes during pregnancy because it does not cross placenta.	AAP compatible. Any insulin ingested would be destroyed in infant's gastrointestinal tract.
Oral hypoglycemic agents	Contraindicated. Cross placenta and may cause prolonged neonatal hypoglycemia.	Safety not established for most. Observe for infant hypoglycemia if used.
ANTIFUNGALS		
Fluconazole (Diflucan), miconazole (Monistat), nystatin (Mycostatin), terconazole (Terazol)	Risk category C, except for nystatin (category B).	Low risk, but not reviewed by AAP. Fluconazole is FDA-approved for treatment of infants ≥6 months and has an FDA safety profile for infants as young as 1 day.

Continued

Drug	Use during Pregnancy	Use during Breastfeeding
ANTIHYPERTENSIVES (SEE ALSO *DIURETICS*)		
ACE inhibitors (benazepril [Lotensin], captopril [Capoten], enalapril [Vasotec], fosinopril [Monopril], ramipril [Altace])	Risk categories D (primarily 2nd and 3rd trimesters). Renal dysplasia leading to oligohydramnios, which results in Potter's sequence: (joint contractures, loose skin, large ears, Potter's facies, death due to pulmonary hypoplasia).	Use with caution. Captopril and enalapril are AAP compatible. Fosinopril is possibly hazardous, and ramipril is possibly hazardous in neonates. Observe for infant hypotension.
Beta-adrenergic blockers (acebutolol [Monitan, Sectral], atenolol [Tenormin], betaxolol [Kerlone], labetalol [Normodyne], metoprolol [Lopressor, Toprol], nadolol [Corgard], penbutolol [Levatol], pindolol [Viskin], propranolol [Inderal]	Risk category C, except acebutolol and pindolol, which are risk category B, and atenolol and propanolol, which are category D. Labetalol, metoprolol, nadolol, penbutolol, and pindolol are category D in the 2nd and 3rd trimesters. Possible fetal or neonatal effects include transient bradycardia, respiratory depression, and hypoglycemia.	AAP compatible, but potentially hazardous based on reported studies: acebutolol, atenolol, labetalol, nadolol, propranolol. Nadolol has a long half-life and would be a less-preferred drug. Observe infant for pharmacologic effects: hypotension, bradycardia, apnea, sedation, fatigue.
Calcium channel blockers (amlodipine [Norvasc], diltiazem [Cardizem], nicardipine [Cardene], nifedipine [Adalat, Procardia], verapamil [Calan, Isoptin])	Risk category C. Hypotensive effects may reduce uteroplacental perfusion and may lead to fetal heart failure and atrioventricular block. Nifedipine has been used on an investigational basis to inhibit preterm labor.	Drugs excreted in breast milk. AAP compatible: diltiazem, nifedipine, and verapamil. Use with extreme caution; overdoses in young children are dangerous. Observe for hypotension and bradycardia. Delaying nursing for 3-4 hr after the *non–sustained-release* form may reduce transfer to infant.
Centrally acting sympatholytics (clonidine [Catapres], guanabenz [Wytensin], guanfacine [Tenex], methyldopa [Aldomet])	Risk category C, except for guanfacine (risk category B).	Methyldopa is AAP compatible. Others should be used cautiously because safety is not established. Observe for hypotension and sedation.
Vasodilators (hydralazine [Apresoline], minoxidil [Loniten], nitroprusside [Nipride, Nitropress])	Risk category C. No adverse fetal effects associated with long-term use. Excessive hair has been reported.	Hydralazine and minoxidil are AAP compatible. Nitroprusside is a concern because of the drug's conversion to a potentially toxic thiocyanate metabolite.
ANTIMICROBIALS		
Aminoglycosides (gentamicin [Garamycin], kanamycin [Kantrex], streptomycin)	Risk categories C or D. Associated with hearing loss and renal toxicity.	AAP compatible: kanamycin and streptomycin. Most drugs in this class are poorly absorbed orally.
Azithromycin (Zithromax)	Risk category B. Chemically related to erythromycin.	Risk low because minimal amount likely to be received by infant.
Cephalosporins (1st through 4th generation drugs)	Most are risk category B.	Secretion into milk is generally poor. Observe for diarrhea. Several cephalosporins prescribed for breastfeeding mothers are also used in infants in children.
Chloramphenicol (Chloromycetin)	Risk category C. Not recommended for use at term because it is associated with neonatal "gray baby syndrome" (rapid respiration, ashen and pale color, poor feeding, abdominal distention, vasomotor collapse, death).	AAP reason for concern. Generally contraindicated in breastfeeding mothers. Can be extremely toxic, especially in newborns. May cause infant sensitivity. Blood levels should be monitored if used.
Erythromycin (E-mycin, Ilotycin)	Risk category B. Little transfer to fetus across placenta, which limits the drugs' usefulness for treating syphilis.	AAP compatible. May cause alteration in gastrointestinal flora, allergies, interference with infant's cultures for infection.
Fluoroquinolones (includes ciprofloxacin [Cipro], norfloxacin [Chibroxin], ofloxacin [Floxin])	Risk category C. Animal studies have shown joint abnormalities.	Potentially hazardous. Possible association with cartilage damage and colitis in animal studies. If used, observe infant for signs of GI distress.
Nitrofurantoin (Furadantin, Macrodantin)	Risk category B. Use should be avoided near term because it may cause hemolytic anemia in newborn.	AAP compatible for older infants. Should avoid if infant is younger than 1 month. Risk for hemolytic anemia if infant has an enzyme (G-6-PD) deficiency.

Drug	Use during Pregnancy	Use during Breastfeeding
ANTIMICROBIALS—cont'd		
Penicillins (includes amoxicillin [Amoxil], ampicillin [Omnipen, Polycillin], penicillin G)	Risk category B. No reported adverse fetal effects. Penicillins combined with beta-lactamase inhibitors (Augmentin, Timentin, and Unasyn) have not been adequately studied, although fetal effects are unlikely.	Several penicillins are AAP compatible. Those combined with beta-lactamase inhibitors may not have been studied as well. Observe for infant diarrhea or development of sensitivity.
Sulfonamides (sulfamethoxazole [Gantanol], sulfisoxazole [Gantrisin])	Risk category C (sulfamethoxazole) or B (sulfisoxazole). Category D if given near term due to theoretic risk for neonatal hyperbilirubinemia.	Potentially hazardous. Sulfisoxazole is considered compatible, but all should be used with great caution in infants with hyperbilirubinemia and an enzyme deficiency (G-6-PD deficiency).
Tetracyclines	Risk category D. Can interfere with tooth enamel formation and cause discolored teeth. Prenatal exposure does not affect permanent teeth.	AAP compatible for short periods.
ANTIRETROVIRAL AGENTS		
Nucleoside analogues (abacavir [Ziagen], didanosine [ddl, Videx], lamivudine [3TC, Epivir], stavudine [d4T, Zerit], zalcitabine [ddC, Hivid], zidovudine [ZDV, Retrovir])	Risk category B (didanosine) or C (abacavir, lamivudine, stavudine, zalcitabine, zidovudine). Zidovudine is recommended for HIV-seropositive women to reduce risk for perinatal transmission of the virus.	Breastfeeding not recommended due to possibility of HIV transmission to infant.
Non-nucleotide analogues (delavirdine [DLV, Rescriptor], efavirenz [Sustiva], nevirapine [NVP, Viramune])	Risk category C.	Breastfeeding not recommended due to possibility of HIV transmission to infant.
Protease inhibitors (amprenavir [Agenerase], indinavir [Crixivan], nelfinavir [Viracept], ritonavir [Norvir], saquinavir [Invirase])	Risk category B (nelfinavir, ritonavir, saquinavir); category C (amprenavir, indinavir).	Breastfeeding not recommended due to possibility of HIV transmission to infant.
		Breastfeeding not recommended due to possibility of HIV transmission to infant.
ANTITUBERCULOSIS AGENTS (SEE ALSO *ANTIMICROBIALS*)		
Ethambutol	Risk category B. No evidence of increased abnormalities. Fetal effects of combinations of ethambutol with other antituberculosis drugs are unknown.	AAP compatible. Concentration in breast milk is similar to that in maternal serum, so caution is indicated.
Isoniazid (INH)	Risk category C.	AAP compatible. Monitor infant for liver toxicity, neuritis. Observe infant for fatigue, weakness, malaise, anorexia, nausea, vomiting.
Pyrazinamide	Risk category C. No adverse experience with this widely-prescribed agent.	No reported concerns, but not AAP reviewed.
Rifampin (Rifadin)	Risk category C.	AAP compatible. No reported adverse effects.
ANTITUSSIVES AND EXPECTORANTS		
Dextromethorphan (Robitussin-DM)	Risk category C.	Unlikely to cause side effects.
Guaifenesin (Robitussin)	Risk category C. Usefulness as an expectorant is questionable.	Unlikely to cause side effects.
ANTIVIRAL AGENTS		
Acyclovir (Zovirax)	Risk category C.	AAP compatible. Few reported toxicities. If topical drug is used on nipples, wash thoroughly before nursing.
Ribavirin (Virazole)	Risk category X. Administered by aerosol. Women who are pregnant or may become pregnant should avoid exposure.	No data available on transfer to breast milk. Should use caution. Drug is most often given to young children hospitalized with respiratory syncytial virus (RSV), so transfer to breast milk is not likely.

Continued

Drug	Use during Pregnancy	Use during Breastfeeding
BRONCHODILATORS		
Albuterol (Proventil, Ventolin)	Risk category C.	Small amounts likely to be secreted. Observe infant for tremors and excitement, mainly when mother takes orally rather than by inhaler.
Terbutaline (Brethine)	Risk category B. Also used in treatment of preterm labor because of its inhibition of uterine contraction.	AAP compatible. Observe infant for tremors, nervousness, and tachycardia.
Theophylline (Aminophylline, Theo-Dur)	Risk category C.	AAP compatible. Excreted in milk. May result in infant nausea, vomiting, irritability, insomnia, and fretfulness.
CARDIAC MEDICATIONS		
Antiarrhythmics for serious arrhythmias: Amidarone (Cordarone, Pacerone), bretylium (Bretylol)	Risk category C. May reduce uterine blood flow.	Used for life-threatening arrhythmias; woman unlikely to be nursing.
Digoxin (Lanoxin)	Risk category C. Has been used to treat fetal cardiac arrhythmias.	AAP compatible.
Local anesthetics (used as antiarrhythmics)	Risk category C.	Lidocaine is AAP compatible with breastfeeding.
DECONGESTANTS		
Ephedrine, epinephrine, oxymetazoline nasal spray (Afrin, Coricidin, Dristan), phenylephrine nasal spray (Neo-Synephrine)	Risk category C. Ephedrine is commonly used to support blood pressure during epidural or subarachnoid block during intrapartum period.	Use with caution. May cause anorexia, irritability in infant.
Pseudoephedrine	Risk category C. Avoid during third trimester.	AAP compatible. Minimal amounts secreted in milk.
DIURETICS		
Carbonic anhydrase inhibitors: acetazolamide (Diamox), methazolamide (Neptazane)	Risk category C.	Acetazolamide is AAP compatible with breastfeeding.
Loop diuretics (ethacrynic acid [Edecrin], furosemide [Lasix], torsemide [Demadex])	Risk category B (ethacrynic acid) or C (furosemide and torsemide).	Effects unknown but probably minimal. Maternal use could suppress lactation.
Potassium-sparing diuretics (amiloride [Midamor], spironolactone [Aldactone], triamterene [Dyrenium])	Risk category B (amiloride), category D (spironolactone, triamterene).	Spironolactone is AAP compatible, but suppression of milk supply is possible.
Thiazide diuretics (chlorothiazide [Hydrodiuril], hydrochlorothiazide [HydroDIURIL])	Risk category D. Decreased intravascular volume may reduce uteroplacental perfusion. Metabolic disturbances and thrombocytopenia may occur in mother and fetus.	Chlorothiazide AAP approved. Infant thrombocytopenia has been reported, but not substantiated.
Thiazide-like diuretics (chlorthalidone [Hygroton], indapamide [Lozide, Lozol], metolazone [Mykrox, Zaroxolyn])	Risk category B.	Use with caution. No data on some.
HORMONES		
Corticosteroids (beclomethasone [Vanceril, Beclovent], betamethasone [Celestone], cortisone [Cortone], dexamethasone [Decadron], prednisone [Deltasone])	Risk category C. Prednisone is common for asthmatic woman who needs steroids. Betamethasone and dexamethasone are used to accelerate maturation of fetal lungs if preterm delivery is likely.	Potentially hazardous in high doses or with long-term use. Delay nursing 4 hr after dose to reduce transfer to infant. Remove from nipples prior to nursing if applied topically.
Estrogens	Risk category X. Diethylstilbestrol (DES) is associated with development of vaginal cancer in female offspring during adolescence or adulthood.	Early use of oral contraceptives may reduce milk volume and protein content. Try to delay drug until breastfeeding is firmly established.
Oral contraceptives (estrogen-progestin combinations)	Risk category X. Doses much higher than those used in oral contraceptives are associated with masculinization of the female fetus' genitalia.	Ideally, avoid until lactation is well established for best quantity and quality of breast milk.

Drug	Use during Pregnancy	Use during Breastfeeding
HORMONES—CONT'D		
Clomiphene citrate (Clomid)	Risk category X. Questionable association with neural tube defects. Drug is discontinued after pregnancy is achieved.	May suppress early lactation. Unlikely to be prescribed during lactation because it is given for infertility.
Danazol (Danocrine)	Risk category X. May cause virilization of female fetus.	Likely to suppress breast milk production.
PSYCHOACTIVE DRUGS		
Lithium (Eskalith, Lithobid)	Risk category D. Slightly increased risk for cardiac abnormalities.	AAP contraindicated.
Benzodiazepines: alprazolam (Xanax), clonazepam (Klonopin), diazepam (Valium), flurazepam (Dalmane), lorazepam (Ativan), midazolam (Versed), oxazepam (Serax), temazepam (Restoril), triazolam (Halcion)	Most are risk category D. Some reports of mild facial abnormalities and developmental delay, but no conclusive studies. The following sedative-hypnotic drugs in this class are risk category X: flurazepam, temazepam, and triazolam.	Potentially hazardous due to the long half-lives of most drugs in this class and the potential development of dependence. Acute use, such as for surgery, is unlikely to cause problems. Preferred drugs in this class are lorazepam or midazolam because of their shorter half-lives and oxazepam is the least lipid soluble. Observe infant for sedation, poor feeding.
Chlordiazepoxide (Librium, Libritabs)	Risk category D.	May be hazardous with long-term use. Observe for infant sedation.
Meprobamate (Equanil, Miltown)	Risk category D. Has been associated with cardiac malformations.	Concentrations in milk are higher than in maternal serum. Observe for infant sedation.
Phenothiazines: chlorpromazine (Thorazine), prochlorperazine (Compazine), thioridazine (Mellaril)	Risk category C. Risk of malformations is uncertain but these are probably safe for use in humans. Use during pregnancy should be carefully evaluated.	AAP reason for concern: chlorpromazine. Some drugs in this class have a long half-life and all are sedating. Young infants are very sensitive to sedation.
Tricyclic antidepressants: amitriptyline (Elavil), amoxapine (Asendin), clomipramine (Anafranil), desipramine (Norpramin), doxepin (Adepin, Sinequan), imipramine (Tofranil), nortriptyline (Aventyl, Pamelor), protriptyline (Vivactil)	Risk category C. Several studies have shown that tricyclic antidepressant use during pregnancy is most likely not teratogenic.	Several are rated AAP reason for concern. Most are probably safe in usual doses. Doxepin is contraindicated because its active metabolite can concentrate in the infant and has a long half-life. Amoxapine may be an alternative in this class.
SSRIs: fluoxetine (Prozac), paroxetine (Paxil), sertraline (Zoloft)	Risk category B.	AAP reason for concern. Sertraline and paroxetine may have more difficulty transferring to milk and may be preferred over fluoxetine for maternal therapy. Observe infant for severe colic, fussiness, and crying.
THYROID DRUGS		
Antithyroids: methimazole (Tapazole), propylthiouracil (PTU)	Risk category D. May result in neonatal goiter or hypothyroidism, although uncommon at usual therapeutic doses. Methimazole has possible association with scalp defects.	AAP compatible. Propylthiouracil is preferred drug.
Potassium iodide (SSKI, Thyro-Block)	Risk category D. Long-term exposure may produce fetal thyroid enlargement.	Use caution. May cause rash or suppress infant's thyroid function. Large quantities of iodides are contraindicated.
Thyroid replacement hormones: levothyroxine (Synthroid)	Risk category A. Crosses placenta only to limited extent.	Apparently safe.

Continued

Drug	Use during Pregnancy	Use during Breastfeeding
VITAMINS AND RETINOIDS		
Retinoids: etretinate (Tegison), isotretinoin (Accutane)	Risk category X. Related to vitamin A. Associated with severe fetal malformations (microcephaly, ear abnormalities, cardiac defects, central nervous system abnormalities). Etretinate has a long half-life and may have fetal effects up to 18 months after drug is stopped.	Contraindicated for use during breastfeeding.
Vitamin A	Risk category A (X at high doses). Excess intake may lead to abnormalities noted for etretinate and isotretinoin.	Breast milk usually supplies sufficient vitamin A to infant. Mother should not take more than 6000 units per day.
Vitamin D	Risk category C (D at high doses). Excess intake associated with malformations, including aortic stenosis, facial abnormalities, and mental retardation.	AAP compatible. Should be supplemented with caution. High doses could cause infant renal toxicity.
MISCELLANEOUS DRUGS		
Nicotine gum; nicotine transdermal	Risk category D (X if overdose; for example, smoking plus use of gum/patch). Nicotine levels from drug may be less than those from smoking, *if* the woman does not smoke at all.	AAP contraindicated. To avoid transfer to infant, delay nursing for 2 to 3 hours after use of gum. Smoking plus use of nicotine-containing drugs could lead to high levels in infant. Observe for infant shock, vomiting, diarrhea, tachycardia, and restlessness.
Herbal and Botanical Preparations		
Black cohosh (Baneberry, Black Snakeroot, Bugbane, Squawroot, Rattle Root)	Risk category X: Large doses may induce miscarriage because it is a uterine stimulant. Has estrogenic activity.	Caution recommended in breastfeeding due to its estrogenic activity.
Blue cohosh (Blue Ginseng, Squaw Root, Papoose Root, Yellow Ginseng)	Risk category X: Stimulates uterine contractions; should not be used early in pregnancy.	Contraindicated in breastfeeding. Contains compounds that are pharmacologically similar to nicotine.
Chamomile (German Chamomile, Hungarian Chamomile, Sweet False, Wild Chamomile)	No pregnancy risk category. Asthmatics should avoid. Allergic reactions reported at high doses. Probably best to avoid during pregnancy and lactation.	Probably safe. Hypersensitization possible.
Echinacea (Echinacea Angustifolia, Echinacea Purpurea, American Cone Flower, Black Susans, Snakeroot)	No pregnancy risk category. Has been used with no apparent ill effects as an immune stimulant for many years. Should not be used longer than 8 weeks.	No data available on transfer to milk. Should not be used longer than 8 weeks.
Evening primrose oil (EPO)	No pregnancy risk category. Studies by manufacturer have shown benefit of preparation in improvement of syndromes such as cardiovascular disease, rheumatoid arthritis, multiple sclerosis, atopic dermatitis with no adverse effects, but these need independent confirmation.	No reported pediatric concerns.
Kava (also known as *kava-kava*) (Awa, Kew, Tonga)	No pregnancy risk category. Heavy users are underweight, have reduced plasma protein levels, facial edema, scaly rashes, elevated HDL cholesterol, bloody urine, and abnormal blood studies. Germany considers kava contraindicated in pregnancy.	No data available, but care should be exercised. Alcohol use with kava increases its toxicity. Germany considers kava contraindicated in breastfeeding.

Drug	Use during Pregnancy	Use during Breastfeeding
Herbal and Botanical Preparations—cont'd		
St. John's Wort	No pregnancy risk category assigned. Because of uterotonic effects, it should not be used.	Has not proven to be safe for use in lactating women. Probably penetrates milk poorly, however.
Valerian (Valerian Root)	No pregnancy risk category assigned. One group of chemicals in the root, the valepotriates, has possible cytotoxic effects. This effect needs added study.	Use caution. The herb's sedative/hypnotic effects may increase the risk of SIDS in the infant.

REFERENCES

American Academy of Pediatrics Committee on Drugs (1994). Transfer of drugs and other chemicals into human milk. *Pediatrics,* 93(1), 137-150.

American Academy of Pediatrics Committee on Drugs (2000). Use of psychoactive medications during pregnancy and possible effects on the fetus and newborn (RE9866). *Pediatrics,* 105(4), 880-887.

Auerbach, K.G. (1999). Breastfeeding and maternal medication use. *Journal of Obstetric, Gynecologic and Neonatal Nursing,* 28(5), 554-563.

Briggs, G.G., Freeman, R.K., & Yaffee, S.J. (1997). *Drugs in lactation.* Baltimore, MD: Williams & Wilkins.

Caldwell, J. (1996). Hyperthyroidism during pregnancy: Nursing care issues. *Journal of Obstetric, Gynecologic and Neonatal Nursing,* 25(5), 395-400.

Centers for Disease Control and Prevention (CDC). (Jan. 23, 1998). 1998 Guidelines for treatment of sexually transmitted diseases. *Morbidity and Mortality Weekly Report,* 47 (RR-1).

Clark, S.L., Porter, T.F., & West, F.G. (2000). Coumarin derivatives and breastfeeding. *Obstetrics and Gynecology,* 95(6), 938-940.

Cunningham, F.G., MacDonald, P.C., Gant, N.F., Leveno, K.J., Gilstrap, L.C., Hankins, G.D.V., et al. (1997). *Williams obstetrics* (20th ed.). Norwalk, CT: Appleton & Lange.

Gal, P., & Reed, M.D. (2000). Medications. In R.E. Behrman, R.M. Kliegman, & H.B. Jenson (Eds.), *Nelson's textbook of pediatrics* (16th ed., pp. 2235-2304). Philadelphia: W.B. Saunders.

Goldaber, K.G. (1997). Psychotropics. *Seminars in Perinatology,* 21(2), 154-159.

Hale, T. (2000). *Medications and mothers' milk* (9th ed.). Amarillo, TX: Pharmasoft Medical Publishing.

Hewitt, J.B., & Tellier, L. (1998). Risk of adverse outcomes in pregnant women exposed to solvents. *Journal of Obstetric, Gynecologic and Neonatal Nursing,* 27(5), 521-531.

Hodgson, B., Kizior, R., & Kingdon, R. (2001). *Nurse's drug handbook 2001.* Philadelphia: W.B. Saunders.

Jones, K.L. (1999). Effects of therapeutic, diagnostic, and environmental agents. In R.K. Creasy & R. Resnik (Eds.), *Maternal-fetal medicine: Principles and practice* (3rd ed., pp. 132-144). Philadelphia: W.B. Saunders.

Lawrence, R.A., & Lawrence, R.M. (1999). *Breastfeeding: A guide for the medical profession.* St. Louis: Mosby.

Lindberg, C.E. (1995). Perinatal transmission of HIV: How to counsel women. *MCN: American Journal of Maternal-Child Nursing,* 20(4), 207-212.

Little, B.B. (1999). Medication during pregnancy: Maternal and embryo-fetal considerations. In D.K. James, P.J. Steer, C.P. Weiner, & B. Gonik (Eds.), *High-risk pregnancy: Management options* (2nd ed., pp. 599-616). Philadelphia: W.B. Saunders.

Malone, F.D., & D'Alton, M.E. (1997). Drugs in pregnancy: Anticonvulsants. *Seminars in Perinatology,* 21(2), 114-123.

Mastrobattista, J.M. (1997). Angiotensin converting enzyme inhibitors in pregnancy. *Seminars in Perinatology,* 21(2), 124-134.

Monga, M. (1997). Vitamin A and its congeners. *Seminars in Perinatology,* 21(2), 135-142.

Ramin, S.M., Ramin, K.D., & Gilstrap, L.C. (1997). Anticoagulants and thrombolytics during pregnancy. *Seminars in Perinatology,* 21(2), 149-153.

Rebar, R.W. (1994). The breast and the physiology of lactation. In R.K. Creasy & R. Resnik (Eds.), *Maternal-fetal medicine: Principles and practice* (4th ed., pp. 144-161). Philadelphia: W.B. Saunders.

Simpkins, S.M., Hench, C.P., & Ghatia, G. (1996). Management of the obstetric patient with tuberculosis. *Journal of Obstetric, Gynecologic and Neonatal Nursing,* 25(4), 305-312.

Skidmore-Roth, L. (2001). *Mosby's nursing drug reference.* St. Louis: Mosby.

Zenk, K.E. (1999). Antiepileptic drugs in pregnancy. *Mother Baby Journal,* 4(4), 45-47.

APPENDIX D

Keys to Clinical Practice: Components of Daily Care

INTRAPARTUM CARE

Text to Prepare You for Clinical Practice

Chapter 15: Nonpharmacologic techniques (see also Figures 15-5 to 15-8)
Figure 12-4: Pelvic divisions and measurements
Table 13-1: Intrapartum assessment guide
Figure 13-2: Vaginal examination during labor
Figure 13-7: Sequence for delivery
Figure 13-8: Vaginal birth
Table 13-3: Apgar score

New Terms

Amniotomy
Bloody show
Crowning
Dilation
EDD (also known as *EDB*)
Effacement
Gravida
Lochia
Multipara
Nullipara
Para
Presentation
Primipara
Station
VBAC

Equipment and Supplies

Sterile and nonsterile gloves
Lubricant
Urine specimen containers
Amniotic membrane perforator (Amnihook)
Emesis basin
Bedpan
Disposable underpads
Extra linens
Fetal monitoring equipment and related supplies
Electronic fetal monitor and supplies
Doppler transducer
IV fluids, tubing, venipuncture supplies, IV pumps
Urinary catheters (indwelling and straight)
Oxygen equipment, including water, tubing, and face masks
Emergency cart
"Precip tray" (for emergency birth)
Neonatal warmer
Neonatal oxygen equipment and resuscitation supplies

Normal Assessments

Fetus

Gestation. 38 to 42 weeks.

Fetal Heart Rate (FHR). Lower limit of 110 to 120 beats/minute and upper limit of 150 to 160 beats/minute at term. The rate may slow during contractions but should return to its original level by the end of the contraction.

Amniotic Fluid. Clear (may have particles of white vernix); no foul odor.

Woman

Temperature. Lower than 38° C (100.4° F).

Blood Pressure. Near baseline levels established during pregnancy. (Report elevations of 140/90 or higher.)

Pulse. 60 to 100 beats/minute.

Respirations. 12 to 20 breaths/minute.

Contractions. No more than 90 seconds in duration, with at least 60 seconds of uterine relaxation between the end of one contraction and the beginning of the next.

Bloody Show. Dark blood mixed with mucus (has a distinct mucous component). The amount varies but increases as full cervical dilation nears.

Lochia (Fourth Stage). No more than one saturated pad in 1 hour. (Perineal pads containing cold packs absorb less and are saturated sooner than standard pads.)

Fundus (Fourth Stage). Firm, between the symphysis and the umbilicus, midline.

Nursing Care

Clinical experiences in the intrapartum setting are primarily observational. The nursing student works with an experienced nurse when caring for the laboring woman. Primary responsibilities of the novice are to promote family attachment, provide comfort and support to the woman and her family, and report maternal or fetal assessments that are not expected.

Personal protective equipment (PPE), such as gloves and water-repellent gowns or aprons, must be worn whenever the possibility of contact with body fluids (amniotic fluid, blood, lochia, colostrum, breast milk, urine, or stool) exists to conform with standard precautions. Protective eyewear also must be worn if splash or spray contamination of the eyes is a possibility.

Assessments

Unless directed otherwise by the experienced nurse, assess the woman and fetus who do not have complications or medications that require special monitoring by the following guidelines:

1. FHR with continuous electronic fetal monitoring or intermittent auscultation: every hour during the latent phase; every 30 minutes during the active phase; every 15 minutes during the second stage of labor.
2. The woman's temperature every 4 hours unless her membranes have ruptured, then every 2 hours.
3. The woman's blood pressure, pulse, and respirations every hour.
4. Contractions: Assess at same time as FHR.
5. If the woman's membranes rupture, assess FHR for at least 1 minute, and observe the color, odor, and amount of fluid. Notify an experienced nurse that the woman's membranes have ruptured.
6. After birth, during the recovery phase, assess the mother's uterine fundus, lochia, blood pressure, pulse, and respirations every 15 minutes for the first hour.

Interventions

1. Assess the woman and the fetus using the guidelines above or according to the facility's policy. Document all assessments, and *report any findings that do not fall within the expected limits.*
2. If no contraindication exists, give the woman ice chips and encourage her to change position as much as she desires. Ask an experienced nurse to be sure.
3. The woman can usually walk to the bathroom if she is not in advanced labor and has not had analgesia or anesthesia that impairs mobility (such as epidural block). Record each time she voids or has a bowel movement.
4. Help the woman cope with labor:
5. A cool, damp washcloth often feels good on her face, arms, and abdomen.
6. If her back hurts, offer to rub it or apply firm pressure in the sacral area. Ask her where and how firmly to press. Encourage her to try alternate positions.
7. Give generous praise and encouragement for her efforts to give birth. Praise the partner's efforts as a coach.
8. Offer a snack to the woman's partner, or encourage the partner to take a break and have a meal.
9. Look at the woman's perineum if she says that the baby is coming or begins making grunting sounds or bearing down. Summon the experienced nurse with the call bell immediately, but *do not leave the woman.*
10. When the infant is born, focus on the respiratory efforts and maintain warmth. Use a bulb syringe (see p. 553) to suction excess secretions. Keep the infant under a radiant warmer or wrap in warmed blankets. Do not get between the radiant heat source and the infant.
11. Observe parent-infant attachment behaviors such as making eye contact, talking in soft, high-pitched tones, and making remarks about the infant.
12. In many facilities, the infant remains with the parents during the recovery period, and the same nurse cares for both the mother and the newborn. If so, continue to observe the infant's respiratory effort and maintain the temperature.

POSTPARTUM CARE: PHYSIOLOGIC ASPECTS

Text to Prepare You for Clinical Practice

Procedure 17-1: Assessing the uterine fundus
Procedure 17-2: Assessing the perineum
Figure 17-2: Estimating volume of lochia
Figure 17-7: Clinical pathway for vaginal birth

Figure 17-8: Assessing Homan's sign
Table 17-1: Characteristics of lochia
Table 17-4: Observations of the fundus requiring nursing actions
Critical to Remember: Signs of a distended bladder

New Terms
Afterpains
Atony
Colostrum
Engorgement
Episiotomy
Fundus
Lochia rubra, serosa, alba
Puerperium
REEDA (redness, edema, ecchymosis, drainage, approximation)

Equipment and Supplies
Thermometer
Blood pressure equipment
Watch
Stethoscope
Flashlight
Nonsterile gloves
Peripads
Clean linen
Disposable underpads or linen liners

Normal Assessments
Vital Signs
Temperature. Lower than 38° C (100.4° F).

Blood Pressure. Near the baseline levels established during pregnancy.

Pulse. 60 to 90 beats/minute. 50 to 60 beats/minute may occur. Bradycardia reflects the increased amount of blood returning to the central circulation.

Respirations. 12 to 20 breaths/minute. Should be unchanged from preconception levels; the lungs should be free of adventitious breath sounds.

Breasts
1. First 24 hours: Soft.
2. Days 2 to 3: Firm to very firm, as milk comes in.
3. Nipples: Free of redness, abraded areas, blisters, bruising, and fissures.

Gastrointestinal System
1. Mother is hungry and thirsty.
2. Abdomen is soft. Temporary constipation may occur because of dehydration and decreased intake during labor.
3. Bowel sounds usually present within 24 to 36 hours after cesarean birth.
4. Hemorrhoids may be obvious, particularly during the first 24 hours.

Genitourinary System
1. Fundus should be firm, midline, and located at the umbilicus (±1 cm).
2. Lochia rubra should be scant to moderate with a fleshy, earthy odor.
3. Episiotomy edges should be approximated and without redness or edema.
4. Perineum, labia, or both may be slightly bruised or swollen.
5. Abdominal dressing for cesarean birth should be dry and intact. When the dressing is removed, the edges of the surgical incision should be approximated and without signs of infection.
6. Diuresis is normal for the first 2 to 3 days. Mothers often are unaware of the need to urinate.
7. After the woman voids, the bladder should not be palpable and the fundus should remain firm and at the level of the umbilicus.

Nursing Care
Preparation before approaching the new mother helps the nurse recognize unusual or abnormal data and initiate the necessary nursing interventions.

Nonsterile gloves must be worn whenever the possibility of contact with body fluids (blood, lochia, colostrum, breast milk, urine, or stool) exists.

The sequence in which postpartum assessments are performed is important because they should progress from areas that are least likely to be contaminated, such as the breasts, to areas that are associated with pathogenic organisms, such as the perineum and anal areas. The following sequence is recommended.

Assessments
1. Explain the purpose of the assessments: "I know we do these assessments several times a day, but they help us determine if everything is progressing as it should. It is also a good time for you to ask any questions you might have."
2. Assess vital signs, usually every 4 to 8 hours, depending on facility protocols and the condition of the mother.
3. Observe and report edema of the face or hands, which may suggest pregnancy-induced hypertension.
4. Auscultate breath sounds and the ability to deep breathe and cough if the woman had a cesarean birth, if she smokes, or if she has a history of respiratory disorders.
5. Ask the mother to unfasten her bra or to lower the bra flaps to assess the nipples for redness, fissures, or blisters that may occur with breastfeeding. Note nipple size and shape that may make breastfeeding more difficult (flat, retracted, in-

verted). Palpate the breasts and ask how well breastfeeding is progressing and whether she has any questions.

6. Lower the top of the bed, and ask the mother to flex her knees for comfort. If the woman had a cesarean birth, auscultate the abdomen for bowel sounds and ask if she is passing flatus. Palpate the abdomen (soft or distended?).
7. Observe the dressing covering the incision for intactness and discharge. If the dressing has been removed, observe the cesarean incision for REEDA and note whether staples or Steri-Strips remain in place.
8. Assess for bladder distention (observable or palpable bulge above the symphysis pubis) and time and amount of last voiding (can be validated from the chart before beginning the assessment). If an indwelling catheter is in place, note the color and amount of urine.
9. Palpate the lower extremities for the presence and extent of edema. Press the thumb on the pretibial area and the feet to determine whether pitting edema is present. Note how long it takes for the pit to disappear.
10. Observe and palpate the lower extremities for signs of thrombophlebitis (areas of redness, warmth, tenderness, swelling). Sharply dorsiflex the foot to elicit Homan's sign.
11. Lower the perineal pad(s) and observe flow of lochia while palpating the fundus for firmness and location.
12. Observe the perineal pad(s) for color, amount of lochia, and presence of unpleasant or foul odor. Ask how long since the peripad(s) was changed to determine the amount of flow.
13. Ask the mother to turn to her side to assess the episiotomy and perineum for REEDA. Note the number and size of hemorrhoids.
14. Evaluate the mother's ability to ambulate, and elicit information about dizziness, weakness, or lightheadedness during ambulation. Observe her gait for steadiness and balance.
15. Ask the mother about particular problems and concerns. How is her appetite? How much rest is she getting? Does she have discomfort (where, when)? Does she require medication?

Interventions

1. Changes in vital signs may be within expected limits, or they may indicate the beginning of serious problems. Tachycardia or lower-than-expected blood pressure may indicate excessive bleeding and should be reported. Blood pressure that is higher than expected may indicate pregnancy-induced hypertension. The blood pressure should be reassessed with the woman in a left lateral recumbent position. *Temperature above 38° C (100.4° F) suggests infection rather than dehydration and should be reassessed. Diminished or abnormal breath sounds (wheezes or crackles), as well as difficulty breathing or coughing, should be reported at once.*
2. Nipple trauma provides a portal for entry of pathogenic organisms and creates discomfort during breastfeeding. The new mother often needs information, guidance, and encouragement with breastfeeding.
3. *Intervene at once if you are unable to locate the fundus, if the fundus feels soft (boggy), or if it is above the umbilicus or displaced from the midline.* Assist the mother to void or catheterize her if she is unable to empty her bladder. Use uterine massage to contract a boggy uterus.
4. Report a positive Homan's sign and areas of redness, edema, or tenderness of the legs. Assist the woman to ambulate if her gait is unsteady or she experiences lightheadedness when she ambulates.
5. If necessary, teach self-care measures such as perineal care and sitz bath to reduce perineal discomfort and prevent infection.
6. Provide medication for afterpains or perineal discomfort according to the physician's orders. Reassure the mother that very little of the medication administered for discomfort crosses into the breast milk and the infant should not be affected.

POSTPARTUM CARE: PSYCHOSOCIAL ASPECTS

Text to Prepare You for Clinical Practice

Table 18-1: Assessing maternal adaptation
Table 18-3: Assessing family adaptation
Critical to Remember: Reciprocal attachment behaviors

New Terms

Attachment
Bonding
En face
Engrossment
Entrainment
Finger-tipping
Letting-go
Reciprocal bonding behaviors
Taking-hold
Taking-in

Normal Assessments

Maternal Touch. During the first 24 hours, the mother progresses from the discovery phase, when she "finger-tips" the infant, to enfolding the infant and demonstrating a range of consoling behaviors.

Verbal Expressions. The mother progresses from referring to the infant as "it" to "he" or "she" and finally to calling the infant by a given name.

Taking-In Phase. Mothers are concerned with their own physical needs and the need to recount details of their labor and delivery.

Taking-Hold Phase. Mothers become more independent and focus on learning how to care for themselves and the infant.

Fathers. Fathers demonstrate intense fascination with the infant and often are observed to respond gently to infant signals such as fussing and crying.

Family. Family support is obvious when the grandparents visit, offer to assist the mother, and demonstrate interest in the newborn.

Nursing Care

To prepare for the psychological assessment, the nurse should review expected maternal behaviors, progression of maternal touch, and verbal interactions before beginning a psychosocial assessment.

Assessments

1. Collect data from the woman's chart or kardex (age, gravida, para, time and type of delivery, sex and weight of infant, unusual characteristics or anomalies of the infant, time mother was last medicated for discomfort) to identify factors that might affect adjustment.
2. Begin the psychosocial assessment during the physical assessment, and continue to make observations throughout the day.
3. Observe maternal mood, general energy level, and activity.
4. Ask about the mother's comfort, how she slept, and whether she has special concerns.
5. Note the focus of the mother's attention—is it on her own needs or care of the infant? Does she require assistance with hygiene and self-care measures? How much does she talk of the birth experience?
6. Observe the mother's interaction with the infant and her readiness to participate in infant care. Note her voice tone and verbal interaction.
7. Watch how the mother touches the infant and how she responds to infant cues, such as crying and fussing.
8. Note the father's participation in infant care and his comfort in handling the infant.
9. Notice infant behavior (awake, sleepy, gazing, response to parents' voices). Watch closely how the infant responds to the parents and whether the parents are successful in consoling the infant.
10. Observe visitors, particularly the grandparents and family, who may provide assistance to the parents during the early weeks at home.

Interventions

1. Anticipate the mother's needs and provide physical care and comfort measures that are particularly important in the early hours following childbirth.
2. Allow time to listen; this is very important in establishing rapport and assisting the mother to integrate the birth experience into her reality system.
3. Promote bonding and attachment by providing long periods of uninterrupted contact between the parents and the infant. Model behaviors such as gently responding when the infant cries and talking to the infant in a high-pitched voice. Point out positive characteristics of the infant to the parents.
4. Prepare to teach basic infant care including explanations, demonstrations, and use of videos.
5. Answer questions or demonstrate care as the mother indicates a readiness to learn.

THE NEWBORN: INITIAL ASSESSMENTS AND CARE

Text to Prepare You for Clinical Practice

Procedure 20-1: Weighing and measuring the newborn
Procedure 20-2: Assessing vital signs in the newborn
Procedure 20-3: Obtaining blood samples from the newborn by heel puncture
Procedure 21-1: Administering intramuscular injections to newborns
Procedure 21-2: Using a bulb syringe
Figure 21-2: Administration of ophthalmic ointment
Table 20-1: Summary of newborn assessment

New Terms

Acrocyanosis
Caput succedaneum
Cephalhematoma
Hyperbilirubinemia
Lanugo
Milia
Molding
Mongolian spots
Vernix caseosa

Equipment and Supplies

Scale
Radiant warmer
Nonsterile gloves
Stethoscope
Thermometer

Tape measure
Vitamin K, syringe, filter needle, alcohol wipes
Eye medication
Bulb syringe

Normal Assessments

Vital Signs

Temperature. Axillary 36.5 to 37.5° C (97.7 to 99.5° F). Rectal 36.5 to 37.6° C (97.7 to 99.7° F).

Heart Rate. 120 to 160 beats/minute.

Respirations. 30 to 60 breaths/minute. Average 40 breaths/minute.

Blood Glucose. Above 40 to 45 mg/dl by screening tests or above 40 mg/dl by laboratory analysis.

Measurements

Weight. 2500 to 4000 g (5 lb, 8 oz to 8 lb, 13 oz).

Length. 48 to 53 cm (19 to 21 inches).

Head Circumference. 33 to 35.5 cm (13 to 14 inches).

Chest Circumference. 30.5 to 33 cm (12 to 13 inches).

Nursing Care

A typical order in which assessments and care are performed in the labor, delivery, recovery unit or the admission nursery is given here. The elements actually included and the order in which they are performed depend on the facility's routine and the circumstances.

Adhere to standard precautions at all times. Wear nonsterile gloves whenever handling the infant until the bath is given and all blood is removed from the skin. After the bath, wear gloves when soiling with body fluids may occur.

Include family members who are present. They often are very interested in explanations of the assessments and care being given. Promote bonding by encouraging them to touch and talk to the infant.

Assessments

Begin with a quick overall assessment of the infant's general condition. Attend to major problems, such as severe respiratory distress, before continuing the more detailed assessment and routine care. Observe for signs of distress or abnormality in the early hours after birth, when they are most likely to appear. Report and take action, as necessary, for any abnormal findings.

1. Perform a quick general assessment to identify gross abnormalities. *Be constantly alert for signs of respiratory distress.*
2. Assess vital signs. *Report and follow up on abnormalities immediately.*
3. Weigh infant and measure length and head and chest circumferences.
4. Assess blood glucose according to signs of hypoglycemia and agency policy.
5. Perform in-depth assessment (see Table 20-1).
6. Continue monitoring vital signs every 30 minutes until infant has been stable for 2 hours. Assess more often if necessary. Once the infant is stable, vital signs should be checked every 8 hours, or more frequently if abnormal.

Interventions

1. Suction the infant as necessary.
2. Take footprints, if not done previously (according to agency routine).
3. Administer antibiotic ointment to the eyes, and administer vitamin K injection. NOTE: Do not give vitamin K until after the bath or the leg is well cleaned if the mother is hepatitis B or HIV positive.
4. Allow the infant to rest quietly under a radiant warmer between assessments and care. When the initial assessment and procedures are completed and the temperature is stable, wrap the infant in two blankets, place a hat on the head, and give the infant to the parents to hold.
5. When the temperature is stable, bathe the infant under a radiant warmer to remove blood and excess vernix. Keep the infant warm by drying as quickly as possible and removing wet linens. Dry the hair thoroughly to prevent heat loss.
6. Assist the mother with the initial feeding. If the infant is formula fed, give no more than 1 oz. Burp the infant halfway through feeding.
7. Watch continuously for circumoral or central cyanosis, or lack of breathing during sucking. Stop the feeding, suction with a bulb syringe, and stimulate the infant by rubbing the back. Continue feeding when the infant has regained color. Place the infant on the right side with a rolled diaper behind the back after feeding, or elevate the head of the bed slightly.
8. Complete a gestational age assessment.
9. Prepare for transfer from the radiant warmer to a crib. Place clothing and blankets under the warmer to heat. Take the last set of vital signs, dress the infant, apply a hat, and wrap the infant in two warmed blankets. Complete all charting.
10. Give report if another nurse is taking over care of the infant. Include gravida, para, length of labor, medications/anesthesia used in labor and delivery, time of rupture of membranes, any complications during birth, any problems in early hours, feeding, voids and stools, and any other pertinent information.

THE NEWBORN: CONTINUED CARE

Text to Prepare You for Clinical Practice

Procedure 21-3: Identifying infants
Parents Want to Know: Caring for the uncircumcised penis
Parents Want to Know: How to care for the circumcision site
Table 21-1: Precautions to prevent infant abduction

New Terms

Erythema toxicum
Hypoglycemia
Nonshivering thermogenesis

Equipment and Supplies

Stethoscope
Thermometer
Alcohol wipes

Normal Assessments

Vital Signs

Temperature. Axillary 36.5 to 37.5° C (97.7 to 99.5° F). Rectal 36.5 to 37.6° C (97.7 to 99.7° F).

Heart Rate. 120 to 160 beats/minute.

Respirations. 30 to 60 breaths/minute. 40 breaths/minute average.

Blood Glucose. Above 40 to 45 mg/dl by screening tests (according to agency policy) or above 40 mg/dl by laboratory analysis.

Nursing Care

Assess and care for infants using the following list as a guide. Keep in mind that the role of the nurse is to continue to observe for abnormalities and complications, as well as to assess progress of mother-infant bonding and the mother's ability to care for the infant.

Assessments

1. *Vital signs.* Assess vital signs once every 8 hours and more often if any abnormalities exist. Before disturbing a sleeping infant, check the respirations and pulse rate. Temperature should be stable after the first day; if not, action is needed. Continue to listen for abnormal heart sounds. Murmurs heard earlier may disappear after the first day as transition to neonatal circulation becomes complete. Note acrocyanosis or central cyanosis. Breath sounds should be clear.
2. *Weight.* Weigh infants daily at the same time of day according to agency routine.
3. *Neurologic.* Note the state of alertness (six stages), movement of extremities, and reflexes (especially Moro, rooting, suck). Observe the eyes for signs of inflammation (redness, drainage); may be due to reaction to eye medication or infection. Cleanse drainage with sterile water from the inner to outer canthus, ensuring that drainage from one eye does not contaminate the other. Watch for signs of hypoglycemia ("jitteriness," tremors). Check fontanelle with the infant in an upright position. It should be soft and flat. *Report fullness, bulging, depression.*
4. *Skin.* Assess all skin areas to observe for new marks or changes in existing ones. Compare with previous assessments. Expect the skin to be dry and peeling. Look for redness, scratches (keep hands covered), rashes, signs of skin breakdown, or infection. Erythema toxicum may become more apparent. Caput succedaneum may resolve as early as 12 hours or may take several days. Cephalhematoma resolves in several weeks. Physiologic jaundice may begin to develop after the first 24 hours. Blanch the skin over the nose and bony prominences, and note color. Check the cord and base of the cord for redness, foul odor, and serosanguineous or purulent drainage. Note how well the cord is drying. Remove the clamp when the end of the cord is dry and crisp (about 24 hours).
5. *Musculoskeletal.* Note the movement of extremities and muscle tone. The infant should resist when the extremities are extended. Note stiffness, arching of the infant's back, or molding of the infant to the caregiver's body.
6. *Gastrointestinal.* The abdomen should be soft and bowel sounds present. If the mother is giving all feedings, observe at least a part of several feedings. Ask the mother how she feels the feedings are going. Assess for suck and swallow coordination, choking, length of time the feeding lasts, amount taken, and any regurgitation. Note the type and number of stools. Know whether the infant has had a stool on the present shift and when the last stool occurred. (The first stool is generally within 12 to 48 hours of birth.)
7. *Genitourinary.* Note the number of voidings and the color of urine on diapers. Know whether the infant has voided on the present shift and when the last voiding occurred. Teach the parents to expect at least 2 to 6 wet diapers per day during the first 2 days of life and 6 to 10 wet diapers per day thereafter. (The first voiding should occur within 12 to 24 hours.) Observe the circumcision site for drainage (purulent, serous, sanguineous, frank bleeding, or oozing). Determine whether the infant is voiding after a circumcision is performed.
8. *Bonding.* Observe bonding behaviors in the mother and infant. Note how the mother holds the infant, whether she talks to the infant, calls the infant by name, and the like. Note response of the infant to the mother's care.
9. *Teaching.* Assess in which areas the mother (or the parents) need teaching.

Interventions

The following care of the infant is typical for every shift. In addition, make rounds frequently (at least every hour) to monitor the mother's progress in infant care and determine the need for further interventions.

1. *Cord care.* Apply alcohol to the cord once or more each shift, according to agency routine. Use an alcohol wipe or an applicator dipped in alcohol. Cleanse all parts of the cord and the crevices of the umbilicus. Do not apply alcohol to the skin around the cord because this is drying to the skin. Some units apply nothing to the cord or use triple dye or other bactericidal agents once daily. Fold the diaper below the cord.
2. *Care of the circumcision site.* Assess the parent's knowledge of care of the circumcision site, and teach as necessary. If a Plastibell was used, no special care is necessary other than observation for complications. If a Gomco clamp was used, instruct parents to squeeze petroleum jelly liberally over the circumcision site (and apply gauze if part of agency routine) at each diaper change for the first 24 hours. Assess the incision throughout the shift for redness, edema, purulent or sanguineous drainage, and odor.
3. *Identification.* If the mother and infant are separated at any time, use the proper identification process each time the infant is reunited with the mother.
4. *Protection.* Maintain vigilance against kidnappers at all times. Follow methods to provide for infant security.
5. *Feedings.* Determine whether the infant is taking feedings adequately (every 2 to 3 hours if breastfed, every 4 hours if formula fed). Record each feeding including the type, amount (or how long the infant nursed at each breast), how feedings are taken, and any regurgitation. Teach the parents as necessary.
6. *Elimination.* Record each wet diaper and stool. Note the color, amount, and consistency.
7. *Continue observation.* Observe for problems throughout the shift.
8. *Continue teaching.* Provide additional parent teaching as needed along with the "scheduled" teaching that was planned at the beginning of the shift.

ASSISTING THE INEXPERIENCED BREASTFEEDING MOTHER

Text to Prepare You for Clinical Practice

Figure 22-3: Cradle hold
Figure 22-4: Football hold
Figure 22-5: Side-lying position
Figure 22-6: C position of hand on breast
Mothers Want to Know: Is my baby getting enough milk?
Mothers Want to Know: Solutions to common breastfeeding problems
Mothers Want to Know: Breastfeeding after the birth of more than one infant
Mothers Want to Know: How to wean from breastfeeding
Table 22-2: The LATCH Scoring Tool

New Terms

Latch-on
Non-nutritive suckling or sucking
Nutritive suckling or sucking

Normal Assessments

1. The infant is positioned facing the breast, and the infant's body is well supported.
2. The mother is comfortable and holds her breast so that the infant can take it into the mouth without interference.
3. The infant's mouth covers the nipple and as much of the areola as possible.
4. Suckling includes audible swallowing.

Nursing Care

This is a summary of information that nurses can use to help the inexperienced mother, especially during the first breastfeeding sessions.

Assessments

1. Assess the mother's knowledge about breastfeeding techniques.
2. Assess the mother's breasts to identify engorgement, flat or inverted nipples, or nipple trauma.
3. Assess the infant's behavior state, sucking reflex, and coordination of sucking and swallowing.

Interventions

1. Plan with the mother when the infant will be fed, and note any questions or concerns that she has about breastfeeding. Be sure that she is comfortable (pain relief needs met) and not in the middle of other care (AM care, meals). However, if the infant must eat immediately because of concerns about hypoglycemia, meet the mother's needs quickly or postpone her care and begin the feeding.
2. Explain that breastfeeding is a learned skill for both the mother and the infant and that practice is required to perfect the skill.
3. Begin the feeding when the infant is awake and showing signs of hunger. Do not wait until the infant is ravenously hungry and upset.
4. Assist the mother to position herself and the infant. Use pillows or blankets for comfort, to protect an abdominal incision, and to raise the infant to nipple level.
   a. *Sitting.* Place the bed in a high Fowler's position. Position a pillow behind the mother's

back and under her elbow to support her arm.

b. *Cradle hold.* Place the infant in the mother's arms, with the head at the antecubital space (or at nipple level) and the mother's arm extending along the infant's body. The mother's other hand positions the breast. The infant should be totally on the side facing the breast so that turning of the head is not necessary.

c. *Football hold.* Place the infant's head in the mother's hand, with the body along her side supported by pillows or blankets.

d. *Side-lying.* Place pillows behind the mother's back and between her legs. Her lower arm may go under her head or around the infant, while her upper hand positions the breast. Place the infant on the side facing the breast, using pillows to pad the siderails and to maintain the position.

5. Demonstrate the proper hand position, with the hand cupped around the breast, the thumb on top, and the fingers supporting the breast below. Keep the fingers and thumb behind the areola.
6. Elicit latch-on. Brush the nipple against the center of the infant's lower lip until the infant opens the mouth wide. Bring the infant toward the breast while inserting the nipple and as much of the areola as possible into the infant's mouth.
7. Assess the mouth position. The infant's lips should be 1 to 1½ inches from the base of the nipple with the lips flared. Remove the infant from the breast and start over if dimpling of the cheeks, clicking, or smacking sounds occur.
8. Assess the infant's suck. Nutritive suckling is smooth and continuous with occasional pauses. A swallow follows every one to three sucks and has a "ka" or "ah" sound. Non-nutritive suckling is choppy with no swallowing. Do not jiggle the breast in the infant's mouth to stimulate suckling or the infant may lose the grip and chew on the nipple.
9. When swallowing stops, remove the infant from the breast and burp, change sides, awaken, or let sleep if the feeding is finished.
10. Demonstrate removal from the breast. Have the mother insert a finger into the corner of the infant's mouth between the gums to release suction. Remove the infant immediately.
11. Instruct the mother to nurse an average of at least 15 minutes per feeding to begin, increasing as the infant shows interest. Burp the infant between breasts. Instruct her to nurse every 2 to 3 hours during the day and at least every 4 hours throughout the night to build the milk supply.
12. Observe the mother at intervals after the feeding begins. Help her switch sides to observe for difficulty. Then observe the mother at other feedings to give reinforcement and correct technique as needed. Offer praise generously because feeding the infant may affect the mother's view of her mothering abilities.

APPENDIX E

Answers to Check Your Reading

Chapter 1

1. Federal involvement and consumer demands for greater involvement in their families' births have created changes in maternity care since the 1960s.
2. Family-centered maternity care provides safe, quality care that adapts to both the physical and the psychological needs of the entire family during reproduction and greatly increases the responsibilities of nurses providing care.
3. Birthing centers provide professional care during pregnancy and childbirth in a homelike environment for women with low-risk pregnancies. They are associated with a nearby hospital to which the woman can be transferred in case of unexpected complications. Although the home setting provides comfort and closeness, it may not have adequate equipment or personnel to handle unexpected developments. LDR and LDRP rooms offer a homelike setting for birth but within the hospital, where emergencies can be handled more easily.
4. Cost-containment strategies have shortened the length of stay in the birth facility for mothers and their infants. This has created concern for nurses, who must provide information for parents in a very short time. Nurses can also use the demand for cost containment to develop innovative programs for family education.
5. Clinical pathways are guidelines that define expected outcomes for clients, including the length of stay and the time and sequence of interventions that will accomplish the outcomes.
6. A variety of standards guide home care, including agency and organizational standards that spell out the preparation and responsibilities of nurses. Legal standards define the scope of practice, and other regulatory bodies such as OSHA, CDC, and FDA provide guidelines. Accrediting agencies such as JCAHO and CHAP give their stamp of approval when standards reach a certain level.
7. Safety is the major concern with the use of complementary and alternative medicine because these modalities are largely unregulated. Additionally, clients usually refer themselves to practitioners and may either delay care from a conventional health care provider or may not tell the conventional provider about substances they are taking that may be harmful when combined with other medications. Some organic substances have active pharmacologic ingredients of varying strengths.
8. Traditional families are headed by a man and a woman, usually married, who view parenting as the major priority in their lives and whose energies are not depleted by poverty, illness, or substance abuse. Nontraditional families are defined by their unique structure and include single-parent families, blended families, extended families, homosexual families, and adoptive families.
9. Families may be identified as high risk if they are below the poverty level; are headed by a single teenage parent; have a preterm, ill, or disabled infant; or have lifestyle problems such as substance abuse or family violence.
10. A healthy family can adapt without undue stress to the changes precipitated by childbirth. Members communicate openly, volunteer assistance, and agree on basic principles of child care.
11. Factors that interfere with family functioning include lack of family resources, absence of adequate family support, birth of an infant who requires specialized care, unhealthy habits (such as smoking, substance abuse), and the inability to make mature decisions.
12. Nurses should examine their own cultural values and beliefs to determine ways in which their beliefs may generate conflict with those who hold different cultural beliefs.
13. Differences in language create the greatest difficulty; however, differences in style add to potential conflicts.

14. Culture is difficult to understand because, like an iceberg, only the tip (the behavior) is visible. Reasons for the behavior (for example, religious beliefs, moral values) are hidden, much like the submerged part of an iceberg, and require serious study.
15. The infant mortality rate is lower today than at the beginning of the twentieth century because of improved health of the population, application of basic principles of sanitation, increased medical knowledge, widespread availability of antibiotics, and improved prenatal care.
16. The higher incidence of poverty among African-American families is associated with inadequate prenatal care and the birth of low-birth-weight infants who are less likely to survive than white children.
17. The infant mortality rate in the United States ranks twenty-fifth among developed nations.

CHAPTER 2

1. Therapeutic communication is purposeful, goal directed, and focused.
2. Major communication techniques include clarifying, paraphrasing, reflecting, silence, structuring, pinpointing, questioning, directing, and summarizing.
3. Major blocks to communication include conveying a lack of interest or haste, displaying a closed posture, interrupting, providing false reassurance, offering inappropriate self-disclosure, giving advice, and failing to acknowledge comments or feelings.
4. Major principles of teaching and learning include readiness to learn, participation, repetition, positive feedback, and acknowledgment of frustration. Effective methods include role modeling, presenting simple tasks before more complex material, and using a variety of teaching methods.
5. Factors that affect learning include developmental level, language, culture, previous experience, environment, and the organization and skill of the instructor.
6. The purpose of critical thinking is to identify and overcome habits or impulses that result in poor decisions or inappropriate actions and to make the best clinical judgments.
7. Steps that may be helpful in learning critical thinking can be organized into an ABCDE pattern. They include a recognition of assumptions, an examination of personal biases, an analysis of pressure felt for closure, an examination of how data are collected and analyzed, and an evaluation of how emotions may interfere with the ability to think critically.
8. *Reflective skepticism* means to suspend judgment to avoid making decisions in haste or with insufficient data.
9. The screening assessment gathers information about all aspects of the client's health. A focus assessment gathers information about an actual health problem or one for which the client appears to have a higher risk.
10. Actual nursing diagnoses reflect health problems that can be validated by the presence of defining characteristics. Risk nursing diagnoses indicate that risk factors are present that make the client vulnerable to the development of a particular problem, which has not yet developed.
11. The terms *goals* and *expected outcomes* (outcome criteria) are often used interchangeably to describe desired endpoints of care, but they are different. Broad goals do not have the specific criteria of outcome criteria. Expected outcomes should (1) be stated in terms of the client, (2) be observable and measurable, (3) have a time frame, and (4) be realistic.
12. Nursing interventions that are not specific and do not spell out exactly what is to be done are difficult to implement. Clearly written interventions that provide detailed, objective instructions correct the problem.
13. Nursing diagnoses describe health problems that nurses can treat independently and for which they are accountable. Collaborative problems are potential complications that nurses cannot treat independently and that require both physician-prescribed and nursing-prescribed interventions.
14. Client-centered goals (or expected outcomes) are inappropriate for collaborative problems because they imply accountability for problems that nurses cannot manage independently.

CHAPTER 3

1. Ethics examines conduct and distinctions between right and wrong. Bioethics applies specifically to the ethics of health care.
2. Deontologic theory applies ethical principles to determine what is right. It does not vary the solution according to individual situations. Utilitarian theory analyzes the benefits and burdens to determine a course of action that provides the greatest amount of good in a given situation.
3. Ethical principles may conflict when the application of one principle violates another.
4. Assessment is used to gather data from all concerned persons. Ethical theories and principles are analyzed to determine whether an ethical dilemma exists. Planning involves identifying as many options as possible and choosing a solution.

Interventions must be identified to implement the chosen solution, and the results are evaluated.

5. The Supreme Court decision in *Roe v. Wade* declared that abortion was legal anywhere in the United States and that existing state laws prohibiting abortion were unconstitutional because they interfered with a woman's right to privacy.
6. The belief that abortion is a private choice conflicts with the belief that abortion is taking a life.
7. States cannot give a husband veto power over his spouse's decision to have an abortion; states do not have an obligation to pay for abortions, physicians are given broad discretion to determine fetal viability, and states may restrict abortions of viable fetuses. In addition, states may require parental consent for minors to obtain abortion if an alternative (e.g., judge's approval) is available, states may require a woman to wait 24 hours before seeking and obtaining an abortion, and states may not require a married woman to inform her husband before obtaining an abortion.
8. At the time they are employed, nurses must disclose their beliefs about caring for women having an abortion. Nurses must inform a supervisor so that appropriate care can be arranged.
9. Punitive approaches are against the ethical principles of autonomy, bodily integrity, and personal freedom. Although the intended plan may be to protect the fetus, such a plan can have unexpected outcomes, causing the woman to avoid prenatal care or be dishonest with care providers, causing far more harm to her fetus.
10. Problems involved in the use of advanced reproductive techniques include high cost, low success rate, limitation to the affluent, control of unused embryos, and problem or unexpected pregnancy outcomes. Another issue is that the offspring of postmenopausal women are more likely to be orphaned than those of younger mothers.
11. Poverty is the underlying factor that causes many other problems such as inadequate access to health care. The lack of access to health care is a major reason for the large number of low-birth-weight infants and the high infant mortality rate.
12. The Balanced Budget Act of 1997 has further reduced income from Medicare and Medicaid (a major source of funding for most health care facilities). This requires an even greater conservation of funds. Its emphasis on disease prevention provides a positive challenge for nurses.
13. The focus has long been on treatment and cure of illness, often with expensive technology. However, prevention is less expensive and provides care for greater numbers.
14. State boards of nursing administer the individual states' nurse practice acts, which establish what the nurse is allowed and expected to do when practicing nursing in that state.
15. Standards of care and agency policies influence judgment about malpractice because they describe the level of care that can be expected from practitioners.
16. Nursing actions that help defend malpractice claims include securing informed consent appropriately, keeping documentation that provides evidence that the standard of care has been maintained, acting appropriately as a client advocate in terms of taking a problem through the chain of command, and maintaining expertise.
17. Concerns about the use of unlicensed assistive personnel include whether this use compromises the quality of care and the nurse's ability to supervise unlicensed personnel adequately with high workloads.
18. Short lengths of stay lead to concerns about the woman's ability to care for herself and her infant, potential complications that new parents may not identify, and the fact that parents will not have had time to absorb the necessary teaching. Follow-up phone calls help alleviate some concerns and identify some problems that develop after discharge.
19. Facilities that use phone-call triage must have regularly reviewed and updated protocols, good documentation forms, and specific instructions to the client about actions to take if further problems develop.

CHAPTER 4

1. Development of the breasts is the first sign of puberty in girls. In boys, growth of the testes is the first sign, followed by growth of the penis about 1 year later.
2. Usually, Asians and Native Americans have less and finer body hair than either whites or African-Americans. African-Americans usually have body hair that is coarser and curlier than Asians, Native Americans, or whites.
3. The female pelvis has a wide, rounded, basinlike shape that favors efficient passage of the fetus during birth. The male pelvis is heavier and narrower and structurally suited for tasks requiring load bearing.
4. Males generally attain a greater adult height than females because they begin their growth spurt about 1 year later than girls and continue growing for a longer period of time.
5. Female secondary sex characteristics include round hips and breasts and growth of pubic hair, finer skin texture, and a higher-pitched voice. Male secondary sex characteristics include the presence of facial and pubic hair, a deeper voice, broader shoulders, and greater muscle mass.

6. The female external reproductive organs are collectively called the *vulva*. The labia majora extend from the mons pubis to the perineum. The labia minora are within and parallel to the labia majora. The clitoris is at the anterior junction of the labia minora. The urinary meatus and vaginal introitus are found within the vestibule (the area enclosed by the labia minora). The hymen partly closes the vaginal opening. The perineum extends from the fourchette (posterior rim of the vaginal opening) to the anus.
7. The three divisions of the uterus are the corpus (body), isthmus, and cervix (neck). The fundus is the part of the corpus that lies above the entry points of the fallopian tubes.
8. Myometrium is the middle layer of thick uterine muscle between the perimetrium and endometrium. The myometrium includes three types of muscle fibers: (1) longitudinal fibers, mostly in the fundus, to expel the fetus during birth; (2) interlacing figure-8 fibers to compress bleeding blood vessels after birth; and (3) circular fibers to provide constrictions near the fallopian tubes and the internal cervical os, enabling the proper implantation of the fertilized ovum and preventing the reflux of menstrual blood into the fallopian tubes.
9. The fallopian tubes are lined with cells with cilia that beat rhythmically toward the uterine cavity to propel the ovum through the fallopian tube. The fertilized ovum undergoes its early cell divisions in the fallopian tube so that implantation is most likely to occur in the uterine fundus.
10. The two functions of the ovaries are to produce hormones (primarily estrogen and progesterone) and mature an ovum for release during each reproductive cycle.
11. The pelvis is located at the lower end of the spine. The true pelvis is located below the linea terminalis. The true pelvis is the most relevant during birth.
12. Pelvic muscles and ligaments enclose the lower pelvis and support internal reproductive, urinary, and bowel structures.
13. The ripening follicle secretes estrogen. After ovulation, the follicle (now called the *corpus luteum*) secretes large amounts of estrogen and progesterone.
14. Three ovarian phases of the female reproductive cycle are the follicular (maturation of an ovum), ovulatory (release of the mature ovum), and luteal (secretion of estrogen and progesterone by the corpus luteum). The length of the follicular phase varies more among women than the other two phases.
15. The three phases are the proliferative, secretory, and menstrual phases. The proliferative phase occurs during the first half of the cycle, during which the endometrium thickens in preparation for a fertilized ovum. The secretory phase occurs during the last half of the cycle and is characterized by continued growth of the endometrium, growth of blood vessels and glands, and secretion of substances to nourish a fertilized ovum. If pregnancy does not occur, the endometrium becomes ischemic and necrotic as secretion of estrogen and progesterone from the corpus luteum falls. The old endometrium is shed in the menstrual phase.
16. The cervical mucus becomes thin, clear, and elastic during ovulation to facilitate entrance of sperm from the vagina into the uterus and fallopian tube, thus enhancing the chances for conception.
17. Montgomery's tubercles secrete a substance during pregnancy and lactation that keeps the nipples soft.
18. A woman's breast size is not related to the amount of milk she can produce. Breast size is influenced by the amount of fatty tissue in the breast.
19. Milk secretion does not occur during pregnancy because estrogen and progesterone produced by the placenta inhibit its production.
20. As a urinary organ the penis transports urine from the bladder to outside the body during urination. As a reproductive organ, it carries and deposits semen into the vagina during coitus.
21. The two types of erectile tissue in the penis are the corpus spongiosum that surrounds the urethra and the two columns of corpus cavernosum tissue on each side of the penis. The function of erectile tissue is to facilitate entry of the penis into the female's vagina.
22. The scrotum holds the testes away from the body to keep them cooler than the core body temperature, thus facilitating sperm production.
23. The testes function as endocrine glands to produce testosterone and the male gametes (spermatozoa).

CHAPTER 5

1. DNA is the building block of genes. A varying number of genes in turn make up each chromosome.
2. Genes are too small to be seen under a microscope. They can be studied by analysis of the products they instruct cells to produce, direct study of the DNA, or their close association with another gene that can be studied by one of these other methods.
3. Chromosomes can be seen under a microscope when living nucleated cells are dividing. They may be photographed under the microscope and the resulting picture of chromosomes arranged in a karyotype. Fluorescent in situ hybridization is a newer technique that uses DNA probes to identify numerical chromosomal makeup. Spectral karyotyping assigns a color to each chromosome to better identify rearrangements and small additions

or deletions of chromosome material that may cause abnormalities.

4. 46,XY describes the chromosome makeup of a normal human male. 46,XX describes the chromosomes of a normal human female. Abnormalities are described beginning with the total number of chromosomes, followed by the sex chromosome complement, and followed by the abbreviation that describes the chromosome abnormality.
5. The child of a parent with an autosomal dominant disorder has a 50% chance of having the same disorder.
6. Blood relationship (consanguinity) of parents increases the likelihood that both share some of the same harmful autosomal recessive genes, increasing the chance that their offspring will be affected with a disorder.
7. If both parents carry an abnormal gene for an autosomal recessive disorder, each child has a 25% chance of receiving both copies of the defective gene and having the disorder. Each child also has a 50% chance of receiving only one copy of the defective gene and being a carrier like the parents. Each child also has a 25% chance of receiving the normal gene from each parent, thus being neither a carrier nor affected and having no chance of passing the gene to future generations.
8. Males are more likely to have X-linked recessive disorders because they do not have a compensating X chromosome with a normal gene. Each son of a female carrier has a 50% chance of having the trait and a 50% chance of being unaffected. Each daughter of the female carrier has a 50% chance of being a carrier and a 50% chance of being unaffected.
9. A trisomy exists when each body cell contains an extra copy of one chromosome. Down syndrome is the most common trisomy and involves 3 copies of chromosome 21 for a total of 47 chromosomes in each cell.
10. A monosomy exists when each body cell is missing a chromosome. Turner's syndrome (a female with a single X chromosome) is the only monosomy compatible with postnatal life.
11. Genetic material can be lost or duplicated when a chromosome has a structural abnormality. Also, the position of genes on the chromosome may be altered, preventing them from functioning normally.
12. A parent with a balanced chromosomal translocation may have a child with completely normal chromosomes, or the child may have a balanced chromosomal translocation similar to that of the parent. The offspring may also receive an unbalanced amount of chromosomal material (too much or too little), which often results in spontaneous abortion or birth defects.
13. Multifactorial disorders are typically present and detectable at birth. They are usually isolated defects rather than being present with other unrelated defects. However, sometimes the primary multifactorial defect alters further development and results in other related defects.
14. Factors that may affect the likelihood that a multifactorial disorder will occur or recur include the following: the number of affected close relatives, severity of the defect in those affected, gender of the affected person, geographic location, and seasonal variations.
15. The woman may be able to prevent exposing her fetus to teratogens by being immunized against infections such as rubella at least 3 months before pregnancy, eliminating the use of nontherapeutic drugs such as alcohol and illicit drugs, changing therapeutic drugs to those having a lower risk to the fetus, and avoiding x-rays when she may be pregnant.
16. A pregnant woman who has phenylketonuria should return to her low-phenylalanine diet when she is pregnant to prevent buildup of toxic products that would damage the developing fetus.
17. Adequate folic acid intake of at least 0.4 mg (400 mcg) has been associated with a lower incidence of neural tube defects. Because the neural tube begins closure at 4 weeks' gestation, the woman should have adequate intake beginning before conception to ensure the best outcome.

CHAPTER 6

1. Meiosis is a type of cell division that halves the number of chromosomes so that only one of each chromosomal pair goes into each gamete. Meiosis also promotes genetic variation by the process of crossing over, or exchange of chromosomal material between each member of the pair of chromosomes. The union of male and female gametes at conception restores the number of chromosomes to 46 in the offspring.
2. Each oogonium produces one mature ovum after two meiotic divisions. The first meiotic division begins in fetal life and is not completed until shortly before that ovum undergoes ovulation. The second meiotic division begins at ovulation but is not completed unless fertilization occurs.
3. Each spermatogonium undergoes two meiotic divisions to result in four mature spermatozoa. Meiosis begins at puberty and both meiotic divisions are completed before the sperm mature and are ejaculated.
4. Fertilization usually occurs in the distal one third of the fallopian tube (the ampulla), near the ovary.
5. Seminal fluid nourishes and protects the sperm from the acidic environment of the woman's vagina.
6. As sperm approach the ovum, they secrete hyaluronidase to digest a pathway through the corona

radiata and zona pellucida. When one spermatozoon finally penetrates the ovum, changes in the zona pellucida prevent other spermatozoa from entering. The cell membranes of ovum and sperm fuse to allow the sperm to penetrate the ovum. The ovum also completes its second meiotic division.

7. Fertilization is complete when the nuclei of the ovum and spermatozoon unite.
8. Implantation begins 6 days after conception and is complete by the tenth day.
9. The upper uterus is the ideal location for implantation for three reasons: (1) it has a rich blood supply for fetal gas exchange and nutrition, (2) the thick uterine lining prevents the placenta from attaching too deeply, and (3) the strong interlacing muscle fibers contract to limit blood loss after birth.
10. Nutritive fluids produced in the thick decidua pass to the conceptus by diffusion before a placental circulation is established. Primary chorionic villi, which will form the fetal side of the placenta, extend from the conceptus into the decidua basalis, which will become the maternal side of the placenta, to tap these nutrients.
11. During the first 8 weeks after conception, all major organ systems develop. The woman may be unaware that she is pregnant and may inadvertently expose the embryo to harmful substances. These substances may damage organs that are developing.
12. At 4 weeks the trachea develops as a bud of the upper digestive tract. After the trachea separates from the upper digestive tract, it branches into the two bronchi, which then divide to form the three lobes of the right lung and the two lobes of the left. Branching continues until terminal air sacs develop.
13. The intestines are contained mostly within the umbilical cord until 10 weeks because they grow more rapidly than the abdominal cavity and the liver and kidneys are relatively large. By 10 weeks after conception, the abdominal cavity has caught up with the growth of its contents and can accommodate them.
14. Gestational age is calculated from the woman's last menstrual period and is about 2 weeks longer than fertilization age. Gestational age is most commonly used because the menstrual period provides a specific marker.
15. The fetus usually assumes a head-down position because this position best fits the egg shape of the uterus. Also, the head is heavier and tends to go downward with gravity in the pool of amniotic fluid.
16. Vernix caseosa protects fetal skin from constant exposure to amniotic fluid. Lanugo helps vernix adhere to the skin. Brown fat helps the infant maintain temperature stability in the cooler external environment. Surfactant keeps the lung alveoli from collapsing with each expiration, thus making breathing easier after birth.
17. The placenta gradually takes over the function of the corpus luteum and secretes estrogen and progesterone.
18. Exchange of oxygen, nutrients, and waste products between the woman and fetus takes place in the intervillous spaces of the placenta.
19. Maternal and fetal blood may be of incompatible blood types and thus should not mix.
20. The fetus can thrive in a relatively low-oxygen environment because of the following:
    a. Fetal hemoglobin carries more oxygen than adult hemoglobin.
    b. The fetus has a higher hemoglobin and hematocrit level than does the newborn or adult.
    c. Rapid diffusion of carbon dioxide into the maternal blood causes the mother to give up oxygen more readily and causes oxygen to combine with fetal blood more readily.
21. Human chorionic gonadotropin (hCG) causes the corpus luteum of the ovary to persist and secrete estrogens and progesterones, which are essential to maintain the uterine lining for implantation. It also facilitates fetal testosterone secretion in the male fetus. Human placental lactogen promotes normal fetal nutrition and growth and maternal breast development. Estrogens cause enlargement of the woman's uterus and genitalia and enlargement and development of the breasts. Progesterone maintains the secretory endometrium and changes the endometrium into the decidua to nourish the conceptus and reduces uterine contractions to prevent spontaneous abortion. Progesterone facilitates growth and development of the mother's breasts and the cells that will secrete milk. Progesterone may allow immune tolerance of the conceptus.
22. The fetal membranes contain the amniotic fluid that cushions the fetus, maintain a stable temperature, and promote normal prenatal structural development.
23. Oxygenated blood enters the fetus through the umbilical vein. Half the blood goes to the liver, and the rest passes through the ductus venosus to the inferior vena cava. Blood enters the right atrium, where a small amount goes to the right ventricle and the rest goes through the foramen ovale to the left atrium and then to the left ventricle. Some blood from the right ventricle goes to the lungs to nourish their tissue, and the rest goes through the ductus arteriosus, where it joins blood ejected from the left ventricle. After circulation through the body, deoxygenated blood returns to the placenta through the two umbilical arteries.
24. Monozygotic twins occur when one spermatozoon fertilizes one ovum and the resulting conceptus

later divides into two inner cell masses that will become two fetuses.

25. The placentas and chorions may fuse before birth, making it difficult to determine whether the twins are monozygotic or dizygotic.
26. Dizygotic twins develop from two ova that are each fertilized by a spermatozoon and are like other siblings in a family.

CHAPTER 7

1. By 20 weeks' gestation, the uterus generally reaches the level of the umbilicus. By 36 weeks, the uterus extends to the xiphoid process, the highest level of uterine growth.
2. In early pregnancy, most of the blood flow to the uterus is to the endometrium and myometrium. As pregnancy progresses, there is an increase in blood flow into intervillous spaces of the placenta to provide oxygen and nutrients to the fetus.
3. The major purpose of progesterone in early pregnancy is to maintain the pregnancy.
4. The cervical mucus plug blocks ascent of bacteria from the vagina into the uterus, thereby protecting the membranes and the fetus from possible infection.
5. During pregnancy the breasts enlarge and become more vascular; the areola increases in size and becomes more pigmented; the nipples increase in size and become more erect; and Montgomery's tubercles become more prominent.
6. Physiologic anemia of pregnancy is caused by a greater increase in plasma volume than in red blood cells, resulting in a dilution but not inadequate hemoglobin concentration. Iron deficiency anemia is caused by a true lack of iron that affects hemoglobin levels.
7. During pregnancy, increased circulation through the kidneys is needed to remove metabolic wastes generated by the mother and fetus. Increased circulation through the skin is necessary to dissipate heat that is generated by accelerated metabolism.
8. In a supine position, the weight of the gravid uterus on the vena cava and descending aorta impedes blood flow to and from the lower extremities, resulting in decreased cardiac output and a supine hypotensive syndrome.
9. It is important to standardize techniques for taking blood pressure because blood pressure in the pregnant woman is affected by position. It is lowest in a lateral recumbent position and highest when standing.
10. During pregnancy the ribs flare, the substernal angle widens, and the circumference of the chest increases.
11. Progesterone stimulates the minute volume by raising the sensitivity of the respiratory center to carbon dioxide, and breathing becomes thoracic as the uterus lifts the diaphragm.
12. Estrogen causes hyperemia of the gums that may lead to bleeding or gingivitis. Excessive salivation (ptyalism) is a problem for some. Progesterone relaxes smooth muscle in the gastrointestinal tract, allowing additional time for nutrients to be absorbed but also resulting in heartburn and constipation.
13. Expectant mothers are at increased risk for urinary tract infection because of compression of the ureters between the uterus and the pelvic bones, resulting in dilation of the ureters and consequent stasis of urine, which allows prolonged time for bacterial growth.
14. Softening of pelvic ligaments and joints due to relaxin, a maternal hormone, creates instability and results in a wide stance and "waddling" gait. As the uterus increases in size, the woman must lean backward to maintain balance, which creates a progressive lordosis.
15. Progesterone maintains the uterine lining, prevents uterine contractions during pregnancy, and helps prepare the breasts for lactation.
16. Maternal hormones (human placental lactogen, estrogen, and progesterone) create increasing resistance of maternal tissues to insulin during the second and third trimesters. Insulinase speeds up the breakdown of insulin.
17. Most presumptive signs are subjective, probable signs are objective; both can be caused by conditions other than pregnancy.
18. Many things such as gas, peristalsis, or pseudocyesis (false pregnancy) can be mistaken by the woman for fetal movement.
19. The most common causes of false-negative pregnancy tests are pregnancy tests performed too soon, urine that is too dilute, impending spontaneous abortion, ectopic pregnancy, and improper use of the test.
20. A medical-surgical history and an obstetric history are necessary to identify chronic conditions or past trauma that can affect the outcome of the pregnancy.
21. Blood pressure should be obtained while the woman is sitting with the arm supported in a horizontal position at heart level. Documentation should include position of the woman when the blood pressure was taken because the blood pressure may change when the woman changes positions.
22. A gradual, predictable increase in uterine size occurs as gestation advances. From approximately 22 weeks until term, fundal height in centimeters is nearly equal to gestational age in weeks.
23. Major risk factors during pregnancy are age under 16 years, low socioeconomic status, preexisting

medical disorders or infections, and use of substances such as alcohol, tobacco, or illicit drugs.

24. Antepartum visits should begin in the first trimester, every 4 weeks until 28 weeks, every 2 to 3 weeks from 29 to 36 weeks, and weekly from 37 weeks to birth.
25. Maternal adaptation differs in multifetal pregnancies because increased blood volume results in additional work for the heart of the mother. The greatly increased size of the uterus intensifies mechanical effects, such as greater elevation of the diaphragm, and compression of the ureters and bowel.
26. Increased levels of placental hormones, such as estrogen, and hCG plus periodic hypoglycemia are believed to be responsible for "morning sickness."
27. Correct posture and body mechanics as well as exercises such as pelvic rocking can alleviate backache during pregnancy.

CHAPTER 8

1. The fetus seems vague and unreal during the first trimester. Gradually, physical changes (such as uterine growth, weight gain, quickening) confirm that a fetus is developing, and the expectant mother begins to perceive the fetus as a separate though dependent being.
2. Although sexual responses vary widely during pregnancy, the woman may have increased interest in the first trimester unless she has nausea or fears miscarriage. Interest is often increased in the second trimester because of pelvic vasocongestion and a general feeling of well-being. The discomforts of the third trimester may decrease sexual responsiveness. Some expectant fathers are more interested in sex during pregnancy, but others find the pregnant woman unattractive and fear harming the fetus.
3. The pregnant woman explores the role of mother to develop a sense of herself in the role and selects behaviors that confirm her idea of fulfilling the role.
4. The pregnant woman often experiences a temporary sense of sadness when she realizes she must give up certain aspects of her previous self when she moves into the role of mother.
5. The pregnant woman seeks safe passage for herself and the baby when she seeks the care of a physician or nurse-midwife and follows recommendations about diet, vitamins, rest, and subsequent prenatal care.
6. Experiences that make the child more real serve as reality boosters and include hearing the fetal heart tones, feeling the fetus move, and seeing the fetus via ultrasound.
7. Nurses can help men gain recognition as parents by focusing on the father as well as the mother, encouraging the father's questions, and including him in the plan of care.
8. Information about infant behavior and care is more relevant and therefore more useful after the infant is born.
9. Some factors that shape the way grandparents respond to a grandchild are their own ages, the number and spacing of other grandchildren, and their perceptions of their role as grandparents.
10. Toddlers do not understand that a birth is expected and should be told shortly before the expected date. Preschoolers may like to be involved and to help prepare for the birth. Adolescents may be embarrassed by confirmation of their parents' continued sexuality.
11. Parents can make any changes in sleeping arrangements several weeks before the infant is born so that other children do not feel displaced by the newborn. They can increase time and attention to older children and reassure them of their love and acceptance.
12. Priorities of indigent families often focus primarily on present needs such as food and shelter and focus less on preventive activities such as prenatal care.
13. Some health care workers are unsympathetic to the plights of indigent families, who experience long delays at health care facilities, hurried examinations, and rudeness from members of the health care team.
14. Cultural differences that cause conflict between health care workers and families during pregnancy occur most often in the areas of health care beliefs, communication, and time orientation.
15. Cultural negotiation includes acknowledging that the family may hold different views, being sensitive to special concerns, and providing information in an acceptable manner.

CHAPTER 9

1. Weight gain helps determine fetal growth. Too little weight gain may be associated with low birth weight, and too much gain may be associated with large infants.
2. The average woman should gain 11.5 to 16 kg (25 to 35 lb). Underweight women and those carrying more than one fetus should gain more, and overweight women should gain less.
3. The average woman should gain approximately 1.6 kg (3.5 lb) the first trimester and 0.44 kg (slightly less than 1 lb) per week in the second and third trimesters.
4. A woman should eat 300 calories more each day during pregnancy.
5. Approximately 60 g of protein per day, an increase of 10 to 16 g above prepregnancy needs, is recommended during pregnancy.

6. Vitamins B_6, D, E, and folic acid are likely to be low in the diets of pregnant women.
7. Fat-soluble vitamins (such as A, D, E, K) are stored in the fat and available longer than the water-soluble vitamins (such as B_6, B_{12}, folic acid, thiamin, riboflavin, niacin, C), which must be replenished daily. Excessive intake of fat-soluble vitamins may cause toxicity.
8. If all women consumed 400 mcg of folic acid daily, fewer infants would be born with neural tube defects because women would not be deficient in folic acid during the first 4 weeks of a pregnancy, during which time the neural tube is closing.
9. Iron, calcium, zinc, and magnesium are often below the recommended amounts in the diets of pregnant women.
10. Excessive intake of vitamins and minerals may result in toxicity and interfere with absorption of other vitamins and minerals.
11. During pregnancy a woman should drink 8 to 10 8-oz glasses of fluids (mostly water) daily.
12. During pregnancy the following servings from the food pyramid are recommended: seven or more servings of whole grains, five or more servings of fruits and vegetables (with one serving each of vitamins A and C and folic acid sources), three or more servings of dairy products, servings equal to 7 oz of protein, and 3 teaspoons of saturated fats.
13. The nurse should consider traditional foods from the woman's culture, the degree to which she follows the traditional diet, and her inclusion of nontraditional foods in her diet.
14. Both Southeast Asian and Latina women balance yin and yang (cold and hot) foods during pregnancy and may have low intakes of calcium, iron, and vitamin D.
15. The nurse should assess the woman's financial resources for food purchase, need for financial assistance, and education about nutrition.
16. The adolescent may skip meals, eat snacks and fast foods of low nutrient value, and experience peer pressure.
17. The vegan can include nonanimal sources of iron, calcium, and vitamin B_{12} and combine incomplete protein foods to ensure intake of all essential amino acids.
18. Lactose-intolerant women can choose calcium-containing foods like leafy green vegetables, broccoli, corn tortillas, tofu, sunflower seeds, nuts, salmon, and sardines.
19. Other conditions presenting nutritional risk factors during pregnancy are excessive nausea and vomiting, anemia, abnormal prepregnancy weight, eating disorders, pica, grand multiparity, substance abuse, closely spaced pregnancies, and multifetal pregnancy.
20. The lactating woman needs more of most nutrients than the woman who is not pregnant. She needs 200 more calories and slightly more protein and vitamin C than the pregnant woman.
21. The breastfeeding woman should avoid alcohol, caffeine, and foods that seem to cause distress in the infant.
22. The woman who is not breastfeeding should decrease calories by 300 daily, continue to eat a well-balanced diet, and plan to lose extra weight slowly.

CHAPTER 10

1. Major reasons for ultrasonography during the first trimester are to confirm pregnancy, verify gestational age, locate the fetus, determine multifetal pregnancy and fetal growth, confirm fetal viability, and identify and guide chorionic villus sampling (CVS). Indications during the second and third trimesters are to confirm fetal viability, gestational age, and growth; evaluate fetal anatomy, umbilical cord and vessels, and placenta; evaluate multifetal pregnancies; locate the placenta; determine fetal presentation; evaluate amniotic fluid volume; and guide needle placement for amniocentesis and cordocentesis.
2. Transvaginal ultrasonography is most often performed during the first trimester, when the uterus lies within the pelvis. A transabdominal procedure is more common during the second and third trimesters, when the uterus is above the pelvic brim and the contents are clearly visible.
3. Major advantages of ultrasonography are that it allows clear visualization of the fetus and surrounding structures; it is safe, noninvasive, and relatively comfortable; and the results are available immediately. The major disadvantage is the cost. Also, ultrasonography may reveal findings that might indicate a problem but for which data are inadequate to make a clear diagnosis, thus requiring further decisions by the woman and her support person.
4. Maternal serum alpha-fetoprotein (MSAFP) must be viewed as the first step in a series of diagnostic procedures offered if abnormal concentrations are found.
5. Elevated MSAFP may be caused by open neural tube defects, esophageal obstruction, open abdominal wall defects, and undetected fetal demise. Additional causes include multifetal gestation, inaccurate fetal age or maternal weight, maternal diabetes, and threatened abortion.
6. Low levels of AFP suggest chromosomal abnormalities or inaccurate gestational age and maternal weight.

7. Triple marker screening determines maternal serum levels of AFP, human chorionic gonadotropin, and unconjugated estriols. Elevation of human chorionic gonadotropin with low levels of AFP and estriols suggest chromosome abnormalities. Further testing with amniocentesis to positively identify the fetal karyotype will be offered to the woman if triple marker screening is abnormal.
8. CVS is performed slightly sooner than even early amniocentesis, at 10 to 12 weeks' gestation. Obtaining information about fetal anomalies earlier in the pregnancy allows the woman to make a decision about pregnancy termination before the second trimester. CVS is more expensive than amniocentesis and does not provide amniotic fluid for analysis of AFP.
9. Pregnancy loss is slightly higher following CVS than following amniocentesis. The likelihood that chromosome findings will be questionable and lead to additional testing such as amniocentesis is greater.
10. Amniocentesis is most often performed to detect chromosomal abnormalities and other prenatally detectable genetic disorders. Additional indications include investigating abnormal levels of MSAFP, determining fetal lung maturity, and evaluating the fetus affected by Rh isoimmunization.
11. Fetal lung maturity is confirmed by a 2:1 ratio of lecithin/sphingomyelin and the presence of other lipoproteins such as phosphatidylglycerol (PG), and phosphatidylinositol (PI), which comprise pulmonary surfactant. A newer test evaluates the quantity of surfactant phospholipids relative to the quantity of albumin in the amniotic fluid.
12. The degree of bilirubin staining of amniotic fluid reflects the degree of erythrocyte destruction in an Rh-positive fetus whose mother is Rh-sensitized.
13. Early amniocentesis has the same advantage as CVS: information is available early in the pregnancy, allowing parents to make decisions about the pregnancy as early as possible.
14. A nonstress test (so called because the fetus is not challenged or stressed to obtain data) measures acceleration of the fetal heart in response to fetal movement. Acceleration, even without fetal movement felt by the mother, provides reassurance of fetal health.
15. In vibroacoustic stimulation, an artificial larynx is used to stimulate fetal movement and accelerations using sound and vibrations. Fetal accelerations are expected following stimulation. Otherwise, the procedure and interpretation are the same as those in a nonstress test.
16. A contraction stress test indicates fetal response to periodic hypoxia that occurs as a result of uterine contractions. Contractions are initiated by intravenous administration of oxytocin or by breast stimulation. As contractions compress the placental arterioles that supply oxygen to the fetus, a recurrent decrease occurs in fetal oxygen levels.
17. Late decelerations in a CST indicate fetal oxygen reserves are inadequate to tolerate contractions, and fetal acidosis, myocardial depression, or both may result.
18. Loss of fetal tone in a biophysical profile indicates advanced hypoxia and fetal acidosis. Fetal tone develops early in gestation and is the parameter of the biophysical profile that is most resistant to the effects of hypoxia.
19. Decreased amniotic fluid volume is associated with chronic fetal hypoxia, in which blood is shunted away from the fetal lungs and kidneys that produce amniotic fluid, and toward vital organs such as the fetal heart and brain.

CHAPTER 11

1. The goals of perinatal education are to help women and their support persons become knowledgeable consumers and active participants in pregnancy and childbirth.
2. Couples must choose a health care professional, a birth setting, a support person(s), techniques for labor, and a type of education for preparation (if any).
3. Early pregnancy classes emphasize adapting to pregnancy, coping with common discomforts, and learning what to expect in later pregnancy. Later classes discuss preparation for childbirth, the postpartum period, breastfeeding issues, and parenting concerns.
4. The chance that a couple may experience cesarean birth is more than 20%. Therefore all women need to know about cesarean birth.
5. Classes for family members help ease family transition by providing information and opportunities for discussing common feelings.
6. Education, relaxation, and conditioning reduce pain and increase coping ability for childbirth by helping to decrease muscle and mental tension.
7. Cutaneous stimulation and imagery help reduce pain by sending other messages to the brain so that pain messages are not recognized as strongly and perception of pain is reduced.
8. Breathing techniques are used to enhance relaxation during labor.
9. Having a support person during labor increases a woman's satisfaction by helping her deal with stress, focus on her learned techniques, and feel that her experience is being shared.
10. Support roles include active assistance with breathing and relaxation, verbal encouragement,

minimal physical assistance, and presence without active involvement.

11. Specific techniques used by support persons during labor include assistance with relaxation and breathing, encouragement, sacral pressure, massage, and comfort measures.

CHAPTER 12

1. Effacement and dilation of the cervix occur because contractions pull the cervix upward over the fetus and amniotic sac while pushing the fetus and amniotic sac downward against the cervix. The muscle fibers of the upper uterus become shorter to maintain these forces between contractions. In addition, the uterus changes shape and becomes more elongated and narrow to maintain pressure of the fetus and amniotic sac against the cervix.
2. The cervix of the nullipara effaces more before it dilates. The cervix of a multipara is usually thicker than that of a nullipara during the entire labor.
3. Maternal changes occurring during labor include the following:
   a. Cardiovascular system—A slight increase in blood pressure and decrease in pulse rate occurs as each contraction temporarily stops blood flow to her uterus. Supine hypotension may occur if she lies on her back because the heavy uterus compresses her inferior vena cava and reduces blood flow to her heart.
   b. Respiratory system—The depth and rate of respirations increase.
   c. Gastrointestinal system—Although a controversial belief, many authorities think that peristalsis slows during labor.
   d. Renal system—The sensation of a full bladder is reduced.
   e. Hematopoietic system—Leukocyte counts are as high as 25,000 to 30,000, and levels of clotting factors are elevated.
4. Uterine contractions temporarily stop blood flow to the placenta. If the contractions were sustained, the fetus could not receive freshly oxygenated blood and nutrients and dispose of waste products through the placenta.
5. Labor and vaginal birth benefit the newborn by increasing absorption of fetal lung fluid and compressing the upper airways, causing some lung fluid to be expelled. These effects reduce the amount of lung fluid remaining in the newborn's respiratory tract when breathing begins. Labor also stimulates the fetus to secrete catecholamines, which help speed clearance of the lung fluid after birth, stimulate cardiac contraction and breathing, and aid in temperature regulation.
6. The power of labor during the first stage of labor involves uterine contractions. Powers during the second stage include uterine contractions, augmented by the woman's voluntary pushing efforts.
7. The three divisions of the true pelvis are the inlet, midpelvis, and outlet.
8. The vertex presentation, in which the fetal head is fully flexed forward, allows the smallest diameter of the fetal head to enter the pelvis. It also more effectively dilates the cervix.
9. ROP: The fetal landmark is the occiput, indicating a vertex presentation. It is located in the mother's right posterior pelvic quadrant. OA: The fetal landmark is the occiput, which is located in the mother's anterior pelvis and is not directed toward her left or her right. This is often the presentation just before birth. RSA: The fetal landmark is the sacrum, indicating that the fetus is in a breech presentation. It is located in the mother's right anterior pelvis. LMA: The fetal landmark is the mentum, or chin, indicating that the fetus is in a face presentation. The chin is in the mother's left anterior pelvis.
10. If the fetus is in a face presentation, the occiput is not accessible to the examiner's fingers during vaginal examination. For this reason the fetal chin (mentum) is used to describe the position (such as RMA [right mentum anterior]).
11. The woman may note several changes as labor approaches: increased strength and frequency of Braxton Hicks contractions, lightening, increased vaginal mucus, bloody show, an energy spurt, and a small weight loss.
12. False labor tends to differ from true labor in three major ways. True labor is characterized by contractions that progressively become more frequent, last longer, and are more intense. The discomfort of true labor begins in the lower back and sweeps to the lower abdomen. In true labor, progressive effacement and dilation of the cervix occur, which is the most significant difference from false labor.
13. The transverse diameter of the pelvic inlet is slightly larger than the inlet's anteroposterior diameter. The anteroposterior diameter of the fetal head (in line with the sagittal suture) is slightly larger than the transverse diameter. Therefore the fetal head best fits the pelvis if the sagittal suture is aligned with the pelvic transverse diameter.
14. Because the woman's pelvic outlet is usually slightly larger in its anteroposterior diameter than its transverse diameter, the fetal head turns in the mechanism of internal rotation so that the sagittal suture aligns with the anteroposterior diameter.
15. During the first stage, latent phase, the expectant mother is often sociable, excited, and somewhat anxious. During the first stage, active phase, the woman becomes less sociable and is inwardly focused. During the first stage, transition phase, the

woman may become irritable and temporarily lose control. During the second stage, the woman usually concentrates her energy toward pushing her baby out and interacts little with others. She often regains a feeling of control and active participation in the birth during second stage.

16. Contractions vary among women, but the general pattern includes increasing frequency, duration, and intensity throughout labor. In the first stage, latent phase, contractions gradually increase until they are about 5 minutes apart, lasting for 30 to 40 seconds with mild to moderate intensity. In the first stage, active phase, contractions increase to about 2 to 5 minutes apart with a duration of about 40 to 60 seconds and moderate to strong intensity. In the first stage, transition phase, contractions are strong with a frequency of 1.5 to 2 minutes apart and a duration of 60 to 90 seconds. In the second stage, contractions are strong and about 2 to 3 minutes apart and have a duration of about 40 to 60 seconds.
17. Signs that the placenta may have separated include a spheric uterine shape, the rising of the uterus upward in the abdomen, protrusion of the umbilical cord farther outward from the vagina, and a gush of blood.
18. Hemorrhage may occur if the uterus does not remain contracted after birth of the placenta because open blood vessels at the site will not be compressed by the interlacing muscle fibers of the uterus.

CHAPTER 13

1. The nurse should show warmth, concern, and friendliness when the woman and her family enter the hospital or birth center. In addition, a nonjudgmental attitude facilitates communication and shows respect to the woman as an individual.
2. The nurse should try to identify and incorporate beneficial or neutral cultural practices into care during labor and birth by asking about specific practices that are important during birth and facilitating communication by obtaining a fluent interpreter.
3. The nurse should promptly evaluate the maternal and fetal conditions and the nearness of birth when a woman comes to the hospital or birth center. Prompt assessments should include checking the maternal vital signs, fetal heart rate and patterns, and progress of labor.
4. A lower limit of 110 to 120 beats per minute (BPM) and an upper limit of 150 to 160 BPM with a regular rhythm are reassuring. Accelerations and the absence of decelerations from the baseline also are reassuring.
5. Impending birth should be suspected if the woman is grunting, bearing down, sitting on one buttock, or urgently signifying that her baby is about to be born. In that case, the nurse should abbreviate the initial assessment and collect other information after the birth.
6. Two tests assist the nurse, nurse-midwife, or physician to determine whether a woman's membranes have ruptured: the nitrazine test and examination of the amniotic fluid under a microscope for ferning.
7. Hypertonic contractions (too frequent, too long, or an inadequate rest period) reduce blood flow to and from the placenta. This interferes with fetal oxygenation and waste disposal.
8. Routine FHR assessments in uncomplicated labor are performed every hour during latent (early) labor, every 30 minutes during active labor, and every 15 minutes during the second stage. The FHR should be assessed after the membranes rupture to detect whether the fetal umbilical cord was displaced with the gush of fluid and is being compressed between the fetal presenting part and maternal pelvis.
9. Greenish amniotic fluid contains meconium, which may have been passed by the fetus in response to transient hypoxia. Cloudy, yellowish, or foul-smelling fluid suggests infection in the amniotic sac.
10. Frequent vaginal examinations may cause infection because microorganisms from the perineal area can be introduced into the uterus.
11. The woman may specifically request other pain management measures including medication, express ineffectiveness of nonpharmacologic measures, show muscle tension during and between contractions, have a tense facial expression, and express an inability to tolerate the pain.
12. Hypotension reduces blood flow to the placenta and therefore reduces fetal oxygenation because it diverts blood away from the uterus to better supply the mother's brain, heart, and kidneys. Hypertension may result in vasospasm that can reduce exchange of oxygen, nutrients, and waste products in the placenta. Fetal hypoxia and acidosis can be the ultimate result of maternal hypotension and hypertension.
13. The supine position allows the heavy uterus to compress her inferior vena cava, reducing blood return to her heart and reducing placental blood supply. A small wedge under her hip is effective to relieve vena cava compression.
14. General physical comfort measures during labor include soft, dim lighting; a comfortable temperature; maintenance of cleanliness; mouth care; observations for a full bladder; positions for comfort; and a warm bath or shower. Caring for the

support person includes respect for the couple's wishes about partner involvement in birth. The nurse should provide support that the partner cannot and should consider physical needs for food and rest.

15. Shortly before birth, the woman's perineum bulges and the fetal head may become visible during contractions. At this time, birth can occur suddenly.
16. Perineal massage and heat applications to the perineal tissues are considered to facilitate birth of the head and avoid episiotomy and large perineal lacerations. This is not proven, however. Only prelabor perineal massage and stretching by the woman has been shown in controlled studies to be beneficial in this regard.

CHAPTER 14

1. Fetal oxygenation depends on normal maternal blood flow and volume; normal oxygen saturation of the maternal blood; adequate oxygen-carbon dioxide exchange in the placenta; patent umbilical cord vessels; and normal fetal circulatory and oxygen-carrying function.
2. When the umbilical cord is compressed, the umbilical vein is compressed first, resulting in a slight fetal hypotension and acceleration of the fetal heart rate. Continued compression obstructs the umbilical arteries, resulting in fetal hypertension and slowing of the fetal heart rate. As compression is relieved, these changes are reversed.
3. The fetus increases cardiac output, and therefore oxygenation, primarily by increasing the heart rate. Rates lower than 50 BPM may reduce fetal oxygenation. Rates higher than 200 BPM also may reduce fetal oxygenation because the ventricles do not have time to refill with oxygenated blood.
4. Fetal monitoring should be done more frequently if there are risk factors present. These may include antepartum factors in the woman's history or course of pregnancy. They may also include problems in the woman or fetus that develop intrapartally. Although there are no absolute indications for continuous electronic fetal monitoring, most hospitals use it in both low- and high-risk intrapartum care.
5. Intermittent auscultation promotes the laboring woman's mobility and creates a more natural atmosphere. However, it can assess the fetus for only part of labor, may be distracting for some women, and may require more staff. Continuous electronic fetal monitoring provides more data, is often expected by parents, and can assist the nurse to better observe more than one woman. It allows the nurse to devote more time to coaching the woman and her partner. Its primary drawbacks are reduced maternal mobility, adjustments to the equipment, and its technical atmosphere.
6. The upper grid on the paper strip of the electronic fetal monitor records the constant changes in the fetal heart rate. The lower grid records contractions as a series of bell-shaped curves. Other information that may be printed on the strip includes maternal blood pressure and information charted by the nurse by way of data entry devices. Fetal pulse oximetry data may be recorded on monitors equipped with this technology.
7. The Doppler ultrasound transducer senses fetal heart motion and translates the motion into a heart rate.
8. Four factors may affect the accuracy of the external uterine activity monitor: fetal size, maternal abdominal fat thickness, maternal position, and location of the transducer.
9. The two types of internal uterine activity catheters are the solid and the fluid-filled catheter. The solid catheter tends to record higher intrauterine pressures because it senses fluid pressure above its sensor inside the uterus. The fluid-filled catheter can be affected by its height in relation to the mother's transducer.
10. Fetal heart rate accelerations are a reassuring sign of fetal responsiveness and nonacidosis.
11. In early decelerations, the fetal heart rate slows after the contraction begins and returns to the baseline rate by the end of the contraction. They are caused by fetal head compression and are reassuring. Late decelerations are characterized by slowing of the fetal heart rate late in the contraction cycle, often after the peak. They do not return to the baseline until after the contraction has ended. Late decelerations are associated with decreased uteroplacental perfusion and are nonreassuring.
12. Variable decelerations show a fetal heart rate that rises and falls abruptly. They are not consistent in appearance and may not occur at similar times in relation to the contractions. They are caused by compression of the umbilical cord.
13. Fetal scalp stimulation or vibroacoustic stimulation may be done to clarify fetal heart rate patterns as reassuring or nonreassuring when they are vague. The reassuring response to stimulation is an increase in the fetal heart rate of 15 BPM for at least 15 seconds. This suggests that the fetus has a normal oxygen and acid-base balance.
14. Cord blood gas and pH analysis assesses the newborn's oxygen and acid-base status immediately after birth and identifies if the fetus was adjusting to the stresses of labor.
15. Basic nursing actions for nonreassuring fetal heart rate patterns vary according to the pattern. They include identifying the cause of a nonreas-

suring pattern by vaginal examination, taking maternal vital signs, reviewing medications, or applying internal monitoring; increasing placental perfusion by reducing excess uterine activity and positioning the woman on her side; giving the mother oxygen; and reducing cord compression by position changes and amnioinfusion.

16. A tocolytic drug reduces the intensity and frequency of uterine contractions, thus allowing more time for the placenta to be supplied with oxygen-rich maternal blood.
17. Amnioinfusion may be used to replace the fluid cushion around the umbilical cord, reducing compression. It may also be used to dilute thick meconium, which might otherwise cause respiratory distress in the newborn.

CHAPTER 15

1. Childbirth pain differs from other painful experiences because it is part of a normal process, the woman has time to prepare for it, it is self-limited and intermittent, and it ends with the birth of her baby.
2. Excessive, unrelieved labor pain may result in a stress response (diverting blood flow from the uterus and compromising fetal oxygenation), maternal acid-base imbalance, and fetal acidosis. It may increase the length of labor. Poor pain relief can lessen the joy of childbirth for the woman and her partner and may have lasting psychological effects
3. Physical and psychological factors interact to alter the ability to tolerate pain. For example, relaxation and working with the forces of labor enhance the chance that the woman who has a large baby and a small pelvis will give birth vaginally.
4. Four sources of pain present in most labor are cervical dilation, uterine ischemia, pressure and pulling on pelvic structures, and distention of the vagina and perineum.
5. Physical factors that influence pain include the following:
    a. A short, intense labor may be more painful because dilation, effacement, and fetal descent occur rapidly.
    b. A cervix that does not efface or dilate easily is likely to be associated with a longer and more uncomfortable labor.
    c. An abnormal fetal position may cause a longer labor as the woman's body maneuvers it into a better position. Back pain is especially noticeable if the fetus is in an occiput posterior position.
    d. Variations in the mother's pelvic size or shape may result in abnormal fetal presentations or positions and in a longer labor because the fetus does not fit through the pelvis easily.
    e. Fatigue reduces the woman's pain tolerance and ability to use coping skills.
6. Psychosocial factors that influence labor pain include culture, anxiety and fear, previous experiences, preparation for childbirth, and the mother's support system.
7. The gate control theory of pain assumes that there is a gating mechanism in the dorsal horn of the spinal cord that controls the transmission of painful impulses to the brain for interpretation. Pain impulses are transmitted through small-diameter fibers, whereas other sensations, such as tactile (massage, heat, cool) are transmitted more quickly through large-diameter fibers. Therefore the impulses transmitted through the large-diameter fibers interfere with or "close the gate" to transmission of pain impulses. Impulses from the brain, such as auditory stimuli (listening to music, for instance), can also impede pain transmission.
8. Nursing actions to promote relaxation include arranging for environmental comfort, maintaining the woman's general comfort, reducing factors that cause anxiety and fear, and using specific relaxation techniques such as helping the woman focus on relaxing specific tense muscles.
9. Accurate information and a focus on the normal aspects of childbirth help reduce anxiety and fear. Avoid referring to the woman as a "patient," because this word is associated with illness. Empowerment of the birthing partners helps them see themselves as competent to give birth successfully.
10. Self-massage might include effleurage, rubbing the hands together, patting or banging the hands on the rail. Massage by others helps relax tense muscles and aids relaxation. Counterpressure, which may include sacral pressure or other variations, is often used to reduce back pain when the fetus is in an occiput posterior position. Warmth relaxes muscles, promoting relaxation. Cool often feels better to the laboring woman who may be hot, or she may want cool only in a local area, or ice in her mouth.
11. Hydration must be adequate to offset the diuresis that often occurs with immersion in water. Diuresis could reduce placental perfusion if plasma volume is low. Water temperature must be controlled to prevent hyperthermia or hypothermia, which could raise the mother's metabolic rate, increasing her oxygen and glucose consumption. These changes could reduce oxygen and glucose delivered to the fetus.
12. The more complex breathing techniques are more effective for greater pain, but they are tiring. Advancing from simpler to more complex breathing techniques too quickly can cause the mother to become fatigued when she most needs to use these methods.

13. The cleansing breath has 4 purposes: a) release of tension; b) increase oxygen intake to combat myometrial hypoxia; c) clear the woman's mind to focus on relaxing through contraction; and d) signal her labor partner that a contraction has begun.
14. Drugs taken by the mother can affect the fetus directly, such as decreased fetal heart rate variability, or indirectly, such as hypotension that reduces placental blood flow and fetal oxygen supply.
15. (a) Aortocaval compression should be offset by placing a wedge under the woman's hip if a supine position is required. (b) The woman is more sensitive to general anesthesia and may have a greater fall in oxygenation when general anesthesia is induced. (c) The reduced peristalsis and tone of the sphincter at the junction of the esophagus and stomach can lead to regurgitation and aspiration of gastric contents, primarily with general anesthesia. (d) Lower doses of anesthetic agents will be needed for epidural or subarachnoid blocks.
16. Drugs (prescribed, over-the-counter, or illicit), botanical preparations, and alcohol may interact with one another. These interactions may be harmful to the woman, the fetus, or both. Knowledge of exactly what drugs she uses allows the safest choices in pharmacologic pain relief methods.
17. Neonatal respiratory depression is the primary drawback to the use of opioid analgesia. This effect can be reduced by timing the dose to reduce the amount transferred to the fetus (which varies according to the drug) and by giving the narcotic in small, frequent, IV doses at the beginning of the contraction. Naloxone (Narcan) is the drug commonly given to reverse narcotic respiratory depression.
18. Because naloxone's effects are shorter than those of the narcotic, the nurse must observe for a recurrence of respiratory depression.
19. The two major advantages of regional pain management are that the woman can have pain relief and remain alert.
20. Epidural and subarachnoid blocks can cause maternal hypotension. The fall in blood pressure may result in reduced placental blood flow, compromising fetal oxygen supply. Giving the woman IV fluids before the block reduces this effect. Other less serious adverse effects are bladder distention, prolonged second stage of labor (epidural), and postdural puncture headache (usually subarachnoid block).
21. Epidural or intrathecal opioid analgesics may cause nausea, vomiting, itching, or a combination of these. They may also result in delayed respiratory depression (up to 24 hours), depending on the drug used. Management includes promethazine for nausea and vomiting; diphenhydramine, naloxone, or naltrexone for itching; and pulse oximetry and monitoring of respirations while the opioid is given and up to 24 hours after administration ends, depending on the drug.
22. Maternal regurgitation with aspiration of acidic gastric contents is the major potential adverse effect of general anesthesia. The risk may be reduced by limiting intake to clear fluids, giving drugs to raise the gastric pH, giving drugs to reduce gastric secretions or speed emptying of the stomach, and using cricoid pressure (Sellick's maneuver) to block the esophagus while the endotracheal tube is being inserted. Respiratory depression, primarily in the infant, is minimized by delaying general anesthesia until the surgery team is prepared and by keeping the anesthesia level as light as possible until the umbilical cord is cut.

CHAPTER 16

1. Three major risks of amniotomy are prolapsed umbilical cord, infection, and abruptio placentae.
2. The FHR is assessed before the membranes rupture to identify whether the fetus has a normal rate and pattern and establish a baseline. It is checked after the membranes rupture to identify patterns that suggest umbilical cord compression and other problems.
3. Green amniotic fluid contains meconium, passed from the fetal intestines. It may be seen in postterm gestation or placental insufficiency.
4. Signs of chorioamnionitis include fetal tachycardia (often the first sign), elevated maternal temperature, and amniotic fluid that has a foul or strong odor or a cloudy or yellowish appearance.
5. Five precautions that promote safe oxytocin induction or augmentation of labor include the following:
   a. Dilution of the oxytocin in a physiologic electrolyte solution
   b. Piggybacking the oxytocin solution into the port nearest the venipuncture site
   c. Starting the oxytocin infusion slowly
   d. Increasing its rate gradually
   e. Monitoring uterine contractions and FHR
6. Labor may be augmented if it stops or contractions become ineffective. The woman whose labor is augmented with oxytocin usually needs less of the drug than the woman whose labor is being induced because her uterus is more sensitive to its effects.
7. The fetus may have an adverse reaction to oxytocin, manifested by nonreassuring FHR patterns such as bradycardia, tachycardia, late decelerations, or decreased FHR variability.
8. Signs of hypertonic uterine activity include incomplete relaxation of the uterus between contractions or a rest period shorter than 60 seconds

or Montevideo units exceeding 250, which may result in inadequate placental blood flow and a fall in fetal oxygenation.

9. Administration of oxytocin for a prolonged time may lead to postpartum hemorrhage because the fatigued uterus cannot contract properly to compress bleeding vessels at the placenta site (uterine atony).
10. The FHR should be monitored before external version to identify nonreassuring patterns that would preclude the procedure. It should be monitored (by Doppler or real-time ultrasound) as much as possible during and for a short while afterward to detect cord compression that can occur if the umbilical cord becomes entangled during change of the fetal presentation.
11. Uterine activity should be observed after external version for possible onset of labor because this procedure may cause uterine irritability or possible abruptio placentae and is done near term.
12. Forceps and vacuum extraction are used to provide traction to assist the mother in rotation, expulsion, or both, of the fetal head. Special forceps (Piper) can be used to deliver the head of the fetus in a breech presentation, but a vacuum extractor can be used only in a cephalic presentation. Forceps may cause fetal injury such as facial bruising and nerve injury. The vacuum extractor may create an artificial caput called a *chignon.*
13. Catheterization before forceps are used eliminates a full bladder, which would reduce available room in the pelvis. Emptying the bladder also reduces the risk of bladder injury.
14. Use of cold immediately (for the first 12 hours) following episiotomy reduces pain, edema, and formation of hematomas. The nurse should also observe for continuous, bright-red bleeding that suggests a vaginal wall laceration. Warmth after at least 12 hours of cold application promotes resolution of the edema and hematoma.
15. The infant with an asymmetric facial appearance when crying may have facial nerve injury, usually a temporary condition that sometimes occurs when forceps are used to assist birth.
16. The low transverse uterine incision is less likely to rupture during another pregnancy than either of the two vertical incisions. There are, however, valid reasons for the use of vertical incisions.
17. The woman expecting a cesarean birth should be taught the following about the operating room and recovery area:
    a. Preoperative procedures, such as the skin preparation and indwelling catheter
    b. Personnel who will be present and their functions
    c. The narrow table, safety strap, and positioning measures
    d. When her partner or support person can come in
    e. If a regional anesthetic is planned, that she will be awake and feel pulling and pressure sensations but should not expect pain. If a general anesthetic is planned, that all preparations will be made before she is put to sleep but the surgery will not begin before she is asleep and she will not awaken during it.
    f. In the recovery area, use of oxygen, pulse oximeter, and automatic blood pressure cuff and regular checking of her fundus, incision, lochia, and pain relief needs
18. The woman who has cesarean birth needs care similar to the woman who delivers vaginally in terms of vital signs and fundus and lochia assessments. Additional care includes assessment of oxygen saturation and respiratory status, observation of urine output from the indwelling catheter, pain needs, and respiratory care (turning, coughing, deep breathing). Anesthesia-related care includes level of consciousness (primarily if general anesthesia was used) and return of movement and sensation (primarily if epidural or subarachnoid block was used).

CHAPTER 17

1. The three processes involved in involution are contraction of muscle fibers, catabolism, and regeneration of uterine epithelium.
2. The fundus is expected to descend 1 cm (approximately 1 fingerbreadth) per day so that, by the tenth postpartum day, it cannot be palpated.
3. A multipara is expected to experience afterpains because repeated stretching of the uterus makes uterine contraction more difficult. Overdistention of the uterus and breastfeeding also cause afterpains. Afterpains are treated by analgesics. Lying in a prone position with a small pillow under the abdomen also provides relief.
4. Lochia rubra lasts for 3 days after childbirth and consists mostly of blood and is therefore red. Lochia serosa is pink to brown-tinged and usually lasts from the fourth to the tenth day. Lochia alba is white or cream color and may last 3 to 6 weeks.
5. The mother is at risk for urinary retention because she is less sensitive to fluid pressure, decreasing the urge to void even when the bladder is distended. Trauma of childbirth may also make it difficult to void. Urinary tract infection is more likely because stasis of urine allows time for bacteria to multiply. Postpartum hemorrhage may occur because a full bladder displaces the uterus, causing the uterine muscles to relax.

6. Hyperpigmentation decreases because the melanocyte-stimulating hormone decreases rapidly after childbirth.
7. Breastfeeding delays the return of both ovulation and menstruation.
8. The white blood cell count is normally elevated to an average of 14,000 to 16,000 mm^3 after childbirth.
9. Menses will probably resume in the woman who is formula feeding her infant about 7 to 9 weeks after childbirth. The breastfeeding woman may begin menses between 12 weeks and 18 months after childbirth.
10. Women lose approximately 4.5 to 5.5 kg (10 to 12 lb) during childbirth. They often lose another 2.3 to 3.6 kg (5 to 8 lb) during involution.
11. When tachycardia is noted, temperature, blood pressure, location and firmness of the uterus, amount of lochia, estimated blood loss at delivery, hemoglobin, and hematocrit values are necessary. Excitement, fatigue, dehydration, infection, pain, or hypovolemia may cause tachycardia.
12. Orthostatic hypotension, a drop in blood pressure when the mother goes from a supine to standing position quickly, produces symptoms of dizziness, lightheadedness, or feeling faint.
13. Uterine massage is necessary when the uterus is not firmly contracted. The nurse places the nondominant hand above the woman's symphysis pubis to anchor and support the uterus during massage.
14. A cervical or vaginal laceration may cause excessive bleeding even when the uterus is firmly contracted.
15. Frequent respiratory assessments, auscultation of breath sounds and bowel sounds, and inspection of the surgical dressing and wound are necessary for the postcesarean mother.
16. Hypostatic pneumonia can be prevented by frequent turning, coughing, breathing deeply, and ambulating early and frequently.
17. Early ambulation, pelvic lifts, and restriction of carbonated beverages and straws for drinking prevent or minimize abdominal distention.
18. Wearing a snug bra and avoiding nipple stimulation helps prevent lactation. Ice is sometimes used for discomfort.
19. Providing adequate information in a short time is a major problem associated with early discharge. Clinical pathways list guidelines for outcomes and a specific time frame for interventions that will help the new mother achieve the stated outcomes.
20. Before discharge the nurse should be sure that the mother has no complications and all assessments are normal. Ambulation and ability to eat and drink should be normal. The mother should indicate understanding of self-care instructions, signs of complications and proper responses, and infant care. She should have adequate support during the early days after discharge.
21. All methods help meet educational needs by answering parents' questions and providing reassurance. Information lines rely on the family to initiate contact and they usually deal only with the concern that precipitated the call, whereas telephone interviews allow the nurse to guide the interview. Phone calls are relatively inexpensive but nurses must rely on observations made by the family. Home visits allow physical examination of the mother, infant, and environment but are expensive because they require the time of a well-prepared nurse. Outpatient clinics are less expensive and allow direct assessment of the mother and infant. Transportation is a problem for some families, however, and not all families will take advantage of clinics.

CHAPTER 18

1. Bonding describes the initial attraction felt by the parents for the infant. Attachment is the development of an enduring, loving relationship between parents and child. It is progressive and requires response from the infant.
2. Maternal touch may progress from finger-tipping in the discovery phase to enfolding the infant and a full range of consoling behaviors.
3. Parents progress from referring to the newborn as "it" to "he" or "she" and then to using the given name.
4. The mother is focused primarily on her own needs during the taking-in phase. She often is passive and dependent and repeatedly recounts her birth experience. In the taking-hold phase, she becomes more independent, focuses on the infant, and exhibits a heightened readiness to learn.
5. In the letting-go phase, mothers (and fathers) relinquish previous lifestyle patterns to assume the parenting role.
6. The anticipatory stage begins during pregnancy as mothers prepare for the birth of the child. The formal stage begins with birth when parents become acquainted with their child. During the informal stage, parents respond to the unique cues of their child rather than following textbook or health professionals. The personal stage is attained when the parents feel comfortable with their roles as parents.
7. Postpartum blues is believed to be related to hormonal fluctuations that occur during and following childbirth. Nurses can help by focusing on the way the mother is feeling and reassure her that what she is feeling is normal and self-limited.

8. Fathers who are sometimes ignored and not included in infant care may feel left out and unneeded.
9. Siblings may feel jealousy and fear that they will be replaced by the newborn in the affection of the parents.
10. Time must be allowed for the parents to form attachment with each newborn individually.

CHAPTER 19

1. Hypoxia causes decreased Po_2 and pH and increased Pco_2 to affect chemoreceptors that stimulate the respiratory center in the brain. Cool air and handling at birth cause skin sensors to stimulate the respiratory center. Mechanical factors include pressure against the chest that is released, helping air to enter the lungs. These factors all contribute to the initiation of respirations at birth.
2. Surfactant reduces surface tension in the alveoli and allows them to remain partially open on expiration.
3. Fetal lung fluid begins to move into the interstitial spaces shortly before birth owing to changes in the sodium levels. A very small part of the fluid is squeezed out during birth. The rest is absorbed by the lymphatic and vascular systems.
4. The ductus arteriosus closes as a result of increases in blood oxygen levels and decreased prostaglandin E_2 from the placenta. The foramen ovale closes when pressure in the left atrium exceeds that in the right atrium. The ductus venosus closes when the vessels of the cord become occluded.
5. At birth, increasing levels of oxygen cause the pulmonary blood vessels to dilate. In addition, movement of fetal lung fluid into the interstitial tissues allows more room for expansion of the pulmonary blood vessels.
6. Newborns have thinner skin with less subcutaneous fat, blood vessels close to the surface, and a larger skin surface area. These all contribute to greater loss of heat than in older children or adults.
7. Newborns respond to low temperatures by increasing activity and flexion, vasoconstriction, and nonshivering thermogenesis. This increases oxygen and glucose consumption and may cause respiratory distress, hypoglycemia, acidosis, and jaundice.
8. Newborns have higher levels of erythrocytes, hemoglobin, and hematocrit than adults because during fetal life, the available oxygen is lower than after birth. More red blood cells are needed to adequately oxygenate the cells.
9. Stools progress from thick, greenish-black meconium to loose greenish-brown transitional stools to milk stools that are frequent, soft, seedy, and mustard-colored if the infant is breastfed, and pale yellow or light brown, firmer, and less frequent if formula fed.
10. Hypoglycemia is a problem for the newborn because the brain requires a constant supply of glucose and may be damaged without an adequate supply.
11. Infants have an immature liver and more hemolysis of erythrocytes than adults. Trauma at birth, poor early feeding, and an intestinal enzyme that deconjugates bilirubin also increase jaundice.
12. Physiologic jaundice occurs in normal newborns after the first 24 hours of life as a result of hemolysis of red blood cells and immaturity of the liver. Pathologic jaundice is generally a result of excessive destruction of erythrocytes causing bilirubin levels to rise faster and higher than physiologic jaundice. It begins within the first 24 hours and may necessitate phototherapy. Breast milk jaundice begins later than physiologic jaundice and is thought to be due to enzymes in the milk.
13. The newborn's body is composed of a greater percentage of water, with more located in the extracellular compartment, than that in adults.
14. Newborns receive passive immunity to infections when IgG crosses the placenta in utero. After birth, infants produce IgM and IgA to protect against infection. IgM rises in response to infection. IgA lines the gastrointestinal and respiratory tracts to prevent infection and is present in breast milk.
15. During both periods of reactivity, newborns are active and alert, may be interested in feeding, have elevated pulse and respiratory rates, and may have transient signs of respiratory distress.
16. In the quiet sleep state, the infant is in a deep sleep with regular respirations and little response to outside stimuli. In active sleep, infants move about and may have irregular respirations. The drowsy state is the time between sleep and waking. In the quiet alert state the infant is awake and interested in stimuli. The active alert state is a fussy period that may lead to the crying state if the infant's needs are not met.

CHAPTER 20

1. Molding of the head is a change in the shape due to normal temporary overriding of bones during birth. Caput succedaneum is localized swelling from pressure against the cervix, which can cross the suture lines. Cephalhematoma is bleeding between the periosteum and the bone that never crosses suture lines. Molding and caput disappear within a few days, but cephalhematoma may last for several weeks.

2. A quick initial assessment of the infant immediately after birth helps detect serious abnormalities that may need immediate attention. It is followed by a more complete assessment.
3. Measurements of the infant help determine if in-utero growth was adequate for gestational age and if complications are present.
4. The cardiovascular assessment includes history, airway, color, heart sounds, pulses, and blood pressure.
5. Taking a rectal temperature is dangerous because it risks perforation of the rectum, which turns sharply to the right after about 1 inch.
6. Some signs of hypoglycemia are jitteriness, poor muscle tone, respiratory distress (tachypnea, dyspnea, apnea, cyanosis), high-pitched cry, diaphoresis, low temperature, poor suck, lethargy, irritability, seizures, and coma.
7. Using an incorrect site for heel punctures risks damage to the bone, nerves, or blood vessels of the heel.
8. Newborn reflexes provide information about the status of the neonate's central nervous system.
9. The first feeding allows the nurse to evaluate the newborn's ability to suck, swallow, and breathe in coordination and assess for signs of a connection between the trachea and esophagus.
10. Newborns usually pass the first stool within 12 to 48 hours of birth. Feeding and taking a rectal temperature may stimulate stool passage.
11. Infants should void within 12 to 24 hours. Infants void at least 2 to 6 times during the first 2 days and 6 to 10 times a day after that.
12. The nurse documents location, size, color, elevation, and texture of marks on the skin; explains marks to parents; and offers emotional support as needed.
13. The gestational age assessment provides an estimate of the infant's age since conception and alerts the nurse to possible complications related to age and development.
14. The periods of reactivity are important because the infant may need nursing intervention for low temperature, elevated pulse and respirations, and excessive respiratory secretions. During the sleep period, the infant will have relaxed muscle tone and no interest in feeding.

CHAPTER 21

1. All newborns receive vitamin K to prevent hemorrhagic disease of the newborn. The eyes are treated with an antibiotic ointment to prevent ophthalmia neonatorum.
2. Nurses can prevent heat loss in newborns by keeping them dry and covered and away from cold objects or surfaces, drafts, and outside windows and walls.
3. When infants show signs of hypoglycemia, the nurse should check the blood glucose level and temperature, feed the infant, and watch for signs of other complications.
4. Interventions for preventing jaundice include ensuring that the infant is feeding well by working with mothers and infants having difficulty and teaching parents about jaundice and what observations to make.
5. Nurses can prevent a parent from getting the wrong baby by always checking the infant's identification band against that of the mother or support person every time the two are reunited.
6. Nurses and parents can prevent infant abductions by always being alert for suspicious behavior and stopping anyone who might be taking a baby. Parents must know how to identify hospital staff and should never allow anyone without proper identification to remove their infant from them.
7. Scrupulous hand washing by staff and all who come in contact with newborns is the most important way to prevent newborn infections.
8. Parents choose circumcision because of the decreased incidence of urinary tract infections, penile cancer, and some sexually transmissible infections; religious dictates; parent preference; and lack of knowledge about care of the foreskin. Parents decide against circumcision because it causes pain and risk of bleeding, infection, recurrent phimosis, wound separation, urinary retention, meatitis, meatal stenosis, chordee, and inclusions cysts. They also question the need for surgery.
9. Teach parents not to retract the foreskin on an uncircumcised penis until it becomes separated from the glans later in childhood. They can teach the child to retract it to clean after separation occurs. Teach parents of circumcised infants to watch for bleeding and infection and to apply petroleum jelly as instructed unless a Plastibell was used.
10. Planning parent teaching includes coordinating teaching to include all topics, setting priorities based on parents' needs, using a variety of teaching techniques, modeling behavior, including other family members, and considering culture and language.
11. The first hepatitis B vaccine is given at the birth facility to infants whose mothers are hepatitis B positive to prevent them from being infected.
12. Newborn screening tests should be performed as close to discharge as possible as the tests are more sensitive after the first 24 hours of life. If infants are discharged earlier, they should be retested so that any disorders can be diagnosed early.

CHAPTER 22

1. Some infants lose weight after birth because of insufficient intake and normal loss of extracellular fluid.
2. Colostrum is rich in protein, vitamins, minerals, and immunoglobulins. Transitional milk has less protein and immunoglobulin but more lactose, fat, and calories than colostrum. Mature milk appears less rich than colostrum and transitional milk but supplies all nutrients needed.
3. Breast milk nutrients are in an easily digested form and in proportions required by the newborn. Commercial formulas contain cow's milk adapted to simulate human milk. Infants may develop allergies to modified cow's milk and may need other types of formula, but they are not allergic to human milk.
4. Breast milk contains bifidus factor to help establish intestinal flora, leukocytes, lysozymes that are bacteriolytic, lactoferrin to bind iron in bacteria, and immunoglobulins.
5. Commercial formulas include modified cow's milk formula, soy-based or casein-based protein hydrolysate formulas, and special formulas for preterm infants or those with special needs.
6. Cultural influences, employment demands, support from family and friends, knowledge about each method, age, and education may influence a woman's choice of feeding method.
7. Suckling causes release of oxytocin from the posterior pituitary, which produces the let-down reflex. Suckling and removal of milk from the breast cause the anterior pituitary to release prolactin to increase milk production. Therefore the more frequently the infant breastfeeds, the more prolactin is produced. Infrequent feedings decrease prolactin output and milk production.
8. During pregnancy, identification of flat and inverted nipples and possible use of breast shells to help correct them are important.
9. The nurse can help the mother establish breastfeeding during the initial feeding session by initiating early feeding, helping position the infant at the breast, and showing the mother ways to position her hands. The nurse also can help the infant latch on to the breast, assess the position of the mouth on the breast, check for swallowing, and remove the infant from the breast.
10. The mother should feed the infant every 2 to 3 hours (8 to 12 times each day) for about 10 to 15 minutes at the first breast and until the infant is satisfied at the second breast. Length of feedings may vary but should average at least 15 minutes of effective suckling.
11. To wake up a sleepy infant, unwrap the infant's blankets, talk to the infant, change the diaper, rub the infant's back, and express colostrum onto the breast.
12. Sucking from a bottle requires pushing the tongue against the nipple to slow the flow of milk. Suckling from the breast requires drawing the nipple far into the mouth so that the gums compress the areola as the tongue moves over the milk sinus in a wave-like motion.
13. To help the mother who has engorged breasts, the nurse can encourage nursing frequently, applying heat and cold, massaging, and expressing milk to soften the areola.
14. The nurse should advise the mother with sore nipples to ensure proper positioning of the infant at the breast, vary the position of the infant, apply colostrum or compresses to the nipples, and expose the nipples to air.
15. Care available after discharge for the breastfeeding mother includes home visits by nurses, outpatient clinics where nurses assess and teach breastfeeding, and telephone access to nurses.
16. The mother who plans to work and breastfeed should be taught use of a breast pump, proper storage of milk, and ways to maintain her milk supply.
17. A mother might ask about the types of formula available, ways to prepare it correctly, frequency and amount of feedings, and feeding techniques.
18. Propping bottles risks aspiration of milk. Infants who sleep with a propped bottle have more ear infections and may develop cavities when the teeth come in.

CHAPTER 23

1. Parents obtain information about infant care from friends, family, nurses, child care classes, books, and magazines.
2. Nurses may provide follow-up phone calls, home visits, and classes about parenting.
3. All equipment should be checked for safety, and parts should be inspected to see that they are functioning properly.
4. Car seats must be chosen according to the size of the infant and must be used correctly to maintain safety.
5. Infants are not "spoiled" by prompt attention to their needs.
6. Nurses can assist parents of crying infants to determine the cause and appropriate techniques for dealing with a crying infant. Nurses can also use therapeutic communication techniques to help parents deal with negative feelings.
7. Signs of teething include drooling, irritability, decreased appetite and sleep, and red, swollen gums.

8. Diaper rash can be prevented by keeping the area clean and dry and avoiding products to which the infant seems sensitive. If rash occurs, parents should expose the area to air and apply creams sparingly.
9. The amount infants eat during the early weeks will vary but will average about 1 ounce per feeding at first and 5 to 6 ounces per feeding at 12 weeks.
10. Solid foods cannot be digested completely until age 4 to 6 months and may cause allergies, gastric upsets, and decreased intake of needed nutrients from milk. In addition, the extrusion reflex makes it difficult to feed solids to infants younger than 4 months.
11. Understanding the infant's changing capabilities helps parents assess situations to prevent accidents.
12. Well-baby checkups allow the health care provider to assess the infant's growth and development, provide parent teaching, and give immunizations.
13. Immunizations prevent infants from becoming infected with very serious communicable diseases.
14. Immediate help should be obtained if infants have difficulty breathing, show cyanosis, or are hard to arouse from sleep.
15. The cause of sudden infant death syndrome remains unknown, but the risk may be increased with sleeping in a prone position or on soft, loose bedding, overheating, and maternal smoking. Infants should sleep in a supine position and should not sleep with other persons.

CHAPTER 24

1. Pregnancy interrupts developmental tasks such as the achievement of a stable identity, development of a personal value system, completion of educational goals, and achievement of independence from parents.
2. Teenagers experience greater risk for anemia, nutritional deficiencies, and sexually transmissible diseases. Infants are at greater risk of being born prematurely and weighing less than 2500 g. Both infant and maternal mortality rates are higher during the teenage years.
3. A variety of teaching methods such as visual aids, videos, group classes, and one-to-one counseling may be effective for teenagers.
4. Infants develop a sense of trust, which is necessary for future development, when their needs are met promptly and gently. Crying indicates a need and does not mean the infant is "spoiled." Physical growth and development proceed slowly from the head downward.
5. Mature primigravidas often have maturity, problem-solving skills, and emotional and financial resources that are unavailable to younger women.
6. The fetus of a woman older than 35 years is at increased risk for chromosomal anomalies that may be detected by prenatal screening.
7. The older mother may have less energy than younger mothers, and conserving her energy for care of herself and her infant is important.
8. The effects of smoking on the neonate include low birth weight, prematurity, and increased perinatal loss. Later effects include SIDS and delayed neurologic and intellectual development.
9. Fetal alcohol syndrome is characterized by slow growth, central nervous system disorders, and cranial and facial anomalies. Infants with fetal alcohol effect will have fewer and less severe problems than those with fetal alcohol syndrome.
10. The long-term effects of maternal cocaine use on the child include increased risk of SIDS, learning difficulties, slower development of motor skills, and limited interaction with people and objects.
11. Pregnant heroin users are placed on methadone to provide a long-acting, steady drug dose to the fetus to avoid the problems of frequent intrauterine overdosage and withdrawal.
12. Prenatal behaviors that suggest substance abuse include prenatal care sought late in pregnancy, failure to keep appointments, inconsistent follow-through with recommended regimens, poor grooming, inadequate weight gain, needle punctures, thrombosed veins, and signs of cellulitis.
13. Signs and symptoms of recent cocaine use include profuse sweating, high blood pressure, irregular respirations, dilated pupils, increased body temperature, sudden onset of severely painful uterine contractions, fetal tachycardia, and excessive fetal activity. Emotional signs include anger, caustic or abusive reactions to the caregiver, emotional lability, and paranoia.
14. Interventions are focused on preventing maternal or fetal injury and may require setting limits in a firm, nonjudgmental manner with a woman who may be abusive and in great pain.
15. Parents experience less anxiety when they are gently told the condition of the infant and allowed to hold their newborn as soon as possible.
16. Facial and genital defects are believed to affect parenting most.
17. The reaction of parents can be described in terms of a grief response. Initial reactions include shock and disbelief. Denial, anger, and guilt are common.
18. Nurses can promote bonding and attachment by handling the infant gently, emphasizing normal traits, helping parents hold and cuddle the infant, and using communication skills to help parents come to terms with their feelings.
19. Discharge planning for the family of an infant with congenital anomalies should include special feed-

ing and other techniques that the infant may require.

20. The way in which the stillborn infant is presented creates memories that the parents will retain. If necessary, the infant should be washed and lotion or powder applied. If possible, the infant should be presented while still warm and soft, wrapped in a soft, warm blanket.
21. A memory packet that includes a photograph of the baby, footprints, a birth bracelet, and crib card, and if possible, a lock of hair help parents grieve.
22. Mothers see adoption as an act of sacrifice and love when they give up the child to those who can provide a better life.
23. Adoptive parents must be taught the way to care for an infant and what to expect in terms of growth and development.
24. Battering may start or become worse during pregnancy. The abdomen may replace the face and breasts as the target for battery.
25. Nurses can examine their own biases to determine whether they accept a common myth that blames the victim. In addition, nurses can consciously practice in ways that empower women and make it clear that the woman owns her body and no one deserves to be beaten.
26. The battered woman often appears hesitant, embarrassed, or evasive. She may avoid eye contact and appear ashamed, guilty, or frightened. Signs of present and past injury may be present, such as bruising, swelling, lacerations, scars, and old fractures, as well as genital injuries.
27. Nurses can help establish short-term goals by helping the woman acknowledge the abuse, develop a plan for protecting herself and her children, and identify community resources that provide protection.

CHAPTER 25

1. Bleeding is the most common sign of threatened abortion. It may be accompanied by rhythmic cramping, backache, or feelings of pelvic pressure. Gross rupture of membranes and subsequent uterine contractions and bleeding makes the abortion inevitable.
2. Recurrent spontaneous abortions most often occur as a result of genetic or chromosomal abnormalities of the embryo or anomalies of the maternal reproductive tract. Additional causes are believed to be hormonal and immunologic factors or systemic diseases or infections.
3. Nurses can facilitate the grief response by being aware that although many couples grieve over an early pregnancy loss, they often feel a lack of support from family, friends, and health care personnel. When nurses demonstrate empathy and unconditional acceptance of the feelings expressed, they facilitate the grief response. Providing information about the grieving and referrals to additional support groups also may be helpful.
4. Disseminated intravascular coagulation is a life-threatening disorder in which procoagulation and anticoagulation factors are activated simultaneously, resulting in profuse bleeding from any vulnerable area. It may occur with missed abortion (primarily if the pregnancy had reached the second trimester when fetal death occurred), abruptio placentae, severe pregnancy-induced hypertension, amniotic fluid embolism, and other conditions such as sepsis.
5. Ectopic pregnancy remains the leading cause of maternal death because of hemorrhage, and it can reduce the woman's chance of subsequent pregnancies because of damage to a fallopian tube. Also, the condition that caused the ectopic pregnancy in the tube may be present in the opposite tube.
6. The increase in incidence of ectopic pregnancy may occur as a result of pelvic inflammatory disease that may complicate untreated sexually transmitted diseases. Scarring of the fallopian tubes that may result from the infection may make it difficult for the fertilized ovum to pass through the obstructed tube. Treatment for ectopic pregnancy may be medical (chemotherapeutic agent) or surgical (salpingostomy or salpingectomy).
7. Hydatidiform mole is a form of gestational trophoblastic disease that involves abnormal development of the placenta as the fetal part of the pregnancy fails to develop. The first phase of treatment is evacuation of the molar pregnancy from the uterus. The second phase is follow-up to detect malignant changes in remaining trophoblastic tissue.
8. Painless vaginal bleeding in the latter half of pregnancy is the classic sign of placenta previa. Strict bedrest, no sexual intercourse, an adult caregiver present at all times, and availability of emergency transportation to the hospital are essential for home care. The woman must also be taught to monitor fetal movement and to report a decrease in movement or increase in vaginal bleeding.
9. The four classic signs of abruptio placentae are (a) bleeding, which may be evident vaginally or concealed behind the placenta; (b) uterine tenderness; (c) excess uterine activity, with poor relaxation between contractions; (d) abdominal pain.
10. Hemorrhagic shock is the major danger of placental abruption for the mother; anoxia, excessive blood loss, or delivery before maturity are the major dangers for the fetus.
11. Both morning sickness and hyperemesis gravidarum begin in the first trimester. Morning sickness is self-limiting and causes no serious compli-

cations. Hyperemesis is persistent, uncontrollable vomiting that can result in dehydration, and electrolyte or acid-base imbalance.

12. Goals of management are to maintain hydration, replace electrolytes and vitamins, maintain nutrition, and provide emotional support.
13. Nurses must use critical thinking to examine biases that may result in lack of comfort and support for women with hyperemesis.
14. Persistent vasospasm of uterine arterioles may result in fetal hypoxemia, intrauterine growth restriction, or even fetal death.
15. The three classic signs of preeclampsia include hypertension, edema, and possibly proteinuria. Headache, hyperreflexia, visual disturbances, and epigastric pain indicate the disease is worsening. Rest, especially in a lateral position, increases cardiac return and circulatory volume, thus improving perfusion of vital organs. Increased renal perfusion decreases angiotensin II levels, thus lowering blood pressure.
16. Vasospasms cause rupture of cerebral capillaries and small cerebral hemorrhages.
17. Magnesium sulfate prevents seizures by reducing central nervous system irritability and decreasing vasoconstriction. The primary adverse effect is central nervous system depression, which includes depression of the respiratory center.
18. Pulmonary edema, circulatory or renal failure, and cerebral hemorrhage are complications of eclampsia. Disseminated intravascular coagulation is also more likely to occur when a woman has severe preeclampsia or eclampsia.
19. Assessments for the woman with preeclampsia include daily weights, location and degree of edema, vital signs, hourly urinary output, urine for protein, deep tendon reflexes, and subjective signs such as headache, visual disturbances, and epigastric pain. The fetal heart rate should be assessed for nonreassuring patterns. Respiratory rate, level of consciousness, and laboratory data such as creatinine, liver enzymes, and magnesium level should be evaluated. Psychosocial assessment should include the reaction of the woman's family and support system. Nursing assessment is the only way to determine whether the condition is responding to medical management or the disease is worsening.
20. To prevent seizures, maintain a quiet environment, reduce environmental stimuli, and maintain a therapeutic level of magnesium. Nurses must remain with the woman and call for help if a seizure occurs. If time allows, attempt to turn the woman on her side. Note the sequence and time of the seizure. Insert an airway following the seizure and suction the woman's nose and mouth, administer oxygen, administer medications, and prepare for additional medical interventions.
21. To prevent seizure-related injury, the side rails should be padded and raised. The bed should be in the lowest position with the wheels locked. Oxygen and suction should be readily available. Necessary equipment and medications should be kept in the room.
22. Signs of magnesium toxicity include respiratory rate below 12 breaths per minute, hyporeflexia, sweating or flushing, altered sensorium (lethargy, drowsiness, disorientation), and serum magnesium level beyond the therapeutic range. If toxicity occurs, discontinue magnesium and notify the physician so the dose can be altered. Calcium gluconate is the antidote for magnesium toxicity.
23. *H,* Hemolysis; *EL,* elevated liver enzymes; *LP,* low platelets. Major symptoms are pain and tenderness in the right upper quadrant. Additional signs and symptoms may include nausea, vomiting, and severe edema. Laboratory data include a low hematocrit, abnormal liver studies, coagulation abnormalities, and often abnormal renal studies. Palpating the liver could cause trauma, including rupture of a subcapsular hematoma.
24. Preeclampsia occurs only during pregnancy and the early postpartum period. Chronic hypertension is present before pregnancy or before the twentieth week of gestation and persists following the postpartum period. Treatment may be similar during pregnancy; however, chronic hypertension is often treated with antihypertensive medications before and during pregnancy. Preeclampsia may further complicate chronic hypertension.
25. Administration of Rh_0(D) immunoglobulin prevents development of maternal Rh antibodies and is recommended following any procedure that includes the possibility of maternal exposure to Rh-positive fetal blood.
26. Maternal antibodies cross the placental barrier and cause destruction of fetal red blood cells. The fetus becomes anemic, bilirubin increases, and severe neurologic disease can result.
27. Many women with blood type O have anti-A or anti-B antibodies before they become pregnant, so the first pregnancy can be affected. The effects of ABO incompatability are milder than Rh sensitization because fewer antibodies cross into fetal blood.

CHAPTER 26

1. The hormones of pregnancy cause resistance of maternal cells to insulin, which increases the availability of glucose for the fetus.
2. The mother is at risk to develop pregnancy-induced hypertension, urinary tract infections, ketoacidosis, and preterm labor. Possible fetal and neonatal effects include congenital malforma-

tions; small or large fetal size, depending on the placental vascular supply; fetal hypoxemia; and polycythemia. Neonatal effects include hypoglycemia, hypocalcemia, hyperbilirubinemia, and respiratory distress syndrome.

3. Insulin needs decrease during the first trimester and increase sharply during the second and third trimesters (when placental hormones initiate insulin resistance). During labor, insulin needs must be determined by frequent checks of blood glucose. In the postpartum period insulin needs decrease as placental hormones decline.
4. Glycosylated hemoglobin gives an accurate evaluation of blood glucose for the past 4 to 8 weeks and is not affected by recent intake of food.
5. Gestational diabetes mellitus is first diagnosed during pregnancy. It is most often managed by diet and exercise, although insulin may be needed if fasting or postprandial capillary blood glucose values are persistently high.
6. A glucose challenge test is a screening procedure only and requires no preparation. A glucose tolerance test is diagnostic for diabetes mellitus; it requires preparation and 3 hours of testing.
7. Maternal effects of gestational diabetes mellitus include increased incidence of urinary tract infections, hydramnios (excessive amniotic fluid), premature rupture of membranes, and development of pregnancy-induced hypertension. Fetal effects may include macrosomia that can result in shoulder dystocia or cesarean birth. The newborn is at risk for hypoglycemia. Preexisting diabetes has similar maternal effects as gestational diabetes, but fetal and infant effects differ. The infant may have IUGR if the woman's diabetes has caused vascular impairment, or macrosomia if her glucose is poorly controlled and no vascular impairment exists. Congenital anomalies are increased in preexisting diabetes, especially if the diabetes is poorly controlled at conception and during early gestation.
8. Increased intravascular volume and increased cardiac output (particularly stroke volume) place an added burden on the heart of a woman who has a cardiac defect.
9. Rheumatic and congenital heart disease are the two major categories of heart disease. Functional classification depends on the person's ability to tolerate activity. Class I indicates no limitation on activity. Class II indicates slight restriction if necessary. In Class III there is marked limitation, and Class IV indicates that the person has symptoms such as dyspnea even at rest.
10. Goals of treatment are to prevent anemia so there is an adequate supply of red blood cells to transport oxygen and thus reduce the demands on the heart, limit physical activity so cardiac demand does not exceed the capacity of the heart, and limit weight gain, which would add further demands on the heart.
11. With every contraction, blood is shifted from the uterus and placenta into the central circulation; this can lead to fluid overload if fluids are administered rapidly.
12. An additional 500 ml of blood are added to the central circulation with delivery of the placenta. Also, the compression of the vena cava that characterized much of pregnancy is gone. This increases the load on the heart and can lead to further compromise of the heart.
13. Most women begin pregnancy with marginal iron stores, do not have adequate iron stores to meet the demands of pregnancy, and it is difficult to meet the high iron needs of pregnancy by diet alone.
14. The fetus usually receives adequate iron, even at a cost to the mother. Therefore, neonatal effects of moderate maternal anemia are rare. With very severe anemia, the fetus may become hypoxic however.
15. The fetal and neonatal effects of folic acid deficiency are increased risk of spontaneous abortion, abruption of the placenta, and fetal anomalies (particularly neural tube defects).
16. Pregnancy may worsen sickle cell disease, and the risk of "sickle cell crisis" is increased.
17. Frequent evaluations of hemoglobin, blood count, serum iron, and iron-binding capacity as well as folate are necessary to determine the degree of anemia. Frequent fetal surveillance and monitoring for signs of sickle cell crisis are also necessary. The nurse must also be aware that the woman's pain could be a pregnancy complication rather than due to sickle cell crisis.
18. Thalassemia is associated with increased iron absorption and storage, making women with this disorder susceptible to iron overload.
19. The maternal and fetal effects of systemic lupus erythematosus are increased incidence of abortion, preterm delivery, and fetal death. Pregnancy can exacerbate the disease and renal complications pose a special risk.
20. There is often marked improvement of rheumatoid arthritis during pregnancy; however, relapse often occurs soon after childbirth.
21. Anticonvulsant drugs are often teratogenic. However, generalized seizures may also have adverse fetal effects, so maintaining the anticonvulsant dose as low as possible is important.
22. The recommended supportive care for women with Bell's palsy includes eye patching, applying ointment or drops to prevent trauma to the cornea, facial massage, and psychological support. Corticosteroids may also be given.

23. Approximately 2% of all live neonates are infected with cytomegalovirus; 90% of these are asymptomatic and appear normal. The most serious complications of those affected are deafness, mental retardation, seizures, blindness, and dental abnormalities.
24. The first trimester is the time of organogenesis, when damage can be done to all developing organ systems.
25. A vaccine is available to prevent rubella; however, it cannot be given during pregnancy. During pregnancy, a woman can only avoid situations where she is likely to contract rubella.
26. Immunization with varicella-zoster immune globulin is recommended. Infected mothers and infants must be isolated from those who are not immune.
27. Vertical transmission of herpesvirus occurs when organisms ascend following rupture of membranes and during birth when the fetus comes into contact with infectious tissue and secretions.
28. The fetal and neonatal effects of parvovirus 19 infection are failure of red blood cell production, severe fetal anemia, hydrops, and heart failure.
29. Hepatitis B virus is transmitted by contact with infected blood, saliva, vaginal secretions, semen, or breast milk. A newborn whose mother is known to carry the hepatitis B surface antigen should receive hepatitis B immune globulin soon after birth, followed by hepatitis B vaccine. The infant should receive the second and third doses of vaccine at regularly-scheduled times.
30. Avoid sexual transmission by abstinence, avoiding intercourse with infected persons, or using recommended barrier methods. Intravenous drug users who refuse rehabilitation must avoid transmission that occurs when needles are shared with those who are infected.
31. Several combinations of antiretroviral medication regimens may be administered to delay replication of the virus. Medications are also available to prevent *Pneumocystis carinii* pneumonia. Opportunistic diseases are treated. Good hygiene reduces transmission of infectious organisms to the susceptible person, and nutritious meals reduce the risk for opportunistic infection.
32. Toxoplasmosis can be prevented by cooking meat thoroughly, not touching mucous membranes while handling raw meat, washing kitchen surfaces and hands thoroughly after handling raw meat, avoiding uncooked eggs and unpasteurized milk, washing vegetables and fruit before consumption, and avoiding contact with materials that may be contaminated with cat feces.
33. Risk factors for GBS include a prior infant with GBS infection, presence of GBS organisms in the urine in the present pregnancy, preterm birth (before 37 weeks), maternal fever in labor, prolonged membrane rupture (≥18 hours). Intravenous antibacterial therapy is used to prevent colonization.
34. Isoniazid, ethambutol, and rifampin given for 9 months are used to treat tuberculosis in the mother. Pyridoxine is added to prevent neurotoxicity. The infant is skin tested at birth and may be started on INH therapy until the skin test, which will be repeated, remains negative.

CHAPTER 27

1. Hypotonic labor dysfunction usually occurs during the active phase of first-stage labor (4 cm cervical dilation or more), whereas hypertonic dysfunction usually occurs during the latent phase (within the first 3 cm of cervical dilation). Uterine contractions become weaker, shorter, and less frequent in hypotonic dysfunction. In hypertonic dysfunction, contractions are painful but inefficient and the uterine resting tone is high. Hypotonic dysfunction is not painful because the contractions decrease, although the woman may become tired. Hypertonic dysfunction is characterized by a cramping type of pain. Management of both depends on the identified cause. Hypotonic dysfunction often is managed by ensuring adequate intake of fluids and electrolytes, position changes, amniotomy if the membranes are not ruptured, and oxytocin augmentation. Hypertonic dysfunction may be managed by mild sedation or tocolytic drugs to reduce excess uterine activity. Oxytocin in very low doses may be used occasionally to help coordinate uterine activity.
2. Maternal position changes encourage the fetus to rotate from an occiput transverse or occiput posterior position to an occiput anterior position, similar to nesting two spoons together. The convex surface of the rounded fetal back rotates toward the convex surface of the anterior uterus. The squatting position also increases pelvic diameters and straightens the pelvic curve to facilitate both fetal rotation and descent.
3. Other complications are associated with a fetus in a breech presentation that may cause problems, regardless of the method of birth. These include low birth weight, fetal anomalies, and associated pregnancy or labor complications.
4. The staff must be prepared for care of multiple infants. Duplicate staff and equipment should be ready for every infant expected.
5. Bladder distention during labor can consume available room in the woman's pelvis, thus impeding labor progress and fetal descent. In addition, it is a potential source of discomfort.

6. Psychological support reduces stress that otherwise can consume energy the uterus needs, inhibit uterine contractions, reduce placental blood supply, impair the woman's pushing efforts, and increase the woman's pain experience.
7. The average nullipara's cervix dilates about 1.2 cm per hour; minimal fetal descent is 1.0 cm per hour. The average parous woman's cervix dilates about 1.5 cm per hour, with minimal descent of 2 cm per hour.
8. Nursing care for the woman who has prolonged labor is similar to that for dysfunctional labor. Promoting comfort, energy conservation, position changes, and assessments for related complications such as infection should be done.
9. Trauma is the primary maternal risk of a precipitate labor and may include uterine rupture, cervical lacerations, and hematomas. Fetal risks may include trauma, such as intracranial hemorrhage or nerve damage, and hypoxia.
10. Premature rupture of the membranes (PROM) occurs before true labor any time during pregnancy. Preterm premature rupture of the membranes (PPROM) occurs before 37 weeks of gestation are completed and may be accompanied by contractions. PPROM is more likely to be associated with preterm labor and birth.
11. Infection may be both a cause and result of premature rupture of the membranes.
12. Labor is usually induced if a woman with ruptured membranes is near term and has a favorable cervix and if labor does not spontaneously begin within at least 12 to 24 hours. Prostaglandin in the form of Cervidil or Prepidil may be used to soften the unfavorable cervix if she is at least 36 weeks of gestation. If she is slightly preterm (32 to 35 weeks), the physician will deliver the infant if infection is present, the fetal lungs are mature, or both. If no infection exists and the fetal lungs are not mature, expectant care with periodic tests for fetal lung maturity and fetal well-being are done. Steroids and antibiotics are given to mothers at earlier gestations.
13. The nurse should assess the woman's vital signs and FHR, teach her to avoid any breast stimulation, avoid insertion of anything into the vagina, avoid breast stimulation, maintain activity restrictions, note any uterine contractions, and teach the mother how to observe fetal kick counts.
14. Symptoms of preterm labor often are vague. They include uterine contractions that may often be painless, the fetus "balling up," menstrual-like cramps, backache, pelvic pressure, change or increased vaginal discharge, abdominal cramps, thigh pain, and a sense of "feeling bad."
15. Early identification of preterm labor enables management that may delay birth and allow further maturation of the fetus or permit transfer to a facility equipped to care for an immature infant.
16. β-adrenergics such as terbutaline or sometimes ritodrine, magnesium sulfate, prostaglandin synthesis inhibitors (indomethacin), and calcium channel blockers (nifedipine) may be used to stop preterm labor.
17. Corticosteroids are given to the woman who expects to deliver prematurely to accelerate maturation of the fetal lungs and reduce the incidence of intraventricular hemorrhage. The greatest benefits occur if steroids are in the mother's system at least 24 hours.
18. The three potential fetal or newborn risks are reduced placental function and umbilical cord compression before birth and meconium aspiration after birth.
19. If umbilical cord prolapse occurs, the priority of care is to reduce compression of and restore normal blood flow through the cord while giving the mother oxygen to maximize her blood oxygen concentration. At the same time, the nurse should summon help to expedite delivery.
20. Stimulated contractions are potentially more powerful than natural ones and may cause the pressure in the uterus to exceed the uterine wall's ability to withstand that pressure.
21. Shock and hemorrhage are rapidly developing complications of uterine inversion. They are managed by rapid IV fluid and blood replacement, often using two IV lines. A drug that relaxes the uterus is given to allow uterine replacement, and general anesthesia may be needed. Oxytocin is given *after* the uterus is replaced in the proper position.
22. Amniotic fluid contains fetal particulate matter that may obstruct pulmonary capillaries. Also, the fetal cells in maternal blood are antigens that set up an anaphalactoid response.
23. For intrapartum emergencies, nursing considerations include the following: *Prolapsed umbilical cord*—Relieve pressure on the cord to restore adequate blood flow through it. *Uterine rupture*—Attempt to prevent by cautious intrapartum use of uterine stimulants and close monitoring of uterine contractions. *Uterine inversion*—Avoid pressure on the poorly contracted fundus after birth; assess for and correct shock. *Amniotic fluid embolism*—Respiratory support; observe for coagulation deficits.

CHAPTER 28

1. The nurse examines a woman's prenatal record and her labor and delivery record to determine whether any factors predispose her to postpartum hemorrhage.

2. Overdistention of uterine muscles makes their contraction more difficult and predisposes them to excessive bleeding.
3. The nurse cannot be certain that bleeding is controlled because concealed bleeding can occur in soft tissue and produce a hematoma.
4. Initial management of uterine atony focuses on measures to contract the uterus, such as massaging, expressing clots, and emptying the bladder. Pharmacologic measures include fluid replacement and administration of dilute oxytocin, methylergonovine, or other drugs such as Hemabate.
5. Large hematomas may require incision and evacuation of clots, as well as ligation of the bleeding vessel. Small hematomas do not require treatment.
6. Recognizing that the woman is becoming hypovolemic is sometimes difficult because of compensatory mechanisms, such as carotid and aortic baroreceptors that are stimulated to constrict peripheral blood vessels. This shunts blood to central circulation and maintains blood pressure. Catecholamines promote constriction in nonessential organs, increasing the heart rate and raising blood pressure.
7. The major signs of subinvolution are prolonged lochial discharge, irregular or excessive uterine bleeding, pelvic pain, feelings of pelvic heaviness, backache, fatigue, and persistent malaise.
8. Nurses must teach the mother how to locate and palpate the fundus and how to estimate fundal height in relation to the umbilicus. They also teach the mother to report any deviation from the expected pattern or duration of lochia, a foul odor, or pelvic pain.
9. Venous stasis increases during pregnancy because of compression of the large vessels by the enlarging uterus. Venous stasis also may occur if the woman spends a prolonged period of time in stirrups during labor and birth. Pregnancy and the postpartum also are characterized by changes in the coagulation and fibrinolytic systems that elevate the factors that favor coagulation and decrease the factors that favor lysis of clots.
10. Superficial venous thrombosis occurs most often in the calf area with signs and symptoms that include swelling, tenderness, warmth, and redness.
11. Heparin remains the long-term treatment of the pregnant woman with deep venous thrombosis because warfarin (Coumadin), which crosses the placental barrier, may be teratogenic and it predisposes the fetus to hemorrhage. If the woman is in the postpartum period, heparin is changed to warfarin after several days of treatment.
12. Strict bedrest is prescribed for the woman with deep vein thrombosis to decrease interstitial swelling and to promote venous return from that leg.
13. When the mother is receiving anticoagulation medicine, the nurse assesses the mother for unexplained bruising, petechiae, or bleeding from the nose, bladder, gums, or increased vaginal bleeding. Signs of hemorrhage, such as tachycardia, falling blood pressure, or other signs of shock also should be noted.
14. The home care nurse should assess family structure and function that will need to change as a result of prolonged treatment for the mother. The nurse should evaluate mother-infant interaction and determine what support system may be available to provide assistance.
15. Cesarean birth, the use of forceps, or vacuum extraction may result in trauma that provides a portal of entry for infectious organisms.
16. Every part of the reproductive tract is connected to every other part, and organisms can move from the vagina through the cervix, uterus, fallopian tubes, and out into the peritoneal cavity. Alkalinity of the vagina during labor, necrosis of the endometrium, and the presence of lochia encourage bacterial growth.
17. Infection is more likely to develop in a woman who had prolonged labor because organisms have time and opportunity to ascend from the vagina into the uterus during prolonged labor. Also, she may have more vaginal examinations and ruptured membranes for a longer time.
18. Fever, chills, lethargy, malaise, anorexia, abdominal pain and cramping, uterine tenderness, and purulent foul-smelling lochia, tachycardia, and subinvolution are signs and symptoms of metritis. It usually is treated by IV administration of antibiotics, antipyretics, and oxytocin to promote involution.
19. Wound infection most often occurs in sites of episiotomies, lacerations, and incisions performed for cesarean birth.
20. Incisions and lacerations should be inspected for redness, tenderness, edema, and approximation of the edges of the wound, which may pull apart with infection.
21. To prevent urinary tract infection, the woman should be advised to drink at least 2500 to 3000 ml of fluid each day, empty her bladder every 2 to 3 hours during the day, and practice meticulous hygiene. Cystitis is treated with oral antibiotics on an outpatient basis. Pyelonephritis requires readmittance to the hospital and IV administration of antibiotics.
22. Measures to prevent mastitis include correct positioning of the infant, frequent emptying of the breasts, and avoiding nipple trauma and supplemental feedings. In addition, the woman should avoid continuous pressure on the breasts caused by tight bras or infant carriers.

23. The symptoms of postpartum depression differ from those of postpartum "blues" by the number, intensity, and persistence of symptoms. They are present daily for at least 2 weeks. These symptoms include a loss of interest in one's surroundings, a loss of a usual emotional responses, and feelings of unworthiness, guilt, and shame.
24. Nurses can demonstrate care, provide anticipatory guidance, help the mother verbalize her feelings, and make appropriate referrals.
25. Postpartum psychosis usually requires hospitalization, psychotherapy, and appropriate medication.

CHAPTER 29

1. Poor women are at risk for preterm birth because they may have impaired general health and may receive little or no prenatal care.
2. Preterm infants appear frail and weak and are small, with limp extremities, poor muscle tone, red skin, and immature ears, nipples, areola, and genitals.
3. Factors that increase respiratory problems in preterm infants include lack of surfactant, poor cough reflex, small air passages, and weak muscles.
4. Nursing responsibilities for preterm infants with respiratory problems include working with respiratory therapists to manage equipment, monitoring the infant's changing oxygen needs, positioning infants to promote drainage, and suctioning.
5. Nurses wean infants to the open crib by making gradual changes in the environmental temperature, dressing the infant, and using blankets and a hat when the infant is out of the incubator.
6. To measure intake and output for infants, all fluids (IV and oral), including medications, are measured. Diapers are weighed to calculate urine output.
7. Preterm infants' kidneys do not concentrate or dilute urine well, and they have large insensible water losses. They lack passive antibodies from the mother and have an immature immune system. Pain causes physiologic responses such as vital signs changes and decreases in oxygenation.
8. The nurse can diminish overstimulation by organizing care to provide for rest periods, reducing environmental stimuli, minimizing pain, and discussing the plan of care with others.
9. Feeding tolerance is assessed by checking gastric residual before gavage feedings, measuring abdominal girth, testing stools for reducing substances and blood, and observing for regurgitation. During nipple feedings, the nurse watches for signs of respiratory difficulty, decreased oxygenation, and fatigue.
10. The nurse can help breastfeeding mothers of preterm infants by teaching them ways to pump and store milk and breastfeeding techniques adapted to the preterm's needs and by providing support and encouragement.
11. The nurse can help parents feel comfortable with preterm infants by providing warm support, realistic encouragement, and information about the NICU environment, the infant's condition and characteristics, and the equipment and care.
12. Helping parents take on partial responsibility for care, beginning early in hospitalization, and gradually increasing their responsibility will help them prepare for discharge of their infant.
13. Postmature infants may be thin and have loose skin folds, cracked and peeling skin, minimal vernix or lanugo, and meconium staining. They look hyperalert and worried.
14. Postmature infants may have polycythemia, meconium aspiration, hypoglycemia, and poor temperature regulation.
15. In symmetric growth restriction, all body parts are proportionately small. In asymmetric growth restriction, the head is normal in size but seems large for the small body.
16. Large-for-gestational age infants may have birth injuries such as fractures, nerve damage, cephalhematoma, hypoglycemia, and polycythemia.

CHAPTER 30

1. Asphyxia before or during birth may cause meconium aspiration, apnea, acidosis, failure of the ductus arteriosus and foramen ovale to close, brain damage, and death.
2. The nurse's role in asphyxia is to begin resuscitation promptly, assist the team, and provide follow-up and parental support.
3. Transient tachypnea of the newborn is caused by failure of fetal lung fluid to be absorbed completely in full-term or preterm infants. Respiratory distress syndrome occurs in preterm infants as a result of inadequate surfactant.
4. Meconium in amniotic fluid enters the lungs before birth or is drawn in during the first breaths after birth, causing obstruction, air trapping, and inflammation.
5. When meconium-stained amniotic fluid is seen during labor, the nurse must notify the physician, prepare equipment, assist with intubation, and observe for infection or other problems.
6. Jaundice is considered pathologic when it occurs in the first 24 hours of life or lasts longer than the 10th to 14th days of life, when total bilirubin is above 12 mg/dl in full term infants or 10 to 14 mg/dl in preterm infants, or when it rises more than 5 mg/dl in 24 hours.
7. In caring for infants receiving phototherapy, the nurse must prevent cold stress, hypoglycemia, inadequate intake, and injury caused by improper

use of lights. Monitoring for complications also is important.

8. Vertical infection is transmitted from the mother to the infant during pregnancy or birth. Horizontal infection is transmitted from other people to the infant after birth.
9. The role of the nurse in sepsis is to identify early signs, notify the physician, coordinate treatment, observe for change, and support the family.
10. Problems of infants of diabetic mothers include congenital anomalies, macrosomia or intrauterine growth restriction, respiratory distress syndrome, hypoglycemia, hypocalcemia, and polycythemia.
11. Care of the infant of a diabetic mother includes identifying complications, performing glucose screenings, providing early feedings, and supporting parents.
12. Infants who are exposed to drugs in utero are subject to congenital defects, neonatal abstinence syndrome, behavior and feeding problems, failure to gain weight, and abnormal social interaction.
13. Infants with neonatal abstinence syndrome need decreased environmental stimuli and assistance with feeding. Their mothers need help with bonding and learning to care for them.
14. Cyanotic heart defects allow unoxygenated blood flow into the systemic circulation, producing cyanosis. Acyanotic heart defects cause impairment of blood flow or circulation of oxygenated blood into the pulmonary system, usually without cyanosis. Other categories are by blood flow including increased or decreased pulmonary blood flow, obstruction to blood flow, or mixing of venous and oxygenated blood.

CHAPTER 31

1. Almost all contraceptive methods are used by women, and failure will most affect women.
2. The nurse's role in helping women with contraception is to provide information so that women can choose contraceptives appropriately and use them correctly.
3. Important considerations in choosing contraceptive techniques include safety, protection from sexually transmissible diseases, effectiveness, convenience, education needed, side effects, interference with spontaneity, availability, expense, preference of the woman and her partner, and culture.
4. Sterilization, hormonal contraceptives, and intrauterine devices may require signed informed consents.
5. Adolescents may have incorrect beliefs such as that they cannot conceive during first intercourse, without orgasm, or without having menstruated a certain length of time or that douching will prevent pregnancy.
6. Adolescents may not seek contraception because they may fear lack of acceptance, loss of sexual privacy, pelvic examination, or adverse effects of contraception on their health.
7. The nurse can increase teach adolescents effectively by showing sensitivity to their feelings, being accepting, and providing extensive teaching without hurry, using understandable terms and audiovisual materials.
8. Women can conceive until menstruation has ceased for 2 years, but pregnancy is rare after age 50. Perimenopausal women who do not smoke and have no other contraindications can use any method of contraception.
9. Important factors to consider when choosing a method of sterilization include time involved, cost, need for hospitalization, and feelings of each partner about a permanent end to having more children.
10. Hormonal contraceptives alter normal hormone changes, preventing ovulation, altering the endometrium, and making the cervical mucus unfavorable to sperm.
11. Menstrual changes are the reason some women stop using DepoProvera.
12. Women using OCs need to know that the pills must be taken consistently and in the right order every day, what to do if pills are missed, common side effects, and signs that may indicate a problem.
13. The first dose of ECP should be taken as soon as possible after unprotected intercourse and within 72 hours. The second dose is taken 12 hours later.
14. Education for women choosing intrauterine devices includes information about side effects, when and how to check the strings, and when to seek medical treatment.
15. Barrier methods kill sperm and prevent them from entering the cervix.
16. Natural family planning methods avoid drugs, chemicals, and devices; are inexpensive; and are acceptable to most religions. Couples need extensive education and high motivation, however, and they risk pregnancy if they make an error.

CHAPTER 32

1. *Infertility* is strictly defined as the inability to conceive after 1 year of unprotected regular intercourse. A more workable definition that considers the age and other individual factors is the inability of a couple to conceive when desired. Primary infertility is that which occurs in couples who have never conceived. Secondary infertility occurs in those who have conceived before and are not able to conceive again.
2. The normal average number of sperm released at ejaculation is 400 million. Twenty million per ml

is probably the minimum required for unassisted fertility. At least 30% of the sperm must be living and normal and half must have normal forward movement. The amount of seminal fluid should be 2 to 6 ml and it should liquefy within 10 to 30 minutes. Seminal fluid should have fewer white blood cells than 1 million/mL.

3. Erection problems exist if the man cannot initiate and maintain a penile erection that is sufficient to allow intercourse and deposit of seminal fluid with sperm near the woman's cervix. Ejaculation abnormalities may result from retrograde ejaculation, hypospadias, or abnormal ejaculation response (premature, slow, or absent).
4. Abnormalities of the sperm, ejaculation, or the seminal fluid can result from factors such as systemic illness, infections or abnormalities of the reproductive tract, exposure to toxins, excessive alcohol consumption, illicit drug use, elevated scrotal temperature, obstruction, and immunologic factors.
5. Abnormal ovulation can occur because of hormone disruptions caused by cranial tumors, stress, obesity, anorexia, systemic disease, and abnormalities in the ovaries or other endocrine glands.
6. Ovulation disorders often are associated with abnormal menstrual periods because hormone abnormalities associated with the ovulation problem interfere with normal buildup and decline of the endometrium. Menstrual periods may be absent, scant, or very heavy.
7. Fallopian tube obstruction may be caused by scarring or adhesions secondary to infections, endometriosis, or pelvic surgery. Congenital anomalies of the reproductive structures also can cause mechanical interference with successful pregnancy.
8. Abnormal cervical mucus can trap sperm and prevent them from entering the uterus and fallopian tube or prevent their preparation (capacitation) for fertilization.
9. Anatomic abnormalities of the woman's reproductive tract may prevent normal fertilization or implantation. They also may prevent normal placental or fetal growth.
10. Endocrine abnormalities associated with repeated pregnancy loss include inadequate progesterone secretion, inadequate endometrial response to progesterone, hypothyroidism and hyperthyroidism, and maternal diabetes.
11. Immunologic causes of repeated pregnancy loss include an intolerance of the embryo's foreign tissue and lupus erythematosus.
12. Elements included in the history and physical examination include a reproductive history, past medical history, examination for undiagnosed endocrine disturbances, tumors, chronic disease, and abnormalities of the reproductive organs. Chromosome analysis is sometimes done.
13. Medications used to induce ovulation include clomiphene citrate, chorionic gonadotropin, gonadotropic-releasing hormone, menotropins, and urofollitropin. Clomiphene is a common drug for this purpose.
14. Screening tests related to use of donor sperm include those for blood type and Rh factor, possible genetic defects, and infection. In addition, the man's history, physical examination, and lifestyle are reviewed for possible problems that might not be revealed by standard tests. Donor sperm are frozen for 6 months to allow identification of infections or other problems that are evident at the time of collection.
15. In vitro fertilization mixes the male and female gametes outside the body and places embryos back into the uterus. Gamete intrafallopian transfer retrieves ova, then places the ova and sperm into the fallopian tubes, where fertilization takes place. Tubal embryo transfer mixes male and female gametes to allow fertilization and places the fertilized ova into the fallopian tubes.
16. Factors that couples consider when seeking infertility help include their age, the length of their attempt to conceive, their desire for a biologic child, and their feelings about adoption or a child-free life. Financial constraints often are another consideration.
17. When deciding about infertility evaluations and treatments, the couple considers their social, cultural, and religious values; how difficult treatment may be; the probability of success with treatment; and financial concerns.
18. Psychological reactions to infertility include guilt, isolation, depression, or stress on the relationship.
19. Parenthood after infertility may be marked by anxiety about the pregnancy, loss of support from infertile couples, or unrealistic expectations about their parenting abilities.
20. Couples considering adoption must confront their personal preferences, limitations, and prejudices.
21. Couples who lose a pregnancy after a period of infertility often experience grief, but sometimes the grief is mixed with optimism because they were able to achieve pregnancy.

CHAPTER 33

1. The Women's Health Initiative will study the 4 major diseases that kill women: heart disease, breast cancer, colorectal cancer, and osteoporosis.
2. Family history is an important part of a health history to assess risk factors for conditions such as heart disease, breast and colon cancer, and osteoporosis.
3. When taking a sexual history, the nurse should ask about sexual activity, number of partners, age

when sexual activity began, method of contraception, and knowledge and measures used to protect self from sexually transmitted diseases (STDs).

4. Three screening procedures for cancer of the breast are breast self-examination, professional breast examination, and mammography.
5. Vulvar self-examination is recommended to detect signs of precancerous conditions or infections.
6. A Pap test is a cytology specimen of the superficial layers of the cervix and endocervix to detect precancerous and cancerous cells of the cervix.
7. Fecal occult blood testing is important to detect colon or rectal cancer.
8. Medical treatment of fibrocystic breast changes is rare because side effects of the drugs may be more distressing than the breast discomfort. If drugs are used, they may include medroxyprogesterone, tamoxifen, or danozol. Evening primrose oil is a botanical preparation that may help some women.
9. Ultrasound examination, fine needle aspiration biopsy, core needle biopsy, or surgical biopsy are used to determine whether a breast disorder is benign or malignant.
10. Major risk factors for breast cancer are gender (female), age (increases with age), mutations in certain genes (BRCA1, BRCA2, and p53) and a prior history of breast cancer.
11. Staging of breast cancer is important to determine the extent of the breast cancer and to plan appropriate therapy.
12. Adjuvant therapy is supportive or additional therapy recommended following surgery to improve the chance of long-term survival. Adjuvant therapy includes radiation therapy, chemotherapy, hormonal therapy, and immunotherapy.
13. Breasts may be reconstructed during the initial surgery or later. Two major methods are the tissue expansion method and autogenous grafts.
14. Preoperative teaching should include a description of the pressure dressing, portable suction apparatus, the wound, and any special exercises that may be recommended.
15. Discharge planning should emphasize the need for follow-up care, expected adjuvant therapy and its side effects, and signs and symptoms that should be reported to the physician. Referral to local support groups also may be helpful.
16. Although a woman may have the "classic" crushing chest pain that is associated with a myocardial infarction, she is more likely to have atypical pain that often is confused with other conditions, even by professionals. These symptoms include: fatigue, weakness; angina or pain at rest; dyspnea; dizziness or faintness; upper abdominal pain, heartburn, or loss of appetite; nausea, vomiting, or sweating; and pain in the upper body other than the chest (arm, neck, back, jaw, throat, tooth).
17. Measures to reduce the risk for coronary artery disease include: control of hypertension; diet and glucose control to maintain normal weight and optimum fat/cholesterol intake; increasing activity level; and for some women, low-dose aspirin therapy.
18. Primary amenorrhea describes menstruation that fails to occur within 2 years of breast development, usually between the ages of 10 and 16 years. Causes include hormonal imbalances, congenital anomalies, chromosomal defects, and systemic diseases as well as rigorous dieting and exercise. Treatment is aimed at identifying and treating the underlying cause. Secondary amenorrhea describes cessation of menstruation for a period of at least 6 months in a woman who has an established pattern of menstruation. Pregnancy is the most common cause. Added causes include systemic disorders, hormonal imbalances, low weight for height, stress, poor nutrition, drugs (such as oral contraceptives, antidepressants), and tumors of the ovary, pituitary, or adrenal gland. Once pregnancy is ruled out, treatment may include correction of the underlying cause, hormonal replacement therapy, and ovulation stimulation.
19. Possible causes of dysfunctional uterine bleeding include complications of pregnancy, malignant disorders, and systemic diseases, which require prompt treatment.
20. Primary dysmenorrhea is caused by excessive endometrial prostaglandin that diffuses into endometrial tissue, causing abnormal uterine contractions, uterine ischemia, and tissue hypoxia. Effective treatment includes rest, application of warmth, oral contraceptives, and prostaglandin inhibitors. Herbal remedies include black or blue cohosh, black haw, and valerian, but these should only be used with supervision because some are contraindicated in pregnancy.
21. Endometriosis lesions grow and proliferate during the follicular and luteal phases of the menstrual cycle and then slough during menstruation. The menstruation from endometriosis lesions occurs in a closed cavity, which causes pressure and pain on adjacent tissue. Endometriosis often is treated by interrupting the menstrual cycle and thus preventing bleeding into the pelvic cavity.
22. Side effects of danazol include headache, dizziness, irritability, decreased libido, and masculinizing effects. Most common side effects of GnRH agonists are hot flashes, vaginal dryness, decreased libido, and loss of bone mineral density.

23. Symptoms of premenstrual syndrome (PMS) must be cyclic and recur in the luteal phase of the menstrual cycle; the woman should be symptom free during the follicular phase; symptoms must be severe enough to alter the work, lifestyle, and relationships of the woman; and the diagnosis must be based on the woman's charting of her symptoms in a diary rather than by recall.
24. After clearance from their health care provider, the nurse may teach women exercise measures, dietary measures to reduce fluid retention (such as restricting salty or sweet foods), educating the family about how to relate to a woman who is very irritable, and helping the woman to make arrangements so that she can avoid harming her child.
25. Mifepristone, methotrexate, prostaglandins, and misoprostol may be used to induce a medical abortion.
26. The nurse should teach the woman self-care measures: observation for excessive bleeding or signs of infection, information about follow-up visits, and contraception information.
27. Without estrogen, the reproductive organs begin to atrophy and the vagina and labia are thinner and more fragile. The breasts become smaller and atrophy. Bladder changes associated with atrophy make the woman more vulnerable to cystitis. Total cholesterol and low-density lipoproteins ("bad" cholesterol) increase, while high-density lipoproteins ("good" cholesterol) decrease, increasing the woman's risk for coronary artery disease. Hot flashes occur because of vasomotor instability. Bone mineral loss accelerates in the first few years of the climacteric. Loss of estrogen also appears to increase the risk for Alzheimer's disease.
28. Depression, mood swings, and irritability are the most common psychological symptoms of menopause.
29. Estrogen replacement controls hot flashes, alleviates genital atrophy, and protects against coronary heart disease and osteoporosis. Estrogen replacement must begin early in the perimenopause to provide significant protection against osteoporosis. If the woman has a uterus, progesterone is given for part of the cycle to prevent excessive buildup of the endometrium.
30. Osteoporosis is called the "silent thief" because there are no signs or symptoms until fractures occur.
31. Osteoporosis can be prevented by hormonal replacement therapy, calcium and vitamin D supplementation, and exercise.
32. Nurses can help women with osteoporosis avoid falls by making their environment as safe as possible.
33. With a cystocele, the weakened upper anterior wall of the vagina cannot support the weight of urine, and the bladder protrudes downward into the vagina, resulting in incomplete emptying of the bladder and consequent cystitis and stress incontinence. With a rectocele, the rectum protrudes into the vagina as the upper posterior wall of the vagina becomes weakened, which may result in difficulty emptying the rectum.
34. Uterine prolapse is caused when the cardinal ligaments are unduly stretched during pregnancy and do not return to normal. This condition generally is treated surgically according to severity.
35. Pelvic exercises and bladder training may alleviate symptoms of pelvic floor relaxation and urinary incontinence. Additional measures include teaching about the need to maintain hydration, restrict alcohol and caffeine, and use of commercial products to protect the skin and prevent odor.
36. Signs and symptoms of leiomyomas are increased uterine size and excessive vaginal bleeding, which often results in anemia. Treatment depends on size, symptoms, and whether the woman desires more children. Treatment options include removal of the fibroids or hysterectomy.
37. Ultrasound is used to distinguish a fluid-filled ovarian cyst from a solid tumor, which necessitates additional evaluation.
38. Signs and symptoms that suggest cancer of the reproductive organs are irregular vaginal bleeding, unexplained postmenopausal bleeding, unusual vaginal discharge, dyspareunia, persistent vaginal itching, elevated or discolored lesions of the vulva, abdominal bloating, persistent constipation, anorexia, or nausea.
39. Cancer of the cervix can be treated by cryosurgery, destruction of tissue by laser, loop electrosurgical excision procedure (LEEP), surgical conization, or hysterectomy with chemotherapy for more advanced cases. Endometrial cancer is best treated with hysterectomy and bilateral salpingo-oophorectomy plus radiation. Radiation only may be used if the woman is a poor surgical candidate, as many are. Ovarian cancer is often treated by chemotherapy to reduce the tumor's size, followed by oophorectomy and more chemotherapy.
40. Pregnancy, diabetes mellitus, oral contraceptive use, and antibiotic therapy may result in vaginitis caused by *C. albicans.*
41. Candidiasis causes a thick, white discharge, often with "cottage-cheese" characteristics. Trichomoniasis causes a thin or frothy, malodorous, and yellow green or dirty gray discharge.
42. Barrier methods of contraception (particularly condoms) prevent potentially infected ejaculate from entering the genital tract and prevent contact between the penis and vagina.
43. The major symptom of primary syphilis is a painless chancre that disappears in about 6 weeks; the

disease is highly infectious at this time. Symptoms of secondary syphilis are enlargement of the liver and spleen, headache, anorexia, and skin rash. Condylomata lata that contain numerous spirochetes and are highly contagious may develop.

44. Condylomata acuminata (genital warts) are caused by human papillomavirus (HPV), which is associated with cervical cancer.
45. *Chlamydia trachomatis* and *Nisseria gonorrhoeae* cause more than 40% of the cases of pelvic inflammatory disease. Several other pathogens, including *E. coli, Gardnerella* species, and bacterial vaginosis, cause other cases.
46. The risk of toxic shock syndrome can be reduced by changing tampons every 1 to 4 hours, avoiding use of superabsorbent tampons, using pads rather than tampons during hours of sleep, and careful hand washing before and after inserting tampons or changing perineal pads.

Glossary

Abortion A pregnancy that ends before 20 weeks' gestation, either spontaneously or electively. **Miscarriage** is a lay term for a spontaneous abortion.

Abruptio placentae Premature separation of a normally implanted placenta.

Abstinence syndrome A group of symptoms that occur when a person who is addicted to a specific drug withdraws or abstains from taking that drug.

Acidosis A condition resulting from accumulation of acid (hydrogen ions) or depletion of base (bicarbonate). The pH measures acid-base balance.

Acme Peak, or period of greatest strength, of a uterine contraction.

Acquired immunodeficiency syndrome (AIDS) Syndrome caused by the human immunodeficiency virus (HIV), resulting in loss of defense against malignancies and opportunistic infections.

Acrocyanosis Bluish discoloration of the hands and feet due to reduced peripheral circulation.

Addiction Physical or psychological dependence on a substance such as alcohol, tobacco, or drugs, either legal or illicit.

Adjuvant therapy Additional treatment that increases or enhances the action of the primary treatment.

Adnexa Accessory organs of the uterus, such as the fallopian tubes and ovaries.

Afterpains Cramping pain following childbirth caused by alternate relaxation and contraction of uterine muscles.

Agonist A substance that causes a physiologic effect.

Alcoholism A chronic, progressive, and potentially fatal disease characterized by tolerance for and physical dependence on alcohol or by pathologic organ changes due to alcohol abuse, or both.

Allele An alternate form of a gene.

Alpha-fetoprotein (AFP) Plasma protein produced by the fetus.

Ambiguity (ambiguous) Lack of clarity or certainty; having more than one meaning.

Ambivalence Simultaneous conflicting emotions, attitudes, ideas, or wishes.

Amenorrhea Absence of menstruation. **Primary amenorrhea** is a delay of the first menstruation. **Secondary amenorrhea** is cessation of menstruation after its initiation.

Amniocentesis Transabdominal puncture of the amniotic sac to obtain a sample of amniotic fluid that contains fetal cells and biochemical substances for laboratory examination.

Amnioinfusion Infusion of lactated Ringer's solution or isotonic saline into the uterine cavity during labor to reduce umbilical cord compression; also done to dilute meconium in amniotic fluid, reducing the risk that the infant will aspirate thick meconium at birth.

Amnionitis See **Chorioamnionitis.**

Amniotic fluid embolism An embolism in which amniotic fluid with its particulate matter is drawn into the pregnant woman's circulation, lodging in her lungs.

Amniotomy Artificial rupture of the amniotic sac (fetal membranes).

Amphetamines Central nervous system stimulants that create a perception of pleasure that is unrelated to external stimuli.

Analgesic A systemic agent that relieves pain without loss of consciousness.

Anencephaly Absence of the cranial vault and all or most of the cerebral hemispheres; a form of neural tube defect.

Anesthesia Loss of sensation, especially to pain, with or without loss of consciousness.

Anesthesiologist A physician who specializes in administration of anesthesia.

Anorexia nervosa Refusal to eat because of a distorted body image and a concern about obesity.

Anovulatory (or **Anovular**) Menstrual cycles occurring without ovulation.

Antagonist A drug that blocks the action of another drug or of body secretions.

Antepartum Term describing the pregnant woman before the onset of labor.

Antiphospholipid antibodies Autoimmune antibodies directed against phospholipids in cell membranes; associated with recurrent spontaneous abortion, fetal loss, and severe pregnancy-induced hypertension.

Apneic spells Cessation of breathing for more than 15 seconds, accompanied by cyanosis or bradycardia.

Asphyxia Insufficient oxygen and excess carbon dioxide in the blood and tissues.

Aspiration pneumonitis A chemical injury to the lungs that may occur with regurgitation and aspiration of acidic gastric secretions.

Assumptions Beliefs taken for granted without examination.

Atony Absence or lack of usual muscle tone.

Atrophic vaginitis Inflammation that occurs when the vagina becomes dry and fragile, usually as a result of estrogen deficit after menopause.

Attachment Development of strong affectional ties as a result of interaction between an infant and a significant other (mother, father, sibling, caretaker).

Attenuate To weaken.

Attitude Relationship of fetal body parts to one another.

Augmentation of labor Artificial stimulation of uterine contractions that have become ineffective.

Autogenous graft Tissue that is moved from one part of the body to another part of the same person's body.

Autosome Any of the 22 pairs of **chromosomes** other than the **sex chromosomes.**

Axillary tail Wedge of tissue extending from the breast into the axilla (also called the *tail of Spence*).

Azoospermia Absence of sperm in semen.

Baroreceptors Cells that are sensitive to blood pressure changes.

Basal body temperature Body temperature at rest.

Baseline data Information that describes the status of the client before treatment begins.

Bias A prejudice that sways the mind.

Bicornuate (Bicornate) Malformed uterus having two horns.

Bilirubin Unusable component of hemolyzed erythrocytes.

Bilirubin encephalopathy Brain damage resulting from deposits of unconjugated bilirubin in the brain tissue.

Bioethics Rules or principles that govern right conduct, specifically those that relate to health care.

Biophysical profile (BPP) Method for evaluating fetal status during the antepartum period based on five variables originating with the fetus: fetal heart rate, breathing movements, gross movements, muscle tone, and amniotic fluid volume.

Birth defect An abnormality of structure, function, or body metabolism that often results in a physical or mental handicap, shortens life, or is fatal (according to the March of Dimes Birth Defects Foundation).

Birth plan A plan describing a couple's preferences for their birth experience.

Bloody show Mixture of cervical mucus and blood from ruptured capillaries in the cervix; often precedes labor and increases with cervical dilation.

Body image Subjective image of one's physical appearance and capabilities, derived from own observations and from the evaluation of significant others.

Bonding Development of a strong emotional tie of a parent to a newborn; also called *claiming* or *binding-in.*

Braxton Hicks contractions Irregular, mild uterine contractions that occur throughout pregnancy; they become stronger in the last trimester.

Bronchopulmonary dysplasia (BPD) Chronic pulmonary condition in which damage to the infant's lungs requires prolonged dependence on supplemental oxygen.

Brown fat (or brown adipose tissue) Highly vascular specialized fat found in the newborn that provides more heat than other fat when metabolized.

Bulimia Eating disorder characterized by ingestion of large amounts of food, followed by purging behavior such as induced vomiting or laxative abuse.

Café au lait spots Light brown birthmarks.

Calorie See **Kilocalorie.**

Caput succedaneum Area of edema over the presenting part of the fetus or newborn resulting from pressure against the cervix. Often called simply *caput.*

Carcinoma in situ Malignant neoplasm in surface tissue that has not extended into deeper tissue.

Cardiac decompensation Failure of the heart to maintain adequate circulation to the tissues. See also **Congestive heart failure.**

Catabolism A destructive process that converts living cells into simpler compounds; process involved in **involution** (changes) of the uterus after childbirth.

Caudal regressive syndrome A severe malformation that results when the sacrum, lumbar spine, and lower extremities fail to develop.

Cephalhematoma Bleeding between the periosteum and skull from pressure during birth. It does not cross suture lines.

Cephalopelvic disproportion (CPD) Fetal head size that is too large to fit through the maternal pelvis at birth. Also called *fetopelvic disproportion.*

Cerclage Encircling of the cervix with suture to prevent recurrent spontaneous abortion caused by early cervical dilation.

Cerebrospinal fluid (CSF) Clear fluid that bathes and cushions the brain and spinal cord.

Certified nurse-midwife (CNM) A registered nurse who has completed a nurse-midwifery program approved by the American College of Nurse-Midwives (ACNM) and passed the ACNM National Certification Examination.

Cervical cap A small cup-like device placed over the cervix to prevent sperm from entering, thus preventing pregnancy.

Cesarean birth Surgical birth of the fetus through an incision in the abdominal wall and uterus.

Chadwick's sign Bluish discoloration of the cervix, vagina, and labia during pregnancy as a result of increased vascular congestion.

Chemoreceptors Cells that are sensitive to chemical changes in the blood, specifically changes in oxygen and carbon dioxide levels, and in acid-base balance.

Chignon Newborn scalp edema created by a vacuum extractor.

Chloasma Brownish pigmentation of the face during pregnancy; also called "mask of pregnancy."

Choanal atresia Abnormality of the nasal septum that obstructs one or both nasal passages.

Chorioamnionitis Inflammation of the amniotic sac (fetal membranes); usually caused by bacterial or viral infection. Also called **amnionitis.**

Chorionic villus sampling Transcervical or transabdominal sampling of chorionic villi (projections of the outer fetal membrane) for analysis of fetal cells.

Chromosomal sex See **Genetic sex.**

Chromosome Thread of DNA (deoxyribonucleic acid) in the cell nucleus that transmits genetic (hereditary) information.

Cilia Hair-like processes on the surface of a cell. Cilia beat rhythmically to move a cell or to move fluid or other substances over the cell surface.

Cleansing breath A deep breath taken at the beginning and end of each labor contraction.

Climacteric Endocrine, body, and psychic changes occurring at the end of a woman's reproductive period. Also informally called **menopause.**

Coitus Sexual union between a male and a female.

Coitus interruptus Withdrawal of the penis from the vagina before ejaculation.

Colostrum Breat fluid secreted during pregnancy and the first 2 to 3 days following childbirth.

Colposcopy Examination of the vaginal and cervical tissue with a colposcope for magnification of cells.

Complete protein food Food containing all the essential amino acids.

Compliance Stretchability or elasticity of the lungs and thorax that allows distention without resistance during respirations. Also, adherence of the client to a therapeutic plan.

Conceptus Cells and membranes resulting from fertilization of the ovum at any stage of prenatal development.

Condom Latex, polyurethane, or natural membrane shield covering the penis or lining the vagina to prevent sperm from entering the cervix or to prevent infection, or both.

Condyloma A wart-like growth of the skin seen on the external genitalia, in the vagina, on the cervix, or near the anus; may be caused by human papillomavirus (condyloma acuminatum) or by syphilis (condyloma latum).

Congenital Present at birth.

Congenital anomaly Abnormal intrauterine development of an organ or structure.

Congestive heart failure Condition resulting from failure of the heart to maintain adequate circulation; characterized by weakness, dyspnea, and edema in body parts that are lower than the heart.

Containment A method of increasing comfort in infants by using swaddling or other methods to keep the extremities in a flexed position near the body.

Contraception Prevention of pregnancy.

Contraction stress test (CST) Method for evaluating fetal status during the antepartum period by observing response of the fetal heart to the stress of uterine contractions that may induce recurrent episodes of fetal hypoxia.

Cordocentesis See **Percutaneous umbilical blood sampling.**

Corpus luteum Graafian follicle cells remaining after ovulation that produce estrogen and progesterone.

Corrected gestational age Gestational age that a preterm infant would be if still in utero. May also be called *developmental age.*

Couvade Pregnancy-related rituals or a cluster of symptoms experienced by some prospective fathers during pregnancy and childbirth.

Crack A highly addictive form of cocaine that has been processed to be smoked.

Cradle cap See **Seborrheic dermatitis.**

Craniosynostosis Premature closure of the sutures of the infant's head.

Crowning Appearance of the fetal scalp or presenting part at the vaginal opening.

Cryotherapy Destruction of tissue using extreme cold.

Cryptorchidism Failure of one or both testes to descend into the scrotum.

Cul-de-sac See **Fornix.**

Culdocentesis Needle puncture through the upper posterior vaginal wall (cul-de-sac of Douglas) to aspirate blood or fluid from the pelvic cavity.

Culture Sum of values, beliefs, and practices of a group of people that are transmitted from one generation to the next.
Cystocele Prolapse of the urinary bladder through the anterior vaginal wall.
Decidua Name applied to the endometrium during pregnancy; all except the deepest layer is shed after childbirth.
Decrement Period of decreasing strength of a uterine contraction.
Delegated nursing interventions Physician-prescribed nursing actions that require nursing judgment because nurses are accountable for correct implementation. See also **Independent nursing interventions.**
Deontologic theory Ethical theory holding that the right course of action is the one dictated by ethical principles and moral rules.
Developmental task A necessary step in growth and maturation that one must complete before additional growth and maturation are possible.
Diabetes mellitus A disorder of carbohydrate metabolism caused by a relative or complete lack of insulin secretion. Characterized by *glycosuria* (glucose in the urine) and **hyperglycemia.**
Diabetogenic Condition, such as pregnancy, that produces the effects of diabetes mellitus.
Diagnostic statement A phrase that describes a health problem; usually ocnsists of a category label plus the etiology or contributing factors. It may also describe manifestations.
Diaphragm A contraceptive device consisting of a latex dome that covers the cervix and prevents entrance of sperm; must be used with spermicide to be effective.
Diastasis recti Separation of the longitudinal muscles of the abdomen (rectus abdominis) during pregnancy.
Dilation and curettage (D&C) Stretching of the cervical os to permit suctioning or scraping of the walls of the uterus. The procedure is performed in abortion, to obtain samples of uterine lining tissue for laboratory examination, and during the postpartum period to remove retained fragments of placenta.
Dilation and evacuation (D&E) Wide cervical dilation followed by mechanical destruction and removal of fetal parts from the uterus. Following complete removal of the fetus, a vacuum curet is used to remove the placenta and remaining products of conception.
Diploid Having a pair of chromosomes (46 in humans) that represents one copy of every chromosome from each parent; the number of chromosomes normally present in body cells other than **gametes.**
Disturbance in body image Negative feelings about characteristics, functions, or limits of one's body.
Duration Period from the beginning of a uterine contraction to the end of the same contraction.
Dysmenorrhea Painful menstruation.
Dyspareunia Difficult or painful coitus in women.
Dysplasia Abnormal development of tissue.
Dystocia Difficult or prolonged labor; often associated with abnormal uterine activity and **cephalopelvic disproportion.**
Dysuria Painful urination, often associated with urinary tract infection.
Early deceleration Slowing of the fetal heart rate that occurs during the uterine contraction.
Eclampsia Convulsive form of pregancy-induced hypertension.
Ectopic pregnancy Implantation of a fertilized ovum in any area other than the uterus; the most common site is in the fallopian tube.
EDD Abbreviation for estimated date of delivery; this date may also be abbreviated **EDB** (estimated date of birth)
Effleurage Massage of the abdomen or other body part performed during labor contractions.
Egocentrism Interest centered on the self rather than on the needs of others.
Ejaculation Expulsion of **semen** from the penis.
Embolus A clot, usually part or all of a **thrombus,** brought by the blood from another vessel and forced into a smaller one, thus obstructing circulation.
Embryo The developing baby from the beginning of the third week through the eighth week after conception.
Endometrial hyperplasia Excessive proliferation of normal cells of the uterine lining; may be due to administration of estrogen during the postmenopausal period.
Endometriosis Presence of tissue resembling endometrium outside the uterine cavity.
Endometrium Lining of the uterus.
Endorphins Morphine-like substances that occur naturally in the central nervous system and modify pain sensations.
En face Position that allows eye-to-eye contact between the newborn and a parent; optimal distance is 20 to 22 cm (8 to 9 inches).
Engagement Descent of the widest diameter of the fetal presenting part to at least a zero **station** (the level of the ischial spines in the maternal pelvis).
Engorgement Swelling of the breasts resulting from feedings that are delayed, too short, or not frequent enough.
Engrossment Intense fascination and close face-to-face observation between father and newborn.
Enternal feeding Nutrients suupplied to the gastrointestinal tract orally or by feeding tube.
Entrainment Newborn movement in rhythm to adult speech, particularly high-pitched tones, which are more easily heard.
Epidural space The area outside the dura, between the dura mater and the vertebral canal.
Episiotomy Surgical incision of the perineum to enlarge the vaginal opening.
Epispadias Abnormal placement of the urinary meatus on the dorsal side of the penis.
Erythema toxicum Benign rash of unknown cause in newborns with blotchy red areas that may have white or yellow papules in the center.
Erythroblastosis fetalis Agglutination and hemolysis of fetal erythrocytes due to incompatibility between maternal and fetal blood. In most cases, the fetus is Rh-positive and the mother is Rh-negative.
Esophageal atresia Condition in which the esophagus is separated from the stomach and ends in a blind pouch.
Essential amino acids Amino acids that cannot be synthesized by the body and must be obtained from foods.
Ethical dilemma A situation in which no solution seems completely satisfactory.
Ethics Rules or principles that govern right conduct and distinctions between right and wrong.
Ethnic Pertaining to religious, racial, national, or cultural group characteristics, especially speech patterns, social customs, and physical characteristics.
Ethnicity Condition of belonging to a particular **ethnic** group; also refers to ethnic pride.
Ethnocentrism Opinion that the beliefs and customs of one's own ethnic group are superior.
Euglycemia Normal blood glucose level.
Extrusion reflex Automatic nervous system response that causes an infant to push anything solid out of the mouth.
Familial Presence of a trait or condition in a family more often than would be expected by chance alone.
Fantasy Mental images formed to prepare for the birth of a child.
Ferning (or **fern test**) Microscopic appearance of amniotic fluid that resembles fern leaves when the fluid is allowed to dry on a microscopic slide. Used to determine whether the woman's membranes have ruptured. Also describes the microscopic fern-like appearance of dried cervical mucus that is most apparent at the time of ovulation.

Fertilization age Prenatal age of the developing baby calculated from the date of conception. Also called **post-conceptional age.**
Fetal alcohol syndrome A group of physical and mental disorders of the offspring associated with maternal use of alcohol during pregnancy.
Fetal lung fluid Fluid that fills the fetal lungs, expanding the alveoli and promoting lung development.
Fetus The developing baby from 9 weeks after conception until birth. In everyday practice, this term is often used to describe a developing baby during pregnancy, regardless of age.
FHR Abbreviation for fetal heart rate.
Finger-tipping First tactile (touch) experience between mother and newborn; the mother explores the infant's body with her fingertips only.
First period of reactivity Period beginning at birth in which newborns are active and alert. It ends when the infant first falls asleep.
Fontanelle Space at the intersection of sutures connecting fetal or infant skull bones.
Foremilk First breast milk received in a feeding.
Fornix (pl. **fornices**) An arch or pouch-like structure at the upper end of the vagina. Also called a **cul-de-sac.**
Fourth trimester First 12 weeks following birth; a time of transition for parents and siblings.
Frequency Period from the beginning of one uterine contraction until the beginning of the next.
Fundus Part of the uterus that is farthest from the cervix, above the openings of the fallopian tubes.
Gamete Reproductive cell; in the female an **ovum,** and in the male a **spermatozoon.**
Gametogenesis Development and maturation of the **sperm** and **ova.**
Gastroschisis Protrusion of the intestines through a defect in the abdominal wall. Intestines are not covered by a peritoneal sac or skin.
General anesthesia Systemic loss of sensation with loss of consciousness.
Genetic Pertaining to the genes or the chromosomes.
Genetic sex Sex determined at conception by union of two X chromosomes (female) or an X and a Y chromosome (male). Also called **chromosomal sex.**
Genogram See **Pedigree.**
Genotype Genetic makeup of an individual.
Gestational age Prenatal age of the developing baby (measured in weeks) calculated from the first day of the woman's last menstrual period. Also called **menstrual age.** About 2 weeks longer than the **fertilization age.**
Gestational diabetes Impared glucose tolerance that is induced by pregnancy and diagnosed during pregnancy. Usually disappears after childbirth.
Gestational surrogate A woman who carries the embryo of an infertile couple and relinquishes the child after birth.
Gestational trophoblastic disease A spectrum of diseases that includes benign hydatidiform mole and gestational trophoblastic tumors, such as invasive moles and choriocarcinoma.
Gluconeogenesis Formation of glycogen by the liver from noncarbohydrate sources, such as amino or fatty acids.
Gonad Reproductive (sex) gland that produces gametes and sex hormones. The female gonads are *ovaries;* the male gonads are *testes.*
Gonadotropic hormones Secretions of the anterior pituitary gland that stimulate the gonads, specifically follicle-stimulating hormone and luteinizing hormone. Chorionic gonadotropin is secreted by the placenta during pregnancy.
Goodell's sign Softening of the cervix, uterus, and vagina during pregnancy.
Graafian follicle A small sac within the ovary that contains the maturing ovum.
Gravida A pregnant woman. Also refers to a woman's total number of pregnancies, including the one in progress, if applicable.
Gynecologic age The number of years since menarche (first menstrual period).
Habituation Decreased response to a repeated stimulus.
Haploid Having one copy of a chromosome from each pair (23 in humans, or half the diploid number). **Gametes** normally have a haploid number of chromosomes.
Hematoma Localized collection of blood in a space of tissue.
Heme iron Iron obtained from meat, poultry, or fish sources; the form most usable by the body.
Heterozygous Having two different **alleles** for a genetic trait.
Hindmilk Breast milk received nearer the end of a feeding; contains higher fat content than **foremilk.**
Homozygous Having two identical **alleles** for a genetic trait.
Hormone implant Small capsules of progestin inserted subcutaneously to provide contraception.
Human immunodeficiency virus (HIV) A retrovirus that results in the development of AIDS (see **Acquired immunodeficiency syndrome**).
Hydatidiform mole Abnormal pregnancy resulting from proliferation of chorionic villi that give rise to multiple cysts and rapid growth of the uterus.
Hydramnios Excess volume of amniotic fluid (more than 2000 ml at term). Also called **polyhydramnios.**
Hydrops fetalis Heart failure and generalized edema in the fetus secondary to severe anemia resulting from destruction of erythrocytes.
Hyperbilirubinemia Excessive amount of bilirubin in the blood.
Hypercapnia Excess carbon dioxide in the blood, evidenced by an elevated P_{CO_2}.
Hyperemia Excess of blood in a part of the body.
Hyperglycemia An abnormally high blood glucose level.
Hypertonic contractions Uterine contractions that are too long or too frequent, have too short a resting interval, or have an inadequate relaxation period to allow optimal uteroplacental exchange.
Hypertonic labor dysfunction Ineffective labor characterized by erratic and poorly coordinated contractions. **Uterine resting tone** is higher than normal.
Hypoglycemia An abnormally low blood glucose level.
Hypospadias Abnormal placement of the urinary meatus on the ventral side of the penis.
Hypotonic labor dysfunction Ineffective labor characterized by weak, infrequent, and brief but coordinated uterine contractions. **Uterine resting tone** is normal.
Hypovolemia Abnormally decreased volume of circulating fluid in the body.
Hypovolemic shock Acute peripheral circulatory failure due to loss of circulating blood volume.
Hypoxemia Reduced oxygenation of the blood, evidenced by a low P_{O_2}.
Hypoxia Reduced availability of oxygen to the body tissues.
Iatrogenic An adverse condition resulting from treatment.
Impotence Inability of a man to achieve or maintain an erection of the penis that is sufficiently rigid to permit successful sexual intercourse.
Incompetent cervix Inability of the cervix to remain closed long enough during pregnancy for the fetus to survive.
Incomplete protein food Food that does not contain all the essential amino acids.
Increment Period of increasing strength of a uterine contraction.
Independent nursing interventions Nurse-prescribed actions used in both nursing diagnosis and collaborative problems. See also **Delegated nursing interventions.**
Induction of labor Artificial initiation of labor.
Infant mortality rate Number of deaths per 1000 live births that occurs within the first 12 months of life.

Inference The act of drawing a conclusion or making a deduction.

Infertility Inability of a couple to conceive after 1 year of regular intercourse (two to three times weekly) without using contraception; also, the involuntary inability to conceive and produce viable offspring when the couple chooses. **Primary infertility** occurs in a couple who has never conceived; **secondary infertility** occurs in a couple who has conceived at least once before.

Intensity Strength of a uterine contraction.

Intermittent monitoring A variation of electronic fetal monitoring in which an initial strip is obtained on admission. If patterns are reassuring, the woman is remonitored for 15 minutes at regular intervals (about every 30 to 60 minutes).

Interval Period between the end of one uterine contraction and the beginning of the next.

Intrapartum Term describing the time of labor and childbirth.

Intrauterine device (IUD) A mechanical device inserted into the uterus to prevent pregnancy.

Intrauterine growth restriction (IUGR) Failure of a fetus to grow as expected for gestational age. May also be called *intrauterine growth retardation.*

Intraventricular hemorrhage (IVH) Bleeding into the ventricles of the brain.

Introversion Inward concentration on oneself and one's body.

Involution Retrogressive changes that return the reproductive organs, particularly the uterus, to their pre-pregnancy size and condition.

Jaundice Yellow discoloration of the skin and sclera caused by excessive bilirubin in the blood.

Judgment An opinion.

Karyotype A photomicrograph of a cell's chromosomes, arranged from largest to smallest pairs.

Kegel exercises Alternate contracting and relaxing of the pelvic muscles; these movements strengthen the pubococcygeal muscle, which surrounds the urinary meatus and vagina.

Kernicterus Staining of brain tissue caused by accumulation of unconjugated bilirubin in the brain.

Ketosis Accumulation of ketone bodies (metabolic products) in the blood; frequently associated with acidosis.

Kilocalorie A unit of heat; used to show the energy value in foods; commonly called **calorie**

Lactation Secretion of milk from the breasts; also describes the time when a child is breastfed.

Lacto-ovovegetarian A **vegetarian** whose diet includes milk products and eggs.

Lactose intolerance Inability to digest most dairy products because of a lack of the enzyme lactase.

Lactovegetarian A **vegetarian** whose diet includes milk products.

Laminaria Slender cones of prepared seaweed or a similar substance inserted into the cervix to dilate it as they absorb water.

Lanugo Fine, soft hair covering the fetus.

Laparoscopy Insertion of an illuminated tube into the abdominal cavity to visualize contents, locate bleeding, and perform surgical procedures.

Laparotomy Incision through the abdominal wall to examine the abdominal or pelvic organs.

Large-for-gestational age (LGA) infant An infant whose size is above the 90th percentile for gestational age.

Latch-on Attachment of the infant to the breast.

Late deceleration Slowing of the fetal heart rate after the onset of a uterine contraction and persisting after the contraction ends.

Lecithin/sphingomyelin ratio (L/S ratio) Ratio of two phospholipids in amniotic fluid that is used to determine fetal lung maturity; an L/S ratio greater than 2:1 usually indicates fetal lung maturity.

Let-down reflex See **Milk-ejection reflex.**

Letting-go A phase of maternal adaptation that involves relinquishment of previous roles and assumption of a new role as a parent.

Libido Sexual desire.

Lie Relationship of the long axis of the fetus to the long axis of the mother.

Lightening Descent of the fetus toward the pelvic inlet before labor.

Linear salpingostomy Incision along the length of a fallopian tube to remove an ectopic pregnancy and preserve the tube.

Lipogenic Substance, such as insulin, that stimulates the production of fat.

Lochia Vaginal drainage after birth.

Lochia alba Whitish or clear vaginal discharge that follows **lochia serosa;** occurs when the amount of blood is decreased and the number of leukocytes is increased.

Lochia rubra Reddish vaginal discharge that occurs immediately after childbirth; composed mostly of blood.

Lochia serosa Pinkish or brown-tinged vaginal discharge that follows **lochia rubra** and precedes **lochia alba;** composed largely of serous exudate, blood, and leukocytes.

Low-birth-weight (LBW) infant An infant weighing less than 2500 g at birth.

Maceration Discoloration and softening of tissues and eventual disintegration of a fetus that is retained in the uterus after its death.

Macrosomia Unusually large fetal size; infant birth weight more than 4000 g.

Malpractice Negligence by a professional person.

Mammogram Study of breast tissue using very-low-dose x-ray; primary tool in the discovery of breast tumors.

Marfan's syndrome A hereditary condition that involves weakness in connective tissue, bones, and muscles; the vascular system is affected, particularly the aorta.

Mastitis Inflammation of the breast, usually caused by stasis of milk in the ducts or by infection.

Maternal mortality rate Number of maternal deaths from births and complications of pregnancy, childbirth, and puerperium (the first 42 days after termination of the pregnancy) per 100,000 live births.

Mature milk Breast milk that appears after the first 2 weeks of lactation.

Meconium aspiration syndrome Obstruction and air trapping due to meconium in the infant's lungs, which may cause severe respiratory distress.

Meiosis Reduction cell division in **gametes** that halves the number of chromosomes in each cell.

Menarche Onset of menstruation; average age is 13 years.

Meningocele Protrusion of the meninges through a defect in the vertebrae; a form of **neural tube defect.**

Menometrorrhagia Uterine bleeding that is irregular in frequency and also excessive in amount.

Menopause Permanent cessation of menstruation during the **climacteric.**

Menorrhagia Excessive bleeding at the time of menstruation in number of days' duration, amount of blood lost, or both.

Menstrual age See **Gestational age.**

Methadone A synthetic compound with opiate properties. Used as an oral substitute for heroin and morphine in the opiate-addicted person.

Metrorrhagia Bleeding from the uterus at any time other than during the menstrual period.

Milia White cysts, 1 to 2 mm in size, from distended sebaceous glands.

Miliaria (prickly heat) Rash caused by heat.

Milk-ejection reflex Release of milk from the alveoli into the ducts; also known as the **let-down reflex.**

Mimicry Copying the behaviors of other pregnant women or mothers as a method of "trying on" the role of advanced pregnancy or motherhood.

Miscarriage See **Abortion.**

Mitosis Cell division in body cells other than the **gametes.**

Mittelschmerz Low abdominal pain that occurs at **ovulation.**

Molding Shaping of the fetal head during movement through the birth canal.

Mongolian spots Bruise-like marks that occur mostly in newborns with dark skin tones.

Monosomy Presence of only one of a chromosome pair in every body cell.

Motor block Loss of voluntary movement caused by **regional anesthesia.**

Multifetal pregnancy A pregnancy in which the woman is carrying two or more fetuses. Also called **multiple gestation.**

Multipara A woman who has given birth after two or more pregnancies of at least 20 weeks of gestation. Also informally used to describe a pregnant woman before the birth of her second child.

Multiple gestation See **Multifetal pregnancy.**

Mutation Variation in a gene that affects its function.

Myelomeningocele Protrusion of the meninges and spinal cord through a defect in the vertebrae; a form of **neural tube defect.**

Myometrium Uterine muscle.

Narcissism Undue preoccupation with oneself.

Natural family planning Method of predicting **ovulation** based on normal changes in a woman's body.

Necrotizing enterocolitis (NEC) A condition of injury, invasion by bacteria, and possible necrosis of the intestines.

Negligence Failure to act in the way a reasonable, prudent person of similar background would act in similar circumstances.

Neonatal abstinence syndrome A cluster of physical signs exhibited by the newborn who was exposed in utero to maternal use of substances such as methadone or heroin. See also **Abstinence syndrome.**

Neonatal mortality rate Number of deaths per 1000 live births occurring at birth or within the first 28 days of life.

Neonatologist A physician who specializes in the care of newborn infants (from birth until the 29th day of life).

Neural tube defect A congenital defect in closure of the bony encasement of the spinal cord or of the skull. Neural tube defects include **anencephaly, spina bifida, meningocele, myelomeningocele,** and others.

Neutral thermal environment Environment in which body temperature is maintained without an increase in metabolic rate or oxygen use.

Nevus flammeus Permanent purple birthmark. Also called *port wine stain.*

Nevus vasculosus Rough red collection of capillaries with a raised surface that disappears with time.

Nidation Implantation of the fertilized ovum **(zygote)** in the uterine endometrium.

Nitrazine paper Paper used to determine pH; helps to determine whether the amniotic sac has ruptured.

Noncompliance Resistance of the lungs and thorax to distention with air during respirations. Also, failure of the client to adhere to a therapeutic plan.

Non-heme iron Iron obtained from plant sources.

Non-nutritive sucking Sucking during which no milk flow is obtained.

Nonshivering thermogenesis Process of heat production, without shivering, by oxidation of **brown fat.**

Nonstress test A method for evaluating fetal status during the antepartum period by observing the response of the fetal heart rate to fetal movement.

Nuchal cord Umbilical cord around the fetal neck.

Nullipara A woman who has not completed a pregnancy to at least 20 weeks' gestation.

Nurse-anesthetist A registered nurse who has advanced education and certification in administration of anesthetics. Also *certified registered nurse anesthetist* (CRNA).

Nurse-midwife See **Certified nurse-midwife.**

Nurse practice acts Laws that determine the scope of nursing practice in each state.

Nutrient density The quality of protein, vitamins, and minerals per 100 calories in foods.

Nutritive suckling or sucking Steady rhythmic suckling at the breast or sucking at a bottle to obtain milk.

Occult prolapse See **Prolapsed cord.**

Oligohydramnios Abnormally small quanitity of amniotic fluid (less than 500 ml at term).

Oligospermia A decreased number of sperm in semen, usually considered to be under 20 million per milliliter.

Omphalocele Protrusion of the intestines into the base of the umbilical cord. Intestines are covered by a peritoneal sac. May be associated with other anomalies.

Oogenesis Formation of **gametes (ova)** in the female.

Opiate Any narcotic containing opium or a derivative of opium.

Oral contraceptive Drug that inhibits ovulation; contains progestins alone or in combination with estrogen.

Osmotic diuresis Secretion and passage of large amounts of urine as a result of increased osmotic pressure that can result from **hyperglycemia.**

Osteoporosis Increased spaces (porosity) in bone; process greatly accelerates following menopause.

Ovovegetarian A vegetarian whose diet includes eggs.

Ovulation Release of the mature **ovum** from the ovary.

Ovum (pl. **ova**) Female **gamete,** or sex cell.

Oxytocin Hormone produced by the posterior pituitary gland that stimulates uterine contractions and the **milk-ejection reflex;** also prepared synthetically.

Paced breathing Learned breathing technique used during labor contractions to promote relaxation and increase pain tolerance.

Pain threshold (or **pain perception**) The lowest level of stimulus one perceives as painful. Pain threshold is relatively constant under different conditions.

Pain tolerance Maximum pain one is willing to endure. Pain tolerance may increase or decrease under different conditions.

Para A woman who has given birth after a pregnancy of at least 20 weeks' gestation. Also designates the number of a woman's pregnancies that have ended after at least 20 weeks of gestation. (A multifetal gestation, such as twins, is considered one birth when calculating parity.)

Parenteral nutrition Intravenous infusion of all nutrients needed for metabolism and growth.

Peau d'orange Dimpled skin condition that resembles an orange; associated with lymphatic edema and often seen over the area of breast cancer.

Pedigree A graphic representation of a family's medical and hereditary history and the relationships among the family members. May be called a **genogram.**

Percutaneous umbilical blood sampling (PUBS or **cordocentesis)** Procedure for obtaining fetal blood through ultrasound-guided puncture of an umbilical cord vessel to detect fetal problems such as inherited blood disorders, acidosis, or infection.

Perinatologist A physician who specializes in the care of the mother, the fetus, and the infant during the perinatal period (from the 20th week of pregnancy to 4 weeks after childbirth).

Periodic breathing Cessation of breathing lasting no more than 10 seconds without changes in color or heart rate.

Periventricular-intraventricular hemorrhage (PIVH) Bleeding into and around the ventricles of the brain.

Persistent fetal circulation Failure of the pulmonary vessels to dilate and the ductus arteriosus to close; caused by low blood oxygen levels.

Persistent pulmonary hypertension Vasoconstriction of the infant's pulmonary vessels after birth; may result in right-to-left shunting of blood flow through the ductus arteriosus, the foramen ovale, or both.

Phenotype The outward expression of one's genetic makeup.

Phosphatidylglycerol (PG) A major phospholipid of **surfactant;** its presence in amniotic fluid indicates fetal lung maturity.

Phosphatidylinositol (PI) A phospholipid of **surfactant;** produced and secreted in increasing amounts as the fetal lungs mature. Its presence in amniotic fluid indicates fetal lung maturity.

Physiologic anemia of pregnancy Decrease in hematocrit values caused by dilution of erythrocytes by expanded plasma volume rather than by an actual decrease in erythrocytes or hemoglobin.

Pica Ingestion of a nonfood substance, such as laundry starch, dirt, or ice.

Placenta Fetal structure that provides nourishment and removes waste from the developing baby and secretes hormones necessary for the pregnancy to continue.

Placenta accreta A placenta that is abnormlly adherent to the uterine muscle. If the condition is more advanced, it is called **placenta increta** (the placenta extends into the uterine muscle) or **placenta percreta** (the placenta extends through the uterine muscle).

Placenta previa Abnormal implantation of the placenta in the lower uterus.

Point of maximum impulse (PMI) Area of the chest in which the heart sounds are loudest when auscultated.

Polycythemia Abnormally high number of erythrocytes.

Polydactyly More than 10 digits on the hands or feet.

Polydipsia Excessive thirst.

Polyhydramnios See **Hydramnios.**

Polymorphism Common variation in a gene that does not affect its function or the individual's health negatively.

Polyphagia Excessive ingestion of food.

Polyploidy Having additional full sets of chromosomes.

Polyuria Excessive excretion of urine.

Position Relation of a fixed reference point on the fetus to the quadrants of the maternal pelvis.

Postconceptional age See **Fertilization age.**

Postmaturity syndrome Condition in which a **postterm infant** shows characteristics indicative of poor placental functioning before birth.

Postneonatal mortality rate Number of deaths between 28 days and 1 year of life per 1000 live births.

Postpartum Term describing the first 6 weeks following childbirth.

Postpartum blues Temporary, self-limiting period of weepiness experienced by many new mothers within the first few days following childbirth.

Postterm birth A birth that occurs later than 42 weeks of gestation.

Postterm infant An infant born after 42 weeks of gestation.

Precipitate birth A birth that occurs without a trained attendant present.

Precipitate labor An intense, unusually short labor (less than 3 hours).

Pre-eclampsia A hypertensive disorder induced by pregnancy that usually includes a triad of signs and symptoms: hypertension, edema, and proteinuria.

Premature infant See **Preterm infant.**

Premature rupture of the membranes Spontaneous rupture of the membranes before the onset of labor. The gestation may be term, preterm, or postterm.

Presentation Fetal part that enters the pelvic inlet. Also, the **presenting part.**

Presenting part See **Presentation.**

Preterm birth A birth that occurs after the 20th week and before the 38th week of gestation.

Preterm infant An infant born before the beginning of the 38th week of gestation. Also called **premature infant.**

Preterm labor Onset of labor after 20 weeks and before the beginning of the 38th week of gestation.

Primary infertility See **Infertility.**

Primigravida A woman who is pregnant for the first time.

Primipara A woman who has given birth after a pregnancy of at least 20 weeks of gestation. Also used informally to describe a pregnant woman before the birth of her first child.

Progestin Any natural or synthetic form of progesterone.

Prolactin Anterior pituitary hormone that promotes growth of breast tissue and stimulates production of milk.

Prolapsed cord Displacement of the umbilical cord in front of or beside the fetal presenting part. An **occult prolapse** is one that is suspected on the basis of fetal heart rate patterns; the umbilical cord cannot be palpated or seen.

Prune-belly syndrome An absence of abdominal muscles that results in a flabby, distended, and creased abdomen that may occur in the infant exposed to cocaine in utero.

Pseudomenstruation Vaginal bleeding in the newborn, resulting from withdrawal of placental hormones.

Psychoprophylaxis Method of prepared childbirth that emphasizes mental concentration and relaxation to increase **pain tolerance.**

Psychosis Mental state in which a person's ability to recognize reality, communicate, and relate to others is impaired.

Puberty Period of sexual maturation accompanied by the development of secondary sex characteristics and the capacity to reproduce.

Puerperium Period from the end of childbirth until **involution** of the uterus is complete; approximately 6 weeks.

Pulse oximetry Method of determining the level of blood oxygen saturation using sensors attached to the skin.

Reciprocal bonding behaviors Repertoire of infant behaviors that promote attachment between parent and newborn.

Recommended dietary allowances (RDA) Levels of nutrient intake considered to meet the needs of healthy individuals.

Rectocele Herniation (protrusion) of the rectum through the posterior vaginal wall.

REEDA Acronym for redness, ecchymosis, edema, discharge, and approximation; useful for assessing wound healing or the presence of inflammation or infection.

Reflection Meditation, attentive consideration.

Reflux A condition in which stomach contents enter the esophagus and may be aspirated into the lungs.

Regional anesthesia Anesthesia that blocks pain impulses in a localized area without loss of consciousness.

Respiratory distress syndrome (RDS) Condition caused by insufficient production of **surfactant** in the lungs; results in atelectasis (collapse of the lung alveoli), **hypoxemia,** and **hypercapnia.**

Resting tone See **Uterine resting tone.**

Retinopathy of prematurity (ROP) Condition in which interference with blood supply to the retina may cause decreased vision or blindness.

Retrograde ejaculation Discharge of **semen** into the bladder rather than from the end of the penis.

Role transition Changing from one pattern of behavior and one image of self to another.

Ruga (pl. **rugae**) Ridge or fold of tissue, as on the male's scrotum and in the female's vagina.

Salpingectomy Surgical removal of a fallopian tube.

Seborrheic dermatitis (cradle cap) Yellowish, crusty area of the scalp.

Second period of reactivity Period of 4 to 6 hours after the first sleep following birth when the newborn may have an elevated pulse and respiratory rate and excessive mucus.

Secondary infertility See **Infertility.**

Secondary sex characteristics Physical differences between mature males and females that are not directly related to reproduction.

Semen **Spermatozoa** with their nourishing and protective fluid; discharged at **ejaculation.**

Sensory block Loss of sensation caused by **regional anesthesia.**

Seroconversion Change in a blood test result from negative to positive, indicating the development of antibodies in response to infection or immunization.

Sex chromosome The X or Y **chromosome.** Females have two X chromosomes; males have one X and one Y chromosome.

Sexually transmissible (or **transmitted**) **disease (STD)** A disease that is passed to others primarily through sexual contact.

Shoulder dystocia Delayed or difficult birth of the fetal shoulders after the head is born.

Sibling rivalry Feelings of jealousy and fear of replacement when a young child must share the attention of the parents with a newborn infant.

Skepticism Doubt in the absence of conclusive evidence.

Small-for-gestational age (SGA) infant An infant whose size is below the 10th percentile for gestational age.

Somatic cells Body cells other than the **gametes,** or germ cells.

Somatic sex Gender assignment as male or female on the basis of form and structure of the external genitalia.

Sperm See **Spermatozoon.**

Spermatogenesis Formation of male **gametes (sperm)** in the testes.

Spermatozoon (pl. **spermatozoa** or **sperm**) Male **gamete,** or sex cell.

Spermicide A chemical, such as nonoxynol 9, that kills **sperm.**

Spina bifida Defective closure of the bony spine that encloses the spinal cord; a type of **neural tube defect.**

Spinnbarkeit Clear, slippery, stretchy quality of cervical mucus during ovulation.

Standard of care Level of care that can be expected of a professional. This level is determined by laws, professional organizations, and health care agencies.

Standardized procedures Procedures determined by nurses, physicians, and administrators that allow nurses to perform duties usually part of the medical practice.

Station Measurement of fetal descent in relation to the ischial spines of the maternal pelvis. See also **Engagement.**

Sterility Total inability to conceive.

Stork bites See **Telangiectatic nevi.**

Strabismus A turning inward ("crossing") or outward of the eyes due to poor muscle tone.

Striae gravidarum Irregular reddish streaks resulting from tears in connective tissue; during pregnancy, these streaks generally appear on the woman's abdomen, breasts, or thighs.

Subarachnoid space Space between the arachnoid mater and the pia mater containing **cerebrospinal fluid.**

Suckling Giving or taking nourishment from the breast. Sometimes used interchangeably with sucking, which refers only to drawing into the mouth with a partial vacuum, as with a bottle or pacifier.

Sudden infant death syndrome (SIDS) Sudden death of an infant that is unexplained by autopsy, examination of the scene of death, or history.

Surfactant Combination of lipoproteins produced by the lungs of the mature fetus to reduce surface tension in the alveoli, thus promoting lung expansion after birth.

Surrogate mother A fertile woman who is inseminated with the purpose of conceiving and relinquishing a child to an infertile couple.

Suspend To delay or to bring to a stop temporarily.

Sutures Narrow areas of flexible tissue that connect fetal skull bones, permitting slight movement during labor.

Syndactyly Webbing between fingers or toes.

Tachypnea Respiratory rate above 60 breaths per minute in the newborn after the first hour of life.

Taking-hold Second phase of maternal adaptation during which the mother assumes control of her own care and initiates care of the infant.

Taking-in First phase of maternal adaptation during which the mother passively accepts care, comfort, and details of the newborn.

Telangiectatic nevi (stork bites, nevus simplex) Flat pink areas on the nape of the neck and over the eyelids resulting from dilation of the capillaries.

Telemetry Transmission of electronic fetal monitoring data to the bedside monitor unit with radio signals.

Teratogen An agent that can cause defects in a developing baby during pregnancy.

Term A birth that occurs between the 38th and 42nd week of gestation.

Thermogenesis Heat production.

Thermoregulation Maintenance of body temperature.

Thrombus Collection of blood factors, primarily platelets and fibrin, that may cause vascular obstruction at the point of formation.

Tocolytic A drug that inhibits uterine contractions.

Total parenteral nutrition (TPN) Intravenous infusion of all nutrients needed for metabolism and growth.

Toxemia An old term occasionally used to denote pregnancy-induced hypertension, **pre-eclampsia,** and **eclampsia.**

Toxic shock syndrome Rare, potentially fatal disorder caused by a toxin produced by *Staphylococcus aureus;* has been associated with improper use of tampons.

Tracheoesophageal fistula Abnormal connection between the esophagus and the trachea.

Transcutaneous oxygen/carbon dioxide monitoring Method of continuous noninvasive measurement of oxygen and carbon dioxide levels in the blood by transducers attached to the skin.

Transducer A device that translates one physical quantity to another, such as fetal heart motion to an electrical signal for rate calculation or generation of sound or of a written record.

Transient tachypnea of the newborn Condition of rapid respirations due to inadequate absorption of **fetal lung fluid.**

Transitional milk Breast milk that appears between secretion of **colostrum** and **mature milk.**

Translocation Attachment of all or part of a **chromosome** to another chromosome.

Trimester A division of pregnancy into three equal parts of 13 weeks each.

Triple-marker screening Analysis of maternal serum for abnormal levels of **alpha-fetoprotein,** human chorionic gonadotropin, and estriols that may predict chromosomal abnormalities of the fetus.

Trisomy Presence of three copies of **chromosome** in each body cell.

Tubal ligation Occluding of the fallopian tubes to prevent passage of **ova** or **sperm,** thus preventing pregnancy.

Ultrasonography Technique for visualizing deep structures of the body by recording the reflections (echoes) of sound waves directed into the tissue.

Uterine inversion Turning of the uterus inside out after birth of the fetus.

Uterine resting tone Degree of uterine muscle tension when the woman is not in labor or during the interval between labor contractions.

Uterine rupture A tear in the wall of the uterus.

Uteroplacental insufficiency (UPI) Inability of the placenta to exchange oxygen, carbon dioxide, nutrients, and waste products properly between the maternal and fetal circulations.

Utilitarian theory Ethical theory stating that the right course of action is the one that produces the greatest good.

Vacuum curettage (vacuum aspiration) Removal of the uterine contents by application of a vacuum through a hollow curet or cannula introduced into the uterus.

Validate To make certain that the information collected during assessment is accurate.

Valsalva's maneuver Increasing pressure within the abdomen and thorax by holding the breath and pushing against a closed glottis.

Variable deceleration Slowing of the fetal heart rate having an inconsistent relationship to uterine contractions.

Varicocele Abnormal dilation or varicosity of veins in the spermatic cord.

Vasectomy Occluding the vas deferens to prevent passage of **sperm**, thus preventing pregnancy.

Vasoconstriction Narrowing of the lumen of blood vessels.

VBAC Acronym for vaginal birth after cesarean.

Vegan A complete **vegetarian** who does not eat any animal products.

Vegetarian An individual whose diet consists wholly or mostly of plant foods and who avoids animal food sources.

Vernix caseosa Thick white substance that protects the skin of the fetus.

Version Turning the fetus from one presentation to another before birth, usually from breech to cephalic.

Very-low-birth-weight (VLBW) infant An infant weighing 1500 g or less at birth.

Vibroacoustic stimulation test Use of sound stimulation to elicit fetal movement and acceleration (speeding up) of the fetal heart rate.

Withdrawal syndrome See **Abstinence syndrome.**

Zygote The developing baby from conception through the first week of prenatal life.

Index

A

D

J

M

S

Critical to Remember *cont'd*

Want to Know